THE
BREAST

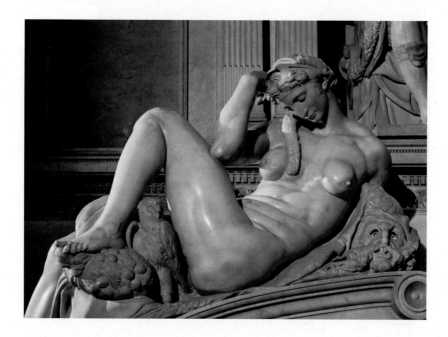

Carved in the 1520s by Michelangelo, the sculpture *Night* has been on display in the Medici Mortuary Chapel in the Church of San Lorenzo in Florence, Italy for hundreds of years. After nearly 500 years and many comments on its appearance, the left breast of *Night* has undergone renewed scrutiny. Close observation reveals a mass in the medial aspect of the breast, slight skin puckering adjacent to the mass, and diffuse swelling of the nipple-areola complex—characteristics of locally advanced breast cancer. None of Michelangelo's numerous other depictions of the female breast share these characteristics. Stark and Nelson[a] concluded that Michelangelo knew that breast cancer was a fatal illness and that he therefore chose it to memorialize his patron Giuliano de' Medici, whose remains reside in the crypt covered by the sculpture. Giuliano died from a protracted wasting illness, possibly tuberculosis; *Night*, they concluded, was an allegory to that illness. Referring to *Night* and its three companion sarcophagi, Michelangelo imagines them conversing: "Day and Night speak, and say, 'We with our swift course have brought Duke Giuliano to death.'" In a sonnet written in 1545, Michelangelo has *Night* say, "I prize my sleep, and more my being stone/As long as Hurt and Shamefulness endure."

Michelangelo was known to have access to human autopsy specimens and, no doubt, had observed the gross morphology of breast cancer. His depiction of breast cancer in *Night* represents one of the first works of art to accurately depict this disease.

James J. Stark, MD, FACP
Professor of Clinical Internal Medicine
Eastern Virginia Medical School
Medical Director, Cancer Program, Maryview Medical Center
Suffolk, VA

Art credit:

Michelangelo Buonarroti (1475-1564)

The figure of Night, from the tomb of Giuliano de' Medici (1478-1516) Duke of Nemours and son of Lorenzo il Magnifico. Marble, 1521-1534.

S. Lorenzo, Florence, Italy

©Erich Lessing/Art Resource, NY

[a]Stark JJ, Nelson JK. The breasts of "Night": Michelangelo as oncologist. *N Engl J Med.* 2000;343: 1577-1578.

THE BREAST

COMPREHENSIVE MANAGEMENT of BENIGN and MALIGNANT DISEASES

Fifth Edition

SENIOR EDITORS

Kirby I. Bland, MD
Professor and Chair Emeritus
Department of Surgery
University of Alabama at Birmingham
Birmingham, Alabama

Edward M. Copeland III, MD
Emeritus Distinguished Professor
Department of Surgery
University of Florida College of Medicine
Gainesville, Florida

V. Suzanne Klimberg, MD, PhD
The Courtney M. Townsend, Jr., M.D. Distinguished
    Chair in General Surgery
Vice Chair for Administration
Professor of Surgery
University of Texas Medical Branch
Galveston, Texas

William J. Gradishar, MD
Betsy Bramsen Professor of Breast Oncology
Professor, Department of Medicine-
    Hematology/Oncology
Northwestern University Feinberg School of Medicine
Chicago, Illinois

ASSOCIATE EDITORS

Julia White, MD
Professor
Department of Radiation Oncology
The Ohio State University Comprehensive Cancer Center
Columbus, Ohio

Soheila Korourian, MD
Professor
Department of Pathology
University of Arkansas for Medical Sciences
Little Rock, Arkansas

ELSEVIER

ELSEVIER

1600 John F. Kennedy Blvd.
Ste 1800
Philadelphia, PA 19103-2899

THE BREAST: COMPREHENSIVE MANAGEMENT OF BENIGN AND   ISBN: 978-0-323-35955-9
MALIGNANT DISEASES, FIFTH EDITION

Previous editions copyrighted 2009, 2004, 1998, and 1991.

Library of Congress Cataloging-in-Publication Data

Names: Bland, K. I., editor. | Klimberg, V. Suzanne, editor. | Copeland,
  Edward M., III, 1937- editor. | Gradishar, William J., editor.
Title: The breast : comprehensive management of benign and malignant diseases
  / senior editors, Kirby I. Bland, V. Suzanne Klimberg, Edward M. Copeland
  III, William J. Gradishar ; associate editors, Julia White, Soheila Korourian.
Other titles: Breast (Bland)
Description: Fifth edition. | Philadelphia, PA : Elsevier, [2018] | Includes
  bibliographical references and index.
Identifiers: LCCN 2017021495 | ISBN 9780323359559 (hardcover : alk. paper)
Subjects: | MESH: Breast Diseases—therapy | Breast Neoplasms—therapy
Classification: LCC RC280.B8 | NLM WP 900 | DDC 618.1/906—dc23 LC record
  available at https://lccn.loc.gov/2017021495

Executive Content Strategist: Michael Houston
Senior Content Development Manager: Kathryn DeFrancesco
Publishing Services Manager: Catherine Jackson
Book Production Specialist: Kristine Feeherty
Design Direction: Maggie Reid

Printed in China

Last digit is the print number: 9   8   7   6   5   4   3   2   1

To our spouses and their dedication, and with appreciation for the generous support they have provided to our careers, which has allowed the development of this book; to our many clinical and scientific mentors; to physicians, nurses, and healthcare providers of all oncologic disciplines who care for patients with diseases of the breast; and most of all, to our patients

Contributors

Balkees Abderrahman, MD
Postdoctoral Research Fellow, Department of Breast Medical
  Oncology, The University of Texas MD Anderson Cancer
  Center, Houston, TX; Medical Advisory Board, Infinity
  Medical Engineering, LLC, Orlando, FL
  21 Steroid Receptors in Breast Cancer

Stefan Aebi, MD
Professor of Medicine, Luzerner Kantonsspital, Cancer Center
  LUKS, Luzern; University of Bern, Bern, Switzerland
  61 Locoregional Recurrence After Mastectomy

Prasanna Alluri, MD, PhD
Chief Resident, Department of Radiation Oncology, University
  of Michigan, Ann Arbor, MI
  49 Postmastectomy Radiotherapy

Benjamin O. Anderson, MD
Director, Breast Health Clinic, Seattle Cancer Care Alliance;
  Professor of Surgery and Global Health Medicine, University
  of Washington School of Medicine, Seattle, WA
  38 Lobular Carcinoma in Situ of the Breast

Cletus A. Arciero, MD, MS
Associate Professor of Surgery, Department of Surgery, Emory
  University School of Medicine, Atlanta, GA
  18 Clinically Established Prognostic Factors in Breast Cancer

Raheela Ashfaq, MS, MD
Director, Breast Pathology; Medical Director, Miraca Research
  and Development Services, Miraca Life Sciences, Irving, TX
  4 Discharges and Secretions of the Nipple

Thomas Aversano, MD
Associate Professor, Department of Medicine, Johns Hopkins
  University, Baltimore, MD
  74 Management of Pericardial Metastases in Breast Cancer

Jennifer Axilbund, MS, CGC
Adjunct Assistant Professor, Oncology, Johns Hopkins
  University, Baltimore, MD
  *17 Breast Cancer Genetics: Syndromes, Genes, Pathology,
    Counseling, Testing, and Treatment*

Ebrahim Azizi, PhD, PharmD
Department of Internal Medicine, Division of Hematology/
  Oncology, Comprehensive Cancer Center, School of
  Medicine, University of Michigan, Ann Arbor, MI
  23 Stem Cells in Breast Development and Cancer

Rajesh Banderudrappagari, MD
University of Arkansas for Medical, Hematology/Oncology,
  Little Rock, AR
  81 General Considerations for Follow-Up

Andrea V. Barrio, MD, FACS
Assistant Attending, Breast Service, Department of Surgery,
  Memorial Sloan Kettering Cancer Center, New York, NY
  75 Bilateral Breast Cancer

Lawrence W. Bassett, MD
Professor Emeritus, Radiology, David Geffen School of
  Medicine at UCLA, Los Angeles, CA
  26 Breast Imaging Screening and Diagnosis

Isabelle Bedrosian, MD
Professor, Breast Surgical Oncology, Division of Surgery, The
  University of Texas MD Anderson Cancer Center, Houston,
  TX
  *59 Surgical Procedures for Advanced Local and Regional
    Malignancies of the Breast*

Alyssa Berkowitz, MPH
Research Assistant, Yale University School of Medicine, New
  Haven, CT
  84 Psychosocial Consequences and Lifestyle Interventions

Therese B. Bevers, MD
Professor, Clinical Cancer Prevention; Medical Director, Cancer
  Prevention Center; Medical Director, Prevention Outreach
  Programs, The University of Texas MD Anderson Cancer
  Center, Houston, TX
  *80 Clinical Management of the Patient at Increased or High
    Risk*

Kirby I. Bland, MD
Professor and Chair Emeritus, Department of Surgery,
  University of Alabama at Birmingham, Birmingham, AL
  1 History of the Therapy of Breast Cancer
  *2 Anatomy of the Breast, Axilla, Chest Wall, and Related
    Metastatic Sites*
  *3 Breast Physiology: Normal and Abnormal Development and
    Function*
  5 Etiology and Management of Benign Breast Disease
  7 Gynecomastia
  *9 In Situ Carcinomas of the Breast: Ductal Carcinoma in Situ
    and Lobular Carcinoma in Situ*
  28 Indications and Techniques for Biopsy
  *29 General Principles of Mastectomy: Evaluation and
    Therapeutic Options*
  30 Halsted Radical Mastectomy
  31 Modified Radical Mastectomy and Simple Mastectomy
  32 Breast Conservation Therapy for Invasive Breast Cancer
  34 Wound Care and Complications of Mastectomy
  45 Surgical Management of Early Breast Cancer

Cristiano Boneti, MD
Assistant Professor, Surgery, Divisions of Plastic Surgery and
Surgery Oncology, University of Miami, Miami, FL
*29 General Principles of Mastectomy: Evaluation and
Therapeutic Options*
33 Breast Reconstruction and Oncoplastic Surgery

Zeynep Bostanci, MD
Chief Resident in Surgery, Penn State Milton S. Hershey
Medical Center, Hershey, PA
*3 Breast Physiology: Normal and Abnormal Development and
Function*

Ursa Brown-Glaberman, MD
Assistant Professor, Department of Internal Medicine, Division
of Hematology/Oncology, University of New Mexico
Comprehensive Cancer Center, Albuquerque, NM
68 Management of Bone Metastases in Breast Cancer

Adam Brufsky, MD, PhD
Professor of Medicine, University of Pittsburgh School of
Medicine, Pittsburgh, PA
57 Bisphosphonates in Early Breast Cancer

Gwendolyn Bryant-Smith, MD
Department of Radiology, University of Arkansas for Medical
Sciences, Little Rock, AR
65 Neoadjuvant Chemotherapy and Radiotherapy

Oren Cahlon, MD
Assistant Attending, Vice Chair for Clinical Operations,
Department of Radiation Oncology, Memorial Sloan
Kettering Cancer Center, New York, NY
48 Radiotherapy and Regional Nodes

Benjamin C. Calhoun, MD, PhD
Director, Breast Pathology, Department of Pathology, Cleveland
Clinic; Assistant Professor, Department of Pathology,
Cleveland Clinic Lerner College of Medicine, Cleveland,
OH
8 Benign, High-Risk, and Premalignant Lesions of the Breast

Kristine E. Calhoun, MD
Associate Director, Breast Health Clinic, Seattle Cancer Care
Alliance; Associate Professor, Department of Surgery,
University of Washington School of Medicine, Seattle, WA
38 Lobular Carcinoma in Situ of the Breast

Ryan J. Carr, MD
Fellow in Dermatopathology, Department of Pathology, The
Ohio State University Wexner Medical Center, Columbus,
OH
13 Primary and Secondary Dermatologic Disorders of the Breast

Helena R. Chang, MD, PhD
Professor, Department of Surgery, David Geffen School of
Medicine at UCLA; Director, Revlon/UCLA Breast Center,
Los Angeles, CA
31 Modified Radical Mastectomy and Simple Mastectomy
*41 Therapeutic Value of Axillary Node Dissection and Selective
Management of the Axilla in Small Breast Cancers*

Steven L. Chen, MD, MBA
Director, Surgical Oncology, OasisMD, San Diego, CA
35 Quality Measures and Outcomes for Breast Cancer Surgery

Alice Chung, MD
Assistant Professor of Surgery, Division of Surgical Oncology,
Cedars-Sinai Medical Center, Los Angeles, CA
*42 Lymphatic Mapping and Sentinel Lymphadenectomy for
Breast Cancer*

Maureen A. Chung, MD, PhD
Medical Director, Southcoast Breast Program, Southcoast
Health, Dartmouth, MA
*41 Therapeutic Value of Axillary Node Dissection and Selective
Management of the Axilla in Small Breast Cancers*

Hiram S. Cody III, MD
Attending Surgeon, Breast Service, Department of Surgery,
Memorial Sloan Kettering Cancer Center; Professor of
Clinical Surgery, Weill Cornell Medical College, New York,
NY
*43 Detection and Significance of Axillary Lymph Node
Micrometastases*
75 Bilateral Breast Cancer

Edward M. Copeland III, MD
Emeritus Distinguished Professor, Department of Surgery,
University of Florida College of Medicine, Gainesville, FL
1 History of the Therapy of Breast Cancer
*2 Anatomy of the Breast, Axilla, Chest Wall, and Related
Metastatic Sites*
5 Etiology and Management of Benign Breast Disease
*29 General Principles of Mastectomy: Evaluation and
Therapeutic Options*
30 Halsted Radical Mastectomy
31 Modified Radical Mastectomy and Simple Mastectomy
*44 Intraoperative Evaluation of Surgical Margins in Breast
Conserving Therapy*
*77 Local Recurrence, the Augmented Breast, and the
Contralateral Breast*

Ricardo Costa, MD, MSc
Instructor in Medicine, Hematology/Oncology, Northwestern
University, Chicago, IL
63 Locally Advanced Breast Cancer
*73 Management of Central Nervous System Metastases in Breast
Cancer*

Jorge I. de la Torre, MD
Professor and Chief, Division of Plastic Surgery, University of
Alabama at Birmingham; Staff Surgeon, Surgery,
Birmingham VA Medical Center, Birmingham, AL
*29 General Principles of Mastectomy: Evaluation and
Therapeutic Options*
33 Breast Reconstruction and Oncoplastic Surgery

Amy C. Degnim, MD
Associate Professor of Surgery, Department of Surgery, Mayo
Clinic, Rochester, MN
*20 Risk Factors for Breast Carcinoma in Women With
Proliferative Breast Disease*

Mary L. Disis, MD, MS
Professor of Medicine, Adjunct Professor, Pathology and
　Obstetrics and Gynecology, University of Washington,
　Seattle, WA
　71 Immunologic Approaches to Breast Cancer Therapy

William D. Dupont, PhD
Professor of Biostatistics and Preventive Medicine, Department
　of Biostatistics, Vanderbilt University School of Medicine,
　Nashville, TN
　*20 Risk Factors for Breast Carcinoma in Women With
　Proliferative Breast Disease*

Melinda S. Epstein, PhD
Clinical Research Scientist, Hoag Memorial Hospital
　Presbyterian, Hoag Institute for Research and Education,
　Newport Beach, CA
　39 Ductal Carcinoma in Situ of the Breast

Francisco J. Esteva, MD, PhD
Professor of Medicine, NYU Perlmutter Cancer Center, NYU
　Langone Medical Center, New York, NY
　*66 Detection and Clinical Implications of Occult Systemic
　Micrometastatic Breast Cancer*

David M. Euhus, MD
Professor, Department of Surgery, Johns Hopkins University,
　Baltimore, MD
　*17 Breast Cancer Genetics: Syndromes, Genes, Pathology,
　Counseling, Testing, and Treatment*

Suzanne Evans, MD, MPH
Associate Professor, Department of Therapeutic Radiology, Yale
　University School of Medicine, New Haven, CT
　46 Biological Basis of Radiotherapy of the Breast

Oluwadamilola M. Fayanju, MD, MA, MPHS
Assistant Professor, Department of Surgery, Duke University,
　Durham, NC
　19 Molecular Prognostic Factors for Breast Carcinoma
　*59 Surgical Procedures for Advanced Local and Regional
　Malignancies of the Breast*

Gary M. Freedman, MD
Associate Professor, Radiation Oncology, Perelman School of
　Medicine of the University of Pennsylvania, Philadelphia, PA
　50 Breast Conserving Therapy for Invasive Breast Cancers
　52 Radiation Complications and Their Management

Patrick Bryan Garvey, MD
Associate Professor, Department of Plastic and Reconstructive
　Surgery, The University of Texas MD Anderson Cancer
　Center, Houston, TX
　*59 Surgical Procedures for Advanced Local and Regional
　Malignancies of the Breast*

Abby Geletzke, MD
Department of Surgery, Penn State Milton S. Hershey Medical
　Center, Hershey, PA
　5 Etiology and Management of Benign Breast Disease

Mary L. Gemignani, MD, MPH
Breast Service, Department of Surgery, Memorial Sloan
　Kettering Cancer Center, New York, NY
　78 Carcinoma of the Breast in Pregnancy and Lactation

Armando E. Giuliano, MD
Executive Vice Chair of Surgery, Chief of Surgical Oncology,
　Cedars-Sinai Medical Center, Los Angeles, CA
　*42 Lymphatic Mapping and Sentinel Lymphadenectomy for
　Breast Cancer*

Mehra Golshan, MD
Medical Director, International Oncology Programs, Dana
　Farber Cancer Institute/Brigham and Women's Hospital, Dr.
　Abdul Mohsen and Sultana Al-Tuwaijri Chair in Surgical
　Oncology, Brigham and Women' Hospital; Director, Breast
　Surgical Services, Dana Farber Cancer Institute/Brigham and
　Women's Cancer Center; Associate Professor of Surgery,
　Harvard Medical School, Boston, MA
　*25 Examination Techniques: Roles of the Physician and Patient
　in Evaluating Breast Disease*

William J. Gradishar, MD
Betsy Bramsen Professor of Breast Oncology, Professor,
　Department of Medicine-Hematology/Oncology,
　Northwestern University Feinberg School of Medicine,
　Chicago, IL
　*55 Adjuvant and Neoadjuvant Systemic Therapies for Early-
　Stage Breast Cancer*
　63 Locally Advanced Breast Cancer
　76 Male Breast Cancer

Jill Granger, MS
Research Area Supervisor, Department of Internal Medicine,
　Division of Hematology/Oncology, University of Michigan,
　Ann Arbor, MI
　23 Stem Cells in Breast Development and Cancer

Caprice C. Greenberg, MD, MPH
Morgridge Distinguished Chair in Health Services Research,
　Vice Chair of Research, Department of Surgery, University
　of Wisconsin, Madison, WI
　35 Quality Measures and Outcomes for Breast Cancer Surgery

Lars J. Grimm, MD, MHS
Assistant Professor, Radiology, Duke University, Durham, NC
　28 Indications and Techniques for Biopsy

Stephen R. Grobmyer, MD
Professor, Department of Surgery, Cleveland Clinic Lerner
　College of Medicine; Director of Surgical Oncology,
　Department of Surgery, Cleveland Clinic, Cleveland, OH
　6 Mastitis and Breast Abscess
　8 Benign, High-Risk, and Premalignant Lesions of the Breast
　34 Wound Care and Complications of Mastectomy
　*44 Intraoperative Evaluation of Surgical Margins in Breast
　Conserving Therapy*

Nora Hansen, MD
Chief, Division of Breast Surgery, Professor of Surgery, Feinberg
    School of Medicine, Northwestern University, Chicago, IL
63 Locally Advanced Breast Cancer

Ramdane Harouaka, PhD
Research Fellow, Department of Internal Medicine, University
    of Michigan, Ann Arbor, MI
23 Stem Cells in Breast Development and Cancer

Eleanor E. Harris, MD
Professor and Chair, Radiation Oncology, Brody School of
    Medicine, East Carolina University, Greenville, NC
51 Partial Breast Irradiation: Accelerated and Intraoperative

Lynn C. Hartmann, MD
Professor of Oncology, Department of Oncology, Mayo Clinic,
    Rochester, MN
*20 Risk Factors for Breast Carcinoma in Women With
    Proliferative Breast Disease*

Tina J. Hieken, MD
Associate Professor, Department of Surgery, Mayo Clinic,
    Rochester, MN
12 Paget Disease of the Breast

Susan Higgins, MD
Professor, Department of Therapeutic Radiology, Yale University
    School of Medicine, New Haven, CT
46 Biological Basis of Radiotherapy of the Breast

Dennis Holmes, MD, FACS
Medical Director, Los Angeles Center for Women's Health, Los
    Angeles, CA
51 Partial Breast Irradiation: Accelerated and Intraoperative

Kelly K. Hunt, MD
Professor, Breast Surgical Oncology, The University of Texas
    MD Anderson Cancer Center, Houston, TX
*59 Surgical Procedures for Advanced Local and Regional
    Malignancies of the Breast*

E. Shelley Hwang, MD, MPH
Professor, Surgery, Duke University, Durham, NC
28 Indications and Techniques for Biopsy

Reshma Jagsi, MD, DPhil
Professor and Deputy Chair, Department of Radiation
    Oncology, University of Michigan, Ann Arbor, MI
49 Postmastectomy Radiotherapy

Sarika Jain, MD
Department of Medicine, Robert H. Lurie Comprehensive
    Cancer Center of Northwestern University, Chicago, IL
76 Male Breast Cancer

Bharti Jasra, MBBS
Assistant Professor, General Surgery, University of Florida,
    Jacksonville, FL
*77 Local Recurrence, the Augmented Breast, and the
    Contralateral Breast*

Jacqueline S. Jeruss, MD, PhD
Associate Professor, Department of Surgery, Pathology, and
    Biomedical Engineering, Director, Breast Care Center,
    Director, Breast Surgical Oncology Fellowship, University of
    Michigan, Ann Arbor, MI
58 Oncofertility Options for Young Women With Breast Cancer

Rafael E. Jimenez, MD
Associate Professor, Department of Laboratory Medicine and
    Pathology, Mayo Clinic, Rochester, MN
12 Paget Disease of the Breast

Veronica Jones, MD
Clinical Assistant Professor, City of Hope, Department of
    Surgical Oncology, Duarte, CA
64 Inflammatory Breast Cancer

V. Craig Jordan, OBE, PhD, DSc, MDhc
Dallas/Fort Worth Living Legend Chair of Cancer Research,
    Department of Breast Medical Oncology, The University of
    Texas MD Anderson Cancer Center, Houston, TX
21 Steroid Receptors in Breast Cancer

Himanshu Joshi, MBBS, PhD
Research Associate, Department of Pathology, Norris
    Comprehensive Cancer Center, University of Southern
    California, Los Angeles, CA
22 Molecular Oncology of Breast Cancer

Virginia Kaklamani, MD
Professor, Department of Medicine, University of Texas Health
    Science Center, San Antonio, TX
*79 Unknown Primary Presenting With Axillary
    Lymphadenopathy*

Nina J. Karlin, MD
Consultant, Division Hematology Oncology, Mayo Clinic
    Arizona, Phoenix, AZ
*11 Mesenchymal Neoplasms and Primary Lymphomas of the
    Breast*

Meghan S. Karuturi, MD
Assistant Professor, Breast Medical Oncology, The University of
    Texas MD Anderson Cancer Center, Houston, TX
*59 Surgical Procedures for Advanced Local and Regional
    Malignancies of the Breast*

Rena B. Kass, MD
Associate Professor of Surgery, Director of Breast Center, Penn
    State Hershey Breast Center, Penn State Milton S. Hershey
    Medical Center, Hershey, PA
*3 Breast Physiology: Normal and Abnormal Development and
    Function*
5 Etiology and Management of Benign Breast Disease

Kenneth Kern, MD, MPH, MS
Senior Medical Director, Early Drug Development, Pfizer
    Oncology, San Diego, CA
86 Delayed Diagnosis of Symptomatic Breast Cancer

Seema A. Khan, MD
Professor of Surgery, Breast Surgery, Northwestern University, Chicago, IL
67 Management of the Intact Breast Primary in the Setting of Metastatic Disease

Jennifer R. Klemp, PhD, MPH
Associate Professor of Medicine, Division of Clinical Oncology; Director, Cancer Survivorship, University of Kansas Cancer Center, Kansas City, KS
85 Breast Cancer Survivorship

V. Suzanne Klimberg, MD, PhD
The Courtney M. Townsend, Jr., M.D. Distinguished Chair in General Surgery, Vice Chair for Administration, Professor of Surgery, University of Texas Medical Branch, Galveston, TX
1 History of the Therapy of Breast Cancer
2 Anatomy of the Breast, Axilla, Chest Wall, and Related Metastatic Sites
3 Breast Physiology: Normal and Abnormal Development and Function
5 Etiology and Management of Benign Breast Disease
9 In Situ Carcinomas of the Breast: Ductal Carcinoma in Situ and Lobular Carcinoma in Situ
14 Breast Biomarker Immunocytochemistry
27 Design and Conduct of Clinical Trials for Breast Cancer
28 Indications and Techniques for Biopsy
29 General Principles of Mastectomy: Evaluation and Therapeutic Options
30 Halsted Radical Mastectomy
32 Breast Conservation Therapy for Invasive Breast Cancer
36 Lymphedema in the Postmastectomy Patient: Pathophysiology, Prevention, and Management
45 Surgical Management of Early Breast Cancer

Soheila Korourian, MD
Professor, Department of Pathology, University of Arkansas for Medical Sciences, Little Rock, AR
10 Infiltrating Carcinomas of the Breast: Not One Disease
14 Breast Biomarker Immunocytochemistry

Henry M. Kuerer, MD, PhD
PH and Fay Eta Robinson Distinguished Professor of Research, Department of Breast Surgical Oncology, MD Anderson Cancer Center; Executive Director, Breast Programs, MD Anderson Cancer Network, Houston, TX
60 Solitary Metastases

Asangi R. Kumarapeli, MD, PhD
Assistant Professor, Department of Pathology, University of Arkansas for Medical Sciences, Little Rock, AR
14 Breast Biomarker Immunocytochemistry

Priya Kumthekar, MD
Assistant Professor of Neurology and Hematology/Oncology, Northwestern University, Chicago, IL
73 Management of Central Nervous System Metastases in Breast Cancer

Maryann Kwa, MD
Instructor of Medicine, NYU Perlmutter Cancer Center, NYU Langone Medical Center, New York, NY
66 Detection and Clinical Implications of Occult Systemic Micrometastatic Breast Cancer

Michael D. Lagios, MD
Director, The Breast Cancer Consultation Service, Tiburon, CA
39 Ductal Carcinoma in Situ of the Breast

Jeffrey Landercasper, MD
Director, Breast Cancer Clinical Outcomes Research, Department of Research Gundersen Medical Foundation, Gundersen Health System, La Crosse, WI; Clinical Adjunct Professor of Surgery, Department of Surgery, University of Wisconsin School of Medicine and Public Health, Madison, WI; Chairman, Patient Safety and Quality Committee, American Society of Breast Surgeons, Columbia, MD
35 Quality Measures and Outcomes for Breast Cancer Surgery

Kate I. Lathrop, MD
Assistant Professor, Medical Oncology and Hematology, Cancer Therapy and Research Center at University of Texas Health Science Center at San Antonio, San Antonio, TX
79 Unknown Primary Presenting With Axillary Lymphadenopathy

Gordon K. Lee, MD
Associate Professor of Plastic and Reconstructive Surgery, Department of Surgery, Stanford School of Medicine, Stanford, CA
33 Breast Reconstruction and Oncoplastic Surgery

Stephanie Lee-Felker, MD
Assistant Professor, Radiology, David Geffen School of Medicine at UCLA, Los Angeles, CA
26 Breast Imaging Screening and Diagnosis

A. Marilyn Leitch, MD
Professor of Surgery, Department of Surgery, University of Texas Southwestern Medical Center, Dallas, TX
4 Discharges and Secretions of the Nipple

D. Scott Lind, MD
Professor and Chairman, Department of Surgery, University of Florida, Jacksonville, FL
77 Local Recurrence, the Augmented Breast, and the Contralateral Breast

Charles L. Loprinzi, MD
Regis Professor of Breast Cancer Research, Department of Oncology, Mayo Clinic, Rochester, MN
82 Management of Menopause in the Breast Cancer Patient

Anthony Lucci, MD
Professor of Surgery, Departments of Breast Surgical Oncology and Surgical Oncology, The University of Texas MD Anderson Cancer Center, Houston, TX
19 Molecular Prognostic Factors for Breast Carcinoma

Tahra Kaur Luther, MS
Assistant Research Program Manager, Department of Internal Medicine, Division of Hematology/Oncology, University of Michigan, Ann Arbor, MI
23 Stem Cells in Breast Development and Cancer

Neil Majithia, MD
Mayo Foundation for Medical Education and Research, Department of Oncology, Mayo Clinic, Rochester, MN
82 Management of Menopause in the Breast Cancer Patient

Issam Makhoul, MD
Professor of Medicine, Hematology/Oncology, University of
    Arkansas for Medical Sciences, Little Rock, AR
    24 Therapeutic Strategies for Breast Cancer
    65 Neoadjuvant Chemotherapy and Radiotherapy
    81 General Considerations for Follow-Up

Melissa Anne Mallory, MD
Resident in General Surgery, Brigham and Women's Hospital/
    Harvard Medical School; Multidisciplinary Image-Guided
    Therapy Breast Surgical Research Fellow in the Advanced
    Multimodality Image-Guided Operating Suite, Department
    of Surgery and Radiology, Dana-Farber Cancer Institute/
    Brigham and Women's Hospital and National Center for
    Image Guided Therapy, Boston, MA
    *25 Examination Techniques: Roles of the Physician and Patient
        in Evaluating Breast Disease*

Anne T. Mancino, MD, FACS
Associate Professor, Surgery, University of Arkansas for Medical
    Sciences; Chief, General Surgery, Surgery, Central Arkansas
    Veterans Healthcare System, Little Rock, AR
    *3 Breast Physiology: Normal and Abnormal Development and
        Function*
    7 Gynecomastia

Sanjay Maraboyina, MD
Department of Radiation Oncology, University of Arkansas for
    Medical Sciences, Little Rock, AR
    65 Neoadjuvant Chemotherapy and Radiotherapy

Aju Mathew, MD, MPhil
Assistant Professor, Medical Oncology, University of Kentucky
    Markey Cancer Center, Lexington, KY
    57 Bisphosphonates in Early Breast Cancer

Damian McCartan, MB, BCh, BAO, PhD
Breast Service, Department of Surgery, Memorial Sloan
    Kettering Cancer Center, New York, NY
    78 Carcinoma of the Breast in Pregnancy and Lactation

Susan A. McCloskey, MD, MSHS
Assistant Professor, Radiation Oncology, University of
    California at Los Angeles, Los Angeles, CA
    47 Radiotherapy and Ductal Carcinoma in Situ

Beryl McCormick, MD, FACR
Attending, Department of Radiation Oncology, Clinical
    Director and External Beam Service Chief, Memorial Sloan
    Kettering Cancer Center; Attending Radiation Oncologist,
    Weill Cornell Medical College, New York, NY
    48 Radiotherapy and Regional Nodes

Karishma Mehra, MD
Fellow, Medical Oncology, Yale University School of Medicine,
    New Haven, CT
    84 Psychosocial Consequences and Lifestyle Interventions

Jane E. Mendez, MD
Chief, Breast Surgery; Attending, Miami Cancer Institute,
    Miami, FL
    60 Solitary Metastases

Priya V. Mhatre, MD
Attending Physician, Shirley Ryan Ability Lab; Assistant
    Professor, Department of Physical Medicine and
    Rehabilitation, Northwestern University Feinberg School of
    Medicine, Chicago, IL
    83 Rehabilitation

Michael D. Mix, MD
Assistant Professor, Radiation Oncology, Upstate Medical
    University, Syracuse, NY
    *53 Radiation Therapy for Locally Advanced Breast Cancer:
        Historical Review to Current Approach*

Meena S. Moran, MD
Professor, Department of Therapeutic Radiology, Yale University
    School of Medicine, New Haven, CT
    46 Biological Basis of Radiotherapy of the Breast

Molly Moravek, MD, MPH
Assistant Professor, Director, Fertility Preservation Program,
    Associate Fellowship Director, Division of Reproductive
    Endocrinology and Infertility, University of Michigan,
    Obstetrics and Gynecology, Ann Arbor, MI
    58 Oncofertility Options for Young Women With Breast Cancer

Leigh Neumayer, MD, MS
Professor and Chair of Surgery, Department of Surgery,
    University of Arizona College of Medicine, Tucson, AZ; Salt
    Lake City, UT
    37 Assessment and Designation of Breast Cancer Stage

Samilia Obeng-Gyasi, MD, MPH
Assistant Professor, General Surgery, Indiana University Melvin
    and Bren Simon Cancer Center, Indianapolis, IN
    28 Indications and Techniques for Biopsy

Patience Odele, MD
Breast Surgery Fellow, Department of Surgery, Division of
    Breast Surgery, Northwestern McGaw Medical Center,
    Chicago, IL
    *67 Management of the Intact Breast Primary in the Setting of
        Metastatic Disease*

Maureen O'Donnell, MD
Clinical Associate, Department of Surgery, Johns Hopkins
    Sibley Memorial Hospital, Washington, DC
    *17 Breast Cancer Genetics: Syndromes, Genes, Pathology,
        Counseling, Testing, and Treatment*

Colleen M. O'Kelly Priddy, MD
Breast Surgeon, Surgery, United Health Services, Johnson City,
    NY; Clinical Instructor, Surgery, University of Southern
    California, Los Angeles, CA
    *40 The New Paradigm: Oncoplastic Breast Conservation
        Surgery*

Ruth M. O'Regan, MD
Chief, Division of Hematology, Oncology, University of
    Wisconsin and Carbone Cancer Center, Madison, WI
    70 Endocrine Therapy for Breast Cancer

Sonal Oza, MD
Resident Physician, Shirley Ryan Ability Lab, Department of
Physical Medicine and Rehabilitation, Northwestern
University Feinberg School of Medicine, Chicago, IL
83 Rehabilitation

Holly J. Pederson, MD
Director, Medical Breast Services, Cleveland Clinic, Cleveland,
OH
85 Breast Cancer Survivorship

Angela Pennisi, MD
Department of Internal Medicine, Hematology/Oncology
Division, University of Arkansas for Medical Sciences, Little
Rock, AR
65 Neoadjuvant Chemotherapy and Radiotherapy
81 General Considerations for Follow-Up

Margot S. Peters, MD
Professor, Department of Dermatology and Department of
Laboratory Medicine & Pathology, Mayo Clinic, Rochester,
MN
12 Paget Disease of the Breast

Sara B. Peters, MD, PhD
Director of Dermatopathology Division, Department of
Pathology, The Ohio State University Wexner Medical
Center, Columbus, OH
*13 Primary and Secondary Dermatologic Disorders of the
Breast*

Lindsay F. Petersen, MD
Breast Surgical Oncology, Henry Ford Health System, Detroit,
MI
58 Oncofertility Options for Young Women With Breast Cancer

Melissa Pilewskie, MD
Assistant Attending, Breast Service, Department of Surgery,
Memorial Sloan Kettering Cancer Center, New York, NY
*43 Detection and Significance of Axillary Lymph Node
Micrometastases*

Raquel Prati, MD
Associate Clinical Professor of Surgery, Revlon/UCLA Breast
Center, Department of Surgery, Division of Surgical
Oncology, University of California at Los Angeles, Los
Angeles, CA
*41 Therapeutic Value of Axillary Node Dissection and Selective
Management of the Axilla in Small Breast Cancers*
45 Surgical Management of Early Breast Cancer

Michael F. Press, MD, PhD
Professor, Harold E. Lee Chair in Cancer Research, Department
of Pathology, Norris Comprehensive Cancer Center,
University of Southern California, Los Angeles, CA
22 Molecular Oncology of Breast Cancer

Erik Ramos, MD
Oncology, University of Washington, Seattle, WA
71 Immunologic Approaches to Breast Cancer Therapy

Amy E. Rivere, MD
Breast Surgical Oncologist, Ochsner Medical Center, New
Orleans, LA
32 Breast Conservation Therapy for Invasive Breast Cancer
*36 Lymphedema in the Postmastectomy Patient: Pathophysiology,
Prevention, and Management*

Arlan L. Rosenbloom, MD
Division of Pediatric Endocrinology, University of Florida,
Gainesville, FL
*3 Breast Physiology: Normal and Abnormal Development and
Function*

Kathryn J. Ruddy, MD, MPH
Associate Professor and Director of Cancer Survivorship,
Department of Oncology, Mayo Clinic, Rochester, MN
82 Management of Menopause in the Breast Cancer Patient

Kilian E. Salerno, MD
Associate Professor, Radiation Medicine, Roswell Park Cancer
Institute, Buffalo, NY
*53 Radiation Therapy for Locally Advanced Breast Cancer:
Historical Review to Current Approach*

Melinda E. Sanders, MD
Associate Professor of Pathology, Microbiology, and
Immunology, Department of Pathology, Microbiology, and
Immunology, Vanderbilt University School of Medicine,
Nashville, TN
*20 Risk Factors for Breast Carcinoma in Women With
Proliferative Breast Disease*

Tara Sanft, MD
Assistant Professor of Medicine, Yale University School of
Medicine, New Haven, CT
84 Psychosocial Consequences and Lifestyle Interventions

Cesar A. Santa-Maria, MD, MSCI
Assistant Professor, Northwestern University, Chicago, IL
*55 Adjuvant and Neoadjuvant Systemic Therapies for Early-
Stage Breast Cancer*

Jennifer Sasaki, MD
Department of Surgery, Penn State Milton S. Hershey Medical
Center, Hershey, PA
5 Etiology and Management of Benign Breast Disease

Nirav B. Savalia, MD
Clinical Assistant Professor of Surgery, Plastic Surgery,
University of Southern California/Keck School of Medicine,
Los Angeles; Director of Oncoplastic and Aesthetic Breast
Surgery at Hoag Memorial Hospital Presbyterian, Newport
Beach, CA
*40 The New Paradigm: Oncoplastic Breast Conservation
Surgery*

Chirag Shah, MD
Associate Staff, Department of Radiation Oncology, Taussig
Cancer Institute, Cleveland Clinic, Cleveland, OH
51 Partial Breast Irradiation: Accelerated and Intraoperative

Samman Shahpar, MD
Attending Physician, Cancer Rehabilitation Program, Shirley
Ryan Ability Lab; Assistant Professor, Department of
Physical Medicine and Rehabilitation, Northwestern
University Feinberg School of Medicine, Chicago, IL
83 Rehabilitation

Yu Shyr, PhD
Director, Center for Quantitative Sciences; Director, Vanderbilt
Technologies for Advanced Genomics Analysis and Research
Design; Harold L. Moses Chair in Cancer Research and
Professor, Biostatistics, Biomedical Informatics, Cancer
Biology and Health Policy, Vanderbilt University Medical
Center, Nashville, TN
27 Design and Conduct of Clinical Trials for Breast Cancer

Melvin J. Silverstein, MD
Clinical Professor, Department of Surgery, University of
Southern California, Los Angeles, CA; Medical Director,
Breast Program, Hoag Memorial Hospital Presbyterian,
Newport Beach, CA
39 Ductal Carcinoma in Situ of the Breast
40 The New Paradigm: Oncoplastic Breast Conservation
Surgery

Jean F. Simpson, MD
President, Breast Pathology Consultants, Inc., Nashville, TN;
Adjunct Professor, Department of Pathology, University of
South Alabama, Mobile, AL
8 Benign, High-Risk, and Premalignant Lesions of the Breast
20 Risk Factors for Breast Carcinoma in Women With
Proliferative Breast Disease

George W. Sledge, Jr., MD
Professor of Medicine, Department of Medicine; Chief,
Division of Oncology, Stanford University, Stanford, CA
56 HER2-Positive Breast Cancer

Karen Lisa Smith, MD, MPH
Assistant Professor of Oncology, Breast Cancer Program, Johns
Hopkins Sidney Kimmel Comprehensive Cancer Center,
Baltimore, MD
54 Adjuvant Endocrine Therapy

Stephen M. Smith, MD
Clinical Instructor and House Staff, Department of Pathology,
The Ohio State University Wexner Medical Center,
Columbus, OH
13 Primary and Secondary Dermatologic Disorders of the Breast

George Somlo, MD
Professor, Departments of Medical Oncology & Therapeutics
Research and Hematology & Hematopoietic Cell
Transplantation, City of Hope, Duarte, CA
64 Inflammatory Breast Cancer

Sasha E. Stanton, MD, PhD
Acting Instructor, Department of Medicine, University of
Washington, Seattle, WA
71 Immunologic Approaches to Breast Cancer Therapy

Vered Stearns, MD
Professor of Oncology, Breast Cancer Program, Johns Hopkins
Sidney Kimmel Comprehensive Cancer Center, Baltimore,
MD
54 Adjuvant Endocrine Therapy

Matthew A. Steliga, MD
Associate Professor of Surgery, Division of Cardiothoracic
Surgery, University of Arkansas for Medical Sciences, Little
Rock, AR
72 Diagnosis and Management of Pleural Metastases and
Malignant Effusion in Breast Cancer

Alison T. Stopeck, MD
Professor of Medicine, Chief, Division of Hematology/
Oncology, Associate Director for Translational Research,
Stony Brook Cancer Center, Stony Brook University, Stony
Brook, NY
68 Management of Bone Metastases in Breast Cancer

Toncred M. Styblo, MD, MS
Associate Professor of Surgery, Department of Surgery, Emory
University School of Medicine, Atlanta, GA
18 Clinically Established Prognostic Factors in Breast Cancer

Susie X. Sun, MD
Resident in Surgery, Penn State Milton S. Hershey Medical
Center, Hershey, PA
3 Breast Physiology: Normal and Abnormal Development and
Function

Melinda L. Telli, MD
Assistant Professor of Medicine, Department of Medicine,
Division of Oncology, Stanford University School of
Medicine, Stanford, CA
62 Principles of Preoperative Therapy for Operable Breast
Cancer

Amye J. Tevaarwerk, MD
Associate Professor, Hematology/Oncology, University of
Wisconsin and Carbone Cancer Center, Madison, WI
70 Endocrine Therapy for Breast Cancer

Parijatham S. Thomas, MD
Assistant Professor, Clinical Cancer Prevention; Assistant
Professor, Breast Medical Oncology, The University of Texas
MD Anderson Cancer Center, Houston, TX
80 Clinical Management of the Patient at Increased or High Risk

Nicholas D. Tingquist, MD
Resident Physician, Department of Surgery, University of
Arkansas for Medical Sciences, Little Rock, AR
72 Diagnosis and Management of Pleural Metastases and
Malignant Effusion in Breast Cancer

Jacqueline Tsai, MD
Breast Oncology Fellow, Stanford University School of
Medicine, Stanford, CA
61 Locoregional Recurrence After Mastectomy

Stephanie A. Valente, DO, FACS
Assistant Professor of Surgery, Cleveland Clinic Lerner College
   of Medicine, Breast Surgical Oncology, General Surgery,
   Cleveland Clinic, Cleveland, OH
   6 Mastitis and Breast Abscess
   *44 Intraoperative Evaluation of Surgical Margins in Breast
      Conserving Therapy*

Astrid Botty Van den Bruele, MD
University of Florida, Jacksonville, FL
   *77 Local Recurrence, the Augmented Breast, and the
      Contralateral Breast*

Luis O. Vasconez, MD, Doctor Honoris Causa
Prof. (Emeritus) Plastic Surgery, Surgery, University of Alabama
   at Birmingham Medical Center, Birmingham, AL
   *29 General Principles of Mastectomy: Evaluation and
      Therapeutic Options*
   33 Breast Reconstruction and Oncoplastic Surgery

Frank A. Vicini, MD
Michigan Healthcare Professionals/21st Century Oncology,
   Department of Radiation Oncology, Farmington Hills, MI
   51 Partial Breast Irradiation: Accelerated and Intraoperative

Rebecca K. Viscusi, MD
Assistant Professor, Department of Surgery, University of
   Arizona College of Medicine, Tucson, AZ
   37 Assessment and Designation of Breast Cancer Stage

Daniel W. Visscher, MD
Professor, Department of Laboratory Medicine and Pathology,
   Mayo Clinic, Rochester, MN
   12 Paget Disease of the Breast

Victor G. Vogel, MD, MHS
Director, Breast Medical Oncology/Research, Geisinger Health
   System, Danville, PA
   15 Epidemiology of Breast Cancer
   16 Primary Prevention of Breast Cancer

Adrienne G. Waks, MD
Instructor in Medicine, Harvard Medical School; Fellow,
   Medical Oncology, Dana-Farber Cancer Institute, Boston,
   MA
   *69 Chemotherapy and HER2-Directed Therapy for Metastatic
      Breast Cancer*

Irene L. Wapnir, MD, FACS
Professor of Surgery, Stanford University School of Medicine,
   Stanford, CA
   61 Locoregional Recurrence After Mastectomy

Thomas Wells, MD
Professor, Department of Pediatrics, University of Arkansas for
   Medical Sciences, Little Rock, AR
   27 Design and Conduct of Clinical Trials for Breast Cancer

Julia White, MD
Professor, Department of Radiation Oncology, The Ohio State
   University Comprehensive Cancer Center, Columbus, OH
   47 Radiotherapy and Ductal Carcinoma in Situ

Max S. Wicha, MD
Department of Internal Medicine, Division of Hematology/
   Oncology, Comprehensive Cancer Center, School of
   Medicine, University of Michigan, Ann Arbor, MI
   23 Stem Cells in Breast Development and Cancer

Eric P. Winer, MD
Chief, Division of Women's Cancers, Susan F. Smith Center for
   Women's Cancers, Dana-Farber Cancer Institute; Professor
   of Medicine, Harvard Medical School, Boston, MA
   *69 Chemotherapy and HER2-Directed Therapy for Metastatic
      Breast Cancer*

Kari B. Wisinski, MD
Associate Professor, Department of Medicine, University of
   Wisconsin and Carbone Cancer Center, Madison, WI
   70 Endocrine Therapy for Breast Cancer

Debra A. Wong, MB, BCh, BAO
Department of Hematology & Medical Oncology, Mayo Clinic,
   Scottsdale, AZ
   *11 Mesenchymal Neoplasms and Primary Lymphomas of the
      Breast*

Teresa K. Woodruff, PhD, DSc
Vice Chair for Research, Thomas J. Watkins Memorial Professor
   of Obstetrics and Gynecology, Department of Obstetrics and
   Gynecology, Northwestern University Feinberg School of
   Medicine, Chicago, IL
   58 Oncofertility Options for Young Women With Breast Cancer

Eric J. Wright, MD
Assistant Professor of Plastic and Reconstructive Surgery,
   Department of Surgery, University of Arkansas for Medical
   Sciences, Little Rock, AR
   33 Breast Reconstruction and Oncoplastic Surgery

Melissa Young, MD, PhD
Department of Therapeutic Radiology, Yale University School of
   Medicine, New Haven, CT
   46 Biological Basis of Radiotherapy of the Breast

Zachary T. Young, MD
General Surgery, University of Arkansas for Medical Sciences,
   Little Rock, AR
   7 Gynecomastia

Preface

All industrialized countries readily acknowledge the impact of breast disease in human society as a major epidemiologic issue that continues to expand exponentially. Additionally, a demographic statistic supported by the Biometry Branch of the National Cancer Institute in the United States recognizes breast cancer as the most frequent and second most lethal carcinoma that occurs in women. Furthermore, one of every three American women will consult a physician for breast diseases, and approximately one of every four women will undergo a breast biopsy. Of distinct demographic importance, the lifetime risk for one of every eight American women and for many Western industrialized societies to develop an invasive carcinoma of the breast is significant and continues to grow. Moreover, current estimates suggest that the rapidly evolving diagnosis of ductal carcinoma in situ may represent as great as one-fourth of all breast cancers diagnosed within the next two decades. All these demographic features support the concern of the epidemiologic increase for diagnosis of this neoplasm, and thus the implementation of state-of-the-art screening and therapies that impact this neoplasm.

With publication of the first edition of *The Breast* in 1991, the authors placed the diagnosis and therapy of breast disease in a working perspective, integrating contemporary, multidisciplinary oncologic principles and therapeutic approaches. These disciplines include surgery, radiation oncology, pathology, medical oncology, radiology, pharmacokinetics, genetics, transplantation, and biostatistics. Each discipline is synergistic in the support for the missions of hospice, social services, and psychosocial support teams to holistically treat all aspects of breast disease. Moreover, practitioners of each medical discipline have pursued an evolutionary process as new therapeutic modalities were added, which has enhanced clinical outcomes and patient care.

With publication of the second edition in 1998, the third edition in 2004, and the fourth edition in 2009, the medical disciplines have noted unprecedented progress in the therapy of breast diseases. Surgery and medicine have, in general, evolved very rapidly as a consequence of notable scientific achievements that include the following:

- Breakthrough of the molecular and genetic subdisease process that expands the formidable knowledge base for phenotypically normal and abnormal (proliferative) disease processes (e.g., cancer genetics, cellular regulatory events in carcinogenesis, carcinoma initiation and disease progression, invasion and metastasis, and molecular diagnostic and prognostic markers)
- DNA sequencing of the human genome with identification of mutational variance that affects genetic progression and phenotypic expression
- Therapeutic innovative advents such as immunotherapy, gene therapy, bone marrow transplantation, angiogenesis inhibitors, and other technical approaches that employ (and exploit) novel biologic discoveries

- The emerging perspective that properly guides clinical outcomes research
- Advancement in surgical techniques and technology

At present, no other human organ system has witnessed the integration of multimodal diagnostic and therapeutic approaches that are recognized to be as focused and successful as those that have been developed for breast neoplasms.

The fifth edition of *The Breast* has evolved into a more refined comprehensive text that was designed as a contemporary readable tome for all medical researchers and clinicians. The fifth edition reviews the basic tenets essential for diagnosis and therapy of the various benign and malignant disorders of the breast. The editors have sought to develop the proper address of many recognized abnormalities presenting in the diagnosis and therapy of metabolic, physiologic, and neoplastic derangements of the organ. When we compare this edition with the first through fourth editions, we consider the present edition to be even more definitive, inclusive, comprehensive, and relevant to scientific and clinical achievements.

Our view and expectations are that this new edition provides the requirements necessary for young clinicians (residents) and scientists in training to acquire fundamental knowledge of basic, clinical, and laboratory concepts and techniques that will complement their oncology education. Integration of these principles with advancements in technologic, molecular, cellular, and biologic sciences represents the 21st century definition of each specialty involved with the care of breast diseases. However, the ultimate measure of professional skill and effectiveness expected of us as clinicians in the management of breast diseases will be the quality that this text brings to bear upon patient outcomes, as well as emotional and physical morbidity.

As a comprehensive treatise of breast diseases, the fifth edition is *not* intended to replace standard textbooks of surgery, medicine, or biology, nor is this edition considered an encyclopedic recitation of the myriad of pathologic permutations that exist with various disorders of this organ site. Rather, the fifth edition of *The Breast* should coexist with other major medical and surgical reference books. Each chapter is selectively organized and supported with notations of carefully selected journal articles, monographs, or chapters within major reference texts that the contributors of these specific subjects consider a valuable resource. Thus this work represents a distillation of the herald contributions of innumerable physicians, physiologists, anatomists, geneticists, clinical scientists, and noted health-related workers who have devoted their careers and research to the management of various disorders of the breast.

The fifth edition comprises 18 sections and 86 chapters, with at least 30% additional and/or revised information when compared with the fourth edition. The opening section documents the historical aspects of breast disease, incorporating the major scientific contributions of investigators and surgeons of the 19th and 20th centuries. The sections that follow include pertinent physiology, anatomy, pathology, genetics, molecular biology, targeted biologics, pharmacokinetics, surgery, radiation biology, medical oncology, and biostatistics. Throughout the fifth edition, authors and coauthors have supplemented the text with supportive history of the evolution and chronology of therapeutic principles. In addition, special sections are dedicated to the management of unusual and advanced presentations of the disease.

Additional chapters provide new approaches to the management of breast pain and the risk for carcinoma of the breast following hormonal replacement therapy; one chapter defines patterns of recurrence. The evolution of precise staging evident with lymphatic mapping and sentinel lymph node biopsy has been addressed in depth and provides a new level of precise documentation of technique and outcomes as a consequence of the international experience with the technique since the completion of the second edition. The authors have also incorporated new approaches for gene therapy and counseling for genetic mutations, angiogenesis, immunology, and the evolving role for the immunotherapy of breast cancer. Furthermore, applications of nutritional management and evolving psychologic principles are incorporated in the text. One chapter, again, is dedicated to addressing legal implications that relate to the management of breast disease. Chapters are also dedicated in this edition to covering the psychologic considerations of breast disease and its implications, which affect the patient, spouse, and family members. Also, an explicit discussion is added in the survivorship chapter to expectations of quality-of-life issues post-therapy.

With the evolution of this comprehensive reference, overlap will continue to exist among several chapters as a consequence of the dynamic interplay and expectations of medical and surgical practitioners involved with the diagnostic and therapeutic management of the cancer patient. However, the editors have made every effort to minimize repetition of data and principles and dedicated comments except where controversial or "state-of-the-art" issues for management exist.

A salient attribute of the text includes the integration of basic science with translational research to emphasize efforts for transfer of knowledge from the bench laboratory to the bedside and the clinic. Only with evolving applications of phase II and phase III trials can the clinician objectively assess the therapeutic value of evolving technical and therapeutic management strategies that arise from state-of-the-art phase I developmental trials. These translational research objectives will continue to evaluate promising chemotherapeutics, immunologic agents, inhibitors of angiogenesis, and additional molecularly engineered products that show promise in inhibiting neoplastic progression in this organ.

As previously noted, the authors are truly hopeful that the fifth edition of *The Breast* has achieved its developmental and scientific goals for assimilating and collating evolving contemporary basic and clinical scientific data. These developmental principles provide clinicians and researchers with multidisciplinary tools used in their clinical practice for the treatment of diseases of the breast. The editors gratefully acknowledge the opportunity provided by the immense challenge that has been entrusted to us by the publisher and are, again, hopeful that our diligence to this task has been properly served.

Kirby I. Bland
Edward M. Copeland III
V. Suzanne Klimberg
William J. Gradishar

Acknowledgments

The editors are deeply indebted to the authors who have contributed to the fifth edition of *The Breast: Comprehensive Management of Benign and Malignant Diseases*. It is the view of the editors and associate editors that this edition remains the most comprehensive international reference provided in the scientific literature that is dedicated to diseases of the breast. Both the editors and associate editors have embellished pertinent clinical trials with basic and translational surgical science that has appropriate outcomes when applied in the clinics. Therefore we are deeply indebted to the associate editors for their efforts toward the completion of this comprehensive tome.

The untold hours essential to properly prepare this treatise represent time taken from busy clinical practices, research laboratories, and our families. Thus the diligent efforts of the contributors to provide insightful state-of-the-art presentations are gratefully acknowledged. Furthermore, the updating of proper scientific knowledge by these contributors through their choice of selective illustrations, tables, and references to bring this text to its readable state of completeness and comprehensiveness is also praiseworthy.

The genesis of the fifth edition began with the encouragement and extensive support of Edward Wickland at Saunders in 1990. Special appreciation should also be paid to Louis Reines, former President of W.B. Saunders, who provided strong encouragement and support for initiation of the first through third editions of this text. The editors wish to pay tribute to the diligent work by the staff members of Elsevier, Inc., who have made publication of the fifth edition possible. Executive Content Strategist Michael Houston provided strong support for complication of this fifth edition, which has been supervised in an extraordinary and skillful manner by Kathryn DeFrancesco and Kristine Feeherty as developmental editors for the book, and who were instrumental in overseeing the editorial process, procuring manuscripts, and scheduling. For these noteworthy contributions, the editors and associate editors are most appreciative.

We further thank our internal editorial staff: Carol Ann Moore at the University of Alabama at Birmingham (UAB) and Laura Adkins at the University of Arkansas, who examined materials to ensure they were as flawless as possible. We are also grateful to all editorial assistants in the Department of Surgery at the UAB, as well as our (KIB, EMC) former secretary and editorial assistant, Ervene Katz, of the University of Florida, who has retired since the publication of the third edition. We also express gratitude to Louis Clark and Jonathan Bland, the principal artists of earlier editions who skillfully prepared the illustrations and line drawings used throughout various chapters of the text.

The editors and associate editors are all deeply appreciative of our residents, research fellows, and colleagues in Surgery, Medicine, Pathology, and Radiation Oncology for their intellectual stimulation and their continual encouragement to proceed with development of the fifth edition. To the faculty and residents who have reviewed manuscripts, rendered opinions, and offered suggestions, we gratefully acknowledge their critiques, enlightening commentary, and sustained interest.

Finally, to all who were involved with the development of this text, inclusive of our immediate families and friends who expressed interest and encouragement in the completion of this textbook, we greatly appreciate your indulgence for the time allowed for us to pursue the ambitious goal of preparing what we consider to be a readable, comprehensive text that properly embraces the tenets essential for the diagnosis and therapy of breast diseases. The editors and associate editors further realize that the goals organized and accomplished by the editorial staff and Elsevier for the fifth edition could have been achieved only with the immense dedication to task that is evident in the contributions of the authors of each chapter, the artists, and our dedicated editorial assistants.

Kirby I. Bland
Edward M. Copeland III
V. Suzanne Klimberg
William J. Gradishar

Contents

Video Contents

1

History of the Therapy of Breast Cancer

KIRBY I. BLAND, EDWARD M. COPELAND III, AND V. SUZANNE KLIMBERG

With their uncertain etiology, breast diseases have captured the attention of physicians throughout the ages. Despite centuries of theoretical meanderings and scientific inquiry, breast cancer remains one of the most dreaded of all human diseases. The historical account of the efforts to cope with breast cancer is complex, and there is no definitive causation as there is in diseases for which cause and cure have been defined. However, progress has been made in lessening the horrors that formerly devastated the body and psyche.

This chapter was developed to examine the history of breast diseases/cancer. It records key milestones in the development of the current progress of the biology and therapy of these presentations, which is based on the achievements and contributions of multiple physicians and scientists over many hundreds of years. Although the milestones listed here are important ones, the list should not be considered comprehensive. This chapter is meant to be a useful reference to all who desire knowledge of the historical background of breast cancer and that of evolving breast cancer therapy.

Ancient Civilizations

Chinese

Huang Di, the Yellow Emperor, was born in 2698 BCE and subsequently wrote the *Nei Jing*, the oldest treatise of medicine, which gives the first description of tumors and documents five forms of therapy: spiritual care, pharmacology, diet, acupuncture, and the treatment of specific diseases.

Egyptian

Imhotep, an Egyptian physician, architect, and astrologer, was born in 2650 BCE. He designed the first pyramid at Saqqara and was deified as the god of healing. The early Egyptians documented many cases of breast tumors, which were treated with cautery. To preserve their findings, the Egyptians etched their cursive script on thin sheets of papyrus leaf and also engraved or painted hieroglyphics on stone. Among six principal papyri, the most informative one with respect to diseases of the breast is that acquired by Edwin Smith (b. 1822) in 1862 and presented to the New York Historical Society at the time of his death. Dating to about 1600 BCE, it is a papyrus roll 15 feet long, with writing on both sides.[1] The front contains 17 columns describing 48 cases devoted to clinical surgery. References are made to diseases of the breast such

as abscesses, trauma, and infected wounds. Case 45 is perhaps the earliest record of breast cancer, with the title *Instructions Concerning Tumors on the Breast* (Fig. 1.1). The examiner is told that a breast with bulging tumors, very cool to the touch, is an ailment for which there is no treatment.

Babylonian

The Code of Hammurabi (ca. 1750 BCE) was commissioned in Babylon. Its 282 clauses provided the first laws that regulated medical practitioners and dealt with physicians' responsibilities and fees. At that time, internal medicine consisted mainly of a recitation of litanies and incantations against the demons of the earth, air, and water. Surgery consisted of opening an abscess with a bronze lancet. If the patient died or lost an eye during treatment, the physician's hands were cut off.

Classic Greek Period (460–136 BCE)

Medicine in Europe had its origins in ancient Greece. The scientific method and clinical advancement of medicine are credited to Hippocrates (b. 460 BCE), who also defined its ethical ideals. His basic philosophy was the linkage of four cardinal body humors (blood, phlegm, yellow bile, and black bile) with four universal elements (earth, air, water, and fire). Perfect health depended on a proper balance in the dynamic qualities of the humors. It was generally believed that blood was in the arteries and veins, phlegm in the brain, yellow bile in the liver, and black bile in the spleen. Hippocrates divided diseases into three general categories: those curable by medicine (most favorable), those not curable by medicine but curable by the knife, and those not curable by the knife but curable by fire. The *Corpus Hippocraticum* deals with the treatment of fractures, tumors, surgical procedures, asthma, allergies, and diseases of the skin. A well-documented case history of Hippocrates describes a woman with breast cancer associated with bloody discharge from the nipple. Hippocrates associated breast cancer with cessation of menstruation, leading to breast engorgement and indurated nodules.

Alexandria on the Nile, founded by Alexander the Great in 332 BCE, became the focal point of Greek science during the third and second centuries BCE. More than 14,000 students studied various elements of Hellenistic knowledge there. This knowledge was contained in 700,000 scrolls in the largest library in antiquity, which was subsequently destroyed by Julius Caesar. Rudimentary

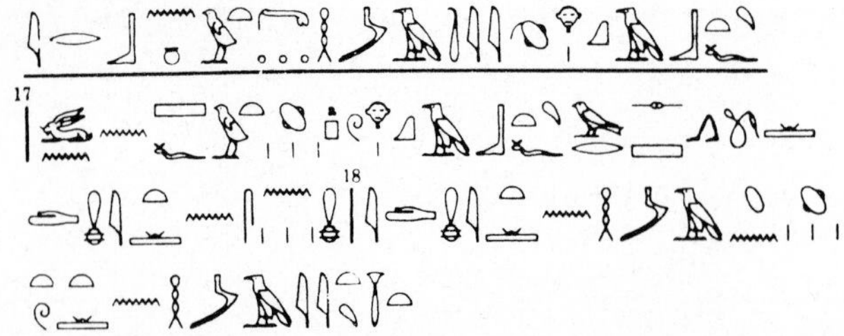

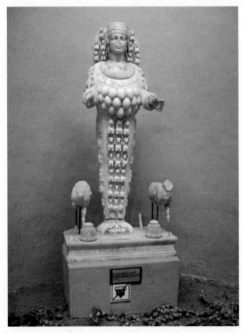

• **Fig. 1.1** Recording of the earliest known case of breast cancer (1600 BCE). (From the Edwin Smith Papyrus. Published in facsimile and hieroglyphic transliteration with translation and commentary by James Henry Breasted. Birmingham, AL: The Classics of Medicine Library; 1984. Reprinted with permission.)

• **Fig. 1.2** Statue of Diana of Ephesus, a fertility deity invoked by Roman women, displaying 20 accessory pectoral breasts. (Photo by David Bjorgen. Available at: https://commons.wikimedia.org/wiki/File:Statue_of_Artemis_Ephesus.jpg. Accessed June 2016.)

anatomic studies were conducted and led to progress in the tools and techniques of surgery.

Greco-Roman Period (150 BCE–AD 500)

After the destruction of Corinth in 146 BCE, Greek medicine migrated to Rome. During the preceding six centuries, the Romans had lived without physicians. They depended on medicinal herbs, assorted concoctions, votive objects, religious rites, and superstitions (Fig. 1.2).

Aurelius Celsus, a Roman born in 25 BCE, described the cardinal signs of inflammation (calor, rubor, dolor, and turgor). He wrote *De Medicina* around AD 30, which contains an early clinical description of *cancer* and likened the lesion to a *crab*. In it he notes that breasts of women as one of the anatomic sites of cancer and describes a fixed irregular swelling with dilated tortuous veins and ulceration. He also delineates four clinical stages of cancer: (1) early cancer, *cacoethes;* (2) cancer without ulcer; (3) ulcerated cancer; and (4) ulcerated cancer with cauliflower-like excrescences that bleed easily. Celsus strongly advised against the treatment of

the last three stages by any method because aggressive measures irritated the condition and led to inevitable recurrence.

The Greek physician Leonides is credited with the *first operative treatment for breast cancer* in the first century AD. His method consisted of an initial incision into the uninvolved portion of the breast, followed by applications of cautery to stop the bleeding. Repetitive incisions and applications of cautery were continued until the entire breast and tumor had been removed and the underlying tissues were covered with an eschar. With Roman influence and support, surgical instruments became highly specialized, as witnessed by the finding of more than 200 different instruments in the excavations of Pompeii and Herculaneum (Figs. 1.3 and 1.4).

The greatest Greek physician to follow Hippocrates was Galen (b. AD 131). He was born on the Mediterranean coast of Asia Minor, studied in Alexandria, and practiced medicine for the remainder of his life in Rome. He is credited as the founder of experimental physiology, and his system of pathology followed that of Hippocrates.

Galen considered black bile, especially when it was extremely dark or thick, to be the most harmful of the four humors and the ultimate cause of cancer. He described breast cancer as a swelling with distended veins resembling the shape of a crab's legs. To prevent accumulation of black bile, Galen advocated that the patient be purged and bled. He claimed to have cured the disease in its early stage when the tumor was on the surface of the breast and all the "roots" could be extirpated at surgery. The roots were not derived from the tumor but were dilated veins filled with morbid black bile. When removing these superficial (anterior) lesions, the surgeon had to be aware of the danger of profuse hemorrhage from large blood vessels. On the other hand, the surgeon was advised to allow the blood to flow freely for a while to allow the "black bile" (blood) to escape.

Middle Ages

The Middle Ages may be considered the period between the downfall of Rome and the beginning of the Renaissance. The doctrine of the four humors, which formed the basis of Hippocratic medicine, was endowed with authority by Galen and governed all aspects of medical thinking throughout and beyond the Middle Ages. This influence can be traced in the Christian, Jewish, and Arabic traditions.

Christian

From the Christian standpoint, the monks and clerics who constituted the educated class maintained medicine in the Middle Ages. In 529, with the founding by Saint Benedict of the Monastery on Monte Cassino in central Italy, there arose a heightened interest in medicine in the scattered cloisters of the Roman Church. Monte Cassino fostered the teaching and practice of medicine, along with the copying and preserving of ancient manuscripts. Many satellite monasteries developed throughout Christendom in which the monks treated the sick and copied medical manuscripts. Subsequently, monastic schools spread under the Benedictines to England, Scotland, Ireland, France, Switzerland, and most of the European continent. The patron saint for breast disease was Saint Agatha. She had been a martyr in Sicily in the middle of the third century when her two breasts were torn off with iron shears because of resistance to the advances of the governor Quinctianus (Fig. 1.5). On Saint Agatha's day, two loaves

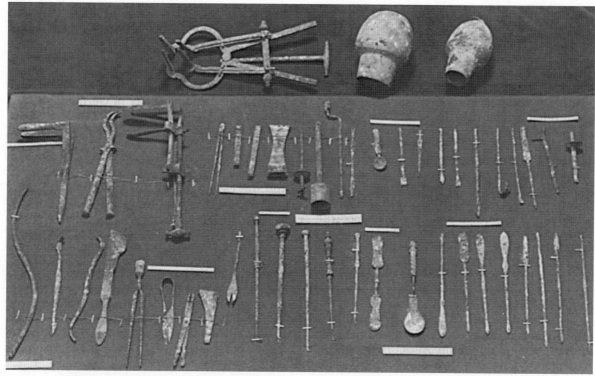

• **Fig. 1.3** Surgical instruments (AD 79) from excavations of Pompeii and Herculaneum. (Courtesy the Archives of Thomas Jefferson University, Philadelphia, PA.)

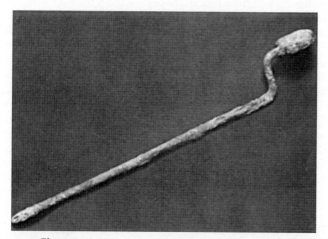

• **Fig. 1.4** Roman cautery (AD 79) depicted from Fig. 1.3.

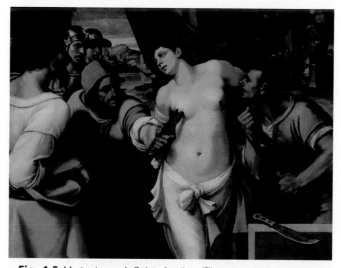

• **Fig. 1.5** Martyrdom of Saint Agatha. (Photo available at: https:// commons.wikimedia.org/wiki/File:Sebastiano_del_Piombo_-_ Martyrdom_of_St_Agatha_-_WGA21109.jpg. Accessed June 2016.)

of bread representing her previously mutilated breasts are carried in procession on a tray.

The Council of Rheims (1131) excluded monks and the clergy from the practice of medicine. From that time on, laymen increasingly preserved the tradition of medical teaching and practice. Cathedral schools, although in clerical hands, profited from greater freedom than the monasteries had provided and enjoyed the intellectual contacts of the large cities. Further growth of cities in the 11th and 12th centuries led to the rise of universities with academic approaches to science; this movement freed the teaching and control of medicine from monastic influence.

Paul of Aegina (b. 625) was an Alexandrian physician and surgeon famed for his *Epitomae Medicae Libri Septem*, which contained descriptions of trephining, tonsillotomy, paracentesis, and mastectomy. Lanfranc of Milan (b. 1250) was an Italian surgeon who worked in Paris and wrote *Chirurgia Magna*, which contained sections on anatomy, embryology, ulcers, fistulas, and fractures, as well as sections on herbs and pharmacy and on cancer of the breast.

Jewish

Jewish physicians were active at Salerno, Italy, as early as the ninth century. They achieved great distinction not only in the art of healing but also in their literary efforts. Popes, kings, and noblemen sought their services. In a time when poisoning of enemies and rivals was common, the Jews were considered the safest medical advisers. The Arabian rulers and Egyptian caliphs also preferred them to their Mohammedan physicians, who practiced magic and astrology in their treatment of disease.

Under the tolerant Moors of Spain and the early Christian rulers of Spain and Portugal, the Jews became leaders in the medical profession. The foremost among them was Moses Maimonides. Born in Cordova, Spain, in 1135, he studied medicine at Cairo and became the physician to Saladin, the Sultan of Egypt. In addition to his own medical treatise, he translated from Arabic into Hebrew the five volume *al-Quanum fil-Tib* of the Iranian physician Avicenna (b. 980), which was the authoritative encyclopedia of medicine during the Middle Ages. Maimonides also made a collection of the aphorisms of Hippocrates and Galen.

Jewish physicians remained prominent in Spain under the Western Caliphate until they were banished from the country in 1492. The Salerno School exploited them as teachers until it had enough indigenous talent to proceed without them. Even at Montpellier in southern France, the Jews were excluded in 1301. It would not be until the onset of the modern industrial age that they would again be admitted to citizenship throughout Europe and given university freedom, which once more liberated their brilliant medical talent.

Arabic

Western society is indebted to Arabic scholars and physicians who valued and preserved the teachings and writings of their Greek predecessors. Without the intervention of the Arabs, the writings of the Greek physicians might have been lost. Baghdad, the capital of the Islamic Empire in Iraq, became the center for translation of the Greek authors. The library at Cordova had 600,000 manuscripts, and the one at Cairo had 18 rooms of books. The Tartars raided the library in Baghdad in 1260 and threw the books into the river.

Rhazes (b. 860), one of the great Arabic physicians, condoned excision of breast cancer only if it could be completely removed and the underlying tissues cauterized. He warned that incising a breast cancer would produce an ulceration. Haly ben Abbas, a Persian who died in 994, authored an encyclopedic work in medicine and surgery based on Rhazes and the Greek sources. He endorsed the removal of breast cancers with allowance for bleeding to evacuate melancholic humors, which were widely believed to predispose to cancer. He did not tie the arteries and made no notation of wound cautery. Avicenna was the successor to Haly ben Abbas and was known as the "Prince of Physicians." He was chief physician to the hospital at Baghdad and was the author of a vast scientific and philosophical encyclopedia, *Kitab-Ash-shifa,* as well as the *al-Quanum fil-Tib,* both of which remained authoritative references for centuries.

Renaissance

The transition from the medieval to the modern era occurred in the latter part of the 15th century, with the introduction of gunpowder into warfare, the discovery of America, and the invention of the printing press. During this period, medical teaching flourished in universities in Montpellier, Bologna, Padua, Paris, Oxford, and Cambridge.

Andreas Vesalius (b. 1514) was a Flemish physician who revolutionized the study of medicine with his detailed descriptions of the anatomy of the human body, based on his own dissection of cadavers. His masterful observation and anatomic descriptions and illustrations were instrumental in opening scientific query and pathologic anatomy in medical science. While at the University of Padua, he wrote and illustrated the first comprehensive textbook of anatomy, *De Humani Corporis Fabrica Libri Septem* (1543). He recommended mastectomy for breast cancer and the use of sutures rather than cautery to control bleeding.

Ambrose Paré (b. 1510) studied medicine in Paris and, through his war experience, became the greatest surgeon of his time. His conservative surgical approach to cancer was detailed in *Oeuvres Complètes* (1575). He encouraged the use of vascular ligatures and the avoidance of cautery and boiling oil. He supported the excision of superficial breast cancers but attempted to treat advanced breast cancers through application of lead plates, which were intended to compress the blood supply and arrest tumor growth. He made the important observation that breast cancer often initiated enlargement of the axillary "glands." Michael Servetus (b. 1509), a Spaniard who studied in Paris, was burned at the stake for his heretical discovery that blood in the pulmonary circulation passes into the heart after having been mixed with air in the lungs. For cancer of the breast, Servetus suggested that the underlying pectoralis muscles be removed en bloc, together with the axillary glands, as described by Paré. This recommendation predated, by nearly four centuries, the anatomic basis of the radical mastectomy espoused by Halsted and Meyer.

Wilhelm Fabry (b. 1560) is held in esteem as the "Father of German Surgery." His name was honored by the placement of a wreath at his statue in Hilden near Düsseldorf, Germany, by members of the International Society of the History of Medicine in 1986 (Fig. 1.6). He devised an instrument (Fig. 1.7) that compressed and fixed the base of the breast so that a scalpel could amputate it more swiftly and less painfully.[2] His text, *Opera,* included clear descriptions of breast cancer operations and illustrations of amputation forceps. He stipulated that the tumor should be mobile so that it could be removed completely, with no remnants left behind. The other famous German surgeon of this period was Johann Schultes (b. 1595), known as Scultetus, who was an illustrator of surgery and inventor of surgical instruments. His book, *Armamentarium Chirurgicum,* which was published posthumously in 1653, contained illustrations of surgical procedures, one of which represented amputation of the breast. He used

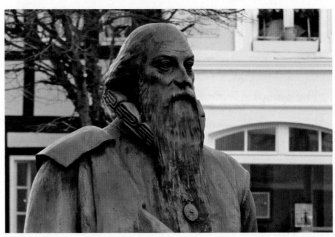

• **Fig. 1.6** Statue of Wilhelm Fabry in Hilden, Germany. (Available at: https://commons.wikimedia.org/wiki/File:Wilhelm_Fabry_Denkmal_02.jpg. Accessed June 2016.)

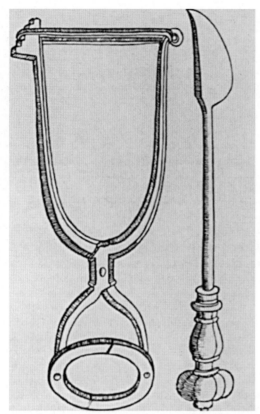

• **Fig. 1.7** Mastectomy instruments of Fabry von Hilden in the late 16th century. (From Robinson JO. Treatment of breast cancer through the ages. *Am J Surg.* 1986;151:317-333.)

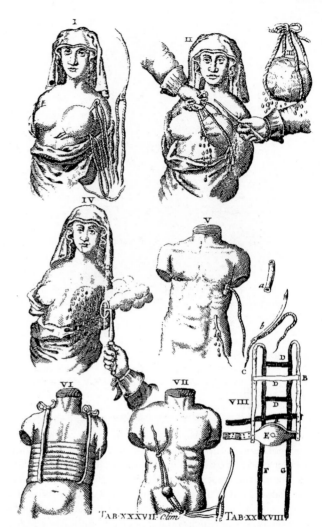

• **Fig. 1.8** Mastectomy procedure of Scultetus in the 7th century. (From Robinson JO. Treatment of breast cancer through the ages. *Am J Surg.* 1986;151:317-333.)

heavy ligatures on large needles, which transfixed the breast so that traction would facilitate its removal by the knife. Hemostasis was secured by cauterization of the base of the tumor (Fig. 1.8).

Because of the morbidity and mortality of breast cancer surgery and a paucity of competent surgeons, few breast amputations were actually performed. Nonsurgical remedies for breast cancer appeared in rudimentary scientific journals that were published toward the end of the 17th century (Fig. 1.9).

Eighteenth Century

The 1700s were slow to develop significant new concepts in pathology and physiology. The arbitrary separation of scirrhus and breast cancer in the doctrine of Galen was still thought to be correct. Many considered scirrhus to be a benign growth that under adverse circumstances could undergo malignant degeneration, whereas others regarded it as an existing stage of cancer. Most believed that scirrhus originated in stagnation and coagulation of body fluids within the breast (local cause). Others believed it to occur from a general internal derangement of the body juices (systemic cause). In accepting both causes, some authors wrote that the local cause could be a precipitating factor in a predisposed patient. Hermann Boerhaave (b. 1668) taught that Galen's yellow bile was blood serum rather than bile itself, that phlegm was serum that had been altered by standing, and that black bile was a part of a clot that had largely separated and had a darkened coloration. Thus the four humors of Galen were only different components of the blood. Pieter Camper (b. 1722) described and illustrated the internal mammary lymph nodes, and Paolo

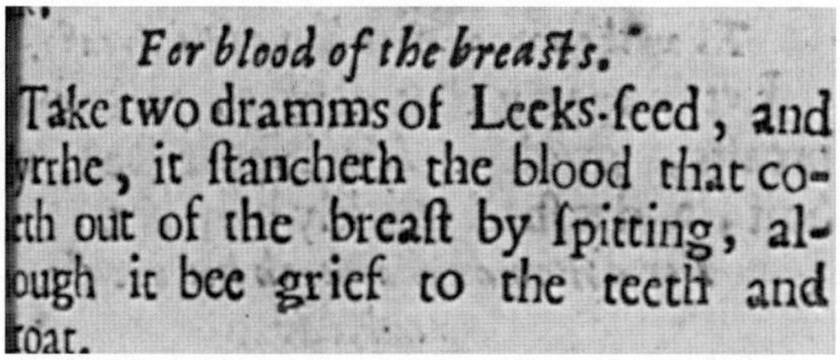

For blood of the breasts.
Take two dramms of Leeks-feed, and yrrhe, it stancheth the blood that cometh out of the breast by spitting, although it bee grief to the teeth and roat.

• **Fig. 1.9** Home remedy "for blood of the breasts" (1664).

Mascagni (b. 1752) did the same for the pectoral lymph nodes. Death caused by metastasis from breast cancer was not yet understood. If death was not caused by hemorrhage, it was ascribed to a general decomposition of the humors.

The surgeon Henri François Le Dran (b. 1685) of France (Fig. 1.10) concluded that cancer was a local disease in its early stages and that its spread to the lymphatic system signaled a worsened prognosis.[3] This was a courageous *contradiction* to the humoral theory of Galen, which had persisted for a thousand years and was to be upheld by many for two centuries to come. A colleague

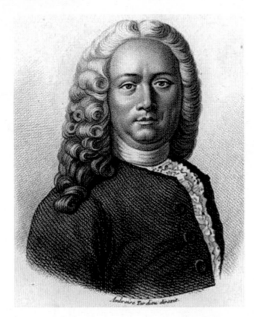

• **Fig. 1.10** Henri François Le Dran (1685–1770) noted that lymphatic spread worsened the prognosis of breast cancer. (Available at: https://commons.wikimedia.org/wiki/File:Henri_Fran%C3%A7ois_Le_Dran.jpg. Accessed June 2016.)

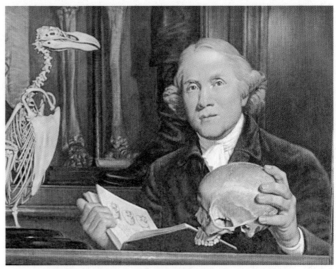

• **Fig. 1.11** John Hunter, Scottish Surgeon (1728–1793).

of Le Dran, Jean Petit (b. 1674), first director of the French Academy of Surgery, supported these principles. As recommended by the martyred Servetus, Le Dran also advocated en bloc removal of the breast, the underlying pectoral muscle, and the axillary lymph nodes.[4] Petit removed skin directly involved by cancer but returned skin closure over the noninvolved breast. In his book, *Traites des Operations,* which was not published until 24 years after his death, Petit recommended total removal of the breast and any enlarged axillary lymph nodes, as well as the pectoralis major muscle if it was involved by cancer.[4–8] He asserted, "the roots of a cancer were the enlarged lymphatic glands." Although Petit recognized the necessity of removing any skin directly involved by a breast cancer, he advised leaving most of the overlying skin, including the nipple, and dissecting breast tissue out from beneath it.[4]

Petit's pupil and colleague, Rene Garangeot (1688–1760), was largely responsible for preserving and disseminating the teachings of Petit. Garangeot explained the rationale for skin preservation in his book, *Traites des Operations de Chirurgie* (1720):

Sewing up the lips of the wound immediately after operation, as was practiced by J.L. Petit, is not only the safest method of arresting hemorrhage but is also the quickest way of healing the wound and preventing the return of the cancer.

Lorenz Heister (1683–1758), a famous German surgeon, used a guillotine device to amputate the entire breast. He was aware of the prognostic implications of axillary lymph node enlargement. In conjunction with mastectomy, he recommended removal of axillary lymph nodes, the pectoralis major muscle, and portions of the chest wall, if necessary, for complete excision of the cancer.[7,9] Another French surgeon, Bernard Peyrilhe (1735–1804), embraced the concept that breast cancer began locally and spread by way of the lymphatics.[10] Peyrilhe unsuccessfully attempted to

transmit cancer by injecting human breast cancer tissue into dogs. Following the practice of Petit and Heister, Peyrilhe advocated total mastectomy along with removal of the axillary lymph nodes and the pectoralis major muscle.[11,12]

In Edinburgh, Scotland, which was strongly oriented to university teaching, the separation of surgeons from barbers occurred by 1718. In London, where barber-surgeon guilds had existed, the separation occurred in 1745. A new era of British surgery began when William Cheselden (b. 1688), surgeon to St. Thomas' and St. George's Hospitals, first established private courses in anatomy and surgery. The Hunter brothers, John (b. 1728) and William (b. 1718), of Scotland followed suit. These courses attracted students from all over the country, the continent, and America. John Hunter is credited as being the founder of experimental surgery and surgical pathology (Fig. 1.11).

Samuel Sharpe, an English surgeon, advocated an approach similar to those of Petit, Heister, and Peyrilhe in his *Treatise on the Operations of Surgery,* which was published in 1735. For small cancers, he recommended removing the entire breast through a longitudinal incision. However, for larger cancers, he recommended removing an oval segment of skin to facilitate the mastectomy. He claimed that mastectomy was impractical if the breast cancer involved the underlying pectoral muscles but removed any "knobs" in the axilla.[7,13,14]

Benjamin Bell (1749–1806), surgeon at the Edinburgh Royal Infirmary, advocated a radical surgical procedure for all breast cancers and emphasized the importance of early diagnosis.[6–8,15] He echoed Petit's views in his book *A System of Surgery* (1784)[16]:

When practitioners have an opportunity of removing a cancerous breast early, they should always embrace it, that as little skin as possible should be removed, and that the breast should be dissected off the pectoral muscle, which ought to be preserved. If any indurated glands be observed, they should be removed and particular care should be given to this part of the operation. For unless all the diseased glands be taken away, no advantage whatever will be derived from it.

Henry Fearon (1750–1825), a British surgeon, recognized the importance of early detection and treatment of breast cancer but acknowledged the difficulties inherent in such an approach. In 1784 he wrote, "the early period of the complaint is beyond all doubt the most favorable period for extirpating it, however patients can seldom be convinced that there is any necessity for an operation while the disease continues in a mild state."[17]

In the late 18th century and the first half of the 19th century, pessimism toward breast cancer pervaded the medical literature, primarily as a result of the poor outcome after radical breast cancer surgery. The first hospital ward for indigent cancer patients opened in Middlesex Hospital in London in 1792 with the acknowledgment that it provided an opportunity to study the natural history of breast cancer.[12] In 1757, Petrus Camper commented on the reluctance of most of the surgeons in Amsterdam, which had a population of 200,000, to perform a mastectomy for breast cancer: "not six times a year a breast was amputated with reasonable chance of cure."[7,12,18] Large numbers of mastectomies were performed during the early 18th century, but this number decreased during the second half of the century because of poor results and the indiscriminate mutilation that occurred with improper patient selection and physician bias.

Alexander Monro Senior (1697–1767) reviewed 60 patients with breast cancer who underwent a mastectomy and found that only 4 of these patients were free of cancer after 2 years. Operative mortality, primarily from sepsis, was reported to be as high as 20%.[19] In 1842, the Scottish surgeon James Syme (1799–1870) wrote in his *Principles of Surgery* that surgical procedures for breast cancer should be abandoned when axillary lymph nodes were involved or when the cancer was too large for complete removal.[6,7,20] He found that surgery was likely to "excite greater activity" from the cancer that was left behind, echoing the comments of Celsus nearly 1900 years earlier.

In 1856, Sir James Paget (1814–1899) wrote that breast cancer was so hopeless that the mortality and morbidity associated with its treatment could not be justified.[21] He reported that women with "scirrhous" breast cancer lived longer if they avoided surgical intervention.[12] On reviewing his 235 breast cancer cases, Paget reported no cures and an 8-year recurrence rate of 100%.[6,7]

Nineteenth Century

Breast surgery changed dramatically in the 1800s. William Morton introduced anesthesia in the United States in 1846 at the Massachusetts General Hospital, and Joseph Lister introduced the principle of bacterial antisepsis in England in 1867. Lister implemented its transfer and development to operating theaters throughout Europe and America. These two pivotal advances were responsible, in part, for this dramatic change in surgical management and outcomes.

European Surgery

At the beginning of the 19th century, the treatment for breast cancer remained in the status quo. In 1811 Samuel Young in England revived the method of Paré, in which compression was used to cut off the blood supply of the tumor.[22] Nooth, another English surgeon, sprayed the breast with carbolic acid, which was a modified form of the ancient practice of cauterization.

James Syme (b. 1799) was a famous Scottish surgeon. His daughter married Sir Joseph Lister. Much of Syme's breast surgery was performed before the use of anesthesia.[20] His third surgical apprentice, John Brown (b. 1810), wrote *Rab and His Friends* (1858), which contains a vivid description of breast surgery as

performed by the then 28-year-old Syme in the Minto House Hospital of Edinburgh, Scotland[23]:

> The operating theater is crowded; much talk and fun and all the cordiality and stir of youth. The surgeon with his staff of assistants is there. In comes Ailie [the patient]: one look at her quiets and abates the eager students. Ailie stepped upon a seat, and laid herself on the table, as her friend the surgeon told her; arranged herself, gave a rapid look at James [her husband], shut her eyes, rested herself on me [Brown], and took my hand. The operation was at once begun; it was necessarily slow; and chloroform—one of God's best gifts to his suffering children—was then unknown. The surgeon did his work. The pale face showed its pain, but was still and silent. Rab's [the family's dog, a mastiff] soul was working within him; he saw that something strange was going on—blood flowing from his mistress, and she suffering; his ragged ear was up, and importunate; he growled and gave now and then a sharp impatient yelp; he would have liked to have done something to that man. But James had him firm, and gave him a glower from time to time, and an intimation of a possible kick—all the better for James, it kept his eye and his mind off Ailie. It is over: she is dressed, steps gently and decently down from the table, looks for James; then turning to the surgeon and the students, she curtsies— and in a low, clear voice, begs their pardon if she has behaved ill. The students—all of us—wept like children; the surgeon helped her up carefully—and resting on James and me, Ailie went to her room, Rab following. Four days after the operation what might have been expected happened. The patient had a chill, the wound was septic, and she died.

Later in life Syme was able to operate with the patient under anesthesia. He felt it incumbent on the surgeon to search carefully for axillary glands in the course of the operation but stated that the results were almost always unsatisfactory when the glands were involved, no matter how perfectly they seemed to have been removed. Sir James Paget (b. 1814) reported an operative mortality of 10% in 235 patients and among survivors, recurrence within 8 years. In 139 patients with scirrhous carcinoma, those who did not undergo surgery lived longer than those who did.[21] In 1874 Paget published *On Disease of the Mammary Areola Preceding Cancer of the Mammary Gland,* which described cancer of the nipple accompanied by eczematous changes and cancer of the lactiferous ducts (Paget's disease of the breast).[24]

In 1867, Charles Hewitt Moore (b. 1821) of the Middlesex Hospital in London championed the belief that the only possibility of cure for breast cancer was through wider and more extensive surgery, despite the frequent disastrous results (Fig. 1.12). His seminal paper, *On the Influence of Inadequate Operation on the Theory of Cancer* (1867), was widely accepted.[25] He appropriately stressed that the tumor should not be divided or incised and that recurrences originated as a result of dispersion from the primary growth and were not independent in origin. His operation called for removal of the entire breast, with special attention to removal of the skin in continuity with the main mass of the tumor en bloc with enlarged axillary lymphatics. Moore did not advocate removal of the pectoralis major muscle. In 1858 Moore was the first to advocate placement of drainage tubes through the axilla.[25]

The father of surgical antiseptic technique and one of Great Britain's most respected surgeons, Sir Joseph Lister (b. 1827) of Edinburgh Scotland, agreed with Moore's principles and in 1870 advocated division of the origins of both pectoral muscles to gain better exposure of the axilla for the axillary gland dissection. His

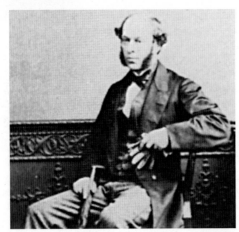

• **Fig. 1.12** Charles Moore, British surgeon of the mid-19th century, advocated wider and more extensive breast surgery. (From Robinson JO. Treatment of breast cancer through the ages. *Am J Surg.* 1986;151: 317-333.)

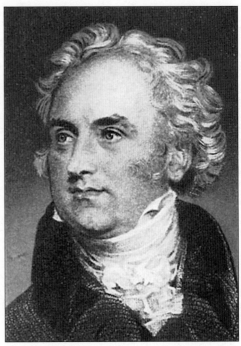

• **Fig. 1.13** Sir Astley Cooper (1768–1841).

contribution of carbolic acid spray was not widely accepted for 15 to 20 years.[26] In 1877 Mitchell Banks of Liverpool, England, advocated removal of the axillary glands in all cases of surgery for breast cancer. He washed the wound with carbolic acid solution but avoided the spray because of its cooling effect on the patient.

Alfred-Armand-Louis-Marie Velpeau (b. 1795) of France, originally apprenticed to the blacksmith trade, later rose to become professor of clinical surgery at the Paris Faculty, which was established in 1834. In his *Treatise on Diseases of the Breast* (1854), he claimed to have seen more than 1000 benign or malignant breast tumors during a practice of 40 years.[27] In those times, once the cancer had been excised, the patient and surgeon parted company and follow-up was scanty. In 1844 Jean-Jacques-Joseph Leroy d'Etiolles (b. 1798) conducted a study of 1192 patients with breast cancer. He concluded that mastectomy was more harmful than beneficial. The 1854 Congress of the Académie de Médecine discussed whether cancer should be treated at all.

Emerging innovative surgical practices developed in Germany in 1875, when Richard von Volkmann (b. 1830) advocated the en bloc resection of the entire breast, no matter the size of the primary tumor. He further recommended resection of the pectoral fascia, with an occasional thick layer of the underlying muscle, together with the axillary nodes.[28] The eminent surgeon Theodor Billroth (b. 1829) of Vienna also removed the entire breast but questioned the value of local excision of the tumor with a surrounding zone of normal tissue. For fixed tumors, Billroth's resections included the pectoral fascia, along with a thick layer of the underlying muscle.[28] His mortality rate of 15.7% with mastectomy alone and 21.3% when axillary dissection was also performed was praised as superior in the 19th century.[29,30] Ernst Küster (b. 1839) of Berlin, Germany, recommended that the axillary fat be removed along with the axillary glands. Lothar Heidenhain (b. 1860), a pupil of Volkmann, recommended removal of the superficial portion of the pectoralis major muscle even if the tumor was freely mobile, but he also recommended that the entire muscle, with its underlying connective tissue, be removed if the tumor was fixed.[31] Concerning benign breast disease, Sir Astley Cooper (b. 1768) (Fig. 1.13), an eminent English surgeon, published *Illustrations of the Diseases of the Breast* in 1829, which clearly differentiated fibroadenomas from chronic cystic mastitis.

Other important milestones of the 19th century are as follows. In 1829 French gynecologist and obstetrician Joseph Récamier introduced the term *metastasis* to describe the spread of cancer. In 1830 the English surgeon Everard Home (b. 1756) published a book on cancer that contained the first illustrations of the appearance of cancer cells under the microscope. Heinrich von Waldeyer-Hartz (b. 1836) cataloged a histologic classification of cancers showing that carcinomas come from epithelial cells, whereas sarcomas come from mesodermal tissue. In 1865 Victor Cornil (b. 1837) described malignant transformation of the acinar epithelium of the breast. In 1893 the first description of loss of differentiation by cancer cells ("anaplasia") was made by David von Hansemann, a German pathologist.

American Surgery

In the 19th century, Philadelphia was the medical center of the United States. It harbored the country's oldest medical college, the University of Pennsylvania (founded in 1765), the Jefferson Medical College (founded in 1824), and more than 50 other medical schools. It had a permanent medical college for women, as well as one in homeopathy and one in osteopathy.

Joseph Pancoast (b. 1805) was a dexterous surgeon-anatomist, who in the flowery language of his era, was said "to have an eye as quick as a flashing sunbeam and a hand as light as floating perfume." His *Treatise on Operative Surgery,*[31] published in 1844 in the preanesthetic and preantiseptic era, illustrates a mastectomy (Fig. 1.14). The patient is awake, with eyes open, and is semireclining. An assistant compresses the subclavian artery above the clavicle with the thumb of one hand. Larger vessels in the wound are compressed with the thumb and index finger of the assistant's other hand. Ligatures are left long and brought through the lower pole of the wound, where they act as a drain and can be pulled out later as they slough off. In one of the smaller sketches, the axillary glands are shown in continuity with the breast, visualized through a single incision that extended into

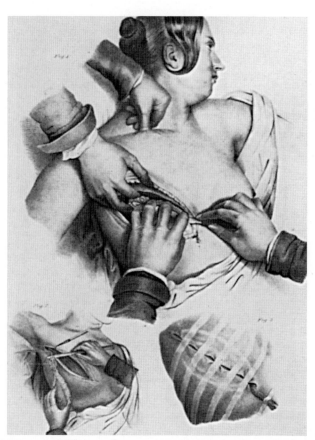

• **Fig. 1.14** Mastectomy (1844) by Dr. Joseph Pancoast in the preanesthetic and preantiseptic era. En bloc removal with axillary lymphatic drainage.

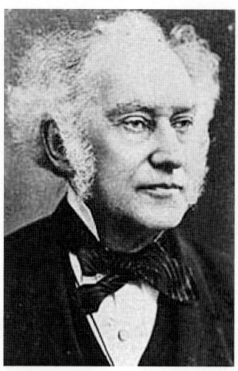

• **Fig. 1.15** Samuel David Gross (1805–1884). (From Bland KI. Preserving surgical academia in the centenary of the Flexnerian Academic Health Center. *Ann Surg.* 2011;254:393-409.)

the axilla. This was the first illustration of en bloc removal of the breast with its axillary lymphatic drainage. Skin removal was scanty, with easy approximation of the wound using five wide adhesive strips.

Samuel David Gross (b. 1805) (Fig. 1.15) was designated as "the greatest American surgeon of his time." His approach to cancer of the breast, however, was more conservative than that of Pancoast, his colleague. He described extirpation of the breast as "generally a very easy and simple affair." Using a small elliptical incision, he attempted to save enough skin for easy approximation of the edges of the wound. He aimed for healing by first intention, which was less likely if the wound were permitted to gape. In dealing with inordinately vascular tumors, he ligated each vessel but generally considered this as awkward and unnecessary. Glands in the axilla were removed only if grossly involved, in which case they were removed through the outer angle of the incision or through a separate one. The glands were enucleated with the finger or handle of the scalpel. It was his rule not to approximate the skin until 4 or 5 hours after the operation, "lest secondary hemorrhage should occur, and thus necessitate the removal of the dressings." In the sixth edition of his *System of Surgery* (1882), he devoted 30 pages to diseases of the breast.[32]

Samuel W. Gross (b. 1837) took a much more aggressive approach than that of his eminent father. He stated in 1887 that "no matter what the situation of the tumor may be, or whether glands can or cannot be detected in the armpit, the entire breast, with all the skin covering it, the paramammary fat, and the fascia of the pectoral muscle are cleanly dissected away, and the axillary

contents are extirpated. It need scarcely be added that aseptic precautions are strictly observed."[33] Removal of all the skin of the breast led to its designation as the "dinner plate operation." Against the criticism that an open large wound resulted in granulations from which cancer would again develop, he said, "When fireplugs produce whales, and oak trees polar bears, then will granulations produce cancer, and not until then."

The younger Gross personally examined all the tumors he removed under the microscope. In 1879 he helped his father found the Philadelphia Academy of Surgery, the oldest surgical society in the United States. After his premature death in 1889, his widow married William Osler. In her will of 1928, Lady Osler bequeathed an endowment for a lectureship at the Jefferson Medical College in honor of her first husband and his special interest in tumors.

D. Hayes Agnew (b. 1818) of the University of Pennsylvania wrote *Principles and Practice of Surgery* (1878), which endorsed Listerian antisepsis.[34] He shared the pessimistic view of many eminent surgeons of the time that few cancers were ever cured with surgery. *The Agnew Clinic* by Thomas Eakins (b. 1844) is the masterpiece of American art depicting a mastectomy performed in 1889 under conditions that would have been considered ideal for the time (Fig. 1.16)

Evolution of a Standardized Radical Mastectomy

Toward the later part of the 19th century, Philadelphia had to share its limelight with a number of other cities throughout the country, especially with Baltimore, where the recently organized (1889) Johns Hopkins Hospital Medical School produced a revolution in medical education and research. At that institution, a standardized surgical procedure for the treatment of breast cancer

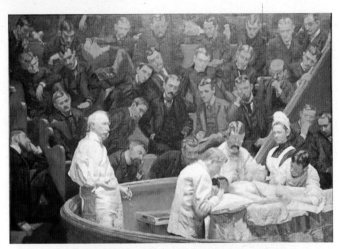

• **Fig. 1.16** Eakins' Agnew Clinic (1889) depicting mastectomy under ideal conditions of the time. (Courtesy University of Pennsylvania School of Medicine, Philadelphia, PA.)

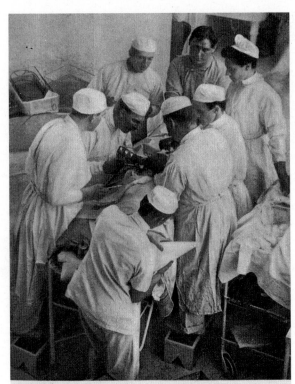

Dr. Halsted's First Operation in the New Surgical Amphitheatre in 1904

• **Fig. 1.18** Dr. William S. Halsted performing a radical mastectomy. Note the absence of masks. (Courtesy of College of Physicians of Philadelphia, Philadelphia, PA.)

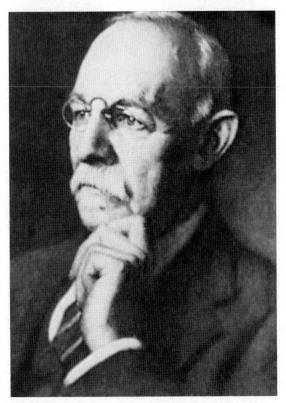

• **Fig. 1.17** William Stewart Halsted shortly before his death at age 70. (Courtesy Johns Hopkins Hospital.)

evolved through the efforts of William Stewart Halsted (1852–1922). Having completed his undergraduate education at Yale in 1874 and his medical education at Columbia in 1877, Halsted spent 2 years in Europe observing the practices of several noted surgeons (Fig. 1.17). For much of this time, he worked in Vienna with Billroth, whose experience he later reviewed, along with that of the other European surgeons. On the basis of analysis of others' results, Halsted returned to New York with a firm idea of what the best surgical procedure for breast cancer should encompass.[30] Believing in the local origin of breast cancer, he extended the

boundaries of wide excision. He believed that the high rates of local recurrence and low rates of survival after the breast cancer procedures used by prominent European surgeons must be caused by an inadequate removal of the tissues surrounding the cancer. He pronounced Volkmann's surgical procedure "a manifestly imperfect one."[35]

Influenced by Lothar Heidenhain's studies, (b.1840), which showed a high incidence of microscopic involvement of the pectoral muscles with cancer cells, Halsted advocated routine removal of the pectoralis major muscle, in addition to the entire breast and meticulous axillary dissection.[36] He also advocated an en bloc resection to avoid cutting across any cancerous tissues. Halsted's first "complete operation" was performed at the Roosevelt Hospital in New York City in 1882 (Fig. 1.18). By 1883, he was performing this complete operation, which became known as the Halsted radical mastectomy, in "almost every case" of breast cancer thereafter.[30] In 1891, his first 13 radical mastectomies were summarized in an article he published on wound healing.[36]

In 1894, Halsted published his landmark study, which described in detail both the radical mastectomy he had developed and the results from his first 50 procedures.[35] There were no operative deaths. The local recurrence rate was 6% (three patients) and the 3-year survival rate was 45%, both of which stood in stark contrast to the results of Halsted's contemporaries, whose work he meticulously analyzed in the same report (Table 1.1). The results he achieved were in a patient population where 27 patients had been labeled "hopeless" or "unfavorable." All 50 patients had axillary lymph node metastases, and 10% had supraclavicular

TABLE 1.1 Results of Surgical Treatment of Breast Carcinoma Up to 1894

Surgeon	Time	Cases (*n*)	Local Recurrence (%)	3-Year Cure (%)
Banks	1877	46	—	20
Bergmann	1882–1887	114	51–60	20
Billroth	1867–1876	170	82	4.7
Czerny	1877–1886	102	62	18.8
Fischer	1871–1878	147	75	—
Gussenbauer	1878–1886	151	64	—
Konig	1875–1885	152	58–62	—
Küster	1871–1885	228	59.6	21.5
Lucke	1881–1890	110	66	16.2
Volkmann	1874–1878	131	60	11
Halsted	1889–1894	50	6	45

Data from Halstead WS. The results of operations for the cure of cancer of the breast performed at the Johns Hopkins Hospital from June 1889 to January 1894. *Johns Hopkins Hosp Rep.* 1894–1895;4:297.

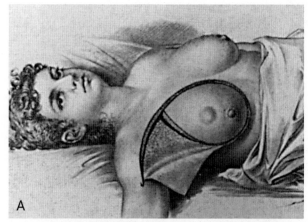

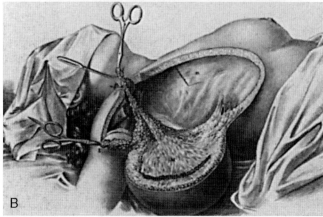

• **Fig. 1.19** (A) and (B) Plates X and XI from Halsted's landmark 1894 paper (from Johns Hopkins Hospital Reports. 1894–1895;4:297) showing his incision and dissection for the radical mastectomy. (Courtesy Johns Hopkins Hospital.)

lymph node metastases. A follow-up study by Lewis and Rienhoff in 1932 reported that the local recurrence rate had increased to 31.5%.[37] In 1980, Henderson and Canellos reanalyzed Halsted's data and demonstrated a disease-free survival (DFS) rate of 8% at 4 years.[38]

Halsted's radical mastectomy involved wide excision of skin via a teardrop incision extending across the deltopectoral groove, excision of the entire pectoralis major muscle, and division of the pectoralis minor muscle to expose the axillary contents for dissection (Fig. 1.19A and B). By 1898, he had extended the surgical procedure to include excision of the supraclavicular lymph nodes and pectoralis minor muscle, with immediate skin grafting of all wounds, a technique he had learned from Thiersch in Germany.[39] Halsted also described the removal of mediastinal nodes in three cases of recurrent breast cancer treated by his house surgeon, Harvey Cushing.

In 1907, before the American Surgical Association, Halsted presented an update of the results from a series of 232 patients who underwent his radical mastectomy at Johns Hopkins, where he had served as professor of surgery since 1891.[40] All 232 patients had been followed for at least 3 years. The operative mortality rate was 1.7% (four patients). Eighteen patients (7.8%) had been lost to follow-up. Sixty-four patients without axillary lymph node metastases (27.6%) did better than those patients with axillary lymph node metastases. Halsted was pessimistic concerning the efficacy of routine supraclavicular node dissection and abandoned the practice in cases where there was no clinical evidence of axillary or cervical lymph node metastases.

Halsted's presentation contained some foundational breast cancer surgery concepts. The number of recurrences after 3 years of follow-up led Halsted to advance the idea that 5-year survival rates were a more appropriate measure of "cure." His data clearly demonstrated the importance of axillary lymph node metastases

as an important prognostic factor. He suggested that the prognosis of a patient with breast cancer related to the extent (stage) of the breast cancer at the time of diagnosis and treatment. Halsted also suggested that the poor outcome of patients with supraclavicular node metastases resulted from systemic dissemination.

Halsted strongly espoused the importance of early detection of breast cancer[35]:

But women are now presenting themselves more promptly for examination, realizing that a cure of breast cancer is not only possible, but, if operated upon early, quite probable. Hence the surgeon is seeing smaller and still smaller tumors, cancers which give not one of the cardinal signs…. It would undoubtedly be possible for the expert to discover of the scirrhous growth earlier stages than he encounters, but unfortunately the tumor must first be recognized by the patient, and a scirrhous cancer large enough to attract her attention has quite surely already gone afield. Our problem, therefore, is to discover these tumors before the afflicted one can do so.

In the evolution of the surgical management of breast cancer, Halsted's radical mastectomy was the first surgical procedure universally embraced for the treatment of breast cancer. However, Halsted was troubled by the knowledge that 23% of node-negative patients in his series died of disseminated cancer. Subsequent studies reiterated the fact that more extensive local excision does

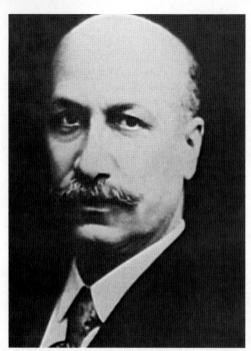

• **Fig. 1.20** Willy Meyer (1858–1932). German-born New York surgeon who conceived of and performed radical mastectomy independently of Halsted in 1894. (From Ravitch MM. *A Century of Surgery*. Vol 1. Philadelphia: JB Lippincott; 1980.)

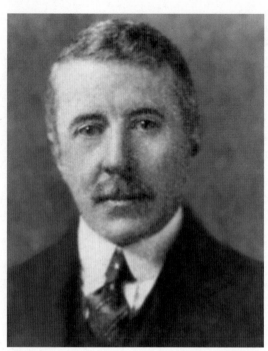

• **Fig. 1.21** William Sampson Handley (1872–1962), surgeon to Middlesex Hospital, whose permeation theory of breast cancer dissemination was embraced by Halsted. (Courtesy Professor Irving Taylor, Department of Surgery, Middlesex Hospital, London.)

not improve the approximate 20% relapse rate in patients with stage I breast cancer.[41]

In the late 19th century, Thiersch and Waldeyer demonstrated that metastases occurred through seeding of distant organs by way of embolization through the lymphatics and bloodstream.[11] This observation formed the basis of the mechanical theory of cancer dissemination that was widely accepted at the beginning of the 20th century.

Another scholar of breast cancer and mastectomy techniques, Willie Meyer (b. 1854) (Fig. 1.20) of the New York Graduate School of Medicine, described a similar technique only 10 days after Halsted's published paper.[42] He advocated removal of the pectoralis minor muscle in addition to the major. His operation has been referred to as the *Willie Meyer modification of the Halsted procedure*. At the close of the 19th century, the Halsted radical mastectomy had been established as state-of-the-art for surgical treatment of breast cancer. This procedure was unchallenged for 70 years, until the advent of breast conservation methods.

In 1895, I. Cullen credited William Welch (b. 1850), a pathologist at Johns Hopkins, as being the first to use frozen section in the diagnosis of breast lesions.[43] Welch is stated to have used this procedure in 1891 on a patient who was found to have a benign breast tumor.

Twentieth Century

At the beginning of the 20th century, it was evident that a higher cure rate for breast cancer would not be achieved through surgery alone. This lowering of surgical expectations stimulated scientific inquiry through epidemiologic studies, laboratory investigation research, and statistical analysis of practical experiences with breast cancer surgery in its various pathologic stages.

Surgery

The radical mastectomy described simultaneously by Halsted and Meyer, although extensive, did not include the supraclavicular and internal mammary nodes. In 1907 Halsted reported the removal of supraclavicular nodes in 119 patients.[40] In 44 patients with metastatic deposits, only 2 were alive and well after 5 years. In 1910 C. Westerman reported surgery involving a patient with local recurrence in which he disarticulated the arm and resected three ribs.[44] The thoracic wall defect was repaired with a pedicled flap. In two other cases, he carried out a partial excision of the thoracic wall and closed the defect with tissue from the contralateral healthy breast. These last two patients died within weeks, and the follow-up on the first was only for 1.5 years. The surgeons discontinued these extensive operations within a few years because of the increased operative mortality and poor survival rates.

Evolving Concepts Regarding Metastases in Breast Cancer

The internal mammary nodes were neglected until the third decade of the century. In 1927 British surgeon William Sampson Handley (b. 1872) of the London's Middlesex Hospital (Fig. 1.21) directed attention to the frequency of internal mammary node involvement, especially when axillary lymph nodes were enlarged.[45] He reported the removal of internal mammary nodes as an extension of the radical mastectomy.

Handley conducted a meticulous study of the pathologic anatomy of the lymphatic circulation and cancer dissemination and applied his observations to the clinical management of breast cancer. He believed that the lymphatics were the sole route through which cancer dissemination occurred, referring to earlier studies indicating that bloodborne cancer cells were routinely destroyed because they stimulated a thrombotic process.[11,14]

According to Handley's theory, regional lymph nodes acted as filters for permeating cancer cells. Only after the cancer cells grew beyond the regional lymph nodes were they capable of reaching the bloodstream for embolic spread. This theory was the conceptual basis for radical mastectomy. It was also the conceptual basis for excising all tissues in continuity so as not to cut across regional lymphatics. Halsted endorsed Handley's theory, which was published in Handley's first book on breast cancer in 1906.[7,9,46] Handley recommended modifying Halsted's radical mastectomy to include excision of a greater portion of the deep fascia, thereby encompassing more fully the at-risk lymphatics.[5]

One of Halsted's concerns, derived from the mechanical theory of cancer dissemination, was the inherent danger of manipulating a breast cancer, which could cause dissemination. Moore had voiced this same concern 30 years earlier. Halsted asserted the following[41,47]:

> *Tumors should never be harpooned, nor should pieces even be excised from malignant tumors for diagnostic purposes. Think of the danger of rapid dissemination of the growth from ... snipping off a piece of the tumor with scissors.*

Halsted's insistence on a one-stage surgical procedure that encompassed both the diagnostic biopsy and the definitive surgical procedure led to the development of frozen section examination at Johns Hopkins. William H. Welch first used this technique in 1891 during breast surgery performed by Halsted.[7]

Handley's permeation theory eventually was discredited.[14] J.H. Gray showed, in an extensive series of observations, that cancer cells could only rarely be found along the entire course of a lymph channel, an observation that Handley postulated was a consequence of an obliterative lymphangitis that obscured cancer cells.[48,49] Gray also found that the deep fascia was virtually devoid of lymphatics, contrary to Handley's assertion. Evidence also accumulated that cancer cells existed in the circulating blood.[50]

After World War II, Jerome Urban of New York and Owen Wangensteen of Minnesota, among others, advocated a "supraradical mastectomy," in which the dissection was carried into the mediastinum and the neck.[51,52]

Cushman Haagensen (Fig. 1.22) of Columbia-Presbyterian Medical Center in New York City dedicated his life to the surgical and pathologic study of breast diseases. He classified breast cancers in his patients according to size, clinical findings with "grave signs," and nodal status while establishing a breast unit where comprehensive data were maintained.[53] He was the first to propose self-examination of the breast and to suggest that lobular neoplasia (lobular carcinoma in situ) was not actual cancer. He distinguished this "marker of risk" from ductal carcinoma in situ.

During the first decade of the 20th century, several surgeons published their experience with the radical mastectomy (Table 1.2). In 1904 J. Collins Warren of Boston presented one of the most comprehensive reports, which described his results in 100 consecutive breast cancer cases, accumulated during a 20-year period, for which at least 3 years' follow-up was available.[54] There was a 2% operative mortality rate and DFS rates of 12% at 5 years and 5% at 10 years. These findings led Warren to assert that "the 3-year limit does not by any means constitute an infallible test of cure." He found that 37% of the locoregional recurrences occurred within 2 years of surgery, whereas 56% occurred within 5 years. A unique contribution was Warren's insistence that a pathologist be present in the operating room throughout the surgical procedure to confirm that all margins were free of cancer.

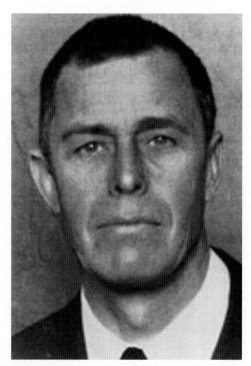

• **Fig. 1.22** Dr. Cushman D. Haagensen, a strong advocate of radical mastectomy, who classified and analyzed breast cancer for half a century. (Courtesy Dr. Gordon Schwartz.)

TABLE 1.2 Results of Radical Operation for the Treatment of Breast Carcinoma Since 1904

Author	Date	No. of Cases	Operative Mortality (%)	Locoregional Recurrence (%)
Warren[50a]	1904	100	2	6
Meyer[48]	1905	72	1.4	9
Greenough[52a]	1907	376	3.6	47.7
Halsted[18]	1907	232	1.7	19.5
Ochsner[51a]	1907	98	3	—
Lee et al.[64]	1924	75	—	—
Harrington[66]	1929	2083	0.76	—
Jessop[103]	1936	217	3.2	—
Taylor and Wallace[55]	1950	2000	0.65	—

[a]Includes a mixture of cases, some of which were subjected to "complete" operations, others to lesser procedures.

In 1907, Albert J. Ochsner of Chicago published the results of his surgical treatment of breast cancer in 164 patients, of whom 98 were followed for a significant period of time after surgery.[55] He reported 54 patients (55.1%) as being alive at intervals of 1 to 13 years after surgery but that only 36 patients had had a 5-year follow-up. Five patients (5.1%) were alive 10 years or more after surgery. There was a 3% (five patients) operative mortality rate (see Table 1.2).

Robert B. Greenough, a Boston surgeon on the faculty of Harvard Medical School, reported on 416 primary surgical procedures for breast cancer. A little more than 90% (376 patients) had long-term follow-up.[56] The operative mortality was 3.6%, but it decreased from 5.1% in the first 5 years to 2% in the last 5 years. The DFS rate at 3 years, excluding a "palliative group," was 21%. In the last 5 years of the study, the DFS rate rose to 26%. The author documented several clinical features associated with a poor prognosis.[57,58] These included skin involvement, ulceration, axillary lymph node metastases, supraclavicular lymph node metastases, bilateral breast cancer, and chest wall or axillary vein invasion.

In 1950, Taylor and Wallace reported their experience at the Massachusetts General Hospital.[59] They analyzed 2500 cases of primary breast cancer, 2000 of which had been treated by radical mastectomy. Patients with Greenough's unfavorable factors were eliminated from study. The operative mortality rate was less than 1%. Five-year DFS was 51%. Patients without axillary lymph node metastases had a 77% 5-year DFS rate, whereas patients with axillary lymph node metastases had a 33% 5-year DFS rate. Although the presence of axillary lymph node metastases was again shown to be prognostically significant, the number of lymph nodes involved was also shown to be important. There was a 76% 5-year DFS rate when only one or two axillary nodes were involved.

The previously mentioned survival rates must be viewed in the context of the natural history of breast cancer. In 1962 Bloom and associates reviewed the clinical course of 250 women with a confirmed diagnosis of breast cancer who had been admitted to the Middlesex Hospital Cancer Ward between 1805 and 1933 but were not treated.[60] They found that there was a median survival of 2.7 years from the onset of symptoms; 20% of the women were alive at 5 years, 5% at 10 years, and 1% after 15 years (Fig. 1.23).

In 1937, London surgeon Geoffrey Keynes demonstrated that less radical surgery was needed in breast cancer, with radiation giving equally good results. However, at the close of World War II, radical mastectomy remained the standard operation for breast cancer. In 1948 two reports appeared that were destined to change the management of breast cancer and become accepted as general principles in the management of localized disease. The first was the concept of modified radical mastectomy by D. Patey and W. Dyson from the Middlesex Hospital in London.[21] The second was treatment with simple mastectomy and radiotherapy, introduced by R. McWhirter of the University of Edinburgh.[61] Subsequent studies of patients treated with simple, radical, and modified radical mastectomies with or without radiotherapy revealed a striking similarity in survival rates. The contemporary trend (since 1970) has been breast conservation surgery followed by irradiation. Axillary dissection was confined to level I and II lymph nodes.

In the later years of the 20th century, Donald Morton (Fig. 1.24) and associates at the John Wayne Cancer Center in Santa Monica, California, developed the sentinel lymph node biopsy technique. It was originally proposed as an alternative to elective lymph node dissection for staging regional lymphatics in patients with cutaneous melanoma.[62] In 1994, Armando Giuliano investigated its use as an alternative to elective axillary lymph node dissection in patients with breast cancer.[63] Sentinel lymph node biopsy has now revolutionized breast cancer staging and is redefining the indications for axillary dissection. In this application the technique uses lymphoscintigraphy and vital blue dye to localize the "sentinel" axillary lymph node, which is the node most likely to contain breast cancer metastases.

Radiotherapy

Two months after the discovery of x-rays in 1895 by Wilhelm Roentgen (b. 1845), Emil Grubbe (b. 1875), a second-year medical student in Chicago, irradiated a patient with cancer of the breast. He protected the skin surrounding the lesion with tinfoil. He subsequently became the first professor of roentgenology at the Hahnemann Medical College of Philadelphia. In 1896 Hermann Gocht (b. 1869) of Hamburg, Germany, irradiated two patients with advanced cases of breast cancer while protecting the adjacent skin with flexible lead.[64] In 1898 Marie Curie and her husband Pierre discovered and isolated the radioactive elements

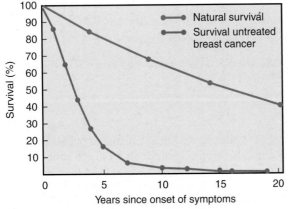

• **Fig. 1.23** Survival of women with untreated breast carcinoma. (Modified from Bloom HJF, Richardson WW, Harries EJ. Natural history of untreated breast cancer (1805–1933). *BMJ*. 1962;2:213.)

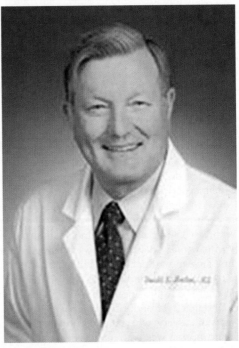

• **Fig. 1.24** Dr. Donald L. Morton. (Courtesy John Wayne Cancer Center, Santa Monica, CA.)

polonium and radium. Their skin was burned as a result of working near these compounds, and in 1904 it was demonstrated that radium rays destroyed human cells.

In 1902, Guido Holzknecht (b. 1872) of Vienna, Austria, introduced a practical dosimeter. The therapeutic application of ionizing radiation soon followed. In 1902 Russian physician S. Goldberg successfully used radium in the treatment of cancer. In 1903 one of the first departments of radiotherapy for cancer was established at the Cancer Hospital in London, under the direction of J. Pollock. Georg Perthes (b. 1869), professor of surgery in Leipzig, Germany, in 1903 ascribed the "curative effect" of x-rays secondary to their inhibition of cell division.[65] Postoperative radiotherapy was initiated in many hospitals in America and Europe in the years before World War I. The equipment of the day permitted a maximum voltage of only 150 kV. Immediately after the war the voltages used increased, ranging from 170 to 200 kV.

In 1929, S. Harrington of the Mayo Clinic reported his follow-up of 1859 breast cancer cases irradiated between 1910 and 1923.[66] After analyzing his results, he expressed doubts about the value of ancillary radiotherapy. Even with improved equipment, controversy continued between enthusiasts and opponents of radiotherapy. George Pfahler (b. 1874) of Philadelphia recommended postoperative radiotherapy in all cases of breast cancer, starting 2 weeks after surgery. In his report of 1022 cases, he found no significant improvement in survival with stage I disease but did document an improved 5-year survival rate for patients with stage II disease.[67]

Radiotherapy as the sole therapeutic modality for breast cancer had been used for inoperable cases since the beginning of the 20th century, but it was not until 1922 that a claim was made for its sole use in operable cases. William Stone (b. 1867) of New York City claimed the superiority of radiotherapy over radical surgery for the treatment of operable breast cancer. He based his conclusions on his experience with 10,000 cases. Geoffrey Keynes (b. 1887) of St. Bartholomew's Hospital in London reported in 1932 that radium could be used as a source of therapeutic irradiation.[68] After experience with this modality as an adjunct to surgery for breast cancer, Keynes extended its use to being the sole treatment. He claimed a 5-year survival rate of 77% in the absence of enlarged axillary nodes and 36% with axillary involvement.

Supervoltage x-rays became available in the 1930s. At that time, François Baclesse (b. 1896) of Paris championed local excision of breast cancer, followed by radiotherapy. He reported cases studied between 1937 and 1953 at the Curie Foundation and concluded that for stage I and II cancers, his results were equal to those of radical mastectomy. In 1948 Robert McWhirter (b. 1904) proposed simple mastectomy followed by radiotherapy.[69] He argued that radical mastectomy for stage I disease was an overkill but was often inadequate for stage II disease, in which distant metastatic disease commonly developed. In the 1960s, even higher voltage x-rays were developed, along with the cobalt beam. In the late 1970s the development of the linear accelerator allowed the delivery of whole-breast radiotherapy of 4000 to 5000 cGy, with focal boost to the tumor bed to 6000 to 7000 cGy.

During the later part of the 20th century, partial or segmental mastectomy (i.e., "tylectomy," "lumpectomy"), axillary node dissection, and adjuvant breast irradiation played an increasingly important role in the therapy of early-stage breast cancer. The validity of breast conservation therapy was demonstrated through a series of carefully designed and controlled clinical trials coordinated through the National Surgical Adjuvant Breast and Bowel

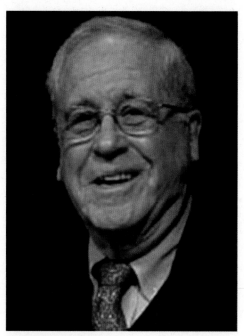

• **Fig. 1.25** Dr. Bernard Fisher. (Courtesy National Surgical Adjuvant Breast and Bowel Project, Pittsburgh, PA.)

Project (NSABP). An American surgeon, Bernard Fisher (Fig. 1.25), served as chairman of the NSABP from 1967 to 1994 and since 1995 has been its scientific director. Fisher's systematic analyses brought breast cancer therapy into a new era and has set a standard for the investigation of therapies for other solid tumors.[70]

Hormonal Therapy

Hormonal treatment for breast cancer was considered even before the beginning of the 20th century. In 1889 Albert Schinzinger (b. 1827) of Freiburg, Germany, proposed oophorectomy before mastectomy to produce "early aging" in menstruating women. This was based on his belief that the prognosis of breast cancer was worse in younger patients. In 1896 and again in 1901, George Beatson (b. 1848) of Glasgow, Scotland, reported three cases of advanced breast cancer that responded favorably to oophorectomy.[71] In 1900, S. Boyd performed the first combined oophorectomy and mastectomy for breast cancer. In 1905 the findings from a series of 99 patients with breast cancer treated by oophorectomy were presented at the Royal Medical and Chirurgical Society by a surgeon at the London Hospital, Hugh Lett.

In 1953, the late Nobel laureate and surgeon/urologist Charles Huggins (Fig. 1.26) of the University of Chicago advocated oophorectomy and adrenalectomy to remove the major sources of estrogens in the body.[72] Some patients with breast cancer responded with dramatic remissions, whereas others remained unaffected. In the early 1950s, hypophysectomy for advanced breast cancer was recommended, with results similar to those of adrenalectomy. Clinical administration of hormones started in 1939, when P. Ulrich reported the beneficial effect of testosterone in two cases of breast cancer.[73] In 1944, Alexander Haddow (b. 1912) of Edinburgh, Scotland, and his collaborators observed a favorable effect of synthetic estrogen in advanced breast cancer.[74] Edward Dodds of London synthesized stilbestrol in 1938.[75] I. Nathanson

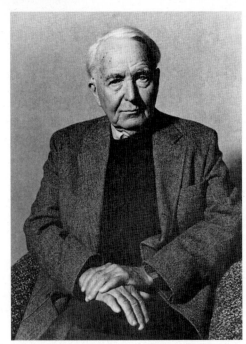

• **Fig. 1.26** Dr. Charles B. Huggins, Nobel Laureate. (Courtesy University of Chicago, Chicago, IL.)

reported its effect on advanced breast cancer in 1946.[76] In the 1950s and 1960s estrogens and androgens remained in active use. In 1973 W. McGuire demonstrated estrogen receptors in human breast tumors.[77] In 1975, K. Horowitz identified progesterone receptors in hormone-dependent breast cancer.[78] Since the 1980s, tamoxifen and other selective estrogen receptor modulators (SERMs) have been used for the treatment and prevention of breast cancer.

Chemotherapy

Adjuvant

The use of chemical compounds, especially arsenic, in the treatment of breast cancer dates to ancient times. However, Paul Ehrlich (b. 1854) is credited as being the "father of chemotherapy." He coined the designation chemotherapy and by 1898 had isolated the first alkylating agent. In a series of historic experiments, he methodically studied a group of compounds that led to the discovery of arsphenamine (Salvarsan) in 1910, which successfully treated syphilis in rabbits.[79] It was not until just after World War II that his work was applied to the treatment of cancers.

During World War II, the US Office of Scientific Research produced nitrogen mustard, an alkylating agent. A ship containing this substance blew up in the harbor at Naples, Italy, and the sailors who were exposed developed marrow and lymphoid hypoplasia. Experimental work with nitrogen mustard for the treatment of lymphosarcoma began at Memorial Hospital in New York City, but the results were withheld until the war secrecy ban was lifted in 1946. That same year Frederick Phillips and Alfred Gilman demonstrated that nitrogen mustards could cause regression of certain lymphomas and leukemias.

Other antineoplastic drugs brought into clinical use were the purine and pyrimidine antagonists. In 1957 C. Heidelberger and collaborators reported the action of 5-fluorouracil, which has remained useful in the treatment of breast cancer.[80] In addition, the National Institutes of Health organized a cancer and chemotherapy national service. In 1958 patients were entered into a randomized, double-blind study using thiotriethylenephosphoramide, an alkylating agent. In 1963 E. Greenspan and his group in New York City were some of the first to engage in multidrug trials using the antimetabolite methotrexate in combination with the alkylating agent thiotepa.[81]

Neoadjuvant

In the late 1970s and early 1980s, researchers first published the results of preliminary reports for induction chemotherapy (neoadjuvant chemotherapy) for locally advanced breast cancer. De Lena, Zucali, and Viganotti reported their findings of 110 patients with inoperable cancer treated with induction neoadjuvant regimens consisting of doxorubicin and vincristine.[82] Approximately 90% of patients had an objective response, of which 16% was complete, 55% was partial, and 19% was an "improvement." The 3-year overall survival rate of the treated patients was 53% in contrast to 41% for the historical control group not receiving chemotherapy.

Importantly, the trial by De Lena and associates[82] initiated interest in other neoadjuvant trials, principally for patients with inoperable disease.[79,83–85] In the 1983 report from the MD Anderson Cancer Center for a series of 52 patients with locally advanced breast cancer, three-cycle treatment with neoadjuvant chemotherapy that contained anthracyclines, the local therapy together with adjuvant therapy rendered 94% of patients free of disease for 2 years. Thereafter, Swain and colleagues[79] at the National Cancer Institute reported on the institute's experience with 76 patients with locally advanced disease treated with induction therapy until maximum clinical response was achieved. As previously, all these patients received adjuvant chemotherapy for at least 6 months with an objective response of 93%, with 43% complete, 44% partial, and 7% stable.

Similar induction chemotherapy response with neoadjuvant therapies has been compared with adjuvant chemotherapy trials in multiple randomized studies that included patients with locally advanced disease.[86–91] Importantly, the neoadjuvant chemotherapy arms had longer overall survival with a median follow-up of 34 months ($p = .04$). This trial[79] was one of the first to confirm that improved survival may reflect the benefit of chemotherapy in general rather than the specific application of the neoadjuvant chemotherapy protocol. Thus outcomes of patients treated with neoadjuvant cytoreductive therapy were not worse than those who received adjuvant chemotherapy. Similar outcomes have been confirmed by Scholl and associates[87] from the Institut Curie, France, and Powles and colleagues[89] of the Royal Marsden Hospital, England, as well as the largest trial of neoadjuvant chemotherapy reported to date in the NSABP B-18, which randomized 1523 women with $T_{1–3}$, $N_{0–1}$ operable breast cancer.[90,91] Overall, complete clinical responses were observed in 35% of patients, a clinical partial response in 44%, and stable disease in 17%. In comparison to the NSABP trial of adjuvant and neoadjuvant therapies, no differences in 5-year survival rates of DFS, distant DFS, or overall survival were evident. Patients with T_3 disease had a survival rate equivalent to the rates of patients treated with adjuvant and neoadjuvant approaches. These similar outcomes have also been reported by the European Organization for Research and Treatment of Cancer Breast Cancer Cooperative Groups in an additional large randomized neoadjuvant chemotherapy trial of women with operable breast cancer.[92] These trials have demonstrated that neoadjuvant and adjuvant therapies produce equivalent outcomes. Although most studies have been conducted in patients with early-stage disease, some have included patients with locally advanced malignancies. The report by Hutcheon and colleagues[93] suggests that the addition of docetaxel to neoadjuvant regimens will improve survival for patients with locally advanced disease.[60]

Finally, the role of neoadjuvant hormonal therapy for locally advanced disease has been assessed in several studies, including those led by Veronesi,[94] Gazet,[95] Hoff,[96] and Ellis,[97] which have typically compared aromatase inhibitors and SERMs with ovarian ablation by medical and surgical measures. The majority of these studies have clearly demonstrated the benefit of neoadjuvant hormonal therapies in the subset of patients not treated with chemotherapy. For patients who can tolerate chemotherapy, however, it remains the standard of care. Although the role of ovarian suppression or ablation has been identified in the premenopausal patient, tamoxifen remains the standard endocrine therapy for the premenopausal individual with breast carcinoma with early-stage hormonal receptor–positive breast cancer. Bao and Davidson[98] acknowledge the uncertainty that exists regarding the optimal applications of endocrine therapy for premenopausal women who are estrogen receptor–positive. Clarke[99] documented in 1998 the journey along a hierarchy of evidence to show why research in ablation remains relevant in the management of these patients.

Mammography

Before and after World War I, early diagnosis of breast cancer was difficult. Patients sought advice only when they felt a hard lump. Surgeons looked for skin retraction and inversion of the nipple and palpated the breast and axilla for masses. In 1913 a German surgeon, A. Salomon, used mammography to study 3000 amputated breasts and was able to differentiate scirrhous forms of breast cancer from nodular types.[100] He noted the microcalcifications in intraductal carcinomas but failed to appreciate their significance. In 1927 O. Kleinschmidt wrote a book in which he described mammography as an aid in diagnosis.[101]

Jacob Gershon-Cohen of Philadelphia studied x-ray mammary patterns from 1937 to 1948 and made notable progress in the accurate diagnosis of breast cancer. He tirelessly advocated the use of x-rays as an aid to clinical diagnosis and in 1948 was the first to demonstrate the feasibility of detecting occult carcinomas.[102] In 1962 at the MD Anderson Hospital and Tumor Institute, R. Egan described imaging of the breast with only two radiographic views. He reported a study of 2522 mammograms in which differentiation between benign and malignant tumors was made without the aid of clinical findings.[103] Since then, mammography has become the most important diagnostic tool for breast cancer.

Breast Reconstruction

Iginio Tansini, Professor of Surgery at the University of Pavia in Italy, first described the latissimus dorsi flap in 1896.[104,105] In the early 20th century, surgeons completed procedures performed without elevation of skin flaps, principally because the skin and subcutaneous tissue were sacrificed with en bloc resections. This left large circular defects centrally, which were repaired by skin grafts on occasion. The innovative approach of Tansini, which involved elevating the flap, allowed the early application of plastic surgical techniques after expiration measures of the Halsted radical procedure. Surgeons typically transposed anteriorly myocutaneous flaps with skin and latissimus dorsi for wound closures. In the early 1900s, it became evident that practitioners of rudimentary skin graft techniques more commonly favored using this technique rather than managing a large circular defect, which ultimately required prolonged wound packing to allow for granulation to occur.[106] Later in the 20th century, the enhancement of diagnostic techniques (e.g., radiographic, nuclear imaging, ultrasound) and downstaging of the primary tumor with chemotherapy allowed the use of extirpative procedures with primary closures.

Brown and McDowell[107] introduced the motorized dermatome in 1958, allowing very large skin grafts that could be meshed to expand for coverage of large surface area. This seminal innovation permitted surgeons to realize the sacrifice of involved skin and, with introduction of adjuvant radiotherapy, allowed enhancement of local control.

The Tansini latissimus dorsi myocutaneous flap was the prevailing reconstruction methodology after mastectomy in Europe until about 1920. However, Halsted made a grand tour of medical centers in Europe and stated: "Beware of the man with the plastic operation" because he considered the latissimus flap both "unnecessary and hazardous."[108] For several reasons, principally the lack of the advent of blood transfusions, anesthetics, antibiotics, and intravenous fluids, Tansini's method did not further breast reconstructive surgery until the 1970s, when the pioneering efforts of McCraw, Vasconez, Hartramph, and others reintroduced the myocutaneous flap. This seminal contribution in pathophysiology and anatomy by McCraw and colleagues represented the single most important contribution to plastic surgery for reconstruction of ablative procedures in the past 75 years (Table 1.3). In 1982 Hartramph and associates first described application of the abdominal myocutaneous flap, which was an abdominal transverse rectus abdominis myocutaneous (TRAM) pedicle flap.[109] Thus for 54 years (1920–1974), the Tansini procedure was completely abandoned, and myocutaneous flaps were not used for immediate reconstruction of the breasts until 1982.

Today substantive remodeling of tissues for esthetic, contour, and functional purposes is the primary goal of the plastic surgeon. The advancement in myocutaneous breast reconstruction followed introduction of silicone breast implants by Cronin and Gerow in 1964 and was thereafter popularized by a number of surgeons for 20 years.[110–114] The pioneering work of these two investigators was conducted in collaboration with Dow Chemical Company using silicone polymers. It was evident early that subpectoral placement of these implants enhanced results over those of the fibrous encapsulation of the implant placed beneath the thin mastectomy skin flaps. Early implant reconstruction failures were principally related to distortion of the breast contour (shape) referred to as *half grapefruit,* which describes the elevated, rounded, and firm implant. Subsequently, silicone implants were abandoned for several years because of concerns about fibromyalgia and immunologically related disorders. Although no firm, statistically objective reviews have confirmed silicone's harmful effects, this concern prompted a resurgence of the use of saline implants in the late 1980s and early 1990s. Today a reentry of silicone implants into the market with superior soft tissue coverage of shaped implants has allowed an improvement in outcomes, both physiologically and esthetically.

The rapid evolution of breast reconstruction techniques among international plastic surgery clinics has allowed women receiving devastating surgical defects from surgery and irradiation, the meaningful improvement in tissue quality, breast contour, and

TABLE 1.3   Historical Evolution of Breast Reconstruction

Date	Reconstructive Procedure
1895	Lumbar lipoma transplant (Czerny)
1896	Latissimus dorsi autogenous flaps (Tansini)
1900	Split/full-thickness skin grafts (Halsted, Meyer)
1957	Racquet-shaped abdominoplasty flap (Gilles, Millard)
1958	Motorized Brown dermatome for split-thickness skin graft (Brown and McDowell)[74]
1960s	Tubed skin flaps
1961	Silicone breast implants (subpectoral/suprapectoral; Cronin, Gerow)
1970s	Reintroduction of Tansini myocutaneous flap rectus abdominis (Mathes and Bostwick)
1973	Free flap one-stage iliofemoral island transfer (Daniel, Taylor)
1979	Free SIEA flap (Holmstrom)
1982	TRAM flap and pedicled TRAM flap (Hartrampf et al.)
1987	Free TRAM with DIEP (Carramenha e Costa et al.)
1989	Free abdominoplasty flap with SIEA (Grotting et al.)[121]
1994	DIEP (Allen, Treece)
1995	Superior gluteal artery perforator flap (Allen, Tucker)

DIEP, Deep inferior epigastric perforator; *SIEA*, superficial inferior epigastric artery; *TRAM*, transverse rectus abdominis myocutaneous.

enhancement of esthetic outcomes with autologous breast reconstruction tissues. This reconstructive advent and advancement contrasts in superiority with the latissimus dorsi myocutaneous flap designed in 1896 by Tansini and the prosthetic implants of the 1960s, first introduced by Cronin and Gerow. The introduction of autologous reconstruction for breast defects was first reported in 1979 by Holmstrom as a "free flap"[115] and was subsequently popularized by Hartrampf and colleagues[116] as the patient-centric cosmetically superior "pedicled" TRAM flap (see Table 1.3). This original flap had improved postoperative body wall contour, flattening of abdominal fat, with hidden scars. This technique provided the transfer of autologous fat and skin into a major tissue deficit with superior esthetic outcomes. However, this previously valued advance had major morbidity postoperatively, including hernia, incisional bulge, and major abdominal wall muscular weakness. The latter side effect with muscular atrophy and weakness prevented former activities including heavy lifting, rapid change in body torque, and aggressive physical activity (e.g., skiing, horseback riding, climbing). Although the TRAM flap gained popularity in the 1980s, it has evolved into a free muscle-sparing transfer with the development of the free TRAM of the deep inferior epigastric perforators (DIEPs) originally introduced by Koshima and Sodea in 1989.[117] With realization that anatomically the "DIEP flap" was physiologically supportive of a large volume of skin and subcutaneous tissue,[118] plastic surgeons saw its advancement with clinical application for breast reconstruction

by Allen and Treece in 1994.[119] This surgical paradigm shift followed the 1991 report by Grotting for breast reconstruction[120]; the DIEP and superficial inferior epigastric artery (SIEA) flaps were used and robustly endorsed by multiple plastic surgeons. The advantage of the SIEA flap is the transfer of large volumes of lower abdominal tissue without excision or incision of the rectus abdominis muscle or fascia; this technique eliminated abdominal donor site morbidity. Although the same lower abdominal skin and subcutaneous tissue of the TRAM and DIEP are used in the SIEA, the disadvantage of the SIEA flap is its shorter pedicle length for transfer and smaller pedicle diameter than either of the aforementioned flaps.

Cancer Biology

The 20th century saw unprecedented growth in our understanding of cancer biology, especially breast cancer biology. In the first part of the century, numerous observations were made concerning the development and behavior of cancer. In 1900 Leo Loeb experimentally transmitted cancer through several generations of animals. In 1911 Jean Clunet of France demonstrated the experimental production of cancer using x-rays. In 1920 an American pathologist, Albert Borders, classified cancers with regard to malignant potential on the basis of the state of differentiation of cancer cells. In 1932 the French physician Antoine Lacassagne demonstrated that breast cancer could be produced in animals with estrone benzoate. In 1944 P. Denoix of the Institut Gustav-Roussy in France proposed the tumor, node, metastasis (TNM) classification for cancer. In 1959 M. Macklin performed a comprehensive analysis of the role of hereditary factors in the predisposition to breast cancer.

The latter part of the 20th century saw the development of molecular biology and the explanation of breast cancer development and behavior in terms of human genetics. In 1926 American geneticist Hermann Müller exposed fruit flies to x-rays and produced mutations and hereditary changes. He demonstrated that the mutations were the result of breakages in chromosomes and changes in individual genes. Hugh Cairns (b. 1922), a molecular biologist and virologist from Oxford University, showed that cancer developed from a single abnormal cell as a result of DNA mutation. Peter Vogt (b. 1932), a German-born American microbiologist from the University of Southern California, discovered oncogenes, which play a role in the normal growth of mammalian cells but can cause cancer through mutation. In 1970 David Baltimore, a New York City oncologist, announced his discovery of the enzyme reverse transcriptase, which can transcribe RNA into DNA, contributing greatly to our understanding of how viruses participate in the development of cancer. In 1978 David Lane, a professor of oncology at Dundee, Scotland, discovered the tumor-suppressor gene p53. Bert Vogelstein (b. 1949), a Baltimore oncologist and a pioneer in the study of the molecular basis of cancer, analyzed DNA from colon cancer cells and described mutation of three tumor suppressor genes: *APC, DCC*, and *p53*. Judith Folkman (b. 1933), an American surgeon, elucidated the importance of angiogenesis and opened the way for new therapy. In 1994 the first breast cancer gene, *BRCA1*, was identified, and in 1996, *BRCA2* was discovered; *HER2* neu positive cell receptor therapy followed, described by Slamon and colleagues. Building on these and other discoveries, the 21st century will undoubtedly see the development of genetically based therapies for breast cancer that will complement or replace the empirical therapies of the past.

Suggested Readings

Bordley J III, Harvey AM. *Two Centuries of American Medicine, 1776 to 1976*. Philadelphia: WB Saunders; 1976.

de Moulin D. *A Short History of Breast Cancer*. The Hague: Martinus Nijhoff; 1983.

Garrison FH. *An Introduction to the History of Medicine*. Philadelphia: WB Saunders; 1929.

Grubbe EH. *X-Ray Treatment: Its Origin, Birth and Early History*. St Paul, MN: Bruce Publishing; 1949.

King LS. *The Medical World of the Eighteenth Century*. Huntington, NY: RE Krieger; 1971.

Lee HSJ. *Dates in Oncology. Landmarks in Medicine Series*. New York: Parthenon; 2000.

Levens P. The pathway to health, London, 1664. In: *Special Collections of Thomas Jefferson University Library*. Philadelphia.

Pancoast J. *Treatise on Operative Surgery*. Philadelphia: Carey & Hart; 1844.

Riesman D. *Medicine in the Middle Ages*. New York: Paul B Hoeber; 1935.

A full reference list is available online at ExpertConsult.com.

2

Anatomy of the Breast, Axilla, Chest Wall, and Related Metastatic Sites

KIRBY I. BLAND, EDWARD M. COPELAND III, AND V. SUZANNE KLIMBERG

Paired mammary glands, or breasts, are a distinguishing feature of mammals. These glands evolve as milk-producing organs to provide nourishment to the offspring, in a relatively immature and dependent state with embryonic development in utero. The organ develops from the primordially derived breast tissue, which anatomically matures as a modified sweat gland. The act of nursing the young provides physiologic benefits to the mother by aiding in postpartum uterine involution and to the newborn with nutritional feeding and the transfer of passive immunity. The nursing of the offspring is also of significance in the emotional bonding between the mother and her infant.

With embryologic development, there is growth and differentiation of the breasts in both sexes (for a review, see Morehead[1]). Embryologically, the nascent paired glands develop along parallel lines, the "milk lines" (Fig. 2.1), extending between the limb buds of the developmental axilla to the future inguinal region. Among the various mammalian species, the number of paired glands varies greatly and is related to the number of fetuses in each litter. In humans and most other primates, only one gland develops ipsilaterally on each side in the pectoral region. An extra breast (*polymastia*) or nipple (*polythelia*) may occur as a heritable condition with frequency of 1% in the female population. These relatively rare conditions also may occur in the male gender. When present, the supernumerary breast or nipple usually forms appendages along the milk lines; about one-third of the affected individuals have multiple extra (supernumerary) breasts or nipples.

With hormonal steroidal influence of the female gender, the breasts undergo extensive postnatal development, which is correlated with age and regulated by ovarian hormones that influence reproductive function. By about 20 years of age, the female breast has reached its developmental maturity, and by age 40, it begins atrophic changes, even before formal presentation of menopause. During each menstrual cycle, structural changes occur in the breast under the influence of fluctuations of ovarian hormone levels. During *pregnancy* and *lactation,* striking changes occur not only in the functional activity of the breast but also in the volume of glandular tissue. The actual secretion and production of milk are induced and enhanced by prolactin from the pituitary and by somatomammotropin from the placenta. With the changes in the hormonal environment that occur at *menopause,* the glandular

component of the breast regresses, or involutes, and is replaced by fat and connective tissue stroma[2] (see Fig. 2.1).

Gross Anatomic Structure: Surface Anatomy

Form and Size

The mammary gland is located within the superficial fascia of the anterior thoracic wall. It consists of 15 to 20 lobes of glandular tissue of the tubuloalveolar type. Longitudinal fibrous connective stroma forms a latticed framework that supports the lobes; adipose tissue fills the space between the lobes.[3] In the premenopausal female, structure and stroma are dense; the organ remains mobile on the chest wall residing on the mammary bursae. Subcutaneous connective tissue surrounds the gland and extends as septa between the lobes and lobules, providing support for the glandular elements; however, the septae does not form a distinctive capsule around any component of the breast. The deep layer of the superficial fascia lies upon the posterior (deep) surface of the breast and resides upon the pectoral (deep) fascia of the thoracic wall. A distinct space, the *retromammary bursa,* can be identified surgically on the posterior aspect of the breast between the deep layer of the superficial fascia and the deep investing fascia of the pectoralis major, and contiguous muscles of the thoracic wall (Fig. 2.2). As noted, the retromammary bursa contributes to the mobility of the breast on the thoracic wall. Fibrous thickenings of the connective tissue interdigitate between the parenchymal tissue of the breast. This connective tissue extends from the deep layer of the superficial fascia (hypodermis) and attaches to the dermis of the skin. These suspensory structures, called *Cooper ligaments,* distinctively insert perpendicular to the delicate superficial fascial layers of the cutis reticularis of the dermis, or corium, permitting remarkable mobility of the breast, while providing central support.

At maturity, the glandular portion of the breast has a unique and distinctive protuberant conical form. The base of the cone is roughly circular, measuring 10 to 12 cm in diameter and 5 to 7 cm in thickness. Commonly, breast tissue extends into the axilla as the axillary tail (tail of Spence). There is tremendous variation in the size of the breast with frequent asymmetry in any individual. A typical nonlactating breast weighs between 150 and 225 g, whereas the lactating breast may exceed 500 g.[4,5] In a study of

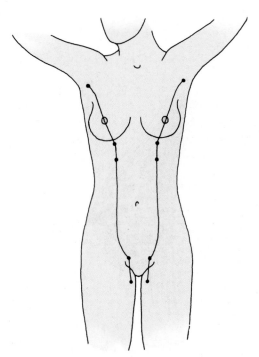

• **Fig. 2.1** Mammary milk line. After development of the milk bud in the pectoral area of ectodermal thickening, the "milk streak" extends from the axilla to the inguinal areas. At week 9 of intrauterine development, atrophy of the bud has occurred except for the presence of the supernumerary nipples of breast.

breast volume in 55 women, Smith and colleagues[6] reported that the mean volume of the right breast was 275.46 mL (SD = 172.65, median = 217.7, minimum = 94.6, maximum = 889.3) and the left breast was 291.69 mL (SD = 168.23, median = 224, minimum = 106.9, maximum = 893.9).

The breast of the nulliparous female has a typical hemispheric configuration with distinct flattening above the nipple.[7] The multiparous breast, which has experienced the hormonal stimulation associated with pregnancy and lactation, is usually larger, more dense, and more pendulous. As noted, during pregnancy and lactation, the breast increases dramatically in size, and with weight of milk assumes a more pendulous configuration. With increasing age, the *postmenopausal* breast usually decreases in volume, becoming somewhat flattened and gravitationally pendulous; thereafter, the organ is less dense, second to replacement of parenchyma with fat.

Extent and Location

The mature female breast extends inferiorly from the level of the second or third rib to the inframammary fold, which is at about the level of the sixth or seventh rib, and laterally from the lateral border of the sternum to the anterior or midaxillary line. The deep or posterior surface of the breast rests on portions of the deep investing fasciae of the pectoralis major, serratus anterior, and external abdominal oblique muscles and the uppermost superior extent of the rectus sheath. The axillary tail (tail of Spence) of the breast extends into the anterior axillary fold. The upper half of the breast, and particularly the upper outer quadrant, contains more glandular tissue than does the remainder of the breast. This anatomic fact accounts for the higher frequency of breast cancer in this quadrant.

Microscopic Anatomic Structure

Nipple and Areola

The epidermis of the nipple and areola is highly pigmented and somewhat wrinkled. It is covered by keratinized, stratified squamous epithelium. The deep surface of the epidermis is invaded by unusually long dermal papillae that allow capillaries to bring blood perfusion to its surface, giving the nipple-areola a pinkish color in young, fair-skinned individuals. At puberty, the pigmentation of the nipple and areola increases, and the nipple becomes more prominent. With the gravid state, the areola enlarges, and the degree of pigmentation increases. Deep to the areola and nipple, bundles of smooth muscle fibers are arranged radially and circumferentially in the dense connective tissue and longitudinally along the lactiferous ducts that extend up into the nipple. These muscle fibers are responsible for the erection of nipple that occurs in response to various stimuli (for a review of the anatomy of the nipple and areola, see Giacometti and Montagna[8]). The areola contains sebaceous glands, sweat glands, and accessory areolar glands (of Montgomery), which are intermediate in their structure between true mammary glands and sweat glands. The accessory areolar glands produce small elevations on the surface of the areola. The sebaceous glands (which usually lack associated hairs) and sweat glands are located along the margin of the areola. Whereas the apex of the nipple contains numerous free sensory nerve cell endings and Meissner corpuscles in the dermal papillae, the areola contains fewer of these structures.[9] In a review of the innervation of the nipple and areola, Montagna and Macpherson[10] reported observing fewer nerve endings than described by other investigators. They reported that most of the sensory endings were at the apex of the nipple. Neuronal plexuses are also present around hair follicles in the skin peripheral to the areola, and palpatory pacinian corpuscles (vibratory pressure sensation and touch) may be present in the dermis and in the glandular tissue. The rich sensory innervation of the breast, particularly the nipple and areola,[11] is of great functional significance. The suckling infant initiates a reflex chain of neural and neurohumoral events, resulting in the release of milk and maintenance of glandular differentiation that is essential for continued lactation.

Inactive Mammary Gland

The adult mammary gland is composed of 15 to 20 irregular lobes of branched tubuloalveolar glands. The lobes, separated by fibrous bands of connective tissue, radiate from the mammary papilla, or nipple, and are further subdivided into numerous lobules. Those fibrous bands that connect with the dermis are the suspensory ligaments of Cooper. Abundant adipose tissue is present in the dense connective tissue of the interlobular spaces. The intralobular connective tissue is much less dense and contains little fat.

Each lobe of the mammary gland ends in a lactiferous duct (2–4 mm in diameter) that opens through a constricted orifice (0.4–0.7 mm in diameter) onto the nipple (see Fig. 2.2). Beneath the areola, each duct has a dilated portion, the lactiferous sinus. Near their openings, the lactiferous ducts are lined with stratified squamous epithelium. The epithelial lining of the duct shows a gradual transition to two layers of cuboidal cells in the lactiferous sinus and then becomes a single layer of columnar or cuboidal cells through the remainder of the duct system. Myoepithelioid cells of ectodermal origin are located within the epithelium between the surface epithelial cells and the basal lamina.[12] These

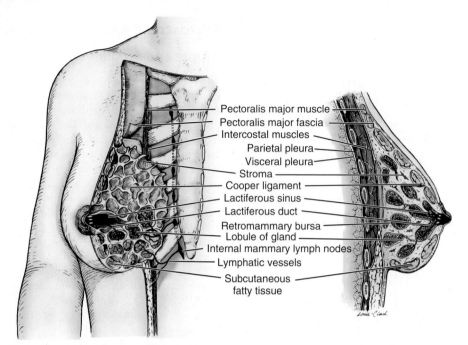

Pectoralis major muscle
Pectoralis major fascia
Intercostal muscles
Parietal pleura
Visceral pleura
Stroma
Cooper ligament
Lactiferous sinus
Lactiferous duct
Retromammary bursa
Lobule of gland
Internal mammary lymph nodes
Lymphatic vessels
Subcutaneous
fatty tissue

• **Fig. 2.2** A tangential view of the breast on the chest wall and a sectional (sagittal) view of the breast and associated chest wall. The breast lies in the superficial fascia just deep to the dermis. It is attached to the skin by the suspensory ligaments of Cooper and is separated from the investing fascia of the pectoralis major muscle by the retromammary bursa. Cooper ligaments form fibrosepta in the stroma that provide support for the breast parenchyma. From 15 to 20 lactiferous ducts extend from lobules composed of glandular epithelium to openings located on the nipple. A dilation of the duct, the lactiferous sinus, is present near the opening of the duct in the subareolar tissue. Subcutaneous fat and adipose tissue distributed around the lobules of the gland give the breast its smooth contour and, in the nonlactating breast, account for most of its mass. Lymphatic vessels pass through the stroma surrounding the lobules of the gland and convey lymph to collecting ducts. Lymphatic channels ending in the internal mammary (or parasternal) lymph nodes are shown. The pectoralis major muscle lies adjacent to the ribs and intercostal muscles. The parietal pleura, attached to the endothoracic fascia, and the visceral pleura, covering the surface of the lung, are shown.

cells, arranged in a basketlike network, are present in the secretory portion of the gland but are more apparent in the larger ducts. They contain myofibrils and are strikingly similar to smooth muscle cells in their cytology.

Under light microscopy, epithelial cells are characteristically seen to be attached to an underlying layer called the basement membrane. With electron microscopy, the substructure of the basement membrane can be identified. The inner layer of the basement membrane is called the basal lamina. In the breast, the parenchymal cells of the tubuloalveolar glands, as well as the epithelial and myoepithelial cells of the ducts, rest on a basement membrane or basal lamina. The integrity of this supporting layer is of significance in evaluating biopsy specimens of breast tissue. Changes in the basement membrane have important implications in immune surveillance, transformation, differentiation, and metastasis.[13–16]

Morphologically, the secretory portion of the normal mammary gland varies greatly with age and during pregnancy and lactation (Fig. 2.3). In the *inactive gland,* the glandular component is sparse and consists chiefly of duct elements (Fig. 2.4). Most investigators believe that the secretory units in the inactive breast are not organized as alveoli and consist only of ductules. During the menstrual cycle, the inactive breast undergoes slight cyclical changes. Early in the cycle, the ductules appear as cords with little or no lumen. Under estrogen stimulation, at about the time of ovulation, secretory cells increase in height, lumina appear as small amounts of

secretions accumulate, and fluids and lipid accumulate in the connective tissue. Then, in the absence of continued hormonal stimulation, the gland regresses to a more inactive state through the remainder of the cycle.

Active Mammary Glands: Pregnancy and Lactation

During pregnancy, in preparation for lactation, the mammary glands undergo dramatic proliferation and development. These changes in the glandular tissue are accompanied by relative decreases in the amount of connective and adipose tissue. Plasma cells, lymphocytes, and eosinophils infiltrate the fibrous component of the connective tissue as the breast develops in response to hormonal stimulation. The development of the glandular tissue is not uniform, and variation in the degree of development may occur within a single lobule. The cells vary in shape from low columnar to flattened. As the cells proliferate by mitotic division, the ductules branch and alveoli begin to develop. In the later stages of pregnancy, alveolar development becomes more prominent (Fig. 2.5). Near the end of pregnancy, the actual proliferation of cells declines, and subsequent enlargement of the breast occurs through hypertrophy of the alveolar cells and accumulation of their secretory product in the lumina of the ductules.

The secretory cells contain abundant endoplasmic reticulum, a moderate number of large mitochondria, a supranuclear Golgi

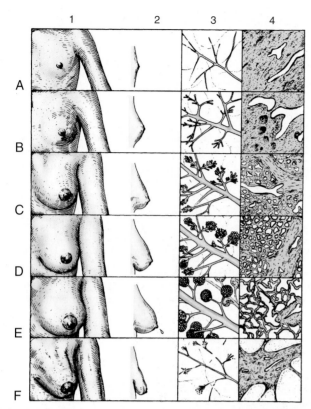

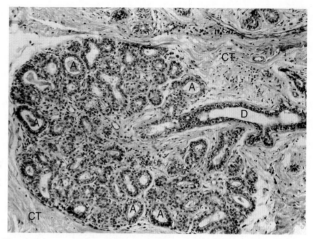

• **Fig. 2.3** Schematic drawing illustrating mammary gland development. Anterior and lateral views of the breast are shown in columns 1 and 2. The microscopic appearances of the ducts and lobules are illustrated in columns 3 and 4, respectively. (A) Prepubertal (childhood); (B) puberty; (C) mature (reproductive); (D) pregnancy; (E) lactation; (F) postmenopausal (senescent) state. (From Copeland EM III, Bland KI. The breast. In: Sabiston DC Jr, ed. *Essentials of Surgery*. Philadelphia: WB Saunders; 1987.)

• **Fig. 2.5** Proliferative or active (pregnant) human mammary gland. The alveolar elements of the gland become conspicuous during the early proliferative period (compare with Fig. 2.4). Within the lobule of the breast, distinct alveoli *(A)* are present. The alveoli are continuous with a duct *(D)*. They are surrounded by highly cellular connective tissue *(CT)*. The individual lobules are separated by dense connective tissue septa. ×160. (Courtesy Michael H. Ross, PhD, University of Florida College of Medicine, Gainesville, FL.)

complex, and a number of dense lysosomes.[17,18] Depending on the secretory state of the cell, large lipid droplets and secretory granules may be present in the apical cytoplasm. Two distinct products produced by the cells are released by different mechanisms.[19] The protein component of the milk is synthesized in the granular endoplasmic reticulum, packaged in membrane-limited secretory granules for transport in the Golgi apparatus, and released from the cell by fusion of the granule's limiting membrane with the plasma membrane. This type of secretion is known as merocrine secretion. The lipid, or fatty, component of the milk arises as free lipid droplets in the cytoplasm. The lipid coalesces into large droplets that pass to the apical region of the cell and project into the lumen of the acinus before their release. As they are released from the cell, the droplets are invested with an envelope of plasma membrane. A thin layer of cytoplasm is trapped between the lipid droplet and plasma membrane as lipid is being released. It should be emphasized that only a very small amount of cytoplasm is lost during this secretory process, classically known as apocrine secretion.

The milk released during the first few days after childbirth is known as colostrum. It has low lipid content but is believed to contain considerable quantities of antibodies that provide the newborn with some degree of passive immunity. The lymphocytes and plasma cells that infiltrate the stroma of the breast during its proliferation and development are believed to be, in part, the source of the components of the colostrum. As the plasma cells and lymphocytes decrease in number, the production of colostrum stops and lipid-rich milk is produced.

Hormonal Regulation of the Mammary Gland

Physiologically enhanced production of estrogens and progesterone by the ovary at puberty induces the initial growth of the mammary gland. Subsequent to this nascent development, slight changes occur in the morphology of the glandular tissue with each ovarian, or menstrual, cycle. With pregnancy, the corpus luteum

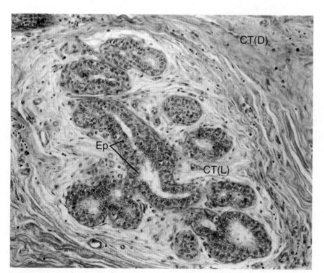

• **Fig. 2.4** Inactive or resting human mammary gland. The epithelial *(Ep)* or glandular elements are embedded in loose connective tissue [*CT(L)*]. Within the lobule the epithelial cells are primarily duct elements. Dense connective tissue [*CT(D)*] surrounds the lobule. ×160. (Courtesy Michael H. Ross, PhD, University of Florida College of Medicine, Gainesville, FL.)

and placenta continuously produce estrogens (estrone, estradiol, estriol) and progesterone, which further stimulate proliferation and development of the mammary gland (see Fig. 2.5). The growth of the glands is also dependent on the presence of prolactin, produced by the adenohypophysis; somatomammotropin (lactogenic hormone), produced by the placenta; and adrenal corticoids. The level of circulating estrogens and progesterone diminishes acutely at *parturition* with the degeneration of the corpus luteum and loss of the placenta. The secretion of milk is then brought about by increased production of prolactin and adrenal cortical steroids. A neurohormonal reflex regulates the high level of prolactin production and release. The act of *suckling* by the infant initiates impulses from receptors in the nipple; these impulses provide feedback regulation for cells in the hypothalamus. The impulses also cause the release of oxytocin in the neurohypophysis. The oxytocin stimulates the myoepithelial cells of the mammary glands, causing them to contract and eject milk.[20] In the absence of the suckling reflex stimulus, secretion of milk ceases and the lobular glands regress and return to an inactive state. After *menopause*, the gland atrophies, or involutes. As the

release of ovarian hormones is diminished, the secretory cells of the alveoli degenerate and disappear, but some of the ducts remain. The connective tissue also demonstrates degenerative changes that are marked by a decrease in the number of stromal cells and collagen fibers.

Thoracic Wall

The thoracic wall is composed of both skeletal and muscular components. The skeletal components include the 12 thoracic vertebrae, the 12 ribs and their costal cartilages, and the sternum. The spaces between the ribs, the intercostal spaces, are filled with the external, internal, and innermost intercostal muscles and the associated intercostal vessels and nerves (Fig. 2.6). Some anatomists refer to the innermost layer as the intima of the internal intercostal muscle. The terminology chosen is of no particular consequence; the relationship that should be appreciated is that the intercostal veins, arteries, and nerves pass in the plane that separates the internal intercostal muscle from the innermost (or intimal) layer. The endothoracic fascia, a thin fibrous layer of

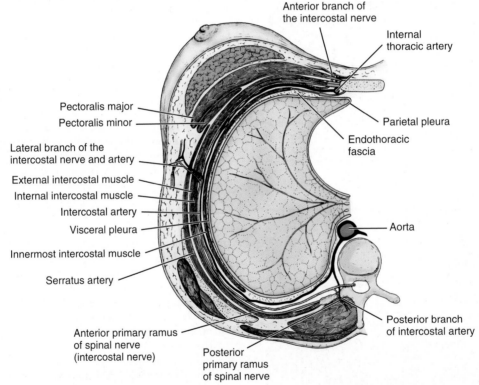

• **Fig. 2.6** Cross section of the breast and chest wall illustrating the layers of the thoracic wall and paths of blood vessels and nerves. The intercostal muscles occur in three layers: external, internal, and innermost. The intercostal vessels and nerves pass between the internal and innermost layers. The posterior intercostal arteries arise from the aorta and pass anterior to anastomose with the anterior intercostal arteries that are branches of the internal thoracic artery. The veins are not shown but basically follow the course of the arteries. The intercostal nerves are direct continuations of the anterior primary rami of thoracic spinal nerves. They supply the intercostal muscles and give anterior and lateral branches that supply the overlying skin, including that of the breast. The breast lies superficial to the pectoralis major muscle and the underlying pectoralis minor muscle. The serratus anterior muscle originates from eight or nine fleshy digitations on the outer lateral surface of the ribs and inserts on the ventral surface of the medial (vertebral) border of the scapula. Parietal pleura attaches to the endothoracic fascia that lines the thoracic cavity. Visceral pleura covers the surface of the lungs. The thin channels in the substance of the lung represent lymphatic channels that convey lymph to pulmonary lymph nodes located in the hilum of the lung. Lymphatic channels draining the thoracic wall and overlying skin and superficial fascia are not illustrated but follow the path of the blood vessels that supply the region (see text).

connective tissue forming a fascial plane continuous with the most internal component of the investing fascia of the intercostal muscles and the adjacent layer of the periosteum, marks the internal limit of the thoracic wall. The parietal pleura rests on the endothoracic fascia.

It is important to recognize that the muscles and skeletal girdles of the upper extremities almost completely cover the thoracic wall anteriorly, laterally, and posteriorly. For the surgeon concerned with the breast, knowledge of the anatomy of the axilla and pectoral region is essential.

The 11 pairs of external intercostal muscles whose fibers run downward and forward form the most superficial layer (see subsequent section on the innervation of the breast and Fig. 2.12 later). The muscle begins posteriorly at the tubercles of the ribs and extends anteriorly to the costochondral junction. Between the costal cartilages, the muscle is replaced by the external intercostal membrane. The fibers of the 11 pairs of internal intercostal muscles run downward and posteriorly. The muscle fibers of this layer reach the sternum anteriorly. Posteriorly, the muscle ends at the angle of the ribs and then the layer continues as the internal intercostal membrane. The innermost intercostal muscles (intercostales intimi) form the most internal layer and have fibers that are oriented more vertically but almost in parallel with the internal intercostal muscle fibers. The muscle fibers of this layer occupy approximately the middle half of the intercostal space. This is the least well developed of the three layers. It can best be distinguished by the fact that its fibers are separated from the internal intercostals by the intercostal vessels and nerves.

The subcostalis and transversus thoracis muscles are located on the internal surface of the thoracic wall. They occur in the same plane as the innermost intercostal muscles and are considered anterior and posterior extensions of this layer. The subcostal muscles are located posteriorly and have the same orientation as the innermost intercostal muscles. They are distinct because they pass to the second or third rib below (i.e., they pass over at least two intercostal spaces). Anteriorly, the transversus thoracis muscles form a layer that arises from the lower internal surface of the sternum and extends upward and laterally to insert on the costal cartilages of the second to sixth ribs (Fig. 2.7). These fibers pass deep to the internal thoracic artery and accompanying veins.

All of these muscles are innervated by the intercostal nerves associated with them. These nerves also give branches to the overlying skin. In a similar fashion, the intercostal vessels supply intercostal muscles and give branches to the overlying tissues. The intercostal nerves are direct continuations of the ventral primary rami of the upper 11 thoracic spinal nerves. As the nerves pass anteriorly, they give branches to supply the intercostal muscles. In addition, each nerve gives a relatively large lateral cutaneous branch, which exits the intercostal space along the midaxillary line near the attachment sites of the serratus anterior muscle on the ribs. The lateral cutaneous nerves then give branches that extend anteriorly and posteriorly. As the intercostal nerve continues anteriorly, it gives additional branches to the intercostal muscles. Just lateral to the border of the sternum the upper five intercostal nerves pierce the internal intercostal muscle and the external intercostal membrane to end superficially as the anterior cutaneous nerves of the chest. These nerves give rise to medial and lateral branches that supply the overlying skin. The lower six intercostal nerves continue past the costal margin into the anterior abdominal wall and are therefore identified as thoracoabdominal nerves.

The intercostal arteries originate in two groups: the anterior and posterior intercostal arteries. The posterior intercostal arteries,

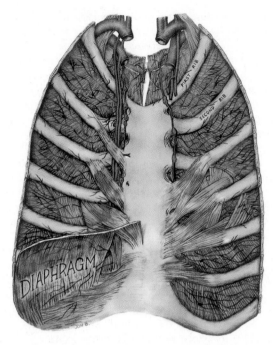

• **Fig. 2.7** The anterior thoracic wall as viewed internally. The internal thoracic arteries and veins can be seen as they pass parallel to and about 1 cm from the sternal margin. Except in the upper two or three intercostal spaces, the transversus thoracic muscle lies deep to these vessels. The internal thoracic lymphatic trunks and associated parasternal lymph nodes accompany these vessels. Lymphatic channels located in the intercostal spaces convey lymph from the thoracic wall anteriorly to the parasternal nodes or posteriorly to the intercostal nodes.

except for the first two spaces, arise from the thoracic aorta. The posterior intercostals for the first two spaces arise from the superior intercostal arteries, which on the left and right sides branch from the costocervical trunk. The anterior intercostals are usually small paired arteries that extend laterally to the region of the costochondral junction. The anterior intercostal arteries of the upper five intercostal spaces arise from the internal thoracic (or mammary) artery; those of the lower six intercostal spaces arise from the musculophrenic artery. The anterior and posterior intercostal veins demonstrate a similar distribution. Anteriorly, they drain into the musculophrenic and internal thoracic veins. Posteriorly, the intercostal veins drain into the azygos and hemiazygos systems of veins.

The superficial muscles of the pectoral region include the pectoralis major and minor muscles and the subclavius muscle. The pectoralis major muscle is a fan-shaped muscle with two divisions. The clavicular division (or head) originates from the clavicle and is easily distinguished from the larger costosternal division that originates from the sternum and costal cartilages of the second through sixth ribs. The fibers of the two divisions converge laterally and insert into the crest of the greater tubercle of the humerus along the lateral lip of the bicipital groove. The cephalic vein serves as a convenient landmark defining the separation of the upper lateral border of the pectoralis major muscle from the deltoid muscle. The cephalic vein can be followed to the deltopectoral triangle, where it pierces the clavipectoral fascia and joins the axillary vein. The pectoralis major muscle acts primarily in flexion, adduction, and medial rotation of the arm at the shoulder joint. This action brings the arm across the chest. In climbing, the pectoralis major muscles, along with the latissimus dorsi muscles, function to elevate the trunk when the arms are fixed. The pectoralis major muscle is innervated by both the *medial* and the *lateral pectoral nerves,* which arise from the *medial and lateral cords* of the brachial plexus, respectively. Located deep to the pectoralis major muscle, the pectoralis minor muscle arises from the external surface of the second to the fifth ribs and inserts on the coracoid process of the scapula. Although its main action is to lower the shoulder, it may serve as an accessory muscle of respiration. It is innervated by the medial pectoral nerve.

The subclavius muscle arises from the first rib near its costochondral junction and extends laterally to insert into the inferior surface of the clavicle. It functions to lower the clavicle and stabilize it during movements of the shoulder girdle. It is innervated by the nerve to the subclavius muscle, which arises from the upper trunk of the brachial plexus.

Axilla

Knowledge of the anatomy of the axilla and its contents is of paramount importance to the clinician. It is also essential that the surgeon be thoroughly familiar with the organization of the deep fascia and neurovascular relationships of the axilla.

Boundaries of the Axilla

The axilla is a pyramidal compartment between the upper extremity and the thoracic walls (Fig. 2.8). It is described as having four walls, an apex, and a base. The curved base is made of axillary fascia and skin. Externally, this region, the armpit, appears dome-shaped (and covered with hair after puberty). The apex is not a

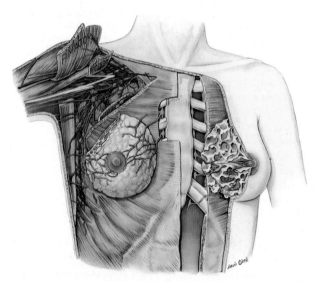

• **Fig. 2.8** The anterior chest illustrating the structure of the chest wall, breast, and axilla. See text for details of the structure of the axilla and a description of its contents. On the right side, the pectoralis major muscle has been cut lateral to the breast and reflected laterally to its insertion into the crest of the greater tubercle of the humerus. This exposes the underlying pectoralis minor muscle and the other muscles forming the walls of the axilla. The contents of the axilla, including the axillary artery and vein, components of the brachial plexus, and axillary lymph node groups and lymphatic channels, are exposed. On the left side, the breast is cut to expose its structure in sagittal view. The lactiferous ducts and sinuses can be seen. Lymphatic channels passing to parasternal lymph nodes are also shown.

roof but an aperture that extends into the posterior triangle of the neck through the cervicoaxillary canal. The cervicoaxillary canal is bounded anteriorly by the clavicle, posteriorly by the scapula, and medially by the first rib. Most structures pass through the cervical axillary canal as they course between the neck and upper extremity. The anterior wall is made up of the pectoralis major and minor muscles and their associated fasciae. The posterior wall is composed primarily of the subscapularis muscle, located on the anterior surface of the scapula, and to a lesser extent by the teres major and latissimus dorsi muscles and their associated tendons. The lateral wall is a thin strip of the humerus, the bicipital groove, between the insertions of the muscles of the anterior and posterior walls. The medial wall is made up of serratus anterior muscle that covers the thoracic wall in this region (over the upper four or five ribs and their associated intercostal muscles).

Contents of the Axilla

The axilla contains the great vessels and nerves of the upper extremity. These, along with the other contents, are surrounded by loose connective tissue. Fig. 2.8 illustrates many of the key relationships of structures within the axilla. The vessels and nerves are closely associated with each other and are enclosed within a layer of fascia, the axillary sheath. This layer of dense connective tissue extends from the neck and gradually disappears as the nerves and vessels branch.

The *axillary artery* may be divided into three parts within the axilla:

1. The first portion, located medial to the pectoralis minor muscle, gives one branch—the supreme thoracic artery that supplies the thoracic wall over the first and second intercostal spaces.
2. The second portion, located posterior to the pectoralis minor muscle, gives two branches—the thoracoacromial artery and the lateral thoracic artery. The thoracoacromial artery divides into the acromial, clavicular, deltoid, and pectoral branches. The lateral thoracic artery passes along the lateral border of the pectoralis minor on the superficial surface of the serratus anterior muscle. Pectoral branches of the thoracoacromial and lateral thoracic arteries supply both the pectoralis major and minor muscles and must be identified during surgical dissection of the axilla. The lateral thoracic artery is of particular importance in surgery of the breast as it supplies the lateral mammary branches.
3. The third portion, located lateral to the pectoralis minor, gives off three branches—the anterior and posterior circumflex humeral arteries, which supply the upper arm and contribute to the collateral circulation around the humerus, and the subscapular artery. Although the latter artery does not supply the breast, it is of particular importance in the surgical dissection of the axilla. It is the largest branch within the axilla, giving rise after a short distance to its terminal branches, the subscapular circumflex and the thoracodorsal arteries, and it is closely associated with the central and subscapular lymph node groups. In the axilla, the thoracodorsal artery crosses the subscapularis and gives branches to it and to the serratus anterior and the latissimus dorsi muscles. A surgeon must use care in approaching this vessel and its branches to avoid undue bleeding that obscures the surgical field.

The *axillary vein* has tributaries that follow the course of the arteries just described. They are usually in the form of *venae comitantes,* paired veins that follow an artery. The cephalic vein passes in the groove between the deltoid and pectoralis major muscles

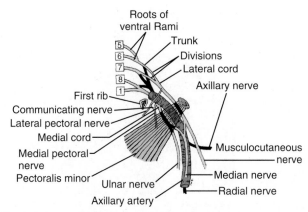

• **Fig. 2.9** Schematic drawing of the brachial plexus illustrating its basic components. The cords are associated with the axillary artery and lie behind the pectoralis minor muscle. The names of the cords reflect their relationship to the artery. Compare with Fig. 2.8 to identify the course of these structures in more detail.

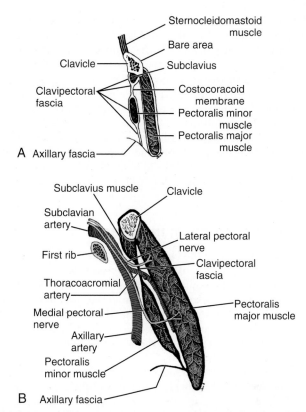

• **Fig. 2.10** Sagittal sections of the chest wall in the axillary region. (A) The anterior wall of the axilla. The clavicle and three muscles inferior to it are shown. (B) Section through the chest wall illustrating the relationship of the axillary artery and medial and lateral pectoral nerves to the clavipectoral fascia. The clavipectoral fascia is a strong sheet of connective tissue that is attached superiorly to the clavicle and envelops the subclavius and pectoralis minor muscles. The fascia extends from the lower border of the pectoralis minor to become continuous with the axillary fascia in the floor of the axilla.

and then joins the axillary vein after piercing the clavipectoral fascia.

Throughout its course in the axilla, the axillary artery is associated with various parts of the brachial plexus (Fig. 2.9). The cords of the brachial plexus—medial, lateral, and posterior—are named according to their relationship with the axillary artery. A majority of the branches of the brachial plexus arise in the axilla. The *lateral cord* gives four branches, namely, the lateral pectoral nerve, which supplies the pectoralis major; a branch that communicates with the medial pectoral nerve, which is called the ansa pectoralis[21]; and two terminal branches, the musculocutaneous nerve and the lateral root of the median nerve. Injury to the medial or lateral pectoral nerves, or the *ansa pectoralis*,[21] which joins them, may lead to atrophy with loss of muscle mass and fat necrosis of the pectoralis major or minor muscles,[22] depending of the level of nerve injury. The ansa pectoralis lies anterior to the axillary artery, making it vulnerable to injury during lymph node dissection in the axilla.

The *medial cord* usually gives five branches, the medial and minor, the median brachial cutaneous nerve, the medial antebrachial cutaneous nerve, and two terminal branches, the ulnar nerve and the lateral root of the median nerve. The *posterior cord* usually has five branches. Three of these nerves arise from the posterior cord in the superior aspect of the axilla—the upper subscapular, the thoracodorsal, and the lower subscapular; the cord then divides into its two terminal branches, the axillary and radial nerves.

Two additional nerves are of particular interest to surgeons because they are vulnerable to injury during axillary dissection: the *long thoracic nerve,* which is a branch of the brachial plexus, and the intercostobrachial nerve. The long thoracic nerve is located on the medial wall of the axilla. It arises in the neck from the fifth, sixth, and seventh roots of the brachial plexus and then enters the axilla through the cervicoaxillary canal. This nerve lies longitudinally on the surface of the serratus anterior muscle, which it innervates. The long thoracic nerve is invested by the serratus fascia and is sometimes accidentally removed with this membrane of fascia during surgery of the axilla. This anatomic feature requires preferential dissection in a longitudinal plane of the course of the nerve to abrogate surgical injury. This results in paralysis of part or all of the serratus anterior muscle ("winged

scapula deficit"). The functional deficit is an inability to raise the arm above the level of the shoulder (or extreme weakness when one attempts this movement). A second nerve, the *intercostobrachial,* is formed by the joining of a lateral cutaneous branch of the second intercostal nerve with the medial cutaneous nerve of the arm. This nerve supplies the skin of the floor of the axilla and the upper medial aspect of the arm. Sometimes a second intercostobrachial nerve may form an anterior branch of the third lateral cutaneous nerve. This nerve is also commonly injured in axillary dissection, resulting in numbness of the skin of the floor of the axilla and the medial aspect of the arm.

Lymph nodes are also present in the axilla. They are found in close association with the blood vessels. The lymph node groups and their location are described in the section on the lymphatic drainage of the breast.

Axillary Fasciae

The anterior wall of the axilla is composed of the pectoralis major and minor muscles and the fascia that covers them. The fasciae occur in two layers: (1) a superficial layer investing the pectoralis major muscle, called the pectoral fascia, and (2) a deep layer that extends from the clavicle to the axillary fascia in the floor of the axilla, called the clavipectoral (or costocoracoid) fascia. The clavipectoral fascia encloses the subclavius muscle located below the clavicle and the pectoralis minor muscle (Fig. 2.10).

The upper portion of the clavipectoral fascia, the costocoracoid membrane, is pierced by the cephalic vein, the lateral pectoral nerve, and branches of the thoracoacromial artery. The medial pectoral nerve does not pierce the costocoracoid membrane but enters the deep surface of the pectoralis minor muscle, supplying it, and passes through the anterior investing layer of the pectoralis minor muscle to innervate the pectoralis major muscle. The lower portion of the clavipectoral fascia, located below the pectoralis minor muscle, is sometimes called the suspensory ligament of the axilla. *Halsted ligament,* a dense condensation of the clavipectoral fascia, extends from the medial end of the clavicle and attaches to the first rib (see Figs. 2.8 and 2.10A). The ligament covers the subclavian artery and vein as they cross the first rib.

Fascial Relationship of the Breast

The breast is located in the superficial fascia in the layer just deep to the dermis, the hypodermis. In approaching the breast, a surgeon may dissect in a bloodless plane just deep to the dermis. This dissection leaves a layer 6 to 8 mm in thickness in thin individuals in association with the skin flap. The layer may be several millimeters (8–10 mm) thick in obese individuals. The blood vessels and lymphatics passing in the deeper layer of the superficial fascia are left undisturbed.

Anterior fibrous processes, the *suspensory ligaments of Cooper,* pass from the septa that divide the lobules of the breast to insert into the cutis of the skin. The posterior aspect of the breast is separated from the deep, or investing, fascia of the pectoralis major muscle by a space filled with loose areolar tissue, the retromammary space or bursa (see Fig. 2.2). The existence of the suspensory ligaments of Cooper and the retromammary space allows the breast to move freely against the thoracic wall. The space between the well-defined fascial planes of the breast and pectoralis major muscle is easily identified by the surgeon removing a breast. Connective tissue thickenings, called posterior suspensory ligaments, extend from the deep surface of the breast to the deep pectoral fascia. Because breast parenchyma may follow these fibrous processes, it has been common practice to remove the adjacent portion of the pectoralis major muscle with the breast.

It is important to recognize, particularly with movements and variation in the size of the breast, that its deep surface contacts the investing fascia of other muscles in addition to the pectoralis major. Only about two-thirds of the breast overlies the pectoralis major muscle. The lateral portion of the breast may contact the fourth through seventh slips of the serratus anterior muscle at its attachment to the thoracic wall. Medial to this anatomic area, the breast may contact the upper portion of the abdominal oblique muscle, where it interdigitates with the attachments of the serratus anterior muscle. The breast extends fully to the axilla; it has contact with the deep fascial envelope present in this region.

Blood Supply of the Breast

Parenchyma and skin of the breast receive their blood supply from:
1. perforating branches of the internal mammary artery;
3. lateral branches of the posterior intercostal arteries; and
4. several branches from the axillary artery, including highest thoracic, lateral thoracic, and pectoral branches of the thoracoacromial artery (Fig. 2.11). For reviews of the blood supply of the breast, see Cunningham,[23] Maliniac,[24] and Sakki.[25]

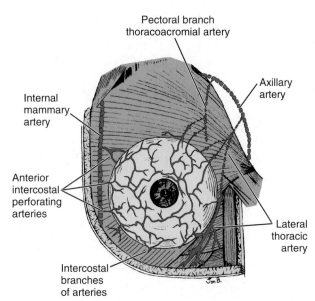

• **Fig. 2.11** Arterial distribution of blood to the breast, axilla, and chest wall. The breast receives its blood supply via three major arterial routes: (1) medially from anterior perforating intercostal branches arising from the internal thoracic artery, (2) laterally from either pectoral branches of the thoracoacromial trunk or branches of the lateral thoracic artery (the thoracoacromial trunk and the lateral thoracic arteries are branches of the axillary artery), and (3) from lateral cutaneous branches of the intercostal arteries that are associated with the overlying breast. The arteries indicated with a *dashed line* lie deep to the muscles of the thoracic wall and axilla. Many of the arteries must pass through these muscles before reaching the breast.

Branches from the second, third, and fourth anterior perforating arteries (see Figs. 2.11 and 2.12) pass to the breast as *medial mammary arteries.* These vessels enlarge considerably during lactation. The lateral thoracic artery gives branches to the serratus anterior muscle, both pectoralis muscles, and the subscapularis muscle. The lateral thoracic artery also gives rise to lateral mammary branches that wrap around the lateral border of the pectoralis major muscle to reach the breast. In the second, third, and fourth intercostal spaces, the posterior intercostal arteries give off *mammary branches;* these vessels increase in size during lactation.

The thoracodorsal branch of the subscapular artery is not contributory to the supply of blood to the breast, but it is important to the surgeon who must deal with this artery during the dissection of the axilla. The central and scapular lymph node groups are intimately associated with this vessel. Bleeding that is difficult to control may result from cutting of branches of these vessels.

A fundamental knowledge of the pattern of venous drainage is important as carcinoma of the breast may metastasize through the veins and because lymphatic vessels often follow the course of the blood vessels. Venae comitantes of the breast closely accompany the path of the arteries, with net venous drainage toward the axilla. The superficial veins demonstrate extensive anastomoses that may be apparent through the skin overlying the breast. The distribution of these veins has been studied by Massopust and Gardner[26] and Haagensen[27] using photographs taken in infrared light. Around the nipple-areolar complex, venae comitantes form an anastomotic circle, the *circulus venosus.* Veins from this circle and

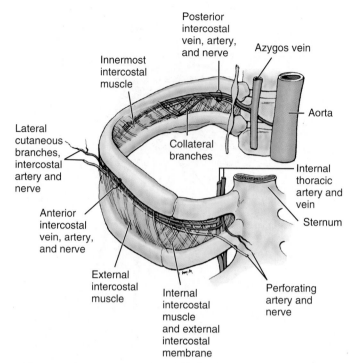

• **Fig. 2.12** A segment of the body wall illustrating the relationship of structures to the ribs. Two ribs are shown as they extend from the vertebrae to attach to the sternum. The orientation of the muscle and connective tissue fibers is shown. The external intercostal muscle extends downward and forward. The muscle layer extends forward from the rib tubercle to the costochondral junction, where the muscle is replaced by the aponeurosis, called the external intercostal membrane. The internal intercostal muscle fibers with the opposite orientation can be seen through this layer. The innermost intercostal muscle fibers are present along the lateral half of the intercostal space. The intercostal nerve and vessels pass through the intercostal space in the plane between the internal and innermost (or intima of the internal) intercostal muscle layers. Anterior intercostal arteries arise from the internal thoracic artery; anterior intercostal veins join the internal thoracic vein. Posterior intercostal arteries arise from the aorta; posterior intercostal veins join the azygos venous system on the right and the hemiazygos system on the left. Lymphatics follow the path of the blood vessels. Anteriorly, lymphatics pass to parasternal (or internal mammary) nodes that are located along the internal mammary vessels; posteriorly, they pass to intercostal nodes located in the intercostal space near the vertebral bodies.

from the substance of the gland transmit blood to the periphery of the breast and then into vessels joining the internal thoracic, axillary, and internal jugular veins.

Three principal groups of veins are involved in the venous drainage of the thoracic wall and the breast:
1. perforating branches of the internal thoracic vein,
2. tributaries of the axillary vein, and
3. perforating branches of posterior intercostal veins.

Metastatic emboli traveling through any of these venous routes will pass through the venous return to the heart and then be stopped as they reach the capillary bed of the lungs, providing a direct venous route for metastasis of breast carcinoma to the lungs.

The *vertebral plexus of veins (Batson plexus)* may provide a second route for metastasis of breast carcinoma via veins.[28–30] This venous plexus surrounds the vertebrae and extends from the base of the skull to the sacrum. Venous channels exist between this plexus and veins associated with thoracic, abdominal, and pelvic organs. In general, these veins do not have valves, making it possible for blood to flow through them in either direction. Furthermore, it is known that increases in intraabdominal pressure may force blood to enter these channels. These vessels provide a route for metastatic emboli to reach the vertebral bodies, ribs, and central nervous system. These venous communications are of particular significance in the breast, where the posterior intercostal arteries are in direct continuity with the vertebral plexus.

Innervation of the Breast

Miller and Kasahara[31] have described the microscopic anatomic features of the innervation of the skin over the breast. They suggest that the specialization of the innervation of the breast, areola, and nipple is associated with the erection of the nipple[11] and flow of milk mediated through a neurohormonal reflex. The infantile suckling reflex initiates impulses from receptors in the nipple that regulate cells in the hypothalamus. In response to the impulses, oxytocin is released in the neurohypophysis. Oxytocin stimulates the myoepithelial cells of the mammary glands, initiating contraction and ejection of milk from the glands. In the dermis of the nipple, Miller and Kasahara[31] found large numbers of multibranched free nerve endings and, in the dermis of the areola and peripheral, Ruffini-like endings and Krause end bulbs. The latter two receptor types are associated with tactile reception of stretch and pressure.

Sensory innervation of the breast is supplied primarily by the *lateral and anterior cutaneous branches of the second through sixth intercostal nerves* (see Fig. 2.12). Although the second and third intercostal nerves may give rise to cutaneous branches to the superior aspect of the breast, the nerves of the breast are derived primarily from the fourth, fifth, and sixth intercostal nerves. A limited region of the skin over the upper portion of the breast is supplied by nerves arising from the cervical plexus, specifically, the anterior, or medial, branches of the *supraclavicular nerve*. All of these nerves convey sympathetic fibers to the breast and overlying skin and therefore influence flow of blood through vessels accompanying the nerves and secretory function of the sweat glands of the skin. However, the secretory activity of the breast is chiefly under the control of ovarian and hypophyseal (pituitary) hormones.

Lateral branches of the intercostal nerves exit the intercostal space at the attachment sites of the slips of serratus anterior muscle. The nerves divide into anterior and posterior branches as they pass between the muscle fibers. As the anterior branches pass in the superficial fascia, they supply the anterolateral thoracic wall; the third through sixth branches, also known as lateral mammary branches, supply the breast. The lateral branch of the second intercostal nerve is of special significance because a large nerve, the *intercostal brachial*, arises from it. This nerve, which can be seen during surgical dissection of the axilla, passes through the fascia of the floor of the axilla and usually joins the medial cutaneous nerve of the arm. However, it is of limited functional significance. If this nerve is injured during surgery, the patient will have loss of cutaneous sensation from the upper medial aspect of the arm and floor of the axilla.

The anterior branches of the intercostal nerves exit the intercostal space near the lateral border of the sternum. These nerves send branches medially and laterally over the thoracic wall. The branches that pass laterally reach the medial aspect of the breast and are sometimes called *medial mammary nerves*.

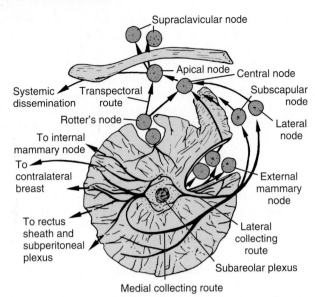

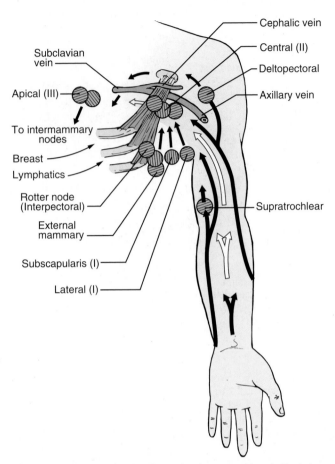

• **Fig. 2.13** Schematic drawing of the breast identifying the position of lymph nodes relative to the breast and illustrating routes of lymphatic drainage. The clavicle is indicated as a reference point. See the text and Fig. 2.15 to identify the group or level to which the lymph nodes belong. Level I lymph nodes include the external mammary (or anterior), axillary vein (or lateral), and scapular (or posterior) groups; level II, the central group; and level III, the subclavicular (or apical). The arrows indicate the routes of lymphatic drainage (see text).

• **Fig. 2.14** Schematic drawing illustrating the route of lymphatic drainage in the upper extremity. The relationship of this drainage to the major axillary lymph node groups is indicated by the arrows. All the lymph vessels of the upper extremity drain directly or indirectly through outlying lymph node groups into the axillary lymph nodes. The outlying lymph nodes are few in number and are organized into three groups: (1) supratrochlear lymph nodes (one or two, located above the medial epicondyle of the humerus adjacent to the basilic vein); (2) deltopectoral lymph nodes (one or two, located beside the cephalic vein where it lies between the pectoralis major and deltoid muscle just below the clavicle); and (3) variable small isolated lymph nodes (few and variable in number; may be located in the cubital fossa or along the medial side of the brachial vessels). Note that the deltopectoral lymph node group drains directly into the subclavicular, or apical, lymph nodes of the axillary group.

Lymphatic Drainage of the Breast

Lymph Nodes of the Axilla

Principal routes for lymphatic drainage of the breast is via the axillary lymph node groups (see Figs. 2.8, 2.12, and 2.13). Therefore it is essential that the clinician understand the anatomy of the grouping of lymph nodes within the axilla. Unfortunately, the boundaries of groups of lymph nodes found in the axilla are not well demarcated. Thus there has been considerable variation in the names provided to the lymph node groups. Anatomists usually define five groups of axillary lymph nodes[32,33]; surgeons usually identify six primary groups.[27] Both professions define these lymphatic groups based on anatomic boundary and contiguous neurovascular structures. The most common terms used to identify the lymph nodes are indicated as follows:

1. The *axillary vein group (lateral group),* usually identified by anatomists as the lateral group, consists of four to six lymph nodes that lie just medial or posterior to the axillary vein in level I. These lymph nodes receive most of the lymph draining from the upper extremity (Fig. 2.14; also see Fig. 2.16 later). The exception is lymph that drains into the deltopectoral lymph nodes, a lymph node group sometimes called infraclavicular. The deltopectoral lymph nodes are not considered part of the axillary lymph node group but rather are outlying lymph nodes that drain into the subclavicular (or apical) lymph node group (see later discussion).

2. The *external mammary group* (see Figs. 2.14 and 2.16) in level I, usually identified by anatomists as the anterior or pectoral group, consists of four or five lymph nodes that lie along the lower border of the pectoralis minor muscle in association with the lateral thoracic vessels. These lymph nodes receive the major portion of the lymph draining from the breast. Lymph

drains primarily from these lymph nodes into the central lymph nodes. However, lymph may pass directly from the external mammary nodes into the subclavicular lymph nodes.

3. The *scapular and subscapular group* (see Figs. 2.14, 2.15, and 2.16), also level I, is usually identified by anatomists as the posterior or subscapular group, consists of six or seven lymph nodes that lie along the posterior wall of the axilla at the lateral border of the scapula in association with the subscapular vessels. These lymph nodes receive lymph primarily from the inferior aspect of the posterior region of the neck, the posterior aspect of the trunk as far inferior as the iliac crest, and the posterior aspect of the shoulder region. Lymph from the scapular nodes passes to the central and subclavicular nodes.

4. The *central group* (see Figs. 2.14 and 2.16) (both anatomists and surgeons use the same terminology for this group) consists of three or four large lymph nodes that are embedded in the fat of the axilla, usually posterior to the pectoralis minor

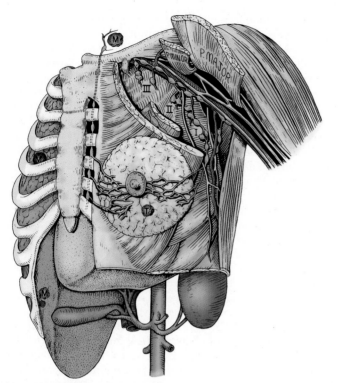

• **Fig. 2.15** Lymphatic drainage of the breast. The pectoralis major and minor muscles, which contribute to the anterior wall of the axilla, have been cut and reflected. This exposes the medial and posterior walls of the axilla, as well as the basic contents of the axilla. The lymph node groups of the axilla and the internal mammary nodes are depicted. Also shown is the location of the long thoracic nerve on the surface of the serratus anterior muscle (on the medial wall of the axilla). The scapular lymph node group is closely associated with the thoracodorsal nerve and vessels. The Roman numerals indicate lymph node groups defined in Fig. 2.16.

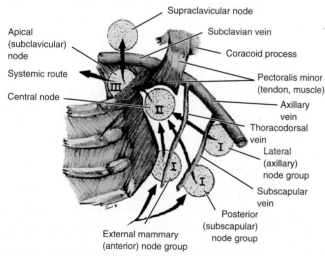

• **Fig. 2.16** Schematic drawing illustrating the major lymph node groups associated with the lymphatic drainage of the breast. The Roman numerals indicate three levels or groups of lymph nodes that are defined by their location relative to the pectoralis minor. Level I includes lymph nodes located lateral to the pectoralis minor; level II, lymph nodes located deep to the muscle; and level III, lymph nodes located medial to the muscle. The arrows indicate the general direction of lymph flow. The axillary vein and its major tributaries associated with the pectoralis minor are included.

muscle. This level II group receives lymph from the three preceding groups and may receive afferent lymphatic vessels directly from the breast. Lymph from the central nodes passes directly to the subclavicular (apical) nodes. This group is often superficially placed beneath the skin and fascia of the midaxilla and is centrally located between the posterior and anterior axillary folds. This nodal group is commonly palpable because of its superficial position and allows the clinical estimation of metastatic disease.[27,34]

5. The *subclavicular* (see Fig. 2.14) group, level III, usually identified by anatomists as the *apical group,* consists of 6 to 12 lymph nodes located partly posterior to the upper border of the pectoralis minor and partly superior to it. These lymph nodes extend into the apex of the axilla along the medial side of the axillary vein. They may receive lymph directly or indirectly from all the other groups of axillary lymph nodes. The efferent lymphatic vessels from the subclavicular lymph nodes unite to form the subclavian trunk. The course of the subclavian trunk is highly variable. It may directly join the internal jugular vein, the subclavian vein, or the junction of these two; likewise, on the right side of the trunk, it may join the right lymphatic duct, and on the left side, it may join the thoracic duct. Efferent vessels from the subclavicular lymph nodes may also pass to deep cervical lymph nodes.

6. The *interpectoral* or *Rotter lymph nodes* (see Figs. 2.14 and 2.16),[35] a group of nodes identified by surgeons[27] but considered less prominent by anatomists, is anatomically level I group and consists of one to four small lymph nodes that are located between the pectoralis major and minor muscles in association with the pectoral branches of the thoracoacromial vessels. Lymph from these nodes passes directly into central and subclavicular nodes.

Surgeons also define the axillary lymph nodes with respect to their relationship with the pectoralis minor muscle. These relationships are illustrated schematically in Fig. 2.16. Lymph nodes that are located lateral to or below the lower border of the pectoralis minor muscle are called *level I* and include the *external mammary, axillary vein (lateral), and scapular lymph node groups.* Those lymph nodes located deep or posterior to the pectoralis minor muscle are called *level II* and include the *central lymph node group* and possibly some of the *subclavicular lymph node* group. Those lymph nodes located medial or superior to the upper border of the pectoralis minor muscle are indicated as level III and include the subclavicular or apical lymph node group (see Figs. 2.14–2.16).

Surgeons use the term *prepectoral* to identify a single lymph node that is only rarely found in the subcutaneous tissue associated with the breast or in the breast itself in its upper outer sector.[27] Cushman Haagensen reported finding only one or two prepectoral nodes each year among the several hundred mammary lesions studied.[27]

Sentinel Lymph Node Biopsy

Several reviews[36–54] have discussed the potential benefits and risks of sentinel lymph node (SLN) identification and biopsy in breast cancer surgery and treatment. The basic tenet of SLN biopsy is that the first lymph node that receives drainage from a tumor is the first site of lymphatic metastasis. The status of the SLN reflects the status of the more distal lymph nodes along the lymphatic chain. The report by Lee and colleagues[38] on several studies confirmed that should only one lymph node have metastatic involvement, it is almost always the SLN; furthermore, in early stages of breast cancer it is often the *only site* of metastasis.

The three most important pathologic determinants for the prognosis of early breast cancer are the status of the axillary lymph nodes, histologic grade, and tumor size. Currently, molecular and genetic profiling of tumor and/or archival specimens constitutes the indices of metastatic risk and outcomes assessment. For the past century, axillary lymph node dissection (ALND) has been an integral component of breast cancer management. The presence of axillary metastasis is associated with reduced disease-free and overall survival, and the number of involved axillary nodes has an inverse order of prognostic significance. Both are defining of optimal therapeutic strategies. SLN biopsy further defines the probability of true pathologic staging with anatomic sampling of the involved axillary lymph nodes for the staging of breast cancer.

A number of techniques have been reported to optimize the identification of the SLN. The two proven methods used are blue dye (isosulfan blue [Lymphazurin]/methylene blue) and/or technetium radiolabeled sulfa colloid protein. In both techniques, the dye or radiolabeled material is injected around the tumor or deep in the overlying skin. With the blue dye, the location of the SLN is not known preoperatively, and the blue-stained lymphatics are followed intraoperatively to locate the SLN. Use of radiolabeled material (Tc99msulfa colloid) allows the tracer to be detected preoperatively with lymphoscintigraphy, or intraoperatively with a gamma probe, or the combination of both. Lee and colleagues[38] reported that in recent large studies, the SLN was identified 93% to 99% of the time. They also reported that in the larger series of studies, the false-negative SLN with metastasis elsewhere in the axilla was in the range of 1% to 11%.

Before SLN biopsy can be used to determine specific surgical approaches and the extent of adjuvant chemotherapy and regional radiation therapy, there must be consensus on the sensitivity of the method and the accepted false-negative rates. In his review, Von Smitten[40] reported rates of detection of sentinel nodes ranging from 66% to 100%, and false-negative rates of 17% to 0% have been reported. Von Smitten[40] suggested that a theoretical false-negative rate of 2% to 3% may be acceptable; Cody[36] suggested that a goal for surgeons and institutions using SLN biopsy may be at least 90% successful in finding the SLN with no more than 5% to 10% false-negative findings. In the case of SLN biopsy, as is true in most areas of medicine, the skill, expertise, and thoroughness of the pathologist who reads the specimen is of utmost importance.

Numerous recent reviews provide insight into the controversy with respect to SLN biopsy.[38,39,41-55] Many investigators have supported the positive aspect of more limited lymph node dissection by taking advantage of information gained via findings from carefully assessed SLN biopsy. The reader of this text is further referred to Chapter 42 for contemporary SLN identification techniques and outcomes.

Lymph Flow

Anatomic familiarity and physiologic conceptualization of lymphatic drainage of the breast is essential to the student of breast pathophysiology. Metastatic dissemination of breast cancer occurs predominantly within the rich and extensive lymphatic routes that arborize multidirectionality via skin and mesenchymal (intraparenchymal) lymphatics. The delicate lymphatics of the corium are valveless; flow encompasses the lobular parenchyma and thereafter parallels major venous tributaries to enter the regional lymph nodes. This unidirectional lymphatic flow is pulsatile as a consequence of the wavelike contractions of the lymphatics to allow rapid transit and emptying of the lymphatic vascular spaces that interdigitate the extensive periductal and perilobular networks. As a consequence of obstruction to lymph flow by inflammatory or neoplastic diseases, a reversal in lymphatic flow is evident and can be appreciated microscopically as endolymphatic metastases within the dermis or breast parenchyma. This obstruction of lymphatic flow accounts for the neoplastic growth in local and regional sites remote from the primary neoplasm. Lymphatic flow is typically unidirectional, except in the pathologic state, and has preferential flow from the periphery toward larger collecting ducts. Lymphatic capillaries begin as blind-ending ducts in tissues from which the lymph is collected; throughout their course these capillaries anastomose and fuse to form larger lymphatic channels that ultimately terminate in the thoracic duct on the left side of the body or the smaller right lymphatic duct on the right side. The thoracic duct empties into the region of the juncture of the left subclavian and left internal jugular veins, whereas the right lymphatic duct drains into the right subclavian vein near its juncture with the right internal jugular vein.

Anson and McVay[34] and Haagensen[27] acknowledged two accessory directions for lymphatic flow from breast parenchyma to nodes of the apex of the axilla: the *transpectoral* and *retropectoral* routes (see Fig. 2.13). Lymphatics of the transpectoral route (i.e., interpectoral nodes) lie between the pectoralis major and minor muscles and are referred to as *Rotter nodes*. The transpectoral route begins in the loose areolar tissue of the retromammary plexus and interdigitates between the pectoral fascia and breast to perforate the pectoralis major muscle and follow the course of the thoracoacromial artery and terminate in the subclavicular (level III) group of nodes.

The second accessory lymphatic drainage group, the *retropectoral pathway,* drains the superior and internal aspects of the breast. Lymphatic vessels from this region of the breast join lymphatics from the posterior and lateral surfaces of the pectoralis major and minor muscles. These lymphatic channels terminate at the apex of the axilla in the *subclavicular (level III) group*. This route of lymphatic drainage is found in approximately one-third of individuals and is a more direct mechanism of lymphatic flow to the subclavicular group. This accessory pathway is also the major lymphatic drainage by way of the external mammary and central axillary nodal groups (levels I and II, respectively).[27,34]

The recognition of metastatic spread of breast carcinoma into internal mammary nodes as a primary route of systemic dissemination is credited to the British surgeon R.S. Handley.[55] Extensive investigation confirmed that central and medial lymphatics of the breast pass medially and parallel the course of major blood vessels to perforate the pectoralis major muscle and thereafter terminate in the internal mammary nodal chain.

The internal mammary nodal group (see Figs. 2.7 and 2.15) is anatomically situated in the retrosternal interspaces between the costal cartilages approximately 2 to 3 cm within the sternal margin. These nodal groups also traverse and parallel the internal mammary vasculature and are invested by endothoracic fascia. The internal mammary lymphatic trunks eventually terminate in subclavicular nodal groups (see Figs. 2.7, 2.13, and 2.16). The right internal mammary nodal group enters the right lymphatic duct and the left enters the thoracic duct (Fig. 2.17). The presence of supraclavicular nodes (stage IV disease) results from lymphatic permeation and subsequent obstruction of the inferior, deep cervical group of nodes of the jugular-subclavian confluence. In effect,

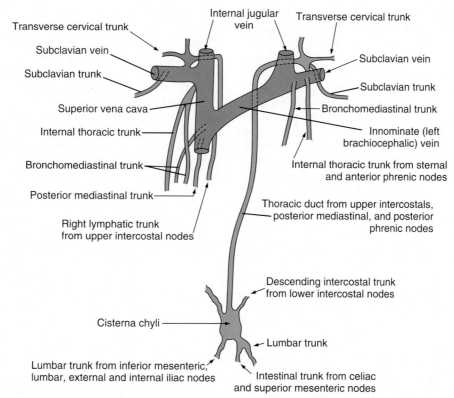

Internal jugular vein

Transverse cervical trunk

Transverse cervical trunk

Subclavian vein

Subclavian trunk

Subclavian vein

Subclavian trunk

Superior vena cava

Bronchomediastinal trunk

Internal thoracic trunk

Innominate (left brachiocephalic) vein

Bronchomediastinal trunk

Internal thoracic trunk from sternal and anterior phrenic nodes

Posterior mediastinal trunk

Thoracic duct from upper intercostals, posterior mediastinal, and posterior phrenic nodes

Right lymphatic trunk from upper intercostal nodes

Descending intercostal trunk from lower intercostal nodes

Cisterna chyli

Lumbar trunk

Lumbar trunk from inferior mesenteric, lumbar, external and internal iliac nodes

Intestinal trunk from celiac and superior mesenteric nodes

• **Fig. 2.17** Schematic of the major lymphatic vessels of the thorax and the root of the neck. The thoracic duct begins at the cisterna chyli, a dilated sac that receives drainage from the lower extremities and the abdominal and pelvic cavities via the lumbar and intestinal trunks. Lymph enters the systemic circulation via channels that join the great veins of the neck and superior mediastinum. The lymphatic vessels demonstrate considerable variation as to their number and pattern of branching. A typical pattern is illustrated here. Most of the major trunks, including the thoracic and right lymphatic ducts, end at or near the confluence of the internal jugular with the subclavian veins.

the supraclavicular nodal group represents the termination of efferent trunks from subclavian nodes of the internal mammary nodal group. These nodes are situated beneath the lateral margin of the inferior aspect of the sternocleidomastoid muscle beneath the clavicle and represent common sites of distant metastases from mammary carcinoma.

Cross-communication from the interstices of connecting lymphatic channels from each breast provides ready access of lymphatic flow to the opposite axilla. This observation of communicating dermal lymphatics to the contralateral breast explains occasional metastatic involvement of the opposite breast and axilla. Structures of the chest wall, including the internal and external intercostal musculature (see Fig. 2.12), have extensive lymphatic drainage that parallels the course of their major intercostal blood supply. As expected, invasive neoplasms of the lateral breast that involve deep musculature of the thoracic cavity have preferential flow toward the axilla. Invasion of medial musculature of the chest wall allows preferential drainage toward the internal mammary nodal groups, whereas bidirectional metastases may be evident with invasive central or subareolar cancers.

The lymphatic vessels that drain the breast occur in three interconnecting groups[56]: (1) a primary set of vessels originates as channels within the gland in the interlobular spaces and along the lactiferous ducts; (2) vessels draining the glandular tissue and overlying skin of the central part of the gland pass to an interconnecting network of vessels located beneath the areola, called the

subareolar plexus[57]; and (3) a plexus on the deep surface of the breast communicates with minute vessels in the deep fascia underlying the breast. Along the medial border of the breast, lymphatic vessels within the substance of the gland anastomose with vessels passing to parasternal nodes.

Using autoradiographs of surgical specimens, Turner-Warwick[56] demonstrated that the main lymphatic drainage of the breast is via the system of lymphatic vessels occurring within the substance of the gland and not through the vessels on the superficial or deep surface. The main collecting trunks run laterally as they pass through the axillary fascia in the substance of the axillary tail. The subareolar plexus plays no essential part in the lymphatic drainage of the breast.[56] Using vital dyes, Halsell and coworkers[58] demonstrated that this plexus receives lymph primarily from the nipple and the areola and conveys it toward the axilla. The lymphatics communicating with minute vessels in the deep fascia play no role in the principle lymphatic drainage of the breast and provide an alternative route only when the normal pathways are obstructed. More than 75% of the lymph from the breast passes to the axillary lymph nodes (see Fig. 2.13). Most of the remainder of the lymph passes to parasternal nodes. Some authorities have suggested that the parasternal nodes receive lymph primarily from the medial part of the breast. However, Turner-Warwick[56] reported that both the axillary and the parasternal lymph node groups receive lymph from all quadrants of the breast, with no striking tendency for any quadrant to drain in a particular direction.

Other routes for the flow of lymph from the breast have been identified. Occasionally, lymph from the breast reaches intercostal lymph nodes, located near the heads of the ribs (see later discussion). Lymphatic vessels reach this location by following lateral cutaneous branches of the posterior intercostal arteries. Lymph may pass to lymphatics within the rectus sheath or subperitoneal plexus by following branches of the intercostal and musculophrenic vessels. Lymph may pass directly to subclavicular, or apical, nodes from the upper portion of the breast. SLN biopsy has confirmed the direct metastasis from the breast to the supraclavicular nodes.

The skin over the breast has lymphatic drainage via the *superficial lymphatic vessels,* which ramify subcutaneously and converge on the axillary lymph nodes. The anterolateral chest and the upper abdominal wall above the umbilicus demonstrate striking directional flow of lymph toward the axilla. Lymphatic vessels near the lateral margin of the sternum pass through the intercostal space to the parasternal lymph nodes, which are associated with the internal thoracic vessels. Some of the lymphatic vessels located on adjacent sides of the sternum may anastomose in front of the sternum. In the upper pectoral region, a few of the lymphatic vessels may pass over the clavicle to inferior deep cervical lymph nodes.

The SLN biopsy identification is also providing better evidence of the paths of axillary lymphatic drainage of the breast. This technique is especially useful in identifying the lymphatic drainage into the parasternal or internal mammary lymph nodes.[37] The lymphatic vessels from the deeper structures of the thoracic wall drain primarily into parasternal, intercostal, or diaphragmatic lymph nodes (see subsequent discussion).

Lymph Nodes of the Thoracic Wall

The lymphatic drainage of the skin and superficial tissues of thoracic and anterior abdominal walls is described in the section on the lymphatic drainage of the breast. Three sets of lymph nodes and associated vessels—parasternal, intercostal, and diaphragmatic—are involved in the lymphatic drainage of the deeper tissues of the thoracic wall:

1. *The parasternal, or internal thoracic, lymph nodes* consist of small lymph nodes located about 1 cm lateral to the sternal border in the intercostal spaces along the internal thoracic, or mammary, vessels (see Figs. 2.2 and 2.7). The parasternal nodes lie in the areolar tissue underlying the endothoracic fascia that borders the space between the adjacent costal cartilages. The distribution of the nodes in the upper six intercostal spaces has been the subject of several studies since Stibbe's report in 1918 of an average total of 8.5 internal mammary nodes per subject, including both sides.[59] Stibbe reported that they usually occurred in the pattern of four on one side and five on the other. Each of the three upper spaces usually contained one lymph node, as did the sixth space. Often there were no lymph nodes in the fourth or fifth space; an extra node usually was found in one of the upper three spaces on one of the sides. Soerensen[60] reported finding an average of seven nodes of minute size per subject in 39 autopsies, with an average of 3.5 on each side. Ju (as reported by Haagensen[27]) studied 100 autopsy subjects and found an average of 6.2 parasternal nodes per subject, with an average of 3.1 per side. A majority was found in the upper three spaces. However, in contradiction to Stibbe's findings, a lower but similar frequency of nodes was seen in all three of the lower intercostal spaces. Putti[61] studied

47 cadavers and found an average of 7.7 nodes per subject—again, with a majority of the nodes in the upper three spaces and many fewer in the lower spaces. Araño and Abraño[62] studied 100 autopsy specimens and found a much higher frequency of lymph nodes than had been previously reported. They found an average total of 16.2 per subject, with an average of 8.9 on the right side and 7.3 on the left. In 56.6% of the subjects, they found retromanubrial nodes between the right and left lymphatic trunks at the level of the first intercostal space. An average of 6.6 nodes were seen when the retromanubrial nodes were present.

2. The *intercostal lymph nodes* consist of small lymph nodes located in the posterior part of the thoracic cavity within the intercostal spaces near the head of the ribs (see Fig. 2.12). One or more may be found in each intercostal space in relationship with the intercostal vessels. These lymph nodes receive the deep lymphatics from the posterolateral thoracic wall, including lymphatic channels from the breast. Occasionally, small lymph nodes occur in the intercostal spaces along the lateral thoracic wall. Efferent lymphatics from the lower four or five intercostal spaces, on both the right and the left sides, join to form a trunk that descends to open into either the cisterna chyli or the initial portion of the thoracic duct. The upper efferent lymphatics from the intercostal nodes on the left side terminate in the thoracic duct; the efferent lymphatics from the corresponding nodes on the right side end in the right lymphatic duct.

3. The *diaphragmatic lymph nodes* consist of three sets of small lymph nodes (anterior, lateral, and posterior) located on the thoracic surface of the diaphragm.

The *anterior group of diaphragmatic lymph nodes* includes two or three small lymph nodes (also known as *prepericardial lymph nodes*) located behind the sternum at the base of the xiphoid process, which receive afferent lymphatics from the convex surface of the liver, and one or two nodes located on each side near the junction of the seventh rib with its costal cartilage, which receive afferents from the anterior aspect of the diaphragm. Afferent lymphatics also reach the prepericardial nodes by accompanying the branches of the superior epigastric blood vessels that pass from the rectus abdominis muscle and through the rectus sheath. Efferent lymphatics from the anterior diaphragmatic nodes pass to the parasternal nodes. This lymphatic channel is a potential route by which metastases from the breast may invade the para-sternal region, with the potential for spread to the liver. As Haagensen[27] suggests, metastasis via this (rectus abdominis muscle) route most likely occurs only when the internal mammary lymphatic trunk is blocked higher in the upper intercostal spaces. When blockage occurs, the flow of lymph may be reversed, and carcinoma emboli from the breast may reach the liver. It is significant to note that the autopsy subjects studied by Handley and Thackray,[55] who demonstrated this route of metastasis, had locally advanced breast carcinoma. Handley and Thackray[55] described the importance of the parasternal lymph nodes in carcinoma of the breast. Clearly, as Haagensen[27] and others have suggested, this route is not of importance in early cancer of the breast unless the primary tumor is located in the extreme lower inner portion of the breast where it overlies the sixth costal cartilage.

The *lateral group of diaphragmatic lymph nodes* consists of two or three small lymph nodes on each side of the diaphragm adjacent to the pericardial sac where the phrenic nerves enter the diaphragm. On the right side, they are located near the vena cava, and on the left side, near the esophageal hiatus. Afferent lymphatic vessels reach these nodes from the middle region of the diaphragm; on the right side, afferent lymphatics from the convex surface of the liver also reach these nodes. Efferent lymphatics from the lateral diaphragmatic nodes may pass to the parasternal nodes via the anterior diaphragmatic nodes, to posterior mediastinal nodes, or to anterior nodes via vessels that follow the course of the phrenic nerve.

The *posterior set of diaphragmatic lymph nodes* consists of a few lymph nodes located adjacent to the crura of the diaphragm. They receive lymph from the posterior aspect of the diaphragm and convey it to posterior mediastinal and lateral aortic nodes.

Lymph Nodes of the Thoracic Cavity

Three sets of nodes are involved in the lymphatic drainage of the thoracic viscera—*anterior mediastinal (brachiocephalic), posterior mediastinal,* and *tracheobronchial.* Although a knowledge of the lymphatic drainage of the thoracic viscera may not be particularly significant in treating carcinoma of the breast, it is important that one understand the system of collecting lymphatic trunks in this region (see Fig. 2.17), and that lymphatic flow converges into the confluence of the internal jugular and subclavian veins.

For better comprehension of the pattern of lymphatic drainage in this region, a brief description of the regions and organs drained by the three thoracic lymph node groups is provided. The anterior mediastinal group consists of six to eight lymph nodes located in the upper anterior part of the mediastinum in front of the brachiocephalic veins and the large arterial trunks

arising from the aorta. These correspond to the retromanubrial nodes as identified by Araño and Abraño.[62] The *anterior mediastinal nodes* receive afferent lymphatics from the thymus, thyroid, pericardium, and lateral diaphragmatic lymph nodes. Their efferent lymphatic vessels join with those from the tracheobronchial nodes to form the *bronchomediastinal trunks.* The *posterior mediastinal group* consists of 8 to 10 nodes located posterior to the pericardium in association with the esophagus and descending thoracic aorta. They receive afferent lymphatics from the esophagus, the posterior portion of the pericardium, the diaphragm, and the convex surface of the liver. Most of their efferent lymphatic vessels join the thoracic duct, but some pass to *tracheobronchial nodes.*

The tracheobronchial group consists of a chain of five subgroups of lymph nodes—tracheal, superior tracheobronchial, inferior tracheobronchial, bronchopulmonary, and pulmonary—located adjacent to the trachea and bronchi, as is indicated by the descriptive names. The bronchopulmonary nodes are found in the hilus of each lung; the pulmonary nodes are found within the substance of the lung in association with the segmental bronchi. The tracheal nodes receive afferent lymphatics from the trachea and upper esophagus. The remaining nodes within this group form a continuous chain with boundaries of lymphatic drainage that are not well defined. The pulmonary and bronchopulmonary nodes receive afferent lymphatic vessels from the lungs and bronchial trees. The inferior and superior tracheobronchial nodes receive afferent lymphatic vessels from the lungs and bronchial

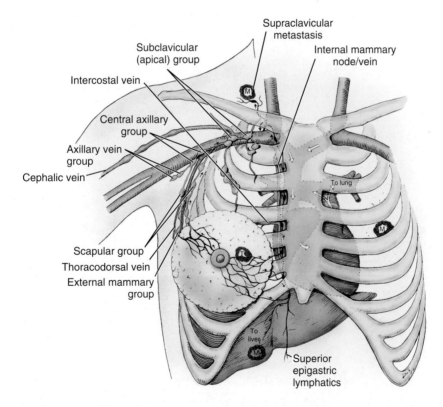

• **Fig. 2.18** Venous drainage of the breast and its relationship to the lymphatics. Lymphatic vessels parallel the course of the three major groups of veins serving the breast and provide routes for metastasis: intercostal, axillary, and internal mammary veins. Visceral metastases to the liver or lungs are possible via vessels providing venous or lymphatic drainage of the breast because these structures communicate with the major venous trunks. (From Copeland EM III, Bland KI. The breast. In: Sabiston DC Jr, ed. *Essentials of Surgery.* Philadelphia: WB Saunders; 1987.)

trees. The inferior and superior tracheobronchial nodes receive nodes; the inferior tracheobronchial nodes also receive some afferent lymphatic vessels from the heart and posterior mediastinal organs. Efferent vessels from the subgroups of the tracheobronchial group pass sequentially to the level of the tracheal nodes. Efferents from the latter unite with efferents from parasternal and anterior mediastinal nodes to form the right and left bronchomediastinal lymphatic trunks. The left trunk may terminate by joining the thoracic duct, and the right trunk may join the right lymphatic duct. However, it is more common for the right and left trunks to open independently into the junction of the internal jugular and subclavian veins, each on their own side (see Fig. 2.17).

Venous Drainage of the Mammary Gland

Lymphatic drainage of the epithelial and mesenchymal components of the breast is the primary route for metastatic dissemination of adenocarcinoma of this organ. However, the vascular route for tumor embolization via venous drainage systems plays a major role in dissemination of neoplasms to the lung, bone, brain, liver, and so forth. The three groups of deep veins that drain the breast (Fig. 2.18) and serve as vascular routes include the following:

1. The *intercostal veins,* which traverse the posterior aspect of the breast from the second to the sixth intercostal spaces and arborize to enter the vertebral veins posteriorly and the azygos vein centrally to terminate in the superior vena cava.

2. The *axillary vein,* which may have variable tributaries that provide segmental drainage of the chest wall, pectoral muscles, and the breast.

3. The *internal mammary vein perforators,* which represent the largest venous plexus to provide drainage of the mammary gland. This venous network traverses the rib interspaces to enter the brachiocephalic (innominate) veins. Thus perforators that drain the parenchyma and epithelial components of the breast allow direct embolization to the pulmonary capillary spaces to establish metastatic disease.[27,34]

Selected References

4. Spratt JS. Anatomy of the breast. *Major Probl Clin Surg.* 1979;5:1-13.
7. Montagu A. Natural selection in the form of the breast in the female. *JAMA.* 1962;180:826-827.
9. Sykes PA. The nerve supply of the human nipple. *J Anat (Lond).* 1969;105:201.
27. Haagensen CD. Anatomy of the mammary glands. In: Haagensen CD, ed. *Diseases of the Breast.* 3rd ed. Philadelphia: WB Saunders; 1986.
49. Veronesi U, Viale G, Paganelli G, et al. Sentinel lymph node biopsy in breast cancer: ten-year results of a randomized controlled study. *Ann Surg.* 2010;251:595-600.
A full reference list is available online at ExpertConsult.com.

3

Breast Physiology: Normal and Abnormal Development and Function

SUSIE X. SUN, ZEYNEP BOSTANCI, RENA B. KASS, ANNE T. MANCINO, ARLAN L. ROSENBLOOM, V. SUZANNE KLIMBERG, AND KIRBY I. BLAND

The mammary gland is composed of an epithelial system of ducts and lobuloalveolar secretory units embedded in a mesenchymally derived fat pad. The growth and morphogenesis of the epithelial structures of the breast occur in various stages and are associated with concurrent hormonal changes and affected by genetic mutations. Each stage reflects the effects of systemic hormones on the glandular epithelium as well as the paracrine effects of locally derived growth factors and other regulatory products produced in the stroma. Appreciating the relationship of epithelium to mesenchyme in normal growth is essential for understanding developmental abnormalities and factors that may lead to disease.

This chapter discusses the morphologic, hormonal, paracrine, and genetic changes of the breast. It also discusses the clinical correlates of the various stages of breast development, including that of the embryo, infancy and childhood, puberty, pregnancy, lactation, and menopause.

Embryology to Childhood

Morphology

The breast of the human newborn is formed through 10 progressive fetal stages that begin in the sixth week of fetal development.[1] During the fifth or sixth week of development, two ventral bands of thickened ectoderm, called the mammary ridges, are present in the embryo. These multilayered epithelial ridges, named the milk lines, extend from the axilla to the groin and give rise to a single pair of placodes (cluster of primitive mammary epithelial cells) in humans over the thorax.[2,3] (Fig. 3.1). After this, the ectoderm invaginates into the surrounding mesenchyme and enters the cluster of preadipocytes that become the mammary fat pad, with subsequent epithelial budding and branching forming a rudimentary ductal tree.[4] During the latter part of pregnancy, this fetal epithelium further canalizes and ultimately differentiates to the end-vesicle stage seen in the newborn.[1] If the structure fails to undergo its normal regression, accessory nipples (polythelia) or accessory mammary glands (polymastia) may occur along the original mammary ridges or milk lines (Fig. 3.2).

Each gland develops as the ingrowth of the ectoderm forms a primary bud of tissue in the underlying mesenchyme (Fig. 3.3A). Each primary bud gives rise to 15 to 20 secondary buds, or outgrowths (Fig. 3.3B). During the fetal period, epithelial cords develop from the secondary buds and extend into the surrounding connective tissue. By the end of prenatal life, lumens have developed in the outgrowths, forming the lactiferous ducts and their branches (Fig. 3.3C). At birth, the lactiferous ducts open into a shallow epithelial depression, known as the mammary pit. The pit becomes elevated and transformed into the nipple shortly after birth as a result of proliferation of the mesenchyme underlying the presumptive nipple and areola (Fig. 3.3D). Failure of elevation of the pit results in a congenital malformation known as inverted nipple.

In a term birth, the breast has six to eight widely patent ducts that empty at the nipple. Recent anatomic studies confirm a parallel bundle of an additional 25 smaller ducts with distinct openings at the nipple surface.[5] All of these initial ducts contain one layer of epithelium and one layer of myoepithelial cells, terminating in a dilated blind sac. These so-called ductules are the precursors of future lobuloalveolar structures, the ultimate milk-producing units of the breast. Interestingly, despite the large number of actual ducts that drain onto the nipple, one-fourth of the breast is drained by one duct and its branches, and one-half of the breast is drained by only three ducts.[5] Similar to the development of the ductal system, the subareolar lymphatic plexus also develops from the ectoderm.[6]

From birth until 2 years of age, there is wide individual variability in the morphologic and functional stages in the breast, with some neonates having more well-developed lobular structures and others with more secretory epithelial phenotypes.[7] The degree of morphologic differentiation does not correlate with functional ability. The ability of the entire ductal structure to respond to secretory stimuli may even occur in the rudimentary ductal systems.[7] Ultimately, in normal infant development, the differentiated glandular structures involute and only small ductal structures are left remaining within the stroma.[8]

During childhood, the ductal structures and stroma grow isometrically at a rate similar to that of the rest of the body until puberty.[7,9] The lymphatics grow simultaneously with the duct system, maintaining connection with the subareolar plexus.[6] As in the fetal stage, there are no morphologic differences between the sexes.[7]

Hormones

The initial fetal stages of breast development are relatively independent of sex steroid influence. At birth the withdrawal of

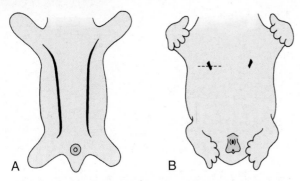

• **Fig. 3.1** The mammary ridges and their regression. (A) Ventral view of an embryo at the beginning of the fifth week of development (about 28 days), showing the mammary ridges that extend from the forelimb to the hind limb. (B) A similar view of the ventral embryo at the end of the sixth week, showing the remains of the ridges located in the pectoral region.

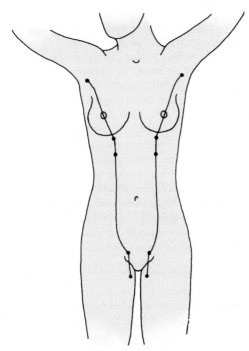

• **Fig. 3.2** Mammary milk line. After development of the milk bud in the pectoral area of ectodermal thickening, the "milk streak" extends from the axilla to the inguinal areas. At week 9 of intrauterine development, atrophy of the bud has occurred except for the presence of the supernumerary nipples or breast.

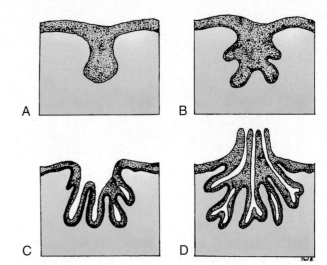

• **Fig. 3.3** Sections through evolutionary development and growth of the mammary bud. (A–C) Similar sections showing the developing gland at successive stages between the 12th week and birth. The mammary pit develops, and major lactiferous ducts are present at the end of gestation. (D) A similar section showing the elevation of the mammary pit by proliferation of the underlying connective tissue forming the nipple soon after birth.

maternal steroids results in secretion of neonatal prolactin (PRL) that stimulates newborn breast secretion.

Regulatory Factors and Potential Genes

It is currently accepted that epithelial ductal proliferation into the mesenchyme is modulated by local factors, which regulate the epithelial-mesenchymal interaction. Many genes have been expressed in either the epithelium or mesenchyme during mammary embryogenesis, including fibroblast growth factor-7 (FGF-7),[10] FGF,[11] HOX,[12,13] tenascin-C,[14] syndecan-1, hedgehog network genes,[15,16] t-box family of transcription factors,[17] androgen receptor,[18] estrogen receptor,[16] transforming growth factor-α (TGF-α), TGF-β,[19] BCL-2,[7] and epidermal growth factor (EGF)

receptor.[5] Mammary epithelial cell line differentiation or milk line specification occurs under the influence of embryonic mammary mesenchyme.[2] For example, NRG3 (a ligand for the receptor tyrosine kinase ERBB4/HER4) appears to be involved in milk line specification by functioning as a mesenchymal paracrine signal and may have roles in mammary epithelial lineage commitment and promoting placode formation.[3] Wnt signaling emanating from the mesenchyme is also necessary for initiating mammary line specification. Formation of placodes occurs subsequently and is regulated by TBX3 (T-box transcription factor), and BMP4 (bone morphogenic protein 4) expression.[2] In addition Lef-1,[20] parathyroid hormone–related protein (PTHrP),[21] and the type 1 parathyroid hormone (PTH)/PTHrP receptor (PTHR-1) are also required for mammary branching and nipple development.

Clinical Correlates

In the human embryo, the mammary ridge first becomes apparent in the 7- to 8-mm-long embryo and atrophies before birth. It is the persistence of mammalian tissue along the milk line that results in ectopically displaced or accessory breast tissue (see Figs. 3.1 and 3.2). This congenital anomaly is commonly bilateral and is often unaccompanied by the areola or the nipple (Fig. 3.4). A classification system to characterize accessory breast tissue was developed in 1915 that is still used: (1) the presence of a complete breast with mammary gland tissue and the nipple-areola complex, (2) the presence of gland tissue and nipple, (3) gland tissue and areola, (4) solitary gland tissue, (5) nipple-areola with fat replacement of the mammary gland tissue (pseudomamma), (6) the nipple alone (polythelia), (7) the areola alone (polythelia areolaris), and (8) the presence of a small patch of hair-bearing tissue (polythelia pilosa).[22]

Polythelia

Polythelia represents the most common variant of supernumerary breast components and occurs predominantly between the breast

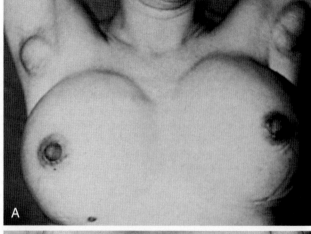

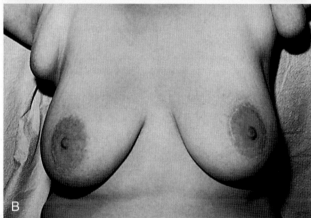

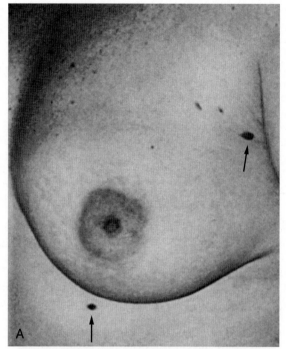

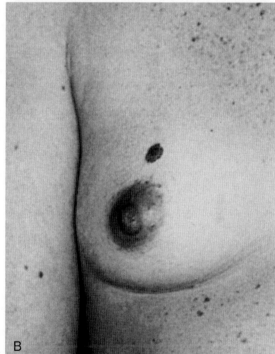

• **Fig. 3.4** (A) and (B) Supernumerary breasts presenting as accessory (ectopic) breast tissue bilaterally in the axilla. Note right supernumerary inframammary nipple presenting in the mammary milk line (A). ([A] From Greer KE. Accessory axillary breast tissue. *Arch Dermatol.* 1974;109:88-89. Copyright © 1974, American Medical Association. All rights reserved. [B] Courtesy Dr. Michael M. Meguid, SUNY Health Sciences Center, Syracuse, NY.)

and the umbilicus.[23] However, glandular tissue compatible with complete or variable components of breast parenchyma can occur within the mammary ridge at sites between the axilla and the groin. The embryology, clinical presentation, diagnosis, treatment, and clinical significance of supernumerary nipples, supernumerary breasts, and ectopic breast tissue have been reviewed and important considerations concerning these common anomalies include the following:[24]

• Supernumerary nipples, supernumerary breasts, and ectopic breast tissue most commonly develop along the milk lines.
• Whereas polythelia is evident at birth, supernumerary and ectopic breast tissue is evident only after hormonal stimulation that occurs at puberty or during pregnancy.
• Ectopic breast tissue is subject to the same pathologic changes that occur in normally positioned breasts.
• Axillary ectopic breast tissue may be confused with other malignant and benign lesions occurring in the area.
• Polythelia may indicate associated conditions, most notably urologic malformations or urogenital malignancies.

The presence of supernumerary or accessory nipples (Fig. 3.5) is a relatively common, minor congenital anomaly that occurs in

• **Fig. 3.5** Supernumerary nipple. (A) A 38-year-old woman with supernumerary nipples *(arrows)* above (in axilla) and below the normal left breast in the mammary milk line. (B) Supernumerary nipple and areolar complex (rudimentary) in upper right breast of a 22-year-old woman. Excisional biopsy was the preferred treatment.

both sexes, with an estimated frequency of 1 in 100 to 1 in 500 persons.[25] The frequency of supernumerary nipples as 0.22% in a white European population, which is significantly lower than the incidence of 1.63% found in African American neonates.[26,27] In the newborn Jewish population, the higher incidence of 2.5% for polythelia was observed.[28] This high frequency of supernumerary nipples could possibly be related to ethnic differences but may be related to a systematic technique for examination of the newborn.

Congenital supernumerary nipples may occur in any size or configuration along the mammary milk line extending from the nipple to the symphysis pubis. As noted earlier, the supernumerary nipple anomaly may be easily overlooked in young infants, in whom these ectopic lesions often appear only as a small spot with a diameter of 2 to 3 mm. Supernumerary nipples usually develop just below the normal breast in the white population, with less common occurrence in abdominal or inguinal sites.[29,30] Bilateral supernumerary nipples occur in approximately half of patients with polythelia.[31] In the ectopic sites, polythelia takes origin from the extramammary buds that are present along the ventral embryonic mammary ridges (see Fig. 3.3). Only a minority of persons with this clinical anomaly have more than two extra nipples.[29]

Polythelia should be searched for in the routine physical examination of every newborn, and the presence of the condition should be reported to the parents. This is important for the following reasons[28]:

- Supernumerary breasts in females may respond to fluctuations in hormones in a physiologic manner such that pubertal enlargement, premenstrual swelling, tenderness, and lactation during pregnancy and parturition may occur.
- Patients with polythelia may be subject to the same spectrum of pathologic diseases observed in normal breasts (e.g., neoplasms, fibroadenomas, papillary adenomas, cysts, or carcinomas).[32–35]
- The supernumerary nipples may be associated with other congenital diseases such as vertebral anomalies,[36–37] cardiac arrhythmias, or renal anomalies.[32,38–43]

In embryogenesis, polythelia occurs during the third month of gestation, when the embryonic mammary ridge fails to regress normally—an event coincident with the development of the urogenital and other organ systems. Although various malformations have been associated with polythelia (Table 3.1), attention has been drawn to the high incidence of renal anomalies and malignancies in children with supernumerary nipples.[44] The association between supernumerary nipples and occult anomalies of the urogenital system has been reported in at least two non–US pediatric populations. Studies from Hungary and Israel have reported that 23% and 40%, respectively, of children with polythelia had obstructive renal abnormalities or duplications of the excretory system.[45,46] Studies in Hungarian children have shown no link between polythelia and renal anomalies. Studies have cited the prevalence of supernumerary nipples to be 4.29% among healthy newborns and 5.86% among healthy schoolchildren.[47] Ultrasound was used to examine the urogenital system of 496 children with supernumerary nipples and 2367 control patients. The prevalence of renal anomalies was 3.74% in children with supernumerary nipples and 3.17% in the control group; 2.86% in newborns with supernumerary nipples and 1.89% in control newborns. The differences were not statistically significant. The association of polythelia with urogenital malformations continues to be controversial. Recommendations vary from no screening to the screening of all children with polythelia. The true association of these two entities likely has not been elucidated completely.[48,49]

Polythelia has also been associated with cancers of the testis and kidney.[26,50–52] Familial as well as sporadic occurrences of polythelia with renal cancer, urogenital anomalies, and germ cell tumors have been reported.[37,52–54] The authors suggest that this may represent a genetic or developmental link between renal adenocarcinoma and polythelia.

Intraareolar polythelia represents a nipple-areola unit within the mammary ridge such that a dichotomy of the vestigial breast and nipple-areola complex exists. Only a few cases of bilateral intraareolar polythelia have been recorded. Multiplicity of nipples is not uncommon, and they are bilateral in approximately half of patients so affected. As many as 10 nipples have been recorded in a single patient.[55] Atypical locations have been noted secondary to the displaced embryonal primordium.[56]

The presence of supernumerary nipples may necessitate operative therapy in instances in which discharge, tumor, or cyst formation is evident. Simple elliptical excision placed in lines of cleavage or skin folds is preferred to achieve maximum cosmesis. Primary closure is usually possible and allows the surgeon to achieve a superior cosmetic result.

Polymastia

Polymastia also results from the embryonic mammary ridge (see Fig. 3.1A) failing to undergo normal regression (see Fig. 3.1B). Causal factors are as yet unknown. The prevalence of polymastia was 0.1% in the Collaborative Perinatal Project, although another study suggested a frequency approaching 1%.[57,58] Similar to polythelia, reports on polymastia suggest an association between renal adenocarcinoma and renal malformations.[44,59]

A familial occurrence of the polymastia anomaly has been observed.[58,60] The association of polymastia with congenital cytogenetic syndromes, especially those involved with chromosomes 3 and 8 has been reported.[61] Furthermore, other congenital anomalies, notably Turner syndrome (ovarian agenesis and dysgenesis with chromosomal karyotypes of 45,X, but mosaic patterns [45,X/46,XX or 45,X/46,XX/47, XXX] are seen) and Fleisher syndrome (lateral displacement of the nipples to the midclavicular lines with bilateral renal hypoplasia[62]) may include polymastia as a component (Fig. 3.6).

A 1995 case presentation and review of the literature regarding carcinoma of ectopic breast tissue reported that of a total of 90 cases of carcinoma of ectopic breast tissue, 64 occurred in the axilla.[63] The combined survival beyond the 4-year posttreatment

TABLE 3.1	**Polythelia and Associated Conditions**	
Urinary Tract Abnormalities	**Cardiac Abnormalities**	**Miscellaneous Abnormalities**
Renal agenesis	Cardiac conduction disturbances, especially left bundle branch block	Pyloric stenosis
Renal cell carcinoma		Epilepsy
Obstructive disease		Ear abnormalities
Supernumerary kidney(s)	Hypertension Congenital heart anomalies	Arthrogryposis multiplex congenita

From Pellegrini JR, Wagner RF Jr. Polythelia and associated conditions. *Am Fam Physician.* 1983;28:129-132.

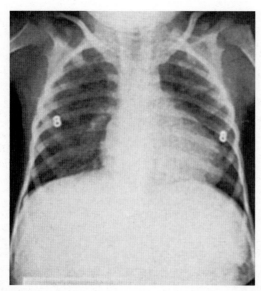

• **Fig. 3.6** Fleisher syndrome. Posteroanterior chest roentgenogram of a 5-year-old with bilateral renal hypoplasia. Although the clavicles are not horizontal, the lateral displacement of the nipples (designated by the lead markers 8) is apparent. (From Fleisher DS. Lateral displacement of the nipples, a sign of bilateral renal hypoplasia. *J Pediatr.* 1966;69:806-809.)

period was 9.4%. No survival advantage was found for radical or modified radical mastectomy over local excision combined with axillary dissection or radiation. The researchers found that the correct preoperative diagnosis was rarely made, and they suggested that improved prognosis requires diagnostic suspicion and early biopsy of suspicious ectopic masses that occur along the embryonic milk lines. In related studies, fine-needle biopsy has been found to be useful in the diagnosis and management of ectopic breast tissue.[55,64,65]

Accessory (Ectopic) Axillary Breast Tissue

Ectopic axillary breast tissue is a relatively uncommon occurrence but is a relatively common variant of polymastia.[66] The presence of accessory axillary breast tissue most commonly becomes apparent at or after puberty, with the most rapid growth observed during pregnancy.[23] It has been suggested that axillary breast tissue may represent true ectopic tissue not contiguous with the breast but more commonly represents an enlargement of the axillary tail of Spence.[67] Thus to determine the presence or absence of accessory axillary breast tissue, one must distinguish between an enlargement of the axillary tail and ectopically displaced mammary tissues of the milk line. The occurrence of ectopic breast tissue *outside the axilla* is exceedingly rare, although a hamartoma of ectopic breast tissue in the inguinal region has been reported.[68,69] The finding, confirmed with histopathologic examination, occurred in a 50-year-old woman suspected of having a chronic incarcerated hernia.

The discovery of accessory axillary breast tissue usually occurs during the first pregnancy as a consequence of the secondary changes initiated with hormonal stimulation by ovarian estradiol and placental estriol. The symptomatic axillary breast tissue becomes painfully enlarged and, on rare occasion, may develop galactoceles with milk secretion via contiguous skin pores.[70] Although these anomalies may not become evident until the first pregnancy, once the lesions are recognized, they continue to recur

with subsequent pregnancies and may undergo cyclical changes during menstruation. Often, the clinician identifies the lesion as excess axillary fat, although lymphadenitis, lymphoma, metastatic carcinoma, and hidradenitis suppurativa are common misdiagnoses. After identification of the hormonal dependency with pregnancy or menstruation, the clinician can often establish the diagnosis, especially if a history of lactation during the puerperium is confirmed.

Management consists of reassuring the patient of its common benignity and its embryologic origin. However, accessory axillary tissue may be misdiagnosed as the symptomatic alterations inherent with pathologic changes of breast tissue (e.g., carcinoma and the benign breast tissue spectrum). Treatment of symptomatic accessory breast tissue during the puerperium and pregnancy involves conservative management for most clinical presentations. The presence of dense, nodular masses suggestive of malignant transformation necessitates aggressive approaches to rule out carcinoma.[71] As this hormonally dependent accessory breast tissue rapidly regresses when lactation ceases, the patient can be reassured but should be admonished that enlargement and painful, lactating, accessory tissue may recur with subsequent pregnancy. Elliptically placed incisions in skin folds of the axilla allow complete dissection and removal of the breast tissue beneath the skin and over the underlying fascia. The cosmetically oriented resections of the accessory tissue are usually curative, although the lesion may recur if excision is incomplete.

Amastia

The congenital absence of one or both breasts (amastia) is a rare clinical anomaly.[72] Unilateral absence of the breast (Fig. 3.7) is more common than bilateral amastia, and such subjects are most commonly female. This rare physical defect occurs as a result of complete failure of the development of the mammary ridge at about the sixth week in utero. Most often, abnormalities are not associated with bilateral absence of nipple and breast tissue. However, association with cleft palate; hypertelorism and saddle nose; and anomalies of the pectoral muscle, ulna, hand, foot, palate, ears, genitourinary tract, and habitus have been observed.[73] Occasionally, several members of a family may be affected. At least four reports[73–76] document the transmission of this anomaly with pedigree penetrance consistent with dominant inheritance. For example, mutations in TBX3 result in autosomal dominant *ulnarmammary syndrome,* characterized by malformation of upper limb structures, apocrine/mammary hypoplasia and/or dysfunction, dental abnormalities and genital abnormalities. Apocrine abnormalities may be as significant as complete absence of breasts (amastia).[17]

Poland Syndrome

Poland syndrome is characterized by unilateral congenital absence of the pectoralis major and minor muscles, associated absence of the external oblique and partial absence of the serratus anterior. Additionally, hypoplasia or complete absence of the breast or nipple, costal cartilage and rib defects, hypoplasia of subcutaneous tissue of the chest wall, and brachysyndactyly may also be observed. Poland syndrome is rare with incidence estimated to be 1:20,000 to 1:50,000. The etiology of this malformation is unknown but believed to be related to improper development of the subclavian axis with a resulting impedance of blood flow to the affected structures.[77,78]

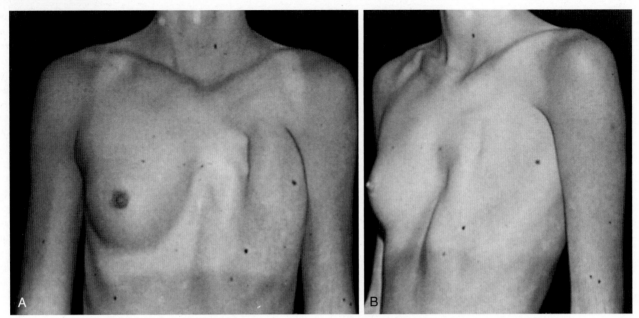

• **Fig. 3.7** (A) and (B) Unilateral amastia in 20-year-old woman with concomitant chest wall deformity of ipsilateral ribs 3 to 6 and cartilage. In contrast to those with Poland syndrome, this patient has accessory musculature of the shoulder, including pectoralis major and minor, latissimus dorsi, and serratus anterior muscles. (Courtesy Dr. John McCraw, Norfolk, VA.)

Clinical manifestations of Poland syndrome are extremely variable, and rarely can all features be recognized in a single individual.[79-82] At least two reports confirm a variant of the disorder associated with large melanotic spots. Because breasts and melanocytes both originate from the ectoderm, abnormalities of breast hypoplasia and hyperpigmentation probably develop from within this germinal layer. Patients often do not request treatment of the pigmented abnormalities, and standard methods used in the therapy of hyperpigmentation often yield unsatisfactory results. Such hyperpigmented areas appear to have no neoplastic risk.

Poland syndrome is invariably unilateral, with a higher incidence in female than in male patients. When a chest wall defect (ribs, cartilage, or both) is evident, there is usually a deep concavity on expiration and lung herniation with inspiration (see Fig. 3.7). The right side is more commonly affected than the left.[83] The most common defect, breast hypoplasia, is readily recognized, and the rudimentary breast tissue is usually higher on the involved side and medially displaced from its normal anatomic position.

Although the cause is unclear, this syndrome is seldom familial. Despite hypoplastic breast tissue, several cases of breast cancer have been documented on the side affected by Poland syndrome. Standard techniques for sentinel lymph node biopsy can be used in these patients even though they have altered anatomy.[77,84] Leukemia has been associated with the syndrome, as have other rare congenital anomalies. Similar defects have been noted with exposure to drugs, such as thalidomide.

Treatment of patients with Poland syndrome varies with the number of anomalies and their physical expression. With the presentation of one or two typical characteristics of Poland syndrome, patients usually complain only about their appearance. These patients are not functionally embarrassed by their lack of anterior chest wall muscle mass or the small size of their breast. Only in extreme cases, as with total absence of the costal cartilage or segments of the anterior ribs, are patients physically impaired and emotionally disturbed by their deformity. Indications for operative intervention include progression of chest depression, lack of protection of the heart and lung, and paradoxical chest wall movement.[85] Surgery may also be needed for cosmetic reconstruction of the breast or chest wall musculature. Surgical procedures to correct the deformities of the chest wall have been documented and include (1) subperiosteal grafts from adjacent ribs with free flaps of latissimus dorsi or external oblique, (2) autologous split-rib grafts, (3) split-rib grafts with periosteum that has been detached posteriorly and rotated from the anterior aspect of the defective rib to the sternum, (4) heterologous bone grafts, (5) metallic mesh implants followed by rib grafts from the opposite chest wall, and (6) customized silicone breast and chest wall prostheses to reconstruct both structures in difficult cases.[82,86–91] In the 1970s, the use of split-rib grafts from the opposite chest wall that are placed across the defect and reinforced with Teflon felt was popularized.[92] Another technique used autologous tissue of the latissimus dorsi myocutaneous flap to augment the hypoplastic breast and to contour the anterior chest wall while simultaneously augmenting the involved hypoplastic breast.[93] When this procedure was initially attempted using free latissimus dorsi flaps, it was unsuccessful because the transplanted muscle atrophied as a result of the omission of the neurovascular pedicle from the transplant, emphasizing the value of preservation of the pedicle when employing this technique.[86] In 1950, the use of a latissimus dorsi muscle flap transferred through the axilla for anterior chest wall reconstruction with preservation of the neurovascular bundle was described.[94] This, too, was abandoned.

The value of a single-stage reconstruction has since been emphasized.[95] The high success rate and the reliability of this technique, which uses the latissimus dorsi myocutaneous flap, represents remarkable advance over the aforementioned methods. Latissimus dorsi myocutaneous flaps continue to be the most commonly used flap for breast and chest wall reconstruction in patients with Poland disease. This procedure is now being performed with an endoscopic approach for flap harvest and reconstruction. Additionally, tissue expanders followed by replacement with permanent prosthetic implants is a technique commonly employed for these patients.[96–98]

Computed tomography (CT) provides useful information in planning reconstructive surgery in patients with Poland syndrome.[99] A three-dimensional CT scan may be used as an adjunct for planning chest wall and breast reconstruction in Poland syndrome.[100] Follow-up with three-dimensional magnetic resonance imaging (MRI) reformation is valuable to demonstrate the results of the implant reconstruction. The authors suggest that these imaging techniques can be used to accurately portray the three-dimensional tissue deficit and assist in the selection of muscle transposition flaps and reconstructive technique.

Newborn Nipple Discharge

As previously described, PRL stimulates newborn breast secretion. This secretion, called *witch's milk,* contains water, fat, and debris; it occurs in 80% to 90% of infants, regardless of sex.[101,102] The secretion dissipates within 3 to 4 weeks as the influence of maternal sex hormones and PRL decreases. It should not be mechanically expressed, which could predispose to staphylococcal infection and result in breast bud destruction. The secretion may sequester at the nipple epithelium and resemble a pearl. This is called a lactocele and will resolve with time.[102]

Premature Thelarche

Premature thelarche is breast development before 8 years of age without concomitant signs of puberty. Usually bilateral, it is most commonly seen within the first 2 years of life. It is believed to be the result of the persistence or increase in the breast tissue present at birth, and it resolves within 3 to 5 years with no adverse sequelae.[103] It has been suggested that although the initial stimulation of the infant breast may be secondary to maternal influences, the persistence of breast tissue may be related to infant hormones that may support breast growth. Persistent elevations of follicle-stimulating hormone (FSH), luteinizing hormone (LH), and estradiol in infants support this hypothesis (Fig. 3.8).[104]

A second period of premature thelarche may occur after 6 years of age.[105] The reason for breast bud formation is unclear; because it can occur before the rise in estrogen levels, it is unlikely that estrogen is the key signal. Serum androgen levels,[106] free estrogen level,[107] altered FSH secretion,[108] and altered serum insulin-like growth factor-I (IGF-I)–to–IGF-binding protein-3 ratios have been implicated as potential factors.[109] The breast tissue may persist or regress, but puberty occurs at the usual time and progresses normally. If assessment of bone age reveals no evidence of precocious puberty, no further evaluation is needed.[105]

Precocious Puberty

Breast development before 8 years of age that is accompanied by other signs of puberty defines precocious puberty. Altered or premature gonadotropin-releasing hormone (GnRH) secretion may cause central precocious puberty (Fig. 3.9). Although more commonly idiopathic, central precocious puberty can be caused by cerebral infections and granulomatous conditions. Certain tumors, in particular hypothalamic hamartomas, can contain GnRH and disrupt the inhibition of GnRH, or release TGF-α (a stimulant of GnRH), resulting in precocious puberty. Peripheral precocious puberty may result from the effects of estrogen from food,[110] from ovarian cysts, from constitutionally activated ovaries in McCune-Albright syndrome (a triad of café-au-lait spots, long-bone fibrous dysplasia, and precocious puberty), or in primary hypothyroidism (Fig. 3.10).[102] In addition to a history and physical examination, serum gonadotropin and sex steroid levels should be obtained in the workup of precocious puberty. High levels of both gonadotropins and sex steroids indicate central precocious puberty. MRI or CT scanning of the head can be performed to rule out a central lesion before treatment with

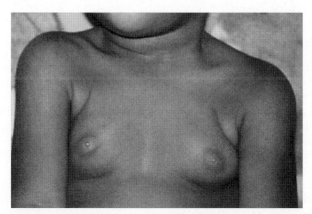

• **Fig. 3.8** Premature thelarche. Fourteen-month-old child with breast development from birth. Height was at the 50th percentile without acceleration, and no other signs of sexual maturation were present. Breast development was considered Tanner stage 3 without nipple maturation. There had been some regression over the several months before this picture was taken.

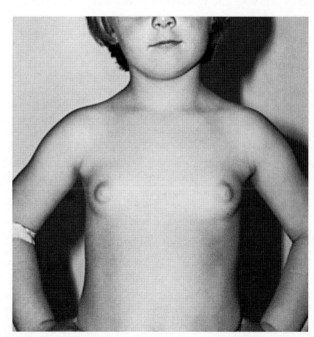

• **Fig. 3.9** Three-and-a-half-year-old girl with central precocious puberty (adolescent levels of gonadotropins and estrogen). Breast development had been present for only a few months but included nipple maturation. Facial maturation was that of a 5- to 6-year-old child. Height age was 4½ years, and osseous maturation was 5 years, 9 months.

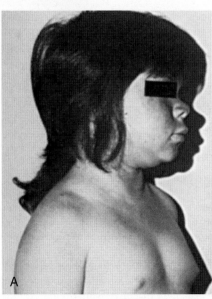
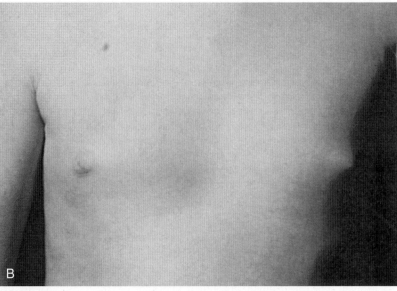

• **Fig. 3.10** (A) Thirteen-year-old girl with acquired hypothyroidism of approximately 5 years' duration, with Tanner stage 2 breast development despite osseous maturation of 8 years and comparable height age. (B) Regression of breast development occurred within months of treatment with thyroid hormone. (Courtesy Dr. A. Rosenbloom, Division of Pediatric Endocrinology, University of Florida, Gainesville, FL.)

GnRH analogs. Suppressed (low) levels of gonadotropins and high levels of sex steroids are consistent with peripheral precocious puberty.[111]

Exposure to toxins early in life may increase the mammary glands' susceptibility to future carcinogenic exposure as well as have direct carcinogenic effects.[112] For example, diethylstilbestrol (DES), a synthetic estrogen used to prevent miscarriage from the 1940s through 1970s, has been associated with breast cancer in women who were directly exposed as well as their daughters.[113,114]

Puberty

Morphology

Thelarche, the beginning of adult breast development, marks the onset of puberty in the majority of white women and occurs at a mean age of 10 years; in African American women, it occurs at 8.9 years and is usually preceded by the appearance of pubic hair.[115] Changes in the breast contour and events in nipple development characterize the milestones in the staging system detailed by Tanner[116] (Fig. 3.11). However, these outward changes in the breast do not necessarily correlate with underlying structural events occurring with the new hormonal milieu of puberty.

The immature ductal system before puberty is believed to undergo a sequential progression to a mature lobuloalveolar system during adolescent development (Fig. 3.12). In the *ductal growth phase,* ducts elongate, ductal epithelium thickens, and periductal connective tissue increases forming an extensive mammary tree. Lateral branches lead to terminal ducts ending with terminal ductal lobular units (TDLUs).[7] These units comprise numerous acini (ductules) embedded in fibroblastic stroma.[2] Mammary gland stroma includes vascular supply, lymphatic drainage, immune barrier, adipose-rich fat pad, and an extracellular matrix working together to promote mammary epithelial cell growth, differentiation, and regression during branching morphogenesis.[117]

In early puberty, the TDLU is termed a *virginal lobule or lobule type 1* (Lob 1).[118] Lob 1 is the predominant lobule found at this stage of development. Under the cyclic influence of ovarian hormones, some of the Lob 1 will undergo further division and differentiate into a lobule type 2 (Lob 2). In Lob 2 the alveolar buds become smaller but four times more numerous than those in Lob 1; these buds are termed *ductules* or *alveoli.* Lob 2 are present in moderate numbers during the late teens but then decline after the mid-20s.[119] Ultimately, the greatest number of lobules will be found in the upper outer quadrant.[120,121]

In the mature breast, the subareolar lymphatic plexus contains communications with both deep and superficial intramammary lymphatics and provides a high volume of lymphatic outflow to regional lymph nodes. In lymphatic studies, there appears to be a consistent channel that originates from the subareolar plexus and extends to the regional lymph nodes, termed the *sentinel lymphatic channel.*[4]

Hormones

The pattern of release of GnRH from the hypothalamus initiates and regulates the secretion of FSH and LH seen with puberty. The initial immaturity of the hypothalamic-pituitary axis results in anovulatory cycles for the first 1 to 2 years after menses begins, subjecting the breast and the endometrium to the effects of unopposed estrogen. It is during this period of unopposed estrogen stimulation, considered an "estrogen window,"[122] that the *ductal growth phase* occurs (see Fig. 3.11).

The major hormonal influence on the breast at the onset of puberty is estrogen. A potent mammogen, estrogen primarily stimulates ductal growth but also increases fat deposition and contributes to later phases of development. Impaired ductal growth has been demonstrated in both mice lacking the functional gene for the estrogen receptor and mice treated with tamoxifen, an estrogen receptor modulator.[123] The estrogen receptor ERα is thought to be the key mediator of estrogen effects, and

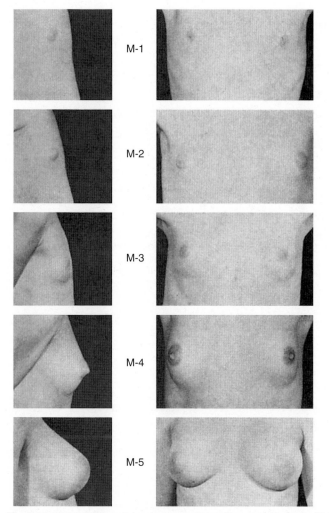

M-1

M-2

M-3

M-4

M-5

• **Fig. 3.11** Stages of breast development. Stage 1 is preadolescent, with slight elevation of the papilla. In stage 2, there is elevation of the breast and papilla as a small mound, with an increase in size of the areola. Stage 3 is characterized by further enlargement of the breast. In stage 4, the areola and papilla form a secondary mound above the level of the breast. In stage 5, the areola recedes into the general contour of the breast. (From van Wieringen JD et al. Growth diagrams 1965 Netherlands, Second National Survey on 0–24 year olds. Netherlands Institute for Preventive Medicine TNO. Groningen, Netherlands: Wolters-Noordoff; 1971.)

has only been documented in luminal epithelium in humans.[124] Despite its influential role, estrogen is unable to work independently. Lyon's classic experiments using oophorectomized, adrenalectomized, and hypophysectomized rodents demonstrated that a minimum combination of estrogen, growth hormone (GH), and corticoids are necessary to induce ductal growth.[125]

The effects of GH may be mediated by enhancing stromal secretion of IGF-I. IGF-I synergizes with estrogen to increase elongation and growth at the terminal end bud (TEB)[126] in a paracrine manner. In some reviews, glucocorticoids contribute to the maximal growth of ducts, but extensive ductal growth can occur in its absence.[127] Progesterone does not appear to be necessary in early ductal growth but appears to be essential for lobuloalveolar development.[128-130] The ratio of the progesterone receptor (PR) isoforms PGR-A and PGR-B may play a critical role in modulating the effect of progesterone.[129,130] PRL, GH,

estrogen, and glucocorticoids, in addition to progesterone, have been found to be necessary for full lobuloalveolar development.[125]

PRL-deficient knockout mice with adequate progesterone levels exhibited incomplete lobule formation.[131] PRL also works indirectly by facilitating progesterone's actions on the breast. PRL increases progesterone secretion from the corpus luteum by inhibiting progesterone's degradation enzyme, 20α-hydroxysteroid dehydrogenase.[132] In addition, PRL upregulates the PR in the mammary epithelium.[133] Estrogen contributes to lobuloalveolar development by upregulating PRs.[134] Insulin can bind to IGF-I receptors and may contribute to ductal or lobuloalveolar development, but it is not essential.[127,135,136]

Menstrual Cycle

During the human menstrual cycle the breast progresses through five histologic phases: *early follicular, follicular, luteal, secretory,* and ultimately the *menstrual phase,* according to the characterizations of Vogel and colleagues[137] (Fig. 3.13). Estrogen rises throughout the first half of the menstrual cycle and peaks at midcycle. After the LH surge, ovulation occurs with subsequent production of progesterone by the corpus luteum in the latter half of the menstrual cycle.

The *early follicular phase* occurs from day 3 to day 7 in a 28-day cycle. The alveoli are compact, with poorly defined lumina, and sit within a dense stroma. There appears to be only one epithelial cell type at this point. According to some, minimum volume is seen 5 to 7 days after menses.[138] However, a pilot study using MRI demonstrated the minimum volume to occur at day 11.[139] The *follicular phase* follows from day 8 through day 14 and marks the progression of epithelial stratification into three cell types: the luminal cell, basal myoepithelial cell, and an intermediate cell. *Ovulation* initiates the *luteal phase,* which lasts from day 15 to day 29. The precise mechanism that initiates ovulation is unclear, but it is postulated to be a combination of critical estrogen levels from the ovaries and alterations in FSH, LH, and gonadotropin levels.[140] In luteal phase progesterone is secreted from the corpus luteum that exposes the breast to the complete cyclic hormonal milieu of adulthood and facilitates the second phase of glandular growth, which is termed *lobuloalveolar growth* and characterized by an overall increase in the size of the lobules resulting from alveoli luminal expansion with secretory products, an increase in the number of alveoli, ballooning of the myoepithelial cells with increased glycogen content, and stromal loosening. The maximum size of the lobules and number of alveoli within each lobule is reached in the *secretory phase,* from day 21 to day 27. This is consistent with MRI breast-volume data.[139] During this phase, there is active protein synthesis and apocrine secretion from the luminal epithelial cells. Peak mitotic activity occurs near day 22 to 24, after the progesterone peak and second estrogen peak.[141,142] The *menstrual phase* occurs on days 28 through 32 and is associated with the withdrawal of estrogen and progesterone. Apocrine secretion lessens and the lobules decrease in size, with fewer alveoli. Russo and Russo suggest that each menstrual cycle fosters new budding that never fully returns to the baseline of the previous cycle. This positive proliferation continues until the mid-30s and plateaus until menopause, when regression is evident.[119]

A more recent meta-analysis of studies of mammary gland changes during the menstrual cycle reflects a trend of peak physiologic and histologic changes that chronologically follow the peak in progesterone. These changes include a peak in mitosis within 24 hours of the progesterone peak and estimated peaks of

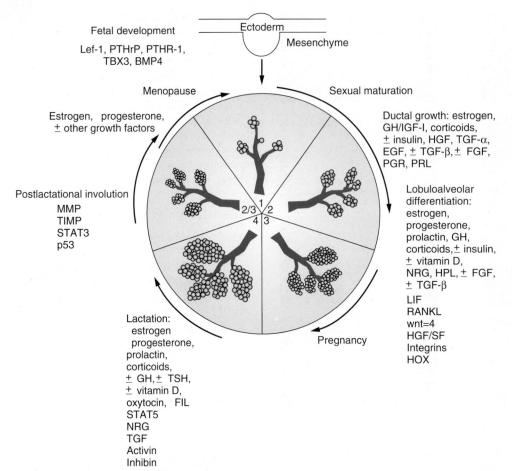

• **Fig. 3.12** Regulatory influences on breast development. Numbers (1, 2, 3, etc.) correspond to lobule type (1, 2, 3, etc.). Ectoderm invaginates into mesenchyme during fetal development. Sexual maturation begins with the onset of puberty through periods of ductal and lobuloalveolar growth and is reflected in the formation of lobules type 1 and 2. Pregnancy initiates the formation of lobule type 3. Lactation, which follows, is associated with lobule type 4. Postlactational involution follows, with regression of lobules. Menopause is characterized by a majority of lobules type 1 and 2, similar to the virgin state. *EGF,* Epidermal growth factor; *FGF,* fibroblast growth factor; *FIL,* feedback inhibitor of lactation; *GH,* growth hormone; *HGF,* hepatocyte growth factor; *HPL,* human placental lactogen; *IGF-I,* insulin-like growth factor-I; *Lef-1,* transcription factor Lef-1; *MMP,* metalloproteinase; *NRG,* neuregulin; *PTH,* parathyroid hormone; *PTHR-1,* PTH/PTHrP receptor type 1; *PTHrP,* parathyroid hormone–related peptide; *TIMP,* tissue inhibitor of metalloproteinase; *TGF-α,* transforming growth factor-α; *TGF-β,* transforming growth factor-β; *TSH,* thyroid-stimulating hormone. (Modified from Russo IH, Russo J. Role of hormones in mammary cancer initiation and progression. *J Mammary Gland Biol Neoplasia.* 1998;3:49; and Dickson R, Russo J. Biochemical control of breast development. In: Harris JR, Lippman ME, Morrow M, Osborne CK, eds. *Diseases of the Breast.* Philadelphia: Lippincott Williams & Wilkins; 2000.)

breast volume, epithelial volume, and surface temperature within 2 to 4 days after the progesterone peak.[143] These changes may in part explain the clinical signs and symptoms of fullness and tenderness that occur premenstrually. Apoptosis peaks just before menses, approximately 5 days after the progesterone peak[144] (see Fig. 3.13).

Regulatory Factors and Potential Genes

The effects of the aforementioned systemic hormones may be mediated through production of local growth factors (see Fig. 3.12). It has been suggested by Anderson and associates[124] that the effects of estrogen and progesterone are mediated by paracrine and juxtacrine factors such as leukemia inhibitory factor (LIF), RANKL, wnt-4, and EGF-like factors secreted by hormone receptor–containing cells as well as stromal-derived factors such as IGF-I and IGF-II and FGF. This hypothesis is supported by the documentation that proliferating cells within the mammary epithelium contain neither ERα nor PR but instead are located commonly adjacent to the steroid receptor expressing cells.[145] The continued importance of the mesenchyme in epithelial proliferation and differentiation is evident in ductal and lobuloalveolar growth during puberty.

Hepatocyte growth factor (HGF)/scatter factor (SF) stimulates proliferation of luminal cells and induces branching morphogenesis in myoepithelial cells, resulting in enhanced ductal growth.[146,147] The mammary fibroblast in the breast mesenchyme is the likely source of HGF/SF, whereas its receptor, c-met, is localized to the ductal epithelium, illustrating its potential paracrine role.[148] Adhesion molecules, in particular $\alpha_2\beta_1$ integrins,

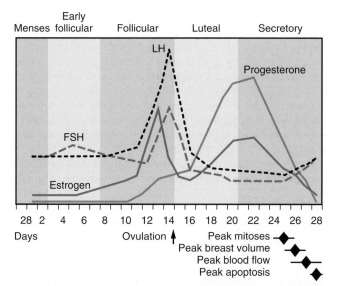

• **Fig. 3.13** Hormonal and histologic changes of the breast during the menstrual cycle. Maximal number of mitosis, breast volume, blood flow, and apoptosis follow the peak in progesterone. *FSH*, Follicle-stimulating hormone; *LH*, luteinizing hormone. (Modified from Speroff L, Glass R, Kase N. Regulation of the menstrual cycle. In: Speroff L, Glass RH, Kase NG. *Clinical Gynecologic Endocrinology and Infertility.* Baltimore: Lippincott Williams & Wilkins; 1999; and Simpson H, Cornélissen G, Katinas G, Halberg F. Meta-analysis of sequential luteal-cycle-associated changes in human breast tissue. *Breast Cancer Res* Treat. 2000;63:171-173.)

may facilitate HGF-induced branching.[147,149] Hydrocortisone, possibly through induction of the c-met receptor, enhances the tubulogenic effect of HGF and also enhances luminal formation.[146] This may partially explain the finding of Lyons, Li, and Johnson[125] that corticoids are necessary for ductal growth. Tubulogenic activity is not restricted to HGF. TGF-α and EGF induce an increase in duct length, but to a lesser degree.[150]

Neuregulins (NRGs), members of the EGF family of growth factors, are also secreted from the stroma. A specific NRG, heregulin, can activate the EGF receptor and contribute to lobuloalveolar growth and secretory activity.[151,152]

Diet may influence the composition of the mammary fat pad and may also affect glandular and ductal growth. Diets deficient in essential fatty acids result in impaired ductal growth and alveolar regression; in contrast, diets rich in unsaturated fat promote parenchymal growth and tumorigenesis and enhance the proliferative effects of EGF.[153–155] Diets deficient in zinc (Zn) during puberty alter mammary gland microenvironment causing oxidative stress, resulting in impaired ductal expansion in mice.[156] The vitamin D receptor, expressed in low levels in the mouse pubertal gland, is upregulated in pregnancy and lactation,[157] at the time of lobuloalveolar development (in mice), and is upregulated in response to cortisol, PRL, and insulin.[158] One study has showed that vitamin D, acting through its receptor, appears to be essential in lobuloalveolar development because vitamin D receptor knockout mice had higher numbers of undifferentiated TEBs.[159]

The progression of the ductal epithelium through the mesenchymal stroma is also modulated by a constantly changing ratio of metalloproteinases (MMPs) that degrade the extracellular matrix and tissue inhibitors of metalloproteinase (TIMPs) that inhibit degradation of the extracellular matrix. MMPs may facilitate branching morphogenesis by releasing growth factors

sequestered in the matrix. MMP can process TGF-α[160] and cleave IGF,[161] increasing their bioavailability. Continual basement membrane and stromal matrix remodeling are necessary to allow for ductal growth and lobuloalveolar expansion.

Finally, it has been suggested by some, that PTEN, a tumor suppressor gene, plays an essential role in controlling the proliferation and differentiation of mammary epithelial cells. Gang and colleagues[162] demonstrated that the mammary tissue of mice with a PTEN-deleted gene exhibited accelerated ductal extension, excessive side branching, and early lobuloalveolar development with subsequent early mammary tumors.

Clinical Correlates

Several *normal variants* may occur during pubertal development that may cause unnecessary concern. Development may be initially unilateral and can mimic an isolated breast mass. Biopsy should not be performed because it may result in permanent breast damage. It is also normal that final breast size may be asymmetric; this finding may be secondary to handedness.[105] Rapid growth of the breast may result in pink or white skin striae; these marks should not be confused with the purple striae of *Cushing syndrome,* particularly if other classic signs of Cushing syndrome are lacking. Periareolar hair is common but should not be removed, because infection and irritation may ensue.[105]

Adolescent, Juvenile, or Virginal Hypertrophy

Adolescent, juvenile, or virginal hypertrophy is a postpubertal continuation of epithelial and stromal growth that results in breasts that can weigh 3 to 8 kg. This clinical presentation denotes the adolescent breast that does not cease its rapid pubertal growth and continues to enlarge even into mature years. There can be ancillary breast tissue within the axilla.[163] The diagnosis should be limited to severe breast enlargement that results in skin ulceration or physical limitations. Most patients with juvenile hypertrophy of the breast have symmetric, bilateral involvement (Fig. 3.14), although unilateral juvenile hypertrophy has been described.[164] This type of hypertrophy is typically postpubertal but can also be seen with pregnancy or severe obesity.[165]

Several conditions may initiate breast asymmetry, including maldevelopment, neoplasms, incisional or excisional biopsies, trauma, and radiotherapy.[166] Juvenile hypertrophy, also referred to as macromastia, may occur secondary to a primary defect of the breast or an endocrinologic disorder.[167,168] The general tenet has been that an augmented plasma level of estrone or estradiol may induce hypertrophy of the breasts. However, the measurement of various mammotropic hormones as the etiology for the disorder has not yielded precise clinical correlates with breast enlargement. Nonetheless, substantial decreases in plasma progesterone levels have been documented for juvenile hypertrophy in the presence of normal plasma estrogen and GH values. These substantial decreases of progesterone in the hormonal milieu may be causing the abnormality. One could also postulate that target organ tissues (ductal epithelium, collagen and stroma of the adolescent female breast) may have estrogen receptors that are highly responsive to minimal concentrations of the mammotropic steroid hormones (e.g., estrogens, progesterone) that regulate breast growth and development.[169] Hypertrophy usually involves both breasts but can be unilateral, suggesting the role of local factors in its cause. Estrogen receptor hypersensitivity,[170] use of the drug penicillamine,[171] and an inherited mutation in the PTEN gene[83] have been implicated in its etiology, with the latter being associated with a higher risk of malignant transformation (Cowden disease).[172]

Workup should include serum estradiol, PRL, FSH, LH, cortisol, somatomedin C, thyroid, and liver function tests, as well as urine 17-keto and hydroxysteroid levels. Typically, however, tests reveal no systemic hormonal imbalances. Discretely palpable masses should be worked up radiographically.

The use of the antiestrogen drugs dydrogesterone and medroxyprogesterone acetate have been recommended in the treatment of virginal hypertrophy.[167,173] Partial success for prevention of regrowth was achieved with tamoxifen citrate. Treatment with

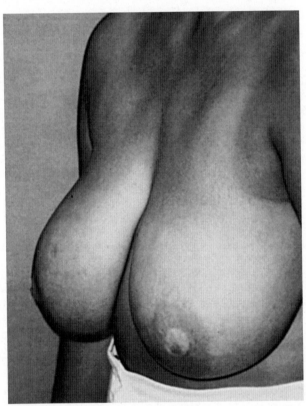

• **Fig. 3.14** Bilateral juvenile hypertrophy in a 17-year-old nulliparous Hispanic girl. The patient presented with mastodynia related to her large breast size. She was not taking any medications known to induce breast gigantism. Therapy consisted of reduction mammaplasty. (Courtesy Dr. Hollis H. Caffee, Division of Plastic and Reconstructive Surgery, University of Florida College of Medicine, Gainesville, FL.)

tamoxifen may be of value after reduction mammaplasty (subcutaneous mastectomy) in patients with strongly positive estrogen receptor profiles in the removed breast tissue. Using an escalating dose of 10 to 40 mg of tamoxifen citrate per day, these authors were able to achieve reduction of breast bulk with the drug. Theoretically, with the use of this compound, estrogen receptors can be converted to a negative profile status. Bromocriptine has also been used in virginal hypertrophy, similar to treatment of pregnancy-induced gigantomastia, but has been shown to be unsuccessful in juvenile hypertrophy.[174]

The most commonly applied technique for the treatment of adolescent (juvenile) hypertrophy continues to be the subcutaneous mastectomy as a reduction mammaplasty.[84] Currently, it is the definitive therapy for juvenile hypertrophy with the possibility of tamoxifen as an adjunct to surgical treatment.[170]

Tuberous Breast Deformity

Tuberous breast deformity was first described in 1976 by Rees and Aston but has been described in many other studies with various names.[171,175] The malformation causes the affected breasts to resemble the root of a tuberous plant, which was the basis of the original description (Fig. 3.15). The incidence of this condition is unknown. There is a large spectrum of this disease; many women are not likely to seek treatment. It has been documented that a high percentage of women presenting with asymmetric breast suffer from tuberous deformity.[176] The abnormality can be seen as a unilateral or bilateral phenomenon and is first noticed at puberty with development of the breast tissue.

In an effort to better characterize this deformity, the following classification system for the tuberous deformities was composed[177]:

Type I—hypoplasia of the lower medial quadrant
Type II—hypoplasia of the lower medial and lateral quadrants; sufficient skin in the subareolar region
Type III—hypoplasia of the lower medial and lateral quadrants; deficiency of skin in the subareolar region
Type IV—severe breast constriction; minimal breast base

There is associated decreased breast tissue and milk ducts of the lower quadrants, especially the lower medial quadrant. Other modifications of this classification system have been proposed, but most descriptions of the deformity agree that the resulting features are from skin shortage and herniation of breast tissue through the nipple-areolar complex.[176,178]

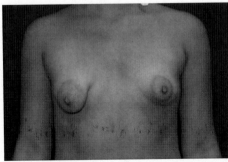
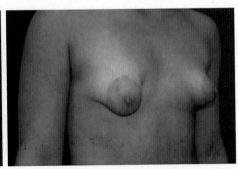

• **Fig. 3.15** A 19-year-old girl with bilateral severe tuberous breast deformity. (From Latham K, Fernandez S, Iteld L, Panthaki Z, Armstrong MB, Thaller S. Pediatric breast deformity. *J Craniofac Surg.* 2006;17:454-467.)

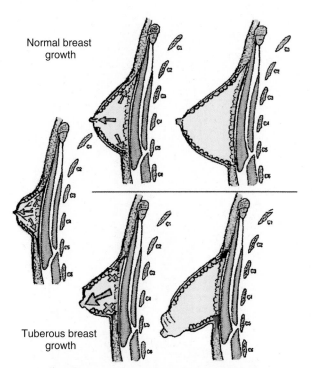

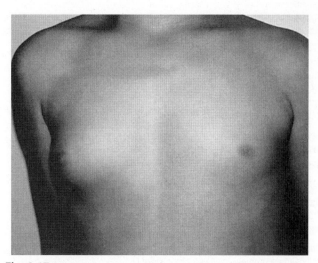

• **Fig. 3.17** Nine-year-old boy with a 1-year history of right-sided gynecomastia. Health, growth, and hormone profile were all normal. Mastectomy was performed for psychological reasons, and there was no recurrence of problems.

• **Fig. 3.16** Depiction of normal and tuberous breast growth. (From Grolleau JL, Lanfrey E, Lavigne B, Chavoin JP, Costagliola M. Breast base anomalies: treatment strategy for tuberous breasts, minor deformities, and asymmetry. *Plast Reconstr Surg.* 1999;104:2040-2048.)

Several theories have been proposed for the cause of the tuberous breast defect. The first hypothesis proposed a strong adherence between the dermis and muscular plane along the lower pole of the breast. As the breast develops, it is unable to separate this adherence, and the peripheral expansion of the breast is restricted (Fig. 3.16). The breast tissue then develops forward, enlarging and sometimes herniating into the areola.[179] Another theory described a fibrous band at the periphery of the nipple-areola complex, representing a thickening of the superficial fascia that inhibits normal breast development. The fibrous ring does not allow for the growing breast tissue to expand inferiorly. Because there is no superficial fascia underneath the areola, the breast tissue herniates toward the nipple-areola complex.[178]

Although many techniques have been proposed, the fundamental principles remain the correction of breast tissue herniation and lowering of the inframammary fold.[175,176] Single-staged procedures with either reduction mammoplasty or breast augmentation have yielded excellent results in less severe malformations.[177] Simple augmentation of severe deformities has frequently resulted in an unsatisfactory "double bubble" appearance, further accentuating the tuberous deformity. In these patients, multiple procedures with tissue expansion and flaps have been proposed.[175,177] Newer single-staged techniques are now consistently and reproducibly giving satisfactory results, with excellent symmetry of the breasts, conveying a better understanding of the disease process.[176,178]

Gynecomastia

In the adolescent male, gynecomastia occurs at age 13 to 14, when male pubertal changes and the sex hormones have established the male pattern.[180] It occurs in 70% of pubertal boys but rarely

exceeds the Tanner B2 stage (elevation of the breast and papilla as a small mound)[104,111,181] (Fig. 3.17). Pubertal gynecomastia is usually resolved within several months to 2 years.[105] Generalized obesity can sometimes mimic gynecomastia. The primary complaint is concentric enlargement of breast tissue, but breast and nipple pain can occur in 25% of cases, with tenderness found in 40%. There is rarely a pathologic cause of adolescent gynecomastia, and histology typically reveals proliferation of the ductal and stromal tissue without evidence of lobuloalveolar formation.[7] An initial rise in estrogen levels, altered ratios of peripheral and central androgens to estrogens, increased diurnal periods of estrogen excess, peripheral aromatization of androgen,[104] and cyclo-oxygenase 2–induced aromatase overexpression[182] have been considered causal.

Higher circulating levels of leptin have been measured in pubertal boys with gynecomastia and may play a role in its pathogenesis either through stimulation of aromatase enzyme activity or producing a direct effect on mammary epithelial cells through the leptin or estrogen receptor.[183] Marijuana can cause gynecomastia, and its use should be ruled out.[184] Endocrinopathies, including *testosterone deficiency, LH receptor deficiency,* and *incomplete androgen insensitivity,* may result in breast formation Rarely, when treated with glucocorticoids, a genetic female completely virilized by congenital adrenal hyperplasia and raised as a male, will undergo adrenal androgen-directed release of suppression of gonadotropins and have breast development).[102] Diagnosis begins with a good breast examination. Breast lipomas, neurofibromas, and carcinomas are more typically nonpainful and eccentrically located. Pubescent gynecomastia may also be the first sign of gonadal tumors[185,186]; therefore, an examination of the testes should also be performed. Serum levels of human chorionic gonadotropin, LH, testosterone, and estrogen can be obtained, with additional levels of PRL and thyroid function tests if initial tests are abnormal. However, laboratory evaluation is typically reserved for prepubertal or postpubertal males. Cosmetic concerns may lead to consideration of a subcutaneous mastectomy but should be performed only after any underlying organic cause has been ruled out. Although hormonal manipulation has been effective in some cases of post pubertal gynecomastia,[187] hormonal

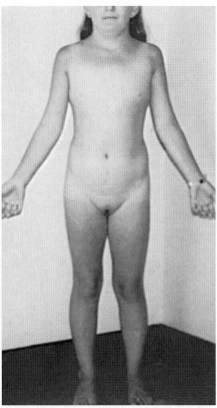

• **Fig. 3.18** Fifteen-year-old girl with Turner syndrome (XO) demonstrating a shieldlike chest with widely separated hypoplastic nipples and lack of sexual maturation.

manipulation through the use of an aromatase inhibitor has not been found to be effective in pubertal boys.[188] The failure to respond to hormonal treatment may be secondary to histologic differences as well as to differences in Ki-67 activity seen between pubertal and postpubertal gynecomastia, which may confer sensitivity to treatment.[189]

Hypogonadotropism

Failure of estrogen production leads to insufficient development of the ductal system. Lack of estrogen can be related to primary ovarian failure or may result from hypogonadotropism. Primary ovarian failure may be the result of direct injury or torsion or may be associated with certain genetic syndromes (Box 3.1). Decreased estrogen levels result in abnormal elevation of gonadotropin levels. The most common cause of primary ovarian failure is the Turner syndrome of gonadal dysgenesis. To prevent osteopenia and psychological problems from sexual infantilism, cyclical estrogen therapy should not be unduly delayed (Fig. 3.18).[190] Intrinsic errors may also occur in aromatase activity and adrenal steroid biosynthesis resulting in failure of female development and virilization; most commonly caused by the $P-450_{c21}$–hydroxylase deficiency[190,191]

Hypogonadotropism may be caused by isolated gonadotropin insufficiency, brain tumors, and several genetic abnormalities. Chronic illness such as diabetes, hypothyroidism, Cushing syndrome, or hyperprolactinemia can cause a functional hypogonadotropism. Malnutrition or low weight, such as that seen in high-performance athletes, can also cause a functional hypogonadotropism and delayed onset of puberty[192] (see Box 3.1).

Recent studies have demonstrated a positive correlation between tallness in pubertal girls (age 7–15) and increased risk of future breast cancer. It has been suggested that this may be related to persistently high serum IGF levels in tall women.[193] Conversely, overweight children seem to have a decreased risk of breast cancer. It is possible that the fat-derived estrogens cause an earlier differentiation of the breast, decreasing malignant potential.[193]

Pregnancy

Morphology

Numerous changes occur in the mammary gland during pregnancy in preparation for lactation primarily regulated by PRL and progesterone. Alterations are seen involving both alveologenesis and gland maturation.[2] Two phases occur during pregnancy to ultimately prepare the gland for lactation. The first phase, which occurs during early pregnancy, is the proliferation of the distal ducts to create more lobules and more alveoli within each lobule. There is considerable heterogeneity within the pregnant breast. Some lobular units may be resting while others expand with proliferative activity. This proliferation leads to the formation of more differentiated forms of lobules, lobule type 3 (Lob 3) and lobule type 4 (Lob 4). Lob 3 outnumbers the more primitive lobules by the end of the first trimester and can have up to 10 times the alveoli per lobules compared with Lob 1.[194] If the first term pregnancy occurs before the third decade of life, the number of Lob 3 significantly increases.[1] Lob 3 remains the dominant structure in all parous women until the fourth decade of life, after which it starts to decline and involute to Lob 1 and 2 after menopause (see Fig. 3.12).

By the midpoint of pregnancy, the lobuloalveolar framework is in place and differentiation of the lobular units into secretory units begins. Cell proliferation and formation of new alveoli are minimized, and the alveoli differentiate into acini. During the last trimester, the epithelial cells are filled with fat droplets, the acini distend with colostrum (an eosinophilic and proteinaceous secretion), and fat and connective tissue have largely been replaced by glandular proliferation. The increase in breast size during this period is secondary to distention of acini and increased vascularity.[195,196]

Hormones

In the pregnant state, estrogen, progesterone, estrogen, and PRL work in concert to prepare the breast for lactation (Fig. 3.19). Progesterone initiates side branching and alveologenesis, which, in concert with PRL and estrogen, promotes differentiation of the alveoli in preparation for lactogenesis.

As in puberty, PRL plays a continued role in lobuloalveolar differentiation. PRL increases beginning at 8 weeks and continues to rise throughout gestation and postpartum.[197,198] Human placental lactogen (HPL), a member of the PRL family, is secreted during the second half of pregnancy. Although HPL has less bioactivity than PRL, by the end of gestation, the HPL concentration is approximately 30 times the concentration of PRL.[197] This suggests that HPL may contribute to the PRL effects on lobuloalveolar development and final maturation of the gestational gland.[139]

The estrogen increase during gestation parallels that of PRL.[198,199] Estrogen is believed to be a direct and indirect modulator of PRL secretion. First, estrogen induces the differentiation of anterior pituitary lactotrophs, which secrete PRL. Second, estrogen, through interaction with an estrogen-responsive element and an adjacent transcription factor–binding site, enhances PRL gene expression.[199–202] Finally, estrogen suppresses the secretion of the PRL inhibitory factor dopamine.[203]

With pregnancy, PRL primes the breast for lactation; however, initiation of lactogenesis is inhibited by the presence of progesterone. Although estrogen and progesterone are necessary for PRL receptor expression, paradoxically, progesterone reduces the binding and antagonizes the positive effects of PRL at its receptor.[204–206] Progesterone can directly suppress production of the milk protein casein by stimulating the production of a transcription inhibitor.[207]

Regulatory Factors and Potential Genes

Studies on progesterone receptors have found two receptor isoforms (PGRA and PGRB). Although both isoforms are expressed in the mammary gland, PGRA levels exceed those of PGRB in mouse models during pregnancy.[208] Interestingly, knockout models have shown that although phenotype is unchanged with loss of PGRB, significant decrease in side-branching and alveologenesis during pregnancy was seen with loss of PGRA.[2] RANKL (receptor activator of NFKB1 ligand), also known as TNFSF11 (tumor necrosis factor ligand superfamily, member 11) was recently identified as a key paracrine regulatory factor in progesterone-induced mammary proliferation. Mice models without RANKL have failed to undergo alveologenesis during pregnancy.[209] Progesterone-induced mammary gland proliferation by RANKL has been associated with increase cell growth in progesterone receptor positive breast cancers.[210]

As seen in puberty, NRG is expressed in the stroma of the mouse mammary gland during pregnancy.[153] In some in vivo models, NRG stimulated alveoli development and secretory activity, suggesting a potential role in mediating PRL. In other models (MMTV mice), however, NRG halted the progression of the lobuloalveolar system at the TEB stage, consistent with PRL deficiency.[153,211] Heregulin-α (HRG), a specific NRG, may play a critical role in lobuloalveolar development and subsequent lactogenesis.[152] Activins and inhibins, STAT5[212] (members of the TGF-β family) may also play a role in modulating glandular development. Mutations in these factors result in an inhibition of alveolar development during pregnancy.[212,213] Certain intracellular signaling molecules, including the transcription factors A-myb, c-erbB, hox9a, hox9b, hox9d, cell cycle protein cyclin D1,[214–217] RANK-L,[129] slug transcription factor,[218] and Wnt4 may play a role in the regulation of lobuloalveolar development.[219] Deletions of the genes coding for several of these factors have caused impairment of lobuloalveolar development.[187–190]

With physiologic progression to puberty, proper balance between matrix-MMP,[220,221] and its inhibitor TIMP-1[193] initiates an important role in lobuloalveolar development during pregnancy and subsequent ability to lactate. For example, overexpression of TIMP caused a reduction in extracellular matrix remodeling and resulted in inhibition of lobuloalveolar development during pregnancy.[220]

Clinical Correlates

Gravid hypertrophy of the breast with pregnancy is a rare condition of unknown cause and is often referred to as gigantomastia of pregnancy.[221] This condition may affect women of all races during the childbearing years; however, Caucasian women are more likely to experience this phenomenon than African American women.[222] The disorder is less common than juvenile (virginal) hypertrophy of the breast, which classically progresses independent of pregnancy and occurs usually between the ages of 11 and 19 years. Gigantomastia of pregnancy usually occurs during the first few months of pregnancy and may progress to necrosis, incapacity, and possibly death.[223] Bilateral breast gigantism is usually observed, although unilateral gigantomastia of pregnancy has been reported.[224]

The typical history is that of a healthy pregnant woman who observes gradual bilateral massive enlargement of her breasts within the first few months of pregnancy. The breasts may enlarge to several times their normal weight and size to become massive, disfiguring, and debilitating. The skin and parenchyma become firm, edematous, and tense and may have prominent subcutaneous veins with a diffuse peau d'orange appearance. As a consequence of rapid breast enlargement and skin pressure, insufficient vascularity of the skin may initiate ulceration, necrosis, infection, or hemorrhage.

In the immediate postpartum period, the hypertrophied breasts recede to approximately their previous volume. With delivery of the fetus, the breasts regress in size but almost always hypertrophies again with succeeding pregnancies. Most authors agree that this condition is hormonal in etiology, but its precise mechanism is unclear. Multiple inciting factors have been proposed as possible causes for this problem, including hormonal abnormalities, tissue receptor sensitivity, malignancy, and autoimmune disorders.[222] Whether there is an overproduction of mammotropic hormone from the pituitary or an enhanced sensitivity of breast parenchyma to the hormones of pregnancy (e.g., estriol, estradiol, human chorionic gonadotropin, progestins) has not been firmly established.

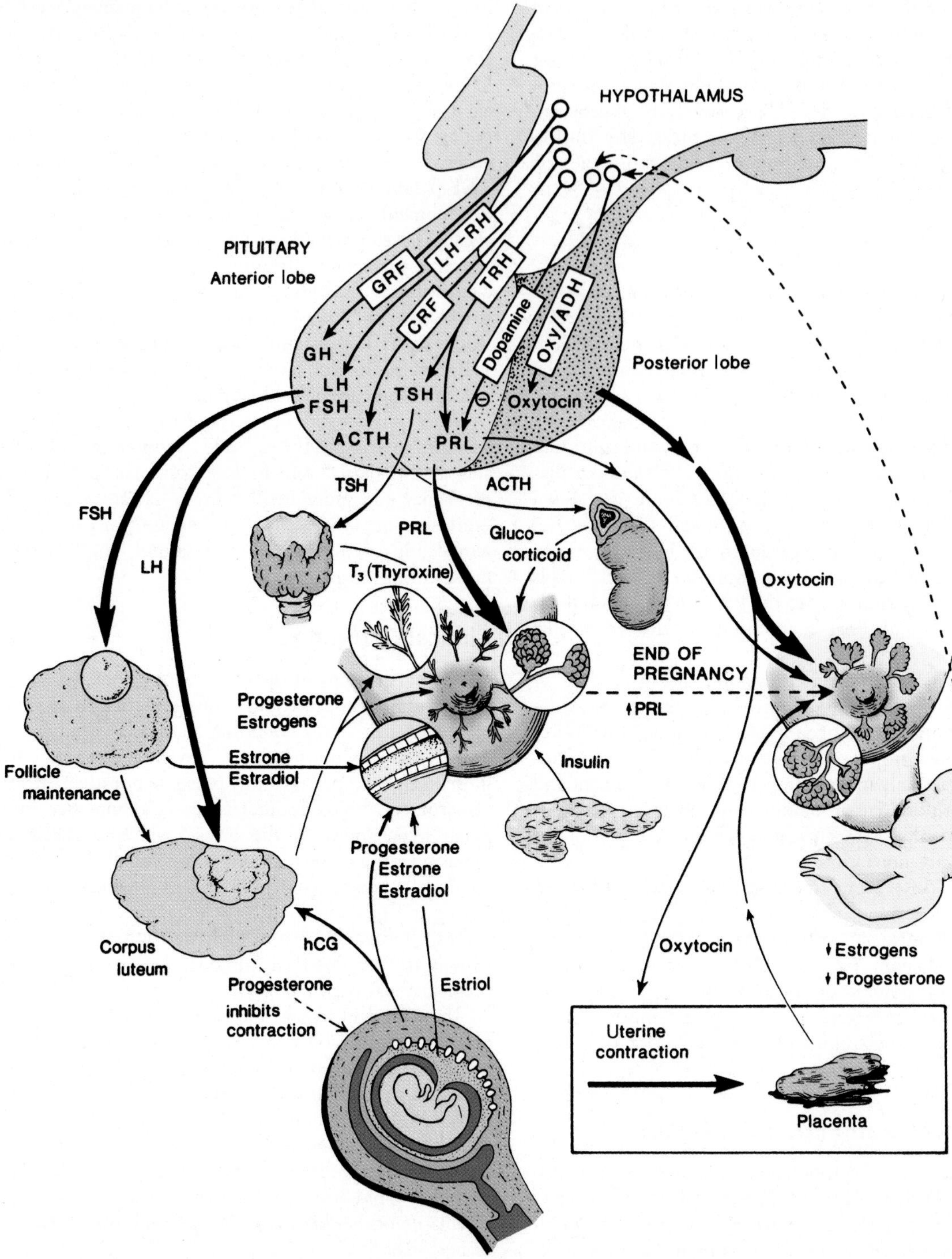

• **Fig. 3.19** Neuroendocrine control of breast development and function. Luteinizing hormone–releasing hormone *(LH-RH)*, also known as gonadotropin-releasing hormone *(GnRH)*, from the hypothalamus stimulates the pituitary secretion of luteinizing hormone *(LH)* and follicle-stimulating hormone *(FSH)*. Thyrotropin-releasing hormone *(TRH)* from the hypothalamus stimulates the release of prolactin *(PRL)*, against the inhibitory control of dopamine from the hypothalamus. The pituitary gonadotropins stimulate ovarian synthesis and the release of progesterone and estrogen, which have mammotrophic effects. Pregnancy enhances the secretion of estrogen and progesterone from the corpus luteum during the first 12 weeks and subsequently from the placenta. After delivery, PRL secretion increases. Neural stimuli from suckling stimulates prolactin and oxytocin release. Milk let-down occurs. Other hormones are depicted that contribute to the growth and function of the mammary gland, including glucocorticoid, growth hormone *(GH)*, insulin, and thyroxin. *ACTH,* Adrenocorticotropic hormone; *ADH,* antidiuretic hormone; *CRF,* corticotropin-releasing factor; *GRF,* growth hormone–releasing factor; *hCG,* human chorionic gonadotropin; *TSH,* thyroid-stimulating hormone.

Although liver dysfunction and the inability to metabolize estrogenic hormones have been theorized to be a possible cause for the disorder, it must be noted that many normal pregnancies are accompanied by severe liver failure without the development of gigantomastia.[225] Bromocriptine is the most widely used medical treatment of this problem. It has shown variable results with arrested breast hypertrophy or mild breast size regression; the agent does not return breast to pregestational size.[222] Although the medical approach has variable results, it should be the first line of treatment in an effort to avoid surgical intervention during pregnancy.

In most instances, gigantomastia is self-limiting and does not progress to pyogenic abscesses, skin ulcerations, necrosis, or systemic illness. Breast size will spontaneously regress to its approximate nonpregnant configuration after delivery. The patient should be advised of proper brassiere support, good skin hygiene, and adequate nutrition. Operative intervention may be necessary to relieve severe pain, massive infection, necrosis, slough, and ulceration or hemorrhage if delivery is not imminent. The operative choices include bilateral reduction mammaplasty versus bilateral mastectomies with delayed reconstruction. Gigantomastia is likely to recur with reduction mammaplasty in subsequent pregnancies. Bilateral mastectomies with delayed reconstruction offer the best chance of avoiding recurrence if the patient should become pregnant again. If there is any retained breast tissue, it is likely to hypertrophy with additional pregnancies.[222]

Epidemiologic studies suggest that early parity has a protective effect against breast cancer. In an attempt to explain the protective effect of parity, the proliferative activity, steroid receptors, angiogenic index, protease inhibitors, serpin and mammary-derived growth inhibitor (MDGI) were measured in the three types of lobules, Lob 1, Lob 2, Lob 3, in parous and nulliparous women.[226,227] Lob 1, the most undifferentiated lobule, had the highest rate of proliferation and highest percentage of cells that expressed both estrogen receptors and PRs. Lob 1 also had the highest angiogenic index, the number of blood vessels in relation to number of alveoli, and no expression of the protease inhibitors. In the progression from Lob 1 to Lob 3, proliferation, the percentage of lobules that are receptor positive, and the angiogenic index decreases, and there is expression of the protease inhibitors. Postmenopausal women who were parous ultimately had the same percentage of Lob 1 as the nulliparous women, but the proliferative index of Lob 1 in nulliparous women was higher than that of parous women. This difference persisted through menopause.[228–230] It has been suggested that cancer initiation involves the interaction of a carcinogen with undifferentiated, highly proliferating mammary epithelium,[1] and the Lob 1 of the nulliparous woman would seem to be a prime target.[231] Human chorionic gonadotropin stimulates mammary gland differentiation, reduction in number of TEBs and an increase in the number of alveolar buds and lobules and decrease rat mammary carcinogenesis.

Rat models have shown that the GH–insulin-like growth factor 1 (GH-IGF-1) axis remains suppressed after pregnancy. PRL levels have also been shown to be transiently decreased in humans in the postpartum period. Decreased levels of GH and PRL in rat models lead to regression of mammary tumors, whereas higher levels of the two hormones are associated with increased rates of mammary carcinogenesis. These findings suggest that the effects of pregnancy on PRL and GH levels may be related to the protective effects of parity on breast cancer.[232]

Lactation

Morphology and Product

Whereas the first half of pregnancy is marked by significant ductal and lobuloalveolar proliferation and formation of Lob 3 structures and some Lob 4 structures, the second half of gestation involves the final maturation of the gland into the secretory organ of lactation. The ability to synthesize and secrete the milk product is termed *lactogenesis*. This is composed of two stages. Lactogenesis I is the synthesis of unique milk components. This portion of the phase is accompanied by morphologic changes in the alveolar epithelial cell with an increase in protein synthetic structures (i.e., rough endoplasmic reticulum, mitochondria, and Golgi apparatus). Complex protein, milk fat, and lactose synthetic pathways are activated, but minimal secretion into the alveoli lumina occurs.[101,196] Studies measuring urine lactose, an index of the breast's synthetic activity, have confirmed that this stage begins, in most mothers, between 15 and 20 weeks of gestation.[233] The alveoli distend with colostrum, an immature milk product, and along with increased vascularity contribute to the increase in breast volume seen in the latter part of gestation. Lob 4, formed during pregnancy, persists throughout lactation[134] (see Fig. 3.12).

Lactogenesis II is the initiation of significant milk secretion at or just after parturition[233] and is marked by a rise in citrate and α-lactalbumin.[127] The initial product is colostrum, which combines both nutritional elements and passive immunity for the infant. Transitional milk follows with less immunoglobulin and total protein. The ultimate product is mature milk that is composed of fat and protein suspended in a lactose solution. The fat, lactose, and protein are secreted in an apocrine fashion. Lactose and protein are also secreted in a merocrine fashion[101] (Fig. 3.20). Mature milk secretion begins 30 to 40 hours postpartum[233] and averages 1 to 2 mL/g of breast tissue per day. The rate of lactation remains constant for the first 6 months of lactation.[234–236] During lactation the *stromal lymphatics* increase compared with other periods. Interepithelial gaps widen, allowing for more direct uptake of particles and fluids and improved clearance from the breast.[237]

After weaning, the breast involutes and returns to a state resembling that of prepregnancy. The lobules decrease in size, with a decrease in the number of alveoli per lobule. The ducts are not involved, in contrast with menopausal involution when both the lobules and ducts are reduced in number. There are two phases of postlactational involution. The first phase is reversible, in that suckling will reestablish milk supply, and is associated with the accumulation of milk. It is triggered by either physical distortion of the luminal epithelial cells or by accumulation of apoptosis-inducing factors in the milk; however, no significant morphologic changes occur.[238] The second phase begins after 48 hours without suckling and is characterized by active tissue remodeling and apoptosis, including destruction of basement membranes and alveolar structure. This results in the irreversible loss of lactogenic function of the mammary gland.[239,240] By 6 days, a large portion of the secretory gland is replaced by adipocytes. Even though the remodeled gland appears morphologically similar to the prepregnancy gland, significant differences exist on molecular and genetic levels.[2]

Hormones

The physiologic importance of PRL and related peptides in mammary gland growth and differentiation is seen with lactation,

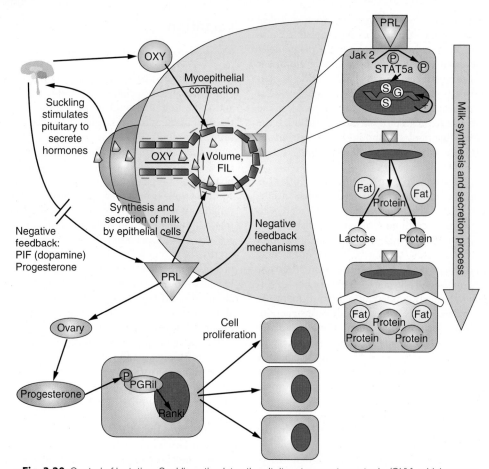

• **Fig. 3.20** Control of lactation. Suckling stimulates the pituitary to secrete oxytocin *(OXY),* which causes myoepithelial contraction and milk release, and prolactin *(PRL),* which promotes synthesis and secretion of milk. Increased alveolar intraluminal volume, milk levels of feedback inhibitor of lactation *(FIL),* and systemic hormone (dopamine and progesterone) levels inhibit PRL action. Expanded view details PRL action on the epithelial cell. PRL binds its transmembrane receptor, activating the Jak-STAT pathway with resultant phosphorylation of STAT5a. A ternary complex of a STAT5a dimer *(S-S)* with a glucocorticoid receptor *(G)* forms and binds DNA in the nucleus, stimulating production of milk proteins. The mRNA of certain milk proteins can positively feedback on further gene expression. Complex protein, milk fat, and lactose synthetic pathways are activated. Lactose and some milk proteins can be secreted in a merocrine fashion. Other milk proteins and fats are stored in vesicles in the apex of the luminal epithelial cell. The proteins and fats are then secreted into the lumen along with the apical portion of the cell (apocrine secretion). Progesterone pathway shows progesterone induced mammary cell proliferation through interaction with progesterone receptors and RANKL. *PIF,* PRL inhibitory factor. (Courtesy Dr. Joshua S. Winder, Department of Surgery, Penn State Hershey Medical Center, Hershey, PA.)

the terminal state of differentiation of the mature mammary gland (see Figs. 3.19 and 3.20). PRL is the principal hormone for the synthesis of milk proteins and the maintenance of lactation.[9] Production of casein, the primary milk protein, does not occur in the absence of PRL.[140] This hormone is secreted in increasing amounts throughout pregnancy and peaks before delivery. However, the presence of the PRL inhibitory factor, luteal, and placental sex steroids, especially progesterone, prohibits PRL from achieving its full lactational effect.

Glucocorticoids work along with PRL to differentiate mammary epithelium and stimulate milk synthesis and secretion. Both glucocorticoids and their receptors are increased in late pregnancy and lactation. Progesterone binds the glucocorticoid receptor and acts as a glucocorticoid antagonist.[196]

After birth, in the background of dissipating progesterone, PRL, in concert with glucocorticoids, is able to initiate lactogenesis II. Neural stimuli from suckling enhance the release of PRL from the anterior pituitary gland. PRL then binds its membrane receptor. An intracellular portion of the receptor associates with Jak2, a tyrosine kinase, which ultimately phosphorylates STAT5a.[241] Isolated disruptions of STAT5a in mice have resulted in failure to lactate.[242] A dimeric complex of STAT5a couples with the glucocorticoid receptor, forming a ternary complex that then translocates to the nucleus and alters mRNA synthesis.[9] The mRNA of certain milk proteins can positively feedback on further gene expression (see Fig. 3.20).[243]

Several stimulatory secretagogues of PRL have been enumerated, including estrogen,[244] hypothalamic peptides, thyrotropin-releasing hormone and vasoactive intestinal peptide,[245,246] and local factors EGF[247] and FGF.[248] Oral thyrotropin-releasing hormone may have benefits in improving lactation in women who occasionally breastfeed by increasing PRL levels. In these women, their baseline PRLs were lower than that of average fully breast-feeding women.[249] Extrapituitary synthesis of PRL occurs in the mammary gland and contributes to the high levels of the hormone secreted into the milk. Maturation of the newborn and fetal hypothalamic neuroendocrine system may be modulated by both PRL in the milk and PRL secreted into the amniotic fluid by the uterine decidua.[250]

Oxytocin is responsible for release of stored milk, commonly referred to as *milk let-down*. Oxytocin is secreted from the posterior pituitary by a sensory stimulation from the nipple-areola complex, via T4, T5, and T6 sensory afferent nerve roots. Uniquely, it can be secreted in anticipation of nursing in the presence of a crying infant[140] and can be inhibited by pain and embarrassment.[102] Oxytocin stimulates contraction of the myoepithelial cells surrounding the acini and small ducts, resulting in an expulsion of milk into the lactiferous sinuses.

Lactogens of GH, PRL, and placental origin are structurally related hormones and may, to some extent, be interchangeable in function. Deficiency in one of them is not sufficient to cause lack of mammary gland development and function. For example, women with pituitary dwarfism who lack detectable GH, women who have had a pituitary adenoma removed with no subsequent rise in PRL during pregnancy or lactation,[251] and women with low levels of HPL[251] had normal pregnancies and were able to breastfeed.

Glucocorticoid and systemic lactogenic hormones act as survival factors both during lactation and through the phase of involution.[252] Decreasing levels of systemic hormones allow for increasing apoptosis and progression into the second phase of involution.

Regulatory Factors and Potential Genes

Cell-cell interactions play a regulatory role in lobuloalveolar development and milk synthesis. Alterations in the expression of E-cadherin in luminal epithelial cells and P-cadherin in myoepithelial cells[253] vary the onset of lobuloalveolar development and milk synthesis.[254,255] The role of hedgehog network genes in lactogenesis is still being elucidated.[15] Certain nuclear factor I proteins may also contribute to the control of lactation and involution.[256]

It has been noted that each breast has an independent rate of milk synthesis, suggesting a more important role for local factors in modulating function. Systemic factors, particularly PRL, do not appear to regulate the rate of milk synthesis. Luminal volume may contribute to synthesis rate by altering the interaction between the basement membrane and the lactocyte, leading to an inhibition of the PRL receptor.[257,258] Breast volume, however, is not the primary control of milk synthesis. Lactating goats, whose full breasts demonstrated a decrease in milk synthesis, had a resurgence of milk production when the milk was emptied and replaced isovolumetrically with a sucrose solution, suggesting that a compound within the milk was providing negative feedback. This intrinsic milk factor, the feedback inhibitor of lactation, is now thought to modulate local control of milk synthesis. This compound has been noted in many species, including women, and has been found to inhibit lactocyte differentiation, disrupt Golgi vesicle secretion, and inhibit protein synthesis in lactocytes.[259]

Involution requires active gene expression. *Milk stasis* is thought to initiate apoptosis of mammary epithelial cells through activation of p53- and Stat 3–mediated pathways (see Fig. 3.12).[260]

During stage 1, there is upregulation of SGP-2, Stat 3, Fas antigen, Westmead DMBA8 nonmetastatic cDNA 1 (WDNM1), and other TIMPs[261,262] and downregulation STAT5a and STAT5b.[262,263] During this first phase, local factors are sufficient to induce alveolar cell death, even in the presence of systemic lactogenic hormones. Insulin, dexamethasone, PRL, and their combinations did not affect expression of WDNM1 and SGP-2 genes. EGF, however, strongly inhibited the expression of WDNM1 and SGP2 in cell culture, and the addition of EGF with insulin completely protected the cells in culture from apoptosis.[264] Thus, EGF acts like a survival factor[264]; it is possible that loss of EGF induces gain of a death signal and leads to stage 1 of involution.

The second stage of involution is characterized by the upregulation of MMPs gelatinase A, stromelysin-1, serine protease urokinase-type plasminogen activator and activation of proteinase-dependent pathways and downregulation of the inhibitor TIMP-1.[239] This change in the ratio of MMP to TIMP, favoring MMP, is thought to correlate with the loss of expression of B-casein, a marker for milk production. The addition of TIMP-1 to change the ratio in the opposite direction favors cell survival and maintenance of secretory phenotype.[265] The role of other genes in lactational involution, TGF-α,[266] are currently being elucidated and may ultimately offer insight into the mechanisms of tumorigenesis.

Clinical Correlates

Delayed Onset of Lactation

Chapman and Perez-Escamilla[267] have identified risk factors for *delayed onset of lactation*. These factors include lack of infant suckling, unscheduled cesarean delivery or vaginal delivery with prolonged stage 2 labor, and obesity. In these women, delay of lactogenesis II may be more than 72 hours postpartum. They should be encouraged to have frequent nursing sessions to potentially enhance the onset of lactation.[267] Progesterone, as described previously, inhibits the onset of lactogenesis II. Women who have portions of *retained placenta* may continue to have sufficient progesterone levels to inhibit their milk synthesis. The delay persists until the fragments are removed.[268,269] As described earlier, the exact role of insulin in lactogenesis is unclear; however, it has been observed that patients with *type 1 insulin-dependent diabetes mellitus* have a 24-hour delay in the onset of lactogenesis II. With assurance and prior knowledge of this information, these mothers can have success with breastfeeding.[268,269] Lactogenesis may also be affected by a high body mass index.[270]

Lactational Success

Although it was once concluded that women with smaller breasts had *inadequate milk production* and less success with breastfeeding, this has now been disproved. New computerized topographic techniques (computer breast measurement) have allowed breast physiologists to study breast growth during pregnancy, short-term milk synthesis (between feeding intervals), and the degree of fullness without interrupting normal breastfeeding patterns.[233] Women with smaller-capacity breasts achieved lactational success by increasing the frequency of feedings and the degree of breast emptying with each feeding. Women with larger-capacity breasts have more flexibility in scheduling their feedings and can go longer at night without compromising their synthesis capabilities.[233]

Women who have minimal breast growth during pregnancy should not be dissuaded from breastfeeding. Women who had only small breast growth during pregnancy, with only a small increase in lactose in their urine, had compensatory growth during the first month postpartum. The growth during this month was equivalent to the growth of other women from conception to delivery.[233] Vigorous aerobic exercise should not be a deterrent to breastfeeding because it affects neither the volume nor the composition of breast milk.[271]

In the small subset of women who have lactational insufficiency secondary to low levels of PRL, drugs such as metoclopramide have been shown to increase the secretion of PRL. Low levels of PRL should be documented and need to be measured 45 minutes after suckling. As mentioned, oral thyrotropin-releasing hormone may improve lactation in insufficient women noted to have low levels of PRL, although hyperthyroidism in the mother may be a side effect.[249] Lactational failure may be the first sign of *Sheehan syndrome* (infarction of the pituitary gland with ensuing insufficiency of PRL and other hormones). Other, rarer causes of lactational failure include lymphocytic hypophysitis, isolated hypoprolactinemia, or hypoprolactinemia as part of a generalized pituitary deficiency.[102]

Impact on Breast Cancer Risk

The association of postlactational involution and breast cancer has been extensively studied. Involution is tightly regulated, and it involves massive apoptosis and tissue remodeling. Analysis of glandular transcription profiles during involution show many similarities to those found during wound healing and tumorigenesis. Although involution usually occurs without malignant transformation of mammary cells, the inflammatory process and cell turnover may create a microenvironment that promotes the development of preneoplastic cells. These findings may be associated with the transient increase in breast cancer risk seen in the first few years after pregnancy.[2,232,272]

Multiple epidemiologic studies have shown that breastfeeding is associated with lowering breast cancer risk with longer durations predictive of lower risk.[273,274] BRCA1-positive patients who breastfed for more than 1 year were found to be at lower risk for breast cancer compared with their counterparts who never breastfed. Interestingly this association was not uniformly seen with BCRA2 carriers.[275,276] The exact mechanism of the oncoprotective nature of prolonged breastfeeding has yet to be fully understood. It has been hypothesized that breastfeeding leads to greater levels of TDLU involution. TDLU involution have been shown to lower breast cancer risk, whereas lack of involution is associated with risk for basal-like breast cancers.[277–279] Thus by promoting TDLU involution, long-term breastfeeding may lower breast cancer risk.[278]

Menopause

Morphology

As women approach menopause, age-related lobular involution is seen. There is an increased number of Lob 1 and a decline in Lob 2 and Lob 3, with all women by the end of the fifth decade having mostly Lob 1. Independent of age, nulliparous women have 65%

to 80% Lob 1, 10% to 35% Lob 2, and 0% to 5% Lob 3. Parous women, from postlactation involution to the fourth decade, have 70% to 90% of Lob 3. After the fourth decade, their breasts start to involute, and after menopause the breakdown of lobular percentages are equivalent to those of nulliparous women (see Fig. 3.12).

Menopause otherwise progresses in much the same manner in both parous and nulliparous women. The climacteric phase from age 45 to 55 has a moderate decrease in glandular epithelium. This is followed by the postmenopausal phase, which typically occurs after age 50. During the postmenopausal phase, the glandular epithelium undergoes apoptosis, the interlobular stomal tissue regresses, and there is replacement by fat. The intralobular tissue is replaced by collagen. Menopausal involution results in reduction of the number of ducts and lobules. Fat intercalates the fibrous separations, so there are no well-defined quadrants or fascial planes. Lymphatic channels are also reduced in number.[6] Only residual islands of ductal tissue remain scattered throughout the fibrous tissue and fat.[101]

Hormones

During menopause the ovarian hormones, estrogen and progesterone, have declined, and the ovarian androgens, androstenedione, testosterone, and dehydroepiandrosterone, become predominant.

Clinical Correlates

Age is considered a prominent risk factor for the development of breast cancer; most breast cancers (nearly two-thirds) are seen in postmenopausal women. As discussed previously, postmenopausal women return to a high percentage of Lob 1, and in nulliparous women these Lob 1 cells have a higher proliferative index than that of parous women. Thus postmenopausal women have ductile and lobular tissues that are more susceptible to interaction with carcinogens. Furthermore, the more highly proliferative cells in nulliparous women add to this risk. Diminished lymphatic capacity in postmenopausal women may impair localization of the sentinel lymph nodes and limit the utility of this technique in this higher risk group of women.[6]

Acknowledgment

We gratefully acknowledge the contribution of J. Harrison Howard and Lynn J. Romrell who authored this chapter in previous editions.

Selected References

1. Russo J, Hu YF, Silva ID, Russo IH. Cancer risk related to mammary gland structure and development. *Microsc Res Tech*. 2001;52:204-223.
2. Macias H, Hinck L. Mammary gland development. Wiley interdisciplinary reviews. *Dev Biol*. 2012;1:533-557. PubMed PMID: 22844349. Pubmed Central PMCID: 3404495.
A full reference list is available online at ExpertConsult.com.

4

Discharges and Secretions of the Nipple

A. MARILYN LEITCH AND RAHEELA ASHFAQ

Introduction and Definitions

Nipple discharge prompts the majority of women to seek immediate attention from their physician. Women view nipple discharge as a potential indicator of breast cancer. Thus it is critical for a physician caring for women with breast disease to have a comprehensive understanding of the physiology of breast secretions and the clinical significance of secretions and discharges. In this chapter, we review the pathophysiology of nipple discharge as well as the significance of breast secretions with respect to the risk of breast cancer. A review of the clinical management and evaluation of nipple discharge follows. This chapter includes a description of methods for collection and preparation of nipple fluid for analysis, ductoscopy, and surgical management of nipple discharge.

The terms *discharge* and *secretion* of the nipple are defined as follows: *discharge* is fluid that extrudes spontaneously from the nipple. *Secretion* refers to fluid present in mammary ducts that can be collected by nipple aspiration or by other means that include conventional breast pump or massage and expression from the ducts (nonspontaneous secretion). *Ductal lavage fluid* refers to the application of saline washing into individual breast ducts with fluid retrieval via a microcatheter device.

The breast is a secretory gland that shows evidence of secretory activity under influence of maternal hormones initiated in in utero and under sex hormones during puberty and adult reproductive life. With the estrogen-progestin hormonal cycle, breast epithelium undergoes cellular proliferation in the estrogenic phase, followed by secretory activity. Breast tissue studies confirm cyclical changes related to follicular and luteal phases. Similar observations on changes in histologic pattern, cellular morphology, mitoses, and DNA content are evident.[1-3] Longacre and Bartow found excessive lymphocytes, duct epithelial degenerative changes, and sloughing into duct lumens in the late secretory and early menstrual phases.[4] Ferguson and Anderson[1] also confirmed cell depletion through a process of apoptosis in this time interval, which peaks on day 28.

Objective measures of breast epithelial cyclical changes can be determined with image cytometry of fine-needle aspiration (FNA) samples. In FNA biopsies, image cytometry assessing five nuclear features—area, circumference, boundary fluctuation, chromatin granularity, and stain intensity—successfully discriminated samples from women in *follicular phase* and those in *luteal phase*.[5] Because the proliferative changes in the *postovulatory phase* can mimic atypia or malignancy, Malberger and colleagues recommended that FNA be used *only* in the *preovulatory phase*. These potentially confusing histologic changes in the sampled cells

should be taken into account when evaluating cytologic features of nipple discharges and nipple fluid aspirates.

The functional unit of the breast is the terminal duct lobular unit (TDLU) (Fig. 4.1). Mammary secretions originate in the lobules. Lobules are connected by the intralobular ducts to the extralobular ductal system, which empties into the lactiferous sinus and onto the vestibule of the nipple. Anatomically, the breast has 15 to 20 segments, each assumed to have unique drainage (Fig. 4.2). Love and Barsky challenged this anatomic concept.[6] Applying several methodologies to study the nipple ducts, it was shown that 90% of nipples contain five to nine ductal orifices distributed in two groups: central and peripheral. The central ducts extend back from the nipple toward the chest wall, and the peripheral ducts extend radially. The separate ductal systems do not connect or anastomose.

Nipple secretion is usually not clinically evident in nonlactating women because keratotic debris obstructs passage into lactiferous sinuses, but secretory material can be seen in the duct lumen in histologic sections of breast tissue. By removing the keratotic debris, the physician may easily obtain nipple fluid from a large proportion of women using a simple nipple aspirator device breast pump or manual expression.[7-10]

Nipple Aspiration Fluid: Characterization and Significance

Many investigators have an interest in intraductal physiology and cytology as an indicator of risk of breast cancer. It is thought that breast cancer results from a cascade of sequential molecular and morphologic events that occur in the ductal epithelial cells. If that process can be detected before transition to a malignant phenotype, there is the opportunity for prevention strategies (Fig. 4.3). The methodologies for obtaining breast secretions and classifying cellular patterns, as well as the biochemical makeup of nipple aspiration fluid (NAF), are discussed in this section.

NAF is a simple, minimally invasive method of sampling histologic alterations within the breast. After cleaning of the nipple orifice to remove keratin plugs, the breast is massaged from the base to the nipple. Using a modified breast pump (Fig. 4.4), suction is applied to elicit the fluid. NAF appears as droplets on the nipple and is collected with small capillary tubes. Samples are usually pooled for examination to improve cellular yield.

Cytologic examination of the breast fluid has long been considered a potential aid in the detection of breast disease. Saphir (1950)[11] and Ringrose (1966)[12] reported the cytologic criteria for the diagnosis of chronic mastitis, intraductal papillomas,

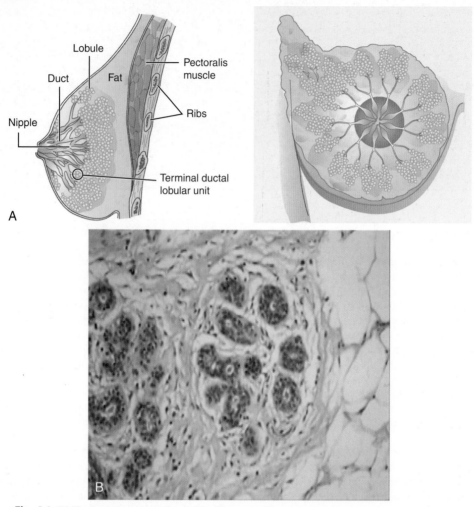

• **Fig. 4.1** (A) The breast duct lobular system. There are 15 to 20 ductal systems per breast. However, more recent studies have determined that the average breast nipple contains five to nine milk pores. Each pore corresponds to a central duct that projects back to the chest wall. Other orifices at the nipple are blind sebaceous glands. The ducts have lateral branches called lobules. At the far end of these branches are the terminal ductal-lobular units, where milk is produced during lactation. Together the duct and the lobules form the ductal-lobular system. During lactation, the system distends with milk. In the absence of lactation, the walls of the empty ducts are collapsed. (B) Histology of the terminal ductal-lobular unit. ([A] Redrawn from art provided courtesy Hologic, Inc. Original images by Jennifer Fairman, CMI.)

and carcinoma based on stained smears of spontaneous nipple discharge.

After the successful application of the cervical smear (Pap smear) for the diagnosis of cervical cancer, George Papanicolaou developed the concept of a "Pap smear" for breast cancer. In 1950 Papanicolaou began a study to investigate normal, atypical, and malignant breast epithelia.[13] In this study, he examined breast aspirates in 917 asymptomatic patients. Using a breast pump, secretions were obtained unilaterally in 171 (18.5%) and bilaterally in 74 (8.1%). Premenopausal women yielded a higher percentage of fluid than postmenopausal women, with the highest percentage found in women 20 to 39 years of age. Four occult carcinomas and one ductal carcinoma in situ (DCIS) were found. Papanicolaou also sought to define "normal" cytologic findings in nipple fluid. The two cell types most often encountered were foam cells and duct epithelial cells. Scant histiocytes and lymphocytes were also present.

In the 1970s, using a modified breast pump, Sartorius and associates attempted nipple aspiration in 1503 women with suspected breast disease and 203 asymptomatic volunteers.[7] They developed the histologic classification to define cytologic changes; it required a minimum of 50 to 100 cells for diagnosis. Diagnostic categories included the following:

- Normal: all duct lining cells uniform in size and staining characteristics
- Hyperplasia: excessive number of ductal groups with multilayering and slight variations in size and shape, but without significant nuclear abnormality and a constant nucleocytoplasmic ratio
- Atypical hyperplasia: criteria similar to that used for hyperplasia but with greater variation in nuclear size and shape, abnormal distribution of chromatin and increased nuclear:cytoplasmic ratio and prominent nucleoli
- Suspected carcinoma: criteria similar to atypical hyperplasia but with marked nuclear abnormality, chromatin clearing, nuclear membrane irregularity, and nucleoli

See Fig. 4.5 for examples of nipple fluid cytology and corresponding histology.

Of the 203 asymptomatic volunteers, NAF was obtained in 163 (80%), with adequate cellular samples obtained in 48.7%. Of the 1503 women with breast disease, NAF with adequate cellularity was obtained in 825 (54.9%); 11.2% yielded fluid without adequate cells. Women 31 to 50 years of age (65%) gave cellular samples, and those older than 60 years of age yielded less fluid. Of the 825 women who yielded fluid, 237 were classified as high risk on the basis of factors such as family history and history of prior breast surgery. A significantly larger percentage of high-risk women had abnormal cytology compared with the normal risk group. This association was seen more frequently in women older than 40 years.

Petrakis and King further validated the association of atypical epithelial cells in NAF of asymptomatic women with histologically confirmed proliferative disease and atypical hyperplasia.[14,15] This finding was particularly evident among women at increased risk for breast cancer. These authors first proposed the finding of atypical cells in NAF as a possible marker to identify women at risk who would need close surveillance.

King and coworkers[16] conducted a cytologic-histologic correlation study of NAF among 82 women with cancer and 237 women subsequently diagnosed with benign breast disease. In this analysis of 134 samples (34 cancer; 100 noncancer), patients met the criteria for the presence of a minimum of 10 cells. Atypical hyperplasia in NAF was present in 80% of cancers and 39% of benign breast diseases. The diagnosis of cancer was made in only 21% of the cases. NAF was proposed as a novel approach to study breast cancer precursors but was not considered a diagnostic tool. Factors that affect NAF production in nonlactating women include age, existing proliferative breast disease, previous breast biopsy, and family history of breast cancer.

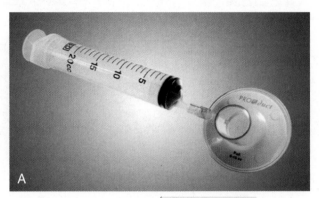

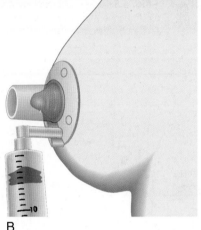

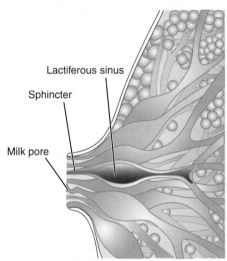

• **Fig. 4.2** Anatomy of the breast duct. Within the duct, 1 to 2 cm beneath the surface of the nipple, is the lactiferous sinus. The duct also has a tiny sphincter. (Redrawn from art provided courtesy Hologic, Inc. Original images by Jennifer Fairman, CMI.)

• **Fig. 4.4** (A) Breast pump used for obtaining nipple aspirate fluid. (B) Nipple aspiration using a modified pump. Gentle suction is applied to draw the fluid. ([B] Redrawn from art provided courtesy Hologic, Inc. Original images by Jennifer Fairman, CMI.)

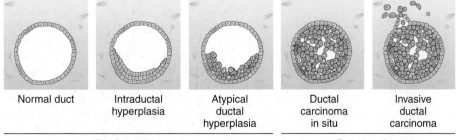

| Normal duct | Intraductal hyperplasia | Atypical ductal hyperplasia | Ductal carcinoma in situ | Invasive ductal carcinoma |

Predict and prevent   Detect and treat

• **Fig. 4.3** Multistep pathogenesis of breast cancer. Breast cancer is believed to be the result of the progressive molecular and morphologic changes that develop in ductal epithelial cells. These changes have been studied extensively. (Redrawn from art provided courtesy Hologic, Inc. Original images by Jennifer Fairman, CMI.)

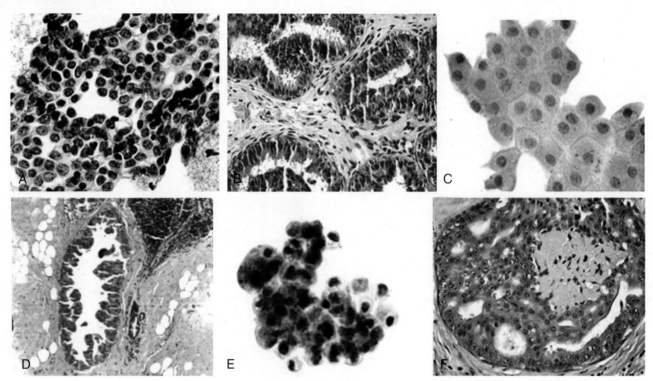

• **Fig. 4.5** Nipple fluid cytology and corresponding histology. (A) and (B) Epithelial hyperplasia. (C) and (D) Apocrine metaplasia. (E) and (F) High-grade ductal carcinoma in situ. (Courtesy David Euhus, MD, UT Southwestern Medical Center.)

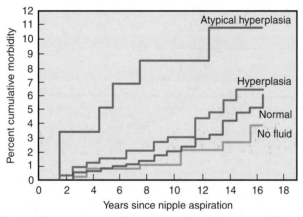

• **Fig. 4.6** The occurrence of breast cancer in relation to the findings on cytology of nipple aspiration fluid. (From Wrensch MR, Petrakis NL, King EB, et al, Breast cancer incidence in women with abnormal cytology in nipple aspirates of breast fluid. *Am J Epidemiol*. 1992;135:130-141.)

In a large prospective trial to determine breast cancer risk in relation to NAF, Wrensch and coworkers enrolled 2701 nonlactating women between 1973 and 1980 and reported their long-term follow-up (average, 12.7 years) in 1991.[17] In this study, women who did not yield any fluid were described as the referent group because they represent the lowest risk of developing breast cancer. With follow-up at 87%, the study confirmed that women with atypical hyperplasia were 4.9 times more likely to develop breast cancer compared with non–NAF-producing patients; this risk was 2.8 times more likely compared with women with normal cytology (Fig. 4.6). The increase in the risk of breast cancer with abnormal cytology was more pronounced in younger (25–54

years) versus older (>55 years) women. Women with atypical NAF and family history of breast cancer were six times more likely to develop breast cancer than women with atypical hyperplasia but without a family history of breast cancer. The study concluded that women with cytologic diagnosis of atypical hyperplasia experienced a significant increase in risk of developing breast cancer.

In 2001 Wrensch and colleagues reported their findings on extended follow-up of 3627 volunteers.[18] This study demonstrated that 3.5% of women developed breast cancer (median of 12 years follow-up), and 7.8% developed cancer in the median of 21 years follow-up. Women with NAF production were more likely to develop breast cancer than the non–NAF-producing group. This long-term follow-up data upheld their previous findings of increased risk for developing breast cancer related to abnormal cytology.

Sauter and associates used a modified breast pump to collect NAF in 177 patients with a success rate of 94%; evaluable cytology was obtained in 95%.[19] NAF cytology correlated with increased risk of breast cancer. Birth control pills, hormone replacement therapy, or phase of menstrual cycle had no influence on NAF production. These authors were successful in obtaining NAF in postmenopausal women and advocated the use of NAF as a screening tool and as a marker for chemoprevention.

Biochemical Composition of Nipple Aspiration Fluid

The noncellular component of the NAF has been studied for a number of biochemical substances and biomarkers. In a prospective study of patients planned for excisional breast biopsy, NAF was evaluated for candidate proteins such as prostate-specific antigen (PSA), human glandular kallikrein (hK2), basic fibroblast growth factor (bFGF), and cellular markers such as S-phase fraction, as well as for DNA index and cytology.[20] The best breast cancer predictive model included cytology, bFGF, and age (88% sensitivity; 57% specificity). Incorporation of menopausal status to predict the optimal model of breast cancer indicates NAF hK2 or PSA and age to be 100% sensitive and 41% specific in premenopausal versus 93% sensitive and 12% specific in postmenopausal women.

Subsequently, the focus for NAF has shifted from studying healthy volunteers or women with benign breast disease for comparison of NAF from a breast with cancer to the healthy contralateral breast. Kuerer and coworkers prospectively determined the concentration of extracellular domain of Her2 in affected versus nonaffected breasts and found NAF Her2 levels to be highly correlative ($r = 0.302$; $p = .038$); tumors that overexpressed Her2 had higher Her2 levels in the affected versus the nonaffected breast.[21] Zhang and colleagues reported that microarray profiling of nipple discharge for microRNAs (miRNAs) revealed that three miRNAs were upregulated and three miRNAs were downregulated in intraductal carcinoma breast cancer patients compared with those with benign papilloma.[22] In addition, NAF contains chemical substances of exogenous origin, such as caffeine, nicotine, pesticides, and orally ingested drugs. Approximately 10% of NAF samples have substances with mutagenic activity that could portend the development of breast cancer.[23] These types of analyses may serve as potential diagnostic tools for breast cancer.

Minimally Invasive Techniques for Determining Risk of Breast Cancer

Ductal Lavage

Although quite promising, NAF cytology has major limitations in clinical screening because of the inconsistency of adequate cellular yield and the presumption that nipple aspiration fails to harvest cells from the distal portion of the duct-lobular system. To overcome these limitations, a new approach was developed in 1999 that allows collection of higher numbers of exfoliated cells from the TDLU. The ductal lavage (DL) procedure involves nipple aspiration using a modified suction cup to localize the NAF-yielding ducts. NAF-yielding ducts can subsequently be localized and cannulated using a microcatheter (Hologic, Bedford, MA). Fluid-yielding ducts are infused with normal saline. Ductal effluent collected through the microcatheter is then analyzed cytologically (Fig. 4.7).

The DL technique was first attempted during a breast duct endoscopy study in which dilators were introduced into the ducts. Thereafter, a cannula (outer diameter, 0.4 mm) was inserted into the duct and saline was injected to wash the ductal lumen.[24] The washings were collected and studied cytologically. The technique was later refined with special development of a double-lumen catheter. Dooley and colleagues designed a prospective multicenter study to compare DL and nipple aspiration with regard to safety, tolerability, and outcomes for detection of abnormal cells.[25] The effluent was collected and cytologic preparations were performed using the Millipore technique (also used in early NAF studies). The study enrolled 507 women, 291 (57%) of whom had a history of breast cancer and 199 (39%) had a Gail risk of breast cancer of 1.7%. The minimum age was 52 years. Overall, the procedure was tolerated well. NAF was obtained in 417 women, and DL was performed in 383. On average, the NAF had 120 epithelial cells compared with 13,200 epithelial cells in the DL samples. Greater cellularity and high diagnostic yield was also noted in DL samples. Importantly, atypia was diagnosed in 24% of the DL versus 10% of NAF

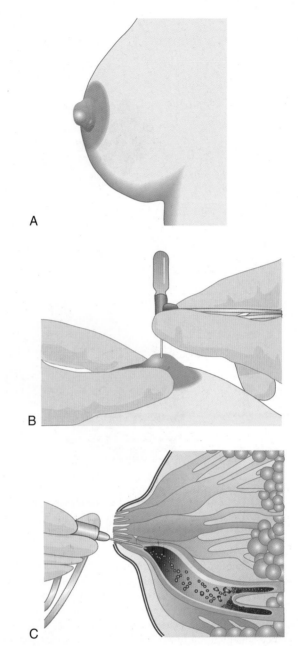

A

B

C

• **Fig. 4.7** (A) to (C) Ductal lavage technique. Once the ductal orifice has been located by the presence of a nipple aspirate fluid droplet, a flexible microcatheter is inserted about 1.5 cm into the duct through the duct's natural opening on the nipple surface. One to two cubic centimeters of lidocaine is then infused intraductally through the catheter to anesthetize the duct. Sometimes, to facilitate cannulation, the ductal orifice is first enlarged with multiple dilators. (Redrawn from art provided courtesy Hologic, Inc. Original images by Jennifer Fairman, CMI.)

samples. Only ducts yielding NAF were targeted for DL (average 1.5 ducts/breast were lavaged).

Ductal Lavage Procedure. Preparation for the DL procedure is labor- and time-intensive; the technique requires breast massage for 30 minutes. A topical anesthetic (2.5% lidocaine and 2.5% prilocaine [EMLA]) is applied. Keratin plugs are removed from the nipple. The nipple suction device is used to obtain NAF and localize the ducts that can be cannulated. A grid can be used to record the location of the ducts for future reference. Usually 5 to 10 mL of saline are infused, collected, and submitted to a cytology

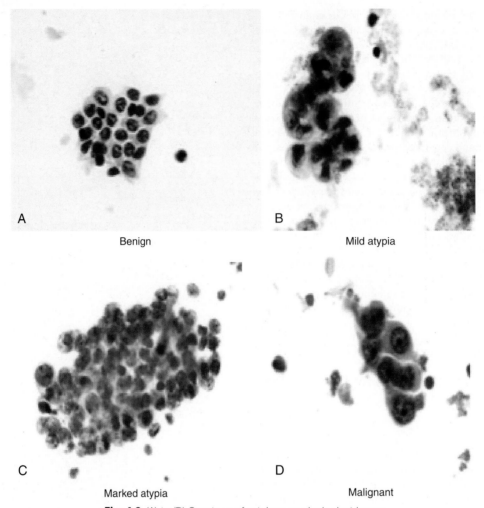

Benign

Mild atypia

Marked atypia

Malignant

• **Fig. 4.8** (A) to (D) Spectrum of cytology on nipple duct lavage.

laboratory in CytoLyt (Cytyc) solution. In the laboratory, a Thin-Prep slide can be prepared and stained using the routine Papanicolaou stain. The diagnostic categories used for reporting DL cytology were developed by Wrensch and coworkers[17] and were further refined using the National Cancer Institute Consensus Conference Statement on breast FNAs.[26] The categories included the following:

- Insufficient cellular material for diagnosis: A minimum of 10 epithelial cells should be present per slide. The presence of macrophages alone does not render a specimen diagnostic.
- Benign: Samples categorized as benign contain 10 or more epithelial cells and variable number of other cellular components such as squamous cells, lymphocytes, and foamy macrophages. The benign duct epithelial cells are 10 to 15 μm in diameter and have a cyanophilic cytoplasm that may contain fine vacuoles. Ductal cells are more easily recognized in groups than in single cells, which are difficult to differentiate from lymphocytes. Cells may be arranged in monolayer sheets or strands.
- Mild atypia: In mild atypia, there is nuclear enlargement 1.5 to 3 times the normal ductal cell, and higher nuclear-cytoplasmic ratio. The nucleus may be hyperchromatic or hypochromatic and there may be nucleoli. Multilayering or complex and papillary architectural groups may be present and usually indicate hyperplastic changes.

- Marked atypia: The preceding abnormalities are more pronounced, nucleoli are more prominent, and nuclear membrane irregularities are easily appreciable.
- Malignant cells: Malignant cells on DL have obvious features of malignancy with high nuclear-cytoplasmic ratio, hyperchromasia, macronucleoli, and dyshesion (Figs. 4.8 and 4.9).

The diagnosis of malignancy on DL is uncommon because the large majority of women who undergo the procedure have no palpable or mammographic abnormality. Occasionally, however, a high-grade DCIS may be diagnosed in this manner. In Dooley's study, less than 1% of cases were diagnosed as malignant.[25]

Limitations of Ductal Lavage. The procedure is not widely available. The cost of disposables is high. Special expertise and training is required for the performance of DL. Cytologic interpretation may be variable and training is required for pathologists to become familiar with DL cytology. DL detects milder atypia than NAF (17% vs. 6%). It remains to be seen, however, as in NAF, whether mild atypia poses an increased risk. The negative predictive value (NPV) of the procedure is not known (i.e., number of women at increased risk with negative DL who will develop breast cancer).

There are also important limitations to the nipple DL (NDL) methodology. Maddux and colleagues evaluated the atypia rate by NDL fluid-producing ducts compared with non–fluid-producing ducts and the atypia rate in high-risk versus low-risk patients.[27]

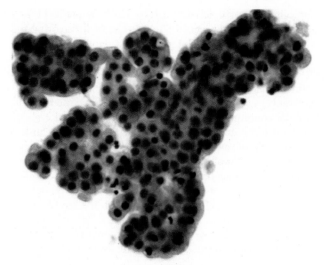

• **Fig. 4.9** Cytologic features of intraductal papilloma on nipple duct lavage.

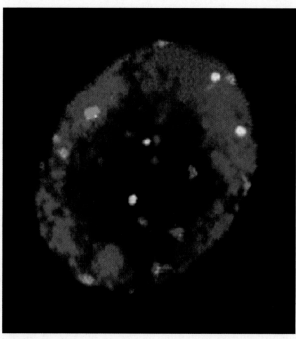

• **Fig. 4.10** Interphase fluorescent in situ hybridization for chromosomes 1 and 8. Chromosomes 11 and 17 can be used to determine aneusomy in breast cells. Normal cells are usually diploid, whereas malignant cells are aneuploid.

Fifty-five women with 226 ducts were lavaged, resulting in 136 ducts producing fluid versus 90 ducts producing no fluid. Of these, 44% had a Gail risk index greater than or equal to 1.7, and 56% had a Gail risk index less than 1.7. Cytologic atypia was diagnosed in 34% of patients. The cytologic atypia rate was not statistically different in low-risk versus high-risk women based on a Gail index (33% vs. 35%; $p = 1$) or fluid-producing versus non–fluid-producing ducts (19% vs. 15%; $p = .61$), respectively. In this study, there was a higher atypia rate for fluid-producing ducts versus non–fluid-producing ducts (32% vs. 11%) in women at high-risk (Gail risk ≥1.7).

Another limitation of NDL is the lack of studies related to the performance characteristics of the procedure. It is possible that some atypical lavages may reflect underlying atypical hyperplasia, whereas others may reflect reversible physiologic changes. Johnson-Maddux and associates proposed that persistent lavage atypia may be related to underlying pathology such as atypical duct hyperplasia, whereas reversible atypia may be associated with physiologic changes.[28] In a reproducibility study for NDL, Maddux and associates found marked atypia in 36% of breasts with incident carcinoma and in 24% of benign breasts ($p = .19$). However, marked atypia was diagnosed more frequently in breasts with an incident carcinoma (22%) than in unaffected breasts (7%; $p = .01$). Interestingly, the insufficient sample rate was higher for ducts in breasts with an incident carcinoma (40%) than for ducts in breasts unaffected with carcinoma (27%; $p = .06$). Thirty-two patients with atypical lavage from the unaffected breast underwent repeat lavage at median 8.3 months, with atypia occurring in only 48%. The number of duct orifices presents a challenge in reidentification with repeat lavage. Reproducibility is also affected by variables such as hormonal changes and number of cells and cytologic interpretation. The insufficient rate on repeat lavage was 29%. The higher prevalence of lavage atypia, along with low reproducibility, limits the use of a single NDL in predicting high risk of breast carcinoma.

Ductal Lavage and Molecular Markers. In addition to routine cytology, DL may permit analysis of molecular markers associated with breast carcinoma.[29] Cytologic preparations of DL can be used for immunocytochemical analysis. Molecular cytogenetics analysis by King and colleagues on 39 paired cases of DL

and surgically excised breast lesions revealed interphase fluorescent in situ hybridization (FISH) cytogenetic changes on chromosomes 1, 8, 11, and/or 17 in 10 of 14 (71%) malignant tumors versus 2 of 18 (11%) from benign neoplasms (Fig. 4.10).[30] This study confirms the potential utility of FISH as a future adjunctive technique. In another study by Yamamoto and associates, DL was performed in women with nipple discharge and abnormal ductography.[31] None of the samples collected from 54 benign cases showed aneusomy for chromosomes 1, 11, and 17, giving a specificity of 100%, whereas aneusomy of at least three of these chromosomes was seen in all six malignant cases. In the future, the adjunctive use of FISH may be helpful in improving the discriminatory value of cytology.

Similarly, Evron and coworkers performed methylation-specific polymerase chain reaction (PCR), or MSP, for cyclin D2, RAR B, and Twist genes on DL specimens.[32] At least one of the genes was methylated in 96% of surgically excised primary tumors and 57% of DCIS, but not in normal breast tissue, resulting in high sensitivity and specificity. Thirty-seven women with biopsy-proven cancers underwent DL. On MSP, 17 of 20 women (85%) also had at least one gene methylated in the DL sample. All four women with negative DL were additionally observed to be negative by MSP. These data demonstrate the feasibility for the early detection of molecular markers in DL, which may play a role in the early detection of breast cancer.

Euhus and colleagues measured the prevalence of tumor suppressor gene methylation by quantitative multiplex methylation-specific PCR (QM-MSP) for cyclin D_2, APC, HIN1, RASSF1A, and RAR-β2.[33] Methylation of at least two genes correlated with marked atypia in univariate analysis but not in multivariate analysis that was adjusted for sample cellularity and risk group stratification. This study concluded that both methylation and marked atypia are independently associated with highly cellular sampling,

Gail index, and personal history of breast cancer. On the basis of cytology and methylation profiles, Euhus and colleagues concluded that NDL ipsilateral to a breast cancer rarely retrieves cancer cells (9%). It is apparent that NDL does not seem to be suitable for early detection of focal lesions such as carcinoma, and addition of molecular biomarkers does not resolve this issue. However, NDL may be useful for detection of more diffuse risk-associated field changes in the breast. Cytologic assessment of QM-MSP analysis of NDL samples may provide an approach for identifying high-risk women for monitoring the effects of chemopreventive strategies to reduce the risk of cancer.

Ongoing investigations are exploring the proteome for unique signatures that can be exploited for diagnosis as well as risk determination. High throughput proteomic technologies such as surface-enhanced laser desorption and ionization time of flight (SELDI-TOF) mass spectrometry have been used in a number of studies to generate unique signatures expressed in cancerous breasts and normal breasts. Using SELDI-TOF to examine NAF in 12 women with breast cancer and 15 healthy control participants, Paweletz and associates identified unique proteomic patterns that were discriminatory between the two groups.[34] Using gel-based proteomics, Kuerer and coworkers detected 30 to 202 qualitative protein expression differences in NAF in the breast with cancer compared with the contralateral breast without cancer in the same patient.[35] Varnum and colleagues identified 64 proteins in NAF, including osteopontin and cathepsin D, which have been previously documented to vary with breast cancer status.[36]

Random Periareolar Fine-Needle Aspiration

Recognizing the limitations of approaching the ductal system for fluid retrieval to assess risk of breast cancer, investigators have looked for approaches to identify cellular predictors of breast cancer risk. Random periareolar FNA (RPFNA) is based on the premise that a widespread proliferative change in the breast might be detected by the technique.[37] Rather than detecting specific ducts that produce NAF, RPFNA detects field effect with the underlying presumption that women with atypia on RPFNA have a high density of proliferative changes and possess a higher *short-term risk* for breast cancer compared with women without atypia. RPFNA can be performed on four quadrants or even two quadrants as proposed by Fabian and associates using local anesthesia, 21-gauge needle and a 12-mL syringe prewetted with RPM1.[38] Four to five aspirations are performed. Samples are pooled and can be expressed directly into CytoLyt solution plus 1% of buffered formalin. The cell pellet is transferred to PreservCyt solution and monolayer slides prepared. In nonproliferative samples, cellularity ranges from 100 to 499 cells, and only one to two slides can be prepared, whereas in proliferative lesions cellularity exceeds 5000 cells. The procedure is low in cost and generally well tolerated with few minor complications.

Fabian found that RPFNA revealed nonproliferative cytology in 30% of cases, hyperplasia in 49%, and hyperplasia with atypia in 21%. Premenopausal women and postmenopausal women on hormone replacement therapy have a higher rate of atypia on RPFNA than postmenopausal women. With a median follow-up of 45 months, women with RPFNA atypical hyperplasia were more likely to have developed DCIS or invasive carcinoma than women without atypia. This incidence, based on Gail risk scores, was 15% for high-risk versus 4% for low-risk groups.[37] The technique is limited by high interobserver variance in the cytologic interpretation. Masood and coworkers developed a six-category cytology scoring index depending on the degree of abnormality.[39]

Nonproliferative samples scored 6 to 10, hyperplasia 11 to 14, and hyperplasia with atypia 15 to 18. Use of this scoring index has been shown to reduce interobserver variability.

Summary

The intraductal approach for diagnosis and risk assessment of breast cancer is a theoretically attractive strategy. The availability of cellular components for cytologic examination and evaluation with novel techniques provide an interesting paradigm in breast evaluation. Nipple aspiration and RPFNA are the least expensive methodologies. Nipple aspiration is limited by low cellularity, whereas RPFNA may have issues related to patient tolerability of the procedure as well as operator skill issues. DL, although more invasive, produces highly cellular material in the sample, has not been widely adopted because the procedure is expensive and dilution of the material may interfere with biomarker assays. These techniques remain investigational for risk assessment.

Clinical Evaluation and Management of the Patient With Nipple Discharge

When a patient presents with nipple discharge, the physician must approach evaluation and treatment in a systematic fashion taking into account the patient's history and presentation features, the probability of an underlying malignancy versus a benign condition, and additional data found on workup.

Frequency and Etiology of Nipple Discharge

Spontaneous nipple discharge is the chief complaint in 3% to 6% of women presenting to breast specialty services.[40] In a series of 10,000 encounters, Seltzer reported that only 3% were the result of nipple discharge.[41] Of those, one-third occurred in women older than 50 years. However, nipple discharge may not always be reported by the patient. Newman and colleagues found spontaneous discharge in 10% of 2685 women seen for routine examination.[42] The great majority of nipple discharges are caused by benign conditions (Table 4.1).[43–57] Papillomas or papillomatosis are the most frequent causes of pathologic nipple discharge, which has been consistent over time from the earliest studies to the present. The frequency of cancer as the etiology of nipple discharge varies in reported series. This may be related to the nature of the institutional practice and whether it is heavily weighted to cancer patients. Also, in some series, the patients ultimately undergoing surgery were highly selected and thus would be expected to have a higher proportion of cancers. In the series reported by Florio and colleagues, only those patients with abnormal cytology had surgical resection of the duct.[49] Cabioglu and coworkers studied patients presenting with nipple discharge to the University of Texas MD Anderson Cancer Center and found that 20% were diagnosed with cancer.[50] The incidence of cancer in patients with nipple discharge is lower in other series.[40,45,51,53] Benign papillomas and duct ectasia are more common in younger women, and cancer is more common in older women.[46]

The clinical significance of nipple discharge and the appropriate decision-making for its management is most important in the absence of a palpable mass. Cancers infrequently present as an isolated discharge. Chaudary and coworkers reported that only 16 of 2476 (0.6%) cancers presented with isolated discharge.[58] Devitt reported discharge associated with 2% of all breast cancers.[59]

TABLE
4.1 **Etiology of Pathologic Nipple Discharge**

Study	No. of Patients	Cancer (%)	Papilloma/ Papillomatosis (%)	Duct Ectasia/ Fibrocystic Conditions (%)	Atypia (%)	Other Benign Conditions (%)
Adair, 1930[43]	108	47.2	45.3	—	—	7.4
Madalin et al., 1957[44]	100	1	58	25	—	16
Urban and Egeli, 1978[45]	435	8	45	36.5	—	10.5
Murad et al., 1982[46]	267	21	35	42	—	—
Leis, 1989[47]	586	14.3	48.1	4.8	18.2	14.6
Dawes et al., 1998[48]	39	12.8	64.1	23.1	—	—
Florio et al.,[a] 1999[49]	94	26.6	59.5	2.1	—	11.8
Cabioglu et al., 2003[50]	94	20.2	66	—	—	13.8
Lau et al., 2005[51]	118	9.3	57.6	—	—	33.1
Adepoju et al., 2005[52]	168	12	48	14	11	16
Vargas et al., 2006[40]	68	5.8	57	32.4	—	4.4
Richards et al., 2007[53]	86	2	29	69	—	—
Montroni et al., 2010[54]	915	23.9	—	—	—	—
Morrogh et al., 2010[55]	287	23	42	15	10	9
Dupont et al., 2015[56]	311	17	56	—	—	—
Yang et al., 2015[57]	208	26	40	19	—	14

[a]Only patients with suspicious cytology had operative intervention.

Seltzer found that 9% of patients older than 50 years of age presenting with nipple discharge had breast cancer compared with only 1% of those younger than 50 years of age.[41]

Intraductal Papilloma

Papillomas are benign epithelial lesions growing within ducts. Most common is the solitary intraductal papilloma located in the major ducts near the nipple. Papillary lesions of the breast represent a spectrum of disease that can be challenging to differentiate on pathology. A papilloma may have an area of atypical hyperplasia. Histologically, papillomas are arborizing lesions with papillary fronds and a fibrovascular core, lined by epithelial and myoepithelial cells (Fig. 4.11).[60] The papillary fronds are friable, accounting for the production of bloody nipple discharge.

Less common are peripheral papillomas. Ohuchi and colleagues reported that 6 of 25 patients with multiple peripheral papillomas had associated DCIS.[61] In their series of 77 patients with papillary lesions, Cardenosa and Eklund found that 18% of patients have multiple peripheral papillomas.[62] Only one of these patients had nipple discharge as a presenting symptom.

Nipple adenoma or florid papillomatosis of the terminal portion of lactiferous ducts is also associated with bloody nipple discharge. Occasionally, intraductal papillary carcinoma and invasive ductal carcinoma may arise in nipple adenomas.

Duct Ectasia

Ectasia is a dilation of ducts with loss of elastin in duct walls and the presence of chronic inflammatory cells, especially plasma cells,

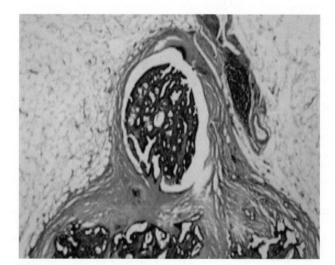

• **Fig. 4.11** Papilloma. Note the arborizing fronds of an intraductal papilloma lined by epithelial cells.

around duct walls. Theories of causation range from transudation of secretions sequestered in ducts dilated from previous pregnancy to primary periductal inflammation. Microscopically, the ductal epithelium is not hyperplastic and may be thinned out or completely absent. Sloughed epithelium may be seen in ductal lumens. Lipid-laden foamy histiocytes can be seen within the duct lumen and in adjacent stroma. Intraepithelial histiocytes can also be

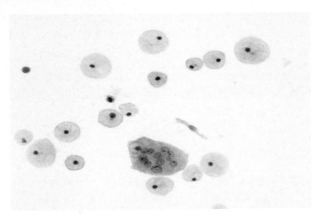

• **Fig. 4.12** Cytologic examination of the nipple discharge may reveal foamy histiocytes only.

seen.[63] Cytologically/histologically, the duct contents comprise proteinaceous debris, lipid-containing histiocytes (Fig. 4.12), cholesterol crystals, and calcification (duct ectasia).

Nipple discharges associated with duct ectasia have been shown to have bacteria (*Enterococcus,* anaerobic *Streptococcus, Staphylococcus aureus,* and *Bacteroides*) in 60% to 88% of cases.[64,65] Whether infection is the primary cause or a secondary colonization is debated. Duct ectasia does not indicate predisposition to cancer.

Lactational Bloody Nipple Discharge

Pregnancy is associated with significant proliferative alterations in the breast tissue. The "normal" cytology of breast secretions during pregnancy is characterized by increased cellularity compared with the resting breast, particularly in the late months of pregnancy. Cell types are the same as those found in the absence of pregnancy but show some differences in the proportions of various cells. Epithelial cell clusters are numerous and sometimes possess a configuration suggesting a papillary structure. In the late third trimester and after childbirth, neutrophils are abundant.

Holmquist and Papanicolaou found an unexpectedly large number of ductal epithelial cells in patients during pregnancy and lactation.[66] The groups of cells were papillary in structure and similar to papillary fronds from intraductal papilloma. Kline and Lash studied the cytology of breast secretions obtained during the third trimester from 50 pregnant women (16–39 years of age).[67] This study was prompted by the erroneous interpretation of cytologic findings during pregnancy based on the papillary groupings and changes similar to those described by Holmquist and Papanicolaou. In the Kline and Lash study, 43 of the 50 women had papillary groupings, whereas the remaining seven had only foam cells and leukocytes. Tissue from four biopsies obtained in the third trimester of pregnancy revealed "tufts" of cells forming "spurs" or invaginations into duct and alveolar lumens with similar structures that were desquamated into lumina and were similar to clusters of cells found in the breast secretions. The observed "spurs" were closely associated with the formation of new alveoli. Delicate capillary networks within these tufts of cells could be easily traumatized, causing blood to appear in breast secretions.

Blood may be found in secretions from pregnant and lactating patients in the absence of clinically significant lesions.[67,68] Thus it is reasonable to observe bloody nipple discharges in pregnant or lactating women but confirmation of the absence of suspicious clinical or radiologic findings is necessary.

Nonbreast Etiology

Prolactinemia from a pituitary adenoma may initiate nipple discharge. Although discharge has been reported in nearly one-half of patients with pituitary adenomas, the incidence of prolactin tumors in patients with discharge is low. A 2.2% incidence of pituitary neoplasms was reported by Newman and colleagues.[42] Normal serum prolactin levels are less than or equal 20 mcg/L. If values are repeatedly elevated, contrasted magnetic resonance imaging (MRI) of the head should be performed, with pituitary images obtained to evaluate for a mass lesion.[69] Patients with only moderate elevation often have normal radiologic results, but they should be followed closely. With advanced prolactin tumors, patients may experience loss of visual fields and report a history of infertility.

Because the breast lacks a biological feedback mechanism, prolonged secretory responses may follow short, often unrecognized, surges in circulating prolactin. Transient rises in prolactin may explain the nipple discharge seen with breast and nipple stimulation, chest trauma, or after thoracotomy. Prolactin elevations can also occur in patients with renal or hepatic failure due to reduced prolactin clearance and with primary hypothyroidism.

Psychotropic drugs (e.g., phenothiazines, reserpine, risperidone, methyldopa, selective serotonin reuptake inhibitors, monoamine oxidase inhibitors) can induce galactorrhea. Other medications such as dopaminergic blockers (e.g., metoclopramide), some antihypertensive agents, reserpine and verapamil, opiates, and H2 receptor blockers may also cause elevation of prolactin. The discharge stops after discontinuation of drug usage and may not return with smaller doses.

History

In assessing the clinical significance of a nipple discharge, it is important to take a detailed history to characterize the nature and origin of the discharge. The most important factor in the history is whether the discharge is spontaneous or elicited. The index of suspicion for a pathologic discharge is greater when the patient complains of a spontaneous discharge, which she may first note as a stain on her clothing. In the past, patient education in breast self-examination has emphasized observation for a nipple discharge as a sign of cancer. Women often manipulate the nipple quite vigorously to check for a discharge. It is common that one or more drops of liquid can be expressed from about half of women during their reproductive years. Generally, a discharge that occurs only with manipulation does not require further evaluation. However, the presence of a significant amount of clear, bloody, or serous fluid on a routine physical examination with compression or during a mammogram requires further evaluation. If the discharge occurred when the patient manipulated the breast, it may be instructive to the examiner to have the patient demonstrate the discharge.

It is also important to ascertain whether the discharge is bilateral or unilateral or comes from a single duct or multiple ducts. The color and consistency of the observed discharge should be noted. The patient should be queried as to whether the discharge was associated with painful swelling of the breast, a mass, skin changes or nipple deformities.

Breast discharge can be a response to a variety of stimuli other than underlying breast disease. It is necessary to query the patient with regard to trauma to the breast or chest wall and to take a detailed history of current medications. The patient should be asked about a known history of endocrine problems.

Examination

Examination should identify the duct or ducts producing the discharge, its color and nature, and the location of the trigger point (quadrant of origin) that on compression causes the discharge. The patient should be carefully examined for other signs of breast pathology such as a mass, skin changes of the nipple-areola complex, nipple inversion, or retraction. The examiner should ascertain whether the discharge is from multiple or single ducts. Discharges from multiple ducts are rarely malignant, whereas a single-duct discharge is more likely to be related to malignancy. Ciatto and colleagues report that single-duct discharge has a relative risk of 4.07 (confidence interval, 2.7–6.0) of malignancy compared with an asymptomatic population.[70] Multiductal or bilateral discharges have breast cancer risk similar to that of the general population. Murad and associates report that none of their patients with cancer had bilateral discharges.[46]

Leis and coworkers describe four types of discharge—serous, serosanguineous, sanguineous, and watery—that in ascending frequency (6.3%, 11.9%, 24%, and 45.5%, respectively) are more likely to be associated with cancer.[47] Although only 24% of bloody discharges were associated with a cancer, 45% of all of the cancers did have a bloody discharge. In a review of 386 nipple discharges without associated mass, 177 (46%) were bloody. Of patients with benign disease, 38% had bloody discharge, compared with 69% in women with carcinoma. Funderburk and Syphax found serous or bloody fluid in 107 of 167 of samples (63%) and milky, colored, or clear fluid in 61 of 167 (37%).[71] The serous or bloody fluids were associated with carcinoma, papilloma or other papillary lesions in 74% of cases (78 of 106); fibrocystic changes in 22%; and duct ectasia, drugs, and other conditions in 4%. The majority (94%) of discharges with secretory components were associated with fibrocystic change and other nonproliferative breast lesions, whereas only 6% (4 of 61) were associated with papilloma.

Elicited fluid should be tested for occult blood even if it appears nonbloody. Chaudary's group tested for heme with laboratory test sticks (as used for urine dip testing).[58] Test sticks detect as few as 5 to 15 red blood cells/mL, which would not be visible as bloody fluid. All 16 patients with cancer had hemoglobin in nipple secretions; however, positive predictive value (PPV) is low because 107 of 132 intraductal papillomas and 67 of 94 duct ectasias also had hemoglobin in the discharge.

Single-duct discharges typically have a trigger point on the breast where pressure induces a discharge. This trigger point should be identified and documented in the patient's chart before planning surgery (see subsequent discussion). The patient is examined in a standard position, preferably supine with the ipsilateral hand behind the head. Direct digital pressure is then applied to sequential points around the areola by the examiner until the site where pressure elicits the maximum discharge is identified. It is rarely necessary to squeeze the nipple to elicit a pathologic nipple discharge. Should the physician be unable to elicit the discharge, the patient can be asked to squeeze the nipple in a final attempt to elicit the discharge. This makes the examination less traumatic to the patient.

Clinical breast examination is important to identify palpable lesions because discharge with an associated mass is more likely to be due to a cancer. Devitt found in his series of patients with discharge that 8 of 10 women with cancer had palpable masses; 1 patient had nipple distortion but no mass.[59] Leis and associates reported palpable masses in 88% of 67 patients with nipple discharge and cancer.[47] Florio and coworkers report cancer in only 10% of women with discharge and a mass.[49] Cabioglu and associates reported that six of 19 women with malignant nipple discharge had a mass on physical examination.[50] Morrogh and coworkers at the Memorial Sloan Kettering Cancer Center identified cancer in 25 of 37 women (62%) with discharge who had a palpable mass.[55]

Imaging Evaluation

Mammography and Ultrasound

There is controversy regarding the extent of radiographic workup that is warranted to evaluate nipple discharge. When radiographic studies are negative, one cannot assume that there is no intraductal pathology. Mammography should be performed in all patients with nipple discharge to seek a focal occult lesion and/or to characterize an abnormality identified on physical examination. The mammogram may be normal in as many as 80% to 93% of patients with spontaneous nipple discharge.[55,57,72] Mammographic findings include benign-appearing circumscribed masses of various sizes (typically retroareolar in location), a solitary dilated retroareolar duct, and calcifications (Fig. 4.13).

Ultrasound. Ultrasound of the central breast can be performed to identify dilated ducts with intraductal lesions. However, it is critical to have confidence that the lesion identified by ultrasound is in fact associated with the discharge. Cabioglu and associates identified sonographic abnormalities in 40% of patients with papilloma and in 60% of patients with cancers.[50] An abnormal ultrasound was associated with a 5.5-fold relative risk for breast cancer in patients with a nipple discharge. Rissanen and coworkers assessed the value of ultrasound in localizing intraductal lesions in patients with nipple discharge.[73] Ultrasound demonstrated intraductal lesions in 36 of 52 patients (69%), ductal dilatation in 6 patients (12%), and no lesion in 10 patients (19%). Although only 20% of malignant lesions demonstrated an ultrasound abnormality, 80% of papillomatous lesions were associated with an ultrasound abnormality. In a study of 198 patients

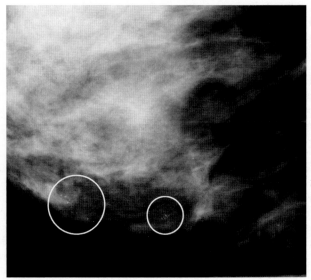

• **Fig. 4.13** Mammogram in a patient with spontaneous copious nipple discharge. Microcalcifications are suspicious and in area of tortuous ducts identified on ductogram. Final pathology is ductal carcinoma in situ. (Courtesy Phil Evans, MD, UT Southwestern Medical Center.)

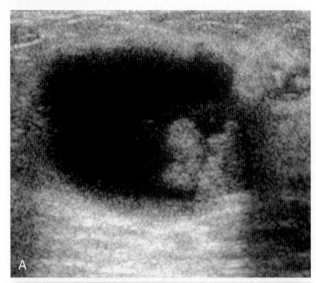

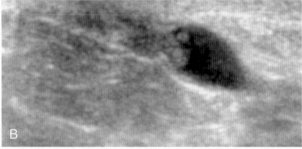

• **Fig. 4.14** (A) Ultrasound showing intracystic papilloma. (B) Ultrasound showing intraductal papilloma filling a duct. (Courtesy Ralph Wynn, MD, UT Southwestern Medical Center.)

with nipple discharge who underwent ultrasound evaluation, the imaging results were negative in 97 (49.0%) and positive in 101 (51.0%) patients. The malignancy rates for the Breast Imaging Reporting and Data System (BI-RADS) categories of the ultrasound were 0.0% for category 1, 5.9% for category 2, 9.4% for category 3, 21.5% for category 4 and 100.0% for category 5.[74] These authors note that 89 (44.9%) of the 198 patients with nipple discharge were able to avoid invasive diagnostic procedures such as galactography or surgery for diagnosis. Pathologic diagnosis was obtained by ultrasound -guided biopsy instead. When ultrasound abnormalities are identified, they should be localized before the surgical procedure to ensure the removal of the lesion. Examples of intraductal lesions seen on ultrasound are shown in Fig. 4.14.

Magnetic Resonance Imaging of the Breast

As there are limitations to both mammography and ultrasound in evaluating for etiology of nipple discharge, the use of MRI of the breast has been evaluated. Van Gelder described MRI findings in 111 patients with bloody nipple discharge who also had conventional imaging with mammogram and ultrasound.[75] MRI was read as suspicious for malignancy in 9 patients; however, DCIS was found in only 2 patients. These authors concluded that the addition of MRI is not warranted in evaluation of bloody nipple discharge. Manganaro and colleagues performed MRI and galactography on a highly selected group of 53 patients with bloody nipple discharge.[76] Galactography showed an overall sensitivity of 48.9%, a specificity of 100%, a PPV of 100%, and an NPV of

25.81% in detecting the presence of ductal pathologies, benign or malignant. For MRI, the sensitivity was 97.8%, with a specificity of 100%, PPV of 88.89%, and NPV of 100%. The sensitivity of galactography was considered to be lower than other series because duct ectasia was not considered a pathologic finding. Papillomas could be seen as an enhancing mass on MRI in a dilated duct, whereas the papilloma might be obscured by duct ectasia on a galactogram.

Lubina and coworkers reported a study comparing the 3.0-Tesla MRI to galactography in the evaluation of nipple discharge with negative conventional imaging among 56 breasts in 50 women.[77] All patients had histologic confirmation of the findings. Sensitivity and specificity of MRI versus galactography for detecting pathologic findings were 95.7% versus 85.7% and 69.7% versus 33.3%, respectively. MRI abnormalities were seen in 71.4% of breasts. Malignant lesions were detected in 14.8%. Bahl and coworkers performed a retrospective review of 91 patients with a nipple discharge who underwent MRI as part of their evaluation.[78] The sensitivity and specificity of MRI for the detection of malignancy only were 100% (11 of 11) and 68% (54 of 80), respectively. The PPV and NPV were 37% and 100%, respectively. This study differed from the others in that 26% of patients had a prior history of breast cancer and 23% were high risk due to family history. In addition, approximately 10% did not have conventional imaging with mammogram or ultrasound.

In all studies evaluating MRI, it is pointed out that additional data are needed to define the role of MRI in nipple discharge evaluation. In evaluating these studies, it is important to note that some calculated sensitivity and specificity including both benign and malignant pathologies.

Ductography-Galactography

Ductography or galactography can be performed to define the intraductal abnormality. Ductography involves cannulation of the discharging duct with a small catheter or 30-gauge blunt tip needle (often with a 90-degree bend near the tip). The cannula is introduced into the discharging orifice after elicitation of the discharge with compression at the edge of the nipple-areola complex. It may be necessary to elevate the nipple between the thumb and forefinger to facilitate cannulation of the duct. The cannula is attached to extension tubing with a 1- to 3-mL syringe. Water-soluble contrast 60% iothalamate meglumine is injected.[79] Typically, the volume required to fill the duct is 0.2 to 1.0 mL, depending on the configuration of the duct arborization and the type of abnormality. The injection should be discontinued if the patient has acute pain and should be done with low pressure to avoid extravasation. The cannula is then taped to the skin. Mammograms are performed immediately while the contrast material is in the breast ducts. Magnification views in the craniocaudal and mediolateral oblique projection are obtained. If an intraductal lesion is not identified, the cannula can be removed from the duct orifice, because it may be obscuring a lesion at the distal duct or nipple ampulla.

Allergic reactions to the injection of contrast into the ductal system are rare compared with intravenous (IV) injections of similar agents. However, patients with a prior history of rash and itching with IV contrast should be premedicated with diphenhydramine and steroids. Patients with a history of anaphylactic reactions to IV contrast should not undergo ductography.

If ductography fails because of inability to cannulate the duct, several strategies can be undertaken. Schwab and colleagues described a technique of applying a local anesthetic (lidocaine)

spray typically used for mucosal anesthesia.[80] The operator waits 5 minutes to attempt cannulation, which allows for relaxation of the nipple and areola. In the series of 47 patients, Schwab reported that cannulation of the duct initially failed in 8 patients. With application of the lidocaine spray, they were able to successfully cannulate the nipple duct all 8 patients. Berna-Serna and associates reported the use of lidocaine and prilocaine cream application 45 to 60 minutes before ductography.[81] With use of anesthetic cream, all 27 patients had successful ductography. Four of 19 patients experienced unsuccessful duct cannulation when no anesthetic cream was used.

Magnification of the nipple-areola complex is another strategy for facilitating duct cannulation. The application of warm moist compresses may augment relaxation of the nipple-areola complex. Another maneuver that can be undertaken involves placement of a 2-0 polypropylene suture into the discharging orifice as a guide over which the cannula is introduced. Hou and coworkers report successful cannulation of discharging ducts in 105 consecutive patients using this technique.[82] However, success with ductography varies significantly. Sharma and colleagues report failure of ductography in 33% of the 148 patients in whom it was attempted.[83]

Ductograms commonly reveal intraductal lesions within several centimeters of the nipple. Ductographic findings include (1) a cutoff sign or ductal obstruction, (2) ductal dilatation, (3) filling defects, (4) irregularity of the ductal wall, (5) ductal narrowing, and (6) distortion of the ductal arborization (Figs. 4.15 to 4.17). Although the duct may have arborization into the deeper breast, the duct excision may be more limited if the lesion is solitary in the distal ductal region. Dawes and associates reported that 20% of ductograms demonstrated one or more lesions greater than 3 cm from the nipple.[48] Blum reported results of successful ductography and correlation with ultrasound and pathology in 56 patients with nipple discharge.[84] They reported a 10% failure rate in cannulating a duct for imaging. Ductal abnormalities were identified in 70% of examinations. Findings included filling defect, duct ectasia, and duct cutoff. A duct cutoff was the most common finding for malignant lesions (56%). They found ductography superior to ultrasound in defining intraductal pathology. However, neither technique successfully differentiated malignant from benign lesions.

Dinkel and associates support the latter view that galactography should be used primarily to estimate the extent of a lesion rather than to rule out cancer.[85] They correlated preoperative galactography with pathology for 143 duct excisions, which included 11 women with cancer. Most commonly, cancer caused a filling defect or cutoff on galactography; however, only 6 of 90 patients with filling defects had cancer. Two cancers caused duct compression, and one was associated with duct ectasia. Importantly, in only 2 of 11 cancers was galactography normal.

Some authors advocate continued observation if the ductogram is negative.[86] However, others conclude that the false-negative rate is not acceptable.[48] Other investigators have combined cytologic examination and galactography to select patients for biopsy.[49,85] They report that combined abnormal cytology and abnormal ductography findings indicate a high likelihood of either malignancy or a papilloma. However, there is minimal information on the patients followed without biopsy.

Ductoscopy

Mammary ductoscopy allows direct visualization of the interior of the discharging duct. The technique has evolved over time with

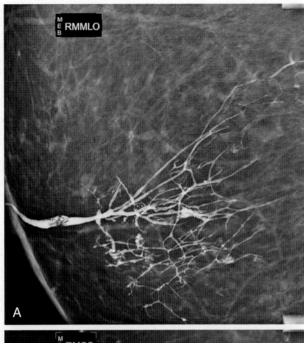

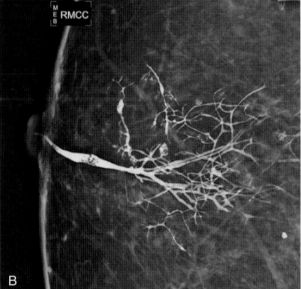

• **Fig. 4.15** (A) Ductogram with multiple filling defects magnified craniocaudal view. (B) Ductogram with multiple filling defects magnified mediolateral oblique view. (Courtesy Phil Evans, MD, UT Southwestern Medical Center.)

better optics, resolution, smaller-caliber scopes and the ability to biopsy under direct visualization. Mammary ductoscopy can be performed under local anesthesia in an office setting or outpatient surgery setting.[87] The orifice of the duct that produces the discharge is dilated either with lacrimal probes or sequentially larger catheters. A fiberoptic scope is introduced into the dilated nipple orifice, manipulated through tortuous sections of the duct in the nipple, and then advanced into the ducts. Fluid is irrigated through the scope as it is advanced. Some scopes can be introduced through a plastic sleeve, which serves both as a dilator and as an access to obtain washings. In a darkened room, the light of the scope can be seen through breast tissue. If a point of interest is identified, the skin can be marked over the spot of light to guide subsequent biopsy.

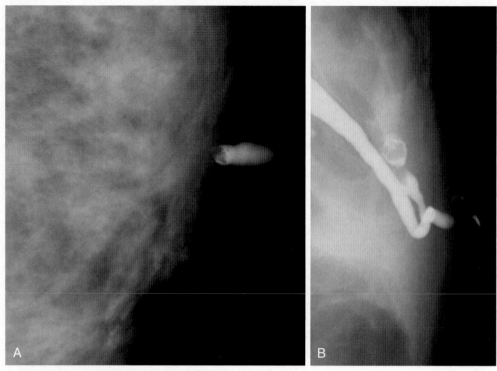

• **Fig. 4.16** (A) Ductogram with "cutoff" or duct obstruction. Diagnosis of papilloma. (B) Ductogram with filling defect. Diagnosis of papilloma. (Courtesy Ralph Wynn, MD, UT Southwestern Medical Center.)

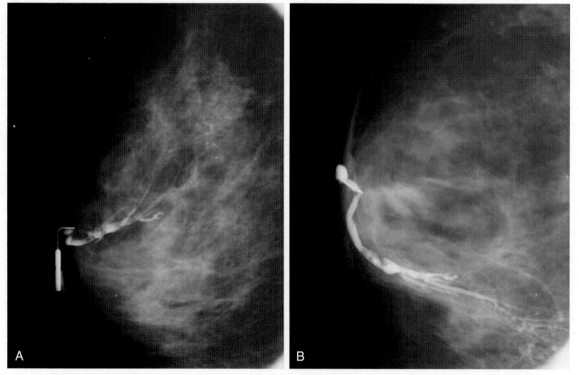

• **Fig. 4.17** Ductal carcinoma in situ. (A) Mediolateral view. Ductogram with filling defect and filling of ducts proximal to lesion, with injecting needle in place. (B) Craniocaudad view. ([A] Courtesy Ralph Wynn, MD, UT Southwestern Medical Center.)

Technical limitations of ductoscopy are related to breast anatomy. Rusby and colleagues performed an anatomic study of 129 breast specimens and found that the median number of ducts was 23 with a range of 5 to 50.[88] They and other investigators have shown that the number of detectable duct orifices on the nipple is 5 to 15. Rusby and associates found that there are shared openings of many ducts in a single cleft on the surface of the nipple and that the caliber of most ducts is narrow close to the nipple tip. This accounts for the observed discrepancy between collecting ducts and orifices on the nipple seen in most studies. This anatomic finding points out the challenge of using mammary ductoscopy and ductography in diagnostic evaluation.

Endoscopic findings may include an intraductal mass, blood staining or injection in the wall of the duct, irregularity of the duct wall, duct obstruction, and scar.[89] Matsunaga and colleagues classified intraductal lesions by type as hemispheric, papillary, and flat protrusion.[90] Intraductal papillomas were more likely to be hemispheric or papillary in shape; the flat protrusion configuration was more common in malignant lesions.[91] The normal duct surface is smooth and shiny.

Kothari and coworkers performed ex vivo mammary ductoscopy on 115 ducts in 35 mastectomy specimens.[92] Abnormalities were seen on 40% of ducts. The authors proposed a morphologic classification of intraluminal lesions. These include (1) obstructing intraluminal lesions; (2) epithelial surface abnormalities subdivided into premalignant and malignant epithelial proliferation versus inflammation; (3) papillomatous lesions, single or multiple; (4) intraductal scars, adhesions, and duct obliteration; and (5) intraductal calcifications. In a series of 88 patients undergoing endoscopy, Dooley and associates noted that 18% of patients had normal-appearing ducts on endoscopic examination.[93] Sauter and colleagues reported a normal intraductal examination in 25% of patients with spontaneous nipple discharge.[94] On the other hand, Vaughan and associates reported abnormal findings in 79 of 80 ductoscopies with a broad definition of abnormal findings.[95] However, 10% had no specific pathologic findings on duct excision.

In the United States, ductoscopy is not widely adopted, but it has become more routinely used in Asia to evaluate nipple discharge. Yang and associates reported a series of 419 patients with successful ductoscopy in 97%.[96] None of the patients had lesions identified on mammogram and ultrasound. Papillary lesions were visualized in 28% of patients. Among those who underwent duct excision, 89% had benign intraductal papilloma and 13% invasive cancer or DCIS. In this series, nipple fluid pathology was positive in only one patient for a sensitivity of 12%.

A meta-analysis of ductoscopy studies included 20 studies with 1994 patients.[97] Median successful cannulation in selective follow-up studies was 85% (range, 81%–100%) compared with 94% (range, 86%–100%) in the surgical reference studies. Sensitivity of DSany (ductoscopy with any findings) was defined as the proportion of women with a positive ductoscopy among all women subsequently diagnosed with malignancy at histologic assessment or follow-up. Specificity of DSany was defined as the proportion of women with a negative ductoscopy among all women with benign outcome at histology or follow-up. Malignancy was found in 151 cases (7.6%). The respective pooled sensitivity of ductoscopy for any findings was 94% with a specificity of 47%. The NPV of DSany ranged from 98% to 100% in these series. Selective follow-up was described for patients with negative ductoscopic (and cytologic) findings and those with endoscopically acquired histologic tissue diagnosis of benign intraductal papilloma. The patients in the selective follow-up studies showed low rates of malignancy (5%). The studies included in the meta-analysis varied with respect to workup before ductoscopy and selection criteria for ductoscopy. Yet it seems that ductoscopy is a tool that can have a role in selecting patients for surgery versus conservative management of nipple discharge.

Cytologic Evaluation of Nipple Discharge

The cytologic examination of nipple discharge is an attractive approach for identifying those patients who require surgical intervention. However, the use of this technique has its pitfalls. An adequate sample is critical for diagnostic accuracy for breast cytologic examination. The preparatory methods for this pathologic technique include direct smears from spontaneous nipple discharge and the membrane filtration of NAF samples. Cytologic examination needs to be systematic and thorough, and a classification system should use terminology related to the anticipated histopathology.

Sample Collection

Spontaneous nipple discharge is expressed directly onto the glass slide, which is held at the opening of the duct, and then it is moved across the drop of fluid at the surface of the nipple to ensure a thin spread. This slide is then smeared with a second slide lengthwise. The slides are immersed immediately in the fixative of 95% ethanol. It is suggested that four to six smears be prepared from each discharge because the material is often more cellular in the last drops of fluid.

Sample Preparation

Two important aspects of specimen preparation include the concentration of cells and recovery of cells. *Cell concentration* refers to increasing the number of cells per unit volume or area. *Cell recovery* is the efficiency of collecting cells per unit volume of sample or the percentage of total cells in a sample. In NAF samples, cell recovery is especially important because of the scant cellularity. NAF samples are concentrated and recovered on membrane Millipore filters. Direct smears require no special laboratory preparation other than appropriate staining with Papanicolaou stain or other stains preferred by the laboratory.

Cytologic Examination

Pathologic examination of NAF, DL fluid, and breast discharge cytology should be performed by a pathologist with training and experience in this specialized area of cytopathology. Qualitative assessment is made of the cellular composition, including types of cells and degree of cellularity. Cytologic evaluation is based on the changes in epithelial cells and accompanying cellular findings. The final interpretation should be made correlating with complete clinical data. It is essential that the clinician understand that a negative cytology does not exclude malignancy.

The cytologic diagnosis of nipple discharge samples is shown from several studies in Table 4.2.[13,71,98–100] Hou and associates reported an improvement in results with cytology of single duct discharge in absence of a mass when they used an intraductal aspiration method.[101] Adequate samples were obtained from 96.6% of patients with intraductal aspiration compared with 76% collected with the conventional method using pressure. Among 27 cancers in the series, 24 (88.9%) were correctly diagnosed with the aspiration sample; 33.3% were diagnosed using the conventional method.

TABLE 4.2   Reported Results With Cytologic Examination of Nipple Discharge

Study	Year	N	With Cancer	POSITIVE CYTOLOGY		FALSE-POSITIVE CYTOLOGY	
				n	%	*n*	%
Papanicolaou et al.[13]	1958	495	45	45	60	3	1
Kjellgren[99]	1964	216	25	21	89	15	8
Funderburk and Syphax[71]	1969	182	7	6	86	—	—
Uei et al.[98]	1980	190	80	53	66	4	4
Kooistra et al.[100]	2009	163	36	5	14	8	6

Carty and coworkers proposed use of a "triple test" for evaluation of nipple discharges.[102] This is similar to the triple test used with FNA cytology of palpable masses. They do not perform a surgical biopsy if clinical examination, mammography, and NAF cytologic examination are negative for suspicious findings. In a series of 56 women, 17 required biopsy using these criteria and 5 had malignancy. The authors followed 38 of the other 39 women for a minimum of 5 years, and the women had no further breast disease. However, 17 had additional nipple discharge on follow-up.

An interesting study from the College of American Pathologists reviewed responses of pathologists and cytotechnologists for interpretation of a slide set of nipple discharge preparations.[103] For the diagnosis of carcinoma, the agreement with that diagnosis was 87.5%, for papillary lesion 84.8% and for benign, 96.6%. The false-positive rate was 12.8%, and the false-negative rate was 3.4%. The most frequent false-negative diagnosis for a cancer was mastitis. The authors concluded that nipple discharge cytology is not a reliable method for diagnosis and that a duct excision specimen is preferred.

Diagnosis and Surgical Intervention

Definitive diagnosis of the etiology of a pathologic nipple discharge is based on biopsy that should first be directed to any suspicious area identified by physical examination, mammography, or other studies. If no specific lesion is identified, duct excision of the discharging duct is undertaken for patients with a pathologic nipple discharge. The initial procedure described by Hadfield involved complete excision of the major ductal system with a conical tissue resection. However, a preferable procedure is microductectomy, which involves a more directed excision of the discharging duct and its arborization into the breast. Surgical duct excision is both diagnostic and therapeutic for nipple discharge. Even benign discharges may be sufficiently bothersome to the patient that she would prefer duct excision to continued drainage of fluid from the nipple.

Technique of Duct Excision

Duct excision is an outpatient procedure that can be performed with the patient under local anesthesia, usually with IV sedation or general anesthetic (Fig. 4.18). A long-acting anesthetic agent is infiltrated at the site of the proposed incision, under the areola, and around the nipple. The discharge is elicited by pressing at the

previously identified trigger point to identify the duct for cannulation with a lacrimal probe. The largest size probe that will accommodate the duct orifice should be used (see Fig. 4.18B). Alternatively, or together with placement of the lacrimal probe, the discharging duct can be injected with methylene blue via a 30-gauge catheter.

A circumareolar incision is made that should not encompass more than 50% of the circumference of the areola to avoid devascularization of the nipple-areola complex. The incision centers on the trigger point or the pathology located by ductography or other studies (see Fig. 4.18C). The epicenter of the periareolar incision lies within the trigger point quadrant of the breast. The direction that the lacrimal probe takes on introduction may also guide the placement of the incision and direction of the dissection. Meticulous hemostasis is maintained. Using fine scissors or a 15-blade allows precise dissection. The edge of the areola is elevated with skin hooks, and dissection proceeds with the blade to raise a thick skin flap of the areolar skin toward the base of the nipple.

There are three methods to find the symptomatic duct: (1) palpation of the lacrimal duct probe through the tissue at the base of the nipple, (2) visually identifying the dilated duct by dissection posterior to the nipple, and (3) visually identifying the blue-stained duct when methylene blue is injected into the duct before making the skin incision. The identified duct is then dissected superficially to the dermis of the nipple. Using a fine-tipped curved right-angle hemostat, the terminal duct is dissected circumferentially (see Fig. 4.18D and E). The lacrimal probe may be left in place to facilitate palpation of the extent of the duct. However, if the lacrimal probe cannot be introduced more than 1 cm, it is preferable to ligate the duct at its termination on the nipple and transect the duct (see Fig. 4.18F and G). A suture can be placed through the proximal duct for gentle traction during the dissection into the deeper breast (see Fig. 4.18H). The dissection in the posterior breast planes involves dissecting out a pyramidal-shaped specimen of surrounding tissue (see Fig. 4.18I).

The duct is usually within a segment of the breast that is denser than the adjacent tissue, often surrounded by either loose connective tissue or fatty tissue. The specimen increases in diameter as dissection extends into the deeper breast parenchyma. The extent of dissection into the posterior breast can be limited if the ductogram has revealed a lesion and the dissection can be tailored to fully encompass the lesion. If a dilated duct containing discharge is transected during dissection, it should be marked with a suture for later identification and excision.

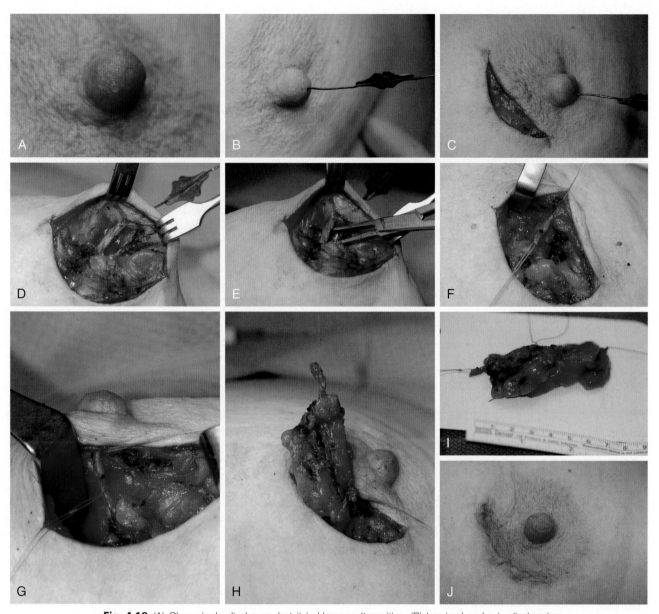

• **Fig. 4.18** (A) Clear nipple discharge, but it is Hemoccult positive. (B) Lacrimal probe in discharging duct. (C) Incision made at areolar edge corresponding to trigger point and palpable course of lacrimal probe. (D) Cannulated duct dissected out. (E) Cannulated duct dissected circumferentially. Duct ligated proximally (F) and distally (G). (G) shows the relationship to the visible nipple. (H) Duct transected and gentle traction applied. (I) Specimen. (J) Circumareolar wound closure.

If methylene blue has been injected into the duct, all blue-stained areas are generally removed. However, if an intraductal lesion has been identified by ductography or ultrasound in the immediate subareolar region, it is unnecessary to complete a segmental resection of the breast.

Van Zee and colleagues confirmed that preoperative injection of dye facilitated excision.[104] With methylene blue, they noted the pathology review explained the discharge in 100% of patients. However, without dye injection, they found pathology to account for the discharge in only 67% of duct excisions.

As wound closure is undertaken, attention should be directed to avoid the collapse of the nipple-areola complex into the soft tissue defect resulting from the resection (see Fig. 4.18J). It is often feasible to mobilize tissue on either side of the defect in the subareolar location and approximate it with absorbable interrupted sutures to repair the defect. The dermis and subcutaneous tissue are closed with interrupted absorbable sutures. The skin is then closed with a running subcuticular, absorbable suture. The patient is advised to wear a bra for support for 72 hours. Vigorous upper body activity should also be avoided during this period.

Technical Modifications for Duct Excision

In the circumstance of surgical biopsy for nipple discharge, there is concern as to whether the lesion is actually retrieved with the surgery. This perhaps results from incorrect estimation of the

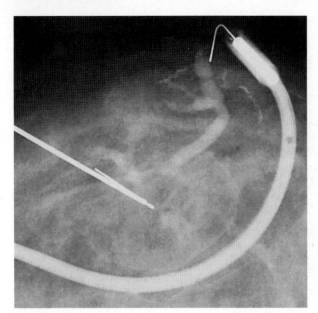

• **Fig. 4.19** Wire localization of filling defect to facilitate localization of deeper lesion. Galactography combined with wire localization biopsy. The duct has an abrupt cutoff at the site of the lesion. The guidewire was placed while contrast media was within the duct. The contrast was not present at the time of the biopsy and could not be seen on the specimen radiograph. The lesion was a benign papilloma. (Courtesy Edward A. Sickles, MD.)

depth of the dissection to encompass the ductal abnormality. Precise measurements to identify the distance of the lesion from the nipple are performed at the time the breast is compressed for mammography. Other proposed methods to ensure resection of the lesion include wire localization of abnormalities identified on ductogram, diagnostic mammogram, sonogram, and the novel application of intraoperative ductoscopy.

Chow and coworkers described the performance of a ductogram on the day of surgery with placement of a localizing wire in the area of the identified ductal abnormality.[105] A localization wire is placed while the contrast is still in the duct (Fig. 4.19). Because water-soluble contrast media do not usually persist in the duct, the specimen radiograph usually does not show any abnormality. Koskela and colleagues described the use of wire localization when there is no mammographic or ultrasound identified lesion.[106] The wire is placed with stereotactic guidance so that the tip is placed in the area of the abnormality identified on ductography. Rissanen and associates reported using wire localization in 11 and 49 patients undergoing surgical resection for nipple discharge.[73] In their technique, the abnormal duct was localized before surgery by either methylene blue staining or sonographically guided wire localization. Methylene blue staining was done with the same cannulation technique as for diagnostic galactography. A 1:2 solution of 1% methylene blue and contrast material (300 mg/mL iopromide) was injected, and 2 orthogonal mammogram views were obtained to confirm that the pathologic duct was filled. Ultrasound-guided wire localization was used in the following circumstances: (1) failure to cannulate the discharging duct, (2) preoperative ductogram identified a duct different from the one identified with the original diagnostic galactography, or (3) a positive ultrasound with a negative ductogram. There is no intraoperative means to verify removal of the pathologic tissue with these techniques, other than confirming that the localizing

wire tip is centrally located within the specimen with a margin of tissue circumferentially. A case study in the workup of nipple discharge (Fig. 4.20) demonstrates our approach to combining techniques to maximize assurance of resection of the pathologic lesions.

Dooley describes the technique for use of ductoscopy for intraoperative visualization of ductal abnormalities.[107] The discharging duct is cannulated with a 2-0 Prolene suture. The duct orifice is sequentially dilated using 26-, 24-, and 22-gauge catheters. Local anesthetic is instilled into the duct. The 0.9-mm fiberoptic endoscope is introduced. The ductal abnormalities are identified. The margin of resection of tissue is guided by transillumination from the scope. Twenty-seven patients with Hemoccult-positive spontaneous nipple discharge and negative mammography were taken to surgery for microductectomy. In 96% of cases, the intraductal lesion responsible for bleeding was identified. Multiple lesions were found in 70% of cases and often were deeper in the breast. Dooley noted coexistence of superficial papillomas with deeper DCIS lesions. Dietz and colleagues described a series of 119 patients undergoing endoscopically guided duct excision.[108] Cannulation of the discharging duct was successful in 88% of women, and endoscopy-directed resection was achieved in 87%. Cancer and hyperplasia were more likely to be correlated with failed duct cannulation. Similar to the report by Dooley, multiple lesions and those more than 4 cm from the nipple were noted in 22% of women. Dietz suggested that these lesions might have been left behind with standard microductectomy. Ductoscopy was more accurate than preoperative ductography in identifying specific intraductal pathology (90% vs. 76%).

Moncrief and associates compared ductoscopy-guided versus conventional surgical duct excision in 117 women with spontaneous nipple discharge.[109] There was good correlation between the endoscopic findings and the pathologic diagnosis when an intraductal tumor was seen on ductoscopy, with 90% of 49 ducts demonstrating a papilloma or more severe pathology. The range of pathologic diagnoses was similar between the two procedures. The authors suggested that the gross appearance of the intraductal lesion cannot reliably distinguish between benign and malignant lesions. In the ductoscopy group, more peripheral lesions were identified, and multiple papillomas were more commonly found in the specimen. The potential advantage of ductoscopy-guided surgery is the identification of more peripheral lesions, which might impart a greater risk of breast cancer. Another potential advantage would be limitation of the extent of subareolar duct excision when resection is focused on the area of the lesion identified at ductoscopy rather than the entire duct. However, the authors did not provide data on the volume of tissue resected or preservation of subareolar ductal tissue.

Fisher and Margenthaler described a series of 121 patients who underwent intraoperative ductoscopy and directed duct excision.[110] They noted that 93% of their patients had normal breast imaging. The ductoscope was introduced into the duct and the lesion identified to direct the extent of resection. As with most series, final pathology revealed papilloma in 53%, duct ectasia in 40% and DCIS in 6%, and atypia in 1%. The ductoscopic interpretation of findings for patients with a final diagnosis of cancer was varied, including papilloma, intraductal inflammation, and intraductal debris or webs. These authors concluded that duct excision is warranted for a pathologic discharge, regardless of ductoscopic findings. The considered benefits of intraoperative ductoscopy are the potential identification of the lesion to reduce extent of dissection, avoidance of additional testing such as

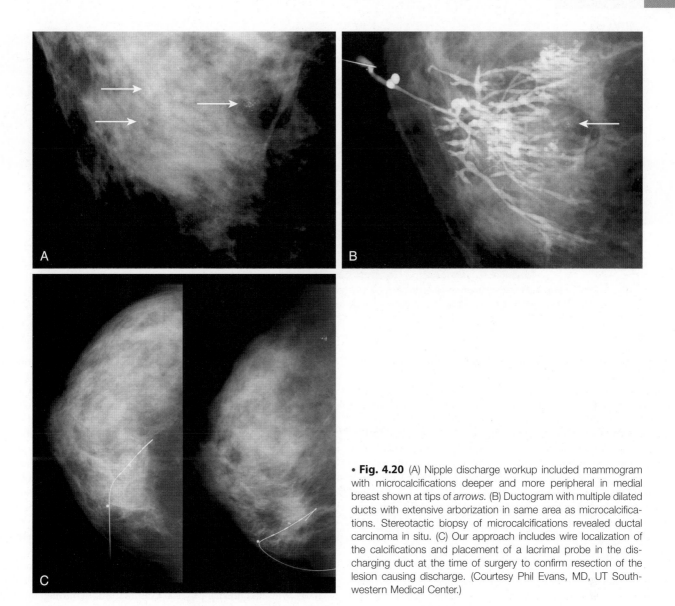

• **Fig. 4.20** (A) Nipple discharge workup included mammogram with microcalcifications deeper and more peripheral in medial breast shown at tips of *arrows*. (B) Ductogram with multiple dilated ducts with extensive arborization in same area as microcalcifications. Stereotactic biopsy of microcalcifications revealed ductal carcinoma in situ. (C) Our approach includes wire localization of the calcifications and placement of a lacrimal probe in the discharging duct at the time of surgery to confirm resection of the lesion causing discharge. (Courtesy Phil Evans, MD, UT Southwestern Medical Center.)

ductography and MRI, and fewer complications of surgery due to directed excision.

Minimally Invasive Techniques for Biopsy of Intraductal Lesions

There is increasing interest in using nonsurgical techniques to biopsy intraductal lesions. Govindarajulu and coworkers reported on the use of ultrasound-guided Mammotome biopsy for 77 patients with pathologic nipple discharge.[111] The biopsy targeted a dilated duct only in 50% of cases and an intraductal lesion in 50%. A 3- to 5-cm segment of the duct was excised with the Mammotome. Pathology results included papilloma (41%), epithelial hyperplasia (23%), chronic inflammation (29%), atypical ductal hyperplasia (1%), and malignancy (6%). Complications included recurrence of symptoms in 5% of patients, requiring duct excision or repeat Mammotome resection. Six percent had a hematoma and a similar number had bleeding from the nipple. Long-term follow-up was not reported.

Beechey-Newman and colleagues used ductoscopy with a microbrush technique to biopsy intraductal lesions in 50 patients presenting with nipple discharge.[112] The microbrush has nylon bristles with a 0.55-mm diameter. The brush was inserted via a working channel in the scope, and DL fluid was obtained after brushing. The patients underwent either microductectomy or total duct excision after ductoscopy. Thirty-three patients (66%) had an intraluminal lesion identified at ductoscopy. The microbrush was used to sample eight presumed papillary lesions. Of these, seven yielded papillary cells (87.5% sensitivity).

Hunerbein and colleagues described a biopsy technique via a rigid ductoscope.[113] The rigid scope has improved optics using fused gradient index lenses. The scope is introduced via a 0.9-mm needle with a lateral port for air insufflation. The introducer needle has a biopsy port to retrieve the specimen with suction. Biopsy via the ductoscope was successfully performed in 34 of 36 patients with nipple discharge and intraductal lesions. The specimen size was typically 1 mm. The results of the ductoscopic

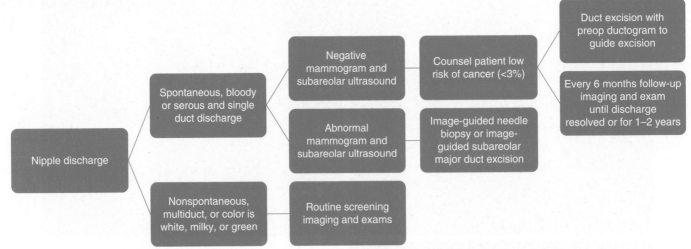

• **Fig. 4.21** Algorithm for evaluation of nipple discharge, Mayo Clinic. (From Ashfaq A, Senior D, Pockaj BA, et al. Validation study of a modern treatment algorithm for nipple discharge. *Am J Surg.* 2014;208:222-227.)

biopsies were more accurate than DL cytology. However, resection of lesions was not feasible.

Matsunaga and associates reported on follow-up greater than 3 years for 70 patients undergoing 75 intraductal breast biopsy (IDBB) procedures with ductoscopy guidance.[114] Thirty-six patients experienced resolution of nipple discharge after IDBB; another 13 had resolution after subsequent repeat IDBB. Thus 70% of patients with nipple discharge had control of their symptoms. In 15 patients in whom bloody nipple discharge persisted, IDBB was repeated on several occasions. IDBB was less likely to be therapeutic in patients with multiple lesions. Two patients (3%) developed breast cancer 3 years after IDBB. Among 89 patients having a negative ductoscopic examination, 3 (4%) developed breast cancer, although the authors indicate that the cancer occurred in a different quadrant of the breast from that of the original lesion seen on ductography. Matsunaga points out that IDBB was less successful in diagnosing carcinoma, with only one-third of patients with breast cancer having a positive IDBB.

Algorithms for Management of Nipple Discharge

There is interest among investigators to develop an algorithm for management of pathologic nipple discharge without surgical duct excision, while establishing an accurate diagnosis and controlling the presenting symptom of discharge. Liu and colleagues from China devised an algorithm with initial workup including mammogram, ultrasound, and ductoscopy.[115] Patients having a positive ductoscopy or BI-RADS 4 or 5 lesions on mammogram or ultrasound were recommended to have surgical duct excision. If ductoscopy was negative, the patients were observed. Ductoscopy was successful in 266 of 271 breasts. Six percent of those with a positive ductoscopy had cancer. Ductoscopy was negative in 98 (37%). Of those with a median follow-up of 48 months, 78% had resolution of nipple discharge, 10% were lost to follow-up, and 12% had recurrent discharge resulting in surgical excision with final benign papillary diagnoses. For most series reporting minimally invasive techniques for diagnosis of nipple discharge, there is no long-term follow-up for the patients who did not have surgical duct excision after ductoscopic examination.

Other investigators have developed algorithms to avoid surgery with conventional imaging screening of patients with nipple discharge. Ashfaq and coworkers at Mayo Clinic validated an algorithm shown in Fig. 4.21.[72] For patients with negative mammogram and subareolar ultrasound, follow-up every 6 months was offered. Among 94 patients offered close follow-up, 20% ultimately underwent duct excision for persistent discharge without a cancer diagnosis, and 1 patient had duct excision for a new imaging abnormality and was found to have DCIS. At a median follow-up of 28 months, the 74 patients who remained in close observation had no cancers diagnosed and 81% had resolution of the discharge. These authors note that they have abandoned ductography due to the high sensitivity of subareolar ultrasound. Sabel and colleagues arrived at a similar approach from a retrospective look at their experience.[116] They noted that 25% of duct excisions could have been avoided by observing patients with nipple discharge who had normal physical examination, mammogram, and ultrasound. These authors did suggest that the number of duct excisions avoided might be greater with the addition of other tools for evaluation, such as ductography and MRI.

The algorithm for management of nipple discharge developed at the University of Texas MD Anderson Cancer Center includes the recommendation for a ductogram if the initial diagnostic mammogram is negative (Fig. 4.22).[117] The National Comprehensive Cancer Network guidelines for evaluation of pathologic nipple discharge recommend both mammogram and ultrasound as initial step. If the imaging evaluation is BI-RADS 1 to 3, then ductogram or MRI are considered optional before proceeding with duct excision for definitive diagnosis.[118]

It is important that patients undergoing minimally invasive biopsy techniques or nonsurgical management to evaluate spontaneous nipple discharge have long-term follow-up that provides a better understanding of the false-negative rate of these technologies.

Outcomes

The long-term outcome after a benign diagnosis of nipple discharge is generally quite good. Early recurrence of the discharge after duct excision may be related to evacuation of a seroma

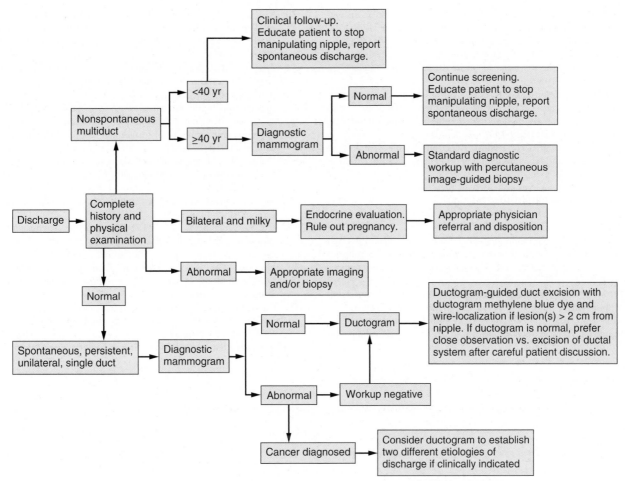

• **Fig. 4.22** Algorithm for evaluation of nipple discharge, University of Texas MD Anderson Cancer Center. (From Lang JE, Kuerer HM. Breast ductal secretions: clinical features, potential uses, and possible applications. *Cancer Control*. 2007;14:350-359.)

through the orifice of the transected duct. Vargas and coworkers described a series of 157 patients presenting with nipple discharge, of whom 82 were deemed to harbor a pathologic discharge.[40] There was no recurrence of nipple discharge at 18 months postoperatively in 63 patients who underwent duct excision. Lau and colleagues performed 118 duct excisions on 116 patients between 1995 and 2002, and none developed recurrent discharge.[51]

Summary

Spontaneous nipple discharge requires a systematic evaluation to ascertain the etiology. Although multiple additional studies, such as mammography, ultrasound, ductography, MRI, and cytologic examination, may be obtained, the definitive diagnosis is established with surgical excision of the involved duct. The marked improvement of imaging technology over the years has increased the sensitivity and accuracy of these studies, and this must be taken into account when comparing outcomes of case series from decades ago compared with today. Ancillary tests, when positive, can provide valuable information for planning the extent of surgical resection. When using imaging tools such as MRI, ductography, and ductoscopy to avoid surgery, physicians must be aware of their institution's false-negative rates for these techniques. Interventions such as ductoscopy require special instrumentation and technical skills that are not readily available in many institutions.

When any of these tests are abnormal, the patient is commonly highly motivated to proceed with duct excision. If negative, the patient may be less inclined for duct excision. As has been shown in many studies, negative imaging or cytology does not guarantee that malignant pathology is not present. The value of minimally invasive procedures to diagnose pathologic nipple discharge is not yet clearly defined; longer follow-up is required to evaluate outcomes. There continues to be interest in the evaluation of breast secretions obtained by NAF or DL to estimate breast cancer risk; however, these approaches remain investigational and at present are not incorporated into the routine management of nipple discharges or risk assessment.

Selected References

1. Ferguson DJ, Anderson TJ. Morphological evaluation of cell turnover in relation to the menstrual cycle in the "resting" human breast. *Br J Cancer*. 1981;44:177-181.
3. Meyer J. Cell proliferation in normal human breast ducts, fibroadenomas, and other ductal hyperplasias measured by nuclear labeling with tritiated thymidine. Effects of menstrual phase, age, and oral contraceptive hormones. *Hum Pathol*. 1977;8:67-81.
4. Longacre TA, Bartow SA. A correlative morphologic study of human breast and endometrium in the menstrual cycle. *Am J Surg Pathol*. 1986;10:382-393.

5. Malberger E, Gutterman E, Bartfeld E, Zajicek G. Cellular changes in the mammary gland epithelium during the menstrual cycle. A computer image analysis study. *Acta Cytol*. 1987;31:305-308.

7. Sartorius OW, Smith HS, Morris P, et al. Cytologic evaluation of breast fluid in the detection of breast disease. *J Natl Cancer Inst*. 1977;59:1073-1080.

8. Petrakis NL, Mason L, Lee R, et al. Association of race, age, menopausal status, and cerumen type with breast fluid secretion in nonlactating women, as determined by nipple aspiration. *J Natl Cancer Inst*. 1975;54:829-834.

9. Wynder EL, Lahti H, Laakso K, et al. Nipple aspirates of breast fluid and the epidemiology of breast disease. *Cancer*. 1985;56:1473-1478.

11. Saphir O. Cytologic examination of breast secretions. *Am J Clin Pathol*. 1950;20:1001-1010.

12. Ringrose CA. The role of cytology in the early detection of breast disease. *Acta Cytol*. 1966;10:373-375.

13. Papanicolaou GN, Holmquist DG, Bader GM, Falk EA. Exfoliative cytology of the human mammary gland and its value in the diagnosis of cancer and other diseases of the breast. *Cancer*. 1958;11:377-409.

14. Petrakis NL. Physiologic, biochemical, and cytologic aspects of nipple aspirate fluid. *Breast Cancer Res Treat*. 1986;8:7-19.

15. King EB, Barrett D, Petrakis NL. Cellular composition of the nipple aspirate specimen of breast fluid. II. Abnormal findings. *Am J Clin Pathol*. 1975;64:739-748.

20. Sauter ER, Wagner-Mann C, Ehya H, Klein-Szanto A. Biologic markers of breast cancer in nipple aspirate fluid and nipple discharge are associated with clinical findings. *Cancer Detect Prev*. 2007;31:50-58.

52. Adepoju LJ, Chun J, El-Tamer M, et al. The value of clinical characteristics and breast-imaging studies in predicting a histopathologic diagnosis of cancer or high-risk lesion in patients with spontaneous nipple discharge. *Am J Surg*. 2005;190:644-646.

90. Matsunaga T, Ohta D, Misaka T, et al. Mammary ductoscopy for diagnosis and treatment of intraductal lesions of the breast. *Breast Cancer*. 2001;8:213-221.

93. Dooley WC, Francescatti D, Clark L, Webber G. Office-based breast ductoscopy for diagnosis. *Am J Surg*. 2004;188:415-418.

94. Sauter ER, Ehya H, Klein-Szanto AJ. Fiberoptic ductoscopy findings in women with and without spontaneous nipple discharge. *Cancer*. 2005;103:914-921.

98. Uei Y, Watanabe Y, Hirota T, et al. Cytologic diagnosis of breast carcinoma with nipple discharge: special significance of the spherical cell cluster. *Acta Cytol*. 1980;24:522-528.

101. Hou M, Tsai K, Lin H, et al. A simple intraductal aspiration method for cytodiagnosis in nipple discharge. *Acta Cytol*. 2000;44:1029-1034.

102. Carty NJ, Mudan SS, Ravichandran D, et al. Prospective study of outcome in women presenting with nipple discharge. *Ann R Coll Surg Engl*. 1994;76:387-389.

A full reference list is available online at ExpertConsult.com.

5

Etiology and Management of Benign Breast Disease

JENNIFER SASAKI,[a] ABBY GELETZKE,[a] RENA B. KASS, V. SUZANNE KLIMBERG, EDWARD M. COPELAND III, AND KIRBY I. BLAND

The aberrations of normal development and involution (ANDI) classification of benign breast disorder (BBD) provides an overall framework for benign conditions of the breast that encompasses both pathogenesis and the degree of abnormality.[1] It is a bidirectional framework based on the fact that most BBDs arise from normal physiologic processes (Table 5.1). The horizontal component defines BBD along a spectrum from normal to mild abnormality ("disorder") to severe abnormality ("disease"). The vertical component defines the pathogenesis of the condition. Together these two components provide a comprehensive framework into which most BBDs can be fit. This scheme was recommended by an international multidisciplinary working group in 1992.[2]

Breast Pain

Although mastalgia is one of the most commonly reported symptoms in women with breast complaints at dedicated breast clinics or general practice,[3] it is still underreported and poorly characterized. In a 2014 general population survey of 1659 women, more than half (51.5%) experienced breast pain, with 17% reporting a severity of pain greater than 7 out of 10.[4] Maddox and Mansel reported that only 50% of women with breast pain had consulted a family physician,[5] and fewer still had visited a dedicated breast clinic. Because of the increasing awareness of breast cancer and the possibility that mastalgia may indicate disease, as well as the effect mastalgia has on the quality of life, more women than ever are seeking help for breast pain. Treatment usually balances management of relatively minor complaints with the side effects of treatment. More than 90% of patients with cyclic mastalgia and 64% of patients with noncyclic mastalgia can obtain relief by using a combination of nonprescription and prescription drugs.[6]

Clinical Assessment

The degree, severity, and relationship of breast pain to the menstrual cycle are best assessed with the use of a daily breast pain chart that uses a visual analog scale. This chart should be kept during at least two menstrual cycles. Mild breast pain (<3 on the scale) that lasts fewer than 5 days before a menstrual cycle is considered normal. The extent to which mastalgia disrupts the patient's normal lifestyle in terms of sleep, work, and intimacy provides a useful assessment of severity. A thorough history that includes diet, methylxanthine intake, and use of new medications (especially hormones, antidepressants such as serotonin reuptake inhibitors, cardiac medications such as digoxin and cimetidine) or illicit drugs such as marijuana should be taken,[7] and a history of recent stress should be recorded. Other conditions should be excluded, such as possible referred pain, such as shoulder bursitis, cervical radiculopathy, costochondritis, myocardial ischemia, lung disease, hiatal hernia, and cholelithiasis.

Patients are reassured that they do not have breast cancer only after clinical examination and mammography are performed and reveal no malignancy.[5] Fortunately, isolated breast pain is an uncommon symptom of malignancy. In a study by Noroozian and colleagues of 1386 women with mammograms performed for breast pain, only 1.8% were found to have breast cancer.[8] Ultrasonography can be a useful adjunct to evaluate focal pain, especially in young dense breasts because 23% of breast pain patients have cysts or benign masses as the root cause.[9]

No study to date has reported an increased risk of breast cancer with cyclic mastalgia. Initial evaluation should exclude breast pain from localized benign lesions of the breast that may require needle aspiration or surgical therapy, such as painful cysts, fibroadenomas, subareolar duct ectasia, lipomas, and fibrocystic changes.

Classification

Classification of mastalgia provides a baseline measurement of pain and severity, dividing symptoms into the categories of cyclic mastalgia, noncyclic mastalgia, and chest wall pain. This distinction is important because presentation, occurrence of spontaneous remission, and likelihood of a response to treatment differs for these three conditions. A useful response is obtained in 92% of patients with cyclic mastalgia, 64% of those with noncyclic mastalgia,[5] and 97% of those with chest wall pain.[10]

Cyclic mastalgia accounts for approximately 67% of cases and usually is first seen during the third decade of life as dull, burning,

---

[a]Jennifer Sasaki and Abby Geletzke share first authorship of this chapter.

TABLE 5.1	Aberrations of Normal Development and Involution Classification of Benign Breast Disease		
	Normal	**Disorder**	**Disease**
Early reproductive years (age 15–25)	Lobular development	Fibroadenoma	Giant fibroadenoma
	Stromal development	Adolescent hypertrophy	Gigantomastia
	Nipple eversion	Nipple inversion	Subareolar abscess/mammary duct fistula
Mature reproductive years (age 25–40)	Cyclical changes of menstruation	Cyclical mastalgia	Incapacitating mastalgia
	Epithelial hyperplasia of pregnancy	Nodularity	
		Bloody nipple discharge	
Involution (age 35–55)	Lobular involution	Macrocysts	
		Sclerosing lesions	
	Duct involution/dilation sclerosis	Duct ectasia	Periductal mastitis/abscess
	Epithelial turnover	Nipple retraction	Epithelial hyperplasia with atypia
		Epithelial hyperplasia	

or aching pain.[10] However, one breast is usually involved to a greater extent than the other, and the pain may be sharp and shooting, with radiation to the axilla or arm because of glandular entrapment of the intercostobrachial nerve. Cyclic mastalgia usually starts in the upper outer quadrant of the breast 5 days or more before the menstrual cycle, although severe pain can persist throughout the cycle. Exacerbation of symptoms just before menopause can occur. Resolution of symptoms at menopause occurs in 42% of women; however, spontaneous resolution before menopause occurs in 14% of patients.[11]

Noncyclic mastalgia tends to occur much less frequently, in 26% of patients, and peaks during the fourth decade of life.[9] The duration of noncyclic mastalgia tends to be shorter, with spontaneous resolution occurring in nearly 50% of patients.[11] In contrast to cyclic mastalgia, noncyclic mastalgia is almost always unilateral. Exacerbations of pain occur for no apparent reason and are difficult to treat.

A careful clinical breast examination should also rule out a small thrombosed vein that can present as persistent breast pain. Mondor disease, superficial thrombophlebitis of the breast, typically presents as a painful, tender, palpable cord. Although the exact etiology is unknown, risk factors include trauma, surgery, local intravenous access, and smoking.[12] Ultrasound is the recommended mode of diagnostic imaging, with sonogram revealing an anechoic, noncompressible, tubular structure with areas of narrowing and absence of flow on Doppler,[13] however, diagnosis can often be made by clinical findings alone. Rates of associated malignancy are low, but underlying cancer should be excluded by imaging and clinical findings. It is generally self-limited with resolution in 2 to 8 weeks, though supportive treatment may include antiinflammatories and warm compresses.[14]

Mastalgia from other origins includes scapular bursitis,[10] costochondritis,[15] lateral extramammary pain syndrome,[16] cervical radiculopathy,[17] or other nonbreast causes. Chest wall pain from these etiologies is almost always felt either on the lateral chest wall or at the costochondral junction.[16] Tietze syndrome, which commonly affects the second and third costochondral junctions, can manifest as focal medial breast pain.[18] Musculoskeletal inflammation, especially scapular bursitis, can present as referred pain to the breast and is often diagnosed by improvement with a scapular trigger point injection anesthetic and treatment with an injection of steroid.[10] Neurogenic pain is much more difficult to diagnose

and treat. If pain of neurogenic origin is suspected, an empirical trial of amitriptyline or carbamazepine may be beneficial for diagnosis and treatment.

Nomenclature

The term *fibrocystic disease,* of which mastalgia is the most common symptom, is unhelpful because it fails to delineate the full spectrum of disease. Postmortem studies of "normal" breast specimens indicate that fibrocystic changes occur in 50% to 100% of individuals.[19–21] The ANDI classification is used to classify BBDs, such as mastalgia, into those arising secondary to abnormalities of breast development, cyclic changes, or involution rather than as disease (see Table 5.1).[1]

Pathophysiology of Mastalgia

Pathogenesis and Etiology

Epithelial and stromal activity, as well as regression, constantly occur within the breast. Fibrosis, adenosis, and lymphoid infiltration, commonly used to characterize mastalgia, cannot be correlated with clinical episodes.[1] Watt-Boolsen and colleagues found no histologic differences between women with cyclic and noncyclic mastalgia and asymptomatic patients.[22] Jorgensen and Watt-Boolsen reported fibrocystic changes in 100% of 41 women with breast pain who underwent breast biopsy.[23] Although a higher incidence of fibrocystic changes was seen in this cohort than in asymptomatic controls, the total incidence of breast abnormalities did not differ between groups. Attempts to demonstrate edema as the main cause of cyclic pain and nodularity have been unsuccessful. Cysts that commonly occur with ANDI and mastalgia are secondary to changes of involution, periductal inflammation, and fibrosis, which may narrow the ducts distally and cause proximal dilation.[1]

Endocrine Influences

The natural history of mastalgia is clearly linked to the reproductive cycle, with onset at the age of menarche, a linear increase in prevalence up to age 50 (prevalence 68%), and cessation of symptoms at menopause. In a prospective study of reproductive factors associated with mastalgia, Gateley and colleagues reported that women with cyclic mastalgia were more likely to be premenopausal, to be nulliparous, or to have been at a young age when they had their first child.[6] However, theories of the exact hormonal events, including progesterone deficiency,[24] excess estrogen,[25] changes in the progestin/estrogen ratio,[26] differences in receptor sensitivity,[27] disparate follicle-stimulating hormone (FSH) and luteinizing hormone (LH) secretion,[28] low androgen levels,[29] and high prolactin (PRL) levels[30] have been difficult to prove or have not abated with hormone therapy.

Under normal circumstances, PRL exerts structural growth and secretory differentiation, mammary immune system development, and initiation and maintenance of milk secretion.[31] PRL secretion is episodic and shows circadian rhythm, with clustering of more intense episodes after midnight. In addition, PRL secretion has menstrual and seasonal variations.[32] These variations may, to some extent, account for the discrepancies in available reports.[29] Mastalgia may be related to an upward shift in the circadian PRL profile, a possible downward shift in menstrual profiles, and loss of seasonal variations.[32] Patients with mastalgia also show a heightened PRL secretion in response to thyrotropin-releasing hormone (TRH) antidopaminergic drugs[28] and may actively sequester iodine within their breast tissue as a result of an alteration in PRL control[33] (Fig. 5.1). In addition, stress can cause a rise in PRL response.[34]

Disturbances in the pituitary-ovarian steroid axis have long been associated with breast pain (see Fig. 5.1). However, numerous studies have not shown differences in estrogen and progesterone between asymptomatic controls and patients with mastalgia.[35–44] Available reports have measured estrogen over various time courses, from single mid-luteal phase samples to daily for an entire cycle. Clearly, circadian, menstrual, seasonal, or episodic changes could have been overlooked. More important, normal breast function is a balance between estrogen and progesterone, which is a part of the neuroendocrine control exerted by the hypothalamic-pituitary-gonadal axis (see Fig. 5.1). The theory of an inadequate luteal phase defect has never been confirmed. Three studies[35–37] demonstrate a significant decrease in luteal phase progesterone in women with mastalgia versus pain-free control subjects; however, four other comparable studies have not confirmed these results.[38–41] Nevertheless, an estrogen-progesterone imbalance could affect PRL secretion. An impairment of the normal ability to counteract estrogen-induced PRL release by increasing the central dopaminergic tone has been suggested as a cause of mastalgia.[45]

Nonendocrine Influences

Serum studies in animals demonstrate that caffeine intake can increase PRL,[46] insulin,[47] and corticosterone[48] and can decrease thyroid-stimulating hormone, free triiodothyronine, and thyroxine.[46] Minton and associates[49,50] originally hypothesized that methylxanthines, either by inhibiting phosphodiesterase and breakdown of cyclic adenosine monophosphate (cAMP) or by increasing catecholamine release, increase cAMP, leading to cellular proliferation in the breast[51] (see Fig. 5.1). Tissue from patients with breast disease showed unchanged phosphodiesterase activity but appeared to have increased adenylate cyclase levels and increased responsiveness to the biochemical-stimulating effects of methylxanthines.[49,50] Caffeine itself has no direct effect on cAMP, but catecholamines can increase cAMP. Studies in Minton's laboratory have shown increased release of circulating catecholamines in response to caffeine consumption[52] (see Fig. 5.1).

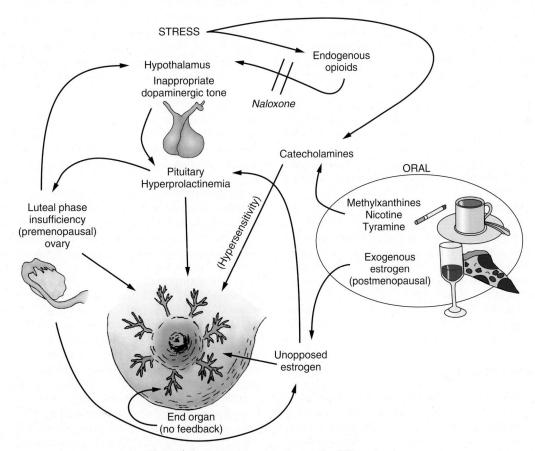

• **Fig. 5.1** Suggested theories of causation of breast pain.

Indeed, studies by Minton and colleagues have shown "catecholamine supersensitivity" in patients with ANDI. There were significantly higher levels of β-adrenergic receptors in symptomatic patients than in asymptomatic controls.[53] The increased activity and sensitivity of the β-adrenergic–adenylate cyclase system in symptomatic patients suggest a genetic predisposition for ANDI that is stimulated by the biochemical or hormonal effects of methylxanthines. Moreover, Butler and colleagues have been able to categorize patients genetically into fast and slow acetylators based on their caffeine metabolism.[54] Like the methylxanthines, a common biochemical effect of nicotine, tyramine, and physical and emotional stress is enhancement of catecholamine release and an increase of circulating catecholamines[53] (see Fig. 5.1). Arsiriy showed that women with mastalgia and ANDI had significantly higher levels of urinary catecholamines than did asymptomatic controls.[55] Studies have shown increased serum epinephrine and norepinephrine and decreased baseline dopamine levels in patients with cyclic as well as noncyclic mastalgia.[53] The increase or stimulation of adenylate cyclase activity in breast tissue appears to be an important step for triggering the intracellular cAMP-mediated events leading to symptomatic ANDI.[53] Randomized studies on smoking, tyramine, or stress reduction have not been performed.

The theory that fat increases endogenous hormone levels, and thus breast pain, has led to the performance of dietary fat-restriction studies.[56] In these studies, women with breast pain show lower levels of plasma essential fatty acid gamma-linolenic acid than do asymptomatic controls. It has been hypothesized that essential fatty acid deficiencies may affect the functioning of the cell membrane receptors of the breast by producing a supersensitive state.[57,58] High levels of saturated fats inhibit the rate-limiting delta-6 desaturation step between linoleic acid and gamma-linolenic acid. Catecholamines, diabetes, glucocorticoids, viral infections, and high cholesterol levels likewise limit this step.[57,58] With both estrogen and progesterone receptors, a supersensitive state can be produced with a higher ratio of saturated to unsaturated fatty acids. Administration of essential fatty acids in the form of evening primrose oil (9% gamma-linolenic acid) bypasses the delta-6 desaturation step, leading to a gradual reduction in the proportions of the saturated fatty acids[57] and diminishing the abnormal sensitivity of the breast tissue. Likewise, Ghent and colleagues have theorized that the absence of dietary iodine may also render terminal intralobular duct epithelium more sensitive to estrogen stimulation.[59]

Anatomic and extrinsic factors may contribute to the development of breast pain. Scurr and associates found breast pain to be related to cup size but not underband size. Women reported increased pain with participation in sports and activities exacerbated by ill-fitting and nonsupportive bras; however, overall breast pain was more common in women with lower activity levels. In a survey conducted in the female runners of the 2012 London marathon, 75% reported bra fit issues, most commonly chaffing and shoulder strap discomfort, suggesting that poor bra fit may be a factor in activity-related breast pain.[60]

Management of Mastalgia

As might be anticipated, there is a long list of suggested modalities for the treatment of a ubiquitous entity whose cause is unknown and whose relationship to fibrocystic breast disease and cancer is poorly understood. Breast pain may resolve spontaneously, and 19% of patients have marked responses to placebo therapy.

TABLE 5.2	Effectiveness of Interventions for Mastalgia			
	MASTALGIA			
Drug	**Cyclical**	**Noncyclical**	**Combined**	**Side Effects**
Methylxanthines[50]	—	—	83%	None
Dietary fat reduction[69]	90%	73%	83%	None
Evening primrose oil[6]	58%	38%	—	4%
Molecular iodine[59]	—	—	65%	11%
Danazol[6,7]	92%	64%	—	30%
Gestrinone[91]	—	—	55%	None
LHRH agonist[9,93]	—	—	67%	37%
Thyroid replacement	—	—	73%	None
Analgesics[11,104]	—	—	92%	None
Tamoxifen[108]	90%	56%	—	65%[a]

LHRH, Luteinizing hormone-releasing hormone.
[a]Regimen is 20 mg of tamoxifen. On 10 mg, side effects and efficacy are lower.

Therefore double-blind, placebo-controlled trials are required to prove the effectiveness of drugs in the treatment of mastalgia.[61] Gamma-linolenic acid, bromocriptine, danazol, LH-releasing hormone (LHRH) agonists, molecular iodine, and tamoxifen have all been shown by such trials to be of use in the treatment of breast pain. The safety and efficacy of these therapies, as well as less proven therapies, are discussed in the next section (Table 5.2).

Nutritional Therapy

Nutritional factors have been less well documented than other modalities in the cause and treatment of breast pain. Although they are the least expensive and least prone to side effects, dietary changes are often the most difficult to institute in the noncompliant patient.

Methylxanthines. Chemicals classified as methylxanthines include caffeine, theophylline, and theobromine. These substances are found in coffee, tea, chocolate, and cola beverages, as well as in many respiratory medications and stimulants. Minton and colleagues reported complete disappearance of all palpable nodules, pain, tenderness, and nipple discharge 1 to 6 months after eliminating methylxanthines from the diet of 13 of 20 women (65%).[62] In a subsequent clinical trial involving 87 women, complete resolution was seen in 82.5%, with significant improvement in 15% of women abstaining from methylxanthines.[50] Resumption of methylxanthines was associated with recurrence of symptoms in this cohort. These data are supported by nonrandomized studies, including retrospective data from 90 pairs of twins[63] in which the twin with breast pain was found to be more likely to consume more coffee than the unaffected twin. Ernster and colleagues randomized 82 of 158 women to abstain from methylxanthine and 76 women to no dietary instruction.[64] Differences in clinically palpable breast findings were significantly less in the caffeine-abstaining group, but absolute changes were minor. Bullough and colleagues studied daily methylxanthine ingestion from drug and dietary sources and found that both breast pain and fibrocystic disease are positively correlated with caffeine and with total methylxanthine ingestion.[65] Minton reported the evaluation of 315 patients with ANDI for a mean of 3 years (range, 1–11 years),[53] demonstrating improvement off caffeine and return of symptoms with resumption of caffeine.

Other case-controlled studies, however, have not confirmed these clinical findings. A study of an age- and race-matched cohort of approximately 3000 women who were a part of the Breast Cancer Detection Demonstration Project demonstrated no association between methylxanthine consumption and breast tenderness in women with fibrocystic disease or in controls.[66] In a single-blind clinical trial of 56 women randomized to a control (no dietary restrictions), a placebo (cholesterol-free diet), and an experimental group (caffeine-free diet) for 4 months, Allen and Froberg showed that caffeine restriction did not lessen breast pain or tenderness.[67] Another factor is the significant difference in the length of withdrawal of caffeine seen between positive and negative studies. Minton's work has been criticized for lack of control subjects and blinding as well as the general instability of findings in patients with mastalgia.[68] An unflawed, large-scale, prospective, long-term study that would count methylxanthines from all sources and use reliable dependent variables to assess pain, either to prove or disprove the value of methylxanthine withdrawal, has yet to be performed. Until then, clinicians may want to suggest a methylxanthine-restricted diet, especially in light of its no-cost, no-side-effect status and the other unwanted health consequences of caffeine.

Low Dietary Fat. As with breast cancer, mastalgia is less common in the global East and in Eskimos, whose diets are notably lower in fat. Reduction of dietary fat intake (to <15% of total calories for 6 months) significantly improves cyclic breast tenderness and swelling.[56] In one study, Sharma and colleagues demonstrated significant elevations in high-density lipoprotein cholesterol and the ratio of high-density lipoprotein cholesterol to low-density lipoproteins, as well as a decrease in the ratio of total cholesterol to high-density lipoprotein cholesterol in 32 cyclic and 25 noncyclic mastalgia patients.[69] Response to a low-fat dietary regimen was significant only in the cyclic mastalgia group, suggesting that cyclic mastalgia may be from cyclic aberrations in lipid metabolism and that dietary management may need to be pursued. A good or partial response was seen in 19 of 21 of the cyclic and 11 of 15 of the noncyclic patients. It is unclear what would lead to such a lipid profile abnormality—whether excessive intake, a genetic predisposition, or both. Nevertheless, dietary manipulation of this kind is difficult to achieve, is difficult to monitor, and requires a high degree of compliance.[70]

Evening Primrose Oil and Gamma-Linolenic Acid. Studies have shown that women with severe cyclic mastalgia have abnormal blood levels of some essential fatty acids,[71] which have been implicated in the control of PRL secretion and steroid hormone receptor alterations.[27] Early clinical experience with evening primrose oil (EPO), a source of gamma-linolenic acid, produced a 58% response rate with cyclic mastalgia and a 38% response rate with noncyclic mastalgia.[6] Symptoms of pain and nodularity were significantly improved with EPO (3 g/day) in a placebo-controlled trial after 4 months, and treatment was associated with an elevation of essential fatty acids toward normal levels.[72] A recent small pilot study of 41 patients randomized to receive EPO (3 g/day), vitamin E (1200 IU/day), or both found an improvement in worst pain in all three treatment groups but no difference with

placebo ($p = .093$) in intent-to-treat analysis.[73] Two more randomized controlled trials have not supported or contradicted this evidence of the efficacy of EPO in the treatment of mastalgia. In a large multicenter trial, Goyal and associates[74] evaluated mastalgia in 555 women and compared EPO plus antioxidants, EPO plus placebo antioxidants, antioxidants plus placebo EPO, and placebo antioxidants and placebo EPO. After 4 months, the investigators found no difference in recorded pain scores between women taking EPO plus vitamins versus placebo plus vitamins (15.2 vs. 14.9; $p = .3$). Similarly, Blommers and colleagues[75] found no significant difference between EPO and placebo in the frequency or severity of pain at 6 months. In this trial, 120 women were studied in four comparison groups: EPO plus placebo oil, fish oil plus placebo oil, fish oil plus EPO, and two placebo oils alone. Furthermore, a large recent meta-analysis performed by Srivastava and associates[76] reviewing the data from all randomized controlled trials using EPO revealed no significant beneficial effect of EPO over placebo. This new evidence in part, questions or refutes the utility of EPO as a first-line agent in the treatment of mastalgia, and the United Kingdom has withdrawn the prescription license for EPO because of its lack of efficacy.[77] Flaxseed oil, a source of alpha-linolenic acid, has also been shown to reduce breast pain. In a small, randomized controlled trial, women receiving 25 g flaxseed daily had reduced cyclical breast pain at both 1- and 2-month time points compared with placebo.[78]

Iodine. The exact influence of iodine on breast tissue is not understood. In contrast to iodides, which are thyrotrophic, Eskin and colleagues demonstrated that iodine is involved primarily in extrathyroidal activities, particularly in the breast.[79] Ghent and coworkers theorized that the absence of iodine may render the epithelium of the terminal intralobular ducts more sensitive to estrogen stimulation and proceeded to perform three studies.[59] In an uncontrolled study with sodium-bound iodide (313 volunteers for 2 years) and protein-bound iodide (588 volunteers for 5 years), subjects had 70% and 40% clinical improvement, respectively. The rate of side effects was high. In a prospective controlled crossover study, 145 patients in whom treatment with protein-bound iodide failed were given molecular iodine (0.08 mg/kg) and compared with 108 volunteers treated initially with molecular iodine. Objective improvement was noted in 74% of the patients in the crossover series and in 72% of those receiving molecular iodine as first-line therapy. The third part of the study was a controlled double-blind study in which 23 patients received molecular iodine (0.07–0.09 mg/kg) and 33 patients received placebo. In the treatment group, 65% had subjective and objective improvement. In the control group, 33% showed subjective placebo effect and 3% showed objective deterioration. Molecular iodine was found to be nonthyrotropic, without side effects, and beneficial for breast pain. In a randomized double-blind, placebo multicenter trial, Kessler[33] has since reported on the efficacy of Iogen for cyclical mastalgia. Iogen is a novel iodine formulation that generates molecular iodine (I_2), a substance thought to be less thyrotoxic on dissolution in gastric juices. In Kessler's study of 111 women with breast pain, 50% of patients reported a significant decrease in pain after 3 months in the 6-mg treatment group but not in the 1.5-mg and placebo groups.

Endocrine Therapy

Although it is difficult to prove, hormonal factors clearly play a role in the cause of cyclic mastalgia. This is evidenced by the fact that the condition manifests itself primarily during the ovulatory years, with symptoms that fluctuate during the course of the menstrual cycle, intensifying premenstrually and subsiding with menses.[80]

Androgens

Testosterone. One of the earliest effective hormonal treatments for mastalgia was testosterone injections. Its use has been limited by its adverse side effects. However, results from a placebo-controlled trial using 40 mg twice daily of the undecenoate oral form of testosterone demonstrated a reduction in mastalgia pain scores of 50%, with acceptable tolerance.[81]

Danazol. Danazol is an attenuated androgen and the 2,3-isoxazol derivative of 17α-ethinyl testosterone (ethisterone). Danazol competitively inhibits estrogen and progesterone receptors in the breast, hypothalamus, and pituitary[82]; inhibits multiple enzymes of ovarian steroidogenesis[83]; inhibits the midcycle surge of LH in premenopausal women; and reduces gonadotropin levels in postmenopausal women.[84] The precise mechanism of danazol in reducing breast pain is unknown. It is the only medication approved by the US Food and Drug Administration (FDA) for the treatment of mastalgia.

In initial studies, a double-blind crossover trial comparing two dosages of danazol (200 vs. 400 mg/day) in 21 patients with mastalgia demonstrated significant decreases in pain and nodularity at both dosages.[85] Onset of response and side effects were higher with the higher dosage. Of the participants, 30% had amenorrhea and weight gain. There was significant reduction in mean pain scores and mammographic density using danazol in a randomized trial with daily treatments of 200 or 400 mg of danazol for 6 months.[86] Patients relapsed more quickly (9.2 vs. 12.2 months) and to a greater extent (67% vs. 52%) in women taking 200 versus 400 mg of danazol. Gateley and colleagues found a clinically useful response to danazol (200 mg/day) in 92% of 324 patients with cyclical mastalgia and 64% of 90 patients with noncyclical mastalgia with 30% experiencing adverse events (mainly weight gain and menstrual irregularity) and 43 patients having to stop treatment despite 19 having an effective response.[87] Because the side effects of danazol are dose related, Harrison and colleagues[88] and Sutton and O'Malley[89] developed low-dose regimens. Patients responding to a dosage of 200 mg/day of danazol after 2 months were given a dosage of 100 mg/day for 2 months and then 100 mg every other day or 100 mg daily only during the second half of the menstrual cycle.[88] If previous reductions were well tolerated, the danazol was discontinued.[89] Symptoms were controlled without side effects at a total average monthly dose of 700 mg. Of 20 women, 13 (65%) of whom had experienced previous side effects, none reported side effects while taking this low dose. Some relief of pain was seen in all women, with a complete response maintained in 55%. Other reported side effects of danazol include muscle cramps, acne, oily hair, hot flashes, nervousness, hirsutism, voice change, fluid retention, increased libido, depression, headaches, and dyspareunia, which usually resolve after discontinuation of treatment. The drug is contraindicated in women with a history of thromboembolic disease. For women of childbearing age, adequate nonhormonal contraception is essential.

Recommendations for the administration of danazol are 100 mg twice daily for 2 months while the patient keeps a breast pain record. If no response or an incomplete response is obtained, the dose may be increased to 200 mg twice daily. If there is still no response, another drug should be tried. Therapy should not continue longer than 6 months (because side effects may develop), and the drug should be tapered, as described by Harrison and associates[88] and Sutton and O'Malley.[89]

Gestrinone. Gestrinone is an androgen derivative of 19-nortestosterone. As such, its mode of action and side effects are similar to those of danazol. However, side effects occur less frequently with the reduced dosage required for treatment (5 mg vs. 1400–2800 mg/wk). With its androgenic, antiestrogenic, and antiprogestagenic properties, gestrinone may inhibit the midcycle gonadotropin surge and act directly on the pituitary gland, in the ovary, directly at the estrogen receptor of the mammary gland.[90]

In a multicenter trial evaluating the safety and efficacy of gestrinone,[91] 105 patients were randomized to receive gestrinone or placebo 2.5 mg twice weekly for 3 months. Of patients treated with gestrinone, 55% had a clinically favorable response, with a placebo effect of 25%. Complete resolution of symptoms with gestrinone occurred only in 22% of patients. Further trials with gestrinone have not been performed.

Others

Luteinizing Hormone–Releasing Hormone Agonist. The mechanisms of LHRH analogs are thought to be their antigonadotropic action and direct inhibition of ovarian steroidogenesis, which almost completely induce ovarian ablation, resulting in extremely low levels of the ovarian hormones estradiol, progesterone, androgens, and PRL. In a nonrandomized trial, Monosonego and colleagues[92] gave intramuscular LHRH agonist (3.75 mg as a monthly depot) to 66 patients during a 3- to 6-month period. A complete response was observed in 44% of the patients treated with an LHRH agonist alone, and a partial response was seen in 45%. Monthly injections of the LHRH analog goserelin resulted in significantly diminished pain in 67% of patients with either cyclic or noncyclic mastalgia in a randomized multicenter study of 147 premenopausal women. Side effects, which included vaginal dryness, hot flashes, decreased libido, oily skin or hair, and decreased breast size, were seen more frequently in patients receiving goserelin (27 of 73 patients) than sham (4 of 74 patients).[93] Significantly, treatment with an LHRH agonist-induced remarkable loss of trabecular bone.[94] For this reason, only short courses of LHRH analogs should be administered and only for acute and severe cases of mastalgia.

Thyroid Hormone. Data from in vitro studies have suggested that thyroid hormones may antagonize the effects of estrogen at the pituitary receptor levels of lactotrophs, such as TRH, although there is no conclusive support for this.[37] Relative estrogen dominance is suggested as a cause for the increase in PRL responsiveness to TRH in patients with mastalgia.

Kumar and colleagues[42] found a generalized abnormality of hypothalamic-pituitary axis in 17 patients with cyclic mastalgia compared with 11 controls by using a combined TRH and gonadotropin-releasing hormone test. The release of PRL, LH, and FSH was significantly greater in patients with cyclic mastalgia than in controls, although estrogen and progesterone levels were normal. Bhargav and colleagues studied 201 women with BBD, none of whom had previously suspected hypothyroidism. The prevalence of hypothyroidism was 23.2%, and relief of BBD symptoms was attained in 83% of patients with hypothyroidism with thyroid replacement alone.[95] A large, randomized, placebo-controlled trial of levothyroxine is needed before any recommendation is made for its use as a standard treatment.

Nonendocrine Therapy

Bromocriptine. Results of recent studies point toward a PRL secretory hypersensitivity for estradiol in patients with cyclic mastalgia (see Fig. 5.1). Watt-Boolsen and colleagues[44] studied 20 women with cyclic mastalgia and compared them with 10 women who were asymptomatic. Basal serum PRL levels were significantly elevated, although within the normal range, in the mastalgia group versus controls. Cole and associates[30] have demonstrated that PRL is involved in the regulation of water and electrolyte balance in the nonlactating breast. An increase in serum PRL levels could possibly cause an influx of water and electrolytes in the breast, thus increasing tension and causing pain. However, in women with true hyperprolactinemia, levels of mammotrophic hormones are entirely different because ovarian steroid levels are suppressed. Bromocriptine is an ergot alkaloid that acts as a dopaminergic agonist on the hypothalamic-pituitary axis. One result of this action is suppression of PRL secretion.

Mansel and colleagues[96] reported a double-blind crossover study using bromocriptine in a group of patients with mastalgia. Lowered PRL levels associated with a significant clinical response were seen in patients with cyclic breast pain but not in those with noncyclic breast pain. In a double-blind controlled trial of danazol and bromocriptine, Hinton and associates[97] reported a clinical response with bromocriptine in two-thirds of patients with cyclic pain but no response in patients with noncyclic pain. In contrast, Pye and coworkers[98] reported a minimal response rate of 20% with bromocriptine in patients with noncyclic mastalgia versus 47% in those with cyclic mastalgia. The European Multi-Center Trial of bromocriptine in cyclic mastalgia confirmed the efficacy of bromocriptine. Side effects occurred in 45% of patients and were severe enough to warrant discontinuation of therapy in 11%. Side effects were reduced by an incremental buildup of doses over 2 weeks. However, reports of serious side effects of bromocriptine prescribed for lactation cessation, including seizures (63), strokes (31), and deaths (9), have resulted in its removal from the indication list of bromocriptine by the FDA.[99] Despite its apparent effectiveness, because of the seriousness and frequency of the reported side effects, we do not recommend bromocriptine for use in mastalgia.

Cabergoline, another long-lasting, potent, dopamine, has been demonstrated to be as effective as bromocriptine with fewer side effects. In a multicenter, open-label study of 140 women with cyclic mastalgia randomized to receive bromocriptine (5 mg/day during the second half of the menstrual cycle) or cabergoline (0.5 mg/wk during the second half of the menstrual cycle), 66.6% of women receiving bromocriptine and 68.4% of women receiving cabergoline has a positive response. Side effects were, however, much lower in the cabergoline group, with less frequent vomiting (4.5% vs. 28%), nausea (20.9% vs. 39%), and headache (6% vs. 23%) when comparing cabergoline to bromocriptine. In this small study, the serious side effects observed with bromocriptine (i.e., seizure, stroke, or death) did not occur.[100]

Analgesics. In a retrospective questionnaire survey of 71 patients, a negligible response was seen to conium cream, phytolacca cream, metronidazole, aspirin, cyproterone acetate, and ibuprofen cream.[101] Recently, a prospective but nonrandomized trial administering nimesulide, an oral analgesic, was reported. All but 2 of 60 patients had a clinically useful response (97%) after 2 weeks of therapy. Of 60 patients, 28 (47%) had complete resolution of their symptoms. Two patients could not take the analgesic because of complaints of gastritis.[102] In a randomized controlled trial of 108 women, Diclofenac, a topical nonsteroidal antiinflammatory drug (NSAID), has been shown to be effective for the treatment of both cyclical and noncyclical mastalgia.[103] Topical NSAID was also shown to be more effective at controlling breast pain than EPO (92% vs. 64% clinically significant pain

TABLE 5.3	Medications Causing Mastalgia	
Category	**Examples**
Cardiac and antihypertensive	Digoxin, methyldopa, minoxidil, spironolactone, other diuretics
Gynecologic	Oral contraceptive pills, hormone replacement therapy
Psychiatric	Selective serotonin reuptake inhibitors, venlafaxine, haloperidol, other antipsychotics
Antimicrobials	Ketoconazole, metronidazole
Other	Cimetidine, cyclosporine, domperidone, penicillamine, methadone

Data from Smith RL, Pruthi S, Fitzpatrick LA. Evaluation and management of breast pain. Mayo *Clin Proc.* 2004;79:353-372.

reduction).[104] However, another small, randomized, double-blind study did not show a benefit or oral NSAIDs over placebo.[105]

Abstention From Medications. Onset of breast pain with the recent prescription of any medication should be suspect (Table 5.3). This is particularly so with estrogen replacement therapy, and withdrawal of such can produce dramatic results. Tenderness caused by this therapy can be circumvented with initial low-dose therapy and dosage escalation or with short "drug holidays" when patients become symptomatic.

Refractory Mastalgia

Tamoxifen. Tamoxifen is an estrogen agonist-antagonist commonly used in the treatment of breast cancer. It is thought to competitively inhibit the action of estradiol on the mammary gland. In 1985 Cupceancu[106] first reported a noncontrolled prospective study of tamoxifen given for 10 to 20 days of the menstrual cycle at a dosage of 20 mg/day for up to six cycles; breast pain disappeared in 71% of patients and symptoms were ameliorated in 27%. Controlled trials at dosages of 10 and 20 mg per day produced greater than 50% reduction in mean pain scores in 90% of patients with cyclic mastalgia and in 56% of those with noncyclic mastalgia.[107,108] The higher dose was no more effective, but side effects were more prominent. In a double-blind, controlled, crossover trial of tamoxifen (20 mg/day) given during a 3-month period, pain relief was seen in 75% of patients receiving tamoxifen and in 22% of those receiving placebo. Major side effects included hot flashes (26%) and vaginal discharge (16%). In an effort to reduce side effects while maintaining efficacy, the tamoxifen dosage was lowered to 10 mg/day for 3 to 6 months. Side effects were seen in approximately 65% of patients taking 20 mg and in 20% of those taking 10 mg.[108] The efficacy of tamoxifen for the treatment of mastalgia is well supported by the recent meta-analysis of randomized controlled trials for mastalgia performed by Srisvastava and associates[76] in which tamoxifen achieved a relative risk of pain relief of 1.92. These results have led these authors to their recommendation that tamoxifen should be used as a first-line agent for the treatment of breast pain. However, possible links between tamoxifen use and endometrial carcinoma have relegated its use only for patients in whom symptoms are severe and in whom all standard therapies have failed.

Gong and colleagues[109] have hypothesized that toremifene, a newer member of the family of selective estrogen receptor modulators (SERMs), may be a better medication than tamoxifen for mastalgia. Compared with tamoxifen as adjuvant endocrine therapy for breast cancer, toremifene has a comparable therapeutic effect yet is associated with fewer adverse effects. In their double-blind, randomized control trial, patients treated for cyclical mastalgia with 30 mg daily of toremifene noted a 76.7% response rate compared with a 34.8% response rate seen in placebo treatment ($p < .001$); patients with noncyclical mastalgia had a 48.1% response rate with toremifene compared with 24% for placebo. The incidence of an intolerable adverse effect was not increased with toremifene therapy. However, toremifene has been reported to cause serious heart arrhythmias.

A recent study by Mansel and coworkers[110] evaluated the safety and efficacy of a topical gel containing the potent tamoxifen metabolite, afimoxifene (4-hydroxytamoxifen) for the treatment of cyclical mastalgia in premenopausal women. In their phase II trial, 130 women were randomized to placebo versus 2 or 4 mg of the transdermal agent for four menstrual cycles. After four cycles, patients in the 4-mg group were more likely to demonstrate improvements in pain ($p = .010$), tenderness ($p = .012$), and nodularity ($p = .017$) compared with placebo. Afimoxifene delivered percutaneously had 1000-fold lower serum levels than levels achieved after oral delivery of tamoxifen. There was no change in plasma hormone levels or any serious side effects in any of the treatment arms.

Ormeloxifene is another SERM, currently not available in the United States, that has recently been compared with tamoxifen in the treatment of mastalgia with equivalent results in pain relief after 3 months, but higher incidence of side effects including dizziness, menstrual irregularity, and ovarian cysts.[111]

Trigger Point Injections for Extramammary Pain (Scapulothoracic Bursitis) Mimicking Noncyclical Breast Pain. Because of the extensive confluence of afferent signals from the shoulder region to the dorsal horn of the spinal cord, the location of symptoms may or may not correspond to the proximity of the pain source. As expected, pain may involve the shoulder, the scapular area, the axilla, the arm, and, more commonly unrecognized, the breast.[112] A thorough history and physical examination is essential for patients presenting with mastalgia. Scapulothoracic bursitis should be ruled out in any postmenopausal woman presenting with breast pain. Trigger points along the medial scapular border are diagnostic of bursitis but may or may not be present. Injections containing a mixture of lidocaine (for diagnostic purposes), bupivacaine, and steroids in the trigger point(s) result in relief within 15 minutes (Fig. 5.2).[10] In conjunction with daily heat to the scapulothoracic bursa (shoulder blade) and nonsteroidal analgesics, this results in long-lasting relief in most patients. In a study of 461 patient with breast/chest pain, 103 were diagnosed with shoulder bursitis, with 83.5% having complete relief of pain after injection of local anesthetic and corticosteroid.[113] Similarly, musculoskeletal chest wall pain, costochondritis with tenderness of the costochondral or chondrosternal joints, and Tietze syndrome with pain and nonsuppurative swelling of the costochondral junctions particularly of the second and third ribs also respond to rest, heat, NSAIDs, and reassurance.[87]

Psychiatric Approaches. Lack of treatment for patients with mastalgia stems from the prevailing belief, as first proclaimed by Sir Astley Cooper, that all unexplained breast pain is a psychosomatic complaint seen in the neurotic female, not a real physiologic entity.[114] Indeed, in states of acute emotional stress, PRL is released

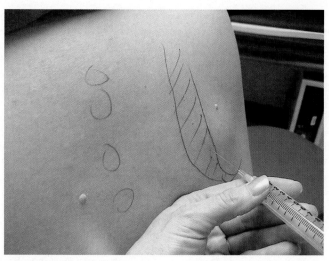

• **Fig. 5.2** The most common site of a trigger point causing severe noncyclical breast pain, which is usually at the junction of the lower third and upper two-thirds of the scapula.

and may form a physiologic basis for mastalgia (see Fig. 5.1). A study by Preece and colleagues found similarly low psychoneurotic scores for patients presenting with cyclical and noncyclical mastalgia and those presenting with varicose veins in comparison to high scores seen with outpatient psychiatric patients. However, a small subgroup of patients (5.4%) with treatment-resistant mastalgia did have characteristics that were similar to those of a psychiatric patient group.[115] Subsequently, Jenkins and associates[116] hypothesized that patients with severe or resistant mastalgia are likely to exhibit psychiatric problems. To investigate this hypothesis, 25 patients with severe mastalgia completed a psychiatric evaluation using the Composite International Diagnostic Interview (CIDI) and a general health questionnaire. On the basis of the CIDI examination, 17 had current anxiety, 5 had panic disorders, 7 had somatization disorders, and 16 had current major depressive disorders. Jenkins suggested that in patients in whom "standard pharmacologic interventions" for mastalgia fail, evaluation by a psychiatrist and a trial of tricyclic antidepressants may be indicated.

Surgical Approaches. Surgery, such as a subcutaneous mastectomy[117] or excisional breast biopsy for mastodynia, is ill-advised and should be a tool of last resort. It should be offered only at the behest of the patient and then only after significant counseling. In general, surgical excision of localized trigger spots without an identifiable breast abnormality is unsuccessful 20% of the time and runs the risk of replacing a painful area with a painful scar.[118]

Ineffective Treatments

Diuretics. Diuretics have never been tested in a double-blind, placebo-controlled trial. However, Preece and colleagues demonstrated that premenstrual fluid retention in patients with mastalgia is no different from that in symptom-free control subjects, limiting the rationale for the use of diuretics.[119]

Progesterones. Studies by Maddox and associates (among others) using a randomized, controlled, double-blind, crossover design with 20 mg of medroxyprogesterone acetate during the luteal phase showed no benefit for the patient with mastalgia.[120]

Vitamins. Abrams[121] reported a favorable response to vitamin E in an uncontrolled trial in 1965. In a small, prospective, double-blind, crossover study of the efficacy of vitamin E or placebo,

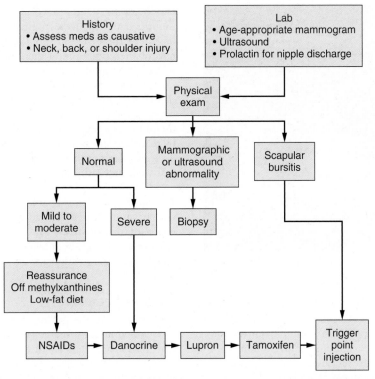

• **Fig. 5.3** Algorithm of a plausible approach to mastalgia. *NSAIDs,* Nonsteroidal antiinflammatory drugs.

10 of 12 patients receiving 300 IU/day and 22 of 26 patients receiving 600 IU/day showed improvement after 4 weeks of taking vitamin E. Serum levels of dehydroepiandrosterone, but not estrogen or progesterone, were significantly higher in the responders to the drug before and normalized after administration of vitamin E. Meyer and associates[122] conducted a double-blind, placebo-controlled, crossover trial that randomized 105 women to receive either vitamin E (600 IU/day) for 3 months or placebo. Although 37% reported improvement while taking vitamin E, versus 19% reporting improvement with placebo, this was not statistically significant. Parsay and colleagues, however, showed a significant improvement in cyclic mastalgia in women treated with vitamin E (400 IU/day) versus placebo in a randomized, double-blind study of 150 women at both 2- and 4-month time intervals.[123] In contrast, double-blind, placebo-controlled trials by London and coworkers[124] (128 patients receiving 150, 300, and 600 IU vitamin E for 2 months) and Ernster and colleagues[125] (73 patients receiving 600 IU for 2 months) reported no benefits from vitamin E.

Supplementation with vitamins B_1 and B_6[126,127] is thought to be of no benefit. A recent report by McFayden and associates[101] retrospectively reviewed treatment of 289 patients with pyridoxine (100 mg/day) for 3 months; 49% had a beneficial response, with only 2% reporting side effects. However, a double-blind controlled trial in 42 patients showed no benefit.

Vitamin A was first used for mastodynia by Brocq and colleagues in 1956 at a daily dose of 50,000 IU for 2 months, which led to significant reductions in pain.[128] In a small, nonrandomized trial in patients with symptomatic breast pain, 9 of 12 patients had marked pain reduction after 3 months of therapy with daily doses of 150,000 IU of vitamin A (all transretinal).[129] These results were associated with toxic effects often severe enough to stop or interrupt treatment. Santamaria and Bianchi-Santamaria developed a protocol of daily doses of 20 mg of beta-carotene interrupted with 300,000 IU of retinol acetate starting 7 days before each menstrual period and continuing for 7 days for each cycle.[130] Twenty-five patients with cyclic mastalgia were treated with this regimen for 6 months. Two patients had a complete response, and the remaining patients had a modest partial response. No side effects were reported. This regimen was not effective for noncyclic mastalgia. Controlled trials have failed to demonstrate a role for vitamins in the treatment of breast pain.

Summary

Fig. 5.3 suggests a plausible algorithm for the treatment of breast pain.

Benign Breast Disorders

The classification system developed by Page separates the various types of BBD into three clinically relevant groups: nonproliferative lesions, proliferative lesions without atypia, and proliferative lesions with atypia. This classification eliminates potentially confusing terminology and incorporates histologic criteria that are associated with an increased risk of the development of breast cancer and was adopted by the American College of Pathologists.[131,132] The histologic features of the breast biopsy specimen, together with the patient's personal and family history, establishes the relative risk of cancer. These data, combined with mammographic and physical examination findings, determine the management strategy and follow-up for the patient.[1]

A study from the Mayo Clinic found that the relative risk of breast cancer in a large cohort of women with benign breast disease was 1.56, and this risk remains for up to 25 years after biopsy. Furthermore, they found that histologic features, age at biopsy and degree of family history were major factors in the risk

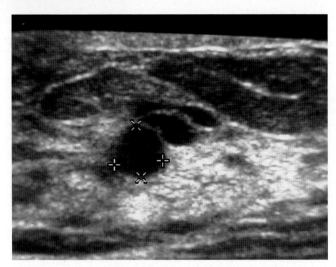

• **Fig. 5.4** Multiloculated cyst.

for developing breast cancer after a diagnosis of benign breast disease. Regarding the histologic classification of benign breast lesions, the relative risk associated with nonproliferative lesions without a family history is 0.89, nonproliferative lesions with a family history is 1.62, proliferative lesions without atypia the relative risk is 1.88, and for atypical hyperplasia it is 4.24.[133]

Nonproliferative Lesions of the Breast

Nonproliferative lesions of the breast account for approximately 70% of benign lesions. Cysts and apocrine metaplasia, duct ectasia, ductal epithelial hyperplasia, calcifications, fibroadenomas, and related lesions are included in this category.

Breast Cysts

Cysts are defined by the presence of fluid-filled, epithelialized spaces (Fig. 5.4).[134,135] Cysts in the breast vary greatly in size and number and can be microscopic or macroscopic. These lesions are almost always multifocal and bilateral, and they are almost never malignant. Cysts originate from the terminal duct lobular unit or from an obstructed duct ectasia. The typical macroscopic cyst is round, appears bluish (blue-domed cyst), and usually contains dark fluid ranging in color from green-gray to brown. The epithelium of the cyst is often flattened, and apocrine metaplasia of the epithelium lining the wall of the cyst is occasionally seen.

Cysts are categorized by their imaging characteristics as simple, complicated, or complex. Simple cysts are typically benign with anechoic content, imperceptible walls, and posterior acoustic enhancement. Complicated cysts are probably benign with hypoechoic content, thin walls, and with or without posterior acoustic enhancement. Finally, complex cysts are of an indeterminate nature and have thick walls, septa, and solid components. Complex cysts should undergo biopsy, percutaneous removal, and/or surgical excision because they can be associated with a wide range of diagnoses from benign to malignant conditions.[136]

Simple cysts do not need to be aspirated by their very presence. If age-appropriate mammography and ultrasound demonstrate a benign cyst, then no further intervention is required. In fact, it is discouraged because it can cause future mammographic and ultrasound artifact. If the cyst is painful or very large, aspiration can be performed under ultrasound guidance. Aspirated fluid that is bloody or contains debris should be sent for cytology. Once the

cyst is aspirated, it can be followed with repeat imaging in 6 months if it remains asymptomatic and cytology is negative. A biopsy of the cyst wall should be obtained if the cyst does not resolve after aspiration, if there is asymmetric wall thickening, or if there is atypical cellularity in the aspirate.[137]

Percutaneous removal is an alternative approach to management of complicated cysts. This approach obtains complete removal as well as tissue for examination. This is particularly useful for large macrocysts where aspiration is sure to be followed by reaccumulation. Percutaneous excision with a vacuum-assisted device can remove all the fluid as well as remove a piece of the cyst wall, preventing reaccumulation.

Multiple cysts and cyst aspirations are clinical markers of associated underlying histologic breast proliferation.[138] Women who have undergone aspiration of multiple breast cysts have an increased risk of breast cancer, and they should be advised to practice regular self-examination, in addition to undergoing periodic clinical examination and age-appropriate mammography and ultrasound.[138,139]

Apocrine Metaplasia

Apocrine metaplasia presents pathologically as dilated ducts and cysts containing inspissated secretions. It is commonly associated with fibrocystic change and does not increase the risk of cancer without atypia. Apocrine metaplasia typically presents as a cluster of microcysts or a microlobulated mass seen sonographically but can also present as thick-walled cysts or complex cystic lesions that may require biopsy.[137,140] In addition, it has been associated with enhancing lesions on magnetic resonance imaging (MRI) and has been responsible for up to 11% of benign MRI biopsies.[141] These lesions may require biopsy or short-term follow-up based on clinical and radiographic findings.

Duct Ectasia and Periductal Mastitis

Duct ectasia is present in nearly half of women older than 60 years of age and is considered part of the normal aging process.[142] Duct ectasia involves the large and intermediate ductules of the breast.[143] Duct ectasia is most often recognized by the presence of palpable dilated ducts filled with desquamated ductal epithelium and proteinaceous secretions. Periductal inflammation is a distinguishing histologic characteristic in this condition. The pathogenesis of duct ectasia is obscure but probably periductal mastitis, leading to weakening of the muscular layer of the ducts and secondary dilation, is the primary process.[144] The presenting symptoms of duct ectasia are nipple discharge, nipple retraction, inflammatory masses, and abscesses. Both duct dilation and duct sclerosis represent disorders of involution. Periductal fibrosis can occur in the absence of duct ectasia or inflammation and alternatively represents part of the normal involutional process.[145] The clinical significance of severe duct ectasia lies in its mimicry of invasive ductal carcinoma, but there is no demonstrated relationship to breast cancer risk.

Mild Ductal Epithelial Hyperplasia

The fundamental feature of epithelial hyperplasia is an increased number of nonstromal cells relative to the normally observed two cell layers along the basement membrane.[131] Subtypes include apocrine, ductal, and lobular types (Box 5.1). Mild ductal epithelial hyperplasia, as opposed to florid ductal epithelial hyperplasia, which is discussed later, does not increase the risk for breast cancer. In general, some degree of epithelial hyperplasia is seen in the majority of women over 70 years of age.[146]

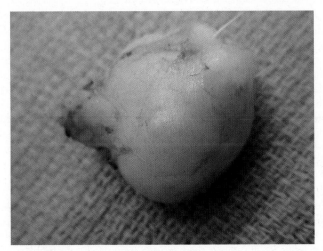

• **Fig. 5.5** A well-marginated multilobulated fibroadenoma.

Fibroadenoma and Related Lesions

Fibroadenoma. Autopsy studies demonstrate that fibroadenomas are present in approximately 10% of women.[147] The peak incidence occurs between the second and third decades of life. However, these lesions are occasionally seen in the elderly. They are often solitary lesions, but 50% of patients will present with multiple masses. Fibroadenomas are benign, well-marginated, pseudoencapsulated tumors (Fig. 5.5). They are a subset of fibroepithelial tumors that comprise stromal and epithelial components.[148] The histologic pattern depends on which of these components is predominant. Common stromal patterns include diffuse myxoid change, hyalinization, and increased cellularity; less commonly foci of smooth muscle differentiation or pseudo-angiomatous stromal hyperplasia can be seen.[149] Other histologic characteristics include biphasic tumor, low cellularity, no pleomorphism, 1 to 2 mitoses per 10 HPF (high-power field), and very low Ki-67 index.[149]

Fibroadenomas are very responsive to hormonal stimulus and may enlarge premenstrually or during pregnancy. Growth beyond 5 cm is considered a giant fibroadenoma. Fibroadenoma fits well into the ANDI classification: small fibroadenomas are normal, clinical fibroadenomas (1–3 cm) are a disorder of the normal process, and giant and multiple fibroadenomas fit in the disease end of the spectrum. The incidence of carcinoma arising in a fibroadenoma is approximately 0.1% to 0.3%, with invasive carcinomas more frequently of the lobular type.[150]

Diagnosis is based on the combination of clinical examination, imaging, and percutaneous tissue aspiration or biopsy (the "triple" test). A clinical diagnosis of fibroadenoma alone is unreliable and does not exclude malignancy, even in younger women. Ultrasound, in combination with mammography in select patients, should be performed. A subsequent core needle biopsy is the most accurate means of establishing the diagnosis. Because of the heterogeneity of fibroadenomas and the overlapping features of fibroepithelial tumors, an accurate diagnosis from core needle biopsy can be challenging. Any atypical epithelial proliferation or unusual stromal changes on biopsy should prompt complete excision to rule out malignant transformation or phyllodes tumor.[149] In the future, gene expression profiling may prove useful in discerning these differences along the spectrum of fibroepithelial lesions. In a recent study, the levels of expression of proliferation-related genes (e.g., CCNB1 and MKI67) and mesenchymal/epithelial-related genes (e.g., CLDN3 and EPCAM) were used to distinguish fibroadenoma from malignant phyllodes tumor.[151]

Traditionally, symptomatic fibroadenomas, as well as those greater than 2 to 3 cm, have been treated by surgical excision.[137,152] Currently, alternatives to surgical excision include percutaneous removal[153] radiofrequency ablation[154] or cryoablation.[155] Core biopsy–proven fibroadenomas in young women (<35 years) that are mobile, less than 2.5 cm, and otherwise clinically benign can be safely observed.[156]

Complex Fibroadenoma. Complex fibroadenomas are fibroadenomas harboring one or more complex features including epithelial calcifications, apocrine metaplasia, sclerosing adenosis, or cysts greater than 3 mm. Imaging features that can help distinguish complex fibroadenomas include irregular shape, noncircumscribed borders, complex echo structure, microcalcifications, and posterior acoustic enhancement.[157] The risk of invasive carcinoma developing in women with complex fibroadenoma was found to be three times that of the general population.[158] The literature supports excision of complex fibroadenomas.[159]

Fibroadenomatosis (Fibroadenomatoid Mastopathy). Fibroadenomatosis is a benign breast lesion with the composite histologic features of a fibroadenoma and fibrocystic changes that may represent a morphologic stage in the development of fibroadenomas. The lesion is characterized by microscopic fibroadenomatoid foci intermingled with dilated ducts, epitheliosis, and adenosis and was found in more than 10% of cases of BBD.[160] Although there is no clear etiology of fibroadenomatosis, there have been case reports of cyclosporine-induced fibroadenomatosis in immunosuppressed patients after renal transplantation.[161,162]

Tubular Adenoma. Tubular adenomas are rare, benign epithelial tumors that usually present in young women of reproductive age. They are well-defined, freely mobile tumors that clinically resemble fibroadenomas being composed of benign epithelial elements with sparse stroma.[163] The sparse stroma is the histologic feature that differentiates adenomas from stromal-rich fibroadenomas.[164] Tubular adenomas or pure adenomas have not been associated with an increased risk of breast cancer development.[165]

Lactating Adenoma. Lactating adenomas present during pregnancy or during the postpartum period. On microscopic examination, lactating adenomas have lobulated borders and are composed of glands lined by cuboidal cells that possess secretory activity identical to that normally observed in breast tissue during pregnancy and lactation. They are usually slow growing and seldom reach a size larger than 3 cm. In rare cases, rapid growth can occur resulting in giant lactating adenomas greater than 5 cm.[166]

Hamartoma. Hamartomas are rare, benign tumors that can lead to unilateral breast enlargement without a palpable, localized mass lesion. On imaging, they appear as rounded, well-circumscribed masses of mixed, heterogeneous densities with a mottled center and a thin capsule. No consensus has been reached on definitive histologic criteria, but characteristic findings include the presence of lobules within a fibrotic stroma that surrounds and extends between individual lobules and obliterates the usual loose stroma.[167] Multiple hamartomas are associated with Cowden disease, which carries a higher risk of breast cancer.[168]

Adenolipoma/Lipoma. Adenolipomas/lipomas are common and consist of sharply circumscribed nodules of fatty tissue that have normal lobules and ducts interspersed.[169] Microscopically the fat is normal, and the lobules and ducts are fairly evenly distributed throughout the tumor. They represent no increased risk of breast cancer.

Pseudoangiomatous Stromal Hyperplasia

Pseudoangiomatous stromal hyperplasia (PASH) generally presents as a painless mass. It is characterized by myofibroblast-lined, slitlike spaces resembling blood vessels surrounded by dense, collagenous stroma that may require differentiation from low-grade angiosarcoma.[170] It presents sonographically as a hypoechoic mass or mammographically as a noncalcified, circumscribed mass.[152] After diagnosis by core needle biopsy, these lesions may be safely followed with routine screening assessment in the absence of interval growth or other suspicious radiologic findings.[171] There have been reports of PASH being responsible for rapid breast enlargement documented in the literature.[172–174]

Proliferative Lesions Without Atypia

Proliferative breast disorders without atypia make up approximately 30% of benign breast disease and include sclerosing adenosis, radial scars and complex sclerosing lesions, florid ductal epithelial hyperplasia, and intraductal papillomas.

The diagnostic workup for each of these lesions is similar and involves stereoscopic or open biopsy depending on the facilities and experience available and the perceived risk of malignancy from the radiologic appearance. It is widely accepted that it is impossible to differentiate these lesions with certainty from cancer by mammographic features.[175]

Sclerosing Adenosis

Sclerosing adenosis is more common in perimenopausal women and is found in approximately 28% of benign biopsies.[176] It is a proliferative lesion characterized by an increased number of acinar structures and fibrosis of the lobular stroma while the normal two-cell population along the enveloping basement membrane is maintained. The borders of the lesion are irregular, while it maintains its lobular architecture. Sclerosing adenosis commonly occurs in the context of multiple microscopic cysts and diffuse microcalcifications that make screening mammography difficult. Recent data suggest that sclerosing adenosis may double the risk for developing breast cancer compared with benign breast disease without sclerosing adenosis.[177]

Radial Scar and Complex Sclerosing Lesions

Radial scars and complex sclerosing lesions of the breast are characterized by central sclerosis and varying degrees of epithelial proliferation, apocrine metaplasia, and papilloma formation.[178] The term *radial scar* is reserved for smaller pathologic lesions (up to 1 cm in diameter), whereas complex sclerosing lesion is used for larger masses. Radial scars originate at the point of terminal duct branching. With the naked eye, the appearance is often unremarkable, but with magnification, the characteristic histologic changes radiate from a central white area of fibrosis, which contains elastic elements. In a review by Degnim and colleagues radial scars appear to have a twofold increased risk for future breast cancer.[179] However, others have suggested that this risk is close to that imparted by proliferative disease overall.[178,180] Short-term follow-up may be appropriate for radial scars without atypia and those that are sampled with 12 or more cores by a large biopsy needle (11-gauge or greater) due to lower reported rates of upgrade to cancer (5% or less).[179]

Florid Ductal Epithelial Hyperplasia

Florid hyperplasia is found in more than 20% of biopsy samples and thus is the most common proliferative lesion of the breast. It is associated with a minor increased risk of breast cancer.[131,133] This entity is characterized by an increase in cell number within the ducts, with a proliferation of cells that occupies at least 70% of the duct lumen. Architecturally, epithelial hyperplasia is either solid or papillary and is characterized by intracellular spaces that are irregular, slitlike, and variably shaped. It has been suggested that the expression of estrogen receptor alpha in adjacent normal lobules may increase the breast cancer risk in patients with epithelial hyperplasia lacking atypia.[181]

Intraductal Papilloma

Solitary intraductal papillomas are tumors of the major lactiferous ducts and are most commonly observed in premenopausal women. Common presenting features include serous or bloody nipple discharge.[182,183] Grossly, these lesions are pinkish-tan, friable, and are usually attached to the wall of the involved duct by a stalk. Microscopically, they are composed of multiple branching papillae with a central fibrous vascular core that is lined by a layer of epithelial cells. Central papillomas tend to be single whereas peripheral papillomas are more likely to be multiple and impart a higher risk of atypia and subsequent carcinoma.[184,185] Lewis and colleagues reported a relative risk of breast cancer of twofold in single papillomas without atypia, fivefold in those with atypia, and a relative risk of threefold and sevenfold in multiple papillomas without and with atypia, respectively.[186]

It is often difficult to differentiate between benign papilloma and papillary cancer on core biopsy due to the heterogeneity of papillary lesions, which often require review of the entire lesion to ensure accurate diagnosis.[179] Standard surgical excision after diagnosis of a papillary lesion reveals an upgrade rate of 10% to 38%[179,187,188]; however, in reviewing only the papillary lesions diagnosed without atypia, others have shown much lower upgrade rates ranging from 0% to 6%.[189–191] Furthermore, some studies have found no pathologic upgrades when patients with nipple discharge or palpable masses are excluded, suggesting that there might be a subset of patients that can be followed with observation rather than excision as long as there is radiographic-pathologic concordance.[189,190,192] Alternatively, small papillomas can be percutaneously removed in their entirety via newer biopsy devices.

Juvenile papillomatosis is a rare subset of papillary breast disease occurring primarily in children and young adults. It generally presents as a firm, well-circumscribed mass, similar to fibroadenoma. Ultrasound reveals ill-defined, heterogeneous masses with surrounding small cystic spaces. Management generally involves complete surgical excision with annual surveillance. More than 25% of patients with juvenile papillomatosis have a family history of breast cancer, suggesting it may be a marker of a familial predisposition for breast cancer. The family of affected patients may also benefit from screening.[184,193]

Proliferative Lesions With Atypia

Atypical proliferative lesions include both ductal and lobular lesions. These lesions have some, but not all, of the features of carcinoma in situ. At times, even the most experienced pathologists disagree as to whether a given lesion is atypical hyperplasia or carcinoma in situ.[194]

Results from the Nurses' Health Study reveal an odds ratio for breast cancer of 4.1 among all women with atypical hyperplasia.[195] Similar results were described by Degnim and colleagues.[196] Their study found an increased risk of breast cancer development in patients with multifocal atypia and younger age, with the risk remaining elevated for more than 20 years.

Atypical hyperplasia has been shown to increase the future cancer risk in both breasts. In a group of nearly 700 women followed for a mean of 12.5 years, approximately 20% developed breast cancer. This study reported a 2:1 ratio of ipsilateral to contralateral breast cancer with ipsilateral predominance in the first 5 years and long-term bilateral risk continuing thereafter.[197]

Atypical Lobular Hyperplasia

Atypical lobular hyperplasia (ALH) fulfills some, but not all, of the criteria of lobular carcinoma in situ.[198] The cytology of ALH is usually quite bland, with round, lightly stained eosinophilic cytoplasm. The uniformity and roundness of the cell population is pathognomonic of ALH. The lobular unit is less than half filled with these cells, and no significant distortion of the lobular unit is present.[199] According to Page and colleagues, the risk of subsequent invasive cancer in women with ALH is four times that of women who do not have this diagnosis and increased if associated with a family history.[200–202] Degnim and associates in the Mayo cohort did not find that family history further increased the risk of this breast lesion and reported a lower relative risk of cancer of 3.67 among women with ALH.[194] More recently, Collins and colleagues reported an odds ratio of 7.3 for breast cancer risk among women with ALH (Table 5.4). There are no clear guidelines on the management of ALH found on percutaneous biopsy. Most recent studies report pathologic upgrade rates ranging from 0% to 22%.[179,203] Although historically, surgical excision has been recommended for cores revealing ALH, some recent reports suggest observation with short-term follow-up may be appropriate for lesions with concordant findings and no other high-risk lesions within the biopsy specimen.[179]

Atypical Ductal Hyperplasia

Atypical ductal hyperplasia is diagnosed when atypia is present and either the cytologic or architectural criteria for ductal carcinoma in situ (DCIS) are absent. Page and coworkers[200] have emphasized that each of the following criteria must be met for a diagnosis of DCIS: (1) a uniform population of cells, (2) smooth geometric spaces between cells or micropapillary formation with

TABLE 5.4 Risk for Development of Invasive Carcinoma	
Lesion	Relative Risk
Nonproliferative lesions of the breast	0[a] to 1.6-fold
Sclerosing adenosis	2-fold
Radial scar	2-fold
Florid epithelial hyperplasia	1.5-fold
Intraductal papilloma	2- to 5[b]-fold
Atypical lobular hyperplasia	4-fold
Atypical ductal hyperplasia	4-fold

Data from references 133, 177, 179, 186.
[a]Relative risk = 0.89.
[b]5-fold increased risk with atypia.

uniform cellular placement, and (3) hyperchromatic nuclei. Atypical ductal hyperplasia has some, but not all, of these features. The natural history of atypical ductal hyperplasia suggests an intermediate risk (approximately fourfold) for the development of invasive cancer[200] with similar results from the Nurses' Health Study (odds ratio 3.1)[195] (Table 5.4). When ADH was diagnosed by percutaneous biopsy, the rate of upgrading to DCIS or invasive carcinoma at surgery was found to be in the range of 13% to 31%,[179,204,205] and subsequent surgical excision is recommended for most patients.[179] Refer to Chapter 8 for further management of atypical hyperplasia.

Flat Epithelial Atypia

Flat epithelial atypia (FEA) is a rare lesion that presents pathologically as nuclear atypia in the setting of columnar cell change or hyperplasia, frequently with microcalcifications seen on imaging. Recent studies suggest it may be a nonobligate precursor to low-grade breast carcinoma.[206] It has been found that, with radiologic-pathologic correlation of FEA diagnosed on core needle biopsy, upgrade rates to carcinoma are up to 13%, although these rates are lower when calcifications are removed. For patients with pure FEA on core needle biopsy, the World Health Organization Working Group advocates radiologic-pathologic correlation, and, in the absence of clinically suspicious indicators, recommends observation.[207] However, others deem surgical excision reasonable given pathologic upgrade rates.[179] Despite one small study in which FEA demonstrated a small increase in future breast cancer risk (relative risk 1.5),[179] there are insufficient data to indicate the need for clinical follow-up or risk-reducing therapies.[152]

Other Benign Breast Disorders

Nipple Discharge

In a study of 10,000 consecutive new surgical consultations for breast complaints, 3% were for nipple discharge alone.[208] Of the population with periductal mastitis/ductal ectasia complex, 15% to 20% have nipple discharge.[209] Nonbloody, nonspontaneous, bilateral nipple discharge, typically from several ducts, is a benign condition with no increased cancer risk and is not normally an indication for surgical treatment.[210] Bloody nipple discharge is associated with a significant risk of cancer, with an odds ratio of 2.27 compared with patients with nonbloody discharge,[211] although benign bilateral bloody nipple discharge can be seen with pregnancy. Duct excision remains the gold standard treatment for pathologic nipple discharge that includes bloody or serous discharge. A few have suggested that there may be a subset of patients that presents without palpable mass and normal examination and imaging for whom observation or ductoscopy or galactography may be an appropriate alternative.[212–214] However, excision is both diagnostic and curative. Reference Chapter 4 for additional information on nipple discharge.

Nipple Inversion

Primary nipple inversion is a disorder of the development of the terminal ducts, preventing the normal protrusion of ducts and areola. Onset later in life can represent periductal fibrosis, but cancer must be excluded.[215] Although the results are usually satisfactory, patients seeking correction for cosmetic reasons should be aware of the possibility of nipple necrosis, interference with sensation, inability to breastfeed, and the possibility that postoperative fibrosis will lead to late recurrent inversion. Because the benign condition results from shortening of the ducts, a complete division of the subareolar ducts is the only procedure that can correct it permanently.

Epithelial Hyperplasia of Pregnancy

Marked hyperplasia of the duct epithelium occurs in pregnancy. The papillary projections sometimes give rise to bilateral bloody nipple discharge. Although this resolves in most cases without consequence, full workup to rule out carcinoma should be pursued.[216]

Adolescent Hypertrophy

Adolescent hypertrophy is associated with gross stromal hyperplasia at the time of breast development and can be categorized by differing growth patterns. Juvenile gigantomastia demonstrates rapid growth over 6 months, followed by a period of slower persistent growth. Adolescent macromastia, an additional subtype, demonstrates a more continuous growth curve. In addition, there appears to be an obesity-related breast hypertrophy. The exact cause of adolescent hypertrophy is unknown; however, there appears to be a hormonal basis to the condition. Proposed theories include hypersensitivity of the mammary estrogen receptors, excess local estrogen production and the presence of estrogen-like substances.[217] The spectrum from a small breast through massive hyperplasia fits the horizontal element of the ANDI concept: an excessively large breast is a disorder, whereas gigantomastia is at the disease end of the spectrum. Reduction mammoplasty can be an effective treatment option and may help relieve the psychological distress and physical strain from this condition.[217]

Fat Necrosis

Fat necrosis usually presents as a firm mass that develops after trauma or surgery that can mimic malignancy. There may be associated skin retraction and tenderness. There is a wide spectrum of pathologic and radiographic findings that evolve over the course of healing. Microscopically, early lesions may have anucleated adipocytes, foamy histiocytes, and multinucleated giant cells along with signs of hemorrhage when viewed microscopically. Signs of hemorrhage may be present grossly as well. Older lesions develop fibrosis and hemosiderin-laden macrophages with dystrophic calcification microscopically with signs of saponification, calcification, and fibrosis when viewed grossly. Mammographic findings may change over time and can include early linear and curvilinear calcifications and later central calcifications, typical for oil cysts. Focal asymmetries and spiculated masses may be other radiographic findings.[218,219]

The tender, acute retroareolar mass of periductal mastitis often resolves spontaneously, so surgery is delayed and antibiotics may be given if biopsy is suggestive of this diagnosis.[209]

Subareolar Abscess and Fistula

A subareolar abscess is confirmed with needle aspiration, which also provides a specimen for bacterial culture.[220] Aspiration can be facilitated by ultrasound guidance. Repeat aspirations are often necessary, and 40% of cases involving anaerobic bacteria recur after a short follow-up period. For recurrent symptoms, some have advocated for a total nipple core biopsy or excision of the central nipple, including the obstructed ducts. This technique achieves a cure rate of 91% and an overall 95% satisfaction rate in the cosmetic outcome of the nipple.[221]

Terminal mammary duct obstruction may result in the formation of a fistulous tract from the lactiferous duct to the skin and predisposes to recurrent subareolar abscesses. In this setting, fistulectomy is recommended for definitive treatment. Smokers are at particular risk, and smoking cessation is recommended. See Chapter 6 for further detail. Nipple inversion or occlusion during lactation are also thought to be causative factors.[222,223]

Selected References

1. Hughes LE, Mansel RE, Webster DJ. Aberrations of normal development and involution (ANDI): a new perspective on pathogenesis and nomenclature of benign breast disorders. *Lancet*. 1987;2:1316-1319.
2. Hughes LE, Smallwood J, Dixon JM. Nomenclature of benign breast disorders: report of a working party on the rationalization of concepts and terminology of benign breast conditions. *Breast*. 1992;1:15.
133. Hartmann LC, Sellers TA, Frost MH, et al. Benign breast disease and the risk of breast cancer. *N Engl J Med*. 2005;353:229-237.
179. Degnim AC, King TA. Surgical management of high-risk breast lesions. *Surg Clin North Am*. 2013;93:329-340.
137. Amin AL, Purdy AC, Mattingly JD, Kong AL, Termuhlen PM. Benign breast disease. *Surg Clin North Am*. 2013;93: 299-308.

A full reference list is available online at ExpertConsult.com.

6

Mastitis and Breast Abscess

STEPHANIE A. VALENTE AND STEPHEN R. GROBMYER

Management of patients with a breast abscess is an art, and each abscess has unique features that require familiarity by the treating physician. Breast abscesses can be frustrating for both the patient and the surgeon. Even for patients referred with chronic, recurring abscesses, the surgeon should initially repeat the breast conservative treatment that may have failed in the past, the purpose of which is to "get to know" the abscess and the patient. Knowing the personality of the patient is important because, on rare occasions, a simple mastectomy may be the last alternative to the patient's ability to live without recurrent breast abscesses.

Mastitis

Mastitis is an infection of the breast that presents as pain, redness, and swelling. An infection of the breast parenchyma that goes unnoticed or untreated can eventually develop into an abscess. Patients with acute mastitis and abscess formation often represent a diagnostic and therapeutic challenge. Some abscesses drain spontaneously, and others require intervention that can include needle aspiration, incision and drainage, or excision. There is currently no consensus on optimal management strategies. The principles that guide successful diagnosis, evaluation, and management of various types of primary breast infections are discussed in this chapter.

Presentation

Patients with acute breast infection typically present with one or more of the following symptoms: skin erythema, palpable mass, tenderness, fever, and/or pain.[1–3] Breast abscesses may occur in both the lactational and nonlactational settings.[4–7] Breast abscesses have been most commonly reported to occur in women between 20 to 50 years of age. However, breast infections have also been reported in men,[8] postmenopausal women,[3,9] and children.[10] Postmenopausal patients with a breast abscess often have a more indolent presentation and may lack many of the classical findings of a traditional breast abscess.[10] Abscesses may occur either centrally (subareolar or periareolar) or peripherally in the breast, usually in the upper outer quadrant where a majority of breast tissue is located.[3] Breast infection can result from recent surgery,[11] tattoos, or nipple piercing,[12] but most causes are unknown. The incidence of breast infection associated with surgery is 5% to 10%[13,14] and with nipple piercing is estimated the be as high as 10% to 20% in the months after the procedure.[15]

Evaluation

Careful clinical examination is the cornerstone of diagnosis for acute breast infection. Findings on examination can include a mass, erythema, skin warmth, skin thickening, and tenderness.[1,2,4] (Fig. 6.1) Ultrasound is a useful modality as an adjunct to physical examination to evaluate for the presence or absence of an associated underlying abscess.[2,16,17] Additionally, ultrasound can help to identify the size and depth of the abscess cavity as well as the presence of multiple abscesses, which may not be appreciated on physical examination (Fig. 6.2). Many patients with a breast abscess also have abnormal mammograms with nonspecific findings, including an irregular mass, focal asymmetry, diffuse asymmetric density, circumscribed mass, or architectural distortion[2] (Fig. 6.3). These findings in the acute setting may be difficult to differentiate from those findings associated with malignancy. In addition, in the acute setting of suspected breast infection, mammography is often not possible secondary to breast pain and tenderness. Importantly, in cases of atypical presentation or patients with recurrent, nonimproving symptoms, a mammogram should be performed to rule out inflammatory breast cancer.[18] After successful medical, percutaneous, or surgical management and resolution of an acute breast infection or abscess, mammography to exclude an underlying or associated malignancy and to ensure complete resolution is recommended.[8,19]

Microbiology

In the management of breast abscess, particular attention should be given to obtaining cultures for specific pathogens to help guide treatment decisions. *Staphylococcus aureus* is the most common organism associated with breast abscess.[3,7,18] Recently, an increase in methicillin-resistant *S. aureus* has been detected in community-acquired breast infections.[18,20] Other commonly reported causative organisms include *Pseudomonas aeruginosa, Staphylococcus epidermidis, Proteus, Serratia, Bacteroides,* and *Kelbsiella.*[1,3,21] Of note, 20% to 40% of breast abscesses are found to be sterile on culture.[1,3,21] Cigarette smoking has been associated with increased rates of anaerobic breast infections and increased rates of recurrent breast abscess.[22,23] Pathologic organisms that have been documented after nipple piercing include aerobic, anaerobic, and mycobacterial infections.[24–26] A variety of unusual pathologic organisms have been documented in association with breast abscess, including *Actinomyces* species,[27] *Brucella,*[28] *Mycobacterium tuberculosis,*[28] *Fusarium solani,*[29] *Echinococcus,*[30] and *Cryptococcus.*[31] Many of these unusual infections are endemic to specific areas and specific patient populations, and they

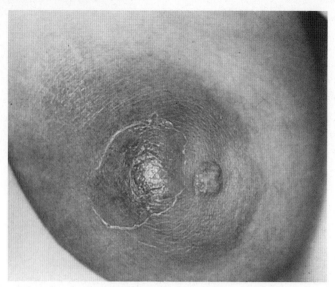

• **Fig. 6.1** A 38-year-old smoker presented with acute onset of right breast pain. A red, hot, tender, fluctuant mass was observed.

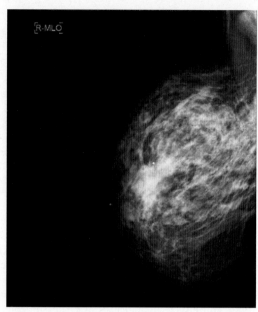

• **Fig. 6.3** Mammogram showing an abnormal, asymmetric breast mass.

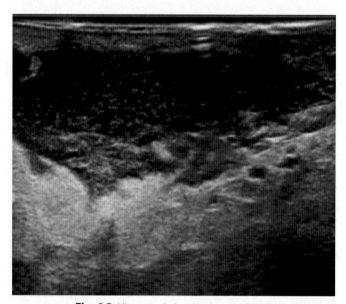

• **Fig. 6.2** Ultrasound showing breast abscess.

require special consideration in the appropriate clinical setting. Necrotizing soft tissue infections and gangrene of the breast have been reported in association with anticoagulant treatment, trauma, and in the postpartum period.[32–35]

Management

Antibiotics

In patients who present with signs and symptoms of mastitis who are clinically suspected of having an underlying breast infection or abscess, ultrasound is useful for the detection of an intramammary fluid collection. For patients with no fluid or a small fluid collection seen on ultrasound, a trial of oral antibiotics is warranted.[21,36] Initial choice of antibiotics is best directed by local antibiograms and to cover the most common pathogen *S. aureus.*[20] Antibiotic recommendations include cephalexin 500 mg four times daily,

dicloxacillin 500 mg four times daily, clindamycin 300 mg four times daily, with the optional addition of metronidazole 500 mg three times daily[7] for 7 to 10 days' duration. Failure to improve should prompt further evaluation with repeat ultrasound to evaluate for the development of an intramammary fluid collection requiring an alteration in the management strategy. In some cases, a tissue biopsy may be necessary to exclude malignancy. The patient should be scheduled for regular follow-up appointments until the infectious process has completely resolved.[3]

Invasive Intervention

Early Abscess. The traditional initial treatment approach of surgical incision and drainage of a breast abscess has been replaced by needle aspiration. Aspirated material should always be sent for microbiological analysis to allow for adjustments of the antibiotic regimen accordingly. Warm compresses placed over the abscess are recommended for comfort.

Aspiration. Numerous authors have suggested aspiration of breast lactational and nonlactational abscesses as the primary management.[1,3,4,7,37–39] Benefits of aspiration as an initial management strategy include improved cosmesis, lack of requirement for general anesthesia, no requirement for wound packing, and decreased cost.[3,8,40] It has been reported to be successful in 54% to 85% of all cases.[3,41,42] The described aspiration technique of several authors involves use a 16-gauge needle (or larger if necessary) with aspiration and irrigation of the cavity through an area where the skin is not thinned from inflammation.[1,21] Use of ultrasound to guide aspiration may be helpful and is associated with higher rates of success but is not required, especially in superficial lesions.[3,43] The addition of oral antibiotics is a necessary component of initial therapy for breast abscess managed with aspiration.[3,43] Cultures of aspirated fluid may be useful to guide antibiotic choice. Although some authors have suggested sending abscess fluid for cytology to exclude malignancy, the value of this practice is not well defined and not widely recommended.[44] Some authors have advocated instillation of antibiotics or saline irrigation into the abscess cavity[1,21]; however, this practice is not widely accepted, and its benefit has not been clearly demonstrated. Some have advocated placement of an indwelling drain at the time of aspiration, but this is also not routinely recommended.[3] After initial management, patients should undergo at minimum biweekly clinical reassessment to determine resolution of the abscess or subsequent requirement for additional treatment (repeat aspiration or surgical drainage).[3] Median time to resolution of breast abscess with aspiration is approximately 2 weeks (range, 1–8 weeks).[3,21] Reported success rates for the aspiration technique are highest with repeated, multiple aspirations. Successful treatment for single and multiple aspirations of breast abscess are 57% to 79% and 90% to 96%, respectively.[1,8,43] Patients who fail to improve with multiple aspirations or whose clinical condition deteriorates, require surgical incision and drainage. Factors that have been associated with failure of aspiration include large size (>3 cm) and presence of multiple loculations.[1,3,43]

Surgical Intervention. Surgical intervention in the form of incision and drainage should be performed for an abscess that has failed repeat aspiration. As with needle aspiration, this technique can be performed in the outpatient setting with use of minimal conscious sedation or local anesthetic. Use of conventional local anesthetic agents (e.g., lidocaine) is seldom effective in providing adequate local analgesia for the incision because of the low tissue pH in the inflamed skin tissue fluid, but should still be used. Additional options to make the patient comfortable include oral sedation in the office, administration of intravenous/intramuscular conscious sedation in the emergency department, or performing the procedure under general anesthesia in the operating room.

To perform incision and drainage, the incision should be made over the site of maximum fluctuance and kept within Langer's lines for optimal cosmesis. The abscess cavity should be explored and all the loculi and septations broken down using either finger fracture technique or a hemostat. The abscess may be extensive or multilocular and must be drained completely, with care to not excise the surrounding indurated tissue so as not to destroy surrounding breast tissue or disfigure the breast. The purulent material should be cultured for both aerobic and anaerobic bacteria, and a Gram stain should be performed. In the appropriate age group, a biopsy specimen of the abscess wall should be taken to rule out carcinoma. The abscess cavity should then be irrigated with normal saline solution. After irrigation of the abscess cavity, a gauze wick packing is placed to assist drainage and prevent premature skin closure. Tight packing should be avoided because it can cause necrosis of the tissue and overlying skin. Postprocedurally, antibiotics should be continued. The patient should be scheduled for biweekly follow-up appointments until the process has resolved. Final follow-up should include an ultrasound to document complete resolution.

Late Abscess. The traditional approach to the large, chronic, deep breast abscess involves taking the patient to the operating room for surgical incision and drainage with disruption of septae and open packing of the wound to heal by secondary intention[1,45] (Fig. 6.4). Options to consider include use of operative ultrasound to identify all subclinical abscess pockets in the breast, pulse lavage, antibiotic-impregnated irrigation (such as gentamycin), and finger fracture or a hemostat to break up intervening loculations in the abscess cavity, packing the wound open with normal saline or iodine-soaked gauze or placement of a temporary dwelling Penrose drain. Planned return trips to the operating room and frequent follow-up should also be considered.

Limitations to this approach include need for general anesthesia, high cost of performing in an operating room, and patient's understanding of potential prolonged healing, need for frequent packing/dressing changes, close follow-up, and risk of cosmetic deformity and recurrence.[21] In addition, surgical incision and

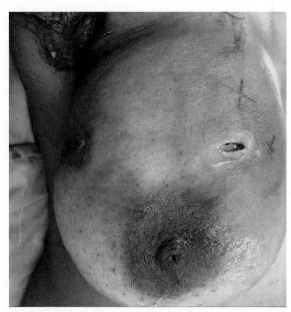

• **Fig. 6.4** Surgical approach to late breast abscess. Ultrasound demonstrated multiple abscesses that were marked and then subsequently incised and drained.

drainage have been associated with recurrence rates between 10% to 38% requiring additional procedures.[46]

Principles of management of necrotizing soft tissue infection of the breast are similar to necrotizing soft tissue infections of other areas and include early diagnosis, early and aggressive surgical management, and systemic antibiotics.[32,33,35,47] Because necrotizing soft tissue infections are most commonly polymicrobial in etiology, broad-spectrum antibiotics represent the best initial choice of antimicrobial coverage.[34]

Lactational Mastitis and Abscess

A breast abscess that develops in the postpartum period is referred to as a lactational or puerperal abscess. This type of abscess tends to occur within the first 12 weeks after birth or at the time of weaning from breastfeeding.[3,4,7] The patient presents with a tender breast mass, and is currently breastfeeding or has recently slowed frequency or stopped. In a lactational associated abscess, the pathogen is most often *S. aureus*.[7,48] It remains unclear whether the staphylococci are derived from the skin of the patient or from the mouth of her suckling infant, and both may be sources of infection. Most lactation mastitis is a result of bacteria entry though a crack or sore in the skin of the nipple from feeding in combination with milk stasis from decreased frequency of breastfeeding.[48,49] In milk stasis, the milk components can create a blockage of a lactiferous duct, resulting in retention of milk in the peripheral lobules creating a milk retention cyst called a galactocele.[50] Usually, a galactocele does not become infected because the milk within the cyst is sterile, but this stagnant milk produces breast engorgement and in some cases can become infected.[3,51]

The general principles for evaluation and management of breast infection, outlined previously, are applicable to lactational abscesses, and underlying malignancy must be excluded.[6,52] Management consists of drainage (percutaneous or open) and systemic antibiotics. During treatment for lactational breast abscess, women are encouraged to continue to breastfeed, and this does not pose a risk to the infant.[48] The breast with the abscess should be fully drained frequently via a breastfeeding or breast pump to prevent milk stasis and engorgement.[1,4,6] Antibiotics given to a breastfeeding mother need to be nontoxic for an infant because these can be passed through the milk. Recommendations include any of the penicillin antibiotic regimens described earlier or ampicillin-sulbactam 875 mg twice daily for 10 days.[6,48] Alternatives for a penicillin allergy include use of clindamycin 300 mg four times daily[48] or azithromycin. If the mother requires antibiotics, which are not safe for a breastfeeding infant, the mother must be instructed to "pump and dump" her breast milk products until she has completed her antibiotic course.

Milk fistula is an uncommon condition, which can occur as a complication after a needle aspiration but more commonly after incision and drainage of a breast abscess in a lactating woman.[3,53] In this situation, a fistula tract forms between the skin surface and the duct in the breast, resulting in spontaneous drainage of milk from this path of least resistance. Most milk fistulas will close primarily with time without the need for surgical intervention.[53] On rare occasions, the mother will need to stop breastfeeding to allow the fistula to heal.

Periductal Abscess/Chronic Subareolar Abscess

In 1951 the association of a chronic, recurring periareolar breast abscess and an associated draining fistula was described by Zuska and colleagues and is often referred to as Zuska disease.[54]

Presentation

Most patients who present are women aged 20 to 58 years,[55,56] with a history of multiple recurrences of a periareolar breast abscess in the same location with the presence of a recurrent, chronic draining fistula at the edge of the areola.[58,59] On occasion, associated nipple discharge[60] or nipple inversion[55,60] is observed. The diagnosis is made on clinical grounds based on presentation and history of recurrences.[61]

On physical examination, the characteristic features are the presence of an acute breast subareolar abscess with accompanying local tenderness, swelling, erythema, and induration. The abscess is characteristically located at the edge of the areola, usually with an associated draining sinus tract located at the vermilion border of the areola[62,63] (Fig. 6.5). On examination, the finger-thumb test can be performed for evaluation of a subareolar mass, nipple discharge, or discharge from the fistula of the involved breast (Fig. 6.6). Intermittent nipple discharge occurs in 8% to 84% of patients. Mammography and ultrasonography are helpful in detecting signs of prominent subareolar mammary ducts and to rule out an underlying mass or malignancy.

Causes

The cause and sequence of this benign disease process appears to be multifactorial, and the exact mechanism of the pathogenesis of this disease has been speculated.[54,59,63–65] The disease progression hypothesis for a subareolar breast abscess is thought to begin with an abnormal change of the normal cuboidal lining of the lactiferous ducts into squamous metaplasia.[29,59] The squamous epithelium then produces keratin, which in turn plugs the ducts, leading to obstruction.[59] This accumulation of cellular debris produces dilatation of the duct and eventual rupture. The debris

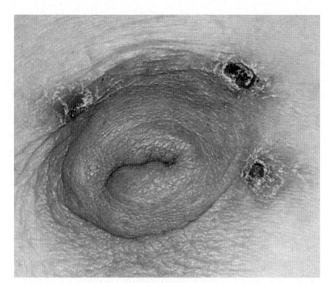

• **Fig. 6.5** Patient with chronic periductal mastits resulting in inversion of the nipple and formation of three fistulas at the vermillion border of the areola.

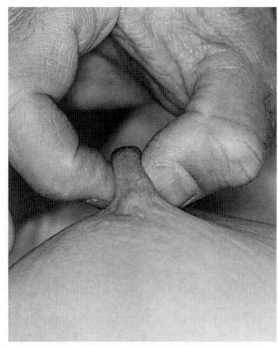

• **Fig. 6.6** The finger-and-thumb test to assess degree of inflammatory involvement and dilation of subareolar mammary ducts.

and secretory material infiltrate the surrounding tissue creating an inflammatory response in the breast tissue, and subsequent bacterial invasion results in abscess formation. Spontaneous drainage of the abscess occurs via the shortest and most direct route of least resistance, which is usually at the edge of the areola (Fig. 6.7). Occasionally, the discharge also exits via the nipple. After the sinus has healed, in the vast majority of cases, the process continues and a recurrent abscess appears and discharges once more along the same route, establishing a permanent fistulous tract.[63,64] Chronic fistulas have been reported to occur in 12% to 67% of patients.[66] This is followed by the hallmark of this disease process—a recurrent subareolar abscess at a later date,

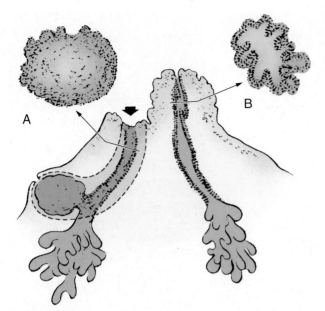

• **Fig. 6.7** Squamous metaplasia (A) often coexists with retraction of the nipple and plugging of the lactiferous duct with epithelial debris. Resulting suppuration breaks out at areolar margin. Dashed line designates margin of dissection recommended in core excision. In the normal situation (B), cuboidal epithelium and ductal continuity are maintained. Note pleating in lactiferous sinus. (From Powell BC, Maull KI, Sachatello CR. Recurrent subareolar abscess of the breast and squamous metaplasia of the lactiferous ducts: a clinical syndrome. *South Med J.* 1977;70:935-937.)

either at the same site or in an adjacent segment of the breast. Until the underlying cause is identified and the entire diseased duct is completely removed, repeated episodes of infection are common and seldom self-limiting.[59] Several authors have reported an association among cigarette smoking, vitamin A deficiency, or hormonal imbalances.[7,61,63]

The main organisms cultured most commonly are mixed flora of aerobes and anaerobes consisting of *S. aureus,* coagulase-negative staphylococci, *Streptococcus,* and anaerobes.[7,56]

Factors

The development of a subareolar abscess is a spectrum of varying degrees of duct ectasia, followed by a primary chemically induced inflammatory reaction, and secondary bacterial growth, subsequently followed by an infection and chronic periductal inflammation. The development of a chronic mammary fistula is thought to be the final stage of a benign but complicated inflammatory process termed mammary duct–associated inflammatory disease sequence (MDAIDS).[63] This concept is supported by the increased recognition and consensus that proper management of this disease entails use of a combination of antibiotics to cover aerobes and anaerobes followed by surgical excision of the involved duct and the associated periductal inflammation. The effect of hormonal (estrogen, prolactin), environmental (smoking), and nutritional (relative vitamin A deficiency) influences, as well as anatomic factors (congenital nipple retraction), is thought to play a contributory role to the development of subareolar abscesses.[63] There is increasing epidemiologic and experimental evidence that vitamin A or retinoids have a significant biologic effect on mammary duct epithelial cell proliferation and differentiation.[63] Many studies have also noted an increased incidence of mammary

duct squamous metaplasia in smokers.[61,67] The molecular mechanisms through which smoking induces squamous metaplasia have yet to be identified, although their association is strong, particularly in heavy smokers (more than 10 cigarettes per day).[68] Interestingly, it has been shown that, within 30 minutes of smoking, nicotine and its metabolite cotinine are detected in the breast milk of lactating women.[69] By its direct toxic effect, smoking can damage the subareolar ductal epithelium, making it easily prone to bacterial invasion from skin flora.[57]

Treatment Plan

The approach to treatment of an active infection with a subareolar breast abscess should be determined by the degree of inflammation and existence of concurrent fistula. For an acute infection with abscess formation, initial treatment with antibiotics and either needle aspiration or incision and drainage is appropriate to clear the purulent infection[58] as described earlier in this chapter. Perioperative antibiotic coverage should be employed, and the treating surgeon must recognize that this is only a temporizing measure. Broad antibiotic coverage should be considered to cover anaerobic and aerobic organisms. One option is using both cephalexin 500 mg four times daily and metronidazole[70] 500 mg by mouth three times a day for 10 days; other options include amoxicillin/clavulanate potassium 875/125 mg twice daily,[56] ciprofloxacin 500 mg twice daily, or sulfamethoxazole/trimethoprim 800/160 mg twice daily. It is anticipated that the infection will improve, but recurrence should be expected because the underlying disease process has not been eradicated.[56] Definitive operative treatment of the abscess and the associated duct should then be planned for 4 to 6 weeks after the acute inflammatory process has subsided.

Surgical Management

When the fistula is chronic and well established, the patient should undergo surgery, usually with general anesthesia and continued antibiotic coverage. Surgical management requires complete excision of the fistula tract; diseased duct and surrounding inflamed tissue. Numerous different surgical techniques have been described.[55,58,59,62,63,71,72]

Ductectomy

When only an isolated single duct appears to be involved in the disease process, the operative procedure recommended is called a ductectomy. With use of general anesthesia, this surgical technique involves placement of a lacrimal ductal probe into the fistula opening to define the fistula tract. This identifies the connection between the discharging duct in the nipple and the draining sinus at the edge of the areola[62] (Fig. 6.8). Alternately, injection of the fistula tract with 1% methylene blue before the start of the dissection is often helpful in identifying the corresponding major subareolar duct that connects with the fistula.[71] Next, a radial elliptical incision is made to include the skin of the nipple and overlying areola including the entire involved duct and fistula tract as well as the inflamed tissue, resected back to normal tissue.[58,59,62] The radial incision is made starting from the middle of the nipple and extending laterally through the areola and the vermilion border. After the entire diseased portion of the duct and surrounding tissue is removed, the nipple areolar complex is carefully reconstructed by placing 4-0 absorbable suture material subcutaneously at three critical sites: (1) the circumferential edge of the apex of the nipple, (2) the base of the nipple, and (3) the vermilion

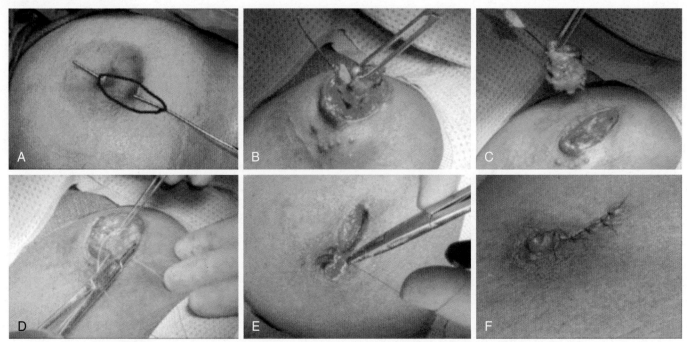

• **Fig. 6.8** Surgical technique. (A) Radial elliptical incision. (B) and (C) Excision of complete duct, fistula tract, and all surrounding inflammatory tissue. (D) Closure of breast tissue. (E) Stitch at base of nipple to cause adequate protrusion. (F) Primary closure of skin. (From Lannin DR. Twenty-two-year experience with recurring subareolar abscess and lactiferous duct fistula treated by a single breast surgeon. *Am J Surg.* 2004;188:407-410.)

border of the areola.[63] In patients who present with inverted nipples or a retracted nipple secondary to a previously drained chronic disease site, the nipple is everted, and a fourth suture consisting of a purse-string or Z-suture is placed inside the base of the nipple to prevent it from collapsing.[63]

Studies have described management of the remainder of the radial incision as the skin being closed primarily,[58] a Penrose drain or gauze packing wick placed in the radial corner to allow for drainage,[62] or the skin left open for daily packing (Fig. 6.9).[55] For open packing, iodoform gauze of appropriate size can be used. It is placed as a wick into the surgically created defect in the subareolar space and is exteriorized beyond the vermilion border through the lateral aspect of the incision.[62] The patient is taught to change the wick daily. Antibiotics suitable for coverage against aerobes and anaerobes are selected and prescribed for a course of 10 to 14 days.

Resection of Major Mammary Ducts

When multiple ducts are involved, or the subareolar abscess reoccurs despite a ductectomy, a resection of all of the major mammary ducts must be performed. For this surgical technique, a radial incision can be used similar to that described previously.[72] Alternatively, a circumareolar incision is made below the areola.[72] Dissection and elevation of the nipple and the areola complex from the underlying breast gland are performed (Fig. 6.10A). The major ducts are isolated and separated from the base of the nipple by passing a curved tonsil forceps or hemostat around the nipple base and dividing the ducts with a knife (Fig. 6.10B and C). The nipple base is cored to carefully remove all ductal tissue from the base of the nipple (Fig. 6.10D). Care is taken to avoid devascularizing the nipple skin. A purse-string or Z-suture of

no. 4-0 Vicryl may be inserted through the nipple base to hold it everted without causing necrosis.[63] The major subareolar duct system is then dissected out from the middle of the underlying breast tissue and removed (Fig. 6.10E and H). The wound is irrigated. Primary closure of the subareolar space is performed to obliterate the dead space, and then either the areolar skin is sutured in position with a subcuticular, interrupted suture, or the skin is left open for drainage with the option to approximate the skin edges with Steri-Strips or sutures to obtain an optimal cosmetic result (Fig. 6.10F and G).[72] A drain or packing is usually not required in the elective setting but can be placed. If a drain is used it should be removed within 24 hours.[72] The operation is performed with antibiotic coverage and antibiotics are continued postoperatively.

Patients undergoing surgery should be warned of the potential for recurrent problems and possibly loss of nipple sensation. Nipple necrosis is an uncommon but potential complication of repeated surgery. Reasons for failure of surgery include inadequate removal of major duct tissue, either from the nipple base or from the breast disk itself.[70,72]

It has been reported that in some cases of repeat recurrences (i.e., more than three), consideration for resection of the entire nipple and ducts is recommended for definitive cure[59] (Fig. 6.11). In these cases, reconstructive surgery may be necessary, and various techniques have been described.[73,74] Mastectomy is rarely necessary to achieve symptom control.[59,70]

Idiopathic Granulomatous Mastitis

Idiopathic granulomatous mastitis (IGM) is a rare, chronic, relapsing, benign inflammatory condition of the breast with an

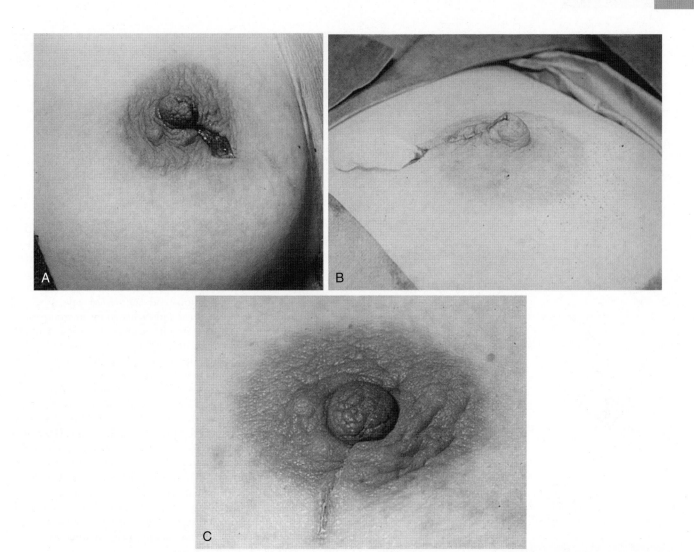

• **Fig. 6.9** Options for managing surgical defect after ductectomy. (A) Leaving radial portion of the incision open, (B) placement of packing and gauze wick at the radial edge, or (C) primary closure of the surgical wound. (From Meguid MM, Oler A, Numann PJ, Khan S. Pathogenesis-based treatment of recurring subareolar breast abscesses. *Surgery.* 1995;118:775-782.)

unknown etiology. First described in 1972,[75] it is also referred to as idiopathic granulomatous lobular mastitis. IGM most commonly affects women of childbearing age (age range 20–60 years)[76–78] with a history of pregnancy and lactation within the past 5 years.[45,76,77,79,80] The most common clinical presentation of IGM is a palpable breast lesion(s) ranging in size from 1 to >5 cm, accompanied by overlying skin induration, tenderness, erythema, sinus tract formation with suppurate drainage, or breast edema that clinically can mimic a bacterial abscess or breast cancer[75–77,81–85] (Fig. 6.12). There tends to be a higher incidence in Hispanics[76,79] and Middle Easterners.[80,86,87] IGM can present in any quadrant of the breast, but the upper outer quadrant is the most common location.[76–78] IGM is more often unilateral[76] but can be bilateral.[80] Nipple inversion or retraction due to the inflammation of Cooper's ligaments can occur,[45] and enlarged palpable reactive axillary lymph nodes are identified in 13% to 40% of women.[76,78,84] The presence of one or more fistulae or sinus formation associated with sterile abscesses or chronic suppuration may be among the key presenting clinical features. Evaluation and management of these patients remains a clinical challenge. Recognizing the

presentation to avoid misdiagnosis is important to avoid unnecessary prolonged antibiotics and numerous disfiguring surgical interventions of IGM's chronic relapsing course.

On mammography, IGM presents as an ill-defined density with speculated margins and associated overlying skin thickening[84,88] (Fig. 6.13). Ultrasound demonstrates a hypoechoic mass or abscess formation with tubular extensions and can show enlarged lymph nodes with mild concentric cortical thickening and preservation of the hila[76,84,88] (Fig. 6.14). On magnetic resonance imaging (MRI), IGM appears as a mass or masses with ring or nodular enhancement.[88] MRIs are helpful in determining the extent of the disease at presentation and allow for following the reduction of lesions over time.[45]

Diagnosis

The differential diagnosis of IGM includes infectious and noninfectious etiologies listed in Box 6.1.[45] The diagnosis of IGM is one of exclusion of all other causes and specific pathologic findings on biopsy.

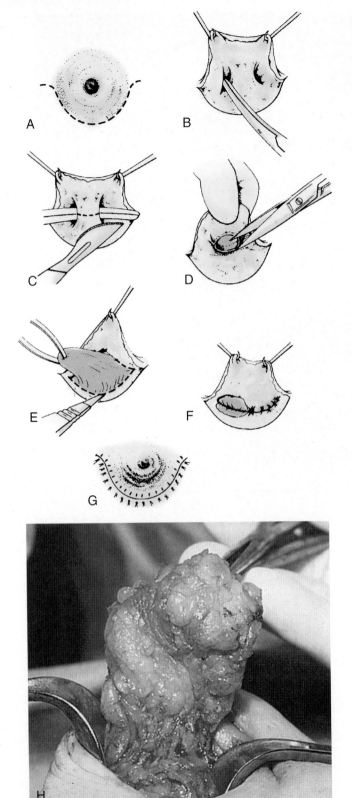

• **Fig. 6.10** (A–G) Technique of subareolar dissection (see text). (H) Close-up view of subareolar tissue dissected in a patient after recurrent abscesses. ([A–G] From Hartley MN, Stewart J, Benson EA. Subareolar dissection for duct ectasia and periareolar sepsis. *Br J Surg.* 1991;78: 1187-1188.)

• BOX 6.1	Differential Diagnosis of Idiopathic Granulomatous Mastitis

Tuberculosis	Diabetic mastitis
Parasitic infection	Autoimmune
Fungal infection	Trauma
Sarcoidosis	Polyarteritis nodosa
Wegener granulomatosis	*Corynebacterium* infection
Giant cell arteritis	Breast cancer
Bacterial abscess	Foreign body reaction
Periductal mastitis	*Mycobacterium* infection

A core needle biopsy of the wall of the mass should be performed and is preferable to a fine-needle aspiration (FNA) or excisional biopsy because a core biopsy completely characterizes the lesion compared with an FNA and is less invasive and disfiguring than an excisional biopsy.[77] All abscesses should be drained, preferably by needle aspiration, and cultures of any associated abscess fluid should be obtained and evaluated for microorganism (Gram), fungal infection (periodic acid–Schiff), and acid-fast bacilli (Zeihl-Neelsen) to exclude an infectious etiology.[76] Additionally, one must rule out other infections, including mycobacterial, mycotic, or parasitic as well as autoimmune causes such as sarcoidosis or foreign material.[45,75,80] To rule out tuberculosis, in additional to staining for the presence of acid-fast bacilli in the tissue, a purified protein derivative (PPD) serum test or skin test and a chest x-ray to check for presence of any concurrent lung granulomas can be performed. To rule out an underlying autoimmune etiology, blood work to check for C-reactive protein, antinuclear antibody (ANA), rheumatoid factor, and alpha-1-antitrypsin can be sent for analysis.[45] Pathologic analysis demonstrates hallmark noncaseating granulomatous inflammation of the lobular units of the breast, presence of multinucleated giant cells, polymorphonuclear leukocytes, plasma cells, lymphocytes, and occasionally sterile microabscessses[76–78,84,89] (Fig. 6.15).

Etiology

The exact underlying cause of IGM is unknown, but an exaggerated autoimmune response has been postulated.[45,75] It is speculated that damage to the ductal epithelium produced by a local trauma, hormonal changes, chemical irritant, or infection allows luminal secretions to leak into the lobular connective tissue triggering lymphocyte and macrophage migration, thereby creating a granulomatous response.[45] There seems to be a correlation with recent pregnancy and lactation[76,77] Some have suggested an association with smoking, oral contraceptives,[77] and corynebacteria,[90] but other studies have found no correlation.[85,87] The natural history of IGM is variable but often characterized by a chronic relapsing course. Management of patients with IGM can be challenging, and numerous therapeutic approaches and management algorithms have been described, including close follow-up, antibiotic therapy, surgical excision, systemic steroids, immunosuppressants, and mastectomy.[80,82]

Treatment

Initial treatment strategies are controversial, and articles published in the literature are case reports or institutional series with various proposed management algorithms.[76–78,80–82,91] Treatment recommendations depend on size of the lesions, severity of the

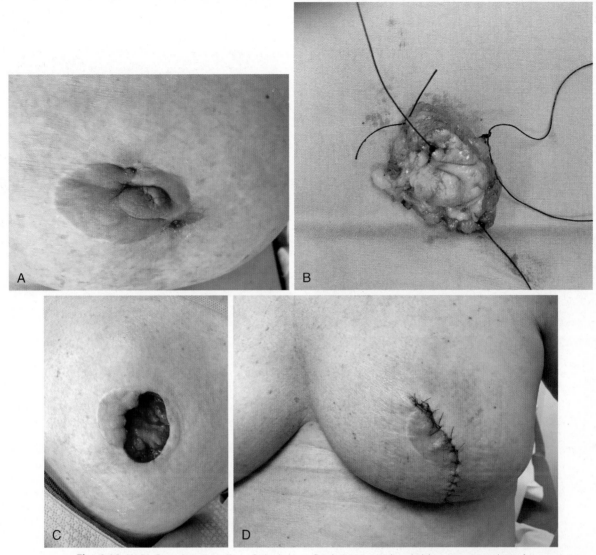

• **Fig. 6.11** (A–D) Complete resection of nipple, two fistula tracts, and underlying mammary ducts for recurrent breast abscess.

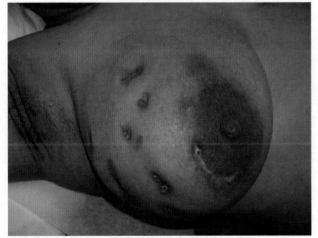

• **Fig. 6.12** Clinical appearance of right breast in a patient with granulomatous mastitis with classic chronic inflammatory changes and sinus formation. (From Wilson JP. Idiopathic granulomatous mastitis: in search of a therapeutic paradigm. *Am Surg.* 2007;73:798-802.)

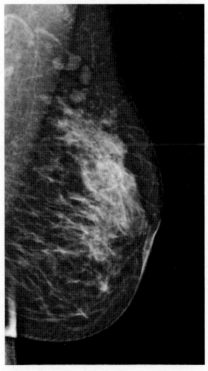

• **Fig. 6.13** Mammogram showing an area of ill-defined asymmetry in idiopathic granulomatous mastitis.

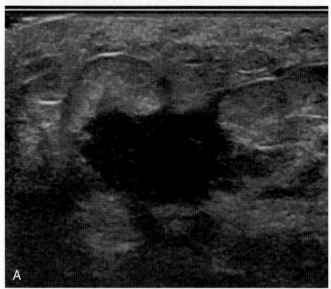

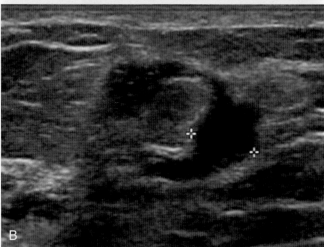

• **Fig. 6.14** Ultrasounds showing idiopathic granulomatous mastitis. (A) Hypoechoic mass consistent with abscess. (B) Lymph node with abnormal cortical thickening.

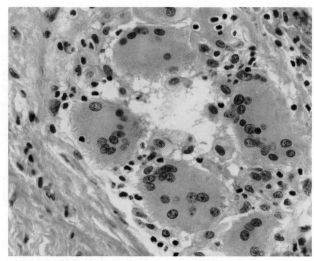

• **Fig. 6.15** Granulomatous lobular mastitis with central multinucleated histiocytes and peripheral lymphocytes.

symptoms, and the patient's overall health, as well as the surgeon's experience with IGM and preferred treatment preference. Despite management algorithms, there is no standard universal treatment and recurrence and relapse rates are high during the time period, with reports of up to 20% to 50%.[76,88,92] Regardless of treatment type, most reports show that, with time, the disease tends to be self-limiting.

Treat Expectantly

Literature has shown that IGM eventually is a self-limiting disease and that approximately half of all cases will improve and resolve usually within 2 to 24 months of onset, regardless of treatment type.[78,88] Conservative management with regular clinical examinations without surgical intervention has been successfully described.[92,93] There have been no reports that IGM progresses to cancer and no deaths from infectious complications have been reported with this disease. However, most women present with a painful abscess-like mass, so initial observation alone in most cases is insufficient.

Antibiotics

The most important facet on initial presentation is to rule out an underling pyogenic infectious cause because bacterial abscesses are more common than IGM. At initial presentation, all abscesses should be treated with percutaneous aspiration.[77] After aspiration of the abscess, prophylactic initiation of a broad-spectrum antibiotic is recommended through the period of diagnostic evaluation. The initial antibiotics of choice can include amoxicillin/clavulanate,[78] sulfamethoxazole and trimethoprim, or metronidazole. Nonsteroidal antiinflammatory drugs help with the inflammatory pain associated with these IGM masses and are usually the most appropriate and helpful pain relief choice.[76] Although IGM looks painful, seldom do these patients require opiates for pain control.[76]

Steroids

Use of oral steroids as first-line treatment has frequently been reported with up to 80% success.[76] Doses of oral steroids prescribed range between 10 and 60 mg/day of prednisone or 30 to 60 mg/day of prednisolone,[80] with a gradual taper over weeks to months.[85] Additional options described include prednisone (1 mg/kg) for 3 weeks[76] or 16 mg prednisolone twice daily for 2 weeks, among others.[94] Despite the high rates of resolution and noninvasiveness of oral steroids, many patients and physicians are reluctant to use high-dose steroids because of the side effects of glucose intolerance, cushingoid features, and insomnia. Unfortunately, up to half of patients treated with oral steroids can potentially have a relapse 1 to 2 months after discontinuing initial treatment.[76] In these cases, a second course of steroids can be prescribed. Topical steroid use with prednisolone (0.125%) for 4 to 12 weeks has been described with all patients achieving complete response and only 10% having a relapse.[94] Case reports are few but appear safe and effective without the side effects of the systemic oral equivalent.

Immune Modulators

Methotrexate has also been used successfully with variable results to treat this disease as an alternative for patients who are unresponsive to steroid therapy.[76] The suggested dose of methotrexate is 15 mg/wk. The side effects that need to be monitored and may cause discontinuation include alopecia and elevated liver enzymes.

Surgical Treatment

Reported surgical approaches include abscess drainage, wide surgical excision, and mastectomy. Although wide excision has been reported successfully,[78,85] recurrence rates in larger series range from 5% to 50%.[85,95] Surgical excision as initial treatment can be considered in patients who present with a single, small lesion, but relapse rates are high with this approach. The goal of wide local excision for IGM is complete excision of the involved area including the affected overlying skin, fistula tract, and obtaining a lesion free margin of 5 to 10 mm.[76,85] Surgical excision has also been reported to have delays in wound healing, fistula formation, and poor cosmetic results.[83,96] Most important, care must be used to avoid repeated surgical interventions because of multiple recurrences, which can cause resultant disfigurement or removal of the breast.[97]

Authors' Recommendations

The understanding in management for IGM is that each case is unique and one size does not fit all. There is a need for a combination approach with watchful waiting, antibiotics, immunosuppressants, and surgical intervention. For example, for patients presenting with mild, localized symptoms of IGM, a trial of antibiotics and observation is recommended.[82] For patients with progressive symptoms or those presenting with severe, generalized involvement of the breast, a trial of oral steroids is warranted and may rapidly alleviate symptoms. Mastectomy should only be indicated for patients with IGM who have intractable, severe symptoms and have failed other therapeutic approaches.[82]

Selected References

7. Trop I, Dugas A, David J, et al. Breast abscesses: evidence-based algorithms for diagnosis, management, and follow-up. *Radiographics*. 2011;31:1683-1699.

8. Scott BG, Silberfein EJ, Pham HQ, et al. Rate of malignancies in breast abscesses and argument for ultrasound drainage. *Am J Surg*. 2006;192:869-872.

11. Indelicato DJ, Grobmyer SR, Newlin H, et al. Delayed breast cellulitis: an evolving complication of breast conservation. *Int J Radiat Oncol Biol Phys*. 2006;66:1339-1346.

13. Olsen MA, Nickel KB, Margenthaler JA, et al. Development of a risk prediction model to individualize risk factors for surgical site infection after mastectomy. *Ann Surg Oncol*. 2016;23:2471-2479.

22. Schafer P, Furrer C, Mermillod B. An association of cigarette smoking with recurrent subareolar breast abscess. *Int J Epidemiol*. 1988;17:810-813.

A full reference list is available online at ExpertConsult.com.

7

Gynecomastia

ANNE T. MANCINO, ZACHARY T. YOUNG, AND KIRBY I. BLAND

Gynecomastia is benign enlargement of the male breast due to proliferation of the glandular component. This common clinical condition, which may be unilateral or bilateral, presents as an incidental finding on routine physical examination, a painless unilateral or bilateral breast enlargement, or a painful and tender mass beneath the areolar region. This chapter focuses on the prevalence, clinical presentation, physiology, histopathology, pathophysiology, diagnosis, and treatment of gynecomastia. Finally, certain specific clinical situations of gynecomastia are reviewed to provide easily understood summaries of the complexities of this topic.

Prevalence

There are three distinct peaks in the age distribution of physiologic gynecomastia. The first peak is during the neonatal period when palpable breast tissue transiently develops in 60% to 90% of newborns because of the transplacental passage of estrogens.[1,2] The second peak is during puberty, with prevalence increasing at approximately 10 years of age and peaking between 13 and 14 years of age, followed by a decline during the later teenage years. Pubertal gynecomastia is estimated to occur within 15 months after an increase in testicular size, the first sign of puberty.[3–6] The third peak is found in the adult population, with prevalence increasing at approximately 50 years of age and continuing into the eighth decade of life.[5–7]

Most patients seeking consultation for gynecomastia have idiopathic gynecomastia (approximately 25%) or acute/persistent gynecomastia due to puberty (25%), drugs (10%–20%), cirrhosis/malnutrition (8%), or primary hypogonadism (8%). A lesser number have testicular tumors (3%), secondary hypogonadism (2%), hyperthyroidism (1.5%), or renal disease (1%).[1]

Clinical Presentation

The patient presents with a swelling of the breast, often unilateral, which is commonly tender. The patient may be concerned about the tenderness, the cosmetic appearance or the possibility of malignancy. Examination reveals a firm "donut" of retroareolar tissue, which is mobile.

There is usually a clear demarcation of the firm breast tissue from the softer adjacent fat. Gynecomastia may be differentiated from pseudogynecomastia or lipomastia (fatty breasts), in which the subareolar tissue is of the same consistency as the adjacent subcutaneous adipose tissue.[8] The hallmark of gynecomastia is concentricity. If an eccentric mass is found, an alternate diagnosis

should be considered, and mammography and biopsy should be performed.

Physiology

Development of the Male Breast

Male breast development in the fetus occurs in an analogous fashion to female breast development. By the ninth week of gestation, a recognizable nipple bud has formed from basal cells in the pectoral region. By the end of the third month, squamous epithelium invades the nipple bud and ducts develop, which connect to the nipple at the skin's surface. These become canalized and form lactiferous ducts. The blind ends of these ducts bud to form alveolar structures.[9]

Neonatal Gynecomastia

Palpable enlargement of the male breast in the neonate is normal and occurs as a result of the action of prolactin, placental estrogens, and progesterone on the neonatal breast parenchyma. At birth, with decline in these hormones, this breast enlargement usually regresses within a few weeks; however, it has been observed to persist for longer periods.[9,10]

Puberty

The breast tissues of both sexes appear histologically identical at birth and remain relatively quiescent during childhood, undergoing further differentiation at the time of puberty.[1,2] In the majority of males, transient proliferation of the ducts and surrounding mesenchymal tissue takes place during the period of rapid sexual maturation, followed by involution and ultimately atrophy of the ducts. In contrast, in females, the breast ductal and periductal tissues continue to enlarge and develop terminal acini, processes that require both estrogen and progesterone.[11]

Because estrogens stimulate breast tissue and androgens antagonize these effects, gynecomastia has long been considered the result of an imbalance between these hormones.[12,13] The transition from the prepubertal to the postpubertal state is accompanied by a 30-fold increase in the concentration of testosterone, with only a threefold increase in estrogen levels.[14] Therefore, a relative imbalance between serum estrogen and androgen levels can exist during a portion of the pubertal process and may result in gynecomastia. In an analysis of tissues from 30 males with gynecomastia,

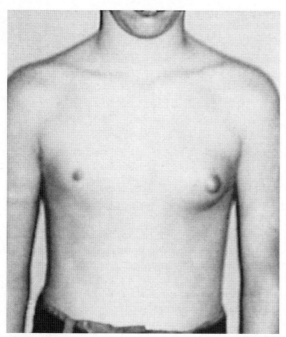

• **Fig. 7.1** An 11-year-old boy with unilateral (left) gynecomastia at puberty.

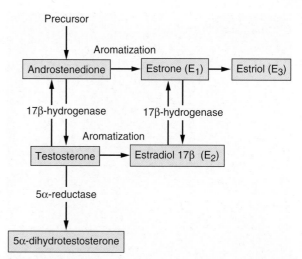

• **Fig. 7.2** Potential pathways for androgen-estrogen interconversion in healthy men. (Modified from Gordon GG, Olivo J, Rafil F, Southren AL. Conversion of androgens to estrogens in cirrhosis of the liver. *J Clin Endocrinol Metab*. 1975;40:1018-1026.)

estrogen, progesterone, and androgen receptors were observed in 100%.[15]

Pubertal Gynecomastia

Up to 70% of all boys will develop some degree of pubertal gynecomastia.[4,5,6] Transient proliferation of the ducts and surrounding mesenchymal tissue takes place during this period of rapid sexual maturation, followed by involution and ultimately atrophy of the ducts. Gynecomastia is evident in as many as 69% of schoolboys in the United States.[16] For many of these boys, the enlarged breast(s) is asymmetric, tender, and psychologically disturbing (Fig. 7.1). However, by age 20, only a small percentage of these boys have a remaining palpable abnormality.

Normal Circulating Male Estrogen Concentrations

The adult testes secrete approximately 15% of the estradiol and less than 5% of the estrone in the circulation, whereas extragonadal tissues produce 85% of the estradiol and more than 95% of the estrone through the aromatization of precursors. The principal precursor of estradiol is testosterone, 95% of which is derived from the testes (Fig. 7.2). Androstenedione, an androgen secreted primarily by the adrenal gland, serves as a precursor of estrone formation. The important extraglandular sites of aromatization are adipose tissue, liver, and muscle. In addition, a substantial degree of interconversion between estrone and estradiol takes place through the action of the widely distributed enzyme 17-ketosteroid reductase, which also catalyzes the conversion of androstenedione to testosterone.[12,17,18]

Senile Gynecomastia

Senile gynecomastia occurs in 32% to 65% of adult males (Fig. 7.3A and B), its prevalence correlates with the body fat content,

and it does not require clinical evaluation unless symptomatic or of recent, rapid onset.[5,6,7,19] Plasma testosterone concentration values begin to fall at approximately 70 years of age.[20] In addition, there is concurrent elevation in the plasma sex hormone-binding globulin (SHBG), which causes a further fall in the free or unbound testosterone concentrations. A simultaneous increase in plasma luteinizing hormone (LH) may cause a concurrent increase in the rate of conversion of androgen to estrogen in peripheral tissues.[21] Hence, relative hyperestrinism is evident with a decrease in the plasma androgen-to-estrogen ratio.

Histopathology

The histologic pattern of gynecomastia progresses from an early active phase (florid) to an inactive phase (fibrous), no matter what the cause. Grossly, there is a relatively sharp margin between breast tissue and surrounding subcutaneous fat. The few ductal structures of the male breast enlarge, elongate, and branch along with the encasing connective tissue.[22,23] This combined increase in glandular and stromal elements provides for a regular distribution of each element throughout the enlarged breast. Often, there is an increase in cell number relative to the basement membrane. A recent study shows a consistent three-layered composition of ducts in gynecomastia, including a myoepithelial, intermediate (hormone receptor positive) luminal and inner (hormone receptor negative) luminal cell layer.[24]

The loose connective tissue that regularly outlines the ducts as a central feature of gynecomastia is prominent only in the earliest stage of the disease. The fibroblasts within this loose tissue are relatively large but lack atypical features and are not clustered, even though they appear more frequently immediately adjacent to the basement membrane of the ducts.

Fibrous gynecomastia describes the later stage of gynecomastia and histologically has a dense collagenous stroma that contains relatively few fibroblasts. This dense collagenous tissue is applied closely to delicate basement membrane regions surrounding sparse epithelial elements in which hyperplasia is usually absent. The loose pattern of periductal stroma that characterizes the florid stage of gynecomastia is lacking. The stromal fibrosis is unlikely

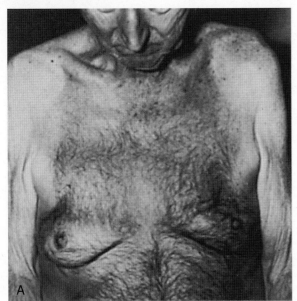

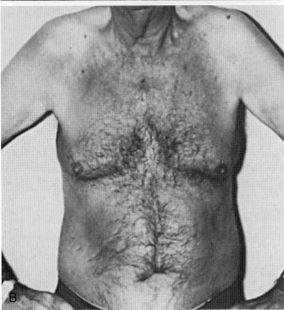

• **Fig. 7.3** (A) Senescent bilateral gynecomastia in an 85-year-old man. The patient had observed a gradual increase in the size of both breasts over the past 4 years. There are no breast masses, and the patient takes no medication. (B) Senescent bilateral gynecomastia in a 72-year-old man with progressive enlargement of breasts over a 6-year period. The patient has no systemic diseases and takes no medications.

• BOX 7.1	Conditions Associated With Gynecomastia

Estrogen Excess	**Androgen Deficiency**
Testicular neoplasms	Primary testicular failure
Adrenal cortex neoplasms	Secondary testicular failure
Ectopic HCG production	Androgen resistance syndromes
Hermaphroditism	Increased aromatase activity
Hyperthyroidism	Chronic renal failure
Liver cirrhosis	
Recovery from starvation	**Drug Related**
	See Box 7.2

HCG, *Human chorionic gonadotropin.*

reported to occur in the male breast, most often the solid and comedo types, although complex cribriform patterns are also demonstrated.[28,29]

Whether the unusual cases of atypical hyperplasia and carcinoma in the male breast are preceded by gynecomastia is unknown. DNA analysis in patients with breast carcinoma, fibroadenoma, and gynecomastia has demonstrated *HER2/neu* amplification in 26.8% of breast carcinoma specimens but not in patients with fibroadenoma or gynecomastia.[30] In addition, recent immunohistochemical studies have shown that inner luminal cells of gynecomastia differ in biomarkers from male DCIS, indicating that gynecomastia does not seem to be an obligate precursor of male breast cancer.[24]

Pathophysiology

As previously stated, most patients who present with possible gynecomastia have idiopathic gynecomastia or acute/persistent gynecomastia due to puberty, drugs, cirrhosis/malnutrition, or primary hypogonadism. A few have testicular tumors, secondary hypogonadism, hyperthyroidism, or renal disease.[1] Box 7.1 presents a comprehensive summary of the conditions commonly associated with gynecomastia. Gynecomastia can occur as a result of a relative or absolute excess of estrogens or a relative or absolute decrease in androgens.

Estrogen Excess

Testicular Tumors

Testicular tumors can lead to increased blood estrogen levels by (1) estrogen overproduction, (2) androgen overproduction with aromatization in the periphery to estrogens, and (3) ectopic secretion of gonadotropins that stimulate otherwise normal Leydig cells.

Leydig Cell Neoplasms. Leydig cell neoplasms are relatively uncommon, constituting approximately 2% to 3% of all testicular neoplasms.[31] Such neoplasms are found in children as young as 2 years of age and in adults as old as 82 years of age.[32] The average age at diagnosis is between 20 and 60 years. Leydig cell tumors account for up to 39% of non–germ cell tumors of the testes and 12% of the testicular neoplasms of children.[33–36] Leydig cell tumors of the testes are most often unilateral.[33,37] Sexual precocity is usually observed in children with these tumors and is accompanied by an increase in muscle mass and stature with advanced bone age in most patients. In children, Leydig cell tumors are almost uniformly benign.

to respond to medical therapy.[23] Researchers used immunohistochemical techniques to show that the majority (89%) of gynecomastia specimens are estrogen receptor positive.[25] The investigators were unable to demonstrate an association between histopathologic staging of gynecomastia or hormonal parameters and estrogen receptor status.

Virtually any benign alteration found in the female breast (in particular, fibroadenoma and sclerosing adenosis) may be found in the male breast, although such changes are rare. Differentiating carcinoma of the male breast from gynecomastia may be difficult clinically, but the problem is easily resolved with histologic or cytologic examination. There are reports of concurrent gynecomastia and breast cancer[26,27]; ductal carcinoma in situ (DCIS) is

In adults, physical changes are less frequent, with endocrine signs noted in approximately 30% of adults with these tumors[38]; painful gynecomastia and decreased libido are the most common manifestations. Symptoms may precede the onset of a palpable testicular mass, particularly with Leydig cell hyperplasia. Approximately 25% of the Leydig cell tumors in adult men secrete predominantly estrogen.[35,36,39,40] For some patients, gynecomastia may be observed despite normal serum estrogen and testosterone levels. In these patients, gynecomastia may occur after in situ conversion of androstenedione to estrone in breast parenchyma, leading to increased tissue estrogen values without increasing serum levels.[41–44]

Malignant transformation of Leydig cell tumors occurs in approximately 10% of patients, predominantly in adults and older men.[45,46] Gynecomastia associated with Leydig cell tumors is more often seen when these tumors are benign, especially when 17-ketosteroid values are normal. Malignant Leydig cell tumors usually demonstrate abnormal estrogen or androgen levels and are associated more frequently with elevated estrogens and 17-ketosteroid levels without gynecomastia.[45–47]

For patients with gynecomastia and increased circulating estrogen levels, pituitary suppression of LH release may initiate atrophy of the contralateral testis.[48] A prolonged plasma estradiol response to human chorionic gonadotropin (HCG) is a useful, although nonspecific, adjunct in the diagnosis of Leydig cell tumors.[49]

Sertoli Cell Tumors. Sertoli cell tumors comprise less than 1% of all testicular tumors and occur at all ages, but one third occur in children younger than 13 years of age, usually in boys younger than 6 months of age. The tumors usually do not produce endocrine effects in children.

Gynecomastia is seen in 26% to 33% of individuals with benign Sertoli cell tumors, and it rapidly regresses after orchiectomy.[50,51] In most cases, there was no elevation of estrogen or testosterone serum concentrations. Of five reported patients with malignant Sertoli cell tumors and gynecomastia, two had elevated gonadotropin levels.[52]

Multifocal Sertoli cell tumors in boys have been associated with the autosomal dominant syndrome of Peutz-Jeghers syndrome.[53–55] The increased risk of gonadal tumors for females with Peutz-Jeghers syndrome was recognized at an earlier date.[56]

The majority of Sertoli cell tumors are benign, but as many as 10% can be malignant. Males with distant metastatic disease have been reported.[57,58]

Germ Cell Tumors. Germ cell tumors are the most common cancers in males between 15 and 35 years of age. They are divided into seminomatous and nonseminomatous subtypes. The theory of a common origin of germ cell tumors of the testes from embryonal carcinoma cells is supported by ultrastructural studies[59] and experimental production of teratoma from embryonal carcinoma explants.[60,61] Estrogen effects in men with germ cell neoplasms occur secondary to increased aromatization of testosterone and androstenedione into estrogens in peripheral sites.[62] Androstenedione, which has low androgenicity and is readily aromatized to estrone peripherally, may be produced in increased concentrations by some tumors, with the result of enhanced estrogen production.[21]

Men with germ cell tumors who exhibit gynecomastia have a higher mortality than those without gynecomastia.[63,64] After orchiectomy and chemotherapy, a 75% reduction in the number of men with gynecomastia is observed.[64]

Use of testicular ultrasound for detection and localization of early testicular masses in males with gynecomastia is essential. Any young adult male with unexplained gynecomastia, loss of libido, or impotence should have diagnostic testicular ultrasound for evaluation of occult tumors.[65,66]

Adrenal Cortex Neoplasms

Feminizing adrenocortical tumors are malignant tumors, which either secrete estrogen or massive amounts of adrenal androgens that are aromatized to estrogen in other tissues.[67] Peak incidence is in young and middle aged males.[68]

Childhood adrenal tumors are rare (0.04% of tumors).[69,70] Adrenal neoplasms should be suspected in any child with premature or inappropriate signs of virilization or feminization, especially if accompanied by evidence of hyperadrenocorticism or gynecomastia. Evidence of premature development of secondary sexual characteristics, such as enlarged penis, axillary hair, and pubic hair, may be seen in children with gynecomastia associated with tumors of the adrenal gland.[70]

An estrogen-producing adrenal tumor in an adult male was first reported in 1919.[71] In men, adrenal carcinomas that result only in feminization are very uncommon.[72] However, neoplasms producing mixed syndromes, such as feminization and Cushing disease, are almost always malignant.[73–75] Successful treatment of the tumor might result in regression of gynecomastia. In unresectable tumors, estrogen blockade with tamoxifen or raloxifene may provide some effect.[68]

Ectopic Human Chorionic Gonadotropin Production

Carcinoma of the Lung. This disease may initiate an increase in serum chorionic gonadotropin values with simultaneous escalation in estrogen secretion.[76] Gonadotropins were identified in the urine of four male patients who died of bronchogenic carcinoma.[77] In three patients, gonadotropins were also present in tissue samples from the primary lung tumor. The appearance of gynecomastia in an adult male smoker should arouse suspicion of an underlying carcinoma of the lung. It has been proposed that the detection of HCG may be an aid in the diagnosis of bronchogenic carcinoma.[78]

Hepatocellular Carcinoma. This can also initiate gynecomastia via elevated serum HCG.[79] Normal hepatic parenchyma and primary hepatic neoplasms carry estrogen receptors. Hepatocellular carcinoma carries androgen receptors, whereas normal liver parenchyma cells do not.[80]

Hermaphroditism

True Hermaphroditism. True hermaphroditism occurs when an ovary and a testis or a gonad with mixed histologic features (ovotestis) is present. Four categories are recognized: (1) bilateral, with testicular and ovarian tissue (ovotestis) anatomically present on each side; (2) unilateral, with an ovotestis on one side and a normal ovary or testis on the contralateral side; (3) lateral, with a testis is evident on one side and an ovary on the opposite side; and (4) indeterminate, in which the clinical syndrome is expressed but the location and type of gonadal tissue is uncertain.[81]

Significant gynecomastia is evident at puberty in approximately 75% of individuals with true hermaphroditism. Approximately 50% of these individuals menstruate. For the phenotypic male with true hermaphroditism, menstruation presents as cyclic hematuria. Excess estradiol secretion relative to androgen production by the ovotestis is common.[82] Gonadal secretion of estradiol is observed in phenotypic men with feminization (gynecomastia and menstruation).[82,83]

Pseudohermaphroditism. 17-Ketosteroid reductase deficiency results in male pseudohermaphroditism with a marked overproduction of androstenedione and estrone as well as a decreased production of testosterone and estradiol. A late-onset form of testicular 17-ketosteroid reductase deficiency can cause gynecomastia and hypogonadism in men.[84]

Altered Androgen-to-Estrogen Ratio

Hyperthyroidism

Gynecomastia may develop in 20% to 40% of hyperthyroidism. In most cases the gynecomastia is bilateral and resolves after restoration of euthyroid state.[85,86] The diffuse toxic goiter of Graves disease is most commonly associated with gynecomastia.[86]

Both elevated estrogen and progesterone serum concentrations can be identified in men with hyperthyroidism.[87,88] These elevations decrease with reestablishment of the euthyroid state. Gynecomastia may also be due to elevated estrogens that results from a stimulatory effect of thyroxin on peripheral aromatase.[89]

Liver Cirrhosis

The evaluation of estrogen, testosterone, androstenedione, and cortisol concentrations, and the percentage of binding of these steroids to plasma proteins, demonstrated that alterations were most marked in patients with cirrhosis.[90] They were also evident to a lesser degree in patients with fatty metamorphosis of the liver and in normal aging patients.[90] Patients with cirrhosis showed an increase in estrone, a smaller increase in estradiol, a decrease in testosterone, and a rise in LH concentration. Cortisol concentration remained unchanged, whereas ratios of estradiol to testosterone and estrone to testosterone were augmented in patients with cirrhosis and were higher than those in healthy young subjects. The combination of elevated estrone and estradiol and reduced testosterone, which is strongly bound by increased SHBG, appeared to be responsible for gynecomastia and hypogonadism in chronic liver diseases. Other investigators have observed that plasma progesterone concentration is increased in 72% of men with nonalcoholic cirrhosis and gynecomastia compared with healthy male controls.[91] However, this increase was not observed in men with alcoholic fatty change and alcoholic cirrhosis.

Gynecomastia is observed in approximately 40% of men with cirrhosis.[92–97] As stated, total plasma testosterone concentrations are lower than normal.[90,98–102] However, there is a far greater decline in the non–protein bound (biologically active) plasma testosterone.[87,93,100,103] This decrease appears to result from an increased concentration of SHBG.[104–106] The decreased concentration of plasma testosterone of men with cirrhosis is initiated by a reduction in testosterone synthesis by the testes; kinetic studies have confirmed that the production of testosterone is reduced by 75%.[107–109] In fact, 15% of the testosterone produced in males with cirrhosis is derived from peripheral conversion of circulating androstenedione.[108] There is disagreement about the relative roles of unbound (biologically active) plasma estradiol in men with cirrhosis and gynecomastia and the changes affecting testosterone concentrations, but the decline in non–protein bound (biologically active) plasma testosterone appears to be the most important factor.[110,111]

Recovery From Starvation

Gynecomastia produced by return to diet after nutritional deprivation is well documented.[112–114] Although initially seen in prisoners of war and refugees, this may also be seen in therapeutic dieting.[115] Starvation and significant weight loss result in secondary hypogonadism; refeeding leads to transient imbalance of estrogen and androgen which leads to gynecomastia.[112] In most cases, gynecomastia is bilateral and resolves within 1 to 2 years of resuming normal diet.[115]

Androgen Deficiency

Primary Testicular Failure

Klinefelter Syndrome. Klinefelter syndrome (XXY) was described more than four decades ago in adult phenotypic males with gynecomastia, hypergonadotropic hypogonadism, and azoospermia.[116] The chromosomal pattern XXY occurs in approximately 1 in 600 live births.[117] Klinefelter syndrome represents the most common variant of male hypogonadism. However, the full spectrum of clinical findings, gynecomastia, eunuchoidism, and macroorchidism does not emerge until the midteens and may never be fully expressed. By midpuberty, affected individuals are uniformly hypergonadotropic and testicular growth ceases. After 15 years of age, serum testosterone concentrations remain in the low-normal range, but serum estradiol values are increased, irrespective of the presence or absence of gynecomastia.[118] Although testicular biopsy during childhood reveals a reduced number of spermatogonia, tubular fibrosis and hyalinization of seminiferous tubules are not observed until midpuberty.[119] Biochemical findings in the adult male include reduced levels of serum testosterone with high-normal or enhanced values of serum estradiol.[120]

It is estimated that carcinoma of the breast is 20 to 66.5 times more frequent in men with Klinefelter syndrome than in the normal male population.[121,122] Bilateral carcinoma of the breast has also been reported.[123]

Hereditary Defects of Androgen Biosynthesis. Multiple hereditary defects have been identified that result in defective androgen biosynthesis with incomplete virilization of the male embryo.[124–128] The enzymes responsible for these failures in biosynthesis include 20,22-desmolase, 17,20-desmolase, 3β-hydroxysteroid dehydrogenase, 17α-hydroxylase, 17β-hydroxysteroid dehydrogenase, and 17-oxosteroid reductase. Each enzyme represents a critical pathway for the conversion of cholesterol to testosterone. As a consequence of the variability in the blockade of these enzymatic biochemical reactions, affected individuals have a profound escalation in gonadotropin secretion after negative feedback. For individuals with complete or partial deficiencies of 17β-hydroxysteroid dehydrogenase, feminization with gynecomastia develops in the early teens. Gynecomastia is also a common occurrence in male patients with 11-β-hydroxylase deficiency.[129] Deficiency of 17-oxosteroid reductase causes elevation in estrone and androstenedione, which is then further aromatized to estradiol.[130]

Secondary Testicular Failure

Gynecomastia is common after testicular injury resulting from trauma, viral orchitis (mumps), or bacterial infections (e.g., tuberculosis, leprosy). The common pathogenic mechanism is functional revascularization of one or both testes. Mumps represents the most common cause of viral orchitis, although echovirus, lymphocytic choriomeningitis virus, and group B arboviruses, among others, have all been implicated in secondary testicular failure.[131]

The use of chemotherapy and local radiation therapy as cancer treatment in children and adolescents can cause testicular failure.[132]

The testes of boys in early puberty are particularly susceptible to injury. Furthermore, radiation therapy to the hypothalamic-pituitary axis in children with brain tumors can result in gonadotropin deficiency or hyperprolactinemia, which, in turn, can result in gonadal insufficiency.

Androgen Resistance Syndromes

The androgen resistance syndromes are characterized by gynecomastia and varying degrees of pseudohermaphroditism. Androgens are not recognized by the peripheral tissues, including the breast and pituitary. Androgen resistance at the pituitary results in elevated serum LH levels and increased circulating testosterone. The increased serum testosterone is then aromatized peripherally, promoting gynecomastia.[133]

Reifenstein Syndrome. First described in 1947, Reifenstein syndrome (XY) is characterized by hypospadias, incomplete virilization, and maturational arrest during spermatogenesis, resulting in azoospermia.[134-137] Affected males have profound gynecomastia. Laboratory studies show elevated plasma LH and estradiol concentrations along with normal to high testosterone concentrations.

Kennedy Syndrome. Individuals with Kennedy syndrome, a neurodegenerative disease, have a defective androgen receptor,[137] caused by an expanded number of CAG (glutamine codon) repeats in exon 1 of the gene that encodes for the receptor. In affected males, gynecomastia is the combined result of decreased androgen responsiveness at the breast level and increased estrogen levels as a result of elevated androgen precursors of estradiol and estrone. A similar increase of CAG repeats has been identified in some phenotypes of Klinefelter syndrome.[138]

Increased Aromatase Activity

Estrogen effects on the breast may be the result of either circulating estradiol levels or locally produced estrogens. Aromatase P450 catalyzes the conversion of the C19 steroids, androstenedione, testosterone, and 16-α-hydroxyandrostenedione to estrone, estradiol, and estriol. Hence, an overabundance of substrate or increased enzymatic activity can increase estrogen concentrations and promote the development of gynecomastia.

The biological effects of overexpression of the aromatase enzyme in male mouse transgenics caused increased mammary growth, histologic changes similar to gynecomastia, an increase in estrogen and progesterone receptors, and an increase in downstream growth factors such as transforming growth factor-β and β-fibroblast growth factor.[23,139] Use of an aromatase inhibitor leads to loss of the mammary gland phenotype.[140]

A familial form of gynecomastia has been discovered in which affected family members had elevated extragonadal aromatase activity.[141] Gain-of-function mutations in chromosome 15 have been reported to cause gynecomastia through the formation of cryptic promoters that lead to overexpression of aromatase.[142] Obesity may cause estrogen excess through increased aromatase activity in adipose tissue.

Chronic Renal Failure

Gynecomastia is common in uremic males, and 50% of males undergoing chronic hemodialysis develop gynecomastia.[143-148] Plasma LH and follicle-stimulating hormone (FSH) concentrations are increased fourfold in men whose creatinine clearance rates are 4 mL per minute or less, whereas testosterone concentrations are only 30% of normal.[145] There is histologic damage to the testes, hypospermia, and a subnormal response to HCG

• BOX 7.2	Drugs Causing Gynecomastia: 2015 Review
Anastrazole	Leuprorelin
Bicalutamide	Lopinavir
Cimetidine	Metoclopramide
Diethylstilbestrol	Nelfinavir
Dutasteride	Nilutamide
Estrogen	Phenothrin
Ethinylestradiol	Prednisone
Finasteride	Ritonavir
Flutamide	Saquinavir
Gonadotropin-releasing hormone	Spironolactone
Goserelin	Stavudine
Indinavir	Tamoxifen
Lamivudine	Zidovudine

administration, suggesting that secondary gonadal failure is the primary cause of gynecomastia.

Drugs Associated With Gynecomastia

Although there are many medications that have case reports of gynecomastia as a side effect, a more thorough evaluation of the literature suggests that the list of medications with moderate or strong relationships is likely much lower.[149] Krause performed a literature review in which 92 medications were reported to have association with gynecomastia.[150] Of those 92, less than half were deemed to be causal or highly probable in relationship to gynecomastia. There does exist evidence that some antiandrogens, antiretrovirals, exogenous hormones, and certain other medications have a higher association with gynecomastia.[150,151] Box 7.2 lists the medications Krause listed as frequently causing gynecomastia[150] and/or causal.[151] Given the numbers of medicines that appear to be implicated in the disease process, a careful review of the patient medication list is imperative. However, one must also weigh the level of evidence supporting each medicine against the likelihood that a particular drug is causing the patient's condition.

In a significant number of cases, gynecomastia is associated with drugs or chemicals that cause an increased estrogen effect on breast tissues. With some drugs or chemicals, the mechanism of action is known (Table 7.1), whereas with others it is unknown (Box 7.3). Known mechanisms include estrogen-like properties or binding of the estrogen receptor, stimulation of estrogen synthesis, supply of estrogen precursors for aromatases, damage to testicles, blockage of testosterone synthesis, blockage of androgen action, and displacement of estrogen from SHBG.

Known Mechanisms

Contact with estrogen vaginal creams can elevate circulating estrogen levels. Some of the creams contain synthetic estrogens; therefore, they may not be detected by standard estrogenic qualitative assays. An estrogen-containing embalming cream has been reported to cause gynecomastia in morticians.[152,153] Abuse of marijuana, a phytoestrogen, has also been associated with gynecomastia. It has been suggested that digitalis causes gynecomastia through its ability to bind to estrogen receptors.[154,155] The appearance of gynecomastia has been described in body builders and athletes after the administration of aromatizable androgens;

TABLE 7.1 **Drugs Associated With Gynecomastia: Known Mechanisms**

Estrogen-Like, or Binds the Estrogen Receptor	Stimulates Estrogen Synthesis	Supplies Precursors for Aromatase	Direct Testicular Damage	Blocks Testosterone Synthesis	Blocks Androgen Action	Displaces Estrogen From SHBG
Estrogen vaginal cream	Gonadotropins	Exogenous androgens	Busulfan	Ketoconazole	Flutamide	Spironolactone
Estrogen-containing embalming cream	Growth hormone	Androgen precursors (androstenedione, DHEA)	Nitrosourea	Spironolactone	Bicalutamide	Ethanol
Delousing powder			Vincristine	Metronidazole	Finasteride	
Digitalis			Ethanol	Etomidate	Cyproterone	
Clomiphene					Zanoterone	
Marijuana					Cimetidine Ranitidine Spironolactone	

DHEA, Dihydroepiandrosterone; *SHBG,* sex hormone-binding globulin.

gynecomastia results from the conversion of androgens to estrogens by peripheral aromatase enzymes.[156]

Drugs or chemicals cause decreased testosterone levels through direct testicular damage or by blocking testosterone synthesis or androgen action. Phenothrin, a component of delousing agents, possessing antiandrogenic activity, has been identified as the cause of an epidemic of gynecomastia among Haitian refugees in the early 1980s.[157] Chemotherapeutic agents, such as alkylating agents, cause Leydig cell and germ cell damage, resulting in primary hypogonadism. Flutamide, an antiestrogen used as treatment for prostate cancer, blocks androgen action in the peripheral tissues, whereas cimetidine blocks androgen receptors. Ketoconazole inhibits steroidogenic enzymes required for testosterone synthesis. Spironolactone causes gynecomastia by several mechanisms. Like ketoconazole, it can block androgen production by inhibiting enzymes in the testosterone synthetic pathway (17-α-hydroxylase and 17-20-desmolase), but it can also block receptor binding of testosterone and dihydrotestosterone.[158] In addition to decreasing testosterone levels and biologic effects, spironolactone also displaces estradiol from SHBG, increasing free estrogen levels. Ethanol increases the estrogen-to-androgen ratio and also induces gynecomastia by multiple mechanisms: (1) increasing circulating levels of SHBG, which decreases free testosterone levels; (2) increasing hepatic clearance of testosterone; and (3) causing testicular damage.[159]

Unknown Mechanisms

Many drugs or chemicals are associated with gynecomastia through unknown mechanisms. They generally are listed by their category of known action: (1) cardiac agents and antihypertensives; (2) psychoactive drugs, including illegal street drugs such as amphetamines; (3) agents for infectious disease, including antivirals for human immunodeficiency virus (HIV); and (4) miscellaneous agents (see Box 7.3).

Management of Gynecomastia

A primary concern in the evaluation of male breast enlargement is the possibility of male breast cancer. Although male breast

• BOX 7.3 **Drugs Associated With Gynecomastia: Unknown Mechanisms**

Cardiac Drugs/Antihypertensives
Calcium channel blockers
ACE inhibitors
Amiodarone
Methyldopa
Reserpine
Nitrates

Psychoactive Drugs
Neuroleptics
Diazepam
Phenytoin
Tricyclic antidepressants
Haloperidol
Amphetamines

Psychoactive Drugs
Neuroleptics

Infectious Disease Drugs
Indinavir
Isoniazid
Ethionamide
Griseofulvin
HIV antivirals

Other Drugs
Theophylline
Omeprazole
Auranofin
Diethylpropion
Domperidone
Penicillamine
Sulindac
Heparin

ACE, Angiotensin-converting enzyme; HIV, human immunodeficiency virus.

cancer is rare, constituting only 0.2% of all male cancers, it must be included in the differential diagnosis of male breast enlargement, which also includes such disorders as neurofibroma, lymphangioma, hematoma, lipoma, and dermoid cyst. The risk of breast cancer in men with gynecomastia secondary to Klinefelter syndrome is more than 20 times higher than in other men. Gynecomastia is otherwise not associated with an increased risk of breast cancer.[160]

On examination of the enlarged male breast, abnormalities such as asymmetry, firmness, or fixation of the breast tissue, dimpling of the overlying skin, retraction or crusting of the nipple, nipple discharge, or axillary lymphadenopathy require mammography and fine-needle biopsy for diagnosis.[161,162]

Evaluation of Male Breast Enlargement

The differentiation of gynecomastia from fatty enlargement of the breasts without glandular proliferation (pseudogynecomastia) is made by clinical examination. With the patient in a supine position, the examiner grasps the breast between the thumb and forefinger and gently moves the two digits toward the nipple. If gynecomastia is present, a firm or rubbery, mobile, disklike mound of tissue arising concentrically from beneath the nipple and areolar region will be felt. However, if the breast enlargement is caused by adipose tissue, no such disk of tissue is apparent.

Tender gynecomastia appearing during mid-to-late puberty requires only a history and physical examination, including careful palpation of the testicles. In the majority of boys, pubertal gynecomastia resolves spontaneously within 1 year. A 6-month return appointment can be scheduled. At times, the cosmetic and emotional consequences of pubertal gynecomastia warrant medical or surgical intervention.

Because gynecomastia is common in adult males, the presence of long-standing, stable breast enlargement requires minimal laboratory evaluation. A careful history, including the patient's use of medications, alcohol, and drugs such as marijuana and amphetamines, along with specific inquiry concerning the symptoms and signs of hepatic dysfunction, testicular insufficiency (decreased libido or impotence), and hyperthyroidism, most often uncovers the underlying cause of the gynecomastia. If no abnormalities are uncovered by a careful history and subsequent physical examination, laboratory assessment of hepatic, renal, and thyroid function is sufficient. As previously stated, medical or surgical intervention may be necessary based on the preferences of the patient.

Routine mammogram and ultrasound are not recommended in the evaluation of clinically apparent gynecomastia; they can prove helpful in determining other benign entities, such as pseudogynecomastia, or fat necrosis, or if physical examination is suspicious for cancer.[163] The American College of Radiology recommends age-based protocols for imaging.[164] For men younger than 25 years of age, ultrasound (US) should be used to evaluate mass and mammogram should be performed only if US is suspicious. Conversely, for men older than 25 years, mammogram is recommended with supplemental US if mammogram is inconclusive or suspicious.

Rapid onset and/or progressive gynecomastia in the adult male may require more extensive laboratory investigation. If no underlying cause of such gynecomastia is apparent from the history, physical examination, or the laboratory screening tests previously discussed, measurements of HCG, testosterone, and LH can determine the underlying cause (Fig. 7.4).

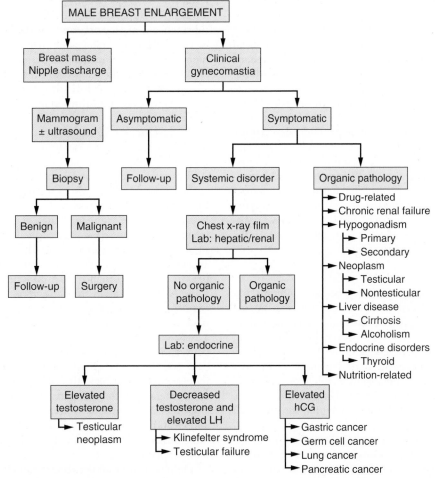

• **Fig. 7.4** An algorithm for diagnostic approaches to the male patient with unilateral/bilateral breast mass(es) suspicious for gynecomastia. *hCG,* Human chorionic gonadotropin; *LH,* luteinizing hormone. (Modified from Lucas LM, Kumar KL, Smith DL. Gynaecomastia: a worrisome problem for the patient. *Postgrad Med.* 1987;82:73.)

Treatment of Male Breast Enlargement

If, during the evaluation process, an underlying cause for gynecomastia is identified, treatment is focused on the underlying cause; treatment can be as simple as stopping a medication. For gynecomastia with no known cause or for persistent gynecomastia after treatment of the underlying cause, medical and surgical therapies may be required.

Medical Therapy

Two concepts are integral to appropriate medical therapy of male breast enlargement: (1) gynecomastia, especially pubertal gynecomastia, has a high rate of spontaneous regression[161]; and (2) medical therapy is most effective during the active, proliferative phase of gynecomastia. After an interval of 12 months, there is increased stromal hyalinization, dilation of the ducts, and a marked reduction in epithelial proliferation.[23,165,166] The resulting fibrotic tissue responds poorly to medical therapy.

Both antiestrogens and antiandrogens have some efficacy in the treatment of gynecomastia. Danazol (antiandrogen) has been studied in several uncontrolled trials and at least one prospective placebo-controlled study. In the latter, gynecomastia cleared in 23% of the patients receiving danazol and 12% of the patients receiving placebo ($p < .05$).[166] Compared with tamoxifen, danazol was less effective in clearing gynecomastia (40% vs. 78.2%) but did have lower relapse rate.[167] The side effects of danazol include weight gain, edema, acne, muscle cramps, and nausea; these limit its usefulness.

Tamoxifen, raloxifene, and clomiphene citrate have been used for their antiestrogenic effects. Studies with clomiphene (50–100 mg/day) have shown reduction in breast size of adolescent boys, but it is less effective than tamoxifen.[168,169] There were no side effects from the use of clomiphene in any of these clinical studies, although nausea, rashes, and visual problems have been noted when this drug is used in other settings. Tamoxifen (10 mg two times daily) has led to significant reduction in breast size and tenderness, without side effects.[170–174] A 3-month course of tamoxifen is a reasonable treatment strategy. Patients in whom tamoxifen is effective usually experience a decrease in pain and tenderness within 1 month. Raloxifene is effective in treating pubertal gynecomastia in 90% of boys.[173] Aromatase inhibitors, such as testolactone and anastrozole, are less effective than antiestrogens in the treatment of pubertal gynecomastia.[175,176]

Surgical Therapy

Gynecomastia is generally accepted to be a benign condition, but it can have a significant adverse effect on those patients afflicted by this condition. Cosmesis, physical discomfort, and uncertainty of underlying pathology can all lead to psychological stress and ultimately a desire for surgical intervention. The well-rounded breast surgeon is wise to have several surgical methods for addressing this condition. Appropriate preoperative evaluation and surgical planning should allow for satisfactory esthetic outcomes in the majority of patients who seek surgical intervention for this often overlooked condition.

Numerous surgical techniques have been described in the literature ranging from minimally invasive options such as liposuction[177] to traditional incision-based surgeries.[178] The choice of procedure type and incision are largely dictated by patient anatomy and surgeon preference. Rohrich described a grading scale for gynecomastia that stratifies patients based on breast tissue hypertrophy, the type of breast tissue hypertrophy, and ptosis.[177] The

American Society of Plastic Surgeons suggests the use of a more subjective grading system that is defined on physical appearance of the breasts.[179]

Once identifiable and correctable sources of gynecomastia have been eliminated and addressed appropriately, surgical correction of excess breast tissue is considered. Special circumstances exist in young men with gynecomastia because these patients should not undergo surgical correction before pubescence to prevent recurrence.[5] Of the patients deemed appropriate candidates for surgical correction, there are many described procedures. Minimally invasive procedures such as liposuction[177] and endoscopic approaches[180] have become increasingly popular, especially for grade I gynecomastia. Historically, the mainstay of surgery for grade II to IV has been subcutaneous mastectomy through various periareolar incisions[181,182] tailored to the individual patient. A periareolar incision along the inferior border of the nipple allows access to the breast tissue for subcutaneous mastectomy in patients with minimal excess skin.[183]

Patients with excess skin present a dilemma as to the most appropriate approach to minimize scarring and maximize esthetic outcome. Patients with excess skin who undergo simple subcutaneous mastectomy can have redundant skin that lessens esthetic outcome. Benelli described the round block approach using a periareolar approach to skin reduction in breast surgery.[184] This has been applied to grade II and III gynecomastia with favorable results.[185,186] The circumareolar[185] approach, or donut technique,[186,187] combines the Benelli round block technique with a subcutaneous mastectomy and has the benefit of limiting the scar to the periareolar region while reducing excess skin. This technique creates a deepithelialized dermal pedicle that serves as the blood supply to the nipple while removing skin between two concentric circles, which results in mastopexy. We have adopted this technique at our institution in select patients with satisfactory results[187] (Fig. 7.5).

To perform the procedure, the entire chest is prepared and draped in a sterile fashion from the shoulders superiorly, the midaxillary lines laterally and the xiphoid process inferiorly. The sternal notch, xiphoid, and center of sternum are clearly marked at the outset. Ideal location of the nipple areolar complex (NAC) from the midline is between 10 and 12 cm. The inner donut is marked along the pigmented edge of the NAC (Fig. 7.6). When bilateral mammoplasty was performed, the NAC was adjusted to sit above the inframammary fold. The distance between the outer and inner donuts for bilateral mammoplasty was chosen to compensate for NAC distance from midline and ptosis. For instance, if the NAC was 14 cm from the midline, a radius of 2 cm from the NAC was marked for the outer donut. The two donuts are made so that the intervening epithelium is removed as part of a mastopexy. In our experience, up to a 4-cm radial distance between inner and outer donuts was tolerated without cosmetic detriment or wound complication. If unilateral reduction mammoplasty is performed, the NAC should be matched to the contralateral side for symmetry. The circumference of the outer and inner donuts was optimized to match the contralateral NAC and creation of the immediate paraareolar donut is chosen based on contralateral nipple size in patients undergoing unilateral mammoplasty.

Deepithelialization between the inner donut and outer donut was then meticulously performed circumferentially. Special care must be taken to not injure the dermis, which provides the NAC with its blood supply after mastectomy is performed. Techniques using tumescence to facilitate deepithelialization

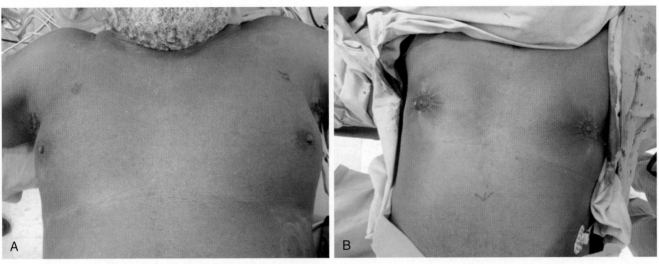

• **Fig. 7.5** Patient with gynecomastia before (A) and after (B) his subcutaneous mastectomy using the "double donut technique."

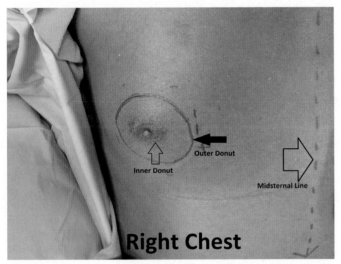

• **Fig. 7.6** Skin markings for the technique with outer donut marked at 10 cm from mid-sternal line and inner donut marked to decrease nipple areolar complex to a diameter of 3 cm.

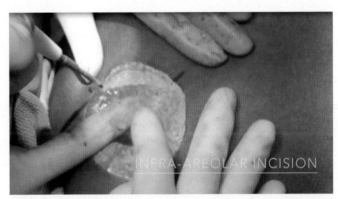

• **Fig. 7.7** Infraalveolar incision made in area of deepithelialized skin.

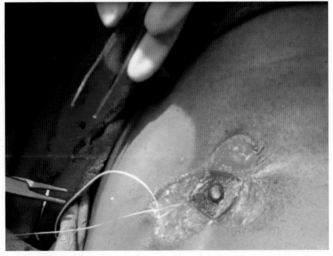

• **Fig. 7.8** Initial closure of skin with "clover-leaf" pattern.

have been described[6]; however, this was not used in our patient population.

Access to the breast tissue was gained through an infraalveolar curvilinear incision from 4 to 8 o'clock along the inferior portion of the deepithelialized skin (Fig. 7.7). Using this area of deepithelialized skin allows for a larger incision to be made than is typical for a similar subcutaneous mastectomy approach. The surgeon will find that the use of this larger incision facilitates ease of mastectomy without sacrificing cosmetic outcomes. The breast tissue superiorly to the clavicle, medially to the sternum, laterally to the latissimus dorsi and inferiorly to the inframammary fold is excised down to the pectoralis muscle for an en bloc breast tissue resection. Great care is taken to ensure hemostasis to mitigate the risk of postoperative hematoma and seroma formation. The decision to leave a surgical drain is not mandatory but may prove useful in some patients.

The last step is approximation of the NAC to the surrounding epithelialized skin. The initial four sutures are placed in such a manner as to create a four-leaf clover pattern (a stitch at 12, 3, 6, and 9 o'clock; Fig. 7.8). Serial bisection with interrupted suture is then placed between the anchoring sutures until the NAC is well approximated against the surrounding tissues. Interrupting this layer allows for even distribution of tension and minimizes

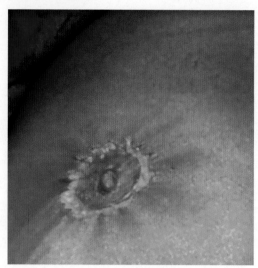

• **Fig. 7.9** Further interrupted sutures before subcuticular stitch.

puckering that can be seen if a purse-string suture is used in this layer (Fig. 7.9). The final step is epithelial approximation, which is performed using a running subcuticular absorbable monofilament suture. We prefer a 4-0 suture for the skin closure. Cutaneous skin glue is used to seal the skin edges. A light compressive wrap is placed over the breast tissue and left in place for 24 to 48 hours after the operation. If a surgical drain is placed in the resultant defect, it is left until the output is less than 30 mL per day.

Grade IV gynecomastia often requires a more aggressive skin resection to correct ptosis and redundancy. This can typically be achieved through vertically or horizontally based incisions. In select cases, large volume skin reductions may be necessary using a Wise-type pattern with free nipple transfer.[188]

Summary

Gynecomastia is a complex clinical entity. In review of some of the key, clinically relevant information presented in this chapter, pubertal gynecomastia and gynecomastia in the aging male are summarized in the following sections. For a more detailed discussion of these topics, see Braunstein.[189]

Gynecomastia in the Pubertal Male

An adolescent presenting with gynecomastia has physiologic pubertal gynecomastia in the great majority of cases. It generally appears at 13 or 14 years of age, lasts for 6 months or less, and then regresses. Fewer than 5% of affected boys have persistent gynecomastia, but this persistence is the reason that young men in their late teens or early 20s present for evaluation. Other conditions to consider in adolescents and young adults with persistent gynecomastia are Klinefelter syndrome, familial or sporadic excessive aromatase activity, incomplete androgen insensitivity, feminizing testicular or adrenal tumors, and hyperthyroidism.[142,190,191] Drug abuse, especially with anabolic steroids, but also with alcohol, marijuana, amphetamines, or opioids, also should be considered.[191]

Laboratory tests to determine the cause of pubertal gynecomastia without a history suggestive of an underlying pathologic cause and with an otherwise normal physical examination are unlikely to be revealing. On physical examination, careful attention must be paid to the testicles; any abnormality must be investigated using ultrasound techniques. If the gynecomastia should progress, evaluation of serum testosterone, LH, and HCG levels are appropriate.

If a specific cause of gynecomastia can be identified and treated, there may be regression of the breast enlargement. This regression most often occurs with discontinuation of an offending drug. If the gynecomastia is drug-induced, decreased tenderness and softening of the glandular tissue will usually be apparent within 1 month after discontinuation of the drug.

Because pubertal gynecomastia is self-limiting, no therapy is required in the great majority of cases. Persistent or progressive pubertal gynecomastia may cause emotional distress. In this circumstance, when there is no known cause after appropriate evaluation, simple surgical excision through a periareolar incision is sufficient. The patient and his family must be made aware that flattening of the involved nipple may occur because of inadvertent removal of subcutaneous fat in addition to the offending breast tissue.

Gynecomastia in the Aging Male

Asymptomatic gynecomastia is found on examination in one third to two thirds of elderly men and at autopsy in 40% to 55% of men.[7] The condition has usually been present for months or years when it is first discovered during a physical examination. Histologic examination of the breast tissue in this setting usually shows dilated ducts with periductal fibrosis, stromal hyalinization, and increased subareolar fat.

The high prevalence of asymptomatic gynecomastia among older men raises the question of whether it should be considered to be pathologic or a part of the normal process of aging. It is likely that many cases of asymptomatic gynecomastia are due to the enhanced aromatization of androgens in subareolar fat tissue, resulting in high local concentrations of estrogens, as well as to the age-related decline in testosterone production.[20,192] Another possible cause is unrecognized exposure over time to unidentified environmental estrogens or antiandrogens.

The first step in the clinical evaluation of the elderly male is to determine whether the enlarged breast tissue or mass is gynecomastia. Pseudogynecomastia is characterized by increased subareolar fat without enlargement of the breast glandular component. The differentiation between gynecomastia and pseudogynecomastia is made on physical examination. In the elderly population, breast cancer is also a concern. Nipple discharge is present in approximately 10% of men with breast cancer, but it is not expected with gynecomastia.[193] If the differentiation between gynecomastia and breast carcinoma cannot be made on the basis of clinical findings alone, the patient should undergo diagnostic mammography, which has 90% sensitivity and specificity for distinguishing malignant from benign breast diseases.[194]

There is no uniformity of opinion regarding what biochemical evaluation, if any, should be performed in an aging male with asymptomatic gynecomastia. In a retrospective study of 87 men with symptomatic gynecomastia, 16% had apparent liver or renal disease, 21% had drug-induced gynecomastia, and 2% had hyperthyroidism, whereas 61% were considered to have idiopathic gynecomastia. Forty-five of the 53 patients in the group with idiopathic gynecomastia underwent endocrine testing, of whom only one patient (2%) was found to have an endocrine abnormality—an occult Leydig cell testicular tumor.[195]

Once the diagnosis of gynecomastia is established, it is important to review all medications, including over-the-counter drugs such as herbal products, which may contain phytoestrogens. Ingestion of sex steroid hormones or their precursors may cause gynecomastia through bioconversion to estrogens. Antiandrogens used for the treatment of prostate cancer, spironolactone, cimetidine, and one or more components of highly active antiviral therapy used for HIV infection (especially protease inhibitors) have been clearly shown to be associated with gynecomastia.[196–201] Several drugs used for cancer chemotherapy, particularly alkylating agents, can damage the testes and result in primary hypogonadism.

If an adult presents with unilateral or bilateral gynecomastia that has a rapid onset and is progressive, and if the patient's history and physical examination do not reveal the cause, HCG, LH, and testosterone should be measured. Many of the available measurements of testosterone have poor accuracy and precision, especially in men with testosterone levels at the low end of the normal range.[202] Measurement of these levels in the morning is recommended, because testosterone and LH secretion have a circadian rhythm, with the highest levels in the morning, as well as secretory bursts throughout the day. If the total testosterone level is borderline or low, free or bioavailable testosterone should be measured or calculated to confirm hypogonadism. Although such laboratory evaluation is prudent, no abnormalities are detected in the majority of patients.

If a specific cause of gynecomastia can be identified and treated during the painful proliferative phase, there may be regression of the breast enlargement. This regression most often occurs with discontinuation of an offending drug or after initiation of testosterone treatment for primary hypogonadism. If the gynecomastia is drug-induced, decreased tenderness and softening of the glandular tissue will usually be apparent within 1 month after discontinuation of the drug. However, if the gynecomastia has been present for more than 1 year, it is unlikely to regress substantially, either spontaneously or with medical therapy, because of the presence of fibrosis. In such circumstances, surgical removal is the best option for cosmetic improvement.

Gynecomastia Associated With Prostate Cancer Therapy

In patients with locally advanced prostate cancer, monotherapy with bicalutamide (Casodex) has been associated with gynecomastia due to increase in the estrogen:androgen ratio in the male breast. Symptoms of gynecomastia usually start in first 6 to 9 months, with risk of discontinuation of therapy. Tamoxifen[203] and radiation therapy have been proposed for prevention and treatment. Although tamoxifen has been used in men treated for prostate cancer, it is not approved by the US Food and Drug Administration for this indication. However, it has been suggested that therapy with tamoxifen may prevent the development of gynecomastia in men receiving monotherapy with high doses of bicalutamide (Casodex) for prostate cancer. In a randomized, double-blind, controlled trial involving men receiving high-dose bicalutamide (150 mg per day),[204] gynecomastia occurred in 10% of patients who received tamoxifen at a dose of 20 mg daily, but it occurred in 51% of those who received anastrozole at a dose of 1 mg daily and in 73% of those who received placebo, over a period of 48 weeks. Mastalgia occurred in 6%, 27%, and 39% of these patients, respectively. In another trial involving 3 months of therapy, gynecomastia, mastalgia, or both occurred in 69.4% of patients receiving placebo, 11.8% receiving tamoxifen ($p < .001$ for comparison with placebo), and 63.9% receiving anastrozole (not significantly different from the rate in the placebo group).[205]

Among patients treated with bicalutamide alone, gynecomastia occurred in 68.6% and mastalgia occurred in 56.8%. These rates were significantly lower among patients receiving one 12-Gy fraction of radiation therapy to the breast on the first day of treatment with bicalutamide (34% and 30%, respectively), and they were further reduced among patients receiving bicalutamide and tamoxifen (8% and 6%, respectively).[206]

A meta-analysis found that tamoxifen 20 mg daily for 48 weeks is efficient prophylaxis for bicalutamide-induced gynecomastia and that definitive radiotherapy is the preferred first-line treatment option for established bicalutamide-induced gynecomastia.[207] Both modalities were found to be well tolerated. However, prophylactic radiotherapy should be reserved for patients who are not candidates for tamoxifen. Aromatase inhibitors are not recommended. Surgery is the treatment of choice only after the foregoing noninvasive modalities fail.

Selected References

8. Narula HS, Carlson HE. Gynecomastia—pathophysiology, diagnosis and treatment. *Nat Rev Endocrinol.* 2014;10:684-698.

149. Nuttall FQ, Warrier RS, Gannon MC. Gynecomastia and drugs: a critical evaluation of the literature. *Eur J Clin Pharmacol.* 2015;71:569-578.

164. Maniero MB, Lourenco AP, Barke LD, et al. ACR appropriateness criteria evaluation of the symptomatic male breast. *J Am Coll Radiol.* 2015;12:678-682.

174. Lapid O, van Wingerden JJ, Perlemuter L. Tamoxifen therapy for the management of pubertal gynecomastia: a systematic review. *J Pediatr Endocrinol Metab.* 2013;26:803-807.

182. Cordova A, Moschella F. Algorithm for clinical evaluation and surgical treatment of gynaecomastia. *J Plast Reconstr Aesth Surg.* 2008;61:41-49.

207. Tunio MA, Al-Asiri M, Al-Amro A, Bayoumi Y, Fareed M. Optimal prophylactic and definitive therapy for bicalutamide-induced gynecomastia: results of a meta-analysis. *Curr Oncol.* 2012;19:e280-e288.

A full reference list is available online at ExpertConsult.com.

8

Benign, High-Risk, and Premalignant Lesions of the Breast

BENJAMIN C. CALHOUN, STEPHEN R. GROBMYER, AND JEAN F. SIMPSON

This chapter presents a histopathologic classification of the wide variety of noncancerous lesions identified in the human female breast, stratified into categories that predict breast cancer risk in broad terms.[1,2] The magnitude of risk in these various groups is based on the following assumption: any change that does not indicate an increased risk of subsequent breast cancer greater than 50% above that for women controlled for similar age and length of time at follow-up is assigned no elevation of risk. Many of these lesions are not associated with cellular proliferation and are designated as nonproliferative. Nonproliferative lesions may result in biopsy or present clinical symptoms without an association of increased risk. Other lesions that maintain an association with subsequent breast cancer risk are defined as proliferative lesions.

Benign Lesions Without Cancer Risk Implications

Benign breast conditions have a diverse array of clinical presentations. The subjective discomfort of mammary pain and clinical signs of lumpiness have little correlation with histologic alterations. Lumpiness on physical examination is common to many benign and malignant situations. The continued use of such broad terms of convenience as *fibrocystic disease* or *fibrocystic change* and *benign breast disease* occurs because these terms are deeply embedded in clinical parlance. Despite their imprecision, these terms have utility precisely because of their imprecision, familiarity, and wide reference. The term *benign breast disease* is an intrinsically imprecise term that refers to all noncancerous lesions of the breast. The use of the term *fibrocystic disease* has been problematic despite its intent of providing a clinicopathologic correlation between lumpiness and histologic alterations.[3] The difficulty probably arises from the use of the word *disease,* which has reinforced the widely held belief that cancer risk was elevated in this setting.[4] With the introduction of *fibrocystic disease* in the 1940s, an association with cancer was implied by concurrent associations.[5,6] Using the term *fibrocystic change* should remove the implication of cancer risk.[7–9] In surgical pathology or histopathology, these terms had no precise reference and provide no clear understanding of pathogenesis. The following discussion highlights anatomic pathology while acknowledging that histopathology is an empty exercise without clinical correlates and predictability.

Although it may be difficult to draw sharp borders of definition for these changes, it is certain that they occur in more than 50% of the immediately premenopausal women in North America. The presence of cysts without hyperplasia and other epithelial proliferation does not identify a group of women who have an increased risk compared with others of the same ethnic or geographically defined group.[7] Hyperplastic changes may be more common in breasts that are clinically lumpy, but no formal recent analysis of co-occurrence of these conditions is available. Similarly, reliable mammographic correlates of epithelial hyperplasia are not at hand. Mammograms with increased density have imperfect associations with histologic findings because fibrosis is as common as hyperplasia, although hyperplastic lesions are somewhat more common in dense breasts.[10–12]

Histopathology of Benign Breast Disease

The most common benign histologic change in the breast is the presence of cysts often lined by pink apocrine cells. Cysts range from approximately 1 mm to many centimeters. Cysts are usually unilocular within the breast, resulting from dilatation, unfolding, and coalescence of individual terminal duct lobular units (Fig. 8.1).[13] Small cysts are often inapparent on gross tissue examination.[14] Associated fibrosis may make smaller cysts palpable or more evident with imaging. These clinical correlates have become less important, particularly when most accept the fact that a biopsy may be appropriate based on clinical or imaging findings, even if histopathology demonstrates no specific abnormality. Understandably, fibrosis is often reported by pathologists in an attempt to explain clinical palpability or mammographic density. The gross appearance of large cysts is often blue, a reflection of the slightly cloudy, brown fluid usually found within.[15]

Many cysts are lined by cells that have characteristic cytologic features of apocrine glands. The cells have many mitochondrial-lysosomal and secretory granules that appear pink with eosin staining. The nuclei are round and often have a prominent round and eosinophilic nucleolus. This epithelium is often columnar, with a single protuberance of the apical aspect of the cytoplasm appearing as a bleb or snout. Such changes may be prominent in enlarged lobular units and may have minor associations with concurrent atypical lesions.[16,17] The apocrine cells are often grouped in tufted or papillary clusters and sometimes produce prominent papillary prolongations from the basement membrane region, which may or may not contain fibrovascular stalks

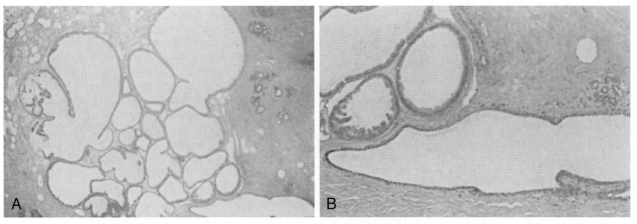

• **Fig. 8.1** (A) Apocrine cysts. Acini of this lobular unit have dilated and become distorted. Note entering lobular terminal duct at lower right. Low magnification (×40). (B) Higher power of part A showing apocrine-like epithelium lining dilated terminal duct and cysts. (Magnification ×80.)

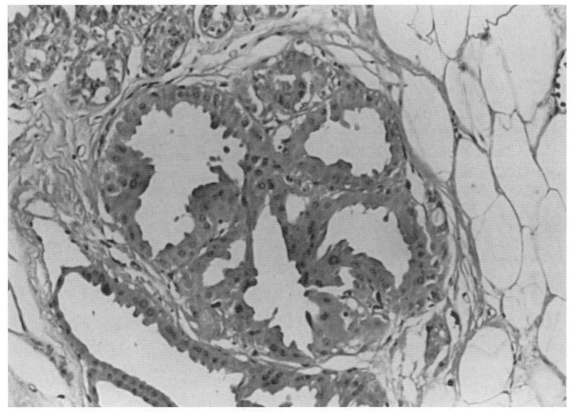

• **Fig. 8.2** These dilated spaces of a lobular unit show prominent coalescent arches. Note prominent apical blebs, or "snouts" (Original magnification ×225.)

(Figs. 8.2 and 8.3). This papillary apocrine change may demonstrate highly complex patterns but is not associated with a significant increased risk of later cancer development unless there is concurrent atypical hyperplasia (AH) (see later discussion).[18] Breast cysts, particularly larger ones, may show no evidence of epithelial lining or may have a simple squamous lining with an extremely flattened and undifferentiated epithelialized surface. Several studies have differentiated these two types of cysts, apocrine and simple, indicating that apocrine cysts have a high potassium content and different steroid hormones.[19] A suggestion of a difference in cancer risk between the two kinds of cysts is unproven.[19,20] Apocrine cysts are probably more commonly associated with multiplicity and recurrence than are nonapocrine cysts.[13,20,21] Whether this alteration of mammary epithelium to resemble that of apocrine sweat glands is a true metaplasia seems a point of practical irrelevance. However, many scholars believe that enzymatic profiles and ultrastructural evidence support a true metaplasia.[22] Slight to marked protuberance of cell groups (papillary apocrine change) rather than a smooth, single cell layer is more frequent in the breast compared with the apocrine sweat glands.

Cysts alone are not associated with risk, even when larger ones are separately analyzed.[7,23,24] Cysts are more common in high-risk geographic groups but are not determinants of cancer risk within geographic groups. Although epithelial hyperplasia is often

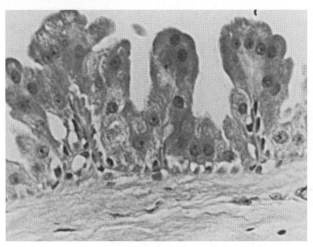

• **Fig. 8.3** Papillary apocrine change. The lining of this cyst shows complex papillary tufts. Note prominent centrally placed nucleoli. (Magnification ×320.)

associated with increased incidence of cysts and increased (albeit slight) cancer risk,[24] either change may be present singly in an individual biopsy specimen or entire breast. The apocrine cytoplasmic alteration is also of no proven importance in breast cancer risk. Apocrine change was found by Wellings and Alpers[25] to be more commonly present concurrently in breasts associated with cancer than those without. However, it is not an indicator of breast cancer risk in a predictive fashion. Moreover, papillary apocrine change without concurrent patterns of proliferative disease is not associated with an increased cancer risk.[18] In summary, neither cysts nor apocrine change significantly elevate cancer risk in an individual woman in the absence of other considerations.[8,9]

Chronic inflammation, edema, pigment-laden macrophages, and fibrosis are often found around cysts. Although duct ectasia and cysts have some histologic similarities, they are usually easily separable based on the general contour of the lesions and the greater degree of inflammation and/or scarring associated with duct ectasia[26]; furthermore, mammographic findings in duct ectasia are distinctive. Duct ectasia is usually present adjacent to the nipple, although it may extend a distance into the breast.

Epithelial Hyperplasia and Proliferative Breast Disease

The classification presented of epithelial hyperplasia in the breast is based on a large follow-up (cohort) epidemiologic study[7] (and subsequently confirmed in other cohorts[27–29]) that sought to link epithelial histologic patterns to magnitudes of risk of breast cancer.[7] The positive relationship of more extensive and complex examples of hyperplasia with carcinoma has been supported in many other prospective studies.[30–35]

Definition and Background

Consistent with its definition elsewhere in the body, epithelial hyperplasia of the breast means an increased number of cells bounded by a basement membrane. Thus the increased number of glands without a concomitant increase relative to the basement

membrane would not constitute hyperplasia but rather adenosis. Hyperplasia represents an increased number of cells above the basement membrane, and because this number is normally two, the presence of three or more cells above the basement membrane constitutes hyperplasia.

The intent of the term *usual* is to denote common patterns of cytology and cell relationships seen when cell numbers are increased within the basement membrane–bound spaces within the human breast. The usual type or common patterns of hyperplasia have also been termed *ductal* largely to contrast them with the lobular series. Because these lesions regularly occur within acini of lobular units, the designation of ductal is imprecise. Proliferative lesions in true ducts are unusual and are often truly papillary, that is, having branching, fibrous stalks (see later discussion).

The stratification of these hyperplastic lesions of usual type depends largely on quantitative changes. When the alterations begin to approximate patterns seen in carcinoma in situ, these lesions must be differentiated from those termed *atypical ductal hyperplasia* (ADH). Note that the features on the lesser end of the spectrum, between mild and moderate hyperplasia of usual type, depend on quantity and that the differentiation of the larger lesions from ADH depends on qualitative features of intercellular patterns and cytology (see later discussion).[36] Mild hyperplasia of usual type is characterized by the presence of three or more cells above the basement membrane in a lobular unit or duct and is not associated with any increased risk of cancer. Hyperplastic lesions that reach five or more cells above the basement membrane and tend to cross and distend the space in which they occur are called *moderate*. *Florid* is used for more pronounced changes, without any firm definition separating the moderate and the florid categories (Fig. 8.4). The reason for this is not to deny that there are quantitatively lesser and greater phenomena but rather that their reliable separation is not accomplishable. Moderate and florid hyperplasia of the usual type is found in more than 20% of biopsies. In follow-up studies, the cancer risk between these two groups was found to be similar (see Chapter 20). The term *papillomatosis,* proposed by Foote and Stewart,[6] may still be infrequently used in North America to indicate the common or usual hyperplasias of moderate and florid degree, and this practice is discouraged to prevent confusion with a diagnosis of a papillary lesion (see later).

Risk categories may be stratified into slight, moderate, and marked, with *slight* indicating a risk of 1.5 to 2 times that of the general population and *marked* indicating about a 10-fold increased risk (see Chapter 20). The assignments of histologic parameters to risk groups is shown in Box 8.1 and has changed little from that presented by a consensus conference that was supported by the American Cancer Society and the College of American Pathologists.[1,2] The clinical significance of usual hyperplasia of moderate and florid degree rests in the positive demonstration of a slightly increased risk (1.5–2 times) of subsequent invasive carcinoma.

The positive histologic features of this group (Figs. 8.5 to 8.7) are as follows:
• There is a mild variation in the size, placement, and shape of cells and, more specifically, nuclei. This feature is of great importance in differentiating these lesions from those of AH and noncomedo ductal carcinoma in situ (DCIS). They are most commonly present within lobular units and terminal ducts.
• The cells often exhibit patterns of swirling or streaming.

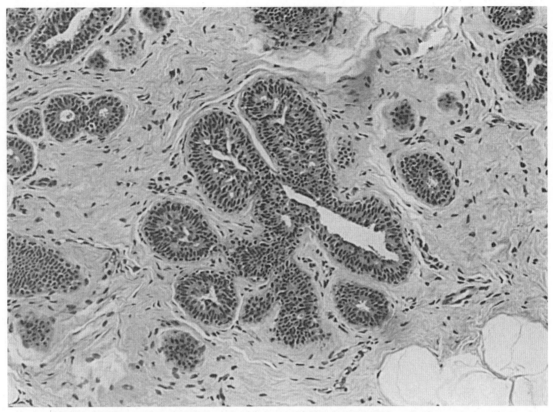

• **Fig. 8.4** Moderate hyperplasia of the usual type. The ductules are partially filled by a heterogeneous population of cells. Note the normally polarized layer of cells just above the basement membrane. (Magnification ×175.)

| • BOX 8.1 | Relative Risk for Invasive Breast Carcinoma Based on Histologic Examination of Breast Tissue Without Carcinoma[a] |

No Increased Risk (No Proliferative Disease)
Apocrine change
Duct ectasia
Mild epithelial hyperplasia of usual type

Slightly Increased Risk (1.5–2 Times)
Hyperplasia of usual type, moderate or florid
Sclerosing adenosis,[b] papilloma

Moderately Increased Risk (4–5 Times)[c]
Atypical ductal hyperplasia and atypical lobular hyperplasia

High Risk (8–10 Times)[d]
Lobular carcinoma in situ and ductal carcinoma in situ (noncomedo)

[a]Women in each category are compared with women matched for age who have had no breast biopsy with regard to risk of invasive breast cancer in the ensuing 10 to 20 years. Note: These risks are not lifetime risks.
[b]Jensen and colleagues[56] have shown sclerosing adenosis to be an independent risk factor for subsequent development of invasive breast carcinoma.
[c]Atypical hyperplasia or borderline lesions.
[d]Carcinoma in situ.
Modified from Fitzgibbons PL, Henson DE, Hutter RV. Benign breast changes and the risk for subsequent breast cancer: an update of the 1985 consensus statement. Cancer Committee of the College of American Pathologists. Arch Pathol Lab Med. 1998;122:1053-1055.

- As the epithelial cells proliferate, there is a varied shape of secondary lumens, which are often slitlike and are present between the cells within individual spaces.
- The secondary lumens, particularly in larger, more cellular lesions, may be present peripherally, immediately above the cells that surmount the basement membrane of the containing space.
- The cells appear to be varied, in cytologic appearance and in placement. Thus nuclei are not evenly separated one from the other, and cell membranes are not distinct. This is concomitant to the swirling or streaming change noted earlier.

Atypical Hyperplasia

The intent of the term *atypical hyperplasia* is to indicate a group of specific histologic patterns that are not generically "atypical" or "unusual" but for which the specific criteria have been shown to implicate an increased risk of later breast cancer development (see Box 8.1).[37] The clinical significance of these specific histologic patterns is that women with AH have an approximately 1% per year risk of breast cancer, whereas women with benign or usual type hyperplasia have 0.5% risk per year.[38,39] Of the tumors that developed after a biopsy diagnosis of AH in a large case-control study, 91% were estrogen receptor–positive, and 24% were lymph-node positive.[40] The cumulative breast cancer risk over decades has clear implications for the consideration of preventive therapy[41,42] (see Chapter 16).

The link of specific histologic patterns to a moderate magnitude of risk of breast cancer depends on the use of defined criteria.

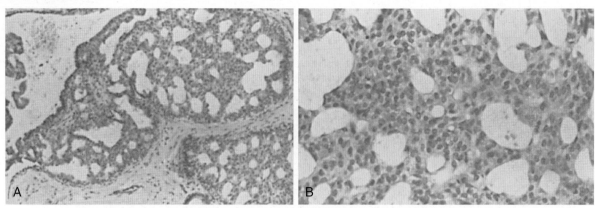

• **Fig. 8.5** (A) Florid hyperplasia of usual type. Ductules are partially filled with irregular arcade of cells. Note the irregularly shaped secondary lumens. (Magnification ×150.) (B) Higher power of part A. There is mild nuclear variability and irregular placement of cells, features supporting the lack of atypia. (Magnification ×280.)

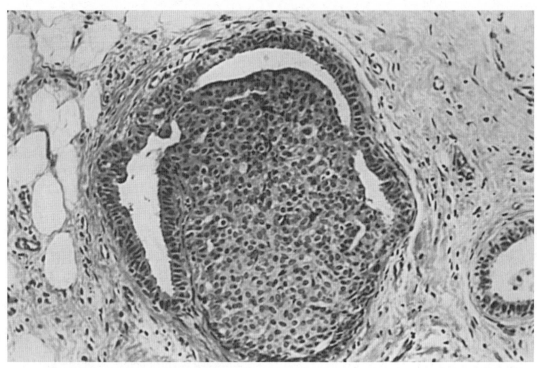

• **Fig. 8.6** Florid hyperplasia of usual type with solid pattern and peripheral placement of secondary spaces. Nuclei are predominantly heterogeneous. (Magnification ×350.)

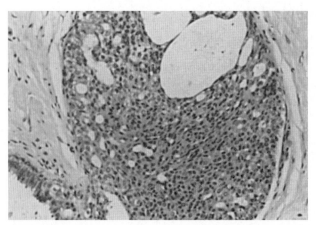

• **Fig. 8.7** Florid hyperplasia of usual type demonstrating prominent nuclear streaming or swirling. (Magnification ×200.)

This link of AH lesions to risk is the result of a group of studies that sought to restrict the term *atypical hyperplasia* to a small number of histologic patterns that have some of the same features as the analogous carcinoma in situ lesions. Many prospective studies have supported the relationship of epithelial hyperplasia to premalignant states.[33–35] There are conflicting data from large case-control studies on whether the extent of AH contributes to breast cancer risk.[39,43]

Atypical hyperplastic lesions have some of the same features as those of carcinomas in situ but either lack a major defining feature of carcinoma in situ or have the features in less developed form.[36,37] The three major defining criteria are cytology, histologic pattern, and lesion extent.[36] Specific histologic features differentiate each of the AHs from lesser categories, as well as from the analogous carcinoma in situ lesions after which they are named: lobular and DCIS. Traditionally, the histologic definitions have not been

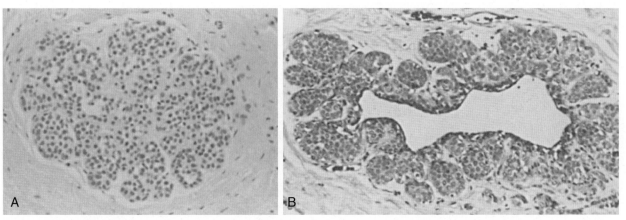

• **Fig. 8.8** (A) Atypical lobular hyperplasia (ALH). There is a resemblance to lobular carcinoma in situ (LCIS), but less than 50% of the individual acini are uniformly distended. (Magnification ×180.) (B) ALH undermining a different luminal cellular population. The same appearance may occur in LCIS; the defining diagnostic features must be present in lobular units to distinguish ALH from LCIS. (Magnification ×180.) (From Page DL, Anderson TJ. *Diagnostic Histopathology of the Breast.* Edinburgh: Churchill Livingstone; 1987.)

viewed as resting within spectra of changes. On the contrary, these histologic categories represented an attempt to accept natural pattern groupings within the complex array of mammary alterations reflected in histologic preparations.

Lobular carcinoma in situ (see also Chapter 9) is recognized when there is a well-developed example of filling, distention, and distortion of over half the acini of a lobular unit by a uniform population of characteristic cells. This follows the intent of the original description.[44] The analogous AH lesion, atypical lobular hyperplasia (ALH), is recognized when fewer than half of the acini in a lobular unit are completely involved, but the appearance is otherwise similar (Fig. 8.8).[45]

Histologically, ALH is characterized by a monomorphic epithelial cell proliferation that lacks cellular cohesion, often contains intracytoplasmic vacuoles, and expands less than 50% of a terminal ductal lobular unit.[37] The separation of ALH and lobular carcinoma in situ imposes stratification on what is otherwise an undivided continuum. Many pathologists prefer to use one diagnostic term for this range of histologic appearances (e.g., lobular neoplasia).[46] This term is valuable because it covers both ALH and lobular carcinoma in situ. However, in diagnostic practice, more clinical guidance is given by the use of the separate designations lobular carcinoma in situ and ALH.[47]

A specific feature of lobular neoplasia is its tendency to undermine an otherwise normal luminal epithelial layer. Because this is the interposition of an abnormal epithelial cell population within another, it has been termed *pagetoid spread* (because of the obvious analogy to Paget disease of the nipple). Some have equated this pattern with lobular carcinoma in situ; however, pagetoid spread does occur when the degree of involvement within lobular units reaches only the diagnostic level of ALH. The histologic patterns produced are usually more subtle in ALH,[48] without the solid pattern of ductal involvement seen in lobular carcinoma in situ. This pattern of involvement of ductal spaces outside of lobular units by the cells of lobular neoplasia in the presence of ALH has been termed *ductal involvement in atypical lobular hyperplasia.*[49] In the past, the cancer risk associated with ALH was thought to be equal for both breasts. However, long-term follow-up from the Nashville cohort and the Nurses' Health Study showed that invasive cancer developed in the ipsilateral breast in approximately two-thirds of patients.[27,50]

The philosophical underpinnings of the diagnostic term *atypical ductal hyperplasia* are the same as those for ALH. Thus the same features present in the analogous carcinoma in situ lesion are evident but in a less developed form. Because the criteria of ADH are derived from those of DCIS, histologic criteria for the latter must be followed (see Chapter 9). Two major criteria are required for the diagnosis of DCIS (low grade, noncomedo). First, a uniform population of neoplastic cells must populate the entire basement membrane–bound space. Furthermore, this alteration must involve at least two adjacent spaces (Figs. 8.9 and 8.10). An adjunct to assessing the extent of involvement has been put forth by Tavassoli and Norris.[51] They consider lesions smaller than 2 or 3 mm as ADH, with a resulting moderate increase in later cancer development. In addition to extent, an intercellular pattern of rigid arches and even placement of cells must be uniformly present. A helpful secondary criterion is hyperchromatic nuclei, which may not be present in all cases.[36] The pattern of comedo DCIS is not discussed here because its characteristic extreme nuclear atypia is far beyond the patterns seen in ADH. Without the uniform application of criteria, consistency in diagnosis is unlikely[52]; however, when standardized criteria are applied, concordance is most often ensured.[53]

Some cases of ADH share features with the so-called clinging carcinoma described by Azzopardi and coworkers.[54] A study from northern Italy indicates a considerable overlap of clinging carcinoma with ADH in histologic patterns and in risk of subsequent cancer development.[32] Many experts do not believe that the diagnosis of clinging carcinoma as a form of DCIS is appropriate because it obviously indicates a different behavior from that expected of widely accepted forms of DCIS (see Chapter 9).

Localized Sclerosing Lesions

The classic example of localized sclerosing lesions is sclerosing adenosis (SA), which has long been accepted as a gross and histologic mimicker of invasive carcinoma. It is in that capacity that

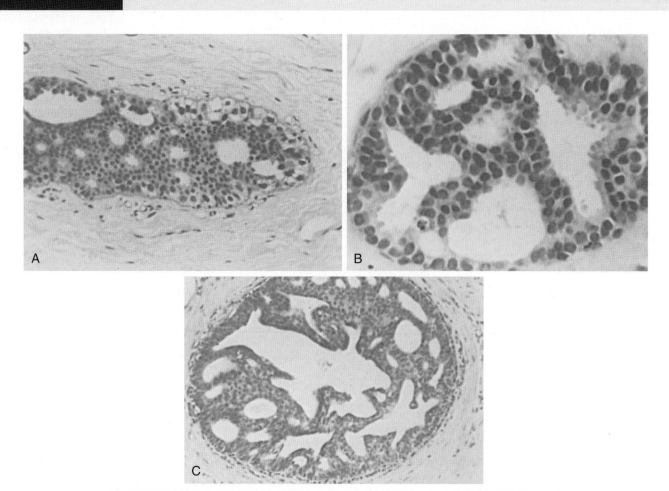

• **Fig. 8.9** (A) Atypical ductal hyperplasia (ADH) is evident in this ductule cut longitudinally. Note the regular placement of hyperchromatic nuclei and the regularity of centrally placed secondary lumens. (Magnification ×190.) (B) Rigid bar crossing the central portion of the photograph suggests ductal carcinoma in situ (DCIS); however, the cell pattern is not maintained throughout the remainder of the space. Note the polarity of the cells at the lower portion of the space, a finding that indicates ADH rather than DCIS. (Magnification ×350.) (C) Although there is some uniformity of some of the intercellular spaces, the cellular prolongations tend to taper, and there is a tendency for peripheral placement of secondary spaces. The pattern and cytologic criteria for DCIS are not clearly uniformly met; therefore this is an example of ADH. (Magnification ×170.) (From Page DL, Anderson TJ. *Diagnostic Histopathology of the Breast.* Edinburgh: Churchill Livingstone; 1987.)

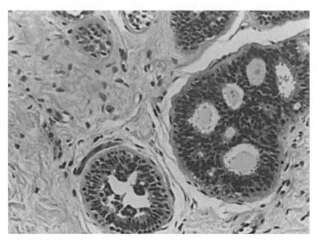

• **Fig. 8.10** Florid hyperplasia of usual type. Although there are hyperchromatism and regularly spaced secondary spaces, there is not a uniform population of evenly spaced cells; this is not diagnostic of atypical ductal hyperplasia. (Magnification ×225.)

it still has its greatest utility as a recognized diagnostic term and histologic pattern in the armamentarium of histopathologists. In its most usual form, SA is present as a microscopic lesion, probably unrecognized in both clinical and gross examination of tissues. SA is diagnosed only when a clearly lobulocentric change gives rise to enlargement and distortion of lobular units with a combination of increased numbers of acinar structures and a coexistent fibrous alteration (Fig. 8.11). The normal two-cell population is maintained above the basement membrane in most areas, and the glandular units are regularly deformed.

Enlarged lobular units that appear otherwise normal or with slight gland deformity may not be recognized as SA but instead be diagnosed using the noncommittal and appropriately descriptive term *adenosis.* A palpable mass may be created by aggregations of microscopic foci of SA (aggregate adenosis). This situation has been termed *adenosis tumor*[55] to indicate that a clinically palpable tumor may be produced. SA also commonly contains foci of microcalcification and, when present in this aggregate form, may be detectable with mammography.

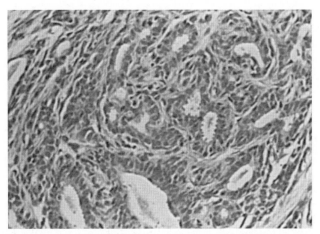

• **Fig. 8.11** Sclerosing adenosis. Glandular elements are deformed and surrounded by stromal fibrous alteration. Two-cell population (basal or myoepithelial and luminal) is focally inapparent. (Magnification ×240.)

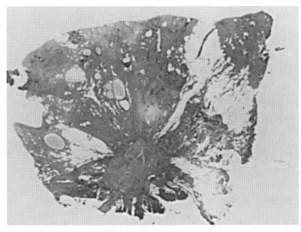

• **Fig. 8.12** Mature radial scar with sclerotic center showing microcystic peripheral parenchyma. (Magnification ×5.)

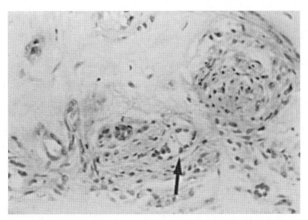

• **Fig. 8.13** Pseudoinfiltration of glandular elements adjacent to a nerve *(arrow)* from a case of radial scar. The entrapped epithelial elements may closely mimic tubular carcinoma. (Magnification ×300.)

There is a favored association of SA with ALH.[56] Diagnostic patterns of ALH are usually present in nonsclerosed lobules elsewhere in the biopsy and are certainly difficult to recognize when present within a focus of SA. This may be because of the maintenance of relatively small spaces within readily identifiable lesions of SA (see discussion of ALH). The cytologic features of apocrine change may also be seen in adenosis, so-called apocrine adenosis.[57,58] The enlarged nuclei and prominent nucleoli of apocrine cells, when present in a deformed, sclerotic lesion, can occasionally mimic invasive carcinoma. Some have used the appellation *atypical* to describe this setting.[59] Atypical apocrine adenosis does not appear to be associated with an increased risk for the subsequent of breast carcinoma.[60]

The differential diagnosis of these lesions includes tubular carcinoma and its variants. Usually, careful attention to the fact that SA is lobulocentric will suffice to correctly identify it. It is also true in SA that adjacent tubules tend to take approximately the same or similar shape as their immediate neighbors, although minor variations become marked if one skips to several tubular structures away. Myoepithelial markers are generally retained in SA, although densely sclerotic foci with glandular atrophy may have reduced or absent myoepithelial cells. This is then a helpful but not an absolute criterion. The spaces of a tubular carcinoma tend to be open, occasionally producing an irregular extension of the cluster of cells at one edge, resembling a teardrop. The cells of an infiltrating tubular carcinoma usually are layered singly, and when they are multilayered, the cells appear similar (see Chapter 10).

A rare condition known as *microglandular adenosis* may also mimic tubular carcinoma.[61,62] In this condition, irregular, nonlobulocentric, small glandular spaces are present in increased numbers and appear to dissect and infiltrate through both stroma and fat, and a clinically palpable mass of several centimeters in diameter may be produced, which may be irregularly demarcated from surrounding tissue. The importance of this rare lesion is its ability to mimic tubular carcinoma.

Radial Scar and Complex Sclerosing Lesions

Radial scar and complex sclerosing lesions have some similarities to SA: carcinoma may be mimicked clinically, histologically, or by breast imaging. Similar lesions were first described by Fenoglio and Lattes[63] as mimickers of carcinoma. The lesions appear

spiculated, hence the term *radial scar*. The lesions are not lobulocentric but evidently incorporate several deformed lobular units within their makeup, having as their probable origin a major stem of the duct system. This is particularly true of very large lesions. These are all characterized by a central scar from which elements radiate. The scar may vary through the full range of histologic appearances of the breast, including cystic dilation and units demonstrating hyperplasia and lobulocentric sclerosis, like that of SA. Myoepithelial markers may be reduced or lost in these sclerosing lesions. The microscopic features are determined by the degree of maturation; the classic appearance (Fig. 8.12) represents the well-developed stage II. Lesions at an earlier stage show noticeable spindle cells and chronic inflammatory cells around the central parenchymal components, which are less distorted. The association of hyperplasia and cystic and apocrine change becomes more evident as the lesion matures.

The progressive nature of these lesions was studied ultrastructurally by Battersby and Anderson.[64] A feature associated with early lesions was myofibroblasts in close proximity to degenerating parenchymal structures. Mature radial scars showed relatively few, sparsely distributed stromal myofibroblasts. Within the central scar, there are entrapped epithelial elements that mimic an invasive process (Fig. 8.13). Although these are the elements that most commonly mimic carcinoma histologically, atypical hyperplastic lesions may be found within the preformed epithelial spaces in the outer portions of the lesion. The entrapped epithelial units may closely mimic tubular carcinoma, especially on core biopsy.

Anderson and Battersby[65] analyzed the qualitative and quantitative features of more than 100 examples of radial scars from cases with and without cancer. Their frequency is similar in both groups and depends heavily on the diligence of search and the amount of tissue assessed. Bilaterality and multifocality were present in both groups, as was the full range of histologic appearance. No premalignant definition of these lesions was supported.

A variety of terms have been proposed for these lesions. However, it is likely that *radial scar* will maintain dominance. We favor the term *complex sclerosing lesion* for the larger examples (i.e., >10 mm) in this series. This is because they tend to have a variety of appearances, and their complexity with regard to mimicry of carcinoma is clearly portrayed by the term *complex*. The term *radial* is also useful to indicate the spiculated nature of the lesions. There are conflicting data on the independent contribution to breast cancer risk by radial scars.[66,67]

Duct Ectasia and Fat Necrosis

Duct Ectasia

Duct ectasia is an entity or group of entities that has somewhat unclear confines of definition.[68] Some recognize only dilated ducts, as the term would indicate, to represent this condition. When this approach is taken, the condition is common but typically not associated with clinical pain or scarring. The separation of this entity into two large groups affecting different age groups and having different causes is becoming widely recognized.[26]

Most observers reserve the diagnostic term for those conditions in which a clinical presentation includes palpable lumpiness in the region of the breast under the areola. Ducts tend to be involved in a segmental fashion; that is, adjacent ducts extending out into the breast from the nipple are involved. Periductal inflammation is a histologic hallmark of this condition.[22] It is generally believed that the process begins with such a change and proceeds by destroying the elastic network to ectasia and periductal fibrosis.[19] Nipple discharge is a common but not invariable accompaniment of this condition, and undoubtedly the periductal scarring attendant to the later stages of this process is responsible for most cases of benign, acquired nipple inversion.[69]

Most cases described are found in the perimenopausal age group. There are also younger women who present with inflammation of the ducts in the region of the nipple, which may produce fissures and fistulas with connections from the nipple ducts to the skin at the edges of the areola. The presentation of fistulas in younger women seems to be clearly connected with infection. This so-called periductal mastitis is commonly associated with a history of previous periareolar inflammation.[26] The more classic appearance of duct ectasia in older women may be a more smoldering infection of the larger ducts, and infection as the basis of this condition has been strongly suggested but remains unproven for most cases.[19,70] Few patients with duct ectasia have a history of periductal mastitis, suggesting that these two conditions are probably unrelated. There is no association with parity or lactation.[71] As is the case with so many of these benign conditions of the breast, the greatest importance clinically is the mimicry of carcinoma. The plaquelike calcifications that occur within the scarred wall are, of course, visible with mammography (Fig. 8.14). Usually, these calcifications can be differentiated from the more

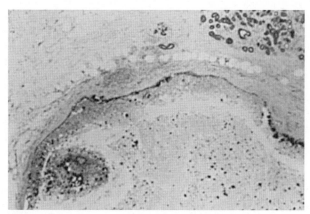

• **Fig. 8.14** Large duct affected by duct ectasia. There is periductal fibrosis and inflammation. Note calcification in the wall of duct. (Magnification ×50.)

irregular punctate calcifications of comedocarcinoma, but this is not always clear. Besides this frequent approximation to the mammographic appearance of comedo DCIS, the localized scarring of duct ectasia can produce lumps that are fixed within inflamed scar in the breast. These lumps can closely mimic carcinoma on occasion. One variant of this condition containing many plasma cells has been termed *plasma cell mastitis*. This is probably not a separate condition but rather part of the spectrum of duct ectasia. This is known to be a close mimicker of breast carcinoma of lobular infiltrating type, both grossly and microscopically.

Fat Necrosis

Fat necrosis is relatively uncommon but may present in a most dramatic fashion, mimicking a well-developed carcinoma or even inflammatory carcinoma. In its late, scarred phase, fat necrosis may not have an identifiable preceding traumatic cause; however, the mammographic appearance in the late stages is characteristic.[72] Most cases seen in the more acute phases, with some inflammatory activity still apparent, are associated with an identifiable recent traumatic event.

The histology of fat necrosis in the breast is no different from its appearance in other organs. The characteristic active chronic inflammatory cells are usually evident, with lymphocytes and histiocytes predominating. In the unusual acute cases presenting within 1 week after an inciting event, polymorphonuclear leukocytes and free, oily lipid material may be most apparent, particularly on needle aspiration. In this stage, the clinical features of swelling, redness, and warmth are present.

In the later stage, collagenous scar is the predominant finding, with seemingly granular histiocytes surrounding oil cysts of varying size. These "oil cysts" contain the free lipid material released by lipocyte necrosis.[73] The greatest clinical importance of fat necrosis is in its mimicry of carcinoma, as noted earlier. There is no known association with carcinoma or carcinoma risk.

Fibroadenoma and Phyllodes Tumor

Fibroadenoma

Fibroadenomas (FAs) most often have a characteristic clinical presentation with an easily movable mass, seemingly unfixed to surrounding breast tissue. The gross appearance is usually characteristic. The sharp circumscription and smooth interface with surrounding breast tissue, usually producing an elevation of the FA on cut section, is also characteristic. The cut surface is white, although one may identify the epithelial elements, if they are numerous, as light-brown areas. The cut surface is shiny and occasionally may seem to present an almost papillary appearance if the clefts lined by epithelium are larger. There may be slight variation from one area to another, with denser fibrosis in the stroma and occasionally calcification. The latter two features are more common in older women.

Although traditionally the risk of subsequent carcinoma in patients with typical FA has not been considered to be higher than that for the general population,[19] one study reported that, overall, FAs were found to be associated with a slight increased relative risk of later cancer.[74] The level of risk varies, depending on the characteristics of the FA itself and the status of the adjacent epithelium. If the adjacent epithelium shows proliferative changes or if the FA is complex, defined as the presence of cysts, SA, epithelial calcifications, or papillary apocrine changes within the FA, the risk is slightly higher than when these changes are absent.[74] Indeed, without these specific features, the women have no increased risk. One of the interesting aspects of this study, also shown by Levi and coworkers,[75] is that the risk identified by FA may not decrease in relative terms in the next 5 or 10 years after identification with biopsy.[74]

Carcinoma arising in FAs is distinctly uncommon. In this setting, lobular carcinoma in situ is the predominant type.[76–78]

Risk implications for lobular neoplasia within an FA are not known for certain but probably are no greater than when lobular neoplasia is seen in the usual setting[74]; indeed, a large study indicates that AH within FAs presents no increased risk of later cancer development.[79] Microscopically, fibrous tissue makes up most of the FA; either the stroma may surround rounded and easily definable ductlike epithelial structures or the epithelium may be stretched into curvilinear arrangements (Figs. 8.15 and 8.16). This

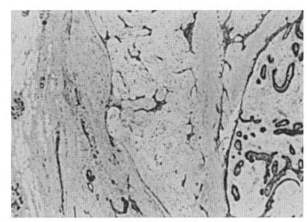

• **Fig. 8.15** Fibroadenoma showing prominent intracanalicular pattern. (Magnification ×30.)

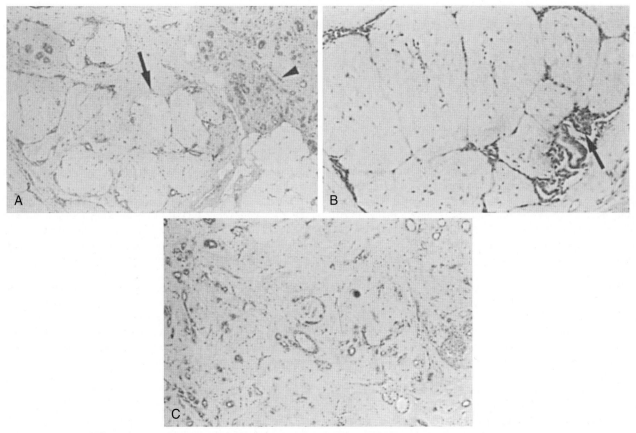

• **Fig. 8.16** (A) Fibroadenoma with irregular border. Both intracanalicular *(arrow)* and pericanalicular *(arrowhead)* patterns are well demonstrated. (Magnification ×30.) (B) Higher power of part A. Fixation artifact gives appearance of hyperplastic epithelium *(arrow)*. (Magnification ×125.) (C) Same case as part A. Complex epithelial patterns are evident. (Magnification ×50.)

latter pattern has been termed *intracanalicular,* and the former pattern has been termed *pericanalicular.* These two terms are still useful as descriptors but are of no practical or prognostic importance and therefore are not used to define supposed subtypes of FA. Smooth muscle is an extremely rare component of FAs.[80] The epithelium within an FA may have the same appearance as elsewhere in the breast, including apocrine metaplasia.[81] Rarely, squamous metaplasia is present.[82]

FAs that are allowed to grow after initial detection usually cease to grow when they reach 2 to 3 cm in diameter.[83] African Americans more commonly develop FAs than Caucasians, and they develop them at a younger age as well. FAs in African Americans are also more likely to recur.[84] Because FAs are more common in African Americans, related lesions are also probably more common in the African American population.[85] Infarcts of the breast may occur during pregnancy or lactation with a resultant discrete mass.[86] Approximately 1 of 200 FAs shows infarction.[87,88] Pain and tenderness may occur during pregnancy, and an inflammatory reaction may be accompanied by lymphadenopathy, leading to the clinical impression of carcinoma.

Fibroadenoma may also be regarded as a generic term, referring to any benign, confined tumor of the breast (mass-occupying lesion) that has a mixture of glandular and mesenchymal elements. When it is viewed as a more specific term, special or specific variants of the general pattern are recognized as being separate entities. These include hamartoma, tubular adenoma, lactating adenoma, adenolipoma, juvenile FA, and giant adenoma.

Hamartomas of the breast have received greater attention with the introduction of mammography.[89,90] These are lesions made up of recognizable lobular units, often present at the sharply demarcated margins of these lesions.[91] Fat is rare in FAs, which are also rarely characterized by well-ordered lobular units throughout their substance. Another feature supporting the recognition of hamartomas as separate entities is that their average age of presentation is almost two decades after that for FAs in general. It is the sharp, smooth borders of these lesions and their intermixture with fat that allows mammographic identification in pronounced examples.[92] A similar lesion is the adenolipoma, which is only one-tenth as common as ordinary lipomas.[93]

Other types of FAs, perhaps better regarded as variants rather than as separate entities, are lesions that tend to occur in women in the younger age range; they are characterized by increased cellularity of stroma or epithelium, or both. Cellular FAs are likely to occur in adolescents and not thought to have a higher likelihood of recurrence than typical FA.[94] The main diagnostic challenge these lesions pose is related to their potential to show histologic features suggestive of a benign phyllodes tumor.[95,96] On the basis of similar outcomes data, the World Health Organization (WHO) Working Group recommends classifying lesions with overlapping features of cellular FA and benign phyllodes tumor as fibroadenoma.[97] *Juvenile fibroadenoma* is a diagnostic term based on clinical grounds.[98] Pike and Oberman[99] characterized these lesions by their tendency to occur around the time of menarche, the common ductal pattern of epithelial hyperplasia, and the defining stromal hypercellularity. Local recurrence was not believed to be a feature of these lesions. Mies and Rosen[100] have also described a series of patients with an average age of 26 years who had an unusual and atypical pattern of epithelial hyperplasia within FAs, which may be misinterpreted as carcinoma in situ. No specific clinical feature was suggested. The practical utility of these interesting approaches to unusual FAs appears to be that rapidly growing lesions in juveniles are usually benign, often have

a densely cellular stroma, and less often have prominent epithelial hyperplasia.

A variant of FA is tubular adenoma. These lesions are uncommon and are recognized as having dominant tubular elements in a circumscribed mass with minimal supporting stroma.[101,102] Grossly tubular adenomas have a fine nodularity.[103] Portions of otherwise characteristic FAs may have the appearance of a tubular adenoma. Uniform tubular structures are seen, and lobular anatomy is usually not evident. Tubular adenomas may have evidence of secretory activity, but when they do not occur in association with pregnancy or lactation, they should not be termed *lactating adenomas.* Lactating adenomas are certainly analogous in some ways to tubular adenomas and may represent a physiologic response of the tubular adenoma to pregnancy.[104] In addition to showing lactational changes, the adenomas presenting in pregnancy have a more evident lobular anatomy than that seen in most tubular adenomas. Some authors have supported the notion that the lesions arising in pregnancy, formerly termed *lactating adenomas,* be termed *breast tumor of pregnancy.*[105] This term is proposed because they are distinct from tubular adenomas and should not be related to lactation (despite histologic changes) because they arise during pregnancy, not during the time of breastfeeding. The microscopic changes seen in the breast tumor of pregnancy are similar to those seen in the normal pregnant breast but are variable in degree and are often out of phase with the normal breast changes resulting from pregnancy.

Phyllodes Tumor

The series of mammary tumors known as *phyllodes tumors* continue to pose challenges for the physician managing breast disease. Phyllodes tumors may show significant overlap with FA in their radiologic and histologic appearance.[106] Two additional problems remain incompletely resolved: (1) the rarity of these lesions has made the distinction between benign and borderline lesions difficult, and (2) there remain a fairly large number of cases, relative to the entire group of lesions, that must continue to be regarded as having borderline malignant potential, presenting obvious problems in patient management, although such "borderline" cases should present a threat of local recurrence only. Malignant phyllodes tumors often grow rapidly and become symptomatic in the interval between screening mammograms.[107]

There is no reliable way to differentiate grossly a giant FA (or the so-called juvenile FA) from a benign phyllodes tumor. Indeed, the tendency to recognize the large size as the dominant characteristic of phyllodes tumor has led to the frequent confusion of these entities. A classic gross pattern for a phyllodes tumor includes sharp demarcation from the surrounding normal breast tissue, with the normal tissue obviously compressed. The connective tissue that makes up the greatest bulk of the mass is firm and varies from dense and white to glistening and edematous. Local areas of degeneration lead to cystic and discolored areas. The classic pattern that gave these tumors their name may be evident with smoothly contoured leaflike areas separated from others by narrow, epithelial-lined spaces. The histologic appearance is characterized by hypercellular stroma in addition to the aforementioned leaflike architecture (Fig. 8.17).

Although it is often stated that histologic criteria are not reliable and that lesions appearing to be benign histopathologically may metastasize, these events are poorly characterized or poorly documented. The current WHO classification recognizes three categories of phyllodes tumors: benign, borderline, and malignant.[97]

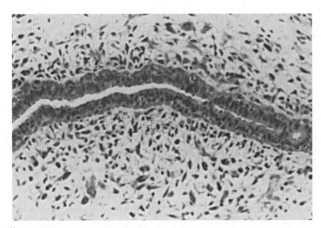

• **Fig. 8.17** Phyllodes tumor. Hypercellular stroma shows nuclear pleomorphism and atypia. (Magnification ×300.)

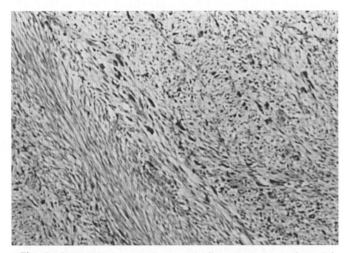

• **Fig. 8.18** Phyllodes tumor. Low-grade fibrosarcomatous element is evident. (Magnification ×110.)

A predominantly circumscribed margin, 5 to 10 mitoses per high-power microscopic field, and moderate nuclear pleomorphism are features distinguishing a borderline phyllodes tumor from a benign phyllodes tumor.[97] With the use of a borderline category, our ability to predict behavior and guide management may be improved. Most malignant phyllodes tumors reported in the literature that have metastasized have had overgrowth of an obvious sarcomatous element (Fig. 8.18). The stroma of a malignant phyllodes tumor may contain areas with a heterologous component (e.g., liposarcoma, rhabdomyosarcoma).

The conventional wisdom has been that incomplete excision of phyllodes tumors (or excision with close margins) is a major determinant for local recurrence, and this may be especially true for malignant tumors.[108,109] However, recent studies show low recurrence rates for benign and borderline phyllodes tumors with close or positive margins.[110,111] Stromal overgrowth remains a predictor of recurrence and survival in malignant phyllodes tumors.[111] It must be noted that local recurrences appear to be unlikely to evolve into malignancy if this feature was not present in the primary tumor.[112]

Pseudoangiomatous Stromal Hyperplasia

Pseudoangiomatous stromal hyperplasia (PASH) is a benign proliferative condition of the breast stromal cells first described by Vuitch and colleagues.[113] Patients with PASH are typically pre- or perimenopausal and may present with a mass on physical examination or a new finding on imaging studies.[114] Most patients with a biopsy diagnosis of PASH may be offered surveillance. Women with enlarging lesions and a high risk of developing breast cancer may be treated with local excision.[114] PASH, by itself, does not appear to confer an increased risk for the subsequent development of breast cancer.[115]

Papilloma

The usual and classic solitary papilloma is a mass lesion of the large ducts most often presenting in the subareolar region. In the periphery, papillary lesions are often multiple and continuous with hyperplastic alterations within lobular units, as shown by Ohuchi and colleagues[116] in three-dimensional reconstruction studies of papillomas. Particularly when they are extensive, these lesions may be associated with AH and ductal pattern carcinoma in situ within and adjacent to the peripheral papillomas.

There is an important clinical correlate of these papillary lesions: they commonly present with ipsilateral, often bloody, nipple discharge.[117] This is true for the more central and larger lesions but may be also seen in smaller, more peripheral lesions. A careful follow-up of women with a solitary papilloma showed an increased risk of subsequent carcinoma development.[118] It was suggested that accompanying epithelial hyperplasia was responsible for further elevating the increased risk (see Box 8.1). From the Nashville series of patients, a nested case-control study evaluated the risk of carcinoma development after having a papilloma identified with biopsy.[119] A papilloma with or without ordinary patterns of hyperplasia was associated with only a slight increased risk, similar to other features of proliferative breast disease without atypia.[119] The presence of AH (pattern and extent analogous to ADH) within a papilloma increased the risk of subsequent development of breast cancer, predominantly near the site of the original papilloma. This single study suggests that women who have papillomas with AH may have a similar or higher cancer risk than others who have patterns of AH within breast parenchyma. Other studies have shown that women with multiple papillomas,[120,121] especially those who also have AH,[121] have an increased risk of subsequent development of carcinoma.

Histopathology

Papillomas are truly papillary lesions with a branching fibrovascular core surmounted by epithelium (Fig. 8.19). They are most often identified on careful gross examination as lying within dilated ductal sacs. The papillomas may attain several centimeters in size, causing them to appear encysted with the continuity of the duct within which they arose, less apparent than in smaller examples. The texture of papillomas varies from soft to firm with dense sclerotic foci. Focal areas of necrosis and hemorrhage are a natural part of the basic elements of papillomas. Infarction may cause compression and distortion of epithelium, producing the appearance of carcinoma.[122] Squamous metaplasia may also be present.[122,123] The epithelial lining in benign papillomas varies greatly but is usually easily identified as benign (see Fig. 8.19). A double cell layer with more rounded cells adjacent to the basement membrane and surmounted by more columnar cells is commonly seen. When the cell numbers are increased beyond that, the same rules for atypia (usually ADH) and carcinoma in situ used for hyperplasia may be applied. Thus there are papillomas with focal atypia that may qualify for AH (see earlier discussion).

When the cell proliferation is uniform and attains the features seen in patterns in DCIS, an encapsulated or intracystic papillary carcinoma may be diagnosed (see Chapter 9).

Other lesions bearing resemblance to papilloma are discussed here for convenience, because they remain a portion of the differential diagnosis of those lesions. These include nipple adenoma (florid papillomatosis of the nipple) and nodular adenosis (ductal adenoma).

Nipple adenoma is a term used to describe a variety of appearances that may present in the nipple or immediately adjacent tissues. Patterns of hyperplasia with pseudoinvasion of dense stroma may be taken to be the basic features of these lesions.

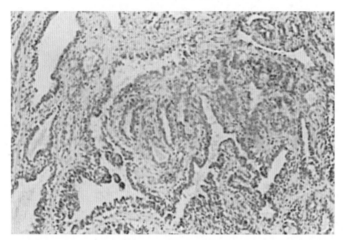

• **Fig. 8.19** Delicate fibrovascular fronds of papilloma covered by single or double epithelial cell layers. (Magnification ×280.)

They may be misinterpreted clinically as Paget disease because of irregularities of the surface of the nipple. However, they rarely ulcerate and therefore do not have the moist, red appearance of the eczematous features of Paget disease. These lesions have localized areas of hyperplasia of slightly varying patterns intermixed with fibrous and cystic changes that may suggest atypia. Nipple adenomas or subareolar papillomatosis usually are diagnosed when they are approximately 1 cm or smaller. Patterns of papilloma are also mimicked. Careful histologic sampling and complete excision are important because foci of carcinoma have been described in such lesions but apparently are rare.[124,125] These lesions often have nuclear hyperchromatism and a relatively high nuclear cytoplasmic ratio, as well as fibrosis—features that may be worrisome. Complex patterns of epithelial hyperplasia enveloped by fibrosis may lead to the mistaken diagnosis of malignancy. Careful attention to these features avoids overdiagnosis of malignancy.[126]

Nodular adenosis and *ductal adenoma* are similar terms for an important group of lesions presenting varied histology. These lesions are most closely related to papillomas with unusual patterns of sclerosis and adenosis.[127] Because these lesions are characteristically surrounded by dense fibrous tissue within which epithelial cells are pseudoinvasive; they may be overdiagnosed as malignancy by the unwary (Fig. 8.20).

Columnar Cell Lesions

Columnar cell lesions are often associated with calcifications detected by screening mammography,[16] and they have been referred to using a variety of essentially synonymous terms[128] (Fig. 8.21). Columnar cell lesions have been classified as

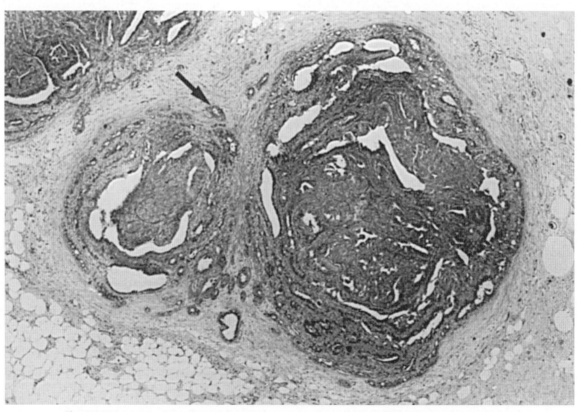

• **Fig. 8.20** Proliferating glandular epithelium of a "ductal adenoma." Irregularities at the interface between adenotic elements and fibrous capsule simulate invasion *(arrow)*. (Magnification ×70.)

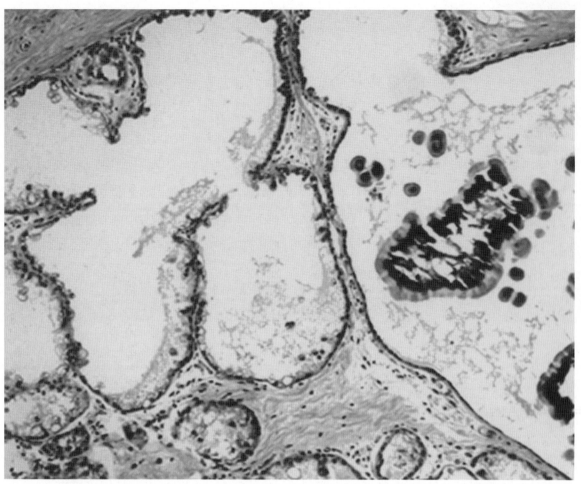

• **Fig. 8.21** A lobular unit with enlarged acinar spaces with columnar alteration of the epithelium (Magnification ×200.)

"blunt duct adenosis,"[6,129] "hyperplastic enlarged lobular units,"[130] "columnar alteration with prominent apical snouts and secretions,"[16] and "enlarged lobular units with columnar alteration."[131] The diagnostic terms for columnar cell lesions with nuclear atypia (flat epithelial atypia [FEA] in the WHO classification,[132,133] discussed shortly) have included "clinging carcinoma, monomorphic type,"[54] ductal intraepithelial neoplasia,[134] and columnar cell change with atypia.[135] The descriptor "flat" has been applied to columnar cell lesions to emphasize absence of architectural complexity typical of classical ADH or low-grade DCIS.

The current WHO classification is limited to three diagnostic categories of columnar cell lesions: columnar cell change, columnar cell hyperplasia, and FEA.[133] FEA encompasses columnar cell change and columnar cell hyperplasia with atypia. The atypia in atypical columnar cell lesions is cytologic atypia alone, whereas a diagnosis of ADH or low-grade DCIS requires a combination of cytologic and architectural features (see Chapter 9).

Multiple morphologic and molecular studies have suggested a potential relationship between FEA and breast neoplasia.[136] Columnar cell change and FEA are often colocalized with ADH and ALH[137,138] and may be associated with low-grade in situ and invasive carcinomas.[139] Analysis of FEA, AH, and low-grade carcinoma from the same tissue section has shown a set of shared genetic alterations, suggesting that FEA may be a nonobligate precursor in a low-grade breast neoplasia pathway.[140,141]

It must be noted that case-control studies of open biopsies indicate that the risk associated with columnar cell lesions and FEA alone is lower than the risk associated with ADH and ALH.[137,138] For patients with pure FEA diagnosed on core needle biopsy, the WHO Working Group recommends radiologic-pathologic correlation.[133] In the absence of any other clinical or radiologic indications for excision, observation may be an acceptable management strategy for pure FEA.[142,143]

Selected References

39. Degnim AC, Dupont WD, Radisky DC, et al. Extent of atypical hyperplasia stratifies breast cancer risk in 2 independent cohorts of women. *Cancer*. 2016;122:2971-2978.
40. Visscher DW, Frost MH, Hartmann LC, et al. Clinicopathologic features of breast cancers that develop in women with previous benign breast disease. *Cancer*. 2016;122:378-385.
42. Morrow M, Schnitt SJ, Norton L. Current management of lesions associated with an increased risk of breast cancer. *Nat Rev Clin Oncol*. 2015;12:227-238.
43. Collins LC, Aroner SA, Connolly JL, et al. Breast cancer risk by extent and type of atypical hyperplasia: an update from the Nurses' Health Studies. *Cancer*. 2016;122:515-520.
50. Page DL, Schuyler PA, Dupont WD, et al. Atypical lobular hyperplasia as a unilateral predictor of breast cancer risk: a retrospective cohort study. *Lancet*. 2003;361:125-129.

A full reference list is available online at ExpertConsult.com.

9

In Situ Carcinomas of the Breast: Ductal Carcinoma in Situ and Lobular Carcinoma in Situ

V. SUZANNE KLIMBERG AND KIRBY I. BLAND

Over the past several decades, the widespread adoption of mammographic screening has had a significant impact on the incidence, diagnosis, classification, and treatment of all breast diseases. These changes have been particularly profound for in situ carcinoma of the breast. As a result, there has been a vast increase in the number of publications in the literature with regard to the definition, diagnostic criteria, and both short-term and long-term risks associated with specific histologic variants or types of in situ carcinoma of the breast. It is estimated that by 2020, approximately 1 million women will be living with DCIS—more than double the number in 2005.[1] In situ carcinomas of the breast were first recognized in the early 20th century and were identified morphologically as cells cytologically similar to those of invasive carcinomas but confined to ductal structures within the breast parenchyma. Such lesions were generally found to be located adjacent to areas of invasive carcinoma. The original definitions given to in situ carcinomas of the breast were arbitrary. Opportunities to study the natural history and behavior of such in situ lesions independent of an invasive component of disease or after a surgical procedure less than that of mastectomy were previously rarely encountered.[2–4] Since that time, several studies relying on the review of archival slide material have demonstrated basic differences between distinct histologic patterns of in situ carcinomas. This subsequently resulted in the distinction between those lesions representing purely markers of increased risk (e.g., lobular carcinoma in situ [LCIS] and atypical hyperplasia, with increased breast cancer risk that was essentially equally distributed to either breast) and committed premalignant lesions (e.g., ductal carcinoma in situ [DCIS], with increased breast cancer risk that was more often reported to be confined to the ipsilateral breast[5–7]).

The classical studies of Wellings and Jensen focused attention on the terminal ductal-lobular unit as a common anatomic site for the development of hyperplastic changes of both the ductal and the lobular type as well as corresponding neoplastic lesions.[8] The terms *DCIS* and *LCIS* were once meant to signify separate anatomic origins, with one originating within the ductal structures and the other originating within the lobular structures. However, this anachronous concept is now recognized to be inaccurate. Unfortunately, the idea of distinct lobular and ductal origins for breast neoplasms continues to persist despite our current understanding of neoplastic development within the breast. Currently, the term *DCIS* refers to patterns of abnormal epithelial cell proliferation associated with a prominent involvement of true ducts within the in situ carcinoma category and has a high risk of local recurrence without adequate local treatment. Thus DCIS is essentially a diagnosis of exclusion, including in its broad sweep any lesion deemed in situ carcinoma that does not exhibit the cytologic features of lobular neoplasia cells.[9–11] In part, this distinction remains important because the distribution of DCIS and LCIS within a breast as well as between the breasts represents a recognized difference between these two in situ carcinoma entities. In that regard, those studies that have specifically addressed the incidence rate or relative risk of developing a subsequent ipsilateral and contralateral invasive breast cancer in women with in situ carcinoma have traditionally shown a higher incidence rate or relative risk of contralateral invasive breast cancer for those women with LCIS compared with those women with DCIS.[12–15] Although these differences between DCIS and LCIS have persisted within the literature, the most recently reported series demonstrate that this difference is likely much smaller than previously thought.[14,15]

Recent Insights Into the Unique Biology of Ductal Carcinoma in Situ and Lobular Carcinoma in Situ

In many respects, DCIS should be regarded as carcinoma of the ductal system, for it possesses all of the molecular and biological abnormalities as frankly invasive carcinoma.[16–19] DCIS is clonal and frequently expresses abnormal p53 and HER2/neu. It has the same loss of heterozygosity patterns as its invasive counterpart. Using comparative genomic hybridization studies, DCIS exhibits no gains or losses of chromosomal regions compared with its invasive counterpart. Rather, DCIS is held in check by a surrounding

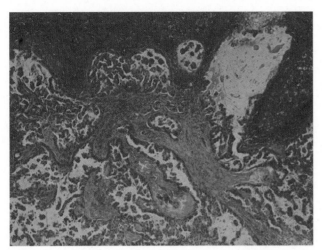

• **Fig. 9.1** The micropapillary type of noncomedo ductal carcinoma in situ is characterized by intraductal papillations projecting into a central lumen.

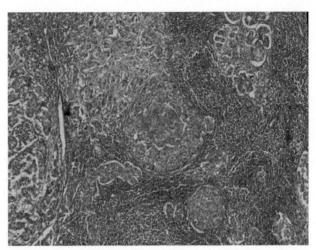

• **Fig. 9.3** The solid type of ductal carcinoma in situ exhibits a solid sheet of intraluminal cells.

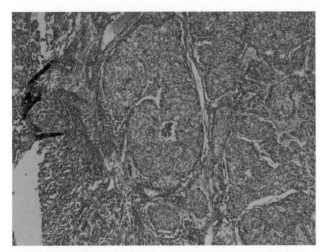

• **Fig. 9.2** The cribriform type of noncomedo ductal carcinoma in situ, in contrast, consists of intraductal proliferations showing bridging and "Roman arch" formation.

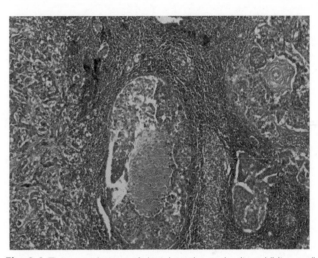

• **Fig. 9.4** The comedo type of ductal carcinoma in situ exhibits a solid pattern of intraluminal proliferation with high nuclear grade and central necrosis.

layer of myoepithelial cells that exert paracrine suppressive effects on invasion.[20–24] Because of this, the histopathologic patterns of DCIS usually strongly correlate with its invasive counterpart, when present in individual cases. For example, papillary DCIS (Fig. 9.1) tends to invade as papillary adenocarcinoma. Cribriform DCIS (Fig. 9.2) and solid DCIS (Fig. 9.3) of intermediate nuclear grades tend to invade as a moderately differentiated adenocarcinoma. Comedo DCIS of high nuclear grade (Fig. 9.4) tends to invade as a poorly differentiated adenocarcinoma. The precursor lesion of DCIS is thought to be atypical ductal hyperplasia (ADH) for the DCIS of low or intermediate nuclear grades. Simple ductal hyperplasia, based on loss of heterozygosity and genomic hybridization studies, is no longer thought to be a precursor lesion of either ADH or DCIS. A recently described lesion, flat epithelial atypia or columnar cell atypia (Figs. 9.5 and 9.6), based on its abnormal nuclear features and its presence juxtaposed to DCIS, especially high-grade DCIS, is thought to be a possible precursor lesion. However, this has not yet been proved in prospective studies. The evidence is incontrovertible that DCIS can and often does progress to frank invasive adenocarcinoma, and clearly, the same clone is involved.

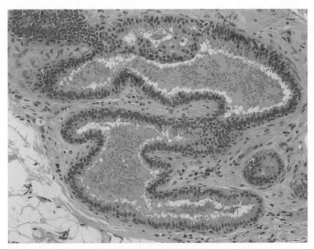

• **Fig. 9.5** The lesion of flat columnar epithelial atypia is characterized by dilated ducts lined by a single luminal cell layer.

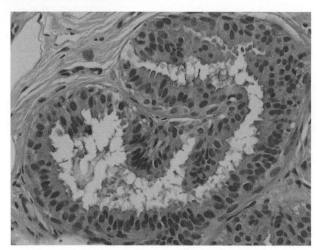

• **Fig. 9.6** At higher magnification, the single luminal cell layer is columnar in shape and manifests marked nuclear atypia.

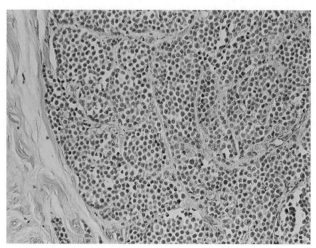

• **Fig. 9.8** Lobular carcinoma in situ of the pleomorphic type exhibits individual cells that are larger and more individually defined.

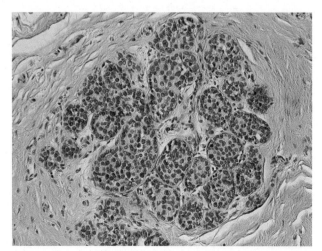

• **Fig. 9.7** Lobular carcinoma in situ of the classic type fills and distends acini.

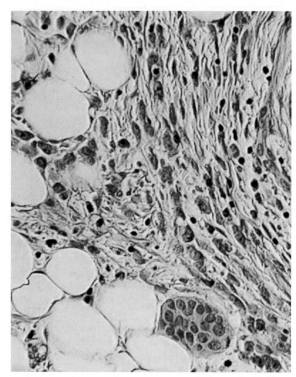

• **Fig. 9.9** Lobular carcinoma in situ, especially of the pleomorphic type *(bottom)*, can directly progress to invasion *(central* and *top)*.

With LCIS, the story is both similar and different. Emerging evidence has suggested that LCIS is a heterogeneous disease.[25] Some types of LCIS are associated with a 4- to 10-fold increased risk of invasive breast carcinoma (Fig. 9.7). The increased risk can be associated with any type of infiltrating breast carcinoma, including both ductal as well as lobular carcinoma. Other forms of LCIS may be more innocuous. Still others, for example, those that express more nuclear pleomorphism such as pleomorphic LCIS (Fig. 9.8), may actually progress to invasive lobular carcinoma (Fig. 9.9). This latter type of LCIS resembles DCIS in its biology. Still other types of LCIS can mimic other features of DCIS. Some LCIS spreads laterally through the ductal system analogous to Paget disease (Fig. 9.10). This spread of LCIS is aptly termed *pagetoid spread*. Preliminary molecular studies of LCIS by loss of heterozygosity and genomic hybridization confirm the molecular heterogeneity of LCIS. Some LCIS has few, if any, obvious chromosomal abnormalities. Other types of LCIS exhibit evidence of genomic instability. Still other types of LCIS exhibit the same clonal abnormalities as its invasive lobular counterpart. This molecular heterogeneity suggests that some forms of LCIS may be innocuous, others may confer increased risk for the development of breast cancer, and still others can directly progress to

invasive lobular breast cancer. This latter type of LCIS is therefore analogous to DCIS. Clearly, the appropriate therapy would depend on the type of LCIS present. So-called innocuous LCIS could be treated by "watchful waiting," genomically unstable LCIS with an increased risk of breast cancer could be treated with tamoxifen, and the LCIS that directly progresses to invasive carcinoma could be treated with surgical extirpation. Prospective randomized studies and not just historical controls are needed to resolve the LCIS question.

One consistent molecular difference between LCIS and DCIS is the loss of epithelial cadherin (E-cadherin) expression by mutation, promoter methylation, or cis/trans promoter silencing in LCIS but the maintenance of expression of E-cadherin in DCIS.

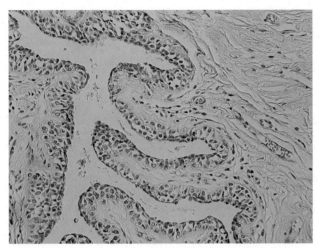

• **Fig. 9.10** Lobular carcinoma in situ can also exhibit pagetoid spread into adjacent ducts.

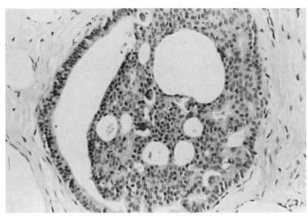

• **Fig. 9.12** Photomicrograph exhibiting a detail of the polarization of luminal cells near the basement membrane that are quite different from the evenly placed and "suspicious" cells present in the central proliferation. This is atypical ductal hyperplasia. Magnification: ×200.

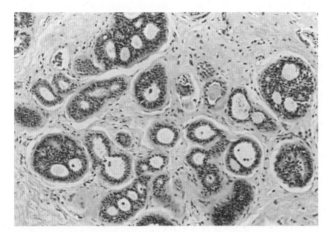

• **Fig. 9.11** Low-power photograph demonstrating the full extent of the evidence supporting a diagnosis of atypical ductal hyperplasia (ADH). Note that there are only three or four spaces in which a central population of uniform cells may be seen. In the others, only narrow bars cross from one side to the other. Thus, there are pattern and cell population features of ductal carcinoma in situ (DCIS). However, in the three largest spaces involved, there are cells adjacent to the basement membrane that appear different; thus a diagnosis of ADH rather than DCIS is made. Magnification: ×75.

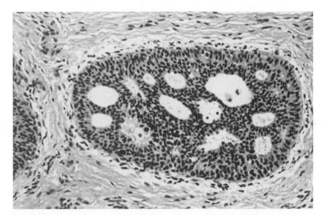

• **Fig. 9.13** This central cribriform pattern of similar cells with outer cells normally polarized (above basement membrane) is probably the most common pattern of atypical ductal hyperplasia. (×150.) (From Anderson TJ, Page DL. Risk assessment in breast cancer. In: Anthony PP, MacSween RNM, Lowe DG, eds. *Recent Advances in Histopathology*. Vol 17. Edinburgh: Churchill Livingstone; 1997.)

This observation can be extended to invasive lobular versus invasive ductal carcinoma as well.

Pathology of Ductal Carcinoma in Situ

DCIS comprises a heterogeneous group of noninvasive neoplastic proliferations with diverse morphologies and risks of subsequent recurrence and invasive transformation (Figs. 9.11 to 9.17). Although DCIS probably arises predominantly in the terminal ductal-lobular unit, it often extends out to involve extralobular ducts. Compared with LCIS, DCIS is generally more variable histologically and cytologically, with larger and more pleomorphic nuclei and a tendency to form microacini, cribriform spaces, or papillary structures. In some cases, the periphery of these lesions may include patterns overlapping with atypical hyperplasia.[26] Pathologists do not agree on whether small lesions should be considered atypical hyperplasia or in situ carcinoma. In general,

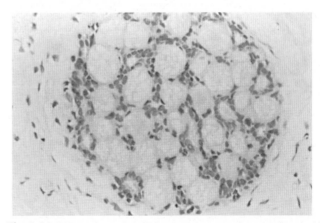

• **Fig. 9.14** Collagenous spherulosis, a pattern sometimes confused with atypical ductal hyperplasia or ductal carcinoma in situ.[98] Note that the spaces are defined by a secreted material that may be seen faintly. The spaces are surrounded by a sparse population of cells that everywhere is tapered or thinned in its extent. Such a pattern is not recognized as atypical. Magnification: ×150.

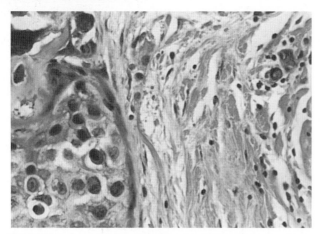

• **Fig. 9.15** High-power view of comedo ductal carcinoma in situ demonstrating necrosis in the upper left-hand corner. Note also that the stroma is altered about this area, which occurs frequently in this type of carcinoma in situ. Magnification: ×700.

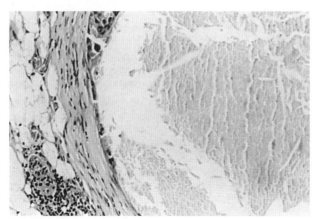

• **Fig. 9.16** Occasionally cellular necrosis in comedo ductal carcinoma in situ is so extensive that very few atypical cells remain. Indeed, the necrosis may appear to extend to the basement membrane. Magnification: ×125.

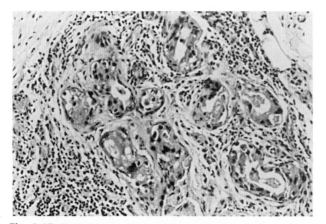

• **Fig. 9.17** Characteristic of more advanced and comedo carcinoma–type examples of ductal carcinoma in situ is the spread of highly atypical cells into lobular units. Here this phenomenon of so-called cancerization of lobules is demonstrated. Magnification: ×200.

• BOX 9.1   Classification Schema for Ductal Carcinoma in Situ[a]

1. Differentiation, mainly based on nuclear morphology and cell polarization[47]
2. Nuclear grade and necrosis[48]
3. Intersection of nuclear grade and extent of necrosis similar to Silverstein, but with separate identification of special types[60]

[a]*It is evident that the classification scheme should promote consistency.*

---

lesions that involve only a few membrane-bound spaces and that measure less than 2 to 3 mm in greatest dimension should be regarded as hyperplastic lesions (with or without atypia) and not in situ carcinoma. There is a greater degree of concordance in larger lesions, however.[27] Pathologists tend to agree about the diagnosis of difficult, smaller, borderline lesions if they have agreed on criteria[28] (Box 9.1). Occasionally, it may be difficult to distinguish DCIS and LCIS histologically, with some forms of DCIS characterized by small uniform cells with a solid growth pattern simulating LCIS. In rare instances, in situ neoplastic proliferations are indeterminate. In such cases, they are presumed to have the prognostic implications of both diagnoses (e.g., local evolution to invasion for DCIS and increased general risk in each breast for LCIS).[10] It has been proposed that E-cadherin stains are useful in such overlap cases,[29,30] but it should be pointed out that no long-term follow-up study has examined the implications of E-cadherin staining or absence thereof for regional breast cancer risk. It has been our approach to diagnose such cases as in situ carcinoma, mixed pattern, and to indicate that a regional risk for local recurrence should be assumed.

Terminology is an important consideration here, and as noted earlier, there are distinct clinical implications concerning the terms *lobular* and *ductal*. Although the inherited terms have a historical legacy that may carry other significance, they have the impelling merit of familiarity. It is for us to develop more specific criteria for subtypes and to accept that it is the criteria linked to clinical end point analysis that guides clinical practice.[27] One significant problem is the wonderfully earthy word *comedo*. It refers to the lowly comedones (e.g., acne) of common experience from our teen years, an unfailing image of the gross appearance of these lesions. Bloodgood coined the term *comedo-adenoma* because when treated with mastectomy in the halstedian era, it was associated with long-term survival.[31] For Bloodgood, the alternative to carcinoma was adenoma, a lesion capable of cure when adequately excised. The term *comedo* remains descriptive and is now somewhat confusingly used to indicate both a type of DCIS with a coagulation-type necrosis and frequent nuclear debris, as well as merely the evidence of necrosis alone (comedo necrosis). Today most students of DCIS use comedo as a modifier for DCIS, signifying high-grade lesions that exhibit necrosis.

A major transition in our thinking regarding DCIS was the idea that perhaps not all DCIS cases were the same and that the different histologic appearances of DCIS might in fact have important clinical implications. Translating this concept into practical terms, it was suggested that if comedo-type DCIS did have a more menacing clinical import, then one should err on the side of including any questionable case within this category.[10] Thus in 1989, the critically important concept of further stratification was introduced[32] as a part of the inception of the modern era of understanding of DCIS. Because minor amounts

TABLE 9.1	**Ductal Carcinoma in Situ Classifications**[a]			
		NUCLEAR GRADE		
	Necrosis	I	II	III
Lagios[32]	+		Intermediate	High
	−	Low		
Silverstein[48]	−		Group 2	Group 3
	−		Group 1	Group 3
Solin[50]	+			Comedo
	−		Noncomedo	

High, intermediate, or low indicates respective nuclear grade.
[a]Based on nuclear grade and necrosis.
Modified from Lagios MD. Ductal carcinoma in situ: controversies in diagnosis, biology, and treatment. *Breast J.* 1995;1:67-78.

of necrosis may be seen in the common hyperplasias without features of atypia, specific guidelines are necessary to make appropriate stratifications. Thus, inclusion of an intermediate-grade category has been adopted by the majority of DCIS classifications put forth since the early 1990s (Table 9.1) to recognize examples with minimal necrosis and a moderate degree of nuclear pleomorphism.

Conventionally, DCIS has been classified on the basis of architectural features, such as comedo, cribriform, papillary, solid, and micropapillary.[33,34] Although comedo-type DCIS includes advanced nuclear abnormalities within the neoplastic proliferation as part of the definition, the diagnosis of other patterns of DCIS were based on architecture alone. These patterns were accepted to be overlapping when DCIS was considered one entity and not held to have separate clinical or biological implications.[34,35] The first indication that distinguishing among comedo, noncomedo, and micropapillary subtypes,[36] as well as separation by grade,[32] was of clinical utility certainly inaugurated the modern era of DCIS in 1989.

The increasing use of breast conserving therapy (BCT) in the treatment of mammographically detected DCIS has permitted studies on factors that predict local recurrences and invasive events in the remaining breast after excisional biopsy. Before a large number of small mammographically detected DCIS cases were found with screening, mastectomy was the only acceptable treatment for DCIS and remains a standard treatment for multifocal and multicentric disease.[37,38]

Three prognostic factors have been shown to be important in local control of DCIS after attempts at BCT[39]: (1) the extent (size) of disease in the breast (and its corollary, the residuum after an attempt at excision), (2) the status of margins (also reflecting residual disease in the breast), and (3) the grade of the DCIS (and possibly pure subtype, particularly micropapillary). The most significant of these factors appears to be margin status, followed by histologic grade.[40-47] High nuclear grade and necrosis together define forms of DCIS at much higher risk of local recurrence and invasive transformation. The grade of a DCIS is largely independent of the conventional pattern classification. For example, lesions of high nuclear grade can exhibit any architectural pattern (although lack of precise patterns is most common).[32,47] However, as recognized in the classification system of Holland and associates[47] (see Box 9.1), ordered intercellular relationships are most

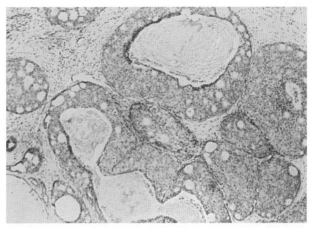

• **Fig. 9.18** This low-power view of a common form of ductal carcinoma in situ shows solid cellular masses distending basement membrane–bound spaces. Within these cellular masses are sharply defined, rounded secondary lumens. There are central areas of necrosis as well as evident distention and distortion of the involved spaces. Magnification: ×75.

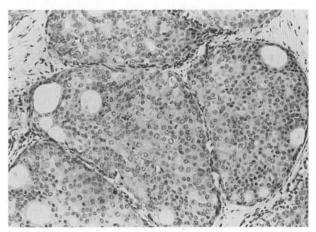

• **Fig. 9.19** This high-power view of Fig. 9.11 demonstrates that the nuclei are of low grade, being similar one to another and without demonstrated irregularity. The presence of necrosis and low-grade nuclei is indicative of a condition intermediate between well-developed comedo ductal carcinoma in situ (DCIS) and the usual noncomedo DCIS. Magnification: ×200.

common in lesions of low nuclear grade. There is a growing consensus that classifications based on nuclear grade and necrosis can identify the majority of patients with DCIS who are at risk for short-term local recurrence and invasive transformation after excision[22,48-51] with or without irradiation. Most of these short-term recurrences are associated with DCIS exhibiting high (3/3 or grade III) nuclear grade morphology and significant coagulative necrosis. Such lesions would be conventionally classified as comedo DCIS. Studies using conventional classification schemes have shown that most short-term failures are associated with comedo-type DCIS.[51-54] It should be recalled that the term *comedo-type DCIS* is not synonymous with high nuclear grade when it is used to indicate necrosis only. Some lesions exhibiting comedo-type necrosis and a solid growth pattern are composed of intermediate-grade and, in rare cases, borderline low-grade nuclei (Figs. 9.18 to 9.27).

Information regarding the potential for recurrence of low-grade (noncomedo-type) DCIS after biopsy or BCT resides in a

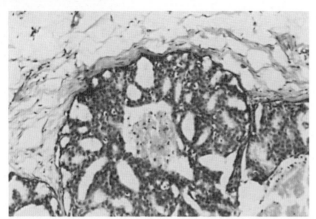

• **Fig. 9.20** This example of ductal carcinoma in situ is characterized by sinuous, interconnecting strands of hyperchromatic cells. Note the few necrotic cells centrally. Magnification: ×100.

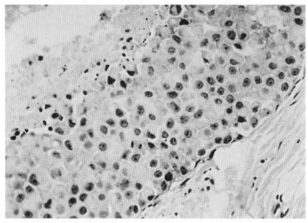

• **Fig. 9.21** This example of intermediate-grade ductal carcinoma in situ (DCIS) presents highly atypical nuclei but not the most advanced, bizarre, and varied cytologic patterns often seen in comedo DCIS. Although one might debate whether these represent intermediate-grade nuclei, the limited luminal necrosis (here at upper left and elsewhere in this case) indicate an intermediate-grade designation. Magnification: ×350.

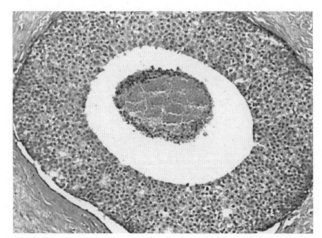

• **Fig. 9.22** In this example of intermediate-grade ductal carcinoma in situ, the presence of necrosis helps define the category. Low- to intermediate-grade nuclei are present (×200). (From Anderson TJ, Page DL. Risk assessment in breast cancer. In: Anthony PP, MacSween RNM, Lowe DG, eds. *Recent Advances in Histopathology*. Vol 17. Edinburgh: Churchill Livingstone; 1997.)

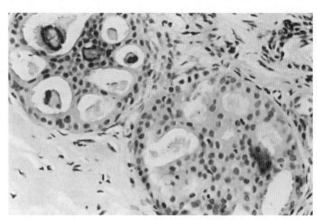

• **Fig. 9.23** Rigid arches of a cribriform pattern variant of ductal carcinoma in situ. Note: calcified material in central spaces is not indicative of cellular necrosis. Magnification: ×225.

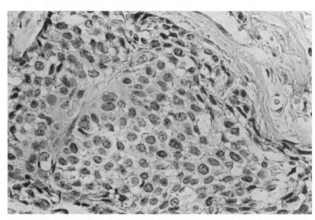

• **Fig. 9.24** An example of a solid pattern variant of ductal carcinoma in situ. There are no evident intercellular spaces, and the slightly irregular placement of cells and sharply defined intercellular contours are not consistent with lobular carcinoma in situ. Magnification: ×450.

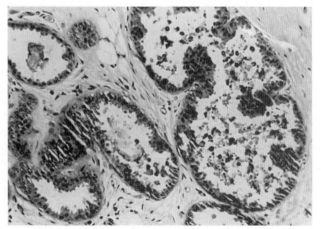

• **Fig. 9.25** Micropapillary ductal carcinoma in situ with necrosis. Although some cells have lighter cytoplasm, the nuclear pattern is similar throughout. Magnification: ×400.

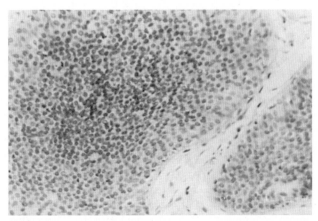

• **Fig. 9.26** This solid variant of atypical ductal hyperplasia (ADH) is diagnostically very similar to solid ductal carcinoma in situ. The more vesicular nuclei in the second population of cells render a diagnosis of ADH. Magnification: ×150.

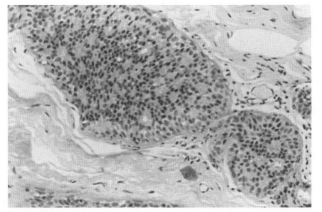

• **Fig. 9.27** The microglandular or "endocrine" pattern of solid ductal carcinoma in situ. Magnification: ×150.

TABLE 9.2	Subclassification of Ductal Carcinoma in Situ of the Breast[a]		
Histology	**Nuclear Grade**	**Necrosis**	**Final DCIS Grade**
Comedo	High	Extensive	High
Intermediate[b]	Intermediate	Focal or absent	Intermediate
Noncomedo[c]	Low	Absent	Low

DCIS, Ductal carcinoma in situ.
[a]Common presentation.
[b]Often a mixture of noncomedo patterns.
[c]Solid, cribriform, papillary, or focal micropapillary.

small number of published studies. It is clear that in the short term (5–10 years), few local recurrences or invasive transformations occur. However, a recent update of the only study of low-grade DCIS present at biopsy (without planned excision[6]) and with extended follow-up[7,55] noted a substantially delayed recurrence rate of invasive lesions (e.g., approximately 37% and 50% at 25 years and more than 40 years of follow-up, respectively). Although the sample is small, it is significant that recurrences were generally in the same quadrant and, in some women, in the site of the prior biopsy, thus representing a biology identical to that of higher-grade DCIS and a risk that does not diminish after menopause. This biology of DCIS should be contrasted with that of risk marker lesions (e.g., ADH and atypical lobular hyperplasia [ALH]), which do not predict the side of involvement and in which risk diminishes postmenopausally (at least for ALH and LCIS).[27,56–58]

There are several published classifications of DCIS,[59] many of which use nuclear grade and necrosis as the major distinguishing features in a general classification applying to most cases of specific subtypes. The separations achieved by these classifications are different and in part may affect the interpretation of outcome results (Table 9.2). DCIS characterized by nuclear morphology (high grade III; e.g., advanced atypia) and necrosis is uniformly classified as high grade.[26,32,48–50,52,60] The European Organization for

Research and Treatment of Cancer (EORTC) classification,[47] although it does not use conventional nuclear grade or necrosis as major discriminates, would also regard this as a high-grade or, in their terminology, a poorly differentiated DCIS. Fisher and colleagues[61] summarized the pathology analysis from the National Surgical Adjuvant Breast Project (NSABP) studies on DCIS and noted that DCIS with grade III nuclei and DCIS that exhibited larger areas of necrosis (greater than one third of ducts involved) had a higher local recurrence rate. The authors reported these results separately, not analyzing the risk associated with the two features in concert. Despite the differences in classification,[59] it would appear that high-grade DCIS can be recognized uniformly, with all investigators showing that the high-grade subtype, so defined, has the highest risk of local recurrence and invasive transformation.

The recognition that necrosis and high nuclear grade usually cluster together[62] may foster agreement between observers by using limited necrosis as a way of defining an intermediate-grade category.[32,60,63] The separate classifications are less consistent with regard to the remainder of the heterogeneous noncomedo-type group (see Table 9.1). DCIS with grade III nuclei but without necrosis, an uncommon situation, is classified as high grade by Silverstein and coworkers[48] but "noncomedo" (a lower grade) by Solin and associates.[50] Lagios and colleagues[32] and Silverstein and coworkers[48] use nuclear grade to separate the remaining DCIS groups. However, Lagios and colleagues[32] classify low-grade DCIS as grade I nuclei without necrosis and intermediate-grade DCIS as grade II with or without necrosis. Silverstein and coworkers[48] separate DCIS with nuclear grades I and II on the basis of necrosis. Group I (low grade) may exhibit grade I or II nuclei but no necrosis, whereas DCIS with grade I or II nuclei but with any necrosis is classified as intermediate (group II). Solin and associates[50] regard all DCIS without grade III nuclei and necrosis as noncomedo-type DCIS. Despite these differences in classification, all investigators have shown a substantially diminished local recurrence rate for DCIS that is not characterized by grade III nuclei and necrosis. Moreover, in those studies in which DCIS is divided into three groups, as opposed to the dichotomous comedo/ noncomedo structure, there is a recognizable intermediate group (intermediate grade, group II, intermediately differentiated) that exhibits a morphology and risk intermediate between low- and high-grade DCIS.

Classification of Ductal Carcinoma in Situ

Although nuclear grade and necrosis would appear to define most of the risk associated with DCIS, certain architectural patterns appear to bear clinical significance independent of the nuclear grade. For example, DCIS with almost pure micropapillary architectural features is strongly associated with extensive disease, that is, within seemingly separate foci of different quadrants.[36,52] This growth pattern makes adequate excision extremely difficult. In some cases, mammographic and histopathologic evidence of disease is present in all four quadrants of the breast. As a result, most clinical studies that define DCIS with micropapillary features and low nuclear grade were based on excisions without theoretically adequate margins of resection.

Conventional classification of DCIS covers perhaps 85% of what is recognized as noninvasive ductal carcinoma. A number of less common subtypes remains to be fully defined morphologically and with regard to risk. Proliferations with apocrine features, bridging the spectrum from minimal atypia to frank DCIS, were the subject of a proposed classification by O'Malley and associates.[64] Because of the difficulty of applying traditional rules regarding cellular atypia and architecture to apocrine lesions, this schema proposed that definitive diagnoses of low-grade apocrine DCIS be limited to cases measuring at least 8 mm in size. In addition, a borderline category was proposed for lesions measuring 4 to 8 mm, with the suggestion that these lesions had the relative risk implications of at least ADH. Furthermore, apocrine DCIS, which is characteristically estrogen receptor negative, progesterone receptor negative, and androgen receptor positive and represents a heterogeneous group of lesions ranging from low-grade lesion (which should be differentiated from atypical hyperplastic apocrine lesions) to obvious malignant, high-grade tumors (which are difficult to recognize as apocrine), was more recently classified into three histologic grades based on nuclear grade and necrosis by Leal and colleagues,[65] similar to schema for classical DCIS. Confirmation of the utility of any of these approaches to classifying such apocrine lesions awaits long-term follow-up analysis of cases treated with conservative surgery.

Another contender for special-type status is the so-called endocrine type of DCIS,[66,67] which presents a particularly low-grade pattern of disease. Similarly, a possible special type characterized by hypersecretory features is discussed subsequently. In all of these less common special types of DCIS, a major limitation is the lack of precise confines of histologic definition that specifically and reproducibly describes the entire spectrum of changes with a linkage to clinical implications corroborated by long-term follow-up studies. With this background of remaining uncertainty, it is generally recommended that all the traditional rules for characterization and classification be applied to these less common entities, so as not to misdiagnose or mistreat such in situ lesions.

The classification of DCIS has been subjected to different approaches, each with advantages and disadvantages. The purpose of any classification scheme for DCIS is to predict the likelihood of recurrences and the likelihood of progression to invasion, and no classification scheme is ideal from these perspectives. For these reasons, newer classification schemes are continually evolving. The classification scheme proposed by Page and Lagios is summarized (see Tables 9.1 and 9.2).[32,60,63] Several other DCIS classifications are presented (see Box 9.1), providing a basis from which to understand the slightly varied approaches. The major differences between Page's classification and most of the other schemes are that Page's uses the intersection of two variables—necrosis and nuclear grade—to foster agreement. It is common to debate between adjacent nuclear grades, viz, 1 or 2, and 2 or 3. The extensiveness of the necrosis is to be used to aid in the resolution of these issues.

In a test set, agreement was fostered by this approach.[60] The second feature of Page's scheme is to separate some special types of DCIS because they present patterns not readily allowing grading. In the special case of pure (not intermixed with solid or cribriform) micropapillary DCIS, Page believes that the usual extensiveness of disease is independent of the nuclear grade. It should be noted that separating special types from the majority of cases is precisely what we do with invasive disease.

Extent of Disease

Clinical concern with the evaluation of size or extent of the area of the breast occupied by DCIS was an early focus during the development of BCT for this disease entity. By using a serial subgross sectioning technique correlated with specimen radiography, developed by Egan and associates,[68,69] a clear association was shown between the likelihood of invasive growth and the extent of disease.[35] Egan's technique permitted correlative studies of radiographic images and pathologic mapping of areas of involvement by DCIS in mastectomy specimens. The initial concern was whether occult invasion might exist in the breast separate from an adequately excised focus of DCIS. This has not generally been shown to be the case. DCIS cases measuring 25 mm or less, completely excised, were not associated with demonstrable occult areas of invasion in those cases that subsequently went to mastectomy and standard pathologic assessment. Silverstein[70] demonstrated a similar correlation between the extent of disease and the likelihood of invasion, as did Patchefsky and coworkers.[36] What was not clearly described at the time was that the invasive focus always occurred within the area occupied by DCIS and that the area occupied by DCIS had a segmental distribution, as clearly noted subsequently.[71,72] Using the same serial subgross technique but applying it to radial segments of the breast, which more closely approximate the true anatomy of the ductal system, Holland and colleagues[72] were able to define more clearly the relationships of DCIS to mammographic microcalcification and to the remaining breast. They identified different distribution patterns among DCIS of different subtypes. High-grade DCIS (poorly differentiated) was more closely defined by the extent of mammographic microcalcifications. Therefore, its extent could be estimated with more certainty preoperatively. It was also associated with fewer discontinuities or "skip areas" in its distribution. In contrast, DCIS of lower grades (intermediate and well differentiated) were poorly associated with microcalcification and often exhibited a discontinuous distribution. However, Faverly and associates[71] note that 85% of low-grade (well-differentiated) DCIS would be excised with a 10-mm margin. Despite the greater likelihood of residual disease, lower grades of DCIS have a much lower frequency of local recurrence after attempts at BCT, at least in the first 10 years of follow-up.[44,54]

Extensiveness, Multicentricity, and Multifocality

The literature on the multicentricity and multifocality of DCIS remains confusing because of the different definitions, methods of tissue processing, and sampling techniques used, as well as differences in the perspective of the investigators. Two groups of investigators, both of which used Egan's serial subgross technique of examination,[68,69] exemplify useful approaches to resolving this problem. The focus of Lagios and coworkers was on the question of residual disease after segmental mastectomy (or lumpectomy), a new and radical direction for American surgeons at the time.[35] They defined as multicentric any focus lying beyond 5 cm of the border of the resection. In most cases, this feature defined involvement in another quadrant. Holland and colleagues[72] and Faverly and associates[71] (although clearly concerned about the success of a surgical resection) were focused more on the distribution of the disease. Multicentric DCIS, by very definition, required a 4-cm zone of uninvolved breast tissue between the primary and any potential multicentric site. Discontinuous foci of DCIS within 4 cm were defined as multifocal. Holland and colleagues noted that only 5% of cases of DCIS were multicentric using this definition.[72] To what extent these data reflect the large size of DCIS in their patient population remains unknown. However, Faverly and associates[71] reported that 63% of the cases of DCIS studied at mastectomy had an extent greater than 5 cm (50 mm), whereas Lagios and coworkers,[35] in a similar mastectomy series, noted that 52% were 25 mm or less and 25% were 50 mm or more. Irrespectively, it is most prudent to clearly describe the extent and distribution of disease within the breast in unequivocal terms that cannot be misinterpreted.

Distribution

The considerations of the extent of DCIS are discussed primarily in Chapter 37. It is generally accepted that there is a somewhat segmental anatomy of the breast. Although these segmental lobes are not precisely placed or sized, they are generally viewed as subtending regions drained by major ducts and are somewhat overlapping in distribution (see Chapter 37). The hallmark of DCIS is its somewhat orderly spread through the large duct system. The segmental lobes are not precisely demarcated anatomically, but rather, the major spread in any given case of DCIS appears to be within the same segmental lobe toward and away from the nipple and in adjacent segmental lobes as well. This clinical situation may be varied in that a major lesion deep within the breast may involve many lobular units, and then a single duct may seem to ascend toward the nipple with few other lobular elements involved. This is demonstrated by Ohtake and colleagues[73] and also illustrated by the three-dimensional reconstruction studies of Moffat and Going.[74]

Mammographic Correlation

The distribution of DCIS within the breast, its association with microcalcification, the types of microcalcification, and the likelihood that DCIS may exhibit an extensive growth pattern with a substantial risk of residual disease after attempts at excision are also correlated with grade and subtype. High-grade DCIS with comedo necrosis exhibits a greater extent, is often segmental[72,74,75] (see Chapter 37) and contiguous in distribution, is more closely associated with microcalcifications, and is less likely to show an intermittent or discontinuous distribution in the breast.[71,76] In contrast, DCIS of intermediate and low grades is less likely to exhibit a contiguous growth pattern, especially on mammography, even if its distribution can be understood to lie within a segmental duct system. DCIS of these lower grades is more likely to exhibit discontinuous but regional growth and to show less association with microcalcification, although many cases are continuous on three-dimensional reconstruction studies. From a clinical and mammographic point of view, high-grade comedo-type DCIS is more likely to be adequately excised, given its association with

microcalcification and contiguous growth pattern. Nonetheless, it is associated with the greatest risk of local recurrence and invasive transformation. An important study of the growth pattern of DCIS in time has come from the group in Nottingham.[77] Rates and direction of change in mammographic calcifications were correlated with DCIS histology. Growth rates increased with increasing nuclear grade of DCIS, and the DCIS growth rate was greatest along an axis toward and away from the nipple. The latter finding demonstrated preferential growth of DCIS along the radiating anatomy of the ducts from the nipple to the end of the breast disk. There may be a special form of DCIS that demonstrates discontinuous spread histologically within ducts[78] and that is associated with recurrence despite performance of an extensive quadrantectomy. Low-grade DCIS is more likely to be inadequately excised unless surgical resection margins are carefully assessed with means other than mammography for residual disease in the same quadrant. Nonetheless, it is associated with a lower risk of subsequent recurrence and invasive transformation.

Margin Status

Assessment of the adequacy of surgical resection margins during BCT for DCIS has been a major focus of attention since the inception of BCT in the mid-1970s. The most common method of margin assessment is based on the use of India ink or some other permanent dye or pigment and selective sampling. This method works well for invasive carcinomas in which a likely area of involved margins can be estimated with palpation in most cases and confirmed with a few appropriate sections. This method, although still applicable, is more problematic for DCIS, in which the lesion is generally not palpable, is not grossly visible, may not be uniformly associated with microcalcification, and may have a discontinuous distribution. In these circumstances, margins must be examined more comprehensively. This often substantially increases the number of tissue samples or cassettes (blocks) prepared. However, neither margin involvement nor occult microinvasion can be entirely excluded without more complete tissue processing. Differences in the kind of tissue processing used can contribute significantly to outcome results in BCT for DCIS.[11,79] This is a major limitation of large multicenter clinical trials in which the patients may be randomized but the pathologists and their technique for specimen processing are not.

Considering that careful and precise assessment of surgical resection margin status is likely the most critical variable in determining the recurrence rate for DCIS (e.g., theoretically if the lesion has been completely removed, then further therapy should not make a difference), it is little wonder that carefully designed single-institution studies with consistent and rigorous pathologic assessment of the specimens have proved so useful. Ideally, breast specimens should be oriented by the surgeon in reference to the nipple and axilla and processed such that the extent of the lesion and its proximity to margins in all three dimensions can be determined. Multicolor inking protocols considerably facilitate analysis, along with uniform sectioning of the specimen at 2- to 3-mm intervals. In addition, specimen radiography to aid in lesion identification and in the focused submission of blocks on larger specimens is advocated. However, the histologic appearance of the lesion should never be compromised by compression of the submitted specimen during specimen radiography.

The adequacy of surgical resection margins for DCIS has long been and continues to be an area of ongoing debate. This debate has been fueled by the propensity of DCIS to exhibit a discontinuous distribution within the breast tissue. Early on, the NSABP defined "margins as free when the tumor is not transected."[61,80] As a result, an arbitrary assignment of 1 mm or greater has been considered by many as an acceptable standard.[81] However, many have challenged this minimalistic view to the adequacy of surgical resection margins. Previous work by Holland and colleagues[72,82] and Silverstein and associates[43,83] has suggested that a 1-mm margin may not be adequate for DCIS. In analyzing the results of initial attempts at excision biopsy, Silverstein and associates noted that 45% of cases of DCIS that were thought to be adequately excised had residual disease, either at reexcision or on mastectomy, and that, all other factors being equal, the distance of the free margin was directly related to the probability of local recurrence.[43] However, even using a definition of 1 mm as an adequate margin achieves a better local recurrence-free survival than did the NSABP B-17 criterion of nontranssection of DCIS (e.g., 16% of local recurrence at 124 months' mean follow-up[40] vs. 22% local recurrence rate at 43 months' mean follow-up[80]). There are those that strongly advocate extremely wide margins (≥10 mm) based on the classical findings of Silverstein and associates[43] in which they demonstrated that DCIS patients with margins greater than 10 mm had the lowest local recurrence rate. Conversely, those same particular patients did not receive added benefit from whole-breast radiation therapy compared with those DCIS patients with closer margins who did benefit from whole breast radiation therapy.[43] Most recently, a more moderate viewpoint has been portrayed in the literature with recommendations of margins in the range of greater than 2 mm to up to 5 mm.[84,85] Despite all these differing opinions, there has yet to be a consensus reached or any consensus statements published on setting finite criteria for defining the adequacy of surgical resection margins during BCT for DCIS. Lastly, the contribution of specimen handling (e.g., compressive vs. noncompressive specimen mammogram) as well as specimen and tissue pathology processing to creating artifactually close or positive margins has been long suggested[39] but has never been systematically evaluated. Although such handling and processing variables likely have a significant impact on cases of invasive carcinomas because of the obvious contrast in tissue quality between the invasive cancer "mass" and surrounding fibrofatty tissue within the excised breast tissue, their contribution on cases of DCIS is less likely as a result of the general lack of a masslike quality of DCIS within the excised breast tissue.

Risks of Evolution and Recurrence From Ductal Carcinoma in Situ

It is evident that high-grade, comedo/high-grade DCIS lesions are not easily cured, that recurrences are common even after radiation therapy, and that such lesions have a high risk of evolution to invasive carcinoma.[43,83] In contrast, small, noncomedo DCIS are nonobligate precursor lesions, and it is estimated that only 25% to 50% of such lesions will eventually evolve into invasive carcinomas if left untreated for several decades.[5,7,55] They may be regarded as lesions of increased risk because their relative risk of later invasive cancer development is about 10 times that of the general population. There is strong evidence that DCIS of small size and low histologic grade is easily cured with local excision without radiation therapy.[43,83] This is certainly true of lesions that are smaller than 1 cm in largest dimension. Thus, the best estimate of the size of a DCIS lesion should be stated even for core

biopsy specimens to help facilitate clinical management. The greatest extent of a lesion is assessed most easily with careful pathologic-mammographic correlation, which is essential in such instances. Precisely which concurrence of histologic grade, size, and margin clearance is to be the determinant of therapeutic decision making is an area under ongoing investigation. However, it should be understood that local recurrence in the setting of a low-grade lesion is unlikely to be a life-threatening event and that a woman's desire for breast conservation with a willingness to accept the possibility of local recurrence may be as important with regard to therapeutic decision-making as any other consideration. In contrast, local recurrence in the setting of a high-grade DCIS lesion is much more likely to be associated with invasion, high-grade histology, and development of metastases.[6,51] Thus careful pathologic assessment of DCIS lesions that includes histologic pattern, grade, size, and margin status is essential for optimal clinical management and should be considered an essential part of any breast biopsy report for DCIS.[84–86]

Recently a consensus guideline on margins for DCIS was published by a collaboration of the Society of Surgical Oncology, the American Society for Radiation Oncology, and the American Society of Clinical Oncology.[87] All specialties were represented, including pathologists. The guidelines were based on a meta-analysis by Marinovich and colleagues in patients with DCIS, lumpectomy, and whole breast irradiation.[88] On the basis of 20 studies with 7883 patients and 865 local recurrences, the odds ratio of local recurrence was 0.51 compared with >0 or 1 mm and was not improved significantly with greater margins. Therefore the consensus panel recommended the use of a 2-mm margin as the standard and sufficient margin for DCIS that was not based on the biology of the tumor. The use of such a standard has the potential to decrease reexcision rates, improve cosmetic outcomes, and decrease health care costs.

Receptor Proteins, Oncogenes, Tumor Suppressor Genes, and Ploidy

A wealth of information in the literature describes the presence and distribution of specific oncogenes, receptor proteins, and measures of ploidy and proliferative activity in DCIS. Initially there was an expectation that such investigations would be able to identify DCIS subgroups that are at increased risk for invasive transformation or local recurrence after BCT, particularly among patients at highest risk. In part, these expectations were met but largely by demonstrating a correlation between specific oncogenes or gene products and DCIS subtypes recognized with conventional morphologic analysis as being a high risk for recurrence (e.g., high-grade [poorly differentiated], comedo-type DCIS, or both).

The clearest association between an oncogene and a DCIS subtype is seen with *HER2/neu* oncogene and its *erbB2* product, which is largely restricted to DCIS subtypes characterized by large cell type and higher nuclear grade.[89–94] Bartkova and colleagues[95] have shown that among those cases of DCIS that are of mixed subtypes, *HER2/neu* expression is seen only in the large cell component, and this factor is dramatically evident in cases in which the mixed cell population occurs within single ductules (Fig. 9.28).

DePotter and associates[90] demonstrated a significant association between *HER2/neu*-positive large cell–type DCIS and the extent of disease in the breast, which was independent of mitotic

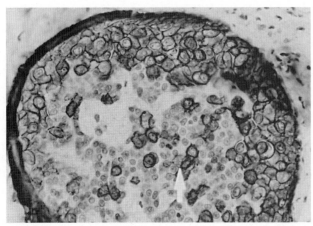

• **Fig. 9.28** Immunocytochemical stain for *erbB2* with strong membrane staining of large cells in a higher grade ductal carcinoma in situ. Note the presence of a negative, small-cell population. Magnification: ×200.

index, and hypothesized that *HER2/neu/erbB2* has a role in motility of in situ carcinomas within the ductal epithelium. Gupta and coworkers[96] have shown that E-cadherin expression is associated with the apparent degree of differentiation or orderliness. The cadherins are related to lateral complex integrity, polarity, and probably cell-to-cell communication.

p53, largely studied with immunoperoxidase techniques in noninvasive lesions, is also correlated with high nuclear grade subtypes.[6,89,94,97] O'Malley and colleagues,[64] among others, have noted that p53 protein overexpression is largely limited to high-grade, comedo-type DCIS. Immunohistochemical studies have shown overexpression in some cases in which p53 mutations were not detected by sequencing in the most highly conserved portion of the gene. Poller and coworkers[97] concluded that there was no relationship between *p53* and *HER2/neu* status; they nonetheless noted that almost all cases of *p53*-positive DCIS were large cell, with 35.8% of large cell DCIS being *p53* positive and only 4.1% of small cell DCIS being *p53* positive.[64] Others have documented similar relationships between high-grade DCIS, *HER2/neu*, and *p53*.[47,89,93,98]

Estrogen receptor and progesterone receptor protein expression, as demonstrated with immunohistochemistry, shows consistent, but not absolute, correlation with DCIS subtypes.[99] Bobrow and coworkers[89] noted an association between cytonuclear differentiation and progesterone status. DCIS with "poor" cytonuclear differentiation, as opposed to "good" differentiation, tended to lack demonstrable progesterone receptors. Similarly, Poller and associates[100] noted that estrogen receptor expression is related to noncomedo architecture, negative *HER2/neu* status, small cell size, and surprisingly higher S-phase fraction on flow cytometry. Wilbur and Barrows[99] noted a similar trend between grade (i.e., cytonuclear differentiation) and receptor status. They noted that 75% of estrogen receptor–negative DCIS exhibited nuclear grade III morphology (high grade), whereas only 14% of estrogen receptor–positive DCIS were nuclear grade III. Leal and colleagues[91] and Zafrani and coworkers[94] noted no relationship between DCIS subtype and receptor status. These studies suggest that there is a weak association between high nuclear grade and negative receptor status similar to that noted in many high-grade invasive carcinomas.

Despite the fact that some investigators used two-tiered classification and others used three-tiered classifications, agreement

between the studies has been substantial. DCIS subtypes characterized by large cell type and high nuclear grade tend to be *HER2/neu* positive, are more likely *p53* positive[97,98] and estrogen receptor negative,[99] are aneuploid, and are more likely to exhibit a higher S-phase fraction or other measurement of proliferation. They are also more likely to exhibit significant comedo-type necrosis, periductal stromal desmoplasia, and a diffuse increase in microvessel density.[49,101,102] In contrast, DCIS of small cell size, and of intermediate or low nuclear grade, or of noncomedo-type architecture tend to be *erbB2* and *p53* negative and diploid and, in most studies, exhibit a lower S-phase fraction and a tendency toward positive receptor status.[103] They also tend to lack significant necrosis and stromal reaction.

Despite concerted efforts using immunohistochemical demonstration of oncogenes and determination of ploidy and S-phase fraction with flow and image cytometry, identification of a subset of morphologically defined high-grade DCIS at even greater risk of invasive transformation remains elusive. Somewhat surprisingly, cyclin D expression was found to be similar and high in all grades of DCIS, with low levels in most ADH lesions.[104] In contrast, most genetic and molecular analyses have shown that the low-grade DCIS lesions are more similar to ADH than they are to high-grade DCIS lesions. The cyclins D, especially cyclin D1, control important transitional events in the cell cycle, especially entrance into DNA synthesis. Morphologic grading achieves as much separation as do numerous ancillary tests. Susnik and associates,[105] using a classification based on nuclear texture features quantified with high-resolution image cytometry, were able to identify 100% of high-grade comedo-type DCIS concurrently associated with invasion and 80% of noncomedo-type lesions associated with invasion. The study design was necessarily retrospective, but the results are suggestive. If further validated, automated quantitative analysis of nuclear texture features in DCIS may be able to identify patients at different levels of risk. However, prospective studies are needed to certify the prospective utility of these approaches.

Simpson and associates[106] compared NM23 expression in situ carcinoma associated with an invasive component with those not associated concurrently with an invasive component and found there was a higher expression of NM23 in comedo-type DCIS unassociated with an invasive component, suggesting that NM23 expression within comedo-type lesions might identify lesions with a lesser risk of evolution to invasion and metastatic capacity. Goldstein and Murphy[107] evaluated nuclear grade in a three-scale system and found grades of invasive and in situ components to agree most of the time.

Similar to the 21-gene recurrence score for invasive cancer, there is a new 12-gene recurrence score (RS) for DCIS (Onco*type* DX Breast DCIS Score (DCIS Score). It is a multigene expression assay that generates individualized 10-year risk estimates of the treatment of DCIS without radiation. It is based on 12 of the 21 genes in the invasive Onco*type* test including *Ki-67*, *STK15*, *Survivin*, *Cyclin B1*, and *MYBL2*, progesterone receptor, the *GSTM1* gene, and 5 reference genes.[108–110] Potential use of this RS could include not only to predict who is more likely to recur but to determine whether there are patients who are unlikely to benefit from radiation therapy.[111] At present, it is estimated that 30% of patients with DCIS are treated with breast conservation alone.[112,113] In a recent study comparing the Van Nuys Prognostic Index,[114] the Memorial Sloan Kettering Cancer Center nomogram,[115] physician estimates showed no strong correlation with the DCIS RS.[111] Use of this RS across 10 centers demonstrated that treatment recommendations changed more than 30% of the time.[116]

Special Types of Ductal Carcinoma in Situ With Special Implications

Hypersecretory Ductal Carcinoma in Situ

Hypersecretory changes in the breast represent a type of cellular presentation and cytoplasmic differentiation. Although they are poorly understood at present, these histologic elements coexisting with atypia appear to be associated with special features in the distribution and perhaps evolution of in situ disease toward malignancy. These lesions tend not to produce a lump within the breast and often have benign-appearing, lobular-type calcifications because it is the central secretion that calcifies. Often the mammogram produces patterns that outline the lobules in an area of the breast. The presentation of the disease is commonly regional but does not have the uniformity of continuity seen in most forms of DCIS.

This entity was first described by Rosen and Scott in 1984.[117] The original paper and the follow-up presentation by the same group in 1988[118] emphasized the cystic dilation of the spaces involved and allowed for a category of atypia without the designation of DCIS. The association with the development of clinically evident malignancy in most of these cases was inapparent or unproved.[119] Often these cases present striking patterns of hugely enlarged nuclei abutting into the lumen, as seen in hypersecretory changes in the endometrium.[120,121]

The approach to these extremely difficult cases is generally to recognize atypicality in a biopsy and recommend careful continued mammographic surveillance. Unfortunately, calcifications may be present in clearly benign secretory alterations in the same region, representing a challenge for mammographic follow-up.[76]

However, there are a certain number of cases in which the diagnosis of DCIS is mandatory, and this diagnostic plateau is reached definitively when true ducts are involved. The recognition of DCIS status is particularly evident when patterns of micropapillary DCIS are reached.[122] It is indeed this favorite association with micropapillary DCIS that may be one of the more interesting elements in this complex of newly recognized diseases.[123] Because of the regional presentation of this disease, it has occasionally been suggested segmentectomy or quadrantectomy, although again the regionality of this disease appears to be not as precise as that seen in more typical cases of DCIS. It is clearly different from ALH and does not often coexist with ALH.

Paget Disease of the Nipple

Paget disease of the breast has been recognized as a specific clinical entity for more than 100 years, but it does not inherently imply any extension of the disease process beyond the nipple.[124] Thus the diversity of disease from within the breast after presentation of Paget disease of the nipple is what needs to be emphasized, and Paget disease of the breast should no longer be viewed as a type of breast cancer. Rather, Paget disease of the nipple should be viewed as a type of initial presentation of a breast cancer. After complete evaluation of the presentation, the overall disease process may be local or extensive within the breast.[125–128]

The classical and still relevant presentation is with an eczematous area of the nipple. This feature may be subtle or evolve to an obviously eroded, weeping lesion. The underlying process is population of the epidermis of the nipple surface with a scattering of neoplastic breast epithelial cells. Often, but not uniformly, these cells are identical with a DCIS lesion in the underlying ducts.[118,119] In advanced cases, the process may extend from the nipple to the pigmented skin of the areolar region and even to the adjacent surrounding, nonpigmented skin of the breast. The terms *pagetoid change* and *pagetoid features* are used for the interspersion of one cell type within another anywhere within the ducts and lobules of the breast. Immunohistochemical stains for *erbB2* (see Fig. 9.28) are useful in demonstrating these cells and are often helpful in the differential diagnosis, because *erbB2* expression is common to virtually all examples of Paget disease of the nipple.[90,129]

Paget disease is usually associated with extensive DCIS within the breast.[130] In the early mammographic era, Paget disease of the nipple was associated with invasive carcinoma and DCIS in 50% of cases. The practical importance with regard to accepting conservation, when possible, is that at present about only 10% of cases are associated with disease confined to the immediate area of the nipple and are amenable to excision of the nipple-areola complex for cure.[131,132] Because of the importance of Paget disease and recently emerging information concerning this disease, there is a separate chapter (see Chapter 12) exclusively devoted to Paget disease of the breast.

Encysted, Noninvasive Papillary Carcinoma

Encysted, noninvasive papillary carcinoma is an entity with features that are otherwise diagnostic for DCIS. These lesions are essentially anatomically confined and probably represent DCIS arising in and overtaking the residual aspects of an intraductal papilloma. The DCIS component usually is low grade, but it can be intermediate. The clinical importance of these lesions was originally clarified by Carter, Orr, and Merino,[133] who introduced the concept of an encysted lesion and reached a conclusion that in the absence of adjacent DCIS in neighboring ducts, local excision of these lesions is curative.[134,135] This valuable study has not been improved on. It is consistent with all the information we have at present about the importance of the extensiveness of regional DCIS with regard to the likelihood of local recurrence. It is widely recognized that a pattern of these lesions has very tall cells similar to those seen in villous adenoma of the colon with enlarged hyperchromatic nuclei. These nuclei are present without an increased cell number above fibrovascular stalks. Such an entity is considered as an encysted, noninvasive lesion within this category (Fig. 9.29).

It should be noted that the cutoff point between papillomas with atypia (analogous to ADH), encysted or otherwise, from the nonencysted and encysted papillary carcinoma lesions is unclear. Reports by Raju and Vertes[136] and Page and coworkers[137] have stated that some degree of atypia similar to that of ADH present within papillomas may increase the likelihood of later cancer occurrence, but the two studies are in disagreement. There is an indication from the study by Page and coworkers[137] that well-developed atypical hyperplasia within papillomas of any size indicates increased likelihood of local occurrence of carcinoma, or at least regional occurrence of carcinoma after local excision for biopsy alone. There is no certainty at this time that wider excision after such a finding is necessary. However, it is recommended that careful mammographic surveillance of the area continue until this situation is better determined.

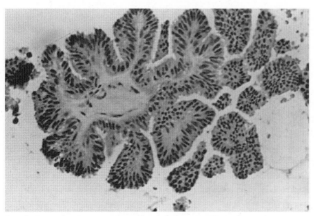

• **Fig. 9.29** The presence of tall and hyperchromatic cells surmounting these papillary fronds supports the possibility of a diagnosis of encysted papillary carcinoma. Usually the epithelium is much more atypical and closely mimics that found in other ductal carcinoma in situ patterns. Magnification: ×125.

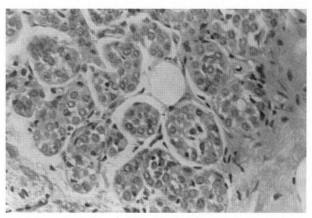

• **Fig. 9.31** Portion of a lobular unit demonstrating some distention and little filling of the involved acini. This is atypical lobular hyperplasia. Magnification: ×300.

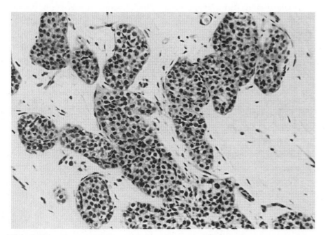

• **Fig. 9.30** An example of lobular carcinoma in situ showing complete distention and filling of the majority of spaces in this area by characteristic population of cells. Magnification: ×200.

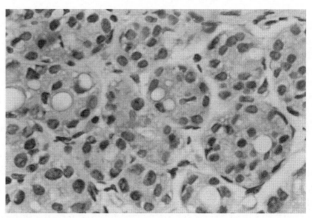

• **Fig. 9.32** The vacuoles or globules in the cytoplasm are characteristic of lobular neoplasia. Note that some of the cells have the appearance of signet ring cells. Magnification: ×400.

Pathology of Lobular Carcinoma in Situ

Epithelial proliferative lesions (noninvasive or in situ) of the human breast termed lobular were inaugurated by the introduction of the term LCIS in 1941 by Foote and Stewart.[138] Critical to the definition and concept was the distinctive caricature of lobular units produced by the diagnostic clustering of three major criteria: distention, distortion, and filling by a population of characteristic cells (Figs. 9.30 to 9.32). Also important to the definition, in all probability, was that more than 60% of invasive cancers presenting with single filing of cancer cells with similar cytology have such in situ lesions present in the same breast. Through the 1970s and 1980s, an important general acceptance of LCIS as an elevated cancer risk marker was established.[34,139] The two important papers of 1978 by Haagensen and colleagues[140] and Rosen and associates[141] concluded that there was generally no difference in risk between more well-developed and less well-developed histologic examples, and the reports included minor histologic examples with little distortion of lobular units in their overall analysis. The Haagensen paper introduced the term *lobular neoplasia* (LN).[140] Page and coworkers in a large Nashville cohort of benign breast biopsies separated lesser lesions, reported lesser risk for such lesser lesions, and continued to vehemently stress the distinguishing features between ALH and LCIS (considering both these two entities to represent stages of LN).[58,142] These distinctions were later further discussed in the work of both Bodian, Perzin, and Lattes[143] and Fisher and associates.[144]

Bodian and colleagues continued to use the term LN to describe the full range of changes from ALH to LCIS.[143] Page and coworkers continued to use separate and different terminology, describing histologically less well-developed examples as ALH because they demonstrated that such lesser entities were associated with a lower risk of cancer.[57,58] Of importance, Bodian and coworkers[143] and the work of the NSABP[144] have divided the LN spectrum into well-developed and less well-developed examples on a numeric basis. It has been suggested by Page and coworkers[142] that the NSABP series by Fisher and associates[144] is a biased series because the cases were originally diagnosed by study pathologists as DCIS. Both of these recent studies[143,144] found a lower risk for less well-developed examples, whether it is called ALH or LN numbers 1 and 2, as opposed to LN 3. In the report by Bodian and coworkers,[143] the incidence of LN in a group of 2134 biopsies was more than 10%. Page and coworkers[142] have suggested that this is a highly selected series and that what the researchers classified as ALH included most of the cases within the broad range of cases in LN. Contrary, using their own restricted criteria for LCIS, Page and coworkers found an incidence of only 0.5% of LCIS in an unselected series of slightly more than 10,000 biopsies.[58,142] In this regard, Page and coworkers continue to stress the point that the term LN should apply to a very wide range of changes from maximal to minimal, with LCIS referring to maximal changes, and that ALH refers to the rest of such lesions.[142] Furthermore, in addition to the fact that the work of both Bodian and colleagues[143] and Page and associates[58,142] supported the belief that less extensive histologic disease has less cancer risk, both series also have recognized that LN identified in patients older than 55 years was of less clinical significance. Lastly, although the work of Bodian and colleagues[143] did not indicate that ductal involvement by LN incurs a greater risk, Page and colleagues (using their own criteria[58]) found that ductal involvement conferred a somewhat increased risk when present in cases of ALH within the lobular units.[145]

Thus the terminology used for ALH, LCIS, and LN continues to signify an increased risk of later cancer development in either breast, and other useful interactive associations remain to be further evaluated. Although the usual and common examples of LN are clearly multifocal with sparing of scattered lobular units, there is a suggestion by Page and associates that the risk of later breast cancer favors the breast that had ALH on biopsy,[146,147] with about 65% of later cancer occurring in the ipsilateral breast. Whatever the terminology, it is clear that lesser examples of histologic involvement (e.g., ALH) are associated with lower risk than more classic and more extensive examples recognized as fully developed LCIS, and most findings are best regarded as ALH.[146–148] The LN spectrum, with LCIS representing the fully developed example, is clearly very different from that of DCIS, although rare examples of local proliferation share features of each category and may be best regarded as exemplifying each lesion for patient care purposes.

With the more recent advent of minimally invasive breast biopsy technology, a developing theme within the literature has been seen with regard to the importance of finding LN (e.g., either ALH and/or LCIS) in such core breast biopsy specimens. There is certainly a wide range of opinions that have been given with regard to the necessity of subsequent formal surgical excision.[149–160] Nevertheless, it is apparent that there is little agreement; no obvious consensus has yet been reached. It is likely that the extent of LN found within the submitted core breast biopsy specimen, as well as the type of minimally invasive breast biopsy device used (e.g., smaller 14-gauge to 18-gauge automated spring-loaded core biopsy devices vs. larger 8-gauge to 11-gauge vacuum-assisted core biopsy devices) and the volume of the sampled tissue that is extracted with such devices, may become important variables in the decision-making process concerning whether a formal surgical excision is warranted.

Acknowledgment

The authors gratefully acknowledge Stephen P. Povoski and Sanford H. Barsky for their contribution of this chapter in the previous edition.

Selected References

87. Morrow M, Van Zee KJ, Solin LJ, et al. Society of Surgical Oncology-American Society for Radiation Oncology-American Society of Clinical Oncology Consensus Guideline on Margins for Breast-Conserving Surgery with Whole-Breast Irradiation in Ductal Carcinoma In Situ. *Ann Surg Oncol.* 2016;23:3801-3810.

88. Marinovich ML, Azizi L, Macaskill P, et al. The association of surgical margins and local recurrence in women with ductal carcinoma in situ treated with breast-conserving therapy: a meta-analysis. *Ann Surg Oncol.* 2016;23:3811-3821.

108. Solin LJ, Gray R, Baehner FL, et al. A multigene expression assay to predict local recurrence risk for ductal carcinoma in situ of the breast. *J Natl Cancer Inst.* 2013;105:701-710.

110. Rakovitch E, Nofech-Mozes S, Hanna W, et al. A population-based validation study of the DCIS Score predicting recurrence risk in individuals treated by breast-conserving surgery alone. *Breast Cancer Res Treat.* 2015;152:389-398.

113. Solin LJ, Gray R, Hughes LL, et al. Surgical excision without radiation for ductal carcinoma in situ of the breast: 12-year results from the ECOG-ACRIN E5194 Study. *J Clin Oncol.* 2015;33:3938-3944.

116. Alvarado M, Carter DL, Guenther JM, et al. The impact of genomic testing on the recommendation for radiation therapy in patients with ductal carcinoma in situ: a prospective clinical utility assessment of the 12-gene DCIS score result. *J Surg Oncol.* 2015;111:935-940.

A full reference list is available online at ExpertConsult.com.

10

Infiltrating Carcinomas of the Breast: Not One Disease

SOHEILA KOROURIAN

Molecular classifications, the availability of targeted therapies, and the emerging observations provided by pharmacogenomics and molecular studies underscore that breast cancer could not, and should not, be treated as one disease.

Since the 1990s, tremendous advances in cancer treatment have been achieved. To achieve a higher cure rate, a comprehensive database on all breast cancers is required. Once all data are integrated into a final report, the results can be more easily retrieved by local and national tumor registries. Currently the national registry for Surveillance, Epidemiology, and End Results (SEER) gathers its information from local tumor registries. Because the original data are incomplete, available data through the SEER registry do not provide a complete summary regarding the outcome of many cancers. Personalized medicine cannot be achieved without a thorough understanding and careful follow-up of a large number of histologically and biochemically well-defined and similar breast cancer subsets. The purpose of this chapter is to highlight the histologic subtype and link morphologic findings to those of biochemical results and potentially to the molecular subtypes of breast cancer.

Traditionally breast cancer has been classified according to the morphologic features. Despite the emerging era of personalized medicine and the availability of molecular testing, the traditional pathologic classification of infiltrating breast carcinoma remains valuable. Pathologists were one of the first groups to recognize that breast cancer was a morphologically heterogeneous group of diseases. Different patterns of breast cancer were noted to have different clinical presentations, and some of the patterns were associated with specific prognoses. In addition, pathologists were able to describe a grading system that seemed to be an independent prognostic indicator. Once tumors were routinely analyzed for the presence of estrogen and progesterone receptors (ER/PR), others in the scientific community realized that breast cancers are quite heterogeneous. During the late 1980s and early 1990s, it was recognized that some breast cancers show HER2/neu protein overexpression or *ERBB2* gene amplification. This group represented a subset of cancers that had a worse prognosis, independent of their clinical or pathologic stage. After all tumors were routinely examined for ER/PR and HER2/neu amplification, another group of cancers emerged. This group of breast cancers did not express hormonal receptors and showed no evidence of HER2 amplification. These tumors were classified as "triple-negative" carcinomas (TNBCs). Recent studies have shown that even TNBCs represent a heterogeneous group of cancers.[1,2]

Molecular classifications, the availability of targeted therapies, and the emerging observations provided by pharmacogenomics and molecular studies underscore that breast cancer could not, and should not, be treated as one disease.

Traditional histopathological classification of breast cancer, including the World Health Organization (WHO) classification remains important; however, other information must be considered before any treatment decision. In this chapter, an attempt is made to delineate how all available information including traditional histopathological classification, the commonly used grading system, and the result of ancillary tests can be incorporated. This approach allows us to better understand the biology of cancer and might allow us to link traditional information to molecular subtyping.

Tremendous advances in cancer treatment have been achieved during the past two decades. To achieve a higher cure rate, more comprehensive data on all breast cancers is required. Once all data are integrated into a final report, the results can be easier to retrieve by the local and national tumor registries. Currently the national registry for Surveillance, Epidemiology, and End Results (SEER) gathers its information from local tumor registries. Because the original data are not complete, available data through the SEER registry do not provide a complete summary regarding the outcome of many cancers. Personalized medicine cannot be achieved without a thorough understanding and careful follow-up of a large number of histologically and biochemically well-defined and similar breast cancer subsets.

Molecular Classification

Molecular classifications have contributed to the paradigm shift that human breast cancer is not one disease. Breast cancer is considered to show at least five major molecular subtypes, each characterized by distinct gene expression profiles.[3-6] This is of paramount importance because the patients with varying subtypes have different clinical outcomes, and each responds differently to treatment (Fig. 10.1).

By definition, luminal type cancers express hormonal receptors (ER/PR). According to this classification, luminal A cancers express both the ER and PR, but HER2 amplification is absent. They are also marked by low levels of proliferation markers.[7,8] The

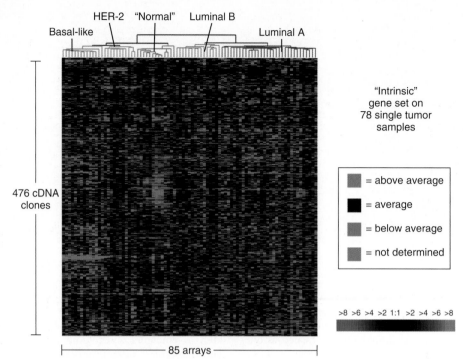

• **Fig. 10.1** The major molecular subclassification for breast cancer based on gene expression profiling. (From Sorlie T, Perou CM, Tibshirani R, et al. Gene expression patterns of breast carcinomas distinguish tumor subclasses with clinical implications. *Proc Natl Acad Sci U S A*. 2001;98:10869–10874. Copyright 2001 National Academy of Sciences, USA.)

TABLE 10.1 Major Subtypes of Breast Cancer Defined by Gene Profiles

Subtype	Percent[145,146]	DDS	Outcome[137,a] OS	Standard IHC[144,145]
Luminal A	51–61	75	90	ER+, PRþ, HER2-
Luminal B	14–16	47	40	ER+ and/or PR+, HER2+
HER2	7–9	34	31	ER and PR-, HER2+
Basal	11–20	18	0	ER, PR, and HER2–, Cytokeratin 5/6 and EGFR+
Unclassified	2–6	NA	NA	Negative for all markers

aPercent of patients without distant metastases or alive with systemic therapy at 5 years.

DDS, Distant-disease free survival; *EGFR*, epidermal growth factor receptor; *ER*, estrogen receptor; *IHC*, immunohistochemistry; *OS*, overall survival; *PR*, progesterone receptor.

From Perou CM, Sorlie T, Eisen MB, et al. Molecular portraits of human breast tumours. *Nature*. 2000;406:747-752; and Sorlie T, Perou CM, Tibshirani R, et al. Gene expression patterns of breast carcinomas distinguish tumour subclasses with clinical implications. *Proc Natl Acad Sci U S A*. 2001;98:10869-10874.

second group is luminal B which also express ER and PR and may, or may not, be HER2. Luminal B tumors have a higher level of expression of proliferation markers compared with luminal A. The great majority of invasive breast cancers belong to one of these two groups. As it has been known for many decades that ER status is a predictive biomarker in the treatment of breast cancer. Luminal A and B subtypes are phenotypically characterized by the expression of ER; the overall survival of patients with luminal A cancers is significantly greater than patients with luminal B cancers.[9,10] The level of ki67, a proliferation marker, plays an important role in luminal B cancers. High levels of proliferation have been shown to be an independent prognostic indicator in lymph node–negative cancers.[11] The HER2 overexpressing subtype occurs in approximately 10% to 20% of breast cancers. These patients respond to HER2-directed therapy such as trastuzumab, a humanized monoclonal antibody directed to the external domain of HER2 (or *ERBB2*) transmembrane tyrosine kinase, and lapatinib, a small molecule inhibitor of HER1 (epidermal growth factor receptor) and HER2.[12,13] HER2 overexpressing cancers and basal-like subtypes have higher initial responses to anthracycline-based chemotherapy than the luminal subtypes and have worse prognosis and shorter disease-free survival.[14–18] As evident from the Table 10.1 TNBC represent 20% to 25% of all invasive cancers. This group does not represent a biologically uniform cancer; in fact it is very heterogeneous.[19] Table 10.1 suggests that a great majority of basal-like tumors express markers such as CK5/6 and P63;

other studies show a more diverse immunoprofile.[20,21] The subtypes defined by gene expression arrays can also be approximated by standard immunohistochemical stains (see Table 10.1). Another study by Cheang and colleagues has confirmed that using additional immunostains, such as CK5/6 and EGFR, could identify a group of TNBCs with a worse prognosis.

The heterogeneity of TNBCs has been known for many years. Recent studies have identified that TNBCs have various types of long noncoding RNAs (ncRNAs), defined as RNA molecules longer than 200 nucleotides in length that do not belong to known categories of small RNAs are involved in a spectrum of biological processes, such as development and maintenance of pluripotency.[21,22] On the basis of this system, Lui and colleagues were able to classify TNBCs into four distinct clusters, including an immunomodulatory subtype (IM), a luminal androgen receptor subtype (LAR), a mesenchymal-like subtype (MES), and a basal-like and immune suppressed (BLIS) subtype.[23]

Increasingly, clinical trials are being designed according to the different molecular subtypes of breast cancer. In contrast, earlier clinical trials required that patients have only histologic confirmation of breast cancer. Nevertheless the initial histologic classification remains important in establishing the initial diagnosis.

Histopathologic Classification

Understanding the histopathologic features of breast cancer remains a necessary element for the appropriate management of breast cancer. This histopathological classification system has been well established for many years.[24–27] The latest WHO classification of breast cancer recognizes 20 subtypes of breast cancer.[28] There have been two general approaches to prognostication via histopathologic analysis. The first categorizes breast carcinomas based on specific features, recognizing the so-called special type of carcinomas. The second parameter evaluates the grade of the cancer. Two grading systems, Bloom-Richardson and Nottingham, are routinely applied to all invasive cancers. Both of these systems consider similar aspects of the tumor including nuclear pleomorphism, extent of gland formation, and mitotic index. Using this approach has allowed the pathologists and clinical teams to categorize patients with a very good prognosis to a very poor prognosis. Classifying tumors based on their morphology and assigning a grade are a standard component of pathology reports.

Histologic Types of Invasive Carcinoma

Invasive Mammary Carcinoma, Not Otherwise Specified

Early classifications of breast carcinomas used the term *lobular* for tumors commonly associated with lobular carcinoma in situ. Because ducts were the other source of epithelium within the breast, lesions that did not have a lobular pattern were referred to as *ductal*. As highlighted in the WHO classification system of invasive breast cancer, 40% to 75% of breast cancers are currently classified as *invasive mammary carcinoma, not otherwise specified* (IDC NOS).[28] Breast cancers are known to originate from terminal duct-lobular structures; the term *ductal* is a misnomer.[29] These tumors are best classified as IDC NOS. Nevertheless the term *ductal* is used by both clinicians and pathologists (hence the acronym *IDC*). These tumors are poorly characterized and represent a heterogeneous group of cancers based on gross appearance, morphologic features, grade, and the prognostic biomarkers. In addition, some familial breast cancers with known *BRCA1* and *BRCA2* mutations are classified as mammary carcinoma, NOS (invasive ductal carcinoma).[30–32] The majority of carcinomas with familial *BRCA1* and *BRCA2* mutation are higher grade.[33] Many familial BRCA cancers are TNBC and show basal subtype differentiation.[34] Despite numerous publications, immunostains for basal subtype markers are not routinely applied to separate basal subtype cancers from the other invasive mammary carcinoma, NOS. Fig. 10.2 shows a composite image of four separate cancers with various morphologic features and grades. All four cancers are classified as mammary carcinoma, NOS. There is clearly a need to further divide this group.

Invasive Lobular Carcinoma

Approximately 5% to 15% of invasive carcinomas are classified as invasive lobular (ILC). More than 90% of the tumor should show lobular features to be classified as such. If 50% to 90% of the tumor shows lobular features, these cancers are currently classified as ductal-lobular carcinoma. The incidence of ILC has been increasing since the 1980s.[35,36] The increase in incidence might be related to hormone replacement therapy.[37–42] An alternative explanation for the increased incidence may be the significant improvement in detection methodology. Many of these cancers are known to grow along the fibrous septae and do not form a distinct mass. On occasion, patients have developed metastatic disease, and the primary site was only subsequently recognized using magnetic resonance imaging (MRI).[43,44] Morphologically, ILCs show single discohesive cells that infiltrate the fibrous connective tissue. Tumor cells often form a concentric pattern around normal ductal structures, showing the characteristic targetoid pattern of ILC. These tumors are known to be more often multicentric.[45,46] The incidence of contralateral tumors, particularly synchronous tumors is reported to be as high as 5% to 19%.[46,47] This rate is higher than those reported for IDC NOS. Several morphologic patterns are recognized. The most common type is the "classic type" composed of a uniform, discohesive cell population.[48] The pleomorphic variant may either grow as single file pleomorphic cells or form globular aggregates.[49,50] The tubulolobular variant shows both evidence of tubule formation and the characteristic lobular feature of single file tumor cells.[51] The last type represents a mixture of ductal carcinoma NOS, admixed with a single file of tumor cells.[52] More than 95% of these tumors are luminal type and strongly express ER.[50–54]

Loss of heterozygosity of the 16q chromosomal regions and the absence of epithelial cadherin (E-cadherin) expression are common findings in invasive lobular carcinomas.[55] ILC and LCIS show a decrease or absence of E-cadherin expression while showing aberrant expression of p120 catenin.[56] Recent studies suggest lack of functionality of E-cadherin with aberrant expression of p120 is more useful in detecting these cancers than absence of E-cadherin alone.[57] The majority of ILC cases do not express basal cell markers such as CK5/6, CK14, or CK17.[58] Fig. 10.3 shows a composite image of invasive lobular carcinoma. Unfortunately pathologists have not uniformly applied criteria for this diagnosis; historically ILC was thought to have a better prognosis than other subtypes[58]; however, recent data do not completely support this assumption. The majority of investigators agree that these tumors are responsive to endocrine therapy and respond relatively poorly to chemotherapy.[59,60] It remains important to clearly separate ER-positive and HER2-negative ILC from rare ILCs that lack ER and/or overexpress HER2.

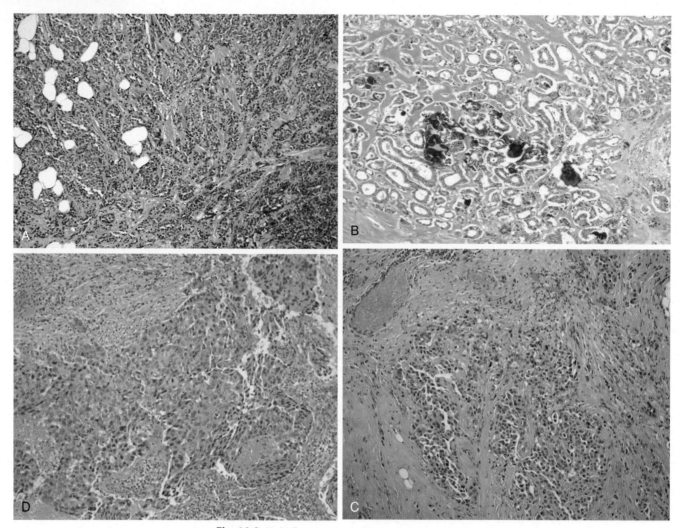

• **Fig. 10.2** (A–D) Four cases of invasive ductal carcinoma.

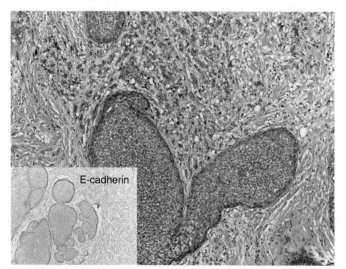

• **Fig. 10.3** Invasive and in situ lobular carcinoma; more than 95% of these tumors express estrogen receptor and do not overexpress HER2/neu. Tumor cells lack epithelial cadherin (E-cadherin) expression.

Tubular Carcinoma

Tubular carcinomas are grade I invasive carcinomas that express ER and PR but not HER2. This pattern strongly correlates with the luminal A molecular subtype.[61] Distant metastatic potential is highly unlikely when this tumor is present in pure form. The diagnosis is made when characteristic angulated tubules, composed of a single layer of relatively uniform cells with no significant pleomorphism, comprise at least 90% of the carcinoma[26] (Fig. 10.4). These neoplastic tubules are haphazardly arranged and are often found infiltrating between existing benign structures. Low-grade ductal carcinoma in situ and atypical ductal hyperplasia are common associated findings.

The prognosis for patients with tubular carcinoma depends on the purity of the histologic pattern.[62,63] In the classic series of 54 cases reported by Cooper, Patchefsky, and Krall, all 12 patients whose carcinoma was composed purely of the characteristic low-grade, angulated tubules survived 15 years, regardless of tumor size.[61]

In screening programs, tubular carcinoma represents 9% of detected carcinomas, whereas in mammographic series, this special type of carcinoma is responsible for as many as 27% of detected carcinomas. Mammographic features include a spiculated mass, with or without associated microcalcifications, or, less

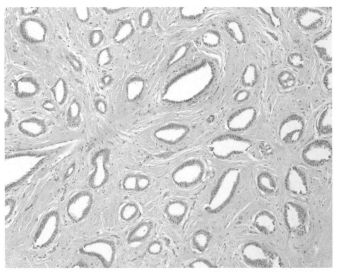

• **Fig. 10.4** Invasive tubular carcinoma.

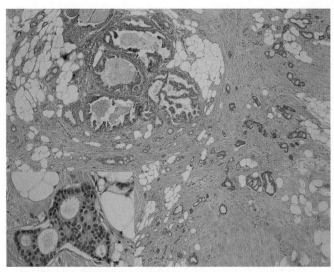

• **Fig. 10.5** Invasive cribriform carcinoma.

commonly, asymmetric density and architectural distortion with associated calcifications.[62–64]

Tubular carcinoma represents only approximately 3% to 5% of all invasive carcinomas; thus the significance may be lost when cases are grouped and analyzed only by stage. The importance of tubular carcinoma lies with therapeutic decisions for individual patients. It is more likely to occur in older patients. The survival of patients with tubular carcinoma is generally similar to that of the general population, and systemic adjuvant therapy may be avoided in these patients. A review of surgical therapy states that for cases of pure tubular carcinoma with an adequate negative margin, mastectomy, radiation, or even axillary lymph node dissection may be unnecessary.[65]

Invasive Cribriform Carcinoma

Closely related, histologically and biologically, to tubular carcinoma is invasive cribriform carcinoma (ICC).[66–68] Histopathologically, these carcinomas infiltrate the stroma as islands of cells that have the same appearance as cribriform-type ductal carcinoma in situ (Fig. 10.5). Differentiating cribriform in situ from ICC may be difficult because of distortion and scarring. Irregular clustering of cellular islands signifies an invasive process. Another helpful feature is that the invasive islands in ICC are usually evenly spaced and often of uniform size.[26] One-fourth of cases have intermixed areas of tubular carcinoma. Because both tubular carcinoma and ICC have equally excellent prognoses, this feature has no bearing on an otherwise excellent prognosis. In studies of pure tubular carcinoma and ICC, the presence of one or two positive low axillary lymph nodes did not adversely affect survival. More than 90% of tumors should show this pattern because the presence of carcinoma that does not conform to special-type criteria increases the likelihood not only of nodal involvement but also of shorter survival.[69] Similar to tubular carcinomas, these tumors are strongly ER/PR-positive, HER2-negative, and ki67 low. They also belong to the luminal A molecular subtype of breast cancer.[70,71]

Mucinous Carcinoma

Mucinous (colloid) carcinoma, when present in its pure form, is also associated with an excellent prognosis. Its defining histologic

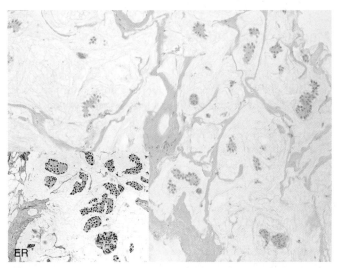

• **Fig. 10.6** Invasive mucinous carcinoma: the majority of these cases are paucicellular. They are luminal type cancer and, without exception, estrogen receptor positive.

characteristic is extracellular pools of mucin in which low-grade tumor aggregates that appear to be suspended (Fig. 10.6). As with tubular carcinoma, the importance of pure patterns is essential to ensure an excellent prognosis (90% 10-year survival) in the absence of adjuvant chemotherapy.[72,73] Other studies confirm that the excellent prognosis of mucinous carcinoma is confined to pure examples of this special type of breast carcinoma.[74–77]

Pure and mixed mucinous carcinomas also have different mammographic appearances. On mammograms, pure mucinous carcinomas have a circumscribed, lobular contour (corresponding histologically to pools of extracellular mucin), whereas mixed carcinomas have an ill-defined, irregular contour. This lack of circumscription corresponds histologically to the interface between invasive carcinoma and the often-fibrotic stroma.[78] Mucinous carcinomas are usually grade I, ER/PR-positive, and HER2-negative. This pattern strongly correlates with the luminal A molecular subtype.[9,10]

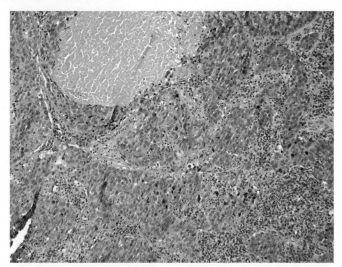

• **Fig. 10.7** Medullary carcinoma: tumor cells grow in syncytia with prominent lymphohistiocytic response.

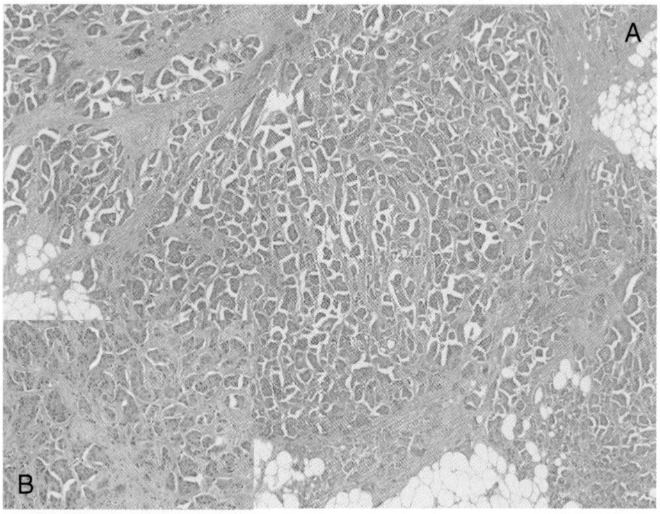

• **Fig. 10.8** (A) Micropapillary carcinoma; (B) *inset* shows higher magnification.

Medullary Carcinoma

Medullary carcinomas (MC) have characteristic mammographic, clinical, and pathologic correlates. Medullary carcinoma is a common phenotype of hereditary breast cancer and is found in women who are at risk for cancer because of mutations in the tumor suppressor gene *BRCA1*.[79] This observation is less common in patients with *BRCA2* and those with no known germline mutation. This pattern is observed in 7.8% to 13% of *BRCA1* patients compared with 2% in the general public.[35] This genetic characteristic is in large part attributable to the young age of the patients.[81] Medullary features have been reported in 35% to 60% of tumors arising in *BRCA1* patients.[77] Multifactorial analysis has shown that high mitotic count, pushing tumor margins, and a lymphocytic infiltrate are independently associated with a *BRCA1* mutation.[78] Medullary carcinoma of the breast is rarely associated with microsatellite instability.[79]

The distinctive smooth, pushing border of medullary carcinoma is reflected mammographically as a sharply circumscribed mass. Grossly, medullary carcinoma has a uniform, soft consistency. The essential histologic features include islands of tumor cells having irregular borders, without sharp edges, that are often connected (Fig. 10.7). These islands do not invade the adjacent breast tissue, but they appear to push against it instead, resulting in a smooth interface with the adjacent normal breast tissue.[26] Unlike the special-type carcinomas discussed earlier, medullary carcinoma is characterized by nuclei that have pronounced anaplastic features. The nuclei are large and pleomorphic, with clumped chromatin, frequent nucleoli, and readily identifiable mitotic figures. The other required histologic feature is a prominent infiltrate of lymphocytes and plasma cells in the loose connective tissue between the cellular islands.

The preceding overview highlights the challenge of correctly diagnosing breast cancer. First, these tumors are known to be triple negative; they do not express ER/PR or HER2 and have very high ki67.[35,81–86] A study conducted on medullary found tumors with high level of ki67 even within this morphology that are more likely to be lymph node positive.[85] This study also showed that many of these tumors show strong staining diffusely for p53. A recent study done by Park and colleagues confirms that the prognosis of these patients does not significantly differ from the other high-grade invasive ductal carcinoma; therefore the same treatment protocol should be considered for these tumors as those with TNBC.[87]

Micropapillary Carcinoma

Micropapillary carcinoma is characterized by small clusters of tumor cells lying within clear stromal spaces, resembling dilated vascular channels (Fig. 10.8). Many of these spaces are not lined by endothelial cells.[88] Micropapillary carcinomas may manifest florid but early lymphovascular invasion.[89] These cancers show relatively high proliferation with moderate to severe cytologic atypia. The majority of these tumors are ER positive, and more than 50% are HER2 positive.[85,86,90,91]

Secretory Carcinoma

This tumor was originally recognized in young patients and represents 0.15% of all invasive cancers; rarely, it can also affect older women. The characteristic histologic feature is the presence of abundant intracellular and extracellular clear areas that contain secretions. Most examples are associated with discontinuous fibrous tissue that is often prominent within the lesion. The secretory material stains with periodic acid–Schiff stain and other mucosubstance stains. Features that correlate with an excellent prognosis include young age, tumor diameter less than 2 cm, and well-demarcated borders with no stromal invasion at the periphery of the lesion.[92] A literature review suggests that some of these cancers express ER and PR and are usually HER2 negative. A 2012 report described this tumor in an 8-year-old female.[88] The majority of investigators suggest no additional systemic treatment for this cancer.[93]

Salivary Gland–Type Breast Carcinoma

These patterns are rare. They display the same morphology as in the salivary gland. The most important salivary gland type of tumor in the breast is adenoid cystic carcinoma.

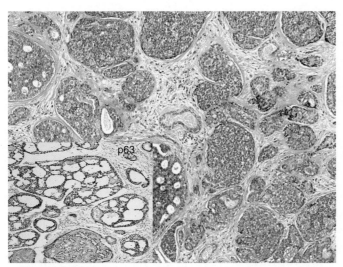

• **Fig. 10.9.** Adenoid cystic carcinoma: tumor cells are usually strongly positive with p63.

Adenoid Cystic Carcinoma

Adenoid cystic carcinoma of the breast is associated with an excellent prognosis.[94–98] These tumors represent less than 0.1% of all invasive breast cancers, and despite showing basal-like features, lack of HER2 gene amplification, and lack of ER/PR expression, they usually remain local and have an excellent prognosis. Fig. 10.9 presents an image of adenoid cystic carcinoma.

Mucoepidermoid Carcinoma

This tumor shows the same histopathologic features as its salivary gland counterpart. The salient features mucin production and squamous differentiation can, however, be a nonspecific feature of mammary carcinoma no specific type (NST). The identification of mucoepidermoid carcinoma is probably important only when it is a low-grade tumor.[99–102] Case reports of high-grade mucoepidermoid carcinoma have demonstrated an aggressive course.

Metaplastic Carcinoma

Metaplastic breast cancer (MBC) encompasses almost 25% of all breast cancers and includes many morphologic patterns, including squamous cell carcinoma, spindle cell carcinoma, adenosquamous cell carcinoma, matrix producing carcinomas, and carcinomas with true malignant mesenchymal component.[103,104] Essentially 100% of these cancers diffusely or focally express basal-like markers and usually lack ER/PR and HER2.[103,104] Fig. 10.10 shows a composite image of several metaplastic carcinomas. The incidence of TNBC is remarkably higher in MBC than in IDC NOS.[105] The presence of certain metaplastic elements has been associated with varying prognoses. The presence of high-grade spindled or pleomorphic components, for example, has been associated with aggressive behavior such as metastases, whereas the low-grade, fibromatosis-like metaplastic carcinomas with bland spindled cells have a high risk of local recurrence but minimal risk of metastatic spread.[106–110] Molecular and genomic analyses have suggested that MBCs are enriched in the epithelial-to-mesenchymal transition and cancer stem cell characteristics.[111,112] Despite aggressive local and systemic management strategies, patients with

MBC have suboptimal breast cancer outcomes.[113,114] A review of a large database has shown that many of these tumors are larger at the time of presentation than IDC NOS. This review also shows that the majority of patients are treated very aggressively; however, the prognosis remains poor, especially compared with other breast cancers.[115,116] A subset of these tumors show prominent squamous differentiation. Primary squamous cell carcinoma of the breast in a pure pattern is distinctly unusual and often cystic; it may also assume a solid pattern with keratinization.[117] The importance in its recognition lies with better understanding in the event of later metastases. Fig. 10.11 shows gross and microscopic images of an invasive squamous cell carcinoma.

Prognosis of Invasive Breast Carcinoma

Predicting outcome for patients with breast carcinoma, especially those whose carcinoma is confined to the breast, is of critical importance. Enormous efforts have been expended to identify predictors of prognosis. Evaluating which of these factors gives significant independent information is difficult because available studies have differences in the end points being evaluated, patient groups, length of follow-up, and treatments, as well as inconsistent inclusion of known prognostic factors to test for independent significance in the final analysis.[117–119]

The College of American Pathologists (CAP) Cancer Committee continues to address the clinical relevance of prognostic markers for solid tumors. Previous CAP conferences have classified prognostic factors into three general categories based on their clinical utility and results of clinical investigation. The most recent CAP conference refined these classifications; the clinically important category includes factors that are well supported by the literature and are in general use in patient management, including TNM staging information, histologic tumor type, histologic grade, mitotic figure count, and hormone receptor and HER2 status.[120–122] The CAP effort has universally been accepted and has been endorsed by both clinicians and pathologists.

Tumor Stage

Tumor stage is the most useful means for predicting survival. The TNM staging system, the mainstay for prognostication for breast cancer, considers three variables: diameter of the primary tumor (T), lymph node metastasis (N), and distant metastasis (M)[123,124] The primary tumor is categorized as T1 if it is 2 cm or smaller in diameter. This stage is further divided as follows: T1a, less than or equal to 0.5 cm; T1b, greater than 0.5 cm but less than or equal to 1 cm[125]; and T1c, greater than 1 cm but less than or equal to 2 cm. T2 indicates the tumor is greater than 2 cm but not greater than 5 cm, and T3 if larger than 5 cm.[125]

The size of the primary tumor and the status of axillary lymph nodes are independent and additive in predicting survival. Both parameters reflect the tumor's ability to spread distantly.[126] As important as the tumor size is, it is important to distinguish the invasive component in establishing the T stage because the in situ component does not have metastatic capacity. Staging is especially useful at the extremes of the scale. Clearly, the prognosis associated with a small carcinoma (<1 cm) that does not involve axillary lymph nodes is significantly better; therefore adjunctive measures might not play a major role.[127–131] On the other hand, most experts would agree that patients with 3-cm carcinomas should receive adjuvant therapy. However, pure special-type carcinomas, such as tubular and mucinous carcinomas, have an excellent

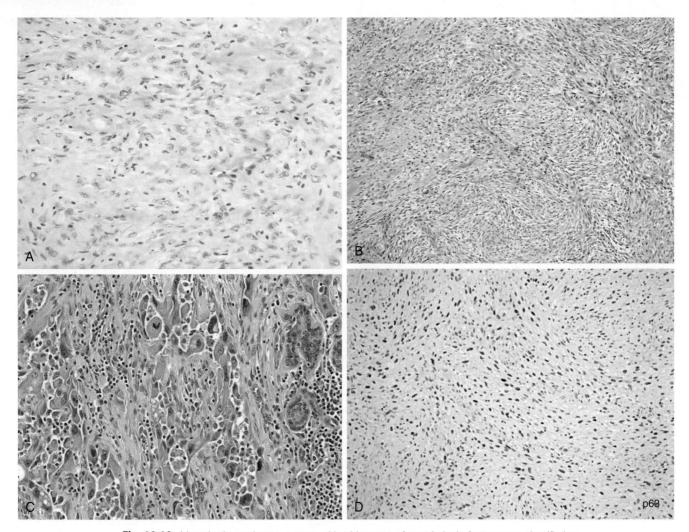

• **Fig. 10.10.** Metaplastic carcinoma; tumors with wide range of morphologic features are classified as metaplastic carcinoma. (A–C) Three separate morphologic patterns that might be seen in a metaplastic carcinoma. The majority of these tumors express a basal cell marker. (D) A metaplastic carcinoma with strong and diffuse p63 expression.

long-term prognosis, even if they are larger in size. The challenge for surgical pathologists is to apply the specific histologic criteria that would allow their recognition consistently, thus ensuring good prognosis.

There have been some recent changes in the TNM staging system that address the status of lymph nodes. These changes are especially timely considering the current emphasis placed on sentinel lymph node examination. A category of pN1mi was created for micrometastasis (>0.2 mm and <2 mm). The category of pN0 is no evidence of regional metastases.[123]

Histologic Grading

Grade of the cancer plays a significant role in prognosis, especially in patients with negative lymph nodes. Grading of the carcinomas may help stratify this group of patients.[128]

The most commonly used grading system endorsed by CAP and the American Joint Committee on Cancer is based on architectural and cytologic features and mitotic index. This system was introduced by Scarff, Bloom, and Richardson and modified by Elston and Ellis and is now known as the Nottingham combined

TABLE 10.2	Combined Histologic Grading System	
Tubule Formation (%)	Nuclear Pleomorphism	Mitotic Activity[a]
>75% = 1	Mild = 1	<10 per 10 HPF = 1
10%–75% = 2	Moderate = 2	10–19 per 10 HPF = 2
<10% = 3	Marked = 3	≥20 per 10 HPF = 3

[a]Based on high-power field (HPF) area of 0.274 mm^2.
Modified from Elston CW, Ellis IO. Pathologic prognostic factors in breast cancer. I. The value of histologic grade in breast cancer: Experience from a large study with long-term follow-up. *Histopathology.* 1991;19:403.

histologic grade.[129,130] This system is a composite of degrees of glandular formation, nuclear pleomorphism, and mitotic activity. Each of these parameters is assigned a numerical score from 1 to 3, based on specific criteria (Table 10.2). The scores from each category are then summed:

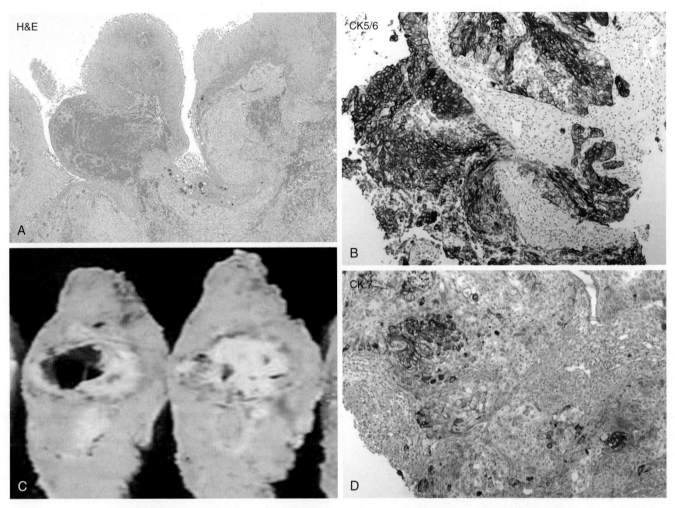

• **Fig. 10.11.** (A) and (B) Squamous cell carcinoma, microscopic image. *H&E,* Hematoxylin and eosin. (C) Central necrosis is often encountered in these tumors. (D) Typical immunoprofile: these tumors often show diffuse and strong CK5/6 expression. They also show CK7 expression, but this is frequently focal and much weaker. (From Nozoe T, Mori E, Ninomiya M, et al. Squamous cell carcinoma of the breast. *Breast Cancer.* 2012;19:177-179.)

- 3 (lowest score possible), 4, or 5—equivalent to grade 1
- 6 or 7—equivalent to grade 2
- 8 or 9—equivalent to grade 3

Graders who use this system are required to evaluate each parameter, fostering interobserver agreement.[132] Although the Scarff, Bloom, and Richardson system has been used for many years, modification and extensive application to more than 2,000 cases of primary operable breast cancer by Elston and Ellis clarified these criteria, strengthening predictive power and reproducibility. Elston and Ellis showed a highly significant correlation between grade and both relapse-free and overall survival.

The three grades of Nottingham combined histological grade are also interesting: 19% were grade I, 34% grade II, and 47% grade III. This is in contrast to other grading schemes that place approximately two-thirds of cases into the poorly differentiated category, thus reducing predictive power.[133,134] Others have shown that grading is predictive of outcome,[135] being second only to lymph node involvement as an independent prognostic factor.[136] Histologic grade of small carcinomas is especially important in prognostication.[137]

Additional Elements Occasionally Helpful

The prognostic significance of vascular invasion has not been completely straightforward. In general, lymphatics are the vessels most often involved in breast carcinoma, although blood vessels sometimes contain carcinoma. Misinterpreting carcinoma in soft tissue spaces or intraductal carcinoma as tumor in lymphatic spaces is often responsible for the overdiagnosis of lymphatic invasion. However, emerging evidence has suggested that these "space artifacts" may not be true artifacts but indicative of true lymphovascular invasion[138] (Fig. 10.12).

These mistakes may be avoided if the physician requires the presence of tumor cell emboli in a space lined by endothelial cells to make the histologic determination of vascular invasion. Studies that have adhered to this criterion for vascular space involvement have found that peritumoral lymphatic invasion portends a worse prognosis. This has been found in lymph node positive cases and in node-negative cases. Moreover, for primary carcinomas that are smaller than 2 cm in greatest diameter, lymphatic involvement was an independent predictor of the presence of axillary lymph node metastasis.[139,140]

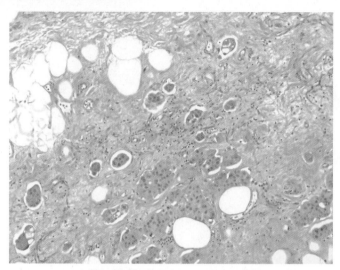

• **Fig. 10.12.** Lymphovascular invasion.

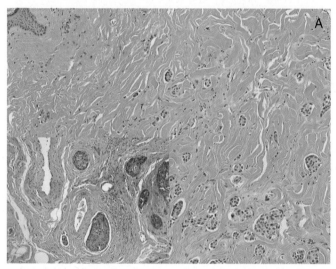

• **Fig. 10.13.** Inflammatory carcinoma with extensive dermal lymphatic involvement; upper left corner shows a small edge of the epidermis. *Inset* shows higher magnification.

Carcinoma involving the lymphatic spaces of the dermis often results in the distinctive clinical entity, inflammatory breast cancer (INBC). This diagnosis is made when a breast containing carcinoma is red, edematous, and warm. Dermal lymphatic invasion can be demonstrated in most patients so affected (Fig. 10.13). Clinical impression is required for diagnosis of inflammatory carcinoma. Although these tumors represent less than 2% to 4% of all breast cancers, they are responsible for 10% of breast cancer mortality. The majority of these cancers are higher grade. The size of the primary tumor does not influence the ultimate prognosis.[140-142]

It is rare for patients with inflammatory carcinoma to survive 5 years, although a multimodality approach multiagent chemotherapy, surgery, and irradiation may improve survival.

In summary, prognostication based on tumor stage, histologic recognition of special types of carcinomas, and careful histologic grading are proven predictive factors. Surgical pathology reporting

is incomplete without them. Likewise, studies of new prognostic factors should include these proven factors in the final analysis.

Prognostic Profiles in Breast Cancer

The improvement in disease-free and overall survival from systemic adjuvant antiestrogen therapy and chemotherapy was proven by the results of randomized clinical trials. Since the late 1990s, international collaboration has resulted in meta-analyses that were updated every 5 years. An online decision tool (www.adjuvantonline.com) developed by Ravdin and others was useful in making treatment decisions regarding the benefits of systemic therapies.[143] Characteristics of the breast cancer such as size, grade, ER, and nodal status are inputted into the model, and results are interpreted as the 10-year absolute benefits on disease-free and overall survival with or without systemic therapy. The results predicted by the decision tool were highly concordant with the long-term follow-up in the British Columbia Breast Cancer Outcomes database of more than 4,000 breast cancer patients,[144] and in clinical practice, it was easy to use for both patients and physicians and both informed and affected decisions about adjuvant chemotherapy.[145]

Predictive Profiles in Breast Cancer

Once breast cancer was classified according to the gene expression profile,[146-148] others began to use this information to stratify breast cancer and predict the prognosis. Three approaches based on gene profiling of breast cancers have been introduced: the 21-gene, 70-gene, and 76-gene profiles (Oncotype DX, Mammoprint, and multicenter profile).[149-155]

The 21-gene profile was first developed by selecting 16 genes, which were apportioned into groups that were associated with proliferation, invasiveness, ER, and HER2, plus five reference genes, and determining their expression by reverse transcription polymerase chain reaction. These expression profiles were transformed into a continuous variable termed the *recurrence score*. This score was used as a prognostic factor for adjuvant tamoxifen in patients with ER-positive/lymph node-negative breast cancers and as a predictive factor in identifying those patients who would benefit most by receiving adjuvant chemotherapy. Six 10-μm sections and one hematoxylin and eosin slide from the standard formalin-fixed paraffin-embedded tissue block was the source material for this assay (www.genomichealth.com). The Oncotype DX test has been validated and endorsed by American Society of Clinical Oncology.[156]

These biomarkers have become important tools in clinical practice for the identification of low-risk patients for whom chemotherapy could be avoided. The Mammoprint test was based on the work of van de Vijver and others at the Netherlands Cancer Institute in Amsterdam.[157-159] This test segregated patients with lymph node–negative breast cancers into "good" versus "poor" prognostic groups based on a 70-gene expression profile. This test originally required that a sample of breast cancer be either fresh-frozen or placed in RNA stabilization solution and a kit provided by the manufacturer (www.agendia.com). The 70-gene profile has also been prospectively validated in a large trial (Microarray in Node-Negative Disease May Avoid Chemotherapy, or MINDACT).[160,161]

The 76-gene profile was developed and validated in a multicenter study to show a "good" versus a "poor" signature. The 21-gene, 70-gene, and 76-gene profiles all show reasonably high concordance (about 80%) despite containing different genes.[162] In addition, studies demonstrate that they function as independent prognostic factors adding additional information to the standard prognostic profiles. Preliminary reports show that these tests influence oncologists' decisions concerning adjuvant chemotherapy recommendations and that they are cost-effective because they identify patients who may not benefit from chemotherapy.[163–166] There is no evidence that their findings can be extrapolated to patients who fall outside of the original "training set." Furthermore, US Food and Drug Administration approval has been slow in coming. Still, these tests illustrate a proof of principle that molecular profiling can predict response to therapy and guide proper therapy. Over the next decade, more molecular tests will emerge that will provide better predictive information as we attempt to personalize breast cancer therapy under the axiom that "one size does not fit all."

Conclusion and Shortcomings of the Current System

We need to develop a more precise classification that incorporates all existing modalities. Currently our reports are incomplete. Various tests are done by different laboratories, and the results are not combined into a complete report, nor are they easily accessible and understandable to the patients or to those who gather data for local tumor registries.

Incorporating the results of all ancillary tests as well as any other tests performed on a cancer in the final surgical pathology report would enable our patients to better understand the biology of their cancer, and if they would like to access additional information, it would empower them to search for the correct class of cancers. It would also allow our biostatisticians to better correlate the results of cancer outcome with treatment and follow patients with more uniform histology and diagnosis.

Selected References

31. Lakhani SR, Schnitt SJ, Tan PH, et al. *WHO classification of tumors of the breast*. Geneva, Switzerland: World Health Organization; 2012.

88. Park I, Kim J, Kim M, et al. Comparison of the characteristics of medullary breast carcinoma and invasive ductal carcinoma. *J Breast Cancer*. 2013;16:417-425.

112. Cimino-mathews A, Verma S, Figueroa-magalhaes MC, et al. A clinicopathologic analysis of 45 patients with metaplastic breast carcinoma. *Am J Clin Pathol*. 2016;145:365-372.

150. Cheang MCU, van de Rijn M, Nielsen TO. Gene expression profiling of breast cancer. *Annu Rev Pathol*. 2008;3:67-97.

154. Paik S, Tang G, Shak S, et al. Gene expression and benefit of chemotherapy in women with node-negative, estrogen receptor positive breast cancer. *J Clin Oncol*. 2006;24:3726-3734.

A full reference list is available online at ExpertConsult.com.

11

Mesenchymal Neoplasms and Primary Lymphomas of the Breast

NINA J. KARLIN AND DEBRA A. WONG

Mesenchymal tumors and primary lymphomas of the breast are rare but distinct entities. Primary breast sarcoma and the fibroepithelial neoplasms, such as fibroadenoma and phyllodes tumor, both arise from mesoderm, the connective tissue of the breast. The first section also describes the more uncommon fibroblastic and myofibroblastic tumors, vascular neoplasms, and lipomatous and neural tumors of the breast and concludes with the myogenic and rare osseous neoplasms that can arise from breast mesenchyme. The second part of the chapter is devoted to discussion of primary breast lymphomas, with a focus on the more prevalent diffuse large B-cell lymphoma.

Mesenchymal Neoplasms of the Breast

Breast Sarcoma

Primary breast sarcoma accounts for less than 1% of all breast malignancies and less than 5% of all soft tissue sarcomas.[1] Estimated annual incidence is 4.6 new cases per million women.[2] Primary breast sarcoma has no known etiology; however, radiation and chronic lymphedema may be associated with secondary breast sarcoma.[3,4] A 90-year review of the Mayo Clinic database revealed that primary breast sarcoma accounted for 0.06% of all breast cancers.[5] Angiosarcoma, fibrosarcoma, and unclassified sarcoma are the most frequent subtypes. Breast sarcoma rarely involves local lymph nodes due to hematogenous spread. Incidence of lymphatic spread is less than 5%, and outcomes are not improved with lymph node dissection.[6] In the absence of palpable axillary lymphadenopathy, routine lymph node dissection should not be undertaken. If axillary lymph node metastasis has been pathologically documented, then lymph node dissection is indicated. With few exceptions, sarcomas require total mastectomy. The most important prognostic factor is negative surgical margins.[7,8]

Fibroepithelial Neoplasms

Fibroadenoma

Fibroadenoma (FA) is a common cause of breast masses that are prone to affect women between 15 and 35 years of age.[9] FA is a painless, mobile lump that is unilateral, bilateral, or infrequently multifocal. The cut surface has a distinctive bulging, firm, off-white nodular look, which is sharply delimited from surrounding breast tissue. Calcification may be present. A homogeneous increase in stromal connective tissue distorts ductal epithelium into long, thin, intersecting compressed strands (intracanalicular pattern) or surrounds ductules in a circumferential manner (pericanalicular pattern).[10] Both patterns may occur in the same mass; neither have biological significance. Stromal nuclei are spindle-shaped and euchromatic with smooth nuclear contours. Ductal epithelium may exhibit a wide range of proliferative and nonproliferative changes.[11] FA is considered a proliferative lesion[12]; however, most simple FAs do not portend an increased risk of breast cancer. If there is an adjoining proliferative lesion, breast cancer family history, or if the FA is complex, then there may be increased risk of breast cancer.[12–14] *Juvenile FA* is a diagnosis reserved for tumors that have a rapid growth rate, are very large (>10 cm), and arise in adolescence.[15] *Complex FA* contains one or more complex features, such as epithelial calcifications, papillary apocrine metaplasia, sclerosing adenosis, and other proliferative changes.[16] Typically, FA is managed with observation alone and tumors often shrink without intervention. However, if the diagnosis is uncertain or if the tumor causes discomfort, lumpectomy or excisional biopsy may be necessary. Cryoablation is another treatment option in certain cases, if the diagnosis is certain.

Phyllodes Tumor

Phyllodes tumor (PT) is an exceptionally rare breast neoplasm representing less than 0.5% of all primary breast tumors.[17,18] After it was first described, it was not known to have malignant potential for almost 100 years.[19] Mean age at diagnosis is 42 to 45 years of age, although a broad age range exists.[20] Tumor size is variable and axillary lymph nodes are uncommonly involved. Grossly, PT has a whorled pattern with visible cracks or fissures. Cystic change, hemorrhage, and necrosis may occur in large neoplasms.[21] The biphasic nature involves a benign epithelial component and an abnormally cellular stromal/mesenchymal component. Although the stroma is generally more cellular than that seen in FA, a more important distinguishing feature is that stromal cellularity is heterogeneous. Frond-like stromal overgrowth (accounting for the term *phyllodes*) produces an exaggerated intracanalicular pattern and is also a more reliable feature of PT (Fig. 11.1A). Like FA, benign PT has a circumscribed edge, cytologically uniform stromal cells, and few mitoses (Fig. 11.1B).

Histologic grading of PT into benign, borderline, and malignant categories is recommended.[12] This classification is based on a constellation of features, including mitotic count, degree of stromal overgrowth (defined as lack of any epithelial component

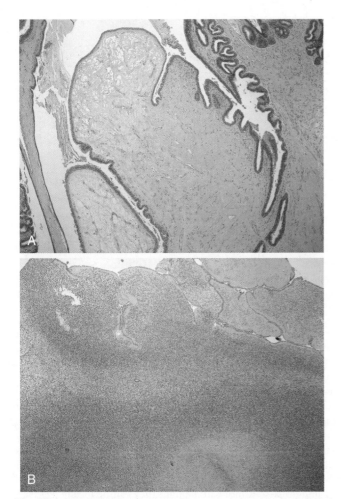

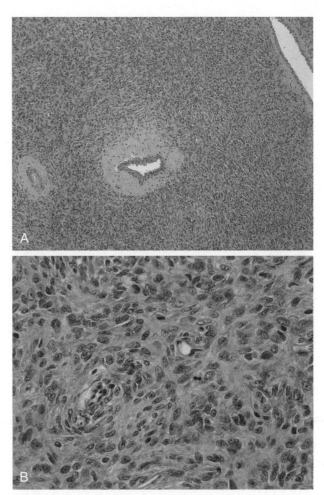

• **Fig. 11.1** (A) Leaflike fronds define the low-power architecture of phyllodes tumor. (B) The stroma underlying these fronds has increased cellularity with varying numbers of mitosis.

• **Fig. 11.2** (A) A borderline phyllodes tumor with increased stromal cellularity. (B) This tumor also exhibits prominent mitoses.

in at least 1 low-power/40× field), and whether the border is infiltrative or circumscribed.[5,22,23] Different authors use different mitotic counts to subdivide PT into various grades, ranging from 1 to 2 per 10 high-power fields (HPFs) for benign PT,[10,24] to up to 10 mitoses per 10 HPFs for borderline PT (Fig. 11.2).[25] The World Health Organization avoids a strict numerical count because of the variability of HPFs among microscopes. Instead, a semiquantitative method of few if any mitoses, intermediate number of mitoses, and numerous mitoses (>10 mitoses per 10 HPFs) is used to help subclassify PT into benign, borderline, and malignant categories, respectively.[26] Classification criteria also include degree of stromal cellularity and atypia, presence or absence of infiltrative margins, and stromal overgrowth.[21] Along with stromal heterogeneity, hyalinization and myxoid change are common.[10] Benign heterologous elements, including chondroid, osseous, squamous, and lipomatous metaplasia, may be seen in benign PT, whereas malignant PT may contain foci of liposarcoma, undifferentiated/unclassified sarcoma, undifferentiated pleomorphic sarcoma, chondrosarcoma, and rhabdomyosarcoma.[27] Distinction between benign PT and FA is imprecise, and it is particularly problematic with core needle biopsy specimens. Lee and colleagues found that higher stromal cellularity (compared with FA in >50% of the cores), stromal overgrowth, fragmentation (defined as stromal fragments with epithelium at one or both ends), and adipose tissue within stroma are statistically

significant features useful in separating PT from FA in needle biopsies.[28]

Malignant PT is recognizable by its cellular pleomorphism, stromal overgrowth, atypical heterologous elements, and mitotic count (Fig. 11.3A). *Ki-67* staining has been used as a proliferation marker but adds little to mitosis counting. Size alone is not a predictor of malignancy. Overexpression of *p53* and the epidermal growth factor receptor gene are not correlated with outcome.[29] Estrogen receptor (ER) and progesterone receptor (PR) expression positivity may be seen in the epithelial component but are rare in the stroma.[30]

Resection of PT with negative histologic margins is recommended.[31] Recurrence correlates primarily with completeness of resection; however, recurrence is not certain even with positive margins.[32] Locally recurrent tumors are usually the same grade as the original. Pseudoangiomatous stromal hyperplasia (PASH) within PT correlates with a decreased risk of recurrence in one study.[33] Lymph node metastasis is rare, and hence axillary lymph node dissection is not routinely performed.[34] Metastases occur in less than 10% of cases and consist of sarcomatous stroma.[34,35] Lung, pleura, and bone are the most common metastatic sites (see Fig. 11.3B).

Adjuvant chemotherapy does not appear to affect survival in PT.[36] However, some advocate for chemotherapy in tumors greater than 5 cm or recurrent malignant tumors.[37] The use of

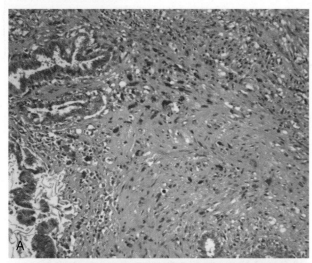

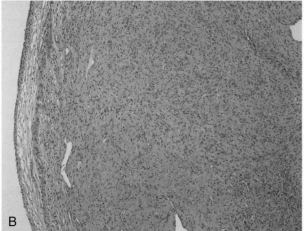

• **Fig. 11.3** (A) Malignant phyllodes tumor (PT). Pleomorphic and spindle-shaped enlarged nuclei concentrate just beneath the hyperplastic ductal epithelium, which is at the left of the field. (B) Metastasis of malignant PT to bronchus confirms its malignant nature.

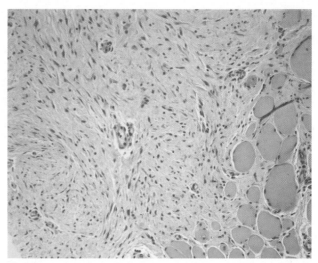

• **Fig. 11.4** Fibromatosis. This example is infiltrating skeletal muscle *(right edge)* of the chest wall. Note the abundant stromal collagen and slender cell nuclei.

radiation therapy remains controversial. Some advocate for radiation therapy in the setting of borderline and malignant PTs because it is associated with decreased recurrence.[38,39] There is no role for endocrine therapy in PT, given the ER negativity of the stromal area.[30]

Mammary Hamartoma

Hamartoma is a well-delimited mass that occurs in perimeno-pausal women as an incidental mammographic finding. It is composed of benign breast lobules, adipose tissue, and fibrous tissue in varying quantity, without the lobular structure of FA, and is outlined by a pseudocapsule of compressed breast tissue. Surgical excision is indicated due to the possibility of coexisting malignancy.[40]

Fibroblastic and Myofibroblastic Neoplasms

Fibromatosis

Fibromatosis is a proliferation of fibroblasts that comprises less than 0.2% of breast lesions.[41] Women of a wide age range (15–80 years of age; median, 40 years) are affected.[42] A unilateral pain-less, firm mass that is mammographically indistinguishable from

carcinoma is typical. Grossly, this is a firm, off-white lesion averaging 2 to 3 cm that deceptively appears to be circumscribed; some cases show irregular stellate borders. Even with circumscribed lesions, radially oriented extensions of tumor subtly infiltrate adjacent tissue, making it difficult to judge adequacy of resection. Light microscopy reveals banal-appearing fibroblasts with oval to spindle-shaped pale nuclei arranged in interlacing fascicles set in a variably dense collagenous matrix (Fig. 11.4). Lymphocyte clusters are common. Fibromatoses are vimentin and β-catenin (80%) positive,[43] and they are cytokeratin, ER, and PR negative.[44] Although these tumors are benign, they can be locally aggressive and locally recurrent.[45] Complete surgical excision with negative margins remains standard treatment.[46]

Myofibroblastoma

Mammary-type myofibroblastoma (MYB) is an uncommon neoplasm that affects men almost as much as women. A unilateral circumscribed mass occurs in patients in their fourth to eighth decades. MYB is a benign, slow growing, stromal tumor. It ranges from 1 to 10 cm in size, although most are 4 cm or less at presentation, and has a homogeneous bulging pink cut surface.[47] Multilobulation and myxoid foci may be seen. There is a broad morphologic spectrum, but typically, features of fibroblasts and myofibroblasts are present.[48] Microscopically, MYB is characterized by a spindle cell proliferation with few mitoses set in a fibrous stroma.[49] Collagen bundles are typically thick and ropy, with cells laid down in short, randomly intersecting fascicles, rather than the long, sweeping fascicles seen in fibromatosis (Fig. 11.5). Cells have small oval/elongated nuclei, small nucleoli, and occasional grooves. Mitoses are rare, but mast cells are usually numerous. Morphologic variations include an infiltrative rather than circumscribed border; myxoid change; multinucleated giant cells; and cartilaginous, osseous, or fatty metaplasia (so-called lipomatous MYB).[50–52] Immunohistochemically, most of these tumors are positive for vimentin, α-smooth muscle actin, bcl-12, and CD99; variable expression can be seen in different tumor areas.[53] Immunohistochemical (ICH) stains for cytokeratin, EMA, S100, HMB-45, and c-kit are consistently negative. There is variable positive staining for ER and PR.[54] Surgical resection is recommended. If margins are negative, recurrence is unlikely.[55]

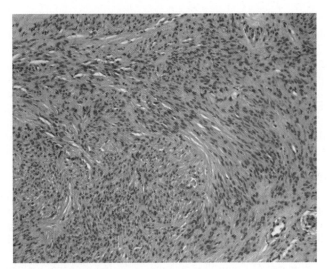

• **Fig. 11.5** Myofibroblastoma. More cellular than fibromatosis, the cells have a short fascicular pattern.

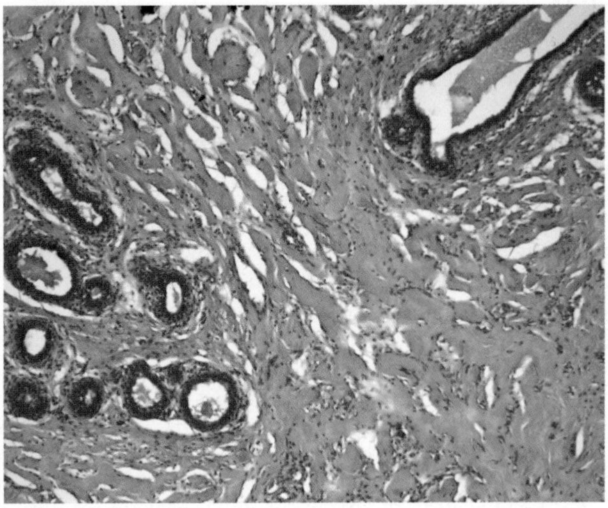

• **Fig. 11.6** Pseudoangiomatous stromal hyperplasia. Widely patent, empty slits partially obscure the proliferating spindle cells as they surround benign lobules.

Hemangiopericytoma

So-called hemangiopericytoma is an older term used to describe a benign spindle cell neoplasm with a branching vascular pattern, which is its most conspicuous feature. This tumor originates from capillary pericytes. Proliferating plump oval- to spindle-shaped cells focally entrap ducts and ductules at the lesion's edge. A thin-walled "staghorn"-type branching vascular pattern is seen throughout the tumor. Its occurrence in the breast is rare.[56] Clinical presentation varies, but most often hemangiopericytoma manifests as a slowly enlarging painless mass.[57] Hemangiopericytomas range in size from 1 to 19 cm and exhibit a firm gray-white cut surface. Surgical resection with negative margins is the recommended treatment and is potentially curative.

Pseudoangiomatous Stromal Hyperplasia

PASH is not a true vascular lesion but a peculiar proliferation of cytologically bland stromal fibroblasts/myofibroblasts that creates empty slitlike spaces mimicking a vasoformative lesion.[58,59] On average, patients are diagnosed in the fourth decade of life, but a wide continuum exists. The clinical spectrum of PASH ranges from an incidental microscopic finding (most common), to a palpable/nodular mass (rare), to breast thickening, to diffuse breast involvement. Nodular forms of PASH resemble FA or mammary hamartoma on imaging and gross pathology examination. Tissue spaces formed by separation of densely hyalinized collagen fibers may or may not be lined by cells (Fig. 11.6). This proliferation may create a concentric perilobular pattern.[60,61] Fibroblasts lack cytologic atypia or mitoses, and necrosis and effacement of normal breast tissue are absent. Gynecomastia-like changes include apocrine metaplasia, ductal hyperplasia, and cystic change.[62] Cells show positive staining for CD34, muscle-specific actin, calponin, and the PR[62]; CD31 and cytokeratin stains are negative. Surgical resection is required only if the lesion enlarges.[63] Other considerations for resection include Breast Imaging Reporting and Data System 4 or 5 lesions on mammography, discordance, or clinically symptomatic lesions.[64]

Inflammatory Myofibroblastic Tumor

Primary breast inflammatory myofibroblastic tumors (IMTs) represent a relatively rare benign mesenchymal disorder and are scarcely reported in the literature. They are generally considered a subtype of inflammatory pseudotumors, and the World Health Organization classifies them as borderline lesions that can variably range from reactive to truly neoplastic.[65] IMTs have been observed to occur in any anatomic region and tend to affect younger individuals. Most lesions are solitary, mobile, slow-growing masses that may or may not be seen on a mammogram; their appearance on ultrasound or magnetic resonance imaging (MRI) is not particularly differentiating, and tissue biopsy is needed for diagnosis. Microscopically, they are characterized by spindle cell proliferation and predominantly lymphocytic or plasmacytic inflammatory infiltrates.[66] Although IMTs were initially thought to develop triggered by inflammatory or infectious stimuli, the pathogenesis is now known to involve cytogenetic aberrations in chromosomes 2 and 9.[67] In addition, nearly half of breast IMTs also have clonal abnormalities in the anaplastic lymphoma kinase (ALK) gene at 2p23, which favors a neoplastic process.[68,69] The clinical and prognostic significance of ALK-positivity remain unclear, however.[70,71] Immunohistochemistry is also important in obtaining the correct diagnosis of IMT because the spindle cells typically express CD34 and desmin but are negative for cytokeratins or S100.[72]

Treatment of IMT of the breast is wide local excision with negative margins.[65] Axillary involvement appears rare, and thus routine sentinel lymph node biopsy is probably unnecessary.[68] Recurrence rates up to 25% have been reported for IMT at other anatomic sites, but there is a paucity of data on recurrence and metastasis of breast IMT.[73] Chemotherapy, radiation therapy, immunotherapy, and antiinflammatory agents have not been consistently effective in the treatment of breast IMT,[74,75] and thus surgery is the mainstay of management.

Malignant Fibrous Histiocytoma

Malignant fibrous histiocytoma (MFH) of the breast is a rare tumor.[76] Approximately 50 cases have been reported.[77] Average size of breast MFH is 6 cm.[78] Mean age at presentation is 57 to 67 years.[78] MFH has been divided into four subtypes: pleomorphic MFH, myxofibrosarcoma, giant cell MFH, and inflammatory MFH.[76] IHC is typically negative for epithelial markers but positive for vimentin.[79] Surgical resection with negative margins is recommended. Axillary lymph node dissection should not be performed if there is a clinically negative axilla. The role of adjuvant radiation therapy and chemotherapy for MFH is unclear.

Vascular Neoplasms

Hemangioma

Vascular neoplasms occur either within the breast parenchyma proper or in the overlying skin/subcutis. Mammary hemangiomas have been described in patients of all ages, ranging from infancy to the elderly.[80] All hemangiomas lack anastomosing connections, endothelial tufting, and atypical mitoses, and they are often an incidental finding. Benign hemangiomas include perilobular, cavernous, and capillary hemangiomas. Of the various subtypes, cavernous hemangioma is most common, consisting of large, widely dilated vessels separated by thin fibrous septa and lined by flattened endothelial cells. These lesions are well circumscribed.[81] Intraluminal thrombi are not uncommon. Capillary hemangiomas consist of numerous small, closely packed vascular channels with a lobular pattern, which often lack luminal red cells. Perilobular hemangiomas comprise a lobular expansion of small- to medium-sized blood-filled vessels within the intralobular stroma. Many examples also extend into extralobular stroma and adipose tissue.[82] Perilobular hemangiomas are not particularly rare, being encountered in 11% of 210 forensic autopsies.[83]

Atypical vascular lesions after radiation therapy are usually restricted to the dermis and, in contrast to angiosarcoma (AS), are well circumscribed and generally less than 1 cm in size. They present as erythematous/bluish papules, nodules, or vesicles. There is a median latency of 3.5 years after radiation therapy.[84] Atypical vascular lesions have a lymphangiomatous quality, with thin-walled, irregular vascular spaces that are empty or filled with proteinaceous material. Focal dissection into dermal collagen is seen. Endothelial cell nuclei are hyperchromatic, with some displaying a hobnail projection into the lumen but lacking the necrosis, mitoses, and dissection into the subcutis that is typical of AS. Their clinical behavior is benign.[84–86] Some experts have proposed that atypical vascular lesions and cutaneous AS represent a morphologic continuum.[84] Ki-67 ICH may be helpful in distinguishing atypical hemangioma from AS.[87] Hemangiomas of the breast are effectively treated with surgical excision, although if vascularity precludes surgical resection, radiation therapy can be considered. Alternatively, transcatheter embolization is an option for tumors that have infiltrated through surrounding muscle layers and are not amenable to surgical removal.

Angiomatosis

Angiomatosis (diffuse hemangioma) of the breast is a rare benign entity. It affects patients from infancy to the sixth decade but typically occurs in young women.[88] A diffuse network of sinusoidal small and large anastomosing vessels affects a large area of the breast. Vessels proliferate around but not into terminal duct lobular units.[89] In contrast to AS, vessels have a uniform distribution; a heterogeneous appearance of large venous, cavernous, and capillary-type channels; and endothelial cells that lack cytologic atypia or tufting. These lesions do not progress to sarcoma.

Hemangioendothelioma

Epithelioid hemangioendothelioma is an exceedingly rare primary breast tumor.[90] Like its soft tissue equivalent, it demonstrates an infiltrative population of epithelioid cells arranged in nests or short cords, with rounded enlarged nuclei and eosinophilic or singly vacuolated cytoplasm. The tumor is set in a chondromyxoid or hyaline matrix. A possible association with breast implants has been reported.[91] Unlike hemangioma, epithelioid hemangioendothelioma can be misinterpreted as a carcinoma because of its epithelioid morphology and positive staining with pan-cytokeratin markers in addition to endothelial markers. However, they are also IHC positive for vascular Ag (CD31, 34, fVIII), which are not positive in breast cancers.[92]

Angiosarcoma and Related Syndromes

AS accounts for 3% to 9% of all breast sarcomas and less than 1% of all breast tumors.[81] AS is divided into two categories: primary AS and secondary AS, the latter of which arises after radiation therapy, mastectomy, and/or chronic ipsilateral lymphedema, in which case it is termed Stewart-Treves syndrome.

Primary AS typically presents as a fast-growing, painless mass. Tumors range from 2 to 20 cm and average 4 to 5 cm in diameter.[93] Macroscopically, the cut surface varies from hemorrhagic and spongy (low-grade AS) to firm, dull-white, and variably necrotic (high-grade AS). The most widely recognized histologic classification subdivides AS into low, intermediate, and high grades, with 5-year overall survival (OS) rates of 91%, 68%, and 14%, respectively.[94] High-grade (grade III) AS is most common in younger patients and consists of more than 50% solid and spindle cell areas. These foci exhibit pleomorphism, hyperchromatic nuclei, macronucleoli, numerous mitoses, endothelial tufting, and papillary formation. A characteristic of AS is infiltration and destruction of preexisting terminal duct lobular units. CD31 staining is nearly always positive in grade III AS; CD34 and factor VIII–related antigen may be negative. There may also be necrosis. Low-grade (grade I) AS is deceptively bland and may be potentially misdiagnosed as hemangioma. It has widely patent interanastomosing vascular channels that dissect within stroma but are lined by hyperchromatic nuclei with few or no mitoses (Fig. 11.7). Solid foci, papillary formations, and blood lakes are absent. Intermediate-grade tumors have less than 25% solid foci and occasional endothelial tufting, but they lack necrosis. A diagnostic pitfall is the bland, almost hemangioma-like appearance at

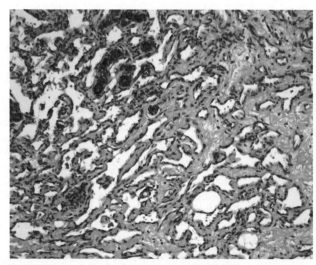

• **Fig. 11.7** Angiosarcoma. A small lobule *(upper left)* is being infiltrated by anastomosing vascular channels lined by hyperchromatic nuclei.

the periphery of low- and intermediate-grade AS. This is particularly challenging when evaluating a small biopsy or incompletely sampled tumor.

Bone, liver, lung, ovary, skin, and brain are common metastatic sites for AS. Contralateral breast involvement may also occur.[95] Because AS has a predilection for microscopic extension beyond the main mass, wide resection margins are required, thereby necessitating mastectomy in most patients. Lymph node metastasis is rare; hence, axillary lymph node dissection is not typically performed. Prognosis is directly related to the histologic grade of the AS.[95]

Development of AS in the ipsilateral arm after radical mastectomy and axillary dissection, described by Stewart and Treves (S-T syndrome), is secondary to long-standing lymphedema.[4] The incidence of S-T syndrome is 0.1 to 0.5%, and it develops, on average, 10 years after mastectomy. Pulmonary metastases are common, yielding a median survival of 19 months.[96] Increased use of breast conservation surgery and sentinel node biopsy has led to a reduction in this clinical form of AS. Secondary AS after radiation therapy has increased, however, with many cases documented in the literature.[97]

AS occurring after radiation therapy is a cancer of postmenopausal women. On average, affected patients are in their sixth to seventh decades of life.[98,99] Postradiation AS can arise either in the chest wall after mastectomy, but currently it is more apt to occur in the breast tissue after conservative treatment. Unlike primary AS, it is primarily a dermal/subcutaneous tumor, with patients commonly complaining of cutaneous violaceous or nonpigmented nodules, plaques, vesicles, and macules.[100] The incidence of AS, which is 5 to 9 times higher in patients with breast cancer who receive radiotherapy,[3,101] is estimated to range from 0.09% to 0.16%.[102] Relative risk ranges from 11 to 15.9,[103] with a latency period of 6 months to 17 years (median 5–6 years) after radiation therapy.[98,99,104] Light microscopy reveals an ill-defined infiltrative neoplasm dissecting within dermal collagen and involving subcutaneous fat. Cells lining slitlike spaces show moderate nucleomegaly, hyperchromasia, and distinct nucleoli. Mitotic figures and papillary tufting are common. Similar to primary AS, these may be subdivided into low-, intermediate-, and high-grade sarcoma. Most patients suffer multiple local recurrences; thus, the mainstay of treatment is wide local excision.[100]

However, other treatment modalities have also been effective in treating AS and should also be considered. A single institution experience showed that patients with secondary AS after breast conserving surgery were effectively treated with hyperfractionated accelerated reirradiation (HART), with or without subsequent surgery. Patients received three radiation treatments per day, 5 days per week at 1 Gy per fraction, to total doses of 45 Gy, 60 Gy, and 75 Gy, depending on the risk for subclinical disease or presence of gross disease. HART was well tolerated, and OS, progression-free survival (PFS), and cause-specific survival rates were higher than in patients treated with surgery alone, conventional radiation therapy, or chemotherapy.[105–107] HART followed by surgical excision and vascularized flap closure can thus be considered in select cases of breast AS arising after breast conserving surgery.

Another novel approach to the treatment of AS includes electrochemotherapy, where chemotherapy such as bleomycin is given intravenously and delivered to tumors via percutaneous electric pulses. This therapy has shown cytotoxic and antivascular effects, and a small study demonstrated that electrochemotherapy can be useful for superficial advanced AS, including of the

breast, with improved local PFS as well as palliation of pain and bleeding.[108]

Lipomatous Neoplasms

Lipoma

Intramammary lipomas are uncommon, with most appearing in women in their fourth and fifth decades. These tumors are well demarcated and thinly encapsulated, showing identical morphology to the surrounding mature adipose tissue. Degenerative changes such as focal fat necrosis, calcification, hyalinization, and myxoid change may be seen. Average size is 2 to 3 cm in diameter. Angiolipoma is typically a subcutaneous lesion composed of small capillary-sized vessels within a lipoma. Intraluminal thrombi are commonly seen.[109] Chondrolipoma contains plates of hyaline-type cartilage randomly distributed within a nodule of adipose tissue. Other types of lipoma include spindle cell lipoma, hibernoma, adenohibernoma, and myolipoma. Lipomas have low potential for malignant transformation. Definitive treatment of breast lipomas is surgical excision, although this can pose reconstructive challenges.

Liposarcoma

Primary pure liposarcoma of the breast is exceedingly rare. Sufficient tumor sampling is required to exclude an underlying malignant PT with secondary liposarcomatous differentiation.[110] There are no distinguishing clinical features. Patients affected range in age from young adults to elderly individuals, but mean age at presentation is 47 years.[111] Tumors are typically slow growing and sometimes painful. Most are firm, well demarcated, and larger than 5 cm (mean 8 cm).[111] All major histologic subtypes (well differentiated, myxoid/round cell, dedifferentiated, and pleomorphic) have been reported.[112] Like their soft tissue equivalent, mammary liposarcoma shows lipogenic differentiation (Fig. 11.8) and has the potential to locally recur and metastasize. Surgical excision is warranted for localized tumors, and adjuvant radiation therapy may be needed if there are high-risk features such as positive margins. Systemic chemotherapy is necessary for metastatic disease. However, adjuvant chemotherapy and its benefit remain controversial. It should be considered for high-grade breast sarcomas with size greater than 5 cm or lymph node involvement.

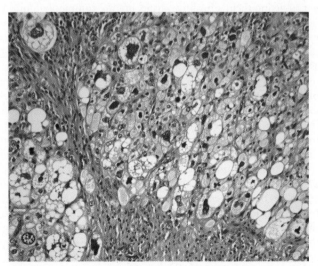

• **Fig. 11.8** Liposarcoma. Cells with monstrously large nuclei contain micro- and macrovacuolated lipid-filled cytoplasm.

Neural Neoplasms

Granular Cell Tumor

Granular cell tumor of the breast is an uncommon lesion that arises from primitive nerve cells and frequently affects African American women in the fourth decade of life or earlier.[113] It can be confused with carcinoma both clinically (very firm to palpation, cutaneous retraction) and radiologically (irregular spiculated mass).[114] Less than 5% of lesions are multifocal. Tumor diameter ranges between 2 and 4 cm.[111] The cut surface shows a spiculated scirrhous gray white/yellow lesion. Microscopically, large cells with an enormous amount of coarsely granular cytoplasm infiltrate a densely collagen matrix. Nuclei are slightly enlarged and rarely display any mitoses. S100 and CD 68 staining by IHC is present in nearly all cases.[115] Rare malignant forms are characterized by high cellularity, large nuclei, mitoses, and spindling.[116]

Idiopathic granulomatous mastitis, a benign breast lesion characterized histologically by noncaseating granulomas, small abscesses, and an inflammatory infiltrate, poses diagnostic and therapeutic challenges and is often confused with carcinoma. Appropriate imaging followed by core biopsy for culture and pathology is needed for diagnosis. A trial of antibiotics is reasonable during workup. Treatment approaches have included observation only, steroids, wide local excision, and mastectomy, depending on the severity of symptoms. In a small case series of 116 patients, idiopathic granulomatous mastitis was successfully managed with observation (n = 9, 56%), steroids (n = 29, 42%), partial mastectomy (n = 75, 79%), and mastectomy (n = 3, 100%).[117] The authors propose an algorithm for management of this condition based on clinical findings and symptom severity: if the tumor is localized and symptoms are mild, excision, steroids, or observation can be considered; if findings are generalized and symptoms are severe, steroids can be tried, but if unsuccessful, mastectomy should be performed.[117]

Benign Peripheral Nerve Sheath Tumors

Neurofibroma. Neurofibromas are benign subcutaneous tumors comprised of Schwan cells, perineural-like cells, and fibroblasts admixed with nerve fibers, collagen, and myxoid matrix.[118,119] The majority of lesions are solitary (90%) and not associated with neurofibromatosis type 1 (NF1).[118] Neurofibromas are classified by location and appearance. They occur alongside any peripheral nerve, giving them a fusiform shape, but are commonly found in skin or subcutaneous tissues. They rarely arise in the breast, but when they do, they usually arise in the setting of NF1 and tend to be periareolar.[72,120] Presentation and size varies, but the NF1-associated lesions are typically larger and are more frequently multiple than the sporadically occurring lesions.[121] Mammography and ultrasound reveal well-defined benign appearing masses. Computed tomography (CT) or MRI can better characterize the lesions; on T2 images, a neurofibroma may have a characteristic hypodense central region, attributed to dense collagen and fibrous tissue in the center of the tumor. Histologic examination reveals spindle cells with thin, often wavy nuclei that stain positive for S100.[72] Treatment of asymptomatic neurofibromas is often not necessary, but local excision can be performed for cosmesis.[72]

Schwannoma. Also called neurilemomas, schwannomas are the most common type of peripheral nerve tumor, although they are exceedingly rare in the breast.[122,123] They are benign encapsulated tumors composed of neoplastic Schwann cells.[118,119] These tumors grow slowly and eccentrically, with the peripheral nerve itself usually incorporated into the schwannoma capsule.[118]

Diagnosis is histologic: schwannomas demonstrate nuclear palisading (Verocay bodies) and biphasic architecture of Antoni A (dense) and B (loose) patterns, and a few pathologic variants have been described.[119,122] Similar to neurofibromas and other tumors of neural origin, schwannomas are diffusely immunoreactive for S100.[124,125] Schwannomas can arise in patients of all ages, and there is no predilection to gender or race. The majority are solitary and sporadic, although they can occur in association with NF2 or other genetic syndromes.[126] Most patients are asymptomatic, although dysesthesia, radicular-type pain, sensory loss, and weakness can occur due to nerve impingement.[127] Schwannomas can have a similar appearance as neurofibromas on imaging—well circumscribed, hypoechoic, and heterogeneous—and frequently the two cannot be distinguished.[118,123] Symptoms from schwannomas prompt surgical removal less often than in neurofibromas, but when surgery is necessary, outcomes are usually successful, with large preservation of neurologic function.[128]

Myogenic Neoplasms

Leiomyoma

An exceedingly rare entity first described by Strong[129] in 1913 and currently only reported in about 30 case studies,[130] leiomyoma of the breast is a benign tumor that tends to occur in women of late middle age and is typically found in the subareolar region, which may be related to the abundance of smooth muscle cells around the nipple and areola.[131,132] For unclear reasons, they occur more often in the right breast. Radiologically, leiomyomas appear as well-circumscribed solid masses without distal attenuation on ultrasound, which distinguishes them from FAs.[131,133,134] Histologically, leiomyomas are characterized by interlacing bundles of spindle-shaped cells with blunt-ended nuclei and eosinophilic cytoplasm.[132] Most stain positive for vimentin, desmin, and muscle-specific actin.[133] Leiomyoma must be differentiated from leiomyosarcoma, which can either occur deep in breast parenchyma or superficially near the nipple-areola complex and has a propensity for local recurrence or distant metastasis. The divergent cytogenetic profiles of these tumors indicate that different molecular genetic mechanisms are at play.[135] Leiomyoma growth may be stimulated by tamoxifen, or antiobesity drugs, such as sibutramine and orlistat.[131,136] Treatment is complete excision to prevent recurrence.

Leiomyosarcoma

Leiomyosarcoma is a rare breast malignancy that develops in women in their fourth to eighth decades of life.[137] Myofibroblasts in the nipple-areolar complex may be a reason these tumors arise in this location.[138] Histologically, leiomyosarcoma demonstrates a spindle cell proliferation with elongated blunt-ended nuclei and merging cytoplasmic processes, which create fascicles and whorled patterns. As in other sarcomas, histologic grade is dependent on cellularity, mitotic count, necrosis, and cellular atypia. Immunohistology shows expression of actin, smooth muscle actin, vimentin, desmin (focal), and occasionally cytokeratin (focal).[111] Treatment is centered on surgical excision, although local recurrence and distant metastases are common, sometimes occurring as late as 15 years after surgery.[139]

Rhabdomyosarcoma

Rhabdomyosarcoma (RMS) of the breast mostly represents a metastasis from an extramammary site. A 25-year review found that only 2% of non-PT primary breast sarcomas were RMS, whereas AS was the most common type.[140] RMS differentiation may develop in malignant PT or metaplastic carcinoma. Both primary and metastatic pure RMS predominantly affect adolescent females, and histology overwhelming (>90%) shows an alveolar subtype, which is known as ARMS.[85] Classic ARMS has loosely cohesive cells, producing spaces surrounded by fibrous septa. Solid-type ARMS consists of a solid sheet of cells. Both types contain small rounded cells with minimal cytoplasm. Immunohistology is required to confidently diagnose RMS. Myogenin is the most sensitive and specific stain; desmin, myoglobin, and myoD1 are also useful. Intracellular glycogen may also be seen. ARMS has a unique cytogenetic abnormality, t(2;13)(q35;q14), detected by fluorescence in situ hybridization, allows distinction of this entity from other sarcomas.[141] Local recurrence and pulmonary metastases are not uncommon. Five-year survival with resected RMS and without metastatic disease is greater than 90% for stage I disease and falls to 80%, 70%, and 30% for stages II, III, and IV, respectively.[142]

Osseous Neoplasms

Pure osteosarcoma of the breast is rare. Mean age in a large study was 64 years.[143] Coarse calcification is seen mammographically. These calcifications produce a gritty sensation when tumor is sectioned. Osteosarcoma is often well demarcated and varies from hard to somewhat firm, depending on the amount of osseous differentiation. Microscopy shows malignant spindle, stellate, and variably pleomorphic cells that are intimately associated with osteoid production.[143,144] Osteoid varies from thin, lacelike eosinophilic stroma to thick, bony trabeculae. Metaplastic carcinoma or malignant PT with heterologous chondro-osseous differentiation must be excluded. Treatment of osteosarcoma of the breast comprises wide local excision with clear margins or mastectomy. There are no standard guidelines on adjuvant radiation or chemotherapy, and given limited breast-specific data, providers should follow those for soft tissue sarcomas in general. Early recurrence and survival less than 2 years is not uncommon.[145]

Primary Breast Lymphoma

Primary extranodal lymphoma has been described for several organs that contain lymphoid tissue, including the skin, bone, brain, gastrointestinal tract, thyroid, testis, Waldeyer ring, and breast. Primary lymphoma of the breast, which arises from resident stromal lymphocytes, is an uncommon entity. Only a few hundred cases of primary breast lymphoma (PBL) have been reported in retrospective series,[146–167] and only two prospective studies has been identified.[168–170] PBL comprises only 0.5% of all breast malignancies and about 1% to 2% of extranodal lymphomas,[161,162,168,171–175] and the most common histology is diffuse large B-cell lymphoma (DLBCL).

PBL may be accurately diagnosed when the breast is the first major site of lymphomatous involvement and there is no evidence of concurrent systemic disease. Morphologically, there are no differences between primary and secondary breast lymphoma, but it is important to distinguish between the two. The definition of PBL, as outlined by Wiseman and Liao[176] in 1972 and modified by Hugh and colleagues in 1990,[200] is still applied widely and requires that several criteria are fulfilled: adequate histopathologic evaluation; the lymphomatous infiltrate must be in close association with mammary tissue; and systemic lymphoma or antecedent extramammary lymphoma must be excluded, although ipsilateral

axillary lymph node involvement is acceptable.[176] Thus PBL is, by definition, limited disease by Ann Arbor staging. However, a strong case can also be made to include patients with regional lymph node (supraclavicular and internal mammary) involvement.[177] In fact, the 2004 World Health Organization reclassification of breast lymphoma determines that disease is primary if the breast is the main lesion, regardless of stage or involvement of other organs.[178] Accordingly, some researchers consider PBL to be lymphoma occurring in or localized to the breast tissue, even though there may be diffuse disease.[179] Breast lymphoma is considered secondary when the breast is involved but not the predominant lesion in the setting of widespread systemic lymphomatous disease. Such would be the case in chronic lymphocytic leukemia/small lymphocytic lymphoma with secondary involvement of the breast (Fig. 11.9A–C). In many situations of advanced lymphoma where there is both breast and systemic involvement, it is impossible to determine which came first.

Clinical Features

PBL most frequently occurs in women (98%) between 60 and 64 years of age in Western countries, although there is a broad range of ages reported in the literature.[161–164,172–174,180,181] The female predominance suggests a hormonal role in the etiology of PBL. However, PBL does rarely occur in men: 1 in 23 patients in an MD Anderson series and 1 in 25 PBL patients at Mayo Clinic were male.[151,153] Although the data are limited, outcomes in men appear similar.[153,162,182–186] Interestingly, when PBL arises in younger or pregnant women, it is more often bilateral and more often exhibits features of a Burkitt or Burkitt-like lymphoma[186] (Fig. 11.10A–C). Contralateral relapse occurs in up to 15% of cases, which suggests a possible malignant clone or a homing mechanism. The mechanism of this organ-specific relapse may be mediated by cellular receptors and tissue chemoattractants such as CXCL12 and CXCL13, which has been described in other extranodal lymphomas.[187]

Most breast lymphomas present as a painless, mobile, enlarging mass in the outer quadrants.[177] Diffuse hypertrophy and noncalcified lumps are usually associated.[179] Breast lymphomas tend to be larger than epithelial breast cancers, and the average size is 4 cm, although they can range up to 20 cm.[162] Interestingly, for unclear reasons, the right breast is more frequently involved than the left breast.[161,162,165,181,188] Although uncommon, patients may present with respiratory symptoms, bulky lymphadenopathy, "B" symptoms, and central nervous system (CNS) symptoms, or other constitutional symptoms usually representative of disseminated disease.[177] Nipple retraction, discharge, and skin manifestations (e.g., peau d'orange, indicating dermal lymphatic infiltration) are rare in PBL.[174,189]

Diagnosis and Staging
Radiologic Features

Lymphoma of the breast is frequently well defined and circumscribed on mammography and may be difficult to distinguish from other tumor types. Some differences in the mammographic appearance of PBL compared with breast carcinoma have been reported, including larger size (4–5 cm in lymphoma vs. 2–3 cm in carcinoma) and absence of spiculation, calcification, and architectural distortion in the surrounding tissue.[189] A typical radiographic appearance of PBL is a well-circumscribed, oval-shaped mass without calcification. However, mammographic findings

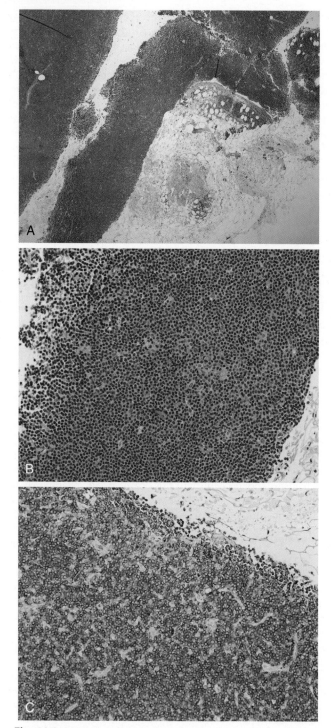

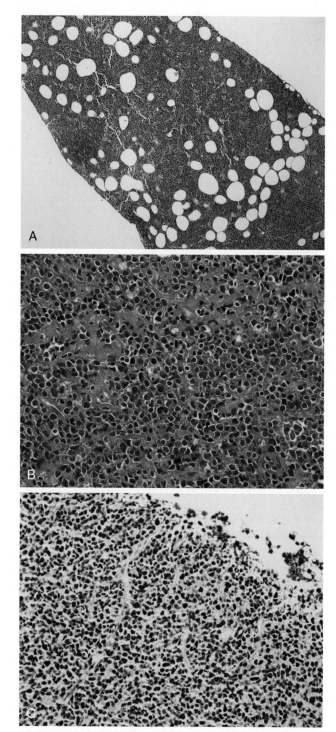

• **Fig. 11.9** Small lymphocytic lymphoma or chronic lymphocytic leukemia manifests also as diffuse involvement of the breast (A), seen at higher magnification as an infiltrate of small round lymphocytes (B), and confirmed by bcl-2 immunoreactivity (C).

• **Fig. 11.10** High-grade primary breast lymphomas (e.g., Burkitt) can also occur. At low magnification, diffuse involvement of the breast is observed (A), confirmed at higher magnification as a highly infiltrative process (B), and marked by a high (>98%) Ki-67 proliferative index (C).

may range from a discrete, well-circumscribed nodule with benign features, to a lesion with spiculated borders, and thus no radiologic features are truly specific for PBL and biopsy remains mandatory.[177] Patients with PBL may even have normal mammography. Breast ultrasound features also can vary and quite often reveal hypoechogenicity with well-defined borders that lack significant acoustic shadowing. It should be stressed, however, that PBL can

have a wide spectrum of appearances on ultrasound. Breast MRI may show characteristic findings, such as strong enhancement with penetrating vessels in masses on early-phase dynamic MRI, strong high intensity on diffusion-weighted imaging, a cerebroid appearance, and septal enhancement.[190] These may offer diagnostic clues, but overall, PBL does not exhibit any obvious radiographic features that help differentiate it from other breast lesions.[179] Fluoro(^{18}F)-2-deoxyglucose positron emission tomography (FDG-PET) imaging is, on the other hand, a useful tool to help ascertain lymph node avidity and stage, and is also used to follow treatment response. PET-CT scans maintain a sensitivity of 89% to 97% and specificity of 100% for non-Hodgkin lymphoma and Hodgkin disease[191,192] and thus has an important role in imaging PBL as well. PET-CT also has a high sensitivity in detecting local recurrence and can thus be used in posttreatment restaging.[171,192]

Excisional biopsy is needed for correct diagnosis of PBL, as in nodal lymphomas. Preservation of architecture is important to determine non-Hodgkin lymphoma subtype. Thus fine-needle aspiration and cytology, although they can differentiate between lymphoma and carcinoma, are insufficient for diagnosis. Imaging-guided core biopsy is acceptable if excisional biopsy is not possible.[177] Histologic, ICH, and increasingly, genetic studies, are necessary to correctly establish the diagnosis of PBL.[193] For example, the *BRAF* V600 mutation has been recently described for positive identification of hairy cell leukemia, and thus tumor genomic analysis can be used in diagnosing this rare subtype of PBL, along with the characteristic nuclear positivity for cyclin D1 and cytoplasmic positivity for annexin, TRAP, and weak CD25.[194]

Staging. PBLs are staged similar to other non-Hodgkin lymphomas, using the Ann Arbor staging system. Because the definition of PBL requires the lymphoma to be limited to the breast or ipsilateral lymph nodes, disease is most commonly classified as stage IE or IIE (i.e., limited stage). Most patients at diagnosis are stage IE (70%), while 30% have regional nodal involvement and are stage IIE.[161,162,181] Clinical and radiographic assessment of the contralateral breast is mandatory because PBL is bilateral in 4% to 13% of patients at diagnosis, and cumulative incidence approximates 30%.[161,162,166,181,195] Bilateral PBL appears to have a more aggressive course and poorer prognosis,[162,166] and expert opinion is divided in terms of classifying bilateral PBL as stage IIE versus stage IV. Moreover, because PBL can occur synchronous with breast carcinoma, appropriate biopsies of any suspicious breast mass should be obtained. Minimum recommended studies of staging include a core or excisional biopsy; PET-CT scan; bone marrow biopsy; and lumbar puncture for CSF for cytology and flow cytometry.[177,196] Basic laboratory studies should include a complete blood count with differential, serum chemistries, liver blood tests, and lactate dehydrogenase. Further imaging such as brain MRI should be obtained if neurologic manifestations are present. Multidisciplinary discussion among pathologists, radiologists, medical oncologists, radiation oncologists, and surgeons is imperative to ensure correct diagnosis and optimal management of these patients.

Risk Factors/Pathogenesis

Many potential risk factors for the development of PBL have been proposed, but none are definitively causative or associative. The presence of breast cancer itself may increase risk for breast lymphoma, given the number of reported cases of synchronous PBL with invasive ductal carcinoma.[197] Case reports of PBL arising after treatment for breast carcinoma imply metachronous disease due to tissue damage, inflammation, and possible changes in the microenvironment and also implicate chemotherapy and/or radiation exposure as possible risk factors for PBL.[198] Histologic transformation from low-grade lymphoma to higher-grade PBL has been proposed, given the presence of overlapping morphologic features in single specimens[199] or based on cytogenetics.[200] Immunodeficiency or an immunosuppressed state, even induced by the

lymphoma itself[201,202] and infection, such as by Epstein-Barr virus[203] or the mouse mammary tumor virus, which induces *WNT1* gene expression in both breast cancer and lymphoma, have also been postulated as risk factors.[177] Autoimmune disease may also have a potential role in the pathogenesis in PBL. Several cases of PBL with antecedent autoimmune disease have been reported,[204,154] and the increased risk of NHL in patients with connective tissues disease and autoimmune disorders is well documented.[205,206]

The strong female predominance in PBL implies a role for estrogen in lymphomagenesis, and although epidemiologic evidence for estrogen as a risk factor for lymphoma are mixed,[171,207–209] a large study by Teras and coworkers revealed an increased risk of almost 30% for NHL (but not specifically PBL) in women treated with estrogen replacement therapy (ERT), compared with women not exposed to ERT.[210] The beta-isoform of the estrogen receptor (ER-beta) is found on lymphoma cell lines, and in vitro and in vivo studies have shown that selective ER-beta agonists have antiproliferative effects in ER-beta expressing lymphomas.[211,212] Further investigation into the clinical effects of ER-beta agonists in PBL is needed. Several cases of anaplastic large cell lymphoma (ALCL, T-cell variant) have been described in association with breast implants; compiled data indicate that women with implants have a very small risk of developing ALCL and should be counseled about this.[177,213,214] The ALCL that arises in the setting of breast implants tends to be more indolent compared with other PBLs.[214]

Pathology

Most PBLs are non-Hodgkin lymphomas, representing approximately 1% of all NHLs.[161,162,171–174] The majority of PBLs are B-cell lymphomas, and the most common histologic type is DLBCL[177,215] (Fig. 11.11A–C). Intermediate- and high-grade histologies predominate. After DLBCL, extranodal marginal zone lymphomas (Fig. 11.12A–C) including those of the mucosa-associated lymphoid tissue (MALT lymphomas), and follicular lymphoma of the breast have been described. Rarer (<1% each) are primary breast mantle cell lymphoma (Fig. 11.13A–C), Hodgkin disease, and hairy cell lymphoma.[216] Peripheral T-cell lymphoma of the breast is extremely rare, but T-cell ALCL is now well described in association with breast implants, as mentioned earlier.[177,213,214,217]

Diagnosis of breast lymphoma is based on cytologic and histopathologic features of this unique neoplasm. Histologically, breast lymphoma typically resembles other anatomic site lymphomas. A uniform population of malignant lymphoid cells densely infiltrates mammary lobules and effaces normal parenchymal architecture (see Figs. 11.9 to 11.13). Cells are round or oval, medium-sized or larger, exhibit little cytoplasm and sometimes have vesicular nuclei, and mitotic count is typically 2 to 6/HPF.[179] Distinguishing PBL from poorly differentiated breast carcinomas and pseudolymphoma is important because treatment differs dramatically. Fine-needle aspiration cytologic examination is a useful but limited tool in PBL, and a core biopsy or excisional biopsy is preferred to preserve tissue architecture.

It can be difficult to distinguish lymphoid cells from reactive lymphocytes. Studies of clonality may be useful. Adequate tissue biopsy for histopathologic evaluation and immunophenotyping remains a key step. However, even after pathologic review of tissue, PBL may be difficult to diagnose. ICH markers can aid conventional histologic examination. Some authors suggest that BOB.1 and Oct2 are overexpressed in PBL and may be useful ICH markers for DLBCL of the breast.[218] Characteristic markers

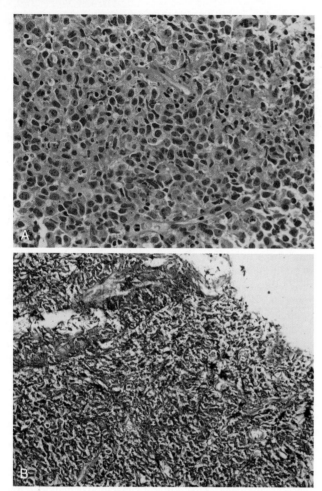

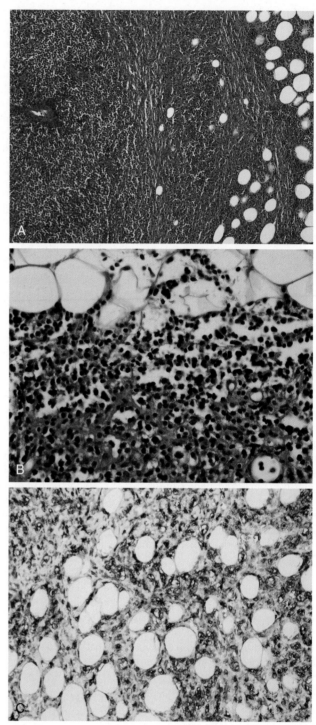

• **Fig. 11.11** Diffuse large B-cell lymphoma is the most common histologic type of primary breast lymphoma (A), confirmed immunohistochemically by positive CD20 (B).

of PB-DLBCL also include BCL-6 and MUM1, and CD20 positivity is seen on flow cytometry in nearly all of the B-cell lymphomas. Other investigators have shown that PB-DLBCLs have high proliferative rates (e.g., Ki-67 and MIB1 index)[179] and characteristics of a nongerminal center phenotype[219] (see Fig. 11.11A). They postulate that these characteristics may contribute to a poorer prognosis. Follicular lymphomas of the breast are positive for BCL-2 and CD10. Mantle cell lymphoma is positive for CD20, CD5, and cyclin D1. Thus applying knowledge about the characteristic immunophenotypes as well as the cytogenetics of nodal lymphomas helps facilitate the diagnosis and histologic subtype of PBL. Researchers are also investigating possible activating mutations in MYD88 or CD79A/B, which leads to chronic B-cell receptor signaling in PBL.[177] Furthermore, the BCL2 and MYC oncogenes are often deregulated in lymphomas, and concurrent IGH-BCL2 and MYC translocations, although rare, have been seen in high-grade PBL.[220] Thus a combination of cytogenetics, fluorescence in situ hybridization analysis, and understanding nuclear factor kappa B pathway signaling along with routine immunophenotyping is important when evaluating PBL. In addition, molecular analysis techniques using cDNA microarrays may facilitate identification of different molecular "signatures" in lymphomas with identical morphology, as has been the case with nodal DLBCLs.

• **Fig. 11.12** Low-grade lymphomas, such as marginal zone lymphomas, can occur as primary breast lymphoma. At low magnification, a "marginal" zone of lymphocytes is seen (A), illustrated at higher magnification as a monotonous sheet of cells (B), and confirmed by intense CD20 immunoreactivity (C).

Natural History and Prognosis

The definition, epidemiology, natural history, appropriate treatment, and prognosis of PBL has varied over time, largely because of the rarity of the disease, and a firm consensus has not been fully established. The majority of information on this entity is culled from case reports and retrospective reviews. Some series

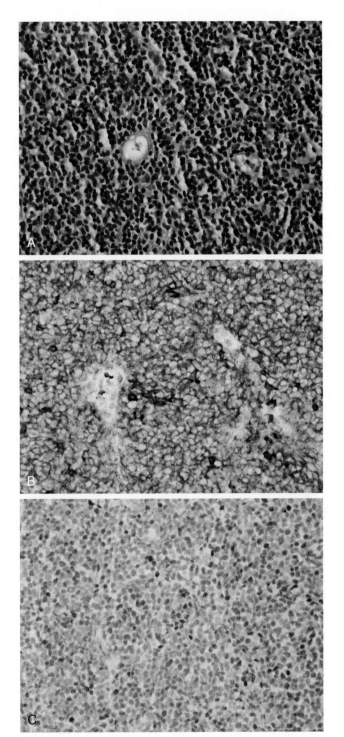

• **Fig. 11.13** Other aggressive primary lymphomas such as mantle cell lymphoma (A) can occur as primary lymphomas in the breast, confirmed immunohistochemically by positive CD5 (B) and bcl-1 (C) staining.

suggest that the breast is an unfavorable primary site and carries a worse prognosis than that of other extranodal lymphomas of the same stage. The 5-year OS rate of PBL with a B-cell phenotype is about 43% to 48%.[215,219] This is worse than that reported for extranodal lymphoma of the thyroid (79%)[221] and Waldeyer ring (70%).[222] However, a more recent 2008 meta-analysis found the 5-year OS rate to be closer to 53%.[172] Broken down by stage, patients with stage IE PBL had a 5-year OS of 78% to 83%,

compared with 20% to 57% 5-year OS in patients with stage IIE PBL,[196] underscoring a poorer prognosis when there is regional nodal involvement.

Although identifying prognostic factors in such a rare disease as PBL has its limitations, some insights have been gained from retrospective studies with some consistency. For example, the International Prognostic Index (IPI) has remained predictive of outcome in PB-DLBCL in several studies[162,223]; an IPI greater than 2 portends worse PFS as well as OS.[166] Other prognostic factors that adversely affect PFS and OS, outlined nicely by Cheah and colleagues[177] include omission of anthracycline or chemoradiation; stage IIE disease (vs. stage IE); more than four cycles of chemotherapy; bilateral involvement of the breasts; and tumor size greater than 4 to 5 cm. Additional poor prognostic factors cited in the literature include poor performance status, increased lactase dehydrogenase, erythrocyte sedimentation rate greater than 30 mm per hour, high tumor microvascular density, and soluble serum interleukin-2 greater than 1000 IU/mL.[163,171,223–225]

Overall, however, it is accepted that stage-for-stage, patients with PBL have a similar prognosis as patients with the same lymphoma histology at other sites.[205] The histologic subtype of PBL (as categorized in the World Health Organization classification) and the clinical stage (as determined by the Ann Arbor staging system) seem to be the most important prognostic factors. Shao and coworkers include age and the IPI along with stage[215] and subtype as prognostic indicators. Clearly, further studies regarding the biology and patterns of spread of extranodal PBL are needed.

Patterns of Relapse

Some studies suggest that PBL has a higher rate of contralateral organ and CNS relapse (in similar fashion to primary testicular lymphoma) than lymphoma at other sites.[226,227] Contralateral breast involvement can be either synchronous or metachronous up to 10 years after the first lesion. Whether PBL exhibits tropism for the CNS remains a contentious and unresolved issue, although more recent reports do support the idea of extranodal tropism at relapse in PB-DLBCL.[189,228] Larger retrospective studies have shown CNS relapse in 5% to 16% of PB-DLBCL patients,[162,164,165,170,172] and higher rates of relapse are reported in PB-DLBCL compared with limited stage nodal DLBCL (23.6% vs. 1.4%, $p < .001$) after uniform treatment with cyclophosphamide, doxorubicin, vincristine, and prednisolone plus rituximab immunotherapy (R-CHOP).[229] Thus there is likely an increased risk of CNS relapse in PB-DLBCL, with most relapses occurring within 2 years of completing therapy.[230] This has implications regarding CNS-directed prophylaxis, which remains a controversial issue. Potential high-risk features for CNS relapse include stage IIE disease, stage-modified IPI score greater than 2, bilateral breast involvement, and tumor size greater than 5 cm.[177] If any of these features are present, strong consideration should be given to CNS prophylaxis.

Treatment

Treatment for PBL has varied widely and is guided by the subtype and stage of lymphoma. Spontaneous regression of PBL has also been reported but remains quite infrequent.[231] Surgical resection or mastectomy is not recommended because these malignancies are extremely sensitive to both multiagent chemotherapy combined with rituximab and/or radiation therapy.[232] It is well documented that surgery in patients with PBL increases all-cause and disease-specific mortality.[162,172,232] Surgery should thus be used for diagnostic purposes only (i.e., excisional biopsy) because breast lymphoma is thought of as an invasive disease. On the other hand, some studies have shown that surgery does have a role in improving local disease control.[184] Nevertheless, surgery alone should be avoided, and it is suggested that patients who undergo surgical excision perhaps because of a misdiagnosis of breast carcinoma should receive chemoimmunotherapy and subsequent radiotherapy as soon as possible.[177]

For aggressive lymphoma limited to the breast, as well as for indolent lymphoma that is stage IIE or higher, systemic chemotherapy remains the treatment of choice. Data from large recent retrospective studies and two prospective trials looking at chemotherapy with or without rituximab in PB-DLBCL form the basis on which chemotherapy is recommended.[161–167,169,170] R-CHOP is the standard of care in nodal DLBCL, and this regimen is becoming routine in PB-DLBCL as well.[177] Patients with PB-DLBCL who received more than four cycles were found to have significantly greater PFS and OS than those who received less than four cycles, and thus four to six cycles of R-CHOP is currently recommended.[164] Chemotherapy followed by radiation therapy yields 5-year PFS and OS rates between 50% and 70%.[161,162,165,170] It should be noted that the evidence for rituximab is mixed, with many studies showing a nonsignificant improvement in PFS and OS[161,164] or no benefit at all[165,223]; one study did show a statistically significant improvement in 5-year PFS in patients who received R-CHOP versus CHOP.[233] Extrapolating from nodal DLBCL, however, it is generally recommended that rituximab should be included in the treatment of PB-DLBCL and CD20-positive PBLs, in combination with anthracycline-based chemotherapy.[171,177,196]

Radiation therapy, which may also be incorporated into the treatment schema, is the treatment of choice for indolent lymphoma limited to the breast. It can be used as sole treatment for stage IE indolent lymphoma and now routinely used as consolidation therapy after chemoimmunotherapy for aggressive stage IE and IIE non-Hodgkin lymphoma. Improvement in local control as well as improved long-term event-free survival and OS after consolidation radiation therapy to the ipsilateral breast has been demonstrated in patients with PB-DLBCL.[17,23] The current approach for consolidation therapy uses involved site radiotherapy (ISRT), again drawing on nodal DLBCL data and treatment practices[234–236]; thus the ipsilateral breast plus any additional sites of known prechemotherapy nodal disease or contralateral breast disease should be irradiated. Smaller radiotherapy volumes with ISRT compared with involved-field radiation therapy, for example, are thought to decrease the risk of radiation side effects without compromising treatment efficacy,[177] especially when patients receive systemic chemotherapy, again recognizing the chemosensitivity of these lymphomas.

CNS prophylaxis should be considered for patients with PB-DLBCL or Burkitt lymphoma of the breast due to the high incidence of CNS relapse with these histologic subtypes.[237–239] CNS-directed prophylaxis should also be considered in patients in whom high-risk features are present, as discussed earlier.[177] However, this remains a contentious issue. Most published case series did not use intrathecal chemotherapy, making it difficult to assess the effect of CNS prophylaxis. Intrathecal methotrexate with each cycle of chemoimmunotherapy, as well as high-dose intravenous methotrexate after chemotherapy, have been used in attempt to decrease the risk of CNS relapse after PBL.[169,240]

Bilateral PBL is particularly high risk, and it is suggested that patients with bilateral PBL who are young and fit be considered for more intensive chemotherapy (e.g., R-hyper-CVAD [rituximab, hyperfractionated cyclophosphamide, doxorubicin, vincristine, and dexamethasone] or R-MA [rituximab, high-dose IV methotrexate, cytarabine].[177] Data on tolerability and efficacy of these regimens is limited, however.

Available data indicate poor outcomes with relapsed PB-DLBCL, including CNS relapse.[161,162,168] Ryan and colleagues reported a median survival of 1 year in the International Extranodal Lymphoma Study Group series after disease relapse, with a 5-year OS of 20%.[162] Options for salvage therapy remain limited, and most patients succumb to progressive lymphoma.

Future Directions and Conclusion

PBL is a rare disease with specific pathologic and clinical features that can present diagnostic and treatment challenges. Histologic diagnosis and full staging are important to guide therapy, and in general, systemic chemoimmunotherapy followed by consolidation radiation therapy are the mainstays of treatment for the majority of primary breast B-cell lymphomas. Surgery rarely has a role in treatment aside from excisional biopsy. Patients with bilateral breast involvement or high-risk features should be considered for more intensive therapy, including CNS prophylaxis. Future direction involves further investigation into the role of sex hormones in lymphogenesis and exploration of estrogen inhibitors in therapy. Additional study into the genomics of PBL, including specific oncogenic mutations and alterations in key molecular pathways that lead to lymphogenesis, is necessary, given the potential of existing targeted therapies or novel small molecule inhibitors in the treatment of PBL.

Acknowledgment

We gratefully acknowledge the contribution of Paul E. Wakely, who authored the mesenchymal portion of this chapter in previous editions.

Selected References

10. Rosen PP. Fibroepithelial lesions. In: *Rosen's Breast Pathology*. 2nd ed. Philadelphia: Lippincott Williams & Wilkins; 2001:163-200.

30. Telli ML, Horst KC, Guardino AE, et al. Phyllodes tumors of the breast: natural history, diagnosis and treatment. *J Natl Compr Canc Netw*. 2007;5:324.

161. Caon J, Wai ES, Hart J, et al. Treatment and outcomes of primary breast lymphoma. *Clin Breast Cancer*. 2012;12:412-419.

162. Ryan G, Martinelli G, Kuper-Hommel M, et al. Primary diffuse large B-cell lymphoma of the breast: prognostic factors and outcomes of a study by the International Extranodal Lymphoma Study Group. *Ann Oncol*. 2008;19:233-241.

177. Cheah CY, Cambell BA, Seymour JF. Primary breast lymphoma. *Cancer Treat Rev*. 2013;40:900-908.

184. Radkani P, Joshi D, Paramo JC, et al. Primary breast lymphoma: 30 years of experience with diagnosis and treatment at a single medical center. *JAMA Surg*. 2014;149:91-93.

215. Shao YB, Sun XF, He YN, et al. Clinicopathological features of thirty patients with primary breast lymphoma and review of the literature. *Med Oncol*. 2015;32:448.

225. Ganjoo K, Advani R, Marippan M, et al. Non-Hodgkin lymphoma of the breast. *Cancer*. 2007;110:25-30.

A full reference list is available online at ExpertConsult.com.

12

Paget Disease of the Breast

RAFAEL E. JIMENEZ, TINA J. HIEKEN, MARGOT S. PETERS, AND DANIEL W. VISSCHER

Paget disease (PD) is histologically defined as the presence of neoplastic cells of glandular differentiation, interspersed between keratinocytes of nipple epidermis, and most often presents as an eczema-like nipple lesion. More than 90% of cases are associated with an underlying in situ or invasive breast carcinoma, detected before, simultaneously with, or after the diagnosis of PD.

Sir James Paget, who described the condition in 1874, considered it a preneoplastic or paraneoplastic process preceding the appearance of breast carcinoma.[1] It was not until 1904 that Jacobaeus described the histopathology of PD and proposed that it represented spread of carcinoma cells into the epidermis of the nipple from an underlying preexisting neoplasm.[2] This is today the most accepted theory regarding its pathogenesis.

PD constitutes approximately 1% of the cases of breast carcinoma diagnosed in the United States.[3,4] According to published data from Surveillance, Epidemiology and End Results (SEER) registry of the National Cancer Institute,[3] despite an increase of 10% in the incidence of both invasive and in situ ductal carcinomas of the breast during 1988 to 2002, the incidence of PD decreased by 45% in the same period of time. Eighty-six percent of cases were associated with an underlying invasive or in situ carcinoma. The median patient age at presentation was 62 years according to the SEER registry, 70 in a Scandinavian study,[4] and 48.1 in a large Chinese series.[5]

Pathogenesis

The most accepted explanation for the development of PD is that the neoplastic cells (commonly referred to as *Paget cells*) result from the migration of cells from the underlying adenocarcinoma through the duct system, and into the epidermis, the so-called epidermotropic theory. This theory is supported by the existence of an underlying carcinoma in about 90% of cases of PD, which usually shares phenotypic similarities with Paget cells.[6,7] Further support for this theory comes from the reported decrease in incidence of PD despite an increase in breast cancer incidence, suggesting that the former is a result of earlier detection of tumors at a point before the spread of malignant cells into the epidermis.[3] The occurrence of secondary PD also supports an epidermotropic mechanism for this phenomenon. In these cases, PD is seen surrounding an area in the skin that has been directly invaded by a tumor,[8] not necessarily in the proximity of the nipple, suggesting a tumoral origin of the Paget cells. A molecular mechanism has been proposed to explain the migration capabilities of Paget cells.[9] According to this model, heregulin-α is produced by keratinocytes, as demonstrated by the presence of heregulin-α messenger RNA in skin keratinocytes. This factor induces spreading, motility and chemotaxis of cultured breast cancer cells, a phenomenon likely mediated through its binding to HER3 or HER4 receptors, which in turn are dimerized to highly overexpressed HER2. Migration capability of cultured cells was inhibited when they were previously exposed to monoclonal antibody AB2 directed against the extracellular domain of HER2.[9] Vimentin expression in breast cancer cell lines has also been associated with increased motility and invasiveness in vitro.[10,11] In one study,[12] vimentin expression was found in 44.7% of cases of mammary PD, suggesting a potential role of this intermediate filament in cell motility and migration. p16, a molecule involved in cell motility, is expressed at similar levels in PD and in underlying ductal carcinoma in situ (DCIS), suggesting a role for this molecule in the intraepithelial spread of Paget cells.[13]

Approximately 10% of cases of PD are not associated with an underlying breast cancer. Some of these cases may represent an undetected breast tumor, resulting from failure to detect a small occult breast cancer in a large, albeit well-sectioned, surgical specimen due to practical limitations (cost and time). However, some data suggest the possibility of a primary neoplastic process localized in the nipple-areola complex epithelium. For example, some studies have shown genotypic differences between Paget cells and underlying carcinoma cells,[14] whereas others have shown that some cases of PD associated with underlying DCIS contain substantial areas of normal-appearing ducts between the two neoplastic processes (i.e., skipped areas).[15] These findings have prompted an alternative explanation of PD histogenesis, which is commonly referred to as the intraepidermal transformation theory. This hypothesis maintains that Paget cells arise in situ from transformation of multipotential cells in the epidermis or from the terminal portion of the lactiferous duct at its junction with the epidermis.[15,16] The occurrence of extramammary PD (i.e., presence of similar histologic findings in other sites of the body) gives further support to this theory, particularly because extramammary PD is much less often associated with an underlying malignancy. At the core of this theory are Toker cells, which are considered by some as precursors of PD. Toker cells are inconspicuous clear cells that are predominantly located in the skin of the nipple-areola complex.[17-20] They are detected in 10% of nipples with routine histology, but in up to 83% of cases when immunohistochemical stains are used,[21] distributed in a dispersed fashion within the epidermis, mainly as scattered individual cells. Their cytomorphologic features are bland, without suggestion of malignancy (Fig. 12.1). Ultrastructurally, Toker cells are globoid with dendritic

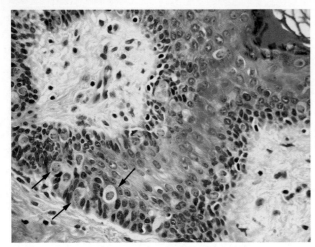

• **Fig. 12.1** Toker cells *(arrows)* are seen in a large proportion of normal nipples. They are believed to be cells of lactiferous duct or sebaceous gland origin, migrating into the epidermis of the nipple. Notice the similarities with Paget cells, except for their bland cytologic features.

cytoplasmic projections and are distinct from surrounding keratinocytes, Langerhans cells, melanocytes, and Merkel cells.[22] Toker cells are immunophenotypically similar to Paget cells in sharing expression of cytokeratin 7 and CAM 5.2 but lack high molecular weight cytokeratin, S100, and HMB45 expression.[18,21–23] They differ in the negative expression of mucin, CD138, HER2, and epithelial membrane antigen.[18,22,24] They are consistently negative for estrogen receptors (ER) and progesterone receptors (PR).[20] Whether Toker cells are the result of upward migration of ductal cells into the epidermis, are of sebaceous gland apparatus origin, or develop through an in situ transformation of keratinocytes is still unresolved.[21,24–27] Independently of the origin, the similarities between Toker and Paget cells have suggested that the former may represent the cell that undergoes malignant transformation in the initial phases of PD.[22,28] A case report of PD confined to the areola associated with multifocal Toker cell hyperplasia suggests that indeed Toker cells play a significant role in the pathogenesis of PD.[29] Yet some authors have suggested that Paget cells derive directly from altered keratinocytes, a theory supported by the finding of desmosomes between Paget cells and adjacent keratinocytes.[16] The referenced study from Chen and colleagues demonstrated that despite steadily decreasing incidence rates of PD with an underlying tumor between 1988 and 2002, the incidence rates of PD without an underlying tumor remained unchanged.[3] These data suggest that although a majority of cases of PD represent epidermotropic extension of preexisting underlying breast tumor cells, a smaller proportion without an underlying malignancy may arise from intraepidermal transformation of Toker cells or keratinocytes.

Histopathology

The hallmark of PD is the presence of neoplastic cells with abundant clear or pale cytoplasm, situated individually or in small clusters between native epidermal keratinocytes (Fig. 12.2A). These cells can be present in any layer of the epidermis, being usually more numerous in the basal and lower spinous strata and can form intraepidermal aggregates and even glandular structures.[30–32] Usually larger than the surrounding keratinocytes, PD cells are

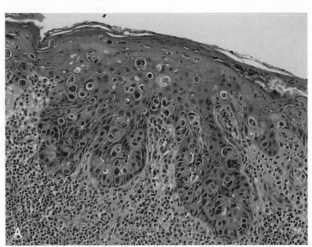

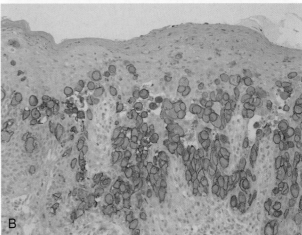

• **Fig. 12.2** (A) Classic histologic picture of Paget disease, as neoplastic cells with clear cytoplasm and pleomorphic nuclei interspersed singly and in clusters among normal-appearing native keratinocytes. Notice the concentration of the neoplastic cells in the basal and lower spinous layers of the epidermis, and mixed chronic inflammation of underlying dermis. (B) Tumor cells are positive for HER2 overexpression.

pleomorphic, display prominent nucleoli and frequent mitoses, and show intracytoplasmic mucin-filled vacuoles in up to 25% to 50% of cases,[8,33] which are highlighted with a periodic acid–Schiff or mucicarmine stain. The epidermis can show hyperkeratosis with parakeratosis, hyperplasia with papillomatosis, or ulceration with crusting. The underlying dermis usually shows reactive changes, including a prominent lymphoplasmacytic infiltrate and hypervascularity.

Paget cells may often be identified in the underlying lactiferous ducts, sometimes merging unperceptively with underlying DCIS, which is more often high nuclear grade, solid, or comedo type. Association with lobular carcinoma in situ has been reported, although it is extremely rare.[34,35] In these cases, bilateral PD may be present.[35]

When an underlying invasive carcinoma is present, it is usually of ductal type and high histologic grade. Most often it is located in the central portion of the breast, occasionally abutting the dermis, as terminal lobular units have been described within the nipple in approximately 25% of entirely examined nipples.[36,37] Relatively distant quadrant peripheral tumors can be seen connected to the PD through ducts involved by DCIS. Multifocality is not uncommon.[7]

Paget cells are usually positive for markers of breast epithelium differentiation. As opposed to the surrounding keratinocytes, Paget cells are frequently positive for cytokeratin 7, CAM 5.2, and other low molecular weight cytokeratins, and negative for high-molecular weight cytokeratins.[38,39] They usually show expression of MUC1, carcinoembryonic antigen, epithelial membrane antigen and occasionally gross fluid cystic disease protein. The vast majority of cases will show strong overexpression of the HER2 protein[40] and amplification of the gene[41] (Fig. 12.2B). This would also explain the relatively low frequency of ER or PR expression in PD.[40] Sek and associates demonstrated a HER2 overexpressing molecular subtype, characterized by HER2-positive, ER-negative immunophenotype, in 86% of cases of PD, whereas "luminal B" (ER-positive, HER2-positive) and "luminal A" (ER-positive, HER2-negative) subtypes represented 12% and 2% of cases, respectively. The underlying in situ or invasive tumors demonstrated a similar distribution of subtypes.[42] Lester and colleagues found different molecular subtypes depending on whether the PD was associated with underlying DCIS (most commonly HER2 overexpressing subtype) or with invasive carcinoma (most commonly luminal B).[43] Up to 18% of Paget cells express S100 protein,[44] in keeping with the occasional expression of this marker by breast carcinomas. However, contrary to cells of melanoma in situ, Melan-A is consistently negative.

On rare occasions, the intraepithelial cells of PD invade into the underlying dermis, a variant commonly referred to as "invasive PD" (Fig. 12.3). This phenomenon has been described in cases of PD associated with an underlying invasive breast tumor, with an in situ carcinoma only, or with no underlying breast neoplasm.[45-49] It is thought to represent a later event in the progression of PD, in which Paget cells acquire invasive capabilities. Reported incidence of this phenomenon ranges from 4% to 11% of cases of PD.[45,47,50] The dermal invasive component is usually small, and by definition, should be distinctively separate from any invasive tumor that may exist in the breast parenchyma. Mean depth of invasion and mean diameter were reported as 0.637 and 1.268 mm, respectively, in the largest series published to date.[47] In this study, no significant difference in prognosis was found between cases with invasive and noninvasive PD. However, lymph node metastases have been reported in cases of invasive PD in the absence of an invasive breast carcinoma.[45,48] Accurate recognition of this variant should avoid overstaging tumors by confusing it with skin involvement (pT4b disease) or tumor satellitosis.[47,49]

The histopathologic differential diagnosis of PD includes conditions that may display intraepidermal clear or pale cells, which appear morphologically distinct from surrounding keratinocytes, a histologic picture also known as a "pagetoid" pattern. These include nonneoplastic conditions, benign pathologic processes, and other malignancies[23,51] (Table 12.1).

Keratinocytes with accumulated glycogen within their cytoplasm, giving them the appearance of clear cells interspersed within more classic keratinocytes, are frequently seen in nipple epidermis. These cells usually show a pycnotic angulated nucleus, and the surrounding cytoplasm appears empty on routine histology. They are predominantly located in the midepidermis.[8] Some authors consider them to be reactive in nature and refer to them as pagetoid dyskeratosis cells[52,53]; in contrast with Paget cells, pagetoid dyskeratosis cells share with epidermal keratinocytes expression of high molecular weight keratins. Toker cells, as described earlier, are benign clear cells seen normally in the nipple epidermis. As discussed, they are immunoreactive with cytokeratin 7 and likely represent benign ductal cells extending into the epidermis. Toker cells differ from Paget cells in that they do not show cytologic features of malignancy and are consistently negative for HER2 and epithelial membrane antigen.

Nipple adenoma is part of the differential diagnosis not only because it may clinically present as an eczematous lesion, but also because it is usually associated with Toker cell hyperplasia,

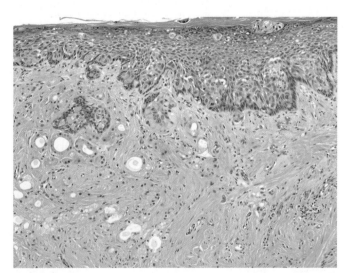

• **Fig. 12.3** Invasive Paget disease. Paget cells are seen in the overlying epidermis, while invasive glandular elements are present in the superficial dermis. This focus of invasion had no spatial relationship with the underlying breast cancer.

TABLE 12.1 Differential Expression of Immunohistochemical Markers in Entities Potentially Confused With Paget Disease

	Cytokeratin 7	CAM 5.2	HMWCK	S100	Melan A	HER2
Paget disease	+++	+++	–	+/–	–	+++
Toker cells	+++	+++	–	–	–	–
Malignant melanoma	–	–	–	+++	+++	–
Squamous cell carcinoma in situ	–/focally +	–	+++	–	–	–

HMWCK, High molecular weight cytokeratin; +++, consistently expressed; –, consistently nonexpressed; +/–, variable expression.

mimicking PD.[24,54] Nipple adenomas are localized lesions characterized by an adenomatous proliferation of ducts and tubules, associated with florid epithelial and myoepithelial cell hyperplasia, usually within a desmoplastic stroma. The architectural complexity of the lesion may be confused with invasive or in situ carcinoma, leading to the erroneous interpretation of the associated Toker cell hyperplasia as PD. If in doubt, a HER2 stain can help in determining the exact nature of these cells.

Squamous cell carcinoma in situ (SCCIS), or Bowen disease, rarely involves the nipple[55] but can present with a pagetoid pattern, with isolated, clustered, and sheets of pale or clear atypical keratinocytes dispersed in the epidermis, usually on a background of more mature-appearing atypical keratinocytes. Contrary to Paget cells, the atypical pagetoid keratinocytes can show single cell keratinization, intercellular bridges and cytoplasmic keratohyalin granules. Frequently, other areas of the tumor will exhibit classic SCCIS. In difficult cases, immunophenotyping often resolves the issue, as the atypical keratinocytes usually are cytokeratin 7 and CAM 5.2 negative, and express high molecular weight-cytokeratins.[38] A so-called acantholytic anaplastic variant of PD may be particularly difficult to differentiate from acantholytic squamous cell carcinoma.[56–58] A battery of immunostains may be necessary to distinguish SCCIS from PD, because SCCIS, particularly the pagetoid variant, may express cytokeratin 7.[59]

Malignant melanoma should be considered in both the clinical and histopathologic differential diagnoses. Paget cells frequently incorporate melanin from adjacent epidermal cells, further complicating the histologic or cytologic picture.[60] However, primary malignant melanoma of the nipple is a rare disease that should not be diagnosed before thoroughly excluding the possibility of PD. Immunohistochemistry is helpful because Paget cells are usually Melan A negative and positive for cytokeratin 7, whereas melanoma cells would show the opposite immunophenotype. As mentioned, S100 protein is not useful in this differential diagnosis because some cases of PD may show positivity for this marker. A recent report of HMB45-positive PD should raise caution over false-positive results with this marker.[61] Concomitant use of another melanocytic marker, such as SOX10, should minimize diagnostic difficulty.

Other diagnoses rarely in the differential algorithm of a pagetoid histologic pattern involving the nipple include clear cell papulosis, sebaceous carcinoma, cutaneous T-cell lymphoma, and Langerhans cell histiocytosis.[23] Adequate histologic sampling and judicious use of immunohistochemistry usually suffice to arrive to the correct diagnosis.

Clinical Presentation

PD characteristically presents as an eczema- or psoriasis-like lesion of the nipple. In advanced cases, adjacent areola and surrounding skin may also be involved (Fig. 12.4). The latter finding is present in 25% to 98% of cases, depending on the series.[4,62–68] Rare cases of extensive skin involvement,[69] including spread beyond the breast to chest wall skin,[70] have been reported. PD also may present with nipple scaling, erythema, ulceration, hyperkeratosis, hyperpigmentation, induration, bloody discharge, crust, inversion, or distortion. New-onset nipple inversion can be present in up to 20% of cases, and nipple discharge has been reported in up to 36% of patients.[67] Symptoms are common, particularly nipple pruritus, pain, or burning sensation.[66] PD may represent tumor persistence or recurrence in patients with breast cancer treated with nipple-sparing mastectomy.[71] Rare cases may center in the

axilla, associated with underlying accessory mammary tissue.[72] Up to 40% of cases have a palpable mass on presentation, and some patients may present with enlarged axillary lymph nodes.[66] A case associated with surrounding ipsilateral eruptive seborrheic keratoses (Leser-Trelat sign) has been reported.[73] One case of pigmented PD presented as unilateral enlargement of the areola.[74] PD is reportedly asymptomatic in 22% to 67% of cases, depending on the series.[36,63–65,68] In these cases, the patient usually has undergone surgery for a clinically detected breast cancer, and histologic changes of PD are found in the resection specimen. Bilateral presentation is rare[35,75]; however, PD may present several years after a contralateral breast cancer.[76,77] To avoid misdiagnosis as delayed radiation dermatitis, it is important to keep in mind that initially occult PD may present with clinical abnormalities months or years after wide local excision or nipple-sparing mastectomy of ipsilateral breast carcinoma.[36,78]

Although the vast majority of cases are seen in female patients, PD of the male breast is occasionally encountered.[79–82] As in the female patient, PD in the male may be associated with an invasive carcinoma,[80] an in situ breast cancer,[81,83] or no underlying breast cancer.[82] A worse prognosis has been suggested for male cases,[79] although no large series exist that control for stage at presentation and diagnosis delay in this population.

Eczematous or other inflammatory dermatoses are necessarily in the differential diagnosis, such as atopic dermatitis, irritant or allergic contact dermatitis, and psoriasis.[54,84,85] In contrast with PD, atopic dermatitis, and often irritant or allergic contact dermatitis, usually presents with bilateral involvement. The differential diagnosis of a scaling, eczematous, or ulcerated lesion of the nipple also includes infections, such as candidiasis, tinea corporis (dermatophyte infection), or syphilis.[54,84–86] Various benign or malignant disorders rarely reported to present with PD-like involvement of nipple and/or areola include erosive nipple adenoma,[54,84,85] nevoid hyperkeratosis,[87] pemphigus vulgaris,[88] sebaceous carcinoma,[88,89] basal cell carcinoma,[90] Langerhans cell histiocytosis,[91] and pagetoid reticulosis–like T-cell lymphoma.[92] Skin changes associated with nipple reconstruction and tattooing may also mimic PD.[93]

A thorough clinical examination may be valuable in differentiating these conditions, because it may reveal systemic abnormalities or extramammary skin lesions that could orient the diagnosis. The finding of a palpable breast mass is an ominous sign that would point to the diagnosis of PD. Primary malignant melanoma of the nipple is rare, as stated, and in most reported cases, PD was a strong consideration in the differential diagnosis.[94,95] PD can mimic malignant melanoma, as pigmentation of Paget cells is common.[74,96–98]

Up to 20% of patients may have symptoms and/or signs of PD for more than a year before seeking medical attention.[4,75] Various factors contribute to a sometimes profound delay in diagnosis. In particular, patients or providers may conclude that the eczema-like appearance or symptoms of pruritus are due to inflammation of the nipple and empirically recommend treatment with topical steroids, which results in transient or sustained improvement in symptoms and/or appearance of the nipple. Indeed, treatment-associated or spontaneous apparent remission—so-called healed PD[78,99,100]—reinforces the false conclusion that the clinical abnormality is insignificant. Inflammatory dermatoses often are considered before PD, particularly when a breast abnormality is not detected by clinical examination or imaging studies. Furthermore, physicians often are reluctant to biopsy the nipple, usually due to the erroneous impression that such a seemingly minor problem

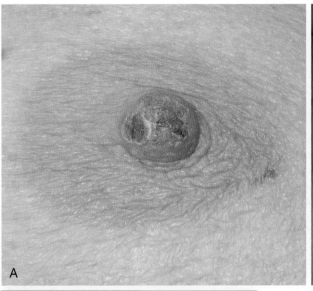

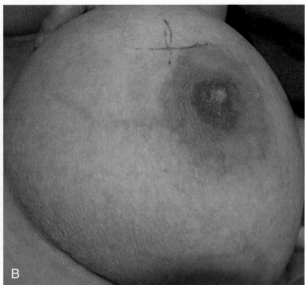

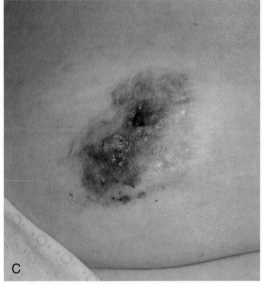

• **Fig. 12.4** Clinical presentation of Paget disease. (A) Early disease, with scaling, crusting, and eczema limited to the nipple. (B) More extensive disease, with eczema extending to the areola. (C) Advanced disease, with destruction of the nipple-areolar complex and extension into skin. ([B] Courtesy Dr. Doreen Agnese, MD, The Ohio State University.)

must be benign, mistaken concern that a carefully performed biopsy will result in nipple disfigurement or impair potential for lactation in a premenopausal woman, or that the patient is too young to have PD (despite reports of its occurrence in women during the third decade of life). Thus timely diagnosis of PD requires a low threshold for obtaining a biopsy: any unilateral nipple abnormality in an adult woman should be considered malignant until proven otherwise.

Clinicians have several options to obtain tissue for diagnosis of PD. Wedge biopsy of the skin and underlying breast tissue renders the most diagnostic material because this excisional specimen includes a well-represented epidermis and underlying lactiferous ducts. Punch biopsy may have a lower diagnostic yield because of its smaller size and the potentially discontinuous nature of Paget cells, but is a convenient, relatively high-yield option[101] for obtaining diagnostic tissue; the punch biopsy site usually heals with limited scarring or distortion of the nipple-areola. In addition, particularly when a larger (5- or 6-mm vs. 3- or 4-mm diameter) punch biopsy is obtained, the resultant tissue specimen may be deep enough to include a lactiferous gland containing the

associated DCIS. In the absence of an imaging abnormality that suggests an abnormality deep within or below the nipple, the narrow diameter of a core needle biopsy makes sampling error with this method more likely than with even a small punch biopsy. Shave biopsies offer breadth of epidermis, but superficial shaves may produce only nondiagnostic serosanguineous keratotic crust. Even when the specimen includes full-thickness epidermis, allowing for exclusion of PD, a superficial shave biopsy is insufficient to reveal an alternative abnormality involving the dermis, such as nipple adenoma. A saucerization-type shave biopsy, which produces a broad and deep tissue specimen, is associated with substantial risk of nipple disfigurement. Scraping or imprint of the nipple surface is an accessible noninvasive method for rapid diagnosis, although data on sensitivity and specificity of the technique are limited,[102–104] this method is likely unreliable because it yields even less material than superficial shave biopsies.

No single method is completely reliable for establishing a diagnosis of PD because most biopsies represent partial samples of the disorder. Any specimen may be false negative, particularly a narrow biopsy (such as a core needle or a 2- to 3-mm punch), a sample from an ulcerated or hyperkeratotic lesion, or those from symptomatic patients with limited or no visible abnormalities. In general, biopsy should be centered on the most clinically abnormal (e.g., most eczematous or indurated) portion of the nipple, except that biopsy of the edge rather than base of an ulcer is preferable because at least a portion of intact epidermis is needed for diagnosis. Additional biopsy is usually indicated when the first specimen fails to yield a specific diagnosis, and in all cases when most or all of the epidermis is absent. For such patients, particularly when clinical suspicion for PD is high and no specific diagnosis can be rendered on the initial biopsy, the second procedure should include a broader and deeper sample than the first (e.g., use of a punch rather than core needle biopsy, larger punch, or wedge incisional or excisional biopsy).

Radiologic Findings

Up to two-thirds of patients presenting with PD without a palpable breast mass have a normal mammogram at diagnosis. Among the remainder, approximately 60% will have findings limited to the nipple-areolar region (including nipple thickening or retraction, or a retroareolar mass or calcifications), and 40% will have a suspicious intraparenchymal breast mass or calcifications.[64,65,105–107] Although the sensitivity of mammography is as low as 34%, a positive mammogram is a relatively robust predictor of the extent of disease within the breast.[105,108] In contrast, more than 90% of patients presenting with a palpable mass in whom PD is detected will subsequently have an abnormal mammogram. Most patients with a normal mammogram and no clinical breast mass will have associated DCIS.[65] In Ikeda's series, invasive carcinoma was present in 5.5% of patients with a negative mammogram, 60% of patients with mammographic microcalcifications, and 82% of patients with a mammographic mass.[65] Zakaria and colleagues reported on 40 patients with PD, no clinical breast mass, and a negative mammogram; at operation, 5% had invasive cancer and 68% had DCIS that extended beyond the nipple.[107] In a more recent study by Morrogh and colleagues, 23 of 34 PD patients without a breast mass on physical examination had a negative mammogram.[105] At operation, 12 (52%) had DCIS, 4 (17%) had DCIS with microinvasion, 5 (22%) had invasive carcinoma, and 2 (8%) had no neoplasm other than the PD.

Ultrasound is recommended as an adjunct to mammography at diagnosis. It can confirm mammographic findings and facilitate diagnostic percutaneous needle biopsy of parenchymal masses. Ultrasound demonstrates a primary breast tumor in up to 67% of cases and can identify unsuspected multifocal disease,[64,109] including in patients with negative mammography. The most frequent sonographic finding is a hypoechoic mass, although more subtle changes such as parenchymal heterogeneity or hypoechoicity may be seen. Changes of the nipple-areola complex, notably skin thickening, are frequently delineated by ultrasound.[110]

Magnetic resonance imaging (MRI) is increasingly recommended particularly in cases without a finding on clinical examination, mammogram, or ultrasound.[62,105] MRI may reveal thickening and enhancement of the nipple-areolar complex, best reported compared with the contralateral side, and may detect underlying parenchymal disease not otherwise evident. In the series of Frei and associates, eight of nine cases of PD with underlying DCIS were associated with abnormal findings on MRI.[111] In the report of Morrogh and colleagues, 7 of 12 cancers (1 invasive, 4 DCIS, 2 DCIS with microinvasion) found at operation were identified on preoperative breast MRI, a sensitivity of 54%.[105] Siponen and colleagues reported on findings from 14 MRI examinations performed for PD and found a sensitivity of 100% for detection of invasive cancer and 44% for detection of DCIS.[112] MRI may be particularly useful to establish extent and centricity of disease in patients for whom breast conserving surgery is being contemplated.[105,108,111]

Management

Historically, PD has been treated with modified radical mastectomy (total mastectomy with axillary dissection).[34,113] Although this is in part a reflection of the historical management of breast cancer, the strong association of PD with underlying DCIS or invasive cancer, its relative rarity, its multicentricity in 20% to 80% of cases[67,108] and esthetic concerns with central lumpectomy and nipple-areolar complex removal, have all been reasons for slow adoption of breast conservation and sentinel node surgery for patients presenting with PD. Breast conservation for PD was first described in 1984 by Lagios and colleagues,[114] who reported partial or complete nipple-areolar complex excision in five patients with no associated mass or imaging abnormality and observed one recurrence in the retained areola at 12 months. Marshall and associates published 15-year results of partial or complete nipple-areolar resection followed by radiotherapy for 36 PD patients, reporting a 17% local recurrence rate.[115] These data support complete resection of the nipple-areolar complex along with all visible disease with a margin of normal-appearing skin and pathologic confirmation of negative margins to maximize local disease control. Pierce and colleagues reported their experience with 30 cases from several collaborative institutions treated with local surgery and radiotherapy.[116] Of these, 29 had noninvasive disease. They found 5- and 8-year local recurrence rates of 9% and 16%, respectively, rates very similar to those reported for DCIS treated with radiotherapy in other parts of the breast. Seven years later, this group updated their data to report recurrence rates at 10- and 15-year posttreatment, which were 17% and 24%, respectively, and a 5-, 10-, and 15-year disease-free survival of 97%, 93%, and 93%, respectively.[115]

The European Organization for Research and Treatment of Cancer 10871 trial is the only published prospective study of breast conserving surgery for PD. Of 61 patients with PD and DCIS (invasive cancers were excluded) treated with breast conserving surgery and radiotherapy, 5.2% showed a local recurrence at 5 years.[115] In all patients in this study, margins were required to be confirmed free by histologic analysis after surgery. Singh and associates reported similar outcome in patients treated with mastectomy and patients treated with breast conserving surgery.[117] Similarly, Kawase and colleagues reported no significant differences in overall, disease-specific, or recurrence-free survival between patients with PD treated with mastectomy and breast conserving surgery.[118] Joseph and coworkers also reported no difference in overall recurrence and mortality rates between patients treated with breast conservation and mastectomy.[119]

Radiotherapy, however, is indicated as adjuvant therapy in cases treated with breast conserving surgery to ensure adequate local control rates. Dixon and colleagues reported that 4 of 10 patients treated with cone excision of the nipple-areola complex and subjacent breast tissue without postoperative radiotherapy had local recurrences, with 2 patients eventually developing metastatic disease.[99] More recently, Polgar reported on 33 patients treated with cone excision without radiotherapy. The local recurrence rate was 33.3%, a much higher rate than that reported in series where adjuvant radiotherapy was used.[120] Despite the data suggesting that breast conserving surgery plus radiotherapy is an effective method of treating PD, mastectomy continues to be the most popular method of treatment. In a SEER study of 1642 women with PD who underwent surgery between 1988 and 2002,[3] 18% underwent central lumpectomy and 82% underwent mastectomy. Eighty-four percent of women with PD and invasive tumors smaller than 2 cm that were centrally located underwent mastectomy rather than central lumpectomy, compared with 52% of patients without PD that had similarly centrally localized, small tumors. Similarly, 64% of centrally localized DCIS associated with PD underwent mastectomy, compared with 37% of patients with centrally localized DCIS without PD during this same period. These data suggest a significant bias to perform mastectomy in PD, even in presence of tumors that would likely be managed with breast conservation had they not presented with PD. In this analysis, the 15-year breast cancer specific survival rate was 92% and 94% for patients who underwent central lumpectomy and mastectomy, respectively, for PD associated with noninvasive tumors. Similarly, the 15-year breast cancer–specific survival rates were 87% for patients who underwent central lumpectomy and 60% for patients who underwent mastectomy among those patients who had PD with an underlying invasive tumor. A more recent report on PD cases in the SEER registry treated between 2000 and 2011 identified that only 23% of the 2631 study patients had breast conserving surgery.[121] In addition, less than half of these patients had adjuvant radiotherapy, raising concerns about undertreatment. Even in this relatively modern patient cohort, modified radical mastectomy remained the initial surgical procedure in 43% of women, and total mastectomy was performed in another 35%. Onoe and colleagues evaluated feasibility of breast conserving surgery in their cohort of 59 women treated with mastectomy for PD. Histopathology revealed that the 55 underlying neoplasms were within 4 cm of the nipple-areolar complex in 85% of patients.[106] For women who are candidates for breast conservation, nipple reconstruction or tattooing can be performed after the initial surgery and adjuvant radiotherapy, as can contralateral mastopexy for symmetry. Discussion of these options with patients is advisable.

Evaluation of the axilla in patients with PD is recommended for all patients with underlying invasive cancer and selectively for patients with DCIS, such as when mastectomy is performed, invasive disease is suspected, or when a second operation is highly undesirable. Three studies have reported sentinel lymph node (SLN) biopsy specifically in patients with PD. Sukumvanich and associates studied a cohort of patients with PD, which they divided into those presenting as PD alone (only nipple skin changes) versus those presenting as PD with associated findings (skin changes plus palpable mass or imaging abnormality). Their success rate for SLN identification was 98%, with a mean number of SLN removed of three. In the first group, 27% of patients had invasive ductal carcinoma, despite the absence of associated findings; in 11% of these cases, the SLN contained metastatic carcinoma.[122] Laronga and colleagues studied 54 patients with PD, 36 who were managed with SLN biopsy. In four of five patients with metastatic carcinoma, the metasasis was detected through SLN biopsy. In three of these, the SLN was the only lymph node positive for tumor, suggesting that SLN biopsy is an accurate technique in this setting.[123] Siponen and associates performed SLN surgery for PD patients from 2002 onward and reported no positive SLN in 6 patients with PD and DCIS undergoing SLN surgery, whereas 5 of 12 patients with PD and underlying invasive

cancer were SLN-positive[112]; four underwent axillary dissection (omitted in the fifth patient who was 95 years of age), and all had additional positive axillary nodes. Thus the limited published data confirm the appropriateness of SLN surgery for PD patients with a clinically negative axilla and suggest it should be used in accordance with guidelines established for usual breast cancer. Despite the widespread adoption of SLN surgery for breast cancer, 40% of lymph node negative patients with PD treated in 2011 in the recent SEER study had axillary dissection as their primary surgery.[121] The role of SLN biopsy in patients with invasive PD (see definition earlier in chapter) with no associated invasive breast neoplasm is still unclear. Although most cases reported have been node-negative, reports of metastatic disease (one case with isolated tumor cells[45] and another one with macrometastases[48]) suggest axillary evaluation with SLN biopsy is reasonable. However, the small number of cases of this uncommon scenario precludes solid conclusions.

Among the more than 90% of PD patients who have an underlying breast neoplasm, approximately 35% to 75% have an underlying invasive cancer.[107,108,121] The invasive cancers associated with PD tend to be more aggressive tumors, frequently high grade (25%–52%),[124,125] ER-negative (41%–71%),[5,124–126] and HER2-positive (39%–82%).[5,124–126] Such tumors, especially when identified as lymph node–positive by axillary ultrasound and fine-needle aspiration (FNA) of a suspicious lymph node at the time of diagnosis, are amenable to treatment with neoadjuvant chemotherapy, but there are no data on this approach in patients with PD. The use of neoadjuvant chemotherapy might downstage both the breast and axilla, permitting more patients to be candidates for breast conservation and SLN surgery.

On the basis of the preceding data, our approach to the patient presenting with nipple-areolar changes and biopsy-proven PD is evaluation with clinical examination of the breast and axilla and radiologic evaluation with mammography and ultrasound. Abnormalities within the breast should undergo image-guided percutaneous needle biopsy, and ultrasound-guided FNA should be done when suspicious axillary lymph nodes are identified. We perform breast MRI selectively, most often for patients with no breast masses and negative conventional imaging. Surgical treatment recommendations are then formulated and patients can be selected for breast conservation, mastectomy with or without immediate breast reconstruction, or either approach and axillary surgery tailored to clinical nodal status. Patients with underlying invasive breast cancer may be offered neoadjuvant systemic therapy based on the approximated biological subtype of the tumor and clinical stage. We treat PD without underlying DCIS or invasive cancer with either wide local excision or mastectomy and SLN surgery, with axillary lymph node dissection limited to patients with pathologically confirmed nodal metastasis.

Prognosis

Prognosis in PD is largely determined by the underlying breast tumor, and it is well known that such tumors are typically of high histopathologic grade. Relatively few data exist on outcome of PD without an underlying breast carcinoma. In the SEER data report mentioned earlier, the 15-year cancer-specific survival for PD without underlying tumors was 88%, compared with 94% for PD associated only with DCIS, and 61% for PD associated with invasive ductal carcinoma.[3] In the same series, patients with PD were more likely to have histologically high-grade tumors, positive lymph nodes, negative ER status, and negative PR status, but only size of tumor and lymph node status were independent prognostic factors for survival on multivariate analysis.[3] Similarly, in Kothari's series, 60% of underlying invasive tumors were histologic grade III, 96.5% of the in situ tumors were high grade, and HER2 overexpression was present in 82.5% and 96.5 of invasive and in situ tumors, respectively.[67] These findings are not unexpected, considering the pivotal role that HER2 may have in the pathogenesis of PD.[9] Whether the development of PD itself changes the prognostic impact of the underlying breast tumor remains controversial. In the same series,[67] PD patients did not have overall survival rates different from controls, when matched for age, tumor size, grade, nodal status, and HER2 status. On the contrary, both Ortiz-Pagan and colleagues and Ling and associates found significant differences in survival between cases with and without PD, even when controlling for tumor size, lymph node status, hormone receptor status, and HER2 status,[125,126] suggesting that additional, as-yet-unidentified factors that favor development of PD may affect tumor behavior and prognosis. Differences in survival based on the presence or absence of a palpable mass may be explained by the fact that patients without a palpable mass are more likely to bear noninvasive tumors, compared with patients with a palpable mass, who mostly have underlying invasive tumors.[68,107] In one study, patients who presented without a palpable mass had a 5-year overall survival of 94%; 73% of these patients had only DCIS with no invasive component, and 84% had N0 nodal status. In contrast, patients who presented with a palpable mass had a 19% 5-year overall survival; 8% of such patients had only DCIS with no invasive component, and 50% were pathologically node-positive.[68]

Selected References

3. Chen CY, Sun LM, Anderson BO. Paget disease of the breast: changing patterns of incidence, clinical presentation, and treatment in the U.S. *Cancer*. 2006;107:1448-1458.

9. Schelfhout VR, Coene ED, Delaey B, et al. Pathogenesis of Paget's disease: epidermal heregulin-alpha, motility factor, and the HER receptor family. *J Natl Cancer Inst*. 2000;92:622-628.

45. Duan X, Sneige N, Gullett AE, et al. Invasive paget disease of the breast: clinicopathologic study of an underrecognized entity in the breast. *Am J Surg Pathol*. 2012;36:1353-1358.

64. Gunhan-Bilgen I, Oktay A. Paget's disease of the breast: clinical, mammographic, sonographic and pathologic findings in 52 cases. *Eur J Radiol*. 2006;60:256-263.

115. Marshall JK, Griffith KA, Haffty BG, et al. Conservative management of Paget disease of the breast with radiotherapy: 10- and 15-year results. *Cancer*. 2003;97:2142-2149.

A full reference list is available online at ExpertConsult.com.

13

Primary and Secondary Dermatologic Disorders of the Breast

RYAN J. CARR, STEPHEN M. SMITH, AND SARA B. PETERS

The skin of the breast consists of keratinizing stratified squamous epithelium overlying a thick fibrocollagenous dermis containing vascular and lymphatic vessels, adnexal structures, and the suspensory ligaments of Cooper. Adnexal structures, including hair follicles, apocrine and eccrine glands, and cutaneous nerves, reside within the dermis. The subcutaneous fatty tissue that constitutes the majority of the breast envelops the mammary ducts and glands, which physiologically proliferate as a result of hormonal influences, particularly at puberty and during pregnancy. The terminal ductal lobular unit, from which the vast majority of epithelial carcinoma and carcinoma in situ arises, comprises both lactiferous ducts of variable calibers and epithelial secretory lobules. The ducts are supported by a dual layer of epithelial cells, and the lobules are composed of a luminal lining of epithelial cells and a supportive layer of myoepithelial cells. Terminal ductal lobular units are supported by variable degrees of subcutaneous fibrous and adipose tissue and undergo secretory changes under normal physiologic circumstances.

The highly specialized skin of the nipple has a papillomatous surface and numerous openings for terminal lactiferous ducts, sebaceous glands, and apocrine glands. Areolar skin demonstrates similar histology but shows occasional vellus or terminal hairs as well as prominent sebaceous gland units associated with lactiferous ducts in the dermis (i.e., Montgomery tubercles). The mammary glands connect to lactiferous ducts and produce milk-like substances and colostrum; these glands are under hormonal influences.[1,2]

Numerous dermal diseases, including congenital anomalies, benign and malignant neoplasms and manifestations of various dermatoses, may involve the skin of the breast. These disorders may involve the breast solely or the breast may be involved as a result of a systemic dermatosis. In reviewing a dermatologic disorder of the breast, one useful approach is to divide these diverse entities into those primary diseases that are specific, nearly specific, or common for the skin of the breast and those secondary disorders that predominantly affect other dermatologic areas of the body but affect the breast incidentally or less commonly. The decision to classify a cutaneous disease of the breast as primary versus secondary may prove difficult and, at times, is best left unstated. Both types of dermatologic disorders may also mimic primary or secondary diseases of the breast parenchyma. For all these reasons, it is important for both the breast generalist as well as the breast specialist to be versed in these primary and secondary dermatologic disorders of the breast.

Primary Breast Dermatologic Disorders

Primary Congenital and Developmental Disorders

Amastia and Athelia

Amastia and athelia represent exquisitely rare conditions in which normal development of either breast or only nipple and areolar tissue do not occur.[3] This does not represent an involutional phenomenon. Development of the embryologic mammary ridge (i.e., milk line), which generally extends from the bilateral axillary tails to the inguinal region, fails to occur. In the case of amastia, there is often evidence of associated ectodermal defects such as cleft palate, isolated pectoral muscle, and upper limb deformities or urologic abnormalities.

Hypoplasia and Associated Conditions

Hypoplasia (or hypomastia), defined as breast size of 200 mg (mL) or less in an adult female, represents a significant decrease in size of breast tissue relative to standard breast size adjusted for age and developmental status. Hypoplasia of mammary tissue may be unilateral or bilateral. Specifically, bilateral hypoplasia of the breast may occur in Turner (XO) syndrome and unilateral hypoplasia has been described in association with the Poland anomaly and anterior thoracic hypoplasia.[4,5] Congenital mammary hypoplasia occurs in utero and has a high association with ipsilateral pectoral muscle hypoplasia. It may also occur as part of a constellation of findings in anterior thoracic hypoplasia syndrome. Acquired mammary hypoplasia may be associated with a number of conditions and comorbidities, including, but not limited to, human immunodeficiency virus (HIV) infection, anorexia nervosa, mitral valve prolapse, and tuberculosis.[6] Unilateral or bilateral acquired hypoplasia may also be associated with high-dose irradiation to the chest and mammary structures, and degree of hypoplasia have been correlated with the dosage of irradiation.[7] Morphea (localized scleroderma) of the chest wall in a prepubertal child may lead to deformity and hypoplasia of the breast in later years.[8] Other congenital neural syndromes may be associated with breast hypoplasia.[9–12]

Rudimentary (absent or maldeveloped) nipples may be present as an isolated congenital defect or as a component of syndromes, such as the scalp-ear-nipple (SEN) syndrome, ectodermal dysplasia complex, or Al-Awadi/Rass-Rothschild/Schinzel phocomelia syndromes.[13–16] Cutaneous manifestations may include aplasia cutis congenital of the scalp, protuberant cupped or folded external ears, and sparse axillary hair; however, variable manifestations are common.

Hyperplasias, Hamartomas and Associated Conditions

Hyperplasia or macromastia refers to inappropriate and excessive growth of mammary tissue. Hyperplasia may occur in a number of settings and may be physiologic (e.g., adolescence, pregnancy), pathologic (e.g., related to neoplasia or malignancy), iatrogenic (e.g., secondary to medications), or idiopathic. Macromastia during adolescence typically occurs secondary to hormonal influences, is usually bilateral and symmetric, and can occasionally be massive (up to 10 kg per breast).[17] The breast may show increased stromal density as a result, with variable degrees of increased dermal collagen and fibrosis. Concomitant pseudoangiomatous stromal hyperplasia may be present and demonstrates pseudovascular spaces in a dense collagenous stroma.[18] Hyperplasia gravidarum (gravid gigantomastia) is a rare complication of pregnancy that occurs secondary to hormonal surges and occurs most often in primigravid individuals, although it is likely to recur in subsequent pregnancies.[19] Iatrogenic causes of hyperplasia often involves medications, such as penicillamine, indinavir, cyclosporine, and various antibiotics subclasses; however, isolated cases of palpation or manipulation macromastia have been documented. Iatrogenic causes may manifest as either unilateral or bilateral breast enlargement and medications are only marginally effective in reducing hyperplasia when attempted.[20,21]

Polythelia (supernumerary nipples) (Fig. 13.1) and polymastia (supernumerary breasts) develop along embryonic mammary lines, from the axillary vaults to the inguinal regions bilaterally. Specifically, polythelia represents the most common anomaly of mammary tissue in both males and females. Polythelia is present in up to 2.1% to 3.7% of individuals and greater than 90% of cases are present in the inframammary region.[22] Accessory nipples require no treatment unless the nipple causes irritation or is excised for cosmetic reasons. Notably, vulvar lesions that previously were termed supernumerary nipples actually represent adenomas of vulvar apocrine gland derivation. Supernumerary breast tissue predominantly occurs in women and often takes the form of insignificant, gently raised, pigmented papules and most commonly is found in the left axillary and inframammary regions.[23,24] Clinically they may be mistaken for acrochordon, nevi, "birthmarks," dermatoses, or fibromas by the novice observer. Histologically, these supernumerary structures may consist of the nipple, areola, glandular tissue, or any combination of these. Microscopic sections of accessory mammary tissue are similar to those of normal mammary tissue. The epidermis may display acanthosis with undulating papillomatosis and basal layer hyperpigmentation. In the dermis, smooth muscle bundles, mammary glands, and lactiferous ducts are seen in conventional configurations.

Becker nevus (pigmented hairy epidermal nevus) represents a hamartoma of pigmented epidermis, terminal differentiated hairs and arrector pili muscles that usually occurs on the chest, shoulder, upper back, and/or upper arm. It is an androgen-dependent lesion that occurs most frequently in males in the second and third decades. It is associated with abnormalities of the underlying musculoskeletal system, including spina bifida, scoliosis, localized lipoatrophy, and hypoplasia of the pectoralis muscle, which can lead to hypoplasia or compensatory hyperplasia of the breast. The rare familial syndrome of hereditary acrolabial telangiectasia, a type of hamartoma, consists of an extensive network of superficial, thin-walled vessels and variable proliferation of vessels in the deeper soft tissues.[15] These superficial vessels impart a bluish hue to the lips, areolas, nipples, and nail beds, which may be mistaken for cyanosis at birth. Varicose veins and migraine headaches may develop in adulthood. No serious vascular or coagulative sequelae have been reported in these cases.[15]

Benign and malignant neoplasms, described later in this chapter, can uncommonly involve accessory or supernumerary tissues like the breast proper. In a study from Japan, benign adnexal polyps of the areola were reported to involve 4% of neonates. These small (1-mm), firm, pink papules contain hair follicles, eccrine glands, and vestigial sebaceous glands. Most wither rapidly and fall off shortly after birth.[25]

Gynecomastia

Gynecomastia occurs in males and refers to inappropriate enlargement of the breasts. Myriad medications and exogenous substances have been associated with gynecomastia, most notably a broad range of estrogens, antiandrogens, antituberculosis medications, proton pump inhibitors, antipsychotics, antidepressants, antihypertensives, and antiretroviral therapy for patients with HIV.[26–28] Approximately 40% to 50% of men with diagnosed prostate cancer develop gynecomastia as a result of treatment and hormonal dysregulation.[29] It may occur after chemotherapy or radiation therapy for visceral malignancies or after bone marrow transplantation for hematopoietic malignancies. Traumatic gynecomastia may occur after an isolated injury to the torso or as an iatrogenic phenomenon, most notably after thoracotomy.[30] Gynecomastia alone is not associated with an increased risk of malignant transformation. Klinefelter syndrome (XXY syndrome) is associated with the development of gynecomastia; there is a slight but significant risk of breast cancer in these patients, particularly the luminal A and B subtypes.[31,32] Gynecomastia is discussed in detail in Chapter 7.

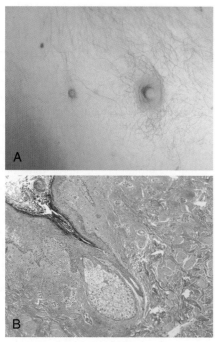

• **Fig. 13.1** (A) Accessory nipple is observed inferior to main nipple. (B) Histologically the accessory nipple may consist of a ductal orifice as well as areolar-type smooth muscle fascicles.

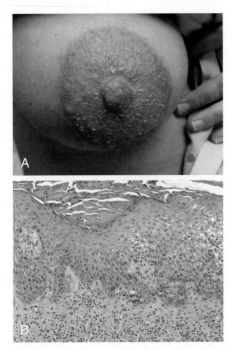

• **Fig. 13.2** (A) Nipple eczema can mimic the appearance of contact dermatitis, as well as Paget's disease or Bowen disease. (B) Histologically, epidermal hyperproliferation and spongiosis is observed together with a lymphocytic infiltrate.

The histologic appearance of gynecomastia transitions from an early active phase into an inactive quiescent phase during the traditional chronology of this disorder. In the active phase, there is ductal proliferation and hyperplasia of stromal parenchyma accompanied by a periductal or diffuse mixed lymphoplasmacytic and mononuclear infiltrate. The ducts may develop papillary and cribriform patterns with a prominent myoepithelial layer. As the lesion develops, the inactive phase is attained; this phase is characterized by ductal epithelial atrophy and stromal fibrosis.

Primary Inflammatory Disorders

Dermatoses of the Nipple and Breast

Eczematous Dermatitis (Nummular Eczema). Eczematous dermatitis (nummular eczema or eczema) (Fig. 13.2) of the nipple clinically presents as ill-defined, erythematous, scaly patches or plaques that may demonstrate total and partial lichenification or excoriation due to associated irritation and pruritus. Bilateral involvement is common. Eczema of the breast or nipple may present as erythema, scale, crusting, fissures, vesicles, erosions, or lichenification.[33,34] Nummular eczema may also present as single or multiple erythematous, slightly raised plaques with fine to moderate scale, slight oozing, and extreme pruritus. Involvement of the nipple may mimic Paget's disease, squamous cell carcinoma in situ (i.e., Bowen disease), and myriad inflammatory or infectious etiologies. Nipple eczema is the most common presentation of atopic dermatitis of the breast and has been considered a minor criterion in the diagnosis of atopic dermatitis.[35–38] At present, it is not included in the diagnostic major criteria for atopic dermatitis[36]; however, it represents an important diagnostic feature, particularly during prepubertal years and periods of breastfeeding.[39,40] All of these disorders typically present as a scaly erythematous, often pruritic nipple-areola complex (Box 13.1).

Eczematous involvement localized to a mastectomy scar may also raise suspicion of breast carcinoma recurrence.

A biopsy specimen of eczema typically shows spongiotic dermatitis with a mixed dermal perivascular and/or interstitial inflammatory infiltrates composed of variable proportions of lymphocytes and histiocytes with occasional eosinophils and neutrophils (see Fig. 13.2B). During an acute flare, the predominant histologic finding is spongiosis that may coalesce to produce microvesicles, vesicles or bullae. Neutrophilic microabscesses in the stratum corneum and focal parakeratosis, along with serum and scale crust, can be observed as lesions become irritated and/or impetiginized. As the lesion progresses, the degree of spongiosis and inflammation recedes and epidermal hyperplasia becomes more prominent, manifesting as either regular psoriasiform hyperplasia or changes consistent with lichen simplex chronicus. Chronic lesions may demonstrate persistent mild patchy lymphocytic inflammation in addition to changes such as dermal fibrosis, pigment incontinence and/or epidermal atrophy. The differential diagnosis includes allergic contact dermatitis,[41–43] irritant contact dermatitis,[44] lichen simplex chronicus, infection with *Candida* spp.[40] and Paget's disease.[45] Nummular eczema may be difficult to distinguish from chronic allergic contact dermatitis; patch testing may prove helpful in identification of an offending allergen. Finally, *Sarcoptes scabiei* mites can directly infest the nipple, areola, and inframammary creases to produce characteristic linear lesions produced by mite burrows. Patients present with extreme pruritus and excoriation secondary to the presence of the mites and/or scybala in the stratum corneum. Manual unroofing of burrow sites during clinical visits allow for scrapings to be produced for microscopy, which will reveal the organism, its eggs, and/or feces. Topical scabicides typically eradicate the mites after multiple applications.

Allergic Contact Dermatitis. Allergic contact dermatitis (Fig. 13.3) is a less common type of dermatitis but should be considered in all cases with appropriate signs and symptoms. Contact dermatitis in the area of the breast and nipple most often results from nickel allergy, and the lesions appear under bra straps and hooks in the shape of the offending metal part. Other common causes of contact dermatitis include topical medications, perfumes, latex, and airborne allergens.[46] Contact dermatitis to lanolin, beeswax emollients, chamomile ointments, and nail polish has been reported.[39,41,42] A careful history of environmental exposures and the use of patch testing usually identifies an offending agent or collection of agents. Histologic examination

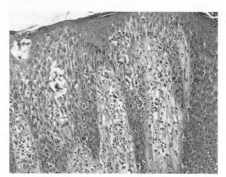

• **Fig. 13.3** Allergic contact dermatitis. Allergic contact dermatitis of the nipple can mimic nipple eczema histologically but shows more spongiosis and more eosinophilic infiltrate.

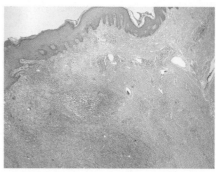

• **Fig. 13.4** Subareolar abscess. The subareolar region is susceptible to abscess formation, sometimes mimicking the appearance of infiltrating carcinoma.

characteristically shows spongiotic dermatitis with eosinophils (see Fig. 13.3). Flask-shaped collections of Langerhans cells, which often open up onto the skin surface, are common findings. Changes resulting from chronic irritation (i.e., lichen simplex chronicus) may also be present histologically if the exposure is long-standing.

Irritant Contact Dermatitis. Irritant contact dermatitis of the nipple (e.g., jogger's nipple, runner's nipple) or breast develops most commonly in physically active adults and occurs secondary to friction with clothing. Treatment of irritant contact dermatitis is tailored to cause and generally consists of gentle cleansers, moisturizers, and topical corticosteroids as needed for symptomatic relief.[47–50] Relief may also be achieved by wearing soft, nonabrasive clothing or applying adhesive tape to protect the nipples. Topical calcineurin inhibitors may be used for maintenance therapy in difficult cases.[48,49] Identification and subsequent avoidance of the triggering factor is the treatment of choice. The most important clinical and diagnostic issue with respect to nipple dermatitis is discerning this benign reactive entity from Paget's disease of the nipple. If a case of suspected nipple dermatitis does not resolve with topical therapy, the diagnosis of Paget's disease should be more seriously entertained. A biopsy may prove necessary for definitive diagnosis in these cases. Histologic features include eosinophilic spongiotic dermatitis with or without a superficial dermal inflammatory infiltrate. Flask-shaped collections of Langerhans cells, which often open up onto the skin surface, are common findings. Abnormal findings, such as nests of melanocytes or malignant epithelial cells, Pagetoid spread of atypical cells, full-thickness epithelial atypia, or tumor formation, are invariably absent.

Dermatoses and Inflammatory Conditions Involving the Dermis

A wide range of reactive and inflammatory conditions can involve the dermal mammary tissue. Their importance cannot be understated not only because of their capacity to cause concern and discomfort for patients but also their ability to simulate neoplastic and malignant conditions on clinical examination and radiography. Benign conditions account for the majority of breast biopsies in the United States, with reactive and inflammatory conditions representing the majority of these nonneoplastic biopsy specimens. An understanding of these reactive and inflammatory conditions will aid in avoiding misdiagnosis and preventing unnecessary treatment.

Mammary Duct Ectasia. Duct ectasia may occasionally be identified in skin biopsies and consists of superficial lactiferous ducts in mammary tissue. Currently, it is hypothesized that duct ectasia results from obstruction of ducts with secondary inflammatory reaction to the stagnant contents. Superimposed changes consistent with ductal rupture are often concomitantly present. Histologically, there is ectasia of medium- to large-sized lactiferous ducts with accumulation of amphophilic secretory material and macrophages in the lumen and fibroelastic thickening of the duct wall. External concentric fibrosis may be seen in subacute or chronic lesions, and eccentric fibrosis, epithelial denudation, and/or fibrous obliteration of the duct may highlight an area of previous rupture and repair. A particularly helpful histologic feature may include the presence of cholesterol crystals in the periductal infiltrate. Mammary duct ectasia can be found in association with fibrocystic diseases; however, these two entities are not thought to be pathogenetically related.[51,52]

Radiation Dermatitis. Multiple manifestations of radiation dermatitis can involve the skin of the breast. The first and most common type is erythema with fine scales that develops during the course of radiotherapy. The patient is typically uncomfortable, but the course is self-limited and generally can be managed with soothing topical treatments; however, in some cases, scarring, atrophy, telangiectasia, and scaling may become superimposed on prior sites affected by radiation therapy. This form of radiodermatitis is rare but chronic and may progress to tissue necrosis, ulceration, and de novo cutaneous malignancies (most commonly squamous cell carcinoma or basal cell carcinoma). Patients with a clinical history of prior radiation therapy may develop radiation recall dermatitis when exposed to subsequent chemotherapy agents. Radiation recall dermatitis often presents as a painful, erythematous maculopapular rash directly overlying or in close approximation to a previous site of irradiation.[53–57] Vitiligo has also been reported after radiotherapy as well.[58]

Hidradenitis Suppurativa. Hidradenitis suppurativa is a congenital state where the apocrine glands do not undergo normal apoptosis and histologically shows a florid mixed inflammatory infiltrate extending deep into dermal tissue usually predominates. In active lesions, collections of abscesses are noted, along with follicular plugging and sinus tract formation. During the course of healing and wound contraction, granulation tissue, broken hair shafts, keratin debris, and ensuing foreign-body giant cell reaction may be evident. Chronic lesions commonly demonstrate extensive scarring and fibrosis along with eradication of normal adnexal structures.

Subareolar Abscess. Repeated or chronic abscess formation (Fig. 13.4) in the subareolar region results in squamous metaplasia of the terminal ends of lactiferous ducts, further sequestering and

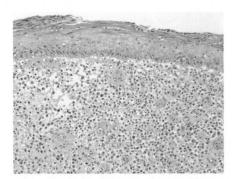

• **Fig. 13.5** Fat necrosis. In the breast, fat necrosis characterized by foamy macrophages and fat digestion can be an insidious and progressive lesion.

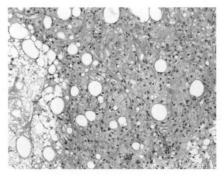

• **Fig. 13.6** Mastitis. This example of mastitis was infectious in nature and caused by *Staphylococcus aureus*.

propagating abscess pockets. The clinical presentation and treatment is discussed in detail in Chapter 6.

Ruptured Epidermal Inclusion Cyst. A ruptured epidermal inclusion cyst can be characterized by intense inflammation and abscess formation, most commonly in subareolar tissue. A ruptured cyst can mimic the superficial appearance of infiltrative carcinomas on physical examination.

Dermatoses and Inflammatory Conditions Involving the Subcutaneous Tissue

Fat Necrosis. Fat necrosis presenting as a palpable mass may raise serious concern for clinicians and patients alike. Clinically significant fat necrosis arising in superficial subcutaneous tissue is most commonly secondary to trauma (Fig. 13.5). Fat necrosis is a benign nonsuppurative inflammatory disease of adipose tissue that was initially described in the breast in 1920.[59,60] It is a sterile process resulting from aseptic saponification of fat by means of blood and tissue lipase. The incidence is estimated to be 0.6% in the breast, representing up to 2.75% of all benign lesions.[59–63] It is found incidentally accompanying 0.8% of breast tumors and 1% of cases of surgical breast reduction.[64] The average age of patients at presentation is 50 years.[62,63] Causes are variable and include trauma,[59,60,62,63] radiotherapy,[61,65,66] anticoagulation therapy (e.g., warfarin administration),[67] cyst aspiration, biopsy, lumpectomy, reduction mammoplasty, implant removal, breast reconstruction with tissue transfer,[68] duct ectasia,[52] and breast infection. Less common causes include polyarteritis nodosa and granulomatous angiopanniculitis. In a significant number of patients, the cause is designated as idiopathic.[61,69]

Fat necrosis can present as a mass on palpation and either as a hyper- or hypoechoic area on ultrasound imaging. Clinically, therefore, it can mimic the appearance of invasive carcinoma. It is obviously important to distinguish fat necrosis from invasive carcinoma, and thus biopsy may be warranted. Core biopsy of breast lesions has been shown to be more sensitive than fine-needle aspiration.[70] Ironically, one of the side effects of biopsy is iatrogenic fat necrosis, which contributes to an additional enlarging mass. Unfortunately, some patients experience biopsy after biopsy only to reveal a diagnosis of ongoing or recrudescent fat necrosis.

Fat necrosis is recognized histologically by lipid-engorged macrophages and foreign-body giant cells surrounded by an interstitial inflammatory infiltrate composed of plasma cells and lymphocytes. Apoptosis and necrosis prevail in adipose lobules. Healing occurs by fibrosis, which begins at the periphery of the cyst-like areas. Depending on the degree of fibrosis, these areas are either replaced completely by fibrous tissue or remain as cavities.[68] Calcification may occur in the area of fibrosis and represents a relatively late finding. Clinical presentations range from an incidental benign lesion to a mass lesion.[64,71] In most instances, fat necrosis is clinically occult; however, it may present as a single or multiple smooth, round, firm nodules or irregular masses and can also be associated with overlying cutaneous ecchymosis, erythema, inflammation, pain, retraction or thickening, nipple retraction, and lymphadenopathy.[64,68,72–74]

Panniculitis. Panniculitis (inflammation of the subcutaneous tissue) may be encountered in the breast secondary to many different causes. Autoimmune phenomena may uncommonly produce lobular panniculitides, such as lupus profundus in patients with established or evolving systemic lupus erythematosus.[75] Ruptured or bleeding breast implants may cause extensive or generalized panniculitis that may extend beyond the confines of the breast, an important clinical sign. Silicone granulomas appear as painful, irregularly shaped lumps or plaques in patients who have received injections of free silicone or whose silicone implants have ruptured.[76] Microscopic examination of this tissue shows a characteristic "Swiss cheese" granulomatous inflammatory pattern where the silicone has dissolved from multinucleated giant cells and extracellular areas during histologic processing.

Factitial panniculitis may arise from mechanical injury to the breast or from repetitive attempts at self-injurious behavior by the patient.[77] Possible presentations may mimic virtually any dermatosis and include excoriation, ulceration, puncture wounds and embedded foreign bodies, eczema, vesiculobullous lesions, and nipple discharge. Factitial disease should be considered when an unusual pattern or presentation is not consistent with established clinicopathologic entities or when the patient exhibits an unusual or strange affect or response to the problem. Careful clinical evaluation with mammography and biopsy, if necessary, should be taken to rule out primary organic disease of the breast. Documented practices that may unfortunately result in panniculitis include acupuncture and cupping.[78,79] Psychiatric evaluation is recommended in cases of suspected self-injurious factitious panniculitis.

Mastitis. Mastitis is defined as inflammation of the breast, irrespective of cause, and can be infectious or noninfectious in origin (Fig. 13.6). The incidence of mastitis is approximately 10% in mothers by 3 months postpartum.[80] Reported rates range from 2% to 33%, and the condition can occur in nonlactating patients. Abscesses occur in about 3% of women who experience breast inflammation and are more likely to occur within the first 6 weeks postpartum.[81–83] A prevalence of 23% has been reported for *Candida albicans* colonization at 2 weeks postpartum, but not all of these women develop an infection.[83] Ductal infections caused by *Staphylococcus aureus* and mixed flora have been documented.[84,85]

Noninfectious mastitis may occur and should be considered as "milk stasis" secondary to ineffective or obstructed milk removal. When breast milk is obstructed, the paracellular pathways open, resulting in increased levels of sodium and chloride, decreased levels of lactose and potassium, and leakage of inflammatory cytokines, which can provoke fever, chills, and muscle aches, clinically mimicking an infectious process. Mastitis can present with no significant redness, fever, or systemic symptoms; however, it may manifest in such a severe fashion to necessitate hospitalization and intravenous antibiotic therapy.[86,87]

Infectious mastitis is most frequently caused by *S. aureus* and coagulase-negative staphylococci.[88,89] Another known cause is streptococci, which should be suspected whenever bilateral mastitis presents early in the postpartum period. Other causes include *Bacteroides* spp., *Escherichia coli*, *Peptostreptococcus* spp., *Moraxella* spp., *Eikenella* spp., *Mycobacterium tuberculosis* (rare), and *Candida* spp. (rare).[86–90] In the case of infectious mastitis, especially candidal mastitis during breastfeeding, both mother and infant need to be treated simultaneously. Infectious mastitis typically presents with a fever greater than 38.5°C, flulike symptoms, and a wedge-shaped area of localized tenderness. Treatment is focused on reversing milk stasis, maintaining milk supply, and continuing breastfeeding, along with providing maternal comfort. Patients with acute pain, severe symptoms, systemic symptoms, and/or fever need prompt medical attention with the appropriate antibiotics and incision and drainage of an abscess.

Special diagnostic subtypes of mastitis exist, all of which may involve an infectious, inflammatory and/or retention etiology: plasma cell mastitis, puerperal/lactational mastitis, lymphocytic mastitis, granulomatous lobular mastitis, and foreign-body mastitis.

Plasma Cell Mastitis. Microscopic sections of lesions demonstrate a florid periductal mastitis characterized by an impressive plasma cell reaction to retained ductal secretions. Key features for diagnosis include ductal epithelial hyperplasia accompanied by an associated intense lymphoplasmacytic infiltrate. Xanthomatous features can often be observed as lymphocytes and plasma cells surround zones of histiocytes engulfing disrupted ductal material. Neutrophils and periductal fibrosis are uncommonly observed.[91]

Puerperal/Lactational Mastitis. The histologic appearance is dependent on the nature and chronicity of these lesions. Acute involvement typically shows neutrophilic influx along with focal necrosis, whereas chronic lesions often display organized abscess formation with variable degrees of fibrosis and secondary fistula formation.[80,90,91]

Lymphocytic Mastitis. This entity is also referred to as sclerosing lymphocytic lobulitis, which characterizes the histologic appearance. There are circumscribed aggregates of lymphocytes within and surrounding terminal ducts and lobules associated with surrounding stromal fibrosis. Perivascular lymphocytic inflammation and germinal centers are also noted. Diabetic mastopathy shares certain clinical and pathologic features.[92]

Granulomatous Lobular Mastitis. This form of mastitis represents a notable mimic of benign or malignant neoplasia in breast lesions, typically in women of young to middle age. A significant number of cases are associated with parity or oral contraceptive pills; however, many cases have no well-defined causes and are designated as idiopathic. It is characterized histologically by multiple

necrotizing granulomata and/or abscesses located in association with or in approximation to segmental and subsegmental lactiferous ducts in a lobulocentric pattern.[93–96] Acid fast and/or Gomori methenamine silver stains may be needed to exclude mycobacterial and fungal infections.

Foreign-Body Mastitis. Paraffin or silicon injections for cosmetic purposes may uncommon induce a prominent foreign-body giant cell reaction with a characteristic histologic appearance.[76,97] The exogenous deposits are often dissolved during tissue processing, subsequently revealing a residual interstitial vacuolar ("Swiss cheese") appearance to the biopsy specimen. Microscopic examination reveals characteristic vacuoles of variable size surrounded by macrophages and foreign-body giant cells. When the reaction is severe, cutaneous ulceration, capsule formation, and sinus tracts may develop. The same histopathology can be produced by ruptured or leaking silicone breast implants, as previously described. Breast implants are discussed in Chapter 33.

Disorders of Keratinization

Reactive changes involving epidermal keratinization (e.g., hyperkeratosis, parakeratosis) are secondarily discussed in other sections on inflammatory and reactive dermatoses, where appropriate.

Axillary Granular Parakeratosis. Axillary granular parakeratosis is an acquired disorder of keratinization, originally detailed by Northcutt and colleagues[98] in 1991, which typically presents as a bilateral pruritic cutaneous eruption involving flexural regions. It occurs most commonly in the axillae and may extend to the skin of the axillary tail and upper outer quadrants of the breasts; however, lesions may occur in any body flexure, including the inframammary folds.[99] The lesions typically appear as hyperpigmented red or brown papules that coalesce over time into dark to violaceous plaques covered by an adherent keratotic scale. The astute clinician may be able to accurately diagnose this disorder in prototypical cases, although the findings may be nonspecific and can mimic a number of inflammatory and neoplastic diseases. The clinical differential diagnosis includes seborrheic dermatitis, lichen planus, acanthosis nigricans, and genodermatoses, such as Darier disease and Hailey-Hailey disease.[100–102] Distinctive features are present on histopathologic examination: broad compact parakeratosis, hyperkeratosis with hypergranulosis that involves the stratum corneum, vascular proliferation in the superficial dermis, and variable degrees of acanthosis and papillomatosis. Inflammation is usually mild, if present, unless there is secondary traumatization or excoriation. The pathogenesis of these lesions is currently believed to be due to inhibition of conversion of profilaggrin to filaggrin in the skin, which leads to disruption of maturation in the stratum corneum. Processing and trafficking of keratohyalin granules is affected and leads to retention of granules in the stratum corneum, producing its characteristic histologic appearance.[103,104] This is reinforced by the demonstration of an absence of filaggrin in keratinocytes from patients with axillary granular parakeratosis. The majority of cases are seen in middle-aged women, although cases have been documented in children and men. There is no obvious racial predilection. Lesions are most commonly associated with mechanical forces (e.g., friction, perspiration, humidity, follicular occlusion), introduction of new medications, and chemical components of antiperspirants and deodorants, but myriad causes have been proposed.[98–104] A significant number of cases are self-resolving within weeks to months after the initial presentation; however, some cases may cause significant discomfort and/or are esthetically displeasing to the patient. Topical or oral retinoids, especially isotretinoin, and topical steroids have shown excellent results in patients with chronic or recurrent disease.[105] Other treatments include keratolytics, topical vitamin D analogs, and cryotherapy.

Primary Neoplastic Disorders

Primary Benign Neoplastic Disorders

Seborrheic Keratosis. Seborrheic keratoses are the most common epithelial neoplasms of the breast. Grossly, the lesions are typically flat-topped or irregular waxy papules and small plaques that sit on the surface of the skin. Occasional lesions may be mounded, polypoid, or pedunculated. They are generally brown or black in color; however, they may present as flesh-colored or erythematous lesions de novo or secondarily as a result of irritation. Bleeding and crusting are not uncommon, usually as a result of excoriation, trauma due to rubbing on clothing or other garments, mechanical removal, or, uncommonly, autoamputation. Patients may present with solitary seborrheic keratosis, but it is extremely common to present with multiple synchronous or metachronous lesions. The Leser-Trélat sign refers to a paraneoplastic phenomenon in which there is an abrupt eruption of numerous seborrheic keratoses in patients with visceral malignancies and is related to high levels of circulating epidermal growth factor receptor.[106,107] Uncommonly, this sign has heralded the diagnosis of an occult malignancy, including carcinoma of the breast. Although many histologic variants of seborrheic keratosis have been described, all subtypes exhibit hyperkeratosis, acanthosis, papillomatosis, pseudohorn cysts, and variable inflammation. These lesions are uniformly benign. Treatment is generally reserved for symptomatic lesions or for cosmetic reasons, which consists of excision, curettage, cryotherapy, or ablation.[107]

Lichen Planus–Like Keratosis. Lichen planus–like keratoses, also referred to as benign lichenoid keratoses, are solitary (rarely multiple) 5- to 20-mm, bright red, violaceous or brown plaques on the chest and upper back. Clinically, they can mimic lentigo simplex and other pigmented lesions, superficial basal cell carcinoma, or squamous cell carcinoma in situ. The histologic features mimic those of lichen planus. Lesions typically demonstrate hyperkeratosis, serrated acanthosis, wedge-shaped hypergranulosis and a dense bandlike lymphocytic inflammatory infiltrate abutting the dermal-epidermal interface. Lichen planus–like keratosis typically demonstrates parakeratosis and the presence of increased eosinophils in the inflammatory infiltrate. These features, along with clinical history and presentation, help to distinguish these benign lesions from traditional lichen planus.

Benign Cysts and Adnexal Tumors. Adnexal tumors of pilosebaceous origin that occur on the breast are predominantly cystic and include epidermal inclusion cysts, trichilemmal cysts (pilar cyst), vellus hair cysts, and steatocystomas.[108–113] Epidermal inclusion cysts are common smooth dome-shaped lesions with an overlying pinpoint punctum that are fluctuant on palpation. These lesions may enlarge and either become inflamed and/or rupture, which often brings them to clinical attention. Histologic examination reveals a unilocular cystic structure lined by keratinizing squamous epithelium with a conspicuous granular layer and filled with lamellated keratin debris. Ruptured cysts are denoted histologically by granulomatous inflammation with a mixed inflammatory infiltrate and multinucleated histiocytes, some of which may contain phagocytosed keratin.

Trichilemmal cysts (pilar cysts) typically present as smooth dome-shaped lesions without an overlying punctum and are notably firm ("rock-like") on palpation. Histology shows a cystic

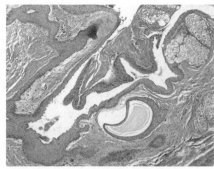

• **Fig. 13.7** Steatocystoma multiplex. This lesion can occur in the breast and consists of a cyst lined by stratified squamous epithelium with mature sebaceous glands in the wall.

nodule lined by keratinizing squamous epithelium without a granular layer and containing densely packed lamellated keratin with or without calcification. Because of their composition, they are easily shelled out by surgical means.

Vellus hair cysts are asymptomatic 1- to 2-mm follicular papules that typically appear in late childhood or early adulthood and may be associated with an autosomal dominant inheritance pattern. Histologic examination reveals a cyst lined by keratinizing squamous epithelium and containing lamellated keratin and one to many small, vellus hair shafts. Rupture with accompanying granulomatous inflammation is not uncommon. Steatocystomas are small, solitary (steatocystoma simplex) or multiple (steatocystoma multiplex), 1- to 5-mm yellowish papules containing a creamy or oily fluid upon expression. These cysts are lined by thin, stratified squamous epithelium with a prominent homogeneous, eosinophilic, crenulated cuticle that mimics a sebaceous duct. Attenuated sebaceous lobules may be seen in contiguity with the epithelial lining. The cysts usually appear empty on histology because the contents dissolve during processing. Steatocystoma multiplex (Fig. 13.7) is an autosomal dominant inherited, or uncommonly, sporadic disorder which presents as multiple asymptomatic cysts on the trunk and proximal extremities.[114–116] Steatocystoma simplex is a sporadic condition that begins in adolescence or young adulthood and affects both sexes equally. This condition has been associated with pachyonychia, acrokeratosis verruciformis, hypertrophic lichen planus, hypohidrosis, hidradenitis suppurativa and natal teeth. A relationship between steatocystomas and vellus hair cysts has been reported, and some hypothesize that eruptive vellus hair cysts and steatocystomas represents variants of the same pathogenetic disease. Hybrid lesions with histologic features of both cyst types have been described. Steatocystoma multiplex express keratins 10 and 17 in contrast to eruptive vellus hair cysts, which express only keratin 17. Treatment usually is not required for these benign conditions; however, treatment may be attempted for inflammatory lesions and may include oral tetracycline antibiotics.[114,115] Isotretinoin therapy also has been shown to be effective in some patients. Cosmetic treatment may be sought for persistent or enlarging lesions. Surgical treatment may include aspiration, extirpation, surgical excision, or laser destruction. Carcinoma may arise from the epidermal portions of these cysts in rare cases.

Adnexal tumors of eccrine and apocrine origin commonly occur on the breast. Given that the mammary gland is a modified sweat gland. Common benign adnexal tumors involving the breast include, but are not limited to, poromas (tumors arising from or differentiating as the intraepithelial portion of the eccrine duct), hidradenomas (tumors of the straight portion of the eccrine duct), spiradenomas, and cylindromas (tumors of the deep coiled eccrine gland).[108–113,117,118]

Poromas appear clinically as raised or polypoid flesh-colored lesions that may ulcerate and, as a result, are often mistaken for pyogenic granulomas. Histologic examination shows a proliferation of broad, anastomosing bands of small, cuboidal cells containing small caliber duct-like spaces beneath a flattened epidermis. The intervening stroma is characteristically edematous and richly vascular. The absence of peripheral palisading is an important distinguishing histologic feature from basal cell carcinoma.

Hidradenomas are primarily intradermal tumors, 0.5 to 2 cm in diameter, with intact overlying skin. Microscopically, well-circumscribed, sometimes encapsulated lobules of polygonal and cuboidal cells within which simple tubular ducts are embedded are present in the dermis. The polygonal cells have round nuclei with basophilic cytoplasm and indistinct cell borders. The cuboidal cells have clear or pale cytoplasm; when clear cells are numerous, the tumor is termed *clear cell hidradenoma.*

Spiradenomas and cylindromas present as solitary, markedly tender, dermal or subcutaneous masses without epidermal connection. Microscopic examination reveals a spectrum of deeply basophilic, sharply demarcated lobules containing variable admixtures of two types of epithelial cells. One cell type consists of cells with relatively large, centrally placed clear nuclei and scant cytoplasm that forms ductular structures, whereas the second cell type consists of cells with small dark nuclei and wispy basophilic cytoplasm found primarily at the periphery of the lobules. Reduplicated basement membrane material, appearing as homogeneous, dull, eosinophilic masses, is also present within and/or surrounding the tumor in hidradenomas, spiradenomas, and cylindromas. Lymphocytes are present in lobules of spiradenomas more commonly than in cylindromas. Mitoses may be present in all cutaneous tumors and, unless atypical in appearance, should not be taken as a sign of malignancy unless other concerning morphologic features are observed. Unless frank carcinoma or lymphovascular or perineural invasion arises in an adnexal neoplasm, histologic features alone may not predict the clinical behavior of individual neoplasm. Consequently, excision of benign adnexal tumors is the currently recommended management. Benign neoplasms of sebaceous gland origin that occur as primary dermatologic neoplasms must be distinguished from invasive breast carcinoma, which may involve the skin of the breast. Adenomas of sebaceous glands consist of well-differentiated sebaceous lobules containing cells with prototypical multivacuolated cytoplasm and small basophilic nuclei.

Syringomatous adenoma of the nipple (syringomatous tumor) represents an uncommon neoplasm of sweat gland derivation that bears a histologic resemblance to conventional cutaneous syringoma. It is found predominantly in adult females with the greatest incidence in the fourth and fifth decades and usually presents as a unilateral firm erythematous or flesh-colored lesion.[119–122] An unusual report of syringomatous adenoma arising in a supernumerary breast has been reported.[123] This is a benign but locally infiltrative lesion typically located in the dermis and/or subcutis subjacent to the nipple or areola. Ulceration is uncommon because these are typically seated deeply in the skin. Gross examination upon sectioning may reveal multiple small cysts in the dermis or subcutis. Histologically, round or irregular open tubules that have been likened to commas or teardrop figures extend in an infiltrative growth pattern to involve dermal collagen, subcutaneous fat,

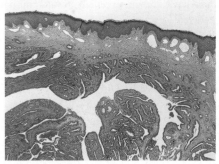

• **Fig. 13.8** Erosive adenomatosis of the nipple, which consists of a benign proliferation of glands within the lactiferous sinuses that is important to distinguish from carcinoma.

or smooth muscle. Tubular lumens may contain amphophilic or eosinophilic secretions or, uncommonly, keratinous debris. The superjacent epidermis is typically acanthotic. Variable amounts of squamous and apocrine differentiation are usually present and do not affect the diagnosis or prognosis of this entity.[119,120] Perineural invasion is not uncommon and does not indicate malignant behavior. Myoepithelial cells are invariably present around the tubules (although these cells may be inconspicuous without immunohistochemistry), differentiating this lesion from invasive carcinoma. Cytologic atypia and necrosis are minimal. Of note, this lesion was once believed to be a superficially located variant of low-grade adenosquamous carcinoma of the breast, although this diagnosis has lost favor. Metastasis has not been reported in association with these lesions. Complete excision is the recommended management of this lesions.[119,120,124,125]

Erosive Adenomatosis of the Nipple. Erosive adenomatosis of the nipple (nipple adenoma, florid papillomatosis of the nipple) (Fig. 13.8) is a rare, benign neoplasm of lactiferous ductal epithelium.[126–130] The peak incidence is in the fifth to seventh decades. This condition usually presents clinically with a unilateral erythematous crusting or oozing lesion with induration of the nipple that may be accompanied by ulceration. A subareolar mass may be present in a significant number of cases, which may provide the impetus for clinical attention. Clinically, this lesion can be mistaken for Paget's disease, nipple eczema, or carcinoma.[131,132] On histologic examination, two patterns of growth are evident. The first pattern, associated with erosive lesions, is adenomatous, a proliferation of round, oval, or irregularly shaped ducts lined by cuboidal to columnar epithelium with an outer myoepithelial layer and embedded in a fibrovascular or centrally hyalinized stroma. The second pattern, associated with a mass effect, is papillomatous-papillary–type hyperplasia of columnar epithelial cells lining the ducts resulting in tufting intraluminal projections without fibrovascular cores. These papillomatous regions may demonstrate distortion and crowding. Occasional mitotic figures and focal necrosis may be present; however, these features in isolation are not indicative of malignancy. Squamous metaplasia may present focally. In both patterns, the superjacent epidermis is acanthotic. Numerous plasma cells may be seen in the dermis. Histologically, nipple adenomas may be mistaken for invasive ductal carcinoma or ductal carcinoma in situ. Important differences from invasive carcinoma and ductal carcinoma in situ include absence of significant cytologic atypia and absence of atypical mitotic figures. Myoepithelial cells are ubiquitously present and true cribriform proliferations are not seen in nipple

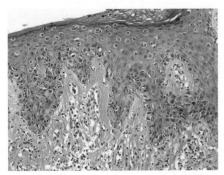

• **Fig. 13.9** Paget's disease of the breast. Paget's disease consists of malignant Paget's cells percolating through the nipple. This disease can mimic nipple eczema or contact dermatitis. With Paget's disease, there is often an underlying malignancy.

adenomas. Cases of nipple adenoma with synchronous and metachronous carcinomas have been reported. Additionally, malignant transformation of a nipple adenoma has rarely occurred, and noncontiguous invasive mammary carcinoma has secondarily involved nipple adenomas of the breast in exceptionally rare cases. Excisional biopsy is most helpful in establishing the diagnosis. Although the morphologic features of this lesion may concern the novice observer, knowledge of this lesion and its typical histologic appearance and configuration will help prevent misdiagnosis of a malignant neoplasm. Complete excision is recommended.

Primary Malignant and Neoplastic Disorders

Paget's Disease of the Breast. Paget's disease of the nipple (Fig. 13.9) represents a malignant neoplasm that is defined pathologically as an intraepidermal carcinoma. Although Paget's disease can occur anywhere along the milk line, the disease is most commonly localized to the breast and therefore it is included here as a primary breast neoplasm. Paget's disease was first described in 1856 by Velpeau[133] and the concept was later refined by Sir James Paget in 1874 as a syndrome in which ulceration of the nipple was associated with an underlying carcinoma.[134] Paget's disease of the breast is an uncommon neoplasm, accounting for 1% to 3% of all breast tumors.[135–137] This disease occurs predominantly in women, although cases in men do occur and are associated with a worse prognosis.[138] Clinically, it presents as eczema, erythema, weeping, ulceration, bleeding, and/or itching of the nipple or areola depending on the chronicity of the lesion. Nipple discharge is not infrequent. The eczematous reaction most often appears initially on the nipple and then subsequently spreads centrifugally toward the areola.[139,140] In advanced cases, the carcinoma can extend to the periareolar skin. The diagnosis of Paget's disease can be easily confused with reactive or inflammatory dermatoses and is often delayed for months before a correct diagnosis is rendered.[141]

Currently, the most widely accepted theory (i.e., epidermotropic theory) regarding the pathogenesis of Paget's disease theorizes that Paget's cells are ductal carcinoma cells that have migrated from the underlying mammary ducts or lobules of the terminal ductal lobular unit to the epidermis.[135,142–144] This theory is strongly supported by the presence of concomitant invasive mammary carcinoma or carcinoma in situ in the vast majority of cases, ranging from 92% to 100% of cases.[135,138,144–148] The underlying carcinoma or carcinoma in situ can be located in any quadrant of the breast and can demonstrate either ductal or lobular morphology. Interestingly, one report found that 45% of palpable invasive carcinomas associated with Paget's disease were located in

the upper outer quadrant of the breast[136]; however, this predilection has not been consistently reproduced. The underlying neoplasm associated with cases of Paget's disease is multifocal or multicentric in 32% to 63% of cases.[144,145,147] This potential for multicentricity renders it crucial to evaluate the entire breast, even if a solitary lesion is noted on physical examination (particularly solitary subareolar masses).[149] Invasive carcinoma may also be clinically occult in a significant number of cases, with Paget's disease heralding its presence.[150] The exceptionally rare diagnosis of invasive mammary Paget's disease involving dermal tissue without definitive evidence of a concomitant invasive ductal or lobular mammary carcinoma is rendered as a diagnosis of exclusion and is of great academic interest.[148]

Paget's disease is characterized histologically by the infiltration of the epidermis with enlarged round and ovoid tumor cells with abundant pale amphophilic cytoplasm and pleomorphic vesicular nuclei. The tumor cells are often arranged in a "buckshot" pattern throughout the epidermis, with individual cells present at all layers. Cytologic atypia is present, including pleomorphism and mitotic figures. Paget's cells show similar immunohistochemical staining pattern as that of conventional mammary carcinomas, with overexpression with low molecular weight cytokeratins (CKs), such as CK7. High molecular weight CKs and CK20 are typically negative.[151,152] Paget's cells typically express other antigens, such as epithelial membrane antigen, carcinoembryonic antigen, gross cystic disease fluid protein 15 (GCDFP-15), and mucicarmine,[153] reinforcing the glandular origin of these cells. Paget's cells also typically overexpress p53 and HER2 and exhibit an increased proliferative rate with ki67 (MIB-1).[154–156] Studies have demonstrated that the HER2 oncoprotein may function in vivo to promote intraepithelial spread of adenocarcinoma cells.[156,157] Invasive carcinoma associated with Paget's disease more commonly exhibits negative estrogen and progesterone receptor immunoreactivity due to the preponderance of underlying carcinomas that possess a higher pathologic grade.[158–160] The RAS oncogene product p21 and c-erbB-2 demonstrate overexpression, and these findings are associated with aggressive disease and with worse prognosis.[161–163]

Diagnosis is accomplished by histologic examination of lesional tissue, although contemporary imaging modalities (e.g., magnetic resonance imaging, ultrasound, or radiographic mammography) continue to prove useful in triaging and characterizing these lesions. Specifically, in cases of noninvasive breast cancer, magnetic resonance imaging has a sensitivity of 95% compared with a value of 70% for mammography.[164] This sensitivity is amplified in cases in which physical examination and mammography are unremarkable.[150,165] Breast conserving surgery combined with irradiation therapy for patients with invasive and in situ mammary carcinoma has become the treatment of choice in many instances. Surgical procedures should immutably include the entire nipple-areolar complex.[159,166] Treatment with breast conserving surgery has demonstrated similar long-term survival rates to those of modified or radical mastectomy.[148,159,160,167] Sentinel lymph node biopsy should be considered to evaluate the axillary lymph nodes in all patients with Paget's disease, although the prognostic utility of categorical sentinel lymph node evaluation is debatable among providers.[159,168–170] Prognosis depends largely on the presence and grade of an underlying carcinoma or carcinoma in situ. Paget's disease and its significance outside of its dermatologic manifestations and pathology are discussed extensively in Chapter 12.

Paget's disease without evidence of underlying invasive or in situ mammary carcinoma most commonly occurs in cases of occult or undetected concomitant disease; however, cases may certainly present in which Paget's disease appears to exist in isolation after an extensive initial battery of clinical, radiologic, and pathologic testing. In the uncommon event that Paget's disease of the breast presents without an initially identifiable underlying invasive or in situ carcinoma component, a more dedicated clinical, radiologic, and pathologic assessment would be prudent. Secondary modalities, such as breast magnetic resonance imaging and fine-needle aspiration, can prove useful.[160,167,168,171] Currently, recommended management for patients with biopsy-proven Paget's disease and without clinical, radiologic, and pathologic evidence of invasive or in situ mammary carcinoma is excision of the nipple-areolar complex and circumferential periareolar skin with conservative clinical follow-up.[160,166–170,172] If invasive carcinoma is subsequently found, sentinel lymph node evaluation and adjuvant therapy can be undertaken at the discretion of the clinician in addition to conventional surgical management. The utility of sentinel lymph node sampling in patients with confirmed Paget's disease and compelling lack of evidence for an invasive carcinoma has been debated, although it is not required for evaluation in these patients at this time.[159,160,166–170]

Inflammatory Breast Carcinoma.

Inflammatory breast carcinoma (Fig. 13.10) represents a primary breast dermatologic malignancy that prototypically presents as diffusely red, warm, slightly indurated, and tender skin overlying at least one-third of the overall surface area of the breast.[173–177] The clinical manifestations noted are required for diagnosis and appropriate

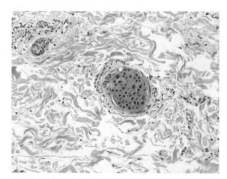

• **Fig. 13.10** Inflammatory breast carcinoma, which consists of lymphovascular tumor emboli within the dermis. This condition often mimics the appearance of mastitis, and dermal biopsy may prove necessary.

categorization, including American Joint Committee on Cancer tumor staging.[177] Histologic sections demonstrate diffuse occlusion or obstruction of dermal and/or subcutaneous lymphatic and vascular channels by tumor emboli, which are cytologically atypical and often similar in appearance to the primary mammary carcinoma. Vascular congestion and tissue edema accompany the presence of lymphovascular tumor emboli. Recurrent metastatic carcinoma, most often found in mastectomy scars, may also manifest as florid lymphovascular tumor embolization (i.e., secondary inflammatory breast carcinoma). Because of the diagnostic and prognostic importance of this condition, it is discussed in greater detail in Chapter 64.

Atypical Vascular Lesion.

After radiation therapy for breast cancer, a variety of vascular proliferations can be found in the overlying skin ranging from benign lymphovascular proliferations to angiosarcomas. Atypical vascular lesion (AVL) is the term given to a lesion of uncertain malignant potential that has histologic features intermediate between benign and malignant tumors. The majority of reported AVLs are considered benign; however, angiosarcoma has been reported to arise in rare AVLs. Typically the time course between radiation and the development of an AVL is relatively short compared with the time course for the development of angiosarcoma. Histologically it can be difficult to distinguish an AVL from low-grade angiosarcoma. Correlation with clinical and radiographic findings is necessary. Consultation with expert pathologists may be necessary for difficult lesions.

Angiosarcoma.

Angiosarcoma is an uncommon malignant neoplasm of endothelial cells that may occur at any site on the body; however, the unique clinicopathologic presentation in the breast (including its typical dermal tumor location) and well-documented association with prior breast irradiation make it appropriate to discuss as a primary breast neoplastic disorder (Fig. 13.11). Angiosarcoma accounts for 0.04% of primary mammary tumors and approximately 8% of all mammary sarcomas.[178,179] Before the use of radiation therapy for breast cancer, angiosarcomas of the breast most commonly occurred during the third and fourth decades of life.[180] Approximately 6% to 12% of the cases were diagnosed during pregnancy.[181,182] Angiosarcoma was historically designated under multiple titles before its current classification, including names such as *hemangioendothelioma, hemangioblastoma, hemangiosarcoma,* and *metastasizing angioma.*[178,183–189] It carries a uniformly poor prognosis regardless of disease associations or comorbidities, with a 5-year survival of 8% to 50%.[190] Metastases from mammary angiosarcomas have been reported in

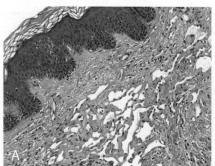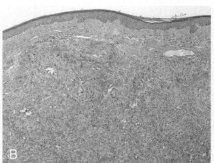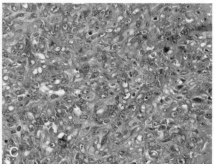

• **Fig. 13.11** Angiosarcoma, its precursors and mimics. (A) Atypical vascular ectasia from irradiation. This lesion may be a possible precursor of angiosarcoma or a mimic, but it is not angiosarcoma. (B) Example of solid vascular proliferation in the breast dermis indicative of angiosarcoma. (C) Higher-power view of angiosarcoma indicating nuclear and cellular anaplasia.

the lung, skin, liver, bone, central nervous system, spleen, ovary, lymph nodes, and heart.[181,182]

Angiosarcomas of the breast have increasingly been associated with radiation therapy that occurs before or after surgical intervention for breast cancer.[180,191,192] The ever-increasing use of breast conserving therapy and neoadjuvant and adjuvant irradiation projects that the incidence of angiosarcomas will continue to increase. They account for more than 50% of all mammary sarcomas identified in patients who had prior radiation therapy but only 20% of sarcomas in those who had no prior radiation therapy.[180] Angiosarcomas can also occur on the upper extremity or axilla as a result of long-standing lymphedema, which is eponymously referred to as Stewart-Treves syndrome.[193] Those angiosarcomas that arise as a result of chronic lymphedema (i.e., swelling resulting from lymphatic obstruction) usually occur as a complication of mastectomy, dedicated lymphadenectomy, and/or radiotherapy for breast carcinoma.[194] Preoperative diagnosis of angiosarcomas of the breast using fine-needle aspiration is often immensely difficult and diagnosis is best established via incisional biopsy.[181] Irradiation of the breast can produce vascular ectasia or vascular proliferations within the superficial dermis that can exhibit atypical features (Fig. 13.11A) but do not meet the histologic criteria for angiosarcoma. These lesions are designated AVLs; however, when a vascular lesion progresses to invade the breast lobules or develops a solid growth pattern (Fig. 13.11B), it is diagnostic for angiosarcoma. AVLs may represent vascular proliferations of a reactive angiogenic nature or precursors of vascular lesions of undetermined malignant potential or angiosarcoma. Currently, characterization and diagnosis of these lesions is difficult, and AVLs lack official prognostic factors and guidelines for surgical management.[195] *MYC* amplification is a consistent feature of radiation-associated angiosarcoma, which can be diagnostically demonstrated via immunohistochemistry or in situ hybridization.[196–198]

Histologic evaluation of angiosarcoma exhibits anaplastic nuclear features in a hypercellular neoplasm (see Fig. 13.11C). Histologic sections from primary angiosarcoma of the irradiated breast and primary angiosarcoma of the axilla secondary to lymphedema show dermal infiltration by ill-defined fenestrated vascular spaces lined by atypical endothelial cells. Well-differentiated lesions show an anastomosing network of vessels lined by a single layer of endothelial cells with mild to moderate nuclear atypia. Poorly differentiated tumors demonstrate sheets of dedifferentiated cells with frank endothelial nuclear pleomorphism, increasing mitotic activity and necrosis without obvious vascular lumens. Focal papillary protrusions may be observed. Angiosarcomas are immunoreactive for endothelial and vascular antigens, specifically CD31, CD34, ERG, Fli-1, factor VIII–related antigen, D2-40 and *Ulex europaeus* antigen.[199,200] Ultrastructural examination can reveal the vascular nature of angiosarcomas by demonstrating Weibel-Palade bodies and pinocytic vesicles.

Treatment involves a multidisciplinary approach because angiosarcomas of the breast are quite resistant to conventional chemotherapy regiments.[201] Angiosarcomas typically extend microscopically beyond their clinical gross margins due to their insidious dermal growth pattern, and therefore simple excision is unacceptable because of its high rate of local recurrence. Surgical treatment of angiosarcoma is usually contraindicated in tumors that extend to vital structures, are of massive size, or are in multicentric tumors; however, early and complete surgical excision of the mass lesion with tumor-free margins should be attempted, if achievable.[200,202] Doxorubicin-based neoadjuvant therapy is reserved for unresectable tumors, tumors invading the chest wall, and tumors larger than 5 cm. Breast angiosarcomas are best treated with a combination of radiotherapy and chemotherapy for local control. Neoadjuvant and adjuvant therapy is being used with increasing frequency, although the benefit of adjuvant therapy remains unclear. Axillary dissection is not indicated because these tumors spread in a hematogenous fashion and nodal involvement is rare. In unconventional cases, modified radical mastectomy may be part of the treatment protocol. Radical mastectomy is generally reserved only for tumors with extension to deep fascial planes or the chest wall. The decision for mastectomy is guided by the following factors: size and location of the tumor, presence of multicentricity, capacity to follow the breast by mammography, and physical examination for evidence of postoperative recurrence and patient preference for treatment.[202,203]

Malignant Adnexal Tumors. Malignant neoplasms of eccrine or apocrine glands are rare, accounting for less than 0.001% of all primary breast cancers. These tumors generally affect a younger population than conventional invasive mammary carcinoma, usually those in the third to fifth decades.[108–113] These neoplasms, in general, represent the malignant counterparts of benign adnexal tumors in that they display typical pathologic features of a particular adnexal tumor. In addition they display lymphovascular and/or perineural invasion, atypical or anaplastic morphology, atypical mitotic figures, extensive necrosis, and/or a destructive invasive pattern of growth.[118,204] Apocrine lesions are postulated to be significantly more common than eccrine lesions, although this distinction is tenuous at best in some cases, and this delineation has generally not been shown to affect prognosis (Fig. 13.12). In some lesions, tumor cells exhibit both eccrine and apocrine differentiation. Malignant adnexal neoplasms usually present as indurated slowly growing plaques with irregular geographic outlines. Malignant adnexal tumors may evolve from benign adnexal tumors or arise de novo. Adnexal carcinomas, like adenomas, may mimic the appearance of breast carcinomas.[118] Both benign and malignant sweat gland tumors can express estrogen receptor, progesterone receptor, and/or *HER2/neu*. Immunoperoxidase stains have not been shown to reliably differentiate sweat gland carcinomas from breast carcinomas. The treatment for adnexal carcinomas is surgical therapy with wide margins. Metastatic potential is high in these lesions and prognosis remains poor, even with the administration of combination chemotherapy and radiation therapy regimens.

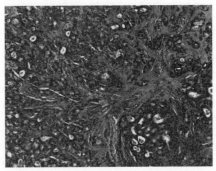

• **Fig. 13.12** Apocrine adenocarcinoma, a malignant adnexal tumor of the breast, can resemble infiltrating ductal breast carcinoma, from which it must be distinguished.

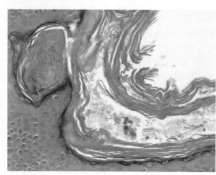

• **Fig. 13.13** Erythrasma. Erythrasma is a secondary infectious disease of the breast resulting from a cutaneous superficial bacterial infection, as evidenced by the appearances of small coccobacilli in the superficial stratum corneum.

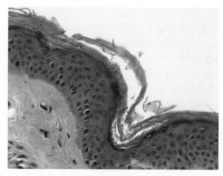

• **Fig. 13.14** In contrast to erythrasma, dermatophytosis (tinea) is caused by a fungus, and fungal hyphae are observed within the stratum corneum.

Secondary Breast Dermatologic Disorders

Secondary Inflammatory Disorders

Infectious Disorders

Erythrasma. Erythrasma is a chronic cutaneous bacterial infection caused by the organism *Corynebacterium minutissimum*. Although usually intertriginous, erythrasma presents as a well-demarcated, oval, reddish brown patch with fine scaling. Clinical forms may be diagnosed by characteristic coral-red fluorescence under Wood light. Biopsies often appear unremarkable with hematoxylin and eosin staining; however, gram-positive coccobacilli in the superficial stratum corneum are diagnostic (Fig. 13.13).[205] It is well established that erythrasma, like acanthosis nigricans, can be a presenting sign of diabetes mellitus.[206,207]

Candidiasis. Candidiasis on routine histology is typically quite subtle. The characteristic histologic clue to the diagnosis is the presence of neutrophils in the stratum corneum, initially resembling impetigo. The underlying epidermis may show variable degrees of spongiosis and mild acanthosis. Yeast and pseudohyphal fungal elements can be better visualized with periodic acid–Schiff or silver stains. Although cutaneous candidiasis can occur anywhere on the skin, the breast is particularly affected in two scenarios: (1) nipple-areolar infection secondary to pregnancy and breastfeeding[208,209] and (2) submammary intertrigo secondary to friction with entry caused by large, pendulous breasts, or obesity.[210] Topical nystatin or clotrimazole is a recommended treatment in the latter condition.

Dermatophytosis (*Tinea*). *Tinea mammae* was first described by Bohmer and colleagues in 1998.[211] *Trichophyton rubrum* is the most common organism isolated in these rare lesions and may occur anywhere on the breast, but most commonly in the inframammary folds. *Malassezia furfur* (tinea versicolor) has been rarely documented in the nipple-areola region as well.[212,213] Clinically these appear similar to candidiasis, with dry, erythematous, flaky/scaling skin present. These lesions tend to be rounded clinically and are quite pruritic. One useful clue to the microscopic diagnosis of tinea is the "sandwich sign," consisting of orthokeratosis or parakeratosis interspersed within normal basket-weave stratum corneum (Fig. 13.14). Some degree of spongiosis or psoriasiform hyperplasia may be present along with a variable inflammatory response. Fungal hyphae are observed in the stratum corneum or within hair follicles and can be best highlighted with periodic acid–Schiff or Gomori methenamine silver stains.

Treatment with topical antifungal medication typically leads to resolution.

Varicella Zoster Virus. Blistering or bullous cutaneous eruptions limited to the breast are rare; when they occur on breast skin, they are generally part of a more widespread eruption. Of these, the most common is *herpes zoster* (shingles), which manifests as severe stinging, burning pain in a dermatomal distribution, followed within a few days by papulovesicular eruption with small, grouped vesicles on an erythematous base. Constitutional symptoms such as fever, headache, and malaise may precede or accompany a severe outbreak. Postherpetic neuralgia is a complication in approximately 2% of patients.[214] A Tzanck smear shows multinucleate keratinocytes with nuclear molding. A biopsy may not be necessary; however, when obtained, it shows characteristic viral cytopathologic features with ballooning and reticular degeneration of keratinocytes, multinucleate keratinocytes with ground-glass nuclei and nuclear molding. Leukocytoclastic vasculitis may be present in the underlying small dermal capillaries. Prompt administration of antiviral therapy leads to resolution of the initial lesion, with a marked decrease in the incidence, severity, and duration of postherpetic neuralgia. Topical capsaicin may also be used to control the pain of postherpetic neuralgia.

Noninfectious Benign Lesions

Lichen Sclerosis et Atrophicus. Lichen sclerosis et atrophicus (LS) is an inflammatory disease of unknown cause and incompletely elicited pathogenesis. Extragenital LS is most common on the neck and shoulders but may occur in the breast. It is usually asymptomatic but may be pruritic. Typically the eruption of LS begins as white, polygonal papules that coalesce into plaques with comedo-like plugs or evenly spaced dells. The dells may disappear, leaving a smooth, often porcelain-white plaque. This is not characteristically a premalignant condition when occurring on the breast. Initial lesions of LS show epidermal atrophy along with superficial dermal edema associated with an underlying bandlike lymphocytic infiltrate associated with effaced rete ridges and necrosis of scattered epidermal keratinocytes. As lesions become more sclerotic, the papillary dermal collagen becomes homogenized and the epidermis is attenuated with flattening of rete ridges. Treatment is with topical steroids.

Seborrheic Dermatitis. Seborrheic dermatitis is characteristically distributed on the scalp, eyebrows, eyelid margins, cheeks, nasolabial folds and paranasal areas, external ear canals, presternal area, or the inframammary folds. Lesions generally present with a dry, powdery scale, but when there is extensive presternal or inframammary involvement, lesions may exhibit coarse scale on an erythematous base with follicular pustules. The clinical

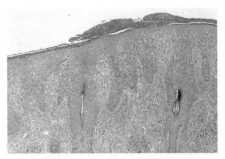

• **Fig. 13.15** Seborrheic dermatitis. Seborrheic dermatitis may secondarily affect the breast and is characterized by parakeratosis, spongiosis, acanthosis, and lymphocytic infiltration.

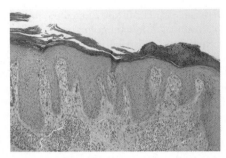

• **Fig. 13.16** Psoriasis. Psoriasis may also secondarily affect the breast and can be similar in appearance to seborrheic dermatitis. However, in psoriasis confluent parakeratosis and neutrophilic exocytosis are present.

course is chronic with remissions and exacerbations. Microscopic examination reveals spongiosis associated with a mild superficial, perivascular, and perifollicular lymphocytic infiltrate. More chronic lesions are often psoriasiform with focal parakeratosis, most prominent around follicular openings. The main histologic differential diagnosis is psoriasis; however, in seborrheic dermatitis, neutrophilic exocytosis, Munro microabscesses, and confluent parakeratosis are absent (Fig. 13.15). Low-potency topical steroids are the treatment of choice. The differential diagnosis includes psoriasis, tinea corporis, tinea versicolor, erythrasma, and contact dermatitis.[215]

Psoriasis. Psoriasis (Fig. 13.16) is distinguished by characteristic lesions on the elbows, knees, and other extensor body surfaces but may also occur on the breast. Psoriasis, especially when it involves the areola or nipple, may be difficult to distinguish clinically from Bowen disease (squamous cell carcinoma in situ).[216,217] A biopsy readily distinguishes the two entities. Chronic plaque-type psoriasis of the breast is characterized by hyperkeratosis with confluent parakeratosis, hypogranulosis, regular acanthosis, suprapapillary epidermal thinning, and neutrophilic exocytosis within the stratum corneum (Munro microabscesses) and the superficial epidermis (spongiform pustules of Kogoj). In the dermis, a mild perivascular lymphocytic infiltrate is present. Tortuous dilated capillaries extending into dermal papillae accounts for the Auspitz sign. Guttate psoriasis differs histologically from chronic plaque-type psoriasis by showing foci of parakeratosis and less acanthosis. Inverse or flexural psoriasis involving inframammary folds or axillae tends to be more spongiotic and has fewer histologic features than chronic plaque type; sudden onset of this subtype may signal infection with HIV.[218,219] Pustular psoriasis is characterized by more prominent aggregates of neutrophils between keratinocytes and within the stratum corneum.

To the breast specialist, psoriasis may manifest as a reactive process. The Koebner phenomenon is the manifestation of psoriasis at a place of cutaneous injury and has been documented in postmastectomy cases.[220,221] Herceptin treatment has also been shown to induce psoriasis.[222] Breastfeeding can also induce the development of psoriasis or be associated with features of existing disease.[208] Low-potency corticosteroids (category V or VI) may be used as treatment in these scenarios.

Drug Hypersensitivity Reactions. Drug hypersensitivity reactions may occur at any body site. A myriad of clinical manifestations of drug hypersensitivity (typically a pruritic maculopapular rash, either diffuse or localized) are associated with equally diverse histopathologic findings. Patterns range from interface dermatitis with perivascular inflammation and minimal epidermal change to lichenoid dermatitis to intraepidermal pustular aggregates. All can be seen with variable degrees of keratinocyte necrosis. Although the presence of eosinophils is a vital clue to a drug reaction, clinicopathologic correlation is essential because contact dermatitis may exhibit identical histologic features. For the breast oncologist, cutaneous drug reactions have been documented to occur within days to months after the administration of tamoxifen.[223] Similar documented reactions to paclitaxel also have been reported in the literature.[222]

Coumadin Necrosis. Coumadin necrosis occurs in patients with inborn or acquired abnormalities of the coagulation cascade, particularly deficiencies of protein C or protein S. These patients develop seemingly paradoxical intravascular coagulation with initiation of warfarin anticoagulant therapy secondary to depletion of vitamin K–dependent clotting factors (factors II, VII, IX, X). Intravascular thrombi form preferentially in relatively cool, fatty areas of the body such as the breasts, buttocks, and abdominal panniculus. Widespread ischemic tissue necrosis is the usual outcome. Discrete lesions appear that are initially erythematous or hemorrhagic and exquisitely tender. Blisters and bullae develop, leading to full-thickness skin loss and eschar formation. Biopsy specimens reveal hemorrhagic necrosis of the epidermis and breast parenchyma along with characteristic noninflammatory fibrin thrombi formation in the dermal vasculature. As the skin attempts to heal, scar tissue and granulation tissue develop.[224]

Pyoderma Gangrenosum. Postsurgical pyoderma gangrenosum (PG) has been described as an idiopathic pustular ulcerative disease.[225–227] In the postoperative setting, PG most commonly occurs on the breast, specifically after mammoplasties and reductions. Histologically, ulcerative, bullous, pustular, and vegetative patterns may be present. Neutrophils are marked in number, forming abscesses and extend into the mid to deep dermis or subcutis. A zone of peripheral lymphocytosis is typically present. The adjacent preserved epidermis may show pseudoepitheliomatous hyperplasia. Granuloma formation may be present adjacent to areas of abscess formation. Recognition of this entity is important to spare the patient unnecessary debridement and to prevent excessive scarring after resolution of the lesions. Most cases of PG respond to oral or systemic steroid therapy alone or in combination with cyclosporine or topical tacrolimus.[226] Of note, several cases of underlying breast malignancy have been associated with the presence of PG[228,229]; however, PG is not currently viewed as a paraneoplastic phenomenon.

Mondor Disease. Mondor disease is a superficial thrombophlebitis of the thoracoepigastric, lateral thoracic, or superior epigastric vein, most commonly presenting on the breast or superficial chest wall. The usual presentation as tender, firm, linear subcutaneous bands or strings usually observed with arm extension. Affected patients are usually in the third to fifth decade, and women are predominantly affected (female-to-male ratio 9:1).[230] Most cases are idiopathic; however, multiple risk factors have been identified, including breast surgery; breast trauma; large, pendulous breasts; multiparous women with long history of pregnancy, breastfeeding, and infections; among others.[231-233] Treatment is symptomatic, with most patients demonstrating improvement on anticoagulant therapy.[234]

Granuloma Annulare. Granuloma annulare, an idiopathic disease of collagen necrobiosis, can occur anywhere on the body, including the breast. Lesions appear as red-brown papules that coalesce to form annular plaques with ulcerated borders and without scaling. Microscopic examination of classic granuloma annulare reveals collections of epithelioid histiocytes and giant cells surrounding a central zone of necrobiosis consisting of degenerated connective tissue and mucin. Epidermal changes are typically minimal. Perivascular lymphocytes and eosinophils may be present. In the interstitial form of granuloma annulare, the histologic changes are more subtle. The dermis appears more cellular than classic forms from an initial low-power assessment. Higher magnification reveals lymphocytes, histiocytes in the dermal interstitium, and mucin deposition that separates collagen bundles. Well-circumscribed areas of necrobiosis are absent in the interstitial variant of granuloma annulare.

Acanthosis Nigricans. Velvety darkened or diffuse brown-pigmented areas of skin typically present in intertriginous and flexural areas, such as the inframammary region and axillae, are termed acanthosis nigricans.[235] The disorder in and of itself is innocuous, signaling only hyperkeratosis of the affected skin on biopsy; however, this clinical finding is important to clinicians because it may herald several disorders including diabetes mellitus[236] and can signal underlying visceral malignancy such as gastrointestinal, gynecologic, and breast carcinomas.[237,238]

Annular Erythema. Also termed *gyrate erythemas, erythema annulare centrifugum,* and *erythema gyratum repens,* annular erythema may serve as cutaneous manifestations of underlying malignancy. Lesions appear as erythematous plaques coalescing together at a rapid rate, with a gyrate "wood-grain" pattern of spread. Several reports have described these lesions in association with primary and recurrent breast malignancies, likely secondary to a hypersensitivity or paraneoplastic reaction.[239-241]

Sarcoidosis. Systemic sarcoidosis can affect any organ, including the skin. Clinically, the lesions may express a wide variety of patterns and may also present as a mass lesion.[242] Biopsy specimens display epithelioid nonnecrotizing granulomas with a minimal to mild surrounding lymphoplasmacytic infiltrate. Occasionally, asteroid or Schaumann bodies can be present within multinucleated giant cells within the granulomas. Rarely, sarcoidosis can be associated with underlying breast malignancy.[243]

Pityriasis Rosea. Pityriasis rosea, with its oval, finely scaling, salmon-colored patches, is an idiopathic papulosquamous disorder. Potential causes include human herpesviruses 6 and 7, as well as medications.[244] It typically occurs in young adults over the back or the trunk and can spontaneously resolve in 6 to 8 weeks. Postinflammatory hypopigmentation may occur. Although a rare case of localized pityriasis rosea to the breast was successfully treated with topical steroids,[245] topical steroid therapy often prolongs the course of pityriasis rosea.

Lupus Panniculitis. Lupus panniculitis (lupus profundus) is an uncommon, benign inflammatory condition characterized by inflammation of deep subcutaneous adipose tissue, typically presenting on the neck, extremities, or buttocks. Lupus panniculitis occurring on the breast is termed as *lupus mastitis.* The erythematous and indurated clinical appearance can mimic inflammatory carcinoma of the breast or carcinoma erysipelatoides.[246] It can be seen in patients with a known history of systemic lupus erythematous or discoid lupus or herald these disorders. Most commonly, lupus panniculitis affects women in the fourth decade of life.[247] The most common histologic findings are the presence of a dense lymphoplasmacytic infiltration of fat lobules, hyaline fat necrosis, and mucin deposition. Calcifications and germinal centers may be present. Radiologic characteristics of lupus panniculitis can mimic a malignant lesion. Interestingly, patients with systemic lupus erythematosus have been found to be at a decreased risk of breast carcinoma, which is thought to be a result of antibody interference with DNA repair mechanisms in malignant cells.[248]

Darier Disease. Darier disease (keratosis follicularis) is an uncommon, autosomal dominant granulomatosis disorder with a seborrheic dermatitis–like distribution that can infrequently occur on the breast. The affected skin develops firm, discrete, 2- to 3-mm, red-brown spiny papules that may coalesce to form large plaques. The disease can be exacerbated by heat, high humidity, exposure to ultraviolet or ionizing radiation, or trauma. Secondary bacterial or fungal infection is common. This disorder has a characteristic appearance: individual keratinocytes in the suprabasal layer detach from their adjacent keratinocytes because of loss of intercellular bridges (acantholysis). These acantholytic cells undergo premature keratinization (dyskeratosis) and appear as shrunken, round, or flattened cells (corp ronds and grains) in hyperchromatic stratum corneum.[249] Oral synthetic retinoids may be used to control primary lesions, although the disease recurs when retinoids are discontinued. Avoiding or minimizing exposure to exacerbating factors is a mainstay of therapy. Appropriate topical or oral antibiotics and antifungals may be used to combat documented secondary infections. Of note, Darier disease overlying the breast may mask Paget's disease.[250] Grover disease, or transient acantholytic dermatosis, exhibits a nearly identical histologic picture but is characterized clinically by an eruption of itchy papules and macules on the upper chest and back of adults. It can also occasionally affect the breast. There is no familial predisposition and the disease is self-limited.

Connective Tissue Disorders. Systemic connective tissue disorders that may manifest on the breast include lupus panniculitis, localized or *systemic scleroderma,* and *dermatomyositis.*

Scleroderma appears as firm, indurated, white plaques with a central depression and faintly violaceous border that can occur anywhere on the body, including the breast. Scleroderma may manifest either as a localized lesion (termed *localized scleroderma, linear scleroderma,* or *morphea*) or as a systemic disorder that may be associated with systemic sclerosis or CREST syndrome (calcinosis cutis, Raynaud phenomenon, esophageal involvement, sclerodactyly, and telangiectasia). The dermatologic differential diagnosis includes scar, sclerotic carcinoma, sclerodermoid graft-versus-host disease and dermatomyofibroma. Importantly, when morphea is present in the breast, it may mimic inflammatory carcinoma of the breast.[251] Biopsy shows thickened sclerotic collagen (Fig. 13.17), particularly at the interface between the reticular dermis and the subcutaneous tissue with a sparse to mild associated lymphoplasmacytic inflammatory infiltrate. Therapy consists of potent topical steroids or steroids under occlusion. Although progression of the lesion may be inhibited, the plaque generally does not resolve. In patients with breast carcinoma, localized postradiation morphea may manifest as an irregular

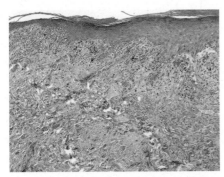

• **Fig. 13.17** Localized scleroderma or morphea is seen as dense collagenous bundles forming a nodule in the breast dermis.

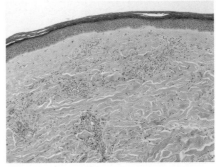

• **Fig. 13.19** Systemic lupus erythematosus can manifest in the skin of the breast and exhibit the characteristic lymphocytic infiltrate with epidermal atrophy and hydropic degeneration of the epidermal basal layer.

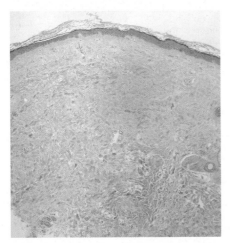

• **Fig. 13.18** Dermatomyositis. This systemic disorder can present in the breast as epidermal atrophy and perivascular lymphocytic infiltration.

erythematous mass and should not be confused with recurrent disease.[252–255]

Dermatomyositis (Fig. 13.18) is a clinical entity important for its paraneoplastic associations with underlying malignancy, including breast carcinoma.[256–259] Clinically, the disorder typically presents with symmetric proximal muscle weakness, heliotrope rash, Gottron papules, and vasculopathy.[260] Microscopic features of dermatomyositis can be subtle and consist of interface changes including basal vacuolar liquefactive degeneration, thickened basement membrane, epidermal atrophy, and presence of interstitial dermal mucin. The inflammation is sparse with few scattered interface and superficial perivascular lymphocytes. Occasionally, dermal or subcutaneous calcification may be noted. The histology of dermatomyositis may be indistinguishable from that of lupus erythematosus (Fig. 13.19).

Body Modification–Associated Dermopathy. Recent publications have documented dermopathies associated with tattooing and piercing. The process of tattooing mechanically injects colored pigments/inks into the dermis of the skin. Depending on the acuity of the user and sterility of equipment and pigments, the risk for associated infection may be high. Associated infections can include *Staphylococcus aureus* (which may be methicillin-resistant), human papillomavirus (which may cause verruca plana or verruca vulgaris), and atypical mycobacteria, among others.[261–263] Painful local inflammation in and adjacent to the pigment with or without axillary lymphadenopathy is the clinical manifestation of tattoo-associated infection. Abscess formation may

occur. Histologic examination of the tissue typically reveals acute inflammation and, with the correct ancillary staining, the presence of microorganisms. Piercing, most typically of the nipple, involves puncturing the skin to insert a foreign body. Metallic rings or jewels are typically used in the procedure. Similar to tattooing, local infection may occur with abscess formation.[264–267] The most frequent pathogens encountered are *Staphylococcus aureus, Streptococcus pyogenes,* and *Pseudomonas aeruginosa.*[261]

Both piercing and tattooing histopathologically may result in foreign-body reactions to the inorganic materials, demonstrated by granulomatous inflammation, multinucleated giant cells, chronic inflammation, and subsequent fibrosis adjacent to the foreign material. Unlike pigment incontinence associated with melanocytic proliferations, tattoo pigment is also present free in dermal tissue. Contact dermatitis may be seen in some individuals, heralded by pruritus associated with the recent piercing or tattoo.[268]

Secondary Neoplastic Disorders

Benign Disorders

Galactoceles. These benign milk-retention cysts may be found anywhere in the breast and in the skin in the nipple-areolar complex. They may form a single mass or multiple masses and should not be confused with malignancy. Microscopically, galactoceles are lined by cuboidal or flattened epithelium with cytoplasmic vacuolization resulting from lipid accumulation. Fibrosis typically surrounds intact cysts, whereas chronic inflammation and foreign-body giant cells may be seen with rupture. The lumen contains inspissated secretions.[269]

Hair Disorders. Vellus hair cysts and trichostasis spinulosa occur most frequently on the chest and abdomen. *Vellus hair cysts* commonly occur in childhood to the third decade of life and appear as multiple small red or brown papules. Histologically, these benign lesions are lined by a thin stratified squamous epithelial layer. The lumen contains small vellus hair arranged in a haphazard manner admixed with loose lamellated keratin debris. *Trichostasis spinulosa* is a follicular disorder resulting from the retention of vellus hairs within sebaceous follicles. It commonly occurs after the third decade of life and appears as spinous comedones or plugs. Histologically, an acanthotic epidermis is seen with multiple small hairs arranged in a keratin plug. Recognition of these lesions is important largely due to their association with other benign and malignant lesions, including syringomas and nodular basal cell carcinomas.[270]

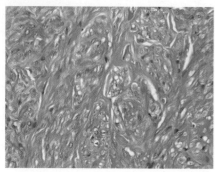

• **Fig. 13.20** Leiomyoma. Leiomyomas or pilileiomyomas are uncommon in the nipple-areola area but can occur and must be distinguished from infiltrating breast carcinomas.

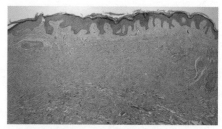

• **Fig. 13.21** Dermatofibroma. Common skin lesions also commonly occur in the breast dermis.

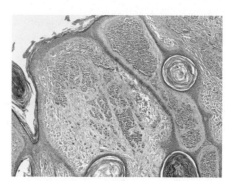

• **Fig. 13.22** Intradermal nevus. Intradermal nevi are common in the breast.

Vascular Neoplasms. *Cherry angiomas* are red to violaceous papules measuring a few millimeters in diameter that are common in adults. Histologic examination shows a cluster of dilated thin-walled vessels in the superficial dermis. *Angiokeratomas* are vascular lesions with ectatic vascular spaces that directly abut the epidermis may be markers for Fabry disease (alpha-galactosidase deficiency) and should prompt a search for clusters of angiokeratomas around the navel and on the genitals (i.e., angiokeratoma corporis diffusum), corneal opacities, and symptoms of anhidrosis or hypohidrosis.[271]

Smooth Muscle Neoplasms. *Pilar leiomyomas* are benign proliferations of smooth muscle bundles resembling those that attach to hair follicles (Fig. 13.20). Arrector pili are especially prominent in the nipple-areolar area, and pilar leiomyomas may occur in this region. Pilar leiomyomas are often exquisitely painful and respond to light touch, stroking, or chilling with painful contraction. Occasionally, these pilar leiomyomas can grow large and present as a nipple or areolar mass lesion. Bilateral smooth muscle tumors arising in the areola and nipple have been reported.[272] Calcium channel blockers have been used to control activation of these muscles when excision is not feasible. Pilar leiomyomas are also a feature of Becker nevus (discussed at the beginning of the chapter) but in this setting are not painful.

Although rare examples of smooth muscle tumors of the breast parenchyma have been reported,[273] most *leiomyomas* of the breast occur in a subareolar location. The etiology of these benign tumors is unclear, and a family history or genetic linkage has not been conclusively reported. Nipple leiomyomas may be asymptomatic for long periods or present with a mass or recurrent attacks of severe pain that occur spontaneously after application of pressure or after exposure to cold. The pain is thought to be related to contractions of the neoplastic smooth muscle. Examination may reveal a single, small, firm dermal or subcutaneous papule. The differential diagnosis includes papilloma, adenoma, and Paget's disease. In contrast to Paget's disease, leiomyomas show characteristic pain without inflammation. Cytologic atypia and mitotic figures are not seen. Surgical excision may be helpful for symptomatic tumors.

Fibrous Neoplasms. Solitary *dermatofibromas* may occur in the breast. These lesions clinically appear as firm, colorless, subcutaneous nodules (Fig. 13.21). Dermatofibromas are histologically defined by a dermal proliferation composed of spindled fibroblasts and histiocytes arranged in fascicles with intervening entrapped dense hyalinized collagen bundles. Variable cellularity is observed. The overlying epidermis may show variable hyperplasia and hyperpigmentation but is generally uninvolved. Simple excision is curative in most cases. *Dermatomyofibroma* and *granular cell tumor* are both uncommon and benign dermal entities that can occur in the breast.

Benign Melanocytic Lesions. Pigmented lesions of the breast are common. The average Caucasian adult has 40 to 100 benign melanocytic nevi scattered over all body surfaces, and these are common in the breast. These lesions range from simple lentigos (basilar hyperpigmentation of keratinocytes with variable numbers of melanocytes) to junctional, compound, and intradermal melanocytic nevi (Fig. 13.22). Nevi are generally smaller than 0.5 cm, oval to round, tan to brown, evenly pigmented, macular or papular lesions with relatively smooth borders. Congenital nevi may be larger, darker, and slightly asymmetric. *Becker nevus syndrome*, detailed earlier, is commonly associated with unilateral breast hypoplasia.[274,275] *Nevoid hyperkeratosis* is a rare benign hyperkeratosis of the nipple[276,277] histologically characterized by orthokeratotic hyperkeratosis, acanthosis, and papillomatosis with occasional keratotic plugging and mild papillary dermal fibrosis. Microscopic differential diagnoses include seborrheic keratosis and epidermal nevus.

Melanosis of the nipple, a benign entity, cannot be clinically distinguished from pigmented Paget's disease of the breast or malignant melanoma. Increased melanin may be seen in basilar melanocytes and keratinocytes, but there is no increase in number or abnormal localization of melanocytes in the biopsy.[278] Dermoscopy may be useful in deciding whether to biopsy a pigmented lesion on the breast or nipple.

Malignant Disorders

Actinic Keratosis and Bowen Disease. Both actinic keratosis (AK) and Bowen disease are considered premalignant lesions with potential to progress to invasive squamous cell carcinoma. Clinically, AKs appear as discrete erythematous rough hyperkeratotic papules with scale. AKs have been documented as a dermatologic side effect of both doxorubicin and capecitabine, chemotherapy

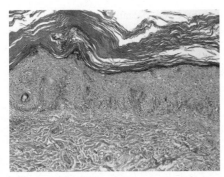

• **Fig. 13.23** Bowen disease. Bowen disease or carcinoma in situ, characterized by crowded atypical squamous epithelium, can occur on the breast, may be related to prior irradiation, and most importantly, may progress to invasive squamous cell carcinoma.[283]

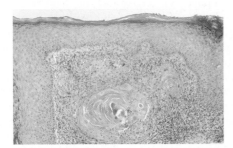

• **Fig. 13.24** Squamous cell carcinoma. Invasive squamous cell carcinoma exhibits keratin pearl formation and an invasive growth pattern and can occur in the breast.

for breast carcinoma.[279,280] Squamous cell carcinoma in situ, also called Bowen disease, clinically appears as a velvety red patch that is sharply demarcated from the adjacent skin (Fig. 13.23). Histologically, full-thickness squamous atypia of the epidermis without extension through the epithelial basement membrane is present. The risk of developing invasive carcinoma from Bowen disease is estimated at 3% to 5%.[281,282] Both AK and Bowen disease generally occur on sun-exposed areas and may regress spontaneously, remain stable, or evolve to invasive squamous cell carcinoma.[283]

Squamous Cell Carcinoma. Squamous cell carcinoma can occur on any mucocutaneous surface. These lesions may have a similar clinical appearance to AK and Bowen disease. Histologically, well-differentiated squamous cell carcinoma is characterized by an infiltrative lobular growth of atypical keratinocytes with variable degrees of pleomorphism and mitoses (Fig. 13.24). The lesional cells are present in the dermis individually and/or in nests and may exhibit intercellular bridges, keratin pearls, and apoptotic cells. Poorly differentiated squamous cell carcinomas are highly infiltrative and lack overt features of their squamous lineage such as keratinization and intercellular bridges. Perineural invasion and sclerotic changes are more common as the tumor becomes more aggressive.

Basal Cell Carcinoma. Basal cell carcinoma is the most common malignancy in both men and women. Fortunately, this tumor typically remains confined to the skin and rarely metastasizes, although local recurrence is not uncommon. Basal cell carcinoma arises most frequently on sun-damaged skin but can occur on a non–sun-exposed breast (Fig. 13.25). Histologic subtypes of basal cell carcinoma are numerous and include superficial, nodular, pigmented, morpheaform, and noduloulcerative variants, the latter of which is the most common on the breast. Clinically, these

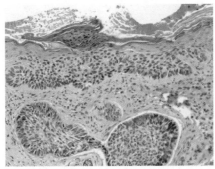

• **Fig. 13.25** Basal cell carcinoma. Basal cell carcinoma, the most common cancer in men and women, can also occur in the breast and is characterized by islands of cells with peripheral palisading.

lesions present as pearly nodules with associated telangiectasia. Histologically, the tumor consists of nests of small, basaloid epithelial cells with peripheral palisading of nuclei at the dermal-epidermal junction and/or in the dermis. A characteristic feature of basal cell carcinoma is retraction of the stroma around the tumor islands, creating artifactual clefts. Ulceration may be present in the overlying epidermis and adnexal differentiation may be seen in the tumor. Multifocality of these tumors is not uncommon and may make evaluation of specimen margins difficult. If incompletely excised, basal cell carcinoma may recur. Histologic features associated with aggressive clinical behavior include perineural invasion, lymphovascular invasion, and micronodular, infiltrative, and morpheaform patterns of growth.

Approximately 40 cases of primary basal cell carcinoma of the nipple-areolar complex have been reported in the literature.[284,285] It is important for the clinician to be aware of this possibility because this lesion may mimic nipple duct adenoma (florid papillomatosis), Paget's disease, and squamous cells carcinoma, as well as underlying primary breast malignancy. Treatment of basal cell carcinoma of the breast or the nipple remains the same as treatment at other body sites.[286,287] Patients with neoplasms at low risk for recurrence (<20 mm in greatest dimension, well-defined borders, nodular/superficial subtype on biopsy) undergo curettage and electrodesiccation or standard excision with 4.0-mm negative margins. Radiation therapy remains a possibility for patients who are not surgical candidates. High-risk of recurrence neoplasms (aggressive histologic subtype, >20 mm, perineural invasion) are offered standard excision with wide surgical margins or Mohs surgery.

Malignant Melanoma. The differential diagnosis of a pigmented lesion on the breast is lengthy and includes nevoid lentigo, melanocytic nevus, pigmented seborrheic keratosis, pigmented basal cell carcinoma, melanoma in situ, and malignant melanoma (Fig. 13.26). Malignant melanomas, like basal cell carcinomas and squamous cell carcinomas, are more commonly observed in sun-exposed areas and are related to sun exposure. Primary malignant melanoma of the skin of the breast accounts for 3% to 5% of melanomas.[288,289]

Pigmented lesions that change, grow, ulcerate, itch, bleed, show significant color variation, or develop border irregularities should be excised (or, if larger than 2.0 cm, biopsied) to rule out melanoma. The initial evaluation of a patient with a suspected melanoma includes a personal history, family history, and appropriate physical examination, which includes a whole-body skin examination and palpation of the regional lymph nodes. The focus of this evaluation is to identify risk factors, signs, or symptoms of metastases, atypical moles, and additional melanomas. Routine

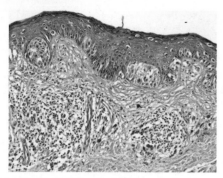

• **Fig. 13.26** Malignant melanoma. Malignant melanoma can also occur in the breast. Although overall its biology is similar to melanomas elsewhere, melanomas of the nipple and areola are thought to have a better prognosis than nonbreast melanomas; the reasons for this are not understood.

screening performed by dermatologists is recommended in high-risk populations.[290] Of note, the most common second malignancy in a person with a biopsy-proven melanoma is a second melanoma.[290] Clinically, the lesions are large, asymmetric plaques of variable color (from white—indicating areas of regression—to black, brown, blue, or red).

All major types of malignant melanoma can occur on the breast. Of these the most common subtype of melanoma that arises on the breast is the superficial spreading type. Superficial spreading melanomas demonstrate atypical proliferations of nested, epithelioid melanocytes often associated with prominent pagetoid spread. A bandlike inflammatory infiltrate is often noted in the superficial dermis. Lentigo maligna melanomas show epidermal atrophy and prominent solar elastosis associated with subtle proliferation of melanocytes along the basal layer with invasion into the superficial dermis. Pagetoid spread is less likely to be found, but there is often extension of tumor cells downward along adnexal elements. Nodular melanomas are predominantly thick dermal lesions with limited intraepidermal spread beyond the dermal component of the lesion. The cytology is epithelioid and similar to that of superficial spreading melanoma. Desmoplastic melanomas show spindled melanocytes embedded within a fibrotic stroma, suggesting the presence of a scar upon initial observation. Further examination reveals spindled cells arranged in haphazard, fascicular, or storiform growth patterns. Melanin pigmentation is often scant or absent. The immunohistochemical profile of melanomas of the breast is identical to that of melanomas at other cutaneous sites. Most melanomas are positive for melanocytic markers such as S100, HMB-45, Melan-A (MART-1), tyrosinase, MITF, and SOX10. Desmoplastic melanomas typically demonstrate only positive immunoreactivity for SOX10. Staining for all other markers is either weak or absent in desmoplastic melanomas.

In situ melanomas are those confined to the epidermis and skin appendages. Invasive melanomas invade into the dermis and provoke a variable inflammatory host response. Depth of invasion is generally reported both by Clark level, which reflects the functional level of invasion, and Breslow thickness, which is the depth of invasion as measured from the top of the granular layer to the deepest lesion cell using a calibrated ocular micrometer.

Tumor staging as described in the seventh edition of the American Joint Committee on Cancer Manual has undergone some significant revisions. Any invasive melanoma 1.0 mm or smaller in thickness is tumor stage I. Without ulceration, such thin melanomas are stage T1a provided there is less than 1 mitosis/mm².

Stage T1b lesions have ulceration and/or demonstrable mitotic activity. Stage T2a and stage T3a lesions are nonulcerated lesions measuring 1.01 to 2.00 and 2.01 to 4.0 mm in thickness, respectively; stage T2b and T3b lesions measure the same respective thickness but exhibit ulceration. pT4 melanomas are greater than 4.0 mm, with T4a having an intact epidermis and T4b exhibiting ulceration.[177]

Standard therapy for melanoma is wide surgical excision. Recommended resection margins for melanoma in situ are 0.5 cm; wider margins are unsupported by current evidence.[291]

The surgical margin should be histologically free of tumor. For invasive lesions, a 1.0- to 2.0-cm negative margin should be sufficient based on current evidence.[286] Elective regional lymph node dissection is not indicated for patients with thin melanomas. Removal and microscopic examination of the sentinel lymph node identified by dye or lymphoscintigraphy for micrometastatic melanoma is "an important staging tool, but has not been shown to improve disease-specific survival among all patients."[286] Extensive diagnostic studies (e.g., computed tomography, magnetic resonance imaging, scintigraphy) are not indicated and should not be performed when staging asymptomatic patients; however, origin of the melanoma from the skin of the breast is an independent but significant negative prognostic factor.[177] An exception is primary melanoma of the nipple and areola, which is exceedingly rare and overall has a better prognosis and lower incidence of metastasis than other melanomas of the breast. Other negative prognostic factors include a Breslow thickness greater than 1.5 mm, ulceration, perineural invasion, and male sex. Regional or distant lymphadenopathy or symptoms suggesting distant organ metastases are grave prognostic indicators.

Dermatofibrosarcoma Protuberans. Dermatofibrosarcoma protuberans (DFSP) is a low-grade cutaneous sarcoma that typically occurs in the extremities of young and middle-aged adults. Sporadic reported cases affecting the breast are noted in the literature.[292–296] Clinically, this lesion appears as a firm nodular or multinodular subcutaneous mass with erythematous plaque-like growth. DFSP exhibits histology similar to dermatofibroma, with dermal proliferation of spindled cells arranged in a storiform or herringbone pattern, interlaced with collagen bundles. Nuclear atypia is often minimal and mitoses may be present. Architecturally, the tumor characteristically is found to infiltrate into the subcutis in a honeycomb pattern, interdigitating between fat lobules. The epidermis is characteristically uninvolved. An important histologic variant of DFSP demonstrates fibrosarcomatous change, which likely represents a progression of disease toward dedifferentiation and portends a poor outcome.[297] The major differential diagnosis is dermatofibroma; by immunohistochemistry, DFSPs are typically positive for CD34 and negative for factor XIIIa, whereas dermatofibromas typically exhibit the opposite phenotype. DFSPs are locally aggressive and, if incompletely excised, may recur with a more aggressive clinical behavior.

Lymphomas. *Cutaneous T-cell lymphomas* (mycosis fungoides) affecting the breast or presenting initially as breast lesions are found in multiple case reports in the available literature.[298–300] Cutaneous T-cell lymphoma typically appears as brownish red patches with fine scale and delicate wrinkling on the skin of the trunk, typically within intertriginous areas such as inframammary folds and axillae (Fig. 13.27). Histologically, the lymphocytic infiltrate is identified in superficial dermis with extension by single and clustered lymphocytes into the overlying epidermis without prominent spongiosis. The epidermal basement membrane is preserved, contrary to that seen in lichenoid or reactive processes.

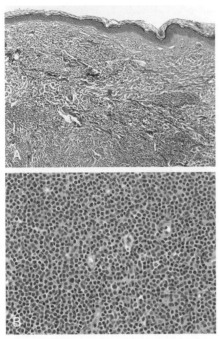

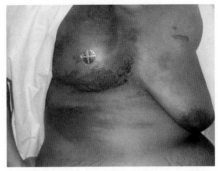

• **Fig. 13.29** Carcinoma erysipeloids. Carcinoma erysipeloids of the breast can be obvious as a hard plaque appearance of the breast due to infiltration of the breast dermis by carcinoma cells.

• **Fig. 13.27** Small lymphocytic lymphoma. A small lymphocytic lymphoma can either arise in the breast or secondarily involve the breast. (A) Here a small lymphocytic infiltrate is observed to infiltrate the dermis of the breast. (B) At higher magnification, the cells consist of relatively mature lymphocytes.

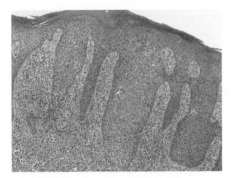

• **Fig. 13.28** Mycosis fungoides. Mycosis fungoides is characterized by atypical dermal lymphocytes showing epidermotropism. It can similarly either arise in the breast or secondarily involve the breast.

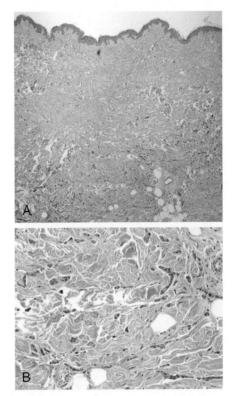

• **Fig. 13.30** (A) Breast carcinoma cells directly infiltrating the dermis of the breast. (B) Higher magnification shows the carcinoma cells percolating through the collagen and adipose tissue. This biology, when present, uniformly confers a poor prognosis.

The hallmark immunohistochemical analysis reveals the lesional cells to be comprised of an overwhelming predominance of CD4+ lymphocytes, with few scattered CD8+ T cells intermixed within. Loss of other pan T-cell antigens, such as CD7 and CD5, may be present.

Subcutaneous panniculitis-like T-cell lymphoma has been documented to affect the breast only rarely,[301] at times as a breast mass.[302] These lesions may be classified in two forms: *alpha-beta* types, which do not express CD4 and CD56 but express CD8, and *gamma-delta* types, which express CD56 but are negative for CD4 and CD8. Patients with alpha-beta subtype demonstrate a significantly better prognosis than those with the gamma-delta subtype (mean survival of 5 years vs. 15 months).[303,304]

Other forms of lymphoma less commonly affect the skin of the breast, including *extranodal natural killer/T-cell lymphoma, nasal type*[305] and *primary cutaneous B-cell lymphomas* (Fig. 13.28).[306,307] Careful clinical evaluation of the patient and ancillary studies, including biopsy tissue submitted for routine processing and for molecular and genetic analysis, allow accurate categorization of most lymphoproliferative disorders. The subject of primary and secondary breast lymphoma is discussed extensively in Chapter 11.

Satellite Skin Metastasis. One should keep in mind at all times that the skin of the breast is a potential site of metastasis for invasive breast carcinoma. When the skin is involved, the breast cancer is staged as a T4, which confers a poor prognosis. Four clinical patterns are observed: inflammatory carcinoma, telangiectatic carcinoma, nodular carcinoma, and carcinoma en cuirasse. One or more types may be present in the same patient. The clinical presentation, with a swollen, hard, or inflamed breast ("peau d'orange") or an inverted nipple, strongly suggests cutaneous involvement by carcinoma, termed as *carcinoma erysipeloides* (Fig. 13.29). Other times, a biopsy is necessary (Fig. 13.30).

Selected References

52. Monifar F. *Essentials of Diagnostic Breast Pathology*. New York: Springer; 2007.

108. Abenoza P, Ackerman AB. *Neoplasms With Eccrine Differentiation: Ackerman's Histologic Diagnosis of Neoplastic Skin Diseases: A Method by Pattern Analysis*. Philadelphia: Lea & Febiger; 1989.

270. Panchaprateep R, Tanus A, Tosti A. Clinical, dermoscopic, and histopathologic features of body hair disorders. *J Am Acad Dermatol*. 2015;72:890-900. doi:10.1016/j.jaad.2015.01.024.

277. Spyropoulou GA, Pavlidis L, Trakatelli M, et al. Rare benign tumors of the nipple. *J Eur Acad Dermatol Venereol*. 2015; 29:7-13.

278. Isbary G, Coras-Stepanek B, Dyall-Smith D, et al. Five patients with melanosis of the nipple and areola clinically mimicking melanoma. *J Eur Acad Dermatol Venereol*. 2014;28:1251-1254.

279. Krathen M, Treat J, James WD. Capecitabine induced inflammation of actinic keratoses. *Dermatol Online J*. 2007;13:13.

A full reference list is available online at ExpertConsult.com.

14

Breast Biomarker Immunocytochemistry

SOHEILA KOROURIAN, ASANGI R. KUMARAPELI, AND V. SUZANNE KLIMBERG

Breast cancer is a heterogeneous disease process. According to the World Health Organization, more than 20 morphologic subtypes of breast cancer have been recognized.[1] By gene expression, invasive breast cancer is classified into at least four major subtypes: luminal A, luminal B, human epidermal growth factor receptor 2 (HER2)/neu-positive, and triple-negative cancers.[2–4] The biology and the prognosis of these subtypes are vastly different.[5] It is well recognized that genetic profiles of these cancer subtypes are also interlinked with the traditional breast biomarkers.[6–8] According to the US National Institutes of Health's (NIH's) Working Group and Biomarkers Consortium, a biomarker is a characteristic that is objectively measured as an indicator of normal biological processes, pathogenic processes, or a pharmacologic response to a therapeutic intervention.[9] For more than 40 years, estrogen receptor (ER) has been recognized to play a crucial central role in the development and progression of breast cancer.[10] This knowledge has been used to develop treatment protocols targeting this biomarker to block the progression and recurrence of breast cancer.[11,12] With the passage of time, additional biomarkers were discovered. Today ER, progesterone receptor (PR), and HER2/neu are considered important biomarkers that can predict not only the response to treatment but also prognosis and potentially disease recurrence.[13–15] The reporting of these biomarkers is now almost completely standardized throughout the United States.[16,17] Other commonly used but less defined biomarkers are Ki67, a proliferation marker, and p53.[18,19] Currently, there is no universal protocol for reporting. The significance of p53 expression is even less defined; therefore, this biomarker will not be discussed.

Epithelial cadherin (E-cadherin) and p120 that are used to confirm diagnosis of lobular differentiation are not traditionally considered breast biomarkers. Because invasive lobular carcinoma is thought to have a different prognosis independent of the stage, these immunohistochemical markers should also be considered in the category of breast biomarkers.[20,21]

Estrogen Receptor: Historical Perspective

ER status has long been recognized as an important predictive and prognostic biomarker in breast cancer. Adjuvant hormonal therapy has shown considerable benefits in terms of reduced overall disease recurrence and 15-year mortality from breast cancer in women of all ages with ER-positive tumors (that generally represents more than 75% of all breast tumors).[22,23] ER assessment by immunohistochemistry (IHC) is now the standard in the management of breast cancer. Like other steroid receptors, ER belongs to the nuclear receptor superfamily. It consists of 553 amino acids

forming an N-terminal domain with transcription activation functions, a central DNA-binding domain and a ligand-binding domain at the carboxy terminal.[24] Two isoforms of ER exist: ERα and Erβ, which are encoded by two different genes with no homology in their amino acid sequences.[25] Although the specific roles of ERβ are still being elucidated, ERα is the most studied and clinically measured isoform. The ligand for ER is the female sex hormone 17β-estradiol (E2) that in the physiologic state mediates growth and differentiation of the breast ducts. Estrogen signaling pathway is activated when the hormone diffuses through the cell membrane and binds to nuclear ER, inducing its dimerization. The ligand-receptor complex then promotes downstream gene transcriptions.[26]

The association between estrogen hormone and breast cancer pathogenesis has been known since the late 1800s. Objective evidence of tumor regression with oophorectomy, adrenalectomy, or hypophysectomy has been documented for metastatic and inoperable breast tumors.[11,27] The initial report on the characterization and measurements of ER was from Jensen and associates in the mid-1960s.[28] A few years later, McGuire and colleagues observed that there was variability in the concentration of ER in primary and metastatic breast cancers and emphasized that an assay for ER must be quantitative.[10] Their studies provided the early insights into this hormone receptor's utility as a biomarker for breast cancer.

Before the era of IHC, ligand-binding assays were used primarily for receptor quantitation. These biochemical procedures were often cumbersome and involved extraction of receptor proteins by homogenization of fresh-frozen tumor tissue, incubation of the homogenate with radioactive and nonradioactive E2, followed by separation of the bound and unbound hormone. Scatchard plots and standard curves were subsequently used to quantify ER and expressed in femtomoles of ER protein per milligram of cytosol protein. Some of the earlier receptor analytic methods included Sephadex gel filtration, protamine sulfate precipitation, sucrose density gradient ultracentrifugation, and dextran-coated charcoal assay.[29] The latter two methods were commonly used, with dextran-coated charcoal assay preferred because of its ease of use and its accuracy.[29,30] Although newer methodologies such as enzyme immunoassays and IHC have made ligand-binding assays obsolete, they were the first assays that broadened our understanding of ER and the response to hormonal therapy, helped determine positive and negative cutoff levels for ER, and were even used to validate the newer assays.[31]

The application of IHC for ER gained widespread acceptance in the 1990s with the development of new monoclonal antibodies to ER and different antigen retrieval techniques. IHC offers many advantages over the traditional biochemical assays; importantly, it can be applied on very small amounts of tumor in formalin-fixed, paraffin-embedded tissue as well as frozen tissue. The immunohistochemical stain can be directly applied to a microscopic slide, which permits direct visualization of anti-ER antibodies binding to tumor cells and helps differentiate ER staining of stromal cells, necrotic tumor, and benign parenchyma from the tumor cells. Furthermore, in situ and invasive components and different morphologic subtypes can be selectively evaluated with IHC.[32] Worldwide, the current practice is to use IHC exclusively on paraffin sections to assess ER status of breast cancers.[33]

Progesterone Receptor: Historical Perspective

Like ER, PR status is an independent predictive factor for benefit from adjuvant endocrine therapy and a prognostic indicator for early recurrence in breast cancer.[34–36] This discovery was preceded by observations that a subset of ER-positive breast cancers failed to respond to hormonal manipulation, indicating that ER presence alone was not a sufficient indicator of hormone dependence in breast cancer. It was shown that ER-positive/PR-positive breast cancers fared better compared with ER-positive/PR-negative tumors to adjuvant treatment.[37] Studies by Horowitz and associates, the same group that extensively studied ER, suggested that the presence of PR might serve as an indicator of the functionality of the estrogen signaling pathway in the breast.[38]

PR, too, is a member of the steroid receptor subgroup of ligand-activated transcription factors within the large nuclear receptor superfamily. It contains 946 amino acids, a DNA-binding domain sandwiched between an N-terminal domain with transcription activation and inhibitory functions and a C-terminal ligand-binding domain. The central DNA-binding domain of PR shows considerable sequence homology to that of ER. The two isoforms, namely PR-A and PR-B, are encoded by the same gene (unlike the isoforms of ER) and are identical except that the truncated PR-A is short of 164 amino acids that are seen at the N-terminal end of PR-B.[39,40] In the normal breast PR-A and PR-B are coexpressed at equal levels in luminal epithelial cells, suggesting that both proteins are required to mediate physiologically relevant progesterone signaling (i.e., formation of lobular-alveolar structures, modulation of milk synthesis and duct development). In breast cancer, however, predominance of one isoform is common, suggesting that the resultant unbalanced expression of PR-A and PR-B may induce aberrant targeting of genes.[41] PRs are under the control of E2 or related estrogens, and in breast cancer, PR is synthesized by tumor cells that are stimulated by estrogens through an interaction with ER.[42] Thus PR is a surrogate marker of ER activity, and it is rare that PR-positive cells do not also express ER.[43,44]

Ligand-binding assays (sucrose gradient ultracentrifugation and dextran-coated charcoal assays) were the gold standard for early characterization and measurement of PR.[45] With the advent of monoclonal antibodies to PR, IHC largely replaced the biochemical assays for PR measurement in the mid-1990s.[46]

Several studies demonstrated that IHC was superior to ligand-binding assays and enzyme immunoassays for assessing ER and PR status in primary breast cancer and had equivalent or better ability to predict response to adjuvant endocrine therapy.[46–50] However, reproducible and reliable IHC assays are essential with proper standardization for meaningful clinical application.

Receptor Status Assessment: Why Is It Important?

The assessment of hormone receptors in primary invasive breast cancer is now mandatory because of its significant clinical therapeutic implications.[51] Both ER and PR are strong predictive factors and relatively weak prognostic factors for response to adjuvant and therapeutic hormonal therapy. The standard of treatment for premenopausal women who have ER-positive breast cancer has been 5 years of tamoxifen. For postmenopausal patients, a minimum of 5 years of adjuvant therapy with an aromatase inhibitor or tamoxifen followed by an aromatase inhibitor (in sequence) had been recommended.[52,53] Findings from several recent phase III randomized control trials have prompted a shift in these practice guidelines. It is now viewed that 10 years of tamoxifen treatment instead of stopping at 5 years can further reduce recurrence and approximately halve breast cancer mortality during the second decade after diagnosis.[54,55] It was noted that the therapeutic benefit was directly proportional to the level of ER, with patients with higher expression of ER in the breast cancers demonstrating the most benefit.[56] Also, low ER or PR is associated with a high risk of recurrence after hormonal therapy.[57] On the other hand, ER-negative cancers respond favorably to chemotherapy and are more likely to achieve a complete pathologic response after neoadjuvant chemotherapy than do ER-positive tumors.[5] Interestingly, single hormone receptor-positive tumors (ER-positive/PR-negative and ER-negative/PR-positive) are known to have less sensitivity to tamoxifen, although some reports claim that patients with ER-negative/PR-positive tumors may derive benefit from tamoxifen.[35,57–59] Such knowledge underscores the importance of properly identifying patients who truly express ER and PR in their tumors, so that they do not lose the opportunity for timely and appropriate treatment.

It was expected that IHC, like ligand-binding assays, was an intrinsically quantitative method that demonstrated a direct linear relationship between the amount of ER protein present in tumor cell nuclei and the amount of ER antigen detected by IHC. However, a number of studies have shown that this is not the case and that ER IHC results are often highly influenced by preanalytic and analytic factors such as tissue fixation time, antigen retrieval methods, and antigen detection methods.[60–63] Hormone receptor IHC has been the topic of numerous controversies due to lack of standardization of the test, poor reproducibility among laboratories, and lack of proficiency testing. Standardization of IHC testing and cutoff values for positive results are hence critical to avoid false-negative results.[64,65] In 2001, an NIH consensus development panel recommended that patients with any expression of hormone receptor in their tumor cells may benefit from hormonal therapy, implying that a mere positive or negative ER status suffices in therapeutic decision-making.[66] Later studies however, emphasized that quantification of hormonal receptors by IHC may help better identify patients who may benefit from adjuvant chemotherapy and also clarify why some patients do not respond to hormonal therapy.[67]

Scoring of Receptor Expression

There has been no uniform method of interpreting IHC results. Although some pathologists use a binary system (completely negative or unequivocally positive), others use a continuous reporting system for ER and PR.[68,69] Also, no uniformly accepted cutoff point for positivity has been determined. Some laboratories use such arbitrary thresholds as more than 5%, more than 10%, and even 20% for ER-positive tumors.[47] To address these issues, quantification systems have been generated that may use only the proportion of positive cell nuclei or may include the intensity of immunoreactivity as well. The proportion of positive staining cells is a visual estimation, usually depicted as a percentage, whereas staining intensity of cells are reported as weak, moderate, or strong based on the degree of staining characteristics. There is heterogeneity of immunoreactivity in most cancers and the intensity of stained cells are often affected by the actual amount of protein present, the concentration and quality of antibodies used (high or low affinity), and other technical aspects, such as antigen retrieval and detection systems.

In 1985, McCarty and colleagues described the H-score semiquantitative scoring system.[70] The H-score consists of the sum of the percent of tumor cells staining multiplied by an ordinal value corresponding to the intensity level (0 = none; 1 = weak; 2 = moderate; and 3 = strong) with a maximum possible score of 300. According to the modified H-score, a score less than 1 is considered negative, a score less than 100 is weakly positive (1+), a score of 101 to 200 is moderately positive (2+), and a score of 201 to 300 is strongly positive (3+).

The Allred score, described by Allred and colleagues, is calculated by adding a proportion score to an intensity score.[71,72] The proportion of positive staining cells is scored on a 0 to 5 scale (0 = no staining; 1 = less than 1%; 2 = 1%–10%; 3 = 11%–33%; 4 = 34%–66% and 5 = 67%–100%). The staining intensity of tumor cells is scored on a 0 to 3 scale (0 = none; 1 = weak; 2 = moderate; 3 = strong). These two scores are then added together for a final score of 0 or 2 through 8. A final score of 0 to 2 is considered negative and a score between 3 and 8 are positive. Studies have shown that cancers with an Allred score of 2 had similar outcome compared with patients whose cancers were completely negative for ER.[47] Most breast cancers fall between Allred scores 7 and 8 that show excellent response to treatment. Tumors with scores 3 and 4, although considered positive, are not well studied.

Both the H-score and Allred score are widely used, and they classify tumors to fairly comparable but not identical groups.[73] Among other scoring systems, a modified J-score, introduced by Japanese investigators, only evaluated the number of positive cells without taking the staining intensity into consideration.[74] The criteria used for J-score was as follows, using both 1% and 10% as their cutoff points; J-score 0: no staining; J-score 1: less than 1% stained cells; J-score 2: stained cells more than 1% but less than 10%, and J-score 3: more than 10% stained cells. The final decision on hormone receptor status was classified as negative (J-score 0), Equivocal (J-score 1 and 2), and Positive (J-score 3). This scoring system did not appear to gain acceptance in the Western world, however.

Larger laboratories use computer-assisted image analysis to aid in quantitation of staining in IHC. This is expected to improve interlaboratory variability. Turbin and associates showed that fully automated quantitation of ER immunostaining yielded results that did not differ from human manual scoring against both biochemical assay and patient outcome gold standards.[75] Their cutoff scores were 0: less than 1% positive tumor nuclei, 1+: 1% to 25% positive nuclei, 2+: 25% to 75% positive nuclei, and 3+: more than 75% positive nuclei). The optimal cutoff point found in their study for automated scoring was 0.4% of positive tumor nuclei, consistent with the findings of Harvey and colleagues.[47]

American Society of Clinical Oncology/College of American Pathologists Recommendations

To improve the accuracy of immunohistochemical ER and PR testing in breast cancer and the utility of these receptors as predictive markers, the American Society of Clinical Oncology (ASCO) and College of American Pathologists (CAP) guideline recommendations were announced in 2010. The expert panel determined that when 1% or more of the tumor cell nuclei are immunoreactive to ER (or PR), the test is considered positive, provided expected reactivity of internal and external controls are met.[76] It has been shown that higher ER levels have a higher probability of response to therapy. Although debatable, ER expression as low as 1% positive staining has been associated with clinical response. Therefore reporting low or weak ER expressions in the range of 1% to 10% will allow the clinician to assess the benefits of hormonal therapy versus risks on a case-by-case basis.[47,49] This was the basis for a ≥1% cutoff choice. According to ASCO/CAP recommendations, less than 1% immunoreactive tumor cells (in the presence of positive internal controls) are considered receptor negative. Allred scores, H-scores, or simply reporting the percentage of positive cells are used for receptor quantitation.

The CAP imposes stringent quality assurance and reporting requirements for ER and PR testing. These include proper validation of tests to ensure accuracy, carrying out laboratory inspections and accreditations, and conducting external proficiency testing surveys. Minimizing cold ischemic time of breast specimens to less than 1 hour and adhering to adequate fixation times (more than 6 hours and less than 72 hours) are also crucial.[51,76] Patient test reports should list antibody and dilutions used, antigen retrieval methods (if performed), and document the use and appropriate staining of controls.

Fig. 14.1 depicts images of four separate invasive breast cancers. Two of them show strong and diffuse ER positivity, the third shows a mixed pattern of ER expression, and the fourth case shows complete absence of ER. Note the presence of ER, marked as nuclear positivity within the benign ductal structure, internal control, confirming antigen preservation.

Correlation With Oncotype Dx

With the new concepts of personalized medicine, the past decade has seen the emergence of several gene classifier tests to assess the risk of disease recurrence and thereby tailor individual treatment in breast cancer patients. Oncotype Dx (GenomicHealth, Redwood City, CA) is one such molecular assay with its 21-gene signature (16 prognostic genes that included ER and PR and 5 reference genes) that has gained worldwide acceptance among oncologists.[77,78] It is a quantitative reverse transcriptase polymerase chain reaction (qRT-PCR) test performed on formalin-fixed paraffin-embedded tissue that generates a recurrence score (ranging from 0 to 100) classifying patients as having low (score <18), intermediate (18–30), or high (>31) risk of disease recurrence. Studies demonstrated that patients with assigned low recurrence score by Oncotype Dx could be spared adjuvant chemotherapy and be treated with tamoxifen alone, whereas patients with higher recurrence scores would benefit from combined tamoxifen and chemotherapy to significantly reduce disease relapse.[77] Ongoing trials attempt to determine the benefits of combined therapy versus hormonal therapy for the Oncotype Dx intermediate

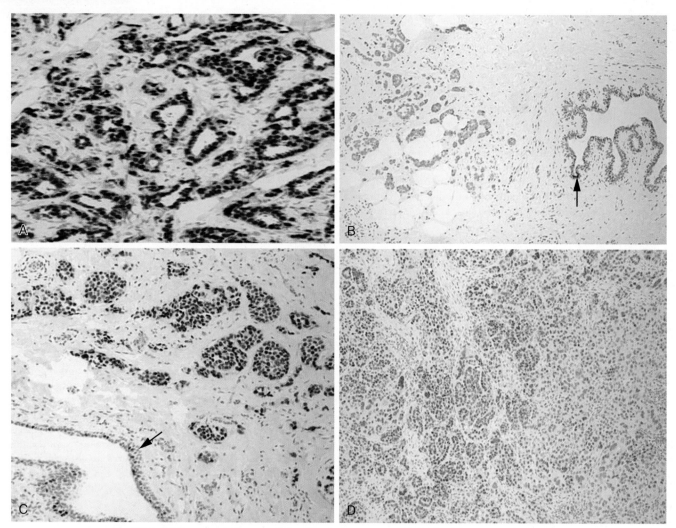

• **Fig. 14.1.** (A) Strong and diffuse positivity with estrogen receptor. (B) Estrogen receptor negative (*arrow*, internal control). (C) Strong and diffuse positivity with estrogen receptor (*arrow*, internal control). (D) Estrogen receptor positive, mixed pattern.

recurrence score patients.[79] The test was originally intended for early stage (stages I, II, and IIIa) ER-positive, node-negative invasive breast cancer. With multiple clinical validation studies, this test is now extended for the use of all newly diagnosed early stage, node-negative, or node-positive (1–3 nodes), ER-positive, and HER2-negative breast cancers, although the test's exact role in the node-positive patients remain controversial.[80,81]

Oncotype Dx assay with its recurrence score is undoubtedly a valuable prognostic tool in therapeutic decision-making. In addition to the recurrence scores, this test also reports quantitative ER and PR RNA expression levels at internally validated positive cutoff levels (≥ 6.5 for ER and ≥ 5.5 for PR). Several studies identified discordance between hormone receptor status detected with IHC and the RT-PCR assay.[82,83] In both studies there was relatively good (~90%) concordance between IHC and RT-PCR. However, Badve and associates noted in their analysis that IHC ER-negative cases that were RT-PCR positive were more common than IHC ER-positive cases that were RT-PCR negative. In regard to PR, Badve and colleagues[82] and Kraus and associates[83] reported that IHC PR-negative cases that were RT-PCR positive were less

common than IHC PR-positive cases that were RT-PCR negative. Kraus and colleagues concluded that IHC was superior to and more sensitive than RT-PCR in detecting low-intensity or heterogeneous expression of hormonal positivity in tumors.[83] They also noted that the technical aspects involved in RT-PCR (RNA extraction techniques, primers, and reagents used as well as tissue microdissection and grinding that could cause potential contamination with normal breast tissue, inflammatory cells, and in situ carcinoma) could result in the discrepancies. In addition, it should be kept in mind that although IHC detects ER and PR at the protein level, RT-PCR detects RNA expression that may or may not always be translated to proteins. Therefore IHC should remain the gold standard in ER and PR analysis in the management of breast cancer patients.

Repeat Immunohistochemical Studies on Recurrent and Metastatic Disease

Hormone receptor testing in all primary breast cancers is now mandatory. However, repeat IHC testing may also be indicated in the settings of recurrent and metastatic breast cancer because alterations of the ER status of tumors have been known to occur over time that could affect treatment decisions.[84,85] Reports show that the ER status of breast cancer could revert from ER-positive to ER-negative and vice versa in as much as a third of cases.[86] Receptor status conversion generally occurs over long periods of time but has rarely been reported under 1 year. Patients with an ER-negative to ER-positive tumor conversion may benefit from hormonal therapy. However, losing ER status in a recurrent or metastatic disease may signify aggressive disease often resistant to treatment. The ER status of the recurrent or metastatic disease is considered the current ER status of a patient for treatment purposes.

For completeness, other instances that warrant repeat testing for ER and PR are mentioned here. It is strongly advocated to repeat IHC on resection specimens when a core biopsy (with or without appropriate internal positive controls) shows negative results. This is mainly because tumor cells express hormonal receptors in a wide dynamic range with resultant staining heterogeneity that could be missed in small biopsy specimens. Likewise, IHC should be repeated when the background normal breast tissue in a biopsy (that serves as internal positive control) is negative.

ER-negative and PR-positive tumors are rare and sometimes a controversial entity. Therefore it is prudent to repeat ER and PR studies before reporting in such cases.

Commonly Used Monoclonal Antibodies

The original monoclonal antibodies for ER and PR IHC were raised in mouse sera.[87–89] The different clones of the established mouse antibodies currently available in the market have shown comparable results.[90] Rabbit monoclonal antibodies for ER and PR were introduced in the mid-2000s with the claims that they had higher affinity than their mouse monoclonal counterparts, allowing the use of the antibodies at higher dilutions and in some instances eliminating the need for heat-based antigen retrieval.[91,92] Cheang and colleagues showed that rabbit monoclonal ER antibody clone SP1 was a better independent prognostic factor than one of the most routinely used mouse monoclonal antibody clone, 1D5.[93] Later studies concluded that the quality and reliability of IHC results achieved with rabbit monoclonal antibodies to ER and PR in invasive breast cancer were comparable to those achieved with established mouse monoclonal counterparts.[94] Newer clones of antibodies are being introduced, and a recent ER rabbit monoclonal clone EP1 was shown to be a highly sensitive and specific antibody. The EP1 resulted in a stronger staining intensity compared with established clone SP1, allowing improved interpretation of ER IHC results.[95]

Tables 14.1 and 14.2 list some of the commonly used monoclonal antibodies for ER and PR. The optimal dilutions for primary antibodies must be determined by the individual laboratories depending on the procedures, antigen retrieval methods, and detection systems used.

Human Epidermal Growth Factor Receptor 2

Historical Perspective

HER2 is a transmembrane tyrosine kinase receptor belonging to a family of epidermal growth factor receptors (EGFRs), encoded by erbB2/HER2-neu oncogene and located on chromosome 17q21.[96] ErbB2 was first discovered as an avian retrovirus

TABLE 14.1 Commonly Used Monoclonal Antibodies for Estrogen Receptor (ER)

ER Clone	Manufacturer	Source	Suggested Dilution
1D5	DakoCytomation, Carpinteria, CA	Mouse	1:10–1:50
SP1	LabVision, Fremont, CA	Rabbit	1:30–1:100
6F11	Novocastra, Newcastle upon Tyne, UK	Mouse	1:20–1:50
EP1	DakoCytomation, Carpinteria, CA	Rabbit	Ready to use

TABLE 14.2 Commonly Used Monoclonal Antibodies for Progesterone Receptor (PR)

PR Clone	Manufacturer	Source	Suggested Dilution
PgR636	DakoCytomation, Carpinteria, CA	Mouse	1:50
SP2	LabVision, Fremont, CA	Rabbit	1:50
1294	DakoCytomation, Carpinteria, CA	Mouse	1:50
1A6	DakoCytomation, Carpinteria, CA	Rabbit	Ready to use

oncogene that could induce erythroid leukemia.[97,98] Researchers found that exposure of neu oncogene transformed NIH 3T3 cells to monoclonal antibodies reactive with the neu gene product p185 resulted in the rapid and reversible loss of both cell surface and total cellular p185. They suggested that p185 was required to maintain the transformation induced by neu oncogene.[99] The erbB/HER2 gene was first sequenced in 1984, and it later was shown that 50% of the amino acids of HER2/neu and the EGFR were identical with greater than 80% homology in the amino acids of their tyrosine kinase domains.[100–102] Studies also revealed that, although related, HER2 was distinct from EGFR. Amplification of erbB/HER2 gene had been recognized in three separate adenocarcinoma cell lines originating from salivary gland, mammary gland, and gastric carcinoma.[103] These observations indicated that this gene might play an important role in cancer progression.

In 1987 Slamon and his colleagues found that HER2/neu gene was amplified 2- to 20-fold in approximately 30% of the primary human breast cancers they studied.[104] They and others identified that this gene amplification was a significant predictor of both overall survival (OS) and time to relapse in patients with breast cancer. Moreover, multivariate analysis showed HER2/neu amplification had greater prognostic value than other prognosticators like hormonal receptor status with the exception of positive lymph node metastases.[104,105] Subsequent studies recognized that some of the methods used to evaluate HER2/neu amplification such as solid matrix blotting techniques (Southern, Western, and Northern) could potentially underestimate the number of cancers with amplified genes due to sample contamination caused by adjacent noncancerous tissue.[106] Immunochemistry can be easily employed to assess HER2/neu expression on formalin-fixed paraffin-embedded tissue sections that appear to correlate well with gene expression.

Fendly and colleagues reported data on treating breast cancer cell lines with monoclonal antibodies directed against the extracellular domain of HER2/neu. They demonstrated that the antibodies inhibited the growth of tumor cells and prevented colony formation.[107] Furthermore they showed that the resistance to cytotoxic effects of tumor necrosis factor was significantly reduced in the cells lines treated with monoclonal HER2/neu antibodies. Transfected NIH 3T3 cell lines expressing HER2/neu gene were used to produce and characterize 10 monoclonal antibodies that could immunoprecipitate p185HER2.[107] These monoclonal antibodies would bind to the extracellular domain of p185HER2 and not cross-react with EGFR.

In 1992, researchers humanized antibodies against the 185 kD glycoprotein of HER2/neu that were previously developed in rodents. However, these antibodies were not sufficiently specific to be used in the treatment of breast cancer.[108] In 1994 Pietras and associates showed that anti- p185 HER2/neu in combination with cytotoxic drugs such as cisplatin promoted drug-induced killing of HER2/neu overexpressed tumor cells.[109] This rationale was used to formulate clinical trials.

Genentech (San Francisco, CA), a private biotechnology company, started the phase I clinical trial with recombinant, humanized monoclonal anti-p185 HER2/neu.[110,111] This antibody was eventually named trastuzumab (Herceptin). After successful enrollment and completion of the phase I clinical trial, the phase II trial was launched in 54 centers in North America, Australia, and New Zealand. Due to amazing success observed in some patients, a phase III trial was initiated before the completion of phase II. However, techniques for identifying HER2/neu-amplified cases were still not standardized.[112-114] Some laboratories promoted IHC to be performed on frozen tumor and the digitalized images of the immunostained slides analyzed by computer-assisted programs.[115] This methodology was cumbersome and not easily adaptable by all pathology laboratories. By the time the phase III clinical trial was completed, Genentech received US Food and Drug Administration (FDA) approval for marketing trastuzumab. Dako (Carpinteria, CA) received FDA clearance for HercepTest, a semiquantitative immunohistochemical assay for determination of HER2/neu protein overexpression in breast cancer tissues routinely processed for histologic evaluation.[110]

In 1997 Press and colleagues published the validation study of fluorescence in situ hybridization (FISH) for HER2/neu gene from formalin-fixed archival blocks. They showed this technique was superior to Southern blot hybridization with sensitivity of 98% and specificity of 100%. They also demonstrated that HER2/neu gene amplification was an independent factor highlighting poor prognosis in patients who had not received any adjuvant treatment.[116,117] Several studies confirmed that accurate assessment of HER2/neu was essential to ensure the effectiveness of Herceptin.[71,118] Multiple studies of metastatic and recurrent breast cancers confirmed that patients with immunohistochemical 3+ or FISH-positive breast cancers gained the greatest clinical benefits.[119-121] It was particularly impressive that the response rate was superior if trastuzumab was given together with cytotoxic drugs.[122-124]

At the same time, several researchers recognized that the results of HER2/neu by IHC were not reliable without proper standardization.[125,126] Treatment of breast cancer was rapidly changing, necessitating standardized surgical pathology reports, including breast biomarker results. At a national consensus conference, breast experts emphasized that the most appropriate methods to identify HER2/neu amplification were IHC and FISH.[127] They also highlighted that PCR-based assays had shown significant association but not complete concordance of HER2/neu results with the preceding methods.[128-130] They felt there was compelling evidence for routine testing for HER2/neu on all invasive carcinoma. They also reiterated the current methodology for testing had not been optimized, and it was not clear whether FISH was superior to IHC; therefore they recommended, if in doubt, to perform both tests and a conservative approach in interpreting the results.[128] Meanwhile other studies showed that the length of formalin fixation could cause loss of nuclear signals and erroneous HER2 FISH result.[131-133] Cell lines grown in culture with specific copy of HER2/neu signals and fixed in formalin were introduced to represent an optimal control for HER2/neu tests.[134] A group conducted a retrospective study comparing the result of two separate available immunoassays using the same antibody at two separate institutions. Only 84% concordance could be achieved by IHC. They felt if the tumor showed strong and diffuse cytoplasmic positivity, it was more likely to show HER2/neu gene amplification; however, if the cytoplasmic membrane staining was not strong and diffuse, only 27% showed HER2 gene amplification. They recommended that all breast cancers showing moderate complete cytoplasmic membrane positivity to be tested by FISH.[135] This method was gaining popularity compared with IHC analysis and seemed to predict more accurately clinical responses to trastuzumab-based therapies.[136,137]

In May 2003 the CAP created a new comprehensive education model, called "Strategic Science," with expert speakers integrating new and evolving basic, clinical, and scientific issues of HER2/neu testing.[138] In 2006 the CAP published the result of interlaboratory comparison of HER2/neu testing from 2004 to 2005. The comparison studies among the laboratories had been excellent with 90% and 91% consensus.[139] Because the majority of general pathologists do not work fluorescence microscopy, investigators tried to identify new methodologies to recognize gene amplification. One such method was introduced by a group as dual chromogenic in situ hybridization (CISH). They described their method to be superior to single CISH. They suggested their method was more user-friendly for practicing pathologists, and the result showed an almost 100% correlation with FISH results.[140-143] In 2007 the ASCO and CAP published joint recommendations stating that all invasive breast cancers required HER2/neu testing. The recommended algorithm was introduced for more accurate and reproducible results. They also established a clear algorithm defining positive, equivocal, and negative values for both HER2/neu protein expression and gene amplification.[144]

Standard Practice and New Challenges

Since the FDA approval of HercepTest in 1998 for identifying HER2/neu amplified breast cancers and trastuzumab for treatment of these patients, the scientific community has made tremendous effort to standardize the HER2 testing in breast tissue. Several studies have been performed, reevaluating the HER2 result by examining microarray slides. In the discrepant cases, the entire slide was reexamined. The result has been promising. The actual false-positive rate was 1.3%, and the false-negative rate 0.7%.[145] This result is encouraging for both patients and oncologists. According to the latest recommendation of ASCO/CAP, all newly diagnosed, recurrent, and metastatic breast cancers should be tested for HER2/neu amplification by IHC or CISH.[146] This recommendation was necessary as more laboratories were evaluating gene amplification by bright field, and the original recommendations did not address scoring methods for bright field, mono-color and dual-color in situ hybridization.[147,148] Additional strategies for detecting HER2/neu amplification were published, including DNA expression by microarray and messenger RNA (mRNA) expression RT-PCR.[149–151] Because the majority of pathology (CAP or Clinical Laboratory Improvement Amendment [CLIA]-certified) laboratories are following the strict updated guidelines by ASCO/CAP, these issues need to be resolved. The reviewers at the 2013 meeting acknowledged that the treatment of HER2-positive breast cancers by trastuzumab as a single drug or in combination with other cytotoxic drugs has become standard practice.[152–154] These studies have shown that using trastuzumab would significantly improve OS. The committee members reported that at this point there is insufficient evidence to support use of mRNA or DNA microarray assays to determine HER2 status in unselected patients.[155,156] The committee members also acknowledged that prior guidelines had not taken into consideration some of the new challenges in evaluating HER2, such as unusual HER2 genotypic abnormalities, aneusomy (monosomy or polysomy) of chromosome 17, colocalization of HER2 and chromosome enumeration probe 17 (CEP17) signals that affect HER2/CEP ratio in dual signal in situ hybridization (ISH) and genetic heterogeneity.[157] Aneusomy 17 (monosomy 17 or polysomy 17) can be detected in approximately 30% of breast cancers. Anomalies in chromosome 17 are common in tumors with discrepant ERBB2 expression and in tumors with discordant ERBB2-protein and ERBB2 gene copy number measurements.[158–161]

Polysomy defined by the presence of extra copies of one or more whole chromosomes provides an alternative mechanism for apparent HER2 gene amplification. Polysomy of chromosome 17 has frequently been reported in breast cancer. In fact, polysomy has been recognized as a major cause of discrepancy between IHC and ISH results.[161] A study published in 2012 confirmed that the absolute number of HER2/neu signals was important in response to the treatment rather than the ratio of HER2/CEP17.[162] Because the ASCO/CAP committee members intended to reduce or possibly eliminate false-positive and false-negative cases, they felt that a change in reporting HER2/neu positivity was necessary. In the United States, this guideline recommends the use of an FDA-approved assay. CLIA-certified laboratories may choose a laboratory developed test, but they are expected to validate them.[163] A list of FDA-approved assays is available at their website.

Table 14.3 reflects the reporting recommendation for IHC. Table 14.4 reflects the reporting recommendation for FISH/dual bright-field in situ hybridization.

To ensure the quality, all specimens used for HER2/neu testing (cytologic sample, biopsy, or resection) must be fixed within 1 hour, in 10% neutral buffered formalin for duration of 6 to 72 hours.[164–168] In addition, the laboratories must conform to standards set for CAP accreditation or an equivalent accreditation authority, including initial test validation, ongoing internal quality assurance, ongoing external proficiency testing, and routine periodic performance monitoring.[157] The committee urged pathologists and the laboratories to be more vigilant in eliminating false results because additional HER2-targeted drugs, such as lapatinib and pertuzumab, are shown to have significantly more side effects. These drugs are also more expensive and associated with other dose-limiting side effects. These drugs have shown

TABLE 14.3	Reporting Recommendation for Immunohistochemistry	
Score	**Pattern**
Negative (0)	No staining observed or Faint/barely perceptible membrane staining in ≤10% of invasive tumor cells
Negative (1+)	Incomplete membrane staining that is faint/barely perceptible within >10% of invasive tumor cells
Equivocal (2+)	Complete circumferential membrane staining in ≤10% of invasive tumor cells Incomplete weak to moderate circumferential membrane staining in >10% of invasive tumor cells
Positive (3+)	**Complete intense circumferential membrane staining in >10% of invasive tumor cells**

TABLE 14.4	Reporting Recommendation for Fluorescence in Situ Hybridization/Dual Bright-Field in Situ Hybridization	
HER2/CEP17	**Average HER2**	**Final Result**
Ratio <2	Average HER2 copy/cell ≥6	**ISH positive**
	Average HER2 copy/cell ≥4 <6	ISH equivocal
	Average HER2 copy/<4	ISH negative
Ratio ≥2	Average HER 2 copy/cell ≥4	**ISH positive**
	Average HER 2 copy/cell <4	**ISH positive**

ISH, In situ hybridization.

no clinical benefit in patients with HER2/neu negative metastatic disease.[169]

Several issues remain unresolved. It is still unclear how patients with HER2/neu heterogeneity respond to the anti-HER2 treatment. Many breast cancers show intratumoral heterogeneity. This becomes a challenge for HER2 testing.[170] Two types of HER2 heterogeneity have been described. One shows cluster or colonies of amplified cells. The second group of cancers shows dispersed HER2/neu-amplified cells. By definition, if more than 5% and less than 50% of the cells should show evidence of HER2/neu amplification, the tumor can be classified as showing HER2/neu heterogeneity. The ratio of HER2/Cep17 should be two or more or the neoplastic cells should show more than six HER2/neu signals.[171] Some studies have shown that tumors with less than 80% HER2 positivity of (3+) by IHC or a HER2/Cep17 gene amplification greater than 2.2 recur faster and have lower OS.[172,173] Evaluation of data published after the 2013 ASCO/CAP recommendation has shown that the number of equivocal and positive cases examined by IHC and CIS had increased.[174] The question remains of how many of these patients will be enrolled in a clinical trial.

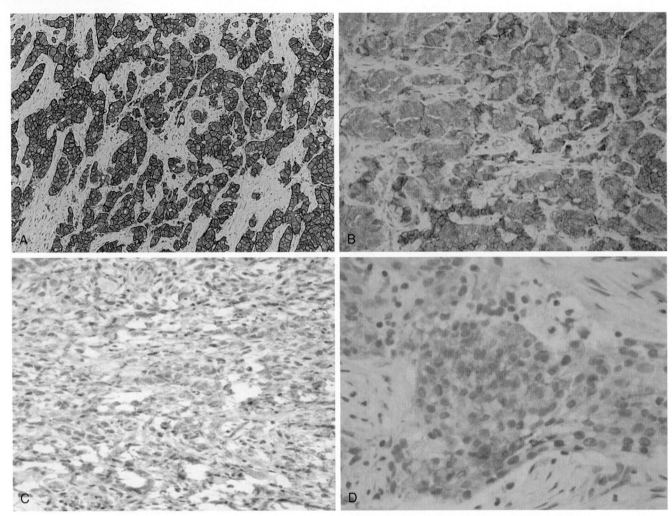

• **Fig. 14.2.** HER2 expression by immunohistochemistry scored according to the current American Society of Clinical Oncology and College of American Pathologists standards. (A) HER2: positive (3+). (B) HER2: equivocal (2+). (C) HER2: negative (0). (D) HER2: negative (1+).

Fig. 14.2 shows a composite image of HER2 expression by IHC scored according to the current ASCO/CAP standards.

Fig. 14.3 shows an image of an invasive mammary carcinoma with heterogeneous HER2 expression. The insert shows higher magnification. In this tumor, there is clear progression from a HER2-negative cancer to a HER2-positive one.

Ki67 (Proliferation Marker)

Decision-making regarding adjuvant treatment for early breast cancer is complex. Presence or absence of hormonal receptor plays a significant factor in this decision. In recent years researchers have recognized that the effect of many chemotherapeutic agents is significantly diminished in estrogen-positive cancers with low proliferation index.[175–180] Ki67 is known to be present in all proliferating cells, and it has been used as a surrogate marker to assess proliferation index. The Ki67 antigen was originally identified by Gerdes and colleagues.[181] This protein, which is associated with all phases of cell cycle except G0, is located in the cortex of the nucleus.[181] The level of expression varies during phases of the cell

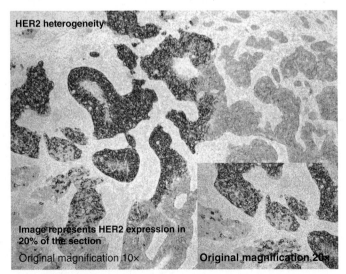

• **Fig. 14.3.** HER2 expression in 20% of the section. Original magnification 10×; inset, original magnification 20×.

cycle. Ki67 levels are low in the G1 and S phases and rise to their peak level in early phases of mitosis; later in the mitotic phase (anaphase and telophase), a sharp decrease in Ki67 levels occurs.[182] This change in level of expression most likely explains the various levels of expression observed in some tumors by IHC.[183] For more than a quarter century, investigators have tried to use Ki67 as a surrogate marker to establish proliferation index in a tumor.[181] Many approaches have been taken to measure this marker in breast cancers.[183,184]

In the late 1980s Bouzubar and associates found that the level of Ki67 expression was an independent prognostic marker of tumor size, lymph node status, or presence or absence of ER. A high level of Ki67 was associated with early recurrence or decreased OS.[185,186] Since then investigators have tried to use this marker as a prognostic and predictive marker.[186–189] Ki67 has also been used as a surrogate marker to monitor response to treatment.[190–193]

Despite numerous publications highlighting the significance of Ki67 expression in OS and disease-free survival of breast cancer patients, Ki67 remains a controversial biomarker. This controversy predominantly originates from lack of reproducibility, secondary to different types of scoring methodology (hot-spot vs. average count; manual vs. automated scoring).[194–196] In 2012–2013 an international group took to the task to standardize Ki67 immunostaining and scoring. The group felt that some of the interobserver variability could be corrected through web-based learning techniques. Although they felt that their results were encouraging, clinically relevant discrepancies continue to persist. They pointed out that some of this discrepancy originated from the nature of the sample (i.e., biopsy vs. excision); the second major factor was the nature of tumors and the heterogeneity within different regions of a tumor. The group felt that these factors remain problematic and required further analysis.[197] In a more recent study, another group scored 500 cells in a zone with the highest Ki67 expression. They found that a Ki67 labeling index of 20 or higher was associated with poor prognosis, in the absence of adjuvant chemotherapy.[198] Honma and colleagues examined more than 400 ER-positive HER2-negative cases. They found that a high level of Ki67, defined at greater than 15% within the hottest area of the section, would identify patients with the poorest clinical outcome.[199] Dodson and associates introduced a new scoring methodology to evaluate ER/PR, HER2, and Ki67. They feel that this method is reproducible.[200] Their methodology needs to be tested in clinical practice.

Nonetheless, the scientific community cannot agree on a specific labeling index to distinguish cancers that might not respond to the chemotherapy from those that clearly require adjuvant chemotherapy. It is clear that a very low Ki67 index (10%) is associated with relatively good prognosis, and these tumors are unlikely to respond to chemotherapy; on the other hand, a tumor with a high labeling index greater than 50% would likely respond to adjuvant chemotherapy. Ki67 as a biomarker might be of value in a subset of ER-positive and HER2-negative breast cancers.

Fig. 14.4 shows strong Ki67 expression in more than 90% of the infiltrating neoplastic cells.

E-Cadherin and p120

Analysis of E-cadherin expression by IHC has greatly advanced our knowledge about lobular carcinoma in situ (LCIS) and invasive lobular carcinomas (ILCs). The lack or decreased level of

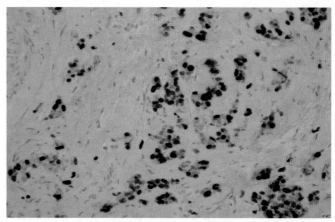

• **Fig. 14.4.** Ki67 expressed in more than 80% of tumor cells.

expression of E-cadherin has facilitated correct classification of pleomorphic variant of lobular carcinomas.[201] Approximately 15% of all invasive carcinomas are lobular (ILC). The true incidence of LCIS remains unknown. LCIS is typically discovered coincidently. It does not usually cause any mammographic abnormalities.[202] LCIS was first described by Foote and Stewart as a neoplastic process composed of discohesive cells with intracytoplasmic vacuoles almost 75 years ago. They also noted that these lesions are often multicentric.[203] The pleomorphic variant of LCIS has been recognized only since the early 2000s. The pleomorphic variant of LCIS often presents with abnormal calcification and can be misdiagnosed as ductal carcinoma in situ because they can show central comedo necrosis (Fig. 14.5).[204,205] Before recognizing LCIS with comedo necrosis as a variant of LCIS, this tumor used to be classified as ductal-lobular carcinomas.[206] Similar to the classic variant of lobular carcinomas, this tumor shows lack or decreased levels of E-cadherin expression. On the genetic level, these tumors also remain closely linked.[7] One of the most important factors is that the incidence of both LCIS and ILC has almost tripled since the 1980s.[207,208]

E-cadherin and p120-catenin have been used to distinguish these tumors from ductal carcinoma in situ.[209–211] Biologically and clinically LCIS and ILCs differ from other cancers. ER positivity is detected in more than 95% of classic pattern of ILC. The rate of ER positivity is lower in pleomorphic variant of ILC.[212–215] Although ILC has shown a relatively good short-term prognosis, its long-term recurrent rate is higher than other invasive mammary carcinomas.[216,217]

The expression of these two molecules is closely interlinked. Disruption of cell adhesion molecule E-cadherin results in the characteristic discohesive growth pattern seen in LCIS and ILC. The E-cadherin molecule has an intracellular domain that binds to α-, β-, and p120-catenins via actin cytoskeleton.[218] These bindings allow formation of adherens junctions. More than 90% of ILC and LCIS show complete absence or significant decrease in E-cadherin expression.[219] This E-cadherin deregulation can even be observed in cases of atypical lobular hyperplasia.[220] Canas and colleagues recently emphasized the importance of recognizing the correct pattern of expression.[221] It is becoming increasingly important to recognize and correctly classify all cancers, especially lobular, because they seem to show a distinct clinical and biological signature.[222] We might be able to individualize the treatment of these patients in future.

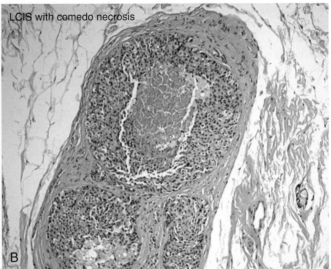

E-cadherin

LCIS with comedo necrosis

A

B

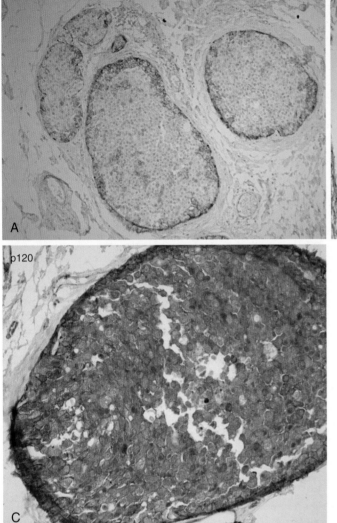

p120

C

• **Fig. 14.5.** (A) E-cadherin. (B) Lobular carcinoma in situ *(LCIS)* with comedo necrosis. (C) p120.

Selected References

8. Kos Z, Dabbs DJ. Biomarker assessment and molecular testing for prognostication in breast cancer. *Histopathology.* 2016;68:70-85.
51. Harris L, Fritsche H, Mennel R, et al. American Society of Clinical Oncology 2007 update of recommendations for the use of tumor markers in breast cancer. *J Clin Oncol.* 2007;25:5287-5312.
69. Collins LC, Botero ML, Schnitt SJ. Bimodal frequency distribution of estrogen receptor immunohistochemical staining results in breast cancer: an analysis of 825 cases. *Am J Clin Pathol.* 2005;123:16-20.
76. Hammond ME, Hayes DF, Dowsett M, et al. American Society of Clinical Oncology/College of American Pathologists guideline recommendations for immunohistochemical testing of estrogen and progesterone receptors in breast cancer (unabridged version). *Arch Pathol Lab Med.* 2010;134:e48-e72.
81. Goldstein LJ, Gray R, Badve S, et al. Prognostic utility of the 21-gene assay in hormone receptor-positive operable breast cancer compared with classical clinicopathologic features. *J Clin Oncol.* 2008;26:4063-4071.

83. Kraus JA, Dabbs DJ, Beriwal S, Bhargava R. Semi-quantitative immunohistochemical assay versus oncotype DX(®) qRT-PCR assay for estrogen and progesterone receptors: an independent quality assurance study. *Mod Pathol.* 2012;25:869-876.
106. Slamon DJ, Godolphin W, Jones LA, et al. Studies of the HER-2/neu proto-oncogene in human breast and ovarian cancer. *Science.* 1989;244:707-712.
157. Wolff AC, Hammond ME, Hicks DG, et al. Recommendations for human epidermal growth factor receptor 2 testing in breast cancer: American Society of Clinical Oncology/College of American Pathologists clinical practice guideline update. *J Clin Oncol.* 2013;31:3997-4013.
199. Honma N, Horii R, Iwase T, et al. Ki-67 evaluation at the hottest spot predicts clinical outcome of patients with hormone receptor-positive/HER2- negative breast cancer treated with adjuvant tamoxifen monotherapy. *Breast Cancer.* 2015;22:71-78.
220. Dabbs DJ, Schnitt SJ, Geyer FC, et al. Lobular neoplasia of the breast revisited with emphasis on the role of E-cadherin immunohistochemistry. *Am J Surg Pathol.* 2013;37:e1-e11.
A full reference list is available online at ExpertConsult.com.

15

Epidemiology of Breast Cancer

VICTOR G. VOGEL

Descriptive Epidemiology

In 2015, an estimated 231,840 new cases of invasive breast cancer were diagnosed among US women, as well as an estimated 60,290 additional cases of in situ breast cancer. In the same year, approximately 40,290 US women died from breast cancer. Only lung cancer accounts for more cancer deaths in women. Breast cancer is the most commonly diagnosed cancer in women in the United States and accounts for 26% of all female cancers (excluding nonmelanoma skin cancers and in situ cancers).[1] Incidence rates of in situ breast cancer rose rapidly during the 1980s and 1990s, largely because of increases in mammography screening. The increase in incidence was greater in women 50 years of age and older than in those younger than 50. Incidence rates of in situ breast cancer have stabilized since 2000 among women 50 and older and since 2007 among younger women. These trends likely reflect trends in mammography screening rates, which peaked in 2000 and then stabilized at a slightly lower rate after 2005.

Some of the historic increase in breast cancer incidence reflects changes in reproductive patterns, such as delayed childbearing and having fewer children, which are known risk factors for breast cancer. Between 2002 and 2003, breast cancer rates dropped sharply (nearly 7%), likely due to the decreased use of menopausal hormones after the publication of clinical trial results that found higher risk of breast cancer and heart disease among users. The decline in incidence occurred primarily in white women, in women 50 years of age and older, and for estrogen receptor (ER)-positive disease. From 2004 to 2012, overall breast cancer incidence rates remained stable.

Overall breast cancer death rates decreased 36% from 1989 to 2012, after slowly increasing (0.4% per year) since 1975.[2] The decrease occurred in both younger and older women, although since 2007, the breast cancer death rate has been level among women younger than 50 years. The decline in breast cancer mortality has been attributed to both improvements in breast cancer treatment and early detection. However, not all segments of the population have benefited equally from these advances. A striking divergence in long-term breast cancer mortality trends between black and white women began in the early 1980s. This mortality difference reflects a combination of factors, including differences in stage at diagnosis, obesity and comorbidities, and tumor characteristics, as well as access, adherence, and response to treatment. The racial disparity may also reflect differences in mammography screening. As treatment for breast cancers has improved, the racial disparity has widened; by 2012 breast cancer death rates were 42% higher in black than white women.

Differences in Subtypes of Breast Cancer by Race, Ethnicity and Geography

Since 2010, Surveillance, Epidemiology, and End Results (SEER) registries have collected human epidermal growth factor 2 (HER2) receptor status for breast cancer cases. Breast cancer subtypes can be defined by both hormone receptor (HR) (ER and progesterone receptor [PR]) and HER2 status. Age-specific incidence rates by subtype differ for non-Hispanic (NH) white, NH black, NH Asian Pacific Islander (API), and Hispanic women.[3] Hormone receptor and HER2 status distributions can be summarized by age, race/ethnicity, county-level poverty, registry, stage, Bloom-Richardson grade, tumor size, and nodal status. Among patients with known hormone receptor and HER2 status, 73% were found to be HR-positive/HER2-negative, 12% were triple-negative (HR-negative/HER2-negative), 10% were HR-positive/HER2-positive, and nearly 5% were HR-negative/HER2-positive; 12% had unknown HR/HER2 status. NH white women had the highest incidence rate of the HR-positive/HER2-negative subtype, and NH black women had the highest rate of the triple-negative subtype.

Compared with women with the HR-positive/HER2-negative subtype, triple-negative patients were more likely to be NH black and Hispanic; HR-positive/HER2-positive patients were more likely to be NH API; and HR-negative/HER2-positive patients were more likely to be NH black, NH API, and Hispanic. Patients with triple-negative, HR-positive/HER2-positive, and HR-negative/HER2-positive breast cancer were 10% to 30% less likely to be diagnosed at older ages compared with HR-positive/HER2-negative patients and 6-fold to 20-fold more likely to present with high-grade disease. These data demonstrate that there are differences in breast cancer subtypes presenting at diagnosis among different racial/ethnic groups. The reasons for these differences are not yet well defined.

Breast cancer is the most frequently diagnosed cancer worldwide and is the leading cause of cancer death in females.[4] Breast cancer incidence rates are highest in North America, Australia/New Zealand, and in Western and northern Europe, and lowest in Asia and sub-Saharan Africa. Despite the decreases in incidence rates in North America, breast cancer incidence has been increasing in other parts of the world, such as Asia and Africa.[5] These

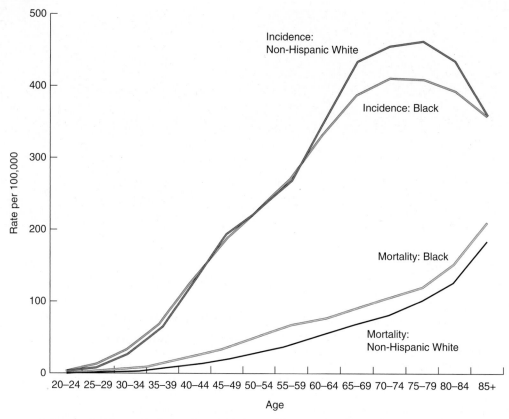

Source: Incidence: North American Association of Central Cancer Registries (NAACCR), 2015. Mortality: US mortality date, National Center for Health Statistics, Centers for Disease Control and Prevention.

American Cancer Society, Inc., Surveillance Research, 2015

• **Fig. 15.1** Age-specific female breast cancer incidence and mortality rates, United States, 2008 to 2012.

international differences are thought to be related to societal changes occurring during industrialization (e.g., changes in fat intake, body weight, age at menarche, and/or lactation, and reproductive patterns such as fewer pregnancies and later age at first birth). Within the United States, breast cancer risk varies substantially among regions. Geographic cluster regions with high breast cancer incidence rates have been identified, such as Cape Cod, Massachusetts; Long Island, New York; and Marin County, California. These clusters are most likely due to regional differences in established breast cancer risk factors.

As shown in Fig. 15.1, breast cancer incidence and mortality are higher in African American and Caucasian women than in women of other races and ethnicities. Incidence data have been available for white and black women since 1975 and for women of other races and ethnicities since 1992. During 2008–2012 (the most recent 5 years of data available), overall breast cancer incidence rates increased among NH black (0.4% per year) and API (1.5% per year) women, but were stable among NH whites, Hispanics, or American Indians/Alaska Natives. Notably, breast cancer rates for whites and blacks converged in 2012, reflecting the slow but steady increase in incidence in black women and relatively stable rates in white women.

Breast cancer incidence in Asians and Pacific Islanders was 93.5 per 100,000 in 1999 to 2003. Incidence in Hispanics was 87.1 per 100,000 for the same period. Incidence in Native Americans and Alaskan Natives was 74.4 per 100,000 for 1999 to 2002.[3]

Mortality rates (per 100,000) for these time periods were 12.6 for Asians and Pacific Islanders, 16.3 for Hispanics, and 13.8 for Native Americans and Alaskan Natives.[6]

A variety of genetic, environmental, and behavioral factors may explain the racial differences in the incidence of breast cancer. Migration studies have documented that the risk of breast cancer is higher in Asian American women born in the West compared with those born in Asia (relative risk [RR] 1.6; 95% confidence interval [CI] 1.2–2.1).[7] Risk of breast cancer is further increased with the number of the woman's grandparents born in the West (RR 1.89; 95% CI 1.2–3 for a woman with one to two grandparents born in the West compared with a woman with all grandparents born in Asia). Risk is decreased in more recent immigrants (RR 0.32; 95% CI 0.18–0.57 for 2–4 years lived in the west) compared with those who have lived in the west their entire lives. Incidence rates for breast cancer in Asian Americans in Los Angeles County rose substantially between 1993 and 1997.[8] Most notably, the incidence rate for breast cancer in Japanese American women in this country is rapidly approaching that of NH white women. Factors such as acculturation and adoption of a Western diet may at least partially explain these recent trends.

Sociodemographic Factors

Poverty, less education, and a lack of health insurance are also associated with lower breast cancer survival.[9–11] Breast cancer

TABLE 15.1 Traditional Risk Factors for Breast Cancer, Relative Risks, and Associated Population Attributable Risks

Risk Factor	Comparison Category	Risk Category	Relative Risk	Prevalence (%)	Population Attributable Risk[a]
Age at menarche	16 years	<12 years	1.3	16	0.05
Age at menopause	45–54 years	>55 years	1.5	6	0.03
Age when first child born alive	Before 20 years	Nulliparous or >30 years	1.9	21	0.16
Benign breast disease	No biopsy or fine-needle aspiration	Any benign disease	1.5	15	0.07
		Proliferative disease	2	4	0.04
		Atypical hyperplasia	4	1	0.03
Family history of breast cancer	No first-degree relative affected	Mother affected	1.7	8	0.05
		Two first-degree relatives affected	5	4	0.14

[a]Population attributable risk = [prevalence × (relative risk − 1)] / {[prevalence × (relative risk − 1)] + 1}.

Modified from Harris JR, Lippman ME, Veronesi U, Willet W. Breast cancer (part 1). *N Engl J Med.* 1992;327:319-328. Copyright © 1992 Massachusetts Medical Society. All rights reserved.

patients who reside in lower-income areas have lower 5-year survival rates than those in higher-income areas at every stage of diagnosis.[12]

Traditional Risk Factors for Breast Cancer

Well-established epidemiologic risk factors for breast cancer are listed in Table 15.1. Age is the most important risk factor for breast cancer, and breast cancer incidence rises sharply with age (Fig. 15.2). The SEER database of the National Cancer Institute allows calculation of the probability of a woman developing breast cancer in the United States through specific attained ages[6]:

- Birth to age 49—1.9 (1 in 53 women)
- Age 50 to 69—2.3 (1 in 44 women)
- Age 60 to 69—3.5 (1 in 29 women)
- Age 70 and older—6.7 (1 in 15 women)
- Birth to death—12.3 (1 in 8 women)

The overall incidence rate of breast cancer is low at younger ages (e.g., 1.4 per 100,000 in women 20–24 years of age).

Benign Breast Disease

Benign breast lesions can be classified according to their histologic appearance (Table 15.2). Benign breast lesions thought to impart no increased risk of breast cancer include adenosis, duct ectasia, simple fibroadenoma, fibrosis, mastitis, mild hyperplasia, cysts, and metaplasia of the apocrine or squamous types.[13,14] Lesions associated with a slight increase in the subsequent risk of developing invasive breast cancer include complex fibroadenoma, moderate or florid hyperplasia with or without atypia, sclerosing adenosis, and papilloma. Atypical hyperplasia of the ductal or lobular type is associated with a 4- to 5-fold increased risk of developing subsequent breast cancer, and this risk increases to approximately 10-fold if it is also associated with a family history of invasive breast cancer in a first-degree relative.

Lobular Carcinoma in Situ and Atypical Hyperplasia

Women with a history of lobular carcinoma in situ (LCIS) experience an annual risk of invasive breast cancer of approximately 1.5% per year. Women with atypical hyperplasia also experience an increased risk of subsequent invasive breast cancer. There are two types of atypical hyperplasia, as classified on the basis of microscopic appearance: atypical ductal hyperplasia and atypical lobular hyperplasia; atypical hyperplasia confers a relative risk of 4.0. These risk statistics have been recognized for decades, and the absolute risk among women with atypical hyperplasia has been shown to approach 30% at 25 years of follow-up.[15] The risk of developing invasive disease after a diagnosis of atypia is inversely related to the age at diagnosis, directly related to the number of atypical foci seen on the biopsy, and appears to be slightly higher with atypical lobular compared with atypical ductal hyperplasia.[13] Atypical hyperplasia is found in approximately 10% of biopsies with benign findings. In studies with long-term follow-up, atypical hyperplasia has been shown to confer high relative risks for future breast cancer[16,17] with an absolute risk of approximately 1% to 2% per year of developing invasive breast cancer.[18-21]

Family History

Women who have a first-degree relative with a history of breast cancer are at increased risk of the disease themselves.[22] The risk conferred by family history is further increased if the affected family member was diagnosed with the disease at a younger age. For example, a woman with a first-degree relative diagnosed with breast cancer before 40 years of age has a 5.7 times increased risk (99% CI 2.7–11.8) of being diagnosed with breast cancer before she is 40 compared with a woman of the same age but without a family history of breast cancer.[23] Two genes, *BRCA1* and *BRCA2*, have been implicated in familial breast cancer but account for less than 10% of all breast cancer cases.[24] *BRCA* mutations are most strongly related to breast cancer occurring in younger, premenopausal women. In women diagnosed with breast cancer before age 40, 9% have a *BRCA* mutation, compared with only 2% of women of any age diagnosed with breast cancer.[25]

Reproductive Factors

Early age at menarche and late age at menopause have been found to increase the risk of breast cancer, whereas premenopausal oophorectomy reduces risk. Late age at first and possibly last

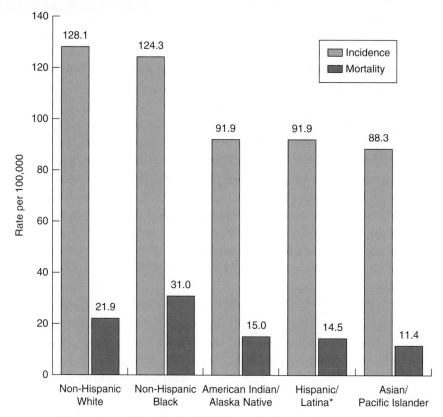

Rates are age adjusted to the 2000 US standard population.
*Persons of Hispanic origin may be any race.
Sources: Copeland et al.[25] Mortality: US mortality date, National Center for Health Statistics, Centers for Disease Control and Prevention.
American Cancer Society, Inc., Surveillance Research, 2015

• **Fig. 15.2** Female breast cancer incidence and mortality rates by race and ethnicity, United States, 2008 to 2012.

TABLE 15.2 Classification of Benign Breast Disease and the Risk of Subsequent Breast Cancer

| Benign Lesion | Description | ASSOCIATED RELATIVE RISK OF BREAST CANCER[a] | |
		With Family History of Breast Cancer	Without Family History of Breast Cancer
Proliferative Disease Without Atypia		2.4–2.7	1.7–1.9
Moderate and florid ductal hyperplasia of the usual type	Most common type of hyperplasia; cells do not have the cytologic appearance of lobular or apocrine-like lesions; florid lesions have a proliferation of cells that fill more than 70% of the involved space		
Additional lesions	Intraductal papilloma, radial scar, sclerosing adenosis, apocrine metaplasia		
Atypical Hyperplasia		11	4.2–4.3
Atypical ductal hyperplasia	Has features similar to ductal carcinoma in situ but lacks the complete criteria for that diagnosis		
Atypical lobular hyperplasia	Defined by changes that are similar to lobular carcinoma in situ but lack the complete criteria for that diagnosis		
Nonproliferative	Normal, cysts, duct, ectasia, mild hyperplasia, fibroadenoma	1.2–2.6	0.9–1

[a]Relative risks represent the range of values reported in the published literature.

Modified from Vogel VG. Breast cancer risk factors and preventive approaches to breast cancer. In: Kavanagh JS, Einhorn N, DePetrillo AD, eds. *Cancer in Women.* Cambridge, MA: Blackwell Scientific; 1998:58-91; and Fitzgibbons PL, Henson DE, Hutter RV. Benign breast changes and the risk for subsequent breast cancer: an update of the 1985 consensus statement. Cancer Committee of the College of American Pathologists. *Arch Pathol Lab Med.* 1998;122:1053-1055.

full-term pregnancy have been associated with an elevated risk; risk decreases with increasing parity.[26] Breastfeeding has also been shown to decrease the risk of breast cancer.[24,27] The timing of the initiation of the carcinogenic process is an important consideration when studying the effect of reproductive factors on the risk of breast cancer.[28] Risk of premenopausal breast cancer decreases about 9% (95% CI 7%–11%) for each 1-year increase in age at menarche, whereas risk of postmenopausal breast cancer decreases only about 4% (95% CI 2%–5%) for each 1-year increase in age at menarche. Risk of breast cancer increases with increasing age at first full-term pregnancy by 5% (95% CI 5%–6%) per year for breast cancer diagnosed before menopause and by 3% (95% CI 2%–4%) for cancers diagnosed after menopause. Each full-term pregnancy is associated with a 3% (95% CI 1%–6%) reduction in risk of breast cancer diagnosed before menopause, whereas the reduction was 12% (95% CI 10%–14%) for breast cancer diagnosed later.

Other Risk Factors for Breast Cancer

The field of breast cancer epidemiology is a vibrant and evolving body of knowledge. Newer and more recently identified risk factors (Table 15.3) and protective factors (Table 15.4) for breast cancer are discussed individually in the sections that follow.

Anthropometry

Obesity has emerged as a significant risk factor for postmenopausal breast cancer and is possibly a protective factor for premenopausal breast cancer. Further, adjustment for measures of obesity attenuates, but does not eliminate, the racial difference in stage at breast cancer diagnosis.[29,30] The most frequently used measure of obesity is the body mass index (BMI). BMI is calculated as weight in kilograms divided by the square of height in meters. In postmenopausal women, some studies report either no association or only a weak association between BMI and risk of breast cancer,[31,32] whereas the vast majority report that increased BMI significantly raises the risk of breast cancer[33-35] (e.g., a 4% increase in the odds of postmenopausal breast cancer for every 1 kg/m^2 increase in current BMI[34]). A meta-analysis of prospective studies found that the risk of breast cancer increased 7% with each 4 kg/m^2 increase in BMI in postmenopausal women.[35] Some studies have reported that the positive association between BMI and risk of postmenopausal breast cancer occurs only or more strongly in women with certain other risk factors, such as a family history of breast cancer[36] or older age.[37] A consistent finding is that elevated BMI increases the risk of postmenopausal breast cancer only in women who have never used postmenopausal hormone therapy.[35,38-40]

Central adiposity, commonly measured by waist circumference or waist-to-hip ratio, has been positively associated with postmenopausal breast cancer,[41,42] and this effect is stronger in women who never used hormone therapy. Finally, multiple studies have reported that weight gain during adulthood increases the risk of postmenopausal breast cancer[43] and that weight loss can reduce this risk.[44,45]

Obesity appears to have an opposite effect on the risk of breast cancer in premenopausal women. Few studies report either a positive association[46] or no association[43] between BMI and premenopausal breast cancer. Many studies, however, have reported that BMI is inversely associated with risk of premenopausal or early-age breast cancer.[33,47,48] For example, the same meta-analysis that reported a positive association between BMI and the risk of postmenopausal breast cancer reported a significant negative

TABLE 15.3 Newer Epidemiologic Risk Factors for Breast Cancer

Characteristic	Menopausal Status[a]	Comparison Category	Risk Category	Estimate of Effect[b]
Genetic Factors				
BRCA1 mutation[c]	Both	No mutation	Mutation present in gene	Lifetime risk 50%–73% by age 50 and 65%–87% by age 70
BRCA2 mutation[c]	Both	No mutation	Mutation present in gene	Lifetime risk 59% by age 50 and 82% by age 70
Hormonal Factors				
Oral contraceptive use[d]	Both	Never users	Current users	RR 1.24 (1.15–1.33)
	Both	Never users	≥10 years since last use	RR 1.01 (0.96–1.05)
Postmenopausal hormone therapy use	Postmenopausal[e]	Nonusers with an intact uterus	Estrogen + progestin users	HR 1.24 (1.01–1.54)
	Postmenopausal[f]	Nonusers with a hysterectomy	Estrogen users	HR 0.80 (0.62–1.04)
Circulating estradiol	Premenopausal[g]	Lowest quartile	Highest quartile	OR 1 (0.66–1.52)
	Postmenopausal[h]	Lowest quintile	Highest quintile	RR 2 (1.47–2.71)
Circulating estrone	Premenopausal[g]	Lowest quartile	Highest quartile	OR 1.16 (1.48–3.22)
	Postmenopausal[h]	Lowest quintile	Highest quintile	RR 2.19 (1.48–3.22)
Testosterone	Premenopausal[e]	<1.13 nmol/L	≥2.04 nmol/L	OR 1.73 (1.16–2.57)
	Postmenopausal[g]	Lowest quintile	Highest quintile	RR 2.22 (1.59–3.10)

Continued

Newer Epidemiologic Risk Factors for Breast Cancer—cont'd

Characteristic	Menopausal Status[a]	Comparison Category	Risk Category	Estimate of Effect[b]
Other Biological Factors				
Mammographic breast density[j]	Both	<5% density	≥75% density	RR 4.64 (3.64–5.91)
Bone mineral density[j]	Postmenopausal	Lowest quartile at each of three skeletal sites	Highest quartile at each of three skeletal sites	RR 2.70 (1.4–5.3)
Circulating IGF-I[k]	Premenopausal	25th percentile	75th percentile	OR 1.93 (1.38–2.69)
	Postmenopausal	25th percentile	75th percentile	OR 0.95 (0.62–1.33)
Circulating IGFBP-III[k]	Premenopausal	25th percentile	75th percentile	OR 1.96 (1.28–2.99)
	Postmenopausal	25th percentile	75th percentile	OR 0.97 (0.53–1.77)
Behavioral Factors				
Body mass index[l]	Postmenopausal	<21 kg/m²	≥33 kg/m²	RR 1.27 (1.03–1.55)
Height[l]	Premenopausal	<1.60 cm	≥1.75 cm	RR 1.42 (0.95–2.12)
	Postmenopausal	<1.60 cm	≥1.75 cm	RR 1.28 (0.94–1.76)
Weight[l]	Postmenopausal	<60 kg	≥80 kg	RR 1.25 (1.02–1.52)
Alcohol use[l]	Both	Never drinkers	>12 g/day	RR 1.10 (1.06–1.14)
Smoking[m]	Postmenopausal	Never smokers	Smoked >40 years	RR 1.5 (1.2–1.9)
Night work[n]	Both	No nightshift work	Any nightshift work	OR 1.48 (1.36–1.61)
Dietary Factors				
Total fat intake[o]	Both	Lowest quantile	Highest quantile	OR 1.13 (1.03–1.25)
Saturated fat intake[o]	Both	Lowest quantile	Highest quantile	OR 1.19 (1.06–1.35)
Meat intake[m]	Both	Lowest quantile	Highest quantile	OR 1.17 (1.06–1.29)
Environmental Factors				
Ionizing radiation[p]	Both	0–0.09 Gy exposure to Nagasaki or Hiroshima atomic bomb	≥0.50 Gy exposure to Nagasaki or Hiroshima atomic bomb	RR varies depending on age at exposure: RR = 9 at age 0–4; RR = 2 at age 35–39

OR, Odds ratio; *RR*, relative risk.
[a]Refers to menopausal status at the time of diagnosis.
[b]Data in parentheses are 95% confidence intervals.
[c]From National Cancer Institute.[25]
[d]From Collaborative Group on Hormonal Factors in Breast Cancer.[86]
[e]From Chlebowski et al.[90]
[f]From Stefanick et al.[91]
[g]From Kaaks et al.[63]
[h]From Key et al.[59]
[i]From McCormack and dos Santos Silva.[101]
[j]From Zmuda et al.[57]
[k]From Renehan AG, Zwahlen M, Minder C, et al, Insulin-like growth factor (IGF)-I, IGF binding protein-3, and cancer risk: Systematic review and metaregression analysis. *Lancet.* 2004;363:1346-1353.
[l]From Ellison et al.[116]
[m]From Cui Y, Miller AB, Rohan TE, Cigarette smoking and breast cancer risk: update of a prospective cohort study. *Breast Cancer Res Treat.* 2006;100:293-299.
[n]From Megdal et al.[134]
[o]From Boyd NF, Stone J, Vogt KN, et al, Dietary fat and breast cancer risk revisited: a meta-analysis of the published literature. *Br J Cancer.* 2003;89:1672-1685.
[p]From Tokunaga et al.[139]

TABLE 15.4 Possible Protective Factors for Breast Cancer

Characteristic	Menopausal Status[a]	Reference Group	Comparison Group	Estimate of Effect[b]
Reproductive Factors				
Parity[c]	Both	Nulliparous	Two live births	OR 0.91 (0.85–0.97)
Breastfeeding[d]	Premenopausal	Never breastfed	Ever breastfed	RR 0.78 (0.66–0.91)
	Postmenopausal	Never breastfed	Ever breastfed	RR 1.04 (0.95–1.14)
Preeclampsia[e]	Both	No preeclampsia	Ever preeclampsia	ORs range from 0.27 (0.08–0.63) to 0.81 (0.61–1.1)
Hormonal Factors				
Estrogen metabolite ratio[f]	Premenopausal	2:16-OH ratio ≤1.80	2:16-OH ratio ≥3.29	OR 0.55 (0.23–1.32)
	Postmenopausal	2:16-OH ratio ≤1.77	2.16-OH ratio ≥3.66	OR 1.31 (0.53–3.18)
Circulating sex hormone–binding globulin	Premenopausal[n]	<31.1 nmol/L	≥64.5 nmol/L	OR 0.95 (0.65–1.40)
	Postmenopausal[o]	Lowest quintile	Highest quintile	RR 0.66 (0.43–1)
Other Biological Factors				
Bone fracture[g]	Postmenopausal	No fracture in past 5 years	History of fracture	OR 0.80 (0.68–0.94)
Behavioral Factors				
Body mass index[h]	Premenopausal	<21 kg/m^2	≥33 kg/m^2	RR 0.58 (0.34–1)
Physical activity	Premenopausal[p]	<9.1 hours/week	≥20.8 hours/week	OR 0.74 (0.52–1.05)
	Postmenopausal[q]	Not currently active	>40 metabolic-equivalent hours per week	RR 0.78 (0.62–1)
NSAID use[i]	Both	Nonusers	Current user of any NSAID	OR 0.80 (0.73–0.87)
Dietary Factors				
Calcium (dietary)[j]	Postmenopausal	≤500 mg/day	>1250 mg/day	RR 0.80 (0.67–0.95)
Folate (total)[k]	Both	150–299 µg/day	≥600 µg/day	RR 0.93 (0.83–1.03)
Soy[l]	Premenopausal	Low intake	High intake	OR 0.70 (0.58–0.85)
	Postmenopausal	Low intake	High intake	OR 0.77 (0.60–0.98)
Vitamin D (total)[m]	Postmenopausal	<400 IU	≥800 IU	RR 0.89 (0.77–1.03)

OR, Odds ratio; *NSAID,* nonsteroidal antiinflammatory drug; *RR,* relative risk.

[a]Refers to menopausal status at the time of diagnosis.

[b]Data in parentheses are 95% confidence intervals.

[c]From Lambe M, Hsieh CC, Chan HW, et al. Parity, age at first and last birth, and risk of breast cancer: a population-based study in Sweden. *Breast Cancer Res Treat.* 1996;38:305-311.

[d]From Newcomb et al.[27]

[e]From Innes and Byers.[93]

[f]From Muti et al.[81]

[g]From Newcomb PA, Trentham-Dietz A, Egan KM, et al. Fracture history and risk of breast and endometrial cancer. *Am J Epidemiol.* 2001;153:1071-1078.

[h]From van den Brandt et al.[33]

[i]From Khuder SA, Mutgi AB. Breast cancer and NSAID use: a meta-analysis. *Br J Cancer.* 2001;84:1188-1192.

[j]From McCullough ML, Rodriguez C, Diver WR, et al. Dairy, calcium, and vitamin D intake and postmenopausal breast cancer risk in the Cancer Prevention Study II Nutrition Cohort. *Cancer Epidemiol Biomarkers Prev.* 2005;14:2898–2904.

[k]From Zhang S, Hunter DJ, Hankinson SE, et al. A prospective study of folate intake and the risk of breast cancer. *JAMA.* 1999;281:1632-1637.

[l]From Trock BJ, Hilakivi-Clarke L, Clarke R. Meta-analysis of soy intake and breast cancer risk. *J Natl Cancer Inst.* 2006;98:459-471.

[m]From Robien K, Cutler GJ, Lazovich D. Vitamin D intake and breast cancer risk in postmenopausal women: the Iowa Women's Health Study. *Cancer Causes Control.* 2007;18:775-782.

[n]From Kaaks et al.[63]

[o]From Key T et al.[59]

[p]From John EM, Horn-Ross PL, Koo J. Lifetime physical activity and breast cancer risk in a multiethnic population: the San Francisco Bay area breast cancer study. *Cancer Epidemiol Biomarkers Prev.* 2003;12:1143-1152.

[q]From McTiernan A, Kooperberg C, White E, et al: Recreational physical activity and the risk of breast cancer in postmenopausal women: the Women's Health Initiative Cohort Study. *JAMA.* 2003;290:1331-1336.

association between BMI and risk of premenopausal breast cancer, with an 11% reduction in risk for every 4 kg/m^2 increase in BMI (RR 0.89; 95% CI 0.81–0.97).[33] The effect of BMI on the risk of premenopausal breast cancer may vary by race, with one study reporting a negative association in Caucasian women but no association in African American women.[31]

Similar relationships between obesity and risk of premenopausal breast cancer are observed when other anthropometric measures are considered. Weight has been reported to be either negatively associated[33,43,] or not associated[49,50] with premenopausal breast cancer. One study reported a positive association between waist-to-hip ratio and risk of premenopausal breast cancer,[42] whereas another reported no association.[41] The effect of weight gain on premenopausal breast cancer may also vary by race, with studies of Caucasian women reporting either no[51,52] or a negative association,[40] whereas a study of Hispanic women reported a nonsignificant positive association.[52] Overall, the totality of the current evidence suggests that obesity reduces the risk of premenopausal breast cancer. The reason for this observation is not clear.

Endogenous Hormones

Exposure to estrogen is closely linked to the etiology of breast cancer. Estrogen is a female sex hormone that is required for a number of processes in the body. The mechanisms through which estrogens contribute to the carcinogenic process are complex; however, evidence exists confirming that estrogens cause both normal and malignant breast cell proliferation.[53] Many established risk factors for breast cancer can be attributed to either some means of elevated estrogen exposure or cyclical ovarian function. For example, both an early age of menarche and a late age of menopause are related to prolonged exposure to the high levels of estrogen that occur during the menstrual cycle, and both are associated with increased risk of breast cancer.[54,55] Surgical menopause, which results in an abrupt arrest of estrogen secretion by the ovaries, is protective against breast cancer.[56] Moreover, the rate of age-specific breast cancer slows around the time of menopause, a time when estrogen levels decline. Increased bone mineral density, a potential reflection of cumulative estrogen exposure, is associated with increased breast cancer development in menopausal women (see discussion later in the chapter).[57] Obesity, which is positively correlated with circulating estrogen levels, is associated with risk of postmenopausal breast cancer.[33,57]

Numerous studies have consistently demonstrated that increased levels of endogenous estrogen are related to increased risk of breast cancer in postmenopausal women.[58,59] For example, a meta-analysis of nine prospective studies examining hormone levels in relation to postmenopausal breast cancer reported a twofold increase (RR 2; 95% CI 1.47–2.71; p for trend < .001) in risk of breast cancer for women in the highest quintile of estradiol compared with those in the lowest quintile.

The association between estradiol and premenopausal breast cancer, however, is far less clear. Estradiol levels fluctuate throughout the menstrual cycle, with peaks occurring toward the ends of both the follicular and luteal phases.[60] Some studies have reported similar positive associations between estradiol and breast cancer in premenopausal women,[61,62] whereas others have reported no association.[63–65] Studies of estradiol and premenopausal breast cancer have been limited by a number of factors, however, including small numbers,[62] failure to control for phase of the menstrual cycle,[62,65] and inclusion of cases that were premenopausal at the

time of the blood sample but not at the time of breast cancer diagnosis.[62,63] The Nurses' Health Study II, an observational study of women's health, reported that free estradiol (RR 2.4; 95% CI 1.3–4.5 for fourth vs. first quartile) and total estradiol (RR 2.1; 95% CI 1.1–4.1 for fourth vs. first quartile) levels during the follicular phase were positively associated with breast cancer, whereas free and total estradiol levels during the luteal phase were not.[61] Although this study was prospective, carefully controlled for phase of the menstrual cycle, and used large numbers, the menopausal status of the cases at the time of diagnosis was unclear.

In addition to the observational studies linking circulating estradiol concentration and risk of breast cancer, convincing data from large clinical trials show that drugs blocking the action of estrogen reduce breast cancer incidence. The risk reduction is more pronounced in women with higher estrogen levels than in those with lower levels, further strengthening the evidence that estrogen exposure is associated with the development of breast cancer.[66,67] In the Multiple Outcomes of Raloxifene Evaluation (MORE) trial, it was found that postmenopausal women with the highest estradiol levels had a 2.1-fold risk of breast cancer compared with women with the lowest estradiol levels.[68] Women in the placebo arm of the trial had nearly seven times the risk of developing breast cancer than women with estradiol levels lower (0.6% per year) than the assay's detection limit, and women with circulating levels of estradiol greater than 10 pmol/L in the raloxifene treatment group had a breast cancer rate 76% lower than women with similar levels of estradiol in the placebo group. Raloxifene is a selective ER modulator, a competitive inhibitor of estradiol binding to its receptor protein. Thus inhibiting the action of estrogen plays an obvious role in reducing the risk of breast cancer.[66]

Dietary Fat and Serum Estradiol

Varying levels of fat consumption may influence incidence of hormonally dependent breast cancer by modifying levels of circulating estrogens,[69–71] and free fatty acids added to plasma can significantly increase levels of estradiol in vitro.[72,73] A meta-analysis of 13 intervention trials found serum estradiol levels to be 23% (95% CI –27.7% to –18.1%) lower in healthy postmenopausal women consuming the least amount of dietary fat compared with women with the highest fat intake.[69] The Diet and Androgens (DIANA) Randomized Trial found a nonsignificant reduction in serum estradiol (–18% in intervention group vs. –5.5% in control group; p = .13) in postmenopausal women consuming a low animal fat and high omega-3 diet.[70] However, not all studies evaluating dietary fat and estrogen levels have observed reductions in circulating estradiol levels; it has been hypothesized that inadequate dietary assessment may be one cause of this contradiction.

Estrogen Metabolism

There is evidence that the way estrogen is metabolized is associated with the risk of breast cancer.[74,75] Estradiol metabolism is predominantly oxidative; it is first (reversibly) converted to estrone, which is irreversibly converted to either 2- or 16-α-hydroxy (2-OH and 16-OH, respectively) estrone to eliminate it from the body. Both 16-OH estrone and 16-OH estradiol strongly activate the classical ER and, like estradiol, can stimulate uterine tissue growth.[76] On the other hand, the 2-OH metabolites do not appear to promote cellular proliferation and may even have antiestrogenic effects.[77] Because the 2-OH and 16-OH metabolites compete for a limited substrate pool, a rise in one pathway will reduce the amount of product in the competing pathway. Thus the relative activity of these two metabolic pathways (2:16-OH) may be an endocrine biomarker for risk of breast cancer.

Despite the biological evidence, however, epidemiologic support is lacking. Only a handful of studies have explored the association between the risk of breast cancer and the 2:16-OH ratio, with mixed results.[78–83] Possible explanations for these disparate findings include small sample sizes, retrospective study designs, and the use of prevalent breast cancer cases. Metabolite levels in women with breast cancer may not reflect the hormonal milieu during the etiologically relevant period. Moreover, the use of prevalent cases may mask any association, because estrogen metabolism may be altered by treatment.[84] Notably, only two prospective studies[80,81] have found a decreased risk associated with a high urinary 2:16-OH ratio; however, the results were not statistically significant in either study. Moreover, in one study,[81] the association was limited to premenopausal women only. In summary, although there is evidence to suggest an association between estrogen metabolism and risk of breast cancer, supporting data from large, population-based studies are lacking.

Diethylstilbestrol Exposure

In the first half of the 20th century, several million women were exposed in utero to diethylstilbestrol (DES), which was given to their mothers to prevent pregnancy complications. Whether these women are also at an increased risk for breast cancer is unclear. A long-term follow-up study of DES-exposed women and unexposed controls reported a nearly twofold increase in the cumulative risk of breast cancer in exposed women aged 40 or older.[85] DES exposure during pregnancy has not occurred in the United States for nearly 50 years.

Exogenous Hormones: Oral Contraceptives and Postmenopausal Hormone Therapy

Exposure to exogenous estrogen has been related to the risk of breast cancer. In the general population, oral contraceptive (OC) use is weakly associated with such risk. The Collaborative Group on Hormonal Factors in Breast Cancer analyzed the worldwide epidemiologic evidence on the relation between risk of breast cancer and use of hormonal contraceptives.[86] This large meta-analysis combined individual data on 53,297 women with breast cancer and 100,239 women without breast cancer from 54 epidemiologic studies conducted in 25 countries. Results showed that women who used OCs had a slight but significant increased risk of breast cancer, compared with nonusers (RR 1.24; 95% CI 1.15–1.33). Reassuringly, the risk diminished steadily after cessation of use, with no increase in risk 10 years after cessation of OC use, irrespective of family history of breast cancer, reproductive history, geographic area of residence, ethnic background, differences in study designs, dose and type of hormone, and duration of use.

More recent population-based studies of the risk of breast cancer in former and current users of OCs do not suggest that these drugs increase risk.[87,88] In women 35 to 64 years of age participating in a population-based, case-control study (the National Institute of Child Health and Human Development

Women's Contraceptive and Reproductive Experiences Study [CARE]), current or former OC use was not associated with a significantly increased risk of breast cancer.[88]

A retrospective cohort study evaluated the effect of OCs in women with a familial predisposition to breast cancer.[89] After accounting for age and birth cohort, any OC use was significantly associated with increased risk of breast cancer in first-degree relatives only (RR 3.3; 95% CI 1.6–6.7). The elevated risk in women with a first-degree family history of breast cancer was most evident for OC use during or before 1975, when formulations were likely to contain higher dosages of estrogen and progestins.

The results of the Women's Health Initiative (WHI) showed that increased risk may occur only in users of combined estrogen and progestin regimens[90] and not in women using unopposed estrogen.[91] The WHI conducted two separate randomized, controlled primary prevention trials of hormone therapy use in postmenopausal women 50 to 79 years of age. One was a trial of conjugated equine estrogens, 0.625 mg daily, plus medroxyprogesterone acetate, 2.5 mg daily, in a single tablet (n = 8506) versus placebo (n = 8102) in women with an intact uterus. The other was a trial of conjugated equine estrogens, 0.625 mg daily (n = 5310) versus placebo (n = 5429) in women with a hysterectomy. Women randomized to take the combination of estrogen and progestin had a 24% increase in risk of invasive breast cancer compared with those randomized to placebo (hazard ratio 1.24; 95% CI 1.01–1.54).[90] However, in the unopposed estrogen trial, women randomized to active treatment had a similar risk of invasive breast cancer as women randomized to placebo.[91] The Nurses' Health Study reported that the risk of breast cancer increased with the duration of unopposed estrogen use. The multivariate RRs and 95% CIs for breast cancer with current hormone therapy use for less than 5 years, 5 to 9.9 years, 10 to 14.9 years, 15 to 19.9 years, and 20 years or more were, respectively, 0.96 (0.75–1.22), 0.90 (0.73–1.12), 1.06 (0.87–1.30), 1.18 (0.95–1.48), and 1.42 (1.13–1.77; p for trend < .001).[92] The relationship was more notable in ER-positive and PR-positive tumors, and it became statistically significant after 15 years of use (RR 1.48).

Preeclampsia

Preeclampsia, a common complication of pregnancy, may be a particularly sensitive marker for endogenous hormonal factors associated with the development of breast cancer. In a review of the connection between preeclampsia and the risk of breast cancer, the data suggest that both a personal and maternal history of preeclampsia are inversely and independently associated with subsequent risk of breast cancer.[93] Preeclampsia may be a novel marker of endogenous hormonal factors that are related to breast cancer development, including reduced levels of estrogens and insulin-like growth factor I (IGF-I), as well as elevated levels of progesterone, androgens, and IGF-I binding protein. These factors may act both individually and synergistically to decrease the risk of breast cancer.

Induced Abortion

It has been hypothesized that an interrupted pregnancy might increase a woman's risk of breast cancer because of proliferation of breast cells without the later protective effect of differentiation. In a cohort of 1.5 million women (28.5 million person-years of observation) and after adjustment for known risk factors, induced abortion as determined by a national Danish registry was not associated with an increased risk of breast cancer. No increases in risk were found in subgroups defined according to age at abortion, parity, time since abortion, or age at diagnosis of breast cancer.[94] The RR of breast cancer increased with increasing gestational age of the fetus at the time of the most recent induced abortion: less than 7 weeks, 0.81 (95% CI 0.58–1.13); greater than 12 weeks, 1.38 (1–1.9; reference category, 9–10 weeks). Induced abortions appear to have no overall effect on the risk of breast cancer.

Mammographic Breast Density

Mammographic density is associated with an increased risk of ER- and PR-positive tumors, which suggests a hormonal etiology for mammographic density. A model that incorporates breast density calculates both the 5- and 10-year risk for breast cancer[95] and shows higher risks are associated with increasing levels of mammographic density. Mammographic density may reflect high levels of circulating sex hormones or sensitivity to hormones but has a stronger predictive association with breast cancer than serum hormone levels alone. Indeed, endogenous sex hormone levels are strongly and independently related to the risk of breast cancer in postmenopausal women.[96] Measurement of sex hormone levels has not gained wide acceptance as a clinical risk assessment tool, however.

Higher-percent breast density is a strong risk factor for breast cancer in women with known *BRCA1/BRCA2* mutations.[97] The odds of breast cancer in mutation carriers with density greater than or equal to 50% is twice that of mutation carriers with less than 50% density (odds ratio [OR] 2.29). In general, the presence of risk factors for breast cancer increases mammographic breast density. For example, nulliparity and later age at first birth have been associated with increased density.[98] On the other hand, breast density has been shown to decrease with increasing age,[98,99] although increased age is a risk factor for breast cancer. This apparent contradiction has been explained by noting that breast density may be related to the rate of change in breast cancer incidence rather than the incidence of breast cancer itself.[100]

A meta-analysis[101] found a consistent association between higher breast density and a greater risk of invasive breast cancer, with four- to fivefold increased breast cancer risk for women in the highest category of breast density compared with those in the lowest. Prospective studies of breast density and subsequent risk of breast cancer reported that women in the highest quartile of percent density (≥28%) have a 3.8-fold greater risk of breast cancer than those in the lowest quartile (≤5.4%). Mammographic breast density is an established, independent risk factor for breast cancer.

Exogenous Hormones and Mammographic Density

Studies have repeatedly shown that increased breast density is related to postmenopausal hormone replacement therapy (HRT).[102–104] The percent of women whose breast density changes after initiating HRT varies by type of HRT used, with increased density occurring more often in estrogen-plus-progestin regimens than with estrogen-alone regimens. In the WHI, investigators reported that 75% of women on active treatment experienced an increase in breast density after 1 year. The mean change in percent density from baseline to year 1 was 6% (95% CI 4.6–7.5) in the treatment group compared with –0.9% (95% CI –1.5 to –0.2) in the placebo group.[104] Short-term cessation of HRT use before mammography results in a decrease in breast density[105] or less

frequent increase in density compared with women who continue to take HRT,[103] and even months after cessation of therapy, there appears to be residual effects of HRT on breast density.[106]

Data on the effect of OC use on breast density are limited, probably because the majority of women for whom screening mammography is recommended (age ≥40) are postmenopausal and would not be currently using OCs. One study has reported, however, that use of OCs before first birth was not related to breast density later in life.[107]

Dietary Fat and Mammographic Breast Density

The few studies that have assessed the role of dietary fat on mammographic density have revealed that diet may influence percent breast density. A 2-year intervention with a low-fat, high-carbohydrate diet reduced breast density by 6.1% in the experimental group compared with 2.1% in the control group (*p* = .02).[108] Positive associations between total fat intake and high mammographic density have been observed.[109,110] However, decreased density and null findings have also been associated with total fat intake.[111–113] As with total fat, positive and null relationships have been found between total polyunsaturated fat intake and breast density.[109–113] Two studies assessed the effects of total meat intake and breast density. A nonsignificant, positive association (OR 1.59; 95% CI 0.83, 3.04) was observed in one study; however, no relationship was found between total meat intake and breast density in the other.[113,114]

Physical Activity

Evidence for an association between physical activity and breast cancer is not entirely consistent. A review of such studies showed that the strength of association between physical activity and breast cancer ranges from 0.3 to 1.6.[115] Thirty-two of 44 studies observed a reduction in the risk of breast cancer in women who were most physically active, and the risk reduction averaged between 30% and 40%. An inverse dose-response relationship between increasing activity levels and decreased risk of breast cancer was found in 20 of 23 studies that examined this trend. Only two studies observed an opposite trend such that breast cancer risk increased with increasing physical activity levels; the remaining studies found no association at all.

Alcohol Consumption

Although the association of alcohol consumption with increased risk of breast cancer has been a consistent finding in the majority of epidemiologic studies, questions remain, nevertheless, regarding the interactions between alcohol and other risk factors and the biological mechanisms involved. A meta-analysis of epidemiologic studies examined the dose-response relation and assessed whether effect estimates differed according to various study characteristics.[116] Overall, there was an increase in the RR of breast cancer with alcohol consumption, but the magnitude of the effect was small; in comparison with nondrinkers, women consuming an average of 12 grams per day of alcohol (approximately one typical drink) had an RR of 1.10. Estimates of RR were 7% greater in hospital-based case-control studies than in cohort studies or community-based case control studies, 3% greater in studies published earlier than later studies, and 5% greater in studies conducted outside of the United States than inside the country. The findings of five US cohort studies published later yielded an increased risk of 6% for consumers of 12 grams per day of alcohol compared with nondrinkers. Cohort studies with less than 10 years of follow-up yielded estimates 11% higher than studies with longer follow-up periods. No meaningful differences are seen by either menopausal status or type of beverage consumed.

Alcohol-related risk of breast cancer may be associated with endogenous hormone levels.[117] Observational results collected from postmenopausal women participating in the Nurses' Health Study are consistent with the hypothesis that the use of alcohol increases the risk of breast cancer through a hormonal mechanism. Risk of breast cancer was about 30% higher in women who currently used postmenopausal hormones for 5 or more years and did not drink alcohol (RR 1.32; 95% CI 1.05–1.66). Those who never used postmenopausal hormones but consumed 1.5 to 2 drinks or more of alcohol daily had a nonsignificantly increased risk of 28%. Current users of postmenopausal hormones for 5 or more years who consumed 20 or more grams of alcohol daily had an RR for breast cancer nearly twice that of nondrinking nonusers of postmenopausal hormones (RR 1.99; 95% CI 1.42–2.79). Women who are making decisions about alcohol and postmenopausal hormone use may want to consider the added risks associated with breast cancer.[118]

Smoking

The role of active and passive smoking in breast cancer remains controversial, largely because breast cancer is hormone-dependent and cigarette smoking appears to have antiestrogenic effects in women.[119,120] Most reports demonstrated no association between smoking and risk of breast cancer; however, many studies included passive smokers within the referent category, possibly diluting any true effect that active or passive smoking exposure might have on risk of breast cancer.[121] In a review of 11 studies, five found significantly increased ORs of at least 1.5 for passive smokers versus unexposed, and six reported significantly increased risk of breast cancer for active smokers versus nonsmoking women, suggesting a similar strength of association between active or passive smoking and risk of breast cancer. Some of the inconsistency in the relationship of breast cancer to cigarette smoking may also result from the influence of age at diagnosis and menopausal status on the response of breast cells to exposure to cigarette smoke.[120]

The risk of breast cancer is significantly higher (70%) in parous women who initiated smoking within 5 years post menarche and in nulliparous women who smoked 20 cigarettes per day or more (sevenfold increase in risk) and for 20 cumulative pack-years or more (OR 7.48; 95% CI 1.59–35.2).[122] On the contrary, postmenopausal women who began smoking after their first full-term pregnancy and whose BMI increased from 18 years of age had half the risk of breast cancer.

Smoking before or after a diagnosis of breast cancer is associated with a higher mortality from both breast cancer and other causes.[123] Active smokers 1 year before breast cancer diagnosis are about 25% more likely than never smokers to die of breast cancer. Women who continue to smoke after diagnosis are more than 70% more likely than never smokers to die of breast cancer. Compared with women who continued to smoke after diagnosis, those who quit smoking after diagnosis have lower mortality from both breast cancer and respiratory cancer. It is not known whether these findings suggest a biological mechanism related to the carcinogenic properties of tobacco smoke on tumor progression and metastasis or are related to demographic, behavioral, or clinical factors.

Bone Mineral Density

Bone contains ERs and is highly sensitive to circulating estrogen levels. Bone mineral density is thus considered a surrogate marker for long-term exposure to endogenous and exogenous estrogen. In multiple studies, women with higher bone density have a higher breast cancer risk.[124–127] In a meta-analysis of eight prospective cohort and two nested-control studies, women in the highest hip bone density category were more than 60% more likely to develop breast cancer compared with women in the lowest density category.[128]

Bisphosphonates

Oral bisphosphonates are used for the treatment of osteoporosis and for women with breast cancer with evidence of bone loss. Whether their use is a true protective factor is unclear. Several studies have suggested a protective effect of oral bisphosphonates,[129–132] but low bone density is associated with a decreased risk of breast cancer. It is not known, therefore, if there is a true causal association between bisphosphonates and breast cancer risk reduction.

Night-Shift Work

Night-shift work is recognized by the International Agency for Research on Cancer and the World Health Organization as a probable carcinogen.[133] A meta-analysis exploring the relationship between night work and breast cancer risk included studies of airline cabin attendants and nighttime shift workers and reported a nearly 50% increase in risk.[134] The risk was similar between both female air cabin crew and female night workers.

A study of nurses reported that working shifts after midnight was associated with an 80% elevated risk of breast cancer with the highest risk noted in nurses working long-term day-to-night rotating shifts (OR 2.6).[135] This association may be related to nocturnal light exposure, which results in the suppression of nocturnal melatonin production by the pineal gland.[136] Evidence to support this comes from the finding that low levels of 6-sulfatoxymelatonin, the major melatonin metabolite, are associated with an increased risk of breast cancer.[136,137]

Ionizing Radiation

There is a well-established relationship between exposure to ionizing radiation and the risk of breast cancer.[138,139] Increased risk of breast cancer has been consistently observed in association with a variety of exposures, such as the Hiroshima or Nagasaki atomic explosions, fluoroscopy for tuberculosis, and radiation treatments for medical conditions (e.g., Hodgkin disease). Although risk is inversely associated with age at radiation exposure, exposures past the menopausal age seem to carry a low risk. Although an estimate of the risk of breast cancer associated with medical radiology puts the figure at less than 1% of the total,[140] certain populations, such as women who are heterozygous for the ataxia-telangiectasia gene *(ATM)*, may be at increased risk from usual sources of radiation exposure.[141]

Women with a history of benign breast disease or a family history of breast cancer appear to have a greater risk of breast cancer after relatively low ionizing radiation exposure compared with other women.[142] Risk of breast cancer is elevated in women exposed to medical radiation before 20 years of age versus women who are not unexposed, and this increased risk is observed only in women with a history of benign breast disease. Overall, risk is not associated with exposure to medical radiation after 20 years of age, although in women with a positive family history of breast or ovarian cancer, exposed women have an increased risk. Importantly, the elevated risks are attributable to exposures and radiation doses that are no longer common, hampering study generalizability to younger cohorts. In theory, patients with breast cancer who are treated with lumpectomy and radiation therapy may be at increased risk for second breast or other malignancies compared with those treated with mastectomy. Outcome studies after a median follow-up of 12 to 15 years show no difference, however, in the risk of second malignancies.[143-144]

Summary of Risk Factors for Breast Cancer

A meta-analysis and systematic review of 66 studies provided data for estimates of risk factors for breast cancer for women aged 40 to 49 years of age.[145] Studies varied by measures, reference groups, and adjustment for confounders, and effects of multiple risk factors were not considered. Extremely dense breasts on mammography or having first-degree relatives with breast cancer are associated with at least a twofold increase in risk for breast cancer. Prior breast biopsy, second-degree relatives with breast cancer, or heterogeneously dense breasts were associated with a 1.5- to 2.0-fold increased risk; current use of OCs, nulliparity, and age 30 years or older at first birth were associated with a 1.0- to 1.5-fold increased risk. Identification of these risk factors may be useful for personalized mammography screening.

Selected References

2. Siegel RL, Miller KD, Jemal A. Cancer statistics, 2016. *CA Cancer J Clin*. 2016;66:7-30.

15. Hartmann LC, Degnim AC, Santen RJ, et al. Atypical hyperplasia of the breast—risk assessment and management options. *N Engl J Med*. 2015;372:78-89.

19. Hartmann LC, Radisky DC, Frost MH, et al. Understanding the premalignant potential of atypical hyperplasia through its natural history: a longitudinal cohort study. *Cancer Prev Res (Phila)*. 2014;7:211-217.

90. Chlebowski RT, Hendrix SL, Langer RD, et al. Influence of estrogen plus progestin on breast cancer and mammography in healthy postmenopausal women: the Women's Health Initiative Randomized Trial. *JAMA*. 2003;289:3243-3253.

91. Stefanick ML, Anderson GL, Margolis KL, et al. Effects of conjugated equine estrogens on breast cancer and mammography screening in postmenopausal women with hysterectomy. *JAMA*. 2006;295:1647-1657.

95. Tice JA, Miglioretti DL, Li C-S, et al. Breast density and benign breast disease: risk assessment to identify women at high risk of breast cancer. *J Clin Oncol*. 2015;33:3137-3143.

145. Nelson HD, Zakher B, Cantor A, et al. Risk factors for breast cancer for women aged 40 to 49 years: a systematic review and meta-analysis. *Ann Intern Med*. 2012;156:635-648.

A full reference list is available online at ExpertConsult.com.

16

Primary Prevention of Breast Cancer

VICTOR G. VOGEL

Identifying Women at Risk

Chemoprevention can be defined as the use of natural or synthetic chemical agents to reverse, suppress, or prevent carcinogenic progression to invasive cancer.[1–5] Epidemiologic data suggesting that breast cancer is preventable through drug intervention include time trends in cancer incidence and mortality, geographic variations and the effects of migration, identification of specific causative factors, and the observation that most human cancers do not show simple patterns of genetic inheritance.

Chemoprevention may be recommended for certain women who are at increased risk of breast cancer. Indeed, the need for effective breast cancer preventive strategies is apparent based solely on the number of women who are at increased risk for the disease. More than 45 million women in the United States are older than 50 years of age, and at least 2.5 million of these women have first-degree relatives with breast cancer. At least 8 million postmenopausal women have undergone biopsy for benign breast disease, and one in four of these women have proliferative changes. At least 10 million older women are obese, and one in six women 40 years of age or older is nulliparous.[6] A substantial proportion of breast cancer occurs in women with these characteristics, and strategies to reduce this risk would have a significant effect on the burden of breast cancer in the United States.

The clinician's role in identifying candidates for chemoprophylaxis should include a detailed assessment of familial breast cancer, the opportunity for genetic testing when appropriate, comprehensive quantitative risk assessment, and a specific management prescription.[7] Clinicians should also address the risks and benefits of screening, prophylactic surgery when indicated, and risk reduction using approved chemopreventive agents.

Familial breast cancer—often in a mother, aunt, and/or sister—is a leading reason why women seek counseling from their physicians about their own risks of developing breast cancer. Well-characterized breast cancer susceptibility genes, including *BRCA1* and *BRCA2,* may account for as many as one in six breast cancers.[8] The cumulative lifetime risk of developing breast cancer approaches 85% for some carriers of *BRCA* mutations, as estimated by the number of relatives with positive breast diagnoses before 50 years of age. If there is a suspicion that one of the susceptibility genes may be involved in the etiology of the breast cancers in a woman's family, further risk assessment is recommended.[9]

Clinicians should strive to ensure that the patient understands her objective risk and its implications for making a decision about chemoprevention. In addition to genetic susceptibility, hormonally linked adult reproductive and anthropometric risk factors have been well established in the etiology of pre- and postmeno-pausal breast cancers,[10,11] and early-life exposures have also been evaluated.[12]

Breast Cancer Risk Models

Multiple quantitative models are available to assess a woman's risk of developing invasive breast cancer, but all of the models are limited by moderate discriminatory accuracy.[13] The quantitative breast cancer risk assessment model developed by Gail and colleagues[14] estimates the probability that a woman who engages in annual mammographic screening will develop invasive or in situ ductal or lobular cancer over a particular age interval. The model has been widely used in clinical trials of pharmacologic agents to reduce the risk of breast cancer. There are six risk factors in the model, and they were adjusted simultaneously for the presence of the other risk factors. They include current age, age at menarche, number of breast biopsies, age at first live birth (or nulliparity), family history of breast cancer in first-degree relatives, and race. Risk of breast cancer may be determined by validated models other than the Gail model[15–17] (including the Tyrer-Cuzick model[18]) or by the eligibility criteria used in the various breast cancer chemoprevention trials.

The Gail model is available online at www.cancer.gov/bcrisktool. The average American woman's Gail score is 0.3%, which represents her estimated risk of developing invasive breast cancer over the next 5 years; the lifetime risk for the average American woman is 10.1%. A previous diagnosis of atypical lobular or ductal hyperplasia nearly doubles the estimated risk, although the model underestimates the risk of women with atypical hyperplasia. The model has high predictive accuracy within populations or among groups of women, and it estimates the absolute risk of developing invasive breast cancer only in women 35 years and older. It was not designed for women with prior diagnoses of breast cancer, lobular carcinoma in situ (LCIS), or ductal carcinoma in situ (DCIS).

The Breast Cancer Risk Assessment tool has validity for estimating risk in African American women.[19] It represents one of the easiest, least expensive, and enduring ways to assess objectively those women who are at greatest risk of developing breast cancer. The tool and model is only appropriate for breast cancer risk estimation in high-risk women who do not present with genetic susceptibility genes.

The 5-year risk has been the standard used for decision-making about chemoprevention because the National Cancer Institute (NCI) breast cancer risk assessment tool, which reports a 5-year risk for invasive breast cancer, was the basis for enrollment onto the two major US prevention trials and forms the basis of the US

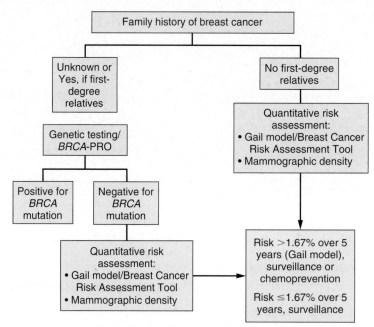

• **Fig. 16.1** Algorithm for clinical management of breast cancer risk.

Food and Drug Administration (FDA) indication for both tamoxifen and raloxifene. The US Preventive Services Task Force (USPSTF) guidelines (discussed later in the chapter) state that, for women with a 5-year risk 3% or greater, and using models such as the NCI breast cancer risk assessment tool, a provider should discuss the use of selective estrogen receptor (ER) modulators (SERMs) for primary prevention. Published estimates show that 27% of women with proliferative benign breast disease have an estimated 5-year risk 3% or greater.

Mammographic Density

The extent of hormonally active and proliferative breast tissue is positively associated with increased breast cancer risk. Women with dense tissue in at least 75% of their breasts have a risk of breast cancer four to six times as high as women with low or normal breast densities. The associations between mammographic density and both DCIS and invasive breast cancer are similar in magnitude.[20]

Mammographic density is also associated with an increased risk of ER- and progesterone receptor–positive tumors, which suggests a hormonal etiology for mammographic density. A model that incorporates breast density calculates both the 5- and 10-year risk for breast cancer.[21] Mammographic density may reflect high levels of circulating sex hormones or sensitivity to hormones but has a stronger predictive association with breast cancer than serum hormone levels alone. Indeed, endogenous sex hormone levels are strongly and independently related to the risk of breast cancer in postmenopausal women.[22] Measurement of sex hormone levels has not gained wide acceptance, however, as a clinical risk assessment tool.

Clinical Risk Counseling

The major steps in risk assessment of breast cancer include (1) assessment of genetic susceptibility via genetic counseling and (2) quantitative risk assessment via the Gail model/Breast Cancer Risk Assessment tool and/or mammographic density analysis. These steps are outlined in Fig. 16.1. Women at lower risk of breast cancer qualify for routine surveillance, including annual mammography for women older than 40 years of age as well as annual clinical breast examinations and self-breast examinations starting at 20 years of age. High-risk women who have a 5-year risk of breast cancer of 1.67% according to the Gail model/Breast Cancer Risk Assessment tool may qualify for chemoprevention in addition to routine or enhanced surveillance. Those options are discussed in the following sections.

Chemoprevention

Three areas unique to the field of chemoprevention must be considered in all stages of the clinical evaluation of a new chemopreventive agent. First, the characteristics of the target population must be clearly defined. For breast cancer chemoprevention, the target is a group of healthy women who may have had a previous diagnosis of breast cancer or who may be known to have a condition that predisposes them to the development of breast cancer. Second, the frequency and severity of side effects of the chemopreventive agent should be acceptable to the individual and ethically justifiable in the target population. Third, the duration of use of the chemopreventive agent must be defined. For most preventable malignancies, this requires a sustained period of drug administration that may be lifelong.

Epidemiologic studies indicate that estrogen-mediated events are integral to the development of breast cancer[23–25] and support the hypothesis that intact ovarian function is required to develop breast cancer. Oophorectomy or radiation-induced ovarian ablation can reduce the incidence of breast cancer by up to 75%.[26] These observations suggest that estrogen antagonists may be instrumental in the primary prevention of breast cancer.

Freedman and colleagues[27] conducted a retrospective analysis that included data from the Study of Tamoxifen and Raloxifene (STAR) and Breast Cancer Prevention Trial (BCPT) trials described later in the chapter. They developed a benefit/risk index

5-year projected risk of IBC (%)	Tamoxifen vs. Placebo (with uterus)				Raloxifene vs. Placebo (with uterus)		
	50–59	60–69	70–79		50–59	60–69	70–79
1.5	−133	−310	−325		21	−11	−15
2.0	−105	−283	−298		43	11	7
2.5	−78	−255	−271		65	33	29
3.0	−51	−228	−244		86	55	51
3.5	−25	−202	−217		108	76	71
4.0	3	−175	−190		128	97	93
4.5	29	−148	−164		150	119	115
5.0	56	−121	−137		172	140	136
5.5	83	−95	−111		193	161	157
6.0	109	−69	−84		214	183	179
6.5	135	−42	−58		236	204	199
7.0	162	−15	−32		256	225	221

Strong evidence of benefits outweighing risks

Moderate evidence of benefits outweighing risks

Benefits do not outweigh risks

5-year projected risk of IBC is ≥1.67%

Using BCPT data and WHI baseline rates

Combining RR from BCPT and STAR using WHI baseline rates

• **Fig. 16.2** Benefit/risk indices for tamoxifen and raloxifene chemoprevention by level of 5-year projected risk for invasive breast cancer *(IBC)* for white non-Hispanic women with a uterus, by age group. *BCPT*, Breast Cancer Prevention Trial; *RR*, relative risk; *STAR*, Study of Tamoxifen and Raloxifene; *WHI*, Women's Health Initiative. (From Freedman AN, Costantino JP, Gail MH, et al. A benefit/risk assessment tool for breast cancer chemoprevention treatment. *J Clin Oncol.* 2011;29:2327-2333.)

to quantify both beneficial and adverse outcomes from chemoprevention with the SERMs tamoxifen or raloxifene. This index helps decide whether to initiate chemoprevention by comparing the benefits and risks of raloxifene versus tamoxifen. Risks and benefits of treatment with raloxifene or tamoxifen depend on age, race, breast cancer risk, and history of hysterectomy. The benefits and risks of raloxifene and tamoxifen are described in tables (Fig. 16.2) that can help identify groups of women for whom the benefits of chemoprevention outweigh the risks. The net benefit index is the expected number of life-threatening events (i.e., invasive breast cancer, hip fracture, endometrial cancer, stroke, and pulmonary embolism [PE]) and severe events (i.e., in situ breast cancer and deep vein thrombosis [DVT]) in 5 years with and without chemoprevention.

On the basis of these data, 9 million of the 65 million women aged 35 to 79 years in the United States with no history of breast cancer were eligible for tamoxifen chemoprevention based on inclusion criteria from the BCPT (described later in the chapter).[28,29] Of these 9 million women, approximately 2.4 million would have derived a net benefit from taking tamoxifen based on their 5-year risk of developing breast cancer. An estimated 58,000 cases of invasive breast cancer would develop over the ensuing 5 years in that population. On the basis of the 49% risk reduction associated with tamoxifen in the BCPT, if all 2.4 million women had taken tamoxifen, more than 24,000 cases of breast cancer may have been prevented.

Tamoxifen

As already noted, hormones, especially estrogens, have been linked historically to breast cancer,[30,31] with their role being attributed to their ability to stimulate cell proliferation. This cellular proliferation leads to the accumulation of random genetic errors that result in neoplastic transformation.[28] According to this concept, chemoprevention of breast cancer is targeted to reduce the rate of cell proliferation through administration of hormonal modulators. Tamoxifen, a triphenylethylene compound, was synthesized in 1966 as a potential fertility agent. Several mechanisms have been proposed regarding tamoxifen's ability to prevent or suppress breast carcinogenesis, including modulating the production of transforming growth factors (TGF-α and TGF-β) that regulate breast cancer cell proliferation; binding to cytoplasmic antiestrogenic binding sites, increasing intracellular drug levels; increasing sex hormone–binding globulin levels, which may decrease the availability of free estrogen for diffusion into tumor cells; increasing levels of natural killer cells; and decreasing circulating insulin-like growth factor-I levels, which may modify the hormonal regulation of breast cancer cell kinetics.[32–35]

Raloxifene

Raloxifene hydrochloride, like tamoxifen, is a SERM that has antiestrogenic effects on breast and endometrial tissue and estrogenic effects on bone, lipid metabolism, and blood clotting.[36] It is a benzothiophene with characteristics similar to but distinct from the triphenylethylene SERMs such as tamoxifen. In vivo studies demonstrated antitumor activity in carcinogen-induced tumors in rodents of a magnitude similar to that observed previously with tamoxifen. In vitro, raloxifene binds to both the alpha and beta subtypes of the ER (α and β, respectively).[37,38]

Chemoprevention Risk-Reduction Trials

Four prospective studies evaluating tamoxifen for reducing the risk of invasive breast cancer have been published: the National Surgical Adjuvant Breast and Bowel Project (NSABP) Breast Cancer Prevention Trial (BCPT, P-1),[28,29] the Royal Marsden Hospital (RMH) Tamoxifen Chemoprevention Trial,[39,40] the Italian Tamoxifen Prevention Study,[41–43] and the International Breast Intervention Study I (IBIS-I).[44,45] A summary of the results of these trials is shown in Table 16.1. Additional trials listed in the table evaluated raloxifene for the reduction of the risk of breast cancer in high-risk postmenopausal women. The findings from the largest of these studies in detail are reviewed in the following subsection. Data regarding arzoxifene and lasofoxifene are not reviewed because these SERMs have not been studied in large-scale, randomized, breast cancer risk-reduction clinical trials, and the agents are not approved by the FDA for this purpose.

Breast Cancer Prevention Trial

The BCPT, a randomized, placebo-controlled, double-blind clinical trial, was initiated in June 1992 by the collaboration of the NCI and the NSABP to evaluate whether tamoxifen reduced risk of invasive breast cancer in women at increased risk. It was the largest, prospective, controlled trial of tamoxifen's risks and benefits in a high-risk population. The primary aim of the trial was to evaluate the effectiveness of 20 mg/day of tamoxifen orally for 5 years in preventing the occurrence of invasive breast cancer in women at high risk. Secondary aims of the trial were to assess osteoporotic fractures and cardiovascular disease in women taking tamoxifen compared with those in the control group.

Between June 1992 and September 1997, 13,388 women deemed at high risk for developing breast cancer were enrolled in the trial. Women were chosen if they were at high risk of developing breast cancer within the next 5 years if they met the following criteria: were 60 years of age or older, were between 35 and 59 years of age with a 5-year predicted risk of breast cancer of at least 1.66% as indicated by the Gail model, or had a history of LCIS. These women were then randomized to receive either 20 mg/day of tamoxifen ($n = 6681$) or placebo ($n = 6707$) for a period of 5 years.

The trial was terminated early when an interim analysis showed that statistical significance had occurred in a number of end points. This decrease was evident only in ER-positive breast cancers, with no significant change seen in ER-negative tumors.

TABLE 16.1 Completed Breast Cancer Prevention Trials

	N	Recruitment Period	Treatment Groups and Daily Dose	Treatment Duration (Years)	Entry Criteria	Median Follow-Up (Months)
NSABP BCPT	13,205	1992–1997	Placebo (6707) Tamoxifen 20 mg (6681)	5	>1%–6% 5-year risk	57.6
IBIS-I	7,109	1992–2001	Placebo (3566) Tamoxifen 20 mg (3573)	5	>2 times relative risk	96.0
Italian	5,408	1992–1997	Placebo (2708) Tamoxifen 20 mg (2700)	5	Normal risk, women with hysterectomy	139.6
Marsden	2,471	1986–1996	Placebo (1233) Tamoxifen 20 mg (1238)	5-S	High risk, family history	171.6
MORE/CORE	7,705/6,511	1994–1998/ 1998–2002	Placebo (2576) Raloxifene 60 mg (2557)/ Placebo (2576) Raloxifene 120 mg (2572)	4/8	Normal risk, postmenopausal women with osteoporosis	71.3
RUTH	10,101	1998–2000	Placebo (5057) Raloxifene 60 mg (5044)	5	Normal risk, postmenopausal women with established or risk of coronary heart disease	66.7
STAR	19,490	1999–2004	Raloxifene 60 mg (9875) Tamoxifen 20 mg (9872)	5	>16% 5-year risk, postmenopausal women	81.0
GENERATIONS	9,354	2004–2009	Placebo (4678) Arzoxifene 20 mg (4676)	4	Normal-risk, postmenopausal with low bone density or osteoporosis	54.3
PEARL	8,856	2001–2007	Placebo (2852) Lasofoxifene 0–50 mg (2852) Lasofoxifene 0–25 mg (2852)	5	Normal-risk, postmenopausal women with osteoporosis	59.6

Data from Cuzick J, Sestak I, Bonanni B, et al. SERM Chemoprevention of Breast Cancer Overview Group. Selective oestrogen receptor modulators in prevention of breast cancer: an updated meta-analysis of individual participant data. *Lancet*. 2013;381:1827-1834.

The median follow-up time at the end point was 48 months, at which time a 49% ($p < .00001$) decreased risk of invasive breast cancer in the total study population was documented, with the greatest benefit seen in women 60 years of age and older. Overall, a total of 264 invasive cases were documented in a total of 13,175 women with measurable end points at the time of the interim analysis. Of the 264 cases, 175 cases occurred in the placebo group, compared with 89 cases in the tamoxifen group, a 49% reduction in the incidence of invasive breast cancer.

Other Outcomes in the Breast Cancer Prevention Trial

Secondary outcomes in the BCPT included osteoporotic fractures and cardiovascular events. Tamoxifen is known to have estrogen agonist–like effects on both mineral density and serum cholesterol levels in postmenopausal women.[46,47] During the BCPT, women in the tamoxifen group had a 19% reduction in hip, spine, and distal radius fractures. Thirty-four of the women enrolled in the trial experienced a hip fracture; when the tamoxifen versus the placebo group were compared, there was a 45% reduction, which failed to reach statistical significance because of the small number of events that occurred. The incidence of cardiovascular events (namely, stroke and transient ischemic attack) revealed no statistically significant difference between the tamoxifen and placebo group likely because only 30% of women in the trial were aged 60 years or older.

Few clinically significant differences in quality-of-life outcomes were seen when comparing the tamoxifen and placebo groups, and tamoxifen was not associated with an increased risk of developing depressive symptoms in the BCPT.[48,49]

Other Unfavorable Outcomes in the Breast Cancer Prevention Trial

Adverse outcomes related to tamoxifen in the BCPT included PE, DVT, endometrial carcinoma, cataracts, and vasomotor symptoms.[50] These outcomes were significantly higher in women older than 50 years of age compared with their younger counterparts. Women on tamoxifen were found to have a statistically significant higher incidence of PE than those on placebo. Although incidences of DVT, stroke, and transient ischemic attack in these women were not statistically significant, incidence in women on tamoxifen was higher.

Women in the tamoxifen arm of the trial were found to have a 2.5 times greater risk of developing invasive endometrial carcinoma than women in the placebo arm, with an annual incidence of 2.3 per 1000 in the tamoxifen arm and 0.9 per 1000 in the placebo arm. This increased risk was greater in postmenopausal women. All cases of endometrial carcinoma that occurred in the BCPT were International Federation of Gynecology and Obstetrics (FIGO) stages 0 or I and had excellent clinical prognoses with treatment. A marginal increase of 14% in the development of cataracts was seen in women who were free of cataracts at initiation of the trial. The number of cataract surgeries was also increased in women taking tamoxifen. Vasomotor symptoms, mainly hot flashes, were reported by 46% of women on tamoxifen and only 29% of women in the placebo arm, whereas an increase in vaginal discharge was reported in 29% of women taking tamoxifen and 13% of women taking placebo.

After 7 years of follow-up in the BCPT,[29] the cumulative rate of invasive breast cancer was reduced from 42.5 per 1000 in the placebo group to 24.8 per 1000 in the tamoxifen group, a 43% reduction in risk, and the cumulative rate of noninvasive breast cancer was reduced from 15.8 per 1000 in the placebo group to 10.2 per 1000 in the tamoxifen group (37% reduction) (Fig. 16.3). Tamoxifen continued to reduce the occurrence of ER-positive tumors by 69%, but no difference was seen in the occurrence of ER-negative tumors. Also after 7 years, risks of PE were approximately 11% lower than in the original report, and risks of endometrial cancer were about 29% higher, but these differences were not statistically significant. The net benefit achieved with tamoxifen varied according to age, race, and level of breast cancer risk. Despite the potential bias caused by the unblinding of the P-1 trial and subsequent crossover between the treatment groups, the magnitudes of all beneficial and undesirable treatment effects of tamoxifen were similar to those initially reported, with notable reductions in breast cancer and increased risks of thromboembolic events and endometrial cancer. The incidence of all osteoporotic fractures was reduced by 19% in women taking tamoxifen compared with those in the placebo group. There was a 45% reduction in fractures of the hip that missed reaching statistical significance because of the small number of events reported.

In summary, the BCPT found that tamoxifen greatly reduced the incidence of ER-positive invasive and noninvasive breast

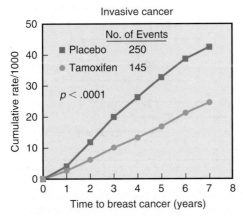
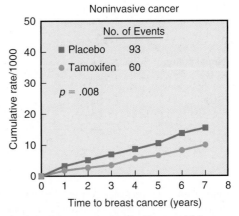

• **Fig. 16.3** Cumulative rates of invasive and noninvasive breast cancer events after 7 years of follow-up in the National Surgical Adjuvant Breast and Bowel Project Breast Cancer Prevention Trial. (From Fisher B, Costantino JP, Wickerham DL, et al. Tamoxifen for the prevention of breast cancer: current status of the National Surgical Adjuvant Breast and Bowel Project P-1 Study. *J Natl Cancer Inst.* 2005;97: 1652-1662.)

cancers compared with placebo over the 84-month follow-up time.

International Breast Cancer Intervention Study I

The IBIS-I trial, a randomized, placebo-controlled study, with design and outcomes similar to that of BCPT, was initiated to evaluate whether tamoxifen reduced the risk of invasive breast cancer in women at increased risk.[44,45] The primary aim of the trial was to evaluate the effectiveness of 20 mg/day of tamoxifen given for 5 years in preventing the occurrence of both invasive and in situ breast cancer in women deemed at high risk compared with placebo.

More than 7000 women 35 to 70 years of age evaluated as high risk for development of breast cancer (invasive or in situ) were enrolled into the trial and randomly assigned to either the tamoxifen or placebo for 5 years. Selection criteria for the trial's high-risk patients required that women 45 to 70 years of age have

at least a twofold relative risk, women 40 to 44 years of age at least a fourfold relative risk, and women 35 to 39 years of age at least a tenfold relative risk of developing breast cancer.[51] Risk factors involved in determining the relative risk of breast cancer development included family history, history of LCIS, history of atypical hyperplasia, benign breast biopsies, and nulliparity. Unlike the BCPT, and like the Italian trial discussed subsequently, women in this trial were permitted use of postmenopausal hormone replacement therapy (HRT), with approximately 40% of women using HRT at some time during the trial. On the basis of the published model, women in this trial were at moderately increased risk of development of breast cancer (Fig. 16.4).

Analysis with a median follow-up of 96 months after randomization in IBIS-I revealed a total of 337 cases of breast cancer that had been diagnosed, 142 breast cancers were diagnosed in the tamoxifen group and 195 in the placebo group, a 42% reduction in risk.[45] The risk-reducing effect of tamoxifen was constant for

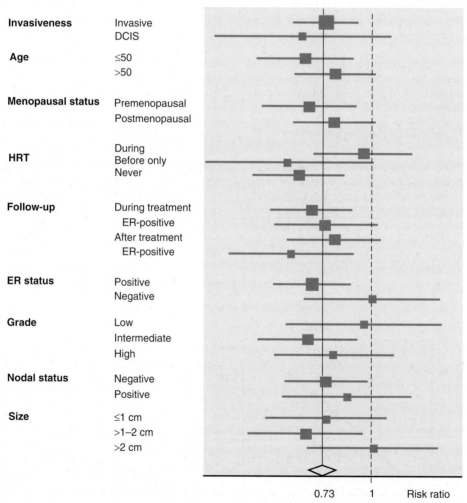

• **Fig. 16.4** Point estimates and 95% confidence intervals for various subgroup outcomes within the International Breast Cancer Intervention Study I trial. Numbers on the left of the vertical dashed line show reduction in the event rate with tamoxifen compared with placebo. The vertical solid line indicates the overall risk ratio of 0.73 for all subsets combined in the entire trial. *DCIS,* Ductal carcinoma in situ; *ER,* estrogen receptor; *HRT,* hormone replacement therapy. (From Cuzick J, Forbes JF, Sestak I, et al. Long-term results of tamoxifen prophylaxis for breast cancer: 96-month follow-up of the randomized IBIS-I trial. *J Natl Cancer Inst.* 2007;99:272–282.)

the entire follow-up period, and no lessening of benefit was observed for up to 10 years after randomization. There was a statistically insignificant interaction between HRT use and treatment with tamoxifen in women in IBIS-I. In women who never used HRT or who used it only before the trial, there was a statistically significant reduction in ER-positive breast cancers in the tamoxifen group compared with the placebo group (a 38% reduction for all breast cancers). For women who used HRT during any point of the trial, no clear benefit of tamoxifen was seen in reducing the risk of breast cancer, either overall (66 vs. 69 cases, relative risk [RR] = 0.92, 95% confidence interval [CI] = 0–1.31) or for ER-positive tumors (40 vs. 43 cases, RR = 0.89, 95% CI = 0.57–1.41). Results were similar regardless of the HRT preparations used (i.e., either estrogen only or combined estrogen and progestin). HRT use was not associated with the development of ER-negative breast cancers, either during the active treatment period or during subsequent follow-up. The risk reduction observed may be smaller that that seen in the BCPT both because patients enrolled onto IBIS-I were allowed to take HRT during the trial and because few women in IBIS-I had atypical hyperplasia, whereas a large reduction in incidence of invasive breast cancer was seen in BCPT.

As in the BCPT trial, adverse outcomes in the tamoxifen arm in the IBIS-I included an increase in thromboembolic events, a marginal increase in risk of endometrial cancer, and an overall increase in risk of death from all causes. The overall risk of clotting events was increased in tamoxifen users, with a 2.5-fold increase in risk of venous thromboembolism. As with the BCPT, this risk was seen predominately in women older than 50 years of age and in those women with a recent history of surgery. There was a marginal, nonstatistically significant increase in the risk of endometrial cancer in women taking tamoxifen, especially in women aged 50 years and older. As observed in the BCPT, all cases of endometrial cancer diagnosed were FIGO stages 0 or I.

Active treatment was discontinued after 5 years. After a median follow-up that extended to 16 years, breast cancers were diagnosed 7.0% of the women in the tamoxifen group versus 9.8% of 3575 women in the placebo group of IBIS-I, an enduring 30% reduction in the risk of all breast cancer.[52] The risk of developing breast cancer was similar between years 0 to 10 and after 10 years. The greatest reduction in risk was seen in invasive ER-positive breast cancer (34%) and DCIS (35%), but no effect was noted for invasive ER-negative breast cancer. These results indicate that tamoxifen offers a long period of protection after treatment cessation and substantially improves the benefit-to-harm ratio of the drug for breast cancer prevention.

Summary of the SERM Chemoprevention Trials

Additional clinical trials that had experimental designs similar to those trials reviewed earlier are summarized in Table 16.2. It should be noted that in the Italian Tamoxifen Prevention Trial, women were eligible for the trial if they were between ages 35 and 70 years and had undergone hysterectomy for benign disease because of the associated risk of endometrial cancer in patients taking tamoxifen. Women in the trial were not required to undergo standard breast cancer risk assessment. Thus some of the participants in the trial were at decreased risk for developing breast cancer at randomization because they had had previous oophorectomy (48.3%) before menopause. Concomitant use of HRT was also permitted. Accrual to the trial was

ended prematurely because of a 26.3% dropout rate for women already randomized secondary to side effects, decreased interest, and fear.

In 2013 a summary of the trials using tamoxifen for breast cancer risk reduction was published by Cuzick and colleagues,[53] and the trials were compared. The investigators performed a meta-analysis with individual participant data from nine prevention trials comparing four SERMs: tamoxifen,[28,29,44,45] raloxifene,[54,55] arzoxifene,[56,57] and lasofoxifene[58,59] with placebo, or, in one study, with tamoxifen. The primary end point was incidence of all breast cancer (including DCIS) during a 10-year follow-up period. Analysis was by intention to treat. There were 83,399 women with 306,617 women-years of follow-up in the trials analyzed. Median follow-up was 65 months. Overall, a 38% reduction in breast cancer incidence, and 42 women would need to be treated to prevent one breast cancer event in the first 10 years of follow-up. The reduction was larger in the first 5 years of follow-up than in years 5 to 10 (42% vs. 25%), but there was no heterogeneity between time periods. Thromboembolic events were significantly increased with all SERMs (odds ratio 1.73, 73%). There was a significant reduction of 34% in vertebral fractures, but only a small effect for nonvertebral fractures (an approximately 7% reduction). Thus for all SERMs, incidence of invasive ER-positive breast cancer was reduced both during treatment and for at least 5 years after completion. Similar to other preventive interventions, careful consideration of risks and benefits is needed to identify women who are most likely to benefit from these drugs.

Tamoxifen and Benign Breast Disease

The incidence of benign breast disease and number of breast biopsies in women taking tamoxifen versus placebo is reduced about 25%,[60] and women taking tamoxifen experience a reduction in risk of benign breast disease of nearly 30% and require fewer breast biopsies. Breast pain is decreased by one-third in women taking tamoxifen. These benefits in decreasing benign breast disease are noted predominately in premenopausal women younger than 50 years of age.

SERMs in Lobular Carcinoma in Situ and Atypical Hyperplasia

Women with a history of LCIS experienced an annual risk of invasive breast cancer of 1.3% per year while assigned to placebo in the BCPT, and tamoxifen reduced this risk by approximately 55%.[28] Women with atypical ductal or lobular hyperplasia experience an increased risk of subsequent invasive breast cancer, and tamoxifen reduced this risk by 86% in BCPT. Women with either LCIS or atypical hyperplasia should therefore be considered candidates for primary reduction of breast cancer risk with tamoxifen if there are no absolute contraindications to its use.

There are two types of atypical hyperplasia, as classified on the basis of microscopic appearance: atypical ductal hyperplasia and atypical lobular hyperplasia. Atypical hyperplasia confers a relative risk of 4.0 and an absolute risk of approximately 1% per year for developing future invasive breast cancer. These risk statistics have been recognized for decades, and the absolute risk among women with atypical hyperplasia has been shown to approach 30% at 25 years of follow-up.[61] The risk of developing

TABLE 16.2 Breast Cancer Incidence in the Chemoprevention Trials

	Overall (Invasive and DCIS)	Annual Rates Per 1000 in Control Group	HR (95% CI) (Tamoxifen vs. Placebo)	ER-Positive Invasive	HR (95% CI)	ER-Negative Invasive	HR (95% CI)	DCIS	HR (95% CI)
Tamoxifen Trials									
Marsden	96 vs. 114	6.4	0.87 (0.63–1.21)	51 vs. 83	0.66 (0.44–0.99)	25 vs. 17	1.66 (0.81–3.40)	14 vs. 9	1.40 (0.44–4.40)
IBIS-I	143 vs. 198	6.7	0.72 (0.58–0.90)	88 vs. 131	0.69 (0.52–0.90)	36 vs. 38	0.97 (0.62–1.54)	16 vs. 27	0.52 (0.27–0.99)
NSABP-P-1	130 vs. 248	6.1	0.52 (0.42–0.64)	44 vs. 134	0.33 (0.23–0.46)	39 vs. 31	1.26 (0.78–2.02)	38 vs. 70	0.54 (0.36–0.80)
Italian	62 vs. 74	4.2	0.83 (0.58–1.19)	36 vs. 48	0.73 (0.45–1.17)	16 vs. 17	0.87 (0.43–1.79)	9 vs. 6	1.80 (0.60–5.38)
Total (0–10 years)	431 vs. 634		0.67 (0.59–0.76)	219 vs. 396	0.56 (0.47–0.67)	116 vs. 103	1.13 (0.86–1.49)	77 vs. 112	0.72 (0.57–0.92)
Total (0–5 years)	256 vs. 409			121 vs. 235	0.62 (0.53–0.73)	78 vs. 76	0.51 (0.41–0.64)	47 vs. 83	1.03 (0.75–1.41)
Total (5–10 years)	175 vs. 225			98 vs. 161	0.78 (0.62–0.97)	38 vs. 27	0.63 (0.47–0.83)	30 vs. 29	1.55 (0.88–2.72)
Raloxifene Trials									
MORE/CORE	57 vs. 65	4.2	0.42 (0.29–0.60)	22 vs. 44	0.24 (0.15–0.40)	15 vs. 7	1.06 (0.43–2.59)	13 vs. 7	0.91 (0.36–2.28)
RUTH	52 vs. 76	4.2	0.67 (0.47–0.96)	25 vs. 55	0.45 (0.28–0.72)	13 vs. 9	1.44 (0.61–3.63)	11 vs. 5	1.7 (0.75–6.25)
STAR (tamoxifen vs. raloxifene)	358 vs. 447	5.9	0.81 (0.70–0.93)	182 vs. 221	0.83 (0.69–1.02)	60 vs. 70	0.79 (0.56–1.11)	111 vs. 137	0.82 (0.64–1.05)
Total (0–10 years)	467 vs. 588		0.66 (0.55–0.80)	229 vs. 320	0.44 (0.34–0.58)	88 vs. 93	1.37 (0.96–1.95)	135 vs. 149	1.07 (0.68–1.68)
Total (0–5 years)	327 vs. 421		0.63 (0.51–0.79)	168 vs. 224	0.40 (0.29–0.56)	62 vs. 71	1.27 (0.83–1.95)	86 vs. 108	1.08 (0.60–1.96)
Total (5–10 years)	140 vs. 167		0.84 (0.51–1.27)	61 vs. 96	0.72 (0.49–1.06)	26 vs. 22	1.70 (0.84–3.47)	49 vs. 41	0.88 (0.45–1.74)
Pearl[a]									
0.25 mg	20 vs. 24	2.0	0.82 (0.45–1.49)	9 vs. 18	0.49 (0.22–1.10)	7 vs. 2	2.83 (0.57–14.02)	4 vs. 4	0.99 (0.25–3.99)
0.5 mg	5 vs. 24	2.0	0.21 (0.08–0.55)	3 vs. 18	0.17 (0.05–0.56)	0 vs. 2		3 vs. 4	0.50 (0.09–2.73)

All Trials[b]

	Annual Rates Per 1000	Overall	HR (95% CI)	ER-Positive Invasive	HR (95% CI)	ER-Negative Invasive	HR (95% CI)	DCIS	HR (95% CI)
Total (0–10 years)	4.7	587 vs. 852	0.62 (0.56–0.69) / 0.61 (0.49–0.75)	287 vs. 543	0.49 (0.42–0.57) / 0.44 (0.33–0.60)	160 vs. 131	1.14 (0.90–1.45) / 1.14 (0.90–1.45)	110 vs. 138	0.69 (0.53–0.90) / 0.79 (0.53–1.19)
Total (0–5 years)	4.6	376 vs. 594	0.58 (0.51–0.66) / 0.58 (0.47–0.73)	174 vs. 360	0.45 (0.38–0.54) / 0.42 (0.29–0.61)	111 vs. 90	1.05 (0.80–1.39) / 1.05 (0.80–1.39)	73 vs. 107	0.66 (0.48–0.90) / 0.73 (0.47–1.14)
Total (5–10 years)	4.9	211 vs. 258	0.75 (0.61–0.93) / 0.75 (0.59–0.94)	113 vs. 183	0.58 (0.45–0.76) / 0.58 (0.45–0.76)	49 vs. 32	1.66 (0.98–2.81) / 1.66 (0.98–2.81)	37 vs. 31	0.94 (0.53–1.66) / 0.94 (0.53–1.66)

CI, Confidence interval; DCIS, ductal carcinoma in situ; ER, estrogen receptor; HR, hazard ratio.

[a]PEARL trial was a randomized comparison of 2 different doses of lasofoxifene vs. placebo.

[b]Upper value is fixed effect; lower value is random effect.

Data from Cuzick J, Sestak I, Bonanni B, et al: SERM Chemoprevention of Breast Cancer Overview Group. Selective oestrogen receptor modulators in prevention of breast cancer: an updated meta-analysis of individual participant data. Lancet. 2013;381:1827-1834.

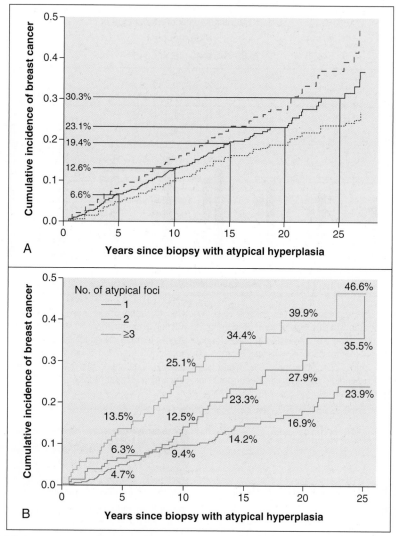

• **Fig. 16.5** Cumulative incidence of breast cancer after a diagnosis of atypical hyperplasia. (A) Shows the cumulative incidence of breast cancer (invasive and ductal carcinoma in situ) after a diagnosis of atypical hyperplasia in the Mayo Clinic cohort (dashed lines in [A] denote 95% confidence intervals). (B) Shows the same cohort stratified according to the number of foci of atypical hyperplasia. (From Hartmann LC, Degnim AC, Santen RJ, et al. Atypical hyperplasia of the breast—risk assessment and management options. *N Engl J Med.* 2015;372:78-89.)

invasive disease after a diagnosis of atypia is inversely related to the age at diagnosis, directly related to the number of atypical foci seen on the biopsy, and appears to be slightly higher with atypical lobular compared with atypical ductal hyperplasia.[62] Atypical hyperplasia is found in approximately 10% of biopsies with benign findings. In atypical hyperplasia, there is a proliferation of dysplastic, monotonous epithelial cell populations that include clonal subpopulations. In models of breast carcinogenesis, atypical hyperplasia occupies a transitional zone between benign and malignant disease because it contains some of, but not all, the requisite features of a cancer and is thus considered to be premalignant.[62–64]

The younger a woman is when she receives a diagnosis of atypical hyperplasia, the more likely it is that breast cancer will develop. The effect of a family history of breast cancer on the breast cancer risk among women with atypical hyperplasia is not clear. Initial reports described a relative risk of breast cancer of approximately 9, compared with a relative risk of 3.5 among women with

atypical hyperplasia but no family history[64]; subsequent data showed no significant difference in risk according to family history among women with atypical hyperplasia.[61]

Overall Risk of Developing Invasive Breast Cancer in Women With Atypical Hyperplasia

In studies with long-term follow-up, atypical hyperplasia has been shown to confer high relative risks for future breast cancer (Fig. 16.5) A longitudinal cohort study described breast cancer risk associated with atypical hyperplasia and was reported in 1985.[65,66] In that study, women with atypical hyperplasia had a relative risk for a later invasive breast cancer of 4.4. Updated information provided confirmation of this absolute risk estimating a 1% to 2% per year risk of developing invasive breast cancer in women with a biopsy showing AH.[67,68] Other investigators have since shown consistently that the relative risk associated with both

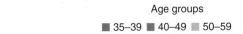

Net benefit or risk from tamoxifen for prevention of breast cancer by 5-year age groups and 5-year quantitative risk of breast cancer (%)

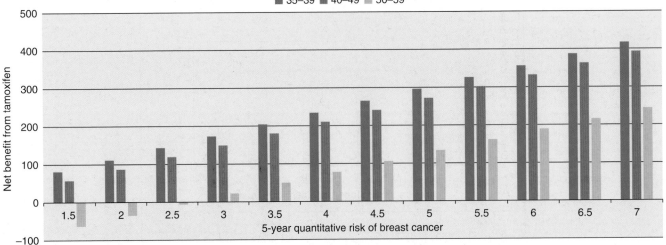

• **Fig. 16.6** Bars represent the net benefit from tamoxifen for each 5-year risk of developing invasive breast cancer among three age groups of women. All women younger than 50 years of age derive net benefit from tamoxifen (i.e., reduction in breast cancer events minus side effect events including thromboses and endometrial cancer), whereas women 50 years and older derive net benefit only when the 5-year risk of breast cancer exceeds 3%. (Data from Gail MH, Costantino JP, Bryant J, et al. Weighing the risks and benefits of tamoxifen treatment for preventing breast cancer. *J Natl Cancer Inst.* 1999;91:1829–1846.)

atypical ductal hyperplasia and atypical lobular hyperplasia is approximately 4.0.[69,70]

Assessing Risks and Benefits of Tamoxifen for Chemoprevention

Breast cancer is the most frequently diagnosed cancer worldwide, highlighting the need and potential global impact of effective breast cancer risk-reduction strategies. Recommendations for chemoprevention are relevant to women without a personal history of breast cancer who are at increased risk of developing the disease. Once women are classified in terms of their risk of breast cancer using quantitative risk modeling, high-risk women should be assessed further to determine their individual specific risk-benefit profile. A woman's risk can change over time, and it is important to revisit risk assessment at multiple stages of a woman's life. Tamoxifen has positive net benefit in women younger than 50 years of age with elevated risk of both invasive and in situ breast cancer (Fig. 16.6). Women older than 70 years of age have adverse events associated with tamoxifen use regardless of race or ethnicity.[71]

Indications and Contraindications for Risk Reduction With SERMs

Women for whom SERMs should be considered for reducing the incidence of invasive breast cancer are listed in Box 16.1. These include history of DCIS or LCIS, history of atypical ductal or lobular hyperplasia, history of *BRCA1* or *BRCA2* mutation who do not elect prophylactic mastectomy (discussed subsequently), or a 5-year predicted risk of invasive breast cancer of

| • BOX 16.1 | Women in Whom Selective Estrogen Receptor Modulators Should Be Considered for Reducing the Incidence of Invasive Breast Cancer |

Women with a history of one of the following:
- Lobular carcinoma in situ
- Ductal carcinoma in situ
- Atypical ductal or lobular hyperplasia

Premenopausal women with mutations in either the *BRCA1* or *BRCA2* genes
Premenopausal women at least 35 years of age with 5-year probability of breast cancer of 1.66%
Women aged 60 years with Gail model 5-year probability of breast cancer of 5%

1.66% or more. Tamoxifen is also indicated as adjuvant therapy in ER-positive breast cancer to prevent contralateral breast cancer.

Absolute contraindications for tamoxifen use include a history of DVT or PE as well as concurrent warfarin therapy. Relative contraindications include history of transient ischemic attack or stroke, poorly controlled diabetes, hypertension, or atrial fibrillation, immobility, mitral valve disease, and ischemic heart disease. Postmenopausal women are at increased risk for adverse events; thus alternate therapy with an agent such as raloxifene should be considered. Women taking oral contraceptives, estrogen, progesterone, or androgens should discontinue these before initiation of tamoxifen therapy. Women should be advised against becoming pregnant while on tamoxifen because the drug has a class D pregnancy recommendation and has been associated with birth defects in rats.

The optimal duration of risk-reducing therapy is unknown, but adjuvant therapy studies with tamoxifen indicate that therapy of less than 5 years is not as effective in reducing the incidence of second contralateral invasive breast cancer as therapy for at least 5 years. In addition, adjuvant treatment of invasive breast cancer with tamoxifen for 10 years is more effective that only 5 years of therapy.[72,73] Whether using tamoxifen for longer than 5 years is more effective in preventing the recurrence of breast cancer than using it for only 5 years is not known; no trials are currently being conducted or planned to examine the ideal duration of therapy in the risk-reduction setting. The optimal age at which to start therapy is unknown. Acceptance of tamoxifen may be poor in eligible subjects who elect prophylactic surgery instead of a chemopreventive risk-reduction strategy. Toxicity is a concern in postmenopausal women.

Effect of Tamoxifen in Carriers of Predisposing Genetic Mutations

Consideration of familial history of breast cancer is an integral component in assessing a patient's lifetime risk of breast cancer. Specific genetic mutations markedly increase the likelihood of breast cancer incidence over the life span. Well-characterized breast cancer susceptibility genes, including *BRCA1* and *BRCA2,* are found in more than 2% of breast cancer cases.[74] Among cases, 2.4% and 2.3% carry deleterious mutations in *BRCA1* and *BRCA2,* respectively. *BRCA1* mutations are significantly more common in white (2.9%) versus black (1.4%) cases and in Jewish (10.2%) versus non-Jewish (2.0%) cases; *BRCA2* mutations are slightly more frequent in black (2.6%) versus white (2.1%) cases. *BRCA1* acts, in part, as a tumor suppressor gene. Reduction in *BRCA1* expression in vitro results in the accelerated growth of breast and ovarian cell lines, whereas overexpression of *BRCA1* results in inhibited growth. *BRCA1* also serves as a substrate for certain cyclin-dependent kinases, and estradiol induces *BRCA1* through an increase in DNA synthesis, which suggests that *BRCA1* may serve as a negative modulator of estradiol-induced growth.[75,76] The cumulative lifetime risk of developing breast cancer can exceed 50% for some carriers of *BRCA* mutations, as estimated by the number of relatives with breast cancer diagnosed before 50 years of age.

Although carriers of *BRCA1* mutations are more likely to develop ER-negative tumors,[77,78] prophylactic oophorectomy reduces the risk of breast cancer by approximately 30% in women who carry mutations in either the *BRCA1* or *BRCA2* gene.[79] More importantly, Narod and colleagues[80,81] compared women with bilateral breast cancer and *BRCA1* or *BRCA2* mutations (bilateral disease cases) with women with unilateral disease and *BRCA1* or *BRCA2* mutations (controls). The reduction in contralateral breast cancer associated with tamoxifen use is approximately 50%. Tamoxifen protected against contralateral breast cancer for carriers of *BRCA1* mutations (35%–60% reduction) and for those with *BRCA2* mutations.[82] The greater apparent benefit of tamoxifen in carriers of *BRCA1* mutations compared with carriers of *BRCA2* mutations is paradoxical given the greater prevalence of ER-positive breast cancer reported in carriers of *BRCA2* mutations. This observation needs to be validated in additional studies.

Women who used tamoxifen for 2 to 4 years had a 75% lowered risk of contralateral breast cancer. The effectiveness of tamoxifen in preventing contralateral, second breast cancers is related to the high concordance of the ER status of the first and second cancers.[83] Other data suggest a 50% reduction in the risk of contralateral, second primary breast tumors in carriers of *BRCA1* mutations who take tamoxifen after a first breast cancer and a 58% reduction of second cancers in *BRCA2* mutation carriers. These results imply that in mutation carriers who develop breast cancer, secondary breast cancers can be prevented using tamoxifen; similar risk reductions are thus likely to be seen for primary breast cancers. However, it remains unclear whether tamoxifen has the greatest efficacy in *BRCA1* or *BRCA2* carriers.

The only prospective evaluation of the effect of tamoxifen in carriers of predisposing mutations was carried out in the BCPT.[84] To evaluate the effect of tamoxifen on the incidence of breast cancer in women with inherited *BRCA1* or *BRCA2* mutations, genomic analysis of *BRCA1* and *BRCA2* was performed in 288 women who developed breast cancer after entry into the trial. Of the 288 cases of breast cancers, 19 (6.6%) inherited disease-predisposing *BRCA1* or *BRCA2* mutations. Of eight patients with *BRCA1* mutations, five received tamoxifen and three received placebo (showing no evidence of primary risk reduction). Of 11 patients with *BRCA2* mutations, however, three received tamoxifen and eight received placebo, a 62% reduction in the incidence of primary breast cancer.

In the BCPT, therefore, tamoxifen reduced the incidence of breast cancer in healthy *BRCA2* carriers, similar to the reduction in incidence of ER-positive breast cancer in all women in the trial. In contrast, tamoxifen use did not reduce breast cancer incidence in healthy women with inherited *BRCA1* mutations. These results must be interpreted with caution, however, because of the small number of women with mutations of either *BRCA1* or *BRCA2* who were identified in the trial. Larger prospective studies of women with predisposing mutations are required to provide conclusive evidence of either protection or lack of effect by tamoxifen in women with these mutations.

Using a simulated cohort of 30-year-old women who tested positive for either *BRCA1* or *BRCA2* mutations, Grann and coworkers[85] estimated that a 30-year-old woman with a mutation of either gene could prolong her survival by undergoing a bilateral oophorectomy and/or bilateral mastectomy, compared with surveillance alone. In their simulation model, chemoprevention with tamoxifen increased survival time by 1.6 years and yielded more quality-adjusted life-years than did prophylactic surgery, even when treatment was delayed until 40 or 50 years of age. All of these procedures were cost-effective or cost-saving procedures compared with surveillance alone. Others have calculated that, compared with surveillance alone, 30-year-old patients with early-stage breast cancer with *BRCA1* or *BRCA2* mutations gain 0.4 to 1.3 years of life expectancy from tamoxifen therapy, 0.2 to 1.8 years from prophylactic oophorectomy and 0.6 to 2.1 years from prophylactic mastectomy. The magnitude of these gains is least for women with low-penetrance mutations and greatest for those with high-penetrance mutations.[86]

Clinical Monitoring of Women Taking Tamoxifen

Endometrial hyperplasia and cancer were more frequent in women taking tamoxifen than in women taking placebo in the BCPT, but there was no evidence of elevated risk from tamoxifen use in women younger than 50 years of age. The utility of endometrial cancer screening with either endometrial biopsy or transvaginal ultrasound in asymptomatic tamoxifen-treated women is limited and is not recommended outside the setting of a clinical trial. Rather, women receiving tamoxifen should have annual cervical cytology and pelvic examinations. Any abnormal bleeding should be evaluated with appropriate diagnostic testing, and women should be counseled about the risk of benign and malignant conditions associated with tamoxifen.

Routine screening with complete blood counts or chemical blood tests is not indicated because no hematologic or hepatic toxicities attributable to tamoxifen were demonstrated in the BCPT or in clinical trials using tamoxifen as adjuvant therapy. Because of the modest increase in risk of cataracts (RR = 1.14) and cataract surgery in women using tamoxifen compared with women taking placebo, women taking tamoxifen should be questioned about symptoms of cataracts during follow-up and should discuss the value of periodic eye examinations with their health care provider.

Tamoxifen Metabolites

Tamoxifen can be considered a classic "prodrug," requiring metabolic activation to elicit pharmacologic activity. The cytochrome P450 (CYP) enzyme 2D6 is the rate-limiting step catalyzing the conversion of tamoxifen into metabolites with significantly greater affinity for the ER and greater ability to inhibit cell proliferation. Both genetic and pharmacologic factors that alter CYP2D6 enzyme activity directly affect the concentrations of the active tamoxifen metabolites and the outcomes of patients receiving adjuvant tamoxifen.[87]

Tamoxifen is hydroxylated by CYP2D6 to the potent metabolites 4-hydroxytamoxifen (4OH-tam) and 4-hydroxy-*N*-desmethyl tamoxifen (4OHNDtam), which are both conjugated by sulphotransferase (SULT)1A1. Clinical studies indicate that CYP2D6 and SULT1A1 genotypes are predictors for treatment response to tamoxifen. The levels of 4OHtam, 4OHNDtam, and *N*-desmethyl tamoxifen are associated with CYP2D6 predicted enzymatic activity ($p < .05$). The SULT1A1 genotype or copy number does not influence the levels of tamoxifen and its metabolites. However, the ratios of *N*-desmethyl tamoxifen/tamoxifen and *N*-dedimethyl tamoxifen/*N*-desmethyl tamoxifen are related to SULT1A1 genotype. CYP2D6 and SULT1A1 genotypes may partly explain the wide interindividual variations in the serum levels of tamoxifen and its metabolites. Use of therapeutic drug monitoring has not been included in studies linking CYP2D6 and SULT1A1 genotypes to clinical outcome.[88]

N-desmethyl tamoxifen, resulting from the *CYP3A4/5*-mediated catalysis of tamoxifen, is quantitatively the major primary metabolite of tamoxifen. Patients homozygous for a *CYP2D6* null allele have significantly lower endoxifen concentrations than patients with one or two *CYP2D6* functional alleles. The *CYP2D6* phenotypes associated with different alleles include poor, intermediate, extensive, and ultrarapid metabolizers.[89] For premenopausal women with breast cancer, there are published data regarding *CYP2D6* genotype and treatment outcomes. None of the published studies indicate a significant influence on treatment outcomes related to CYP2D6 genotype, and routine clinical testing for *CYP2D6* genotype is not required.[90–94]

Clinical caution is required, however, when administering tamoxifen to patients who are concurrently taking selective serotonin reuptake inhibitors that do have a negative effect on circulating concentrations of tamoxifen and its active metabolites.[95,96]

Clinical Data With Raloxifene

A number of clinical trials have been conducted to assess the benefit of the SERM raloxifene on osteoporosis and fracture.[97–100] After the publication of the BCPT, these osteoporosis trials reported data showing a reduced incidence of invasive breast cancer among women taking raloxifene compared with those taking placebo.

Study of Tamoxifen and Raloxifene Trial

The findings of the BCPT and IBIS-I, coupled with the observations from the studies of raloxifene in women with postmenopausal osteoporosis, led the NSABP to design and launch the STAR trial. Eligible women were at least 35 years of age and postmenopausal, and they must have had either LCIS or a 5-year risk of invasive breast cancer of at least 1.67% as determined by the Gail model. Subjects were randomly assigned to receive either tamoxifen 20 mg/day or raloxifene 60 mg/day in a double-blind, double-dummy design. No group of women in the trial received placebo alone.[54,55]

The primary aim of the trial was to evaluate the statistical equivalence of 20 mg/day of tamoxifen orally for over 5 years versus 60 mg/day of raloxifene in decreasing the incidence of breast cancer. Secondary aims were to assess the incidence of noninvasive breast cancer, endometrial cancer, skeletal fractures, and venous thromboembolic events in women on chemoprevention therapy. During 5 years of enrollment, more than 19,000 postmenopausal women (mean age, 58.5 years) with an increased risk of breast cancer were randomly assigned either to receive tamoxifen 20 mg/day or raloxifene 60 mg/day for a period of at least 5 years. Women were evaluated as having an increased risk of breast cancer by using criteria from the Gail model with a mean risk in those randomized equal to 4%.

After a median follow-up of 3.2 years, 331 cases of invasive breast cancer had been reported. Overall, there were 163 cases of invasive breast cancer in women in the tamoxifen arm (4.3 cases/1000 woman-years) compared with 168 cases in the raloxifene arm (4.41 cases/1000 woman-years; RR = 1.02; 95% CI = 0.82–1.28). After a total of 6 years of follow-up, incidence was 25.1 cases/1000 woman-years in the tamoxifen arm and 24.8/1000 woman-years in the raloxifene arm ($P = 0.83$). When subpopulations in the study groups were compared based on categories of age, history of LCIS, history of atypical hyperplasia, 5-year predicted risk of breast cancer, and the number of family members with a history of breast cancer, there was no difference in the incidence of invasive breast cancer between the treatment groups. There was also no difference in tumor size, nodal status, or ER level between compatible subgroups in the two treatment groups. In the tamoxifen arm of the trial, there were fewer incidences of both LCIS and DCIS over a 6-year follow-up. There was a total of 57 cases of noninvasive breast cancer in the tamoxifen arm compared with 80 cases in women on raloxifene (1.51 vs. 2.11 cases/1000 woman-years, respectively; RR = 1.40; 95% CI = 0.98–2).

STAR Results After 81 Months of Follow-Up

An updated analysis of the trial was published with 81 months of follow-up.[55] In contrast with the results in the original report, there was a significant difference between the treatment groups, with 310 cases of invasive breast cancer in the raloxifene group and 247 in the tamoxifen group. The risk of developing invasive breast cancer was 24% higher with raloxifene than with tamoxifen, and for noninvasive disease, it was 22% greater. Compared with initial results, the differences widened for invasive and narrowed for noninvasive breast cancer. Toxicity with raloxifene was 55% less for endometrial cancer compared with tamoxifen (this difference was not significant in the initial results), 81% less for uterine hyperplasia, and 25% less for thromboembolic events. There were no significant mortality differences. Long-term raloxifene retained 76% of the effectiveness of tamoxifen in preventing invasive disease and grew closer over time to tamoxifen in preventing noninvasive disease, with far less toxicity (e.g., highly significantly less endometrial cancer).

As demonstrated in the BCPT, compared with placebo, tamoxifen reduces the risk of invasive breast cancer by about 50%. On the basis of this information and the actual RR of 1.24 observed in the STAR trial, one can extrapolate that raloxifene is about 76% as effective as tamoxifen in reducing breast cancer risk. Then, compared with placebo, raloxifene would reduce the risk of invasive breast cancer by about 38% (50% × 76% = 38%), versus the 50% reduction seen with tamoxifen.

In the initial report of the STAR trial, the difference between treatment groups for the rate of noninvasive breast cancer was of borderline statistical significance. In the updated analysis, the difference between treatment groups for this event was less than originally seen. There were 137 cases in the raloxifene group compared with 111 in the tamoxifen group (22% greater). The difference between treatment groups in noninvasive breast cancer was limited to cases of pure DCIS or cases of mixed DCIS and LCIS. There was no difference between the groups for pure LCIS cases. In parallel with the analysis presented earlier for invasive breast cancer, tamoxifen was shown in the BCPT to reduce the risk of noninvasive breast cancer by about 50%. Therefore, if there were no noninvasive breast cancer risk-reduction effect of raloxifene, the expected rate of noninvasive breast cancer in the raloxifene group would be about twice the rate in the tamoxifen group, yielding an RR of 2 when comparing raloxifene to tamoxifen. On the basis of this information and the actual RR of 1.22 observed in the STAR trial, raloxifene is approximately 78% as effective as tamoxifen in reducing noninvasive breast cancer risk [{(2.00 − 1.22) / (2.00 − 1.00)} × 100 = 78%]. Then, compared with placebo, raloxifene reduces the risk of noninvasive breast cancer by about 39% (50% × 78% = 39%).

The incidence of invasive uterine cancer was significantly lower in the raloxifene group in the STAR trial. The annual average rate per 1000 was 2.25 in the tamoxifen group compared with 1.23 in the raloxifene group in the STAR trial. In the original report, the difference between treatment groups for the rate of invasive uterine cancer was not statistically significant. The average annual incidence rate of uterine hyperplasia, the majority of which was hyperplasia without atypia, was five times higher in the tamoxifen group (4.40 per 1000) than in the raloxifene group. The number of hysterectomies performed in the tamoxifen group (349), including those done for benign disease, was more than double that performed in the raloxifene group.

PE and DVT are other toxicities with a well-recognized association with tamoxifen treatment. The incidence of such events was significantly elevated in the tamoxifen group compared with the raloxifene group in the STAR trial. The average annual rates of thromboembolic events were 3.30 per 1000 (tamoxifen) and 2.47 per 1000, a 25% reduction.

STAR Trial and Potential Population Impact

Raloxifene proved as effective as tamoxifen in reducing the incidence of invasive breast cancer in younger, postmenopausal women at increased risk, with a reduced incidence of both endometrial cancers and thromboembolic events. However, raloxifene is less effective in reducing the incidence of in situ carcinoma compared with tamoxifen. Tamoxifen will prevent 20 invasive and 20 noninvasive breast cancers (based on the long-term data at an 81-month median follow-up—approximately 7 years) in 1000 women at the elevated 5-year risk of 4% (the average risk in STAR) versus causing 2.25 endometrial cancers (in women with an intact uterus at study entry) and 3.3 thromboembolic events in the same group of women over 7 years. Raloxifene will prevent 15 invasive and 16 noninvasive breast cancers over 7 years in 1000 women at an elevated risk (4%) versus causing 2.47 thromboembolic events and no endometrial cancers in the same group over 7 years. For these major effects, tamoxifen causes 40 beneficial versus 5.55 adverse effects (benefit/risk ratio of approximately 7:1) and raloxifene causes 31 beneficial versus 2.47 adverse effects (benefit/risk ratio of approximately 13:1) over 7 years.[101] These ratios indicate a large net gain for women at a 4% 5-year risk of breast cancer and would improve substantially for women at a 4% or higher risk, who number approximately 600,000 in the United States. Symptoms and quality-of-life measures reported by subjects in the STAR trial were similar among women taking tamoxifen compared with those taking raloxifene.[102]

Aromatase Inhibitors

Tamoxifen is not the ideal drug to reduce the incidence of primary invasive breast cancer for a number of reasons, and it has neither the safety nor the efficacy desired to be the optimal agent. Raloxifene is an acceptable alternative for many postmenopausal women, but it is also not ideal. Because of this, several other hormonal agents have been evaluated as possibly more suitable alternatives to tamoxifen for reducing the risk of breast cancer in high-risk women.

In postmenopausal women, the main source of estrogen is the peripheral conversion of androstenedione, produced by the adrenal glands, to estrone and estradiol in breast, muscle, and fat tissue. This conversion requires the aromatase enzyme.[103,104] In postmenopausal women, estrogen is synthesized in these peripheral tissues and circulates at a relatively low and constant level. The selective aromatase inhibitors (AIs) markedly suppress the concentration of estrogen in plasma via inhibition or inactivation of aromatase. The use of AIs is restricted to postmenopausal women, however, because in premenopausal women, high levels of androstenedione compete with AIs at the enzyme complex such that estrogen synthesis is not completely blocked. Moreover, the initial decrease in estrogen levels causes a reflex increase in gonadotropin levels, provoking ovarian hyperstimulation, thereby increasing aromatase in the ovary and consequently overcoming the initial blockade. Unlike tamoxifen, AIs lack partial estrogen agonist activity and are therefore not associated with an increased risk of the development of endometrial cancer.

Anastrozole and letrozole are reversible, nonsteroidal inhibitors of the aromatase enzyme, whereas exemestane is an irreversible steroidal inhibitor. AIs have significant antitumor activity in postmenopausal patients with breast cancer, and a number of randomized trials have evaluated the adjuvant use of AIs in postmenopausal women.[105–107] The ATAC (Arimidex, Tamoxifen, Alone or in

Combination) trial enrolled 9366 postmenopausal women with early breast cancer. The incidence of contralateral breast cancer was reduced by 58% with anastrozole compared with tamoxifen. The updated data at both 47 and 100 months continued to show that anastrozole was superior to tamoxifen in reducing the incidence of new ER-positive breast cancer, but the results were not as dramatic as the initial report.[106,107]

Anastrozole

AIs effectively prevent breast cancer recurrence and development of new contralateral tumors in postmenopausal women. The IBIS-II trial assessed the efficacy and safety of the AI anastrozole for prevention of breast cancer in postmenopausal women who are at high risk of the disease.[108] Between 2003 and 2012, the IBIS-II randomized, placebo-controlled trial recruited postmenopausal women aged 40 to 70 years from 18 countries. Eligible women were at increased risk of breast cancer and were randomly assigned to receive 1 mg oral anastrozole or matching placebo every day for 5 years. The primary end point was histologically confirmed breast cancer (invasive cancers or noninvasive DCIS). Analyses were done by intention to treat. In total, 1920 women were randomly assigned to receive anastrozole and 1944 to placebo.

After a median follow-up of 5 years, 40 women in the anastrozole group (2%) and 85 in the placebo group (4%) had developed breast cancer (hazard ratio 0.47, 95% CI 0.32–0.68, $p <$ .0001). The cumulative incidence of all breast cancers after 7 years was 5.6% in the placebo group and 2.8% in the anastrozole group. These percentages comprised 3.3% invasive, ER-positive cancers in the placebo group compared with only 1.4% in the anastrozole group.

Although many side effects have been associated with estrogen deprivation, they were only slightly more frequent in the anastrozole group than in the placebo group in the IBIS-II trial, indicating that most of these symptoms are not drug related. The most commonly reported side effects were joint stiffness and carpal tunnel syndrome. Some women also reported dry eyes. There were no more fractures in the women taking anastrozole compared with placebo. Importantly, although there was a slightly higher incidence of hypertension among women taking anastrozole compared with placebo (5% vs. 3%), there was no difference in the incidence of myocardial infarction, PE, or DVT. No additional side effects have been reported with anastrozole after adjuvant treatment of breast cancer, and these reassurances likely apply to the preventive setting as well. No more deaths were reported in the anastrozole group compared with the placebo group, and no specific causes were more common in one group than the other.

The reduction in the incidence of breast cancer in the IBIS-II trial was larger than those reported for tamoxifen or raloxifene in the completed risk-reduction trials of these two agents. Anastrozole is therefore a reasonable option for postmenopausal women at increased risk of breast cancer, although it does not yet have approval for this use as a labeled indication in the United States.

Full adherence to the prescribed daily regimen for 5 years was 70% overall in the IBIS-II trial and was only slightly lower in the anastrozole group than in the placebo group. Overall adherence at 3 years was 75%, which is similar to that in the prevention trial with exemestane (discussed next), which had 85% overall adherence at 35 months of follow-up. Adherence to daily oral anastrozole in IBIS-II was slightly better than for tamoxifen in IBIS-I.

Clinicians should advise patients that most side effects were not treatment related. These data indicate that anastrozole effectively reduces incidence of breast cancer in high-risk postmenopausal women. This finding, along with the fact that most of the side effects associated with estrogen deprivation were not attributable to treatment, provides support for the use of anastrozole in postmenopausal women at high risk of breast cancer.

Exemestane

In a randomized, placebo-controlled, double-blind trial of exemestane,[109] eligible postmenopausal women 35 years of age or older had at least one of the following risk factors: 60 years of age or older; Gail 5-year risk score greater than 1.66% of developing invasive breast cancer within 5 years; prior atypical ductal or lobular hyperplasia or LCIS; or DCIS with mastectomy. A total of 4560 women whose median age was 62.5 years and whose median Gail risk score was 2.3% were randomly assigned to either exemestane or placebo. At a median follow-up of 35 months, 11 invasive breast cancers were detected in those given exemestane and in 32 of those given placebo. These observations indicated a 65% relative reduction in the annual incidence of invasive breast cancer by exemestane (0.19% vs. 0.55%). The annual incidence of invasive plus noninvasive (DCIS) breast cancers was 0.35% on exemestane and 0.77% on placebo (53% reduction). The number of women needed to treat with this AI to prevent one case of breast cancer is 94 with 3 years of exemestane therapy and is projected to be only 26 women at 5 years, although the number of women who received treatment for a full 5 years was low.

Toxic effects, health-related and menopause-specific qualities of life were measured in the trial. Adverse events occurred in significantly more women receiving exemestane, but the absolute difference was small (88% of the exemestane group compared with 85% of the placebo group). Arthritis and hot flashes were more common in the exemestane group, but differences between the groups were small (arthritis, 6.5% vs. 4.0%; hot flashes, 18.3% vs. 11.9%). As in the IBIS-II trial, there were no significant differences between the two groups in prespecified secondary end points including new diagnoses of osteoporosis or cardiovascular events. Clinical fracture rates were also similar in the two groups, and the proportion of women in each group who were prescribed bisphosphonate therapy during the trial was also similar (about 24%). There was no significant difference in the number of cancers other than breast cancer or time to detection of these cancers. No significant differences were detected between the two groups with respect to hypercholesterolemia, hypertriglyceridemia, abnormal liver-function tests, acne, alopecia, rash, weight gain, or hair loss. There were no significant differences between the two groups in terms of treatment-related deaths, and minimal quality-of-life differences were observed.

Expert Recommendations on the Use of Pharmacologic Interventions for Breast Cancer Risk Reduction

Three national professional organizations in the United States have made recommendations for the use of hormonal agents to the risk of breast cancer in high-risk women. Those recommendations will be reviewed here. An international consensus statement has also endorsed the use of SERMs and AIs for the reduction of breast cancer risk.[110]

• BOX 16.2 Recommendations From the American Society of Clinical Oncology Clinical Practice Guideline

Underlying facts and assumptions

- Health care providers are encouraged to discuss the option of chemoprevention among women at increased breast cancer risk. The discussion should include the specific risks and benefits associated with each chemopreventive agent.
- Those at increased breast cancer risk are defined as individuals with a 5-year projected absolute risk of breast cancer ≥1.66% (based on the National Cancer Institute Breast Cancer Risk Assessment Tool or an equivalent measure) or women diagnosed with lobular carcinoma in situ.
- In women at increased risk of breast cancer age ≥35 years, tamoxifen (20 mg per day for 5 years) should be discussed as an option to reduce the risk of ER-positive breast cancer.
- In postmenopausal women, raloxifene (60 mg/day for 5 years) and exemestane (25 mg/day for 5 years) should also be discussed as options for breast cancer risk reduction.
- Use of other selective ER modulators or other aromatase inhibitors to lower breast cancer risk is not recommended outside of a clinical trial.

Discussions with patients who are considering the use of selective ER modulators to reduce their risk of breast cancer should include the following key points:

- Assessment and discussion of individual risk of developing breast cancer
- Options for reducing the risk of developing breast cancer (i.e., nonpharmacologic and pharmacologic)
- Potential effect of specific chemoprevention agents on the incidence of both invasive and noninvasive breast cancers
- Potential risks and adverse effects of chemoprevention agents
- Long-term effectiveness of chemoprevention agents
- Chemoprevention studies were not powered to detect differences in mortality because it was considered that a reduction in incidence was itself an important clinical end point
- Accessibility, cost, and insurance coverage
- Resources and materials for consideration (e.g., www.cancer.net, www.cancer.org, http://effectivehealthcare.ahrq.gov)
- Plan for clinical follow-up

ER, Estrogen receptor.

---

recommended for women who are pregnant, women who may become pregnant, or nursing mothers. Tamoxifen is not recommended in combination with postmenopausal HRT. Follow-up while on tamoxifen should include a timely workup of abnormal vaginal bleeding.

The ASCO 2013 Clinical Practice Guideline indicates that premenopausal women older than 35 years of age with Gail model risks of breast cancer greater than 1.67% in 5 years or LCIS should be offered tamoxifen 20 mg orally daily for the reduction of breast cancer risk. The guideline indicates that no study has evaluated the optimal age at which to begin tamoxifen to reduce breast cancer risk; premenopausal women at increased risk derive the greatest net benefit because of the absence of increased risks for either thromboembolic events or uterine cancer in this group. Because the risk of clotting increases with age, and because both stroke and PE are potentially life-threatening consequences of tamoxifen therapy, careful consideration must be given to risks versus benefits in older postmenopausal women who are considering tamoxifen for risk reduction.

The ASCO guideline notes that chemoprevention with a SERM may be particularly beneficial to women with atypical hyperplasia, a 5-year Gail model risk of more than 5%, LCIS, or two or more first-degree relatives with breast cancer based on the published data reviewed in this chapter. There are no primary prevention studies to evaluate the optimal duration of tamoxifen therapy for reducing the risk of breast cancer, but completed clinical trials in the adjuvant therapy setting show that using tamoxifen for 10 years is more beneficial than only 5 years of use.[72,73] No trials are being conducted or are planned to examine the ideal duration of therapy in the risk-reduction setting.

Although the ASCO guideline did not recommend anastrozole, its use should be considered in postmenopausal women based on the favorable results of the IBIS-II trial. Those at increased breast cancer risk are defined as individuals with a 5-year projected absolute risk of breast cancer risk of 1.66% or greater based on the NCI breast cancer Risk Assessment Tool (http://www.cancer.gov/bcrisktool/), using an equivalent measure,[13–21] or women diagnosed with LCIS or atypical lobular or ductal hyperplasia. Use of other SERMs or other AIs to lower breast cancer risk is not recommended outside of a clinical trial.

American Society of Clinical Oncology 2013 Clinical Practice Guideline

The American Society of Clinical Oncology (ASCO) convened clinical experts in 2013 to review the evidence presented here and to make recommendations for the management of breast cancer risk.[111] Clinical practice recommendations for discussing the use of SERMs with patients are summarized in Box 16.2, and specific guidelines for the use of tamoxifen and raloxifene are listed in Table 16.3. In women at increased risk of breast cancer aged 35 years and older, tamoxifen (20 mg/day for 5 years) should be discussed as an option to reduce the risk of ER-positive breast cancer. In postmenopausal women, raloxifene (60 mg/day for 5 years) and exemestane (25 mg/day for 5 years) should also be discussed as options for breast cancer risk reduction.

The risk-reduction benefit with SERMs continues for at least 10 years in both premenopausal and postmenopausal women who include those who had either a natural or an artificial (i.e., surgical) menopause. Tamoxifen is not recommended for use in women with a history of DVT, PE, stroke, or transient ischemic attack or during prolonged immobilization. Tamoxifen is not

US Preventive Services Task Force Recommendations

As previously noted, important risk factors for breast cancer include patient age, race/ethnicity, age at menarche, age at first live childbirth, personal history of ductal or LCIS, number of first-degree relatives with breast cancer, personal history of breast biopsy, body mass index, menopause status or age, breast density, estrogen and progestin use, smoking, alcohol use, physical activity, and diet. Available risk assessment models can accurately predict the number of breast cancer cases that may arise in certain study populations, but their ability to accurately predict which women will develop breast cancer is modest.

The USPSTF believes there is moderate net benefit from use of tamoxifen and raloxifene to reduce the incidence of invasive breast cancer in women who are at increased risk for the disease.[112] A summary of the evidence considered by the Task Force is outlined in Table 16.4. For women who are at increased risk for breast cancer, the USPSTF recommends that clinicians engage in shared, informed decision-making with them about medications to reduce their risk. For women who are at increased risk for breast

TABLE 16.3	Use of Pharmacologic Interventions for Breast Cancer Risk Reduction: American Society of Clinical Oncology Clinical Practice Guideline	
Agent	Recommendations	Strength of Recommendation and Strength of Evidence
Tamoxifen	***Should** be discussed as an option* to reduce the risk of invasive BC, specifically ER-positive BC, in postmenopausal women who are aged ≥35 years with a 5-year projected absolute BC risk ≥1.66% or with LCIS. Risk reduction benefit continues for at least 10 years	Strength of evidence: strong evidence, based on five RCTs with low risk of bias
	Is not recommended for use in women with a history of DVT, PE, stroke, or transient ischemic attack, during prolonged immobilization or in patients with a history of uncontrolled diabetes, hypertension or atrial fibrillation	
	Is not recommended in combination with hormone therapy (estrogen, progesterone, androgen or birth control pills)	
	Is not recommended for women who are pregnant, women who may become pregnant, or nursing mothers	
	Follow-up should include a timely workup of abnormal vaginal bleeding	
	Discussions with patients and health care providers should include both the risks and benefits of tamoxifen in the preventive setting	
	Dosage: 20 mg/day orally for 5 years	
Raloxifene	Should be discussed as an option to reduce the risk of invasive BC, specifically ER-positive BC, in postmenopausal women who are aged ≥35 years with a 5-year projected absolute BC risk ≥1.66% or with LCIS	Strong, evidence-based recommendation
	May be used longer than 5 years in women with osteoporosis, in whom BC risk reduction is a secondary benefit	
	Should not be used for BC risk reduction in premenopausal women	Strength of evidence: strong evidence, based on four RCTs with low risk of bias
	Is not recommended for use in women with a history of DVT, PE, stroke, or transient ischemic attack or during prolonged immobilization	
	Discussions with patients and health care providers should include both the risks and benefits of raloxifene in the preventive setting	
	Dosage: 60 mg per day orally for 5 years	

BC, Breast cancer; DVT, deep vein thrombosis; ER, estrogen receptor; LCIS, lobular carcinoma in situ; PE, pulmonary embolism; RCT, randomized controlled trial.

cancer and at low risk for adverse medication effects, clinicians should offer to prescribe risk-reducing medications, such as tamoxifen or raloxifene. There is high certainty that the net benefit is moderate or there is moderate certainty that the net benefit is moderate to substantial.

For women not at increased risk for breast cancer, the USPSTF recommends against the routine use of medications such as tamoxifen or raloxifene for risk reduction of primary breast cancer. The potential harms of tamoxifen and raloxifene outweigh potential benefits for breast cancer risk reduction in women who are not at increased risk for the disease. Potential harms include thromboembolic events, endometrial cancer, and cataracts.

For a summary of the evidence systematically reviewed in making these recommendations, the full recommendation statement, and supporting documents, see http://www.uspreventiveservicestaskforce.org.

National Comprehensive Cancer Network Recommendations

The National Comprehensive Cancer Network (NCCN) is an alliance of 27 of the world's leading cancer centers in the United States that work together to develop treatment guidelines for most cancers; the alliance is dedicated to research that improves the quality, effectiveness, and efficiency of cancer care. The NCCN has developed an integrated suite of tools to improve the quality of cancer care. The NCCN Clinical Practice Guidelines in Oncology document evidence-based, consensus-driven management to ensure that all patients receive preventive, diagnostic treatment and supportive services that are most likely to lead to optimal outcomes. The guidelines provide recommendations for some of the key cancer prevention and screening topics as well as supportive care considerations. The NCCN guidelines for the use of tamoxifen and raloxifene to reduce the risk of breast cancer are summarized next. The full text of the recommendations is available at https://www.nccn.org/professionals/physician_gls/pdf/breast_risk.pdf.

Tamoxifen Recommendation

The NCCN Breast Cancer Risk Reduction panel recommends tamoxifen as an option to reduce breast cancer risk in healthy pre- and postmenopausal women 35 years of age and older whose life expectancy is 10 years or more and who have 1.7% or greater 5-year risk for breast cancer as determined by the Gail model, or who have had LCIS. The risk/benefit ratio for tamoxifen use in premenopausal women at increased risk for breast cancer is relatively favorable (category 1), and the risk/benefit ratio for tamoxifen use in postmenopausal women is influenced by age, presence of the uterus, or other comorbid conditions. The utility of tamoxifen as a breast cancer risk-reducing agent in women younger than age 35 years is not known. Tamoxifen is a teratogen and thus is contraindicated during pregnancy or in women planning a pregnancy.

TABLE 16.4   Summary of Evidence on the Use of Medications to Reduce the Risk of Primary Breast Cancer, US Preventive Services Task Force, 2013

Studies	Design	Limitations	Consistency	Applicability	Overall Quality
Key Question 1: Benefits of Tamoxifen and Raloxifene When Used to Reduce Risk for Primary Breast Cancer					
Four placebo-controlled trials of tamoxifen and 2 of raloxifene; 1 head-to head trial	RCT	Trials are heterogeneous and lacked data on doses, duration, and timing of use	Consistent	High	Good

Findings: Tamoxifen and raloxifene reduced invasive breast cancer incidence by 30%–68% compared with placebo; tamoxifen had a greater effect than raloxifene in STAR. Noninvasive breast cancer incidence and mortality were not significantly reduced and did not differ between medications. Both reduced fracture incidence.

Studies	Design	Limitations	Consistency	Applicability	Overall Quality
Key Question 2: Harms of Tamoxifen and Raloxifene When Used to Reduce Risk for Primary Breast Cancer					
Four placebo-controlled trials of tamoxifen; 14 trials and 1 study of raloxifene; 1 head-to-head trial	RCT and cohort	Trials are heterogeneous and lacked data on long-term effects	Consistent	High	Fair to good

Findings: Tamoxifen and raloxifene increased incidence of thromboembolic events compared with placebo; tamoxifen had a greater effect than raloxifene in STAR. Tamoxifen increased endometrial cancer incidence compared with placebo and raloxifene and increased incidence of cataracts compared with raloxifene. Both caused undesirable side effects for some women.

Studies	Design	Limitations	Consistency	Applicability	Overall Quality
Key Question 3: Variability of Outcomes in Population Subgroups					
Four placebo-controlled trials of tamoxifen and 2 of raloxifene; 1 head-to head trial	RCT	Trials lacked data for women who are nonwhite, are premenopausal, or have comorbid conditions	Consistent	High	Fair

Findings: Risk reduction was greatest among women with ≥5% 5-year Gail model risk score or atypical hyperplasia for tamoxifen compared with placebo and raloxifene. Thromboembolic events and endometrial cancer were more common in women ≥50 years than younger women using tamoxifen.

Studies	Design	Limitations	Consistency	Applicability	Overall Quality
Key Question 4: Medication Decisions and Concordance, Adherence, and Persistence					
Decisions: 11 studies; adherence and persistence: 4 placebo trials of tamoxifen and 2 of raloxifene; 1 head-to-head trial	RCT and survey	Few decision studies included raloxifene; data on adherence and persistence were lacking	Could not determine	Unclear; data about decisions were descriptive and from small samples	Fair

Findings: Many women elect not to take tamoxifen because of harms. Trials provided limited data about adherence and persistence. Discontinuation rates for tamoxifen and raloxifene were generally slightly higher than placebo.

Studies	Design	Limitations	Consistency	Applicability	Overall Quality
Key Question 5: Methods to Identify Women at Increased Risk for Breast Cancer					
19 studies of 13 models	Diagnostic accuracy	Studies varied by populations and risk parameters	Consistent	High	Good

Findings: Models have modest discriminatory accuracy in predicting the probability of breast cancer in a person.

RCT, Randomized controlled trial.

Raloxifene Recommendation

The NCCN panel felt strongly that tamoxifen is a superior choice as a risk-reducing agent for most postmenopausal women desiring nonsurgical risk-reduction therapy. Consideration of toxicity may still lead to the choice of raloxifene over tamoxifen in some women. If raloxifene is chosen, the panel recommends use of 60 mg per day. Data regarding the use of raloxifene to reduce breast cancer risk is limited to healthy, postmenopausal women older than 35 years who have a Gail model risk score of 1.7% or greater in 5 years or who have a history of LCIS. The risk/benefit ratio for raloxifene use in postmenopausal women at increased risk for breast cancer is influenced by age and comorbid conditions (category 1). Because there are no currently available data

regarding the efficacy of raloxifene for risk reduction in the *BRCA1/2* mutation carriers and women have received prior thoracic radiation, use of raloxifene in these populations is designated as a category 2a recommendation by the NCCN Breast Cancer Risk Reduction panel. Use of raloxifene to reduce breast cancer risk in premenopausal women is inappropriate unless part of a clinical trial.

In the opinion of the NCCN panel, risk-reduction therapy with tamoxifen and raloxifene has been vastly underutilized. Women in whom the benefits of risk-reduction therapy far outweigh harms include those with atypical ductal or lobular hyperplasia and LCIS. Women with atypia or LCIS have a significantly higher risk of developing invasive breast cancer. Considering the opportunity that exists for a significant impact of risk-reduction therapy on reducing incidence of breast cancer, the NCCN panel strongly recommends such therapy in women with atypical hyperplasia.

Aromatase Inhibitor Recommendation

The NCCN experts have included exemestane and anastrozole as choices of a risk-reduction agent for most postmenopausal women desiring nonsurgical risk-reduction therapy (category 1). This recommendation is based on the results exemestane trial reviewed earlier and the IBIS-II trial. The panel recommends use of 25 mg per day of exemestane or 1 mg per day of anastrozole. Data regarding use of AIs to reduce breast cancer risk are limited to postmenopausal women aged 35 years and older with Gail model 5-year risk greater than 1.66% or a history of LCIS. The consensus of the panel is that the risk/benefit ratio for use of an AI in postmenopausal women at increased risk for breast cancer is influenced by age, bone density, and comorbid conditions. Use of an AI to reduce breast cancer risk in premenopausal women is inappropriate unless part of a clinical trial. The utility of an AI as a breast-cancer risk-reduction agent in women younger than 35 years is not known. There are insufficient data on the influence of ethnicity and race on the efficacy and safety of AIs as risk-reducing agents.

Exemestane and anastrozole are not currently FDA approved for breast cancer risk reduction. Currently, there are no data comparing the benefits and risks of AI therapy to those of tamoxifen or raloxifene.

Summary

Despite strong evidence that it is efficacious, chemoprevention has been underused in eligible women. A number of reasons have been put forth to explain why patients may not be willing to adopt a SERM for breast cancer risk reduction.[113] These include the use of HRT along with patients' erroneous perception that the risks of SERM therapy are greater than its benefits. They also perceive the risks of therapy-related side effects to be greater than their risk of breast cancer. This problem is confounded by the fact that they (and perhaps their physicians) are confused by the concept of probabilistic risk. Finally, they fear endometrial cancer out of proportion to its true tamoxifen-related risk, and they do not understand that there is no increased risk of uterine malignancy associated with raloxifene. Additional reasons not to adopt and initiate strategies to reduce the risk of breast cancer include medication costs, lack of reasonably accurate and feasible methods for assessing personal individual risk, and lack of established risk thresholds that maximize benefit and minimize harms.

Regardless of these obstacles, tamoxifen and raloxifene continue to have an important role in the primary prevention of breast cancer. The clinical challenge is to identify those women at highest risk and to offer tamoxifen preferentially to those women who have either had hysterectomy or to those who are at higher levels of risk. These women will derive greater net benefit from using tamoxifen. Raloxifene offers greater safety for postmenopausal women, whose benefit ratio is also related directly to the level of breast cancer risk, as it is for tamoxifen.

Selected References

14. Gail MH, Brinton LA, Byar DP, et al. Projecting individualized probabilities of developing breast cancer for white females who are being examined annually. *J Natl Cancer Inst.* 1989;81:1879-1886.
28. Fisher B, Costantino JP, Wickerham DL, et al. Tamoxifen for prevention of breast cancer: report of the National Surgical Adjuvant Breast and Bowel Project P-1 study. *J Natl Cancer Inst.* 1998;90:1371-1388.
29. Fisher B, Costantino JP, Wickerham DL, et al. Tamoxifen for the prevention of breast cancer: current status of the National Surgical Adjuvant Breast and Bowel Project P-1 study. *J Natl Cancer Inst.* 2005;97:1652-1662.
45. Cuzick J, Forbes JF, Sestak I, et al. Long-term results of tamoxifen prophylaxis for breast cancer: 96-month follow-up of the randomized IBIS-I trial. *J Natl Cancer Inst.* 2007;99:272-282.
50. Gail MH, Costantino JP, Bryant J, et al. Weighing the risks and benefits of tamoxifen treatment for preventing breast cancer. *J Natl Cancer Inst.* 1999;91:1829-1846.
52. Cuzick J, Sestak I, Cawthorn S, et al. Tamoxifen for prevention of breast cancer: extended long-term follow-up of the IBIS-I breast cancer prevention trial. *Lancet Oncol.* 2015;16:67-75.
54. Vogel VG, Costantino JP, Wickerham DL, et al. Effects of tamoxifen vs. raloxifene on the risk of developing invasive breast cancer and other disease outcomes: The NSABP Study of Tamoxifen and Raloxifene (STAR) P-2 Trial. *JAMA.* 2006;295:2727-2741.
55. Vogel VG, Costantino JP, Wickerham DL, et al. Update of the National Surgical Adjuvant Breast and Bowel Project Study of Tamoxifen and Raloxifene (STAR) P-2 Trial: preventing breast cancer. *Cancer Prev Res (Phila).* 2010;3:696-706.
61. Hartmann LC, Degnim AC, Santen RJ, et al. Atypical hyperplasia of the breast—risk assessment and management options. *N Engl J Med.* 2015;372:78-89.
108. Cuzick J, Sestak I, Forbes JF, et al. Anastrozole for prevention of breast cancer in high-risk postmenopausal women (IBIS-II): an international, double-blind, randomised placebo-controlled trial. *Lancet.* 2014;383:1041-1048.
109. Goss PE, Ingle JN, Ales-Martinez JE, et al. Exemestane for breast-cancer prevention in postmenopausal women. *N Engl J Med.* 2011;364:2381-2391.
110. Cuzick J, DeCensi A, Arun B, et al. Preventive therapy for breast cancer: an international consensus statement. *Lancet Oncol.* 2011;12:496-503.
111. Visvanathan K, Hurley P, Bantug E, et al. Use of pharmacologic interventions for breast cancer risk reduction: American Society of Clinical Oncology Clinical Practice Guideline. *J Clin Oncol.* 2013;31:2942-2962.
112. Nelson HD, Smith B, Griffin JC, Fu R. Use of medications to reduce risk for primary breast cancer: a systematic review for the U.S. Preventive Services Task Force. *Ann Intern Med.* 2013;158:604-614.

A full reference list is available online at ExpertConsult.com.

17

Breast Cancer Genetics: Syndromes, Genes, Pathology, Counseling, Testing, and Treatment

MAUREEN O'DONNELL, JENNIFER AXILBUND, AND DAVID M. EUHUS

Not long after the birth of modern medical science at the turn of the 19th century, two prominent physician scientists observed the hereditary nature of cancer and articulated concepts in cancer genetics that hold true to this day. In 1851 Hermann Lebert suggested "children come into this world carrying within them the seeds of a cancerous disease which remains latent for thirty to fifty years, but which, once developed, is fatal in the space of a few years."[1] He recognized the importance of identifying individuals with a cancer predisposition and suggested that these individuals might reduce their risk by relocating to regions with a low cancer incidence. In 1866 Lebert's contemporary, the famed neuroanatomist Pierre Paul Broca, described four generations of a family afflicted with breast and gastrointestinal cancers.[2] Through detailed pedigree analysis, these scientists concluded that major inherited predisposition syndromes account for only 5% to 10% of cases of breast cancer, that women are disproportionately affected with hereditary cancer compared with men, and that identification of high-risk families presents an opportunity to intervene to reduce risk.

The majority of breast cancers are sporadic rather than inherited. It is therefore environmental factors and chance, not germline mutations, that account for a greater number of breast cancers. Twin studies estimate that 12% to 30% of breast cancers have a heritable genetic component.[3–5] However, only 5% to 10% of breast cancers are related to inheritance of major autosomal dominant predisposition genes. Of these, the causative mutation is identifiable in only 35%.[6] Even with whole genome sequencing, we have nearly exhausted the list of identifiable germline mutations responsible for familial breast cancer. *BRCA1* and *BRCA2* still account for the majority of mutations identified in genetic high-risk families. More than a dozen other well-described gene mutations predispose to breast cancer, and the list of rare genes is increasing rapidly (Fig. 17.1). Although genetic predisposition accounts for only a fraction of all breast cancers, identification of gene mutation carriers has great value for breast cancer prevention, diagnosis, and treatment.

The Value of Genetic Testing

For individuals not yet diagnosed with cancer, genetic testing can be the most accurate tool available for cancer risk stratification.

Lifetime breast cancer risk is 57% to 81% for women with pathogenic *BRCA1* mutations and 45% to 85% for *BRCA2* mutations.[7–11] Ovarian cancer risk is 39% by age 70 for *BRCA1* and 17% for *BRCA2*.[11] Mutations in other genes may point to increased risk for gastric, thyroid, endometrial, or other cancers (Table 17.1).[12–22]

Quantitative risk information can guide decisions about enhanced surveillance to diagnose cancers earlier, or prophylactic surgery or chemoprevention to reduce the risk of ever developing cancer. Pathogenic mutations in most of the genes commonly tested today will be associated with at least a 20% lifetime breast cancer risk. These women all meet the risk threshold for consideration of enhanced surveillance with breast magnetic resonance imaging (MRI).[23]

Pathogenic mutations in breast cancer predisposition genes can influence decisions about surgery, radiation therapy, and systemic treatments in the newly diagnosed breast cancer patient. With respect to surgery, second primary breast cancer risk is often elevated in gene mutations carriers. This information is critical for deciding between breast conservation and unilateral or bilateral mastectomy. Most of the known breast cancer predisposition genes serve a role in DNA maintenance and repair. This knowledge can influence radiation therapy decisions. Although therapeutic whole breast radiation is not contraindicated in any other than homozygous *ATM* carriers, it should be used with caution in *TP53* mutation carriers.[24] Partial breast irradiation is classified as "unsuitable outside of a clinical trial" for *BRCA1/BRCA2* gene mutation carrier and is likely ill advised for others with mutations in related DNA repair genes.[25] Pathogenic *BRCA1/BRCA2* gene mutations are increasingly recognized as markers of reduced sensitivity to taxol-based chemotherapy and increased sensitivity to platins[26] and poly(ADP-ribose) polymerase (PARP) inhibitors.[27] Although germline genetic tests are not yet recognized as "predictive tests" for systemic therapy decisions, they can gain patients access to clinical trials that are exploiting the unique biology of *BRCA1/BRCA2*–associated breast cancer.

Role of the Cancer Genetics Counselor

Receiving the results of a genetic test can be emotionally challenging and set in to motion a chain of events with significant

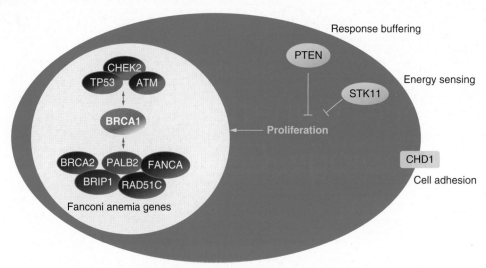

• **Fig. 17.1** Breast cancer predisposition genes.

TABLE 17.1   Hereditary Breast Cancer Predisposition Syndromes

Syndrome	Gene Locus	Neoplasms	Lifetime Breast Cancer Risk	Frequency Among High-Risk Families	Reference
Hereditary breast/ovarian	*BRCA1* (17q12–21)	Female breast, ovarian	57%–81%	5%	18
Hereditary breast/ovarian	BRCA2 (13q12–13)	Male and female breast, ovarian, prostate, pancreatic	45%–85%	4%	18
CHEK2-related	*CHEK2* (22q12.1)	Breast, colorectal, bladder	25%–37%	1.3%	15
PALB2-related	*PALB2* (16p12.1)	Breast, pancreatic, male breast	20%–79%	0.7%	12
ATM-related	*ATM* (11q22.3)	Breast and ovarian	15%–20%	0.7%	14
Li-Fraumeni	*TP53* (17p13.1)	Breast, sarcomas, leukemia, brain tumors, adrenocortical carcinoma, lung	56%–90%	0.2%	19
Moderate risk breast/ ovarian cancer	*BARD1* (2q34-q35)	Breast/ovarian	Unknown	0.2%	21
BRIP1-related	*BRIP1* (17q22-q24)	Breast, ovarian	unknown	0.2%	22
Hereditary diffuse gastric cancer	*CDH1* (16q22.1)	gastric, lobular breast, colorectal	60%	0.1%	17
Cowden	*PTEN* (10q23.3)	Breast, thyroid, endometrial Other: benign hamartomas (of skin, mucosa, GI, GU, CNS, and bones) macrocephaly	67%–85%	<0.1%	13
Peutz-Jeghers	*STK11* (19p13.3)	Breast, ovarian, cervical, uterine, testicular, small bowel, and colon Other: hamartomatous polyps of small bowel and mucocutaneous pigmentation	32%–54%	<0.1%	20
RAD51C	*RAD51C* (17q25.1)	Breast, ovarian	Unknown	<0.1%	16

CNS, Central nervous system; *GI,* gastrointestinal; *GU,* genitourinary.

quality-of-life implications. Some patients simply prefer not to know. Decisions about whether to undergo testing, what test to perform, and then what to do with the results are complex. This complexity is amplified in the era of multigene panel testing, making the involvement of a genetics professional essential. Some have advocated genetic testing by primary care providers, or by those who diagnose and treat breast cancer. The ABOUT study, a survey of 11,159 women who underwent *BRCA1/BRCA2* testing in 2012, found that only 37% received genetic counseling.[28] Those who received genetic counseling had greater knowledge, understanding, and satisfaction than those who did not. In 2012 the American College of Surgeons Commission on Cancer accreditation program mandated that cancer risk assessment, genetic counseling, and genetic testing services be provided to patients by a qualified genetic professional either on site or by referral. This standard was reiterated in 2016 (http://www.facs.org/cancerprogram/index.html). The US Preventive Services Task Force recently completed a systematic review of the literature and concluded that genetic counseling reduces distress, improves risk perception, and reduces intention for testing.[29]

The National Society of Genetic Counselors has outlined the essential functions of the genetic counselor which include (1) estimating cancer risk based on personal and family medical history before genetic testing, (2) offering genetic testing when certain criteria are met, (3) fully informing the individual about the test and the possible results, and (4) disclosing test results in conjunction with a reestimation of cancer risk and a discussion about options for reducing risk.[30] Psychosocial assessment and intervention, when required, is a key function throughout the genetic testing process.

Identifying Mutation Carriers

Mutations in *BRCA1* and *BRCA2* are the most frequently identified cause of hereditary breast cancer predisposition. The prevalence (allelic frequency) of pathogenic *BRCA1/BRCA2* gene mutations is estimated at 0.13% to 0.26% for the general population and 1.3% to 2.7% for Ashkenazi Jewish populations.[31–34] Therefore, considering other genes in addition to *BRCA1* and *BRCA2,* there are 350,000 to more than 500,000 individuals in the United States who carry pathogenic mutations in breast cancer predisposition genes.[35]

Current genetic testing guidelines nearly ensure that genetic high-risk families are only recognized after one or more individuals have already been diagnosed with cancer. Ideally, mutation carriers would be recognized before they develop cancer so they have the opportunity to act to avoid cancer. Nevertheless, current guidelines are based on patterns of personal and family cancer history.[36] Third party payors usually adopt these guidelines, so that financial constraints often limit testing outside of these guidelines. The American Society of Clinical Oncology has recommended genetic testing when the following criteria are met: (1) there is a personal or family history suggesting genetic cancer susceptibility, (2) the test can be adequately interpreted, and (3) the results will aid in the diagnosis or influence the medical or surgical management of the patient or family members at hereditary risk for cancer.[37] A fourth criteria must be considered as well: there must be some provision for paying for the test.

Genetic testing guidelines are directed at recognizing individuals who are reasonably likely to carry a pathogenic mutation. This is currently largely determined by personal and family cancer history unless there is a known gene mutation in the family. National Comprehensive Cancer Network (NCCN) guidelines for recommending genetic evaluation are quite liberal. *BRCA1/BRCA2* testing is recommended, even in the absence of any family history, for women diagnosed with breast cancer at age 50 or younger, triple negative breast cancer at age 60 or younger, bilateral or ipsilateral second primary breast cancer, ovarian cancer, breast or pancreatic cancer at any age in an Ashkenazi Jewish person, or male breast cancer. Combinations of personal or family history of breast, prostate, pancreas, ovarian or other syndrome-associated cancers are also sufficient for pursuing

TABLE 17.2	Criteria for Hereditary Breast/Ovarian Cancer Genetic Risk Evaluation	
Personal History	**Required Family History[a]**
Breast cancer ≤50[b] Triple-negative breast cancer ≤60 Two primary breast cancers (same or opposite side) Ovarian cancer Breast cancer in Ashkenazi Jewish Pancreatic cancer in Ashkenazi Jewish Male breast cancer	None required
Breast cancer (any age)	Breast cancer ≤50 Two or more breast cancers (any age) Ovarian cancer Two or more pancreatic cancer and/or prostate cancer (Gleason score ≥7) Male breast cancer
None required	Two or more primary breast cancers in a single individual Breast cancer ≤45 in a first- or second-degree relative Two or more relatives with breast cancer, one age ≤50 Breast cancer at age ≤50 Ovarian cancer Male breast cancer

Personal of family history of three of the following in any combination: breast cancer, pancreatic cancer, Gleason score ≥7 prostate cancer, melanoma, sarcoma, adrenocortical carcinoma, brain tumor, leukemia, diffuse gastric cancer, colon cancer, endometrial cancer, thyroid cancer, kidney cancer, or phenotypic features of hereditary cancer including macrocephaly, hamartomatous gastrointestinal polyps, macular pigmentation of the glans penis, multiple tricholemmomas, multiple acral keratosis, mucocutaneous neuromas, and oral papillomas.

[a]First-, second-, or third-degree relative in the same lineage.
[b]Breast cancer includes invasive or in situ disease.

Modified from National Comprehensive Cancer Network. Genetic/familial high-risk assessment: breast and ovarian. NCCN Clinical Practice Guidelines in Oncology v2.2016. Fort Washington, PA; 2016.

genetic evaluation (Table 17.2). NCCN guidelines include testing criteria for *TP53* (Li-Fraumeni syndrome) and *PTEN* (Cowden syndrome).

There are more than a dozen genes firmly linked to inherited breast cancer predisposition. Additionally, a step-wise approach to genetic testing may be cost-prohibitive. Generating and maintaining detailed testing criteria for each one may not be practical. In general, hereditary predisposition can be suspected based on early age at breast cancer diagnosis, multiple breast cancers in the same lineage, and the presence of associated cancers such as ovarian, pancreas, or prostate for hereditary breast/ovarian cancer syndrome, and gastric, melanoma, sarcoma, endometrial, or others for the other high penetrance syndromes (see Table 17.1).

The probability that an individual carries a mutation in *BRCA1* or *BRCA2* can be estimated using family history models such as BRCAPRO,[38] Tyrer-Cusick,[39] or BOADICEA.[33] There is no specific mutation probability that is sensitive and specific enough to

TABLE 17.3	A Simple Family History Screening Tool	
Breast cancer at age ≥50		3
Breast cancer at age <50		4
Ovarian cancer at any age		5
Male breast cancer at any age		8
Ashkenazi Jewish heritage		4

Referral recommended for score ≥8. Score all first-, second-, or third-degree relatives.
Modified from Hoskins KF, Zwaagstra A, Ranz M. Validation of a tool for identifying women at high risk for hereditary breast cancer in population-based screening. *Cancer.* 2006;107: 1769-1776.

use as the sole criterion for offering genetic testing. One study found that 6% to 8% of *BRCA1/BRCA2* mutation carriers are missed when the testing criterion is a 10% mutation probability estimated by genetic counselors or the computer model BRCAPRO.[40]

The US Preventive Services Taskforce recommends that primary care providers screen women for personal and family cancer histories that may suggest an inherited predisposition to breast cancer.[41] Numerous screening tools are available.[42–46] The simplest tool is shown in Table 17.3. Despite these recommendations, detailed cancer family history screening is not routinely practiced.[47] One approach for increasing genetic counseling referrals has been to provide physicians with education and tools to facilitate screening, but this approach has not been particularly successful.[48] Many organizations have articulated guidelines for genetics referrals, but providers are often unaware of these guidelines.[49] For all of these reasons, there is interest in moving family history screening out of primary care practices into other venues. A modified Bellcross tool[42] was recently used to screen 96,055 women having mammograms.[50] Five percent of the women met criteria for genetic counseling referral, and 29 mutation carriers identified. This is only 22% of the expected mutation prevalence for a population of this size and composition.

There is reason to question whether self-reported family history screening is the best approach for identifying mutation carriers. In the first place, there are issues with the accuracy of self-reported history,[51] and in the second place, limited family size and structure can contribute to false negatives. A recent study found that half of 306 women with breast cancer diagnosed before age 50, who were seen for genetic risk assessment, had fewer than two first- or second-degree female relatives living past the age of 45.[52] Nevertheless, *BRCA1/BRCA2* mutations were identified in 14% of these women.

These concerns have prompted some to suggest universal mutation testing irrespective of personal or family history.[53] One criticism of this approach is that we may not know how to interpret cancer risks in individuals ascertained in this fashion, and another is that the cost of the testing would need to be less than $250 to get the cost per quality life year gained down to $53,000. A demonstration project among 8195 healthy Ashkenazi Jewish men identified *BRCA1/BRCA2* mutations in 2.2% resulting in the identification of 211 mutation carriers among 629 female relatives.[54] Among mutation carriers identified in this fashion, breast cancer risk to age 80 was 60% for *BRCA1* and 40% for *BRCA2*.

Ovarian cancer risk was 53% for *BRCA1* and 62% for *BRCA2*. This has not yet been evaluated in the general (non–Ashkenazi Jewish) population.

The pathology laboratory may also have a role in the identification of gene mutation carriers. Multigene panel testing was performed in 1824 triple-negative breast cancer patients unselected for family history.[55] Pathogenic *BRCA1* or *BRCA2* mutations were identified in 11.2% and mutations in other genes in 3.7%.

In summary, in the United States alone there are hundreds of thousands of individuals with unrecognized mutations in breast cancer predisposition genes. At a minimum systematic family history screening should be incorporated into primary care, breast care, and cancer screening activities. The limitations of this approach are well recognized. Novel approaches based on histologic and biomarker features of primary tumors may engage pathology laboratories for genetic risk screening in the future. Universal testing generates new social, economic, and political concerns but does offer the opportunity to identify mutation carriers before they develop cancer.

Genetic Testing Technology

Oswald Avery demonstrated that nucleic acids are the medium of genetic transmission in the 1940s. How a mixture of phosphosugars and nucleotides could encode information could not even be guessed at until Watson and Crick worked out the structure of DNA in 1953. It took many years after that to realize that messenger RNAs (mRNAs) were working copies of specific nucleotide sequences that could travel to the cytoplasm and direct ribosomes to assemble amino acids into specific proteins. Frederick Sanger devised methods to determine the sequence of nucleotides in DNA molecules in 1977. Once this was worked out, it was quickly discovered that small differences in nucleotide sequences could generate abnormal proteins that were associated with inherited diseases.

The search for breast cancer genes began in the 1980s with the collection and analysis of family histories. An early modeling study by King, using 1579 pedigrees, concluded there is an autosomal dominant breast cancer predisposition gene with an allelic frequency of 0.0006, that breast cancer risk is 82% with the gene and 8% without, and that the gene accounts for 4% of breast cancers.[56] Using markers for chromosomal regions, the King laboratory eventually determined that this gene was likely located on the long arm of chromosome 17.[57] It was the group at Myriad Genetics that ultimately identified and sequenced *BRCA1* in 1994.[58] Knowing which part of the genome to sequence and being able to reliably sequence that part in any individual using the methods developed by Sanger led to the birth of clinical cancer genetics as a medical discipline.

Sanger Sequencing

For more than a decade, Sanger sequencing was the primary laboratory test performed on DNA extracted from white blood cells or oral mucosal cells to determine whether an individual carried a mutation in a known breast cancer predisposition gene. Sanger sequencing involves separating the two strands of DNA and then defining the region to be sequenced by allowing short complementary sequences (primers) to bind to the DNA at either end of the region of interest. Double-strand DNA is then rebuilt by filling in the gap between the primers with new nucleotides (A, C, T, and G). Included in the mix of new nucleotides are low

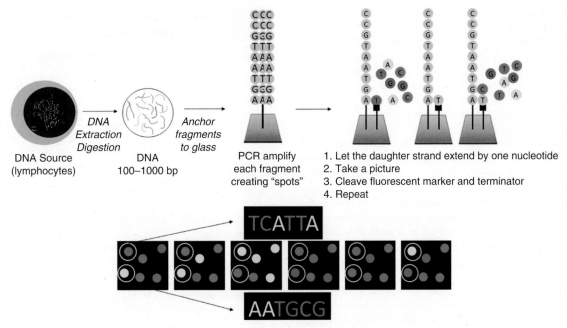

• **Fig. 17.2** The technology behind massive parallel sequencing (next-generation sequencing). *PCR,* Polymerase chain reaction.

concentrations of specially prepared A's, C's, T's, and G's that are labeled with a colored probe that will stop the elongation of the new DNA strand at that point. Several cycles of DNA synthesis in a test tube will produce a mixture of DNA strands of various lengths, each capped with a color marker representing the last nucleotide added to that particular strand. After many cycles of DNA synthesis, the mixture is separated by size using electrophoresis. The order that the colored nucleotides exit the electrophoresis gel will establish the original sequence of nucleotides between the two primer pairs. One limitation of this approach is that only predefined, relatively short (300–900 nucleotides) segments of DNA between the primer pairs will be assessed. A gene like *BRCA2* has 10,254 coding nucleotides so more than a dozen sequencing reactions need to be set up just to assess the coding region. People decide whether other sequencing reactions need to be designed to also assess portions of the promoter region or introns that may contain disease-causing mutations. The point being that sequencing tests in use around the turn of the 21st century may miss important mutations. Another limitation of this approach is that point mutations are recognized by observing two colors coming off of the electrophoresis gel at the same point (one representing the correct nucleotide and one representing the variant nucleotide). If one copy of a particular section of DNA is simply missing (a deletion), only one color will come off of the gel for that section (the normal sequence), and an important genomic alteration will be missed. This is why additional tests to identify insertions, deletions, or rearrangements of entire sections of the DNA have been gradually added to genetic testing protocols over time.

Next Generation Sequencing

Massive parallel sequencing, or next-generation sequencing (NGS), became commercially available in 2005. There are several iterations of the technology, but in general, DNA is minced up to generate short fragments that are then widely distributed across glass surfaces.[59] Each short fragment is duplicated several times to create bundles of DNA with the same sequence. These appear as spots on an imaging screen. Reagents, which include color-labeled nucleotides, are sequentially added and washed away. Each spot is photographed between each cycle. The color of a given spot after any cycle corresponds to the specific nucleotide most recently bound to the immobilized DNA strands at that location. In this way, a nucleotide sequence is generated for each spot (Fig. 17.2). Each sequencing test will include tens of thousands to millions of spots, each generating 50 to 100 base sequences. Translating this enormous data set into nucleotide sequences for specific regions of the genome is a daunting task that is done by computers. First, each individual sequence is aligned to a standard human genome to determine exactly what part of the genome is represented. Because of the random nature of the initial DNA digestion and spot creation, each nucleotide of interest will occur several times on overlapping sequences. Statistical filters are used to assess the quality of nucleotide calls based on the number of replicates generated by the test and the consistency of the calls between replicates. Comparison of the test genome with the standard genome will reveal tens of thousands of sequence variants for any given individual. This very long variant list can be shortened by ignoring known polymorphisms and by focusing only on specific regions of interest (e.g., the *BRCA1* gene). Nevertheless, NGS produces a wealth of sequence variants that pose a problem for interpretation. Technically, NGS is reliable and will identify the same mutations identified by Sanger sequencing.[60–62] NGS can identify large insertions, deletions and rearrangements missed by Sanger sequencing but may have difficulty recognizing small rearrangements.

Large Rearrangements

All of the DNA sequencing technologies are highly sensitive and specific for recognizing single nucleotide changes and short insertions or deletions. Recognizing rearrangement of larger regions is more problematic. These large rearrangements account for up to 17% of pathogenic *BRCA1/BRCA2* gene mutations in individuals of Near East/Middle Eastern ancestry and up to 22% for individuals with Latin American/Caribbean ancestry.[63] In 2012 NCCN guidelines specified that *BRCA1/BRCA2* gene mutation testing should routinely include special tests for large rearrangements. Testing before this may not have included this special testing. NextGen sequencing data files generally include enough information to recognize rearrangements if specific bioinformatics algorithms are used to look for them. Some test providers will supplement NGS "allele dose" calculations with additional tests specifically directed at identifying large rearrangements such as microarray comparative genomic hybridization and multiplex ligation-dependent probe amplification analysis. Thus far sensitivity for detecting these rearrangements seems high, though for some platforms, specificity needs to be improved to reduce the false positive rate.[64] Confirmatory testing using one of the classical assays is currently recommended.

Classifying Variants

DNA sequencing of any kind will always identify small differences between individuals or small differences compared with some standard genome. Each variant must be adjudicated on the basis of available evidence. Variants that occur in greater than 1% of the population are generally considered polymorphisms and easily classified as almost certainly benign. Variants that have previously been definitively linked to breast cancer in family studies are more easily classified as almost certainly pathogenic. In the middle, however, is every shade of gray from "variant likely benign" to "variant likely pathogenic." For some variants there is simply not enough information to make an educated guess. These are reported as "variants of uncertain significance."

The American College of Medical Genetics has published guidelines for reporting DNA sequence variations.[65] There are five possible classifications based on the availability of published data and the type of DNA change (Table 17.4). Classification is straightforward for variants that have previously been reported and for which there are quite a lot of data available. For everything else, it is people who weigh the evidence and initially assign a classification.

There are thousands of distinct rare variants in *BRCA1* and *BRCA2*, and the list is rapidly growing for many other genes as a result of increasing use of multigene panel testing. Each new variant is initially classified somewhere along the spectrum of benign to pathogenic based on features of the specific nucleotide change. Certain types of mutations are more likely to be pathogenic than others. These include single nucleotide changes that result in an early stop codon and a shorter than normal protein (nonsense or truncating variants) as well as insertion or deletion of some number of nucleotides that is not a multiple of three. This will result in a shift in the reading frame and often an early stop codon (frameshift). Missense variants are changes in one nucleotide that result in a different amino acid being added when the mRNA is read. Most of these variants are not pathogenic, although some are.[66] Several additional lines of evidence can move the classification toward or away from pathogenic. Variants that have previously been observed in individuals that have other, definitely pathogenic variants in the same autosomal dominant gene are more likely neutral. A variant that occurs in a region that is normally coded exactly the same across many species (i.e., conserved) may be more likely to be pathogenic, as is a variant

| TABLE 17.4 | American College of Medical Genetics Variant Classification Categories |

Classification	Abbreviated Criteria
Pathogenic	Variant causes loss of protein function, which is known to cause disease.
Likely pathogenic	The bulk of available laboratory and epidemiologic data point to loss of protein function and statistical correlation with disease.
Benign	Known polymorphism that is common in the population. Reliable data do not support loss of protein function or segregation with disease.
Likely benign	Available data suggest no loss of protein function; variant sometimes seen in patients with known pathogenic variants.
Uncertain significance	None of the preceding criteria are met, or available data are contradictory.

From Richards S, Aziz N, Bale S, et al. Standards and guidelines for the interpretation of sequence variants: a joint consensus recommendation of the American College of Medical Genetics and Genomics and the Association for Molecular Pathology. *Genet Med.* 2015; 17:405-424.

that causes a significant change in the type of amino acid that is added to the growing protein chain (e.g., switching from a hydrophilic to a hydrophobic amino acid). Variants that occur near the intron-exon boundary can affect the way that mRNA is spliced together and may also be pathogenic. Fig. 17.3 illustrates the nomenclature used to describe these different types of variants in laboratory reports.

Various informatics tools are available to help classify variants. ClinVar is a publically available list of sequence variations and their current interpretation that is maintained by the National Institutes of Health. The Evidence-based Network for the Interpretation of Germline Mutant Alleles (ENIGMA)[67] is an international group devoted to the collection and interpretation of rare variants in *BRCA1* and *BRCA2*. They have developed a software tool to estimate the probability of pathogenicity for any variant using combined evolutionary sequence conservation, family-based segregation and cancer history,[68] tumor pathology, and RNA splicing effects.[69] Some clinical laboratories use personal and family history weighting to assist in the classification of new variants.[70]

Variants of Uncertain Significance

Every new variant identified in a known breast cancer predisposition gene has uncertain significance until it has been investigated as described in the preceding. Many times, at the conclusion of this investigation there are insufficient data to confidently place it anywhere along the benign-to-pathogenic spectrum. These variants are temporarily classified as variants of uncertain significance (VUS). The natural history of most VUS is definitive reclassification over time as new information becomes available. Sometimes this new information is proactively generated by testing affected and unaffected relatives from the same family or by assessing the

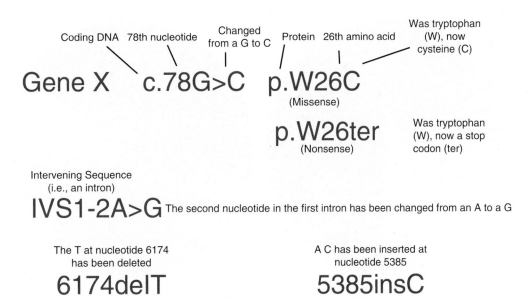

• **Fig. 17.3** Understanding gene mutation reports.

functional significance of the DNA change in the laboratory. Sometimes new information is passively acquired as the same variant is observed in more informative families. The point is that VUS rates are high when a new test begins identifying new variants, but this rate decreases as experience increases. This was observed with *BRCA1* and *BRCA2* gene mutation testing where the VUS rate was 7% to 15% in 2002[71] but had decreased to 2.9% by 2012.[72] VUS rates are somewhat higher for non-Caucasian populations but have declined from 22% to 46%[73,74] to 2.6% to 7.8%[72] in recent years.

The introduction of multigene panel testing has generated a torrent of new variants. VUS rates are currently 20% to 40% for genes that are less well studied than *BRCA1* and *BRCA2*.[75–77] One study that evaluated a 42-gene panel in 175 patients reported an average of 2.1 VUS calls per patient.[60] This degree of uncertainty is understandably unsettling. It will take time to accumulate sufficient clinical and functional data to definitively reclassify these variants. To this end, the Prospective Registry of Multiplex Testing (PROMPT) was established. This is an online registry that collects variant and clinical information from patients who have had multigene panel testing.

Patients whose genetic test result returns a VUS are said to have had a noninformative result. In this case the test was not helpful, and the patient is managed based on the personal and family history. Variant classifications can change over time as more data become available. It is necessary to establish and maintain procedures for recontacting patients if their variant is reclassified.

Multigene Panels

NGS has made it possible to screen numerous genes simultaneously at a significantly reduced cost per nucleotide compared with Sanger sequencing. The first clinical application of multigene panels was in patients with cardiomyopathy.[78] Next-generation multigene panels for hereditary breast cancer first became commercially available around 2010. Early panels did not include *BRCA1* or *BRCA2* because of the Myriad Genetics, Inc. patent on these sequences. On June 13, 2013, the Supreme Court overturned this patent, and subsequent panels included these genes. One effect of this Supreme Court ruling was the introduction of competition into the genetic testing space, which led to multiple choices and significantly reduced costs for patients. Dozens of companies offer hereditary breast cancer panel testing, including several university laboratories. Important questions for the consumer are the following: (1) Are all of these tests equally accurate for mutation detection? (2) Apart from cost, are there any important differences between test providers? (3) To what extent do multigene panels improve the identification of high-risk families?

To measure the sensitivity and specificity of NGS for variant detection, Myriad Genetics, Inc. assessed *BRCA1* and *BRCA2* by NGS for 1864 samples that had previously undergone clinical testing by Sanger sequencing.[62] NGS identified 15,877 variants in these samples, one fewer than had been identified by Sanger sequencing. One polymorphism was missed because a primer for that region happened to overlap the variant. Analytic sensitivity was estimated at greater than 99.96% and specificity at greater than 99.99%. Further validation of an NGS panel that included 25 genes reported 100% concordance with variants identified by Sanger sequencing. In another validation study that included 198 individuals who had undergone standard *BRCA1* and *BRCA2* mutation testing, the InVitae NGS test identified 58 of 59 known pathogenic mutations. One large insertion was missed because no specific deletion-duplication assay was performed at that time and one variant previously classified as pathogenic was considered by InVitae to be a variant of uncertain significance.[60] Other validation studies have reported excellent concordance between NGS and Sanger sequencing[79–81] or between NGS assays performed at different centers.[82]

NGS technology is robust for the identification of single base pair substitutions and small insertions or deletions and can also reliably detect large rearrangements depending on the specific assay design and bioinformatics. Another potential source of variability between test providers is the approach used to manage the very long list of variants generated by NGS to exclude the trivial and recognize the pathogenic. After filtering out polymorphisms, this becomes a very human endeavor that is often more art than

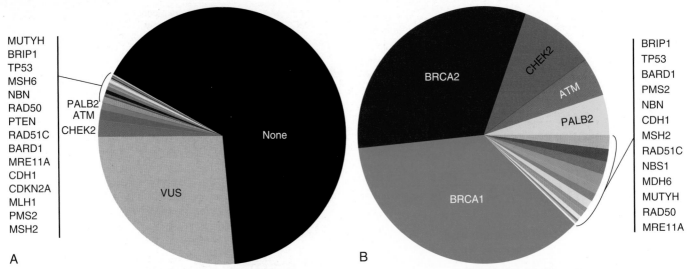

MUTYH
BRIP1
TP53
MSH6
NBN
RAD50
PTEN
RAD51C
BARD1
MRE11A
CDH1
CDKN2A
MLH1
PMS2
MSH2

PALB2
ATM
CHEK2

None

VUS

A

BRCA2

CHEK2

ATM

PALB2

BRCA1

BRIP1
TP53
BARD1
PMS2
NBN
CDH1
MSH2
RAD51C
NBS1
MDH6
MUTYH
RAD50
MRE11A

B

• **Fig. 17.4** (A) Mutations in high-risk families testing negative for *BRCA1* or *BRCA2*. (B) Spectrum of identifiable mutations in hereditary breast cancer predisposition. (Data from references 75–77, 79, 80, and 82.)

science. It is important to understand how each laboratory approaches this process.[70,83] Cost is one straightforward metric for comparing genetic test providers apart from any quality considerations. The cost for hereditary breast cancer predisposition testing can range from less than $500 to nearly $5000 depending on the provider used and the tests performed. On a very practical level, test providers may also be assessed based on the level of service they provide to their clients. This includes legwork for insurance preauthorizations, accurate estimation and constraint of out-of-pocket expenses for the patient, provision for providing testing to the uninsured and underinsured, and vigor with which they pursue VUS reclassification including no-charge testing for family members.

It was anticipated that most apparent familial breast cancer would be explained when testing panels were expanded to dozens of genes beyond *BRCA1* and *BRCA2*. This has not been the case. Multigene panel testing will identify a pathogenic mutation in 4% to 12% of familial high-risk patients who have tested negative for *BRCA1* and *BRCA2* mutation.[75–77,80] *BRCA1* and *BRCA2* mutations still account for 65% to 81% of pathogenic mutations identified on multigene panel testing,[75,79,81,82] with *CHEK2*, *ATM*, and *PALB2* the most frequently affected non–*BRCA1*/*BRCA2* genes. Even with multigene panel testing, most patients with personal and family histories of breast and ovarian cancer will have no identifiable pathogenic mutation, and testing will identify one or more variants of uncertain significance in 19% to 42% (Fig. 17.4).

Managing Cancer Risk

The goal of risk management in mutation carriers is to reduce the probability of developing a breast cancer or to diagnose a breast cancer early when it can be treated with the best outcome and least morbidity. The primary options for managing cancer risk include enhanced surveillance, chemoprevention, and prophylactic surgery. Certain reproductive and lifestyle factors may also modify breast cancer risk in gene mutation carriers. Most available data are derived from studies in *BRCA1* and *BRCA2* gene mutation carriers and may not be relevant to every inherited

TABLE 17.5	Risk-Reducing Interventions by Gene Mutation	
Breast MRI	**Discuss RRM**	**Consider RRSO**
ATM	*BRCA1*	*BRCA1*
BRCA1	*BRCA2*	*BRCA2*
BRCA2	*CDH1*	Lynch syndrome
CDH1	*PTEN*	*BRIP1*
CHEK2	*TP53*	*RAD51C*
PALB2	*PALB2*	*RAD51D*
PTEN		
STK11		
TP53		

MRI, Magnetic resonance imaging; *RRM*, risk-reducing mastectomy; *RRSO*, risk-reducing bilateral salpingo-oophorectomy.
Data from National Comprehensive Cancer Network. Genetic/familial high-risk assessment: breast and ovarian. NCCN Clinical Practice Guidelines in Oncology v2.2016. Fort Washington, PA; 2016.

predisposition syndrome. Table 17.5 lists current recommendations by gene.

Reproductive and Lifestyle Factors

There is evidence that environmental factors, such as parity and alcohol consumption, can modify breast cancer risk associated with common, low penetrance variant alleles (e.g., *LSP1*-rs3817198 and *CASP8*-rs17468277).[84,85] Alcohol consumption is of particular interest because the metabolic byproduct, acetaldehyde, has been shown to damage DNA, leading to *BRCA1* activation.[86] Nevertheless, available epidemiologic data have not identified an association between alcohol consumption and breast cancer risk among *BRCA1* or *BRCA2* gene mutation carriers.[87,88] In general, convincing examples of gene-environment interactions are rare for autosomal dominant breast cancer predisposition syndromes, and where such data exist, the effects are inconsistent. A recent review of the literature and meta-analysis suggested that late age at first live birth and lactation reduced breast cancer risk in *BRCA1* mutation carriers, but data were insufficient for *BRCA2* mutation carriers.[89] An alternative interpretation of the available data is that parity and age at first live birth do not modify breast cancer risk in *BRCA1* mutation carriers,[90–94] although lactation may reduce risk.[94–96] There is also evidence suggesting that, for *BRCA2* mutation carriers, pregnancies do not reduce breast cancer risk the same way they do in nonmutation carriers and may even increase risk with greater risk at later ages at first live birth.[90–92,97] Similar to other women, combined hormone replacement therapy with estrogen and progestin seems to increase breast cancer risk in mutation carriers, whereas estrogen-only therapy does not.[98] Finally, weight gain in adulthood and higher caloric intake have been associated with increased breast cancer risk and earlier age at diagnosis in *BRCA1* and *BRCA2* mutation carriers.[99,100] It seems reasonable to counsel *BRCA1* and *BRCA2* mutation carriers to avoid weight gain in adulthood. However, given the inconsistency of available data and the interpretation of these data, childbearing decisions should be left to the individual, but lactation encouraged as long as it is not considered a substitute for risk-reducing mastectomy.

Enhanced Surveillance

Women with genetic predisposition to breast cancer tend to develop the disease at a younger age when breast tissue is dense and the sensitivity of mammography is low. The sensitivity of MRI ranges from 77% to 100% in high-risk women (compared with 12.5%–40.0% for mammography) and the specificity from 81.0% to 98.9% (compared with 93%–100% for mammography).[101] The false-positive rate is higher for MRI than mammography but not excessively so. Screening MRI increases the diagnosis of smaller, lymph-node-negative breast cancers[102] but has not yet been shown to improve survival.[103,104]

Per NCCN guidelines,[36] women with a genetic predisposition to breast cancer should be familiar with their breasts and report any changes to their health care provider. This breast awareness can include periodic, consistent breast self-examination (BSE) and should begin at age 18. Clinical breast examinations by a health care provider should be done every 6 to 12 months starting at age 20 to 25 years or 5 to 10 years before the earliest known breast cancer in the family (whichever comes first). Enhanced surveillance includes breast imaging starting between ages 20 and 29 years in Li-Fraumeni syndrome, between 25 and 29 years in hereditary breast and ovarian cancer (HBOC) syndrome, and between 30 and 35 years in Cowden syndrome, or 5 and 10 years before the earliest known breast cancer in the family (whichever comes first). Mammography and breast MRI are obtained yearly at 6-month intervals. Annual mammography is generally not recommended before age 30 because of evidence that exposure to diagnostic radiation before age 30 is associated with an increased breast cancer risk.[105–107]

The American Cancer Society supports screening MRI for anyone with lifetime breast cancer risk greater than 20%.[23] This would include most anyone with a pathogenic mutation in any of the established breast cancer predisposition genes included in the modern genetic testing panels. The NCCN guidelines[36] have specifically endorsed enhanced surveillance with MRI for *BRCA1*, *BRCA2*, *ATM*, *CHEK2*, *PALB2*, *TP53*, *CDH1*, *PTEN*, and *STK11*.

There are no established guidelines for ovarian cancer screening. Transvaginal sonography and CA 125 measurements can be performed every 6 months at the physician's discretion, but this approach will not diagnose ovarian cancer at an earlier, more treatable stage and will not improve survival.[108,109] It is not a substitute for bilateral salpingo-oophorectomy.

Men with a *BRCA1* or *BRCA2* mutation should practice breast self-examination starting at age 35. Routine screening mammography is not recommended. Prostate cancer screening with digital rectal examination and PSA measurements is recommended for *BRCA2* mutation carriers beginning at age 40.

Chemoprevention

Tamoxifen has been shown to reduce breast cancer risk by nearly 50% even for women with up to three first-degree relatives with breast cancer[110] but has not yet been shown to improve survival. Because tamoxifen is associated with an increased risk for endometrial cancer and thromboembolic events, especially in postmenopausal women, its safety profile is better in premenopausal women.[111] Chemoprevention options for postmenopausal women also include raloxifene,[112] examestane,[113] and anastrazole.[114] These estrogen response manipulators preferentially reduce the risk of hormone sensitive breast cancer so they may be most appropriate for women with gene mutations associated with a predominance of hormone sensitive breast cancer such as *BRCA2*, *PALB2*, *CHEK2*, and *TP53*. However, there are data showing a 42% to 50% reduction in the risk of contralateral breast cancer in *BRCA1* mutation carriers,[115–117] a group that is at greatest risk for estrogen receptor (ER)-negative breast cancer. It should be noted, however, that data from the NSABP P1 Breast Cancer Prevention Trial suggested that tamoxifen reduced risk in *BRCA2* but not *BRCA1* carriers.[118] The number of mutation carriers included in this trial was quite small so this conclusion may be suspect. Chemoprevention can reasonably be considered for any high-risk woman, but the age distribution of breast cancer risk, the US Food and Drug Administration statements approving tamoxifen for women older than 35 years, and a trend toward later age at childbearing makes chemoprevention an uncommon choice among the genetic high risk.[119]

Oral contraceptive use is convincingly associated with a 50% reduction in ovarian cancer risk among *BRCA1* and *BRCA2* gene mutation carriers.[120–123] The effects of modern, low-dose oral contraceptives on breast cancer risk are uncertain because available data are conflicting.[89] NCCN guidelines do not specifically recommend oral contraceptives for ovarian cancer chemoprevention in mutation carriers, but genetics experts generally support 5 years of oral contraceptive exposure as a way to reduce ovarian cancer risk.

Risk-Reducing Surgery

Bilateral Salpingo-Oophorectomy

Lifetime ovarian cancer risk for *BRCA1* mutation carriers is 39% to 59% and for *BRCA2* carriers 11% to 18%.[8,10,11] Other genes associated with increased ovarian cancer risk include *BRIP1*, *RAD51C*, *RAD51D*, *MSH2*, *MLH1*, *PMS2*, *MSH6*, *PALB2*, and *BARD1*.[124] *BRCA1/2*-associated ovarian cancers are high-grade serous or undifferentiated carcinomas that are typically metastatic at presentation. Most of these tumors arise in one of the fallopian tubes.[125] Median age at ovarian cancer diagnosis for *BRCA1/2* mutation carriers is 51 years.[126] Annual incidence peaks between ages 50 and 59 for *BRCA1* carriers and 60 to 69 for *BRCA2* carriers.[127]

Risk-reducing bilateral salpingo-oophorectomy (RRSO) reduces ovarian cancer risk by 72% to 85% in *BRCA1/BRCA2* gene mutation carriers[127–130] and is also associated with a 60% to 77% reduction in all-cause mortality.[127,130] Specialized protocols for performing the surgery and processing the specimens have been recommended[131–133] as clinically occult cancer can be identified in 4% to 5%.[134]

Case-control and cohort data suggest that bilateral salpingo-oophorectomy also reduces breast cancer risk by 50%.[129,135] There is some evidence that risk reduction is greater when the procedure is performed at a younger age.[135,136] The effect may be larger for *BRCA2* carriers than *BRCA1* carriers.[128] Some have argued that the breast cancer risk reduction observed with RRSO is a statistical aberration resulting from unmanaged bias[137]; others have refuted this.[138] For the time being, it seems prudent to recommend RRSO for the ovarian cancer and mortality benefits without relying too heavily on the procedure for breast cancer risk reduction.

Because it is increasingly recognized that hereditary ovarian cancers most commonly arise in the tubes and not the ovary proper, there is increasing interest in performing salpingectomy alone and leaving the ovaries intact.[139] There are currently no data quantifying the risk reduction afforded by this approach, and it is unlikely that breast cancer risk would be reduced. The current standard of care is to consider bilateral salpingo-oophorectomy after childbearing is complete or about age 35 to 40. NCCN guidelines recommend consideration of risk-reducing salpingo-oophorectomy for women found to carry pathogenic mutations in *BRCA1, BRCA2,* Lynch syndrome genes, *BRIP1, RAD51C,* or *RAD51D.*

Abrupt surgical menopause can adversely affect quality of life due to severe hot flashes, vaginal dryness, sexual dysfunction, sleep disturbances, and cognitive changes. Hormone replacement therapy (HRT) should not be withheld for symptom control because short-term HRT does not seem to negate the risk-reducing effect of RRSO.[140]

Bilateral Prophylactic Mastectomy

A recent meta-analysis that included 2635 *BRCA1/BRCA2* mutation carriers reported a 93% reduction in breast cancer incidence for the 627 women who underwent bilateral risk-reducing mastectomy.[141] On the basis of the four studies included in this meta-analysis, it can be estimated that baseline breast cancer risk was 1.7% to 2.8% per year for *BRCA1/BRCA2* gene mutation carriers (34%–56% after 20 years) and 0% to 0.8% per year after bilateral risk-reducing mastectomy (0%–16% after 20 years). Median follow-up was only 3 to 6 years for these studies, so the durability of these estimates is not certain.

After mastectomy, terminal duct lobular units (TDLUs) can be identified in peripheral skin, in the inframammary crease, and in the nipple-areolar complex. Although removing the nipple-areolar complex reduces the number of residual TDLUs, it is not clear that this is required to achieve an acceptably low breast cancer risk. To date, outcomes for bilateral risk-reducing nipple-sparing mastectomy have been reported for more than 300 *BRCA1/BRCA2* gene mutation carriers.[142–148] Incidental breast cancers were identified in 3% to 6%, and with a median follow-up of 33 months, subsequent breast cancer has developed in 3 patients.

Bilateral risk-reducing mastectomy has not yet been shown to improve breast cancer–specific or overall survival in *BRCA1/BRCA2* mutation carriers, but a 2010 Cochrane review concluded that risk-reducing mastectomy is likely to confer a survival advantage in the highest risk women.[149]

Managing Cancer in Mutation Carriers

BRCA1-associated breast cancer is frequently high-grade basal type breast cancer. One recent meta-analysis found that BRCA1 mutation was associated with worse survival,[150] but a second recent meta-analysis failed to confirm this.[151] It is becoming apparent that *BRCA1/BRCA2*-associated breast cancer is more sensitive to chemotherapy of all types than sporadic breast cancer.[152,153] Outcome for *BRCA1/BRCA2*-associated breast cancer is likely no worse than that for sporadic breast cancer in the era of multimodal treatment.

Breast conservation is an option for nearly all mutation carriers provided they are willing to accept the risk of second primary breast cancer. The risk for ipsilateral breast tumor events ranges from 1.7% to 2.7% per year[154,155] but could be as high as 4% per year for very early-onset breast cancer (e.g., age 42 or younger).[156] This risk is modified downward by hormonal therapy for ER-positive breast cancer[115,116] and by chemotherapy.[154] An exception is homozygous *ATM* mutation carriers in whom radiation is contraindicated and possibly *TP53* mutation carriers who may be at increased risk for radiation-induced malignancies.[24] Lifetime contralateral breast cancer risk is as high as 62% to 83% for *BRCA1/BRCA2* mutation carriers.[10,157] There is some evidence that bilateral mastectomy improves survival in this population.[158,159] It is reasonable to encourage oophorectomy in *BRCA1* and *BRCA2* mutation carriers who are treated for breast cancer because this may reduce mortality by 43% to 70%, an effect that seems greatest for ER-negative breast cancer.[130,160,161]

There is evidence that outcome for *BRCA1/BRCA2* mutation–associated ovarian cancer is better than for sporadic ovarian cancer.[162] This is particularly true for *BRCA2*-associated ovarian cancer, which shows enhanced sensitivity to chemotherapy.[163] Nevertheless, ovarian cancer is the main mortality driver for *BRCA1/BRCA2* mutation carriers and clinicians will sometimes be called on to manage breast cancer risk in patients who have completed ovarian cancer treatment. One recent study that included 364 patients with *BRCA1/BRCA2*–associated ovarian cancer reported a 10-year survival of 11% with 10% of patients developing breast cancer.[164]

There is growing evidence that *BRCA1/BRCA2*-associated breast cancer is less sensitive to taxanes than sporadic breast cancer and more sensitive to DNA damaging agents such as mitomycin-C and platins.[165–167] *BRCA1/BRCA2* mutations also predict sensitivity to PARP inhibition.[168,169] Trials of platin agents and PARP inhibitors consistently identify *BRCA1/BRCA2* mutation as the strongest predictor of response.[168,170] There is a growing list of platin and PARP inhibitor trials open and accruing for *BRCA1* and *BRCA2* mutation carriers. Whether this approach will be equally efficacious for individuals with mutations in other DNA repair genes, such as *PALB2, RAD51C, BRIP, ATM,* and *CHEK2,* is not certain, but it is hoped that the development and validation of predictive homologous recombination assays will make it possible to prospectively identify the right patients for these agents.

The Syndromes

In 1988, Newman reported breast cancer was inherited as a highly penetrant, autosomal dominant trait in some families.[56] Germline mutations in *BRCA1* and *BRCA2* were the first to be identified.

Subsequently, other genes associated with a hereditary susceptibility to breast cancer have been identified. These mutations, such as *CHEK2, PALB2, ATM, CDH1, TP53, RAD51C, PTEN,* and *STK11,* confer breast cancer susceptibility, but with varying levels of penetrance. The following provides a brief update on these genes and their associated syndromes (see Table 17.1).

BRCA1 *and* BRCA2

BRCA1 and *BRCA2* (breast cancer genes 1 and 2) mutations are the most common cause of HBOC. *BRCA1* located on 17q12-21 and *BRCA2* located on 13q12-13 are tumor suppressor genes involved in gene stabilization and homologous DNA repair.[171] As with the majority of inherited breast cancer syndromes, HBOC exhibits classic autosomal dominant transmission and can be transmitted from either the maternal or paternal lineage.

Approximately 1 in 400 to 800 individuals in the general population carries a pathogenic *BRCA1* or *BRCA2* mutation.[31,172] Although *BRCA1/BRCA2* mutations are rare in the general population, approximately 1 in 40 individuals of Ashkenazi Jewish ancestry carries one.[54] Among Ashkenazi Jewish women diagnosed with breast cancer, 1 in 10 carries a *BRCA1* or *BRCA2* mutation.[9] Most *BRCA1* or *BRCA2* mutations in the Ashkenazi Jewish population are one of the three founder mutations: *BRCA1* c.68_69delAG, *BRCA1* c.5266dupC, and *BRCA2* c.5946delT. These mutations can be traced to a small group of people isolated by geographic, cultural, and other factors. Additional founder mutations have been identified in various European and non-European populations.[173]

As addressed earlier, the lifetime risk of breast and ovarian cancer in *BRCA1* and *BRCA2* mutation carriers is variable. In the considerable literature on cancer risk among carriers, risk estimates vary based on ascertainment criteria for the studies. Overall, population-based studies show much lower risk than family-based studies.[174] Overall risk of breast cancer in *BRCA1/BRCA2* mutation carriers is estimated to be about 2.5% per year.[175] Recent data show cumulative breast cancer risk to age 80 for *BRCA1* and *BRCA2* mutation carriers is 67% and 66%, respectively, and cumulative ovarian cancer risk is 45% and 12%, respectively.[176] The mean age at diagnosis is earlier in *BRCA1* carriers (44 years) than *BRCA2* carriers (47 years), but age of onset varies by family, particularly for *BRCA2* families.[177] *BRCA1* and *BRCA2* mutations are associated with an increased risk of contralateral breast cancer and this risk is increased with decreased age of incidence of the first breast cancer.[178]

Most *BRCA1*-related breast cancers are both triple negative and basal-like. Breast cancers in *BRCA1* carriers are also more likely to have medullary histology. *BRCA2*-related breast cancers tend to be more heterogeneous than those related to *BRCA1* but are generally ER and progesterone receptor positive.[179]

Both *BRCA1* and *BRCA2* mutations increase the risk of male breast cancer and prostate cancer, but the risk is greater for *BRCA2*. The lifetime risk of breast cancer for men with *BRCA1* and *BRCA2* mutations is 1% and 8% respectively, compared with 0.1% in the general population.[180] *BRCA1* and *BRCA2* mutations also confer increased risk of melanoma, pancreatic and other cancers, but the risk is not high enough to warrant systematic screening.

PALB2

PALB2 (partner and localizer of *BRCA2*) is a Fanconi anemia gene located on 16q12.22. *BRCA1* and *BRCA2* interact with the PALB2 protein to repair damaged DNA.[181] Biallelic mutations in *PALB2*, similar to biallelic *BRCA2* mutations, cause Fanconi anemia and predispose to childhood malignancies. Monoallelic *PALB2* mutations predispose to breast cancer. *PALB2* mutations are found in 1% to 4% of *BRCA1/BRCA2*-negative familial breast cancer cases depending on the population tested[182–184] and therefore are one of the most common of the rare breast cancer susceptibility genes. As with *BRCA2*, the majority of *PALB2*-associated breast cancers are ER positive. Like *BRCA2*, *PALB2* mutations are associated with pancreatic cancer and male breast cancer, yet an association with ovarian cancer is not clear. The estimated risk of breast cancer in *PALB2* mutation carriers is variable depending on the number of first-degree relatives affected by breast cancer before age 50. Antoniou found a 33% risk of breast cancer by age 70 for those mutation carriers with no first-degree relatives with breast cancer, but 58% risk by age 70 for mutation carriers with two first-degree relatives with breast cancer,[12] thus illustrating the importance of considering family history in determining risk in breast cancer gene mutation carriers. Clinically, breast cancer risk in *PALB2* mutation carriers can be managed the same as *BRCA2* carriers.

TP53

Li-Fraumeni syndrome is a highly penetrant cancer predisposition syndrome caused by an inherited mutation in the *TP53* (tumor protein 53) gene. This tumor suppressor gene is important in cell cycle control, DNA repair, and apoptosis and is somatically mutated in the majority of cancers. Germline *TP53* mutations are rare and associated with a wide spectrum of tumors, including very early-onset breast cancer (before age 35), sarcoma, brain tumors, adrenocortical carcinoma, and other neoplasms. Lifetime risk of any cancer in Li-Fraumeni syndrome is 93% in women and 68% in men. Lifetime breast cancer risk is greater than 60%.[185] *TP53* may be involved in about 1% of hereditary breast cancer cases.[186] Li-Fraumeni syndrome–associated breast cancers are most commonly high grade, ER positive and HER2/neu positive.[187] Per NCCN guidelines, breast cancer surveillance in Li-Fraumeni syndrome includes monthly breast self-examination starting at age 18 and clinical breast examination every 6 to 12 months beginning between age 20 and 25 (or at the age of the earliest breast cancer in the family, if below age 20 years). Breast screening includes annual MRI starting at age 20 to 29, annual mammogram and breast MRI for women 30 to 75, and individual management for women older than 75. Frequent mammography should be avoided before age 30 because of the concern of radiation-induced carcinogenesis. Likewise, *TP53* mutation carriers who develop breast cancer and undergo breast conserving surgery with radiation therapy may be at greater risk for radiation-induced carcinogenesis,[24,188] suggesting that mastectomy may be preferred.

PTEN

PTEN (phosphatase and tensin homolog) is a phosphatase enzyme that functions as a tumor suppressor gene. When mutated, the resultant phosphatase enzyme is unable to restrain cell division or signal abnormal cells to die. A variety of benign and cancerous growths results. Germline *PTEN* mutations are responsible for the PTEN hamartoma tumor syndrome (PTHS), which includes Cowden syndrome. Common features of Cowden syndrome include macrocephaly, with head circumference greater than 58 cm in more than 90%, various skin lesions including facial tricholemmomas or skin tags, hamartomas, and extensive benign breast disease. *PTEN* mutations are associated with increased risk of breast, endometrial, and thyroid cancers. There is an estimated 67% to 85% risk of breast cancer associated with *PTEN* mutations.[13,189] Women with *PTEN* mutations diagnosed with breast cancer should be offered the full range of treatment options with recognition that they have a 29% risk for another primary breast cancer within 10 years,[190] and therefore consideration of prophylactic mastectomy is reasonable. Baseline thyroid ultrasound is recommended as well as annual thyroid palpation. Endometrial management is individualized.

CDH1

CDH1 is the gene that codes for the protein E-cadherin. This protein is found within epithelial cell membranes and is involved in cell adhesion, cell signaling, and tumor suppression. Germline mutations in *CDH1* are known to cause hereditary diffuse gastric cancer (HDGC) syndrome. The risk of gastric cancer by age 80 years is 67% for men and 83% for women with *CDH1* mutations, and the mean age of diagnosis is 40 years.[191] Given the greater than 80% penetrance of HDGC and the limits of endoscopic detection of signet ring cell gastric cancer, prophylactic total gastrectomy is commonly recommended for *CDH1* mutation carriers,[192] although this recommendation may need family history–based modification given the recent identification of many *CDH1* mutations in families without evidence of gastric cancer.[193] Women with germline *CDH1* mutations have a 39% lifetime risk of developing infiltrating lobular carcinoma of the breast.[191] This is not unexpected because loss of CDH1 expression is a cardinal feature of lobular breast cancer, and somatic *CDH1* mutations are frequently found in sporadic lobular breast cancer[194] but only rarely in infiltrating ductal carcinoma. Enhanced surveillance with breast MRI, chemoprevention, and bilateral mastectomy could be considered for *CDH1* mutation carriers. The full range of treatment options should be available to *CDH1* mutation carriers diagnosed with breast cancer.

ATM

Biallelic mutation in *ATM* (ataxia telangiectasia mutated) is responsible for ataxia-telangiectasia (A-T), an autosomal recessive neurodegenerative disorder characterized by progressive cerebellar ataxia, dysarthric speech, immunodeficiency, and an increased risk of malignancy.[195] A-T patients are at increased risk of leukemia and lymphoma and mothers of affected children (i.e., obligate heterozygous carriers of an *ATM* mutation) are at increased risk for breast cancer.[196] Increased breast cancer risk has not been reported in A-T patients, but the disorder is usually lethal by early adulthood. The relative risk of breast cancer in most *ATM* mutation carriers is in the 1.5 to 3 range.[197,198] Certain rare *ATM* mutations are associated with up to a 40% to 60% breast cancer risk by age 80 in some families.[14] Because the penetrance of *ATM* mutations varies so widely, precise management recommendations have not been established. The three-generation cancer family history is useful for estimating penetrance for individual families. In general, the unaffected mutation carrier should consider enhanced surveillance with MRI. The full range of surgical options, including breast conservation, should be available to patients with *ATM* mutations and breast cancer because increased radiosensitivity has not been observed in *ATM* heterozygotes.

CHEK2

Another moderate risk breast cancer gene is *CHEK2* (checkpoint kinase 2). *CHEK2* encodes a cell cycle checkpoint kinase that plays an important role in the DNA damage repair pathway.

Several *CHEK2* mutations are associated with increased breast cancer risk in Eastern and Northern European populations including the 1100delC mutation, the I157T missense mutation, and the IVS2+1G>A mutation. The *CHEK2* 1100delC mutation specifically increases breast cancer risk three- to fivefold.[199] Pathogenic *CHEK2* mutations are found in up to 3% of high-risk individuals, making it the most common of the rare breast cancer genes. There is evidence for variable penetrance between families, thus a family cancer history is particularly important to estimate breast cancer risk. One study that included 277 Polish *CHEK2* mutation carriers estimated lifetime breast cancer risk at 20% if there was no family history of breast cancer, 28% for one affected second-degree relative, 34% for one affected first-degree relative, and 44% for both first- and second-degree relatives.[200] There is evidence that breast cancer patients with *CHEK2* mutations have greater risk of contralateral breast cancer and worse breast cancer–specific survival.[201,202] *CHEK2* mutations may increase the risk of male breast cancer, as well as colon, prostate, thyroid, and kidney cancer.[15]

Unaffected *CHEK2* mutation carriers reach risk thresholds sufficient to consider enhanced surveillance with MRI and chemoprevention, given that the majority of *CHEK2*-associated breast cancers are ER positive.[203] Newly diagnosed breast cancer patients with *CHEK2* mutations should be offered the full range of treatment options available to sporadic breast cancer patients. Given the nearly 30% 10-year risk of a contralateral breast cancer in *CHEK2* mutation carriers, consideration of contralateral risk-reducing mastectomy is warranted.

RAD51C

RAD51C is another Fanconi anemia gene that cooperates with other Fanconi proteins, such as *BRCA2* and *PALB2,* for accurate DNA repair. Pathogenic *RAD51C* mutations are found in 1.3% of high-risk families with both breast and ovarian cancer who are *BRCA1* and *BRCA2* negative.[16] *RAD51C* mutations are more prevalent in families with more than one case of ovarian cancer. Data suggest that *RAD51C* mutation carriers are at significantly increased risk of ovarian cancer, but it is less clear that they are high risk for breast cancer. Management should focus on the ovaries. *RAD51C* mutations have been identified in families with only ovarian cancer in the pedigree yet rarely in families with only breast cancer. Until more data are available regarding breast cancer risk with *RAD51C,* it is reasonable to rely on the pedigree to determine whether the breast is at increased risk of cancer.

STK11

STK11 (serine/threonine kinase 11) mutations allow uncontrolled cell growth and are the cause of Peutz-Jeghers syndrome. Affected individuals can be recognized by the characteristic pigmented mucocutaneous lesions and gastrointestinal hamartomatous polyps. *STK11* mutation carriers are at greatly increased risk for pancreas, gastrointestinal, breast, cervical, uterine, and testicular cancer.[204,205] Enhanced surveillance and chemoprevention are reasonable options for the unaffected STK11 mutation carrier. The full range of treatment options should be available to *STK11* mutation carrier with a new breast cancer. The de novo mutation rate is high for this gene so many affected individuals will have no significant family history of cancer.

BRIP1

BRIP1 (*BRCA1* interacting protein) is a DNA repair gene that contributes to the DNA repair function of *BRCA1.* Similar to

PALB2 and *BRCA2,* biallelic mutations in *BRIP1* result in Fanconi anemia complementation group J (FANC J) and predispose to childhood tumors. Monoallelic *BRIP1* mutations confer an eight-fold increase in the risk of ovarian cancer.[206] Carriers of *BRIP1* mutations may have a 2- to 3.5-fold increase risk of breast cancer.[207] Currently there are no consistent guidelines for managing *BRIP* mutation carriers. Bilateral salpingo-oophorectomy, heightened surveillance, and chemoprevention all warrant consideration.

Selected References

5. Lichtenstein P, Holm NV, Verkasalo PK, et al. Environmental and heritable factors in the causation of cancer—analyses of cohorts of twins from Sweden, Denmark, and Finland. *N Engl J Med.* 2000;343:78-85.

7. Ford D, Easton DF, Stratton M, et al. Genetic heterogeneity and penetrance analysis of the *BRCA1* and *BRCA2* genes in breast cancer families: The Breast Cancer Linkage Consortium. *Am J Hum Genet.* 1998;62:676-689.

8. Antoniou A, Pharoah PD, Narod S, et al. Average risks of breast and ovarian cancer associated with *BRCA1* or *BRCA2* mutations detected in series unselected for family history: a combined analysis of 22 studies. *Am J Hum Genet.* 2003;72:1117-1130.

9. King MC, Marks JH, Mandell JB. Breast and ovarian cancer risks due to inherited mutations in BRCA1 and BRCA2. *Science.* 2003;302:643-646.

10. Mavaddat N, Peock S, Frost D, et al. Cancer risks for BRCA1 and BRCA2 mutation carriers: results from prospective analysis of EMBRACE. *J Natl Cancer Inst.* 2013;105:812-822.

11. Chen S, Parmigiani G. Meta-analysis of BRCA1 and BRCA2 penetrance. *J Clin Oncol.* 2007;25:1329-1333.

23. Saslow D, Boetes C, Burke W, et al. American Cancer Society guidelines for breast screening with MRI as an adjunct to mammography [erratum appears in *CA Cancer J Clin.* 2007;57:185]. *CA Cancer J Clin.* 2010;57:75-89.

76. LaDuca H, Stuenkel AJ, Dolinsky JS, et al. Utilization of multigene panels in hereditary cancer predisposition testing: analysis of more than 2,000 patients. *Genet Med.* 2014;16:830-837.

77. Minion LE, Dolinsky JS, Chase DM, et al. Hereditary predisposition to ovarian cancer, looking beyond BRCA1/BRCA2. *Gynecol Oncol.* 2015;137:86-92.

79. Castera L, Krieger S, Rousselin A, et al. Next-generation sequencing for the diagnosis of hereditary breast and ovarian cancer using genomic capture targeting multiple candidate genes. *Eur J Hum Genet.* 2014;22:1305-1313.

80. Maxwell KN, Wubbenhorst B, D'Andrea K, et al. Prevalence of mutations in a panel of breast cancer susceptibility genes in BRCA1/2-negative patients with early-onset breast cancer. *Genet Med.* 2015;17:630-638.

84. Travis RC, Reeves GK, Green J, et al. Gene-environment interactions in 7610 women with breast cancer: prospective evidence from the Million Women Study. *Lancet.* 2010;375:2143-2151.

89. Friebel TM, Domchek SM, Rebbeck TR. Modifiers of cancer risk in BRCA1 and BRCA2 mutation carriers: systematic review and meta-analysis. *J Natl Cancer Inst.* 2014;106:dju091.

A full reference list is available online at ExpertConsult.com.

18

Clinically Established Prognostic Factors in Breast Cancer

CLETUS A. ARCIERO AND TONCRED M. STYBLO

Nomenclature

Prognostic factors have grown in importance as the options for the treatment of breast cancer have increased. By definition, prognostic factors (Box 18.1) are quantifiable data about the tumor or host that provide information about the expected outcome of a population of patients with similar defining characteristics in the absence of systemic therapy. Several facts that follow from this definition are often overlooked in clinical medicine. The first is that the prognostic value, which may be clearly defined for a population, bears only limited application to any individual within that population. Patients should not be terrorized by membership in a high-risk population, and they should not be made to feel invincible by membership in a favorable risk group. The second fact is that with the broad application of systemic therapy, less and less information will become available about prognostic factors in the absence of such therapy. The best example of a prognostic factor is lymph node status, the degree to which the axillary lymph nodes have been colonized by metastatic breast cancer.[1-5]

Some parameters of a tumor that were measured and originally described as prognostic factors are now considered primarily predictive factors (see Box 18.1). The best example of a predictive factor is estrogen receptor (ER) status. It is of great clinical importance as a predictor of response to hormonal therapy. Certain tumor parameters, such as hormone receptor status, are both prognostic factors and predictive factors and may be considered separately for their contributions to each of these areas.

In the past, prognostic indicators were valued both for their ability to offer a glimpse of risk—desired by both the patient and the physician—and, in a related way, the importance of systemic adjuvant therapy. Prognostic factors can be used to define a population of patients at so little risk of progression or recurrence of breast cancer that systemic therapy may be avoided.[6,7] This is recognized as increasingly important now that the series of overviews from the Early Breast Cancer Trialists' Collaborative Group have demonstrated that the relative value of adjuvant therapy applies to all women with breast cancer.[8-11] Only those with truly minimal risk can be dismissed from consideration because the absolute benefit is so small. On the other hand, studies of the adverse effects of adjuvant therapy that were initially focused on

dose-limiting toxicities are beginning to quantify other toxicities, such as neurocognitive dysfunction associated with cytotoxic chemotherapy.[12-14] With the recognition that an improvement in survival accruing to 2% to 3% of certain subgroups may be achieved at a cost of toxicity accruing to 20% or more of the patients, the need for more precise prognostic factors has grown. Can we divide the most favorable groups of women into those at greater and lesser risk in the future? And of at least as great importance, can we identify predictive factors that will allow us to determine—independent of risk—whether the contemplated therapy will be effective against her tumor?

Clinically established prognostic factors are those that meet the following criteria:

- Are reproducibly associated with a better or worse prognosis at a level of clinical utility
- Provide independent information not available by more easily measured parameters (this requires multivariate analysis with other established factors)
- Are reproducible in multiple clinics or laboratories
- Have demonstrated prognostic value in prospective trials

The literature of prognostic and predictive factors is replete with retrospective analysis of data sets. Although these are useful in generating hypotheses, any of multiple parameters may relate to outcome by play of chance in a given data set. If the data set is large, the statistical significance value of such chance associations may appear great. It is only when evaluated prospectively, at best, or in multiple other data sets retrospectively, that prognostic value may be validated. Of such prognostic values, some may be associated with other values, such as nodal status or tumor size. Unless significant additional prognostic information is added, as evaluated with multivariate statistical methods, they lack clinical utility.

The two best established prognostic factors form the basis of clinical and pathologic staging (Table 18.1). Both nodal status and tumor size represent a summation of biologic effects in both the host and tumor that relate to the rate of tumor progression and the time from the initiation of the tumor or the development of its blood supply. Thus a very indolent cancer biologically, long undetected, may present at an identical stage to an extremely biologically aggressive tumor present for a lesser time. Other prognostic factors, such as markers of proliferation, may distinguish between these two scenarios in a specific individual.

Standard Prognostic Factors

Lymph node status
Tumor size
Histologic grade
Age

Predictive Factors

Estrogen and/or progesterone receptor status
HER2 overexpression

The most powerful adjuvant therapy demonstrated to date—tamoxifen in a premenopausal receptor-positive individual or third-generation aromatase inhibitor in a postmenopausal individual—achieved only a 50% reduction in annual risk of recurrence.[10,15] Although the ability to identify individuals who lack ERs or progesterone receptors (PRs) and who will consequently not benefit at all from tamoxifen therapy is a great triumph, greater still will be the ability to define predictive factors that will identify the responders from the nonresponders in the receptor-positive population. This is even more true in the case of cytotoxic chemotherapy.[6,16] Dose-dense therapy is associated with greater population benefit than less intensive chemotherapy in clinical adjuvant trials. Certain data suggest that this benefit accrues from a subpopulation of individuals who require this greater dose density and that many other individuals would do as well with less aggressive chemotherapy.[6,16] Predictive factors that will reproducibly define these subpopulations are the subject of active investigation.

Prognostic Factors

Axillary Lymph Nodes

The degree of involvement of axillary lymph nodes by metastatic tumor cells is the dominant prognostic factor for later systemic disease.[2,17,18] National Surgical Adjuvant Breast and Bowel Project (NSABP) B-04 and B-06 noted a relationship between survival and the number of nodes involved.[19,20] There is also a well-established relationship between the size of the primary tumor and the axillary nodal burden.[21,22] On the basis of this information and more recent studies, oncologists believe that virtually all women with axillary lymph node involvement should receive adjuvant systemic therapy.[23–25] Other prognostic factors and combinations of such factors have repeatedly been shown to be of equal or greater value in a given retrospective database, but when such factors or a combination of factors have been tested prospectively, axillary lymph node status has been shown to be more predictive. This is understandable because any parameters of the primary tumor are surrogates for the likelihood of metastatic involvement. The potential for metastatic spread also depends on interaction with host resistance. Axillary lymph node status reflects actual end-results data on the interaction between tumor aggressiveness and host defense mechanisms. Therefore it is not surprising that it provides the most important prognostic measure available in clinical decision-making.

In patients with clear axillary metastasis, axillary lymph node dissection (ALND) is often performed providing an absolute number of lymph nodes involved with tumor. However, the extent of surgery is a point of debate in terms of outcomes and prognostic information gained. The early trials of the NSABP failed to show any significant survival benefit based on the extent of axillary surgery. The American College of Surgeons Oncology Group (ACOSOG) Z0011 trial, among patients with limited sentinel lymph node (SLN) metastatic breast cancer treated with breast conservation and systemic therapy, the use of SLN dissection (SLND) alone and ALND did not result in inferior survival.[26] However, when specifically examining patients with a heavy nodal burden, prognosis is poor. A recent examination of the Surveillance, Epidemiology, and End Results Program (SEER) database examining triple-negative breast cancer (TNBC) patients noted N3 patients (undergoing axillary dissection) to have a particularly poor prognosis compared with either lower nodal disease burden or a negative axilla.[27] An additional single institution study of 1711 patients with TNBC also revealed decreased survival for patients with nodal disease, but noted that an additional nodal burden did not further decrease survival in patients with N_2 to N_3 disease.[28]

Clinical staging of axillary lymph nodes is notoriously inaccurate: the difference is 33% in clinical evaluation of axillary nodes, even by experienced clinicians. Cutler and Connelly[29] found that among patients who have clinically negative nodes, 38% had evidence of nodal metastases on pathologic examination, and in those who had clinically suspicious nodes, the nodes were pathologically negative 38% of the time. Fisher and colleagues reported that the false-positive and false-negative clinical evaluation rates for axillary nodes were 24% and 39%, respectively, and the overall error in clinical staging was 32%.[30,31] Smart, Myers, and Gloeckler[32] reported that 35% of clinically negative lymph nodes had metastases detected on pathologic examination, and 87% of those considered clinically positive contained metastases. The increased utilization of preoperative axillary ultrasound has increased the identification rates of diseased nodes, yet the false-negative rate of ultrasound combined with core needle biopsy is still 25%.[33] Because clinical staging of axillary nodes is so inaccurate and accurate staging is so important, histopathologic axillary lymph node staging remains necessary to stage patients accurately and assign population risks for considering adjuvant therapy. To avoid the consequences of axillary dissection for those with negative axillae, a variety of radiologic and nuclear medicine techniques for diagnosis have been attempted. Even though some of the techniques (e.g., positron emission tomography, magnetic resonance imaging) may surpass clinical examination in accuracy, they still remain less accurate than surgical staging of the axilla.

The use of SLN biopsy to limit axillary dissection in those with nodal metastases has revolutionized axillary lymph node staging. The adoption of SLN biopsy has, however, introduced other areas of controversy in prognostic factor research. The first issue concerns the additional value of the number of involved lymph nodes in planning adjuvant systemic therapy. If a patient has a clinically positive node, the risk of systemic failure is roughly 70% at 10 years.[34] Independent of the question of control of axillary disease is the question of additional prognostic information related to the number of involved lymph nodes. For those patients with a low nodal disease burden, the requisite prognostic information can often be obtained with a minimal amount of surgery. The results of the recent ACSOG Z0011 trial established that patients with T_1 or T_2 tumors undergoing breast conservation surgery followed by radiation and chemotherapy could forgo further axillary staging when two or fewer lymph nodes are involved with cancer. The prognostic role of the axillary lymph nodes in these patients is the

TABLE 18.1 **TNM Classification of Breast Cancer**

Classification	Definition
Primary Tumor (T)	
T_X	Primary tumor cannot be assessed
T_0	No evidence of primary tumor
Tis	Carcinoma in situ
Tis (DCIS)	Ductal carcinoma in situ
Tis (LCIS)	Lobular carcinoma in situ
Tis (Paget)	Paget disease of the nipple with no tumor (Paget disease associated with a tumor is classified according to the size of the tumor)
T_1	Tumor ≤2 cm in greatest dimension
T_1mi	Microinvasion ≤0.1 cm in greatest dimension
T_{1a}	Tumor >0.1 cm but ≤0.5 cm in greatest dimension
T_{1b}	Tumor >0.5 cm but ≤1 cm in greatest dimension
T_{1c}	Tumor >1 cm but ≤2 cm in greatest dimension
T_2	Tumor >2 cm but ≤5 cm in greatest dimension
T_3	Tumor >5 cm in greatest dimension
T_4	Tumor of any size with direct extension to chest wall and/or to the skin (ulcerations or skin nodules)
T_{4a}	Extension to chest wall, not including pectoralis muscle adherence/invasion
T_{4b}	Ulceration and/or ipsilateral satellite nodules and/or edema (including peau d'orange) of the skin, which do not meet the criteria for inflammatory carcinoma
T_{4c}	Both T_{4a} and T_{4b}
T_{4d}	Inflammatory carcinoma
Regional Lymph Nodes Clinical (N)	
N_X	Regional lymph nodes cannot be assessed (e.g., previously removed)
N_0	No regional lymph node metastasis
N_1	Metastasis to movable level I, II ipsilateral axillary lymph node(s)
N_2	Metastases in ipsilateral level I, II axillary lymph nodes that are clinically fixed or matted, or in clinically apparent[a] ipsilateral internal mammary nodes in the absence of clinically evident axillary lymph node metastasis
N_{2a}	Metastasis in ipsilateral level I, II axillary lymph nodes fixed to one another (matted) or to other structures
N_{2b}	Metastasis only in clinically detected[a] ipsilateral internal mammary nodes and in the absence of clinically evident level I, II axillary lymph node metastasis
N_3	Metastasis in ipsilateral infraclavicular (level III axillary) lymph node(s), with or without level I, II axillary node involvement, or in clinically apparent[a] ipsilateral internal mammary lymph node(s) and in the presence of clinically evident level I, II axillary lymph node metastasis; or metastasis in ipsilateral supraclavicular lymph node(s), with or without axillary or internal mammary lymph node involvement
N_{3a}	Metastasis in ipsilateral infraclavicular lymph node(s)
N_{3b}	Metastasis in ipsilateral internal mammary lymph node(s) and axillary lymph node(s)
N_{3c}	Metastasis in ipsilateral supraclavicular lymph node(s)

TABLE 18.1   TNM Classification of Breast Cancer—cont'd

Classification	Definition
Regional Lymph Nodes Pathologic (pN)	
pN_X	Regional lymph nodes cannot be assessed (e.g., previously removed, or not removed for pathologic study)
pN_0	No regional lymph node metastasis histologically. *Note:* Isolated tumor cell clusters (ITCs) are defined as small clusters of cells ≤0.2 mm, single tumor cells, or a cluster of <200 cells in a single histologic cross-section; ITCs may be detected by routine histology or by immunohistochemical (IHC) methods; nodes containing only ITCs are excluded from the total positive node count for purposes of N classification but should be included in the total number of nodes evaluated
$pN_0(i-)$	No regional lymph node metastasis histologically, negative IHC
$pN_0(i+)$	Malignant cells in regional lymph node(s) ≤0.2 mm (detected by hematoxylin-eosin stain or IHC including ITC)
$pN_0(mol-)$	No regional lymph node metastasis histologically, negative molecular findings (RT-PCR)
$pN_0(mol+)$	Positive molecular findings (RT-PCR) but no regional lymph node metastasis detected by histology or IHC
pN_1	Micrometastasis; or metastasis in 1–3 axillary lymph nodes, and/or internal mammary nodes, with metastasis detected by sentinel lymph node dissection but not clinically detected[a]
pN_{1mi}	Micrometastasis (>0.2 mm and/or >200 cells, but none >2.0 mm)
pN_{1a}	Metastasis in 1–3 axillary lymph nodes (at least 1 metastasis >2.0 mm)
pN_{1b}	Metastasis in internal mammary nodes, with micrometastasis or macrometastasis detected by sentinel lymph node biopsy but not clinically detected[a]
pN_{1c}	Metastasis in 1–3 axillary lymph nodes and in internal mammary lymph nodes, with micrometastasis or macrometastasis detected by sentinel lymph node biopsy but not clinically detected[a]
pN_2	Metastasis in 4–9 axillary lymph nodes, or in clinically apparent[a] internal mammary lymph nodes in the absence of axillary lymph node metastasis
pN_{2a}	Metastases in 4–9 axillary lymph nodes (at least 1 tumor deposit >2.0 mm)
pN_{2b}	Metastases in clinically detected internal mammary lymph nodes in the absence of axillary lymph node metastases
pN_3	Metastases in ≥10 axillary lymph nodes; or in infraclavicular (level III axillary) lymph nodes; or in clinically detected ipsilateral internal mammary lymph nodes in the presence of ≥1 positive level I, II axillary lymph nodes; or in >3 axillary lymph nodes and in internal mammary lymph nodes, with micrometastases or macrometastases detected by sentinel lymph node biopsy but not clinically detected; or in ipsilateral supraclavicular lymph nodes
pN_{3a}	Metastases in ≥10 axillary lymph nodes (at least 1 tumor deposit >2.0 mm); or metastases to the infraclavicular (level III axillary lymph) nodes
pN_{3b}	Metastases in clinically detected ipsilateral internal mammary lymph nodes in the presence of ≥1 positive axillary lymph nodes; or in >3 axillary lymph nodes and in internal mammary lymph nodes, with micrometastases or macrometastases detected by sentinel lymph node biopsy but not clinically detected
pN_{3c}	Metastases in ipsilateral supraclavicular lymph nodes
Distant Metastasis (M)	
M_0	No clinical or radiographic evidence of distant metastasis
$cM_0(i+)$	No clinical or radiographic evidence of distant metastases, but deposits of molecularly or microscopically detected tumor cells in circulating blood, bone marrow, or other nonregional nodal tissue that are no larger than 0.2 mm in a patient without symptoms or signs of metastases
M_1	Distant detectable metastases as determined by classic clinical and radiographic means and/or histologically proven >0.2 mm

RT-PCR, Reverse transcriptase–polymerase chain reaction.

[a]"Clinically detected" is defined as detected by imaging studies (excluding lymphoscintigraphy) or by clinical examination and having characteristics highly suspicious for malignancy or a presumed pathologic macrometastasis on the basis of fine-needle aspiration biopsy with cytologic examination.

Modified from *NCCN Clinical Practice Guidelines in Oncology: Breast Cancer.* Version 1.2016. National Comprehensive Cancer Network.
<http://www.nccn.org/professionals/physician_gls/pdf/breast.pdf>. Accessed December 30, 2015.

presence or absence of disease rather than the absolutely number of involved nodes, as ~27% of patients in the axillary dissection arm were shown to harbor additional nodal disease even when only one or two on the SLNs were positive. At almost 10 years of follow-up, patients in both arms of the trial have similar survival and similarly low rates of axillary recurrence.[26,35]

The identification of a limited number of SLNs invited a focused pathologic examination of these nodes. This has included multiple histologic sections (vs. one or two),[36] the use of immunohistochemistry (IHC) with cytokeratin stains to identify tiny foci of breast cancer cells that escape notice on hematoxylin and eosin (H&E) staining,[37,38] and the use of polymerase chain reaction (PCR) to search for "breast cancer RNA" in these lymph nodes. Complicating this question is the pervasive use of core needle biopsy for diagnosis with the introduction of tumor cell clumps into local lymphatics. This has been demonstrated to lead to in transit cell clumps in the subcapsular spaces of axillary lymph nodes. Although this is clearly different from an established metastasis in an axillary lymph node, it may also reflect tumor volume, lack of tumor cellular adhesion, or other factors that may be of prognostic influence.

Micrometastases to axillary lymph nodes, defined as metastases less than 2 mm in diameter, have been found in some studies to have the same prognostic significance as negative nodes.[3,39,40] Other authors have suggested a worse prognosis.[41–43] However, any difference in outcome between the populations is not dramatic and calls into question whether this is additional prognostic information that should influence individual therapeutic decision-making. A large meta-analysis of 58 studies and 299,533 patients attempted to determine the significance of H&E identified micrometastasis. They noted an overall decreased survival in patients with micrometastasis but could not prove the independent prognostic value of those micrometastases.[44] The utilization of IHC to examine for additional isolated tumor cells or IHC-only metastasis has been discouraged. Based on the results of two large randomized trials, there is minimal to no benefit in determining the presence or absence of IHC positive only nodal disease. ACOSOG Z-0010 examined 5538 patients who underwent breast conservation surgery and SLN biopsy. Survival for IHC-only positive patients was 95.1%, similar to the survival of patients who were lymph node (and IHC) negative at 95.8% (adjusted hazard ratio 0.88, 95% confidence interval 0.45–1.71, $p = .70$).[45] NSABP B-32 similarly examined patients with occult positive nodal disease. There were 5611 patients randomized to SLN versus SLN and immediate axillary dissection. Survival in patients with occult nodal disease had a 5-year survival rate of 94.6% versus 95.8% for patients who were node negative. Although there was a statistically significant decrease in survival in patients harboring occult nodal disease, the authors noted that isolated tumor cells/micrometastasis do not have the same prognostic value as macrometastatic disease deposits within axillary lymph nodes.[46]

Because virtually all women with axillary lymph nodes involved by breast cancer metastases will be offered adjuvant systemic therapy, it is in advising node-negative patients concerning adjuvant therapy decisions that all the other prognostic and predictive factors are considered.

Tumor Size

Tumor size has historically been the most important single, secondary prognostic factor for risk of recurrence and consequent benefit from systemic therapy in axillary node–negative breast cancer. A recent examination of survival and tumor size noted that survival is improved in patients with tumors less than 5 mm versus tumors only slightly larger at 5 to 10 mm.[47] Colzani and coworkers also noted poorer prognosis in patients with primary tumors greater than 20 mm in size.[48]

Tumor size is also related to nodal status, with the increasing tumor diameter related to increased rates of nodal metastases.[17] The relationship between the size of the primary tumor and prognosis in breast cancer was examined by studies in the 1960s. Fisher and colleagues examined a cohort of patients (2578) from the NSABP files and noted that as the size of the tumor increased, so did the number of positive lymph nodes.[18] They also noted a commensurate drop in survival. However, the authors pointed out that it was not a direct relationship and that both tumor size and nodal positivity had prognostic value individually. In fact, outcomes with a similar number of positive lymph nodes will have decreasing survival with increasing tumor size. Rosen and coworkers noted that tumor size 1 cm or smaller was associated with a very favorable prognosis.[49] Carter and colleagues noted that as tumors increased in size (from 1–2 to 5 cm), survival dropped from 68% to approximately 48% in patients with N$_2$+ disease.[17] Modern series have echoed these earlier conclusions. Axillary nodes were involved in 15% of patients with tumors smaller than 1.1 cm in diameter and in 60% of those with tumors 5.5 cm in diameter or larger. Small tumors associated with positive nodes had a better prognosis than large tumors with positive nodes. Survival decreased with increasing tumor size in all node categories.[50] In examining 1894 patients with tumor ranging in size from 0.1 cm to 5 cm, Narod noted that tumor size was a strong predictor of survival in all groups, but the strongest correlation was noted in node-positive patients.[51]

More recent studies have examined the different subtypes of breast cancer, in terms of hormone receptor status and tumor size as prognostic indicators. When examining ER-negative and HER2-positive tumor, there remains a strong association between tumor size and survival.[52] However, the prognostic value of tumor size and axillary metastases, for that matter, is somewhat altered in patients with triple-negative disease. Although larger tumor size still equates to poorer overall prognosis in TNBC patients, its relationship with node positivity is different. A retrospective examination of TNBC patients noted that the rate of node positivity did not correlate with tumor size in the same manner that non-TNBC patients did.[53] Interestingly, in another study, TNBC patients with smaller tumors and a heavy nodal disease burden (T$_{1a}$N$_2$+) actually exhibited lower breast cancer–specific survival than those with larger primary tumors (T$_{1b}$N$_2$+).[54] Some point to these findings as evidence that tumor size is not as prognostically important as nodal status in TNBC.

Subsequent studies in the chemotherapeutic era have reinforced the importance of a prognostic break at 1 cm for node-negative tumors with 98% to 99% distant disease-free outcomes.[7,55] Node-negative patients with tumors 1 cm or smaller should receive adjuvant systemic therapy only on investigative protocols based on receptor status. Patients with tumors larger than 2 cm benefit significantly from adjuvant therapy, and those with tumors measuring 1 to 2 cm should be evaluated for risks and benefits based on careful examination of other prognostic factors.

Histologic Factors

Histopathologic analysis is based on individual characteristics, such as nuclear grade, gland formation (e.g., tumor grading), or the clustering of various cytologic and histologic features into special types of breast carcinoma. Several histologic grading systems have been described and have prognostic value in the evaluation of breast carcinoma. Two commonly used grading systems were those of Scarff, Blume, Richardson, and Fisher and coworkers.[56,56a] Both evaluated architectural arrangement of cells or tubule formation, degree of nuclear differentiation, and mitotic rate, although each system used distinct and differently weighted histologic criteria. These grading systems have been shown to be poorly reproducible and to have marked interobserver variation. Today the Nottingham combined histologic grade is recommended.[57] Nuclear grading is also subjective, but there is more concordance on grade I of III and grade III of III. Recent examinations of the relationship between Nottingham histologic grade and survival in breast cancer have helped to further solidify its prognostic value. In an examination of 2219 patients with more than 111 months of follow-up, Rakha and colleagues noted improved breast cancer–specific survival and disease-free survival prognostication. In fact, increasing grade from grade I through grade III was noted to lead to decreased breast cancer–specific survival. On multivariate analysis, grade persisted as a strong independent predictor of outcomes.[58] There are indications that the grade of the tumor may reflect the molecular composition of the tumor, portending a much better prognosis with lower grade tumors when combined with other favorable prognostic factors.[59] In fact, regardless of the grading system used, grade I, or its equivalent, identifies a subset of axillary node–negative patients at very low risk of recurrence and death from breast cancer. Grade I cancers up to 2 cm in diameter have a systemic failure rate of only 2% at 5 years.[60]

In addition to nuclear grade, another important indicator of favorable prognosis is histologic tumor type. A number of classifications are aimed at grouping breast cancer according to the histologic growth pattern and structural characteristics.[61–63] Breast cancers generally arise from the two major functional units of the breast: lobules and ducts. Invasive ductal and invasive lobular histologies behave similarly, and the differentiation has no particular prognostic significance. They are further classified as noninvasive or cancers in situ if the malignant cells fail to traverse the basement membrane and as infiltrating or invasive if the malignant cells do invade the basement membrane.

Certain histologic types of breast cancer, even though they are invasive, have a more favorable prognosis. Approximately 20% to 30% of all breast cancers are classified as special, and their frequency has increased as a result of mammographic detection of smaller carcinomas.[64] The histologic features that define special types of carcinomas are present homogeneously throughout more than 90% of the lesion; however, when these features are present throughout only 75% to 90% of the carcinoma, the prognosis may be only slightly better. The three special types of invasive breast cancer are tubular, mucinous (or colloid), and medullary.

Tubular carcinoma has an excellent prognosis.[65,66] It accounts for some 3% to 5% of all breast cancers but may be the most prevalent of the special breast cancers. It is associated with a favorable prognosis when it occurs in its pure form and meets the histologic criteria. Invasive cribriform carcinoma is very similar, both histologically and biologically, to tubular carcinoma.

Colloid carcinoma is a glandular papillary or glandular cystic tumor that demonstrates a high degree of maturity and prominent mucin surrounding the cellular aggregates. It has also been called mucinous or gelatinous carcinoma. A favorable prognosis is associated with colloid carcinoma only when it occurs in the pure form. It accounts for 2% to 4% of all invasive breast cancers and usually affects older women. Women who have pure mucinous carcinomas have a 10-year survival rate of approximately 90%. It is more often seen in the mixed form and, in that context, does not have the favorable prognosis.[30,67–71] Generally, special-type carcinomas are low grade. An exception is medullary carcinoma.

Medullary carcinoma is a parenchyma-rich tumor with little stroma that shows a marked lymphoid infiltrate. These tumors have a favorable prognosis despite a high degree of cellular pleomorphism and a high mitotic rate. Generally, the tumors are well circumscribed and may be large, but size does not seem to affect prognosis adversely.[72,73] Medullary carcinomas account for 5% to 7% of all breast cancers. Bloom, Richardson, and Field,[74] in a 20-year follow-up, reported a 74% survival rate for patients with medullary carcinoma, compared with 14% for those who had other types. Typical medullary breast carcinoma is a favorable histologic type of breast carcinoma with very good prognosis for pathologically node-negative patients.[75]

Pure infiltrating papillary carcinoma is rare, accounting for only 0.3% to 1.5% of all breast cancers. Intraductal papillary growth is a common component of breast cancer of many other histologic types, and like colloid carcinoma, unless the papillary carcinoma is present in the pure form, it is not associated with a more favorable prognosis.[76]

Adverse histologic features such as lymphatic vessel or blood vessel invasion may be noted at the time of diagnosis. These findings are strongly related to the presence of lymph node metastases and are consequently of moderate prognostic significance. There have been studies suggesting lymphovascular invasion (LVI) as a prognostic marker, even calling for its inclusion in the staging of breast cancers.[77] Mirza and coworkers performed a meta-analysis examining prognostic factors for early-stage, node-negative tumors and noted lymphovascular invasion to be significantly associated with survival.[78] A more recent examination placed patients into high- and low-risk categories based on tumor size, age, tumor grade, and receptor status. Although a significant association between LVI and survival was noted for high-risk tumors, there was no association noted for low-risk tumors. The authors concluded that although LVI could provide prognostic information for some subgroups, its role as an independent prognostic factor for all breast cancer patients was not supported.[79] Despite the association with increased risk, LVI is not of independent significance sufficient for them to influence clinical decision-making regarding such things as systemic therapy.

Age and Race

Age at diagnosis has proved to be an important prognostic factor. Younger age is a major risk factor for bad outcome in breast cancer. A multivariate analysis of more than 4000 women younger than 50 years of age demonstrated that the hazard ratio set at 1 for women 40 to 44 years of age and 45 to 49 years of age, was 1.8 for those younger than 30 years of age, 1.7 for those 30 to 34, and 1.5 for those 35 to 39. These differences were highly statistically significant.[80] There have been numerous reviews of population studies examining race as an independent prognostic marker in breast cancer. Using SEER data, Eley noted a higher mortality for African Americans, but this was not statistically significant when other variables were controlled.[81] Simon and Severson did not identify race as an independent predictor of survival in their study.[82] Joslyn and West also used SEER data to examine race and breast cancer survival. Race was an independent predictor of survival in this study and others.[83–85] This epidemiologic observation that race is associated with mortality almost certainly reflects differences in the molecular biology of breast cancer in these populations.[86]

Predictive and Prognostic Factors

Steroid Receptors

The measurement of ERs and PRs is standard practice in the evaluation of patients with primary breast cancer. The measurement can be performed accurately on paraffin-embedded sections of formaldehyde-fixed breast tissue by using immunohistochemical assays, and results correlate well with those of the biochemical (Dextran-coated charcoal) assays. Results from paraffin-embedded sections agree closely with those from frozen sections, so frozen tissue is not needed for optimal results.[87]

Although there is a modest prognostic effect of receptor status, it disappears by 5 years. Much data on the prognostic significance of hormone receptor assays is confounded by the predictive value of receptor positivity. Data from both the NSABP and the National Cancer Institute Breast Intergroup have been confirmed by the Early Breast Cancer Trialists' Collaborative Overview of all randomized trials.[10] These all show that the benefits of tamoxifen, the most potent therapy in preventing systemic failure of breast cancer, are confined to patients with receptor-positive tumors. Thus the treatment benefit prediction confounds the prognostic value except when it is measured in patients who have not received systemic therapy.

DNA and Proliferative Markers

Cell proliferation can also be assessed with immunohistochemical assays that detect and quantify cellular proteins unique to proliferating cells in either single cells or tissue sections.[88] Proliferation-dependent antigens have been identified, including ki67 and proliferating cell nuclear antigen (PCNA), that have been proposed as predictive and/or prognostic markers.[89] Several meta-analyses pointed to an association between ki67, as well as PCNA, with risk of both relapse and overall survival.[90] Inwald and colleagues examined 3658 cases at a single center, noting that ki67 was an independent prognostic factor for both disease-free and overall survival.[91] However, the recurring issue with the utilization of proliferation markers, ki67 in particular, is reproducibility. Examining the reproducibility of ki67 scoring on an international level, Polley and coworkers noted laboratories displayed a high intrareproducibility yet a low interreproducibility.[92] They noted issues such as tumor region selection, counting method as well as subjective assessment of staining as factors in the differential scoring. Similarly, Vörös and coworkers found both inter- and intraobserver reproducibility of ki67 scoring to be poor.[93] Overall, it is unclear whether measures of proliferation (specifically ki67) are superior to the less expensive measure of histologic grade assessed at the time of diagnosis.

Epidermal Growth Factor Receptor Family

Primary breast cancers express a myriad of growth factors, and their receptors are targets for therapy.[94] Some of these are estrogen regulated, some are prognostically important, and the role of many remains unknown.[95] Epidermal growth factor receptors are upregulated in approximately 25% to 40% of breast cancers,

usually ER-negative cases.[96] The upregulation occurs at a transcriptional level. Overexpression of epidermal growth factor receptor is associated with poor prognosis and hormone resistance[80,97] in lymph node–positive and lymph node–negative cases. Another member of the family, HER2, is overexpressed in 20% to 30% of cases, usually as a result of gene amplification.[98] It usually results in overexpression of the encoded transmembrane protein p185. This is associated with poorer prognosis for lymph node–positive cases, and coexpression with epidermal growth factor receptors contributes to a particularly poor outcome.[99] The value of HER2 overexpression is a predictive factor for response to the anti-HER2 drugs trastuzumab (Herceptin) and pertuzumab (Perjeta) and to the small-molecule inhibitor of the tyrosine kinase domains of HER1 and HER2 lapatinib (Tykerb).[100] It is best assayed with fluorescence in situ hybridization (FISH), although immunohistochemical stains can be used to select candidates for FISH analysis. IHC-negative or 1+ tissue is extremely unlikely to overexpress HER2 when studied with FISH. Results may vary among studies depending on the type of assay used and the target of the antibody in IHC assays. Controversy reigns over the role of HER2 overexpression as a predictive factor for tamoxifen resistance, sensitivity to certain cytotoxic agents, or dose density of chemotherapy. In the past, it was suggested that pregnancy-associated breast cancer has a poor prognosis. When pregnant patients are matched stage-for-stage with control subjects, survival seems equivalent, although pregnant patients have more advanced-stage disease.[99,101]

Summary

How can all of these various prognostic factors be used to make rational treatment decisions? The first step in the process is to determine recurrence probability for the subpopulation of patients with a similar profile of established prognostic factors. Oncologists agree that axillary nodal metastases mark a population of breast cancer patients who should receive adjuvant systemic therapy. Within this group of patients the number of involved axillary lymph nodes remains the most powerful predictor of prognosis, overwhelming the results of the other factors.

In the absence of nodal metastases, tumor size and grade or proliferative index, together with the possibility of special histologies, allow patients to be sorted into groups of extremely low risk or increasing risk. The following have a very low risk of distant metastatic disease and hence the most favorable prognosis:

- In situ breast carcinoma: <1% at 10 years
- T_{1a} or T_{1b} N_0 M_0 invasive breast carcinoma: <2% at 10 years
- T_1 N_0 M_0 histologic grade I invasive breast carcinoma: ~2% at 5 years

Some oncologists have suggested that adjuvant systemic therapy is appropriate for all patients with invasive breast cancer, regardless of prognostic factors. With evidence of neurocognitive deficits detectable in roughly 20% of women receiving cytotoxic chemotherapy, it is difficult to propose its use outside of a prospective clinical trial in the subpopulation with only a 2% risk of failure in the next decade who can expect a benefit of 1% or less. For any not in this group with a most favorable prognosis, adjuvant systemic therapy should be considered.

If prognostic factors can identify the populations at risk, predictive factors can identify therapies that will not be effective for certain subgroups. Hormone receptor–negative tumors will not respond to tamoxifen, and tumors that do not overexpress HER2 will not respond to HER2/neu biologics. Decades of basic and clinical research have identified breast cancer as a heterogeneous disease with ever-evolving prognostic and predictive indicators. Targeted therapies have been developed for subclasses of breast cancer, such as hormonal therapies (tamoxifen, aromatase inhibitors) and biologic therapies (trastuzumab, pertuzumab, and lapatinib). These targeted therapies have initiated a molecular revolution in an effort to explain them. Gene expression profiling seems to confirm that the biological heterogeneity of breast cancer has implications for treatment. One such predictor is the intrinsic-subtype classifier, which uses gene-expression profiles to distinguish among breast cancers on the basis of either their cell type of origin—the luminal cell (which is ER positive) or the basal cell (which lacks expression of ER, PR, and HER2)—or whether the tumor is HER2 positive[102] (see Chapter 19).

The prognostic value of several multiple gene expression patterns or signatures using cDNA arrays has been reported. The Amsterdam group identified a 70-gene signature as an independent predicting factor for the risk of early distant metastasis.[103] Another multiple-gene approach has been developed in the United States using multiple reverse-transcriptase polymerase chain reaction (RT-PCR) assays to quantify expression of several genes in formalin-fixed paraffin embedded tissue. The 21-gene signature was analyzed as a prognostic factor and a predictive factor. The results suggest that the high recurrence score group is also predictive of response to chemotherapy (with little or no benefit of chemotherapy in the low and intermediate groups). When the recurrence score was added to age and tumor size in a multivariate Cox model, the recurrence score remains the only independent prognostic factor with a hazard ratio of 3.21 (95% confidence interval 2.23–4.61, $p < .001$).[15] DNA microarrays have made a significant contribution to classifying tumor samples into groups that can predict clinical behavior. In the 21-gene assay, neither size nor patient age were independent prognostic factors.[102]

Can the traditional anatomic prognostic indicators be supplanted by biological ones? At present, it is not clear whether the quantification of the level of expression of dozens or hundreds of genes provides more information about the potential of a cancer for metastasis, virulence,[104] and response to therapy for an individual patient than does an optimal analysis of the standard and readily available histopathologic prognostic factors. These diagnostic advances led to the Microarray in Node-Negative Disease May Avoid Chemotherapy (MINDACT) and the Trial Assigning Individualized Options for Treatment (TAILORx) studies.[105,106] The MINDACT investigators used a 70-gene signature analysis to determine prospectively which patients with ER-positive, node-negative breast cancer benefit from adjuvant chemotherapy and which patients have a risk of recurrence sufficiently low that chemotherapy is unlikely to change their outcome. When specifically examining patients with a high clinical but low genomic risk of recurrence, they noted a 1.5% improvement in 5-year distant metastasis-free survival in patients receiving chemotherapy.[105] These results seemed to echo the early results of the TAILORx study. Examining patients with a low 21-gene recurrence score (0–10) yet otherwise meeting guidelines for systemic therapy, patients treated with hormone therapy alone had low 5-year risk of distant recurrence (<1%) and any recurrence (<2%).[106] The results of these trials use genomic assessment instead of clinical assessment to determine the benefit of chemotherapy and may mark the beginning of a more personalized approach to the application of systemic therapies.

Selected References

9. Systemic treatment of early breast cancer by hormonal, cytotoxic, or immune therapy. 133 randomised trials involving 31,000 recurrences and 24,000 deaths among 75,000 women. Early Breast Cancer Trialists' Collaborative Group. *Lancet.* 1992;339:1-15.

17. Carter CL, Allen C, Henson DE. Relation of tumor size, lymph node status, and survival in 24,740 breast cancer cases. *Cancer.* 1989;63:181-187.

35. Giuliano AE, Ballman K, McCall L, et al. Locoregional recurrence after sentinel lymph node dissection with or without axillary dissection in patients with sentinel lymph node metastases: long-term follow-up from the American College of Surgeons Oncology Group (Alliance) ACOSOG Z0011 Randomized Trial. *Ann Surg.* 2016;264:413-420.

55. Wood WC, Anderson M, Lyles RH, et al. Can we select which patients with small breast cancers should receive adjuvant chemotherapy? *Ann Surg.* 2002;235:859-862.

102. Perou CM, Sørlie T, Eisen MB, et al. Molecular portraits of human breast tumours. *Nature.* 2000;406:747-752.

A full reference list is available online at ExpertConsult.com.

19

Molecular Prognostic Factors for Breast Carcinoma

OLUWADAMILOLA M. FAYANJU AND ANTHONY LUCCI

Survival after breast cancer diagnosis has improved dramatically over the past 50 years with the introduction and refinement of multidisciplinary treatment regimens consisting of surgical resection, radiation treatment, and systemic therapy. In particular, anthracyclines (e.g., doxorubicin, epirubicin), taxanes (e.g., docetaxel), and now anti-HER2/neu therapies (e.g., pertuzumab, trastuzumab) have been exceptionally effective not only in treating locally advanced breast cancer, but also in enabling less radical surgery through tumor downstaging, prevention of local and distant recurrence, and slowing disease progression in the metastatic setting. However, these agents, particularly anthracyclines, are associated with significant morbidity including but not limited to cardiomyopathy and peripheral neuropathy. In addition, hormonal therapy with selective estrogen receptor (ER) modulators (SERMs; e.g., tamoxifen, raloxifene) and aromatase inhibitors (AIs; e.g., exemestane, letrozole, and anastrozole) has been shown to achieve compelling survival and recurrence outcomes in patients with hormone-responsive disease with side effects that are often better tolerated (at least in the short term) than those of traditional chemotherapy agents. Accordingly, increasing attention has been devoted to improving clinicians' collective ability to discern which patients are most and least likely to benefit from receipt of systemic chemotherapy.

Drawing a distinction between prognostic factors and predictive factors remains relevant with regard to distinguishing models that define risk of recurrence as opposed to those that calculate a response to specific interventions.[1] Prognostic factors are those measurable clinical or biological features of a cancer that provide information about potential patient outcomes before initiation of any therapy. These features undoubtedly reflect inherent tumor biology relating to growth, invasion, and metastases. The major prognostic factors associated with breast cancer include the number of involved lymph nodes, tumor size, histologic grade, and hormone receptor status. For example, the presence of cancer in a locoregional nodal basin is a commonly used and robust prognostic factor, one that is associated with an increased risk of recurrence.[2] In contrast, predictive factors provide information about likelihood of response to a particular therapy (Fig. 19.1). The use of the ER modulators, for example, is important clinically as a predictor of the likelihood of response to hormonal therapy. Frequently, factors may be both prognostic and predictive, blurring the distinction between these two entities. One example of this is the use of HER2/neu, which has significant predictive value for

gauging responsiveness to drugs such as trastuzumab, pertuzumab, or lapatinib, but also carries prognostic value in many studies.[3]

However, our current models of prognostic and predictive factors are quite limited. A large number of tumors recur, despite being found at an early stage, and the ability to better characterize tumors has spurred research for other more robust prognostic and predictive markers. The critical objectives of ongoing research are to develop improved prognostic markers, which are sensitive and specific in their ability to identify individuals who do not require adjuvant treatment, as well as to develop robust predictive markers that will aid in identifying optimal treatment regimens. Molecular genomic assays, which can provide both predictive and prognostic information, have thus emerged as important tools in the pursuit of increasingly personalized treatment for breast cancer.

Genomic assays use tissue samples obtained from a given tumor and facilitate analysis of particular tumor genes that are known to correlate with the natural history of a particular malignancy or the likelihood of that malignancy's responding to various forms of treatment. These genes may code for a variety of tumor characteristics, from nuclear receptors to tumor suppressors, and their expression can be detected and quantified through various methods from microarrays to immunohistochemistry. There are now several commercially available genomic assays that have been developed to assess the appropriateness of chemotherapy in the adjuvant setting, and they are contributing to increased understanding of the heterogeneity exhibited by breast cancer even among patients who have similar clinicopathologic characteristics. Although they were developed for and are still primarily used in the adjuvant, postsurgical setting, their use in the neoadjuvant setting is also being explored. For this and other reasons, we believe they are important tools with which medical, radiation, and surgical oncologists should be familiar and should feel comfortable ordering for their patients. There are advantages to having the surgeon, as part of a multidisciplinary approach to care, identify the appropriate patient for genomic testing. For example, the time to a decision about the administration of systemic chemotherapy is much shorter when the surgeon orders the test than when it is ordered by the medical oncologist. At our institution, the University of Texas MD Anderson Cancer Center, this window of time was cut approximately in half when the surgeon ordered the test, which has obvious benefits for both the patient and the multidisciplinary team. The sooner genomic testing can be ordered, the more likely it is that patients can consult with their

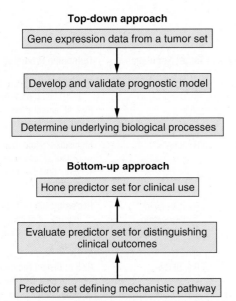

Top-down approach

Gene expression data from a tumor set

↓

Develop and validate prognostic model

↓

Determine underlying biological processes

Bottom-up approach

Hone predictor set for clinical use

↑

Evaluate predictor set for distinguishing clinical outcomes

↑

Predictor set defining mechanistic pathway

• **Fig. 19.1** Two main approaches to the development of predictive markers. (Modified from Liu ET. Mechanism-derived gene expression signatures and predictive biomarkers in clinical oncology. *Proc Natl Acad Sci U S A.* 2005;102:3531-3532. Copyright 2005 National Academy of Sciences, USA.)

medical oncologist with the results of their genomic testing in hand, so that a firm decision on chemotherapy benefit can be made at the time of their initial consultation. Concerns about the surgeon not being qualified to identify appropriate patients appear unfounded.[4]

Here we review the genomic tests that are currently available and/or in development for clinical use in the management of breast cancer and discuss ongoing research related to validating and expanding their utility in different patient populations (Table 19.1).

Genomic Assays

Oncotype Dx

First developed in 2004, Oncotype DX (Genomic Health, Redwood, CA) is a 21-gene (16 breast cancer–related genes and 5 reference genes), reverse-transcriptase polymerase chain reaction (RT-PCR) assay that was developed through a multistep process that involved the following:

1. development of an RT-PCR method that could use formalin-fixed, paraffin-embedded (FFPE) samples;
2. selecting 250 candidate genes based on reviews of the published literature and microarray experiments;
3. conducting studies using three independent cohorts of breast cancer patients (n = 447)—participants in the National Surgical Adjuvant Breast and Bowel Project (NSABP)-20 trial (all node-negative [LN–] and ER+),[5] patients with extensive (≥10 involved nodes) axillary disease who received treatment at Rush University Medical Center (Chicago, IL; included both ER+ and ER– patients),[6] and women treated for breast cancer at Providence St. Joseph's Medical Center (Burbank, CA; included LN+, LN–, ER+, and ER– patients)[7]—to examine the association between the candidate genes and breast cancer recurrence; and

4. using the results of these studies to select the 21 genes for the panel and to develop a genome-based algorithm for predicting recurrence.[8]

The assay was retrospectively validated in 668 tumor samples from women who received adjuvant tamoxifen as part of the NSABP-14 trial, the participants of which all had ER+, HER2/neu nonamplified (HER2–), LN– breast cancer. It was shown to be able to quantify both the likelihood of distant recurrence within 10 years (i.e., is prognostic) and also the likely magnitude of improved distant recurrence–free survival that would occur with receipt of adjuvant hormonal and chemotherapy as opposed to only receiving hormonal therapy (i.e., is predictive).[8,9] Although not formally approved by the US Food and Drug Administration (FDA), Oncotype DX is currently the only genomic assay recommended in treatment guidelines published by the American Society of Clinical Oncology (ASCO) and the National Comprehensive Cancer Center Network (NCCN) and is also recommended by both the European Society for Medical Oncology and the St. Gallen International Breast Cancer Conference for management of invasive carcinoma. A 12-gene version has also been shown to exhibit predictive and prognostic reliability for ductal carcinoma in situ (DCIS), but the small size of its validation cohort size has limited broader adoption.[10,11]

Oncotype DX uses FFPE from surgical specimens to categorize patients into one of three tiers based on a calculated recurrence score (RS)—low (<18), intermediate (18–30), and high (≥31–100)—reflecting their likelihood of distant recurrence in 10 years. In the Trial Assigning IndividuaLized Options for Treatment (Rx), also known as TAILORx, women with an RS of less than 11 were found to have a <1% risk of recurrence in 10 years with receipt of endocrine therapy alone, further bolstering support for a paradigm shift away from mandatory chemotherapy within the context of multimodal treatment.[12] Results from the West German Study Group Phase III PlanB Trial provided additional, prospectively generated evidence that patients with an Oncotype Dx RS 11 or less could avoid chemotherapy without compromising outcomes, even if said patients had clinicopathologic characteristics that would otherwise point toward a high risk of recurrence.[13] The RxPONDER Trial (Rx for Positive Node, Endocrine Responsive Breast Cancer) was initiated in 2011 to explore whether ER+, HER2– patients with limited nodal disease (1–3 LNs) and low to intermediate Oncotype Dx scores would experience decreased survival if chemotherapy were omitted from their regimens; another aim of this trial is to determine whether there is an optimal RS cutoff point for these patients, above which chemotherapy should always be recommended.[14] The 21-gene Oncotype Dx assay is mentioned in the NCCN guidelines as a possible consideration to help guide the addition of chemotherapy in patients with limited (1–3) positive nodes because there is ample data from the Southwest Oncology Group (SWOG) 8814,[15] the NSABP B-28,[16] and the other studies just mentioned to suggest that it provides predictive utility of chemotherapy benefit in patients with limited nodal involvement. The eagerly awaited results from the RxPONDER trial will clarify the role for genomic testing with Oncotype Dx in node-positive patients.

In the meantime, Oncotype Dx continues to be the most commonly used genomic test for breast cancer in the United States. Even though the test can be performed on core biopsy specimens, at our institution, we prefer to order the test on the final pathology specimen rather than the core biopsy sample to minimize the chances we will unexpectedly identify multiple positive nodes at

TABLE 19.1 Genomic Assays for Breast Cancer

Name	Company	Type	Tissue	Laboratory	Target Population	Outcomes Predicted
Breast Cancer Index	bioTheranostics	2-gene HI/ five-gene MGI RT-PCR	FFPE	Reference	ER+, LN–	Risk of distant recurrence 5–10 years post-Dx Risk of benefit from 10 years adj endocrine Rx
BreastOncPx	LabCorp	14-gene RT-PCR	FFPE	Reference	ER+, LN–	Metastasis Score: risk of distant recurrence 10 years post-Dx (low, moderate, high)
BreastPRS	Signal Genetics	200-gene microarray	FF, FFPE	Reference	ER+, LN– with intermediate Oncotype Dx RS	Reclassification into high or low risk of distant recurrence 10 years post-Dx
EndoPredict	Sividon Diagnostics	8-gene RT-PCR	FFPE	Local	ER+, HER2–	Risk of distant recurrence 10 years post-Dx (low or high)
Genomic Grade Index (GGI)	MapQuant Dx	97-gene microarray *or* 4-gene RT-PCR	FF, FFPE	Reference	ER– or ER+, grade II	ER +: Reclassification → low or high risk ER–/ER+: high GGI assoc with ↑ chemosensitivity and ↓ relapse-free survival
IHC4 (conventional)	N/A	4-biomarker IHC	FFPE	Local	ER+	Risk of distant recurrence 10 years post-Dx
IHC4 (NexCourse)	Genoptix	4-biomarker AQUA	FFPE	Reference	ER+	Four categories estimating risk of distant recurrence 10 years post-Dx (low, low-mid, mid, and high)
MammaPrint	Agendia	70-gene microarray	FF, FFPE	Reference	ER– or ER+, LN– or LN+	Risk of distant recurrence 10 years post-Dx (low: <0.4, high: ≥0.4)
MammaTyper	BioNTech	4-gene RT-PCR	FFPE	Local	ER– or ER+, LN–	Improved intrinsic subtyping (especially between luminal A and luminal B)
Mammostrat	Clarient	5-biomarker IHC	FFPE	Local	ER +, LN–, receiving endocrine Rx	Risk of relapse if chemotherapy omitted (low, moderate, high)
NPI +	N/A	4-biomarker IHC; Multivariate model	FFPE	Local	All	Seven biological classes (i.e., refined subtypes) stratified into prognostic groups
Oncotype Dx	Genomic Health	21-gene RT-PCR	FFPE	Reference	ER+, LN–, HER2–	RS: risk of distant recurrence 10 years post-Dx; low: <18, intermediate: 18–30, high: >30
Prosigna (PAM50)	NanoString Technologies	50-gene microarray	FF, FFPE	Local	ER+, LN–, or LN+, postmenopausal, receiving endocrine Rx	Intrinsic subtyping risk of RS (low, intermediate, high)

Dx, Diagnosis; *ER*, estrogen receptor; *FF*, fresh frozen, *FFPE*, formalin fixed paraffin embedded; *HER2–*, HER2/neu nonamplified; *HER2+*, HER2/*neu* amplified; *IHC*, immunohistochemistry; *LN*, lymph node; *RS*, recurrence score; *RT-PCR*, reverse transcriptase polymerase chain reaction; *Rx*, prescription.

operation, thus minimizing the chances of a "wasted" or inappropriate test. Also, Oncotype DX issues separate reports for node-negative and node-positive (N1–3) patients.

MammaPrint

MammaPrint, which was first described in 2006, is a 70-gene DNA assay developed by Agendia (Irvine, CA), a commercial spinoff of the Netherlands Cancer Institute (NKI) and Antoni van Leeuwenhoek Hospital in Amsterdam.[17] It consists of a customized microarray slide that assesses in triplicate the messenger RNA (mRNA) expression of 70 genes initially identified in 78 tumors from a cohort of T1–2, LN– breast cancer patients all under the age of 55 years at diagnosis and treated at NKI; 50% of these patients were ER+.[18] The assay can use either fresh-frozen tumor samples or FFPE. The MammaPrint Index (i.e., score) ranges from –1 to + 1; tumors with a MammaPrint Index less than 0.4 are classified as having a low risk of distant metastasis in 10 years, and those tumors with scores of 0.4 or higher are at high risk for developing distant metastases in 10 years.[19,20]

Initially, MammaPrint was internally validated using only 19 tumors, and its development was criticized for the small size of both the reference and test cohorts. However, its prognostic value was subsequently validated through a retrospective series using 61 node-negative patients from the initial reference group as well as 144 new node-positive patients and 90 new node-negative patients and was found to better predict 5-year overall survival and the likelihood of developing distant metastases at 5 years than the clinicopathologic risk criteria for recurrence found within the then-current guidelines of both St. Gallen and the National Institutes of Health; 77% of the 295 patients in this study were ER+.[18] Retrospective validation was again performed as part of the international multicenter trial by the TRANS-BIG consortium, which included 302 T1–2, LN– patients diagnosed before 1999 who were less than 61 years old at diagnosis and whose treatment was limited to locoregional therapy (i.e., did not receive systemic therapy); 70% of these patients were ER+. The trial was conducted to determine which of three candidate microarrays—MammaPrint, the 76-gene Rotterdam/Veridex signature, or the Genomic Grading Index—should be selected for prospective validation in what would eventually become the MINDACT trial. No significant difference was found between the three methods, and the TRANSBIG consortium ultimately decided to use MammaPrint for prospective validation.[17,19]

The primary objective of the MINDACT trial, which was launched in 2007, was to determine whether patients with ER+ or ER– disease and a low MammaPrint score but who were deemed high risk for recurrence according to traditional clinicopathologic characteristics (as determined through use of Adjuvant Online!) could safely be spared chemotherapy.[19] It was estimated that 10% to 20% of women who would have received adjuvant chemotherapy based on clinicopathologic criteria would be able to forgo systemic therapy without having any adverse effect on their survival. A total of 6693 patients were enrolled in the study between 2007 and 2011 across nine countries; 80% were LN–, 88% were hormone-receptor (HR)-positive (HR+), and 10% were HER2/neu-amplified (HER2+). Patients with concordant high-risk (n = 1806) and low-risk (n = 2745) assessments underwent chemotherapy or did not receive chemotherapy, respectively. Of the remaining patients with discordant evaluations, 592 were deemed low risk by Adjuvant Online! and high risk by MammaPrint, whereas 1550 were deemed high risk by Adjuvant Online! and low risk by MammaPrint. Among the latter cohort of 1550 patients, 748 were randomized to receive no chemotherapy, and of these 748 patients, 644 were confirmed to have no change in risk postenrollment and therefore received no chemotherapy. The primary analysis of these 644 patients in the MINDACT study was presented at the 2016 American Association for Cancer Research meeting, and the full results were published in 2016.[21] The authors reported that after a median follow-up of 5 years, distant metastasis–free survival was greater than 94% in the patients with discordant evaluations regardless of the treatment arm to which they were randomized. Also, 48% of the patients in the group deemed high risk using Adjuvant Online! and low-risk according to MammaPrint had involved lymph nodes. Thus MammaPrint might show promise as a reliable prognosticator for breast cancer patients, regardless of ER or LN status. The study authors found no added value for MammaPrint in patients who were identified as clinically low risk but had a high MammaPrint result. Notably, the MINDACT study was not powered to predict differential responses to chemotherapy, and the results of the trial should be understood in that context.

Mammostrat

First launched in 2010, Mammostrat (Clarient Diagnostic Services, Aliso Viejo, CA) is a five-biomarker, immunohistochemistry (IHC) assay that measures levels of SLC7A5, HTF9C, p53, NDRG1, and CEACAM5 in FFPE tumor samples to stratify patients receiving endocrine therapy for HR+ tumors into three groups, low, moderate, and high, that reflect risk of relapse if chemotherapy is omitted from adjuvant treatment.[22] It has been retrospectively validated in multiple cohorts of patients with ER+, ER–, LN+, and LN– breast cancer; however, its application in the United States remains limited, and it is not approved by the FDA.[22]

Prosigna Breast Cancer Prognostic Gene Signature Assay

Prosigna (formerly called the PAM50 test; NanoString Technologies, Seattle, WA) is based on a 50-gene RT-PCR microarray (PAM50 test) that uses its proprietary nCounter digital technology to process postoperative FFPE samples of invasive carcinoma and assign tumors to one of four intrinsic subtypes: Luminal A, Luminal B, HER2+, and Basal-like. In addition, the Prosigna gene signature also generates an individualized risk of RS (high, intermediate, or low) representing an estimate of the likelihood of developing recurrent disease through an algorithm that takes into account intrinsic subtype, correlation between molecular subtype and a subset of proliferative genes, and tumor size on final pathology. It has been retrospectively validated in postmenopausal women receiving adjuvant endocrine therapy for both LN+ and LN– breast cancer and was cleared by the FDA for marketing as a prognostic tool in 2013.[23]

Breast Cancer Index

The Breast Cancer Index (bioTheranostics, San Diego, CA) represents a combination of two diagnostic tests, the two-gene, HoxB13/IL17BR ratio index and the Molecular Grade Index, a real-time RT-PCR, five-gene microarray assay. It has been retrospectively validated to predict the likelihood of late (i.e., 5–10 years after treatment) recurrence as well as the likelihood of benefit from a 10-year course of adjuvant endocrine therapy in women with early-stage, LN–, ER+ breast cancer.[24,25] Specimens can be FFPE or fresh-frozen. It is not currently approved by the FDA for marketing in the United States.

EndoPredict Test

The EndoPredict Test (Sividon Diagnostics, Köln, Germany) combines EndoPredict, an eight-gene, mRNA-based assay that uses RT-PCR on FFPE tumor samples, with patients' tumor size and nodal status to assign patients with early-stage, ER+, HER2– breast cancer, a score that reflects the likelihood of distant recurrence within 10 years of diagnosis. Patients with a score less than 3.3 are at low risk for recurrence, and those with a score of 3.3 or higher are at high risk for recurrence.[26] The EndoPredict Test is not currently approved by the FDA for marketing in the United States but is approved for use in Europe.

Genomic Grade Index

The Genomic Grade Index (GGI; MapQuant Dx, Ipsogen, France) is a DNA microarray-based assay that uses FFPE tumor samples to measure the expression of 97 genes and assign the tumor a molecular grade. The assay was developed by comparing the gene expression profiles of grade I (i.e., low grade, well-differentiated) and grade III (i.e., high-grade, poorly differentiated) tumors and has also been streamlined into an RT-PCR version that can also use FFPE samples. The test reclassifies grade II (i.e., intermediate grade) ER+ cancers into high- or low-grade categories and thereby confers significantly different prognoses on otherwise similar tumors.[27] High GGI is associated with decreased relapse-free survival in patients who do not go on to receive adjuvant chemotherapy and is also associated with increased sensitivity to neoadjuvant chemotherapy in both ER– and ER+ patients.[28]

IHC4

The IHC4 assay incorporates a semiquantitative assessment of ER, PR, HER2, and ki67 expression using IHC with clinicopathologic factors into a multivariate model for predicting risk of distant metastasis. As originally described, it uses FFPE samples, can theoretically be performed locally, and is a potentially cost-effective method of improving prognostication of early-stage breast cancer with a validated recurrence risk signature.[29] However, its accuracy may be difficult to reproduce in clinical practice given the interobserver variability in IHC assessment, especially with regard to ki67.[29]

The NexCourse IHC4 assay (Genoptix, Carlsbad, CA) purports to minimize this potential variability through use of its internally developed Automated Quantitative Analysis (AQUA) technology for quantification of ER, progesterone receptor, and ki67 expression, although HER2 expression continues to be assessed using IHC or fluorescence in situ hybridization in their assay. In the recently published results of the OPTIMA Prelim trial, there was no significant difference between the conventional IHC4 assay and NexCourse IHC4 with regard to risk assessment for women with ER+ breast cancer.[30] The applicability of this method to clinical practice continues to be a subject of investigation.

Nottingham Prognostic Index/NPI+

The Nottingham Prognostic Index (NPI) is a clinical tool that has been used for more than 30 years to predict prognosis after breast cancer diagnosis. Using a formula that incorporates tumor grade, tumor size, and nodal involvement, patients can be categorized into one of four groups associated with different overall survival estimates, with higher NPIs being associated with worse likelihood of survival at 5 years.[31] More recently, a more granular method of molecular subtyping using 10 vetted biomarkers has expanded the four-tiered intrinsic subtype system, resulting in the identification of seven new breast cancer subtypes: three luminal (Luminal-A, Luminal-N, and Luminal-B), two basal (Basal p53 altered, Basal p53 normal), and two HER2+ (HER2+/ER+, HER2+/ER–).[32] The NPI formula, individualized for each subgroup to only include the most significant clinicopathologic prognostic factors, was then used to further stratify these seven subgroups into prognostic groups, thereby generating a new prognosticator, NPI+ that may prove helpful in clinical decision-making.[32,33]

MammaTyper

MammaTyper is an in vivo diagnostic test (BioNTech, Mainz, Germany) launched in 2015 that categorizes tumors into intrinsic subtypes through quantitative measurement of ER, PR, HER2, and ki67 using RT-PCR of mRNA from FFPE samples. It was developed to improve discrimination between luminal A and B subtypes.[34] The accuracy of subtype classification with MammaTyper has not yet been compared with PAM50 or IHC, and it is not currently approved for use by the FDA.

BreastPRS

BreastPRS (Signal Genetics, Carlsbad, CA) is a molecular assay that uses an algorithm based on 200 genes sourced from a meta-analysis of publicly available genomic databases to stratify patients into groups at low or high risk for recurrence. It can use RNA extracted from either fresh frozen or FFPE samples and was shown to be able to reclassify patients with intermediate Oncotype Dx RS into low- and high-risk designations.[35] It has not been validated in further studies.

BreastOncPx

The Breast Cancer Prognosis Gene Expression Assay (BreastOncPx, LabCorp, Burlington, NC) is a 14-gene RT-PCR assay that uses FFPE samples to assign patients with ER+, LN– breast cancer a low-, moderate-, or high-risk metastasis score that represents an estimated risk of distant metastases at 10 years after diagnosis.[36] It has not been validated in any further studies.

Summary

There is a large and growing cadre of molecular genomic tests to assist physicians in the management of patients with breast cancer, and there are benefits and limitations to all of them. Notably, a recent trial comparing the performance of Prosigna, Oncotype Dx, MammaPrint, MammaTyper, the NexCourse IHC4 assay, and the conventional IHC4 assay demonstrated significant discordance in risk assessment, with approximately 60% of trial participants being assigned to different categories (high vs.

intermediate/low).[30] In this trial, Oncotype Dx assigned the highest proportion of tumors to the low-risk category, thereby potentially sparing the greatest number of women from overtreatment with chemotherapy. Arguments that some of these patients might be undertreated based on low scores appear unfounded based on recent data showing that patients with low Oncotype RSs had recurrence rates of around 1% at 10 years.[12,37,38]

Oncotype Dx is the most widely used genomic assay for breast cancer in the United States and has been the most thoroughly vetted in independent patient cohorts and cost analyses.[39] It is the only test recommended by the NCCN and ASCO for both prognostic and predictive estimations in the management of breast cancer. However, it has been demonstrated to have a high false-negative rate for tumors that are HER2+ and therefore is not indicated for use in HER2+ patients.[40] Furthermore, the intermediate RS category sometimes represents a clinical conundrum for providers, and its accuracy in the neoadjuvant setting has yet to be prospectively demonstrated. MammaPrint was the first genomic assay approved by the FDA and is the most widely used breast cancer–specific genomic assay in Europe. The MINDACT results again confirm that genomic assays trump anatomy for prognostication of breast cancer outcomes.

In summary, a substantial body of evidence supports the use of genomic testing in the clinical management of patients with breast cancer. Judicious use of genomic testing in the context of multidisciplinary care has the potential to expedite the time to treatment and improve personalization of care. HR+, LN– patients with low Oncotype Dx RS derive no benefit from chemotherapy and should be spared the morbidity of this treatment. Future investigation of the prognostic and predictive power of Oncotype Dx and other tools needs to be pursued to help us collectively refine the management of patients along the entire spectrum of breast disease from DCIS to metastatic disease. Development of these tools would allow us to not only determine who would or would not benefit from chemotherapy but also who is most likely to benefit from radiation or even selective metastectomy. It will be important for all physicians involved in the care of breast cancer patients not only to be a part of these investigations but also to be the standard bearers for their application in clinical practice.

Selected References

12. Sparano JA, Gray RJ, Makower DF, et al. Prospective validaof a 21-gene expression assay in breast cancer. *N Engl J Med*. 2015;373: 2005-2014.

21. Cardoso F, van't Veer LJ, Bogaerts J, et al. 70-Gene signature as an aid to treatment decisions in early-stage breast cancer. *N Engl J Med*. 2016;375:717-729.

28. Liedtke C, Hatzis C, Symmans WF, et al. Genomic grade index is associated with response to chemotherapy in patients with breast cancer. *J Clin Oncol*. 2009;27:3185-3191.

29. Cuzick J, Dowsett M, Pineda S, et al. Prognostic value of a combined estrogen receptor, progesterone receptor, Ki-67, and human epidermal growth factor receptor 2 immunohistochemical score and comparison with the Genomic Health recurrence score in early breast cancer. *J Clin Oncol*. 2011;29:4273-4278.

30. Bartlett JM, Bayani J, Marshall A, et al. Comparing breast cancer multiparameter tests in the OPTIMA Prelim Trial: no test is more equal than the others. *J Natl Cancer Inst*. 2016;108.

A full reference list is available online at ExpertConsult.com.

20

Risk Factors for Breast Carcinoma in Women With Proliferative Breast Disease

WILLIAM D. DUPONT, AMY C. DEGNIM, MELINDA E. SANDERS, JEAN F. SIMPSON, AND LYNN C. HARTMANN

The histology of benign breast biopsies is highly variable, and biopsied tissue may range from physiologically normal at one extreme to in situ carcinoma at the other. It thus made sense to subdivide these lesions into biologically meaningful categories and to attempt to determine the cancer risk associated with these different categories. This task has proved to be difficult because the studies must be large, and numerous classification schemes have been proposed to address this question. Many of the authors[1-6] of these schemes have performed concurrent studies in which the malignant potential of benign lesions was judged by the frequency of their association with breast carcinoma in the same biopsy. The problem with such studies is that it is impossible to infer whether the implicated benign lesions are true precursor lesions for cancer, markers of risk elevation, or themselves a consequence of the malignancy. Thus to prove that a benign lesion increases a woman's risk of breast cancer, it is necessary to establish a temporal relationship between the occurrence of the benign lesion and the later development of breast cancer. Several investigators have performed such studies, most notably investigators from the Mayo Clinic,[7-14] the Harvard Medical School,[15-18] the Henry Ford Health System,[19] the Albert Einstein College of Medicine (studying women from Toronto, Canada; Portland, Oregon, United States; and London, United Kingdom),[20] Vanderbilt University (studying the Nashville Breast Cohort),[21-30] and the Breast Cancer Detection Demonstration Project.[31] All these studies used Page's histologic classification scheme for breast disease.[32-37]

The other major challenge with studies of premalignant breast disease is establishing reproducible and biologically meaningful diagnoses. The Nashville Breast Cohort investigators approached this problem with extensive pretesting and devised a preliminary classification scheme that could distinguish between fine differences in breast morphology and cytology and yet be reproducible. This classification scheme was first evaluated in 1978.[24] After revision, it was then applied to more than 10,000 benign breast biopsies, and follow-up was obtained from a suitable sample of the biopsied women. Relative risk estimates associated with the different benign lesions were derived and compared. Our published benign disease categories represent groupings of lesions that are associated with consistent and clinically meaningful levels of cancer risk. These categories and the cancer risks associated with them have been endorsed by the College of American Pathologists.[33,34] The results of our studies are discussed in the next two sections. The relationship between our results and those of other investigators is described subsequently.

Nashville Breast Cohort Studies

At Vanderbilt, we initially evaluated 10,366 consecutive benign breast biopsies performed between 1950 and 1968 at three hospitals in Nashville, Tennessee.[21] These analyses indicated that 70% of women who undergo biopsy revealing benign breast tissue are not at increased risk for breast cancer. The remaining 30% of the 10,000 evaluated biopsies contained proliferative lesions. These lesions are characterized by at least moderate epithelial hyperplasia[38] and are associated with an approximately twofold increase in risk of breast cancer. The lesions within this disease category include, most prominently, hyperplasia of usual type (ductal) of moderate and florid degree, as well as sclerosing adenosis and papillomas. Mild hyperplasia of usual type is excluded from the proliferative disease category because it is not associated with increased risk of cancer and thus is not considered a disease. Clinical correlates of proliferative disease are unproven[39] except for dense mammographic patterns that are positively correlated with the presence of proliferative disease.[39,40]

The proliferative lesions can be further dichotomized into those with and without atypia. The former (atypical hyperplasia [AH]) are characterized by meeting some but not all the criteria needed for a diagnosis of carcinoma in situ. These lesions had a prevalence of 4% in the premammographic era and today are diagnosed in approximately 10% of mammographically detected benign lesions. They are associated with a fourfold to fivefold increase in breast cancer risk. There are two morphologically distinct subtypes of AH: atypical lobular hyperplasia (ALH) and atypical ductal hyperplasia (ADH) (see Chapter 8). However, women with these lesions have roughly comparable breast cancer risks.[25] Minor differences include a shorter average period between biopsy and invasive carcinoma diagnosis for ADH (8 years) than for ALH (12 years). There are also differences in the age distribution,[16,25] with

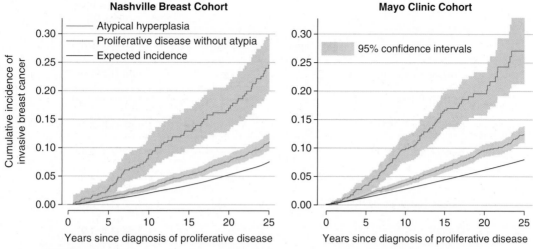

• **Fig. 20.1** Cumulative incidence of invasive breast cancer in the Nashville Breast and Mayo Clinic Cohorts. Incidence is shown for women with atypical hyperplasia and proliferative disease without atypia.[10] The expected incidence is derived from Surveillance, Epidemiology and End Results data and estimates breast cancer incidence from the general population whose age and year of biopsy was similar to that of study subjects.

both types predominating in the perimenopausal period but with ALH even less common in younger and older women. Proliferative disease without atypia (PDWA) was associated with a 60% increase in risk of breast cancer (1.6 times) compared with women from the Third National Cancer Survey and was associated with a 90% increase (1.9 times) compared with women without such changes from our study. The Nashville Breast Cohort currently contains 12,693 women, 708 of whom have developed invasive breast cancer over a median of 20 years of follow-up. Follow-up is available on 430 women with AH and 3941 women with PDWA. Our estimates of the relative risk of invasive breast cancer in this cohort associated with PDWA and AH are 1.58 (95% confidence interval [CI] 1.3–1.9) and 3.56 (95% CI 2.8–4.6), respectively.

Mayo Clinic Studies

The results of the Nashville Breast Cohort have been replicated by several authors, most notably by our studies at the Mayo Clinic.[7,9,10,12–14] The Mayo Clinic Cohort consists of 13,485 women who were diagnosed with benign breast disease and who were followed for a median of 15.8 years.[41] Of these women, 4311 and 711 had PDWA or AH, respectively, diagnosed from their entry biopsy. On follow-up, 1273 breast cancers have developed. The relative risks for PDWA was 1.94 (95% CI 1.78–2.12), whereas that for AH was 4.18 (95% CI 3.53–4.90). These findings are remarkably consistent with those of the Nashville Breast Cohort. The Mayo studies also found that the diagnoses of ADH and ALH were associated with similar levels of breast cancer risk. In the Mayo cohort, the relative risk of breast cancer was 3.93 (95% CI 3.0–5.1) in women with ALH and was 4.76 (95% CI 3.7–6.0) in women with ADH.[10]

Fig. 20.1 shows the cumulative incidence of invasive breast cancer in women from the Nashville or Mayo breast cohorts whose entry biopsies contained AH or PDWA. For reference, the black curves in this figure show the cumulative incidence of invasive breast cancer for women from the Surveillance, Epidemiology and End Results (SEER) data. These curves estimate breast cancer incidence in women from the general population whose age and

year of biopsy was similar to that of study subjects.[42] The Atlanta and Iowa SEER registries were used for the Nashville and Mayo cohorts, respectively. Ninety-five percent confidence bands on these curves show a marked and significant difference between the cancer risks associated with AH and PDWA. The increase in cumulative breast cancer incidence is approximately linear over the first 25 years following the patient's initial diagnosis.

Other Studies

Page's histologic classification scheme[32] has been evaluated in four other studies[18–20,31] in addition to those of Nashville and Mayo Clinic patients. Dupont and colleagues[31] studied women who underwent benign biopsy as part of the Breast Cancer Detection Demonstration Project. Page was not consulted during the pathology review of this study, although he did review his classification scheme with the study pathologists before their reading any of the slides. Collins and colleagues[18] studied women from Harvard's Nurse's Health Study, and Kabat and colleagues[20] studied the combined risk among cohorts of women from three cities, as noted earlier: Toronto, Canada; Portland, Oregon; and London, United Kingdom. Worsham and colleagues[19] studied women from an ethnically diverse cohort of women from Detroit, Michigan. Figs. 20.2 and 20.3 show the relative risks of breast cancer for women with PDWA and AH, respectively. The area of the gray boxes surrounding the relative risk estimates in these figures is proportional to the information content of these studies (larger boxes imply greater precision in the risk estimates). The horizontal black lines give 95% CIs. These studies have overlapping confidence intervals within each diagnostic category and are consistent. The combined relative risk for breast cancer associated with AH is 4.19 (95% CI 3.71–4.74), whereas the relative risk associated with PDWA is 1.65 (95% CI 1.46–1.86). The fact that six groups of pathologists have found similar levels of breast cancer risk associated with these lesions supports the reproducibility and credibility of these findings.[34]

Before the distinction of PDWA and AH as distinct histologic categories, all patients in our study cohorts would have been

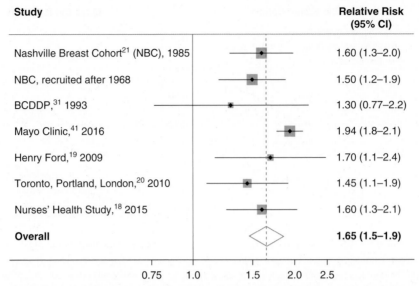

• **Fig. 20.2** Relative risks of breast cancer associated with proliferative disease without atypia reported in the literature. The horizontal lines give 95% confidence intervals (*CIs*). The size of the gray boxes surrounding the relative risk estimates are proportional to the information content of each study. The dotted vertical line marks a weighted geometric mean of the relative risks from all studies. *BCDDP*, Breast Cancer Detection Demonstration Project.

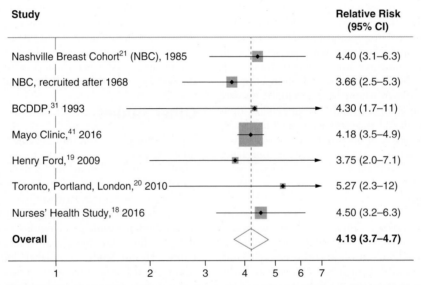

• **Fig. 20.3** Relative risks of breast cancer associated with atypical hyperplasia reported in the literature. The components of this figure are described in the legend to Fig. 20.2. *BCDDP*, Breast Cancer Detection Demonstration Project; *CI*, confidence interval.

diagnosed as having fibrocystic disease. It is clear from Figs. 20.1, 20.2, and 20.3 that this term has little prognostic value and should be replaced by more precise terminology.

Marshall and colleagues[16] have also studied the difference in risk of breast cancer between women with ALH and ADH in the Harvard-based Nurses' Health Study. The estimate of the relative risk of breast cancer in women with ALH was 5.3 (95% CI 2.7–10.4), whereas for women with ADH this risk was 2.4 (95% CI 1.3–4.5). Although the estimated risk was higher for women with ALH than with ADH, the CIs are wide, and these estimates are not significantly different. The researchers also observed a higher estimated relative risk for premenopausal women with ALH than for postmenopausal women with ALH. Overall, the

Nashville, Mayo Clinic, and Harvard cohorts provide consistent estimates of the breast cancer risks associated with AH and its subtypes. On the basis of data available through 1998, the College of American Pathologists Consensus Conference[34] stated that women with PDWA had a slight elevation in risk ranging from 1.5 to 2 times that of the general population; women with AH had a moderately increased relative risk ranging from 4.0 to 5.0.

Extent of Atypical Hyperplasia

Table 20.1 is adapted from Hartmann and colleagues[10,13] and Collins and colleagues[18] and shows the effect of extent of atypia on breast cancer risk. In reading this and subsequent tables, it is

TABLE 20.1	Relative Risk of Breast Cancer Associated With Extent of Atypical Hyperplasia					
Study	Patient Group	No. of Women	No. Cancers[a]	Relative Risk	95% Confidence Interval	p for Trend
Mayo Clinic[13]						
	SEER women from Iowa[42]			1 (reference)		<.001
	Foci of atypical hyperplasia					
	1	410	65	3.19	(2.5–4.1)	
	2	161	40	5.53	(4.0–7.5)	
	≥3	133	37	7.61	(5.4–10)	
Nurses' Health Study[18]						
	Nonproliferative lesions			1 (reference)		.22
	Foci of atypical hyperplasia					
	1	37	66	3.8	(2.4–6.1)	
	2	26	42	4.5	(2.6–7.7)	
	≥3	56	74	5.3	(3.5–8.1)	

[a]Includes both invasive cancer and carcinoma in situ.

important to bear in mind that the estimated relative risks may differ from their true values because of chance by the amount indicated in the 95% CIs. Hartmann and coworkers[10] have found that the risk of breast cancer in women with AH increases as the number of foci of atypia increases. Women with only one focus had a risk of breast cancer that was 3.19 (95% CI 2.46–4.07) times that of the general population. This relative risk increased to 5.53 (95% CI 3.95–7.53) and 7.61 (95% CI 5.36–10.5) in women with two foci or three or more foci, respectively. Collins and colleagues found a similar trend that was not statistically significant. This lack of significance may have been due to insufficient power. Degnim and colleagues have published a joint paper by the Mayo Clinic and Vanderbilt groups that combines the data from both cohorts to address this question.[42a]

Age, Family History, and Proliferative Disease

Table 20.2 is adapted from Dupont and Page.[21] The p values given in these tables are with respect to the null hypothesis that the true relative risk equals 1. The table shows the effect of family history, calcification, and age on the risk of breast cancer in women with and without proliferative disease. The interaction between proliferative disease and age at biopsy is particularly interesting. Women with proliferative disease have approximately twice the risk of breast cancer compared with women of similar age from the general population regardless of whether they are in the premenopausal, perimenopausal, or postmenopausal age group. In contrast, the relative risk of breast cancer falls with increasing age in patients lacking proliferative disease, with postmenopausal patients having about one-third the risk of postmenopausal women in general. This result suggests that women undergoing age-related involution whose breasts lack any hyperplastic activity may be at reduced risk of developing breast cancer.

Radisky and colleagues[43] found that breast cancer risk diminished with increasing involution in the entry biopsy of study subjects. Women whose terminal ductal lobular units (TDLUs) were 26% to 50% and 51% to 75% involuted had breast cancer relative risks of 0.50 (95% CI 0.33–0.76) and 0.16 (95% CI 0.10–0.26), respectively, compared with women whose TDLUs were 0% to 25% involuted.

The literature on how the interaction between AH and a family history of breast cancer affects breast cancer risk is inconsistent. Table 20.3 summarizes the findings of Dupont and Page,[21] Hartmann and colleagues,[13] and Collins and colleagues.[17] The Nashville Breast Cohort observed an interaction between the effects of AH and a family history of breast cancer risk. However, this interaction has not been confirmed in either the Mayo Clinic studies[7] or in the Nurses' Health Study.[17]

Complex Fibroadenoma and Proliferative Breast Disease

Fibroadenomas exhibit a wide range of cytologic and histologic patterns, with the histologic component of these lesions varying from nonexistent to carcinoma in situ. Also, although fibroadenomas have been traditionally thought to be unrelated to risk of breast cancer, several authors have reported that women with these lesions have a mildly elevated risk of breast cancer.[37,44–48] This led us to investigate whether different histologic types of fibroadenomas were associated with different levels of breast cancer risk.[22] We obtained follow-up on 1835 patients from our Nashville study hospitals who were diagnosed with fibroadenoma between 1950 and 1968. These women represented 90% of eligible subjects. The histologic slides of study subjects were reclassified without knowledge of subsequent cancer outcome. The risk of breast cancer in patients who had had fibroadenomas was 1.61 times that of women from a control group consisting

TABLE 20.2   Relative Risk of Breast Cancer in Women Who Have Undergone Benign Breast Biopsy in Nashville

	No. of Women	No. of Cancers	Relative Risk[a]	95% Confidence Interval	p
All women	3303	134	1.5	1.3–1.8	<.0001
Proliferative disease	1925	103	1.9	1.6–2.3	<.0001
No proliferative disease	1378	31	0.89	0.62–1.3	.51
Family history[b]	369	26	2.5	1.7–3.7	<.0001
No family history	2934	108	1.4	1.2–1.7	.0007
Proliferative disease and					
Family history	234	22	3.2	2.1–4.9	<.0001
No family history	1691	81	1.7	1.4–2.2	<.0001
Calcification	359	23	2.4	1.6–3.6	<.0001
No calcification	1566	80	1.8	1.5–2.3	<.0001
Age[c] 20–45	1205	57	1.9	1.5–2.5	<.0001
Age 46–55	563	35	1.9	1.3–2.6	.0002
Age >55	157	11	2.2	1.2–4	.007
No proliferative disease and					
Family history	135	4	1.2	0.43–3.1	.78
No family history	1243	27	0.86	0.59–1.3	.43
Calcification	174	4	0.80	0.30–2.1	.66
No calcification	1204	27	0.90	0.62–1.3	.59
Age 20–45	1025	23	0.99	0.66–1.5	.96
Age 46–55	247	7	0.83	0.40–1.8	.63
Age >55	106	1	0.30	0.04–2.2	.21
Family history and					
Cysts	246	21	3	1.9–4.5	<.0001
No cysts	123	5	1.6	0.65–3.7	.32
No family history and					
Cysts	1808	73	1.5	1.2–1.9	.0008
No cysts	1126	35	1.2	0.88–1.7	.23

Follow-up was obtained on 3303 of these women, representing 84% of eligible subjects. This sample was weighted in favor of patients with proliferative disease. The median length of follow-up was 17 years.
[a]Risk relative to women from Cutler and Young survey, adjusted for age at biopsy and length of follow-up. See Cutler SJ, Young JL, eds. *Third National Cancer Survey: Incidence Data* (NIH Publication No. 75-787). Bethesda, MD: National Cancer Institute; 1975.
[b]Mother, sister, or daughter with breast cancer.
[c]Age at benign breast biopsy.
Modified from Dupont WD, Page DL. WD, Page DL. Risk factors for breast cancer in women with proliferative breast disease. *N Engl J Med.* 1985;312:146-151.

of women from Connecticut[49] and are adjusted for age and year of fibroadenoma biopsy. This risk increased to 2.24 in patients with complex fibroadenomas, defined as those that contained cysts, sclerosing adenosis, epithelial calcifications, or papillary apocrine changes. The risk of breast cancer was also elevated in patients whose adjacent parenchyma contained proliferative disease (Table 20.4).

Breast cancer risks associated with fibroadenoma have also been studied in the Mayo Clinic cohort by Nassar and colleagues,[50] whose findings are also summarized in Table 20.4. Their relative risk estimates for complex and simple fibroadenomas and for fibroadenomas with adjacent PDWA and AH were similar to those of Dupont and associates.[22] They found, however, that women with complex fibroadenoma were more likely to have other, concomitant high-risk histologic characteristics and concluded that the diagnosis of fibroadenoma does not confer increased breast cancer risk beyond that of the established histologic categories of PDWA and AH.

The clinical significance of fibroadenomas is that women need not be overly concerned about the breast cancer risk associated with these lesions, unless AH or ductal carcinoma in situ is present, in which case it should be managed according to those findings. For the remainder of women with fibroadenomas, at worst, they are associated with a cancer risk that is similar to that for PDWA. Evidence of a synergistic effect of fibroadenomas and other risk factors for breast cancer has not been established.

Although it is not appropriate to unduly concern young women with a family history of breast cancer, a diagnosis of complex fibroadenoma should be a further encouragement for regular mammographic surveillance by 35 or 40 years of age. Although it may occasionally be technically difficult, the inclusion of some adjacent parenchyma when fibroadenomas are surgically removed seems appropriate and will more often reduce anxiety than increase it. Women with simple fibroadenomas who have neither adjacent proliferative disease nor a family history of breast cancer are not at elevated risk of breast cancer. It should be

TABLE 20.3	Relative Risk of Breast Cancer Associated With AH and FH				
Study Patient Group	No. of Women	No. Cancers[a]	Relative Risk	95% Confidence Interval	p
Nashville Breast Cohort[21,a]					
Neither PD nor first-degree FH	1243	27	1 (reference)		
AH without first-degree FH	193	20	4.3	(2.4–7.8)	<.0001
AH with first-degree FH	39	10	11	(5.5–24)	<.0001
Mayo Clinic[13,b]					
SEER women from Iowa[42]			1 (reference)		
Atypical hyperplasia and					
No FH	372	70	3.91	(3.1–4.9)	.23[d]
Weak FH	151	39	5.54	(3.9–7.6)	
Strong FH[c]	106	24	4.19	(2.7–6.2)	
Nurses' Health Study[17]					
Neither PD nor first-degree FH			1 (reference)		
AH without first-degree FH	124[e]	70	4.38	(2.9–6.6)	.57[f]
AH with first-degree FH	36[e]	26	5.19	(3.0–9.6)	

[a]Includes invasive cancer only.
[b]Includes both invasive cancer and carcinoma in situ.
[c]First-degree FH with breast cancer before age 50, or two or more relatives with breast cancer, with at least one first-degree FH. Weak FH is any lessor degree of family history.
[d]p for trend.
[e]Control subjects from nested case-control study.
[f]p comparing AH with and without FH.
AH, Atypical hyperplasia; FH, family history of breast cancer; PD, proliferative disease.

emphasized that two-thirds of patients with fibroadenoma have neither a complex lesion nor a family history, and they may be reassured by the knowledge that their risk of breast cancer is not appreciably affected by their tumor.

We believe that there is clinical value in defining *proliferative breast disease* to mean lesions that have been shown to be markers approaching a twofold to threefold elevation in risk of breast cancer. Using this definition, complex fibroadenomas should be included among the proliferative breast lesions.

Effect of Time Since Biopsy on Risk of Breast Cancer

Most relative risk estimates from longitudinal studies are derived under the assumption that each patient's relative risk remains constant over time. It is possible, however, for the relative risk of an individual patient to vary as a function of either age or time since initial diagnosis. An example of such a change can be found in our studies of benign breast disease. We have previously reported that women who have undergone breast biopsy revealing AH have 5.3 times the risk of breast cancer of biopsied women who lacked proliferative disease and that the corresponding relative risk for women with PDWA is 1.9.[21] These results were obtained using a proportional hazards regression model that assumes that relative risk remains constant over time. Fig. 20.4, however, shows an alternative analysis of these same data. The risk estimates were derived from a hazard regression model

that uses time-dependent covariates.[51,52] Fig. 20.4 shows that the breast cancer risk for women with both AH and PDWA is greatest in the first 10 years after benign breast biopsy. Women with PDWA who remain free of breast cancer for 10 years are at no greater risk than are women of similar age who do not have such a history. The relative risk of breast cancer in women with AH is halved if they remain free of breast cancer for 10 years after their initial biopsy. This supports the hypothesis that not all AHs are obligate precursor lesions for breast cancer and that these lesions may progress to cancer, remain unchanged, or possibly regress over a substantial period. Their presence at time of biopsy may be best regarded as a marker of increased risk, even though some of these lesions, left untreated, do evolve into invasive lesions.

Krieger and Hiatt[45] reported similar findings on the effect of time since biopsy on the risk of breast cancer. Women whose benign breast lesions had a Black-Chabon[53] score of 1 or 2 had a twofold elevation in risk of breast cancer that varied little with time since biopsy. For women with a Black-Chabon score of 4, however, relative risks of breast cancer of 3.5, 2.4, and 1.7 were reported for follow-up intervals of 0 to 17, 10 to 17, and 15 to 17 years, respectively.

The absolute risk for all the women in our study cohorts[10,21] seems to be approximately evenly distributed over the 25-year period of follow-up (see Fig. 20.1). The knowledge that invasive carcinomas were fairly evenly distributed over this time would have led us to predict the finding just described. Thus an approximately constant cancer incidence over a 25-year span,

TABLE 20.4 Relative Risk of Invasive Breast Cancer in Patients With Fibroadenoma

Study	Patient Group	No. of Women	No. Cancers[a]	Relative Risk	95% Confidence Interval
Nashville Breast Cohort[22]					
Control women from Connecticut[49]				1 (reference)	
All fibroadenoma patients		1835	87	1.61	(1.3–2)
Internal diagnosis[b]					
	Simple	1413	58	1.42	(1.1–1.8)
	Complex	422	29	2.24	(1.6–3.2)
External diagnosis[c]					
	No parenchyma	477	21	1.59	(1–2.5)
	No PD	1177	51	1.48	(1.1–1.9)
	PD	181	15	2.43	(1.5–4)
	PD without atypia	162	12	2.16	(1.2–3.8)
	Atypical hyperplasia	19	3	4.77	(1.5–15)
Mayo Clinic[50]					
SEER women from Iowa[42]				1 (reference)	
All fibroadenoma patients		2136	191	1.60	(1.4–1.9)
Internal diagnosis[b]					
	Simple	1835	151	1.49	(1.3–1.7)
	Complex	301	40	2.27	(1.6–3.1)
External diagnosis[c]					
	No PD	1534	100	1.2	(0.97–1.5)
PD without atypia	PD without atypia	295	45	2.49	(1.8–3.3)
Atypical hyperplasia	Atypical hyperplasia	28	5	3.67	(1.2–8.5)

PD, Proliferative disease; *SEER*, Surveillance, Epidemiology and End Results.
[a]Includes invasive cancer only.
[b]Complex fibroadenomas contain cysts, sclerosing adenosis, epithelial calcifications, or papillary apocrine change.
[c]Diagnosis of parenchyma adjacent to the fibroadenoma.

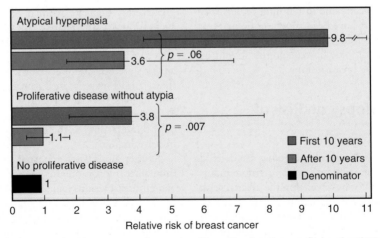

• **Fig. 20.4** Relative risk of breast cancer in women with proliferative disease. Risks of patients with and without atypia are contrasted with risks of biopsied women who did not have proliferative disease. Relative risks of breast cancer drop substantially in women who remain free of breast cancer for 10 years after their proliferative disease biopsy. (From Dupont WD, Page DL. Relative risk of breast cancer varies with time since diagnosis of atypical hyperplasia. *Human Pathol.* 1989;20:723–725.)

together with a rising age-specific incidence in women without proliferative disease (the denominator of the relative risk statistic), implies that a woman's relative risk of breast cancer must fall with increasing time since biopsy. This time-dependent analysis does suggest that one should not presume the constancy of relative risk figures through an entire lifetime when making clinical decisions.

Radial Scar

Jacobs and colleagues[54] from the Harvard Nurses' Health Study evaluated the association between radial scars in benign breast biopsies and risk of breast cancer. They found that women with radial scars had 1.8 (95% CI 1.1–2.9) times the risk compared with women without radial scars. This risk increased to 3 (95% CI 1.7–5.5) in women with both radial scars and PDWA compared with women with neither lesion. In the Nashville Breast Cohort, we found that the relative risk of breast cancer associated with radial scar was 1.82 (95% CI 1.2–2.7) at 10 years.[55] Restricting the analysis to women older than 49 years of age increased the risk to 2.14 (95% CI 0.6–2.8). These risks decreased with increasing years of follow-up. Approximately 92% of women with radial scars also had proliferative disease, but radial scars were present in only 1.3% of biopsies without proliferative disease. Analyses stratifying relative risk with regard to proliferative disease found radial scars to minimally elevate the relative risk of subsequent breast cancer.

Radial scars have also been studied in the Mayo Cohort by Berg and colleagues.[56] Among women with PDWA, the relative risks of breast cancer for women with and without radial scars was very similar: 1.88 (95% CI, 1.36–2.53) and 1.57 (95% CI, 1.37–1.79) for women with and without radial scar, respectively. Among women with AH, there was also no significant difference in breast cancer risk between those with and without radial scars. Women with both AH and radial scars had a relative risk of 2.81 (95% CI, 1.29–5.35), whereas those with atypia but without radial scars had a relative risk of 3.97 (95% CI, 2.99–5.19).

Radial scars in the absence of proliferative disease are uncommon. Although the presence of radial scars in a benign breast biopsy mildly elevates risk of breast cancer, we believe that this risk can be largely attributed to the category of coexistent proliferative disease. In women with both radial scars and AH, recommendations for interventions beyond biopsy should be based on the extent of the AH.

Hormone Replacement Therapy in Women With Proliferative Disease

A question of great importance to women and their physicians is whether hormone replacement therapy (HRT) can be safely given to women with a history of proliferative breast disease. This question has been studied by Dupont and colleagues[57] and by Byrne and colleagues.[58] Both of these studies found no evidence that risk of breast cancer in women with either PDWA or AH was further increased by taking HRT. Although these findings are reassuring, it must be noted that the power of both studies to detect a moderate elevation in risk due to this therapy was fairly low. Hence, these studies cannot rule out such an increase. Also, the majority of women in both studies took HRT for less than 5 years. Hence, the question of risk in these women associated with long-term HRT use cannot be adequately addressed.

It should also be noted that a clinical trial conducted by the Women's Health Initiative[59,60] found HRT to be associated with a relative risk of breast cancer of 1.26 (95% CI 1–1.59). In this trial, women were enrolled after the menopause. The average age at recruitment was 63 years, so the observed increase in breast cancer risk may not be generalizable to perimenopausal women considering HRT for vasomotor symptoms. Therapy consisted of conjugated equine estrogens plus a progestin, which study subjects took for an average duration of 5.2 years. Breast cancer was only elevated in women who had taken HRT before enrolling in this study. The relative risk of breast cancer in women with no prior HRT exposure was 1.06 (95% CI 0.81–1.38).[61] They also found that the risk of breast cancer in women who took unopposed estrogen remained reduced after 10 years of follow-up.[60] Hence, the Women's Health Initiative provides no evidence that taking HRT for a few years to wean women from their endogenous estrogen increases risk of breast cancer. This study also did not address risk of breast cancer in women with a history of benign breast disease. However, in light of these results, it would be prudent for women with a history of AH to avoid taking HRT for more than 5 years. A discussion of pharmacologic risk reduction in women with AH is given by Hartmann and colleagues.[10]

Selected References

7. Hartmann LC, Sellers TA, Frost MH, et al. Benign breast disease and the risk of breast cancer. *N Engl J Med.* 2005;353:229-237.

9. Degnim AC, Visscher DW, Berman HK, et al. Stratification of breast cancer risk in women with atypia: a Mayo cohort study. *J Clin Oncol.* 2007;25:2671-2677.

10. Hartmann LC, Degnim AC, Santen RJ, Dupont WD, Ghosh K. Atypical hyperplasia of the breast—risk assessment and management options. *N Engl J Med.* 2015;372:78-89.

15. London SJ, Connolly JL, Schnitt SJ, Colditz GA. A prospective study of benign breast disease and the risk of breast cancer. *JAMA.* 1992;267:941-944.

20. Kabat GC, Jones JG, Olson N, et al. A multi-center prospective cohort study of benign breast disease and risk of subsequent breast cancer. *Cancer Causes Control.* 2010;21:821-828.

21. Dupont WD, Page DL. Risk factors for breast cancer in women with proliferative breast disease. *N Engl J Med.* 1985;312:146-151.

22. Dupont WD, Page DL, Parl FF, et al. Long-term risk of breast cancer in women with fibroadenoma. *N Engl J Med.* 1994;331:10-15.

31. Dupont WD, Parl FF, Hartmann WH, et al. Breast cancer risk associated with proliferative breast disease and atypical hyperplasia. *Cancer.* 1993;71:1258-1265.

38. Page DL, Anderson TJ, Rogers LW. Epithelial hyperplasia. In: Page DL, Anderson TJ, eds. *Diagnostic Histopathology of the Breast.* Edinburgh: Churchill Livingstone; 1987:120-156.

42a. Degnim AC, Dupont WD, Radisky DC, et al. Extent of atypical hyperplasia stratifies breast cancer risk in 2 independent cohorts of women. *Cancer.* 2016;122:2971-2978.

A full reference list is available online at ExpertConsult.com.

21

Steroid Receptors in Breast Cancer

BALKEES ABDERRAHMAN AND V. CRAIG JORDAN

The nuclear steroid receptor (NSR) superfamily[1] is essential for human life and reproduction. Similarly, the ability of breast cancer to subvert the positive role of NSRs in normal tissues to enhance survival becomes a vulnerability in the application of therapeutics.[2] Not all members of the NSR superfamily are described in this chapter; the focus here is on the estrogen receptor (ER), the progesterone receptor (PR), the glucocorticoid receptor (GR), and the androgen receptor (AR) (Fig. 21.1). However, it is the knowledge of the breast tumor ER that has had the greatest impact on the survival of patients, as the target that is recognized to be the most important[2] in oncology and cancer therapeutics.[3] The agents that bind to the ER and block estrogen-induced cell replication in breast tumors directly are selective ER modulators (SERMs): tamoxifen, raloxifene, and bazedoxifene[4] (Fig. 21.2). Another therapeutic agent that binds to the tumor ER, fulvestrant, is referred to as a "pure antiestrogen," or a selective ER downregulator (SERD) (see Fig. 21.2). The agents that prevent estrogen synthesis in the peripheral tissues of postmenopausal women are aromatase inhibitors (AIs).[5] The translational treatment strategy of long-term adjuvant antihormone therapy—to prevent estrogen action in the tumor—has extended or improved the lives of millions of women worldwide[6] and continues to do so.[7,8]

The PR has debatable value for refining the prediction of a successful outcome of adjuvant antihormone therapy over the ER alone for the treatment of breast cancer.[9] Unlike the ER, which is the principal signal transduction pathway and the driver of breast cancer growth, the understanding of PR biology in breast cancer did not result in successful therapeutic advances to treat breast cancer. Nevertheless, the recent findings from the Women's Health Initiative (WHI), in which estrogen-alone hormone replacement caused a paradoxical decrease in the incidence of breast cancer, whereas the combination of estrogen plus medroxyprogesterone acetate (MPA) causes an increased incidence in breast cancer,[10] must be considered. This mandates a reevaluation of our basic understanding of the mechanism of action and interactions of estrogen and progestin in breast cancer tissue.

It is now clear that estrogen exhibits cytotoxic effects on estrogen-deprived breast cancer cells after menopause.[11] This is placed into clinical context in this chapter, and the molecular modulation of estrogen action by glucocorticoids and androgens is considered. The AR is present in breast cancer.[12] Although no therapeutic agents for breast cancer treatment have yet emerged as the standard of care, the AR is being considered a putative target in triple-negative breast cancer.[13]

Estrogen Receptor

Historical Perspective

The evolution of our understanding of the hormonal control of breast cancer growth has recently been described in detail.[14,15] Nevertheless, it is important to identify the landmark clinical observations and the discovery of the ER as milestones in translational medicine. These observations in the 20th century aided patients' care despite the lack of a clear understanding of the molecular mechanism of estrogen action as the driver of breast cancer growth. Important new biological principles have now been deciphered during the 21st century that provide biological transparency and clinical rules for the care of patients as new standards of health care.

An evaluation of the first successful treatment for breast cancer was conducted by Stanley Boyd in 1900.[16] He accumulated all of the clinical case reports of oophorectomy in premenopausal breast cancer patients to establish a response rate. He noted a 30% response rate to oophorectomy, which has stood the test of time and is noted with all other endocrine ablative, antiestrogenic, or high-dose estrogen therapies.[14] The connection between estrogen and mammary cancer growth in laboratory animals correlated well with ovarian ablation in premenopausal breast cancer patients.[17] Then a paradox occurred. Haddow and coworkers[18] reported that high-dose synthetic estrogen administered to postmenopausal women with metastatic breast cancer (MBC), also had a 30% response rate; but only in patients that were treated more than 5 years past the menopause.[19] This was a completely counterintuitive clinical observation, but despite the fact that there was no understanding of mechanisms, high-dose estrogen therapy became the standard of care for postmenopausal MBC until the discovery and clinical evaluation of tamoxifen in the mid-1970s. Tamoxifen, a nonsteroidal antiestrogen, blocks tumor growth by preventing estrogen binding to the ER.[20] This antiestrogenic treatment strategy reaffirmed the principal role of estrogen to stimulate breast tumor growth.

It is important to state that only a minority of MBC patients during the 1960s and the early 1970s (before tamoxifen) responded to either endocrine ablation (oophorectomy, adrenalectomy, and hypophysectomy) or high-dose estrogen therapy. Responses were transient for a year or two. A predictive test was required for clinicians to decide which patients, who were the majority with MBC, would not respond to endocrine treatment. The goal was to reduce hospitalization and morbidity for those patients who would not respond. The discovery of the ER in estrogen target tissues (uterus,

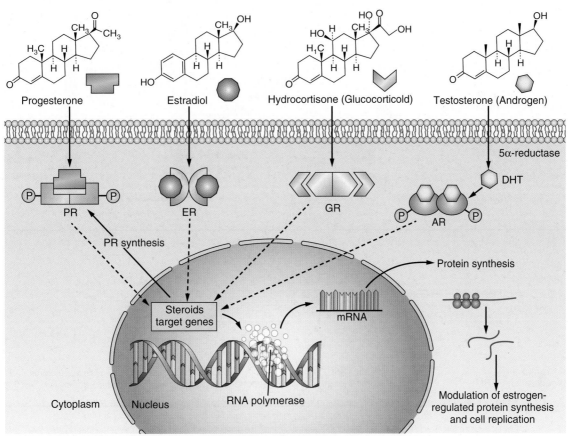

• **Fig. 21.1** Schematic diagram of signal transduction pathways for clones of steroid hormones and their effect on protein regulated synthesis and cellular replication. Progesterone binds to its receptor in the cytoplasm, followed by receptor dimerization and the entry of the complex to the nucleus, where it binds target genes in the DNA to induce transcription with the formation of messenger RNA *(mRNA)* and translation through ribosomes with the production of specific proteins. Estrogens bind to estrogen receptor *(ER)*α in the cytoplasm. The ER then is able to translocate into the nucleus and bind to specific DNA domains to regulate the activity of different estrogen-responsive genes. ER has other functions independent of DNA binding as well. The interplay between the progesterone receptor *(PR)* and ER is shown through estrogen-induced transcription of the PR gene, which is far more complicated than the occupancy of ER. Also, PR functions as a molecular rheostat to control ERα transcriptional activity. It is considered a biomarker of ERα function and indicative of a breast cancer prognosis. However, PR expression has been shown to be an independent prognostic variable in early breast cancer. Glucocorticoids bind their receptor in the cytosol. The activated glucocorticoid receptor *(GR)* complex functions on the cytosolic and the nuclear levels by either upregulating the expression of antiinflammatory proteins in the nucleus or inhibiting the expression of proinflammatory proteins in the cytosol. Androgens bind their receptors in the cytosol, then translocate to the nucleus and bind to DNA-binding transcription factors that are responsible for gene expression. *AR,* Androgen receptor.

vagina, and pituitary gland) in animals[2] and in some breast tumors in women[15,21] created the first understanding of a potential molecular mechanism of estrogen action.

The hypothesis to be tested was straightforward; if there was no ER in the tumor biopsy, then no response would be expected to endocrine ablation therapy. Breast tumor growth would not be dependent on estrogen. The National Cancer Institute convened an international meeting in 1974[21] to review all of the clinical correlations for ER tumor content in biopsies in MBC, with the response of MBC to endocrine additive or ablative therapy (the final conclusions are illustrated in Table 21.1).[21] What was originally a 30% response rate for unselected patients now segregated into a less than 10% response rate for patients with an ER-negative tumor biopsy, whereas patients with an ER-positive tumor biopsy

had more than a 55% to 60% response rate.[22] This conclusion from the meeting resulted in the introduction of the ER assay being required to determine the hormone-responsive status of all women with a diagnosis of breast cancer in the United States. At the time, this was a landmark advance in translational research to aid women's health. However, the strategic targeting of tamoxifen, an antiestrogenic medicine, to the tumor ER, for the long-term adjuvant therapy of breast cancer patients was a life-saving strategy.[23] This innovation with tamoxifen is now credited for extending the lives of millions of women worldwide.[3,6,7] Subsequent advances in the development of AIs for the long-term adjuvant therapy of breast cancer in postmenopausal patients[5,24] improved response rates and decreased the numbers of side effects noted with tamoxifen (thromboembolic events and endometrial cancer)[8]

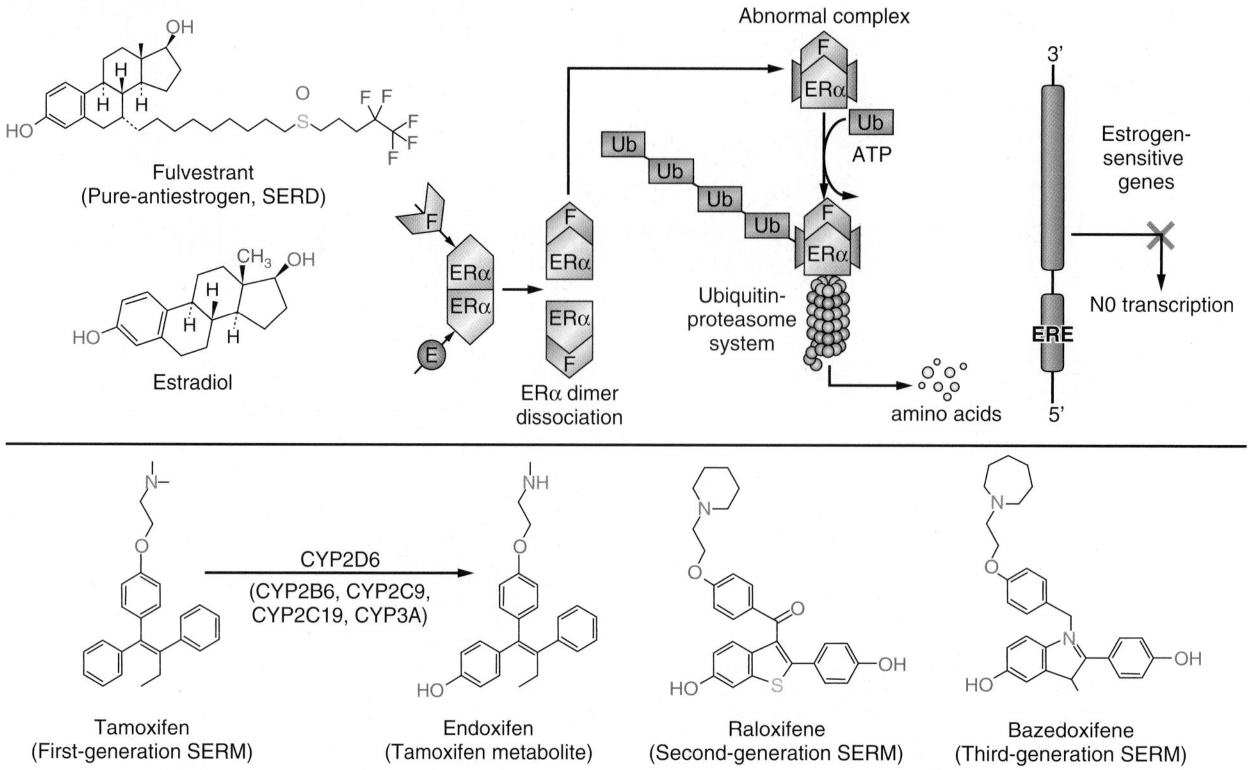

• **Fig. 21.2** Schematic diagram of tamoxifen metabolic activation to a phenolic metabolite "endoxifen," mainly by *CYP2D6* enzyme. The key selective estrogen receptor *(ER)* modulators *(SERMs)* and selective ER downregulators *(SERDs)* that changed breast cancer treatment and women's health: tamoxifen, a first-generation SERM that is used not only in the prevention of breast cancer but also in the treatment of early and advanced breast cancer in pre- and postmenopausal women, is metabolized to endoxifen through the cytochrome p450, chiefly *CYP2D6*. Endoxifen is potent antiestrogen in vitro and binds with a high affinity to the human ER. Fulvestrant is a SERD, or pure antagonist, that destroys the ER and is used in advanced-stage breast cancer in postmenopausal women with ER-positive disease. Raloxifene, a second-generation SERM, is used primarily for the prevention of osteoporosis; it reduces the incidence of breast cancer without increasing that of endometrial cancer. Bazedoxifene, a third-generation SERM, is used for the prevention and treatment of postmenopausal osteoporosis. The molecular mechanism of fulvestrant is also deciphered. Fulvestrant, a SERD or a pure steroidal ERα antagonist, binds competitively and with a high affinity to the ERα. The result is the degradation of the ER by the ubiquitin-proteasome system. Fulvestrant is used in advanced-stage breast cancer in postmenopausal women with ER-positive disease. *ERE,* Estrogen response elements.

TABLE 21.1	Objective Breast Tumor Regressions According to ER Assay and Type of Therapy as Judged by Extramural Review[a]		
Therapy	**ER+**	**ER−**	**ER+/−**
Castration	25/33	4/53	0/2
Adrenalectomy	32/66	4/33	2/8
Hypophysectomy	2/8	0/8	—
TOTAL	55/107 = 55%	8/94 = 8%	2/10 = 30%
Estrogen	37/57	5/58	0/2
Androgen	12/26	2/24	0/1
Glucocorticoid	2/2	—	—
TOTAL	51/85 = 60%	7/82 = 8%	0/3 = 0%

ER, Estrogen receptor.
[a]Out of the outcome of 459 treatment trials meeting the criteria of objective tumor response or failure, ER assays were available in 436 of these trials.

and also prompted the use of a safer SERM, raloxifene,[25] and the use of exemestane (an AI)[26] for the chemoprevention of breast cancer in high-risk postmenopausal women.

A Current View of the Molecular Mechanism of Estrogen Action

The ER is located in the estrogen target tissues around a woman's body, including the majority of breast cancers. It is important to note that the ER is also present in high quantities in male breast cancer, so this mechanism will also apply in that context.[27] The first ER discovered[2] is now referred to as ERα. A second ER, known as ERβ, prompted an intense investigation of the role of both receptors in physiology and breast cancer.[28] At present, ERα is considered to be the principal driver of ER-mediated breast cancer growth and the site of mutations responsible for acquired antihormonal resistance.[29] An exact role for ERβ for breast cancer prognosis and therapy is yet to be defined.[30]

The NSRs for consideration are illustrated in Fig. 21.3, and their structural similarities are compared and contrasted. The domains[1] are named from the N-terminus, A through F. The

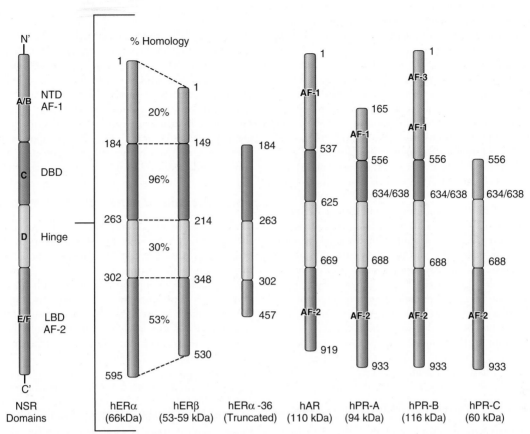

• **Fig. 21.3** Schematic diagram of structural and functional domains of the nuclear steroid receptor (NSR) superfamily. The structural domains of estrogen receptor (ER)α and ERβ are depicted in A through F with the amino acid numbers indicated on the right. The percentage of amino acid homologies between wild-type ER-α and ERβ are shown. In addition, the diagram demonstrates molecular weight. The amino-terminal A/B regions contain a transactivation domain (activation function [AF]-1), which contributes to the transcriptional activity of the ER through the ligand-independent function and a coregulatory domain that is responsible for the recruitment of coactivators and corepressors; ERβ lacks AF-1. The C region corresponds to the DNA-binding domain (DBD), which is the most highly conserved region between ERα and ERβ, C region is required for binding to specific estrogen response elements in the proximal promoter region or at distal regulatory elements of estrogen-responsive genes. The D region corresponds to the hinge region, part of ligand-dependent activating domain and the nuclear localization signal. The carboxy-terminal regions E and F contain the ligand-binding domain (LBD), a coregulatory binding surface, the dimerization domain, the second nuclear localization signal, and AF-2. Human ERα and ERβ variant isoforms are expressed in malignant tissues and influence cancer biology. The ERα-36 isoform,[31] known as the "dwarf or truncated ER," lacks both transactivation domains. It has been identified and cloned. ERα-36 maintains a "nongenomic" signaling pathway through mitogen-activated protein kinase and is shown to be resistant to tamoxifen treatment. The structural domains for hAR and hPR are depicted in A through F with the amino acid numbers indicated on the right. The diagram demonstrates the molecular weight of hAR and hPR. The amino-terminal A/B regions contain a transactivation domain (AF-1). The C region corresponds to the DBD. The D region corresponds to the hinge region. The carboxy-terminal regions E and F contain the LBD and AF-2. C, C terminus; hAR, human androgen receptor; hER, human estrogen receptor; hPR, human progesterone receptor; N, N terminus; NTD, N terminal domain.

important area that allows communication of the ligand-activated ER with the promoter region of ER-responsive genes is described as the DNA-binding domain (DBD), or region C. The ligand-binding domain (LBD) is toward the C-terminus and is referred to as region E, which also encompasses the F region. Domain F modulates the function of the ER in a ligand-, promoter-, and cell-specific fashion. Deletion analysis of the ER has identified two regions with activating functions that are important for the biological activity of the estradiol (E2)-ER complex. Activation function (AF)-1 is in the A/B region of ERα, but this is a truncated region in ERβ (see Fig. 21.3).[31] As a result, the E2-ERβ

complex does not have the same estrogenic efficacy of the E2-ERα complex. Indeed, laboratory experiments demonstrate that ERβ can block the estrogen-like action of the E2-ERα complex.[32] This is because, within the E2-ER complex, AF-1 and AF-2 collaborate with each other at the promoter region for full estrogen-like activity.

The LBD of ERα, has been studied in great detail and crystallized with numerous ligands, eg: estradiol, diethylstilbestrol, and the SERMs: 4-hydroxytamoxifen[33] and raloxifene[34] (see Fig. 21.2). The LBD of ERβ only differs to that of ERα by 2 amino acids. The amino acids Leu384 and Met421 in ERα are replaced by Met336 and Ile373, respectively, in ERβ. Despite the similarities in the LBD, considerable efforts continue to discover ERα and ERβ specific agonists and antagonists.[35]

Estrogen action is triggered by the diffusion of E2 from the circulation into estrogen target tissues, where the ligand binds with high affinity $K_d = 10^{-10}$ M within the unoccupied LBD of ERα. The 3′ phenolic hydroxyl of estradiol is tethered through amino acids glutamic acid (Glu353) and arginine (Arg354), and the 17′ alcoholic hydroxyl at amino acid histidine (His524). This interaction causes a conformational change in the ER with helix 12 sealing the ligand within the LBD. As a result, the external surface of the E2-ER complex exposes AF-2, which allows coactivator molecules (SRC-1, SRC-2, or SRC3)[36] to bind and to construct a transcription complex at the promoter region of estrogen responsive genes. AF-1 and AF-2 cooperate in building the transcription complex. However, the transcription complex is not a static trigger but is required to "breathe" through the destruction of the complex by the proteasomal ubiquitination system[37] (the process is illustrated for estradiol and fulvestrant action shown in Fig. 21.2). The promoter sites are recharged to continue the function of the transcription complex. In this way, the cell is guided through the cell cycle of checkpoints, protein synthesis, and division.

The central position of ER in breast cancer growth has identified this receptor protein as the preeminent target for the therapeutic agents referred to as SERMs and SERDs.

The Molecular Mechanism of Action of SERMs

The important pharmacologic property of the SERMs tamoxifen and raloxifene (see Fig. 21.2) is the different intrinsic estrogenic activity of the respective ER complexes. For example, tamoxifen-ER complexes are estrogenic and thus build bone in postmenopausal women and lower circulating low-density lipoprotein cholesterol (LDL). However, the promiscuous estrogenicity of the tamoxifen-ER complex that accumulates in the nucleus also increases the risk of estrogen-like side effects, such as thromboembolic events and endometrial cancer.[25] Raloxifene has a short biological half-life because it is a polyhydroxylated compound in contrast to tamoxifen, which is lipophilic and heavily protein-bound. The raloxifene molecule is the active agent at the ER, but the tamoxifen molecule is required to be hydroxylated and demethylated to form 4-hydroxytamoxifen and endoxifen (see Fig. 21.2) before receptor binding. The argument has been made that mutations in the *CYP2D6* gene impair tamoxifen's efficacy; however, this is not proven, and clinical testing is not a standard of care.

Early molecular pharmacology studies of the structure-function relationships of nonsteroidal antiestrogens related to tamoxifen[38] demonstrated that the bulky antiestrogenic side chain of nonsteroidal antiestrogens prevented the sealing of the ligand within the LBD. This mechanism was confirmed by x-ray crystallography, which showed both 4-hydroxytamoxifen[33] and raloxifene prevented helix 12 from closing. The SERM-ER complex can bind to the promoter region of estrogen responsive genes, but the conformation of the complex now prevents coactivator binding and the building of a transcription complex (Fig. 21.4). The important aspect of SERM pharmacology is that the ligand binding within the LBD can alter the external surface of the ER complex, which in turn influences the proportion of coactivators or corepressors that can bind. These molecular maneuvers predetermine the balance of estrogen and antiestrogen-like properties of the SERM-ER complex at the target site (see Fig. 21.4).

A recent report that 27-hydroxycholesterol (27-HC) is a "natural SERM"[39] deserves a comment. The synthetic SERMs, by definition,[4] provide beneficial effects in building bone, lowering LDL cholesterol to reduce the risk of coronary heart disease, reduce the risk of strokes, and reduce the risk of breast and endometrial cancers. By contrast, 27-HC increases breast cancer cell growth, increases the risk of coronary heart disease, and does not build bone in estrogen-deprived animals. Indeed, it blocks estrogen from building bone.[39] Thus 27-HC appears to be bad everywhere in a woman's body, and strategies to reduce obesity, and consequently reduce 27-HC, should be a clinical priority.

The Molecular Mechanism of Action of SERDs

The changing trend from the use of long-term adjuvant tamoxifen therapy to long-term adjuvant AI treatment has improved patient prognosis, with a decrease in thromboembolic events and endometrial cancer in postmenopausal patients.[40] Nevertheless, there is an increase in osteoporotic fractures with AIs.

Estrogen deprivation with AIs also causes an upregulation of the ER protein in breast cancer cells, presumably in an attempt to scavenge for low levels of estrogen. Indeed, acquired supersensitivity to estrogen has been noted experimentally as a possible mechanism of AI failure during therapy.[41] An alternative successful approach to complete estrogen deprivation, is the clinical development of the "pure antiestrogen," or SERD, fulvestrant (ICI 182,780) (Fig. 21.2). The steroidal fulvestrant is administered by intramuscular (IM) injection once monthly. Recent clinical trials (COmparisoN of Faslodex In Recurrent or Metastatic Breast Cancer—CONFIRM) compared the standard dose of 250 mg IM once a month with 500 mg IM once/month and found that high-dose fulvestrant was superior to the standard formulation. This dose regimen is now the standard of care.[42]

Fulvestrant binds to the ER, and the long lipophilic side chain produces an inappropriate conformation for the complex. As a result, the aberrant complex is targeted for ubiquitination and rapid destruction by the proteasomal enzyme system (see Fig. 21.2). The success of fulvestrant for the treatment of MBC, despite the unpleasant administration of the monthly depot injection, has encouraged a current search for orally active SERDs that could be employed as long-term adjuvant therapies.[43]

The Mechanisms of Drug Resistance to Long-Term Antihormone Therapy

Numerous recent reviews have focused on the role of growth factor crosstalk with the ER signal transduction pathway system. This molecular adaptation subverts the effectiveness of antihormone therapy during breast cancer treatment.[44] As a result, combinations of growth factor inhibitors have been proposed to overcome intrinsic resistance to antihormone therapies or to subvert the development of acquired resistance.[44] This important topic is not discussed here, but rather we focus on the recent reports of mutations in the ER of breast cancer metastasis and the evolution of acquired resistance to SERM and to AI therapies, during long-term adjuvant treatment.

Breast cancer metastases harbor numerous mutations, but the majority is noted at Asp538 and Tyr537 at helix 12 of the LBD.[29] Primary tumors have low numbers of mutations, whereas it is believed that mutations in metastases arise as a consequence of antihormonal resistance (Fig. 21.5). This form of resistance of the

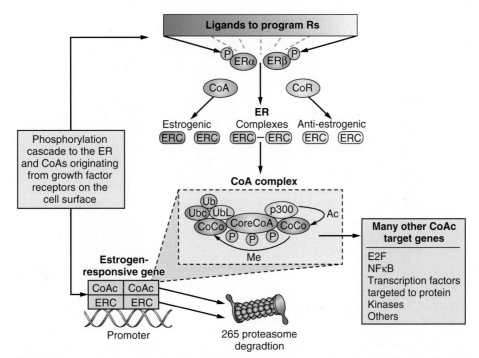

• **Fig. 21.4** Molecular networks potentially influence the expression of selective estrogen receptor *(ER)* modulator action in a target tissue. The shape of the ligands that bind to ERα and ERβ programs the complex to become an estrogenic or antiestrogenic signal. The context of the ER complex *(ERC)* can influence the expression of the response through the numbers of corepressors *(CoR)* or coactivators *(CoA)*. In simple terms, a site with few CoAs or high levels of CoRs might be a dominant antiestrogenic site. However, the expression of estrogenic action is not simply the binding of the receptor complex to the promoter of the estrogen-responsive gene, but a dynamic process of CoA complex assembly and destruction43. A core CoA, for example, steroid receptor coactivator protein 3 (SRC3), and the ERC are influenced by phosphorylation cascades that phosphorylate target sites on both complexes. The core CoA then assembles an activated multiprotein complex containing specific coco-activators *(CoCo)* that might include p300, each of which has a specific enzymatic activity to be activated later. The CoA complex *(CoAc)* binds to the ERC at the estrogen-responsive gene promoter to switch on transcription. The CoCo proteins then perform methylation or acetylation to activate dissociation of the complex. Simultaneously, ubiquitinylation by the bound ubiquitin-conjugating enzyme *(Ubc)* targets ubiquitin ligase *(UbL)* destruction of protein members of the complex through the 26S proteasome. The ERs are also ubiquitinated and destroyed in the 26S proteasome. Therefore a regimented cycle of assembly, activation, and destruction occurs on the basis of the preprogramed ER complex. However, the coactivator, specifically SRC3, has ubiquitous action and can further modulate or amplify the ligand-activated trigger through many modulating genes that can consolidate and increase the stimulatory response of the ERC in a tissue. Therefore the target tissue is programed to express a spectrum of responses between full estrogen action and antiestrogen action on the basis of the shape of the ligand and the sophistication of the tissue-modulating network. *NFκB,* Nuclear factor kB.

metastatic cell that requires a specialized receptor mechanism to survive can be rationalized as darwinian survival through genetic trial and error. The mutant amino acids in helix 12 (Ser537 and Gly538)[45] interact with the anchor amino acid (Asp 351) to close the LBD, thereby forming a ligand-free constitutively activated ER, which promotes tumor growth in an estrogen-free environment.[29] It is known that the amino acids Asp 538, Tyr 537, and Asp 351 play key roles in ER turnover and in the estrogenic or antiestrogenic properties of the ER complex.[29]

Other important mechanisms of acquired resistance resulting from antihormonal self-selection have been deciphered during the past 20 years. It appears that acquired antihormone resistance evolves over time.[46] Laboratory studies described different evolutionary phases. In phase I acquired resistance, which occurs within a year or two, tumor growth control can fail with tamoxifen, and the tumors now can grow with either E2 or SERMs. This is a

unique form of drug resistance to any anticancer therapy. Recent studies have elucidated the cellular growth regulation for resistant cell lines, now stimulated with either estrogen or a SERM.[47] Successful antihormone therapy of ER-positive MBC is only effective for 2 to 3 years. A "tamoxifen withdrawal response"[48,49] and "raloxifene withdrawal response"[50] have been noted clinically. It is now clear that the translational research for SERM treatment in MBC has successfully translated from the laboratory to the clinic.

The laboratory studies on phase I acquired resistance to SERMs present a conundrum for the clinical realities of current successful antihormone adjuvant therapy. Adjuvant therapy with tamoxifen or AIs is effective for 5 to 10 years and does not universally fail after 2 to 3 years. Clearly, the low-tumor burden of micrometastatic disease does not have the genetic variability present in MBC with a high tumor burden. Neither tamoxifen nor AIs are

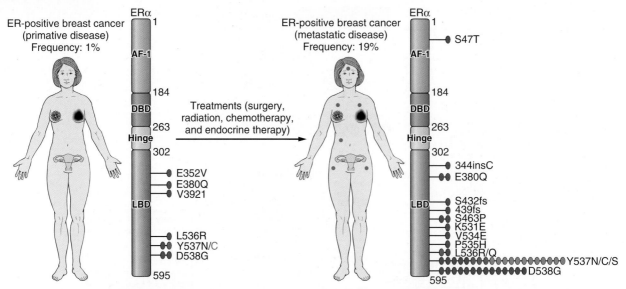

• **Fig. 21.5** Schematic diagram of *ESR1* mutations and their frequency in primary and metastatic advanced estrogen receptor *(ER)*-positive breast cancer, the potential drivers that influence their evolution and the development of ESR1 mutations in ER-positive breast cancer with progressive endocrine treatment. Vast majority of the mutations localize to the ligand-binding domain in helix 12. Nearly all *ESR1* mutations affect the ligand-binding domain *(LBD)* of the ER and often lead to constitutive activation of the ER and DNA-binding domain *(DBD)*. *ESR1* mutations are rare in primary breast tumors but significantly enhanced in metastatic breast cancer by a mutation rate of 12% and in heavily pretreated metastatic breast cancer (heavily pretreated included seven lines of previous treatment, at least two endocrine treatments) by 20%. *AF-1*, Activation function. (From Jordan VC. Chemoprevention of breast cancer with selective estrogen-receptor modulators. *Nat Rev Cancer.* 2007;7:46-53.)

cytotoxic, and the original laboratory studies proposed that long-term adjuvant therapy with tamoxifen[51] should be given forever. The rationale behind this was that tamoxifen is classified as a competitive inhibitor of estrogen action at the tumor ER, and stopping tamoxifen prematurely would allow estrogen to reactivate tumor growth. A similar rationale is used today for the treatment of gastrointestinal stromal tumors with imatinib,[52] which is not cytotoxic and suppresses tumor recurrence as long as it is given.

Be that as it may, the findings of the Early Breast Cancer Trialists Collaborative Group (EBCTCG) demonstrate that mortality decreases dramatically when tamoxifen is stopped after 5 years of adjuvant tamoxifen therapy.[9] In the Adjuvant Tamoxifen Longer Against Shorter (ATLAS) trial, it is estimated that in the 10 years after 10 years of adjuvant tamoxifen, mortality is decreased by 50%, compared with historical no treatment controls.[7] If tamoxifen or AI therapy is not cytotoxic but is just presumed to stop breast cancer growth by blocking E2-stimulated cell replication, where does the cytotoxicity come from to decrease mortality profoundly, only after endocrine therapy stops?

Laboratory evidence in vivo[53] of the evolution of acquired resistance to tamoxifen over a 5-year period (i.e., the equivalent to the then standard of care of adjuvant tamoxifen therapy) noted that physiologic estrogen now causes dramatic tumor regression experimentally after tamoxifen is stopped at 5 years. This form of acquired resistance to tamoxifen is referred to as phase II acquired resistance. Similarly, estrogen deprivation of ER-positive breast cancer cells in vitro,[54] which model long-term AI therapy in patients, also show that low-dose estrogen exhibits antitumor effects through an apoptotic mechanism. These discoveries not only provided an explanation for the

mechanism of action of high-dose synthetic estrogen therapy,[18] used for the treatment of MBC from the 1940s to the introduction of tamoxifen in the 1970s, but also provided an explanation for the profound decreases in mortality that occurs with tamoxifen and AIs after 5 years or more of long-term adjuvant therapy.[33]

It has been suggested[53] that the evolution of long-term antihormone adjuvant therapy develops micrometastatic disease with acquired resistance to long-term estrogen deprivation, which exposes a vulnerability after adjuvant therapy to a woman's own estrogen, which triggers estrogen-induced apoptosis. These laboratory data are consistent with the recent report that either high (30 mg/daily) or low (6 mg/daily) administration of oral estradiol will cause a 30% response rate in breast tumors after failure of AI adjuvant therapy.[55]

Estrogen-Induced Apoptosis

The rediscovery of the antitumor effects of estrogen occurred in the laboratory in the decade between 1991 and 2000.[53,54] The study by Song and coworkers[54] on the long-term effects of estrogen deprivation in ER-positive breast cancer cells demonstrated that both physiologic and pharmacologic concentration of estrogen triggered apoptosis. The authors[54] used these data to suggest a mechanism for the antitumor effects of high-dose of estrogen, first noted by Haddow and colleagues.[18] Nevertheless, these data supported the fact that physiologic estrogen was effective at triggering apoptosis in long-term estrogen-deprived breast cancer cells. These laboratory data illustrate that rigorous estrogen deprivation, prolonged for more than 5 years, and produced by either tamoxifen or estrogen withdrawal under laboratory conditions, was far superior

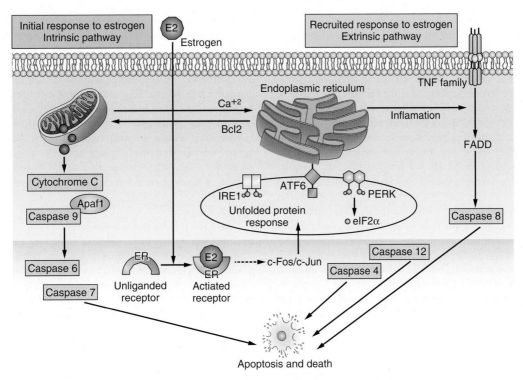

• **Fig. 21.6** Schematic diagram of the mechanism of estrogen-induced apoptosis through an unfolded protein response that triggers the intrinsic pathway of apoptosis in the mitochondria and ultimately recruits the extrinsic pathway. Estradiol *(E2)* activates nuclear estrogen receptor *(ER)* to activate multiple nuclear transcriptional factors including activating protein (AP)-1 family members. c-Fos/AP-1 associates with endoplasmic reticulum to activate unfolded protein response with the function to maintain homeostasis in the endoplasmic reticulum. Overaccumulation of unfolded proteins will cause endoplasmic reticulum stress, which first activates intrinsic (mitochondrial) and then recruits extrinsic (death receptor) apoptosis pathways to cause cell death. Endoplasmic reticulum is a joint regulatory site to integrally modulate growth or apoptosis-associated pathways. E2 activates nuclear ER to cause endoplasmic reticulum stress, which activates a set of signaling pathways including three sensors (protein kinase R–like endoplasmic reticulum kinase *[PERK]*, IRE1α, and ATF6), inflammatory responses, and adenosine monophosphate–activated protein kinase. The biological result in long-term estrogen-deprived ER-positive breast cancer cells is initial cell growth followed by events that lead to estrogen-induced apoptosis. *FADD,* FAS-associated via death domain; *TNF,* tumor necrosis factor.

to the "five-year rule" postmenopause noted by Haddow.[19] This is necessary for optimal breast cancer therapy with high-dose synthetic estrogens. These concepts have been translated into clinical treatment studies in the 21st century,[55,56] mechanistic applications to describe the reduction in the incidence of adverse effects seen in the estrogen-alone WHI trial (discussed in the next section), and an explanation for mortality decreases after long-term antihormone adjuvant therapy.[33]

Laboratory studies starting in the early 2000s, both in vivo[57,58] and in vitro,[59–61] have dissected the mechanism of action of estrogen-induced apoptosis in estrogen-deprived breast cancer cells (Fig. 21.6). The ER is the principle target required to trigger estrogen-induced apoptosis but unlike cytotoxic chemotherapy, which causes complete apoptosis within 2 days, E2 takes much longer. Structure-function relationship studies of estrogen-binding ligands to the ER demonstrate that planar estrogens initially cause growth of breast cancer cells, and after 2 days, cells are committed to apoptosis. Angular estrogens based on the triphenylethylene structure initially cause a perturbation of the ER, which remains in an "antiestrogenic" conformation that evolves over time to an "estrogenic conformation" to produce delayed apoptosis a week later. These events are described in detail in recent reviews.[62,63] It

is, however, appropriate to describe the step-wise events in cell biology that cause an apoptotic death (see Fig. 21.6).

The initial growth spurt observed with estrogen action in long-term estrogen-deprived cells causes increased protein synthesis and an unfolded protein response (UPR) in the endoplasmic reticulum. The UPR detected by the protein kinase R–like endoplasmic reticulum kinase (PERK) sensor triggers the apoptotic cascade. The survival system of the cell is impaired with the loss of Akt and the involvement of mechanistic target of rapamycin (mTOR) pathway, pushing the equilibrium from survival toward apoptosis. Estrogen initially activates the mitochondrial pathway (the intrinsic pathway) to trigger apoptosis by causing leakage of cytochrome c and subsequent activation of caspases. The death receptor Fas/FasL pathway (extrinsic pathway) is then activated to ensure cellular execution. These events are all summarized in Fig. 21.6.

Estrogen-Induced Apoptosis as an Interpretation of the Mortality Decreases After Long-Term Adjuvant Therapy and the WHI

The hypothesis[53] that the cytotoxic component of tamoxifen that causes mortality decreases after long-term adjuvant therapy was most dramatically illustrated in the ATLAS trial,[7] which compares stopping at 5 years of tamoxifen or extending therapy for another 5 years, for a total 10 years adjuvant tamoxifen therapy. The mortality decreases observed with tamoxifen are noted most dramatically during the 10 years after a decade of tamoxifen treatment was stopped. A comparison[7] during tamoxifen treatment and after tamoxifen treatment showed that during years 5 to 9 (relative risk [RR] 0.97; 0.78–1.18), there was little benefit, but in the decade after tamoxifen treatment had stopped (RR 0.71; 0.58–0.88; $p = .002$), there were major survival gains. The Adjuvant Tamoxifen—To Offer More? (aTTom) trial[64] had a similar design as ATLAS, and during years 5 to 9 (RR for mortality 1.08; 0.85–1.38), there was little survival gain, but in the decade after tamoxifen was stopped (RR 0.75; 0.63–0.9; $p = .007$), there were major survival gains. A combined analysis of aTTom and ATLAS demonstrated no benefit of continuing tamoxifen in the 5 years after extending tamoxifen to 10 years; the carryover effect for 5 years of tamoxifen was strong, but the RR for mortality after 10 years of tamoxifen was 0.75 (0.65–0.86; $p = .00004$).

The WHI trial consisted of two placebo-controlled trials: the first recruited women without a uterus and used conjugated equine estrogen (CEE) alone; the second trial, in women with a uterus, used CEE plus MPA. The study population average age for both trials was approximately 63 years. The CEE alone trial had a sustained decrease in breast cancer incidence, and there was a survival advantage for breast cancer versus placebo.[65,66] The CEE patient population had an overall survival advantage compared with placebo. The fact that these women were more than a decade past the menopause suggests long-term estrogen deprivation for any nascent breast tumors. These would be subsequently killed by the administration of CEE.[66] In the CEE plus MPA trial, there was the predicted increase in breast cancer. This raises the question: "How does MPA reverse the cytotoxic effect of estrogen in breast cancer?" In laboratory studies, estrogen-induced apoptosis was found to be preceded by an inflammatory response.[60] Synthetic glucocorticoids completely inhibit estrogen-induced apoptosis,[67] and it was suggested that because MPA is not a pure synthetic progestin but has significant glucocorticoid activity, this particular steroid was blocking the beneficial cytotoxic effect of estrogen.[67] It was further suggested that a 19-nortestosterone derivative could be used in the future as the synthetic progestin to protect the uterus from endometrial cancer, caused by unopposed estrogen action.[67] It is interesting to note that epithelial ovarian cancer has been studied to determine the safety of hormone replacement to improve the quality of life for women after surgery. Unexpectedly, women receiving hormone replacement had an improved survival from the recurrence of their epithelial ovarian cancer.[68] Some women also received norgestrel, a synthetic progestin without glucocorticoid activity; it seems that this synthetic progestin was not detrimental to the beneficial effect of estrogen therapy on survival.

The Progesterone Receptor

The PR is an estrogen-dependent protein in estrogen target tissues[69]; for this reason, it was suggested that assays of ER and PR would further refine the definition of hormone responsiveness in breast cancer. During the 1970s,[70] PR assays were included with an ER assay, for the prediction of therapeutic outcomes in MBC.[71] However, the overview of clinical trials by the EBCTCG did not find that PR assays on primary tumors added further advantage over ER assays alone for prognosis.[9]

Progesterone acts through two isoforms of the PR (see Fig. 21.3), referred to as PR-A, which lacks the first 164 amino acids at the N-terminus of PR-B[72] and PR-B. A single PR gene is situated with two promoter regions on exon 1 that encodes for those two isoforms.[72] Recent studies show that tumors that confer poor patient prognosis have an altered ratio between the two PR isoforms.[73] There is an increase in PR-A and a loss of PR-B, which confers poor prognosis.[72,74] Breast cancer tumors that have PR demonstrate slower growth, better differentiation, and a much better overall short-term prognosis. Previously, PR was only thought to be a surrogate marker of ER expression. However, it is now apparent that the lack or loss of PR expression indicates an underlying epidermal growth factor pathway or the methylation of PR gene.[72]

The PR has been evaluated as a therapeutic target in nonresectable meningioma, which is known to express PR in 70% of cases. The antiprogestin mifepristone had no effect on patient outcomes.[75] High-dose mifepristone (200–400 mg daily) has been evaluated for the treatment of MBC, but few objective responses were reported.[76] Although numerous antiprogestins have been studied, none has entered clinical practice for the treatment of MBC. It is suggested that at high-doses, mifepristone therapy is actually acting as an estrogen in MBC.[77] These data overall confirm that the PR is not a major therapeutic target in cancer.

Androgen Receptor

The AR is present in breast cancer, but its prognostic significance is unclear. The AR is a ligand-activated nuclear transcription factor and a member of the NSR superfamily (see Fig. 21.3). The full-length androgen receptor mRNA is coded from eight exons,[78] and the receptor protein contains four functional domains (see Fig. 21.3). Constitutively active AR variants (AR-Vs) contain the N-terminal domain and the DBD but lack the LBD. The AR-Vs are considered to play a role in tumor progression.[78] In one recent study[79] of 1467 breast cancers, 79% were classified as AR-positive. Among the 1164 ER-positive cases, 88% were AR-positive. The authors[79] concluded that ER status was associated with breast cancer survival but was dependent on ER status. By contrast, in a meta-analysis of 7693 women with breast cancer, AR expression was noted in 61% of patients, and ER-positive tumors tended to express AR rather than ER- negative tumors (75% vs. 32%).[12] The authors[12] concluded that expression of AR in a patient's breast cancer was associated with better disease-free and overall survival, independent of the ER coexpression. There is current interest in using antiandrogens targeted to the AR in breast cancer, except for current investigations of triple-negative breast cancer (TNBC). Triple-negative primary breast cancer that is AR-positive increases with age, and any TNBC primary tumor that is AR-positive also has AR-positive lymph nodes. This has been classified as a unique breast cancer subtype.[80] The role of AR in TNBC has recently been reviewed.[13]

Summary and Conclusions

The NSR superfamily, including the members ER, PR, AR, and GR (see Fig. 21.3), is a finely regulated system, designed to support target cell survival. The ER is a signal transduction pathway, primarily designed for cell replication and the regulation of estrogen responsive genes. The AR, PR, and GR modulate estrogen action under specific circumstances. In breast cancer, the ER has proved to be the most successful therapeutic target.[3]

Selected References

5. Jordan VC, Brodie AM. Development and evolution of therapies targeted to the estrogen receptor for the treatment and prevention of breast cancer. *Steroids.* 2007;72:7-25.

7. Davies C, Pan H, Godwin J, et al. Long-term effects of continuing adjuvant tamoxifen to 10 years versus stopping at 5 years after diagnosis of oestrogen receptor-positive breast cancer: ATLAS, a randomised trial. *Lancet.* 2013;381:805-816.

10. Anderson GL, Chlebowski RT, Aragaki AK, et al. Conjugated equine oestrogen and breast cancer incidence and mortality in postmenopausal women with hysterectomy: extended follow-up of the Women's Health Initiative randomised placebo-controlled trial. *Lancet Oncol.* 2012;13:476-486.

25. Vogel VG, Costantino JP, Wickerham DL, et al. Update of the National Surgical Adjuvant Breast and Bowel Project Study of Tamoxifen and Raloxifene (STAR) P-2 Trial: preventing breast cancer. *Cancer Prev Res (Phila).* 2010;3:696-706.

45. Toy W, Shen Y, Won H, et al. ESR1 ligand-binding domain mutations in hormone-resistant breast cancer. *Nat Genet.* 2013;45:1439-1445.

50. Lemmo W. Anti-estrogen withdrawal effect with raloxifene? A case report. *Integr Cancer Ther.* 2016;15:245-249.

A full reference list is available online at ExpertConsult.com.

22

Molecular Oncology of Breast Cancer

HIMANSHU JOSHI AND MICHAEL F. PRESS

Cancer is a complex disease that involves progressive accumulation of diverse alterations in genetic and epigenetic regulatory programs of cells in interaction with the host stromal environment. Characterization of cancer-driving alterations that confer specific hallmark traits[1] and thereby transform the normal cell into a malignant cell is essential for linking the molecular pathology of cancers to the molecular fingerprint of cancers. This process is not limited to understanding cancer biology but also involves distinctions between driver and passenger alterations, causal and secondary alterations of clinical significance, and actionable and nonactionable alterations in genes and pathways. Molecular heterogeneity has been an element underlying the complexity of cancer biology and thereby also a challenge for effective clinical management. Molecular heterogeneity is composed of intratumoral (presence of multiple clones representing different molecular profiles within the tumor) and intertumoral (presence of different molecular characteristics between cancers of the same tissue) heterogeneity. Intratumoral heterogeneity can vary across the spatial and temporal dimensions as the clones compete for host resources, and under selective pressure clones with mutations that confer increased advantage for growth and proliferation survive, driving cancer progression. Availability of high throughput technology platforms including next-generation sequencing (NGS) has provided an opportunity to study the cancer genome in high resolution to discover the molecular alterations that are key to disease progression and clinical management.

While focused on clinical utility, understanding the genetic and epigenetic alterations at multiple "omic" levels (genome, transcriptome, and epigenome) provides an understanding of major biological pathways that transform normal cells to acquire malignant characteristics and forms the core of molecular discovery. In this chapter, we summarize the biology of breast cancer development, molecular classification of the disease, and subsequently the molecular oncology of clinical significance.

Hallmarks of Cancer

The processes underlying tumor initiation, progression, and metastasis involves altered activity of multiple signaling pathways, including the pathways that regulate key physiologic functions such as growth and proliferation, differentiation, stress response, DNA repair, metabolism, and cell survival. The recruitment of these pathways in neoplastic transformation and cancer progression is a multistaged process. Precise characterization of these

processes is, however, a complex task, especially given the multiple levels of complexity. Intratumoral, intertumoral, and temporal heterogeneity defines cancer as a highly dynamic process. Changes in biological interactions and rewiring of the signaling pathways in response to the environment[2,3] is another aspect that potentially confounds the understanding of carcinogenesis at the molecular level. The pattern and extent of alterations in genes and pathways are also in part contributed by the interactions of cancerous cells with the stromal microenvironment.

Therefore it is important to describe carcinogenesis as a set of signature traits of cancer cells or hallmarks of cancer[1] (Fig. 22.1). These characteristic traits, described as distinctive and complementary, form a conceptual basis to understand functional organization of cancer cells. Different hallmark traits and known molecular markers having their potential role in acquisition of the cancer hallmark characteristics are illustrated in Fig. 22.1.

Sustaining Proliferative Signaling

A core cancer-driving trait is acquisition of sustainable growth signaling. Under normal conditions, growth factors bind to specific receptors localized on the cell membrane, leading to release of signal transducers and second messengers in the cell that transmit the signal to the nucleus. As a consequence, nuclear transcription factors are activated and initiate transcription of specific proteins that induce cell division and growth. Regulation of normal cells is related either to their dependency on other cells for growth factors or by an overproduction of a specific growth receptor required to respond to the corresponding growth factor.

Through bypassing the normal regulatory mechanisms, cancer cells acquire self-sufficiency of growth by one of the following common mechanisms:

1. Secreting growth factor ligands themselves (autocrine)
2. Inducing the normal stromal cells to secrete the growth factors (paracrine)
3. Overexpression of growth inducing receptors
4. Altering the structure or type of the receptor, causing ligand-independent activation of proliferative signaling

In addition to these mechanisms, altered activity of one or more downstream pathways may eliminate dependence on growth receptor-mediated proliferative signaling.

Abnormal activation of multiple alternative pathways may confer self-sufficiency of growth signaling in breast cancer. Estrogen receptor (ER) signaling, human epidermal growth factor

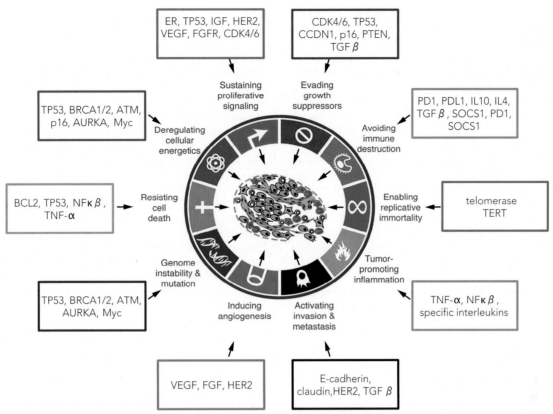

• **Fig. 22.1** Cancer hallmark traits. Cancer-associated traits are caused by altered activity of multiple genes. The figure illustrates key markers associated with respective hallmark traits in context of breast cancer. (Modified from Hanahan D, Weinberg RA. Hallmarks of cancer: the next generation. *Cell.* 2011;144:646-674.)

receptor-2 (HER2) membrane receptor signaling, and vascular endothelial growth factor (EGF) receptor family signaling are the most common known proliferation-inducing pathways in breast cancer.

Approximately 70% of breast cancers express ERα, and therefore ER signaling is a key signaling pathway of diagnostic and therapeutic interest. Estrogen could induce proliferation in ERα-mediated and ERα-independent mechanisms.[4] The classical ERα-mediated proliferative response involves estrogen binding to ERα, followed by modulation of target gene regulation through binding to estrogen response elements (ERE) in target gene promoters. In nonclassical activity, ERα can interact with transcription factors, such as SP1 or Fos/Jun, to modulate transcription of genes that do not possess the ERE in their promoter.[5] In addition, ER activates mitogen-activated protein kinase (MAPK) by forming a complex with it in the nucleus to mediate transcription of specific target genes. An increased rate of cell proliferation results in increased mutagenesis.[6] ER-independent proliferative mechanisms, not widely accepted yet, propose genotoxic damage by estradiol metabolites generated by cytochrome P450.[7]

EGF receptor family member HER2, also known as ERBB2 (avian erythroblastosis oncogene B2), is another common proliferative signaling pathway in breast cancer. *HER2* gene amplification[8] results in overexpression of the HER2 transmembrane receptor, which is involved in growth signaling. Approximately 15% to 25% of invasive breast cancers have amplification of *HER2*, and these cancers are associated with aggressive disease behavior and poor prognosis.[9–11] The overexpressed HER2 protein forms both homodimers and heterodimers with other epidermal

growth factor receptor family receptor tyrosine kinases, and these activate downstream signaling. In addition to homodimerization, HER2 can form heterodimers with other members of the EGF receptor family and activate downstream growth signaling pathways, including but not limited to mitogen-activated protein kinase and phosphatidylinositol 3-kinase (PI3K) signaling.

Other upstream growth pathways involved in proliferative signaling in breast cancer are vascular endothelial growth factor (VEGF) signaling, fibroblast growth factor receptor (FGFR) signaling,[12] and autocrine activation of wingless and integration site growth factor (Wnt) signaling pathway signaling.[13] Although somatic mutations are known to activate downstream signaling pathways, a recent study in breast cancer showed amplifications of *PIK3CA, KRAS, BRAF,* and *EGFR,*[14] thereby contributing to the abnormal activation of Ras-Raf-MAPK signaling.

Inactivation of negative-feedback mechanisms known to attenuate self-sufficient proliferative signaling is an alternative way by which cancer cells enhance proliferative signaling. PTEN is an example of negative feedback, known to antagonize PI3K signaling.[15] In addition, nuclear PTEN downregulates cyclin D1 and prevents the phosphorylation of MAPK,[16] thus loss of function alterations in PTEN promotes proliferation because of loss of its negative feedback.

Evading Growth Suppressors

Cancer cells are capable of evading a variety of growth suppression mechanisms located in the extracellular matrix or on the surface of nearby cells.

Retinoblastoma gene (RB) is considered a gatekeeper and prototype tumor suppressor protein that has a pivotal role in cell cycle progression because of its role as transducer of extracellular growth inhibitory signals.[17,18] Alterations in RB signaling can lead to persistent proliferation. Cell proliferation in breast cancer cell lines may be reversed through inhibition of G1 cyclin-dependent kinases (CDKs) with CDK 4/6 inhibitors leading to hypophosphorylation of pRb and a G1/S-phase cell cycle arrest. Studies of breast cancer cell lines show the most sensitive cell lines have elevated expression of Rb and cyclin D1 but decreased expression of CDKN2A (p16[INK4a]).[19] These observations have been confirmed in clinical trials of CDK 4/6 inhibitors (palbociclib, ribociclib, and abemaciclib) in patients with metastatic ER-positive, HER2-negative breast cancer.[19-21]

Transforming growth factor (TGF)β signaling, another growth suppressor pathway, has been shown to have antiproliferative activity in early breast cancers by downregulation of *c-myc* oncogene.[22] Altered TGFβ receptors or mutations of components of the signaling pathway might lead to evasion of growth suppression by TGFβ. Mutation or altered expression of SMAD4 protein, which is involved in transducing the TGFβ signals could alter the growth suppression by TGFβ.

Resisting Cell Death

Programmed cell death or apoptosis is an essential pathway for maintaining tissue homeostasis and elimination of cells with irreversible damage. Apoptosis mechanisms are divided into two components: First, an extrinsic pathway, which receives and processes extracellular death signals involving Fas ligand and tumor necrosis factor-α (TNFα); second, an intrinsic pathway that integrates intracellular signals, such as release of mitochondrial cytochrome C. Both pathways result in activation of downstream effector caspases. The intrinsic pathway is regulated by the B-cell lymphoma 2 (BCL2) family proteins.[23] Sensing DNA damage, TP53, a checkpoint regulator,[24] can induce apoptosis by activating BH3-only proteins, activating survival pathways such as PI3K-AKT/PKB pathway, increasing insulin-like growth factor (IGF)1/2 and interleukin 3. Cancer cells evade apoptosis by acquiring loss of function mutations in *TP53*, observed in approximately 37% of breast cancer samples,[14] downregulating proapoptotic factors (BH3 only proteins) and inducing antiapoptotic proteins, for instance, BCL2.

Enabling Replicative Immortality

In contrast to normal cells, which are capable of passing through a finite number of growth and division cycles before becoming senescent, cancer cells must acquire replicative immortality. It has been proposed that for cancer cells to acquire this hallmark trait, they upregulate telomerase, a specialized DNA polymerase enzyme that is involved in maintaining telomere length[25] or can add nucleotide repeats—TTAGGG oriented 5′-to-3′ toward and at the end of the chromosomes.[26] More recently a protein subunit of telomerase, known as telomerase reverse transcriptase or TERT, has been shown to possess other functions, even after elimination of the canonical telomerase activity.[27]

Telomerase expression observed in approximately 53% of breast cancers was associated with poor outcomes in patients treated with chemotherapy, while the opposite effect was observed with endocrine therapy.[28] ERα can increase the telomerase activity, whereas the anti-ER tamoxifen is known to suppress telomerase activity.[29]

Inducing Angiogenesis

In contrast to transient activity of angiogenesis in normal tissues, activation of an "angiogenic switch" in cancer cells underlies sustained angiogenesis, thereby stimulating abnormal and sustained angiogenesis in cancer[30] that transports oxygen and nutrients to cancer cells and evacuates the waste and carbon dioxide. An imbalance between the factors that promote and oppose angiogenesis results in activation of persistent angiogenesis. In response to hypoxia or oncogenic stimuli, prototype angiogenesis initiator VEGF is expressed[31] and binds to VEGF receptors (VEGFR1, VEGFR2, and VEGFR3) on cell membrane of endothelial cells. In addition, fibroblast growth factor 1/2 are potent proangiogenic factors, whereas TSP-1 (thrombospondin-1) counteracts the proangiogenic factors by binding the transmembrane receptors on endothelial cells.[32] Although initial clinical trial results using humanized anti-VEGF-A monoclonal antibodies (bevacizumab) in breast cancer patients appeared promising,[33] subsequent clinical trials failed to demonstrate a significant improvement in either progression-free (PFS) or overall (OS) survival.[34]

Additionally, hematopoietic progenitors such as bone marrow–derived progenitor cells may potentially play a role in cancer angiogenesis.[35-37] However, more comprehensive evidence is necessary to understand migration and invasion of these cells into developing breast tumors in vivo.

Activation of Invasion and Metastasis

Transformation of well-differentiated normal epithelial cells into often poorly differentiated cancer cells with migratory and invasive properties is a consequence of specific molecular alterations. The multistep process of invasion and metastasis is described as the invasion-metastasis cascade,[38] which results in local invasion, intravasation of cancer cells, transit, extravasation at distant tissue sites, followed by colonization with a small fraction of the cancer cells, resulting in formation of disseminated cancer nodules (micrometastasis) and, lastly, some proportion of micrometastatic nodules adapt to the local microenvironment and proliferate to become mature metastases.[39] The invasion-metastasis cascade is regulated by a multifaceted program, referred as *epithelial-mesenchymal transition* (EMT), which permits transformed epithelial cells to acquire mesenchymal features including motility, invasiveness, and resistance to apoptosis.[40] The entry of cancer cells into EMT may be transient, stable, or partial.

E-cadherin is a key protein involved in formation of cell-to-cell adherens junctions that assembles adjacent epithelial cells and maintains quiescence of the cells. Loss of functional E-cadherin by transcriptional repression, mutation, chromosomal deletion, or protein degradation may confer metastatic potential and ultimately provoke EMT, in addition to loss of cell-to-cell adherens junctions.[41]

Among other factors, specific members of the integrin family, matrix metalloproteinases, and crosstalk between tumor and stromal cells contribute to invasion and metastasis.

Genome Instability and Mutation

Unlike normal cells, which only infrequently contain mutations, cancer cells have significantly high rates of acquired mutations. Initial occurrence of mutations in gatekeeper genes result in genomic instability, and multiple genomic alterations are a key feature of cancer cells because of their role in developing other

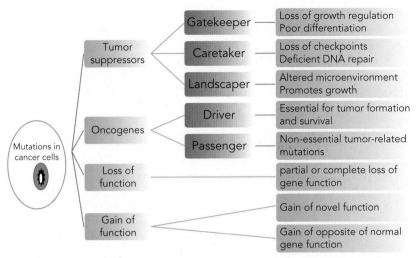

• **Fig. 22.2** Classifications of mutations in cancer: mutations with diverse functional roles in acquisition of cancer hallmark traits by the cancer cells.

cancer hallmark capabilities. Whereas most cancers originate from a single ancestor cell due to a specific mutation(s), their progression is attributed to clonal evolution of the cells with acquisition of additional genomic alterations that confer selective growth advantages and lead to more aggressive behavior.[42–44]

Mutations in DNA repair genes can lead to a *mutator phenotype* that subsequently gives rise to more mutations and eventually genomic instability. Genomic instability is a primary event in hereditary cancers with germline mutations in genes, such as *BRCA1* and *BRCA2,* that are linked to DNA repair. In sporadic cancers, oncogene-induced collapse of DNA replication forks may lead to DNA double strand breaks and genomic instability.[45]

Occurrence of mutations may have diverse, often overlapping or linked functional contributions in conferring hallmark traits including genomic instability, resulting in cancer progression (Fig. 22.2). Tumor suppressor genes are of prominent interest in development of cancer hallmarks. The gatekeeper mutations occur in early cancers and contribute to loss of growth regulation and poor differentiation of cancer cells. *TP53* is a well-studied gene involved in direct regulation of cell cycle, apoptosis, and DNA repair, thereby maintaining genomic integrity. Germline or early occurring somatic mutations of *TP53* drive cancer by loss of their gatekeeper function. Mutation in E-cadherin is another such example. Caretaker genes are involved in DNA repair and checkpoint control; however, they cannot initiate carcinogenesis as a direct consequence of mutations.[46] Mutations in *BRCA1* and *BRCA2* in breast cancer represent good examples of caretaker mutations. The landscaper mutations modulate the microenvironment and can promote cell proliferation. No comprehensive evidence is available that identifies any mutations in the role of a landscape mutation. However, among hereditary *BRCA1/2* mutant cases, alterations in stromal cells have been proposed to contribute as landscape mutations.[47] In addition, mutations may be broadly categorized as driver and passenger mutations. The driver mutations are capable of conferring selective advantage to cancer cells promoting carcinogenesis and survival of the cancerous cells. Mutations in *TP53, PIK3CA, MAP3K1, GATA3, CDH1, BRCA1, PTEN, PIK3R1, AKT1,* and *RB1*[14] are among the prominent driver mutations in breast cancer. Passenger mutations are other nonsynonymous mutations that do not play a direct role in carcinogenesis or progression. Mutations could also cause partial or complete loss of function that applies to tumor suppressor functions. Specific mutations of *TP53* cause gain of novel functions. For instance, interference with the p53 function preventing DNA damage and promoting genetic instability, is the opposite of its wild-type role.

In addition to mutations, loss of telomeric DNA and specific copy number alterations are other factors that may contribute to genomic instability.

Tumor Promoting Inflammation

Cancers induce immune response, resulting in immune infiltration and inflammation. Inflammation could contribute to cancer progression by expression of growth factors, survival factors, and proangiogenic factors to the local microenvironment to promote tumor formation.

Reprogramming Energetics

Normal cells favor glycolysis under anaerobic stress. In contrast, cancer cells, even under aerobic conditions, favor metabolism of glucose to lactate, a state referred as *anaerobic glycolysis*.[48,49] This means that the usual preference for oxidative phosphorylation (OXPHOS) in normal cells is shifted to metabolically inefficient glycolysis despite the presence of oxygen, mainly attributed to mitochondrial malfunction and a hypoxic microenvironment. Cancer cells face two challenges: first, the need to continue support for proliferation and growth by reprogramming metabolism and, second, achieving metabolic adaptation to survive metabolic stress. Regulation of adenosine triphosphate (ATP) synthesis by regulating substrate uptake and glycolytic enzymes is a possible mechanism that enables cells to adapt to the microenvironment.[50]

Mutations in cancer cells also play a role in reprogramming of cancer cell energetics. Mutations in *PIK3CA* are common in breast cancer. Mutant *PIK3CA* or loss of its regulator PTEN can promote PI3K/Akt signaling and ultimately changes in metabolism, by increased expression of nutrient transporters, stimulation of hexo-/phosphor-fructokinase to drive glycolysis, enhanced transcription of genes involved in glycolysis, and/or by an enhanced rate of protein synthesis through Akt-dependent mTOR activation.[51]

Considering reprogramming of metabolism as a consequence of oncogenic activity brings up the question of whether it is a core hallmark of cancer. Regardless, it remains a potential target for novel therapeutic strategies.

Evading Immune Destruction

Cancer cells evade the immunosurveillance and thereby continue to grow locally, metastasize to distant tissues and ultimately result in a macroscopic tumor. There are two potential mechanisms underlying dissemination of cancers: First, mutations accumulated either in a subpopulation of primary tumor or in disseminated cells to confer metastatic potential to a fraction of cells[52] and second, expression of immune mediators (i.e., TGFβ, TP53, HIF, VEGF) by the tumor cells[53] could modulate immune response. T regulatory cells (Tregs) that normally suppress T-cell response and natural killer (NK)-cell activity are observed to be significantly associated with larger tumor size and trend toward an association with estrogen receptor negativity. In addition, the same study observed an association with ER/progesterone receptors (PR)/HER2-negative or triple-negative breast cancer (TNBC) and Nottingham grade III cases that were significantly associated with high number of FOXP3 (fork-head/winged-helix transcription factor, which is involved in the development in Treg cells).[54]

The presence of immune cells in breast cancers may also reflect the potential for harnessing the patients' own immune system to eliminate tumor cells. The presence of tumor-infiltrating lymphocytes (TILs), especially in lymphocyte-predominant breast cancers, has been associated with significant improvements in pathologic complete response to chemotherapy.[55,56] The potential protective role of lymphocytes has been appreciated in cancers with microsatellite instability. The inability of these cancers to efficiently repair errors in exons leads to expression of proteins containing neo-antigens that may be identified by a patient's own immune system ostensibly leading to a high density of TILs. These neo-antigens expressed in proteins on the cell surface are speculated to be most likely to have this effect. This concept has led to the development of novel immunomodulatory therapies, such as programmed cell death 1 inhibitors for the treatment of metastatic cancers, including breast cancers.

Normal Mammary Development and Carcinogenesis

Endogenous hormones have been shown to be key nongenetic factors underlying breast carcinogenesis. Endogenous hormones, on one hand, have essential roles in normal development of the breast, whereas on the other hand, they also increase the risk of breast cancer. Epidemiology studies have shown that early menarche, late menopause, nulliparity, lack of lactation and breastfeeding, and delayed childbearing are associated with increased risk of developing breast cancer, underscoring the profound role endogenous hormones play in cancer development.

Endogenous Hormones and Growth Factors

Understanding breast carcinogenesis requires an understanding of the normal development of the breast. Breast tissue is composed of epithelial and mesenchymal components. Opening onto the skin surface and lined by squamous cells, breast ducts are lined by a double-layered epithelium composed of luminal and myoepithelial cells for the vast majority of the ductal system throughout the breast. The luminal epithelial cells are most prone to malignant transformation. During development steroid hormone receptors, especially ER and PR, facilitate cellular responses to hormones that, among other activities, lead to proliferation of the luminal cells.

Although all mammals are born with a rudimentary mammary gland, after birth, through a process of cyclical growth and involution coupled to body hormone status (Fig. 22.3), the primitive breast undergoes extensive morphogenesis through invasion of the surrounding fat pad and progressive branching to the outer limits of the mesenchymal fat pad to create an extensive treelike structure, the terminal duct lobule unit (TDLU), specialized for milk production during pregnancy.[57]

The branching of large ducts eventually leads to the TDLUs that are composed of terminal ducts and blind-ended ductules. TDLUs in adult women branch into small acini to form the lobules. During adulthood, TDLUs demonstrate proliferative activity, predominantly during the second half of each menstrual cycle, and subsequent epithelial apoptosis at the conclusion of each cycle. Presumably as a result of this repetitive proliferative activity with each menstrual cycle, it is the TDLUs that are responsible for the development of the vast majority of breast cancers.[58]

Estradiol and other estrogens interact with two specific intracellular (nuclear) receptors, which are both inducible transcription factors, ERα and ERβ. Some normal luminal epithelial cells express the ERα[59] and are considered relatively mature cells that infrequently cycle in the adult breast.[60] ERα is expressed in infant, pubertal, and cycling adult breast epithelial cells.[61] ERβ is expressed in most luminal, myoepithelial cells, fibroblasts, and lymphocytes.[62] PR is expressed in the breast as two isoforms, PR-A and PR-B, based on alternative initial transcription start sites from a single PGR gene. PR is expressed in a minority of cells in the luminal epithelium concentrated in the terminal bud cells. Expression of PR is induced by estrogen action at the transcriptional level and is decreased by progestins at both transcriptional and translational levels.[63] In addition to ER/PR-mediated proliferation, a paracrine or juxtacrine mode of regulation of proliferation has been proposed.[64]

Multiple stages of mammary development[65] are depicted in Fig. 22.3. Here we briefly present an overview of the process, the factors involved in it, and the role of stem cells in breast morphogenesis, the details of which are described in other chapters.

Prenatal or Fetal

Mammary glands originate from mammary buds, which are ectodermal ingrowths along the mammary lines and are present in 4-week-old embryos.[66] Between 14 to 18 weeks of gestation, the mammary gland appears as an epithelial anlage resulting from focal ingrowth of the epidermis into the underlying mesenchyme. It subsequently undergoes branching and ductal morphogenesis into the mesenchyme. BCL2 expression is observed at 18 weeks and is known to prevent apoptosis and permit expansion of the epithelial cell population.[67] Differentiation of nipple and areola and development of a rudimentary ductal system occurs during the second half of fetal life.[66] Prolactin is involved in ductal budding by sensitizing the cells to insulin, resulting in a mitogenic effect. By week 28, the luminal cells are separated from the basement membrane by an outer layer of myoepithelial cells. The basal cells express EGFR and TGFα.[68] BCL2 is expressed in stromal cells at this stage and protects them from apoptosis, permitting

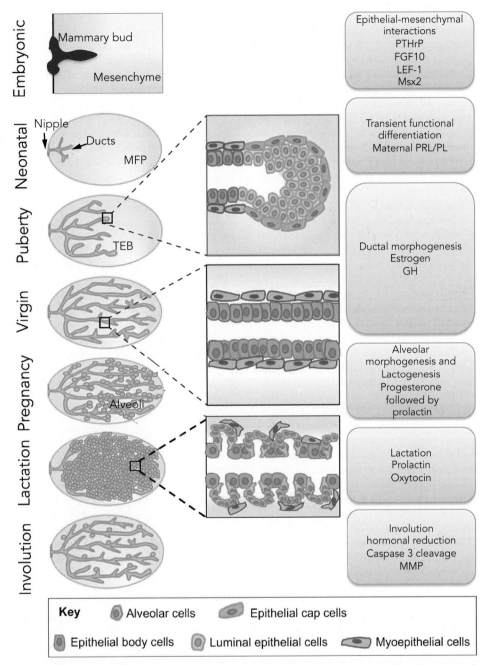

• **Fig. 22.3** Multistage development from fetal to menopausal stages. Appearance of alveoli, increase in their number with increased degree of branching followed by the decrease in both at involution. *GH,* Growth hormone; *MFP,* mammary fat pad; *MMP,* matrix metalloproteinase; *TEB,* terminal end bud. (Modified from Inman JL, Robertson C, Mott JD, Bissell MJ. Mammary gland development: cell fate specification, stem cells and the microenvironment. *Development.* 2015;142:1028-1042.)

their expansion as future fibroblasts.[67] Parathyroid hormone-related protein (PTHrP), together with bone morphogenic proteins (BMP), have been shown to have a role in the development of mammary buds and induction of Msh Homeobox 2 (MSX2).[69]

Postnatal

At birth, the ductal system opens onto the skin surface, through the breast pit. With birth, estrogen, progesterone, and prolactin levels decline, resulting in involution of the breast.[66] From 2 years of age until puberty, the mammary gland is composed of small ductal structures in fibroblastic stroma in both sexes.[68]

Puberty

As a response to a surge in hypothalamic-pituitary-ovarian activity, also referred to as *gonadarche,* increased secretion of gonadotrophins and estrogen initiate the development of the breast glandular architecture, referred as *thelarche.* Apart from estrogen, other factors, including insulin, cortisol, thyroxin, prolactin, and growth hormone, are involved in the gradual process of gland differentiation.[70] An increase in growth hormone secretion occurring in adolescence sensitizes the mammary cells to the mitogenic effects of insulin. The mammary gland at puberty contains multiple types of stem and progenitor cells, including bipotent mammary associated stem cells (MaSCs), which then differentiate into luminal and myoepithelial cells of the duct.[65] The terminal end buds undergo branching, forming blind-ended ductules, known as acini. Collection of acini arising from a terminal duct form a functional unit, terminal ductal-lobular unit (TDLU),[68] a site where most cancers arise.[64] After menarche, the mammary gland continues cyclic epithelial proliferation with an associated increase in the number of alveoli in the TDLU, especially during the luteal phase, when levels of estrogen and progesterone are high, followed by apoptosis with menses during each successive cycle.[71] This association of hormonal levels and proliferation supports the role of a hormonal stimulation in mitotic cell division, thus increasing the chance of errors in DNA replication and repair, leading to carcinogenesis. Luminal cell type is a primary target for carcinogenesis because luminal cells account for more than 90% of epithelial proliferation, as well as the observations that more than 90% of breast carcinomas synthesize cytokeratins and 70% are positive for hormone receptors.[72]

Pregnancy and Lactation

Under the influence of estrogens and progesterone, mammary stem cells induce controlled ductal and alveolar proliferation during pregnancy. The number of TDLUs and alveoli increase as well. Increased rate of proliferation and potential errors in DNA synthesis and accumulation of mutations contributes to transient elevation of breast cancer risk. Human placental lactogen results in increased secretion of fluid and protein causing alveolar dilation. During the late stages of pregnancy, increased DNA synthesis and mitosis occur, related to extensive lobuloalveolar growth.[73] Estrogen and progesterone in the presence of prolactin induce differentiation of alveolar epithelial cells into milk-secreting lobular alveolar epithelial cells, after prior exposure to cortisol, growth hormone, thyroxine, and insulin.[74] After delivery, estrogen, progesterone, and human placental lactogen decrease, resulting in elimination of their inhibitory effect on prolactin, initiation of lactation, and inhibition of proliferation. Weaning is a gradual process, involves apoptosis of alveolar cells, alveolar collapse, and ensuing involution of the breast tubule-alveolar glands. The ability of mammary epithelium to undergo proliferation and differentiation with each pregnancy provides an indication of the important role of stem cells in this process.[75]

Postmenopausal Involution

During postmenopausal involution, both ducts and lobules are reduced in number, in contrast to the postlactational involution that is limited to lobules.[68] The intralobular stroma is replaced by collagen. The glandular epithelium and intralobular and interlobular connective tissue is replaced by fat, leading to reduced mammographic density.[68] Lobular involution and a decreased mitotic rate reduces the rate and number of mutations, thus a relative protective effect of menopause as expressed in the reduced slope of breast cancer induction with age,[76,77] although the majority of breast cancer occurs in postmenopausal women.

Stem Cells

Normal mammary stem cells (MaSC), a type of somatic stem cell, are multipotent cells with a unique capacity for self-renewal as well as the potential to differentiate into all specialized mammary epithelial cell types. MaSCs are key to pubertal elongation of ducts and gestational lobuloalveolar differentiation. Just as normal stem cells are essential for maintaining tissue homeostasis and functional integrity given their properties of self-renewal and

differentiation in the normal gland, cancer stem cells (CSCs) are, similarly, a subpopulation of cancer cells that are proposed to have a tumorigenic role in addition to characteristics of "stemness" displayed by normal stem cells. A small number of cancer stem cells may act as potential reserve cells for cancer recurrence, relapse, and metastasis. Cancer stem cells may (but do not necessarily) originate from normal stem cells[78] and can be one of the origins of cancers.[79] MaSCs with suitable genomic alterations may initiate cancer. The potential role of MaSCs is explained by a parity-associated protective effect against breast cancer, attributable to a decrease in MaSCs during breast epithelial involution after pregnancy and lactation. The MaSCs do not express steroid hormone receptors (ERα and PR) or HER2, the key clinical predictive molecular markers for contemporary breast cancer treatment,[80] favoring their association with specific subsets of breast cancer. Mutations altering key regulatory pathways and epigenetic aberrations[81] could potentially transform stem cells into CSC. Stem cell niches, or stroma associated with cancer stem cells, represent distinct regions of the tumor microenvironment. These niches may play a key role in maintaining stemlike characteristics, which could promote cancer progression and metastasis. Both MaSCs and CSCs express aldehyde dehydrogenase 1 (ALDH1), and ALDH1 expression correlates with proliferation index and *HER2/ERBB2* overexpression in breast carcinomas.[82] In addition, CSCs are known to express CD44 with low/nonexpressed CD24 and Lin proteins.[83] The potential tumorigenic[82] and metastatic[84] roles of CSCs have inspired substantial clinical interest and investigation.

Stemness and Clonal Evolution

Genomic instability and the occurrence of mutations as cancer hallmarks, described in the previous section of this chapter, comply with the classic clonal evolution model. The cancer stem cell model is different from the clonal evolution model, which proposes that any cell accumulating specific genomic alterations has the capability to initiate cancer development and stemness. In contrast, the CSC hypothesis proposes that only the CSCs that have the property of self-renewal can differentiate into cancer cells that are both tumorigenic and nontumorigenic when transplanted to animals. The tumorigenic CSCs are responsible for tumor relapse, recurrence, and metastasis. The two models are not considered mutually exclusive, given available evidence. CSCs have not been detected in all cancers. Cancers that do not show evidence of hierarchical organization (undifferentiated precursor—differentiated descendant relationship), or heterogeneity resulting from a therapeutic response may be explained by clonal evolution, rather than by epigenetic differences between CSCs and their progeny.[85]

Clinical Perspective on Carcinogenesis and Progression

Initiated as premalignant or preinvasive lesions, such as atypical ductal or lobular hyperplasia, ductal carcinoma in situ (DCIS), and lobular carcinoma in situ (LCIS), breast carcinomas acquire multiple hallmarks of cancer in multiple stages and evolve into invasive carcinomas, as demonstrated by the modified Wellings-Jensen-Marcum model.[58] This model provides a context for identification of the underlying molecular alterations in the cancer hallmarks theory and, thereby, the study of cancer progression is viewed as a consequence of acquisition of driver and passenger mutations, copy number aberrations, and other genomic and

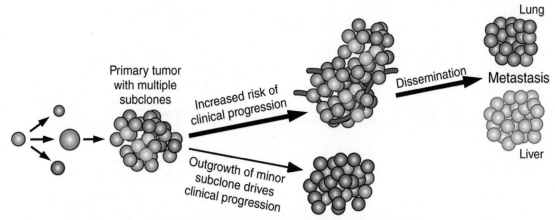

• **Fig. 22.4** Clonal evolution model: multistage progression of cancer originating from a founder cell evolves into localized tumor (niche) and ultimately a mature primary tumor. Under the selective pressure, dominant clone(s) grow and metastasize to distant organs. The minor subclone may potentially drive clinical progression. (Modified from Kleppe M, Levine RL. Tumor heterogeneity confounds and illuminates: assessing the implications. *Nat Med.* 2014;20:342-344.)

epigenomic changes in the terminal duct lobular unit (TDLU). In addition, the intertumor, intratumoral spatial and temporal heterogeneity, as explained by the clonal evolution model (Fig. 22.4), provides a broad overview of clinical cancer progression as a phenotypic outcome of interactions within multiple competing clones within the stromal microenvironment under selective pressure, including the dominant and outcome-determinant subclones in combination with minor subclones, in the context of treatment.[86] From a clinical perspective, this implies the need for multimodal diagnostic and therapeutic approaches to achieve effective disease management.

The following are considered priorities for multimodal clinical management:

1. Large studies to identify specific genomic alterations that underlie altered activity of specific biological pathways that can drive tumor progression and clinical outcome.
2. Development of high-resolution, robust, and reproducible tools to identify molecular drivers of breast cancers.
3. Availability of decision-making tools to expand the use of effective targeted therapeutics for particular cancer-driver pathways.

Molecular Profiling

Technological advances in high-throughput methods, as well as parallel improvements in computation over the past 2 decades, have enabled the generation, analysis, and integration of data from multiple biological levels, including the genome, transcriptome, epigenome, and proteome. Studies based on NGS and microarrays have shown breast cancer to be a molecularly heterogeneous disease, with broad diversity in biological characteristics that correspond to differences in clinical outcome.[14] The number of novel biomarker genes and pathways deciphered from NGS data focusing on cancer driver mechanisms, including clinically significant disease variants, copy number changes, pharmacogenomics, and corresponding clinical trials investigating their therapeutic utility, are anticipated to expand in the near future. However, the current 2016 American Society of Clinical Oncology (ASCO)[87,88] guidelines for breast cancer management recommend ER, PR, and HER2 as markers for clinical decision-making. Besides their use

as predictive markers for antiestrogen or anti-HER2 therapy, they are also used as predictive markers for novel mTOR inhibitors and CDK4/6 inhibitors.[19,89] Despite the continuing progress toward gaining insight into potential driver mechanisms in the recent years, translation related to predictive markers for these targeted therapeutic alternatives have been a challenge, probably due to the requirement for large prospective confirmatory studies with a focus on clinical efficacy, safety, and reproducibility of the potential biomarkers.

Estrogen Receptor

ERα, a member of the steroid hormone receptor superfamily and a ligand-dependent transcription factor, is a regulator of various essential developmental and physiologic processes. Estradiol, the predominant form of biologically active estrogen, interacts with ER for physiologic development and regulation of the reproductive system, bone metabolism, and effects on the cardiovascular and central nervous systems.[90] Given its core involvement in growth and proliferation of breast tissue, a dysregulation of the estrogen hormonal axis in developmental aberrations associated with breast carcinogenesis is not surprising. The link between estrogen and breast cancer was observed as early as 1896[91] by George Beatson, who reported regression of advanced breast cancers in patients after oophorectomy. Since then a number of clinical studies have shown that both endogenous estrogen levels and the duration of hormone replacement therapy, especially estrogen plus progestin, are correlated with an increased risk of breast cancer and disease-related mortality,[92–94] which has evolved into the current view of ER and PR signaling as a core determinant of breast cancer biology and patient outcome.

The effects of estrogen are mediated through two receptor proteins, ERα and ERβ, encoded by corresponding genes on chromosome 6q24 and 14q22, respectively. Both receptors share about 97% homology in the DNA binding domain, with relatively low homology in other domains (Fig. 22.5), indicating that they may share specificity for similar estrogen-responsive elements (EREs) on target gene promoters or enhancers.[95] Although the role of ERβ in normal tissue is not known, loss of ERβ expression in breast cancer is associated with increased proliferation.[96]

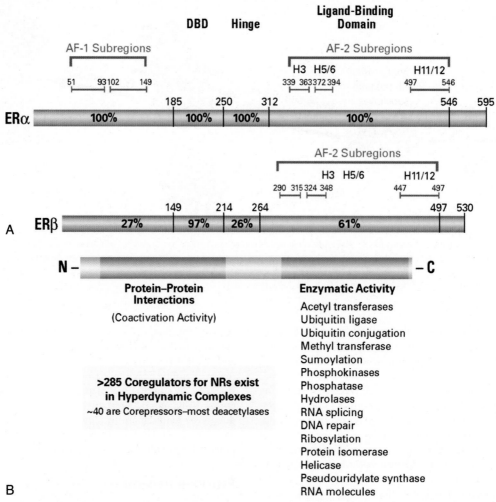

• **Fig. 22.5** The structure of the estrogen receptors, their regulation, and functions. (A) The estrogen receptor contains three main functional domains: the N-terminal activating function 1 (AF1); a DNA-binding domain, a hinge region; and a ligand-binding domain, consisting of activating function 2 (AF2). The AFs bind to the coregulators. (B) Typical domain structure of nuclear receptor with two major functional domains: the protein-protein interactions domain, which binds the coactivators in the coactivator complex, and the enzyme activity domain, with either intrinsic enzymatic activity or an activity by binding the protein. (From Jordan VC, O'Malley BW. Selective estrogen-receptor modulators and antihormonal resistance in breast cancer. *J Clin Oncol.* 2007;25:5815-5824.)

Nevertheless, ERα, but not ERβ, is currently considered to be relevant for patient management and treatment decisions, and therefore only ERα is discussed further.

Upon binding of 17β estradiol, nuclear ER monomers dimerize, bind to EREs, and, in cooperation with coregulators (coactivators and corepressors), facilitate transcription of target genes, referred as classical genomic activity of ER (see Fig. 22.5). The nuclear coregulators modulate transcription through multiple mechanisms, particularly chromosome remodeling and posttranslational modification. The indirect genomic activity involves ER binding to other transcription factors, such as SP1, AP1, and NFκB, and thereby regulation of transcription through their binding to the target gene promoters. Cyclin D1 is a direct ER target that can activate CDK4 and CDK6, which phosphorylate RB with release of E2F, leading to induction of the cell cycle proliferative activity.

In recent years, cytoplasmic/membrane-bound ER cross-talk with HER2, EGFR, IGF1R, and FGFR has been proposed as a trigger contributing to the activation of AKT and downstream signaling components of the PI3K pathway.[97–99] However, the mechanism for this cross-talk is not clear, and comprehensive evidence is needed to establish the presence of significant quantities of cytoplasmic ER, as well as its functional impact in patients.

Breast cancers that express ER are potentially sensitive to endocrine therapy in both primary and metastatic disease settings. ER-positive breast cancer patients have relatively better 5-year survival compared with ER-negative breast cancer patients, although substantially reduced difference in 10-year survival[100] because of the delayed recurrence observed in ER-positive disease. ER expression status is a core predictor of disease aggressiveness, therapeutic response, and patient outcome. The objective of endocrine therapy is to target the key growth-driving pathway—ER signaling—by one of three alternative approaches:

1. Reduction of circulating estrogen levels through surgical ovarian ablation or, more recently, through inhibition of peripheral conversion of steroids to estrogens using drug-mediated inhibition of aromatase with aromatase inhibitor (AI) therapies.
2. Competitive inhibition of estrogen binding to ER using selective estrogen receptor modulators (SERM) such as tamoxifen to inhibit recruitment of activated coregulators through conformational displacement of ER helix 12.[101]
3. Downregulation of ER through irreversible binding of small molecules, such as fulvestrant, to ER with 100 times higher affinity to ER compared with tamoxifen,[102] leading to selective degradation of the ER in breast cancer cells and thereby preventing estrogen-mediated transcriptional activation.

Although AIs are superior to tamoxifen for prevention of contralateral breast cancers as well as prevention of recurrence and metastases in postmenopausal women,[103] tamoxifen is more suitable for adjuvant therapy in premenopausal women. Tamoxifen is also used for prolonged antihormonal therapy beyond the initial 5 years of treatment.[103] A recent meta-analysis demonstrated a 30% reduction in recurrences associated with 5-year therapy with AIs compared with tamoxifen in postmenopausal women with early breast cancers as well as a 15% reduction in mortality.[104]

Approximately 30% of women treated by antihormone therapy may have a recurrence within 15 years. Among the mechanisms of acquired resistance, deregulation of estrogen receptor signaling, either by loss of ERα expression or mutation in the *ESR1* gene encoding ERα, are the most common associations. Loss of ER positivity is a common mode of resistance to endocrine therapy. Mutations clustering in the ligand-binding domain (LBD) are observed in advanced metastatic ER-positive samples (Fig. 22.6A) but are seldom observed in the primary carcinomas,[105,106] suggesting a role for acquisition of *ESR1* point mutations in advanced-stage disease, leading to resistance to endocrine therapy due to constitutive ligand-independent activation of ER.[97,107] Recently a plasma circulating DNA-based prospective-retrospective study focused on patients with ER-positive metastatic cancers who developed disease progression after aromatase inhibitor therapy demonstrated that *ESR1* mutations were predictive of resistance to Exemestane and sensitivity to fulvestrant.[108] Notably, this study observed that a combination of palbociclib (CDK4/6 inhibitor) and fulvestrant was equally effective in patients with or without ESR1 mutations.[108,109] Larger studies are required to further establish the predictive role of ER mutations and their relationship to response to various endocrine treatment options.

In addition, *ESR1* chromosomal translocation, leading to fusion genes with *ESR1*, for instance, *ESR1* (exons 1–6)-*YAP1* (as illustrated in Fig. 22.6B), has been proposed to be another potential mechanism underlying resistance to endocrine therapy.[97]

Progesterone Receptor

The PR is a nuclear receptor closely associated to the ER, being a direct target of ERα as well as its involvement in ERα chromatin binding. Expressed as two highly studied isoforms, PRA (94 kDa) and PRB (116 kDa), and coded from a single gene, PR forms upon hormone binding to form homo/hetero-dimers, binding to the PR response elements (PREs) on target gene promoter regions via the DNA binding domain and thereby modulate transcriptional activation of target genes. PRB has been shown to be the predominant regulator for several of the target genes and uniquely possesses an activation function 3 (AF3) domain in addition to common AF1 and AF2 domains on both isoforms, suggesting

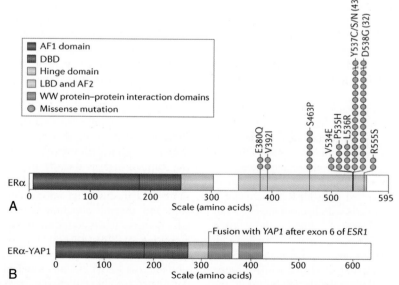

• **Fig. 22.6** Estrogen-independent activation of ERα as a potential mechanism of resistance to endocrine therapy: (A) frequencies of ERα mutations displayed by functional domains ERα in ER-positive metastatic breast cancer after endocrine therapy. (B) The WW protein-protein interaction domains on the ERα-YAP1 fusion protein derived by balanced translocation between 6q and 11q that substituted the ligand-binding domain *(LBD)* of ERα by the carboxyl terminus of YAP1. (Reproduced with permission from Ma CX, Reinert T, Chmielewska I, Ellis MJ. Mechanisms of aromatase inhibitor resistance. *Nat Rev Cancer.* 2015;15:261–275.)

both common as well as unique targets.[110] PRA may suppress PRB activation, although genes regulated uniquely by PRA are known and PRA expression is higher.[110] Both isoforms are equally expressed in normal breast tissues but altered in breast cancer, with higher PRA in many cases.[111]

PR positivity is slightly less common than ER positivity in invasive cancers, although PR positivity indicates active ER signaling. The independent role of PR status in breast cancer phenotypic outcome has been a matter of debate. ER-positive tumors without PR expression are shown to have increased occurrence of copy number changes compared with ER-positive/PR-positive tumors, was well as enrichment of growth factor signaling via PI3K/Akt/mTOR.[112] Loss of PR expression during tamoxifen therapy tends to be dramatic compared with loss of ER and marks potential resistance to therapy.[113] Loss of PR expression is explained by transcriptional inhibition of PR by other growth pathways that can also modify ER functions,[114] thus supporting a potentially beneficial role of SERDs that can effectively block ER signaling or of simultaneous inhibition of other growth pathways. However, a predictive role of PR has not been observed in early breast cancers.[115]

HER2 Membrane Receptor

HER2 or epidermal growth factor receptor 2, a member of the human EGFR family of tyrosine kinases (RTKs), through homodimerization or heterodimerization with other family members, induces tyrosine kinase activity and consequential activation of pathways involved in cell growth, differentiation, and survival. The expression of HER2 is normally found at low levels in all epithelial cells of both fetal and adult tissues,[116] but not in cells of hematopoietic origin. Amplification and/or overexpression of HER2 is found in a number of solid tumors including breast cancer. HER2 protein is a key driver of growth, an aggressive phenotype in cancers and, therefore, a therapeutic target in the subset of breast and gastric cancers that have alterations in the gene encoding this receptor. Amplification of the *HER2* gene (also known as *ERBB2*) is observed in preinvasive breast carcinomas (DCIS)[117] as well as 20% to 30% of invasive breast carcinomas.[8,9] A role for *HER2* gene amplification as a driver alteration that determines biological behavior including progression, resistance to apoptosis, invasion, and metastasis is well established for invasive carcinomas but not DCIS.[117]

Amplification of HER2 is associated with high histologic grade, high proliferative rate, reduced expression of steroid hormone receptors, and lymph node metastases and is a key predictor of shorter patient survival and time to relapse.[9] Besides being a prognostic marker, *HER2* amplification, and the associated directly related protein overexpression, predicts responsiveness to trastuzumab, a humanized anti-HER2 monoclonal antibody, with either anthracycline-based chemotherapy[118,119] or non–anthracycline-based chemotherapy.[120] Another humanized anti-HER2 monoclonal antibody, pertuzumab, as well as an antibody-drug cognate, ado-trastuzumab emtansine (T-DM1), have also been approved for treatment of HER2-positive breast cancer patients. In addition, small molecule inhibitors of the HER2 tyrosine kinase have shown promise in the treatment of HER2-positive breast cancer patients with lapatinib, a dual targeting agent that inhibits both HER2 and HER1 receptors and is Food and Drugs Administration (FDA)-approved for treatment of women with metastatic disease.[121] Other small molecule inhibitors of HER2 are currently in clinical trials.

The downstream consequences of HER2 amplification and its messenger RNA (mRNA) overexpression include formation of active hetero-/homo-dimers of HER2 protein with other RTKs, activation of intracellular tyrosine kinase domain and phosphorylation of the intracellular domain of HER2 and recruitment of adaptor proteins that forms a complex, leading to activation of intracellular signaling pathways, including PI3-kinase/AKT, and RAS/MAPK signaling. HER2 and other downstream signaling pathways increase cell proliferation, cell survival, and loss of apoptosis. Production of VEGF and induction of angiogenesis is one of the downstream consequences of HER2 activation (Fig. 22.7).

Additional therapeutic strategies target this signaling pathway by simultaneously targeting HER2 and HER3 with trastuzumab and pertuzumab, a second humanized anti-HER2 antibody that prevents HER2 dimerization, with concurrent cytotoxic chemotherapy.[122] An antibody-drug conjugate, T-DM1, directed at HER2 has also been developed for treatment of HER2-positive breast cancer patients.

Trastuzumab, a humanized monoclonal antibody was FDA-approved for the treatment of HER2-amplified metastatic breast cancers in 1998 and subsequently for early-stage HER2-positive, node-positive breast cancer in 2006. The antigen-specific site of trastuzumab binds the juxtamembrane portion of the extracellular subdomain 4 of the HER2 receptor (see Fig. 22.7). The mechanism of action of trastuzumab is not completely understood but multiple possible mechanisms include inhibition of the intracellular activation of the HER2 tyrosine kinase domain, antibody-dependent cellular cytotoxicity (ADCC), through binding of trastuzumab with induction of natural killer cell responses against the HER2-overexpressing cells, inhibition of receptor dimerization, receptor degradation through endocytosis, inhibition of shedding of the extracellular domain,[123] and inhibition of ligand-independent, HER2-mediated mitogenic signaling.[124] Trastuzumab activity has been shown in early as well as metastatic breast cancers with *HER2* amplification.[123] HER2 activity is ligand independent. Among the possible heterodimers, the HER2-HER3 pair has been shown to be the most potent in activation of cell proliferation.[125] HER3, upon binding to its ligand, dimerizes with HER2 and activates the phosphatidylinositol-4,5-bisphosphate 3-kinase (PI3-K) signaling pathway. The clinical benefit of trastuzumab therapy can be improved by simultaneously blocking both ligand-independent and ligand-dependent activity. Accordingly, therapy with trastuzumab and pertuzumab could achieve more comprehensive control of HER2 signaling. The CLEOPATRA trial showed significantly reduced risk of disease progression (improved PFS) or death with trastuzumab, pertuzumab, and a docetaxel regimen compared with placebo plus trastuzumab with the same docetaxel therapy in metastatic breast cancers.[125,126] Resistance to trastuzumab remains an important issue. One or more mechanisms could activate alternate growth signaling pathways and, thereby, overcome the HER2 or HER2-HER3 blockade. Factors such as activation of other members of HER family, activation of PI3K/AKT/mTOR by alternative pathway, IGF1 activation, increased activity of VEGF or src, c-MET overexpression or loss of PTEN are some of the potential mechanisms considered possible underlying mechanisms of resistance. Conjugation of trastuzumab with maytansine (DM1), a tubulin inhibitor, also referred as T-DM1, has demonstrated activity against the HER2-overexpressing cells that were resistant to trastuzumab and lapatinib.[127] The combination of T-DM1 with pertuzumab provided superior pathologic complete response rate compared with the paclitaxel with trastuzumab in the I-SPY 2 (Investigation of

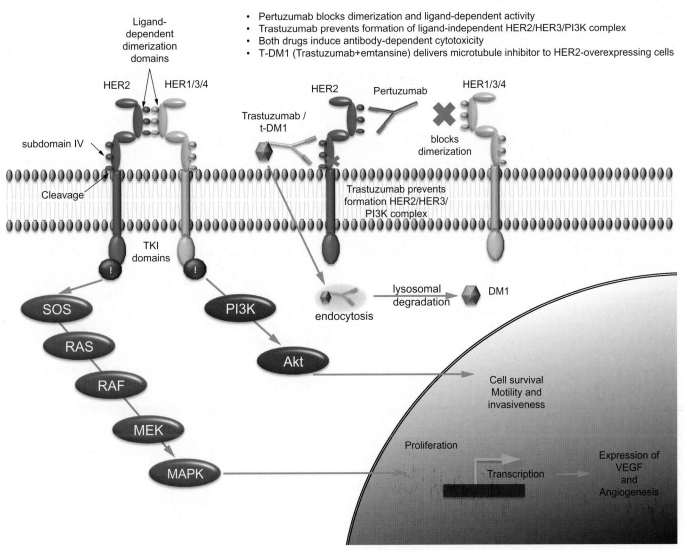

• **Fig. 22.7** HER signaling and core mechanism of action of trastuzumab. Homo/hetero-dimerization of HER family members is followed by the phosphorylation of their intracellular tyrosine kinase domains. The activated domains activate the lipid kinase phosphoinositide 3-kinase (PI3K), which phosphorylates a phosphatidylinositol that in turn binds and phosphorylates the enzyme Ak transforming factor (Akt), driving cell survival. In parallel, a guanine nucleotide exchange factor, the mammalian homologue of the son of sevenless (SOS), activates the rat sarcoma (RAS) enzyme that, in turn, activates receptor activation factor (RAF) and then the mitogen-activated protein kinase (MAPK) and mitogen extracellular signal kinase (MEK). MEK phosphorylates, among others, the MAPK, driving cellular proliferation. Expression of vascular endothelial growth factor (VEGF) is one of the downstream effects of HER signaling, which induces angiogenesis. Trastuzumab binds to the juxtamembrane domain of HER2. It thus inhibits the dimerization involving HER2. Trastuzumab may also recruit Fc-competent immune effector cells and the other components of antibody-dependent cell-mediated cytotoxicity, leading to tumor-cell death (not shown in the figure). The binding reduces shedding of the extracellular domain (proteolytic cleavage), thereby reduces the availability of p95. In addition, potent microtubule inhibitor emtansine (DM-1) in conjugation with trastuzumab provides antimitotic activity on HER2 overexpressing cells.

Serial Studies to Predict Your Therapeutic Response With Imaging And moLecular Analysis 2) trial.[128,129]

Molecular Subtypes of Breast Cancer

In addition to ER, PR, and HER2, which are the key predictive biomarkers, advances in high-throughput technologies have shown breast cancer to be a molecularly, highly heterogeneous disease. The initial aim of classifying breast cancers had been for prognostication and prediction of response to chemotherapy, which with technological advances, has evolved into a broader aim of defining molecular classes by causal or driver alterations that determine patient outcome, disease aggressiveness, metastatic potential, or drug responsiveness.

Molecular expression subtypes were initially based on microarray-based differential mRNA expression patterns across the spectrum of breast cancer samples.[130] A set of 496 genes, defining the subtypes, was composed of genes that showed significantly greater variation in expression between different cancers than between paired samples from the same tumor. These genes also represented the biological characteristics of the cancers and were referred as an intrinsic gene set.[130] The expression clusters were separated into five subtypes: luminal A, luminal B, basal, ERBB2-enriched (HER2-positive) and normal-like. Subsequently, using a 50-gene predictor gene set (PAM50) in a study of 710 node-negative cancers, the molecular subtypes were shown to be associated with differential relapse-free survival and were associated with response to chemotherapy.[131] A randomized trial (MA.12 study) of 672 premenopausal, stage I–III breast cancer patients receiving adjuvant tamoxifen showed the PAM50 subtype to be prognostic for both disease-free survival (DFS; $p = .0003$) and overall survival (OS; $p = .0002$). This study also showed the luminal subtype to be predictive of response to tamoxifen therapy compared with the nonluminal cases.[132] Using a large sample set of 10,000 pooled samples from multiple studies, immunohistochemistry-based expression of ER, PR, HER2, and basal markers (cytokeratins CK5/6, and EGFR) was applied to identify six subtypes: luminal 1 (HER2-negative) with or without expression of basal markers, luminal 2 (HER2-positive) with or without expression of the basal markers, nonluminal HER2-positive, and TNBC. This classification distinguished breast cancers by their short and long-term survival.[133] Overlapping largely with TNBC with high frequency of metaplastic and medullary differentiation, a novel class of tumors, the claudin-low subtype, was identified that are characterized by low or absent expression of luminal differentiation markers, high expression of EMT markers, immune response genes, and CSC-like features.[134]

Although expression subtypes have improved our understanding of molecular heterogeneity, the known expression subtypes do not represent the complete spectrum of the biological variation. Subtype characterization has been based on mRNA expression using microarrays in small sample sets, but its clinical utility is limited, given the lack of reproducibility and robustness, technological difficulties, and insufficient consideration to tumor heterogeneity. These limitations in clinical utility are discussed in greater detail elsewhere.

The concept of molecular subtyping has continued to evolve with advances in identifying the underlying somatic and germline mutations, copy number alterations and other alterations. Five types of data, including mRNA expression, DNA methylation, single nucleotide polymorphism (SNP) arrays, microRNA (miRNA) sequencing, whole-exome sequencing, and protein expression (reverse phase protein array or RPPA) from tumor and germline DNA showed consensus patterns between samples by unsupervised consensus clustering analysis. The four major clusters obtained from these analyses have been correlated with the mRNA expression-subtypes as well as clinical characteristics. Frequent mutation of *PIK3CA* (45%), *MAP3K1, GATA3, TP53, CDH1,* and *MAP2K4* has been observed in luminal A subtype breast cancers, whereas the luminal B subtype most frequently showed mutations in *TP53* and *PIK3CA* (29% each). The highest occurrence (80% samples) of *TP53* mutations was observed in the basal-like cancers. The HER2-positive subtype showed frequent HER2 amplification (80%) and a high rate of mutations of *TP53* (72%) and *PIK3CA* (39%)[14] (Fig. 22.8).

Molecular Subtypes of Triple-Negative Breast Cancers

TNBCs are a heterogeneous group. Using the k-means clustering and consensus clustering on gene expression data of 587 TNBC of which 386 samples were used as a discovery data set compiled from 14 breast cancer data sets and 201 samples were used as a validation data set compiled from 7 data sets, six TNBC subtypes were identified: basal-like 1 (BL1), basal-like 2 (BL2), immunomodulatory (IM), mesenchymal (M), mesenchymal stem–like (MSL), luminal androgen receptor (LAR), and unstable (UNS).[135] The BL1 and BL2 subtypes showed high ki67 proliferation scores and higher response rates after taxane chemotherapy. The BL1 subtype showed enrichment of cell cycle genes, whereas the BL2 subtype showed enrichment of growth factor signaling (IGF1R, MET, EGF, NGF pathways) and showed features suggestive of basal/myoepithelial origin as demonstrated by higher expression levels of TP63 and MME (CD10). The IM subtype showed overlap with the medullary signature and was enriched with genes from immune cell signaling pathways, antigen; processing and presentation, and signaling through core immune signal transduction pathways (NFKB, TNF, and JAK/STAT signaling). The M subtype displayed enrichment of cell motility, extracellular matrix receptor interaction, and cell differentiation pathways. The MSL subtype shared enrichment of similar biological processes as with the M subtype and in addition was enriched by inositol phosphate metabolism, EGFR, platelet-derived growth factor, calcium signaling, G-protein coupled receptor, and ERK1/2 signaling as well as ATP-binding cassette transporters and adipocytokine signaling. The LAR subtype expressed luminal markers CK18 and was enriched with androgen receptor signaling and therefore corresponded to the apocrine variety of tumors.

Although precision in discovery of cancer drivers and propagating events is the key for clinical utility, discovery of more molecular subtypes based on less common driver events will be the result of the ongoing effort.

Hereditary Breast Cancers

Although approximately 20% of breast cancers may be associated with a familial inheritance pattern, only 10% to 12% are considered hereditary with inheritance of alterations in known susceptibility genes or loci. Hereditary breast cancers have been frequently associated with an autosomal dominant pattern of inheritance.

Fig. 22.9 depicts known susceptibility genes and loci. Mutations in high-penetrance genes confer fivefold or greater breast cancer risk, whereas the mutations in moderate-penetrance genes may confer two- to fourfold risk, compared with the reference population. Mutations in low-penetrance loci confer low risk ranging between one- and twofold increased risk (Table 22.1).[136,137]

The functional implications of mutations in susceptibility genes and loci mainly involve DNA repair mechanisms, cell cycle checkpoints, and cell death pathways. These mechanisms are closely linked, and their functional defects may lead to lack of genome stability. Fig. 22.10 summarizes the key genome stability pathways that underlie the hereditary breast and ovarian cancers.[138]

BRCA1 and BRCA2

The breast cancer susceptibility types 1 and 2 (*BRCA1* and *BRCA2*) genes encode proteins that are critically important in DNA double-strand break repair by homologous recombination. Loss of function alterations in these genes create genomic instability through an increase in mutagenesis as a result of alterations introduced through nonhomologous end joining and single-strand annealing. Breast cancers associated with *BRCA1* mutations are frequently medullary-like, high nuclear grade, aneuploid, and triple negative.[139] Unlike *BRCA1, BRCA2* cancers

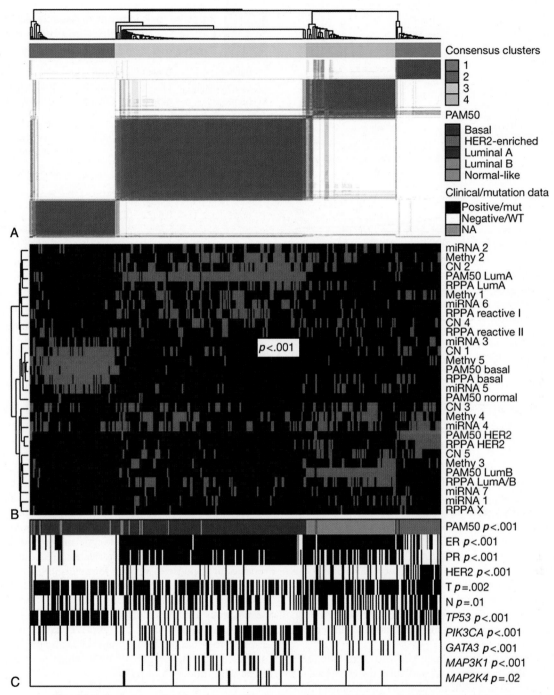

• **Fig. 22.8** Consensus of clusters representing the breast cancer subtypes using different genomic and proteomic data. (A) Sample consensus results in four major clusters (shown as blue biclusters) for breast tumors (samples, n = 348) by unsupervised consensus clustering of the data from multiple platforms. (B) Concordance patterns of miRNA expression, DNA methylation, copy number (CN), PAM50 mRNA expression, and RPPA (protein) expression is displayed in red bar representing the cluster membership. (C) Molecular and clinical features that show significant association (by chi-square *p* values) with the clusters representing the molecular subtypes. (Reproduced with permission from the Cancer Genome Atlas Network. Comprehensive molecular portraits of human breast tumors. *Nature.* 2012;490:61-70.)

are heterogeneous, share similarities with sporadic cancers, and may have more favorable features (Table 22.2).[140] Average risk of developing breast cancer among the *BRCA1* and *BRCA2* mutation carriers by age 70 is 65% (95% confidence interval 44%–78%) and 45% (95% confidence interval 33%–54%), respectively.[141]

BRCA1

BRCA1 is a nuclear phosphoprotein that functions as a gatekeeper in the regulation of gene transcription and DNA repair. Since its discovery in 1994, *BRCA1* has been known to be a classic tumor suppressor gene, which consists of 24 coding exons distributed over approximately 81 kb on 17q21 and the canonical

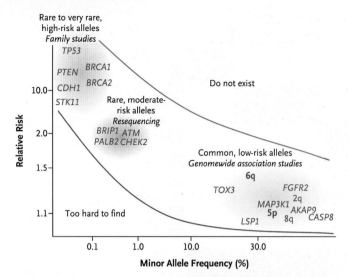

• **Fig. 22.9** Breast cancer susceptibility genes and loci. Known breast cancer susceptibility genes are shown between the red and blue lines. High-risk genes are highlighted in green. *TP53, BRCA1,* and *BRCA2* are well known high-risk germline mutations. Mutations in *STK11, PTEN,* and *CDH1* could confer high risk according to some studies, although some studies report intermediate risk (refer to Table 22.1). The moderate-penetrance genes (highlighted in red) have an approximate relative risk of 2.0. The common, low-risk genes are shown in orange. Single nucleotide polymorphisms in *FGFR2* and *TOX3,* and those on chromosomes 5p and 2q specifically, increase the risk of estrogen receptor–positive breast cancer. (From Foulkes WD. Inherited susceptibility to common cancers. *N Engl J Med.* 2008;359:2143-2153.)

TABLE 22.1	Relative Risk Estimates Associated With Known Cancer Susceptibility Genes With the Syndromes/Conditions Caused by Them	
Cancer Susceptibility Gene	Breast Cancer RR (90% CI, If Available) or Inclusion Criteria	Associated Syndromes /Conditions
BRCA1	200-fold <40 y; 15-fold 40–60 y	Familial breast and ovarian cancer syndrome[137]
TP53	105 (62–165)	Li-Fraumeni syndrome
BRIP1	2.0 (1.3–3.0)	
CDH1	6.6 (2.2–19.9)	Diffuse gastric and lobular breast cancer syndrome
CHEK2	3.0 (2.6–3.5)	(Most data for 1100delC)
PALB2	5.3 (3.0–9.4)	
PTEN	(2.0–5.0)	Cowden syndrome
STK11	(2.0–4.0)	Peutz-Jeghers syndrome
ATM	2.8 (2.2–3.7)	Ataxia-telangiectasia
NBN	2.7 (1.9–3.7)	Nijmegen breakage syndrome

CI, Confidence interval.
Relative risk estimates define the genes into high, moderate and low risk genes.[136]

transcript encodes a protein of 1863 amino acid residues. Mutations in *BRCA1* gene occur predominantly in the N-terminal RING domain (E3 ubiquitin ligase), exons 11 to 13 (protein-binding domains), and tandem *BRCA1* T domain involved in binding phosphoproteins phosphorylated by ATM/ATR kinases. Out of more than 1700 mutations, approximately 850 mutations are known to be of clinical significance.[142] Exon 11 frequently harbors the deleterious mutations that can prevent nuclear localization of *BRCA1.* The majority of *BRCA1* mutations (approximately 80%) are associated with the introduction of a premature stop-codon, leading to expression of a truncated protein product. The clinical significance of several missense variants still remains uncharacterized.

Certain *BRCA1* mutations have been associated with a "founder effect" in which high frequencies of particular disease-associated mutations are identified in specific populations. Two founder mutations 185delAG and 5382insC are, respectively, observed in 0.8% to 1% and 0.1% to 0.4% of Ashkenazi Jewish populations and represent the majority of germline *BRCA1* mutations found in this ethnic group. Interestingly, the 185delAG mutation has also been identified among patients having Spanish ancestry in frequencies similar to the Ashkenazi Jews,[143] presumably dating to religious "conversion" during the Spanish inquisition. In addition, *BRCA1* mutations are also found in Germany, Sweden, and Norway.

BRCA1 acts as a key regulator of genomic stability by its central role in a variety of DNA damage repair processes, including double-stranded DNA break repair via homologous recombination, single strand annealing, and nonhomologous end joining[144] nucleotide-excision repair and base-excision repair.[145] The DNA damage recognition mechanism known as *BRCA1*-associated genome surveillance protein complex (BARC) includes DNA

damage sensors, tumor suppressors, and other signal transducers important in DNA repair, including MSH2, MSH6, MLH1, ATM, BLM, and the RAD50-MRE11-NBS1.[146] Phosphorylation of *BRCA1* by CHK2 at serine-988 after DNA damage results in recruitment of downstream repair kinases such as ATM, ATR, and CHK2, necessary for the cell cycle arrest and DNA damage repair.[147,148] Each kinase phosphorylates *BRCA1* at different serine residues in response to varying forms of DNA damage.[147] ATM/ATR also mediates phosphorylation of CHK2, which in turn phosphorylates *BRCA1.*[147] Activated *BRCA1* mediates error-free homologous recombination while repressing the error-prone nonhomologous end joining.[149,150] *BRCA1* plays a role in cell cycle arrest in response to DNA damage by facilitating the ATM/ATR-mediated phosphorylation of p53, which is essential for G1/S arrest with induction of p21.[151]

BRCA2

Like *BRCA1,* breast cancer susceptibility type 2 *(BRCA2)* encodes a gatekeeper protein involved in maintaining genomic integrity by regulating DNA repair and transcription. Coded by 27 exons spanning over 84 kb on 13q12, BRCA2 is a protein of 3418 amino acid residues. More than 1800 mutations have been found in the *BRCA2* gene, including frameshift deletions, insertions, and nonsense mutations resulting in deleterious effects due to a truncated protein. Among the founder mutations, 6174delT is found among Ashkenazi Jews both in Israel and the United States.[143] Among other ethnicities, 9254del5 and 999del5 mutations have been found among 1% of Spanish high-risk families and 10% Icelandic female breast cancer cases, respectively.[143]

BRCA2 mediates recruitment of the RAD51 recombinase to double strand breaks for homologous recombination.[152]

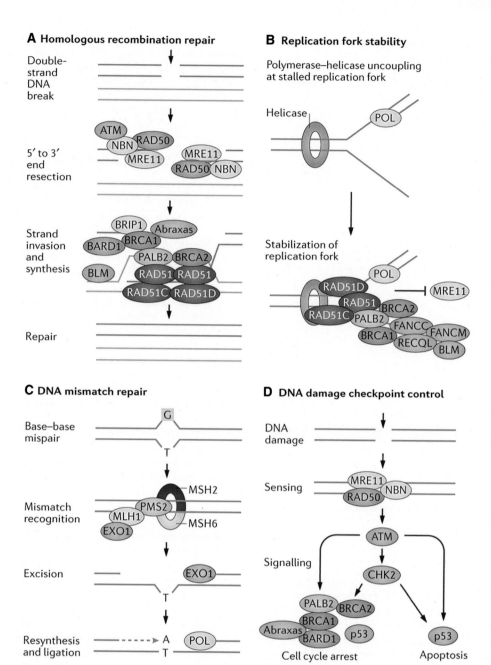

A Homologous recombination repair

Double-strand DNA break

5' to 3' end resection

Strand invasion and synthesis

Repair

B Replication fork stability

Polymerase–helicase uncoupling at stalled replication fork

Helicase

Stabilization of replication fork

C DNA mismatch repair

Base–base mispair

Mismatch recognition

Excision

Resynthesis and ligation

D DNA damage checkpoint control

DNA damage

Sensing

Signalling

Cell cycle arrest

Apoptosis

• **Fig. 22.10** Genome integrity pathways affected in hereditary breast and ovarian cancer syndromes (HBOC). The HBOC genes and their major functional roles are depicted. Alterations in one of these pathways may potentially influence the functioning of the others: defective replication fork stability leads to activation of DNA damage checkpoints and induce homologous recombination repair (HRR). (A) DNA end resection cuts back the 5'-strand leaving a 3'-single strand, a process promoted by ATM and the MRN complex. MRE11 (nuclease), RAD50, and NBN are required for the formation and localization of the MRN complex. *BRCA2* and *PALB2* then load RAD51 onto the resected DNA strand, forming the nucleoprotein filament. Using the complementary sequence on the sister chromatid, RAD51 filament pairs with the complementary DNA sequence, followed by resolution and ligation of the DNA ends. (B) Replication fork protection guards stalling forks from DNA nuclease-mediated degradation of the newly synthesized DNA. HBOC genes may limit degradation mainly by counteracting MRE11 nuclease activity. (C) Mismatch repair corrects erroneous base pairing. HBOC factors are MLH1, MSH2 and PMS2. (D) In DNA damage checkpoint control, the MRN complex recruits ATM via NBN, thereby initiating kinase cascades together with its downstream target CHK2, leading to cell cycle inhibition in G1, S, and G2 phases of the cell cycle, allowing time for DNA repair. *Abraxas,* BRCA1-A complex subunit; *BARD1,* BRCA1-associated RING domain protein 1; *BLM,* Bloom syndrome protein; *BRIP1,* BRCA1-interacting protein C-terminal helicase 1; *EXO1,* exonuclease 1; *FANC,* Fanconi anemia factor; *POL,* DNA polymerase; *RECQL,* ATP-dependent DNA helicase Q1. (Reproduced with permission from Nielsen FC, van Overeem Hansen T, Sørensen CS. Hereditary breast and ovarian cancer: new genes in confined pathways. *Nat Rev Cancer.* 2016;16:599-612.)

TABLE 22.2 Immunophenotypes of *BRCA1*, *BRCA2*, and Sporadic Breast Cancers

Antibodies	BRCA1	BRCA2	Sporadic
ER, PR	–	+	+
BCL-2, BAX	–	+	+
Cyclin D1	–	+	+
p16, p27, p21	–	+	+
RAD50	–	+	+
RAD51 (cytoplasm)	–	+	–
HER-2	–	–	+
CHEK2	+	+	–
RAD51 (nucleus)	+	–	+
p53, ki67	+	–	–
Cyclins (E, A, B1)	+	–	–
Skp2	+	–	–
CK5/6, 14, 17	+	–	–
EGFR, P-cadherin	+	–	–

EGFR, Epithelial growth factor receptor; *ER,* estrogen receptor; *PR,* progesterone receptor.
From Honrado E, Osorio A, Palacios J, Benitez J. Pathology and gene expression of hereditary breast tumors associated with BRCA1, BRCA2 and CHEK2 gene mutations. *Oncogene.* 2006;25:5837-5845.

BRCA2-deficient cells accumulate DNA damage because of a failure to recruit RAD51.[153]

PTEN

Phosphatase and tensin homolog *(PTEN)* is a tumor suppressor and component of PI3K-AKT-mTOR signaling. Cowden syndrome is an inherited, autosomal dominant phenotype composed of multiple hamartomas typically found in the skin, mucous membranes including the gastrointestinal tract, thyroid, and breast. Germline loss of function mutations in *PTEN* predispose to breast cancer as part of Cowden syndrome. Deficient PTEN function may accelerate cellular senescence.[154] With an estimated risk of 85% for breast cancer by age 70,[155] *PTEN* is one of the high penetrance susceptibility genes.

CDH1

CDH1 (E-cadherin) is a component of adherence junction pathway. Germline mutations of *CDH1* predisposes to lobular breast cancer, as a part of the diffuse gastric cancer and lobular breast cancer syndrome with a 42% cumulative risk for lobular breast cancer by the age of 80.[156]

Molecular Profiles of Sporadic Breast Cancers

As described in the previous sections, breast cancer is a heterogeneous group of molecular entities. Moving from the conventionally used clinical variables, such as histopathologic type, grade, tumor size, lymph node involvement, and stage, to a classification inclusive of the steroid hormone receptors (ER and PR), and *HER2* gene amplification/overexpression status improves clinical treatment decision-making, and ultimately clinical outcomes. Here we describe the disease-associated alterations that are of clinical value.

Genetic Abnormalities in Breast Cancer

Genetic alterations can be either inherited (germline), present in all cell types of a patient including the tumor, or they can be acquired during the patient's lifetime and present only in the cancer cells. The latter are referred to as *somatic alterations* and are more commonly associated with breast cancer than are germline alterations. Genetic alterations are classified as mutations at the base-pair sequence level, amplifications (multiple repeats of large regions of a chromosome), deletions (loss of a large chromosome region), aneuploidy (alterations in chromosome number), and translocations (a portion of one chromosome transferred to a nonhomologous chromosome or to another site on the same chromosome).

The occurrence of somatic mutations can be described as a consequence of endogenous and/or exogenous mutagen exposures, aberrant DNA editing, replication errors, and defective DNA maintenance.[157] Studying the pattern of occurrence of gene mutations and their associations with clinical variables can help in understanding disease causation as well as potential clinical utility. As described previously for the clonal evolution model (see Fig. 22.4), carcinogenesis follows natural selection of clones that acquire new mutations potentially conferring survival advantage, metastasis and resistance to treatment.

Oncogenes

Oncogenes are typically genes that encode growth factors, growth factor receptors, downstream effectors of signal transduction pathways, and enzymes responsible for the metabolism of activating proteins. Oncogenes are generated from proto-oncogenes, commonly by acquisition of a gain-of-function mutation or gene amplification, leading to growth factor overexpression. In addition, chromosomal translocation of a region coding a growth-regulatory gene under the regulation of a new promoter can lead to aberrant expression of a gene and its corresponding protein. Oncogene activation usually confers self-sufficiency of growth signaling,[1] which is achieved through endogenous activation of growth signaling with abnormally expressed growth factor to provide independence from exogenous growth regulatory signals (see Fig. 22.1).

Tumor Suppressor Genes

In contrast to the function of oncogenes, the tumor suppressor genes typically inhibit cell proliferation or survival signaling by encoding or regulating cell proliferation and differentiation proteins. Some tumor suppressor genes regulate entry to apoptosis in case DNA damage is irreversible. Most tumor suppressor genes are cell cycle regulators, such as retinoblastoma susceptibility 1 *(RB1)* and *TP53,* that protect cells with DNA damage from proliferative activity that could lead to clonal expansion of an altered phenotype, thereby contributing to maintaining genome integrity. Loss-of-function mutations enable cells to acquire two major traits: resistance to antigrowth signals and evasion of apoptosis.[1] Both alleles can be modified by somatic mutations, combined with loss of heterozygosity or DNA methylation, to interfere with production of the protein that inhibits tumorigenesis.

As described previously as a hallmark of cancer, germline or early occurring somatic mutations in *TP53* drive cancer by loss of its gatekeeper function. Mutations in genes involved in variety of DNA repair mechanisms can lead to chromosome instability, which may give rise to a mutator phenotype. One consequence of chromosomal instability is a loss-of-function mutation in tumor suppressors by loss of heterozygosity through deletion of the normal allele as a result of deletion of a large chromosomal area or inactivation of a promoter by abnormal DNA methylation. During the process of DNA repair after these events, the mutant allele is duplicated, thus resulting in multiple defective copies of the gene and expression of protein having a loss of tumor suppressor function.

Driver and Passenger Alterations

Driver alterations play a direct causal role in carcinogenesis, mainly by conferring selective growth advantage in the microenvironment. Vogelstein and colleagues[158] proposed that identifying the driver genes based on mutation frequency and context alone cannot be sufficient because of the variations in background rates of mutation among different patients and genomic regions. Rather, multiple recurrent mutations for oncogenes or inactivating mutations for tumor suppressors define typical driver genes. The impact of mutations may vary by location and codon altered, thus significantly contributing to interpatient heterogeneity.[158]

Out of 173 genes sequenced, 40 somatic driver genes were identified in a set of 2433 breast cancer profiles. Among the putative driver genes identified by this study, *PIK3CA, TP53, AKT1, KRAS, ERBB2, AGTR2,* and *SF3B1* were estimated to have a high oncogene score. Whereas *PTEN, RB1, CDKN2A, CDKN1A, ARID1A, BRCA1, BRCA2, CHEK2, FOXO3, GATA3, CDH1,* and *CTNNA1* had higher tumor suppressor scores.[159] In addition to the type of potential functional effect, this study showed that *ERBB2, GATA3, KRAS, CDKN1B, PIK3CA, FOXO3,* and *AKT1* are activated predominantly through amplification, whereas mutation coinciding with loss of heterozygosity constitutes most of the alterations found in *TP53, CDH1, CBFB, MAP2K4,* and *PIK3CA*. Homozygous deletions are most common in *CDKN2A, CDKN2B, MAP2K4,* and *PTEN* (Fig. 22.11).

In contrast to the driver alterations, passenger alterations do not occur under selective pressure and typically cannot confer a selective growth advantage. Therefore passenger alterations probably do not contribute to cancer development and are present in cancer cells due to clonal expansion.[158,160] These somatic mutations may occur before the acquisition of driver alterations or as a result of genomic instability and therefore tend to be nonrecurrent.

The majority of mutations and translocations may be passengers according to this definition. Many of the translocations occur in intergenic or noncoding regions of the genome and may occur adjacent to sites that are prone to breakage. Although occurring in cancer cells, the cells with passenger alterations may survive because of deficient DNA repair. The concept of noninvolvement of passenger mutations in carcinogenesis is, however, contradicted by suggestions that some of the passenger mutations can be deleterious by a variety of mechanisms, including loss of function and formation of potentially cytotoxic aggregates, inducing an immune response; therefore they may contribute to cancer progression and

patient outcome.[161] Evidence of passenger alterations with deleterious effects is lacking to date.

Actionable Alterations

Detection of alterations in breast cancer that have a putative driver role in the disease and may predict response, if targeted by a corresponding targeted therapeutic agent, is referred to as an actionable alteration. It is worth noting that factors that are predictive of actionability are poorly characterized for many putatively actionable alterations, thus creating a lack of precision in the definition of actionability. These factors include decisive models for target prioritization in the case of multiple driver alterations present in a tumor, representativeness of subclonal alterations, tissue-specificity of response, functional impact for mutations in driver genes located outside mutation hotspots, epigenomically mediated mechanisms underlying the response, and pharmacogenomic variations of response.

A characteristic example of an actionable alteration is *HER2/ERBB2* amplification in breast cancer, which predicts responsiveness to trastuzumab or ado-trastuzumab. Approximately 20% of TNBCs have potentially actionable somatic alterations that include BRAF V600E, high-level amplifications in EGFR, and mutations in *HER2/ERBB3* genes.[162] Among other instances of potentially actionable alterations in breast cancer are PIK3CA, FGFR, AKT1, RAS, and MET.[163]

Common Somatic Mutations

p53 Tumor Suppressor

Mutations in *TP53* leading to perturbation in the p53 signaling pathway is the most common alteration in breast cancers as well as variety of other cancers.[164] Approximately 75% of *TP53* mutations lead to loss-of-function alterations, often with dominant-negative inhibition of the remaining wild-type p53.[165] Located on the short arm of chromosome 17, *TP53* encodes p53 protein with 393 amino acid residues. There are seven functional domains in the p53 protein: two transactivation domains, a proline-rich domain, a DNA-binding domain, a nuclear localization signal, a tetramerization domain, a basic domain, sterile-alpha-motif (oligomerization) domain.[166] As a transcription factor, p53 is involved in regulating key signaling pathways activated by variety of cellular stress pathways and plays an important role in preventing the proliferation of damaged cells. Fig. 22.12 summarizes a variety of stresses that can induce the p53 activity and downstream pathways. After activation, p53 binds to specific DNA promoter sites and acts as a transcriptional activator of genes involved in inhibition of angiogenesis, inhibition of the cell cycle, apoptosis, DNA repair, and autophagy.[167] In case DNA damage is irreparable, it induces apoptosis. Germline mutations in *TP53* (Li-Fraumeni syndrome) follow a similar positional distribution as sporadic cancers with *TP53* mutations[168] and represent a familial disorder associated with early onset of multiple cancers, including carcinomas of the breast, adrenal gland, stomach, colon, and pancreas as well as soft tissue malignancies such as osteosarcoma.

The COSMIC database reports more than 1000 variants in *TP53*, of which 437 are pathogenic variants reported from tumor tissue. Mutations occur predominantly in the DNA-binding domain. Approximately 30% of mutations in this domain occur at "hotspot" residues (R175, G245, R248, R249, R273, and R282).[169] Another important site is located at codon 72 on

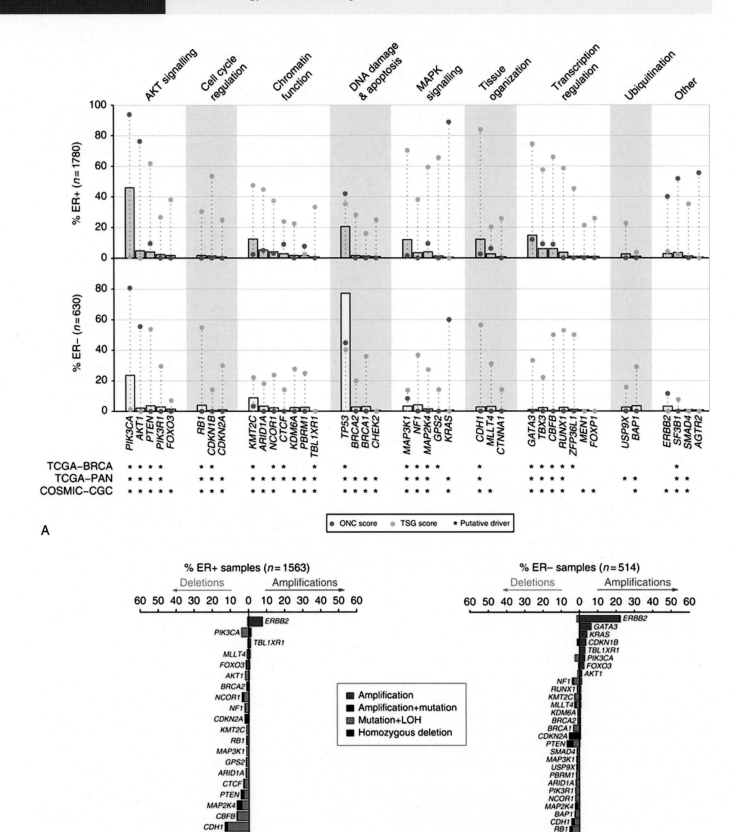

• **Fig. 22.11** Putative driver genes and pathways by ER status. (A) Driver mutations grouped by pathways identified based on the analysis of 2410 breast cancers displayed as red and blue points by the proportions of recurrent (oncogene; ONC score) and inactivating (tumor suppressor gene; TSG score) mutations, respectively. *Gene highlighted by previous studies: *COSMIC,* Cancer gene census from the Catalog of Somatic Mutations in Cancer; *MAPK,* mitogen-activated protein kinase; *TCGA-BRCA,* TCGA breast cancer study; *TCGA-PAN,* TCGA pan-cancer analysis. (B) Barplot showing the proportion of cancers with copy number alterations in genes altered in at least 1% of estrogen receptor (ER)-positive or ER-negative samples. The percentages of cancers with amplifications, simultaneous amplification and mutation events, homozygous deletions, and simultaneous mutations and loss of heterozygosity events are shown. (From Pereira B, Chin SF, Rueda OM, et al. The somatic mutation profiles of 2433 breast cancers refines their genomic and transcriptomic landscapes. *Nat Commun.* 2016;7:11479.)

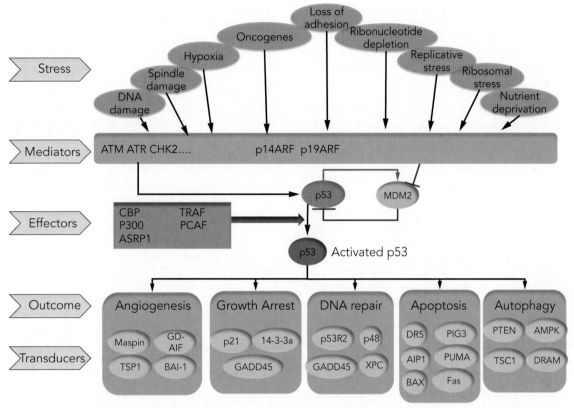

• **Fig. 22.12** Central role of p53 as a switch to determine the fate of damaged cells: a variety of stresses induce the activity of p53 via mediators of stress. On activation, p53 binds to the DNA and regulates the transcription of genes involved in inhibition of angiogenesis, inhibition of cell cycle, apoptosis, DNA repair, and autophagy.

exon 4, where a single nucleotide transversion of G to C results in two different alleles (Arg and Pro). The resultant genotypes may alter transcription factor binding capacity, induce apoptosis,[170] and increase protein turnover.[171] Mutations in the DNA binding domain impairs activity as a transcription factor. Deletions of the C-terminal oligomerization domain may prevent tetramerization.[172]

Somatic mutation frequency in breast cancer is approximately 30% to 35%,[159] depending on cohort composition. However, perturbations in p53 signaling pathway may occur in almost half of the breast cancers.[14] In addition, the dominant negative phenotype as well as the loss of heterozygosity[173] may inactivate the remaining wild-type allele in the presence of a single mutant allele. Accumulation of mutant p53 is often observed in cancer cells.[165] Approximately 75% of *TP53* mutations are single nucleotide substitutions resulting from substitutions of G-C to A-T sites (40%) and are predominantly (85%) associated with missense mutations and positive nuclear p53 protein overexpression by IHC. The remaining 25% of mutations, which include nonsense mutations, especially single base pair insertions and deletions, are associated with positive p53 immunostaining in only approximately 30% of cases with this type of mutation.

Somatic mutations are known to be an early event in carcinogenesis that has been observed in DCIS, both alone and as accompanied with invasive disease.[174–177] Mutations of p53 are frequent in hormone receptor–negative breast cancers, and the mutation signature gene set shows enrichment of cell cycle, ESC, and EMT genes,[177] highlighting a potential role in stemlike properties. The

link of functional p53 with stemness is highlighted by the regulatory role of NUMB, a NOTCH signaling inhibitor, in regulation of p53 activity[178] and its role in inhibiting dedifferentiation and formation of CSCs.[179] In addition, p53 mutations are also found to be associated with *BRCA1/BRCA2* mutations,[180] suggesting that defective DNA repair due to *BRCA1/BRCA2* alterations may influence acquisition of mutations in p53 in breast cancer.[181]

Mutations of *TP53* in breast cancers are associated with shorter DFS in both node-negative and node-positive patients.[182] There is also an association of *TP53* mutations with response to therapy. Although tumors with gain-of-function mutations have been known to be associated with resistance to chemotherapy,[172] increased survival rates have been observed in women with node-negative, *TP53* mutant breast cancers who were treated with local radiotherapy, compared with women who have node-negative breast cancers with wild-type *TP53*,[183] suggesting that *TP53* mutations have potential for selection of treatment in breast cancer management.

Among the other most frequent somatic mutations, alterations in *PIK3CA, PTEN, RB1, MAP3K1, CDH1,* and *NF1* all have been implicated as potential driver mutations.[159]

Copy Number Alterations

Copy number alterations are described as sequence variations that result from either reduplication or deletion of DNA segments larger than 50 base pairs in length.[182] DNA recombination, replication, and repair-associated processes may lead to copy number changes. Approximately 50% of breast cancer samples are considered "amplifying" in terms of genome-wide copy number assessment.[183] Functional impact of copy number change is significant when associated with high mRNA expression and protein overexpression. Amplification of regions encoding proto-oncogenes in the breast cancer genome results in oncogenic activation of corresponding growth signaling. For example, amplification of 17q12, which contains HER2/neu (ERBB2) gene, occurs in 15% to 25% of breast cancers and is one of the most common pathogenic driver amplification units known.

HER2

The human epidermal growth factor receptor 2 (HER2), also known as the neu oncogene or human homolog for the avian erythroblastosis oncogene B2 (ERBB2), encodes a 185-kilodalton tyrosine kinase membrane receptor protein in the epidermal growth factor receptor (HER, ERBB, EGFR) family. Amplification of the HER2-containing region of chromosome 17q is observed in approximately 15% to 25% of invasive breast carcinomas[9,11] and is directly associated with p185HER2 overexpression at both the messenger RNA and protein levels.[8,11] HER2 amplification/overexpression is associated with shorter DFS and OS in women whose axillary lymph nodes are free of metastases[10] as well as those whose axillary nodes are involved with metastases.[9,11]

Because HER2 amplification/overexpression is an important determinant of poor patient outcomes and because the extracellular domain of p185HER2 is accessible to circulating anti-HER2 monoclonal antibodies directed to the extracellular domain, p185HER2 has become an important target for treatment of women with either metastatic[121,184] or early invasive breast cancers that have not disseminated.[118-120] Breast cancer patients treated with chemotherapy plus a monoclonal humanized anti-HER2 antibody, known as trastuzumab, have shown significant improvements in both DFS and OS compared with patients receiving the same chemotherapy alone. Other anti-HER2 antibodies (pertuzumab), antibody-drug conjugates (T-DM1), and small molecule inhibitors of HER2 tyrosine kinase activity (lapatinib, neratinib) are in various stages of clinical development and testing in clinical trials.[125,127]

Although the predominant mechanism of HER2 activation in cancers appears to be gene amplification (approximately 20% of breast cancers), a small proportion (approximately 2% of breast cancers) have activation of HER2 through mutations in either the tyrosine kinase domain[185] or extracellular domain.[186] Because few of these breast cancers also have HER2 overexpression, the most effective treatment appears to be use of small molecular inhibitors, which are currently being evaluated in clinical trials.

Because currently approved HER2-targeted therapeutics are approved only for treatment of women whose breast cancers have HER2 amplification/overexpression, companion diagnostics to identify these cancers are important so the appropriate patients can be treated. ASCO–College of American Pathologists (CAP) and National Comprehensive Cancer Network (NCCN) guidelines[87,88] recommend that HER2 status be determined as a routine in all primary or metastatic breast cancers using either protein overexpression by immunohistochemistry (IHC) and/or gene amplification by in situ hybridization. In an effort to improve and standardize HER2 testing strategies, the ASCO-CAP have created guidelines for HER2 testing.[187,188] These guidelines have not only led to greater standardization in the processing of breast cancer specimens and in the interpretation of FDA-approved tests but

have also raised questions about whether some of the current approaches are optimal.[189,190]

Although the amplicon on chromosome 17q12 appears to invariably include HER2,[191] the size and distribution of this amplicon is variable, resulting in variability in the number of genes that are also amplified with HER2.[192,193] The potential for these coamplified genes to be important in patient outcome and treatment decisions is illustrated by coamplification of the topoisomerase II-α (TOP2A) gene along with HER2. Although several studies reported an association between HER2 amplification/overexpression and increased responsiveness to anthracycline-based chemotherapy,[194-198] it appears from subsequent retrospective evaluation of large clinical trials that it is the potential for TOP2A to be coamplified along with HER2 that determines patients' response to anthracycline-containing chemotherapy.[199] In vitro and in vivo studies have demonstrated that HER2 overexpression alone does not alter anthracycline sensitivity. Because HER2 is located on the long arm of chromosome 17 (17q11.2–12) in close proximity to TOP2A at 17q21-22, TOP2A is coamplified along with HER2 in approximately 35% of HER2-positive breast cancers. It is these patients, whose cancers have HER2–TOP2A coamplification, who have dramatic responses to inclusion of an anthracycline in their chemotherapy regimen. Nevertheless, inclusion of an anthracycline with trastuzumab does not appear to contribute any additional therapeutic improvement over the use of either agent alone in HER2-positive breast cancer patients.[199] These observations raise the possibility that other "passenger" genes in amplification events may contribute survival benefits for the cancer or treatment resistance, which may prove to be important in patient treatment decisions.

FGFR1 and FGFR2

The FGFRs (fibroblast growth factor receptors) are high-affinity transmembrane tyrosine kinase receptors that constitute a key component of the FGF signaling pathway. FGFR1, located on the short arm of chromosome 8 (8p11), encodes an 822-amino-acid residue protein. FGFR2, located on the long arm of chromosome 10 (10q26), encodes a 821-amino-acid membrane receptor protein. Activation of these receptors by their corresponding ligands leads to phosphorylation of specific tyrosine residues that mediate interaction with intracellular adaptor proteins downstream signaling by a variety of intracellular signaling pathways (Fig. 22.13).

Amplicon 8p11-12, which consists of FGFR1, is amplified in approximately 10% of human breast cancers. FGFR1 is associated with poor metastasis-free survival.[200] In another study of 880 breast cancers, in which FGFR1 amplification was assessed by chromogenic in situ hybridization-based tissue microarrays observed amplification of FGFR1 infrequently in HER2-positive cases and was associated with early relapse and poor survival, particularly in ER-positive breast cancers.[201] Turner and colleagues demonstrated the activation of MAPK and PI3K-AKT signaling pathways in FGFR1 amplified breast cancer cells, with evidence of both ligand-dependent and ligand-independent activity.[202] Remarkably, these cells also showed resistance to tamoxifen, reversible by FGFR1 inhibition. The same study also observed 16% to 27% of luminal B breast cancers to be associated with FGFR1 amplification and poor prognosis.[202] FGF2 ligand expression has been observed in basal-like cancers as well as the basal-like breast cancer cell lines. Demonstration of autocrine loop of FGF2-FGFR1 and sensitivity to FGFR inhibitor in these cell lines

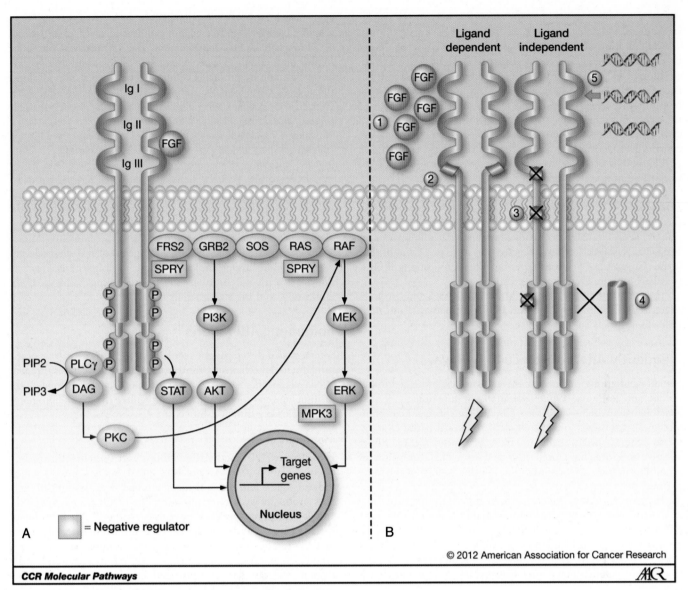

• **Fig. 22.13** Fibroblast growth factor receptor (FGFR) structure, signaling, and dysregulation in cancer. (A) Basic structure of an FGFR and downstream signaling. FGFRs are single-pass transmembrane receptor tyrosine kinases with an extracellular domain that comprises three immunoglobulin-like domains (IgI-III) and an intracellular split tyrosine kinase domain. A complex is formed among the FGF ligand, heparan sulfate, and FGFR to cause receptor dimerization and transphosphorylation at several tyrosine residues in the intracellular portion of the FGFR. Subsequent downstream signaling occurs through two main pathways: via the intracellular receptor substrates FRS2 and PLCg, leading ultimately to upregulation of the Ras-dependent MAPK and Ras-independent PI3K-Akt signaling pathways. Other pathways can also be activated by FGFRs, including STAT-dependent signaling. Negative regulation of the FGFR signaling pathway is mediated via FGF-regulated inhibitory factors such as SPRY and MKP3. (B) FGFR dysregulation in cancer. Ligand activation of FGFRs can be dysregulated when a cell overproduces FGF ligand (1) that activates a corresponding FGFR, or when a cell produces splice-variant FGFRs (2) that have altered specificity to endogenous FGF ligands. Ligand-independent dysregulation of FGFRs can occur when an FGFR becomes mutated (3), leading to receptor dimerization or constitutive activation of the kinase, or when a gene translocation occurs (4), whereby the FGFR fuses with a transcription factor or promoter region resulting in overexpression or activation of the FGFR. A third mechanism is when a gene amplification for the receptor occurs (5), resulting in grossly exaggerated expression of the receptor. Other mechanisms of FGFR dysregulation include germline single nucleotide polymorphisms, which are associated with increased cancer risk or a poor prognosis, and impairment of the normal negative feedback mechanisms, such as reduced expression of the negative regulator SPRY. (Reproduced with permission from Brooks AN, Kilgour E, Smith PD. Molecular pathways: fibroblast growth factor signaling: a new therapeutic opportunity in cancer. *Clin Cancer Res.* 2012;18:1855-1862.)

provided a novel clue about therapeutic targeting of FGFR signaling.[203]

Amplification of *FGFR2* is observed in approximately 2% of breast cancer overall and in approximately 4% of TNBCs.[204] In addition to its role in mammary gland development, FGFR2 has been found essential in sustaining the breast tumor initiating pool by promoting of self-renewal and maintaining the biopotency of the tumor initiating cells.[205] As a transforming oncogene, FGFR2 can confer an invasive phenotype.[206] *FGFR2*-amplified cells are constitutively activated and have demonstrated high sensitivity to FGFR inhibition, by cell death and decrease in the pool of the tumor-initiating cell population.[205,207]

Among the other members of FGFR family, amplification of *FGFR3* and *FGFR4* may occur in 1% to 2% cases depending on the cohort. In vitro evidence has demonstrated increased expression of FGFR3 in MCF7 cells linked to tamoxifen and fulvestrant resistance via MAPK and PI3K activation mediated by phospholipase C gamma.[208] Occurrence of mutations among FGFR members is a rare event in breast cancer.

Therapeutic strategies targeting the FGFR signaling involves selective FGFR inhibitors and anti-FGFR antibodies[209] and multiple clinical trials are in progress.

Frequently Altered Molecular Pathways

Somatic mutations, mainly in driver genes occur in a limited number of pathways. Often alterations in functionally related genes across a patient cohort are observed to cluster in common biological pathway(s) and thereby lead to altered pathway activity to acquire specific hallmark traits of cancer. Genes, under selective pressure, have been proposed to avoid acquisition of mutations in presence of a mutation in other gene(s) of the same pathway.

The term *mutual exclusivity* has been applied to the occurrence of somatic mutations in genes with related function exclusively in either stromal or cellular compartments. Mutually exclusive occurrence of somatic mutations in *PTEN* and *TP53* in cells and stroma has been reported, providing an indication that gene-gene interactions parallel interactions between the stroma and cancer cells.[210]

Pathway-based approaches can help create novel, clinically useful taxonomies by ranking the actionable alterations by overall functional effect of the pathway, given their involvement in each pathway rather than using the individual gene approach and thereby help prioritization of potential targets in precision medicine. An example of the importance of a pathway approach is provided by the observation that high mutation frequency of *PIK3CA* in luminal/ER-positive breast cancers in the absence of elevated protein expression of pAKT, pS6, and p4EBP1—key markers of PI3K pathway activation—indicates relatively lower PI3K pathway activity compared with the basal-like and HER2-enriched expression subtypes, which show not only the higher expression of these markers, but also a correlation with INPP4B and PTEN loss and to some degree with *PIK3CA* amplification. The HER2-enriched subtype also showed higher frequency of PIK3CA mutations.14 The same study identified mutually exclusive alterations in the receptor tyrosine kinase (RTK)/PI3K pathway and mutually exclusive occurrence of mutations in MAP3K1 and MAP2K4.

Among other commonly altered key signaling pathways in breast cancer is p53 signaling. Luminal A expression subtype shows the highest frequency of functional p53 activity, whereas aggressive luminal B subtype, that includes a subset of *HER2* amplified tumors, showed higher occurrence of *TP53* mutations, ATM loss and *MDM2* amplification. The RB1 pathway was intact in the luminal A subtype, whereas *CCND1* amplification was more common in luminal B tumors.[14] The basal-like group shows the highest frequency of amplifications in the PI3K and RAS-RAF-MEK pathways, with alterations in *PIK3CA* (49%), *KRAS* (32%), *BRAF* (30%), and *HER1/EGFR* (23%).[14]

Using a 77-sample data set of luminal breast cancers, Ellis and colleagues identified key somatic alterations in pathways including the caspase cascade/apoptosis, ErbB signaling, Akt/PI3K/mTOR signaling, P53/RB signaling, and MAPK/JNK pathways with frequent mutations in *TP53, MAP3K1, PIK3CA,* and *CDH1*. Less frequently altered genes involved apoptotic cascade, calcium/phospholipase signaling, and G-protein coupled receptors. However, cancers without mutations in frequently mutant genes often shared mutations in other genes of the same relevant pathway. More importantly, aromatase inhibitor resistance was associated with mutations in the p53 signaling pathway, DNA replication, and mismatch repair.[211]

Epigenetic Alterations

Alterations in the epigenetic regulatory mechanisms are one of the fundamental mechanisms contributing to carcinogenesis. Epigenetic mechanisms such as alterations in methylation, histone modification, and microRNA expression regulate the genetic programs involved in key functions of cells.

Methylation

Five distinct DNA methylation groups have been identified based on methylation array data of 802 breast cancers, one of which showed significant enrichment of luminal B expression subtype. This group showed fewer mutations in *PIK3CA* and *MAP3K1*, and lower expression of Wnt-pathway genes.[14] Methylation of specific genes may be predictive of clinical response. Abnormal methylation of *BRCA1* observed in cancer samples has been proposed as an important mechanism of *BRCA1* inactivation. Experimental evidence has demonstrated equal sensitivity to PARP inhibitors compared with response in *BRCA1* mutant cells. Approximately one-third of TNBCs have *BRCA1* methylation,[212] making it potentially important as a group that may respond with therapeutic benefit.

Histone Acetylation

Balance between the histone acetyltransferase and histone deacetylase (HDAC) determine the histone acetylation status of genes. Although the primary role of HDACs is to inhibit transcription, they have a fundamental role in regulating transcription of genes involved in survival, proliferation, differentiation, and apoptosis. Hypoacetylation associated with high expression of HDACs has been observed in cancers. Concurrent inhibition of BRD4/JAK, mainly in the TNBC cells has been demonstrated to sensitize the cancer cells to HDAC inhibitors.[213] Additional research is required to assess the potential therapeutic value of HDAC inhibition.

MicroRNAs

miRNAs are short (20–24 nt) noncoding RNAs that are involved in posttranscriptional regulation of gene expression. Among the short noncoding mRNAs, miRNAs constitute a fundamental mechanism involved in RNA silencing and posttranslational regulation of gene expression. In cancer, oncogenic miRNAs typically target their specific genes that may include transcription factors with oncogenic potential, tumor suppressor genes. In contrast, miRNAs with tumor suppressor, antimetastatic and antiangiogenic activities suppress the expression of oncogenes and genes involved in various aspects of metastasis, including cell migration, motility, EMT, and angiogenesis. In breast cancer, loss or underexpression of tumor suppressor miRNAs, such as miR-17-5p, miR-17-92, miR-206, miR-125a/b, miR-31, miR-34, miR-200, and let-7 have been reported.[214] Tumor suppressor miR-206 has been implicated in suppression of cyclin D2 and Cx43, and can thereby influence proliferation, migration, and invasion. MiR-125b is one of the most downregulated miRNAs, and it may target HER2, erythropoietin, and its receptor. Expression of miR-17-92 cluster is associated with triple negative breast cancer.[215] The miR-200 family has been implicated in EMT via E-cadherin expression by targeting several EMT inducers. miR-31 and miR-335 can target metastasis-related genes.[214]

In contrast, miRNAs with oncogenic activity are usually overexpressed. Among oncogenic miRNAs miR-10b, miR-21, miR-373 target HOXD10, HIF1A, SOCS1, respectively. miR-21 has been found associated with invasive and metastatic breast cancers and has a role in regulating EMT.[216] Both miR-373 and miR-520c have been implicated in targeting CD44, which has a role in migration, invasion, and metastasis.[217] Context-dependence in activation of some miRNAs is potentially important. For instance, miR-146, which may inhibit of NF-κB signaling and thus act as a tumor suppressor, can inhibit *BRCA1,* an important DNA repair mechanism in another context.[214]

One of the main potential clinical utilities of miRNAs is in the area of diagnostics.[214] Circulating miRNAs in patient serum may be useful as a diagnostic tool and for monitoring clinical response. Overexpression of serum miRNAs- miR-21, miR-106a, and miR-155 and underexpression of miR-126, miR-199a, and miR-335 have been observed in tumor samples compared with normal controls. Identification of microRNAs in circulating tumor cells in the peripheral blood is another potential diagnostic application.

Predictive utilities of miRNAs have also been investigated. Study on the sensitizing effect of miR-375 to tamoxifen response via direct targeting of metadherin (MTDH) showed that loss of MTDH restored sensitivity to tamoxifen and could influence patient outcome in tamoxifen-treated patients.[218] Increased expression of plasma miR-210 was found to be associated with resistance to chemotherapy regiment combined with trastuzumab in a study of patients with HER2-positive breast cancers.[219]

Tumor Microenvironment

Apart from the tumor cells, the tumor microenvironment, which is composed of the extracellular matrix and multiple types of stromal cells, mainly fibroblasts, tumor-associated macrophages, T cells, mesenchymal cells (including mesenchymal stem cells), and adipocytes, has been recognized as a major contributor in carcinogenesis.[220] The microenvironment plays an important role in allowing the escape of cancer cells from immune surveillance, inhibiting proapoptotic signaling and promoting cell invasiveness and migration. The microenvironment can also play an important role in inducing resistance to chemotherapy. Studying microenvironmental influences may help formulate novel modes of therapy, particularly immunotherapy that can block immune checkpoints and facilitate antitumor immune response. A variety of interactions between the cancer cells and stromal cells can influence tumor resistance to therapy.[221]

Programmed Cell Death 1 and Programmed Death Ligand 1

Programmed cell death 1 (PD-1), an inhibitory immune checkpoint receptor, is a key component of programmed death signaling. The expression of PD-1 has been observed on a wide variety of immune response cells present in the cancer microenvironment, including activated T cells, B cells, NK cells, and activated monocytes.[222] Programmed death ligand (PD-L1) is a PD1 ligand, involved in suppression of immune response. Expression of PD-L1 is present in tumor infiltrating lymphocytes of 81% ductal carcinoma in situ lesions, but none of the DCIS cells were found to express PD-L1, highlighting the effect of PD-1 signaling at an early stage of carcinogenesis and the potential role of the microenvironment.[220] Expression of PD-L1 correlates to the loss of ER expression and higher expression has been observed in approximately 20% of triple-negative tumors and therefore implicates potential benefit from immune therapy. PD-L1, together with tumor infiltrating T-lymphocytes have been found to correlate with clinical response.[223] A phase Ib trial evaluating pembrolizumab (a PD-1 inhibitor) monotherapy in metastatic TNBC has been completed.[224]

Integrins

Integrins are membrane receptor adhesion molecules that interact with extracellular matrix molecules and modulate a variety of signaling pathways. The type of role of integrins in carcinogenesis may vary. Integrins such as α2β1 may function as tumor suppressor, whereas many others, such as α6β4 and αvβ3, have been implicated for their role in cancer progression.[224] Integrins may cross-talk with growth signaling pathways including the PI3K-AKT, ERK, and NF-κB signaling and can induce resistance and can thus be relevant in understanding the resistance to kinase-targeted therapy.[224,225] β1-integrin expression is a marker of responsiveness to trastuzumab in HER2-positive metastatic breast cancer.[226]

BCL2 and Survivin

VEGF expressed by endothelial and cancer cells can induce BCL2 and survivin (BIRC5). Overexpression of BCL2 further induces the expression of VEGF,[227] whereas downregulation of BCL2 and BIRC5 has been demonstrated to improve sensitivity to treatment.[228]

Biomarkers Used in Clinical Management of Breast Cancer

On the basis of novel molecular insights, special multigene tests have been developed and are commercially available. Use of almost all of these tests is restricted to lymph-node-negative early breast cancers. These tests are mainly used for selecting patients who are not likely to benefit from aggressive chemotherapy, according to the recommendations made by panels of experts.

With the advancement of targeted therapeutics, accurate detection of actionable gene alterations is an emerging priority. Novel diagnostic panels with proven clinical utility based on deep sequencing of cancer genome are under development. Efforts of developing clinically useful disease-specific assays with coverage of genomic regions of interest are in progress.[229,230]

TABLE
22.3 **Biomarkers Endorsed for Clinical Use by Panels of Experts**

Endorsement for Target Group	Biomarker Test	Clinical Utility	Recommendation Source
Node negative breast cancers that are ER positive, PR positive, and HER2 negative	Oncotype DX	21-gene recurrence score to guide decisions on adjuvant systemic therapy	ASCO, NCCN, St. Gallen
	EndoPredict	12-gene risk score to guide decisions on adjuvant systemic therapy	ASCO, St. Gallen
	PAM50	PAM50 risk of recurrence score in conjunction with other clinicopathologic variables to guide decisions on systemic therapy	ASCO, NCCN, St. Gallen
	Breast Cancer Index	To guide decisions on systemic therapy	ASCO, St. Gallen
	Urokinase plasminogen activator and plasminogen activator inhibitor type I	To guide decisions on systemic therapy	ASCO
Node negative Hormone receptor positive or negative	MammaPrint	Risk stratification for recurrence but not for treatment decision-making	NCCN[a]
Hormone receptor positive, HER2 negative	Ki-67 Immunohistochemistry	Distinguish between Luminal A and Luminal B like cancers and for guiding the clinical decisions on endocrine and systemic therapy	St. Gallen
All patients with age of diagnosis <40 years	BRCA mutation testing for germline mutation	To guide decisions with respect to the locoregional or neoadjuvant therapy	St. Gallen

ASCO, American Society of Clinical Oncology[87]; *ER,* estrogen receptor; *NCCN,* National Comprehensive Cancer Network[231]; *PR,* progesterone receptor; *St. Gallen,* Report of 2015 St. Gallen Consensus Conference for early breast cancers.[232]
[a]St. Gallen recommends the use for treatment decisions.

Markers for the Management of Early Breast Cancers

For early breast cancers with known ER and PR status as well as HER2 status determined by immunohistochemistry and/or fluorescence in situ hybridization, multigene tests based on a variety of biomarkers can be helpful in guiding therapeutic decision-making or in assessment of risk of recurrence and prognosis. Table 22.3 provides commonly available tests that are endorsed by one or more expert panels.[87,231,232]

Markers for the Management of Advanced/ Metastatic Breast Cancers

According to the ASCO recommendations, biomarkers, including carcinoembryonic antigen (CEA), cancer antigen 15-3 (CA 15–3), and cancer antigen 27-29 (CA 27-29) can be used for making assessments that contribute to clinical decisions in treating patients with metastatic breast cancers, but these may not be used alone for the purpose of therapeutic decisions.[233] NCCN recommends that significant increases in these serum markers may indicate disease progression but may also occur in cases of responding disease. Corroboration with patient symptoms and bone scans can be useful in bone dominant disease.[231]

Circulating Tumor DNA

Although the markers described in the previous section (e.g., CEA or CA19-9) are expressed in normal and cancer cells, clonal alterations in tumor cells are associated with the presence of circulating cancer-specific mutant genes that are only found in cancer cells. Noninvasive assessment of tumor DNA is possible with cell-free circulating tumor DNA (ctDNA) as well as from circulating tumor cells. In contrast to the circulating intact tumor cells in blood, ctDNA consists of small fragments of nucleic acid that are free of cell fragments or cells. ctDNA is found in approximately 50% to 80% of invasive breast cancers and the frequency of identified ctDNA expression is correlated with the stage of disease.[234] Moreover, increasing levels of ctDNA has been observed to be significantly associated with poor survival and has demonstrated higher sensitivity than circulating tumor cells or serum based markers.[235] A prospective study on a cohort of early breast cancer patients (n = 55) receiving neoadjuvant chemotherapy, predicted metastatic relapse with high accuracy based on mutation tracking by single or serial samples. In addition, this study also demonstrated that sequencing of the minimal residual disease can predict genetic events in subsequently metastatic relapsed disease more accurately than sequencing of the primary cancer and thus may be a valuable tool for identifying early breast cancer patients at high risk of relapse.[236] However, relapse and recurrence is delayed by more than 10 years in many hormone receptor–positive patients, and more studies are required to investigate ctDNA as a tool for assessment of long-term risk of relapse and resistance to therapy.

Conclusion

Advancements in DNA sequencing technology, gene expression microarrays, and other "omic" platforms provide unprecedented power for detection and classification of disease. The use of these technologies for identification of important diagnostic, predictive, and prognostic alterations is expected to increase. With prospective implementation of the Cancer Moonshot initiative, several initiatives related to data sharing and sharing of expertise in precision medicine will facilitate improved statistical power in identifying the less frequent alterations, which nevertheless have clinical utility. These developments are expected to change the landscape of breast cancer diagnostics and therapeutics in the foreseeable future.

Acknowledgment

This work was supported by grants from the Breast Cancer Research Foundation and Tower Cancer Research Foundation (Jessica M. Berman Senior Investigator Award), and a gift from Dr. Richard Blach.

Selected References

1. Hanahan D, Weinberg RA. Hallmarks of cancer: the next generation. *Cell*. 2011;144:646-674.
14. The Cancer Genome Atlas Network. Comprehensive molecular portraits of human breast tumours. *Nature*. 2012;490:61-70.
97. Ma CX, Reinert T, Chmielewska I, Ellis MJ. Mechanisms of aromatase inhibitor resistance. *Nat Rev Cancer*. 2015;15:261-275.
139. Foulkes WD. Inherited susceptibility to common cancers. *N Engl J Med*. 2008;359:2143-2153.
159. Pereira B, et al. The somatic mutation profiles of 2,433 breast cancers refines their genomic and transcriptomic landscapes. *Nat Commun*. 2016;7:11479.

A full reference list is available online at ExpertConsult.com.

23

Stem Cells in Breast Development and Cancer

EBRAHIM AZIZI, JILL GRANGER, RAMDANE HAROUAKA, TAHRA KAUR LUTHER, AND MAX S. WICHA

The concept of the stem cell of origin for cancers was first proposed more than 100 years ago. In this theoretical model, certain cells with self-renewal capacity would form tumors from "embryonic rests."[1] More evidence has accumulated since that time as a result of extensive research that strongly supports the *cancer stem cell (CSC) hypothesis*, suggesting the existence of self-renewing cells that generate heterogenous populations of cells within the tumor mass.[2,3] The preponderance of evidence now suggests that the majority of cancers are hierarchically organized and sustained by a population of cells that display stem cell properties—CSCs.[4] As the case for normal tissue stem cells, CSCs are able to self-renew and differentiate, generating cells that comprise the tumor bulk. Furthermore, preclinical and clinical studies demonstrate that CSCs mediate tumor metastasis and contribute to resistance to chemotherapy and radiation therapy. The CSC hypothesis has fundamental biological and clinical implications that are discussed in detail in this chapter.

Stem Cells in the Normal Breast

Embryologic studies of the normal mammary gland indicate that stem cells in the mammary bud develop into early progenitors and then late progenitors, which then differentiate into either ductal epithelial cells or myoepithelial cells.[5–7] Ductal and alveolar epithelial cells express MUC1 and epithelial keratins, whereas myoepithelial cells express common acute lymphoblastic leukemia antigen (CALLA) and other keratins including CK14.[8,9] Ductal and alveolar epithelial cells are fundamentally different from myoepithelial cells. Ductal and alveolar epithelial cells can proliferate, secrete casein, and express hormonal receptors. Myoepithelial cells, in contrast, synthesize a basement membrane, do not express hormone receptors, and undergo only limited proliferation. Both cell lineages are thought to be derived from undifferentiated mammary stem cells. These normal mammary stem cells characterized as CD49f+/EpCAM− are capable of self-renewal and differentiation both in vitro and in vivo.[10] In fact, obligate features of stem cells are their ability both to self-renew and to differentiate. Self-renewal may consist of either symmetric cell division (into two daughter stem cells) or asymmetric division (into one daughter stem cell and one proliferating cell capable of subsequent differentiation). This differentiation may occur across several different lineages, and thus breast stem cells are characterized as multipotent.[11–13] For example, a normal mammary stem cell can differentiate into either a ductal or alveolar epithelial cell or myoepithelial cell. The ability of mammary stem cells to exhibit evidence of "stemness" can be assayed in two-dimensional culture, three-dimensional culture, and via transplantation into the cleared mammary fat pad of syngenic mice. In in vitro assays, predetermined growth conditions with serum, growth factors, and Matrigel are used. One important in vitro property exhibited by mammary stem cells is the property of forming mammospheres,[14–16] tight aggregates of cells in suspension culture in serum-free media supplemented with growth factors. Single mammary stem cells also have the ability to exhibit alveolar and ductal morphogenesis when cultured in three-dimensional structures in Matrigel. In the developing normal breast, aldehyde dehydrogenase 1 (ALDH1)-positive stem cells, which are also thought to be estrogen receptor (ER) negative, are thought to generate ER-positive progeny.[17]

Markers of Normal Stem Cells

The normal mammary tissue consists of luminal and mesenchymal stem cells that are responsible for self-renewal and expansion associated with cycles of pregnancy that form mammary structures containing luminal, alveolar, and myoepithelial cells.[18] Studies have demonstrated that mammary stem cells are enriched within a CD49f+/EpCAM− population that is also more closely associated with a basal phenotype.[19,20] Another marker that is commonly used to define normal mammary stem cells is the enzyme aldehyde dehydrogenase (ALDH).[21–23] Increased ALDH activity also characterizes hematopoietic and neuronal stem/progenitor cells, where it has been demonstrated to play a functional role in stem cell differentiation. The activity of ALDH can easily be determined by an enzymatic assay termed the Aldefluor assay (Stemcell Technologies, Vancouver, Canada), and a monoclonal antibody detecting the ALDH1 protein can also be used for immunodetection. Studies of normal breast have revealed that approximately 6% of the epithelial cells within the ductal-lobular units were Aldefluor positive.[24] Only ALDH+ cells generated mammospheres in suspension culture. In nonobese diabetic mice with severe combined immunodeficiency, only ALDH+ cells formed ductal structures. Recent studies have shown that different ALDH isoenzymes characterize different mammary stem cell populations. ALDH1a3 is predominantly expressed in stem cells in alveolar "cap" cells, whereas ALDH1a1-expressing stem cells are predominantly found in mammary ducts at branch points.[25]

Mammary Stem Cell Regulatory Pathways

A number of signaling pathways have been implicated in the regulation of normal stem cell self-renewal, lineage commitment, and differentiation. These signaling pathways are activated via ligand activation of membrane receptors, which signal through cytoplasmic intermediaries ultimately regulating gene transcription. Key stem cell signaling pathways include hedgehog (Hh), Notch, WNT, and AKT pathways.[26–29] Hedgehog signaling regulates mammary stem cell self-renewal, as demonstrated by an increase in mammosphere formation after hedgehog pathway activation. Furthermore, increased expression of hedgehog pathway ligands and receptors are found in mammospheres compared with two-dimensional cultures. Notch signaling is initiated via binding of Notch receptors to ligands expressed on adjoining cells. This results in Notch activation via gamma secretase mediated cleavage. The resulting Notch intracellular domain (NICD) then translocates to the nucleus where it activates a number of bHLH transcription factors including HES1, HES5, HEY1, and HEY2. This results in increased stem cell self-renewal as measured by mammosphere formation. Hedgehog and Notch pathways may regulate stem cell self-renewal through regulation of the polycomb gene BMI-1. These signaling pathways do not operate in isolation but are thought to interact with each other as well as other regulatory pathways.

A number of signal transduction pathways may regulate mammary stem cell fate decisions via modulation of microRNAs (miRNAs), which are small, noncoding RNA sequences that can act as potent regulators of stem cell fates. miRNAs have been shown to be involved in several key stem cell regulatory pathways that affect the proliferation and differentiation of normal mammary stem cells.[30,31] For example, Mir 93 regulates mammary stem cells via modulation of TGFBR2, whereas Mir 200 regulates these cells via modulation of BMI-1.[32]

Stem Cells in Breast Cancer

Despite compelling evidence that all cancers, including breast cancer, are monoclonal in origin, established tumors display marked cellular heterogeneity. In fact, this heterogeneity represents the greatest challenge to the development of effective cancer therapeutics. Several models have been proposed to explain this cellular heterogeneity. The stochastic model proposes that cancers develop through a process involving random "stochastic" mutation followed by clonal selection. The term *stochastic* emphasizes that the mutations that develop are random. Multiple rounds of mutation and clonal selection generate genetically heterogenous tumors through a process resembling darwinian evolution. In this model, all of the tumor cells are equally malignant. The CSC model, in contrast, posits that tumors are hierarchically organized and driven by a subpopulation of cells that display stem cell properties. The stochastic model governed our thinking about cancer in the 1980s, whereas the stem cell model has been gaining in popularity since the mid-2000s. However, it is important to emphasize that these two models of carcinogenesis and tumor heterogeneity are not mutually exclusive, and in fact there is now substantial evidence that elements of both apply to most tumors. In such a "hybrid model," tumors arise in self-renewing cell populations, but the resulting CSCs are themselves genetically unstable and subject to mutation and clonal selection. As a result, tumors may be composed of genetically diverse CSCs as well as their more differentiated progeny (Fig. 23.1).

Evidence supporting the stem cell model in breast cancer is based on studies with established human breast cancer cell lines, and more recently in patient-derived xenograft (PDX) models that were sorted on the basis of putative stem cell markers such as CD44+/CD24$^{low/-}$/LIN. Cells expressing the stem cell markers

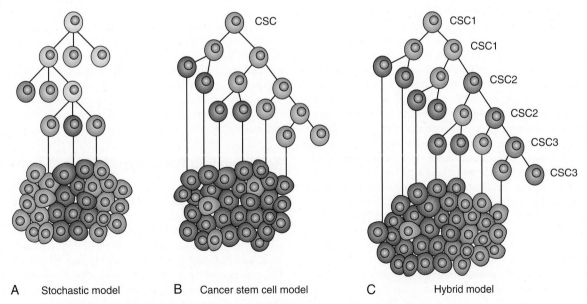

• **Fig. 23.1** Models of tumor heterogeneity. (A) Stochastic model: cancer cells are heterogeneous, but most cells can proliferate extensively and form clones within the new tumor. (B) Cancer stem cell *(CSC)* model: cancer cells are heterogeneous, and only rare CSCs have the ability to proliferate extensively and form new tumors. (C) Hybrid model: cancer cells are heterogenous, and there are several types of CSCs that each one can proliferate to form clones within the tumor.

TABLE 23.1	Normal and Embryonal Stem Cell Markers Expressed by Cancer Stem Cells	
Stem Cell Type	**Molecular Marker**	**Significance**
Embryonic stem cells (ES) or pluripotent stem cells (PS)	Oct-4	Transcription factor essential for establishment and maintenance of undifferentiated PS
	Pax-6	Transcription factor expressed as ES differentiates into neuroepithelium
	Stellar	Specific marker of undifferentiated ES
	Alpha-fetoprotein (AFP)	Reflects endodermal differentiation of PS
	Rex-1	Specific marker of undifferentiated ES
	Germ cell nuclear factor (GCNF)	Transcription factor expressed by PS
	Sox-2	Transcription factor essential for establishment and maintenance of undifferentiated PS
	H19	Marker developmentally regulated in skeletal muscle, smooth muscle, and fetal liver
	Nanog	Transcription factor unique to PS; essential for establishment and maintenance of undifferentiated PS
Hematopoietic stem cells (HS)	CD34	Indicative of HS and EP
	c-kit	Cell surface receptor on bone marrow cell types that identifies HS and MS
	Stem cell antigen (Sca-1)	Indicative of HS and MS in bone marrow and blood
Mesenchymal stem and progenitor cells (MS)	Bone morphogenetic protein receptor (BMPR)	BMPR identifies early mesenchymal lineages (MS)
	Stro-1 antigen	Cell surface glycoprotein on subsets of bone marrow MS
Neural stem cells (NS)	CD133	Identifies NS and HS
	Nestin	Identifies NS
Endothelial progenitor cells (EP)	Fetal liver kinase-1 (Flk-1)	Cell surface receptor protein that identifies EP

More resources are available on the National Institutes of Health website: http://stemcells.nih.gov/info/scireport/appendixE.asp.

were demonstrated to be more tumorigenic compared with the cells lacking expression of these markers.[15] Similar results were obtained using a different stem cell marker, ALDH, where ALDH$^+$ cells were considerably more tumorigenic than ALDH$^-$ cells when introduced into immunosuppressed NOD-SCID mice.[13] Some researchers argued, however, that these experiments were biased toward selecting for cells with the capacity to grow in the immunocompromised mouse microenvironment rather than characteristics of stemness per say. It was argued that if one did the same experiment with a murine tumor in a syngeneic murine host, this differential tumorigenicity might not be observed. However, a number of studies using genetically engineered mouse mammary tumor models have demonstrated that these tumors contain subpopulations of CSCs capable of generating tumors when transplanted into immunocompetent syngeneic mice.[33,34] Although these immune competent mice may represent a more physiologically relevant microenvironment, these studies are still open to the criticism in that serial transplantation of tumor cells disrupts the microenvironment in which these tumors naturally develop. However, three recent landmark studies addressed these arguments by using lineage tracing to demonstrate in three tumor types that tumors originate in self-renewing stem cell populations generating tumors containing CSCs.[35–37] The relevance of these findings to human cancers was further demonstrated using NextGen (Illumina, San Diego, CA) sequencing of CSC populations in human leukemia demonstrating signatures common to normal hematopoietic stem cells.[38]

Markers of Cancer Stem Cells

As noted previously, CSCs display a number of markers that are shared by normal stem cells. This includes CD44$^+$/CD24$^{low/-}$

and ALDH. In addition, embryonal stem cell markers often expressed by CSCs include stellar, rex-1, nestin, and H19, as well as transcriptional factors such as nuclear β-catenin. In addition, OCT4, NANOG, and SOX2 the core transcription factors involved in iPS stem cell reprogramming, are also expressed in a number of CSC populations.[39,40] This raises the interesting possibility that activation of these factors reprograms more differentiated tumor cells into a stemlike state during carcinogenesis. An ever-growing list of cancer stem markers is being described and characterized (Tables 23.1–23.3). One stem cell marker is the ATP-binding cassette transporter protein ABCG2, which facilitates efflux of lipophilic dyes such as Hoechst 33342, identifying a population of cells that is termed the side population on flow cytometric analysis.[41,42] This transporter is also thought to efflux chemotherapeutic drugs from CSCs rendering them resistant to chemotherapy.

Key Signaling Pathways of Cancer Stem Cells

The same signaling pathways that regulate normal stem cells are thought to play similar roles in CSCs. However, in CSCs, these pathways may be constitutively activated through genetic or epigenetic events. Developmental pathways that have been demonstrated to play an important role in CSC function include Hh, Notch, WNT, and Akt pathways. Evidence for the importance of these pathways in CSCs has been derived from experiments showing that pathway activation increases and pathway inhibition reduces the proportion of CSCs. The similarities between signaling pathways in normal and malignant stem cells presents a potential challenge for the development of CSC targeted therapeutics.

Many of the genes implicated in breast carcinogenesis including BRCA1, HER2, and PTEN have also been demonstrated to

TABLE 23.2 Cancer Stem Cell Markers Observed in Human Cancers

Human Cancer Type	Phenotypic Marker	Side Population
Leukemia	CD34$^+$/CD38$^-$, CD44$^+$	Yes
Breast cancer	CD44$^+$/CD24$^{low/-}$, ALDH$^+$, mammosphere formation	Yes
Prostate cancer	CD44$^+$/$\alpha_2\beta_1^{hi}$/CD133$^+$, Sca-1$^+$	Yes
Melanoma	CD20$^+$, spheroid formation	Yes
Brain cancer	CD133$^+$, neurospheroid formation	Yes
Retinoblastoma	ABCG2$^+$, ALDH1 positive	Yes
Colon cancer	CD133$^+$	Yes
	CD44$^+$/CD133$^+$/CD24$^{low/-}$, spheroid formation	No

TABLE 23.3 Summary of Stem Cell Properties Exhibited in Vitro by Cancer Stem Cells

	Stem Cell Properties Exhibited in Vitro
Stem cell–specific markers	Transcriptional determinants as well as specific markers (e.g., oct-4, sox-2, nanog, rex-1) known to be restricted to normal embryonal or tissue stem cells detected within cancer stem cells
Self-renewal and proliferation	Ability of single cancer stem cell to generate secondary spheroids (mammospheres) without initial cell aggregation/cell-cell contact; spheroids containing as few as 100 cells are fully tumorigenic.
Multipotency	Ability of single cancer stem cell cultured in Matrigel to manifest multipotency or differentiation

play important roles in mammary stem cell self-renewal and differentiation. This supports the hypothesis that breast cancers originate in self-renewing cell populations through aberrant activation of these pathways. *BRCA1* is a gene in which a germline mutation can confer an 80% risk of breast cancer. In addition, the majority of breast cancers occurring in *BRCA1* cancers are "triple negative," with significant expression of basal markers (CK5 and CK6). In addition to hereditary breast cancers, a subset of sporadic triple-negative breast cancers (TNBCs) may result from inhibition of somatic *BRCA1* expression via gene methylation. *BRCA1* plays an important role in mammary stem cell differentiation and downregulation of *BRCA1* in normal breast cells increases the proportion of stem cells as evidenced by increased mammosphere formation and ALDH expression.[43] In women with germline *BRCA1* mutations, expansion of ALDH-expressing cells in mammary lobules is associated with loss of heterozygosity of the normal allele.[43] Together these studies demonstrate that in addition to its well-known role in DNA repair, *BRCA1*'s role in

mammary carcinogenesis may also relate to its importance in mammary stem cell regulation.

HER2/neu is amplified in 20% of breast cancers and is associated with a more aggressive clinical course. The development of HER2 targeted therapies for the treatment of HER2-positive tumors represents one of the most significant advances in clinical oncology.[44,45] The clinical efficacy of these agents may relate to the role that HER2 plays in the regulation of breast CSCs. In vitro and in mouse models, HER2 overexpression increases the CSC population, and trastuzumab targets and reduces this population.[46] More recently we have reported that in luminal breast cancers, HER2 may be selectively expressed in CSCs in the absence of HER2 gene amplification.[47] This might account for the surprising finding that HER2 blockade in the adjuvant setting might extend to women whose breast tumors do not display HER2 gene amplification. In addition, this might account for the report of detection of HER2-expressing cells in the blood circulation of women with HER2-"negative" breast cancers.[48,49] The most frequent genetic alteration associated with trastuzumab resistance is PTEN deletion. We have recently demonstrated that *PTEN* deletion activates an inflammatory loop mediated by the cytokine interleukin (IL)-6.[50] This suggests novel strategies to target trastuzumab resistant breast cancer via IL-6 blockade.

Relationship of Epithelial-Mesenchymal Transition and Cancer Stem Cell States

A number of studies have suggested similarities between the CSC phenotype and acquisition of an *epithelial-mesenchymal transition* (EMT) state.[51,52] The EMT is a developmental process that occurs during embryogenesis and tissue formation, which involves loss of epithelial and acquisition of mesenchymal characteristics of migrating cell populations.[53] EMT is a reversible process and through the reverse process mesenchymal-epithelial transition (MET) mesenchymal cells may reacquire an epithelial phenotype. There is evidence that tumor cells may undergo both EMT and MET during the process of metastasis.[53,54] A number of transcription factors, including SNAIL, SLUG, and TWIST have been reported to be involved in EMT. It has been shown that breast CSCs express a number of genes involved in EMT, and conversely breast cancer cells that undergo EMT become stemlike.[55] Researchers have demonstrated that conditions that induce EMT in human breast cancers, such as hypoxia or addition of transforming growth factor beta (TGFβ), also increase the proportion of cells expressing the CSC phenotype CD44$^+$/CD24$^{low/-}$.[55] We have recently demonstrated that in human breast cancer, CSCs exist in alternate states that are characterized by expression of different markers and properties. EMT-like CSCs that have been characterized as CD44$^+$/CD24$^{low/-}$ are highly invasive but relatively quiescent. In contrast, the more epithelial or "MET"-like CSCs, which are characterized by ALDH expression, are more proliferative and capable of "self-renewal." Furthermore, CSCs display plasticity, being able to transition between EMT-like and MET-like states in a process regulated by the tumor microenvironment.[56] As determined by immunohistochemistry, the EMT-like CD44$^+$/CD24$^{low/-}$ CSCs are primarily found at the tumor invasive front, whereas MET-like ALDH$^+$ CSCs are primarily located more centrally. This suggests a model in which EMT CSCs at the tumor invasive front enter the circulation, where they travel to generate metastases at distant sites. These EMT-like micrometastases are nonproliferative and remain dormant until they are induced to convert to an MET "self-renewing" state in which they generate additional CSCs as well as the more differentiated cells that form the tumor bulk. This model is supported by studies demonstrating that both circulating tumor cells as well as disseminated micrometastatic cells in the bone marrow of breast cancer patients are enriched in nonproliferative (KI67 neg) CD44+/CD24low/− cells. In contrast, both primary tumors and macrometastases contain both CD44+/CD24low/− and ALDH+ CSCs.

Cancer Stem Cells and the Tumor Microenvironment: Clinical Implications

Cancer Stem Cells and the Immune System

The complexities of CSC biology outlined thus far in this chapter illustrate the potential, unique challenges for the design of effective therapies to combat tumor development and breast cancer reoccurrence. Indeed, the tumor microenvironment presents a formidable ecological niche that was once considered insurmountable. The immune responses and alterations that occur within this microenvironment involve an intricate network of signaling pathways, immune cell interactions, mediators, cytokine loops, and epigenetic alterations as immune cells interplay between tumor cells and the stroma (Fig. 23.2). To further complicate the process, all of these events occur against the backdrop of dynamic EMT-MET transitions associated with the CSCs. However, it is this very diversity, and the dynamic nature of this process, that also presents a multitude of therapeutic opportunities (Box 23.1).[57,58] Furthermore, the elegant balance between the hosts' innate immune activation and suppression, as well as

commonalities of immune regulation shared between various disease states, could potentially be leveraged to elicit immune responses aimed not only at reducing the tumor bulk but also at targeting and destroying the cancer stem populations responsible for tumor metastasis.

Historically, cancer immunotherapy has focused on stimulating the immune response with subsequent direction toward the tumor target. Most recently, these efforts have centered around several basic strategies; immune checkpoint blockade, the use of monoclonal antibodies, vaccine development, and T-cell-based therapies with chimeric antigen receptors.[59] Each of these therapeutic options has both advantages and limitations. In the context of CSCs, this is particularly challenging because of the heterogeneous nature of CSC populations within a tumor that might require targeting of a number of pathways to achieve an effective therapeutic outcome. However, CSCs also express characteristic surface proteins that may make them more amenable to specific targeting with minimal side effects.[60]

• BOX 23.1 Breast Cancer Diagnosis and Treatment

Diagnosis

Histologic analysis: ER, PR, HER2, BRCA, PTEN
Reverse-phase protein array
Genomic platforms
Proteomic platforms
Tumor-infiltrating lymphocyte (TIL) assessment
Single CSC genomics, transcriptomics and proteomics
Cancer stem cell markers: CD44+/CD24low/−, ALDH+
Embryonal stem cell markers: STELLAR, REX1, NESTIN, H19
Transcription factors: nuclear β-catenin, OCT4, NANOG, SOX2
Side population marker of CSCs: ABCG2

Treatment

Radiation therapy
Surgical resection: removal of tumor bulk
Chemotherapy: docetaxel, HER2-targeted therapy
Immunotherapy:
    Immune manipulation: dendritic cell–based vaccines to prime T cells
    Immune checkpoint blockade affecting pathways for T regulatory cells, APC, signaling: CTLA-4/B7, PD-1/PDL-1, TIM3
    T-cell therapy: chimeric antigen receptor (CAR)
    Monoclonal antibody therapy: trastuzumab, trastuzumab-emtasine, pertuzumab
Endocrine therapy: tamoxifen, aromatase inhibitors, fulvestrant
Small molecule targeted therapy: inhibition of PARP, MAPK, PI3K, JAK/STAT
CSC targeting:
    Antibodies against CSC markers: ALDH1, CD44, ESA (EpCAM), CD133
    Inhibition of signaling pathways for CSC self-renewal:
        NOTCH signaling: γ-secretase inhibitor
        Hedgehog signaling (ER+, ER−): metformin acts to reduce CSC self-renewal, cell survival and invasiveness
        lncRNA silencing results in activated Shh-GLI1 signaling, reduced CSC-associated SOX2 and OCT4
    Reversal agents: resistance to chemotherapy and radiotherapy via surviving CSCs
    Inducers of cellular differentiation: terminal differentiation of CSCs (e.g., salinomycin)
    Drive quiescent stem cells to enter cell cycle
    Tumor microenvironment: epigenetic silencing, repression of T-helper chemokines
    Mitochondrial biogenesis inhibitors: antibiotics (e.g., doxycycline)

CSC, Cancer stem cell; ER, estrogen receptor.

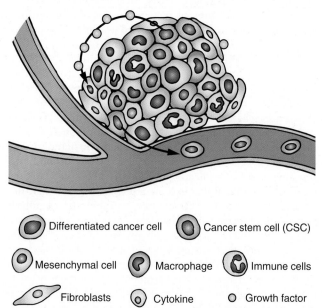

Differentiated cancer cell   Cancer stem cell (CSC)

Mesenchymal cell   Macrophage   Immune cells

Fibroblasts   Cytokine   Growth factor

• **Fig. 23.2** The tumor microenvironment of a metastatic tumor. Similarly to normal stem cells, cancer stem cells (*CSCs*) are regulated by, and in turn regulate, their tumor microenvironment, which consists of mesenchymal stem cells, tissue-associated fibroblasts, and endothelial cells that interact with CSCs via cytokine networks and growth factors. These increased levels of cytokines and growth factors produced by tumor cells recruit tumor-associated macrophages, neutrophils, and mast cells, which secrete additional growth factors and create a positive feedback loop which promotes tumor cell growth and metastases.

Immune checkpoint blockade involves exploiting the immune system's ability to self-regulate through suppression of an immune response.[61] This immune suppression occurs during the process of peripheral tolerance and the minimization of tissue damage that occurs during healing. In the context of the tumor microenvironment, these inhibitory pathways are "hijacked" for the tumor not only to escape immune surveillance but also to promote tumor growth and aid resistance to treatment. This process of "tolerizing" refers to an imbalance in the ratio of effector T cells to regulatory T cells, modifications to antigen presenting cell (APC) activities that signal immune distress, as well as alterations in stimulatory and inhibitory signaling molecules.[62] The regulatory T cells are key players in the suppression that enables tumors to escape immune detection, drawn to the tumor site through tumor-produced CCL22.[63,64] Several pathways have been implicated as key checkpoints in this regulatory process: CTL antigen 4 (CTLA-4)/B7, programmed death 1 (PD-1/PDL-1), and T-cell immunoglobulin and mucin protein 3 (TIM3).[59] It has been suggested that T-cell immunity may be downregulated by CSCs acting through the PD-1/PDL-1 pathway. Furthermore, recent studies in ovarian cancer suggest another mechanism for reduced immune response in which epigenetic silencing may result in repression of T-helper 1 (Th1) chemokines, slowing the trafficking of effector T-cell trafficking into the microenvironment of the tumor.[65]

Monoclonal antibodies represent another possible therapeutic option. In the context of breast CSCs, a variety of monoclonal antibodies that target BCSCs have been described in mouse models. The monoclonal antibody P245, targeting human CD44, has shown promise for inhibiting breast CSCs in xenograft mice. The monoclonal antibody acting against delta-like 4 ligand a ligand involved in Notch signaling, demcizumab (OncoMed Pharmaceuticals, Redwood, CA), effectively reduced breast CSCs in TNBC xenografts, with concomitant inhibition of tumor growth. This antibody is currently being tested in early-phase cancer clinical trials.[66] The Wnt pathway has been targeted using vantictumab (OMP-18R5; OncoMed Pharmaceuticals) with a reduction in tumor growth and CSCs in breast cancer xenografts. B6H12.2 (anti CD47) has likewise been shown to inhibit tumor growth in xenografts.[60,67] This agent also has entered early-phase clinical testing.[68] Our group has shown the effectiveness of using the IL-8 receptor (CXCR1) as a means for targeting breast CSCs in xenograft models.[69] A small molecule CXCR1 inhibitor, reparixin, was administered in combination with the chemotherapeutic agent docetaxel to women with advanced breast cancer with little added toxicity[70] and early signals of efficacy that currently is being tested in a phase III randomized clinical trial.

Another approach is the development of CSC-based vaccines. These vaccines exploit the properties of antigen-presenting cells to promote T-cell immune responses that are specific for tumors. Recent studies using CSC-DC vaccines in syngeneic immunocompetent mouse tumor models for melanoma prevented lung metastasis and inhibited tumor growth of squamous carcinoma.[71] Such vaccines may be useful as an adjuvant treatment after surgical resection of the bulk tumor mass or in combination with other conventional therapies to eliminate micro-metastasis. It has been suggested that T-cell immunity may be downregulated by CSCs acting through the PD-1/PDL-1 pathway, another promising area for vaccine development. Other CSC antigens have been targeted as well, with promising results, in an attempt to eradicate CSCs specifically, including ALDH1, CD44, and CD133.[71]

The advent of single cell technologies will permit examination of the genomic, metabolomic, and proteomic aberrations within the CSCs that are responsible for metastasis, angiogenesis, immune suppression, and growth and proliferation as the tumor becomes established at distant sites. Treatment efficacy may be improved through strategies not only treating the tumor bulk, but combining with those that incorporate the targeting of the unique CSC niche coupled with the stimulation and manipulation of adaptive and/or innate immune responses. Indeed, some effective therapeutic agents may come from "old familiar friends." One example of this is a recent study using antibiotics to selectively target CSCs that resulted from a search for a common phenotypic characteristic that was conserved across many types of cancer.[72] This study, used antibiotics that targeted mitochondrial biogenesis for clonal expansion that was conserved across a variety of CSC types from various tumors. Five classes of drugs were tested, including azithromycin, doxycycline, tigecycline, pyrvinium pamoate, and chloramphenicol. In particular, doxycycline may be an attractive candidate because it has a longer half-life and has been shown to reduce tumor growth. The incorporation of such antibiotics has the potential to be clinically beneficial from premalignancy to advanced disease states.

The ultimate test to prove the CSC hypothesis will be the demonstration that patients' clinical outcomes significantly improve after effective targeted therapy against CSCs. Furthermore, because CSCs may account for growth of micrometastasis, CSC-targeted therapies may have maximal efficacy when they are deployed in the adjuvant setting.

Cancer Stem Cell–Targeting Therapeutics

Selective targeted therapies against CSCs that have no harmful effects on normal stem cells will have great potential in the treatment of many human malignancies.[73] These targeted strategies may include (1) antibodies against CSC-surface markers, (2) inhibitors of signaling pathways that are essential for CSC self-renewal, (3) reversal agents that overcome innate resistance to chemotherapy and radiotherapy in CSCs, and (4) inducers of cellular differentiation to terminally differentiate CSCs.

Inhibiting the Notch signaling pathway is potentially promising in targeted CSC therapy. Small molecules with γ-secretase inhibitory activities or monoclonal antibodies against NOTCH ligands and or receptors are currently in clinical development.[74,75]

Cyclopamine, a plant-derived alkaloid, acts through inhibition of canonical (i.e., classical pathway involving Hh ligands binding to the Smoothened receptor) and noncanonical (Smoothened-independent pathway involving PI3K/AKT activation) Hh signaling pathway that reduces cell proliferation and invasiveness in both ER-positive and ER-negative breast cancer cells.[76] Furthermore, studies have shown that metformin, an antidiabetic drug, inhibits Hh signaling pathway in breast and some other types of cancers. In breast cancer, metformin reduces CSC self-renewal, cell survival, and invasiveness via inhibiting Hh signalling.[77] In addition, studies have shown that lncRNA-Hh silence in a model of Twist-positive mammosphere attenuates the activated Shh-GLI1 signaling that reduces the CSC-associated SOX2 and OCT4 levels. These results explain the role of lncRNAs as an important regulator endowing Twist-induced EMT in breast cancer cells to gain the CSC-like stemness properties that can be a considered as a candidate for targeted therapy of CSCs.[78]

Another possible approach in CSC-specific targeting is inhibition of signals that induce resistance to chemotherapy and/or radiation therapy. Efflux activity of ABC transporters such as BCRP in CSCs has been used in side-population experiments to identify CSC populations. In melanoma, antibodies were used to inhibit the activity of these membrane transporters.[79] Finally, CSC-specific therapy using differentiation inducing compounds might be an effective strategy in converting CSCs to terminally differentiated tumor cells lacking self-renewal capability. In this context, salinomycin has been described as the first compound with the ability to induce terminal epithelial differentiation in breast CSCs.[80] It is well established that certain types of CSCs exist in a quiescent state and thus are resistant to DNA-damaging agents. Induction of these quiescent stem cells to enter the cell cycle to become targets of conventional chemotherapy has been successfully demonstrated in a mouse model for acute myeloid leukemia by treatment with colony-stimulating factors (e.g., granulocyte colony-stimulating factor).[81]

Because of commonalities between the pathways regulating CSCs and normal tissue stem cells, patients on these studies require careful monitoring for potential toxicities related to these agents. Fortunately, limited toxicities have been reported so far in the preliminary results from phase I trials of these agents. Of course, more will be known about efficacies versus harmful effects of these targeting agents during phase II and III studies.

The CSC paradigm has important implications for the assessment of treatment efficacy. Because CSCs constitute only a minor population within a tumor, therapies that target this cell population would not be expected to induce tumor regression. Thus classical criteria such as the RECIST (response evaluation criteria in solid tumors) are not well suited to assess the efficacy of CSC therapeutics. This highlights the need to develop technologies to isolate and characterize these cells. One method that holds great promise is the use of circulating tumor cell technologies to capture and molecularly interrogate tumor cells. A number of studies have demonstrated that circulating tumor cells are highly enriched in cells expressing breast CSC markers, including CD44+/CD24[low/−] and ALDH+.[82] Our group has used Fluidigm's microfluidic platforms (C1 and BioMark HD, South San Francisco, CA) to study the gene expression signature of single tumor cells; this has enabled us to unravel significant heterogeneity among both CSCs and nonstem tumor cells that would not be discernable by conventional bulk cell analysis.[83] These new technologies involving both genomic and proteomic analysis at single cell resolution may allow for the deconvolution of cellular heterogeneity.

Because this heterogeneity presents a major challenge for effective therapeutic development, these technologies may facilitate identification of personalized combinatorial therapeutic strategies.

It is important to note that along with the advancement in single cell "omics" technologies, improved bioinformatic data analysis of huge amount of data being generated from single tumor cells and adopting these methods for clinical use represents a major challenge.

Multifactorial combination therapy, incorporating a variety of elements to alter the tumor microenvironment and harness the power of innate immunity, will change the way we view cancer; the complexity of this disease is no longer overwhelming, but rather a field of opportunity. This new concept will transform the way cancer is diagnosed, treated, and monitored, opening exciting new opportunities for the development of more effective immunotherapies that may result in sustained treatment for our patients.

Acknowledgment

We gratefully acknowledge the contribution of Sanford H. Barsky, who authored this chapter in previous editions.

Selected References

11. Al-Hajj M, Wicha MS, Benito-Hernandez A, Morrison SJ, Clarke MF. Prospective identification of tumorigenic breast cancer cells. *Proc Natl Acad Sci USA*. 2003;100:3983-3988.

13. Ginestier C, Hur MH, Charafe-Jauffret E, et al. ALDH1 is a marker of normal and malignant human mammary stem cells and a predictor of poor clinical outcome. *Cell Stem Cell*. 2007;1:555-567.

43. Liu S, Ginestier C, Charafe-Jauffret E, et al. *BRCA1* regulates human mammary stem/progenitor cell fate. *Proc Natl Acad Sci USA*. 2008;105:1680-1685.

56. Liu S, Cong Y, Wang D, et al. Breast cancer stem cells transition between epithelial and mesenchymal states reflective of their normal counterparts. *Stem Cell Reports*. 2014;2:78-91.

60. Naujokat C. Targeting human cancer stem cells with monoclonal antibodies. *J Clin Cell Immunol S*. 2012;5:007.

A full reference list is available online at ExpertConsult.com.

24

Therapeutic Strategies for Breast Cancer

ISSAM MAKHOUL

No cancer has seen so many dramatic changes in its care and so much passion in the discussions surrounding these changes as breast cancer.[1] In one century, we moved from the aggressive widely mutilating Halstedian surgery[2] to the Z-11 era where up to 25% of patients are left with lymph node metastasis in the axilla without any added recurrence or mortality risk,[3] provided that radiation is given to them. It is clear that we have come a long way in our practice but also in our understanding of this cancer. This magnificent progress occurred most of the time incrementally, as a result of slow scientific discoveries in basic and clinical sciences, but occasionally in bursts that resulted from the advent of scientific breakthroughs, new ideas, and new paradigms to explain cancer in general and the natural history of breast cancer in particular.

Epidemiology of Breast Cancer

Globally, breast cancer is the most common cancer in women and the second most common cancer in the world. More than 1.67 million new breast cancer cases were diagnosed in 2012 (25% of all cancers). Incidence rates range from 27 per 100,000 in developing areas (Middle Africa and East Asia) to 92 in more developed areas (North America).[4] Several epidemiologic studies have linked these different rates to reproductive (parity) and breastfeeding differences[5] in addition to lower screening rates and incomplete reporting.[6] If women in developed countries had the average number of births and lifetime duration of breastfeeding that women in developing countries have had until recently, the cumulative incidence of breast cancer would be reduced by more than half, from 6.3 to 2.7 per 100 women by age 70. The protective effect of parity was restricted to estrogen receptor (ER)-positive/progesterone receptor (PR)-positive breast cancer with each birth reducing the risk of ER-positive PR-positive cancer by 11% (relative risk per birth = 0.89, 95% confidence interval [CI] 0.84–0.94).[7]

Even though incidence rates are much lower in developing countries, mortality rates are practically equal across the world due to less favorable health conditions and limited access to care in the developing countries (324,000 deaths, 14.3% of total, in developing countries vs. 198,000 deaths, 15.4% of total, in developed countries).[4] Worldwide, the incidence of breast cancer has been going up in most regions but at faster rates in developed than developing countries. Trends in mortality from breast cancer, however, show steady decrease in most developed countries and stagnation or slight increase in developing countries.[4]

Incidence rates and mortality from breast cancer in the United States have gone through different phases of increase and decline starting in 1943.[8,9] The increase was slow between 1943 and 1979 by 1% a year, then more rapid from 1980 to 1999 at 4%. It plateaued after 2003 after a gradual (2000–2002) then sharp decline between 2002 and 2003. The rapid increase after 1980 is likely related to increased use of hormone replacement therapy (HRT) and the wide introduction of screening mammography,[9] and the drop after 2002–2003 was explained by a 38% drop in the use of HRT after the publication of the Women's Health Initiative study.[10,11] This increase in incidence was practically exclusively related to in situ and localized ER-positive/PR-positive cancers.[12,13] In the Connecticut experience, which mirrors the whole US experience, in situ and localized cancers increased by 1023% and 86%, respectively. This increase was not associated with a proportional decrease of regional and distant disease (−15% and −20%, respectively).

Between 1975 and 1990, mortality rates continued rising by 0.4% a year, then started declining starting in 1990 by 2.2 % annually until now.[14] Until 1970, mortality rates in the United States were similar for blacks and whites and have been declining since the late 1980s, among whites first, then during the 1990s among blacks.[15]

Breast Cancer Risk Factors

Breast cancer risk factors include age, reproductive factors, breastfeeding, oral contraceptives, HRT, diet, obesity, smoking, alcohol, and heredity (Table 24.1).[16–21]

A rapid review of these risk factors would classify them into three categories: (1) increased and prolonged estrogenic stimulation (early menarche, late menopause, nulliparity, late first full-term pregnancy, oral contraceptives, HRT, obesity in postmenopausal women) increases the risk of breast cancer. Decreased estrogenic stimulation (multiparity, breastfeeding, early menopause, obesity in premenopausal women) decreases the risk of breast cancer. (2) Increased exposure to carcinogens (tobacco, alcohol, others) leads to increased risk of breast cancer. (3) Decreased ability to repair genetic damage or to eliminate cells that harbor them (mutation of *BRCA1* and *BRCA2, PTEN,* p53, and others) leads to higher incidence of breast cancer.

The Natural History of Breast Cancer

Traditional Models for Breast Cancer Natural History

In the beginning of the 20th century, the prevailing model for the natural history of breast cancer at the time of Halsted was the

TABLE 24.1	Risk Factors for Breast Cancer With Relative Risk and the Predominant Type of Breast Cancer	
Relative Risk	**Reproductive Factors**	**Cancer Type**
1.4	Age >40	Luminal A
1.5	Age >40	HER2
1.48	Nulliparous	Luminal type
>4	Postmenopausal breast density	>4
0.5	Full-term pregnancy before age 20	0.5
Increased	Younger age at menarche (<12 y)	
0.03 for every additional year	Older age of menopause (>55 y)	
0.74	Breastfeeding	Less luminal
	Oral contraceptives:	
1.5	Lifetime use ≥15 y	
1.6	Current user ≥5 y	
3.5	Current use for ≥5 y among ages 20–39	Especially TNBC
1.9	HRT (>5 y) especially E-P > E	Luminal A
2.2	Hormone replacement therapy (>5 y) especially E-P > E	HER2
	Overweight (BMI 25–30); obesity (BMI >30)	
1.89	Premenopausal	TNBC
0.63	Premenopausal	Luminal
Increased	Postmenopausal	Luminal
Decreased	Oophorectomy at age <40 y is protective	
Increased	Diet (high fat)	
Increased	Smoking	
1.2	Alcohol ≥2 drinks a day	
Increased	Heredity Hereditary breast cancer syndromes	
6	*BRCA1*	TNBC
5	*BRCA2*	Same as sporadic
Increased	Familial syndromes	Same as sporadic

BMI, Body mass index; *E,* estrogen; *HRT,* hormone replacement therapy; *P,* progesterone; *TNBC,* triple-negative breast cancer.
Data are from references 16 through 21.

centrifugal model.[2,22] This model stipulates that cancer starts in the breast and moves slowly but surely in an orderly, defined manner to invade the breast tissue and surrounding structures then to the lymph nodes, and, if it is not radically removed, then it will spread out from the locoregional basin to distant organs,[23] always by contiguous spread. The involvement of the lymph nodes was conceived to happen by direct extension, and the lymph nodes were viewed as a true barrier to the progression of the cancer. Hematogenous spread was given little importance, and tumors were considered independent of the host. This gradual stepwise progression and understanding of the biology of cancer borrowed from infectious diseases dictated an approach to the management of breast cancer that was based on "en bloc" wide surgical resection of the breast, muscles, fat, and lymph nodes to remove all the cancer without "contaminating" healthy tissues on the side of the affected breast.[2,22] This is the radical mastectomy promoted by Halsted and Meyer at the turn of the 20th century. The success of breast cancer surgery was determined by the extent of tissue removed. Women undergoing this surgery were left with horrendous morbidities such as limited arm mobility, severe lymphedema, and major deformities of body anatomy and image. Despite increasingly aggressive surgeries, women kept progressing to metastatic stages and dying of breast cancer. In the 1950s and 1960s, clinical and basic research led many investigators to question this model.

Debunking the centrifugal model occurred after demonstrating that many of its premises were inaccurate. The first to be discredited was the idea that lymph nodes are effective barriers that stop the spread of tumor cells. Cancer cells injected in the afferent lymphatic of the leg lymph nodes of an animal were collected in the efferent lymph draining from the node.[24] This crude experiment evaluated the question from a mechanical standpoint and did not take into consideration the possibility of interaction between the immune system and the cancer cells that may need time and other conditions to occur. Nevertheless, it was adequate to start shattering the model by causing the first crack in it. The role of the blood as a "highway" for cancer cell dissemination was ascertained in other experiments and led to the conclusion that recurrences are not the result of local treatment failure but of reactivation of dormant disseminated tumor cells that develop from the interaction between the tumor and the host.[25] An "alternative hypothesis" was proposed to account for the aspects that the Halstedian model was unable to explain and to take into consideration these findings. This is the "systemic hypothesis" that suggested that breast cancer is a systemic disease from its inception. The involvement of the lymph nodes is nothing else but an indication that the cancer cells can metastasize and colonize distant organs rather than the instigator of disseminated disease (Table 24.2).[26]

The systemic model stipulates that the stage of the local disease at diagnosis and the extent of local therapy do not alter the natural history of the disease and are unlikely to change the incidence of metastatic recurrences. Several observations with longitudinal follow-up have suggested otherwise. The likelihood of distant metastasis was found to highly correlate with tumor size and the number of involved lymph nodes.[27,28] On the other hand, the optimization of local surgical treatment by the addition of radiation therapy decreased both local and distant metastasis.[29] The sharp dichotomy between the centrifugal model and the systemic model left a large number of tumors out of either model, which suggested to many investigators a different model, the spectrum hypothesis, to account for these discrepancies.[1] The main premise of the

TABLE 24.2	Comparison Between the Halstedian and Alternative Hypotheses	
TWO DIVERGENT HYPOTHESES OF TUMOR BIOLOGY		
Halstedian	**Alternative**	
Tumors spread in an orderly defined manner based on mechanical considerations.	There is no orderly pattern of tumor cell dissemination.	
Tumor cells traverse lymphatics to lymph nodes by direct extension supporting en bloc dissection.	Tumor cells traverse lymphatics by embolization challenging the merit of en bloc dissection.	
The positive lymph node is an indicator of tumor spread and is the instigator of distant disease.	The positive lymph node is an indicator of a host-tumor relationship, which permits development of metastases rather the instigator of distant disease.	
Regional lymph nodes are barriers to the passage of tumor cells.	Regional lymph nodes are ineffective as barriers to tumor cell spread.	
RLNs are of anatomic importance.	RLNs are of biological importance.	
The bloodstream is of little significance as a route of tumor dissemination.	The bloodstream is of considerable importance in tumor dissemination.	
A tumor is autonomous of its host.	Complex host-tumor interrelationships affect every facet of the disease.	
Operable breast cancer is a locoregional disease.	Operable breast cancer is a systemic disease.	
The extent and nuances of operation are the dominant factors influencing patient outcome.	Variations in locoregional therapy are unlikely to substantially affect survival.	

RLN, Regional lymph nodes.
From Fisher B, Redmond C, Fisher ER. The contribution of recent NSABP clinical trials of primary breast cancer therapy to an understanding of tumor biology—an overview of findings. *Cancer.* 1980;46(suppl 4):1009-1025.

spectrum hypothesis is the fundamental biological heterogeneity of breast cancer with variable progression speeds and possibilities to metastasize at different sizes. Some tumors are metastatic from their inception, and early local treatment does not affect the ultimate outcome (these tumors follow the systemic model); others may grow to large sizes, gaining the ability to spread to lymph nodes or distant organs only later during their course (these follow the centrifugal model). Early local treatment is likely to cure those patients. However, most tumors reach the metastagenicity stage at different points that vary depending on the specific biology of the tumor. Those tumors follow the progressive model and can be cured with local treatment only if detected early enough. Finally, some tumors never get there (Fig. 24.1).

The relationship between tumor size and the probability of metastatic dissemination is linear with a median (V50) of 23.6 mL (diameter = 3.56 cm) and a 95% CI 0.14 to 4000 mL.[27] This volume is smaller if the lymph nodes are involved and if tumor grade is high. The spectrum hypothesis suggests that metastatic dissemination is possible at any tumor size and it is influenced by growth rate. The inverse correlation with the number of lymph nodes involved is the result rather than the cause of the early and more vigorous dissemination that leads to lymph node seeding at small volumes. The variability of V50 is responsible for the different models presented in Table 24.3.[30]

This descriptive modeling does not explain the relationship between size and dissemination potential (why do tumor cells disseminate when the tumor reaches certain size?), nor does it tell us why for certain tumor size and growth rate only 50% of the tumors would disseminate not all of them. However, these models were crucial to help physicians design screening and treatment strategies to manage patients. Their validity (albeit partial) was confirmed by the results of modern screening and treatment protocols.

The Estrogen Paradox

From the review of its risk factors, it is clear that breast cancer is an estrogen-driven cancer. However, breast cancer as a disease does not appear until estrogen secretion is depleted in a woman's body. The peak incidence of breast cancer is age 62 years—10 years after the median age of menopause—and fewer than 5% of all breast cancers occur below age 50 when estrogen levels are the highest. Several hypotheses may be formulated to explain this paradox.[31,32] Every menstrual cycle is an opportunity to induce proliferation in the mammary epithelial cell compartment with a possibility for genetic and epigenetic errors (gain of function mutations of oncogenes, loss of function of tumor suppressor genes, methylation of tumor suppressor genes) the probability of which gets higher with higher proliferation rate and higher number of proliferation cycles. The presence of a defect in the DNA repair system (*BRCA* or p53 mutations) increases this probability. A classical autopsy series discovered small foci of subclinical breast cancers (mostly in situ) in 39% of women age 40 to 49 years who died from accidental death, whereas the incidence of clinical breast cancer in this age group is around 1%.[33] Interestingly, many of these patients had multiple foci of preclinical cancers, and yet lifetime breast cancer incidence is not higher than 12% to 13% in our country. Why do these cancers remain silent and not progress to the open disease state?

To progress to clinically open disease, initiated tumor cells have to overcome multiple internal and systemic resistance mechanisms (apoptosis, lack of angiogenic switch, microenvironmental suppression or immune suppression of cancer cells). Indeed, DNA lesions induced by the estrogenic overdrive or carcinogens are necessary to induce malignant transformation but insufficient to induce progression to cancer disease. The progression of these lesions to become open cancers may require more DNA damage (that occurs over time from increased inflammatory response secondary to aging or obesity), initiation of angiogenesis (inflammatory cells may help initiate angiogenesis) and/or weakening of the immune system (Fig. 24.2).

From Descriptive Models to Biologically Informed Carcinogenesis

Breast Cancer Initiation

Epidemiologic and experimental evidence lend a strong support to the role of estrogen in the initiation and progression of breast

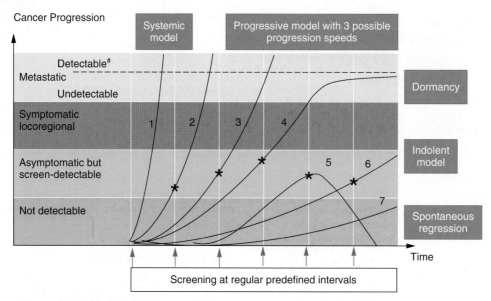

* Cancer detectable by screening
# Cancer detectable by imaging or symptoms

• **Fig. 24.1** Different types of cancer follow different courses. In the systemic model (1), the interval between tumor initiation and widespread dissemination is short, occurring between two screenings. Some cancers in the progressive model move faster than others to disseminate tumor cells to distant organs. In some cases, disseminated tumor cells remain dormant (4) and in other cases (2, 3) they progress to become detectable by imaging or symptoms leading ultimately to patients' death. Some tumors (5) regress spontaneously and unless detected by mammography they will never get noticed. Some tumors (6) are only detectable by available screening methods but do not ever progress to cause any clinical problems to the patients. These are the overdiagnoses that the patients would die with, not of. Finally, there are tumors (7) that appear and remain undetectable even with the most sensitive screening methods. (Modified from Gates TJ. Screening for cancer: concepts and controversies. *Am Fam Physician.* 2014;90:625-631.)

TABLE 24.3 Volume (V50) for Which 50% of the Tumors Metastasize, in Different Groups of Patients

Group	No. Patients	V50 (mL)	Corresponding Diameter (cm)	Variation Interval (mL)	Median Delay Between Diagnosis and Detection of First Distant Metastasis (Months)
Overall	2648	23.6	3.56	19.3–28.8	
Histologic grade known (total)	1596	41.0	4.27	30.5–54.8	
1	298	584.0	10.4	191–1765	65
2	766	29.5	3.83	19.5–44.7	44
3	532	23.0	3.53	14.6–35.0	21
No. axillary lymph nodes invaded known (total)	1722	32.8	3.97	24.5–43.8	
0	560	690.0	11.0	217–2180	69
1–3	657	30.3	3.87	19.0–48.4	43
>3	505	7.2	2.40	4.0–13.1	30

From Koscielny S, Tubiana M, Le MG, et al. Breast cancer: relationship between the size of the primary tumour and the probability of metastatic dissemination. *Br J Cancer.* 1984;49:709-715.

cancer.[34,35] Cells in the normal mammary gland are subject to high turnover orchestrated by endocrine factors (estrogen, progesterone, prolactin, and others) in preparation for lactation during reproductive age. Every menstrual cycle is marked by significant proliferative changes of the ductal-lobular units; in the absence of pregnancy, massive cell death ensues. The process requires the recruitment of normal mammary stem cells that reside in the ducts. These cells are capable of asymmetric division in which one cell rejoins the pool of stem cells, and the other continues proliferating and differentiating to give rise to all the component

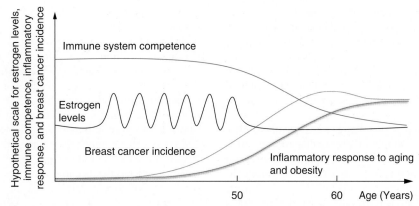

• **Fig. 24.2** The estrogen paradox. Breast cancer is an estrogen-driven cancer. However, fewer than 5% of all breast cancers occur in women younger than age 50 when estrogen levels are highest. Breast cancer rate increases after menopause and peaks at about 10 years later. After 50, the competence of the immune system declines, and the inflammatory response due to aging and overweight/obesity increases.

of the mammary gland: the luminal and myoepithelial cells.[36,37] Random or inherited genetic and epigenetic changes confer proliferative and/or survival advantages on certain mammary cells. These cells are believed either to belong to the stem cell compartment or to the progenitor cells after they have acquired stemness characteristics.

These incipient cancer cells face internal and external control mechanisms that, when successful, lead to the correction of the abnormalities, growth suppression of the cells, or their elimination altogether. The immune system plays a host-protective role in cancer control by detecting transformed cells and eliminating them, but it can, in certain circumstances, be tumor promoting.

Under the pressure of the immune system, transformed cells undergo many changes called *immunoediting*. There are three phases of immunoediting: elimination, equilibrium, and escape.[38,39] Elimination is the process of eradication of the new cancer cells by a normal immune system and is supported by a wealth of experimental evidence in animals and humans. The innate and adaptive arms of the immune system recognize incipient cancer cells by the neoantigens (resulting from mutations or translocations) presented on their surface or by the distress signals that are expressed by transformed cells that have undergone chromosomal changes (aneuploidy or hyperploidy) and eliminate them.[40,41] Equilibrium is reached when the immune system fails to eliminate the transformed cells but stop them from progressing further. It can be conceived as the *dormancy phase* of cancer development. This phase is mediated by equilibrium between cells and cytokines that promote elimination (interleukin [IL]-12, interferon [IFN]γ, tumor necrosis factor [TNF]α, CD4 Th1, CD8+ T cells, natural killer cells, γδT cells) and those that promote persistence of the nascent tumor (IL-23, IL-6, IL10, transforming growth factor-β, natural killer T cells, CD4 Th2, Foxp3+ T regulatory cells (Tregs), and myeloid-derived suppressor cells).[42–44] Monocytes play an important role in this process. Under the influence of tumor microenvironment, they may differentiate into proinflammatory M1 or antiinflammatory M2 types, which play a role in the angiogenic switch (discussed in the next section).[45,46]

Immune escape of cancer cells occurs by different mechanisms. In hormone receptor (HR)-positive breast cancer, the absence of strong tumor neoantigens and low expression of MHC1[47] allow the tumor to progress unnoticed by the immune system. Estrogen plays an immunosuppressive role in the tumor microenvironment

that promotes tolerance of the weakly immunogenic cancer. In HER2 breast cancer, MHC1 presentation is inversely correlated with HER2 expression.[48] Triple-negative breast cancer (TNBC) exhibits a spectrum of MHC1 presentation and strong tumor antigen expression but immune escape in this subtype is mostly related to the development of immunosuppressive tumor microenvironment by expressing immune checkpoints such as CTLA4 or PD-L1.

However, it is still unclear how the balance established during the equilibrium phase gets tilted toward tumor progression. The answer to this question is very likely multifactorial. Aging is associated with reduced production of new B and T lymphocytes in the bone marrow and the thymus, respectively and with decreased function of the mature ones.[49] Systemic inflammation associated with aging and local proinflammatory microenvironment in the breast are incriminated in promoting cancerous progression of mammary stem cells that have been primed by losing tumor suppressor genes.[50,51] Proinflammatory cytokines (TNFα and IL-6) were associated with overexpression of COX2 and the aromatase enzyme,[52] which lead to increased local concentrations of estrogens. Estrogens induce the expansion of Tregs and the inhibition of antigen presenting cells.[53–55] In addition to the gradual decline of the immune system, dietary, commensal microbiota, use of antibiotics, procreational, and hormonal factors, all play some role of variable importance in tilting the balance from equilibrium to escape.[56–59]

The Vascular Phase of Tumor Development: The Angiogenic Switch

The prevascular stages of breast cancer precursor lesion, such as carcinoma in situ, can usually be seen only with microscopic examination. These tumor cells are also usually separated from host microvessels by a basement membrane. From experimental studies, we know that these prevascular lesions exist in a steady state of tumor cell proliferation balanced by cell death[60] and may remain in this state for months to years. The onset of neovascularization, however, can be relatively sudden and is called the *angiogenic switch*.[61,62] In most human breast cancers, angiogenesis is initiated after the emergence of the invasive malignancy, but it can also start at the preinvasive phase.[63] It is understood as a shift in the net balance between positive regulators of angiogenesis (e.g., basic fibroblast growth factor [FGF], vascular endothelial growth factor [VEGF]) and negative regulators of angiogenesis (e.g., thrombospondin-1, 16-kD prolactin, IFN-α, IFN-β, platelet factor 4, angiostatin, endostatin, and others such as IL-12).[64] Tumor-associated macrophages that were polarized to the M2 phenotype and other cells (fibroblasts and adipocytes) participate in generating proangiogenic factors that participate in the angiogenic switch.

Four mechanisms for angiogenic switch were identified. First, direct recruitment of blood supply by prevascular tumors. After the basement membrane is breached, invasive cells enter the stroma and induce neighboring endothelial cells to proliferate toward the source of proangiogenic factors following a concentration gradient. Multiple cell layers form a microcylinder (the radius of which is restricted by the oxygen diffusion limit) that surrounds every new capillary vessel.[65] Second, recruitment of endothelial stem or progenitor cells. VEGF receptor-1–positive bone marrow cells are recruited from the blood to the invasive focus. However, the contribution of these cells in breast cancer angiogenesis is limited. Third, vessel cooption; cancer cells surround preexisting blood vessels.[66] The last mechanism of angiogenic switch is vascular mimicry; the tumor cells dedifferentiate into an endothelial phenotype and make tubelike structures.[67]

Angiogenesis is credited with allowing the tumor to grow from microscopic to macroscopic sizes and to facilitate the shedding of isolated cells or clusters of cells into the bloodstream, which leads to metastasis.[68,69] New blood vessels provide the tumor with oxygen and the necessary nutrients and removal of waste products. Endothelial cells, even without blood flow, can provide the tumor with paracrine growth and survival signaling.[70,71] The final effect of angiogenic switch is decreased apoptosis in the tumor by up to sevenfold while proliferation rates remain similar to the ones in the prevascular stage, which allows the rapid expansion of the tumor mass.[72]

The inability of a tumor to turn the angiogenic switch on results in small microscopic tumors that remain dormant (*angiogenic dormancy*). Tumor dormancy is common in primary breast cancer and in metastatic disease and may extend to several years or decades. Chronic inflammation and the decline of the immune system in addition to the accumulation of genetic/epigenetic hits ultimately break the equilibrium that maintains the dormant state and allows the tumor to take off.

Blood markers (VEGF, FGF, placental growth factor, angiostatin, endostatin, and others) and microvessel density are used in the assessment of angiogenesis, but there is no agreement between investigators about the best methods. None of these methods is used in routine practice.

Relationship Between Primary Tumor and Breast Cancer Metastases

Four patterns of metastatic presentation have been proposed. The first pattern, in which metastases grow after removal of the primary tumor, is seen in animal models and believed to be related to suppressive substances released by the primary tumor (angiostatin) that maintain the metastases in dormancy, but they grow rapidly after the primary tumor is removed.[73] The evidence for the existence of this pattern in humans is scant at best. Rapid progression of micrometastases after surgery may be seen in rare cases but may be explained by the postoperative inflammatory state and the dumping of large amounts of cytokines and growth factors in the blood rather than the removal of a putative suppressive substance with the surgical resection of the tumor.[74]

In the second pattern, the metastases grow concomitantly with the primary tumor. The third pattern, known as the occult primary, could be based on metastatic cells that outgrow the primary tumor and suppress its growth by immunologic or other mechanisms such as angiogenesis. The fourth pattern, in which metastases remain dormant for years after removal of the primary tumor, is observed in breast cancer, colon cancer, Ewing sarcoma, and many other tumor types. Again, the mechanism of this prolonged dormancy is unknown. However, recent reports indicate that once metastases become clinically detectable, they display a similar rate of growth that is independent of the number of years of dormancy. This observation is consistent with a model of microscopic dormant metastases that do not expand until sometime within a year of becoming clinically detectable. One explanation is that these metastases were controlled in their new environment by the immune system that was able to overcome their proliferative and angiogenic drive. The regression of metastases after removal of the primary is not known to happen in breast cancer, although it was described in resected renal cell carcinoma.

Disseminated Tumor Cells

Tumors that have acquired the invasive and angiogenic phenotype start shedding malignant cells in the bloodstream (called disseminated tumor cells [DTCs]). DTCs have to overcome multiple resistance mechanisms that lead to the destruction of the majority of them. Only very few can survive this journey and reach distant organs. Once they have colonized these organs, they go through a phase of dormancy that may last for years before they start growing again, causing metastatic cancer that is responsible for 90% of mortality in breast cancer.[75,76] Breast cancer DTCs have a propensity to relocate to bone.[77–79] The process is not linear and requires the interaction of DTCs with cells in the destination niche and the immune cells.

The bone marrow offers DTCs two nurturing environments normally occupied by hematopoietic stem cells (HSCs): the osteoblastic (for dormant HSCs) and the vascular (for actively dividing HSCs) niches.[80] Breast cancer DTCs interact through their surface receptor CXCR4 (the same receptor expressed by HSCs) with bone marrow stromal cells such as osteoblasts, endothelial cells, and fibroblasts that express stromal derived factor-1 (SDF-1 or CXCL12), CXCR4 ligand.[80] After relocating to the hematopoietic niche the intruding breast cancer cells may secrete cytokines that suppress hematopoiesis, which may explain the anemia seen in this cancer and others. The predilection to the hematopoietic niche also explains why bone metastases do not arise in the parts of the skeleton that do not harbor red bone marrow. Osteoblasts secrete many cytokines such as angiopoietin-1 and stromal cell factor that help retain HSCs and cancer cells in the niche and by activating the Notch pathway they promote HSC and cancer cell stemness and block their differentiation.[81] New drugs targeting CXCL12 or CXCR4 are used to mobilize HSCs for stem cell transplant but also to "expulse" cancer cells out of the bone marrow. Once out of their protective environment, they become more vulnerable to chemotherapy and/or radiation therapy.[82]

It is possible that complete estrogen deprivation induced by aromatase inhibitors (AIs) has two opposed effects on DTCs in the bone marrow. On one hand, it leads to decreased proliferation or apoptosis of highly estrogen-dependent breast cancer cells. On the other hand, estrogen deprivation induces high bone turnover, resulting in the release of many growth factors embedded in the bone, which may rescue estrogen-deprived cancer cells (insulin-like growth factor) or suppress the immune cells infiltrating and surrounding the tumor (transforming growth factor-β). The net effect is favorable in most patients. This may explain why antiresorptive therapy with bisphosphonates decreases recurrences only in postmenopausal women on AIs. This observation was validated in an animal model.[83]

Tumor Heterogeneity

Molecular Subtypes of Breast Cancer

Oncologists have acknowledged early the heterogeneity of breast cancer based on HR expression. By the beginning of the 1990s, it had become clear that at least three types of breast cancer exist, with distinct clinical behavior and responsiveness to therapy: HR-positive, HER2-positive, and triple-negative breast cancers. The advent of genomic sequencing and the possibility to assess gene expression in cancer ushered in a new era of classifying these diseases based on biologic rather than histologic similarity. On the basis of gene expression profiling, five intrinsic subtypes were identified: the basal-like, the HER2 positive, the luminal A and B, and the normal-like[84]; subsequent analysis led to the identification of the Claudin low subtype[85] (Table 24.4). This original work led to the development of the PAM50 and PAM50 risk of relapse (PAM50-ROR) assays.[86] The first allows the classification of breast cancers into different intrinsic subtypes, and the second provides important information about their prognosis. In the next decade, other gene expression profile (GEP)-based prognostic assays were developed including the Oncotype Dx and MammaPrint. All of these assays generate a score that assigns a low, medium, or high risk of recurrence (PAM50-ROR, Oncotype Dx) or good-bad prognosis (MammaPrint) to each individual cancer. Attempts at using a grouping of traditional classifiers such as HR, HER2, and ki67 yielded a good approximation of the intrinsic subtypes (luminal A: HR positive/HER2 negative/ki67 low; luminal B: HR positive/HER2 negative/ki67 high; luminal B: HR positive/HER2-positive; HER2 positive: HR negative/HER2 positive; triple negative: HR negative/HER2 negative)[87] that fell short of fully recapitulating the subtypes defined by GEP.[88]

Other tools of genomic analysis have been developed (Oncotype Dx, EndoPredict, Breast Cancer Index, and urokinase plasminogen activator and plasminogen activator inhibitor type 1).[89] They provide information about the prognosis and potential benefit from chemotherapy or its ability to lead to pathologic complete response (pCR).[90,91]

Limitations of Gene Expression Profiling Platforms

GEPs suffer from what we may call *static original determinism*. The immune system and many stromal and bone marrow–derived cells are involved in carcinogenesis, but they have not been integrated in modern prognostic models (except for the wound-gene signature). GEPs are snapshots of the tumor's gene expression at one point in time that may not even reflect all the information contained in the tumor due to intratumor heterogeneity.[92] GEPs provide an assessment of interpatient heterogeneity by dividing a group of patients into good and poor prognostic groups. However, it assumes that DTCs in the same patient will carry the same signature as the primary tumor forever and will either progress unavoidably to full-blown metastases (poor prognosis group) or not (good prognosis group). In reality GEPs have had variable success at achieving this task.

TABLE 24.4	Molecular Subtypes of Breast Cancer							
Molecular Subtype	Frequency (%)	ER/PR/HER2	CK5/6 EGFR	Genes of Proliferation	Characteristic Genes	Histologic Grade	TP53 Mutation	Prognosis
Basal-like	10–20	ER– PR– HER2–	+	High	KRT5, CDH3, ID4, FABP7, KRT17, TRIM29, LAMC2	High	High	Poor
HER2-enriched	10–15	ER– PR– HER2 +	+/–	High	ERBB2, GRB7	High	High	Poor
Normal breast-like	5–10	ER–/+ HER2–	+	Low	PTN, CD36, FABP4, AQP7, ITGA7	Low	Low	Intermediate
Luminal A	50–60	ER+ PR+ HER2–	–	Low	ESR1, GATA3, KRT8, KRT18, XBP1, FOXA1, TFF3, CCND1, LIV1	Low	Low	Excellent
Luminal B	10–20	ER+/– PR+/– HER2+/–	–	High	ESR1, GATA3, KRT8, KRT18, XBP1, FOXA1, TFF3, SQLE, LAPTM4B	Intermediate/ High	Intermediate	Intermediate/ poor
Claudin-low	12–14	ER– PR– HER2–	+/–	High	CD44, SNAI3	High	High	Poor

Modified from Eroles P, Bosch A, Pérez-Fidalgo JA, Lluch A. Molecular biology in breast cancer: Intrinsic subtypes and signaling pathways. *Cancer Treat Rev.* 2012;38:698-707.

The TAILORx trial used the Onco*type* Dx test to classify node-negative/HR-positive breast cancer patients into three groups (low 0–10, intermediate 11–25, and high >25 recurrence scores [RS]). The first results from the TAILORx trial were recently released regarding patients with low recurrence score (0–10). Of the 10,253 patients enrolled, 1629 (15.9%) had low RS. Five-year distant disease–free survival is 99.3%, and 5-year survival is 98% for these patients. Seventy percent of the patients (70%) had intermediate RS (11–25), and the rest (14.1%) had high RS.[93] The latter group would benefit from chemotherapy, whereas the first group would not. In one way, this is great news for patients with low RS because they will be spared the side effects of chemotherapy. However, the amount of uncertainty remains high for a large subset of patients that fall into the intermediate RS group. The original validation of this test used the cutoff of 18 to define the low recurrence group.[94] Even the "gene dormancy signature"[95] relies on genes of the primary cancer and its predictions rely on the presence or absence of proliferation-promoting genes and they do not do better than the other GEPs.

Intrapatient Heterogeneity and Clonal Evolution

Genetic[96] and epigenetic[97,98] alterations of breast cancer change over time under the pressure of the microenvironment and the immune system.[99–102] The treatments used in the adjuvant and neoadjuvant settings add their selection pressure and lead to genetic and epigenetic changes that underlie therapeutic resistance and recurrence.[103] Genetic instability increases over time, leading to the emergence of diverse subclones.[104] This diversity comes at a cost but ultimately offers the cancer a significant survival and dissemination advantage.[105,106] As tumor cells land in distant organs, cells emerging from some subclones are likely to survive in these new environments and colonize them.[78] Representatives of these subclones can be detected by the analysis of circulating tumor cells in the blood.[107] Colonization may be associated with additional genomic and epigenetic changes. The clonal evolution that began in the primary tumor continues in the secondary metastatic sites leading to further evolution and succession of periods of therapeutic control and failure then ultimately to patient's death.[108]

Breast cancers vary in their proliferative potential with high proliferation being associated with worse survival outcomes.[109] The drivers for proliferation are different depending on breast cancer subtypes. More than two-thirds[110] of breast cancers express the ER and remain dependent on estrogen for their proliferation for a long time. Estrogen deprivation leads to decreased proliferation and apoptosis of many cells in the tumor mass. This explains the sensitivity of these cancers to estrogen deprivation strategies of long duration. Ultimately, some estrogen-dependent breast cancer cells become resistant to estrogen deprivation by mutating their ER or by activating other proliferation-promoting pathways.[111–113] The rest of breast cancers do not express ER and depend for their proliferation on activated oncogenes (HER2) or express activated oncogenes in addition to ER. Proliferation of HR-negative breast cancers is cell-autonomous and largely depends on internal drivers. The assessment of proliferation has yet to find reliable and agreed on markers. ki67 has been historically used but the best measurement method and the best cutoff to stratify patients remain to be determined. A cutoff of more than 25% was found to be associated with a greater risk of death compared with lower expression rates in a meta-analysis that included 64,196 patients.[114]

The hallmarks of cancer[75] are expressed to different degrees in different subtypes of breast cancer.[91] At one extreme, estrogen-dependent breast cancers of the luminal A subtype are usually well differentiated (organ-like), and their proliferation rate is low.[115] They are resistant to chemotherapy-induced apoptosis.[116] Their energy metabolism is mixed, aerobic and anaerobic, and they depend little on VEGF. Their mutational and neoantigen loads are low, and their way of immune escape is by immunoediting rather than immune suppression. These cancers may follow an indolent or progressive course. Many of them may remain small, may be detected by screening mammogram, and are responsible of the phenomenon of overdiagnosis seen with the widespread of mammography screening. In TNBC, genomic instability is high[117] and clonal evolution has progressed with multiple clones in the tumor or in distant sites. Proliferation is high, and dependence on external stimuli is minimal if any. Early in the progression of this type, breast cancer cells are highly proliferative and are susceptible to apoptosis (cancer cells with functional apoptotic machinery). Their energy metabolism is becoming more anaerobic[118,119] and they depend heavily on VEGF.[120] Cells in this subtype are poorly differentiated. Immune escape is achieved by cancer-induced immunosuppression with activation of checkpoints (CTLA4, PD1/PD-L1) and Th2 and M2 polarization of the immune response. These tumors may follow and a systemic model. However, it is clear that there are many possible combinations of different hallmarks of cancer that may lead to the different courses described in the previous section (Fig. 24.3).

Therapeutic Strategies for the Management of Invasive Breast Cancer

Strategies that have been developed to manage breast cancer span the spectrum of the disease from its inception to its diagnosis and treatment than to the posttreatment phase and take advantage of the weaknesses of the cancer. Initiation and progression of breast cancer require (1) a strong estrogenic drive and/or (2) genetic and epigenetic alterations; (3) loss of intracellular control and decreased apoptotic predisposition; (4) weak immune surveillance and chronic inflammatory milieu; and (5) a permissive microenvironment. Inherited factors act by magnifying one or more of the previous disturbances.

Surgery leads to the physical elimination of the tumor and radiation and chemotherapy induce DNA damage or interrupt the cell cycle, which would overwhelm cancer cell repair mechanisms leading to active cell death. In all of these cases, it is possible that the end result is the eradication of cancer cells. Hormone blockade or estrogen depletion may lead to the induction of dormancy of tumor initiating cells. This strategy does not lead to complete elimination of cancer cells that may wake up if the treatment is interrupted. Angiogenesis inhibitors did not prove effective in the adjuvant setting. The failure of targeting angiogenesis in the adjuvant/neoadjuvant setting is one of the most important lessons in the late 2000s that suggest clearly that angiogenesis is not an important mechanism for the maintenance of DTCs or micrometastatic disease. Targeted therapy resulted in a major shift in the treatment of HER2-positive cancer. Recent discoveries suggest that this modality works through activation of the immune system rather than the interruption of the oncogenic drive of HER2. The recently rediscovered immune therapy may induce either one of these outcomes—eradication or dormancy—and is a promising method for opening new horizons in the treatment of cancers, including breast cancer.

The most important principle in clinical management of breast cancer patients is the need for close collaboration among the

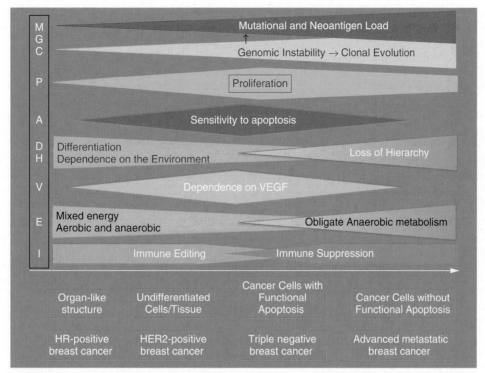

• **Fig. 24.3** Interpatient and intratumor heterogeneity. Cancer may start on the left end and progress to the right while becoming aggressive and resistant, or it may start at any point along this continuum. Multiple subclones may exist in the same tumor at different evolutionary stages. This heterogeneity is the source of treatment failure and should be accounted for as we move forward in the treatment of the cancer. However, cancer can start anywhere on this continuum and may progress toward increased autonomy and independence from the constraints of multicellularity. *A,* Apoptosis; *C,* clonal evolution; *D,* differentiation; *E,* energy metabolism; *G,* genomic instability; *H,* hierarchy; *I,* immune status; *M,* mutational load; *P,* proliferation; *V,* vascular supply.

members of a multidisciplinary team that includes surgeons, medical oncologists, radiation oncologists, radiologists, pathologists, and representatives of different support services. Patients are stratified according to the TNM staging. The TNM stage is one of the first prognostic factors that would determine the prognosis and the type of treatment. Early-stage breast cancers are those with stage I, IIA, and IIB (T2N1). Locally advanced breast cancers are those with stage IIB (T3N0) and stage IIIA though IIIC. This chapter focuses mainly on the multidisciplinary management of early invasive breast cancer. For detailed discussion of the management of locally advanced breast cancer see Chapter 65.

Surgical Treatment

The main stay of surgical treatment of breast cancer is the complete resection of the cancer en bloc with a rim of normal tissue while preserving function and cosmesis. Progress in understanding the biology of breast cancer and improvement of surgical techniques led a revolutionary reversal of the increasingly mutilating surgeries that were performed in the first half of the 20th century. Radical mastectomy was replaced by modified radical mastectomy then lumpectomy (breast conservation surgery [BCS]) with radiation therapy (RT) (BCS + RT + breast conserving therapy [BCT]). This change became possible with the increased usage of screening mammography and the detection of tumors at very small sizes.[121]

National Surgical Adjuvant Breast and Bowel Project (NSABP) B-4 was a seminal trial that propelled BCS forward in the 1970s.

It was the first trial to randomize patients with clinically negative or positive lymph nodes to radical mastectomy (RM) or total mastectomy (TM) with RT. The trial accrued its 1665 patients between 1971 and 1974. They were randomized to the planned procedures and were followed for up to 6 years (average of 36 months). At the time of the publication of the study results, 14% of those with clinically negative lymph nodes who underwent TM (without axillary lymph node dissection [ALND]) had a regional axillary lymph node failure. Patients with clinically negative lymph nodes who underwent RM or TM + RT had no axillary recurrences. Patients who had locoregional failure were rescued with ALND. Disease-free survival did not significantly differ between patients with clinically node-negative axilla on the three arms including those who had a locoregional recurrence and were subsequently rescued with surgery.[122]

Veronesi and coworkers demonstrated equivalence between BCT and RM by showing that all-cause mortality was practically the same (BCT 41.7%, RM 41.2%) in the two groups after 20 years of follow-up. The slight increase in locoregional recurrence in the BCT group compared with RM (8.8% vs. 2.3%) did not affect long-term survival.[123] The need for RT was explored by NSABP B-6, which demonstrated that BCS alone is associated with ipsilateral breast tumor recurrence (IBTR) in 39.2% compared with 14.3% when RT was added to BCS.[124] These seminal studies established the role of BCT that became the predominant form of surgery performed in the developed countries. The Early Breast Cancer Trialists' Collaborative Group (EBCTCG) reviewed the data on 10,801 women in 17 randomized trials and concluded that RT reduces the risk of locoregional recurrence after BCS by half.[125] Several observational studies have shown that BCT offers equivalent—and even superior—long-term survival to patients compared with TM.[126–128] However, it was argued that the observational studies by their nature carry implicit and explicit biases that may be responsible for these results.[129]

Patients who are not eligible for BCT include the following: (1) pregnant women, (2) patients who have had prior RT, (3) patients with multicentric disease or diffuse calcifications on mammography, (4) those with large tumors relative to the breast size, and (5) persistent positive margins after reexcision. Patient preference should be added.

Modified radical mastectomy with axillary lymph node sampling of level I and/or II may be needed to remove all cancer. Otherwise, simple mastectomy is performed if the lymph nodes are clinically negative.

Lymph nodes evaluation is performed with fine-needle aspiration or core needle biopsy if the nodes are clinically positive or with sentinel lymph node biopsy (SLNB) if they are clinically negative. If the SLNB is negative for cancer involvement, no further action is undertaken; if it is positive, ALND is performed. On the basis of the American College of Surgeons Oncology Group trial Z-11, forgoing ALND in patients with clinical T1–2N0 and one or two positive sentinel LNs after undergoing BCS is oncologically safe and is associated with less morbidity.[3] A 10-year follow-up of this study showed no significant difference between the group that received the ALND and the observation group with locoregional recurrence-free survival at 93.2% for the ALND arm and 94.1% for the SNB arm.[130]

Debate regarding margin width continued for years and led to many surgical reexcisions—many of which were not necessary—until a working group of experts from the Society of Surgical Oncology and the American Society for Radiation Oncology met and reviewed the evidence in 2014. They reviewed data from 33 eligible studies published between 1965 and 2013 and included 28,162 patients, of whom 1506 had an IBTR. The conclusion of this meta-analysis was that a "positive margin, defined as ink on invasive cancer or ductal carcinoma in situ (DCIS), is associated with at least a 2-fold increase in IBTR." RT, systemic therapy, or favorable biology do not nullify this increased risk.[131]

Radiation Therapy

RT is based on the induction of massive DNA damage in cancer cell genomes that lead to apoptosis. RT is a locoregional treatment modality that helps limit the extent of surgery, although RT works better in the context of minimal residual disease. The EBCTCG and the St. Gallen International Expert Consensus Group recently updated their findings/guidelines regarding RT.[132]

1. Partial mastectomy and whole breast irradiation (WBI) are equivalent to total mastectomy.
2. Patients who undergo BCS are offered WBI because it decreases the risk of LRR and IBTR and may lead to improved survival. The EBCTCG overview showed that for every four local recurrences prevented, one breast cancer death is avoided at 15 years of follow-up after diagnosis.[125]
3. Patients who undergo mastectomy with negative SLNB do not require RT. However, some patients who underwent mastectomy still benefit from RT if they had a tumor greater than 5 cm, chest wall invasion, positive macrometastatic sentinel node biopsy but no axillary dissection, patients with one to

three involved nodes and adverse pathology, involvement of four or more lymph nodes, or in presence of extranodal extension.[132,133]
4. Regional nodal irradiation (RNI) is not indicated if lymph nodes are negative. If the lymph nodes are positive, the addition of RNI to whole breast RT decreases IBTR without changing long-term survival in an RCT.[134] An observational study showed that radiating the internal mammary LNs (IMLNs) might be associated with survival advantage if IMLNs were positive.[132,135]
5. Women older than 70 with HR-positive stage I breast cancer may forgo RT and be offered tamoxifen after lumpectomy with excellent long-term results. Although local recurrence was higher in the no RT group there was no negative effect on survival.[136–138]
6. Hypofractionated RT using 15 to 16 fractions is considered standard of care by many experts.[139]
7. Partial breast irradiation (PBI) is at least equivalent to WBI in selected patients and it may be associated with lower nonbreast cancer and overall mortality (up to 25% relative decrease in mortality).[140]

Medical Treatment

The major lesson learned from the surgical management of breast cancer since the 1960s was that the type of local management does not affect long-term outcome of the disease that depends on the presence of DTCs/micrometastases outside of the breast. This realization paved the way to systemic therapy with the goal to eradicate DTCs and micrometastases. Major advances in systemic therapy have benefited from better understanding of the biology of breast cancer.

Several strategies have been used to eradicate the hidden reservoir of DTCs and thus prevent recurrence of the disease.
1. The first strategy was based on endocrine manipulations to induce estrogen deprivation. It is possible that this strategy leads to maintaining tumor dormancy instead of its complete eradication.
2. The second strategy was the use of chemotherapy to induce cytotoxicity and cell death. Many chemotherapeutic drugs have been tried since the 1960s to achieve this goal. As we will see, some of the effects of chemotherapy may be related to its immunomodulatory effect.
3. The third strategy emerged in the 1990's after the discovery of oncogenes and tumor suppressor genes. This was the golden age of targeted therapy that allowed major advancements to cure certain types of breast cancer through the targeting of activated oncogenes.
4. Targeting tumor angiogenesis did not result in any significant improvement of outcomes in the adjuvant/neoadjuvant setting.
5. Finally, we are transitioning now to the era of immunotherapy.

Chemotherapy

The success of chemotherapy in childhood leukemia ushered in a new era for the treatment of cancer. Many of the drugs that had shown efficacy in hematologic malignancies were tried in solid tumors including breast cancer. The success of cyclophosphamide, methotrexate, and 5-fluorouracil (CMF) designed by Bonadonna[141] was followed by other combination regimens with equal or superior efficacy (Tables 24.5 and 24.6).

Considering the heterogeneity of breast cancer, there is no single optimal chemotherapy regimen for all subtypes of this

TABLE 24.5	Classification of Adjuvant Chemotherapy Regimens	
Generation	Benefit	Regimens With Substantial Evidence Base
First	35% reduction in breast cancer mortality compared with no adjuvant chemotherapy	CMF ×6, AC ×4, FEC50 ×6
Second	20% reduction in breast cancer mortality compared with first generation regimen	FEC100 ×6, CAF ×6, FAC ×6 AC ×4, T ×4 (every 3 wk) DC ×4, E ×4-CMF ×4
Third	20% reduction in breast cancer mortality compared with second generation regimen	FEC ×4, D ×3, FEC ×4 weekly T ×8 Concurrent DAC Dose-dense AC ×4, T ×4 AC ×4 weekly paclitaxel AC ×4 docetaxel (every 3 wk)

AC, Doxorubicin, cyclophosphamide; *CAF*, cyclophosphamide, doxorubicin, 5-flourouracil; *CMF*, cyclophosphamide, methotrexate, 5-flourouracil; *D*, docetaxel; *DAC*, docetaxel, doxorubicin, cyclophosphamide; *DC*, docetaxel, cyclophosphamide; *E*, epirubicin; *FAC*, 5-flourouracil, doxorubicin, cyclophosphamide; *FEC50*, 5-flourouracil, epirubicin (50 mg/m²), cyclophosphamide; *FEC100*, 5-flourouracil, epirubicin (100 mg/m²), cyclophosphamide; *T*, paclitaxel.
From Anampa J, Makower D, Sparano JA. Progress in adjuvant chemotherapy for breast cancer: an overview. *BMC Med.* 2015;13:195.

disease. However, a few general principles have been established to guide the oncologist and the patient in their shared decision process[142]:

1. The decision to offer chemotherapy to the patient should integrate cancer characteristics (stage, HR, and HER2 statuses, grade and lymphovascular invasion) and patient factors (expected benefit, possible toxicity, age, life expectancy, and patient preference).
2. The use of genomic analysis (Onco*type* Dx, EndoPredict, PAM50, Breast Cancer Index, and urokinase plasminogen activator and plasminogen activator inhibitor type 1) or online calculators to assess benefit and risks may add significant information to help the patient reach a decision.[89]
3. Polychemotherapy is more effective than monochemotherapy.[143,144]
4. Anthracycline-containing regimens have become standard of care but carry the risk of cardiac toxicity, which should be weighed against their benefit.[145]
5. The additional benefit of taxanes should be weighed against their true risk for long-lasting neuropathy.[145]
6. Dose-dense chemotherapy (short intervals between treatments) is slightly superior to traditional schedules (longer interval between treatments with the same agent and doses), but it requires the use of growth factor support that would add significantly to the cost.
7. Toxicity from chemotherapy affects many organs. Major side effects include chemotherapy-induced nausea and vomiting, myelosuppression, fatigue, hair loss, mucositis, and neuropathy. Modern supportive care and antibiotics have improved the control of these side effects in most patients. The probability

for major toxicity should always be considered when making the decision to offer chemotherapy to patients especially the elderly.

Chemotherapy for TNBC

Indications. Patients with tumors greater than 5 mm and/or any lymph node involvement regardless of the size of the primary are offered chemotherapy as the only modality we have available to decrease their risk of recurrence. Tumors 4 to 5 mm in size carry a small risk of recurrence, and the decision to offer chemotherapy to these patients should be weighed against the potential risk for major toxicities that may offset the small benefits. Patients with tumors less than 4 mm are not considered for chemotherapy.

Regimens. Dose-dense adriamycin/cyclophosphamide × 4 cycles followed by weekly taxol × 12 (ddAC-T) is considered the standard of care.[146,147] Taxol can be replaced by docetaxel every 3 weeks for 4 cycles. DAC (docetaxel, adriamycin, and cyclophosphamide every 3 weeks × 6 cycles) is an acceptable alternative option.[148] Docetaxel and cyclophosphamide every 3 weeks × 4 cycles is an acceptable alternative regimen for small tumors with no lymph node involvement.[149] The addition of platinum compounds (carboplatin) has shown efficacy in the neoadjuvant setting (GueparSixto, Cancer and Leukemia Group B 40603)[150,151] and is being tested in the adjuvant setting (NRG-BR003).[152]

Chemotherapy for HR-Positive/HER2-Negative Breast Cancer

Indications. This group of patients is heterogeneous, and the benefit from chemotherapy is not uniform. Patients with tumors 5 mm or less and no lymph node involvement do not need chemotherapy because of their excellent long-term outcome and very low risk of recurrence. Patients with tumors greater than 5 mm and no lymph node involvement may be considered for chemotherapy. The use of one of the validated tools for assessment of prognosis and benefit from chemotherapy can be helpful. Onco*type* Dx, the most commonly used tool in the United States, generates a recurrence score (RS) that helps guide the decision for chemotherapy. Patients with high-RS (>30) derive significant benefit from chemotherapy (absolute decrease in 10-year distant recurrence rate: mean 27.6%, standard error 8.0%). Patients with low RS (<18) derive no benefit from chemotherapy (absolute decrease in distant recurrence rate at 10 years: mean −1.1%; standard error 2.2%). Patients with intermediate RS (18–30) are in the gray zone because current information does not exclude a clinically important benefit.[94] The TAILORx trial used the Onco*type* Dx test to classify lymph node–negative/HR-positive breast cancer patients into three groups (RS: low 0–10, intermediate 11–25, and high >25). The first results from this trial for patients with low RS (0–10) are now available. Of the 10,253 patients enrolled, 1629 (15.9%) had low RS. Five-year distant disease-free survival is 99.3%, and 5-year survival is 98%. Seventy percent (70%) of the patients had intermediate RS (11–25), and the rest (14.1%) had high RS.[93]

Most patients with HR-positive/HER2-negative and LN-positive breast cancer are offered chemotherapy. Data generated from prospectively conducted-retrospectively analyzed clinical trials with similar patients suggest that RS is prognostic, but it is not clear whether it helps select patients for benefit from chemotherapy.[153] The RxPONDER trial (a large phase III randomized clinical trial of standard adjuvant endocrine therapy with or without chemotherapy in patients with one to three positive nodes, hormone receptor–positive/HER2-negative breast cancer

TABLE 24.6 Select Phase III Trials of First-, Second-, and Third-Generation Trials

Generation	Comparison (Reference)	Nodal Status	Patient N	Median Follow-Up (Years)	HR for DFS	HR for OS
First	CMF vs. no chemo[156,157]	+	386	28.5	0.71 (p = .005)	0.79 (p = .04)
	CMF + Tam vs. Tam (B20)[158]	−	2306	5	0.65 (p = .001)	0.64 (p = .03)
	AC vs. CMF (B15)[159,160]	+	2194	3	p = .5[a]	p = .8[a]
	AC vs. CMF (B23)[161]	−	2008	5	p = .9[a]	p = .4[a]
	FEC50 + Tam vs. Tam[162]	+	457	9.4	0.46 (p = .0008)	0.65 (p = .07)
Second	FEC100 vs. FEC50[163]	+	546	5.6	0.63 (p = .02)	0.45 (p = .005)
	ACx4-T ×4 vs. AC ×4 (C9344)[164]	+	3121	5.8	0.83 (p = .002)	0.82 (p = .006)
	ACx4-T ×4 vs. AC ×4 (B28)[165]	+ 0–3	3060	5.4	0.83 (p = .006)	0.93 (p = .46)
	DC ×4 vs. AC ×4[166]	+	1016	7	0.74 (p = .033)	0.69 (p = .032)
	Ex4-CMF ×4 vs. CMF ×6/CMF ×8[167]	+ −	2391	4	0.69 (p < .001)	0.67 (p < .001)
Third	DAC vs. FAC[168,169]	+	1491	10.3	0.80 (p = .004)	0.74 (p = .002)
	DAC vs. FAC[170]	−	1060	6.4	0.68 (p = .01)	0.76 (p = .29)
	FEC-D vs. FEC[171,172]	+	1099	7.8	0.85 (p = .036)	0.75 (p = .007)
	FEC-weekly T vs. FEC[173]	+	1246	5.5	0.77 (p = .022)	0.78 (p = .11)
	FAC-weekly T vs. FAC[174]	−	1925	5.3	0.73 (p = .04)	0.79 (p = .31)
	Q3 vs. q2wk ACT[175,176]	+	2005	5.8	0.80 (p = .01)	0.85 (p = .04)
	AC-T vs. AC-weekly T[146]	+	4954	12.1	0.84 (p = .011)	0.87 (p = .09)
	AC-T vs. AC-D				0.79 (p = .001)	0.86 (p = .054)
	AC-D vs. DAC[177]	+	5351	6.1	0.80 (p = .001)	0.86 (p = .09)
	AC-D vs. AD				0.83 (p = .01)	0.83 (p = .03)

[a]HRs were not reported in the manuscript; however, p values did not reveal any statistical significance between study arms.

AC, Doxorubicin, cyclophosphamide; *CAF,* cyclophosphamide, doxorubicin, 5-flourouracil; *CMF,* cyclophosphamide, methotrexate, 5-flourouracil; *D,* docetaxel; *DAC,* docetaxel, doxorubicin, cyclophosphamide; *DC,* Docetaxel, cyclophosphamide; *E,* epirubicin; *FAC,* 5-flourouracil, doxorubicin, cyclophosphamide; *FEC50,* 5-flourouracil, epirubicin (50 mg/m^2), cyclophosphamide; *FEC100,* 5-flourouracil, epirubicin (100 mg/m^2), cyclophosphamide; *HR,* hazard ratio; T, paclitaxel.

From Anampa J, Makower D, Sparano JA. Progress in adjuvant chemotherapy for breast cancer: an overview. *BMC Med.* 2015;13:195.

with RS of ≤25) completed accrual in 2015, and its results are anxiously awaited.[154]

Regimens. Dose-dense adriamycin/cyclophosphamide × 4 cycles followed by weekly taxol × 12 (ddAC-T) is considered standard of care.[146,147] Taxol can be replaced by docetaxel every 3 weeks for 4 cycles. DAC (docetaxel, adriamycin, and cyclophosphamide every 3 weeks × 6 cycles) is an acceptable alternative regimen.[148] Other alternatives are available (see Tables 24.5 and 24.6).[155–177]

Chemotherapy for HER2-Positive Breast Cancer. Amplification of the *HER2* gene leads to overexpression of the HER2 receptor in 20% to 25% of breast cancer.[178–180] This event plays a major role in the aggressiveness of this type of breast cancer; its targeting changed the outlook of this subtype of breast cancer and led to a dramatic shift in our ways of treating it. Two classes of drugs were developed to target HER2, monoclonal antibodies (trastuzumab and pertuzumab) and tyrosine kinase inhibitors (lapatinib, afatinib, and neratinib). After the success of trastuzumab success in prolonging survival in the metastatic setting,[181] several trials were designed to assess its efficacy in the adjuvant (Table 24.7)[182–194] and neoadjuvant settings.

The major conclusions that were established from these clinical trials are as follows:

1. The benefit from trastuzumab is specific and restricted to patients with breast cancer overexpressing the surface membrane receptor HER2. Overexpression is established by immunohistochemistry (3+ by this method) or by fluorescence in situ hybridization (HER2:CEP 17 ratio > 2).

2. Anthracycline and nonanthracycline regimens were studied. The nonanthracycline regimens are equivalent to the anthracycline regimens.

3. It is preferable to use trastuzumab concurrently with chemotherapy (taxane) due to a slight advantage over sequential use.

4. The duration of trastuzumab therapy is of 1 year. Two years of treatment would add more cardiac toxicity with no additional benefits (HERceptin Adjuvant [HERA] trial). The PHARE trial failed to show that 6 months of trastuzumab was noninferior to 12 months.

5. The magnitude of the benefit in disease-free survival (DFS) from adding trastuzumab to chemotherapy varied from 24% (HERA) to 23% to 28% (BCIRG006), to 37% (NSABP B-31/NCCTG N9831 combined analysis) in large RCTs with the largest effect being associated with concurrent administration of trastuzumab and chemotherapy. Smaller trials showed either a larger significant benefit (47% in the FinHer trial) or smaller nonsignificant benefit (16% in the PACS-04 trial).

6. Trastuzumab is effective for tumors less than 2 cm and negative LNs.[182]

7. There is no role for the tyrosine kinase inhibitor lapatinib in the adjuvant therapy of HER2-positive breast cancer.[183,184]

A joined committee from the American Society of Clinical Oncology and the College of American Pathologists updated the recommendations for HER2 testing in 2013[185]:

1. HER2 status should be determined in every breast cancer as a part of the routine evaluation.

TABLE 24.7 Trastuzumab Adjuvant Trials

Study	Median FU (Months)	Treatment Regimen per Arm	Timing[b]	Duration of Administration (Weeks)	DFS (95% CI)	OS	HR	Cardiac Events	Pt N
BCIRG 006[186,187]	120	AC →D			67.9%	78.7%			1073
		AC→D + T → T	C	52	74.6% (p < .001)	85.9% (p < .0001)	HRR 0.72		1074
		D + Carbo + T→T	C	52	73% (p = .0011)	83.3% (p = .0011)	HRR 0.77		1075
FinHer[188,189]	62	D/V→FEC			73%	82.3%		1.7%	116
		D/V + T → FEC	C	9	83.3%	91.3%	HRR 0.57, (p = .047)	0.9%	115
HERA[190–192]	108	CT +/–RT → observation						0%	1698
		CT +/–RT → T × 1 y	S	52	76%		HRR 0.76, p < .0001	0.5%	1703
		CT +/–RT → T × 2 y	S	104	75.8% (0.85–1.14) p = .86		0.76, p = .0005	1.7%	1701
NCCTG N9831[193,194]	~100	AC → P			75.2%	62.2%		0.1%	1087
		AC → P + T → T	C	52	84%	73.7%	HRD 0.63 (p < .001)	0.3%	949
		AC → P → T	S	52					1097
NSABP B31[194]	~100	AC → P			75.2%	62.2%			872
		AC → P + T → T	C	52	84%	73.7%	HRD 0.63 (p < .001)		864
PACS 04[189]	47	FEC/ED +/– RT			78% (72.3–82.5)				268
		FEC/ED +/–RT →T	S	52	81% (75.3–85.4)		HRR 0.86 p = .41		260
PHARE[195]	42.5	Any chemo + T	S (44.2) C (55.8)	26	91.1 (89.7–92.4)		HRR 1.28 (p = .29)[a]	1.9%	1693
		Any chemo + T	S (43.1%) C (56.9)	52	93.8% (92.6–94.9)			5.7%	1691

AC, Doxorubicin and cyclophosphamide; *BCIRG,* Breast Cancer International Research Group; *C,* concurrent; *Carbo,* carboplatin; *CT,* chemotherapy; *D,* docetaxel; *ED,* epirubicin and docetaxel; *FEC,* fluorouracil, epirubicin, and cyclophosphamide; *FinHer,* Finland HerceptinH study; *HERA,* HerceptinH Adjuvant trial; *NCCTG,* North Central Cancer Treatment Group; *NSABP,* National Surgical Adjuvant Breast and Bowel Project; *P,* paclitaxel; *PACS,* French Protocol Adjuvant dans le Cancer du Sein; *RT,* radiotherapy; *S,* Sequential; *T,* trastuzumab; *V,* vinorelbine.
[a]The trial failed to show that 6 months of trastuzumab was noninferior to 12 months.
[b]Timing of trastuzumab initiation with respect to study chemotherapy.

2. Using either immunohistochemistry or fluorescence in situ hybridization, the results should be expressed as positive, negative, or equivocal.
3. All equivocal results by one method should automatically trigger testing with the other method.
4. The technical requirements for the conduct of the tests were defined, and providers were urged to cooperate to ensure the highest quality testing (the laboratory should demonstrate high concordance rate and must be College of American Pathologists accredited).

Endocrine Therapy

The mainstay of endocrine therapy is the induction of estrogen deprivation at the level of the tumor by blocking access to the ER (selective estrogen receptor modulator [SERMs]: tamoxifen, toremifene) or by depleting estrogen via ovarian ablation in premenopausal women (chemical, surgical, or radiation) with or without AI (anastrozole, letrozole, or exemestane) or by the use of AI in postmenopausal woman.

1. Endocrine therapy is recommended to most patients with invasive tumors greater than 5 mm regardless of the type of surgical treatment.
2. SERMs (tamoxifen and toremifene) can be used in pre- and postmenopausal women.
3. AIs are used for postmenopausal women only.
4. Five years of tamoxifen are better than 2 years, which are better than placebo.[196,197]
5. Ten years of tamoxifen are superior to 5 years of tamoxifen in terms of DFS.[198,199] However, the benefit is more pronounced in patients who had high-risk disease upfront (large tumors or LN involvement).
6. Tamoxifen decreases the risk of recurrence by about a half and the risk of death by one-quarter. The relative risk reduction from tamoxifen is similar regardless of the size of the primary tumor or nodal status.[144,200]

7. In postmenopausal women, 5 years of an AI are better than 5 years of tamoxifen in terms of DFS. Overall survival (OS) is similar.[201,202]

8. In premenopausal women, 5 years of an AI and ovarian suppression are better than 5 years of tamoxifen in terms of DFS, with a similar effect on OS.[203]

9. After 5 years of tamoxifen, an AI decreases the risk of distant recurrence if given for 3 to 5 years.[204]

10. After 5 years of AI or 3 years of tamoxifen and 2 years of AI, extending AI treatment for more than 2 to 3 year is not beneficial.[205–207]

11. Several tools have been designed to help clinicians and their patients make the decisions about long-term endocrine therapy such as the Breast Cancer Index and adjuvant chemotherapy and endocrine therapy sensitivity (ACES) tool.[208,209]

Both tamoxifen and AIs increase the incidence of vasomotor symptoms (tamoxifen > AIs) and musculoskeletal symptoms (AIs > tamoxifen). Tamoxifen increases the risk of thromboembolic events and cancer of the uterus, more so in postmenopausal than premenopausal women. It has a neutral or negative effect on bone mass in premenopausal women and bone-preserving effect in postmenopausal women. AIs have a negative effect on bone mass and may double the risk of osteoporotic fractures. AIs inhibit the conversion of androgens to estrogens in the fat and muscle with an efficiency approaching 96% to 99% in postmenopausal women.[210] Because of their better preventive effect on breast cancer recurrence compared with tamoxifen and their lower risk of thromboembolic events and endometrial cancer, AIs have become the drugs of choice for postmenopausal patients with HR-positive breast cancer.[211] Their negative effects on bone mineral density (BMD) and fracture risk are the highest if they are started immediately after menopause and in patients with low BMD or serum estradiol levels at baseline. The increased fracture risk varies by individual agents and trials between 15% and 115%.[212]

Angiogenic Therapy

Bevacizumab, a humanized monoclonal antibody that was designed to target VEGF-A, was first approved for breast cancer in the metastatic setting in 2008 based on the results of the E2100 Intergroup phase III trial comparing paclitaxel with or without the addition of bevacizumab as first-line therapy.[213] The approval was contingent on the results of further studies, which ultimately did not demonstrate significant improvements in overall survival.[214–220] Thus US Food and Drug Administration (FDA) approval of bevacizumab for breast cancer was officially withdrawn in 2010.[221] Since the withdrawal of bevacizumab approval for breast cancer, 2 adjuvant and 4 neoadjuvant trials have been published.[222–227] The adjuvant trials did not show any improvement of DFS or OS, whereas all the neoadjuvant trials showed modest but statistically significant improvement of pCR. Again, no improvement of DFS or OS was seen in three of the neoadjuvant trials, and the improvement in pCR was seen in HR-negative cancers only. NSABP B-40 was the only neoadjuvant trial that showed improvement of pCR in HR-positive breast cancer and statistically significant improvement of DFS in the bevacizumab arm. Most of these studies were designed for all comers because no specific target for bevacizumab efficacy was identified. For this reason, biomarkers are urgently needed to identify patients most likely to benefit from bevacizumab or other angiogenesis inhibitors.

Immunotherapy

The success of immunotherapy in several solid tumors raised interest in using these treatments in breast cancer. Several strategies were used to harness the power of the immune system and redirect it to eradicate the cancer or to induce immune dormancy.

1. Breast cancer vaccines
2. Checkpoint inhibitors
3. Monoclonal antibodies
4. Enhance the immune-mediated effect of chemotherapy

Breast Cancer Vaccines. Breast vaccines are designed using tumor-associated antigens (TAAs) to stimulate an intrinsic antitumor response to help treat the cancer rather than to prevent it from happening. TAAs that are specifically recognized by T cells include HER2, mucin 1 (MUC-1), carcinoembryonic antigen (CEA), sialyl-Tn (STn), human telomerase reverse transcriptase (hTERT), and Wilms tumor gene *(WT1)*.[228] The antigens where current studies are primarily focused around include HER2 and MUC-1.

As for HER2, there have been a few developments with vaccines involving the E75, GP2, and AE37 peptides. Nelipepimut-S (NeuVax) is an E75 vaccine that, in combination with granulocyte macrophage colony-stimulating factor (GM-CSF), has been shown in phase I/II trials to prolong DFS in HER2 patients.[229] One issue that arose with the E75 vaccine was that the immunity waned after 6 months from the completion of the primary vaccination series. However, a booster given at 6 months from completion of the primary vaccination series was found to be safe and effective in stimulating E75-specific immunity.[230] The work with E75 has led to the current PRESENT trial, which is focused on breast cancer patients with low to intermediate HER2 expression. This phase III trial compares DFS in patients with early-stage, node-positive breast cancer who receive standard of care treatment plus NeuVax with GM-CSF versus patients who are simply given standard of care therapy plus the adjuvant, GM-CSF. It will also use a booster vaccine that will be given every 6 months for five doses after the primary vaccination series has been completed. Work with the GP2 peptide is currently ongoing in a phase II clinical trial where vaccines containing GP2 or AE37 are combined with GM-CSF and then compared with treatment of patients with GM-CSF only. Interim analysis presented in 2009 was already showing a decreased recurrence rate at 17.9 months in a group of patients treated with GP2 and GM-CSF versus GM-CSF alone.[231] The premise behind the AE37 vaccine is that it stimulates a CD4+ T lymphocyte response that could potentially result in a more sustained immune response. The current data from clinical trials does suggest that this vaccine has an effect on the risk of recurrence.[232]

The presence of high levels of antibodies to specific glycoforms of the MUC-1 antigen has been shown to be associated with reduced rates and delay to metastasis in patients who have early-stage breast cancer.[233] One of these particular glycoforms, STnMUC1, has already been used in a phase III trial in the form of the vaccine Theratope (STnMUC1, keyhole limpet hemocyanin, and the adjuvant Detox-B). Given as a single agent, Theratope did not show any improvement in survival. However, when given along with endocrine therapy, there was a demonstrated improvement in time to progression and OS.[234]

Tumor-associated carbohydrate antigens (TACAs) are used by certain vaccines. TACAs are poor immunogens, but certain investigators succeeded in eliciting cytotoxic antibodies reactive with naturally occurring forms of TACA using molecular mimicry to generate peptide mimotopes of TACA. Vaccination of mice with

TACA peptide mimotopes reduced tumor growth and prolonged host survival in a murine tumor model.[235] The first reports of this strategy in humans are promising and trials exploring their role in different types of breast cancer are underway.[236]

Checkpoint Inhibitors. Targeting programmed death-1 and programmed death-ligand 1 (PD-1/PD-L1) in breast cancer appears increasingly appealing after the success of such an approach in other cancers. The PD-1 receptor inhibits innate and adaptive immunity when upregulated on immune cells.[237] Cancers take advantage of this mechanism to induce a local immunosuppression by overexpressing PD-L1. The prognostic significance of PD-L1 is still unclear because some studies have described its value as potentially being a positive and other as negative prognostic factor.[238,239] Regardless, the concept of inhibiting the PD-1/PD-L1 pathway is based on the idea of "inhibiting the inhibition" of the immune system. The agents being tried in breast cancer draw from those already being used in melanoma and other malignancies including nivolumab and pembrolizumab (anti-PD-1 antibodies). Currently, results from a phase I study in heavily pretreated TNBC patients who received pembrolizumab demonstrated an acceptable toxicity and good safety profile, and it is now in a phase II study.[240] More trials using PD-1/PD-L1 inhibitors are being planned in TNBC because this is the breast cancer subtype in which PD-1 + TILs and PD-L1 + cancer cells are more commonly seen.[241]

CTLA-4 is another immune checkpoint that is being targeted in breast cancer. Similar to the PD-1/PD-L1 inhibitors, most ongoing clinical trials involving CTLA-4 generally revolve around melanoma. Ipilimumab is a CTLA-4 monoclonal antibody that is FDA approved for the treatment of unresectable melanoma.[242] It is currently being used in a phase I study examining its safety in combination with a new anti-B7-H3 mAb, enoblituzumab, to patients with multiple refractory cancers, including TNBC.[243] Ipilimumab is also being combined with entinostat and nivolumab in a phase I study for metastatic HER2-negative breast cancer as well as with just nivolumab in a phase II study for patients with recurrent stage IV HER2-negative breast cancer.[244] There are other ongoing trials evaluating the combination of a CTLA-4 inhibitor, with additional treatments. There is a phase II study of tremelimumab (CTLA-4 inhibitor) with a PD-L1 inhibitor, MEDI4736, in patients with HER2-negative breast cancer to look for the safety and efficacy of this regimen.[245] A phase I study has already been completed with the combination of tremelimumab and exemestane in patients with hormone-responsive advanced breast cancer.[246] Besides demonstrating that this treatment regimen is tolerable, the study showed that there was an associated increase in T cells with inducible costimulators (ICOS) and that more of the patients with stable[247] disease tended to express higher levels of ICOS + T cells versus the patients with progressive disease.[246] CTLA-4 inhibitors have been evaluated in combination with other interventions as well. A phase I trial evaluating preoperative intervention in the form of ipilimumab and/or cryoablation in early-stage breast cancer showed these treatments to be safe and tolerable and plans are being made for a phase II trial with this regimen.[248]

Future development of these treatments should balance their benefit with their potential toxicity. CTLA-4 mAbs have been shown to have immune-related adverse events mostly affecting the skin and gastrointestinal tract.[242] Other toxicities include hepatitis, thyroiditis, colitis, and hypophysitis.[247] Compared with treatments targeting CTLA-4, therapy targeting PD-1/PD-L1 appears to have a lower frequency of immune-related adverse events.[249]

The combinations of anti-PD-1/PD-L1 mAbs and anti-CTLA-4 mAbs are more effective than single agents, but they may be associated with increased incidence of pneumonitis that responds to holding the drug and/or using immunosuppressive agents; the rate of pneumonitis was 5% in one study.[250]

Monoclonal Antibodies. Trastuzumab is a standard component of our treatments for HER2-positive breast cancer. Its development in the 1990s was considered a landmark achievement in the field of targeted therapy. When combined with chemotherapy, it improves progression-free survival and OS in metastatic HER2-positive breast cancer and DFS and OS in early-stage HER2-positive breast cancer (Table 24.7).

Trastuzumab's mechanism of action remains elusive. It targets HER2 and leads to its internalization and degradation. It inhibits downstream signaling pathways leading to decreased proliferation and increased apoptosis of cancer cells. Recently its role in activating the immune system against tumor cells emerged as the main mechanism of action by establishing the predictive role of TILs of its action. The FinHer investigators found that every 10% increase in TILs was associated with decreased distant recurrence[251] and other studies found that TILs had a prognostic and predictive value because their presence predicted for higher pCR to trastuzumab-containing chemotherapy and better DFS.[43,252] A meta-analysis of neoadjuvant RCTs showed that the pCR rate was significantly higher in patients with lymphocyte-predominant breast cancer (LPBC) in HER2-positive breast cancer settings, with an absolute difference of 33.3% (95% CI 23.6%–42.7%).[253]

The nature of tumor infiltrating immune cells is more important than the mere presence or absence of TILs. Using CIBERSORT (leukocyte gene matrix LM22) to characterize immune cell composition of 7270 unrelated breast cancer samples from their gene expression profiles, Bense and colleagues showed that the composition of the immune cell types differed per breast cancer subtype and interacted with the treatment. Increased fraction of regulatory T cells in HER2-positive tumors was associated with a lower pCR rate (odds ratio [OR] 0.15) as well as shorter DFS (hazard ratio [HR] 3.13) and OS (HR 7.69). Increased fraction of $\gamma\delta$T cells in all breast cancer patients was associated with a higher pCR rate (OR 1.55), prolonged DFS (HR 0.68), and, in HER2-positive tumors, with prolonged OS (HR 0.27). A higher fraction of activated mast cells was associated with worse DFS (HR 5.85) and OS (HR 5.33) in HER2-positive tumors. Furthermore, a high CD8+ T-cell exhaustion signature score was associated with shortened DFS in patients with ER-positive tumors regardless of HER2 status (HR 1.80).[254]

The implications of these findings are substantial. Sorting out the antioncogenic from the immune stimulating roles of trastuzumab may be very difficult. However, the available data from the Adjuvant Lapatinib and/or Trastuzumab Treatment Optimisation (ALTTO) study suggest that interrupting HER2 downstream signaling using lapatinib does not add any benefit in early-stage breast cancer. It is not clear whether all TKIs will behave like lapatinib, but if this observation is confirmed, other tyrosine kinase inhibitors may not add more benefit either. The challenge for future development of novel drugs is to augment the immune mechanism.

The Immune-Mediated Effect of Chemotherapy. Traditionally, the effect of chemotherapy has been explained by the induction of apoptosis of cancer cells after damaging their DNA or interrupting their cell cycle apparatus. However, alternative mechanisms involving the immune system have been recently invoked.[255,256] Taxanes, doxorubicin, and cyclophosphamide, which are standard chemotherapeutic agents in the treatment of breast cancer, are known to have major effects on the immune system in animals and human experiments.[256–261]

The immune effects of chemotherapy may be mediated by (1) rendering dying cancer cells visible to the immune system by exposing their TAAs, (2) stimulating the innate immune system, (3) stimulating T-cell differentiation, (4) promoting a cytokine profile that increases the likelihood of Th1 polarization, (5) inhibition of myeloid-derived suppressor cells and M2 macrophages, and (6) suppression of FOXP3$^+$ Tregs.[260] Acknowledging these mechanisms is of major importance to optimize their benefit and minimize toxicity to the immune system that becomes an important executioner of chemotherapy effect. Furthermore, integrating chemotherapy with vaccines or checkpoint inhibitors is promising.[262,263]

Conclusion and Future Directions

The different strategies that we have used over the past century took advantage of the progress of our understanding of the biology of breast cancer. Each strategy is based on one aspect of this disease; however, none is adequate to help all the patients. With time, we moved away from the goal of "destroying" or "eradicating" all cancer cells to trying to induce long-lasting dormancy of DTCs that would be the equivalent of a cure as the patients live to the natural end of their lives without a relapse of their cancer by avoiding the awakening of dormant DTCs.

Initiation and progression of breast cancer require (1) a strong estrogenic drive and/or (2) carcinogen-induced genetic and epigenetic alterations, (3) loss of intracellular control and decreased apoptotic predisposition, (4) weak immune surveillance and chronic inflammatory milieu, and (5) a permissive microenvironment. Inherited factors act by magnifying one or more of the previous disturbances. The diversity of risk factors and host responses is the source of interpatient heterogeneity. Host factors and treatments used lead to continued evolutionary pressure that is responsible for intrapatient heterogeneity and clonal evolution that unfolds over time. This inter- and intrapatient heterogeneity is the most important challenge to curing breast cancer. Genomic tools added a major contribution to patient selection for a specific treatment, which helped decrease treatment-related morbidity and mortality. However, better tools and biomarkers are still needed to improve our assessment of prognosis and to predict benefit from a specific therapy for the individual patient. Also, detecting intrapatient heterogeneity over time will add a significant contribution to our knowledge of the ever-changing tumor makeup. Liquid biopsies may bring some answers to this important question.

Surgery leads to the physical elimination of the tumor and has become less aggressive over time with no loss of benefit. Radiation induces DNA damage, which would overwhelm cancer cell repair mechanisms leading to active cell death. Chemotherapy also induces DNA damage or interrupts the cell cycle; current regimens are more effective and less toxic than the old ones. Advancement of chemotherapy seems to have plateaued over the past decade with no new or major advancement. The immune-mediated effect of chemotherapy has emerged as a new mechanism that warrants investigation to maximize it and allow the immune system to turn against the tumor. In all of these cases, it is possible that the end result is the eradication of cancer cells.

Hormone blockade or estrogen depletion may lead to the induction of dormancy of tumor initiating cells. This strategy does not lead to complete elimination of cancer cells that may wake up if the treatment is interrupted. Angiogenesis inhibitors did not prove effective in the adjuvant setting. The failure of targeting angiogenesis in the adjuvant/neoadjuvant setting is one of the most important lessons of the 2000s and suggests clearly that angiogenesis is not an important mechanism for the maintenance of DTCs or micrometastatic disease.

Targeted therapy resulted in a major shift in the treatment of HER2-positive cancer. Recent discoveries suggest that this modality works through activation of the immune system rather than the interruption of the oncogenic drive of HER2. The recently rediscovered immune therapy may induce either one of these outcomes—eradication or dormancy—and may open a promising new era in the treatment of cancers, including breast cancer.

Selected References

44. Dieci MV, Griguolo G, Miglietta F, Guarneri V. The immune system and hormone-receptor positive breast cancer: is it really a dead end? *Cancer Treat Rev.* 2016;46:9-19.
84. Perou CM, Sorlie T, Eisen MB, et al. Molecular portraits of human breast tumours. *Nature.* 2000;406:747-752.
132. Coates AS, Winer EP, Goldhirsch A, et al. Tailoring therapies—improving the management of early breast cancer: St Gallen International Expert Consensus on the primary therapy of early breast cancer 2015. *Ann Oncol.* 2015;26:1533-1546.
144. Early Breast Cancer Trialists' Collaborative Group (EBCTCG). Effects of chemotherapy and hormonal therapy for early breast cancer on recurrence and 15-year survival: an overview of the randomised trials. *Lancet.* 2005;365:1687-1717.
185. Wolff AC, Hammond MEH, Hicks DG, et al. Recommendations for human epidermal growth factor receptor 2 testing in breast cancer: American Society of Clinical Oncology/College of American Pathologists clinical practice guideline update. *Arch Pathol Lab Med.* 2013;138:241-256.

A full reference list is available online at ExpertConsult.com.

25

Examination Techniques: Roles of the Physician and Patient in Evaluating Breast Disease

MELISSA ANNE MALLORY AND MEHRA GOLSHAN

Breast disease encompasses a variety of benign and malignant disorders. Although the majority of breast complaints are ultimately noncancerous, breast carcinoma remains the second most common cause of cancer among women and the second leading cause of cancer-related deaths in the United States. In 2015 there was an estimated 234,190 new cases of invasive breast cancer and 60,290 new cases of ductal carcinoma in situ (DCIS) diagnosed nationwide, with more than 40,000 breast cancer–related deaths.[1] The majority of breast cancer in the United States is detected as an abnormality on imaging; however, patients and clinicians can play an important role in initially identifying and evaluating a suspected lesion. The goal in detecting breast cancer at an early stage is ultimately to improve overall breast cancer survival and patient outcomes. To this end, several strategies exist to help in early detection of breast cancer, including breast self-examination (BSE), clinical breast examination (CBE), imaging, and biopsy.

Breast Self-Examination

Breast cancer can be diagnosed after self-detection; however, the relative contributions of systematic self-examination and incidental discovery is not definitively established. BSE formerly played a larger role in breast cancer screening recommendations, but it is no longer recommended by the American Cancer Society (ACS) or by the US Preventive Service Task Force (USPSTF) because of a lack of clear evidence supporting its benefit.[2–5] The limitations of breast cancer self-screening are based largely on a study of 266,000 female factory workers in Shanghai, China. One group was instructed in BSE, and the control group was given instructions about lower back pain. Neither group had routine conventional breast imaging or clinical examination. In both cohorts, the size of the tumor and mortality for breast cancer was similar, whereas a higher rate of benign breast biopsies was seen in the BSE group.[6] In another study of 27,421 women enrolled in a health plan in the Pacific Northwest, 75% reported performing BSE, with 27% being reported as having performed an adequate examination. Participants ultimately diagnosed with breast cancer were significantly less likely to report performing BSE. Tumor size and stage were also not associated with the performance of BSE.[7]

Although the USPSTF goes as far as to discourage teaching of BSE based on an unfavorable risk/benefit ratio (with the risks of potential psychological harm, inconvenience, and possibility for overdiagnosis and unnecessary procedures outweighing potential benefits), the ACS maintains that although regular BSE is not warranted for women of average risk, women should become familiar with their own breast examination so that they may report any changes to their health care provider.[4,5] With this in mind, any discussion between clinician and patient regarding BSE should primarily emphasize the importance of becoming familiar with how one's breasts normally look and feel. Patients may continue to inquire about and perform when comfortable BSE; clinicians should address both the limitations and potential benefits of BSE as part of a woman's routine self-awareness and health care. Women who wish to use BSE as a method for becoming more familiar with their breasts' normal appearance and physical examination should have a systematic approach to looking at and examining their breasts. Instruction on BSE should be prefaced with a discussion of risk factors for development of breast cancer, including patient age, family history (both paternal and maternal) for breast and ovarian cancer, menarche, menopause, obesity, alcohol consumption, and hormone replacement. During this discussion, clinicians should mention that most early-stage breast cancers do not produce symptoms. The most common sign is a painless mass. All women should be informed of the importance of reporting breast changes, including alterations in the contour of the breast, swelling, dimpling, nipple retraction, skin thickening, nipple discharge, or a palpable finding and bring them to the attention of a health care provider. In the premenopausal setting, a lump may be normal if it appears and regresses with the menstrual cycle. A lump that persists past one or two cycles should be brought to the health care provider's attention. A lump that persists for more than a few weeks in the

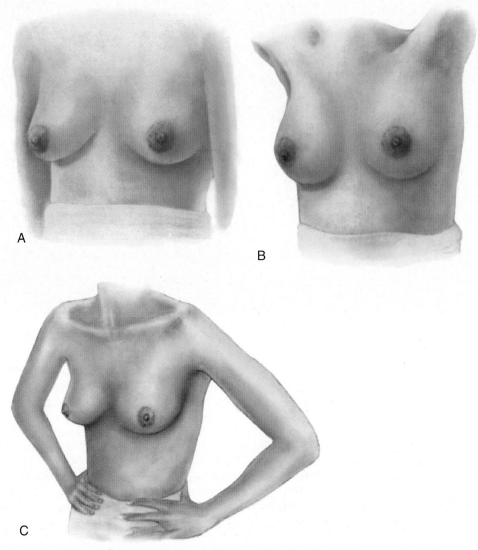

A

B

C

• **Fig. 25.1** Technique for breast inspection. Standing in front of the patient, the physician should inspect the patient with the patient's arms at the sides (A), arms straight up in the air (B), and hands on hips (C).

postmenopausal setting should also be brought to a care provider's attention.

The actual technique for performing a BSE varies but should involve the woman looking at herself in a full-length mirror, with her arms to her side, then over her head, and then to her side with flexion against the side to look for symmetry, dimpling, and retraction (Fig. 25.1). Most women have a slight asymmetry in breast size, and this should be considered normal. A progressive change in size in one breast, whether an increase or decrease, should be brought to the attention of the health care provider. A BSE should also be performed lying down with the arm over the head to allow the breast tissue to splay out evenly over the chest. The examination should be performed with two or three fingers using a circular approach with three degrees of pressure (light, moderate, and deep) and should cover the entire breast from the clavicle to the inframammary fold, laterally to the latissimus, medially to the sternum, and also the low axilla. The entire breast should be examined either in a spoke-wheel fashion or using a vertical-horizontal blind or circular method, covering the entire surface area (Fig. 25.2). This technique should be performed in the same manner on both sides.

Clinical Breast Examination

The role of CBE has a stronger foundation in the early detection of breast carcinoma than BSE; however, limitations in the evidence supporting its routine use are recognized by both the USPSTF and the ACS. The ACS notably shifted their stance away from recommending CBE for women at average risk of breast cancer regardless of age in their 2015 guidelines, citing a lack of evidence showing benefit for CBE performed either alone or in conjunction with mammography, concurrent with an increase in false-positive rates (based on moderate-quality evidence).[5] The most recent USPSTF guidelines in 2009 concluded that the current evidence was insufficient to assess the additional benefits and harms of CBE beyond screening mammography in women 40 years or older; the USPSTF is in the process of updating the breast cancer screening guidelines; however, these are not yet available, and it remains to be seen how CBE will be regarded in their revisions.[2] We continue to recommend CBE as part of our practice in our patient population.

The technique of breast examination should include a thorough inspection and palpation of the entire breast and

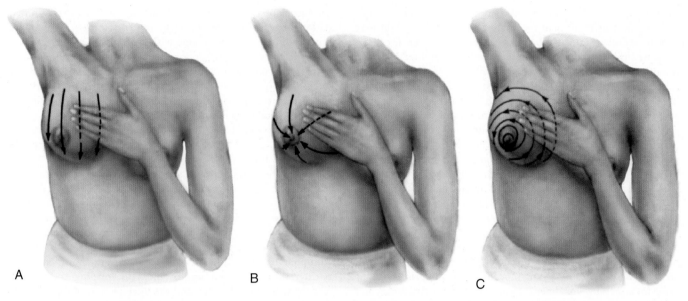

• **Fig. 25.2** Self-examination of the breast; palpation in the vertical or horizontal (A), spoke and wheel (B), and circular directions (C).

the draining lymph node–bearing areas. To perform a CBE, the physician should stand in front of the gowned patient. In a manner that allows for minimal disrobement of the patient, both breasts should be inspected with the patient's arms by her side, with her hands over her head, and finally with her arms to her side with contraction of the pectoralis major muscle. Notes should be taken with regard to size, shape, and symmetry of the breasts. Attention should be made to any changes to the skin, including indentation, protrusions, or skin thickening. The nipple should be inspected for retraction, thickening, flaking, or erosions. After inspecting both breasts, palpation should be performed with the patient in both the sitting and supine position. The entire breast should be examined from the clavicle superiorly to the rectus sheath insertion inferiorly, extending from the latissimus laterally to the sternum medially. Palpation is performed using the pads of the fingers and may again be in the spoke-wheel, vertical-horizontal blind, or circular fashion and should be performed with light, moderate, and deep pressure. Special attention should be made to the lymph nodes in the sitting position. With one arm supporting the woman's hand, the other hand examines the axilla. The supra-clavicular and infraclavicular lymph nodes are best examined from behind with the woman in a seated position. Lymph nodes that measure greater than 1 cm in diameter or that are fixed or matted warrant further diagnostic workup. If a mass is found, a tape measure or caliper is used to estimate its size in two dimensions. The location should be either drawn on a diagram or referenced to a clock time and measured in centimeters from the nipple in a spoke-and-wheel fashion. For a woman who presents with a palpable lump, the detailed history should include length of time present, whether pain is associated with the mass, whether the lump has changed in size since identification, and, in a premeno-pausal woman, whether the mass changes after menses.

During the examination of the breast, focused attention should be given to the nipple-areolar complex. Manipulation of the nipple should occur only if the patient reports nipple discharge. If present, the clinician should note whether the discharge occurs spontaneously or only with mild manual compression and indi-cate whether the discharge is unilateral or bilateral, involving one

or many ducts. The color of the discharge can help with diagnosis and should always be noted, and accompanied with a description of the offending duct(s). A written description, which may also include a diagram or photograph, may be useful for objective reporting in the patient's progress notes. Common discharge colors include clear, white, green, brown, black, and red (bloody). Fluid that is brown or black should undergo guaiac testing at the time of the examination to look for breakdown products of hemo-globin. Discharge that is unilateral and bloody or guaiac-positive has a malignancy risk of approximately 20% to 25%; however, the vast majority is caused by benign entities, such as papillomas.[8] Discharge that is bilateral, multiductal, and milky, clear, green, or bluish in color is almost always benign. As many as 50% to 80% of women in their reproductive years may elicit discharge, and 7% of women referred for surgical evaluation have nipple dis-charge as their primary complaint.[9,10]

At the time of CBE, risk factors for breast cancer should be reviewed with patients, and the physician should perform a detailed assessment of breast cancer risk by obtaining relevant medical and family histories. It is estimated that 7% to 10% of carcinomas diagnosed in the United States result from an inher-ited predisposition to breast and ovarian cancer, the vast majority being *BRCA1* and *BRCA2* mutations.[11] Clinicians should partner with their patients to keep accurate and updated family histories, including maternal and paternal incidences of breast and ovarian cancer dating back two or three generations. Reviewing this infor-mation will help identify patients who may benefit from genetic counseling.

Age is an important risk factor for breast carcinoma; currently, a woman living in the United States has a 12.3% chance of devel-oping breast carcinoma.[12] Patients should inform their clinicians of any previous personal history of carcinoma or breast biopsy, and records should be obtained if needed to determine whether prior biopsy specimens contained atypia.[13] A woman's age at men-arche and menopause, as well as parity should be recorded.[14] The use of exogenous estrogen and/or progesterone in the premeno-pausal and postmenopausal setting should be ascertained.[15] Physi-cians should discuss the importance of a healthy lifestyle with their patients, emphasizing the role that postmenopausal obesity[16] and excessive or more than moderate alcohol consumption may play in the development of breast cancer.[17] Although no direct evidence links inactivity to an increased risk of breast cancer, intensive physical activity has been linked to a reduced breast cancer risk, with a 2011 review suggesting a 25% risk reduction for the most physically active women compared with the least active women. Although results have varied widely regarding the role of smoking on breast cancer risk, numerous studies have suggested an increased risk of breast cancer among active smokers, and a 2013 meta-analysis found early-age at smoking onset (before menarche and before the first birth) was significantly associated with increased risk of breast cancer development.[18] Clinicians should counsel their patients on the numerous adverse risks of smoking and alcohol use and provide counseling regarding cessation when appropriate.

Once a palpable complaint has been interrogated or at the time of a woman's CBE at age 40, diagnostic imaging should be initiated. Numerous breast imaging modalities exist to assist the clinician in screening for breast cancer and for diagnosing and managing breast abnormalities detected by both palpation and imaging.

Imaging Modalities

Breast imaging has emerged as a critical component for the early detection of breast cancer and includes but is not limited to mammography, tomosynthesis, ultrasound, and breast magnetic resonance imaging (MRI). Investigative modalities designed to overcome limitations with existing technologies are under development, and the field of breast imaging is constantly being advanced. The most conventional imaging modality for breast evaluation is mammography, which has been shown in numerous randomized and population-based studies to help improve early detection of carcinoma, patient outcomes, and survival.[19] Despite these trials, there have been some who suggest against routine screening based on a meta-analysis of a few of the trials, however. The majority of the data and leading organizations with panels on women's health who comment on cancer screening agree that regular screening mammography should be a part of women's routine health care.[2-5,20-23]

Mammographic screening guidelines have remained a highly debated topic over the past decade, after the release of the USP-STF's 2009 guidelines. These guidelines recommend biennial screening for women age 50 to 74, a shared decision-making process for screening women aged 40 to 49 (taking risks and patient values into account), and insufficient evidence to support screening in women older than 75.[2] Recently the ACS updated its recommendations for screening, suggesting that although a shared decision-making process should be used for women 40 to 44, all women age 45 to 54 should undergo annual screening; biennial screening is reserved for women age 55 and older, continuing as long as estimated life expectancy is at least 10 years. These are "qualified recommendations" as opposed to "strong recommendations," indicating that although clear evidence of the benefit of screening exists, there is less certainty about the balance of benefits and harms or about patients' values and preferences in these situations, which could lead to different decisions. The ACS also recommends that all women be provided with information about risk factors, risk reduction, and the benefits, limitations, and harms associated with mammography screening. Despite these recent changes from the ACS, the American College of

Obstetricians and Gynecologists maintains its current recommendations that women should begin annual screening mammography beginning at age 40 (along with CBE, for all women aged 19 and older) and strongly support shared decision-making between patients and physicians for breast cancer screening practices.[24] The most recent American College of Radiology screening guidelines are similar, calling for annual mammography starting at age 40 for the general population.[25]

Although widespread screening mammography has been in place in the United States for several decades now, screening rates are still far from ideal. The National Health Interview Survey found that in 2010, only 72.4% of women 50 years and older had obtained a mammogram within the past 2 years, with lower rates for women of Asian, American Indian, or Alaska Native race or Hispanic ethnicity.[26] Screening mammograms can detect more than 80% of all breast carcinomas in women without symptoms, establishing a means for early cancer detection and treatment. Although mammograms are more accurate in the postmenopausal setting, there has been improvement in imaging the younger woman with dense breasts after the introduction of digital mammography and more recently tomosynthesis (which is a modification of digital mammography that allows for the acquisition of three-dimensional (3D) thin section data, improving visualization in dense breasts by reducing limitations created by overlapping structures).[27,28] The vast majority of practices use digital mammography, with accredited full-field digital mammography units making up 97.3% (14,564/14,963) of total accredited mammography units in the United States as of September 1, 2015, and many centers are now obtaining both two-dimensional (2D) digital mammography and 3D tomosynthesis for screening purposes.[28-30]

In general, mammography should be performed at the same center where films can be serially compared for changes. Expertise in breast imaging is important, especially during the workup of abnormal imaging findings. Recent studies have suggested that radiology image consultation by dedicated breast imagers can influence final management for women with breast cancer, and physicians should consider a specialist's review in addition to generalist interpretation for appropriate cases.[31,32] A screening mammogram can detect more than 80% of all breast carcinomas in women without symptoms. Imaging is more accurate in the postmenopausal setting, although with the use of digital mammography, there has been improvement in the younger woman with dense breasts.[17] In the diagnostic setting, it is paramount for the ordering physician to provide the radiologist or breast imaging center with all appropriate information on the location and size of the mass or abnormality, so that appropriate attention and correlation can be made to the concerning region during radiologic assessment.

In addition to mammography, ultrasound plays an integral role in the radiologic assessment of the breast and should be used in the diagnostic setting or to work up an abnormality during the screening process. Focused ultrasound is a valuable tool for the workup of a palpable complaint or mass identified by mammography, and it can be used to help distinguish between the cystic and solid nature of mammographically detected nonpalpable lesions. Ultrasound is particularly useful in evaluating for underlying abnormalities in the premenopausal setting of dense breasts, especially in evaluation of palpable breast lesions. It should be the primary imaging tool for women with palpable lumps who are pregnant, lactating, or younger than 30 years old, and it is the overall procedure of choice during pregnancy.[33] The widespread implementation of whole breast ultrasound screening in the United States has not been successful because of limitations associated with the modality, including the length of time needed to perform the study, operator variability in expertise of the technique, and a high rate of false-positive findings at biopsy.[29] Increasingly, surgeons are becoming more adept at the use of ultrasound in the office as an adjunct to physical examination, and care must be taken in terms of training, qualification, and interpretation before a surgeon implements this in his or her practice. In this respect, the American Society of Breast Surgeons and the American College of Surgeons have taken a leading role in the establishment of guidelines and standards in the use of ultrasound by the surgeon.[34-36]

Digital breast tomosynthesis (DBT) is a relatively new imaging modality (with US Food and Drug Administration approval granted in 2011) designed to overcome limitations associated with conventional 2D mammography.[37] DBT can contribute to increased cancer detection and reduced recall rates regardless of breast density but is especially useful in the setting of increased breast density.[37,38] Data from recent studies highlight additional benefits of tomosynthesis, including significantly reduced false-positive recalls and improved cancer detection when 3D tomosynthesis is added to screening.[39-41] A recent study in the *Journal of the American Medical Association* demonstrated increases in the positive predictive values for recall and for biopsy, and a decrease in overall recall rates when DBT was used in combination with full-field digital mammography (FFDM), compared with FFDM alone.[42] DBT's limitations, however, including longer interpretation times, increased radiation doses, additional costs, and difficulties with insurance reimbursements, prevent it from widespread use in breast cancer screening protocols. The American Society of Breast Surgeon's breast screening recommendations state that breast tomosynthesis may be considered for breast cancer screening, recognizing that neither the ACS nor the USPSTF currently provide specific recommendations regarding mammography-type to be used.[28]

Contrast-enhanced breast MRI is a highly sensitive test with moderate specificity. In the screening population, its use can be justified in certain very high-risk settings, in conjunction with, but not as a substitute for mammography. Women who have an inherited predisposition to breast and ovarian cancer, Li-Fraumeni syndrome, Cowden disease, a lifetime risk of breast cancer of greater than 20% to 25%, history of mantle radiation, or a first-degree relative with an inherited predisposition to breast carcinoma without self-testing are likely to benefit from the addition of breast MRI, and clinicians should consider annual screening with both mammography and breast MRI compliant with ACS and National Comprehensive Cancer Network Guidelines.[28,43,44] In the asymptomatic woman at moderate risk for breast carcinoma based on family history, atypical ductal hyperplasia, atypical lobular hyperplasia, lobular carcinoma in situ, or a lifetime risk of breast cancer of 15% to 20%, the risks and benefits of breast MRI should be discussed.[43] One should note the possibility of findings on MRI that will lead to additional imaging, the majority of which will be biopsy-proven benign.[45] Breast MRI should be performed by dedicated breast imagers using at least a 1.5-Tesla magnet, preferably with a dedicated breast coil and breast biopsy capability. The availability of breast MRI has also raised the possibility of potential assistance in the workup of a known cancer.[46] Unfortunately, prospective and retrospective studies have failed to show that prone preoperative MRI is beneficial in improving breast conserving surgery outcomes in terms of reexcision, local recurrence, or overall survival rates.[46-52]

Other imaging modalities for the evaluation of breast disease are under investigation. Some groups have reported success with scintimammography (molecular breast imaging, MBI) as an adjunct to mammography.[53] This technique uses a breast-specific gamma camera to measure radiotracer uptake of abnormal breast tissue by using technetium sestamibi; with a reported sensitivity approaching up to nearly 70% and an accuracy that is independent of breast density, it has been advocated as a valuable adjunct to mammography, especially for dense breasts.[54,55] However, its widespread use has yet to be validated by prospective randomized trials or widespread availability. Positron emission tomography and positron emission mammography (which focuses exclusively on the breast) are other imaging techniques being studied; however, these have not been shown to be of benefit in screening or early detection of breast carcinoma and are not currently recommended for these purposes.[56,57]

Imaging is also important during the evaluation of nipple discharge. Nipple discharge, especially if bloody or guaiac-positive, requires surgical evaluation and intervention in nearly all circumstances. Physical examination and mammography should be routinely performed, and an ultrasound evaluation of the retroareolar ductal system may also be helpful. Ductogram (or galactography) has traditionally been used for lesion identification if mammogram and ultrasound have failed to detect the cause of concerning nipple discharge.[58] This technique, when performed in centers with expertise using this diagnostic test, can be helpful for lesion localization; specifically, lesions may be identified and then preoperatively marked by methylene blue injection or wire guidance to help locate the abnormality and limit the extent of the terminal ductal unit resection.[59] Contrast-enhanced breast MRI has also been recognized by some groups as helpful in identifying underlying lesions in patients with suspicious nipple discharge.[60] More complex and expensive modalities include ductoscopy, where a fiberoptic camera (diameters ranging from 0.4 to 0.8 mm) is inserted into the offending duct either in the operating room or outpatient setting, which allows abnormalities to be identified and either biopsied or resected. However, its benefits over other, more readily available and conventional techniques have yet to be proven, and studies do not currently support its routine use.[61,62]

Invasive Diagnostic Procedures

Once an abnormality has been identified either by imaging or physical examination, the technique known as image-guided biopsy, freehand core biopsy, or fine-needle aspiration biopsy (FNAB) has become the standard of care. The use of surgical open or wire-localized excisional or incisional biopsy should be used as a last resort when FNAB or core biopsy has failed or is not concordant. Surgical biopsy can also be considered for the uncommon imaging finding not amenable to image-guided biopsy including those lesions that are too close to the nipple, skin, or chest wall. FNAB requires dedicated expertise in cytopathology and, when applicable, provides a moderately high degree of sensitivity and specificity.[63] In the cases of breast carcinoma, cell blocks may be performed to characterize estrogen receptor (ER), progesterone receptor (PR), and HER2/neu receptor status. The main disadvantages of FNAB are the inability to distinguish in situ from invasive carcinoma using FNAB cytology, notably higher rates of nondiagnostic samples, and false-negative results for inexperienced clinicians.[64] The technique of FNAB is also particularly useful in axillary lymph node evaluation under ultrasound guidance, when the diagnosis of breast carcinoma is made to rule out metastatic involvement.[65] More frequently, core needle biopsy is performed, and its diagnostic accuracy and concordance with surgical excision is outstanding; this can be performed under stereotactic, ultrasound, or MRI guidance. The concordance with surgical excisional biopsy specimen is high, between 91% and 100%; sensitivity is 85% to 100%, and specificity is 96% to 100%.[66] In the modern era with larger biopsy devices and the use of vacuum-assisted and en bloc resection devices, the concordance rates will only improve and in certain circumstances obviate the need for surgical resection. Another advantage is the decreased number of surgical procedures required for definitive therapy when a diagnosis of breast carcinoma is made. A study at the Brigham and Women's Hospital showed that women who underwent image-guided core biopsy had 1.25 surgical procedures as opposed to 2.01 in those who underwent wire-localized excisional biopsy for diagnosis.[67] The image-guided core biopsy technique is not without caveats, including its occasional inability to target or adequately sample breast lesions. More importantly, some image-guided diagnoses will ultimately be upstaged at the time of surgical excision, specifically atypical hyperplasia to ductal carcinoma in situ or ductal carcinoma in situ to invasive breast cancer.[68,69] Benign results should prompt the clinician to establish concordance with imaging and/or examination findings. In cases of radiologic-pathologic discordance, excision is mandatory. For example, a mass felt on examination or seen on breast imaging that reveals epithelial hyperplasia is disconcordant and requires surgical excision. Some surgical groups may perform freehand core biopsy with a high rate of accuracy, whereas others find that image-guided core biopsy yields a higher rate of accuracy.[70,71]

Surgical excisional biopsy, either under the guidance of imaging or palpation, should be performed as a diagnostic procedure only on rare occasions. Examples include (1) patient preference for surgical excision regardless of the imaging or core biopsy result, or (2) failed, nondiagnostic, or discordant core biopsy or FNAB. The surgical biopsy is a safe surgical procedure with outstanding results; however, it does leave a scar on the woman's breast that is much larger than a needle core site, and if the lesion proves to be carcinoma, further surgery is required. With an easily palpable finding, surgical excisional biopsy without image guidance may proceed under local or regional anesthesia. Surgical incision planning is important for cosmetic purposes and should consider the possibility of reoperation or eventual mastectomy if a carcinoma is identified. In general, circumareolar incisions provide outstanding cosmesis when excessive tunneling is not necessary, and curvilinear incisions along Langer lines also provide reasonable cosmesis in most cases. In general, radial incisions should be avoided but may be considered for lesions at the 6 o'clock position and occasionally for 3 and 9 o'clock abnormalities. For lesions

that are not easily palpable, wire localization either under mammographic, ultrasound, or MRI-guidance is necessary. Initially described by Bolmgrem in 1977, stereotactic or mammographic guidance has become a standard of care with high accuracy.[72,73] Ultrasound guidance provides another opportunity for wire placement and is often a simpler technique that can be performed quickly, especially for mass lesions.[74] With the advent of contrast-enhanced breast MRI for screening and diagnostic evaluation, abnormalities are identified that may not be correlated by mammography and ultrasound. It is imperative that a center that offers this test has the capability to perform biopsies under either wire guidance and/or needle core.[45,75]

The management of breast disease requires coordinated multidisciplinary care between clinicians and their patients. Over the past decades, extensive progress has been made in the modalities available for the evaluation of breast disease and early detection of breast carcinoma, enabling vast improvements in patient outcomes and survival. Physicians and patients should work together to achieve breast health for each woman, identifying and implementing appropriate guidelines based on personalized risk assessment and diagnostics. The use of appropriate imaging, combined with breast examination and a patient's breast awareness, are critical components for maintaining breast health and evaluating concerning breast problems.

Selected References

1. Siegel RL, Miller KD, Jemal A. Cancer statistics, 2015. *Cancer*. 2015;65:5-29.
2. U.S. Preventive Services Task Force. Screening for breast cancer: U.S. Preventive Services Task Force recommendation statement. *Ann Intern Med*. 2009;151:716-726, W-236.
5. Oeffinger KC, Fontham ET, Etzioni R, et al. Breast cancer screening for women at average risk: 2015 guideline update from the American Cancer Society. *JAMA*. 2015;314:1599-1614.
15. Chlebowski RT, Hendrix SL, Langer RD, et al. Influence of estrogen plus progestin on breast cancer and mammography in healthy postmenopausal women: the Women's Health Initiative Randomized Trial. *JAMA*. 2003;289:3243-3253.
25. Mainiero MB, Lourenco A, Mahoney MC, et al. ACR appropriateness criteria breast cancer screening. *J Am Coll Radiol*. 2013;10: 11-14.
29. Joe BN, Sickles EA. The evolution of breast imaging: past to present. *Radiology*. 2014;273:S23-S44.
33. Lehman CD, Lee AY, Lee CI. Imaging management of palpable breast abnormalities. *AJR Am J Roentgenol*. 2014;203:1142-1153.
49. Houssami N, Turner R, Morrow M. Preoperative magnetic resonance imaging in breast cancer: meta-analysis of surgical outcomes. *Ann Surg*. 2013;257:249-255.

A full reference list is available online at ExpertConsult.com.

26

Breast Imaging Screening and Diagnosis

LAWRENCE W. BASSETT AND STEPHANIE LEE-FELKER

Breast imaging includes all of the imaging modalities used to detect and diagnose breast diseases. The most common breast imaging modality is mammography, which is a radiographic examination of the breasts. Since the first report on mammography in the United States in the 1930s, mammography has undergone striking technological improvements and quality assurance procedures that have improved its sensitivity and accuracy[1,2] (Fig. 26.1). In addition, standardized reporting has been developed to improve the communication of mammography results and management recommendations.[3]

The two major types of mammography are screening mammography and diagnostic mammography. Screening mammography is used to detect unexpected breast cancer in asymptomatic women. Diagnostic mammography is used to evaluate the breasts of patients with symptoms, such as a palpable lump or nipple discharge. Mammography is also used to guide interventional procedures of the breast, including core needle biopsy (CNB)[4] and preoperative needle localization.[5]

Digital mammography is currently the standard screening and diagnostic mammography examination[6]; approximately 95% of mammography units are now digital. Digital mammography stores images electronically in a digital format and displays them on computers. The main advantages of digital mammography are unlimited contrast resolution, computer-aided diagnosis (CAD), and teleradiology. CAD refers to supplementary computer scanning of images to assist in detection of potential imaging abnormalities.[7,8] Teleradiology enables digital images to be transmitted electronically, with the potential to increase access to mammograms.[9]

Digital breast tomosynthesis (DBT) or three-dimensional (3D) mammography is an emerging digital technology that consists of a series of low dose x-rays taken at different angles in a small arc over the breast. DBT can either be performed with or without conventional two-dimensional (2D) digital mammography. When performed without conventional 2D digital mammography, 2D digital views are computer-generated from source images using software. Studies have shown that DBT decreases false-positive interpretation rates and increases cancer detection rates compared with conventional 2D digital mammography.[10]

Breast ultrasound, the use of sonar energy to produce an image of the breast, is used for both screening and diagnostic purposes, as well as for guiding interventional procedures.[11,12]

Magnetic resonance imaging (MRI) is used for screening high-risk women[13] and for diagnostic indications, such as evaluation of extent of disease in newly diagnosed breast cancer.

Other imaging modalities used for the diagnosis of breast diseases include ductography.

Mammography

Screening Mammography

Breast cancer is the most common noncutaneous malignancy in women. Each year, approximately 231,840 new cases of breast cancer are diagnosed, and about 40,290 women die of this disease in the United States.[14] Large randomized controlled screening trials have shown that screening mammography reduces breast cancer mortality by approximately 30%.[15]

For screening mammography, two views of each breast are performed: mediolateral oblique (MLO) and craniocaudal (CC). The MLO view includes the greatest amount of breast tissue and is the only view that includes all of the upper outer quadrant and axillary tail (Figs. 26.2 and 26.3). The CC view provides better image detail because greater compression of the breast is usually possible, as well as better visualization of the inner aspect of the breast (Figs. 26.4 and 26.5).

The importance of proper breast compression during mammography cannot be overemphasized. The compression device helps to (1) immobilize the breast and prevent motion unsharpness, (2) separate overlapping tissues that might obscure underlying lesions, (3) bring the breast closer to the image detector and reduce geometric blur, and (4) decrease the radiation dose by decreasing breast thickness.[16]

Diagnostic Mammography

For diagnostic mammography, imaging is supervised directly by the interpreting physician and is tailored to the specific indication for the examination, such as abnormal screening mammography, findings that require additional imaging, or abnormal clinical findings, including a palpable lump.

In the setting of abnormal screening mammography findings, the diagnostic examination may begin with repeating the view(s) on which the original abnormal finding was visualized to see if it persists. A number of additional mammographic views may be

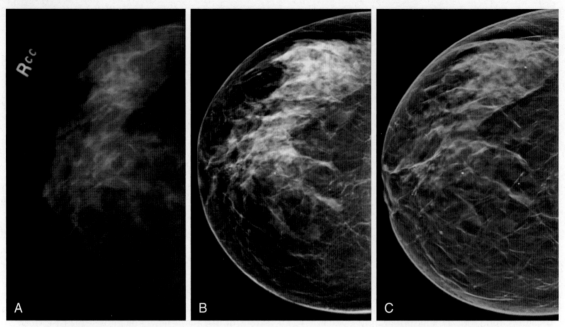

• **Fig. 26.1** These craniocaudal views on screen film mammography (A), digital mammography (B), and digital tomosynthesis mammography (C) depict the striking technological improvements that mammography has undergone over time.

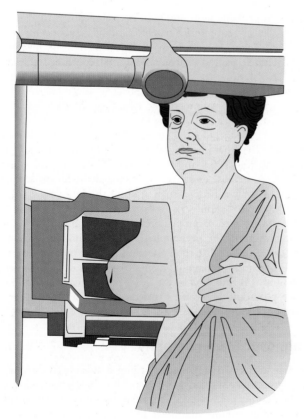

• **Fig. 26.2** This illustration shows positioning for the mediolateral oblique view.

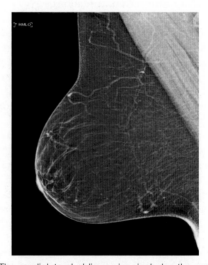

• **Fig. 26.3** The mediolateral oblique view includes the greatest amount of breast tissue, including the upper outer quadrant and axillary tail.

performed to help define the nature of and localize an abnormal finding, the most common of which are the 90-degree lateral and spot compression views.

The 90-degree lateral view is used along with the MLO and CC views to triangulate the location of an abnormal finding. Spot compression involves the use of a small compression device placed directly over the abnormal finding and can be performed in any projection (Fig. 26.6). The smaller compression device allows for greater compression over the area of interest and displaces overlying tissues that could obscure the finding.[17] Magnification technique is often combined with spot compression to better resolve both the margins of masses as well as the character of calcifications. Other projections include rolled, cleavage, and axillary tail views. All of these mammographic views may be performed with either 2D or 3D tomosynthesis technology. Ultrasound targeted to the area of interest is commonly used in conjunction with diagnostic mammography (Fig. 26.6E).

For abnormal clinical findings such as a palpable lump felt on physical examination by a referring health care provider, communication of its location in terms of laterality, clock face, and distance from the nipple is helpful for directing the diagnostic examination, especially when it is not felt by the patient. The mammography technologist palpates the indicated area of palpable abnormality and places a radio-opaque lead marker directly over the area before image acquisition, such that the lead marker indicates the area of concern (see Fig. 26.6). Similarly, the sonographer or physician supervising the examination palpates the indicated area of palpable abnormality before scanning to enable a directed ultrasound examination in the area of concern.

For women 30 years of age and older, both mammography and ultrasound should be performed to better define the nature of the palpable abnormality, to detect concurrent lesions in the ipsilateral or contralateral breast that are clinically occult, and to identify any associated calcifications indicating an intraductal component of a palpable cancer (Fig. 26.7). For women under 30 years of age, ultrasound is the first choice examination, with mammography reserved for cases in which calcifications are suspected (Fig. 26.8).

Standardized Terminology for Mammography Reports

The American College of Radiology (ACR) Breast Imaging Reporting and Data System (BI-RADS) was devised to facilitate uniform reporting of mammographic findings, assessments, and recommendations from different imaging centers, as well as to facilitate outcome monitoring.[3] Every mammography report is required by the federal Mammography Quality Standards Act to include an assessment category, such that management recommendations are as clear as possible. There are seven assessment categories, each associated with a management recommendation. BI-RADS category 0 (incomplete) identifies cases in which additional imaging and/or comparison to prior imaging is needed before a final assessment can be made. Once additional imaging or comparison to prior imaging is accomplished, such cases are assigned one of the six "Final Assessment" categories. Screening mammograms are assigned BI-RADS categories 0, 1, or 2, whereas diagnostic mammograms are assigned BI-RADS categories 1 through 6.

Normal Mammographic Findings

The normal breast has a wide range of mammographic appearances in terms of size, shape, density, and fibroglandular tissue pattern.

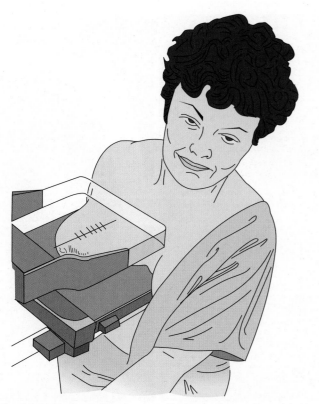

• **Fig. 26.4** This illustration shows positioning for the craniocaudal view.

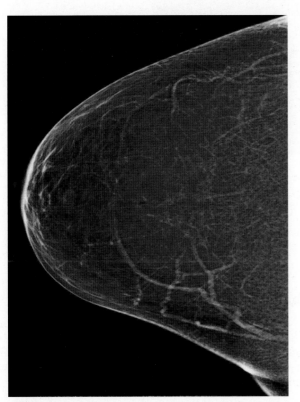

• **Fig. 26.5** The craniocaudal view provides visualization of the inner hemisphere of the breast.

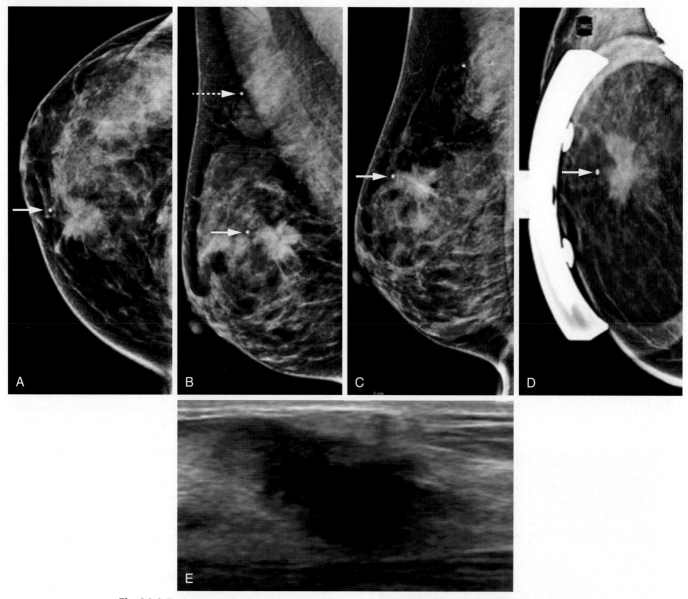

• **Fig. 26.6** Radio-opaque lead markers were placed in the areas of palpable abnormality while the breast was imaged in the craniocaudal (A), mediolateral oblique (B), mediolateral (C), and spot compression craniocaudal (D) views. The lead marker in the upper inner quadrant of the breast corresponds to an irregular mass with spiculated margins (*arrows,* A–D), and another lead marker corresponds to accessory axillary breast tissue (*dotted arrow,* B). Targeted ultrasound in the area of mammographic mass shows a correlative irregular hypoechoic mass with angular margins (E).

Breast density ranges from almost entirely fatty to extremely dense (Fig. 26.9). In the BI-RADS lexicon, breast density is characterized by four categories, with progressively decreased mammographic sensitivity for cancer detection: (1) almost entirely fatty, (2) scattered areas of fibroglandular density, (3) heterogeneously dense, and (4) extremely dense. Because breast cancers are radio-opaque (white on mammograms), they are more easily seen in an almost entirely fatty breast (black on mammograms) compared with an extremely dense breast (white on mammograms).

Increased breast density can be seen in younger women, during pregnancy and lactation (Fig. 26.10), and in response to exogenous hormone therapy due to a higher proportion of fibroglandular tissue.[18]

Abnormal Mammographic Findings

Masses and calcifications are among the most common abnormal findings on mammograms. The BI-RADS lexicon used to describe masses and calcifications indicate their likelihood of malignancy. Other abnormal findings include architectural distortions, asymmetries, and axillary lymphadenopathy.

Masses

A mass is a 3D, space-occupying lesion with convex outward borders that is seen on at least two mammographic projections.

Masses are described by their shape, margin, and density in the BI-RADS lexicon. Shapes are round (spherical), oval (elliptical),

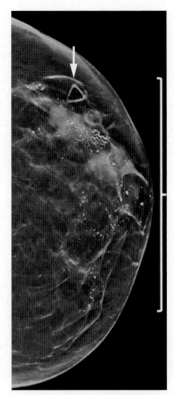

• **Fig. 26.7** A triangular marker was placed in the area of palpable abnormality in the lateral hemisphere on the craniocaudal view *(arrow)*. Unexpected associated fine pleomorphic calcifications are present throughout the breast *(bracket)*, indicating an extensive intraductal component of disease.

or irregular (neither round nor oval) (Fig. 26.11). Round and oval shapes favor benignity.

Margins are circumscribed (with a clear demarcation from surrounding tissue), obscured (hidden by superimposed or adjacent fibroglandular tissue), microlobulated (characterized by short cycle undulations), indistinct (without a clear demarcation from surrounding tissue), or spiculated (characterized by radiating lines) (Fig. 26.12). Circumscribed margins favor benignity. The presence of multiple, bilateral, round or oval, circumscribed masses (Fig. 26.13) is especially suggestive of benign masses such as multiple cysts, fibroadenomas, or intramammary lymph nodes.[19,20] Microlobulated, indistinct, and spiculated margins (Fig. 26.14) are suspicious for malignancy.

Density is determined relative to normal fibroglandular tissue and is described as fat-containing, low, equal, or high. Fat-containing or low densities favor benignity, whereas high density is suspicious for malignancy.[21] Examples of fat-containing masses include oil cysts (Fig. 26.15), lipomas, galactoceles, and hamartomas (Fig. 26.16).

Masses may be associated with other findings, such as microcalcifications (see Fig. 26.7), skin thickening, skin retraction, and nipple retraction, which increase suspicion for malignancy.

Benign Masses. Cysts are solitary or multiple, round or oval, circumscribed, usually equal density masses. They are most commonly seen in women between the ages of 40 and 50 years. Cysts tend to vary in size over serial examinations, usually decreasing in size over time. Targeted ultrasound can be performed in the area of mammographic mass to confirm the presence of a simple cyst (Fig. 26.17). If the characteristic features of a simple cyst are

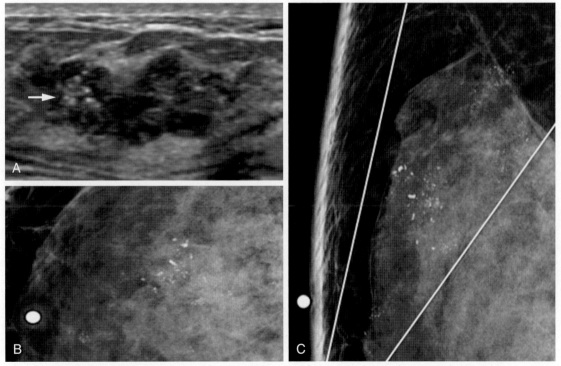

• **Fig. 26.8** A 29-year-old woman presented with a right breast palpable abnormality. Targeted ultrasound showed an irregular hypoechoic mass containing calcifications *(arrow, A)*, after which diagnostic mammography was performed with a radio-opaque lead marker indicating the area of palpable abnormality; fine pleomorphic calcifications are seen in a segmental distribution (B, C).

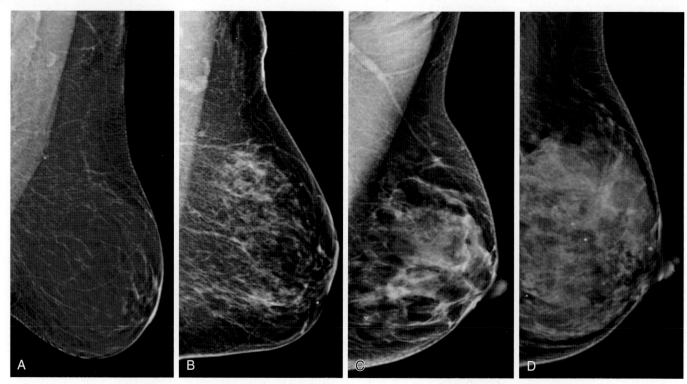

• **Fig. 26.9** These mediolateral oblique views depict the range of normal breast densities: almost entirely fatty (A), scattered areas of fibroglandular density (B), heterogeneously dense (C), and extremely dense (D).

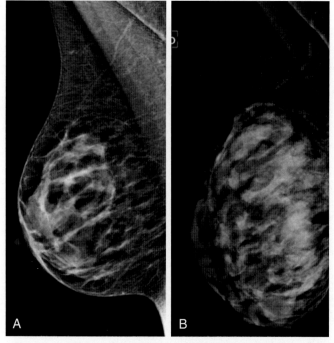

• **Fig. 26.10** These mediolateral oblique views before (A) and during (B) pregnancy show interval increased fibroglandular tissue proliferation, resulting in increased breast density and breast enlargement related to lactational changes.

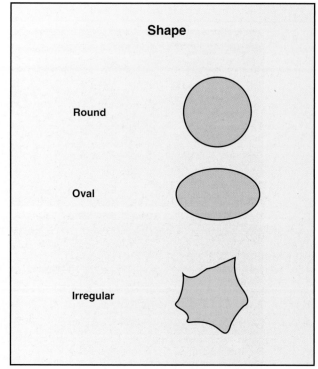

• **Fig. 26.11** These illustrations depict standardized descriptors for mass shapes.

Margins

Circumscribed

Microlobulated

Obscured

Indistinct

Spiculated

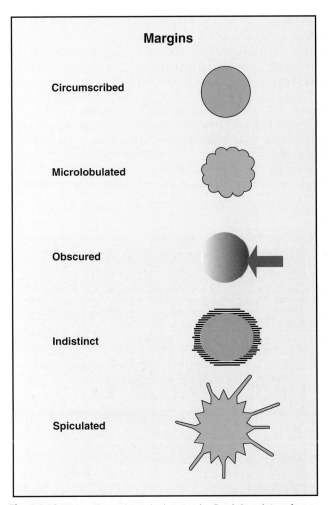

• **Fig. 26.12** These illustrations depict standardized descriptors for mass margins.

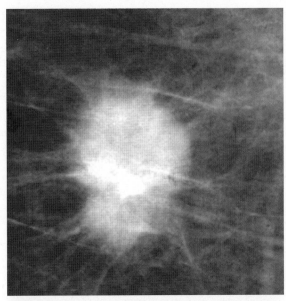

• **Fig. 26.14** Spiculated margins are suspicious for malignancy.

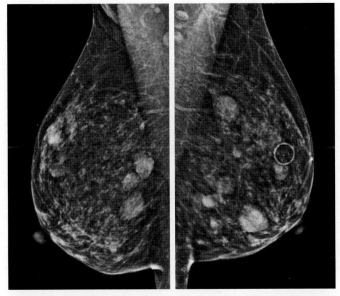

• **Fig. 26.13** Multiple, bilateral, round and oval, circumscribed masses are most likely benign.

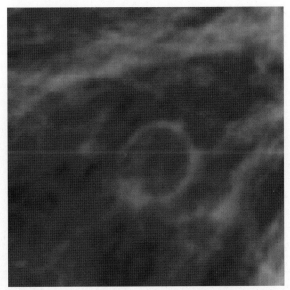

• **Fig. 26.15** Rim calcifications represent calcium deposits on the surfaces of spheres and are seen in cysts and fat necrosis.

present, diagnostic accuracy approaches 100%, thus obviating the need for aspiration or biopsy.[22]

Fibroadenomas are common masses, appearing as solitary or multiple, round or oval, circumscribed masses. As they involute over time, they tend to develop characteristic coarse, "popcorn-like" calcifications (Fig. 26.18).

Intramammary lymph nodes are normal anatomic structures that are most commonly found in the upper outer quadrant of the breast. They have a characteristic reniform shape and central radiolucency representing the fatty hilum. Correlative ultrasound may show central echogenicity representing the fatty hilum and a hilar blood vessel (Fig. 26.19).

Oil cysts result from fat necrosis in the setting of prior trauma or surgery and typically appear as round or oval, fat-containing masses with or without a thin rim of calcification[23] (Fig. 26.20).

Lipomas may be detected incidentally on mammography or present as palpable abnormalities, appearing as oval, fat-containing masses with a thin fibrous capsule in the subcutaneous soft tissue. Lipomas are more difficult to distinguish in a fatty breast; however, their capsules are more easily seen on DBT.[24]

Galactoceles are usually seen in lactating women and are thought to originate from clogged ducts, consisting of milk products including fat. They are variable in density depending on proportion of internal fat contents. When present, a fat-fluid level is pathognomonic.[24]

Hamartomas are round or oval masses with fibrous capsules, variable in density depending on proportions of internal fat and soft tissue components (see Fig. 26.16).

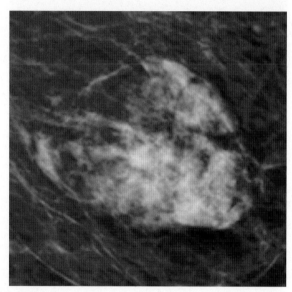

• **Fig. 26.16** Hamartomas are round or oval circumscribed masses with variable density depending on the relative proportions of internal fat and soft tissue components.

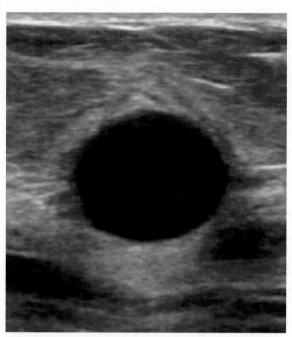

• **Fig. 26.17** Ultrasound of a simple cyst showing characteristic features including round shape, imperceptible wall, and anechoic internal contents with increased posterior acoustic enhancement.

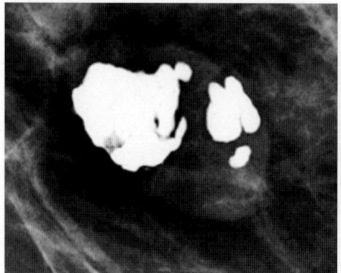
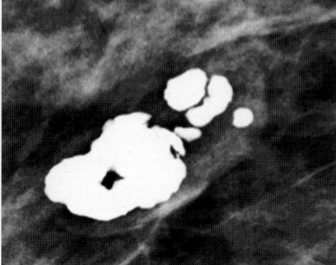

• **Fig. 26.18** Characteristic coarse, "popcorn-like" calcifications in involuting fibroadenomas.

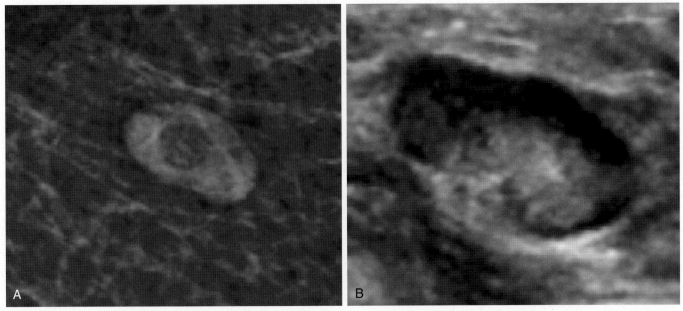

• **Fig. 26.19** Characteristic reniform shape and central radiolucency/echogenicity in intramammary lymph nodes on mammogram (A) and ultrasound (B).

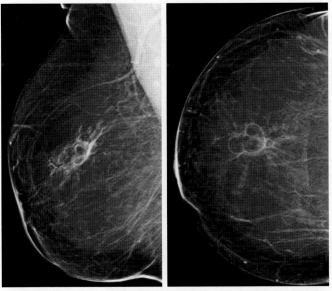

• **Fig. 26.20** Characteristic mammographic appearance of fat necrosis with thin rim calcification in a woman who has undergone ipsilateral reduction mammoplasty.

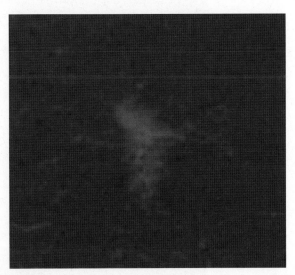

• **Fig. 26.21** Mammographic appearance of a tubular invasive ductal carcinoma with irregular shape and spiculated margins.

Malignant Masses. The most common malignant breast mass is invasive breast cancer. Several subtypes of invasive cancer exist, with varying prognoses.

Invasive Ductal Carcinoma of No Special Type. The most common subtype, invasive ductal carcinoma (IDC) of no special type (NST),[25] usually presents as an irregular mass with indistinct or spiculated margins and high density. Occasionally, this subtype appears to have partially circumscribed margins, which on further diagnostic imaging with spot compression views may reveal partially indistinct margins. Approximately 40% of cases are associated with suspicious microcalcifications, such as fine pleomorphic calcifications (see Fig. 26.7).

Invasive Lobular Carcinoma. Invasive lobular carcinoma (ILC) may appear as an irregular, equal density mass with indistinct or spiculated margins (see Fig. 26.6), as a subtle architectural distortion, or as an asymmetry. However, ILC is often occult on mammography. Because ILC may be unappreciable on clinical palpation or mammography, even when relatively large in size, it may be difficult to diagnose.

Tubular Carcinoma. Tubular carcinomas grow relatively slowly and are usually small when detected on mammography. Other than a characteristically small size, they have the mammographic features of IDC of NST: irregular shape, spiculated margins, and high density (Fig. 26.21). They have an excellent prognosis relative to IDC of NST.

Medullary Carcinoma. Medullary carcinomas are more commonly seen in younger women and tend to have benign mammographic features of oval shape and circumscribed margins (Fig. 26.22). Correlative ultrasound may show internal fluid contents. This combination of apparently benign features may result in delayed diagnosis.

Mucinous Carcinoma (Colloid Carcinoma). Mucinous carcinomas are more commonly seen in older women and tend to have benign imaging features, including oval shape and circumscribed margins on mammogram, posterior acoustic enhancement on ultrasound and T2 hyperintensity on MRI (Fig. 26.23). Mucinous carcinomas usually coexist with other subtypes. Although uncommon, pure mucinous carcinomas have a better prognosis compared with IDC of NST.

Intracystic Papillary Carcinoma/Invasive Papillary Carcinoma. Adenocarcinoma arising from a cyst wall is uncommon and is usually of the papillary subtype. The conglomerate mass is often large and circumscribed on mammography with both cystic and solid components on ultrasound. The solid portions may project centrally from the cyst wall (Fig. 26.24). If the tumor is entirely intracystic, the cancer is noninvasive, and prognosis is excellent. Invasive papillary carcinoma appears similar to

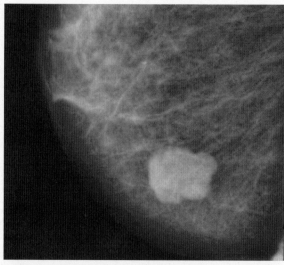

• **Fig. 26.22** Mammographic appearance of medullary invasive ductal carcinoma with oval shape and circumscribed margins.

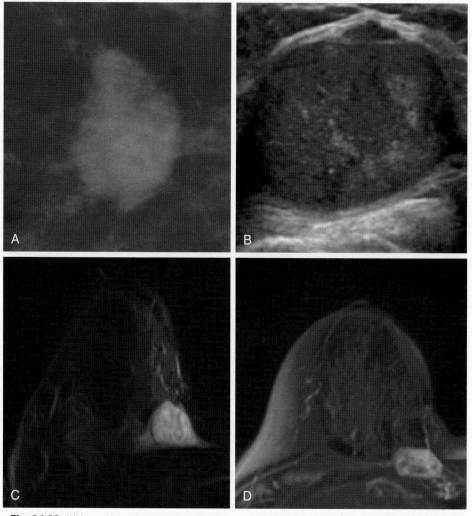

• **Fig. 26.23** (A) Mammographic appearance of a mucinous invasive ductal carcinoma with oval shape and circumscribed margins. (B) Sonographic appearance of a mucinous invasive ductal carcinoma with oval shape and circumscribed margins in a different woman, with corresponding T2 hyperintensity (C) and relatively homogeneous enhancement (D) on magnetic resonance imaging.

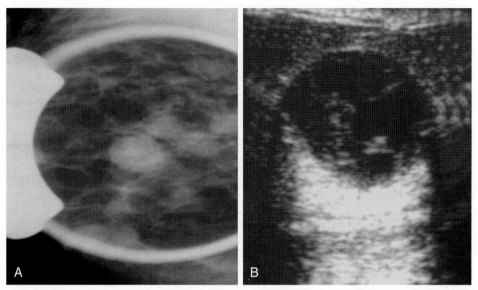

• **Fig. 26.24** Mammographic (A) and sonographic (B) appearances of intracystic papillary carcinoma with oval shape, circumscribed margins, and internal solid components.

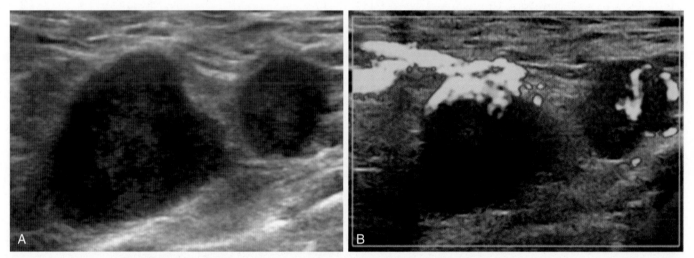

• **Fig. 26.25** Sonographic appearance of biopsy-proven lung cancer metastases to axillary lymph nodes with loss of normal reniform shape and hilar fat (A) and with increased vascular flow (B).

intracystic papillary carcinoma on imaging but shows invasion on histology, with worse prognosis compared with intracystic papillary carcinoma.

Breast Metastases From Extramammary Malignancies. Metastatic involvement of the breast by extramammary malignancies is uncommon. Primary malignancies that metastasize to the breast include lymphoma, melanoma, lung cancer, and ovarian cancer. Metastatic masses are usually solitary with round shape and indistinct margins.[26] Metastatic involvement of the axillary lymph nodes is more commonly seen (Fig. 26.25).

Calcifications. Calcium is a bivalent metallic element of the alkaline earth group. Calcification is the deposition of calcium in soft tissue. In the breast, calcification usually occurs in the form of calcium hydroxyapatite or tricalcium phosphate.[27]

In the BI-RADS lexicon, calcifications are divided into two general groups based on morphology: those that are typically benign and those that appear suspicious. Typically benign calcifications include skin, vascular, coarse, large rod-like, round, rim, dystrophic, milk of calcium, and suture types (Fig. 26.26). Suspicious calcifications include amorphous, coarse heterogeneous, fine pleomorphic, and fine linear or fine-linear branching types[3] (Fig. 26.27).

Calcifications are also characterized by their distribution. Diffuse calcifications are distributed randomly throughout the breast. Regional calcifications occur in a large portion of breast tissue (more than 2 cm) but do not conform to a ductal distribution. Diffuse and regional distributions favor benignity. Grouped (formerly clustered) calcifications include relatively few calcifications in a portion of breast tissue (for example, 5 calcifications within 1 cm). Grouped calcifications may be benign or malignant. Linear calcifications are arrayed in a line and suggest ductal deposition (Fig. 26.28). Segmental calcifications are distributed

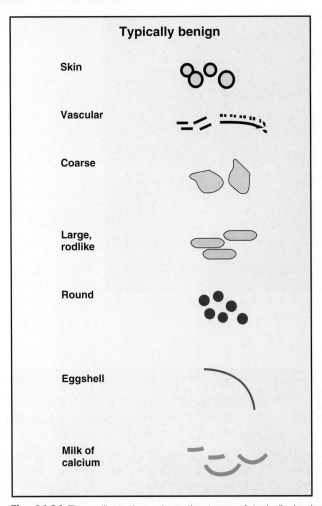

Typically benign

Skin

Vascular

Coarse

Large,
rodlike

Round

Eggshell

Milk of
calcium

• **Fig. 26.26** These illustrations show the types of typically benign calcifications.

in a duct and its branches (Fig. 26.29). Linear and segmental distributions are suspicious for malignancy.

Benign Calcifications. Skin calcifications are usually tightly grouped with lucent centers and are usually located near or within the skin in characteristics distributions, including the inner hemispheres, inframammary folds, periareolar regions, and axillary regions.[28] A tangential view can confirm the dermal origin of such calcifications.

Vascular calcifications are characterized by parallel tubular calcifications resembling railroad tracks in association with blood vessels (Fig. 26.30).

Coarse ("popcorn-like") calcifications are often associated with involuting fibroadenomas (see Fig. 26.18).

Large rodlike (secretory) calcifications represent calcium deposits within ectatic medium and large ducts. These calcifications are usually bilateral and appear as discontinuous, smooth,

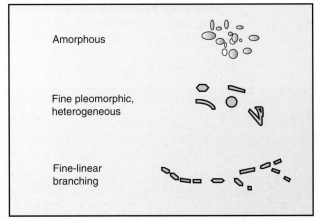

Amorphous

Fine pleomorphic,
heterogeneous

Fine-linear
branching

• **Fig. 26.27** These illustrations show some of the types of typically suspicious calcifications.

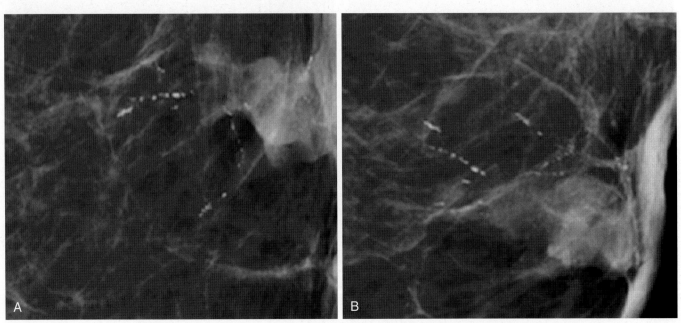

• **Fig. 26.28** Magnification craniocaudal (A) and mediolateral and (B) projections of microcalcifications in a linear distribution, biopsy-proven invasive ductal carcinoma with ductal carcinoma in situ.

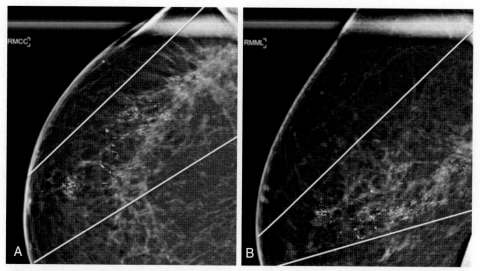

• **Fig. 26.29** Magnification craniocaudal (A) and mediolateral (B) projections of fine pleomorphic micro-calcifications in a segmental distribution, biopsy-proven ductal carcinoma in situ.

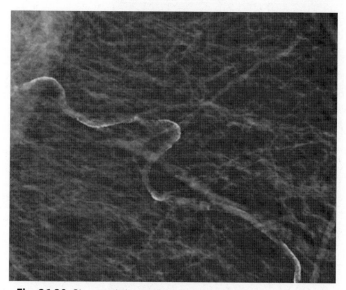

• **Fig. 26.30** Characteristic parallel tubular calcifications resembling rail-road tracks in vascular calcifications.

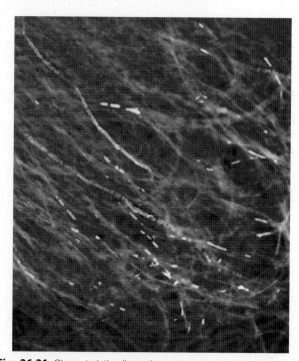

• **Fig. 26.31** Characteristic discontinuous, smooth, thick rods in large rodlike (secretory) calcifications. Vascular calcifications are also present.

thick rods in a ductal distribution extending toward the subareolar region (Fig. 26.31).

Round calcifications are smaller than 1 mm in size and are spherical in configuration.

Rim (eggshell) calcifications represent calcium deposits on the surfaces of spheres and are seen in cysts and in fat necrosis[23] (see Fig. 26.15).

Dystrophic calcifications develop in the setting of prior trauma, surgery, and radiation and are usually larger than 1 mm in size with an irregular shape (Fig. 26.32).

Milk of calcium calcifications represent sedimented calcifications in grouped cysts. The combination of an amorphous appearance on the CC view (Fig. 26.33A and 26.33C) and a curvilinear appearance on the straight lateral view (Fig. 26.33B and 26.33D) is pathognomonic.

Suture calcifications represent calcium deposition on suture material, with a characteristic knotted appearance.

Malignant Calcifications. Suspicious microcalcifications include amorphous, coarse heterogeneous, fine pleomorphic, and fine-linear/fine-linear branching morphologies, with positive predictive values for malignancy of approximately 20%, 20%, 28%, and 70%, respectively.[29] Amorphous calcifications are hazy in appearance, likened to crushed salt crystals, without a particular shape. Coarse heterogeneous calcifications are between 0.5 and 1.0 mm in size and have an irregular shape. Fine pleomorphic calcifications are usually smaller than 0.5 mm in size and have various discrete irregular shapes (Fig. 26.34). Fine-linear/fine-linear branching calcifications are usually smaller than 0.5 mm in size with linear and occasional branching shapes (Fig. 26.35). The

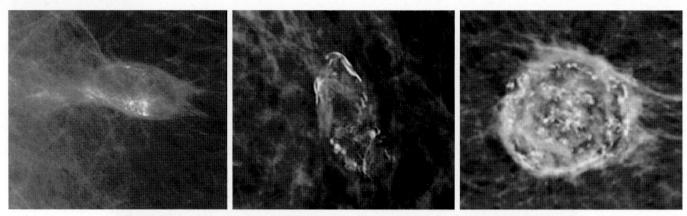

• **Fig. 26.32** Examples of dystrophic calcifications, with various appearances depending on extent of calcium deposition.

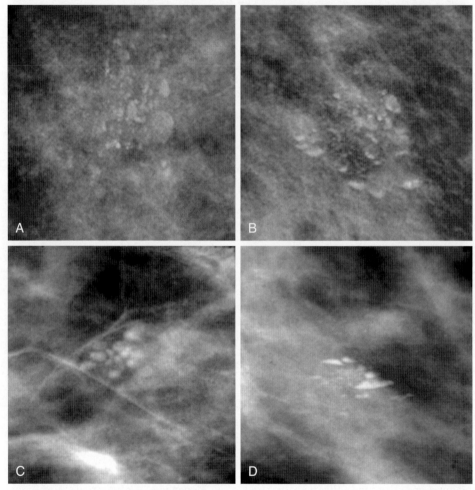

• **Fig. 26.33** The combination of an amorphous appearance on the craniocaudal view (A and C) and a curvilinear appearance on the straight lateral view (B and D) is pathognomonic for milk of calcium calcifications.

distribution of these calcifications is usually grouped, linear (see Fig. 26.28), or segmental (see Fig. 26.29).

Ductal Carcinoma in situ. Ductal carcinoma in situ (DCIS) encompasses multiple subtypes of noninvasive cancer, classically divided between comedocarcinoma and noncomedocarcinoma categories, with varying potential to progress to invasive cancer.

Approximately 75% of cases are diagnosed after detection of suspicious microcalcifications on mammography. Such calcifications tend to appear fine, linear, and branching in the more aggressive comedocarcinomas, representing calcium deposition on necrotic tumor within central portions of ducts. They are variable in appearance in the more indolent noncomedocarcinomas such as micropapillary and cribriform DCIS, representing calcium

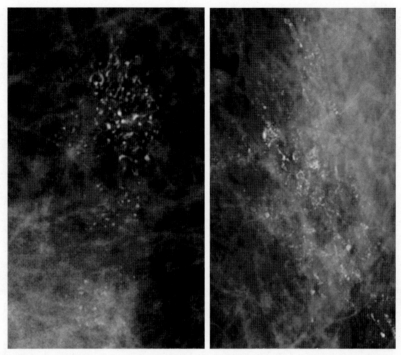

• **Fig. 26.34** Fine pleomorphic calcifications are small in size with various, discernible, irregular shapes.

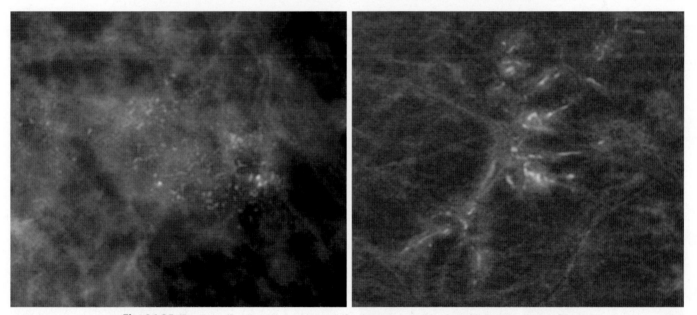

• **Fig. 26.35** Fine-linear/fine-linear branching calcifications are small in size with linear and occasional branching shapes.

deposition on necrotic tumor within noncentral portions of ducts. The mammographic microcalcifications closely match the histologic extent of comedocarcinomas but can underestimate that of noncomedocarcinomas.

Approximately 10% of cases present as mammographic masses (Fig. 26.36). Even less common presentations include architectural distortions, asymmetries, and single dilated retroareolar ducts.

Invasive Carcinoma With Extensive Intraductal Component. When invasive carcinomas are associated with a substantial amount of DCIS, they are qualified as having an extensive intraductal component (EIC) (see Figs. 26.7 and 26.37). Such carcinomas are either primarily invasive with DCIS partially filling involved ducts or with DCIS adjacent to the involved tissue, or they are primarily intraductal with small foci of invasion.[30] Invasive carcinomas with EIC have a higher incidence of local recurrence after lumpectomy and radiation.[31] In cases of DCIS manifesting as microcalcifications, diagnostic mammography with magnification views may be obtained after lumpectomy and before radiation therapy to evaluate for the presence of any residual suspicious calcifications (Fig. 26.38), in which case CNB or reexcision may be considered for further evaluation.[32] The postlumpectomy mammogram also serves as a new baseline for future mammographic comparisons.

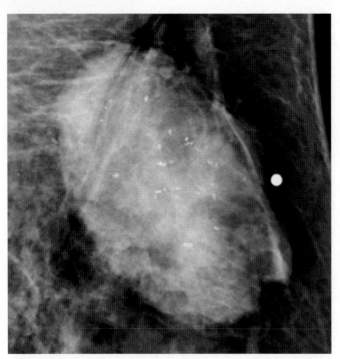

• **Fig. 26.36** Uncommon presentation of ductal carcinoma in situ as a mammographic mass containing fine pleomorphic microcalcifications.

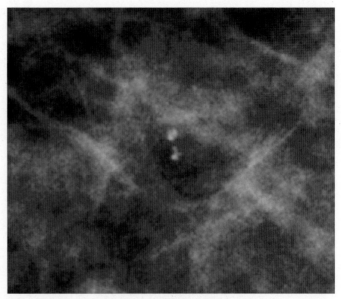

• **Fig. 26.38** A 69-year-old woman with history of ductal carcinoma in situ, treated with lumpectomy. Postlumpectomy, preradiation therapy mammogram showed two residual microcalcifications adjacent to the surgical bed, which underwent stereotactic core needle biopsy. Due to residual atypical ductal hyperplasia on biopsy, the patient underwent reexcision.

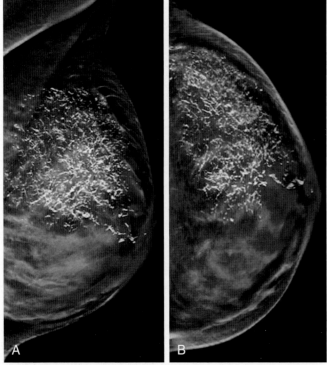

• **Fig. 26.37** Mediolateral oblique (A) and craniocaudal (B) projections showing invasive ductal carcinoma with an extensive intraductal component, involving more than one quadrant of the breast.

Indirect Signs of Breast Cancer

Mammographic evidence of malignancy can be divided into primary, secondary, and indirect signs. Primary signs include masses and calcifications. Secondary signs include associated imaging findings such as skin thickening, skin retraction, and nipple retraction, all of which are usually signs of advanced cancer. Indirect signs include architectural distortions, asymmetries, and abnormal axillary lymph nodes. Such indirect signs may be the only evidence of malignancy in up to 20% of mammographically detected cancers.[33]

Architectural Distortions. Architectural distortions are parenchymal distortions without visible masses, seen as straight lines radiating from a central point (Fig. 26.39). They are associated with invasive breast cancers, postsurgical scars, and radial scars. Wire markers placed directly over surgical scars are useful to communicate the presence and location of any prior breast surgeries because these scars may be confused for malignancies. Postsurgical scars may also be associated with skin thickening and retraction, although such scars and skin changes tend to decrease over time.

Radial scars are benign entities of unknown etiologies that are usually asymptomatic and detected on mammography as straight lines radiating from a radiolucent center with an estimated incidence of 1 in every 1000 screening mammograms.[34] When diagnosed histologically based on CNB, surgical excision is usually recommended to exclude sampling error.

Asymmetries. An asymmetry usually represents normal fibroglandular tissue that is seen in an area of one breast but not in the corresponding area of the contralateral breast. For example, unilateral accessory breast tissue in the axilla is an example of an asymmetry and is a normal variant.[35] The asymmetry is described as global if it involves at least one breast quadrant and as focal if it involves less than one breast quadrant.

If an asymmetry is associated with a palpable abnormality, mass, suspicious microcalcifications, or architectural distortion, or if the asymmetry is new, larger, or more conspicuous than previously (Fig. 26.40), diagnostic imaging including spot compression views and potential CNB should be recommended for further evaluation to exclude malignancy.

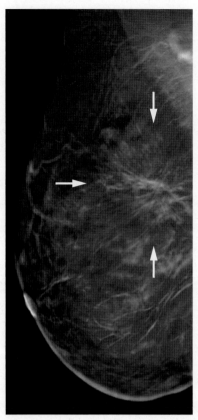

• **Fig. 26.39** Mammographic appearance of an architectural distortion appearing as straight lines radiating from a central point without an associated mass *(arrows)*.

Abnormal Axillary Lymph Nodes. Axillary lymph nodes are commonly seen on the MLO view. Normal lymph nodes are reniform in shape with central radiolucency representing hilar fat. Abnormal lymph nodes are more likely to be round, dense, and larger than 2 cm, although enlarged size itself is not a malignant indicator. Correlative ultrasound may show lymph nodes with eccentrically thickened cortices or loss of normal reniform shapes and fatty hila (Fig. 26.41). In the absence of a known primary malignancy, the presence of unilateral abnormal axillary lymph nodes should prompt imaging evaluation for an occult breast cancer (Fig. 26.42).

Ultrasound

Ultrasound is not only an important adjunct to mammography for screening and diagnostic imaging but is also a primary imaging modality for guiding interventional procedures including cyst aspiration, CNB (Fig. 26.43), preoperative needle localization, abscess drainage, and hematoma/seroma drainage (Fig. 26.44).[12]

Standardized Terminology for Sonography Reports

BI-RADS has been applied to ultrasound to standardize sonography findings, assessments, and recommendations from different imaging centers.

Benign Masses

Sonographic features favoring benignity include absence of any malignant findings; round or oval shape; parallel orientation (the long axis of the mass is parallel to the skin); circumscribed

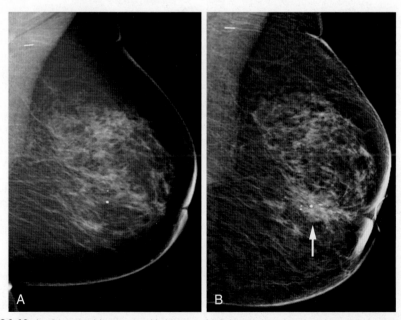

• **Fig. 26.40** An 81-year-old woman with history of left breast invasive ductal carcinoma treated with lumpectomy and radiation therapy in 2001. Routine screening mammogram in 2015 (B) compared with 2006 (A) shows a new asymmetry *(arrow)* in the surgical bed. Stereotactic core needle biopsy showed recurrent invasive ductal carcinoma with ductal carcinoma in situ.

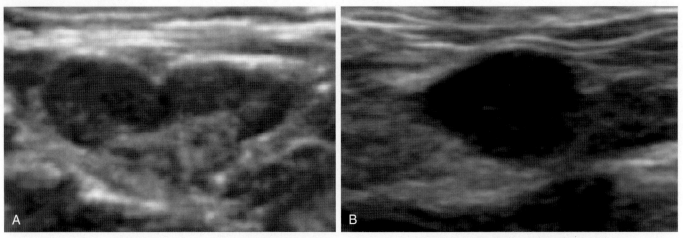

• **Fig. 26.41** Sonographic appearances of abnormal axillary lymph nodes showing eccentrically thickened cortex (A) and loss of normal reniform shape and fatty hilum (B).

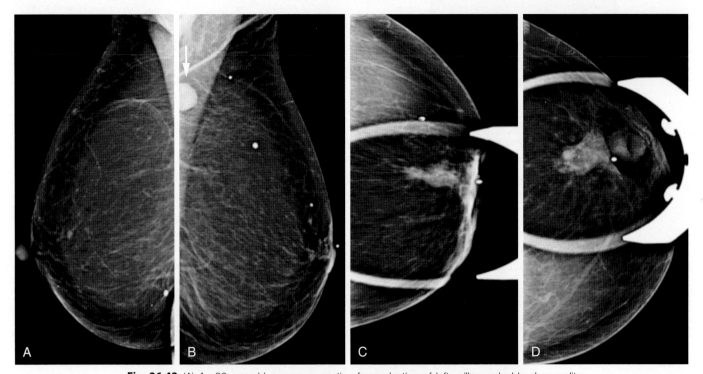

• **Fig. 26.42** (A) An 86-year-old woman presenting for evaluation of left axillary palpable abnormality, corresponding to unilateral abnormally round and dense axillary lymph node (B). Spot compression projections of the ipsilateral breast (C and D) show an irregular dense mass with spiculated margins, biopsy-proven invasive ductal carcinoma with axillary metastases.

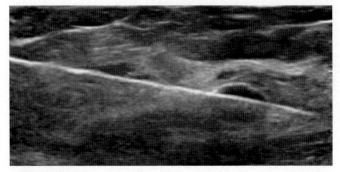

• **Fig. 26.43** Ultrasound-guided core needle biopsy of a small oval hypoechoic mass showing passage of the biopsy needle through the center of the mass, biopsy-proven fibroadenoma.

margins; hyperechogenicity relative to subcutaneous fat; and posterior acoustic enhancement.[36] Examples of benign masses include simple cysts and solid masses such as fibroadenomas (Fig. 26.45).

Malignant Masses

Sonographic features favoring malignancy include irregular shape; nonparallel orientation; not circumscribed margins (indistinct, angular, microlobulated, or spiculated); hypoechogenicity relative to subcutaneous fat; posterior acoustic shadowing (Fig. 26.46); and associated features such as vascularity, calcifications (Fig. 26.47), architectural distortion, ductal changes (Fig. 26.48), and skin changes such as thickening and retraction.

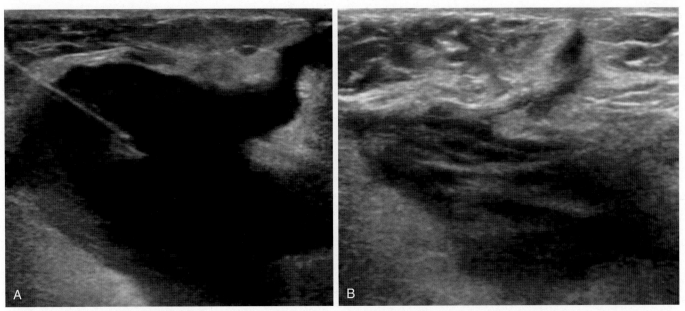

• **Fig. 26.44** (A) Pre– and (B) post–ultrasound-guided seroma drainage showing collapse of fluid collection after aspiration.

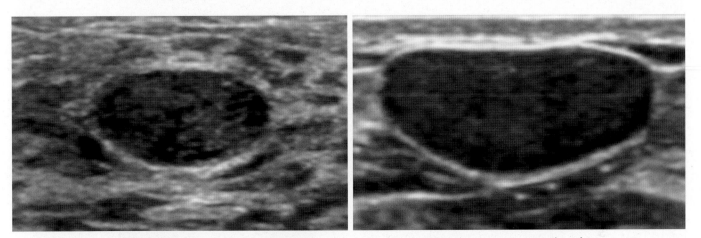

• **Fig. 26.45** Characteristic sonographic appearances of benign-appearing masses suggestive of fibroadenomas with oval shapes, parallel orientations, circumscribed margins, and hypoechoic echogenicities.

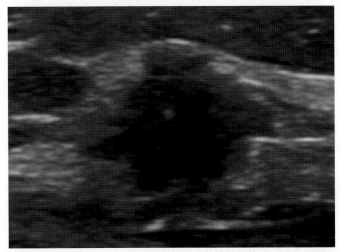

• **Fig. 26.46** Characteristic sonographic appearance of a malignant mass with irregular shape, not parallel orientation, angular margins, and hypoechoic echogenicity, biopsy-proven invasive ductal carcinoma.

Magnetic Resonance Imaging

MRI is a powerful imaging modality used in both screening (in conjunction with mammography) and diagnostic imaging and for guiding interventional procedures.

Screening indications include greater than 20% lifetime risk of developing breast cancer[13]; presence of silicone injections precluding optimal mammographic screening; and history of prior breast cancer.

Diagnostic indications include evaluation of implant integrity (Fig. 26.49); extent of disease in newly diagnosed breast cancer; treatment response to neoadjuvant chemotherapy; residual disease after lumpectomy with positive surgical margins; and occult primary breast cancer in the setting of metastatic axillary lymphadenopathy.[37]

Contrast-enhanced breast MRI is the most sensitive imaging modality for detecting breast cancer but is limited by a relatively lower specificity compared with mammography and ultrasonography due to the propensity for both benign and malignant lesions

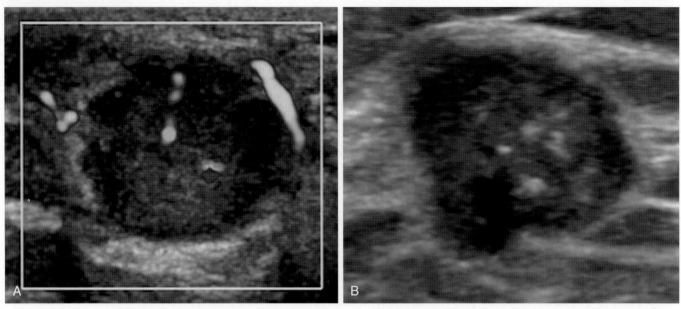

• **Fig. 26.47** Characteristic sonographic appearance of a malignant mass with associated features of increased vascularity (A) and internal calcifications (B).

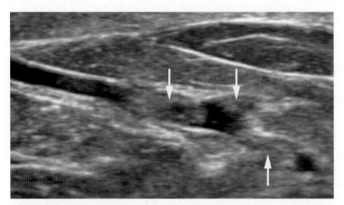

• **Fig. 26.48** Sonographic appearance of ductal changes associated with malignant masses, notable for intraluminal solid components *(arrows)* and obliteration of peripheral ductal branches.

to enhance.[38] Additional limitations include nonvisualization of microcalcifications and potential lack of enhancement in low-grade DCIS.[39]

Standardized Terminology for MRI Reports

BI-RADS has been applied to MRI to standardize MRI findings, assessments, and recommendations from different imaging centers.

Typically Benign Findings

The morphology of a benign mass is similar to that on mammography and ultrasound: round or oval shape with circumscribed margins. A round or oval enhancing circumscribed mass with nonenhancing internal septations especially favors a benign mass, specifically a fibroadenoma (Fig. 26.50).[40] Other typically benign features of enhancing masses include T1 hyperintensity, T2 hyperintensity, and slow initial phase and plateau delayed phase contrast kinetics. However, benign entities such as lymph

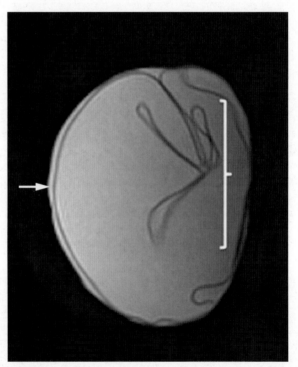

• **Fig. 26.49** Sagittal silicone-specific magnetic resonance imaging sequence showing subcapsular line sign *(arrow)* and linguini sign *(bracket)* in intracapsular silicone implant rupture.

nodes may show fast initial phase and washout delayed phase contrast kinetics. Both morphology and contrast kinetics must be evaluated in conjunction, often with heavier emphasis placed on morphology.

Typically Malignant Findings

The morphology of a malignant mass is also similar to that on mammography and ultrasound: irregular shape with irregular or

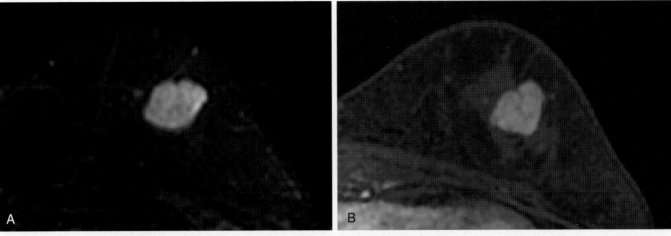

• **Fig. 26.50** Characteristic magnetic resonance imaging appearance of a fibroadenoma with oval shape, T2 hyperintensity (A), and internal nonenhancing septations (B).

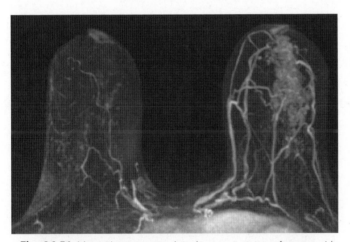

• **Fig. 26.51** Magnetic resonance imaging appearance of asymmetric clumped nonmass enhancement in the left breast, biopsy-proven ductal carcinoma in situ.

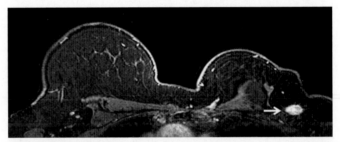

• **Fig. 26.52** Magnetic resonance imaging appearance of abnormal left axillary lymph node *(arrow)* showing loss of reniform shape and fatty hilum and presence of spiculated margins.

spiculated margins. Other typically malignant features include fast initial and washout delayed phase contrast kinetics and associated ipsilateral findings such as asymmetric clumped nonmass enhancement (Fig. 26.51), adjacent skin thickening with enhancement, nipple retraction, pectoralis muscle or chest wall invasion, and abnormal lymph nodes (Fig. 26.52). Unfortunately, some malignant masses, such as mucinous carcinomas, are round or oval in shape, circumscribed in margin, T2 hyperintense, and homogeneously enhancing (Fig. 26.23), features that are typically benign. In such cases, knowledge of clinical information (patient age, *BRCA* status, and family history) and comparison to prior imaging examinations can be helpful to avoid misdiagnosis.

Other Breast Imaging Technologies

Ductography (Galactography)

Indications for ductography include spontaneous, unilateral, clear or bloody nipple discharge from a single orifice. Such nipple discharge is usually caused by benign conditions, such as

intraductal papillomas (Fig. 26.53), ductal ectasia, and fibrocystic changes. However, approximately 15% of cases are caused by DCIS (Fig. 26.54).

Ductography involves the injection of contrast material into the discharging lactiferous duct followed by mammography in two magnification projection views to potentially determine the nature, location, and extent of causative lesions. Ductography is unlikely to be technically successful or diagnostic for nonspontaneous, bilateral, white, yellow, or green nipple discharge from multiple orifices.

Imaging-Guided Interventional Procedures

The most common imaging-guided procedures include CNB and preoperative needle localization.

Imaging-Guided Core Needle Biopsy

Imaging-guided CNB is the primary means for tissue diagnosis, with less common alternatives including fine-needle aspiration and surgical biopsy. Indications for CNB include BI-RADS 4 and 5 lesions, as well as BI-RADS 3 lesions for which patients prefer to undergo CNB rather than return for 6-month follow-up imaging to confirm benignity. Potential precluding factors for CNB include patient body weight exceeding biopsy table threshold, patient body habitus preventing positioning inside MRI

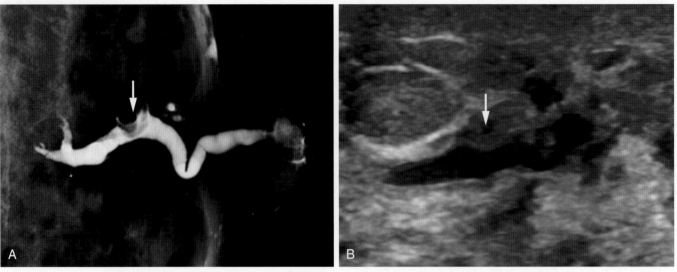

• **Fig. 26.53** Ductogram (A) and ultrasound (B) in a woman presenting for evaluation of unilateral, spontaneous, clear nipple discharge, both showing intraluminal filling defects *(arrows)* and obliteration of peripheral ducts.

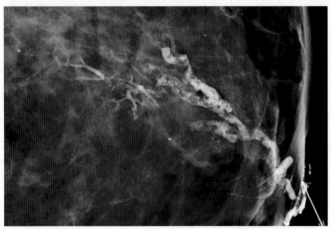

• **Fig. 26.54** Ductogram in a woman presenting for evaluation of unilateral, spontaneous, bloody nipple discharge, showing multiple irregular intraluminal filling defects and obliteration of peripheral ducts, biopsy-proven ductal carcinoma in situ.

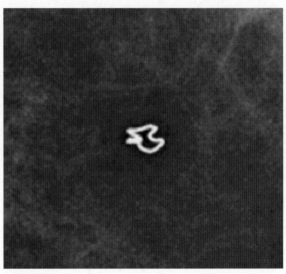

• **Fig. 26.55** Mammographic appearance of a biopsy micromarker indicating area of targeted biopsy.

magnet, lesions that are too close to the skin or chest wall for optimal access, and inadequate breast thickness after compression. In such cases, surgical biopsy may be more appropriate. Other relative contraindications include inability to discontinue anticoagulation therapy, other coagulopathy, and infection of the overlying skin.

CNB can be guided by prone or upright stereotactic mammography with or without DBT capability, ultrasound, and MRI. The imaging modality of choice depends primarily on the nature and location of the biopsy target. For example, suspicious microcalcifications are best seen on mammography, and nonmass enhancement is only seen on MRI. Regardless of the imaging modality used, CNB is followed by metallic biopsy micromarker placement and postprocedural mammography to document the location of the biopsy micromarker (Fig. 26.55), as micromarker migration may occur. The biopsy micromarker serves to help facilitate localization of the biopsy site should histology results require surgical resection.

Radiologists are encouraged to audit their BI-RADS assessment categories and biopsy results to evaluate and improve their practices.[41] Such data outcome analysis involves determining true-positive, false-positive, true-negative, false-negative, positive predictive values, and negative predictive value statistics on a yearly basis.

Of note, high-risk lesions, such as atypical ductal hyperplasia (ADH), are considered benign for such medical audit purposes but are recommended for surgical biopsy because of the difficulty in differentiating ADH from DCIS on CNB. In one series, 20% of cases originally interpreted as ADH based on CNB were upgraded to DCIS after surgical biopsy.[42]

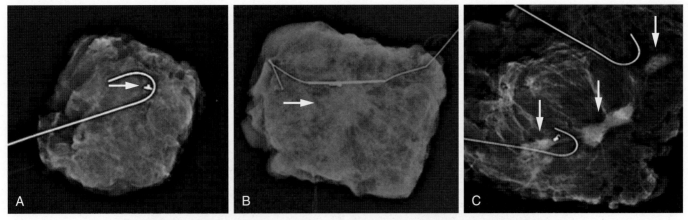

• **Fig. 26.56** Specimen radiographs showing needle/wire localization and removal of a biopsy micro-marker at the site of prior microcalcifications (A, *arrow*), of a mass (B, *arrow*), and of a biopsy micromarker and multiple masses (C, *arrows*).

Imaging-Guided Preoperative Needle Localization

Imaging-guided preoperative needle/wire localization is indicated before surgical excision of biopsy-proven lesions with atypia or malignancy and can be performed using mammographic, ultra-sound, and MRI guidance. The imaging modality of choice depends primarily on the nature and location of the targeted lesion. For example, a biopsy micromarker is best seen on mammography. Regardless of the imaging modality used, the tip of the needle/wire system is placed as close to the target as possible, followed by injection of methylene blue dye through the needle/wire system. Mammograms are obtained to document the location of the needle/wire system in relation to the target. The needle/wire system is left inside the breast before surgery. After surgical biopsy, specimen radiography (Fig. 26.56) or sonography is performed to confirm removal of the target. However, specimen imaging is not a substitute for histologic analysis of surgical margins for residual atypia or malignancy.

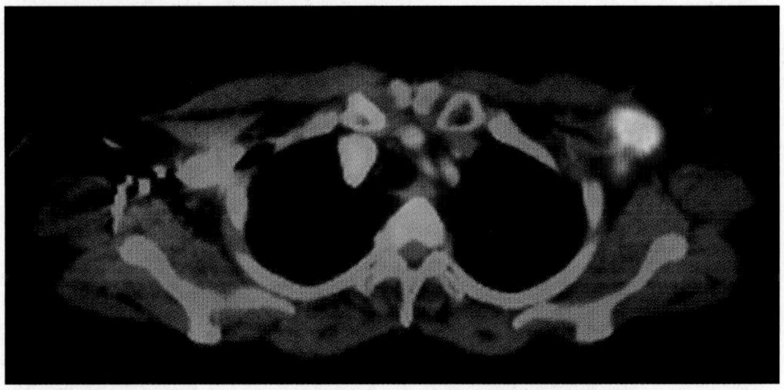

Staging and Imaging Follow-Up of Women With Breast Cancer

Evaluation for Distant Metastases

The most common sites of distant metastases are the bones, lungs, liver, and brain. Women with stage III and IV disease may undergo nuclear medicine bone scan; multidetector computed tomography (CT) of the chest, abdomen, and pelvis; fluorodeoxyglucose positron emission tomography/CT (Fig. 26.57); and/or contrast-enhanced brain MRI depending on the presence of neurologic symptoms.

Follow-Up of the Conservatively Treated Breast

Women who have undergone breast conserving surgery (BCS) receive a diagnostic mammogram of the ipsilateral breast before starting radiation therapy to establish a new baseline for future comparisons, especially if they had DCIS or invasive carcinoma with EIC manifesting as microcalcifications. However, the common practice of repeating such mammograms every 6 months for 2 years after BCS is controversial because most recurrences are unlikely to occur during this interval.[43]

Normal postsurgical findings include skin thickening, skin retraction, edema, hematoma/seroma formation, architectural distortion, and fat necrosis.[44] Such changes should diminish over time (Fig. 26.58).

The typical recurrence rate is 1% to 2.5% per year and typically occurs at or near the site of original tumor 3 to 7 years after BCS. Potential risk factors include young age at the time of initial diagnosis, large tumor size, multifocal disease (more than one lesion within the same breast quadrant), multicentric disease (more than one lesion within different breast quadrants), positive margins after initial BCS, high histologic grade, EIC, and lymphovascular invasion.[45]

The presence of new or increased skin thickening, edema, mass (Fig. 26.59), architectural distortion, asymmetry, suspicious microcalcifications, axillary lymphadenopathy, or enhancement on MRI (Fig. 26.60) is suspicious for recurrence[46,47] and should be followed by recommendation for CNB.

• **Fig. 26.57** A 61-year-old woman with remote history of left breast cancer, presenting for evaluation of a left axillary palpable abnormality, found to have biopsy-proven recurrent invasive ductal carcinoma in a left axillary lymph node. Fluorodeoxyglucose positron emission tomography/computed tomography obtained for staging purposes shows intense tracer uptake in the left axilla at the site of known axillary metastases.

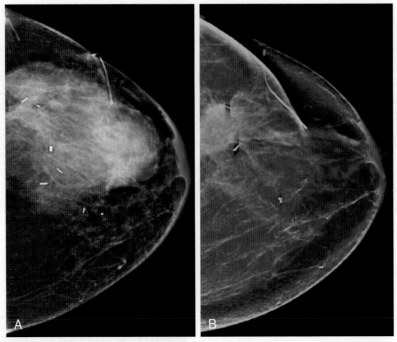

• **Fig. 26.58** Screening mammogram 2 years after lumpectomy and radiation show interval decrease in extent of skin thickening and hematoma/seroma size in (B) compared with (A), with residual skin retraction and architectural distortion, consistent with postsurgical changes.

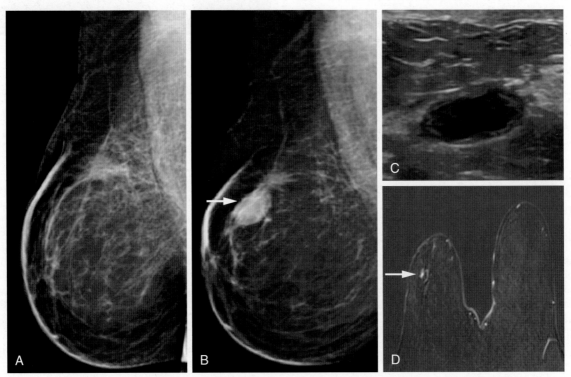

• **Fig. 26.59** (A) A 46-year-old woman with history of invasive ductal carcinoma treated with lumpectomy and radiation, presenting with a new palpable mass at the surgical site 4 years after treatment. Diagnostic mammogram shows a new oval mass in the surgical site (B, *arrow*), with correlative ultrasound showing an oval complex cystic and solid mass with circumscribed margins (C) and magnetic resonance imaging showing an enhancing mass with spiculated margins, biopsy-proven recurrent invasive ductal carcinoma (D, *arrow*).

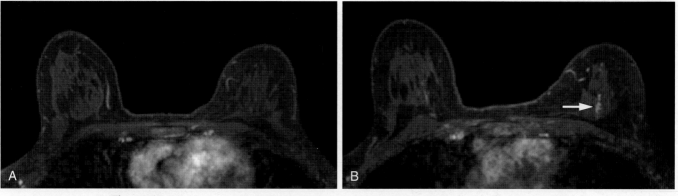

• **Fig. 26.60** Surveillance magnetic resonance imaging shows new linear nonmass enhancement at the surgical site (*arrow,* B) compared with study obtained 1 year prior (A) in a 37-year-old woman with history of invasive ductal carcinoma treated with lumpectomy and radiation 4 years previously.

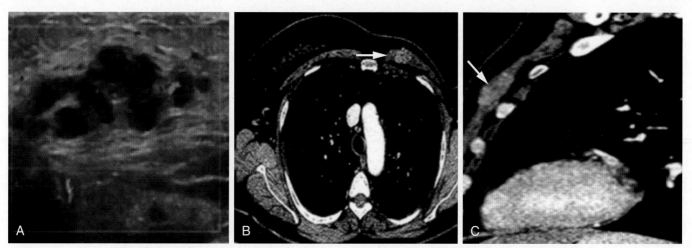

• **Fig. 26.61** A 65-year-old woman with history of left breast invasive ductal carcinoma treated with mastectomy without reconstruction, presenting for evaluation of a palpable left chest wall abnormality. Targeted ultrasound shows an irregular hypoechoic mass with indistinct margins and associated vascularity (A). Computed tomography of the chest obtained for staging shows a corresponding oval enhancing mass in the left chest wall (*arrows,* B and C). Ultrasound-guided core needle biopsy showed recurrent invasive ductal carcinoma.

Follow-Up After Mastectomy

Mammography and MRI of the mastectomy site that has not undergone reconstruction or has undergone implant reconstruction has low added value compared with physical examination, because the majority of recurrences are detected by palpation in this setting.[48] Rather, targeted ultrasound to the area of palpable abnormality is the imaging modality of choice (Fig. 26.61). Mammography is still recommended to screen the contralateral breast and the mastectomy site that has undergone flap reconstruction.[49]

Selected References

3. American College of Radiology (ACR). *Breast Imaging Reporting and Data System (BI-RADS).* 5th ed. Reston, VA: ACR; 2013.

6. Pisano ED, Gatsonis C, Hendrick E, et al. Diagnostic performance of digital versus film mammography for breast-cancer screening. *N Engl J Med.* 2005;353:1773-1783.

10. Skaane P, Bandos AI, Gullien R, et al. Comparison of digital mammography alone and digital mammography plus tomosynthesis in a population-based screening program. *Radiology.* 2013;267: 47-56.

13. Saslow D, Boetes C, Burke W, et al. American Cancer Society guidelines for breast screening with MRI as an adjunct to mammography. *CA Cancer J Clin.* 2007;57:75-89.

38. Wells C, DeBruhl N. Magnetic resonance imaging: indications and interpretation. In: Bassett L, Mahoney M, Apple S, D'Orsi C, eds. *Breast Imaging.* Philadelphia: Saunders; 2011.

A full reference list is available online at ExpertConsult.com.

27

Design and Conduct of Clinical Trials for Breast Cancer

V. SUZANNE KLIMBERG, YU SHYR, AND THOMAS WELLS

The National Institutes of Health (NIH) defines a clinical trial as "a research study in which one or more human subjects are prospectively assigned to one or more interventions (which may include placebo or other control) to evaluate the effects of those interventions on health-related biomedical or behavioral outcomes."[1] One of the more common ways to describe clinical trials is controlled and uncontrolled. Uncontrolled trials lack a comparison group. Controlled trials involve two or more study treatments, at least one of which is a control treatment (i.e., a standard against which new treatments are measured). The main focus of this chapter is noninterventional trials including cohort (cross-sectional, case-control) studies, and interventional trials, that is, intervention(s) applied to the study population synonymous with clinical trials in most texts. Dr. William Thomas Beaver was the clinical pharmacologist at Georgetown University who is credited with drafting the initial regulations defining "adequate and controlled" clinical studies. According to Dr. Beaver, clinical trials are systematic experiments performed on human beings for the purpose of assessing the safety and/or efficacy of treatments or care procedures, and the "function of the controlled clinical trial is not the 'discovery' of a new drug or therapy. Discoveries are made in the animal laboratory, by chance observation, or at the bedside by an acute clinician. The function of the formal controlled clinical trial is to separate the relative handful of discoveries which prove to be true advances in therapy from a legion of false leads and unverifiable clinical impressions, and to delineate in a scientific way the extent of and the limitations which attend the effectiveness of drugs."[2]

Evolving Ethics and Regulation of Clinical Trials in the United States

605 bce—The earliest written account of a clinical trial is from the book of Daniel in the Bible. Daniel did not want to defile himself with King Nebuchadnezzar's food and wine. He asked the head official to give him and three others only vegetables and water for 10 days, while other servants ate the royal food. At the end of 10 days, the four men eating only vegetables and water appeared healthier and better nourished than those that indulged in the king's food.

1667—Diary of Samuel Pepys (member of the English parliament) documented the first mention of a paid research subject.

1747—James Lind offered earliest attempt of a planned controlled trial for the "treatment" of scurvy. Twelve men with similar cases of scurvy ate a common diet and slept together. Six pairs, however, were given different "treatments" for their malady (cider; elixir; seawater; horseradish, mustard, and garlic; vinegar; oranges and lemons). The two who received the oranges and lemons recovered.

1863—Gull and Sutton demonstrated the use of placebo treatment in the natural variability of the course of disease and the possibility of spontaneous cure.

1880—Introduction of "patent" medicines, which represented 72% of drug sales by 1900, including drugs that were both inert and active.

1906—Pure Food and Drug Act provided a legal definition for the terms *adulterated* and *misbranded* as they related to both food and drug products and prescribed legal penalties for each offense. The act also prohibited "false and misleading" statements on product labels. Efforts to prohibit false therapeutic claims on drug labels were defined both by the Supreme Court and the US Congress.

1937—A drug company developed a liquid preparation of sulfanilamide, used to treat strep infections. The product was not tested in animals or humans before marketing. The solvent used to suspend the active drug was diethylene glycol. The US Food and Drug Administration (FDA) was only empowered to act against the deadly product because it was misbranded—it contained no alcohol, whereas the term *elixir* implied that it did contain alcohol. More than 100 people who took the preparation were killed.

1938—Food, Drug, and Cosmetic Act was passed. This act required drug sponsors to submit safety data to FDA officials for evaluation before marketing. The act did not specify any particular testing method(s) but required that drugs be studied by "adequate tests by all methods reasonably applicable to show whether or not the drug is safe." Under this law devices were equal to drugs.

1948—Nuremberg Code developed, outlining 10 basic statements for the protection of human participants in clinical trials. In particular, the code supported the concept of voluntary informed consent.

1962—Kefauver-Harris Drug Amendments. This law, heavily influenced by the 1950 thalidomide incident in Western Europe, required controlled trials that could support claims of efficacy. The law stated that a poorly designed trial not only wasted resources, but unnecessarily put patients at risk.

1964—Declaration of Helsinki outlined ethical codes for physicians and protection of participants in clinical trials all over the world.

1966—Drug Efficacy Study (DES) begun by the FDA. The study required review of all drugs that had been approved under the 1938 Food, Drug, and Cosmetic Act (1938–1962) on the basis of safety alone, this time looking for evidence of efficacy. The results of the study resulted in the removal of more than 1000 ineffective drugs and drug combinations from the marketplace.

1972—Robert Temple noted that as late as the 1960s and early 1970s, "You would be horrified [at the clinical trial data] submitted to the agency. There was often no protocol at all. There was almost never a statistical plan. Sequential analyses were virtually nonexistent. It was a very different world."

1974—National Research Act resulted in the Belmont Report, which laid the foundation for clinical research conducted in the United States (respect for persons, beneficence, and justice). Passing of this act was prompted by the Tuskegee Syphilis Experiment.

1976—Medical Device Amendments Act redefined devices, making them more distinct from drugs. The law established a classification system as well as safety and efficacy requirements for medical devices. It also created new routes to market (premarket notification and premarket approval by the FDA) and Investigational Device Exemptions (IDEs). This act was prompted by the Dalkon Shield Disaster of 1971. Only minimal testing was done on the intrauterine device. The company was warned by scientists of serious design flaws and safety concerns with the device. Despite this warning, safety and efficacy claims were made, and contraindications were ignored and kept quiet. As a result, approximately 8000 injuries were reported, including sepsis, miscarriage, and death.

1987—Introduction of "Treatment IND (Investigational New Drug)" in response to the AIDS epidemic.

1990—Safe Medical Devices Act of 1990 included device tracking for high-risk devices (i.e., implants), required user facilities and manufacturers to report certain adverse events to the FDA, and gave the FDA authority to regulate combination products (drug/device, device/biologic, etc.). It also created incentives for development of orphan or humanitarian use devices (e.g., drugs/devices used to treat diseases or conditions affecting fewer than 4000 people in the United States per year).

1990–1992—Regulations approved by FDA established a "parallel track approval" process in which special categories of drugs would be expedited during the review process and a wider group of patients would have access to the drug than under normal procedures. These regulations gave the agency explicit authority to rely on surrogate markers (measure outcomes that are not clinically valuable by themselves but are thought to correspond with improved clinical outcomes). The FDA is cautious in accepting surrogates and usually requires continued postmarket study to verify and describe continued clinical benefits.

1990—International Conference on Harmonization (ICH) was assembled to help eliminate differences in drug development requirements for three global pharmaceutical markets: Europe, Japan, and the United States.

1997—Food and Drug Administration Modernization Act (FDAMA) recognized changes in the way the FDA would be operating in the 21st century (extended the Prescription Drug User Fee Act, required registration of selected trials in the ClinicalTrials.gov database, established risk-based regulation of medical devices, etc.). Today the FDA is responsible for protecting the public health by ensuring the safety, efficacy, and security of human and veterinary drugs, biological products, medical devices, our nation's food supply, cosmetics, and products that emit radiation.[3]

2002—Medical Device User Fee and Modernization Act (MDUFMA) authorized the FDA to collect monetary fees from companies or sponsors to support the review of certain types of applications. It also established inspections to be conducted by an accredited third-party under certain circumstances and established the Office of Combination Products established to oversee review of products falling under multiple jurisdictions within the FDA.

2007—FDA Amendments Act (FDAAA) and the rules for trial registration.

2016—Final Rule that clarifies and expands the regulatory requirements and procedures for submitting registration and summary results information of clinical trials on ClinicalTrials.gov.

Research Versus Clinical Care

Clinical care involves patients seeking diagnosis and treatment for a disease or condition. Research involves subjects who volunteer to participate in an experiment. Research is conducted to test the safety, effectiveness, dosing, or other use of investigational products. Research according to 45 CFR [code of federal regulation] 46.102(d)) is "a systematic investigation, including research development, testing, and evaluation, designed to develop or contribute to generalizable knowledge." Research may be conducted using unapproved investigational products, approved products for a new indication or in a new population, or approved products in a comparative effectiveness trial. The state Medical Board is empowered to license physicians and other health care practitioners under state statute and to dictate the scope of practice through regulation. Licensure allows physicians to prescribe FDA-approved drugs, biologics, and devices, among other products, and to prescribe approved drugs in an "off-label" manner. Many state medical boards do not regulate research. The FDA does not regulate the practice of medicine. The FDA issues a Drug Label, which is the official description of a drug product and includes what it is used for, who should take it, side effects, instructions for use, and safety information for the patient (aka "package insert").[4] Drug approval takes into account the specific disease or condition (i.e., use), the specific population (e.g., age, gender), the dose and dosage form (formulation, combination drugs), warnings, and contraindications. Physicians may prescribe "off-label" any approved drug, biologic, or medical device. "Off-label use" is defined as the use of an approved drug in a manner that is not consistent with its label and is allowed when treatment-approved drugs have failed, with new drugs based on emerging evidence, and as treatment for orphan conditions. Responsibility falls on the practicing physician to use drugs in a responsible manner (subject to controls through the third party reimbursement and the potential for malpractice claims). However, unapproved drugs, biologics, and medical devices require an IND, IDE, or an exemption. Unlike drugs, devices that have not been cleared by the FDA are sometimes used in routine clinical care.

What Is Not a Clinical Trial

Things that do not fall under the definition of clinical trials are routine clinical care, expanded access programs (emergency treatment, single-patient IND, treatment protocol), humanitarian use devices, observational studies and quality improvement studies (QA/QI). QA/QI studies (e.g., monitoring prescription errors in the pharmacy) may qualify for an exemption and may be published, despite not having institutional review board (IRB) review if it meets preceding criteria. (Example Source: answers.hhs.gov/ohrp/categories/1569; accessed January 22, 2013.)

Why Do Clinical Trials?

Clinical trials can be done for a number of reasons but are research performed on human subjects for the purpose of assessing the safety and/or effectiveness of an intervention. Does the new treatment work in humans? Is it better than what's now being used to treat a certain disease? Is it at least as good while perhaps causing fewer side effects? Or does it work in some people who are not helped by current treatments? Is the new treatment safe? The question to be answered is whether or not the benefits of the new treatment outweigh the possible risks. Assume that a new treatment has potential benefits in a population with a specific disease or condition. Any potential adverse effects resulting from the treatment may not be known. Without adequate and controlled clinical trials, these medicines may be used repeatedly in hundreds of locations before any significant adverse effect is identified and reported. More people will experience the negative effects of the drugs than would have if controlled trials had been conducted.

Designing Clinical Trials

Clinical trials can be observational trials, interventional trials, controlled, uncontrolled trials, or use historical controls, and involve human subjects as defined by 45 CFR 46.102(f) that is "a living individual about whom an investigator (whether professional or student) conducting research obtains: Data through intervention or interaction with the individual, or identifiable private information." The regulatory burden on the investigator is directly proportional to the reason for the study. For example, if the researcher is simply trying to determine whether one surgery is better than another to improve patient outcome, then the burden for conducting the appropriate trial is much lower than if she or he wants to publish the data or than that of the pharmaceutical company that is trying to bring new drugs, biologics, or devices to market. In the later case, planning drug development programs, designing and conducting clinical trials, organizing and analyzing trial data, submitting clinical study reports (CSRs) to the FDA, and manufacturing and marketing products are all necessary tasks to achieve the overall objective.

Types of Clinical Trials

Clinical trials can be categorized by sponsorship (industry-sponsored clinical trials, cooperative group studies, investigator-initiated (investigator sponsor) trials, cooperative group with industry support, multisite federally funded (e.g., subawards), investigator-initiated with industry support), funding source,

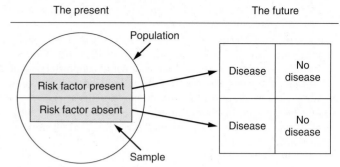

• **Fig. 27.1** Prospective cohort design. (Modified from Hulley SB, Cummings SR, Browner WS, Grady DG, Newman TB. *Designing Clinical Research.* 4th ed. Philadelphia: Lippincott Williams & Wilkins; 2013.)

comparative versus noncomparative, multicenter versus single center, behavioral versus biomedical, preclinical, or purpose that is phase I (safety and efficacy), phase II (single-arm efficacy), phase III (randomized comparison), phase IV (postmarketing), or as a Registry. Clinical trials can be classified into an almost endless set of categories to suit the needs of a particular situation.

Cohort Trials

The purpose of a cohort study is to describe the occurrence of outcomes in a group for subjects over time to analyze associations between predictors and outcomes. Such studies can be prospective or retrospective.

Prospective Cohort Study

A prospective cohort study selects a sample from the population; measures the predictor variables (whether the risk factor is present or absent); and measures the outcome variables at some specified time in the future (Fig. 27.1).

An example of a prospective cohort study would be an investigator who has access to a group of patients without known cancer and wants to examine the relationship between obesity and the development of breast cancer over time. The advantages of this type of study is that it is simple in design, can assess incidence, can measure variables accurately and prospectively, large sample sizes are possible, possible long periods of follow-up allow substantial statistical power, bias in measuring predictors is avoided, and the investigator is able to answer questions that cannot be answered otherwise. Disadvantages include that it is challenging to make causal inference; there can be a multitude of confounding variables (e.g., alcohol intake, *BRCA* incidence within the cohort), a change in predictor variables over time may alter risk for development of the outcome variables (e.g., weight loss or gain with individuals followed for risk of breast cancer with obesity), it is an expensive and inefficient way to study rare outcomes, and long periods of observation may be necessary (more efficient as outcomes become more common and immediate; e.g., measuring incidence of breast cancer in men vs. women).

Retrospective Cohort Study

In a retrospective cohort study (Fig. 27.2), the investigator identifies a cohort that has been assembled in the past, collects predictor variables from existing data (i.e., measured in the past), and measures outcome variables in the present.

For example, suppose that a researcher wanted to describe the natural history of breast cancer and risk factors that lead to breast

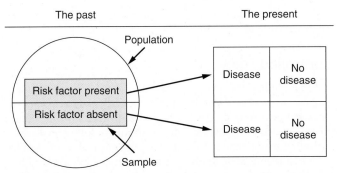

• **Fig. 27.2** Retrospective cohort study. (Modified from Hulley SB, Cummings SR, Browner WS, Grady DG, Newman TB. *Designing Clinical Research*. 4th ed. Philadelphia: Lippincott Williams & Wilkins; 2013.)

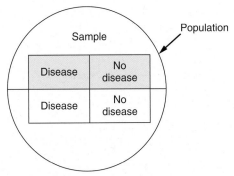

• **Fig. 27.3** Cross-sectional study design. (Modified from Hulley SB, Cummings SR, Browner WS, Grady DG, Newman TB. *Designing Clinical Research*. 4th ed. Philadelphia: Lippincott Williams & Wilkins; 2013.)

cancer death. First the researcher would identify a suitable cohort from the past (hospital records for all patients with breast cancer from 2000 to 2014 and identify all those who had breast cancer listed as their diagnosis). The next step would be to collect data about predictor variables in the past: review medical records of people with the diagnosis of breast cancer and disease-free or overall survival, and collect age, stage, treatment, family history, alcohol intake, obesity, and other factors. The researcher would then gather data on outcome—disease-free or overall survival as measured in the present but not prospectively.

The advantages of a retrospective cohort design is that it can be a very simple design, can have accurate measurement of outcome variables, the long period of follow-up and large sample size can provide substantial statistical power, and study time is often of shorter duration because predictor measurements have already been made and documented. In addition, such studies can be less costly and time-consuming than prospective cohort studies. Disadvantages of this study design are the limited control over sampling of the population; limited control over nature and quality of the predictor variables; retrospective data may have been collected using outmoded technology, poor technique, or other inadequate factors; the predictor measurements that are important or relevant may not have been recorded in the health record; and confounding variables and causality are difficult or impossible to prove (true of all observational studies).

Cross-Sectional Study Design

Cross-sectional studies are used to examine associations between variables. All data (i.e., variables) are collected at the same point in time. These are not longitudinal; there is no present, past, and future as in cohort studies. Labeling which variables are predictors and which are outcomes depends on the cause-and-effect hypothesis put forth by the investigator. The sample is represented by the top half of the circle in Fig. 27.3 and is drawn from the entire population represented by the circle. In a cross-sectional study, the desired sample is selected from the population, and then the variables are measured. Cross-sectional designs are similar to cohort studies except that the measurements are all made at about the same time.

For example, suppose a group of researchers wants to know whether patients with pubertal obesity had a greater risk of breast cancer. First the researchers would select their sample from the population—for example, all women in a gynecology practice. They would then identify and measure the predictor and outcome variables (e.g., the predictor is having had childhood obesity, and

the outcome is history of breast cancer). Note that there are many confounders that one may want to control for (e.g., age, family history). The researchers could then divide patients into quartiles based on body mass index at puberty and then determine whether they were more likely to get breast cancer depending on the quartile. The researchers assume that the sample is representative of the total population. They administer a questionnaire to gather information. The questionnaire is administered, and data for predictors and outcomes is gathered at the same time.

The advantages of this type of study is the immediacy (i.e., data can be collected quickly), no subjects are lost to follow-up, they tend to be inexpensive, and they can be included at the beginning of a cohort study (cross-sectional cohort design). However, it can be difficult to establish causal relationships from observational studies conducted at one point in time, and this design is impractical for rare diseases or conditions. Of note is that this type of study can measure prevalence (number of people with disease out of those at risk) but cannot measure incidence (prevalence over time).

Case-Control Study Design

A case-control study is a retrospective study that identifies patients with and without a disease and looks back to identify the presence or absence of risk factors. In this type of study, the research selects a sample from a population with the disease or condition (cases), then selects a sample from the population at risk that is free of the disease (controls) and then measures predictor variables. It can also be used to look at outcomes (e.g., patients with or without lymphedema after axillary node dissection) (Fig. 27.4).

The advantages of this type of study is that it may involve relatively few subjects; is inexpensive, of short duration, and useful to identify possible risk factors in rare diseases or conditions; may examine large numbers of predictor variables; is useful for generating hypotheses; and can provide an estimate of the strength of the association between predictor variables and the presence or absence of disease (odds ratio). However, case-control studies cannot yield estimates of incidence or prevalence of disease in a population (relatively low sample size); only one outcome variable can be studied; the sequence of events may not be clear; and they are susceptible to bias, including sampling bias, differential measurement bias, and recall bias (i.e., if you have a disease that is suspected of being caused by a drug, you may be more likely to recall exposure). Several strategies for controlling sampling bias that can be used are to select controls from the same hospital or clinic; matching of cases and controls; population-based samples

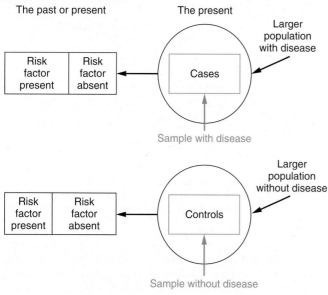

• **Fig. 27.4** Case-control study design.

(have become more common as registries have flourished); using more than one control group selected in different ways.

Interventional Trials

Interventional trials occur when a drug, device, or other treatment is applied to human subjects in a research setting. Interventional trials may be relatively simple uncontrolled trials or may involve more complicated designs, which may employ crossover techniques, masking, placebos, comparators, etc. Some of the more common types are discussed below.

Uncontrolled Trials

Uncontrolled trials are clinical studies in which an intervention is studied without the use of a control group. Common examples would be some phase I studies or phase II trials and pilot studies. Pilot studies are often performed to assess the feasibility of a larger trial, to test methods that will be used in a larger trial, or to generate a new hypothesis for further research. Studies may also be designed without a control group for ethical reasons. The advantages of such studies are that they provide justification for conducting a large-scale randomized controlled trial (i.e., preliminary data), they limit the number of subjects exposed to new drugs or treatments (e.g., no placebo), and it may not be ethically possible to have a control group (e.g., major surgery with anesthesia vs. no anesthesia). Disadvantages include that at the end of the study, it may not be certain that the treatment, rather than a random factor, was responsible for the outcome; the investigator cannot measure any placebo effect; such trials are susceptible to overinterpretation; and it is easy to introduce investigator bias (i.e., the desire of the investigator to see the new treatment work may lead to unconscious—or conscious—bias in selecting subjects).

Historical Controls

An uncontrolled trial may also make use of historical controls—that is, comparison of the results of a new study with results from previous reports (i.e., historical data). There are many potential confounders using this approach, such as differences in diagnostic methodology, ancillary treatments, or complications, for example.

An investigator should consider this design only if there is no other way to compare outcomes.

Controlled Trials

Control implies the use of a randomization scheme (random assignment to one of two or more interventions or sequences of interventions) to reduce the risk of bias. In recent years, clinical trials have demonstrated the value of treatment for many diseases, including breast cancer. With the development of more detailed statistical theories and applications, experimental design and biostatistical analysis have become more important in evaluating the effectiveness of diagnostic techniques, as well as treatments. Several key components of well-performed clinical trials, such as trial design, randomization, sample size determination, interim monitoring, and evaluation of clinical effects, are highly dependent on successful application of biostatistics and an understanding of probabilities. Input from an experienced biostatistician is valuable and highly desirable during the design of the study.

For trials involving FDA-regulated products, the application of biostatistics is relevant throughout phase I, II, III, and IV clinical trials. Phase I trials introduce investigational drugs or devices to humans. The primary objectives of a phase I trial are to generate preliminary information on the biochemical properties of a drug, such as metabolism, pharmacokinetics, and bioavailability, and to determine a safe drug dose, dosing ranges, or schedule of administration. Phase I studies may also provide preliminary evidence of a drug's activity by means of a pharmacodynamic or biomarker response. The focus of the phase I trial is assessment of safety and dose selection; a phase I trial is usually a nonrandomized dose-escalation study with no more than 20 to 80 normal volunteers or patients with disease. For trials involving drugs with significant known toxicity, patients with the target disease or condition are usually used in phase I trials. For less toxic compounds (e.g., an antihypertensive drug), healthy adult volunteers are often used.

In oncology trials, one goal of phase I is usually to determine a safe and/or potentially effective dose to be used in phase II. For cytotoxic agents, the primary objective of the phase I trial is often to determine the maximum tolerated dose (MTD) for a new drug and to evaluate qualitative and quantitative toxicities. For noncytotoxic agents, the primary objective of the phase I trial is to identify the optimal biologically effective dose. For target or novel agents, the phase I trial is designed to determine the minimum effective blood concentration level of the agent or minimum expression level of a molecular target.

Phase II trials provide preliminary information on the efficacy of a drug and additional information on safety and dosing ranges. These trials may be designed to include a control or may use a single-arm design, enrolling 20 to 200 or more patients with disease. It is important that phase II studies provide data on the doses or interventions to be used in phase III, although this may not be as easy as it appears. For phase II oncology trials, tumor response rate is usually the primary end point. Time to progression also may serve as the primary end point, when the estimated median time to progression is relatively short for the study agent. In addition, an early stopping rule is common in phase II oncology trials to prevent the testing of ineffective drugs or agents in more patients.

The phase III trial is a full-scale treatment evaluation, with the primary goal of comparing efficacy of a new treatment with that of the standard regimen. Phase III trials are usually randomized controlled studies enrolling several hundred to several thousand

TABLE 27.1	Probability of Escalating a Dose With a Particular Dose-Limiting Toxicity Rate in the 3 + 3 Trial Design							
True dose-limiting toxicity rate	10%	20%	30%	40%	50%	70%	80%	90%
Probability of escalating	0.91	0.71	0.49	0.31	0.17	0.03	0.01	0.001

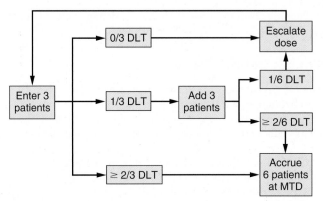

• **Fig. 27.5** The 3 + 3 design, which is the most commonly used phase I oncology trial design. *DLT,* Dose-limiting toxicity; *MTD,* maximum tolerated dose.

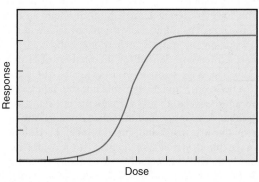

• **Fig. 27.6** Dose-response curve. With the continual reassessment method, the response of interest is toxicity.

patients with disease. For oncology phase III trials, overall survival is usually the primary end point; however, time to progression also may serve as the primary end point if the estimated median overall survival time is relatively long for the study agent. Two distinct treatment regimens might be compared, but often an add-on design is used in which standard therapy and standard therapy plus an investigational agent are compared. Other study designs are possible as well.

To look for uncommon long-term side effects, phase IV or postregistration trials may be conducted after regulatory approval of a new treatment or drug. Thus phase IV trials evaluate agents or drugs already available for physicians to prescribe, rather than new drugs still being developed. These trials can be designed as randomized studies, but they are usually prospective observational studies with thousands of patients.

Trial Design for Phase I Oncology Studies

As mentioned in the previous section, the primary objective of the phase I oncology trial is usually to determine the MTD of a new cytotoxic drug or agent. The most common phase I oncology trial design is the 3 + 3 design (Fig. 27.5). In this design, at least three patients are studied at each dose level and evaluated for toxicity. At any given dose level, three patients are accrued. If none of these patients experiences a dose-limiting toxicity (DLT), the dose is escalated. If one of these patients experiences a DLT, three additional patients are treated. If none of the additional patients develops a DLT, the dose is escalated; otherwise, escalation ceases. If at any time at least two patients (≥2 of 3 or ≥2 of 6) experience a DLT, the MTD has been exceeded. For a dose level at which a patient has a high probability of developing a DLT, the probability of escalation to a higher dose level should be low. As shown in Table 27.1, if the dose level has a true DLT rate of 70%, the probability of escalating a certain dose is only 3%.

Another commonly used phase I oncology trial design is the continual reassessment method, introduced by O'Quigley, Pepe,

and Fisher.[5] Like the 3 + 3 design, the continual reassessment method is designed to determine MTD. This method can be described as a one-parameter Bayesian-based logit model (Fig. 27.6), which describes the association between dose level (x-axis) and toxicity level (y-axis). The investigator picks a target toxicity level for the study agent, for example, 30%. Given this target toxicity, the investigator then selects a first or starting dose associated with this toxicity, using a prior dose-toxicity curve, which may be based on an animal model, results from a similar study, or the investigator's experience. After testing the first dose, the investigator recalculates the dose associated with the target probability of toxicity. This estimated dose is used to treat the next patient(s). The process of treating, evaluating toxicity, statistical model fitting, and dose estimation is repeated until the model converges (i.e., data from additional patients do not improve the model). The advantages of the continual reassessment method are that it is somewhat more efficient than the 3 + 3 design and has an unbiased estimation method. Several other designs, many involving adaptive methods, have been proposed.[5a] The goal of these methods is to improve upon the ability of the 3 + 3 design to identify the dose and toxicity of investigational compounds. No one method for conducting phase I trials has proven to be superior to the others in all instances.

Trial Design for Phase II Oncology Studies

One of the primary objectives of a phase II oncology trial of a new drug or agent is to determine whether the agent has sufficient antitumor activity to warrant more extensive development. Two-stage phase II designs are widely used in oncology studies. Several two-stage designs are discussed in this section: Gehan's, Fleming's, Simon's optimal, Simon's minimax, and Fei and Shyr's balanced two-stage designs.

Gehan's Design

Gehan's design[6] is a two-stage design that estimates response rate while providing for early termination if the drug shows insufficient antitumor activity or effectiveness in the case of a device. The design is most commonly used with the first stage of 14 patients. If no responses (completed or partial) are observed, the trial is terminated. The rationale for stopping is that if the true response probability were at least 20%, at least one response would likely be observed in the first 14 patients; if no responses are seen, it is unlikely that the true response rate is at least 20%. If at least one response is observed in the first 14 patients, then the second stage of accrual is carried out to obtain an estimate of the response rate. The number of patients to accrue in the second stage depends on the number of responses observed in the first stage and the precision desired for the final estimate of response rate. If the first stage consists of 14 patients, the second stage consists of between 1 and 11 patients if a standard error of 10% is desired and between 45 and 86 patients if a standard error of 5% is desired. A common use of Gehan's design is to accrue 14 patients in the first stage and an additional 11 patients in the second stage, for a total of 25 patients. This provides an estimate of response rate with a standard error of about 10%, which corresponds to very broad confidence limits. For example, if three responses are observed among 25 patients, a 95% confidence limit for the true response rate is from about 3% to about 30%.

A limitation of Gehan's design is that a poor drug may be allowed to move to the second stage. For example, if a drug has a response rate of only 5%, there exists a 51% chance of at least one response among the first 14 patients. Thus the first stage of 14 patients will not effectively screen out all inactive drugs.

Fleming's Design

Fleming presented a multistage design for testing the hypothesis that the probability of a true response is less than some uninteresting level (e.g., 5% response rate) against the hypothesis that the probability of a true response is at least as large as a target level (e.g., 20% response rate).[7] Table 27.2 shows two examples of Fleming's design.

As a third example, consider a design with an uninteresting level of a 5% response rate and a clinically interesting (i.e., clinically significant) level of a 20% response rate, for which both error limits (type I and type II) are to be less than 10%. These constraints can be met with a two-stage Fleming's design with 15 patients in the first stage and 20 in the second stage, as follows:
1. If no responses are observed in the first 15 patients, then the trial is terminated and the drug is rejected.

2. If at least three responses are observed in the first 15 patients, then the trial is terminated and the drug is accepted.
3. If one to two responses are observed in the first 15 patients, then 20 more patients are accrued.
4. After all 35 patients are evaluated, the drug is accepted if the response rate is 11.4% or greater (≥4 responses in 35 patients), and the drug is rejected if the response rate is 8.6% or less (≤3 in 35 patients).

Fleming's design is the only two-stage design covered here that may terminate early with an "accept the drug" conclusion.

Simon's Optimal Design

Simon's optimal two-stage designs[8] are optimal in the sense that the expected sample size is minimized if the regimen has low activity subject to type I and type II error probability constraints. The following values provide an example of Simon's optimal design:

Clinically uninteresting level = 5% response rate
Clinically interesting level = 20% response rate
Type I error (α) = 0.05
Type II error (β) = 0.20
Power = 1 − type II error = 0.80
Stage I: Reject the drug if the response rate is ≤0/10
Stage II: Reject the drug if the response rate is ≤3/29

In this example, the first stage consists of 10 patients. If no responses are seen in the first 10 patients, the trial is terminated. Otherwise, accrual continues to a total of 29 patients. If there are at least four responses in the total of 29 patients, the trial may move to a phase III study. The average sample size is 17.6, and the probability of early termination is 60% for a drug with a response rate of 5% (low activity). Simon's optimal design is the most commonly used two-stage design.

Simon's Minimax Design

Simon's minimax two-stage design[8] minimizes maximum sample size subject to type I and type II error probability constraints. The following values provide an example of Simon's minimax design:

Clinically uninteresting level = 5% response rate
Clinically interesting level = 20% response rate
Type I error (α) = 0.05
Type II error (β) = 0.20
Power = 1 − type II error = 0.80
Stage I: Reject the drug if the response rate is ≤0/13
Stage II: Reject the drug if the response rate is ≤3/27

In this example, the first stage consists of 13 patients. If no responses are seen in the first 13 patients, the trial is terminated. Otherwise, accrual continues to a total of 27 patients. If there are at least four responses in the total of 27 patients, the trial may move to a phase III study. The average sample size is 19.8, and the probability of early termination is 51% for a drug with a response rate of 5% (low activity).

Comparisons of the Optimal and Minimax Designs

Simon's optimal two-stage design minimizes expected sample size, but it does not necessarily minimize maximum sample size,

TABLE 27.2	**Examples of Fleming's Two-Stage Design**								
				REJECT DRUG IF RESPONSE RATE		ACCEPT DRUG IF RESPONSE RATE			
P0	P1	n1	n	≤r1/n1	≤r/n	≥r1/n1	≥r/n	α	β
0.05	0.20	15	35	0/15	3/35	3/15	4/35	0.10	0.08
0.05	0.25	15	25	1/15	2/25	3/15	3/25	0.09	0.09

α, Type I error rate; *β*, type II error rate; *n*, total sample size; *n1*, stage I sample size; *P0*, uninteresting response rate; *P1*, clinically interesting response rate; *r*, total number of responses observed at end of stage II; *r1*, number of responses observed in stage I.

subject to error probability constraints. As a result, the minimax design may be more attractive when the difference in expected sample sizes is small and the accrual rate is low. Consider, for example, the case of distinguishing the uninteresting response rate of 10% from the clinically interesting response rate of 30% with $\alpha = \beta = 10\%$. The optimal design has an expected sample size of 19.8 and a maximum sample size of 35. The minimax design has an expected sample size of 20.4 and a maximum sample size of 25. If the accrual rate is only 10 patients per year, it could take 1 year longer to complete the optimal design than the minimax design. This may be more important than the slight reduction in expected sample size.

Fei and Shyr's Balanced Design

As discussed in the previous subsections, Simon's optimal and minimax two-stage designs are commonly used for phase II oncology trials. The optimal design minimizes expected sample size, and the minimax design minimizes maximum sample size. Neither method, however, considers balance between sample sizes in stages I and II (n1 and n2, respectively). For example, with the minimax design, if the investigator is testing a 15% improvement (0.50 vs. 0.65) in response rate, 66 patients are required in stage I but only two patients in stage 2 (n1/n2 = 33). Thus there is little value in early termination; this saves enrolling only two patients. As another example, with the optimal design, if the investigator is testing a 15% improvement (0.35 vs. 0.50) in response rate, 19 patients are required in stage I and 68 additional patients in stage II (n1/n2 = 0.28). In a case such as this, clinical investigators may resist early termination, given that stage I includes only 22% of the total target accrual. To address issues such as these, Fei and Shyr proposed a balanced two-stage design focused on balancing the sample size ratio (n1/n2), subject to type 1 and type 2 error probability constraints.[9] With Fei and Shyr's balanced two-stage design, expected sample size is less than that of the minimax design, and/or maximum sample size is less than that of the optimal design. Tables 27.3 and 27.4 provide examples of balanced design, with comparison to optimal design (see Table 27.3) or minimax design (see Table 27.4). Tables 27.5 and 27.6 provide a more detailed comparison of stage I sample sizes, total sample sizes, expected sample sizes, probability of early termination, and sample size ratios for optimal, minimax, and balanced designs.

Balanced design provides an additional two-stage design choice. This choice allows investigators to stop a trial near the halfway point.

Trial Design for Phase III Randomized Controlled Studies

The most common types of randomized controlled study design are the parallel design, crossover design, and factorial design. Fig. 27.7 illustrates *parallel design*. After patients are recruited, they are randomly assigned to either the intervention group or the control group (i.e., placebo group or standard groups); after the course of therapy is completed, outcomes are measured in each group. There are many variations of the parallel design employing more than two groups, dose escalation within an arm, re-randomization, equivalence, etc. Advantages of this study design are that (1) randomization tends to produce comparable groups and removes bias in the allocation of participants to intervention group versus control group and (2) the validity of statistical tests of significance is likely guaranteed. One major problem with parallel design is that patients vary both in their initial disease state and in their response to therapy. Because of this interpatient variability, the investigator needs substantial groups of patients in each treatment to estimate reliably the magnitude of any treatment difference (see the next section, "Sample Size Determination and Power Analysis," for a discussion of sample size determination).

The *crossover design* is also a randomized controlled study design, in which patients cross from one therapy (e.g., intervention) to another (e.g., placebo). The difference between crossover and parallel designs is that patients in crossover trials receive each treatment in sequence, sometimes with a washout before or between treatments. For example, as illustrated in Fig. 27.8, patients assigned to order I receive treatment A (e.g., intervention) followed by treatment B (e.g., placebo). Patients assigned to order II receive treatment B followed by treatment A. Between the two treatment periods, all patients enter a washout, to ensure they

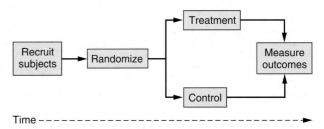

• **Fig. 27.7** Parallel design. Patients are randomized to either treatment or control.

| TABLE 27.3 | Examples of Balanced Two-Stage Design, With Comparison to Optimal Design |

				OPTIMAL DESIGN			BALANCED DESIGN		
P_0	P_1	α	β	n_1	n_2	n_1:n_2	n_1	n_2	n_1:n_2
0.75	0.95	0.05	0.20	3	19	0.16	11	11	1
0.35	0.50	0.10	0.20	19	68	0.28	43	44	0.98
0.70	0.90	0.05	0.20	6	21	0.29	14	14	1

α, Type I error rate; β, type II error rate; n_1, stage I sample size; n_2, stage II sample size; P_0, uninteresting response rate; P_1, clinically interesting response rate.

| TABLE 27.4 | Examples of Balanced Two-Stage Design, With Comparison to Minimax Design |

				MINIMAX DESIGN			BALANCED DESIGN		
P_0	P_1	α	β	n_1	n_2	n_1:n_2	n_1	n_2	n_1:n_2
0.45	0.60	0.05	0.10	93	2	46.5	58	58	1
0.50	0.65	0.05	0.20	66	2	33	39	39	1
0.70	0.90	0.05	0.20	6	21	0.29	14	14	1

α, Type I error rate; β, type II error rate; n_1, stage I sample size; n_2, stage II sample size; P_0, uninteresting response rate; P_1, clinically interesting response rate.

TABLE 27.5 Optimal, Minimax, and Balanced Designs for Independent Data, $p^1 - p^0 = .15$

		OPTIMAL DESIGN					MINIMAX DESIGN					BALANCED DESIGN				
		REJECT DRUG IF RESPONSE RATE					REJECT DRUG IF RESPONSE RATE					REJECT DRUG IF RESPONSE RATE				
p_0	p_1	$\leq r_1/n_1$	$\leq r/n$	EN (p_0)	PET (p_0)	$n_1{:}n_2$	$\leq r_1/n_1$	$\leq r/n$	EN (p_0)	PET (p_0)	$n_1{:}n_2$	$\leq r_1/n_1$	$\leq r/n$	EN (p_0)	PET (p_0)	$n_1{:}n_2$
0.05	0.20	0/12	3/37	23.5	0.54	0.48	0/18	3/32	26.4	0.4	1.29	1/19	3/38	23.7	0.75	1
		0/10	3/29	17.6	0.6	0.53	0/13	3/27	19.8	0.51	0.93	0/14	3/28	21.2	0.49	1
		1/21	4/41	26.7	0.72	1.05	1/29	4/38	32.9	0.57	3.22	1/21	4/42	26.9	0.72	1
0.10	0.25	2/21	7/50	31.2	0.65	0.72	2/27	6/40	33.7	0.48	2.08	2/24	7/48	34.5	0.56	1
		2/18	7/43	24.7	0.73	0.72	2/22	7/40	28.8	0.62	1.22	2/21	7/42	28.4	0.65	1[a]
		2/21	10/66	36.8	0.65	0.47	3/31	9/55	40	0.62	1.29	4/32	10/64	38.8	0.79	1[a]
0.20	0.35	5/27	16/63	43.6	0.54	0.75	6/33	15/58	45.5	0.5	1.32	6/32	16/62	45.9	0.54	1.07
		5/22	19/72	35.4	0.73	0.44	6/31	15/53	40.4	0.57	1.41	7/31	17/62	39.4	0.73	1[a]
		8/37	22/83	51.4	0.69	0.8	8/42	21/77	58.4	0.53	1.2	8/39	21/78	53.7	0.62	1[a]
0.3	0.45	9/30	29/82	51.4	0.59	0.58	16/50	25/69	56	0.68	2.63	12/39	28/78	53.9	0.62	1[a]
		9/27	30/81	41.7	0.73	0.5	16/46	25/65	49.6	0.81	2.42	11/34	26/68	44.4	0.69	1[a]
		13/40	40/110	60.8	0.7	0.57	27/77	33/88	78.5	0.86	7	18/53	39/106	64.4	0.78	1[a]
0.4	0.55	16/38	40/88	54.5	0.67	0.76	18/45	34/73	57.2	0.56	1.61	19/44	40/80	56.2	0.72	1[a]
		11/26	42/88	46.2	0.67	0.42	28/59	34/70	60.1	0.9	5.36	17/39	38/78	49.3	0.73	1[a]
		19/45	49/104	64	0.68	0.76	24/62	45/94	78.9	0.47	1.94	23/53	50/105	66.7	0.74	1
0.5	0.65	18/35	47/84	53	0.63	0.71	19/40	41/72	58	0.44	1.25	20/39	44/78	53.6	0.63	1[a]
		15/28	48/83	43.7	0.71	0.51	39/66	40/68	66.1	0.95	33	21/39	46/78	49.2	0.74	1[a]
		22/42	60/105	62.3	0.68	0.67	28/57	54/93	75	0.5	1.58	25/50	58/100	72.2	0.56	1[a]
0.6	0.75	21/34	47/71	47.1	0.65	0.92	25/43	43/64	54.4	0.46	2.05	24/38	50/76	49	0.71	1
		17/27	46/67	39.3	0.69	0.68	18/30	43/62	43.8	0.57	0.94	22/34	46/67	41.7	0.77	1.03
		21/34	64/95	55.6	0.65	0.56	48/72	57/84	73.2	0.9	6	28/45	61/90	59.7	0.67	1[a]
0.7	0.85	14/20	45/59	36.2	0.58	0.51	15/22	40/52	36.8	0.51	0.73	18/26	40/52	38	0.54	1
		14/19	46/59	30.3	0.72	0.47	16/23	39/49	34.4	0.56	0.88	21/28	44/56	34.2	0.78	1[a]
		18/25	61/79	43.4	0.66	0.46	33/44	53/68	48.5	0.81	1.83	28/38	59/76	47.7	0.74	1[a]
0.80	0.95	5/7	27/31	20.8	0.42	0.29	5/7	27/31	20.8	0.42	0.29	5/7	27/31	20.8	0.42	0.29
		7/9	26/29	17.7	0.56	0.45	7/9	26/29	17.7	0.56	0.45	7/9	26/29	17.7	0.56	0.45
		16/19	37/42	24.4	0.76	0.83	31/35	35/40	35.3	0.94	7	18/22	39/44	29.3	0.67	1

[a]Balanced design has both expected and maximum sample sizes between those of optimal and minimax designs.

EN, Expected sample size; *n*, total sample size; n_1, stage I sample size; p_0, uninteresting response rate; p_1, clinically interesting response rate; *PET*, probability of early termination; *r*, lower bound for total number of responses observed at end of stage II; r_1, lower bound for number of responses observed in stage I.

From Fei Y, Shyr Y. Balanced two-stage designs for phase II clinical trials. *Clin Trials.* 2007;4:514–524.

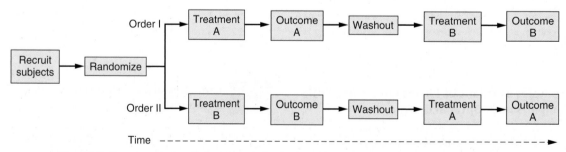

• **Fig. 27.8** Crossover design. Patients are randomized to either treatment A followed by treatment B or treatment B followed by treatment A.

return to their pretreatment baseline before starting the second assigned treatment. The advantages of this design are that (1) interpatient variability is reduced because each patient serves as his or her own control and (2) study sample size tends to be reduced. Disadvantages include (1) a fairly strict assumption about treatment carryover must be made (i.e., the effects of the

intervention during the first period must not carry over into the second period), and (2) it is difficult to design a crossover study for oncology trials.

The other commonly used randomized controlled study is the *factorial design.* Fig. 27.9 shows the details of the factorial design. The patients in this design are randomized to one of multiple

TABLE 27.6 Optimal, Minimax, and Balanced Designs for Independent Data, $p^1 - p^0 = .20$

		OPTIMAL DESIGN					MINIMAX DESIGN					BALANCED DESIGN				
		REJECT DRUG IF RESPONSE RATE					REJECT DRUG IF RESPONSE RATE					REJECT DRUG IF RESPONSE RATE				
p_0	p_1	$\leq r_1/n_1$	$\leq r/n$	EN (p_0)	PET (p_0)	$n_1:n_2$	$\leq r_1/n_1$	$\leq r/n$	EN (p_0)	PET (p_0)	$n_1:n_2$	$\leq r_1/n_1$	$\leq r/n$	EN (p_0)	PET (p_0)	$n_1:n_2$
0.05	0.25	0/9	2/24	14.5	0.63	0.6	0/13	2/20	16.4	0.51	1.86	0/11	2/22	15.7	0.57	1[a]
		0/9	2/17	12	0.63	1.13	0/12	2/16	13.8	0.54	3	1/12	3/25	13.5	0.88	0.92
		0/9	3/30	16.8	0.63	0.43	0/15	3/25	20.4	0.46	1.5	1/15	3/30	17.6	0.83	1
0.10	0.3	1/12	5/35	19.8	0.66	0.52	1/16	4/25	20.4	0.51	1.78	2/17	5/34	21	0.76	1
		1/10	5/29	15	0.74	0.53	1/15	5/25	19.5	0.55	1.5	1/13	5/26	17.9	0.62	1[a]
		2/18	6/35	22.5	0.73	1.06	2/22	6/33	26.2	0.62	2	3/22	8/44	25.8	0.83	1
0.20	0.4	3/17	10/37	26	0.55	0.85	3/19	10/36	28.3	0.46	1.12	4/20	11/40	27.4	0.63	1
		3/13	12/43	20.6	0.75	0.43	4/18	10/33	22.3	0.72	1.2	4/18	11/36	23.1	0.72	1
		4/19	15/54	30.4	0.67	0.54	5/24	13/45	31.2	0.66	1.14	5/24	14/48	32.3	0.66	1
0.3	0.5	7/22	17/46	29.9	0.67	0.92	7/28	15/39	35	0.36	2.55	6/21	16/42	30.4	0.55	1[a]
		5/15	18/46	23.6	0.72	0.48	6/19	16/39	25.7	0.67	0.95	7/21	17/42	26.8	0.72	1
		8/24	24/63	34.7	0.73	0.62	7/24	21/53	36.6	0.56	0.83	9/28	22/56	36.9	0.68	1
0.4	0.6	7/18	22/46	30.2	0.56	0.64	11/28	20/41	33.8	0.55	2.15	10/24	23/48	32.4	0.65	1
		7/16	23/46	24.5	0.72	0.53	17/34	20/39	34.4	0.91	6.8	12/25	25/50	28.8	0.85	1
		11/25	32/66	36	0.73	0.61	12/29	27/54	38.1	0.64	1.16	13/30	30/60	38.6	0.71	1
0.5	0.7	11/21	26/45	29	0.67	0.88	11/23	23/39	31	0.5	1.44	12/23	27/46	30.8	0.66	1
		8/15	26/43	23.5	0.7	0.54	12/23	23/37	27.7	0.66	1.64	12/21	26/43	25.2	0.81	0.95
		13/24	36/61	34	0.73	0.65	14/27	32/53	36.1	0.65	1.04	16/29	35/59	35.9	0.77	0.97[a]
0.6	0.8	6/11	26/38	25.4	0.47	0.41	18/27	24/35	28.5	0.82	3.38	10/18	25/36	28.1	0.44	1[a]
		7/11	30/43	20.5	0.7	0.34	8/13	25/35	20.8	0.65	0.59	11/18	26/36	24.7	0.63	1
		12/19	37/53	29.5	0.69	0.56	15/26	32/45	35.9	0.48	1.37	16/25	35/50	31.8	0.73	1[a]
0.7	0.9	6/9	22/28	17.8	0.54	0.47	11/16	20/25	20	0.55	1.78	11/15	24/30	19.5	0.7	1
		4/6	22/27	14.8	0.58	0.29	19/23	21/26	23.2	0.95	7.67	10/14	23/28	19	0.64	1
		11/15	29/36	21.2	0.7	0.71	13/18	26/32	22.7	0.67	1.29	13/17	31/39	21.4	0.8	0.77

[a]Balanced design has both expected and maximum sample sizes between those of optimal and minimax designs.

EN, Expected sample size; *n*, total sample size; n_1, stage I sample size; p_0, uninteresting response rate; p_1, clinically interesting response rate; *PET*, probability of early termination; *r*, lower bound for total number of responses observed at end of stage II; r_1, lower bound for number of responses observed in stage I.

From Fei Y, Shyr Y. Balanced two-stage designs for phase II clinical trials. *Clin Trials*. 2007;4:514–524.

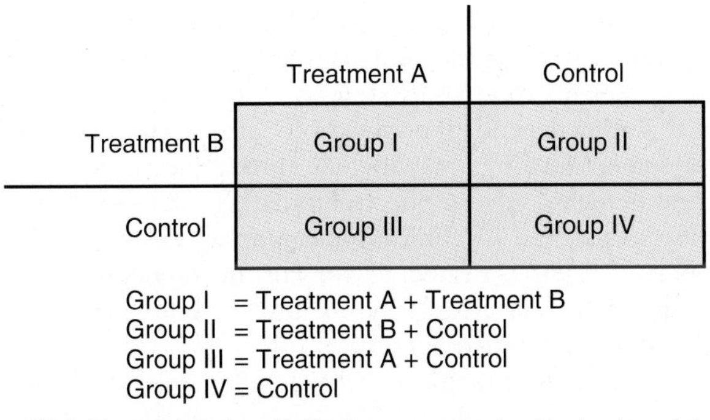

	Treatment A	Control
Treatment B	Group I	Group II
Control	Group III	Group IV

Group I = Treatment A + Treatment B
Group II = Treatment B + Control
Group III = Treatment A + Control
Group IV = Control

• **Fig. 27.9** Factorial design. Patients are randomized to treatment A plus treatment B, treatment A only, treatment B only, or control.

study groups in this illustration: patients assigned to group I receive treatment A (e.g., chemotherapy) and treatment B (e.g., radiation therapy) together; patients assigned to group II or group III receive treatment B or treatment A only, respectively; and group IV is the true placebo or control group. This design is often used in an attempt to identify the most effective dosing combination of two or more treatments. Advantages of this study design are that (1) the investigator is able to evaluate multiple interventions compared with a control in a single experiment, and (2) study sample size tends to be reduced. A concern with factorial design is the possibility of interaction between the two interventions and the effect of potential interaction on the sample size.

Randomization Process

One of the strengths of randomized clinical trials is reduction in bias. Bias may be defined as systematic error or the difference between the true value and that obtained due to all causes other than sampling variability. The randomization process is one of the best tools to reduce bias in clinical trials. Through randomization, each subject has the same chance of being assigned to either intervention or control; to remove investigator bias, neither the subject nor the investigator should know the treatment assignment before the subject's decision to enter the study. Randomization tends to produce groups that are comparable with respect to known or unknown risk factors, prognostic variables, and covariates; it also tends to guarantee the validity of statistical tests.

There are several methods for making random treatment assignments. Many attempt to balance treatment groups over time, over stratification factors, or both. In the following, we assume equal allocation of patients to each treatment (i.e., 1:1 randomization). Complete randomization is the most elementary form of randomization. One simple method of complete randomization is to toss an unbiased coin. Another common method is to generate a random-digit table using a computer program and assign patients with even digits to treatment A and odd digits to treatment B. The advantage of complete randomization is that it is easy to implement; the disadvantage is that, at any point in time, there may be an imbalance in the number of subjects on each treatment. For instance, with n = 20, the chance of a 12:8 split or worse is approximately 50%; with n = 100, the chance of a 60:40 split or worse is still greater than 5%. Thus it may be desirable to restrict randomization to ensure similar treatment numbers throughout the trial. Here we look at three approaches to restricting randomization: replacement randomization, random permuted block randomization, and biased coin randomization.

In replacement randomization, the investigator prespecifies an amount of imbalance that would be unacceptable during the trial. For example, with n = 100 patients on each treatment, the treatment imbalance (number on treatment A minus number on treatment B) should be less than six at any point in time. A simple randomization method is then used to generate a randomization list. If the imbalance is unacceptable based on the prespecified criterion, a new list is generated. This process is repeated as necessary until an acceptable list is obtained.

Random permuted block randomization was described by Hill.[10] This technique is used to avoid serious imbalance in the number of participants assigned to each group and to equalize the number of subjects on each treatment. A block of size b is specified. For each block of b subjects enrolled in the study, b/2 are assigned to each treatment. In the case of block size four, there are six possible combinations of group assignments: AABB, ABAB, BAAB, BABA, BBAA, and ABBA. One of these arrangements is selected at random, and the four participants are assigned accordingly. This process is repeated as many times as needed. The advantage of blocking is that balance between the numbers of participants in each group is guaranteed throughout the course of randomization; thus, if the trial is terminated before enrollment is completed, balance exists in terms of number of participants randomized to each group.

Biased coin randomization is a baseline adaptive randomization procedure, originally discussed by Efron.[11] This technique attempts to balance the number of participants in each treatment group on the basis of previous assignments, but it does not take participant responses into consideration. The purpose of the algorithm is basically to randomize the allocation of participants to groups A and B with equal probability, as long as the number of participants in each group is equal or nearly equal. If an imbalance occurs and the difference in the number of participants is greater than some prespecified value c, the allocation probability p needs to be adjusted to increase the probability of allocation to the group with fewer participants. In other words, if the number of subjects already on each treatment (n_A and n_B) is equal ($n_A \approx n_B$), then we randomize to either treatment with the probability of assignment to each group being equal ($p = \frac{1}{2}$). If $n_A > n_B + c$, then we increase the probability of allocation to treatment B to be greater than 50%. If $n_B > n_A + c$, then we increase the probability of allocation to treatment A to be greater than 50%. Advantages

of this method include that (1) the next treatment assignment cannot be predicted and that the (2) statistical power is greater with equal allocation.

Sample Size Determination and Power Analysis

Clinical trials should have sufficient statistical power to detect differences in treatment outcomes considered to be of clinical interest. Therefore calculation of sample size to ensure statistical significance and adequate power is an essential part of planning. Power can be defined as the probability of rejecting the null hypothesis if a specific alternative (e.g., clinically significant improvement) is true. The biggest danger of low study power (i.e., insufficient sample size) is that no conclusion can be made if a statistically significant difference is not found. Instead of discussing the statistical techniques involved in calculating power, this section focuses on the principles that may affect power analysis. The following questions should be considered before the power analysis:

- What is the desired outcome of the trial? Is it a superiority trial, equivalence trial, or noninferiority trial? Superiority trials are designed to detect a difference between treatments (i.e., that one treatment is superior to another based on a measurable difference in a predetermined outcome). Noninferiority trials are designed to show that a new treatment is not much worse than an existing treatment (i.e., active control). Equivalence trials are designed to confirm the absence of a difference between study groups.
- What study design will be used to achieve the study goal? How many arms are needed? Will the study use a parallel design, crossover design, or factorial design, or some other design? Adaptive designs are gaining in popularity and present unique advantages and challenges. In adaptive trials, data collected during the experiment is used while the trial is underway to modify the design without compromising the integrity of the trial.
- What is the study's principal measure of interest (i.e., primary end point)? What is the study's primary outcome variable? Is it an interval variable, categorical variable, or time-to-event variable? Defining the primary outcome variable is critically important for most study designs. The success or failure of a trial is often dependent on the choice of an appropriate primary outcome. Outcomes may include clinical measures, laboratory measurements, adverse effects, biomarkers, etc. Good outcome measures should be clinically meaningful, easily measured by validated means, related to the disease or condition under study, and occur frequently enough to limit the number of subjects to a reasonable number.
- What result is anticipated with standard treatment, possibly based on other similar studies? For example, in an add-on study design often used in oncology trials, the standard treatment is defined. Subjects may be randomized to receive standard treatment or standard treatment *plus* the experimental intervention. A careful review of the literature, perhaps including the ClinicalTrial.gov database, should be done prior to designing and initiating a clinical trial to ensure that the study has not already been done, or if it has been done, that there is justification for repeating the trial.
- How small a treatment difference is it important to detect (i.e., what is the smallest clinically significant level of difference

between treatments)? With what degree of certainty must this difference be detected? This factor will be an important determinant of sample size. The smaller the clinically meaningful difference in an outcome measure and the greater the variability in that measure, the larger the sample size will be needed to detect the difference with a reasonable degree of certainty.

- Which statistical method will be used to estimate sample size? Is the method to be used a statistical test, confidence interval method, or computer simulation? It is usually wise to engage a biostatistician in this aspect of study design. A statistical plan should be completed prior to the initiation of the study in almost all instances.
- What is the ratio of treatment assignments? Will patients be randomized to intervention and control in a 1:1 ratio, or will more participants be assigned to the intervention group than to the control group? There may be good reasons to select a randomization rate different from the standard 1:1 ratio. In studies with multiple interventions, the randomization schedule may be 1:1:1:1. … In some instances, it may be desirable to skew randomization to increase the number of subjects in the intervention group (e.g., 2:1). The biostatistician can help to determine how such alternate allocations affect the power of the study and the number of subjects required to complete it.
- How will the data be analyzed? Is there any drop-in or drop-out adjustment? Various studies use intention-to-treat or per protocol methods. In intention-to-treat designs, all randomized subjects are used in the data analysis. In per-protocol analysis, only those subjects who completed the protocol are included in the analysis. Intention-to-treat designs generally are more robust because all data are included in the analysis, which is especially important in examining the reasons that subjects may have been discontinued from the study (e.g., if they experienced a significant adverse effect prior to completing the study, they would be included in the intention-to-treat analysis but not in the per-protocol analysis). This may skew the outcome of the study, especially if there are many subjects who were dropped from the study prior to its completion. Another significant issue is whether subjects who discontinue participation in the study prior to collection of the primary outcome measure should be replaced or not. If this is important to the study, most investigators will estimate the dropout rate prior to the initiation of the study.

Sample size calculations are approximate. They are often based on roughly estimated parameter values from mathematical models, which only approximate truth. Because of the approximate nature of sample size calculations, it is best to be liberal when estimating sample size (i.e., overestimate rather than underestimate).

Monitoring Response Variables

Industry sponsored trials, cooperative group studies, and many large, investigator-initiated trials will be monitored by the sponsor. Monitoring is done to assure that the data are captured and reported correctly and that adverse events are reported according to guidelines established by the FDA, NIH, sponsors, and local IRBs. Interim monitoring is used to assure that subjects have been properly enrolled, check protocol compliance, review appropriate regulatory submissions, make sure that data management and forms submission are up to date, and report adverse effects (e.g., treatment toxicity) and summary statistics (e.g., numbers of patients enrolled, completed, etc.). In addition, if treatment

TABLE 27.7	Type I Error Rates With Repeated Testing
No. of Tests	P(rejection) Under H_0 With $\alpha = .05$
1	.05
2	.08
5	.14
10	.19
20	.25
50	.32
1000	.53
∞	1

groups are combined, overall outcome results may be reported. More importantly, interim analyses should monitor the response variables of interest to identify early dramatic benefits of the new treatment, potential harmful effects, or an outcome difference between treatments so unimpressive that showing a statistically significant difference at the end of the trial is very unlikely; any of these results should be reported to the study's data safety and monitoring committee only, not to study investigators or to the public.

This section focuses on techniques for interim monitoring of treatment differences. One of the problems of interim analysis is the repeated testing for significance. Under the null hypothesis H0 (no difference between treatment groups), repeated testing at a type I error level of α yields a probability of finding a significant result greater than α, as shown in Table 27.7 (the figures in Table 27.7 hold for either a test for equality of binomial proportions or a t-test for the difference in means between two normal populations, assuming that roughly equal numbers of patients are added between each interim test). In this section, we look at three techniques for addressing the problem of repeated testing for significance: the group sequential method, the alpha-spending function, and the curtailed sampling procedure.

The Haybittle-Peto procedure[12] is one of the group sequential methods that favors using a large critical value, such as Zi = ± 3, for all interim tests (where i < k, with k = total number of patient groups that will be monitored over the course of the trial, and i = number of groups with completed data at a given point in time). With this method, any adjustment for repeated testing at the final test (i = k) is negligible, and the conventional critical value can be used. This method is ad hoc in the sense that no precise type I error level is guaranteed. It might, however, be viewed as a precursor to the more formal procedures described in the following section.

Pocock[13] modified the repeated testing methods of McPherson and Armitage[14,15] and developed a group sequential method for clinical trials that avoids many of the limitations of the Haybittle-Peto procedure. Pocock's method divides the participants into a series of k equal-sized groups with 2n participants in each, n assigned to intervention and n to control. The number of groups, k, is the number of times that data will be monitored during the course of the trial, and the total expected sample size is 2nk. The test statistic used to compare control and intervention is computed as soon as data for the first group of 2n participants are

<table>
<tr><td>**TABLE 27.8**</td><td colspan="3">**Normal Significance Level Required to Achieve Overall α = .05 or .01 With Repeated Two-Sided Significance Testing**</td></tr>
</table>

No. of Tests	Significance Level for Each Test to Achieve Overall α = .05	Significance Level for Each Test to Achieve Overall α = .01
2	.0290	.0056
3	.0220	.0041
4	.0180	.0033
5	.0160	.0028
10	.0106	.0018
15	.0086	.0015
20	.0075	.0013

<table>
<tr><td>**TABLE 27.9**</td><td colspan="2">**Values of Z* Required to Achieve Overall α = .05 With Repeated Testing**</td></tr>
</table>

No. of Tests	Z
1	1.96
2	1.98
3	2
4	2.02
5	2.04
6	2.05
7	2.06
8	2.07
9	2.08
10	2.09

<table>
<tr><td>**TABLE 27.10**</td><td colspan="2">**Sample Sizes Required to Maintain 90% Power to Detect a Difference of $P^1 = 0.50$ Versus $P^2 = 0.70$ With α = .05 After Repeated Testing**</td></tr>
</table>

No. of Tests	Sample Size
1	262
2	264
3	266
4	267
5	268
10	271

available, and recomputed when data from each successive group become known. Under the null hypothesis, the distribution of the test statistic, Z_i, is assumed to be approximately normal with zero mean and unit variance, where i indicates the number of groups ($i \leq k$) with completed data. This statistic Z_i is compared with the stopping boundaries, $\pm Z'_k$, where Z'_k has been determined such that for up to k repeated tests, the overall significance level for the trial will be α. Table 27.8 shows the normal significance levels required for repeated two-sided significance testing. For example, for k = 5 and α = 0.05 (two-sided), we use a normal significance value of 0.0160 for each test, yielding $Z'_k = 2.413$ (instead of Z_1 = 1.96 for a single test at α = 0.05).

O'Brien and Fleming also discussed a group sequential procedure.[16] Using the preceding notation, their stopping rule compares the statistic Z_i with $Z^*(k/i)1/2$ where Z^* is determined so as to achieve the desired significance level. Table 27.9 shows the values of Z^* for overall α = 0.05. For example, if k = 5 and α = 0.05 (two-sided), $Z^* = 2.04$. One attractive feature of the O'Brien-Fleming procedure is that the critical value used at the last test (i = k) is approximately the same as that used if a single test were done.

The O'Brien-Fleming model is unlikely to lead to stopping in the early stages of a trial. Later on, however, this procedure leads to a greater chance of stopping before the end of a study than does the Pocock or Haybittle-Peto procedure. Both the Haybittle-Peto and the O'Brien-Fleming boundaries avoid the awkward situation of accepting the null hypothesis when the observed statistic at the end of the trial is much larger than the conventional critical value (i.e., 1.96 for a two-sided 5% significance level). There is a slight loss of power with multiple testing. For example, if the investigator is testing a binomial hypothesis (H0: P1 = P2 versus Ha: P1 ≠ P2) and wants 90% power to detect a difference of P1 = 0.50 versus P2 = 0.70 with α = 0.05, the required sample size for a single test is 262. With increasing numbers of tests, the sample sizes required to maintain the same power are shown in Table 27.10.

Lan and DeMets introduced the alpha-spending function.[17] This function allows the investigator to determine how he or she wants to "spend" the type I error (i.e., alpha) during the course of a trial. The alpha-spending function guarantees that at the end of the trial, the overall type I error will be the prespecified value of α; thus this approach is a generalization of the group sequential method, such that the Pocock and O'Brien-Fleming monitoring procedures become special cases. To understand the alpha-spending function, we must first distinguish between calendar time and information fraction. At any particular calendar time t in the study, a certain fraction t^* of the total information is observed. The value for t^* must be between 0 and 1. The information fraction is more generally defined in terms of the ratio of the inverse of the variance of the test statistic at the particular interim analysis to that at the final analysis. The alpha-spending function, $\alpha(t^*)$, determines how the pre specified α is allocated at each interim analysis as a function of the information fraction. At the beginning of the trial, $t^* = 0$ and $\alpha(t^*) = 0$, whereas at the end of the trial, $t^* = 1$ and $\alpha(t^*) = \alpha$. The relationships between the alpha-spending function and the O'Brien-Fleming method and the Pocock method are described as follows:

$$\text{O'Brien-Fleming method: } \alpha_{O-F}(t^*) = 2 \text{ to } 2\Phi(Z_{\alpha/2}/t^*)$$

$$\text{Pocock method: } \alpha_P(t^*) = \alpha \bullet \ln[1 + (e-1)t^*]$$

The advantage of the alpha-spending function is that neither the number nor the time of interim analyses needs to be specified in advance, thereby giving group sequential monitoring the flexibility that is often required in the actual clinical trial setting.

Whereas group sequential methods focus on existing data, curtailed sampling methods consider future data. With curtailed methods, multiple checks for the possibility of early curtailment do not cause problems of repeated testing. Two curtailed sampling procedures are discussed in this section: the simple curtailment method and the stochastic curtailment method.

The principle of simple curtailment is that a study should be stopped as soon as the result is inevitable (i.e., the trend toward a final outcome cannot be reversed). For example, in a two-sample *t* test, suppose all values must be between A and B (A < B), and that after sampling n* out of n total observations, we have observed no significant result. We may assign values to the remaining n − n* observations as follows:

1. Assign all As to group 1, all Bs to group 2, and recompute the test statistic.
2. Assign all Bs to group 1, all As to group 2, and recompute the test statistic.

If both recomputations yield no significance, we can be sure that the final result of all sampling will not reach statistical significance, and the trial may be stopped.

Similarly, if a significant difference is observed after sampling n* out of n total observations, we also may perform the preceding recomputations. If both lead to significance, then the trial may be stopped. With this method, the requirement of absolute certainty is very conservative and does not give much opportunity for early stopping.

By contrast, stochastic curtailment is less conservative, allowing the trial to be stopped as soon as the result is highly probable based on calculation of conditional power; if the conditional power is very low, the trial may be stopped. For example, let S(t) be the test statistic at time t. If T = the end of the trial, then S(T) is the final test statistic. There are two conditions to consider:

1. Suppose the result in the intervention group is significantly better than that in the control group at t < T. Then compute $\pi 0 = P$ (rejecting H0 | H0 true and observed data from the study).
   $\pi 0$ is equal to the probability of still rejecting H0 if the rest of the data come in reflecting no treatment effect. If $\pi 0$ is large (≈ 1), then the trend is unlikely to disappear.
2. Suppose the result in the intervention group is not significantly different from that in the control group at t < T. Then compute, for a set of reasonable values of difference (δ) between the intervention group and control group $\pi 1 = P$ (rejecting H0 | H1 true and observed data from the study).

How large must the true effect (δ) be to reverse the current decision? If δ must be unrealistically large and the probability of reversal is small, then terminating the trial may be considered.

Because there is a small probability that the results will change, a slightly greater risk of type I or type II error will exist if a trial is curtailed than would exist if the trial continued to the scheduled end; however, the type I error is bounded by $\alpha/\pi 0$, and the type II error by $\beta/\pi 1$.

Judging Quality of Clinical Trials: Level of Evidence

Researchers and journals assign a level to the papers they publish about clinical trials. Table 27.11 is the from the Centre for Evidence-Based Medicine that describes the designated level from the highest quality level, Level I, to Level V, which is the lowest

TABLE 27.11	Levels of Evidence for Therapeutic Studies
Level	**Type of Evidence**
1A	Systematic review (with homogeneity) of RCTs
1B	Individual RCT (with narrow confidence intervals)
1C	All or none study
2A	Systematic review (with homogeneity) of cohort studies
2B	Individual cohort study (including low quality RCT, e.g., <80% follow-up)
2C	"Outcomes" research; ecological studies
3A	Systematic review (with homogeneity) of case-control studies
3B	Individual case-control study
4	Case series (and poor quality cohort and case-study control)
5	Expert opinion without explicit critical appraisal or based on physiology bench research or "first principles"

RCT, Randomized controlled trial.
© 2016 Centre for Evidence-Based Medicine. <http://www.cebm.net>; Accessed July 2016.

rating in terms of level of evidence. However, the level of evidence does not always guarantee the quality of research. Not all randomized clinical trials (RCTs) are conducted properly, as has been described in this chapter, due to bias, poor conduct, or being underpowered such that a Level I trial may show a negative result because of poor design or conduct when in fact the opposite may be true. Bhandari and colleagues published a paper assessing the quality of surgical RCTs.[18] The authors evaluated 72 RCTs that had a mean score of 68% with papers scoring greater than 75% being high quality. Sixty percent of the papers had a score less than 75%. Therefore researchers should not automatically assume an RCT is of high quality.

Reporting of Adverse Events for Clinical Trials

The National Cancer Institute and National Institutes of Health, which require that all US clinic trials be listed on clinicaltrials.gov, has published standardized definitions for adverse events. These describe the severity of organ toxicity for patients receiving cancer care and has specific parameters according to the organ system involved. An adverse event does not require causality but is defined as any abnormal clinical finding associated with the therapy.[19]

Common Terminology Criteria for Adverse Events or Common Toxicity Criteria:

Grade 1—mild
Grade 2—moderate
Grade 3—severe
Grade 4—life-threatening
Grade 5—death

The global index of safety is an adverse event–based instrument that evaluates the safety profile of drugs compiling a total score for all adverse events.[20] For example, in the Women's Health Initiative (WHI) trial, the global index contained all the known complications from estrogen plus progesterone ingestion (E + P). These complications compile the global index, and if the figure from the global index (generated by the reporting of adverse events) is surpassed without the drug under study resulting in the anticipated positive result, the study is terminated. In the WHI several known adverse events from the use of E + P compiled the global index (e.g., breast cancer, deep vein thrombosis, pulmonary embolism). The global index was exceeded before any positive influence on cardiovascular disease was identified from the use of E + P. Thus the study was stopped. Because breast cancer was part of the global index already accepted by the study coordinators, the results of the WHI study were interpreted as proving that E + P was a "cause" of breast cancer. Multiple lawsuits were filed against Wyeth laboratories, and an enormous amount of money was spent on this subject. Academic careers were made with articles in prestigious journals decrying the use of E + P because it caused breast cancer. An understanding of adverse events and why they are reported to the central office and an understanding of the meaning of the global index could have prevented much of this turmoil.

Conclusions

Bull indicated that the clinical trial is "the most definitive tool for evaluation of the applicability of clinical research," representing "a key research activity with the potential to improve the quality of health care and control costs through careful comparison of alternative treatment."[19] Study design, randomization, appropriate controls, well-chosen outcome measures, sample size determination, and interim monitoring analysis are key factors for a successful trial. Without solid biostatistical support during the design, conduct, and analysis of the trial, these trial features may not be addressed in full. In other words, without careful and adequate biostatistical input, clinical trials are unable to answer the research questions for which they are designed.

Selected References

1. National Institutes of Health. Notice of revised NIH Definition of "Clinical Trial." http://grants.nih.gov/grants/guide/notice-files/NOT-OD-15-015.html.
3. US Food and Drug Administration. About FDA: what we do: FDA mission, http://www.fda.gov/AboutFDA/WhatWeDo/; Accessed 15 November 2016.
5. O'Quigley J, Pepe M, Fisher L. Continual reassessment method: a practical design for phase I clinical trials in cancer. *Biometrics*. 1990;46:33-48.
13. Pocock SJ. *Clinical trials: A practical approach*. New York: Wiley; 1984.

Suggested Readings

Hulley SB, Cummings SR, Browner WS, Grady DG, Newman TB. *Designing Clinical Research*. 4th ed. Philadelphia: Lippincott Williams & Wilkins; 2013.
Wilke LG, Ballman KV, McCall LM, et al. Adherence to the National Quality Forum (NQF) breast cancer measures within cancer clinical trials: a review from ACOSOG Z0010. *Ann Surg Oncol*. 2010;17:1989-1994.

A full reference list is available online at ExpertConsult.com.

28

Indications and Techniques for Biopsy

SAMILIA OBENG-GYASI, LARS J. GRIMM, E. SHELLEY HWANG, V. SUZANNE KLIMBERG, AND KIRBY I. BLAND

Currently there are multiple modalities available to obtain a tissue diagnosis for a patient who presents with a breast abnormality on physical examination or imaging. Due to advances in breast imaging and biopsy devices, the latter part of the 20th century saw a shift from open surgical biopsy to percutaneous biopsy as the initial tissue acquisition procedure.[1] This paradigm shift was propelled by the multiple benefits and equivalent accuracy to open surgical biopsy offered by percutaneous biopsy.[2] The International Breast Cancer Consensus Conference in 2009 and the American Society of Breast Surgeons have released consensus statements supporting the use of percutaneous biopsy as the initial method for tissue retrieval for breast disease diagnosis.[3,4] A 2009 report by the Agency for Healthcare Research and Quality (AHRQ) comparing image-guided core needle biopsy to open surgical biopsy revealed an excellent safety profile for both modalities. Specifically, their comparative effectiveness review showed a less than 1% absolute incidence of adverse events for both biopsy techniques.[5] However, it should be noted that the majority of patients who are referred for biopsy have benign lesions thus supporting the use of minimally invasive procedures over more invasive surgical procedures.[6]

In the literature, percutaneous biopsies are also called minimally invasive breast biopsies. These biopsies include fine-needle aspiration (FNA) and core needle biopsies (CNB). Open surgical biopsies are sometimes referred to as excisional biopsies or incisional biopsies. *Excisional biopsy* indicates complete removal of the lesion, whereas *incisional biopsy* indicates removal of part of the lesion.[7] For nonpalpable lesions, imaging modalities such as ultrasound (US), mammography, and magnetic resonance imaging (MRI) are useful adjuncts for identifying and localizing the lesion of interest.

The decision of when to perform a breast biopsy is dependent on the patient's history, physical examination findings, and radiologic imaging. The main objective of the biopsy is to obtain a tissue diagnosis that can help dictate treatment and preoperative planning, if indicated. As a result, it is imperative to choose a biopsy technique optimizing the chances for an accurate diagnosis while minimizing costs, limiting patient discomfort, and reducing the need for a repeat procedure.

Fine-Needle Aspiration Biopsy

Fine-needle aspiration of breast masses is a safe and reliable diagnostic technique that can be performed in the office using local anesthesia.[8,9] Compared with CNBs, FNA biopsies have less morbidity, lower cost, and faster turnaround time, with results often available immediately after aspiration. The recent trends away from FNA in favor of CNB can be attributed to the increasing importance of obtaining tumor biomarkers of estrogen receptor (ER), progesterone (PR), and human epidermal growth factor receptor-2 (HER2) status on needle biopsy samples for treatment planning of cancers. Nevertheless, there remains a role for FNA, primarily in the evaluation of palpable masses of low to intermediate suspicion for cancer and in resource-constrained settings where FNA may be more feasible than CNB.

Procedure

The skin overlying the palpable lesion is infiltrated with a local anesthetic. The breast lump is held relatively immobile, using one hand to gently but firmly stabilize the quadrant containing the mass. If the mass is not well defined, the procedure should be performed with ultrasound or mammographic guidance. FNA is facilitated using an "aspiration gun" to allow the operator to apply suction while maintaining the position of the needle tip in the mass (Fig. 28.1). The procedure uses a 10- to 20-mL syringe and 22- or 25-gauge needle. The needle is inserted into the mass, and suction is applied to the syringe. Moving the needle into the lesion at various angles allows clumps of cells to be dislodged from the tumor, aspirated into the syringe, and submitted for cytologic examination. Local pressure is applied after the procedure. The procedure is well tolerated; hematoma is the most common complication but is rare.

Accuracy

The sensitivity of FNA ranges from 80% to 90%[9,10] with a pooled sensitivity on meta-analysis of 92% (95% confidence interval 91%–93%).[11] False-negative results have been shown to range from 6% to 11%.[12,13] It is important to note that these rates do not differ markedly from results of CNB; in one study that directly compared FNA to CNB, the sensitivity of FNA was 93.8% compared with 90.1% for CNB.[14] Furthermore, FNA has been shown to be more cost-effective than CNB without compromising diagnostic accuracy.[15]

The diagnostic performance of the FNA technique relies more strongly on the skill and experience of the operator and cytologist

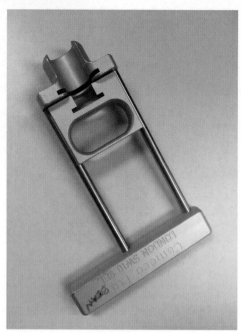

• **Fig. 28.1** Aspiration of a solid breast mass is best performed by using a cytology fine-needle "aspiration gun."

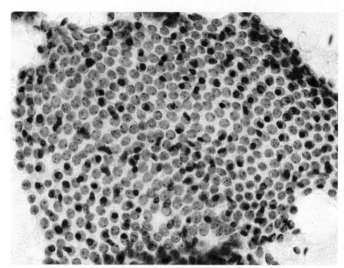

• **Fig. 28.2** High-power view of well-organized sheet of luminar cells with prominent sprinkling of myoepithelial cells (small dark oval nuclei). This type of arrangement of the epithelial components of the duct system of the breast is characteristic of benign lesions including fibroadenomas and fibrocystic change. Papanicolaou stain, 40×.

than CNB.[16] Thus the routine use of FNA requires local institutional expertise, including specialized training and close multidisciplinary communication among the cytopathologist, referring physician, and radiologist. False-positive results are unusual when the aspirated specimen is properly prepared and reviewed by a qualified cytopathologist. Thus lumpectomy may be safely performed on the basis of FNA confirmation of cancer. However, caution would dictate that mastectomy should not be undertaken without further tissue confirmation of malignancy due to the small risk of a falsely positive result.

False-negative results from FNA are much more common, and it must be emphasized that the absence of malignant cells in the aspirate does not rule out the presence of cancer. A recent meta-analysis reported that more than a quarter of all FNA samples may result in insufficient material for diagnosis.[11] Thus any clinically or mammographically suspicious breast mass investigated with FNA where cytology is disconcordant with radiologic findings must be subjected to further diagnosis by means of CNB or surgical excision.

Cytopathology

The National Cancer Institute recommendation for the diagnosis of breast aspiration cytology has divided FNAB findings into five categories: C1 = unsatisfactory; C2 = no suspicious features; C3 = cells suspicious but probably benign; C4 = cells suspicious but probably malignant; and C5 = definitely malignant. Clinically, category C2 is defined as negative, and categories C3 through C5 are defined as positive, indicating additional workup or treatment[8] (Figs. 28.2 and 28.3).

Biomarker evaluation for ER, PR, HER2, and other markers can often be performed on fine-needle aspirate by centrifuging the cellular material and performing immunohistochemical (IHC) staining on the resulting cell block. Several studies have shown that ER and PR can be successfully evaluated on FNA alone, and

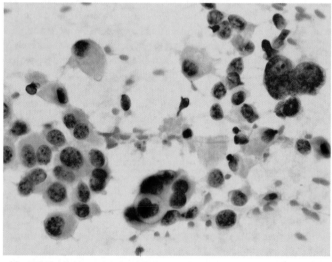

• **Fig. 28.3** High-power view of cancer with high nuclear grade. Note the marked variation in nuclear size and hyperchromasia (dark and clumped chromatin). Papanicolaou stain, 40×.

HER2 IHC testing as well as fluorescence in situ hybridization (FISH) have been performed.[17] However, because of the loss of tissue architecture on a cellular aspirate, FNA cannot distinguish between in situ and invasive cancer. Because this determination is often critical to treatment planning, CNB may often be required to differentiate between these two diagnoses.

FNA remains the most cost-effective diagnostic procedure for the evaluation of breast masses in developing countries.[18] As a procedure that is less invasive than CNB, there are clinical settings in which FNA can be considered a definitive procedure to confirm a diagnosis. However, FNA requires a more specialized expertise and coordinated multidisciplinary approach than CNB and thus may not be readily available at some centers. Radiologic concordance with cytologic findings is essential and this assessment should be performed as a routine component of FNA.

Direct Smear

Specimens for exfoliative cytologic analysis in the patient with suspected Paget disease of the breast may be obtained with direct smear of the weeping eczematoid lesion of the nipple. If the areola and surrounding skin are scaly and encrusted, a sterile glass slide can be used to scrape this area gently. The direct smear technique is simple and can be performed as an office procedure. The technique is rapid and inexpensive; however, histologic confirmation is required for definitive diagnosis. Comprehensive management of nipple cytology and secretions is reviewed in other chapters in this textbook.

Fluid Aspiration

Fluid aspiration is indicated for those masses that on US evaluation are found to have a cystic component. Fluid from palpable breast cysts is simple to aspirate with a needle and syringe. If the cyst is not palpable, ultrasound can be used as a guide to direct the depth and location of the biopsy needle. The return of nonbloody fluid confirms the diagnosis of benign (nonproliferative) cystic disease, and, unless otherwise indicated, this fluid should not be submitted for cytologic examination. Bloody cystic fluid, on the other hand, is more likely to indicate malignancy and therefore should be examined cytologically, either by direct smear or after centrifugation of the aspirated contents. Cystic masses should not be palpable after aspiration because the walls of the cyst collapse and conform to the surrounding breast tissue. If fluid is not obtained or the mass persists, further workup is required. If the mass resolves and later recurs, clinical and mammographic evaluations are also indicated (Fig. 28.4).

Core Needle Biopsy

Image-guided CNBs are currently the primary means by which a pathologic diagnosis is made for suspicious abnormalities identified by screening or diagnostic workups. Image guidance allows precise tissue sampling of the area of interest and ensures that the abnormality identified during diagnostic workup is correctly biopsied. Compared with surgical biopsies, image-guided biopsies have comparable sensitivity and specificity, are associated with fewer adverse events, have shorter recovery times, provide better cosmetic results, and are preferred by patients.[5,19–22] Cost savings of image-guided biopsies are dependent on the specific equipment used but are considered to be significant compared with surgical excision.[5,23] Finally, women who have cancer detected via image-guided biopsy are 15 times more likely to have their cancer treated with only a single surgical procedure.[5] Biopsies may be performed via US, stereotactic, or MRI-guided approaches; strengths and weaknesses have been described with each approach (Table 28.1). Digital breast tomosynthesis (DBT)-guided biopsies are also possible but are not currently performed with any frequency because of the recent implementation of DBT and limited availability of biopsy-capable devices.[24]

Several general principles apply to all forms of image-guided biopsy. First, before the start of the procedure, it is important to have a firm understanding of acceptable concordant and discordant pathology results. This aids in discussions with patients about potential outcomes and also ensures that all necessary noninvasive diagnostic steps are performed before the patient is subjected to a biopsy. Second, there are a large and steadily growing number of biopsy devices, clip deployment devices, and guidance systems.

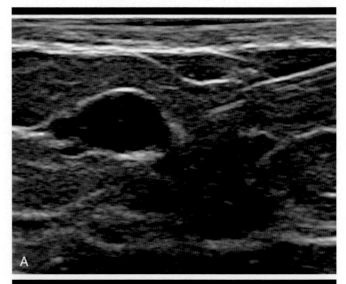

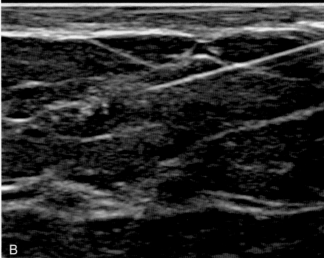

• **Fig. 28.4** Cyst aspiration. (A) Cyst with needle positioned in upper right corner of image. (B) Cyst collapse after aspiration.

It is mandatory to fully understand the strengths and limitations of all biopsy equipment before use because failure to do so can result in increased procedure time, decreased accuracy, and need for additional open biopsies.[5,25–27] Finally, deciding which image-guided modality to use should be based on the modality most likely to obtain a diagnostic tissue sample while also incorporating any special needs of the patient (i.e., inability to lay flat).

Complications related to image-guided biopsy procedures are usually uncommon and minor. The most common complaint from patients is soreness and bruising, especially the day after the procedure. Hematoma formation is common but usually small and self-limited.[28] Antithrombotic usage is associated with an increased risk of nonclinically significant hematoma formation, thus the benefits of continuing antithrombotic therapy often outweigh the very low risk of severe bleeding.[28] The risk of hematoma formation is associated with additional tissue sampling and smaller needle gauge.[28,29] Patients are usually instructed to avoid any strenuous lifting or exercising after the procedure to avoid rebleeding. The likelihood of a vasovagal reaction has been reported to be as low as 1% and is more commonly seen when patients are positioned upright.[5,30] Although image-guided biopsies are

TABLE 28.1 Comparison of Indications, Advantages, and Disadvantages of Fine-Needle Aspiration, Core Needle Biopsy, and Surgical Biopsy

Biopsy Type	Indications	Advantages	Disadvantages
FNA	Palpable masses	Cost-effective compared with CNB and open surgical biopsy 80%–90% diagnostic accuracy Minimal patient discomfort Therapeutic for cyst aspiration Short turn-around time	Cannot distinguish between in situ and invasive diagnoses May require additional sampling by core needle or surgical biopsy for definitive histologic diagnosis Reliant on institutional cytologic expertise
CNB	Image-detected abnormalities	Less invasive than surgical biopsy Better cosmesis compared with surgical biopsy Women diagnosed with cancer on CNB have fewer surgical procedures Helpful in preoperative planning due to clip placement	Discordance in radiologic and pathologic findings warrants additional biopsies, which increase costs
Ultrasound-guided CNB	Preferred CNB approach Axillary lymph nodes	Flexibility of patient and operator positioning Real-time imaging and biopsy	Calcifications typically not visible on ultrasound
Stereotactic guided CNB	Calcifications and other lesions seen only on mammography	Only option available for most calcifications Specimen radiographs can confirm sample contains calcifications	Requires breast compression and ability to lie prone for duration of procedure Not feasible for some chest wall or subareolar lesions Breasts that compress to less than 1.5–2 cm may not be amenable to biopsy
MRI-guided CNB	Lesions only seen on MRI	Only option available for lesions seen only on MRI	Not feasible for some chest wall or subareolar lesions Requires contrast administration Most expensive CNB approach
Surgical biopsy	Lesions close to chest wall, nipple, or breast implant High-risk lesions on CNB (i.e., ADH, ALH) Discordant radiologic imaging and pathology results Inadequate tissue sampling by FNA or CNB	Most definitive of the three biopsy types	More likely to result in multiple surgical procedures if used as index biopsy More costly than CNB and FNA Often requires intravenous sedation Higher risk of postprocedure complications compared with FNA and CNB

ADH, Atypical ductal hyperplasia; *ALH*, atypical lobular hyperplasia; *CNB*, core needle biopsy; *FNA*, fine-needle aspiration; *MRI*, magnetic resonance imaging.

typically clean but not sterile, the risk of infection is extremely low. Among 40 studies including 25,688 procedures, the range of procedures with an infection was 0 to 2.91%.[5] Finally, although injury to the regional structures including the development of a pneumothorax is possible, this risk should be negligible by maintaining a needle position parallel or near-parallel to the chest wall at all times. The reported risk of pneumothorax has been reported to be less than 1 in 2500 patients.[5]

Ultrasound-Guided Biopsy

US is the preferred imaging-guided breast biopsy approach and is the only true real-time imaging approach.[31] US is inexpensive, uses no radiation, requires no compression, does not require contrast, and takes less time than other image-guided biopsy approaches.[5,31–33] Compared with FNA, the increased size of the tissue sample is associated with improved accuracy in some

studies.[34,35] Ultrasound is also the only image-guided modality capable of safely sampling axillary lymph nodes, although very deep nodes may be inaccessible.[36]

Before starting a US-guided biopsy, the patient is scanned in a supine or anterior oblique position to identify the suspicious abnormality. A primary advantage of US-guided biopsies is the ability to position the patient and operator in the most comfortable orientation possible. The biopsy approach can be planned from any direction, and color Doppler can be used to avoid major blood vessels. Once the approach is decided, the site is cleaned and dressed in the usual fashion. The skin is anesthetized, and then under direct visualization anesthetic medication is administered along the proposed biopsy tract and around the abnormality to be biopsied. At any point during the procedure, if the patient complains of inadequate analgesia, additional medication can be administered. After a skin nick, typically an introducer needle with a coaxial sheath is advanced adjacent to the abnormality. The introducer needle is then replaced with the biopsy device.

Either a vacuum-assisted device or a spring-loaded device may be used, typically with an 11- or 14-gauge size. Smaller needles are associated with a decrease in diagnostic accuracy.[34] Samples are obtained under direct visualization and can be obtained from multiple sites within the same abnormality to reduce tissue under sampling. In addition, if multiple adjacent abnormalities need to be sampled, they can often be biopsied through the same skin incision. After sufficient samples have been obtained, typically at least 5, a biopsy marking clip is placed in the center of the abnormality. The patient is then bandaged, and two orthogonal mammogram pictures are obtained to document the position of the biopsy site.

There are few disadvantages and complications unique to US-guided biopsies. Compared with stereotactic and MRI-guided biopsies, US-guided biopsies require a great deal of technical expertise and thus successful sampling and complication rates will be more highly influenced by the experience of the operator.[33] US-guided biopsies are theoretically at greater risk for complications such as pneumothorax or implant rupture because the biopsy device is typically held freehand by the operator and not in a fixed position parallel to the chest wall.[36] Ultrasound is rarely able to identify mammographically detected microcalcifications unless there is an associated mass.[37] Abnormalities initially identified via MRI may undergo a second look US to determine whether they are visible and amenable to US-guided biopsy, but many small lesions or areas of vague enhancement will not be seen on US and must undergo MRI-guided biopsy.

Stereotactic Core Needle Biopsy

Stereotactic-guided biopsies are primarily performed for mammographically detected microcalcifications. Less common indications for stereotactic CNB (SCNB) include asymmetries, architectural distortions, and masses that are seen only on mammography without a US correlate. There are two primary units used in a stereotactic biopsy: prone or upright.[31,36] With a prone unit the patient lies on her abdomen and her breast falls through a hole in the table with the stereotactic unit positioned underneath. A prone unit is preferred because it provides the greatest flexibility for the operator to plan the biopsy approach, and with the breast is positioned in a pendant fashion, it allows sampling of more posterior lesions. With an upright unit the patient is seated, and an add-on device is attached to a mammography unit. An upright unit is typically reserved for facilities that do not have access to a prone table or for patients who are unable to lie flat, typically because of back pain or respiratory difficulties.

Whether the patient is positioned prone or upright, the shortest distance to the abnormality is typically chosen as the direction of approach. Of note, a caudal-cranial approach is not possible with an upright unit because the patient's bent legs will interfere with the biopsy device. A small windowed paddle is used to compression the breast in the area of interest. Images are taken and adjustments in the positioning of the paddle are made until the abnormality of interest is identified (Fig. 28.5). A pair of stereotactic images is then obtained at +15 and −15 degrees to triangulate the lesion. Using the stereotactic software, the computer calculates X and Y coordinates as well as the Z depth. The breast is locally anesthetized, and the biopsy device is lined up with the calculated coordinates and fired into final position. Prefire or postfire images may be obtained and small adjustments to the

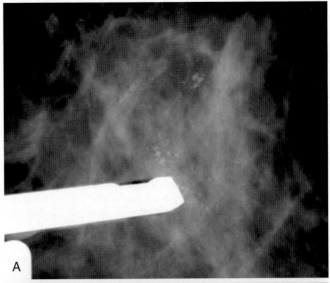

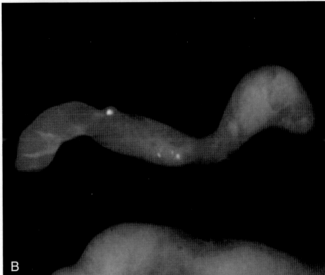

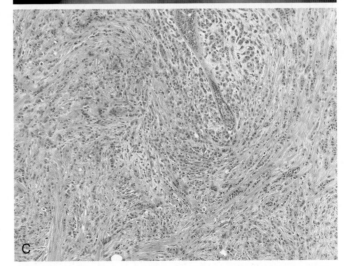

• **Fig. 28.5** Image from a 45-year-old woman with suspicious calcifications seen on mammography. (A) Stereotactic prefire image demonstrating the biopsy device appropriately positioned in front of the calcifications. (B) Specimen radiograph reveals calcifications within one of the tissue samples. (C) Pathology image of hematoxylin and eosin stain of invasive lobular carcinoma.

needle can be made secondary to displacement from the administration of medication or patient motion. Vacuum-assisted samples are then obtained circumferentially or directionally as needed. Typically an 11- or 14-gauge biopsy device is used, and 6 to 12 samples are obtained. If calcifications were biopsied, the specimens can be radiographed to ensure that there was adequate tissue sampling; however, the goal of the biopsy is to sample the calcifications and not remove all of them.[33] If needed, additional samples can be taken at the same site or adjustments to the position of the biopsy device can be made accordingly. A clip is then placed and imaged while the patient is still in place to confirm clip deployment. The patient is then bandaged, and two orthogonal mammographic images are obtained to document the position of the clip. This is especially important in the case of biopsied calcifications, which may be completely removed during the procedure.

There are several disadvantages to stereotactic breast biopsies. Patients must also be able to lie still for the duration of the procedure because precise calculations made initially will have to be repeated if the breast is moved. Calcifications that are very close to the chest wall may not be amenable to stereotactic biopsy because the biopsy device cannot be positioned completely flush with the chest wall. These women may require wire localization followed by surgical excision. Women with breasts that compress very thinly may not be eligible for a stereotactic biopsy because there must be sufficient space for the needle biopsy well and the needle cutting tip. Small or petite needles are available for thinner breasts, but there is a minimum thickness of approximately 1.5 to 2.0 centimeters, depending on the vendor.

Magnetic Resonance Imaging–Guided Biopsy

MRI-guided biopsies are typically reserved for abnormalities seen only via MRI. Abnormalities initially identified on MRI will often undergo a second-look US to see whether they can instead be biopsied via US.[38] Lesions identified via second-look US are more likely to be larger, more suspicious (Breast Imaging Reporting and Data System [BI-RADS] 5 vs. BI-RADS 3 or 4), and described as a mass versus nonmass enhancement.[38–40] However, among lesions with no US correlate, the malignancy rate is 6% to 27%.[38] In preparation for an MRI-guided biopsy, the patient needs to have an intravenous line placed, and routine MRI safety precautions need to be addressed (e.g., pacemaker). Sedating medications can be administered if claustrophobia is a problem. The patient is placed prone on the MRI scanner equipped with a dedicated breast coil. The breast with the abnormality in question is cleaned and compressed between a plate and grid. A lateral approach is preferred because it is much easier to approach the patient from the side rather than having to reach underneath. It is imperative that patients be correctly positioned within the scanner to reduce artifacts that may obscure the lesion in question.[41]

Specific imaging sequences will vary among institutions, but typically localizer scans are obtained followed by axial dynamic postcontrast T1-weighted sequences. Using dedicated biopsy software, the abnormality is identified by the user, and coordinates are calculated by the computer. Local anesthesia is then administered, and an obturator is advanced into position. After confirming appropriate positioning, a vacuum-assisted biopsy device is advanced and samples are obtained. Typically 6 to 12 samples are obtained and a clip is deployed at the biopsy site. The patient then undergoes a two-view mammogram of the breast to confirm the

clip is appropriately placed. Clip deployment in MRI-guided biopsies is especially important because many abnormalities will only be visible via MRI.[42] If the patient needs subsequent surgical excision, then the clip can be localized via a mammographic approach. For patients with a benign biopsy result, most authors recommend a 6-month follow-up.[43,44]

The primary advantage of an MRI-guided biopsy approach is that it is the only modality capable of sampling abnormalities seen only on MRI. MRI has the highest sensitivity of all breast-imaging modalities, but this comes at the cost of false-positive biopsies due to the lower specificity of MRI.[45–47] The disadvantages of MRI-guided biopsies are the high cost, use of breast compression, possibility of patient claustrophobia, and the need for contrast administration. Patient with renal failure may not undergo contrast-enhanced MRI due to the risk of nephrogenic sclerosing fibrosis.

The multiple CNB techniques available provide operators with great flexibility for obtaining diagnostic tissue samples. Choosing the appropriate technique and method of approach are the most important first steps to ensure successful tissue sampling, maximize patient and operator comfort, and reduce the risk of complications. As with most procedures, CNB techniques are highly influenced by operator experience, and all users should be intimately familiar with the preprocedure diagnostic workup, mechanics of the biopsy devices, and postprocedure follow-up imaging.

Open Surgical Biopsy

The advent of percutaneous needle biopsy (CNB and FNA) has limited the use of open surgical biopsy as the initial tissue-acquisition procedure for the workup of palpable and nonpalpable breast lesions. According to the special report from the 2009 International Breast Cancer Consensus Conference, 35% of initial diagnostic biopsies conducted in the United States were still performed with open surgical biopsy.[4] Historically, open surgical biopsy was considered the gold standard for biopsy methods.[5] However, a systematic literature review by the AHRQ showed similar sensitivity and specificity for US and stereotactic biopsies compared with open surgical biopsies.[5] The aforementioned findings, in conjunction with the recommendation of using needle biopsy as a quality measure by the National Quality Forum and the American College of Surgeons, has furthered the paradigm shift toward using percutaneous biopsy over surgical biopsy for initial diagnosis.[48]

The expert panel at the 2009 International Breast Cancer Consensus Conference III recommended percutaneous needle biopsy replace open surgical biopsy as the new gold standard and best practice for the initial diagnostic workup for breast lesions. Further recommendations from the panel include limiting the rate of open surgical biopsy as the initial diagnostic biopsy for breast lesions to less than 5% to 10% of a surgeon's practice.[4]

A recent study evaluating open surgical biopsy versus percutaneous biopsy use among Medicare patients discovered African-American race, low socioeconomic status, residence in a rural area, and living more than 8 miles from a radiologic facility that performs percutaneous biopsies resulted in a higher likelihood of having an open surgical biopsy for initial diagnosis.[6] The authors also noted surgeon factors such as lack of board certification, foreign medical training, lack of specialization (i.e., surgical oncology training), low volume of breast patients, and longer years out of

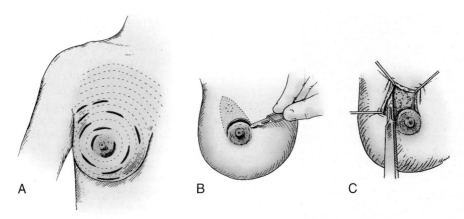

• **Fig. 28.6** Recommended locations of incisions for performing breast biopsy. (A) The most cosmetically acceptable scars result from circumareolar incisions that follow Langer lines. (B and C) Technique for dissection of breast masses within 2 cm of the areolar margin. Thick skin flaps are advised to ensure cosmetically contoured and viable tissues around the areola.

training were associated with surgical biopsy as the first diagnostic biopsy.[6]

On the basis of current consensus guidelines and medical literature, it can be argued the only indication for using surgical biopsy as the initial diagnostic biopsy would be if a facility lacks the structural capability, necessary equipment, and staff expertise to perform a percutaneous biopsy or if a less invasive procedure fails to yield a diagnosis that is concordant with clinical findings. Open surgical biopsy should be used as an adjunct to percutaneous biopsy. Specifically, inadequate tissue or cytologic sampling by percutaneous biopsy warrants further analysis with surgical biopsy. To rule out concomitant invasive or in situ carcinoma, high-risk lesions such as papillary lesions, radial scar, and atypical ductal hyperplasia should undergo surgical biopsy. In addition, patients who have discordant biopsy pathology and radiologic imaging results require further inquiry with surgical biopsy.[4]

Open surgical biopsy can be image-guided or performed with the aid of palpation. Image-guided modalities for nonpalpable lesions include intraoperative US, preoperative image-guided (US, mammogram, or MRI) wire localization, or radioactive seed localization. The choice of incision site depends on the location of the lesion. Final postprocedure cosmesis should be taken into consideration when making decisions about incision placement (Fig. 28.6).

Choice of Anesthesia

The following factors should be considered in the choice of anesthesia (local, local with sedation, or general) for a breast biopsy:

• General medical condition of the patient
• Specific type of biopsy (FNA, core needle, incisional, excisional)
• Size of the breast
• Size and location of the lesion within the breast
• Personal preference of the patient and the physician

Options for anesthesia should be discussed with the patient and recommendations made on the basis of several factors. FNA and CNB are performed under local anesthesia alone or with mild sedation. In most cases, efforts should be made to avoid general anesthesia for open surgical biopsies. Lesions that lie deep in the breast may be best excised with the patient under general anesthesia. In addition, a patient who is apprehensive about undergoing the biopsy with local anesthesia may elect a general anesthetic if his or her medical condition is compatible with this technique. Even primary tumor resection with sentinel lymph node biopsy can be safely performed under local anesthesia with sedation.[49–52] Hypnosis has been shown to be a useful adjunct to anesthesia in breast procedures.[49]

Contraindications to local anesthesia and/or sedation for breast biopsy generally include the following:

• Previous history of problems with local anesthetic agents or the process of intravenous sedation
• Resections in which it is anticipated that the volume of local anesthetic will exceed limits of toxicity
• Procedures lasting more than 1 hour

Wire-Guided Localization

For nonpalpable lesions, wire-guided localization has been the standard for identification of lesions before surgical excision.[53] On the day of surgery, a patient presents to the radiology suite for placement of the wire. On completion of the wire placement, the patient is transported to the operating room with the wire and postplacement images. In the operating room, the wire serves as a marker for the lesion of interest (Fig. 28.7). When prepping the patient the external portion of the wire is included in the prep. The incision is placed directly over the lesion of interest based on its location on mammography. Care must be taken to ensure that the wire is not accidentally cut or displaced during dissection of the breast abnormality. The mammographic images and radiology notes should be used as guides for the location of the lesion relative to the wire. After removal of the specimen, an x-ray is taken to ensure removal of the entire length of the wire and previously placed clip (if the patient underwent percutaneous biopsy before excision) (Fig. 28.8).

Complications from wire-guided localization include improper placement of the wire, displacement of the wire during patient transport, and accidentally cutting the wire intraoperatively.[54,55] The patient should be transferred via a stretcher to the operating room to prevent displacement of the wire during transportation.[56] If the wire is inadvertently cut intraoperatively, it should be retrieved with the assistance of a C-arm fluoroscope.[56]

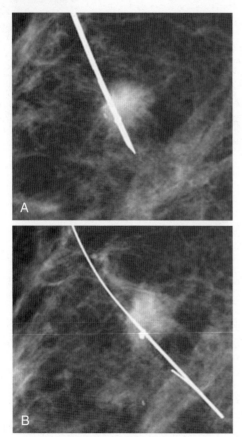

• **Fig. 28.7** Operative technique for needle localization biopsy. (A) The suspicious lesion is "localized" on the mammogram immediately before surgery. During the operation the needle serves as a guide for the surgeon to perform the biopsy. (B) Sagittal view of breast with localization needle in tumor.

Intraoperative Ultrasound Guidance

The use of intraoperative US to guide surgical excision of nonpalpable lesions requires the surgeon to be properly trained in the use of US. The surgeon must ensure that he or she can easily identify the lesion of interest in the clinic setting before taking the patient to the operating room. Under US guidance, an incision is made directly over the lesion, which is excised and sent for pathologic evaluation. Postprocedure intraoperative US should be conducted to ensure the correct lesion has been biopsied.

In a systematic review comparing intraoperative US to wire-guided localization of nonpalpable lesions, Ahmed and colleagues concluded intraoperative US was equally effective in localizing lesions compared with wire-guided localization. Moreover, the study noted that intraoperative US was superior to wire-guided localization in reducing reoperation rates secondary to positive margins.[57]

Radioactive Seed Localization

The use of liquid radioactive tracer for the localization of nonpalpable lesions was first published by Luini and colleagues in 1998.[53,58] The technique, radioguided occult lesion localization (ROLL), involved injection of a liquid radioactive tracer (^{99m}TC) into the tumor. Luini's technique was modified by Gray and coworkers with substitution of a radioactive titanium seed containing 3.7 to 10.7 MBq of ^{125}I into the tumor instead of a liquid radioactive tracer.[53,59]

Preoperatively, ^{125}I is placed in the lesion of interest under image guidance (US, mammography, or MRI). Per National Regulatory Commission guidelines, seeds may be placed a

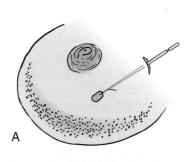

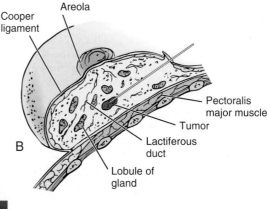

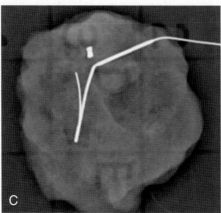

• **Fig. 28.8** Wire localization: image from a 58-year-old woman with newly diagnosed invasive ductal carcinoma undergoing wire localization before surgical excision. (A) Localization needle traverses the mass overlying the biopsy marking clip. (B) Localization needle has been replaced by wire. (C) Specimen radiograph confirms the localization wire, biopsy marking clip, and mass.

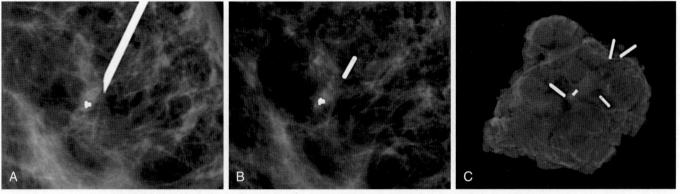

• **Fig. 28.9** Seed localization: 66-year-old woman with atypical ductal hyperplasia undergoing seed localization before surgical excision. (A) Localization needle positioned adjacent to the biopsy marking clip. (B) Radioactive seed has been deployed adjacent to the biopsy marking clip. (C) Specimen radiograph confirms the radioactive seed, biopsy marking clip, and some residual calcifications. Surgical clips are also noted.

maximum of 5 to 7 days before surgery.[60] Before incision, a standard handheld gamma probe is used to find the location of the seed. An incision is made directly over the lesion, and the tissue is excised to achieve a spherically shaped specimen. Upon removal of the lesion, the gamma probe is held over the tissue specimen and subsequently in the lumpectomy cavity to ensure the seed has been removed. An x-ray of the specimen is taken to confirm removal of the seed (Fig. 28.9).

For patients undergoing concomitant sentinel lymph node biopsy with ^{99m}TC, the different gamma radiation emission peaks of ^{99m}TC and ^{125}I enable standard handheld gamma probes to distinguish between both tracers. Specifically, the gamma radiation peak for ^{99m}TC is 140 keV compared with 27 keV for ^{125}I.[61] Furthermore, the half-life for ^{125}I is 60 days versus 6 hours for ^{99m}TC.[60]

Potential complications of radioactive seed localization include failure to retrieve the seed intraoperatively and failure to excise the lesion of interest due to an improperly placed seed. If the seed is not retrieved intraoperatively, the patient must undergo mammographic imaging to locate the seed to make sure it has not migrated. If the seed is improperly placed, another seed must be placed to localize the lesion of interest, and both seeds need to be removed intraoperatively.[60]

Proponents of seed localization argue that the 5- to 7-day window for seed placement reduces scheduling conflicts among radiology, surgery, and the patient by allowing flexible preoperative placement dates compared with wire localization.[60] A comparison of radioactive seed localization to wire-guided localization by Jakub and colleagues showed similar positive margin and reoperation rates for both modalities. However, they noted that operative times were shorter for radioactive seed localization.[59] Before using this biopsy technique, it is important to be aware of the institutional policies concerning the handling and disposal of radioactive material.[60]

Open surgical biopsy offers the most definitive tissue diagnosis of the biopsy techniques presented in this chapter. However, of the modalities discussed, it is the least cost-effective, most likely to result in additional operative procedures, and has an increased risk of postprocedure complications when used as an index tissue acquisition modality. Consequently, open surgical biopsy is best used as an adjunct to FNA or CNB rather than the preferred first choice of biopsy technique.

Conclusion

An accurate tissue diagnosis is essential for the evaluation of a suspicious breast mass or new mammographic finding. Tissue for evaluation may be obtained with FNA, CNB, or surgical biopsy. All may have a role in the evaluation of a breast abnormality, with specific advantages offered by each technique (Table 28.1). Institutional workflow and local expertise can affect the choice of biopsy. Although there are certain clinical settings when surgical biopsy is indicated, open surgical biopsy should be avoided as a first diagnostic procedure. It is important that a breast specialist have clear knowledge of the options available as well as the indications and limitations of each, to achieve the best outcome for the patient. Future directions will allow better discrimination of those conditions requiring biopsy, but the current options allow for minimally invasive, accurate diagnoses with little morbidity.

Acknowledgment

We gratefully acknowledge the contribution of Marshall M. Urist, who authored this chapter in previous editions.

Selected References

6. Eberth JM, Xu Y, Smith GL, et al. Surgeon influence on use of needle biopsy in patients with breast cancer: a national medicare study. *J Clin Oncol.* 2014;32:2206-2216.

16. Ljung BM, Drejet A, Chiampi N, et al. Diagnostic accuracy of fine-needle aspiration biopsy is determined by physician training in sampling technique. *Cancer.* 2001;93:263-268.

24. Schrading S, Distelmaier M, Dirrichs T, et al. Digital breast tomosynthesis-guided vacuum-assisted breast biopsy: initial experiences and comparison with prone stereotactic vacuum-assisted biopsy. *Radiology.* 2015;274:654-662.

38. Chevrier MC, David J, Khoury ME, et al. Breast biopsies under magnetic resonance imaging guidance: challenges of an essential but imperfect technique. *Curr Probl Diagn Radiol.* 2016;45:193-204.

53. Lovrics PJ, Goldsmith CH, Hodgson N, et al. A multicentered, randomized, controlled trial comparing radioguided seed localization to standard wire localization for nonpalpable, invasive and in situ breast carcinomas. *Ann Surg Oncol.* 2011;18:3407-3414.

A full reference list is available online at ExpertConsult.com.

29

General Principles of Mastectomy: Evaluation and Therapeutic Options

KIRBY I. BLAND, JORGE I. DE LA TORRE, EDWARD M. COPELAND III, V. SUZANNE KLIMBERG, CRISTIANO BONETI, AND LUIS O. VASCONEZ

The treatment of a presumably surgically operable mammary carcinoma may be reinforced by two methods: radiation alone and combined radiation and operation. The outlook upon the adoption or otherwise of the reinforcing methods depends on the experience and judgment of the surgeon.

—G.L. CHEATLE AND M. CUTLER (1933)

With pathologic confirmation of the diagnosis of breast cancer, a complete history, physical examination, and accurate clinical staging evaluation are requisite to therapy of the primary invasive neoplasm. Mammary adenocarcinoma that is 5 cm (T2) or less (T1) in transverse diameter and limited to the central or lateral aspect of the breast with the absence of pectoral fascia, skin fixation, and axillary lymphadenopathy can usually be treated with conservation surgery or total mastectomy with or without node dissection alone. Lesions smaller than 4 cm in diameter may be optionally treated with segmental mastectomy (partial mastectomy, lumpectomy, or tylectomy) and postoperative irradiation, with results comparable to those achieved with radical surgical techniques. Conservation approaches are discussed in Chapter 32. For cancers larger than 5 cm (T3) in transverse diameter (stage IIIA or IIIB), a combination of radical surgery and radiation therapy, often after neoadjuvant therapy, is essential to achieve locoregional control of the breast, axilla, and chest wall (see Chapters 49, 63, and 65).

The significant contributions of investigators to the management of breast cancer in the 20th century established the outcome results for conservation surgical techniques to be equivalent to those of radical approaches with regard to disease-free and overall survival. Thus the procedure to be completed and the anatomic site to receive irradiation for stages 0, I, and II disease depend on the location of the primary neoplasm in the breast, the presence or absence of axillary metastases, phenotype of the index cancer, and the growth characteristics of the index tumor (e.g., extension to musculature of chest wall, skin, axilla).[1]

Moreover, the increasing importance of the primary tumor characteristics and its phenotype relative to its natural history have been established in clinical trials as important criteria for procedure selection. The integration of cellular, biochemical, immunohistochemical, and molecular biologic features of the tumor phenotype will increasingly direct therapies for future decades.

Lesions in the lateral aspect of the breast drain principally through axillary lymphatic channels (see Chapter 2). Index tumor presentations in this location can be eradicated from the chest wall by using the modified radical mastectomy with sentinel lymph node biopsy (SLNB; see Chapters 31, 42, and 45). This surgical procedure is defined as a total mastectomy with preservation of the pectoralis minor/major muscles and includes dissection of level I and II axillary lymph nodes. These laterally placed neoplasms with histologically positive axillary lymph node metastases may be associated with internal mammary or supraclavicular lymph node metastases in as many as 25% to 30% of patients. Radiation therapy and chemotherapy are used for "grave" presentations of the tumors: skin fixation, nodularity, greater than 20% of nodes dissected histologically involved, more than three histologically involved nodes, and chest wall tumor fixation.[2]

Centrally located lesions that are fixed to the pectoralis major fascia or high-lying (superiorly located) lesions that are fixed to this fascia may be treated with radical mastectomy or with a combination of radical mastectomy and peripheral lymphatic and chest wall irradiation when palpable axillary lymph node metastases smaller than 2 cm are evident. These centrally placed lesions commonly metastasize through lymphatics that parallel the course of the neurovascular bundle medial to the pectoralis minor muscle. This medial neurovascular bundle that contains the lateral pectoral nerve and innervates the pectoralis major muscle is preserved in the modified radical mastectomy to ensure function of the pectoralis major muscle after mastectomy. In the radical mastectomy procedure, this neurovascular bundle, associated lymphatics, and areolar tissue are resected en bloc with the specimen to accomplish adequate surgical extirpation of regional disease.

For medially located neoplasms, the principal lymphatic drainage is through routes that course to lymph nodes near the ipsilateral internal mammary vessels. These medial lesions may be associated with metastasis to the internal mammary lymphatics in 10% to 30% of patients, as previously confirmed by Handley.[3] The presence of pathologically positive axillary metastasis with an associated medial lesion escalates this incidence of internal mammary metastasis to greater than 50%. In the absence of clinically positive axillary metastases, medially located cancers may be adequately treated with segmental (partial) mastectomy or with modified radical mastectomy and peripheral lymphatic irradiation.

Whether the surgeon chooses the conservation or radical approach depends on tumor size and characteristics, general medical status, patient choice, and desire for reconstruction.

Regardless of the operative procedure selected, clearance of pathologically "free" margins about the neoplasm in three dimensions is paramount to enhancement of locoregional disease-free survival. Margins of the tumor resection that invade the costochondrium and periosteum of ribs or sternum or the intercostal musculature (as confirmed with magnetic resonance imaging or a chest computed tomography scan) require full-thickness chest wall resection with immediate myocutaneous flap reconstruction. With "clear" margins pathologically, radiation may be administered concomitant with the treatment regimen and depends on the presenting tumor characteristics and location and the presence (number) of metastatic lymph nodes (see Chapters 48, 49, and 63). Furthermore, it is common to include chest wall irradiation when axillary metastases are identified pathologically in more than 20% of the removed axillary lymphatics. This principle was originally established because of the high incidence of skin flap recurrence evident with metastatic disease that courses to the axilla through the subdermal lymphatics from medially located primary lesions.

The principal determinant of actuarial survival of the patient after therapy of the primary breast lesion is the pathologic stage of the tumor. As established by the American Joint Committee on Cancer (AJCC), the staging system most commonly used is the tumor, node, metastasis (TNM) system. It is the responsibility of surgeons and radiation oncologists to jointly plan an operative procedure that encompasses, en bloc, the extent of the disease and provides the maximum probability for locoregional chest wall control of the tumor. It is also their responsibility to achieve this end result with minimal morbidity and mortality. These principles are best served by avoiding axillary irradiation after the Patey (complete) surgical dissection of level I to III axillary lymphatics; otherwise the incidence of lymphedema of the extremity of the ipsilaterally irradiated axilla will be increased approximately 7- to 10-fold. After radical resection of lymphatic channels with en bloc dissection of levels I to III, the remaining lymphatics are destroyed with radiation therapy, thus increasing the incidence of lymphedema. In principle, operable breast cancer (stages I and II) treated with total mastectomy and axillary node removal with the radical or modified radical mastectomy should not require postoperative irradiation. Currently, in cases where a SLNB demonstrates metastatic disease, control of the axilla can best be achieved with level I and II dissections; clearance of level III (Patey procedure) is required only if nodes are involved clinically at dissection.[4] In contradistinction, for the treatment of stage III disease with axillary metastases that clinically present with large, matted, or multiple nodes, the radiation oncologist should plan the application of tangential fields to the apex of the axilla, including the peripheral lymphatics and chest wall after the extended simple (total) mastectomy. This therapeutic regimen is essential because level III (apical) lymphatics remain intact after a resection that includes only lymphatics lateral to the border of the pectoralis major and minor muscles. With the extended total mastectomy performed for stage III breast cancer, primary cancer or lymphatics, or both, larger than 1 cm in diameter are unlikely to be sterilized with irradiation alone and require surgical extirpation.

Extension of the primary neoplasm into the axillary space with invasion of the axillary artery, vein, or brachial plexus does not technically allow complete surgical removal and is best treated with regional ionizing irradiation to the axilla, breast chest wall, and supraclavicular sites. Radiotherapy should also be added to low or central axillary nodes that are determined pathologically to have extranodal capsular extension into axillary soft tissues because local and regional control rates are enhanced with this modality despite the significantly increased risk of lymphedema in the ipsilateral arm. In the absence of clinically palpable nodes with primary neoplasms that exceed 5 cm in diameter, neoadjuvant chemotherapy with or without preoperative irradiation often (>80%) induces regression of the primary lesion. Preferably, surgery is performed after neoadjuvant induction with tumor regimen to reduce tumor burden before radiotherapy. The selection of surgical technique depends on the extent (volume) of regression of the primary tumor, the presence or absence of fixation to pectoralis major fascia, location, and the presence or absence of local "grave" signs (ulceration, skin edema and fixation, or satellitosis).[5]

Surgeons should plan the operative procedure with the objective of achieving, at minimum, 1- to 2-cm skin margins with subcutaneous and parenchymal margins of 2 to 3 cm in all directions from the index tumor, which can be accomplished with a radical, modified radical, or extended simple mastectomy. Patients with distant metastases, including supraclavicular lymph node metastases, are best treated with systemic chemotherapy with or without locoregional irradiation. Again, it is the responsibility of surgeons and radiation oncologists to achieve locoregional control except when adequate surgical margins are unobtainable in the absence of tumor regression, thereby reducing the probability of radiotherapeutic responses. The choice of these operative procedures must be individualized for each patient after determination of the site, clinical stage, and histologic type of the primary neoplasm. Similar principles guide the management of inflammatory breast cancers, which may be large, fixed, or ulcerated (see Chapters 63, 64, and 65).

As indicated in Chapters 14, 22, and 24, estrogen receptor (ER) and progesterone receptor (PR) activity, ploidy vc11, jy, HER2/neu status, and cytologic and nuclear grading indicators should be obtained for all pathologically invasive breast cancer specimens to aid the therapeutic planning of endocrine replacement or cytotoxic therapy in the event that adverse prognostic indicators are evident. Prospective data available for analysis suggest that mean survival rates for patients receiving either chemotherapy or hormonal manipulation are greater for patients possessing positive ER/PR activity and favorable biochemical and cellular growth phase indicators than those for patients who do not (negative ER/PR; positive HER2/neu). Regardless of the pathologic stage of the tumor or the receptor activity, the optimal chemotherapeutic regimen for patients with metastatic breast cancer continues to evolve (see Chapter 86). Qualitative values for hormone receptor activity of the primary neoplasm and cellular/biochemical and molecular prognosticators are of significant value to the oncologist and should be obtained from the primary lesion and metastatic sites to prospectively guide subsequent therapy.

The proper technique for the processing of tissues that contain ER and PR activity is essential to the design and implementation of future chemotherapy protocols for specific patients; the surgeon's attention to the preservation and processing of biopsy tissue is crucial. Despite the importance of the ER and PR activity and other cellular/biochemical and oncogene markers to guide future therapies, processing of neoplastic tissue for pathologic examination, in all cases, must take precedence over determination of steroid receptor activity, as well as the procurement of additional tissues to determine cellular, biochemical, and molecular prognostic characteristics that evaluate tumor phenotype (see Chapters 14, 22, and 24).

Immunohistologic methodologies have been extensively applied since the mid-2000s with replacement of quantitative

TABLE 29.1	Steroid Hormone Receptor Versus Ischemia Time[a]				
Receptor (n = 11)	ISCHEMIA TIME (MIN)[b]				
	0	30	60	90	150
ER	100	79 ± 10[c]	67 ± 11[c]	54 ± 11[c]	56 ± 13[c]
PR	100	100 ± 21	101 ± 26	94 ± 14	84 ± 27
AR	100	57 ± 12[c]	53 ± 15[c]	28 ± 9	42 ± 12[c]

[a]Ischemia significantly decreased ER levels within the first 30 minutes ($p = .05$). ER values had sustained decrease throughout 150 minutes of ischemia. Similarly, AR levels were significantly lower by 30 minutes of ischemia ($p = .002$) and remained so throughout 150 minutes of ischemia. The largest decrease in ER and AR levels occurred within the first 30 minutes of ischemia. In contrast, PR levels were unchanged throughout 150 minutes of ischemia.

[b]Values in last four columns are mean ± SEM, expressed as percent of control at baseline.

[c]$p < .005$ compared with baseline by analysis of variance.

AR, Androgen receptor; ER, estrogen receptor; PR, progesterone receptor.

steroid receptor analyses with less problematic concern for receptor invalidation. However, surgeons should also be aware of the potential for electrocautery to diminish steroid receptor activity. This was confirmed by Ellis and associates[6,7] and by Bland and colleagues[8] to be dependent on heat inactivation by the ambient temperature and by devascularization (Table 29.1). The procurement of primary breast cancer tissue for pathologic diagnosis and for determination of immunohistologic (qualitative) steroid receptor activity is best accomplished with the cold scalpel. This technique avoids the possibility of heat induction artifact, tissue necrosis, cellular death, and temperature-dependent inactivation of steroid receptor activity of the procured tissues. Nonetheless, tumor excision with cautery can be used if the operator avoids direct contact of tumor specimen with the cautery blade. The indications and techniques for biopsy of suspicious breast masses are comprehensively reviewed later in this chapter.

Topographic Surgical Anatomy

Chapter 2 provides a detailed review of the anatomy of the breast, including discussions of regional vasculature, neurologic structures, and lymphatic drainage. Hollingshead[9] observed that the fibrous and fatty components of breast tissue occupied the interval between the second or third rib superiorly, with extension to the sixth or seventh ribs inferiorly. The breadth of extension includes the parasternal to the midaxillary lines. The glandular portion of the breast rests largely on the pectoral fascia and the serratus anterior musculature; however, mammary tissue extends typically into the anterior axillary fold (tail of Spence) and may be visible as a well-defined superolateral extension from the upper outer quadrant of breast tissue. Extent of the mammary tissue is ill defined and varies considerably with patient habitus and lean muscle mass.

Parenchymal volume of the gland, with anterior and lateral projections, is variable and depends on lean body mass, habitus, age, and ovarian functional status. Because the ductal and lobular components are almost exclusively sensitive to the trophic effects of secretory estrogen and progestational hormones, the breast remains underdeveloped and rudimentary in the male. In men, short ducts with poorly developed acini are evident. Thus a deficiency of parenchymal fat and nipple-areola development are apparent and contribute to the nonspheroidal or flat appearance of the male breast.

Relative to the male breast, the nonparous breast is hemispheric and somewhat flattened above the nipple. The multiparous breast, on the other hand, is large and is replaced in part with fat, which accounts for its lax, soft appearance; it rarely regains its initial configuration until menopause, when atrophy of glandular tissue is initiated. The breast is circumscribed anteriorly by a superficial layer and posteriorly by a deep layer of the superficial investing fascia of the chest wall. The superficial layer of the superficial fascia of the chest wall derives its anterior boundaries from the fibrous tissue of the tela subcutanea. Haagensen[10] observed the deep layer of the superficial fascia to be contiguous with the pectoral fascia.

After loss of estrogen influence on breast parenchyma and ductal structures, the postmenopausal breast is replaced by fat and is consistently noted to lack supportive parenchymal connective tissue and active (proliferative) glandular components. Spratt and Donegan[11] and Spratt and Tobin[12] note that the nonlactating breast weighs between 150 and 225 g, whereas the lactating organ may weigh as much as 500 g.

Neurologic Innervation of the Pectoral Muscles

For purposes of clarity and consistency, the editors have retained the classic anatomic description and nomenclature for the pectoral (anterior thoracic) nerves and the accompanying neurovascular bundles (see Chapter 2). The name of the neurovascular bundle (lateral or medial) is synonymous with its course (position) in the axilla. Classic anatomy teaches that the pectoral nerves are named from the brachial cord (medial or lateral) from which they originate. In the technical description of operative procedures within this chapter and in anatomic descriptions elsewhere in this textbook (see Chapters 36, 41, 45, and 49), we have retained the classic nomenclature.

As evident in major surgical texts, the anatomy of the medial/lateral pectoral nerves and the innervation of the pectoral muscles have evoked only minimal interest. Major textbooks of surgical anatomy have long considered the names of the medial pectoral and lateral pectoral nerves on the basis of origin from the brachial plexus. Therefore the names in classic anatomic teaching are not correlated with their medial or lateral anatomic positions found during surgery (Fig. 29.1). Moosman,[13] however, completed a detailed study of the pectoral nerves by dissection of 100 adult fixed and fresh cadaver pectoral regions (56 male and 44 female), and he transposed the names of the medial and lateral pectoral nerves according to their anatomic relationship to the pectoral muscles and to the anterior chest wall. These nerves, sometimes called anterior thoracic nerves, originate cephalad and posterior to the axillary vein from an anastomotic nerve loop of variable size between the medial and lateral brachial plexus cords.

Moosman[13] noted in his anatomic dissections that the lateral pectoral nerve arises anatomically from the lateral cord and in location is medial to the pectoralis minor muscle. In its course, it divides into two to four branches that pass downward and medial to supply the clavicular, manubrial, and sternal components of the pectoralis major muscle. Thereafter the nerve passes through the costocoracoid foramen with the thoracoacromial vessels and enters the interpectoral space to mix with tributaries of vascular origin to the muscle. Moosman observed that this nerve is larger than the medial pectoral nerve because of the greater volume of muscle it innervates.

The medial pectoral nerve is smaller (approximately 1–2 mm in diameter and 10–15 cm in length) than the lateral pectoral

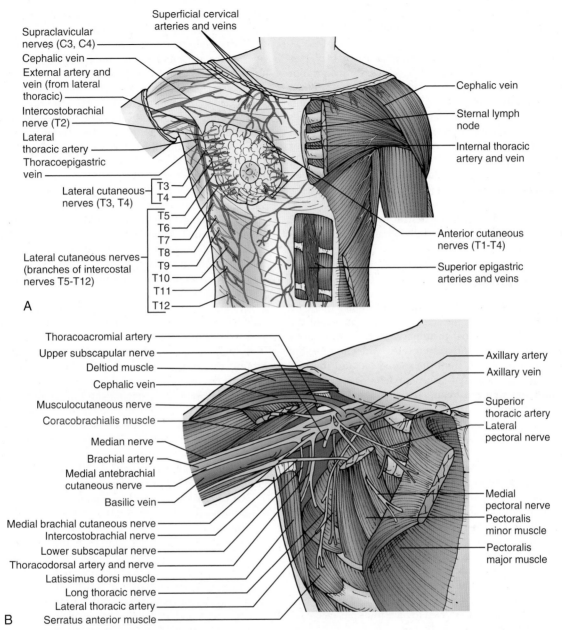

Supraclavicular
nerves (C3, C4)
Cephalic vein
External artery and
vein (from lateral
thoracic)
Intercostobrachial
nerve (T2)
Lateral
thoracic artery
Thoracoepigastric
vein

Superficial cervical
arteries and veins

Lateral cutaneous
nerves (T3, T4)

T3
T4
T5
T6
T7
T8
T9
T10
T11
T12

Lateral cutaneous nerves
(branches of intercostal
nerves T5-T12)

Cephalic vein
Sternal lymph
node
Internal thoracic
artery and vein

Anterior cutaneous
nerves (T1-T4)
Superior epigastric
arteries and veins

A

Thoracoacromial artery
Upper subscapular nerve
Deltiod muscle
Cephalic vein
Musculocutaneous nerve
Coracobrachialis muscle
Median nerve
Brachial artery
Medial antebrachial
cutaneous nerve
Basilic vein
Medial brachial cutaneous nerve
Intercostobrachial nerve
Lower subscapular nerve
Thoracodorsal artery and nerve
Latissimus dorsi muscle
Long thoracic nerve
Lateral thoracic artery
B   Serratus anterior muscle

Axillary artery
Axillary vein
Superior
thoracic artery
Lateral
pectoral nerve

Medial
pectoral nerve
Pectoralis
minor muscle
Pectoralis
major muscle

• **Fig. 29.1** (A and B) Arteries and nerves of the breast. View of nerves of the axilla that provide innervation to the pectoral muscles and muscles of the chest wall and posterior axillary space. The long thoracic nerve is identified and protected at the juncture where the axillary vein passes over the second rib. Injury or division of this nerve will result in "winged scapula" as a result of paralysis of the serratus anterior. The thoracodorsal nerve is found in the posterior axillary space with origin medial to the thoracodorsal vessels. This nerve may accompany the thoracodorsal artery and vein en route to its innervation of the latissimus dorsi. Injury results in weakness of abduction; internal rotation of the shoulder also will result. The medial (anterior thoracic) pectoral nerve is superficial to the axillary vein and lateral to the pectoralis minor muscle, which it variably penetrates en route to its innervation of the pectoralis major muscle. The lateral (anterior thoracic) pectoral nerve lies at the medial edge of the pectoralis minor muscle and superficial to the axillary vein. With origin from the lateral cord of the brachial plexus, this nerve supplies major motor innervation to the pectoralis major.

nerve, and its origin is medial or posterior to the pectoralis minor. This nerve sends branches to the pectoralis minor and descends on its dorsal surface. Typically this nerve crosses the axillary vein and is accompanied by small tributaries from the axillary or thoracoacromial vessels. It enters the interpectoral space and supplies the lower third of the costoabdominal portion of the pectoralis major muscle. In an extensive review of the anatomy of the medial

pectoral nerve, Moosman[13] observed the relationship of this nerve to the pectoralis minor to be one of several variants: (1) as a single descending branch around the lateral border of the lower half of the muscle (38%); (2) division into two branches, with one branch passing through the muscle and the other around its lateral margin (32%); (3) as a single descending branch that passed through the muscle (22%); and (4) as two or three descended branches of varying size, each of which passes through the muscle often at different levels (8%). He observed motor branches to the pectoralis major coursing through the pectoralis minor in 62% of cases.

In rare circumstances the medial pectoral nerve may pass through the medial muscular components of the pectoralis minor or, in other cases, may remain entirely on its medial surface. When numerous branches arise from the major trunks, a more diminutive size can be expected for branches that innervate the pectoralis major. The nerve remains relatively large when it is a single branch, whereas multiple branches passing through the muscle may be of thread size.[13]

Regardless of the anatomic nomenclature used, the surgeon must be cognizant of potential damage to the nerve supply to the pectoralis muscles at all levels of dissection. Manipulation, traction, electrocautery, or resection may destroy the lateral or medial pectoral nerves unless they are carefully separated from nerve branches of variable size.

Vascular Distribution

Nutrient arterial supply to the skin and breast is through branches of the lateral thoracic arteries, the acromiothoracic branch of the axillary artery, and the internal mammary artery.[14] The venous drainage system includes the intercostal veins, which traverse the posterior aspect of the breast from the second or third through the sixth or seventh intercostal spaces to terminate and enter posteriorly into the vertebral veins. The intercostal veins may arborize centrally with the azygos system to terminate in the superior vena cava. The deep venous drainage of the breast in large part parallels the pectoral branches of the acromiothoracic artery and the lateral thoracic artery.

The large epithelial and mesenchymal surface area of the superior, central, and lateral aspects of the breast is drained by tributaries that enter the axillary vein. Venous supply from the pectoralis major and minor muscles also drains into tributaries that enter the axillary vein. Perforating veins of the internal mammary venous system drain the medial aspect of the breast and the pectoralis major muscle. This large venous plexus can be observed to traverse the intercostal musculature and terminate in the innominate vein, providing a direct embolic route to the venous capillary network of the lungs. Each plexus of veins in the lateral and medial aspects of the breast is observed to have multiple, racemose anastomotic connections.

Lymphatic Drainage and Routes for Metastases

The rich and elaborate lymphatic drainage generally parallels the arterial and venous supply of the breast. This lymphatic flow is primarily unidirectional, except in subareolar and central aspects of the breast, or in circumstances in which physiologic lymphatic obstruction occurs as a consequence of neoplastic, inflammatory, or developmental processes that initiate a reversal of flow with bidirectional egress of lymph.[15] This bidirectional lymphatic flow (see Figs. 2.13 and 2.15) may account for metastatic proliferation in sites remote from the primary neoplasm (e.g., the opposite breast and axilla). The delicate lymph vessels of the corium are valveless and encircle the lobular parenchyma to enter each echelon of the regional lymphatic nodes in a progressive and orderly fashion (e.g., level I → level II → level III). As indicated in Chapter 2 (see Figs. 2.15 through 2.17), multiple lymphatic capillaries anastomose and fuse to form fewer lymph channels that subsequently terminate in the large left thoracic duct or the smaller right lymphatic duct (see Figs. 2.8 and 2.16). As a consequence of the predominant unidirectional flow of lymph, two accessory drainage routes exist for lymph en route to nodes of the apex of the axilla and include the transpectoral and the retropectoral routes, as defined by Anson and McVay.[14] First described by German pathologist Rotter, Rotter nodes are lymphatics of the transpectoral or interpectoral routes that occupy the position between the pectoralis major and minor muscles. Cody and coworkers[16] and Netter[17] report Rotter nodes to be present in up to 75% of individuals, with an average of two to three nodes per patient. Cody and coworkers[16] observed that 0.5% patients with negative nodes and 8.2% of patients who had positive axillary nodes had evidence of Rotter lymph node metastases. This observation was rarely reported by Haagensen.[10] Therefore, although the Patey axillary dissection, included in the Halsted radical[18] and in the modified radical mastectomy, removes the interpectoral Rotter group en bloc, this nodal group plays only a diminutive role in the diagnosis and therapy of breast cancer. The retropectoral lymphatics, however, may play a more important physiologic role in drainage of the breast because they are exposed to the superior and internal portions of the mammary glands. These lymphatics arborize lateral and posterior to the surface of the pectoralis major muscle and terminate at the apex of the axilla. To achieve an adequate en bloc resection of major axillary nodal groups, the surgeon must achieve a thorough conceptualization of breast lymphatic drainage. Familiarization with the anatomy of this area is essential for staging and for curative resection.

Chapter 2 deals with the principal axillary nodal groups as described by Anson and McVay.[14] Fig. 29.2 topographically depicts anatomic levels I to III of the axillary contents with relation to the neurovascular bundle, the pectoralis minor, the latissimus dorsi, and the chest wall. The following axillary nodal groups are included in level I:

1. The external mammary group parallels the course of the lateral thoracic artery from the sixth or seventh rib to the axillary vein. This group occupies the loose areolar tissue inferior and lateral to the pectoralis major muscle in the medial distal axillary space.
2. The subscapular group is contiguous with thoracodorsal branches of the subscapular vessels. This group extends from the ventral surface of the axillary vein to the lateral thoracic chest wall and includes loose areolar tissue on the serratus anterior and subscapularis musculature.
3. The lateral axillary vein group is the most laterally placed nodal group of the axillary space. This group also contains the largest number of nodes in the axilla and is observed to be caudad and ventral to the surface of the axillary vein often lateral to the latissimus dorsi muscle. This nodal group is first encountered in the course of proximate dissection on the anteriormost surface of the latissimus dorsi muscle.

Level II, or the central nodal group, is immediately beneath the pectoralis minor muscle and is the most centrally located of the axillary lymphatic groups. This nodal group is located between the anterior and posterior axillary fold and occupies a superficial position beneath the skin and fascia of the midaxilla. The highest and most medially placed of the lymph node groups is the subclavicular (apical group), designated as level III. This is the cephalomedial lymph nodal group that is located just proximate to the termination of the axillary vein at its confluence with the subclavian vein at the level of Halsted's (costoclavicular) ligament (condensation of the clavipectoral fascia). Fig. 29.2 depicts the position of these nodes relative to the pectoralis minor muscle

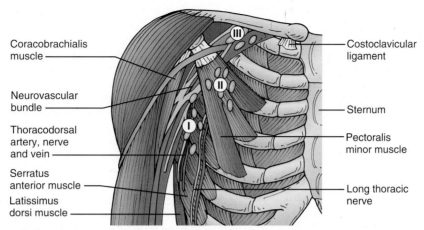

• **Fig. 29.2** Topographic anatomic depiction of levels I, II, and III of the axillary contents with relation to the neurovascular bundle, pectoralis minor, latissimus dorsi, posterior axillary space, and chest wall. Level I comprises three principal axillary nodal groups: the external mammary group, the subscapular group, and the axillary vein (lateral) group. Level II, the central nodal group, is centrally placed immediately beneath the pectoralis minor muscle. The subclavicular (apical) group is designated level III nodes and is supero-medial to the pectoralis minor muscle.

and the posterior axillary space. These nodal groups are described relative to topographic anatomic relationships with the pectoralis minor muscle and the medial, lateral, and posterior axillary space. These lymphatics may be different from the nodal groups described by pathologists to indicate the area of metastatic involvement within the axilla.

Evolution of Surgical Techniques for Mastectomy

In 1894 Halsted[18] and Meyer[19] simultaneously reported their radical operations for treatment of cancer of the breast. By demonstrating superior locoregional control rates using en bloc radical resection techniques, these eminent surgeons established the radical mastectomy as the state-of-the-art modality of that era to control cancer of the breast. Subsequently, many modifications of the original incision developed by Halsted have been reported and include those of Meyer, Kocher, Rodman, Stewart, Warren, Greenough, Orr, Gray, and MacFee, to mention only a few variations of the incision.[20] Many of the original incisions were developed to permit multiple approaches for extirpation of the mammae and to allow access to the axillary contents.

The Halsted[18] and Meyer[19] radical mastectomies differed technically in the sequence in which the breast and nodes were removed. Halsted insisted on primary resection of the breast and pectoral muscles before dissection of the axillary contents. In contrast, the Meyer technique (modified Halsted incision) advised the axillary dissection first, followed in sequence by breast and pectoral muscle resections, respectively. As indicated in Fig. 29.3, the result achieved and the final cosmetic appearance for the Halsted and Meyer mastectomies are similar. Both procedures use a vertical incision to facilitate detachment of the pectoralis major from the clavicle and humerus and removal of the pectoralis minor from the coracoid process of the scapula. Incisions subsequently adopted by various European and American surgeons are indicated in Fig. 29.3 and represent incision modifications for operable breast cancer in each quadrant of the organ. It should be noted that Halsted[18] and Meyer[19] strongly advocated the

necessity of en bloc resections for extirpation of the breast and the contents of the axilla but had little appreciation for clinical staging and the ultimate consequences of systemic disease. In their era, no adjuvant modalities (radiation/chemotherapy) existed to provide effective cytoreduction of the advanced primary lesion; thus, advanced stages of disease could be extirpated only with the use of wider skin margins and larger flaps. For this reason, various incision modifications that incorporate breast resection and wound closure were developed.

Eminent breast surgeons of the late 19th and early 20th centuries appreciated early in the formulation of therapeutic principles that the total mastectomy incision should incorporate both the nipple and the biopsy site to reduce the possibility of tumor implantation in the wound. In original dissections of the axilla, both Halsted[18] and Meyer[19] advocated complete axillary dissection of all three nodal levels from the latissimus dorsi muscle laterally to the thoracic outlet medially. Both surgeons routinely sacrificed the long thoracic nerve and the thoracodorsal neurovascular bundle en bloc with the axillary contents. Therefore it is not surprising that much of the initial criticism leveled at the radical mastectomy in the treatment of breast carcinoma concerned itself with the limitation of motion in the shoulder and the ipsilateral lymphedema that followed surgery. It also could be argued that survival rates for these patients, especially those with advanced locoregional disease, were not increased in proportion to the resultant disabilities (e.g., the "winged scapula" and shoulder fixation) evident with the procedures. Subsequently, Haagensen[10] advocated preservation of the long thoracic nerve to avoid the winged scapula disability and motor apraxia evident with loss of innervation to the serratus anterior. Furthermore, Haagensen[10] advocated removal of the thoracodorsal neurovascular bundle (with neural innervation to the latissimus dorsi muscle) to allow clearance of the subscapular and external mammary lymphatics that follow the course of this neurovascular structure. However, the majority of breast surgeons currently preserve both the long thoracic and the thoracodorsal nerves in the absence of gross invasion by the neoplasm or nodal fixation to these nerves. These principles are strictly enforced to ensure function of the scapula and to preserve viability and motor innervation of the latissimus dorsi,

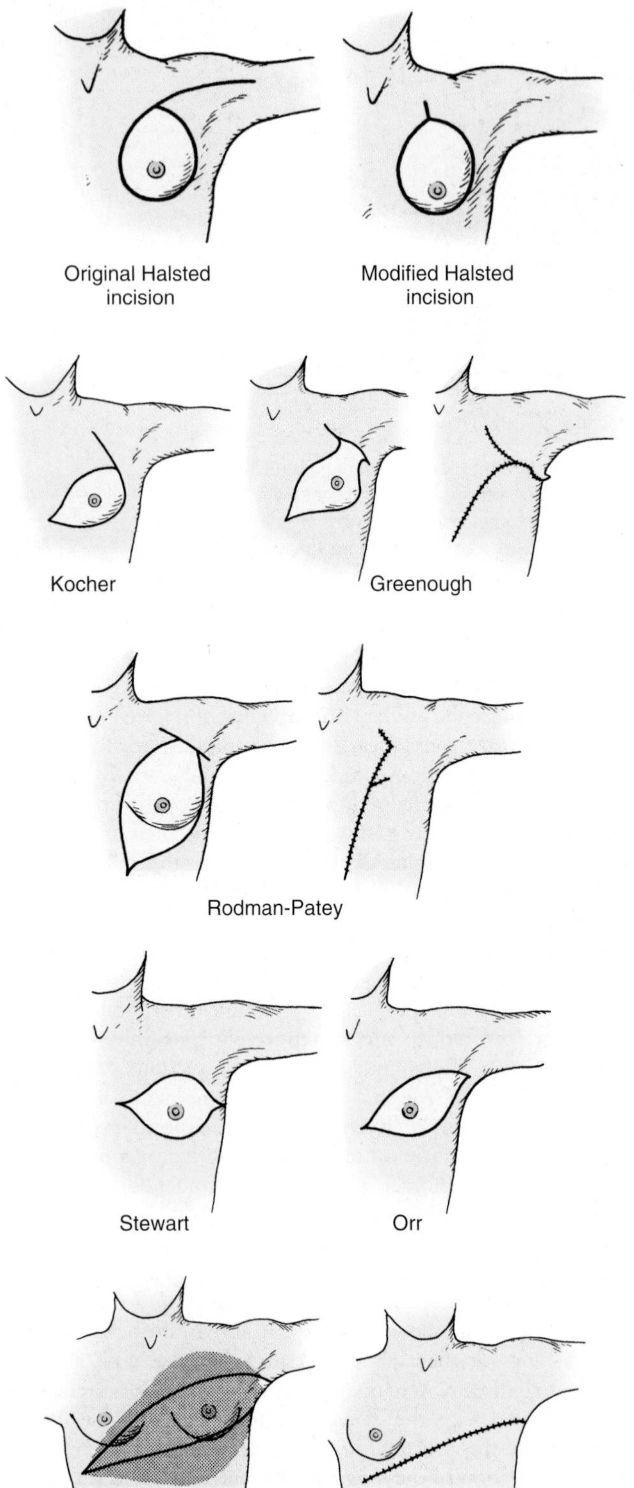

• **Fig. 29.3** Variants of the radical mastectomy incision used in the therapy of primary carcinoma of the breast by various surgeons. The original Halsted incision was revised to avoid encroachment on the cephalic vein, which was preserved in subsequent procedures.

such that myocutaneous breast reconstruction may be a future option.

It should be noted that contemporary modifications of the Halsted or Meyer radical mastectomy, with preservation of the long thoracic nerve, can be performed with little or no increase in morbidity compared with simple mastectomy.[15,21] In addition, any argument of the simple versus the radical procedure should be concerned with the long-term survival of the patient, which is the ultimate goal of therapy. To deny a patient the benefit of an adequate operative procedure on the basis of difficulty in placing cosmetic incisions or difficulty with wound closure is tantamount to disregard of an indisputable tenet that portends locoregional recurrence of disease.

The highly regarded and significant contributions of D.H. Patey[22,23] of the Institute of Clinical Research, Middlesex Hospital, London, should be recognized. His careful clinical development and scientific demonstration of the worth of the "modified radical mastectomy" technique are laudable. In Britain in the 1930s, only a small minority of physicians questioned the absolute necessity of radical mastectomy for carcinoma of smaller size (AJCC stage I–II) with absence of fixation to the pectoral muscles. Three major influences led Patey in the 1930s and 1940s to consider therapeutic alternatives; design of the modified radical mastectomy technique followed. The first and most important consideration was the development and application of modern radiation therapy. The second influence was the growing evidence of dissatisfaction with Sampson Handley's theory of "lymphatic permeation" as the primary process for the dissemination of carcinoma of the breast—a theory that, in its day, provided a logical pathologic basis for some of the technical details of the radical mastectomy.[22] Third, with newer techniques for the study of lymphatic anatomy, Patey was able to scientifically refute the unproven postulates on which the original radical operations were based.[11,15] Thereafter Patey and his colleagues developed the technique for in continuity removal of the breast and axillary contents (levels I, II, and III) with preservation of the pectoralis major muscle. This technique removes the pectoralis minor, like the standard radical operation, as the essential operative maneuver to provide access for complete clearance of the axillary contents. Objective demonstration of the efficacy for removal of axillary lymphatics with the technique was later proven with lymphangiography by Kendall and associates[24] in 1963. Although this operation was performed by Patey for the first time in 1932, it was not adopted as a routine alternative to the standard radical mastectomy until late 1936.[11]

Although Patey is credited with the formulation and implementation of the modified radical mastectomy as a standard approach for operable breast cancer, it was Auchincloss[25] and Madden[26] who described and developed technical variants of the modified radical mastectomy. As described earlier, the Patey mastectomy differs from the Halsted mastectomy in that the pectoralis major muscle is preserved. Patey acknowledged the importance of the complete axillary dissection (levels I, II, and III) and appreciated the anatomic necessity for preservation of the medial and lateral pectoral (anterior thoracic) nerves, which may serve as dual innervation to the pectoralis major. In contrast, Auchincloss[25] and Madden[26] advocated modified radical mastectomies with preservation of both the pectoralis major and minor muscles. The similarities of the approaches were that these techniques required total mastectomy with at least partial axillary lymph node dissection. Because these approaches preserved the pectoralis minor, dissection of the apical (subclavicular, level III) nodes was restricted, and in all cases, nodal recovery was less complete than with the

Patey modified technique. The advantage of the Auchincloss[25] and Madden[26] procedures may be the greater probability for preservation of the medial pectoral nerve, which courses in the lateral neurovascular bundle of the axilla and may course through the pectoralis minor to supply the lateral border of the pectoralis major muscle. Expectantly, the Madden and Auchincloss techniques dissect only level I and II nodes and preserve level III lymphatics. Even currently, some surgeons advocate preservation of the pectoralis minor and simply detach the tendinous portion of the muscle from the coracoid process of the scapula to allow near-complete dissection of level III nodes to Halsted's ligament. On completion of the nodal dissection, the tendon of the pectoralis minor was reapproximated to the coracoid with stainless steel wire or nonabsorbable suture.

Randomized clinical trials have established the safety of breast conservation therapy (BCT) compared with mastectomy. The National Surgical Adjuvant Breast and Bowel Project (NSABP) B0-6 trial compared patients with tumors less than 4 cm undergoing partial mastectomy and axillary node dissection or modified radical mastectomy. At 20 years, the was no different in overall survival (OS) or disease-free survival (DFS), but local recurrence was higher in the BCT group compared with the modified radical mastectomy group.[27] Likewise, the MILAN I trial compared radical mastectomy to partial mastectomy followed by radiation in women with invasive breast cancer <2 cm. Local recurrence reflected those seen in NSABP B-06 with a significant difference of 8.8% for BCT versus 2.3% for radical mastectomy, whereas survival was not different.[28] In the European Organization for Research and Treatment of Cancer 10801 trial, patients with breast tumors less than 5 cm were randomized to BCT or modified radical mastectomy.[29] Results were consistent with the previous similar trials demonstrating an increase in local recurrence with BCT, but no significant difference in OS or time to distant metastasis.[30,31]

Students of breast surgery quickly recognize that incisions for the modified radical mastectomy are less extreme, and wounds are closed primarily. In contrast, radical procedures use wide incision margins, and skin is routinely grafted to wound defects. The application of modern radiobiologic techniques and cytoreductive chemotherapy currently does not require primary incisions that totally ablate the skin of the breast (see Fig. 29.3). Before the application of modern adjuvant techniques, incisions for large tumors that were considered locally advanced (because of ulceration, edema, and other "grave" signs) were designed to encompass these lesions with wide (3- to 5-cm) margins.

All skin flaps should be designed so that the incision incorporates skin and parenchyma at minimum of 1 cm from the periphery of the tumor in three dimensions. In principle, less skin is excised when lesions are located deep within the breast and T size is small in transverse diameter (T1 <2 cm). As indicated in Chapter 2, viable breast tissue is anatomically distributed on the chest wall from the sternum to the axilla and from the clavicle to the aponeurosis of the rectus abdominis tendon. Haagensen[10] demonstrated that small foci of glandular tissue could be histologically identified in close proximity to the dermis just beneath the superficial fascia. Halsted[18] and Haagensen[10] each considered that wide skin excision of at least 5 cm in all directions from the tumor was essential because of the rich superficial lymphatic channels of the central subareolar tissue and subcutaneous dermal lymphatic plexuses of the breast. The rationale of the classic radical and modified radical mastectomies is increasingly being challenged because of the availability of adjuvant modalities that enhance locoregional control with potential lengthening of DFS

and OS rates. These tenets form the anatomic and pathologic basis for the skin-sparing mastectomy, which is comprehensively discussed later in this chapter.

Debate continues regarding the thickness of skin flaps that should be elevated in the planning of the total mastectomy as part of the radical or modified radical procedure. Krohn and colleagues[32] report a two-arm study to evaluate the necessity of the "ultrathin" skin flap and the use of autogenous skin graft as methods to enhance local wound control with 5- and 10-year survival. A similar group of women who underwent radical mastectomy with narrow margins of skin excision with primary wound closure without ultrathin flaps had comparable 5- and 10-year survival and local recurrence rates. Wound complications, duration of hospital stay, and subsequent lymphedema, however, were significantly greater in the patients with thinner skin flaps. Most surgeons acknowledge that superior cosmetic results are achievable with well-vascularized flaps and the avoidance of split-thickness skin grafting. We maintain these basic tenets and avoid development of ultrathin flaps. Flaps developed at the plane of insertion of Cooper's ligament deep to the cutis reticularis with the subcutaneous fat ensure extirpation of the underlying breast parenchyma. In general, flaps of 6- to 8-mm thickness usually ensure generous vascularity and viability of the skin. Subcutaneous fat may be preserved, which is consistent with complete parenchymal resection. Although the deep layer of the superficial investing fascia that intervenes between the subcutaneous fat and the breast tissue is easily identified, the thickness of this well-vascularized flap varies considerably with the patient's habitus and lean body mass.

Total mastectomy for operable cancer that is not amenable to conservation surgical techniques has been addressed previously. In principle, advanced primary lesions (T2 or T3), with pectoralis major fixation, high-lying lesions, and perhaps some lesions with "grave" signs should be treated with radical or modified radical techniques. As discussed previously, the operations designed by Halsted, his predecessors, and his students reflect the necessity of designing wider flaps with large incisions for advanced primary cancers (T3a, T3b, T4) to technically encompass the primary lesion by at least 5 cm. When considering the advanced primary lesions that were treated in that era without adjuvant techniques, the necessity of larger resections can be rationalized as surgery was the only option for locoregional control.

The design of incisions that allow removal of the entire mammary gland (total or simple mastectomy) must incorporate the nipple-areola complex with the primary tumor in a three-dimensional aspect such that deep and peripheral margins are free of disease.[33] Donegan and coworkers[34] previously determined that incisions that resect skin and breast parenchyma at a distance of more than 4 cm from any margin of the palpable tumor achieve no improved therapeutic success. Currently, many surgeons consider a 1- to 2-cm margin adequate to achieve local control without tumor implantation. Intraoperative frozen section for marginal clearance is appropriate, especially margins 1 cm or less from the index neoplasm. As discussed in Chapter 45, incisions placed in the breast for suspicious masses must be planned with consideration for the subsequent need for total mastectomy. Incisions should incorporate the primary biopsy scar, which should be well planned at the time of initial biopsy to allow complete extirpation of the neoplasm with the definitive mastectomy. When the primary breast lesion has been totally removed with the original biopsy as an excisional technique, incisions placed for total mastectomy should incorporate the skin and scar of the biopsy site by a minimal 1-cm margin in all three dimensions of the resection. We prefer incisions (Orr/modified Orr) that are

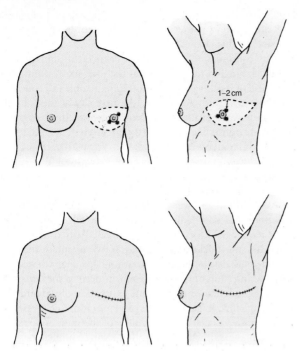

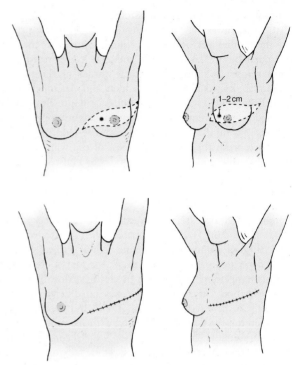

• **Fig. 29.4** Design of the classic Stewart elliptical incision for central and subareolar primary lesions of the breast. The medial extent of the incision ends at the margin of the sternum. The lateral extent of the skin incision should overlie the anterior margin of the latissimus dorsi. The design of the skin incision should incorporate the primary neoplasm en bloc with margins that are 1 to 2 cm from the cranial and caudal edges of the tumor.

• **Fig. 29.5** Design of the obliquely placed modified Stewart incision for cancer of the inner quadrant of the breast. The medial extent of the incision often must incorporate skin to the midsternum to allow a 1- to 2-cm margin in all directions from the edge of the tumor. Lateral extent of the incision ends at the anterior margin of the latissimus.

slightly oblique from the transverse line and that extend cephalad toward the axilla. However, under no circumstance should the cosmetic design of an incision compromise the successful extirpation of the primary neoplasm. Split-thickness skin grafting has virtually been replaced with myocutaneous flap reconstruction after mastectomy for T3 or T4 primary neoplasms when wider margins and larger flaps are required for wound closure after neoadjuvant therapy.

Figs. 29.4 through 29.10 depict the various locations of breast primaries in which adequate therapy, with or without irradiation and chemotherapy, necessitates total mastectomy, which is completed with conventional technique in which reconstruction is not planned. For all mastectomy procedures, note that wide (radical) skin margin (>5 cm) excisions are not considered essential for locoregional disease control. However, skin margins of at least 1 to 2 cm from the gross index tumor or the surgical biopsy (excision) scar are necessary to ensure final pathology-free margins. Margins in excess of 2 cm are technically feasible for most total mastectomies in which reconstruction (early or delayed) will not be completed. Preoperative consideration should be given to the skin-sparing technique (see discussion later in this chapter) when the patient desires reconstruction.

Design of Incisions for Mastectomy in the Treatment of Breast Cancer

Central and Subareolar Primary Lesions

Fig. 29.4 depicts the design of the classic Stewart elliptical skin incision (see Fig. 29.3) that is used for mastectomy of subareolar

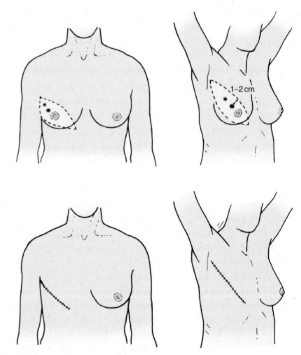

• **Fig. 29.6** Design of the classic Orr oblique incision for carcinoma of the upper outer quadrants of the breast. The skin incision is placed 1 to 2 cm from the margin of the tumor in an oblique plane that is directed cephalad toward the ipsilateral axilla. This incision is a variant of the original Greenough, Kocher, and Rodman techniques for flap development.

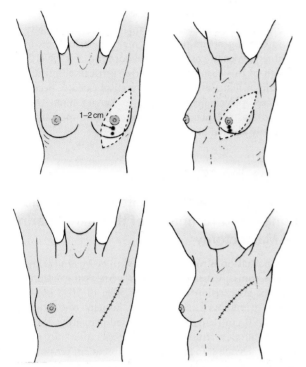

• **Fig. 29.7** Variation of the Orr incision for lower inner and vertically placed (6 o'clock) lesions of the breast. The design of the skin incision is identical to that of Fig. 29.5, with attention directed to margins of 1 to 2 cm.

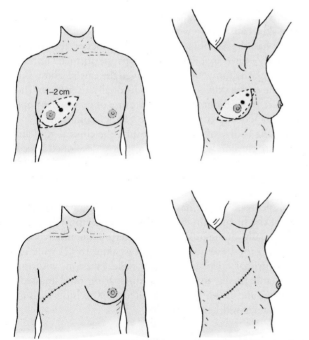

• **Fig. 29.8** Design of skin flaps for upper inner quadrant primary tumors of the breast. The cephalad margin of the flap must be designed to allow access for dissection of the axilla. With flap margins 1 to 2 cm from the tumor, variation in the medial extent of the incision is expectant and may extend beyond the edge of the sternum. On occasion, the modified Stewart incision can incorporate the tumor en bloc, provided that the cancer is not too high on the breast and craniad from the nipple-areola complex. All incision designs must be inclusive of the nipple-areola complex when total mastectomy is planned with primary therapy.

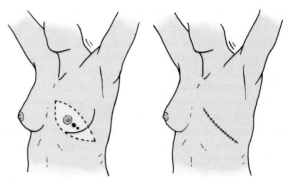

• **Fig. 29.9** Incisions for cancer of the lower outer quadrants of the breast. The surgeon should design incisions that achieve margins of 1 to 2 cm from the tumor with cephalad margins that allow access for dissection of the axilla. The medial extent is the margin of the sternum. Laterally, the inferior extent of the incision is the latissimus.

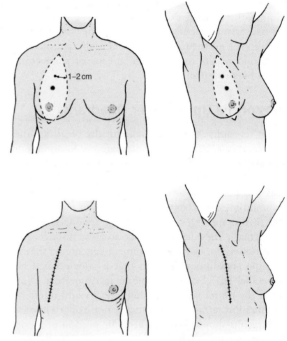

• **Fig. 29.10** Depiction of skin flaps for lesions of the breast that are high lying, infraclavicular, or fixed to the pectoralis major muscle. Fixation to the muscle and/or chest wall necessitates Halsted radical mastectomy with skin margins at least 2 cm. Skin grafting is necessary when large margins of skin are resected for T3 and T4 cancers. Primary closure for T1 and some T2 tumors is often possible.

or central breast primaries. The original biopsy preferably is done through a periareolar incision for lesions in this location. The residual scar should have precise measurements for the cephalad and caudad extents of the incision to include a minimal 1-cm margin. Availability of adequate skin to complete the primary closure is rarely difficult in the pendulous or large breast. For most small breasts, the Stewart (transverse) incision allows primary closure of skin except when more than 4 to 5 cm of skin are encompassed in the primary resection or if evidence of skin devascularization is apparent after completion of the procedure. Loss of skin secondary to loss of vascularity with ultrathin dissection planes or trauma to the flaps may necessitate even wider resections of skin margins.

Fig. 29.5 shows an optional elliptical incision in the contour of the breast for an inner quadrant primary lesion. This incision would perhaps best be described as the modified Stewart incision, which has a predominant extension in a more oblique and cephalad direction toward the ipsilateral axilla. The Stewart incision is commonly preferred by plastic surgeons anticipating delayed reconstruction with myocutaneous flaps, especially when a contralateral simple mastectomy is planned for treatment of high-risk disease or as a prophylactic procedure. Furthermore, this technique is often the choice of oncologic surgeons when radiation to the chest wall is planned before reconstruction.

Lesions of the Upper Outer or Lower Inner Quadrants

Figs. 29.6 and 29.7 denote the incision design for operable breast cancer in the upper outer or lower inner quadrants. Minimal skin margins of 1 to 2 cm from the primary neoplasm are incorporated in a modified Orr incision that is slightly oblique from the transverse line with cephalad extension toward the axilla. Similar to the Orr and Stewart incisions, although somewhat more oblique, these incisions lend themselves to cosmetically satisfactory breast reconstruction results using myocutaneous or subpectoral augmentation breast implants.

Lesions of the Upper Inner Quadrants

Lesions of the upper inner quadrants of the breast are the most difficult to manage because of their anatomic location. Surgeons should recognize the inherent problems encountered with elevation of skin flaps that allow adequate surgical margins and provide cosmesis for wound closure and potential reconstruction. Surgeons should be able to develop a 1- to 2-cm margin for lesions that are in this quadrant, providing the lesion is not cephalad (infraclavicular). These lesions may be accessed through the modified Stewart incision. Commonly, surgeons encounter the dilemma of designing an elliptical incision that is widely based near the cephalomedial aspect of the breast to incorporate a 1- to 2-cm margin of the tumor with extension laterally and inferiorly such that the incision terminates at the anterior axillary line (see Fig. 29.8). Surgeons should plan the cephalic portion of the incision for the superior flap such that adequate access to the pectoralis major and to the axillary contents is ensured.

Lesions of the Lower Outer Quadrants

Lesions of the lower outer quadrants of the breast should have an incision design similar to those of the upper inner quadrant, with margins of 1 to 2 cm around the primary lesion (see Fig. 29.9) and with maximum extension of the cephalad margin to provide access to flaps for dissection of the pectoralis major and the axillary contents.

High-Lying (Infraclavicular) Lesions

With large lesions (T2, T3, T4) that are high lying, infraclavicular, or fixed to the pectoralis major, incisions designed to provide a minimal 1- to 2-cm margin necessitate skin grafting of the defect or coverage with myocutaneous flaps. The original Halsted and Meyer incisions, with subsequent modifications by Greenough, Rodman, and Gray (see Fig. 29.3), were used for treatment of primary lesions of T2, T3, and T4 size.[21] For T1 lesions in this

position, design of an elliptical incision placed in a vertical dimension from the clavicle provides adequate access for axillary dissection and clearing of the pectoralis major muscle when indicated but is unequivocally cosmetically deforming. Fig. 29.10 depicts the design of this cosmetically inferior vertical, elliptical incision for these high-lying lesions and the vertical closure. Because these incisions are placed perpendicular to Langer lines, cosmesis is minimized and the planes of cleavage for the medial breast are subsequently ablated.

Skin-Sparing Mastectomy

Total Mastectomy With Limited Skin Excision: Rationale and Technique of the "Skin-Sparing" Total Mastectomy

Wide skin excision is routinely used with every radical and modified mastectomy. A mastectomy with wide skin excision is often inclusive of an excision in excess of 30% to 50% of the breast skin. This is removed as an ellipse, usually measuring 10 cm (width) by 20 cm (length), and is closed primarily. The elliptical excision facilitates removing the dog-ears that are technically created by the wide skin removal and subsequent tension of excessive tissue at the terminal points of skin closure.

Limited skin excision can be defined as excision of the nipple-areola complex, the skin around the biopsy site, and the skin within 1 to 2 cm of the tumor margin. This technique usually sacrifices 5% to 10% of the breast skin, which is either approximated primarily or closed with an autogenous myocutaneous flap that is used to replace the breast volume. Dog-ears do not occur with this technique because the limited skin removal does not initiate skin contracture with closure. Limited skin excision mastectomy has the advantage of providing better reconstructions, particularly with myocutaneous flaps performed immediately after the mastectomy because it saves the entire chest skin and almost the entire skin envelope. Additionally, excision of the open biopsy site is often not applicable because of increasing popularity of a stereotactically controlled core needle aspiration.[35,36]

Over the course of the 20th century, the clinical guidelines for breast skin excision with mastectomy have developed anecdotally and have been applied by convention. Furthermore, the benefits of wide versus limited skin excision have not been subjected to prospective randomized trials. Because locoregional surgical control of breast cancer has improved over the past 60 years, the extent of the breast skin excision with mastectomy has decreased proportionally. Standards of practice have sequentially evolved as follows: (1) total excision of the breast skin, to (2) wide excision without primary closure, to (3) wide excision with primary closure, and finally to (4) the "skin-sparing total mastectomy." Indications and techniques for limited skin excision with mastectomy are reviewed here.[37–39]

Factors Affecting Local Recurrence

With the increasing acceptance and application of breast conservation techniques for the therapy of ductal carcinoma in situ and invasive neoplasms of lobular and ductal origin, it is essential that the surgeon determines whether adequate excision margins are achieved to confer long-term local control. Gilliland and coworkers[40] and Johnson and associates[41] determined the necessity of total mastectomy with and without node dissection; with the exception of advanced disease (T3 and T4 tumors), immediate breast reconstruction can be completed without any effect on the quality or duration of survival. As noted by Johnson and associates, local recurrence is usually a harbinger of systemic disease, and predictably, factors for local recurrence also represent prognostic indicators of survival.[41] The 1992 report by Kurtz[42] reviewed common host and histologic features that influence local failure after breast conservation and irradiation to the intact breast for clinical stage I and II disease. Kurtz determined that the significant features that correlate with increased risk are young age at time of primary therapy and the presence of an extensive intraductal component within the invasive index (primary) neoplasm. In addition, this clinical study determined that adequacy (volume) of the surgical excision, the use of systemic adjuvant therapy, and high-quality radiation therapy techniques all contribute to a reduction in the risk of locoregional recurrence.

Biologic Factors: Effect on Local Recurrence

Contemporary oncologic treatment planning necessitates the incorporation of biologic factors related to the tumor phenotype and cellular characteristics. Aside from nodal status, these parameters exceed all other considerations in assessing various treatment modalities, including total excision of the breast. With the increasing acceptance and application of breast conservation techniques for treatment of both in situ and invasive neoplasms of lobular and ductal origin, it is essential that the surgeon determine whether adequate excisional margins are achieved to confer long-term locoregional control. Many investigators[43–46] acknowledge the importance of patient selection to achieve optimal DFS relative to locoregional recurrence within the ipsilateral mastectomy site. The large prospective analysis (n = 1036) by the German Breast Cancer Study Group for therapy of T1N0M0 disease concluded that the width of the margin of excision (in centimeters) had no impact on prognosis.[47] However, this analysis of patients who were randomized between breast preservation and mastectomy did establish conclusively that poorer disease-free survival was associated with microscopically involved margins in the conservation technique compared with the mastectomy study group (75% vs. 90% at 3 years). Tumor size and tumor grade were also prognostic factors that accurately predicted recurrence. Age, ER/PR status, menopausal status, histologic tumor type, and type of therapy (mastectomy vs. breast preservation) were not significant predictive factors of recurrence.

The full realization of the impact of contemporary developments in molecular and genetic markers as prognostic indicators of locoregional recurrences has not yet been fully assimilated into oncologic practice.[48] As these tests gain acceptance, recognition of patients with unfavorable disease will be facilitated at the outset after cellular, biochemical, and molecular-genetic analysis of the primary neoplasm. The current method, which uses one variant of the mastectomy for all patients, can then be improved through the design of individual treatment. Moreover, the comprehensive prospective analysis of the NSABP by Fisher and associates[49] suggests that the extent (type) of mastectomy and regional node excision are not associated with significant differences in survival than those from more radical procedures.

Tumor Volume (Size): Effect on Local Recurrence

For patients who are not treated with irradiation after breast conservation surgery, tumor size is an important determinant of risk for local recurrence, as reported in data from the NSABP by Fisher and coinvestigators.[49,50] Fowble and colleagues[51] and Kurtz

TABLE 29.2	Crude Rate of Local Recurrence in the Breast for 1350 Patients With Stage I and II Disease as a Function of Clinical Breast Tumor Size[a]			
TNM Stage	Clinical Tumor Size (cm)	Local Recurrence (%)	p Value	
T1a, T1b	<1	29/255 (11.4)	NS	
T1c	1.1–2	45/438 (10.3)	NS	
T2	2.1–3	40/392 (10.2)	NS	
T2	3.1–4	21/179 (11.7)	NS	
T2	4.1–5	21/86 (13.9)	NS	

[a]Patients were treated at the Cancer Institute and associated clinics in Marseille between 1962 and 1981 (median follow-up 10 years).
NS, Nonsignificant; TNM, tumor, node, metastasis.
Modified from Kurtz JM. Factors influencing the risk of local recurrence in the breast. Eur J Cancer. 1992;28:660-666.

and coworkers[52] note that larger neoplasms (e.g., T3, T4) comprise most of these local failures. These findings are further amplified by the large, long-term study by Kurtz of operable T1 and T2 invasive breast cancers. Within the range of tumor diameter appropriate to breast conservation, Kurtz[42] determined that the size of the primary lesion had no apparent influence on the risk for local recurrence, provided that macroscopically complete resection was achieved (Table 29.2). Although the analysis by Kurtz[42] includes radiation of the intact breast with the goal of preserving the organ, other researchers[53] have come to similar conclusions in patients undergoing mastectomy alone. Dao and Nemoto[53] reiterate that this reduction in the local recurrence rate is evident when the adequacy of resection is confirmed.

Of significance, Holland and coworkers[54] previously determined in serial subgross sectioning of mastectomy specimens that the percentage of breasts harboring residual foci 2 cm distal to the edge of the index tumor was similar for T1 (T1a, T1b, T1c) cancers (≤2 cm) and those between 2 and 5 cm (T2) in transverse diameter. Data from virtually all large series designed to corroborate these findings determined that local failure is not more frequent in operable T2 than in T1 primary tumors. However, from a technical perspective, adequate local excision with macroscopically clear margins is more difficult to achieve in the T2 lesion, especially for patients with diminutive native breast volume.

Breast Skin Excision: Effect on Local Recurrence

The 1963 study by Dao and Nemoto[53] confirmed that the risks associated with skin preservation in mastectomy are in effect more theoretical than actual. In a series of 135 consecutive cases of breast cancer, these investigators observed that skin recurrence was evident in 27.5% of locally advanced tumors, but the incidence was only 2% for patients with nonadvanced disease. This study therefore relates local recurrences to biologic aspects of the tumor more than to extirpative (technical) differences of the procedure. Moreover, Dao and Nemoto[53] concluded that "skin recurrence is nothing more than metastasis at an additional site in patients with widespread disease." These authors further noted that "the frequency of skin recurrence is governed by the pathologic stage of the disease, rather than by the amount of skin that is removed."

Evolution of Breast Skin Excision With Mastectomy

Radical Mastectomy

The halstedian principles of complete mastectomy embodied an anatomic basis for cancer surgery, which presumed an improved survival rate with the more radical extirpative approach (see Chapter 30). Recurrences were usually interpreted as evidence of inadequate locoregional therapy, and therapy was rarely directed to systemic disease.[32] This premise dictated therapy of breast cancers managed in the halstedian era, because the majority were T3 and T4 neoplasms. Extremely wide excision of skin was established as an absolute dictum for the cancer cure; unfortunately, this concept prevailed for 80 years, well into the 20th century. Before World War II, mastectomies for cancer were designed to remove all breast tissue and included the pectoralis major and minor muscles and the axillary lymph nodes. There was some variation, however, in the management of the volume and technique for breast skin excision (see Fig. 29.3).

Near-Total Excision of the Breast Skin Without Undermining to Develop Skin Flaps. In concurrent evolution of the technique of mastectomy, Halsted and Meyer advocated extremely wide skin excision because of the advanced presentation of disease at that time (T3, T4) for most patients.[18,19,55,56] Primary closure was rarely attempted, except by skin grafting. The wound was routinely allowed to granulate.

Wide Dissection of Skin Flaps With Extensive Skin Removal. Handley[57] popularized dissection of the breast skin away from the breast tissue as a thin skin flap. Because the skin removal was much less radical, primary closure of the skin flaps was occasionally attempted.

Wide Dissection of Thin Skin Flaps With Less Extensive Skin Removal. Finney[20] also developed thin skin flaps but with less extensive skin removal.[58] Primary closure of the skin flaps was usually attempted. After World War II, the Finney modification of the Halsted-Meyer mastectomy evolved into the predominant method of radical mastectomy.

Modified Radical Mastectomy

With the evolution of less radical techniques, modified radical mastectomy was popularized by Patey and Dyson[23] in 1948 as an acceptable therapeutic option to the Halsted procedure (see Chapter 30). As stated earlier, Patey began using this method in 1932 and used it routinely after 1936. This conservative approach was a revolutionary departure from the previous time-honored and proven methods espoused by Halsted and Meyer and their surgical pupils in that it preserved the pectoralis major muscle. Patey based his method on the belief that locoregional dissemination of the breast cancer did not commonly involve the pectoralis muscle, unless the tumor was attached to the fascia and/or infiltrated this muscle. However, he did believe that wide skin excision was essential to cancer control because of the histologic proximity of the ductal tissue and the breast skin and their lymphatic-venous connections. In 1969 Handley and Thackray,[59] also from the Middlesex Hospital in London, confirmed the effectiveness of Patey's modified mastectomy. Although the procedure preserved the pectoralis major muscle, all of these surgeons were firmly convinced of the necessity of wide skin excision, as evidenced by the fact that more than 50% of their patients required skin grafting for closure. It was not until the 1960s that primary closure of the Patey mastectomy was routinely attempted. Auchincloss,[25] and later Madden,[26] preserved the pectoralis major and minor muscles and advocated low axillary node dissection (levels I and II) with less extensive skin resection. Auchincloss used a horizontal skin closure, whereas Madden used a vertical skin closure. The Auchincloss-Madden technique routinely allowed the surgeon to close the breast skin, with survival results comparable to those of the operations championed and advocated by Halsted, Meyer, and Patey. As noted by Bland and colleagues[60] (see Chapter 30), the contemporary modified radical mastectomy is essentially the same operation originally described by Moore[61] in 1867, more than a century before it became the worldwide standard of breast cancer therapy.

Currently, the modified radical mastectomy remains the most common surgical therapy for invasive carcinoma of the breast, despite the eligibility of many women for breast conservation techniques or skin-sparing total mastectomy approaches. Furthermore, as of 1991, most patients with ductal carcinoma in situ still had axillary node dissections, despite the low nodal positivity rate that approximates 1% to 2%[4] (see Chapters 39 and 42). Although the 1995 report of the Commission on Cancer of the American College of Surgeons[62] suggests increasing use of breast conserving surgery for in situ disease from 20.9% in 1985 to 35.4% in 1991, modified radical mastectomy represented the principal therapy of the disease and remained constant at 42%. Moreover, the use of radiation for patients with ductal carcinoma in situ after partial mastectomy without node dissection ranged from 24.2% in 1990 to 37.7% in 1985. These contemporary trends suggest an enlightened awareness of the design of the technical procedure to accommodate patient desires while achieving locoregional disease control equivalent to that seen with more radical approaches. However, similar reports emphasize the necessity of inculcation of various objective pathologic and radiologic criteria (e.g., cellular and biochemical variables, oncogenes, mammograms) to integrate risk parameters of the tumor phenotype. These various factors allow the clinician to more accurately determine risk of locoregional recurrence. Future prospective clinical trials will determine the specter of limitations for breast conservation. Regardless, the necessity of total mastectomy with or without regional nodal dissection will maintain primacy as the desired therapeutic modality for various stages of presentation.

Skin Preservation Procedures

With the introduction of the breast conservation treatments of lumpectomy radiation and quadrantectomy radiation, surgeons introduced the concept of minimal skin removal in the quadrant of the tumor and nipple-areola complex preservation, if the latter was clinically uninvolved.[63] Lumpectomy radiation was initially proposed by Mustakallio in 1954 for patients who refused radical mastectomy.[64] This new (but unconventional) treatment proved to be effective in providing DFS, and it evolved as a consequence of the interest and the advocacy of a number of clinical investigators.[65,66] Fisher's concepts of *biological determinism* and hematogenous dissemination acknowledged the ineffectiveness of regional lymphatic systems as tumor "filters." Today both lumpectomy and quadrantectomy are well-accepted variants of treatment options because of the theories developed by Fisher and colleagues[49,50,67] and by Veronesi and coworkers,[63] respectively.

In the late 1970s the mammographic diagnosis of in situ disease and minimal breast cancer (Tmic, T1a, T1b) produced a new subset of patients with early-stage disease. In 1986 Bland and associates[68] described a skin preservation technique in which the nipple is resected and augmentation is achieved with subpectoral prosthetic implants. This procedure described a total "glandular" mastectomy with skin preservation of the entire breast. In 1991 Toth and Lappert[69] described a total mastectomy without extensive skin resection as an appropriate treatment for patients with minimal breast cancer and in situ disease. These authors were first to coin the term *skin-sparing mastectomy* (SSM), which was used primarily in patients with relatively favorable disease indicators. These patients had limited skin resection, which included the biopsy site, the nipple-areola complex, and any additional breast skin adjacent to the tumor needed to provide an adequate histologically free margin of tumor excision. In SSM, skin resection is limited, and all ductal tissue is completely extirpated, as would be completed for any total glandular mastectomy. The technical dictum of complete parenchymal resection is scrupulously observed in this method, including the posterior margins and the axillary tail of Spence. The uninvolved breast skin can be preserved without compromise of oncologic purpose of the procedure. The reconstruction and rehabilitation goal is to provide the patient with breast symmetry, form (cleavage), and contour, which often can be achieved without placement of incisions in medial and upper (infraclavicular) quadrants of the breasts.

SSM has been used primarily for patients with AJCC TNM stages 0, I, and early II disease requiring mastectomy when eligible for immediate autogenous breast reconstruction.[69–71] Most of the patients eligible for the technique of combined mastectomy-reconstruction were selected because they were not candidates for lumpectomy and postoperative radiation. The authors consider the following to be indications for skin-sparing techniques:

- Multicentricity of disease (ductal in situ, any invasive histology)
- Invasive carcinoma associated with an extensive intraductal component that is 25% or more of tumor volume
- T2 tumors (2–5 cm), especially those with unfavorable features on radiographic or physical examination that defy confidence in follow-up examination
- A central tumor that would require removal of the nipple-areola complex

None of the aforementioned indications necessitates wide skin removal to achieve adequate extirpation of the neoplasm. Additional patients have been selected for limited skin resection because of relatively favorable indications, and include the following:

- In situ cancers of lobular and ductal origin
- Multifocal, minimal breast cancer (Tmic, T1a, T1b)
- All T1 and possibly T2a tumors deep within the breast parenchyma, after neoadjuvant therapy, with significant cytoreduction of tumor volume
- A positive family history (first-degree relatives) or genetically confirmed oncogene mutagenesis (e.g., *BRCA1*, *BRCA2*) together with worrisome histologic features such as atypical lobular or ductal hyperplasia
- Patients with and without familial inheritable (genetic) disease when physical or radiographic features, or both, defy confidence in follow-up examination, especially when multiple biopsies are indicated

For the aforementioned patients, extensive removal of breast skin does not enhance treatment control by improving survival or decreasing local recurrences. Conversely, for patients with large tumors (e.g., ≥5 cm, T3, T4), particularly with attachment to the overlying skin and subcutaneous tissues, with or without ulceration, extensive skin removal is clearly justified and advisable; the SSM technique is inadvisable with this stage of presentation of disease.[72–75]

To achieve total glandular mastectomy, some clinics advocate preservation of the areola by nipple-coring to enhance esthetic appearance. Although this practice is acceptable, it may prove ill advised for oncologic procedures that attempt total extirpation of mammary ducts of the nipple-areola complex, because this premise incorrectly assumes that the areola is devoid of mammary ductal tissue. Schnitt and associates[76] performed marginal excision of the nipple (nipple-coring) on eight consecutive mastectomy specimens, excised the areolas, and thereafter submitted all tissues for histologic analysis. Mammary ducts in the areola were extensive and were identical to those of extralobular ducts in the breast parenchyma. Schnitt and colleagues concluded that mammary ducts represent a normal histologic component of the areolar dermis and that nipple-coring alone does not result in complete removal of all mammary ductal tissue from the nipple-areola complex. However, areolar preservation may be an insignificant risk parameter relative to local recurrence because residual breast tissue is evident in all viable skin flaps after total glandular mastectomy.

Technical Aspects of Skin-Sparing Mastectomy

Resection of the previous biopsy scar and wound cavity with skin overlying the neoplasm, the nipple or the nipple-areola complex, and the entire breast parenchymal contents are cardinal technical caveats of the SSM (Box 29.1). Furthermore, Carlson[70] notes that breast symmetry with reconstruction is enhanced with preservation of the native skin because of similar skin color and an improved shape. As indicated previously, technical access to the axilla for lymph node dissection is essential; planning of cosmetically acceptable incisions that allow partial access to sampling (levels I and II) or Patey dissection (levels I, II, and III) are critical to the technical design. Currently, we and others conduct SLNB with the skin-sparing approach. If possible, the SLNB is "frozen" for pathologic analysis by hematoxylin and eosin touch prep technique; axillary node dissection (level I/II) should be completed when the node is histologically positive. This approach is preferred rather than delay the axillary node dissection following transverse rectus abdominis myocutaneous (TRAM) or latissimus dorsi myocutaneous reconstruction. Reentry nodal dissections may injure the vascularity of the tissue transfer or create axillary hematomas with levels I/II node removal.

The anatomy of the breast with regard to SSM has been properly outlined by Carlson.[70] The glandular tissue, including the nipple and areola, is removed en bloc. When the tumor is located within 3 cm or less from the skin surface, the overlying skin is removed en bloc with the specimen. A 1- to 2-cm margin of breast skin is typically removed around the biopsy scar; the remaining breast skin contour is preserved in its entirety.

• BOX 29.1 Technical Features of the Skin-Sparing Mastectomy

- Skin excision (1-cm margins) of the previous biopsy site or scar overlying index neoplasm
- Skin excision (marginal only) of nipple-areola complex
- Total glandular mastectomy, which includes the index tumor or previous biopsy wound cavity en bloc with skin excisions 1 and 2
- Skin incision design must ensure technical access to the axilla when lymph node dissection (sampling, levels I/II; Patey, levels I, II, III) is indicated
- Sentinel lymph node biopsy as indicated; if histologically positive, lymph node dissection to be completed synchronously with skin-sparing mastectomy

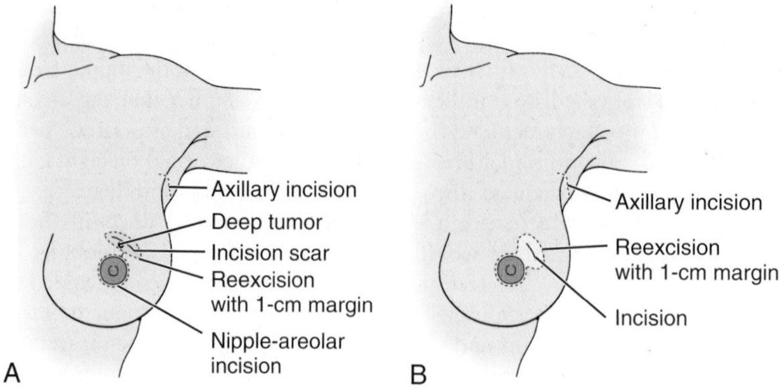

• **Fig. 29.11** (A and B) Breast incisions when the biopsy site is contiguous with the areola. Note that axillary incision is remotely placed.

Incision Design

Ideally, the entire mastectomy should be performed through a keyhole approach, circumscribing the sacrificed nipple and areola, which remain en bloc with the breast parenchyma. Although technically more demanding than the ablative modified/radical approach, this procedure is technically possible in patients with small tumors or minimal breast cancer. This approach is also an option in patients after stereotactically placed core guidance biopsy, where often the cylinder of the needle does not provide complete excision of the tumor. The increasing application of SLNB is diminishing the need for formal axillary node dissections, thus avoiding separate (and deforming) axillary dissections.[77–80] When nodes are histologically positive after sentinel mapping, level I/II dissection should be completed synchronously with the skin-sparing mastectomy.

Figs. 29.11 through 29.25 depict the various therapeutic principles and their application that may exist for patients eligible for skin-sparing techniques. Figs. 29.16, 29.18, 29.21, 29.23, and 29.25 show breast incision variants of SSM for all quadrants when the primary tumors and biopsy sites are located in a site remote from the nipple-areola complex. Essential to completion of the oncologic aspects of this technique are removal of the nipple or the nipple-areola complex and a 1-cm margin of skin about the biopsy site. Lesions that are juxtapositioned to the areola may be excised with a single skin island flap (Figs. 29.26–29.36). Lesions with biopsy scars greater than 4 cm from the areola margin require separate excisions with attention to preservation of a well-vascularized intervening skin bridge. All excisions for both upper and lower hemispheres of the breast are excised through 1-cm margins placed elliptically as nonradical incisions that typically parallel Langer lines.

Placement of superolateral (modified Orr) incisions (see Fig. 29.3) as an extension of the periareolar incision ensures comprehensive exposure for completion of the total mastectomy and axillary lymph node dissection. This incision has value for limited exposure in the course of flap elevation after incision around 1-cm margins of the biopsy scar and marginal excision of the nipple-areola complex. The 1-cm skin margins that circumvent the biopsy site are resected en bloc with the breast parenchyma and are inclusive of the undisturbed (intact) tumor or the biopsy cavity of the index neoplasm.

On occasion, separate axillary incisions designed as indicated in Fig. 29.37 for level I and II nodal sampling or Patey dissection may be used to facilitate exposure with mastectomy. For all presentations of cancer in any quadrant or contiguous with the

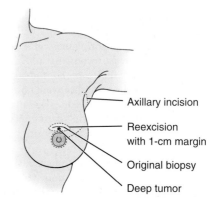

• **Fig. 29.12** Lateral extension of the periareolar incision to enhance exposure for dissection. Remote axillary incision may not be essential if incision is extended toward axilla.

nipple-areola complex, the design of incisions is guided foremost by oncologic principles that place paramount the concern for locoregional disease control. Incision planning jointly by oncologic and plastic surgeons ensures optimal appearance and functional outcome with mastectomy techniques that enhance these disease control measures.

Exposure is gained through ample skin incisions, which are placed precisely parallel to the lines of skin tension. Incisions are placed below the level of the nipple, laterally and inferiorly, passing around the areola. The most satisfactory incisions, both from the standpoint of exposure and the quality of the final scar, extend from the areola at 2 to 3 o'clock and 6 to 8 o'clock. The lateral incision is contoured upward toward the axilla exactly in the lines of skin tension. If the incision is lengthened 10 to 12 cm lateral to the areola, the exposure of the axillary contents should be excellent. Alternatively, a separate 10-cm incision in the axillary hair-bearing skin can be used. The incision inferior to the nipple typically results in a discreet scar, even when it is not placed precisely in the lines of skin tension.

Flap Elevation

After circumscribing the nipple and areola, the skin flaps are elevated widely to reach the axilla and beyond the entire circumference of the peripheral boundaries of breast parenchyma. The flaps are dissected on an avascular plane at the level of the Cooper ligaments to preserve the subcutaneous vascular plexus. If the dissection is somewhat bloody, the level of dissection must

Text continued on p. 414

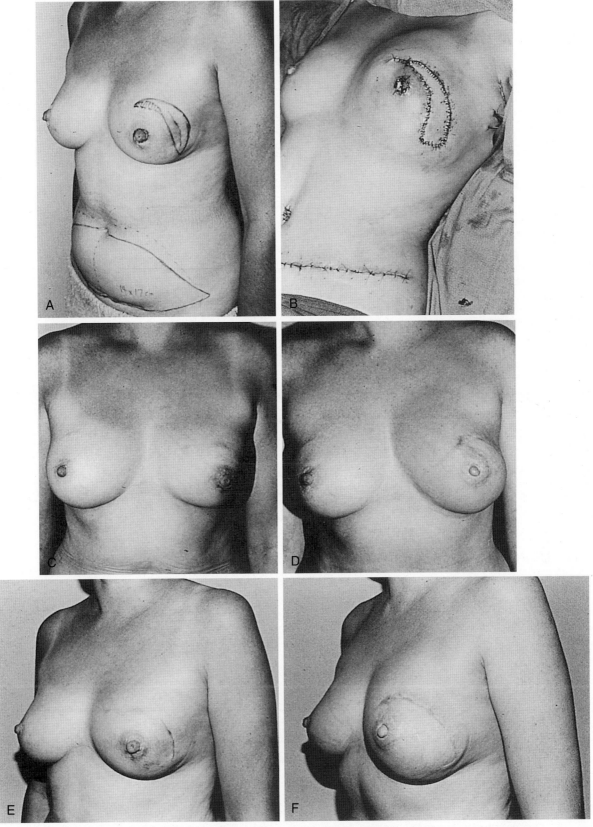

• **Fig. 29.13** (A and B) Preoperative markings of a conservation mastectomy and immediate transverse rectus abdominis myocutaneous (TRAM) flap breast reconstruction. Intraoperative view of the skin replacement of the lateral breast in the area of the previous biopsy. The TRAM flap was used for volume, surface skin replacement, and immediate nipple reconstruction. Preoperative (C) and postoperative (D) views after completion of the left breast and nipple reconstruction. No procedure was completed in the right breast. Without the skin conservation mastectomy, it would not have been possible to match the normal right breast. Oblique preoperative (E) and postoperative (F) views.

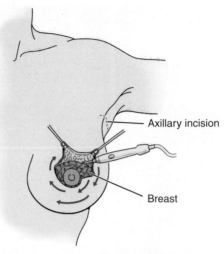

• **Fig. 29.14** Skin flap elevation is above the superficial fascia. Centripetal dissection enhances exposure. Flap contour with thickness of 7 to 8 mm ensures viability. Dissection should not enter breast parenchyma because margins are developed to chest wall en bloc.

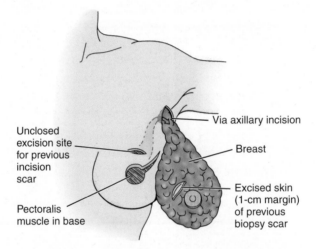

• **Fig. 29.15** After dissection of the flaps and breast parenchyma from the pectoralis major fascia and mammary bursae, the axillary contents are dissected en bloc and delivered through the axillary incision.

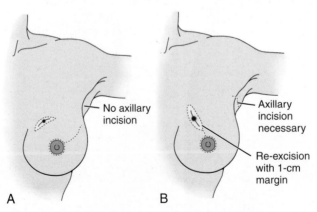

• **Fig. 29.16** Upper inner (medial) quadrant. (A) One-centimeter excision that is remote from periareolar incision with lateral extension of modified Orr incision. No axillary incision is necessary because exposure with this approach is adequate for lymph node sampling. (B) This figure depicts primary tumor and biopsy sites that are vertically placed and radial with 1-cm margins. After incisions at margin of nipple-areola complex, continuous development of incision allows adequate breast parenchymal exposure. When axillary dissection is necessary, remote incision may be planned.

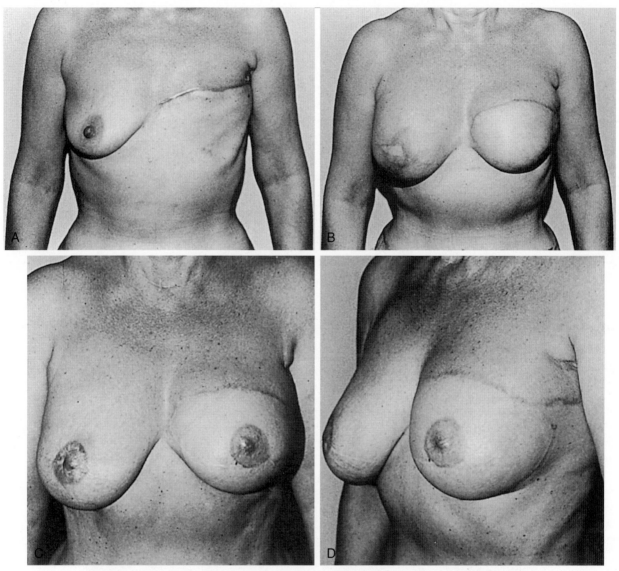

• **Fig. 29.17** Upper inner (medial) quadrant. (A) Patient with a previous left modified mastectomy for stage I disease with no special reason for extensive skin removal. (B) Bilateral transverse rectus abdominis myocutaneous (TRAM) flap breast reconstruction done at the time of the right skin conservation mastectomy. Note the difficult skin replacement in the left breast. It was necessary to replace all of the missing skin below the mastectomy scar with a TRAM flap. In the right breast, all of the TRAM flap was buried except for the part needed to form the nipple and areola. (C) One year after the completion of the breast and nipple reconstructions. (D) Achieving symmetry was difficult because of the radical skin excision of the left breast.

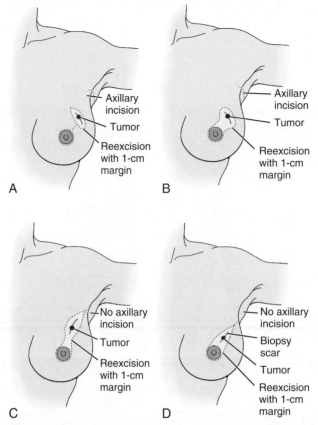

• Fig. 29.18 Upper outer (lateral) quadrant. (A) Nonradial biopsy site excised with 1-cm margins; nipple-areola marginal incision becomes contiguous with biopsy site to give breast exposure for dissection. Remote axillary dissection incision may be essential for proper technical access to level I and II nodes. (B) Nonradial biopsy site excised with 1-cm margins at the most lateral extension of incision with resection of contiguous skin intervening between nipple and areola. Remote axillary incision is usually necessary for adequate sampling exposure. (C) Vertically placed (radial) biopsy site necessitates modified Orr skin flaps inclusive of the 1-cm margins of the biopsy site. Axillary exposure is adequate without remote incision. (D) Has similar radial biopsy site to (C). Periareolar incision in continuity with 1-cm margin of biopsy site gives excellent exposure to breast and axilla.

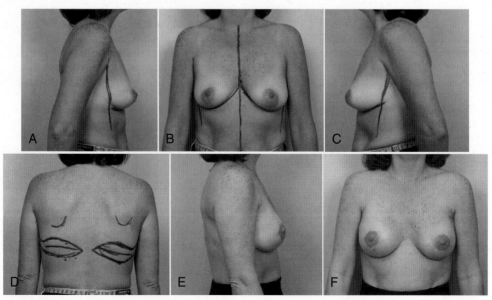

• Fig. 29.19 This image series shows a 40-year-old woman with a history of familial, premenopausal breast cancer who before consultation had six breast biopsies, including three within the past year. This patient underwent bilateral mastectomies and immediate reconstruction using bilateral latissimus dorsi myocutaneous flaps with saline-filled silicone implants to add volume. (A–C) Preoperative markings from anterior and lateral views (note the midline, inframammary, and anterior axillary line markings). (D) A skin island design based on underlying muscle. The skin island is designed as an ellipse to close primarily at the level of the brassiere line. The tips of the scapulae are marked denoting the cephalad extent of the latissimus dorsi muscle bilaterally. (E and F) Postreconstruction anterior and lateral views.

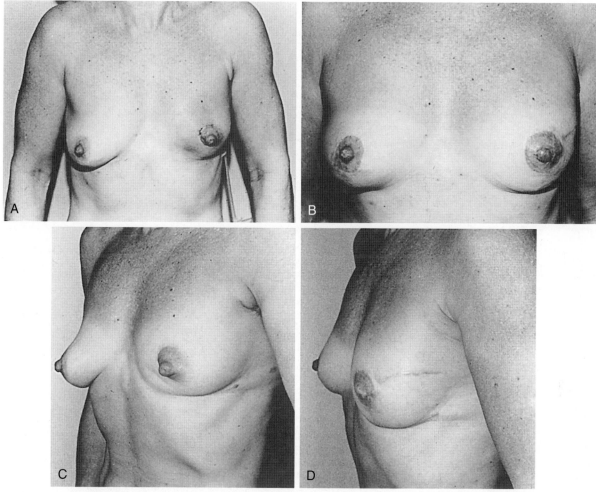

• **Fig. 29.20** Upper outer (lateral). Preoperative (A) and postoperative (B) views after left skin conservation mastectomy for stage I disease. At the time of mastectomy, an immediate free transverse rectus abdominis myocutaneous flap breast and nipple reconstruction were performed in a single stage, with a right mastopexy for symmetry. Oblique preoperative (C) and postoperative (D) views at 1 year. No revision was needed. The areolar tattoo was performed in the office. Note the short lateral skin incision, which was used to encompass the previous biopsy sites.

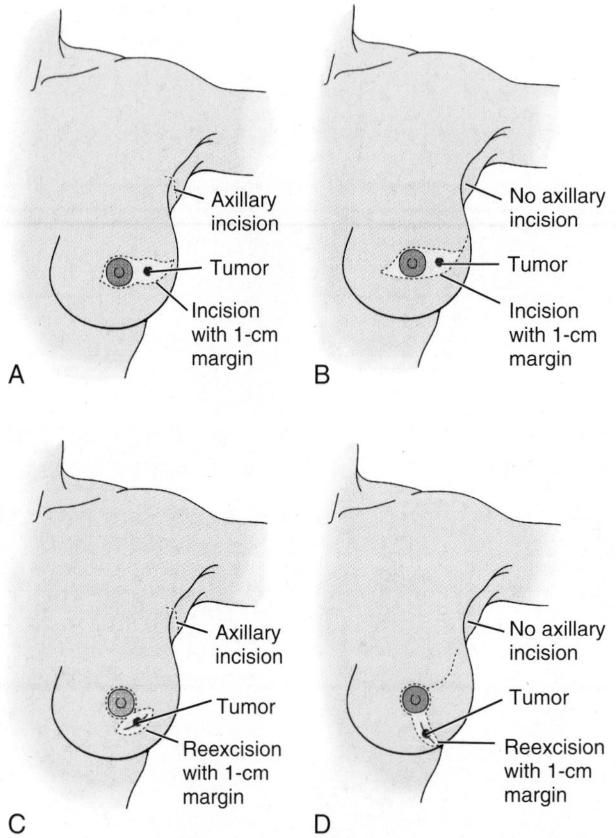

• **Fig. 29.21** Lateral and lower outer (lateral) quadrant. (A) Incision around margin of areolar en bloc with 1-cm tumor margin completed as modified Stewart incision. Separate axillary incision may be required when nodal sampling is indicated. (B) Similar to (A), tumor is noncontiguous with the areola. A modification of the transverse Stewart incision with superolateral extension provides excellent access to breast flap dissection and mastectomy. The axillary dissection can be readily completed with this approach with no need for a separate incision. (C) Nonradial biopsy incision continuous with areolar margin allows adequate breast exposure. Remote axillary incision is necessary. (D) Radial biopsy incision contiguous with areolar. Superolateral extension is necessary to complete flap exposure to parenchyma of breast and axillary dissection.

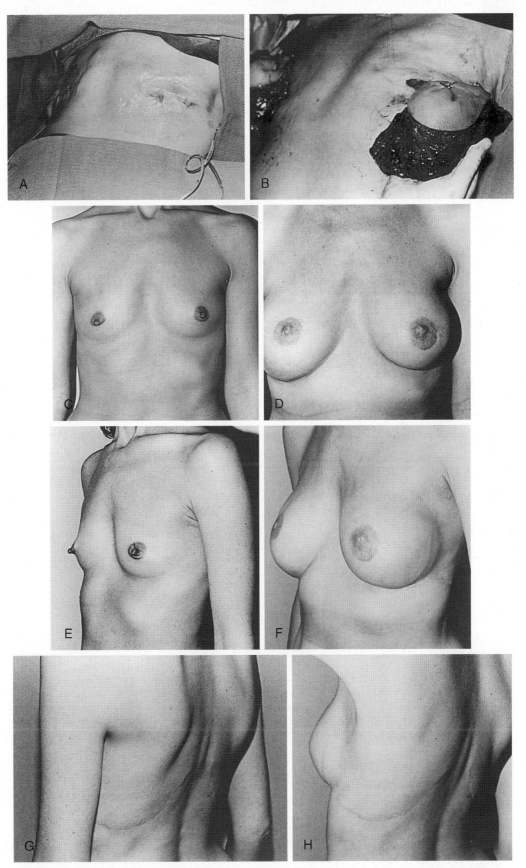

• **Fig. 29.22** (A) Bilateral mastectomy for in situ disease using skin conservation technique through a 10-cm modified transverse (Stewart) incision. (B) Bilateral latissimus flaps are brought out through the incisions before insetting in this immediate reconstruction. Preoperative (C) and postoperative (D) views after completion of nipple-areola reconstructions. Projection was enhanced with 100-mL implants. Oblique preoperative (E) and postoperative (F) views. The excellent result is directly attributable to the skin conservation and the immediate reconstruction. This reconstruction was a prerequisite to the mastectomy in this patient, and there was no reason to delay the reconstruction. Radical skin excision would not have enhanced the extirpation. (G and H) Autogenous latissimus flap donor sites. The scar is usually inconspicuous if placed in the line of a posterolateral thoracotomy.

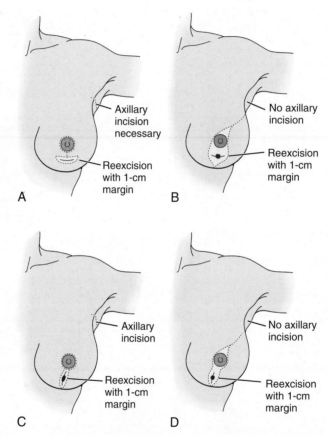

• **Fig. 29.23** Lower half (6 o'clock). (A) Biopsy site may often be placed as a nonradial incision; skin-sparing requires 1-cm marginal excision continuous with periareolar incision. Remote axillary incision is necessary for adequate exposure and dissection. (B) Biopsy site is nonradial in skin-fold contour. Similar to A, reexcision margins are 1 cm and contiguous with skin bridge cephalad toward areola. Superolateral extension of incision allows total mastectomy and axillary dissection (when indicated). (C) Biopsy site is radially placed. Excision of 1-cm biopsy site margin in continuity with areola allows proper breast exposure. Axillary access requires a separate incision. (D) Radial biopsy site excised with tumor inclusion of 1-cm skin-sparing margin. Superolateral extension provides adequate exposure for total mastectomy and axillary dissection.

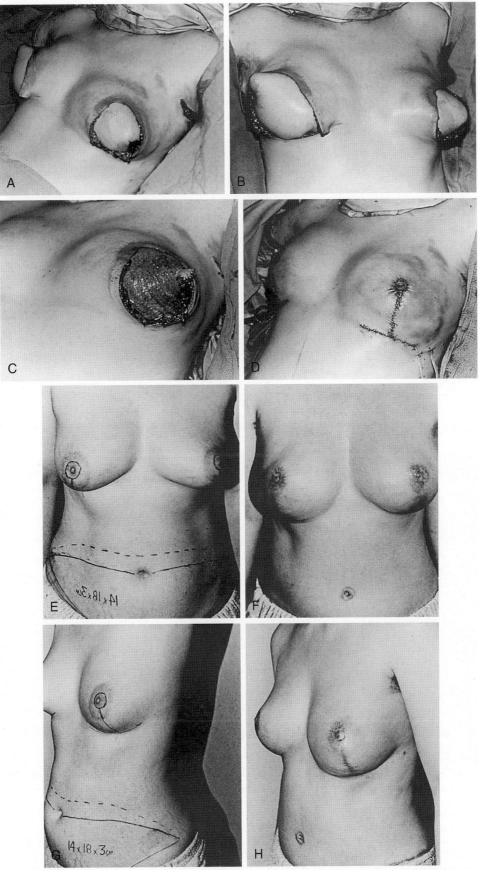

• **Fig. 29.24** (A and B) Bilateral immediate transverse rectus abdominis myocutaneous (TRAM) flap reconstruction of skin conservation mastectomies for in situ disease. No breast skin was excised. (C) View of the de-epithelialized TRAM flap with an immediate nipple reconstruction of the surface of the flap. (D) The mastectomy flaps were closed in the lines of a Wise reduction pattern to remove redundant skin. Preoperative (E) and postoperative (F) views of the bilateral reconstructions. No revision was performed. (G) Oblique views of the preoperative markings. (H) The postoperative results of breast and nipple reconstructions. The areolas and nipples were tattooed in an office procedure.

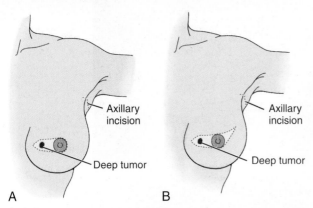

• **Fig. 29.25** Inner (medial) quadrant. (A) Contiguous 1-cm excision of superficial tumor with areolar margin. Remote incision for axillary dissection is always necessary if node sampling is indicated. (B) Similar to A, a 1-cm margin around superficial tumor with lateral and superior extension of incision is essential for breast exposure. Remote axillary incision is necessary when dissection is indicated.

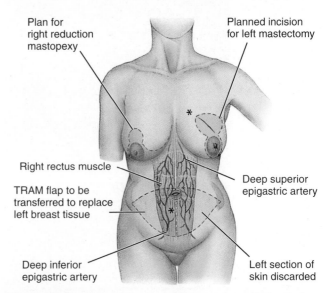

• **Fig. 29.26** The preoperative plan calls for a left modified radical mastectomy; reconstruction with a contralateral, single-pedicle, abdominal flap; and a matching mastopexy on the right. The asterisk indicates the position of the medial edge of the flap after its rotation and transfer to the chest. *TRAM,* Transverse rectus abdominus myocutaneous. (From Copeland EM III. Carcinoma of the breast. In: Copeland EM III, ed. *Surgical Oncology.* New York: John Wiley & Sons; 1983.)

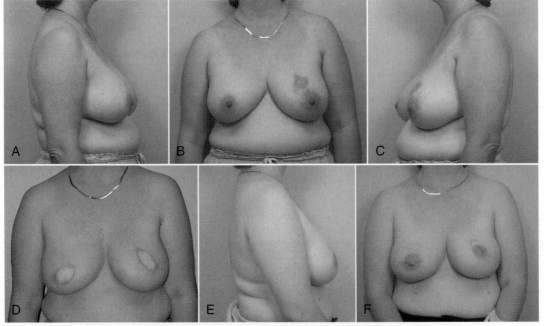

• **Fig. 29.27** This image series shows a 40-year-old woman with a history of a palpable mass in the left breast, which was shown by core biopsy to be invasive lobular carcinoma. Because of the high risk of bilaterality, left modified radical mastectomy in conjunction with prophylactic contralateral mastectomy was selected. Immediate bilateral reconstruction with ipsilateral transverse rectus abdominis myocutaneous flaps was performed. (A–C) Preoperative anterior and lateral views. (D–F) Postoperative results: anterior view before nipple reconstruction and areolar tattooing (D); lateral (E) and anterior (F) views, respectively, after nipple reconstruction and areolar tattooing.

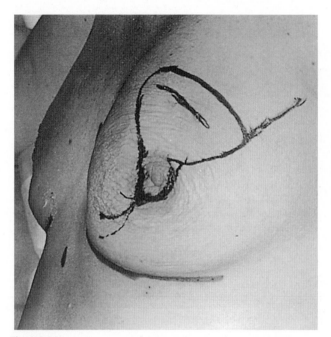

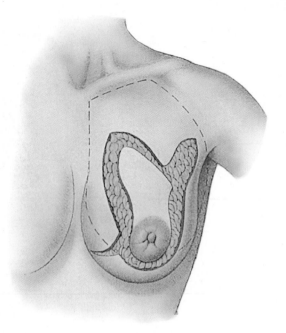

• **Fig. 29.28** General anesthesia has been induced, and the skin incision has been outlined on the left breast. (Nitrous oxide is not used for anesthesia because it could distend the bowel and increase intraabdominal pressure during closure.) The area to be resected includes the biopsy scar and the nipple. Both inframammary folds have been marked to guide the reconstruction and matching mastopexy. (From Copeland EM III. Carcinoma of the breast. In: Copeland EM III, ed. *Surgical Oncology.* New York: John Wiley & Sons; 1983.)

• **Fig. 29.29** The skin has been incised. Skin flaps are raised by electrocautery dissection, and breast tissue beneath the flaps is removed under direct vision. The subcutaneous margins of the flaps *(dashed line)* will extend superiorly to the medial half of the clavicle, superolaterally to the deltopectoral triangle and the cephalic vein, laterally to the anterior edge of the latissimus dorsi muscle, medially to the lateral border of the sternum, and inferiorly to the inframammary fold. (From Copeland EM III. Carcinoma of the breast. In: Copeland EM III, ed. *Surgical Oncology.* New York: John Wiley & Sons; 1983.)

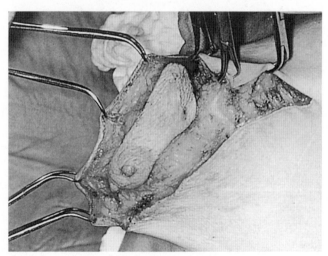

• **Fig. 29.30** For the skin-sparing mastectomy, the superior flap is elevated first by dissection in the plane between the subcutaneous tissue and the investing fascia of the breast. The skin edges are held with towel clips. (From Copeland EM III. Carcinoma of the breast. In: Copeland EM III, ed. *Surgical Oncology.* New York: John Wiley & Sons; 1983.)

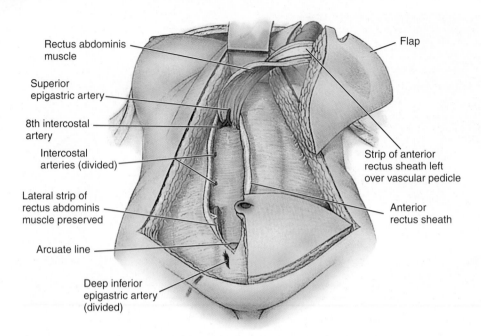

• **Fig. 29.31** After skin-sparing modified radical mastectomy, formation of the transverse rectus abdominis myocutaneous flap and its pedicle is complete. The pedicle of rectus muscle includes sufficient deep epigastric vasculature to ensure the flap's viability. A narrower strip of anterior rectus sheath attached to the muscle helps protect the epigastric artery. A lateral segment of the muscle remains in place from the most inferior tendinous intersection to the arcuate line. (From Copeland EM III. Carcinoma of the breast. In: Copeland EM III, ed. *Surgical Oncology.* New York: John Wiley & Sons; 1983.)

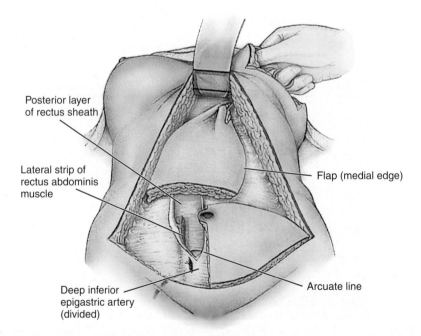

• **Fig. 29.32** The flap is passed through the tunnel into the mastectomy site. Counterclockwise rotation during passage ensures optimal drainage for the flap and avoids kinking of the pedicle. The pedicle is examined to ensure that it is not twisted. The flap will be allowed to perfuse while the abdomen is closed. The left wing of the skin flap is discarded. The right anterior rectus sheath is closed with a running 0-Prolene suture. An opening is left at the cephalad end of the closure to avoid constricting the muscular pedicle. The left sheath is imbricated to centralize the umbilicus. Two large Jackson-Pratt drains are left anterior to the rectus sheath. (From Copeland EM III. Carcinoma of the breast. In: Copeland EM III, ed. *Surgical Oncology.* New York: John Wiley & Sons; 1983.)

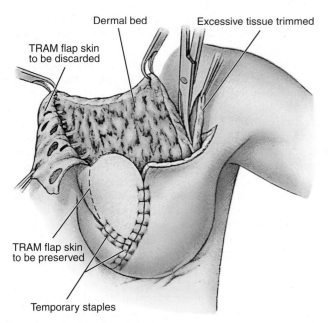

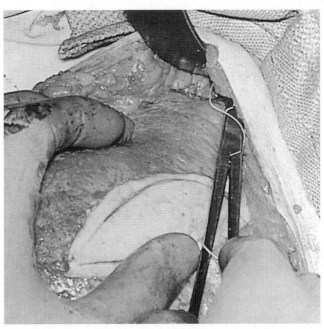

• **Fig. 29.33** Sections of poorly vascularized tissue have been excised from the transverse rectus abdominis myocutaneous *(TRAM)* flap, and the flap is temporarily stapled in place so that it can be trimmed and contoured. As the reconstruction proceeds, any excess skin is deepithelialized, leaving a well-vascularized dermal bed, which will be buried. (From Copeland EM III. Carcinoma of the breast. In: Copeland EM III, ed. *Surgical Oncology.* New York: John Wiley & Sons; 1983.)

• **Fig. 29.34** To fill the infraclavicular hollow, the most superior edge of the flap is set onto the pectoralis major muscle. The buried, deepithelialized portions of the flap are rolled and positioned to create an appropriate degree of projection and ptosis. A symmetric inframammary fold is constructed by tacking the transverse rectus abdominis myocutaneous flap to the periosteum of a rib. (From Copeland EM III. Carcinoma of the breast. In: Copeland EM III, ed. *Surgical Oncology.* New York: John Wiley & Sons; 1983.)

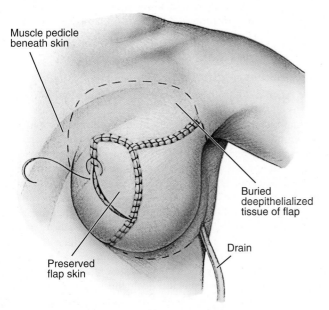

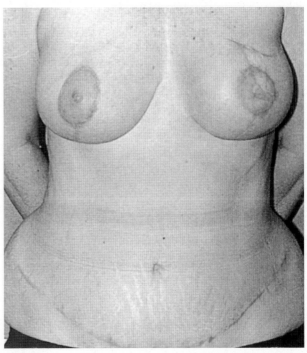

• **Fig. 29.35** The breast skin is closed with a single layer of continuous 5-0 Prolene suture. The axilla will be closed over a drain. (From Copeland EM III. Carcinoma of the breast. In: Copeland EM III, ed. *Surgical Oncology.* New York: John Wiley & Sons; 1983.)

• **Fig. 29.36** Nipple-areola reconstruction has completed the procedure. The left nipple-areola is tattooed for color symmetry. (From Copeland EM III. Carcinoma of the breast. In: Copeland EM III, ed. *Surgical Oncology.* New York: John Wiley & Sons; 1983.)

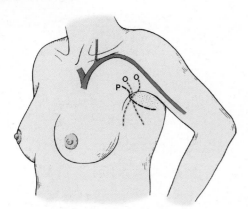

• **Fig. 29.37** Illustration of preferred *(P)* and optional *(O)* incisions used in axillary dissection. Ideally, incisions are placed in skin folds that parallel Langer lines. Incisions are preferably curvilinear with placement just caudal to the hairline of the axilla. Optional incisions depicted are oblique or vertically placed with the chest wall. Because these optional incisions cross the lines of tension (Langer lines), delay in wound repair and inferior cosmetic results may be observed.

be deepened to find this avascular plane. Maintaining the subcutaneous vascular plexus decreases the incidence of skin flap necrosis.[81]

These anatomically distinct boundaries usually extend to the deltopectoral groove and below the clavicle to the subclavius muscle, to the lateral extent of the sternum, and to the anterior border of the latissimus dorsi muscle. Inferiorly, dissection should not extend below the inframammary line, which is tattooed with methylene blue or demarcated with sutures preoperatively. This advice should be heeded because there is no breast tissue below the inframammary line, and the inframammary fold represents an important guideline for breast reconstruction.

Thereafter, skin flaps should be elevated at the subcutaneous tissue level, not at the subdermal level, to preserve the subcutaneous vascular plexus, which nourishes the overlying skin. If elevation is done at the correct level below the subcutaneous plexus, the dissection is bloodless. If profuse bleeding is encountered, the dissection has been conducted in a more superficial plane. It should be noted that the most likely complication of SSM is chest skin flap necrosis (18%–20% in most series).[82–84]

Skin flap mobilization is commenced after elevation of periareolar tissues centrally and those continuous with margins of the excised biopsy scar. Although flap thickness depends on body habitus and fat content, typical thickness of the skin flap is 6 to 8 mm. Electrocautery scalpel using blended cut-coagulation mode may be used for flap elevation but is conducted with extreme caution. Uniform flap thickness that is well vascularized must be fastidiously sought and accomplished; if not, the sole remaining blood supply of the chest skin—the subcutaneous plexus—will be injured. When the white undersurface of the dermis is exposed, the subcutaneous plexus will be injured and flap viability may be harmed distal to the surgical injury. Variation in flap thickness in the process of thinning may devascularize the flap and initiate disastrous wound repair problems. The tumescent technique, which consists of infiltrating a dilute solution of lidocaine with epinephrine at the subcutaneous plane, facilitates the dissection with a knife (electrical dissection with the Bovie is not effective because of the moisture of the tissue). The fluid opens up the avascular plane and makes the wide dissection of the skin and subcutaneous tissue faster and more secure. However, recent data shows that it does not

improve the rate of flap necrosis.[85] Boneti and colleagues have described a technique using dilators to find this avascular plane.[86] Using 14-French cervical dilators, the operator can find the correct plane for any given body habitus. Then by progressively dilating the plane up to 44 French, the operator can easily find the correct plane of dissection or teach the novice.

With completion of flap elevation in superior and medial boundaries, attention is focused to the inferior most extent of the boundary dissection. Preoperative marking of the inframammary fold or fixation with 2-0 silk sutures allows the oncologic surgeon to determine readily the caudad extent of mammary parenchymal resection. The mammary bursa facilitates mobilization of the breast off the pectoralis major fascia. With axillary dissection, when sentinel nodal sampling of levels I and II or Patey dissection (levels I–III) is indicated (see Chapters 30 and 31), preservation of the thoracodorsal neurovascular bundle and the long thoracic nerve are requisite to ensure intact motor innervation of the latissimus dorsi and serratus anterior muscles, respectively. Sensory innervation of the axilla and medial upper inner arm may be preserved when sacrifice of the traversing intercostobrachial cutaneous nerves is avoided. However, transection of these sensory branches creates little long-term morbidity because reinnervation usually occurs within 8 to 10 months. In addition, in the course of axillary lymph node dissection, avoidance of section of the medial pectoral neurovascular bundle ensures motor innervation and function of the pectoralis major and minor muscles. Moreover, it is most important to protect the subscapular vascular pedicle and its thoracodorsal branch, which supplies the latissimus dorsi muscle. Injury of these vessels eliminates the vascular supply and survival of the latissimus myocutaneous flap, which remains as one of the primary reconstructive options. In addition, the subscapular pedicle is an important recipient vessel for free flaps, which may be of value sometime in the future to reconstruct radiation injuries of the chest wall and axilla. It is also helpful, but not essential, to protect the serratus anterior branch of the subscapular pedicle, because this represents the alternative vascular supply to the proximal latissimus dorsi muscle.

Nipple-Sparing Mastectomy

Since the mid-2000s there has been a renewed interest in preserving the entirety of the breast skin envelop for an even better esthetic outcome. Where it is common practice for prophylactic mastectomies, as in high-risk cases with a genetic mutation, nipple-sparing mastectomy (NSM) is now applied for selected breast cancer cases. Since the first long-term follow-up studies were published, there is growing evidence of the oncological safety of these procedures.[87] Most commonly used criteria to consider patients for an NSM include a distance equal or greater than 2 cm from the nipple-areola complex, at least 1-cm distance from the skin, smaller tumors and low axillary burden of disease.

The preservation of the nipple-areola complex makes this procedure more technically challenging because the surgeon needs to accomplish the same oncological goals through a smaller access. Special tools such as lighted retractors are crucial in the success of this technique. There is a steep learning curve, but results are reproducible and reliable when an appropriate level of competence has been reached (Fig. 29.38).

Reconstruction Considerations

Most surgeons would agree that the mastectomy procedure will be the most important determining factor of the final esthetic

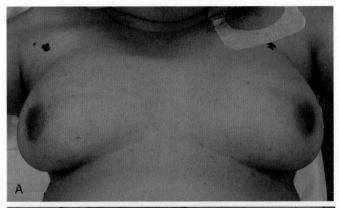

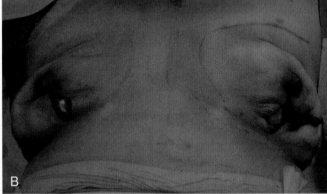

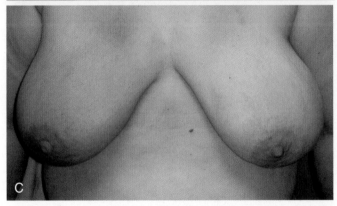

• **Fig. 29.38** (A) Preoperative anterior-posterior view of a breast cancer patient undergoing bilateral nipple sparing mastectomies. (B) Intraoperative view after the mastectomy is completed. Note the entire glandular tissue has been removed through an incision extending from the lower edge of the areola to the inframammary fold. (C) Postoperative view after reconstruction demonstrating the reconstruction result after replacing the breast gland with an implant.

outcome of a breast reconstruction. Considering the breast has a conical shape, any degree of skin resection will require a replacement to restore the natural appearance. Where a Patey incision will require transfer of autologous tissue to avoid a flat and wide appearance to the reconstructed breast, NSMs provide the entire skin envelope corresponding to the opposite breast, leaving only the volume deficit to be filled. A well-performed mastectomy will also preserve the subdermal plexus, maintaining good perfusion to the skin flaps, a critical requirement for immediate breast reconstruction techniques.

The essential factor in breast reconstruction is symmetry between the normal breast and the reconstructed breast. Proper

symmetry requires that the reconstructed breast shape and color "match" the normal appearance of the organ. In practice, it is usually necessary to alter the normal breast with either a mastopexy or reduction mammaplasty to obtain symmetry (Fig. 29.39). An important tenet for the plastic surgeon to follow is the correction of any deformity of the opposite breast rather than to shape the reconstructed breast to match an unattractive, ptotic breast. An increasing number of patients are electing to have bilateral mastectomies that involve prophylaxis of the contralateral breast. There is freedom from concern of developing another cancer in the contralateral breast, assurance of symmetry, and even improvement of the esthetics of the original breast.

Finally, the importance of the skin color provided by the SSM should be emphasized. The native breast skin gives the best possible color match because it is identical to the opposite breast skin. A pale myocutaneous flap on the surface of the breast has the appearance of a "patch" and is remarkably detractive (Fig. 29.40). Use of the autogenous flap on the surface to replace lost breast skin also diminishes the amount of flap that is available for shaping purposes. When implants are used, the breast skin is even more critical for coverage of the implant and subsequent shaping.

The most satisfactory reconstructions are evident in patients with NSMs, particularly in those performed bilaterally (Fig. 29.41). The breast mound is replaced with an implant alone, autogenous tissue alone, or a combination of autogenous tissue and an implant to supplement volume. When resection of the nipple-areola complex is required, a comparable esthetic result can be accomplished by replacing the keyhole skin defect by resection of the nipple and areola with autologous tissue alone or in combination with an implant to supply the extra volume needed (Fig. 29.42). The different-colored skin is later tattooed to simulate the areola. The molding of the breast is simplified because the skin envelope is available and one need only fill the remaining skin envelope that corresponds with that of the contralateral breast from its superior extent to the preserved inframammary fold and anterior axillary line. Increasing experience suggests that no increase in the risk of locoregional recurrence in the reconstituted breast exists; this locoregional failure rate approximates the recurrence rate of the modified radical mastectomies.[84,88]

Overview of Reconstruction

With the evolution of reconstructive techniques and our understanding of breast cancer, the majority of breast reconstructions are now completed synchronously with mastectomy rather than at subsequent intervals. A reconsideration of the placement of improper incisions and the unfounded tenet of extensive breast skin removal in these cases is a byproduct of the preoperative planning by the surgical oncologist together with the plastic surgeon. There are two reasons to consider skin conservation in this setting: (1) little justification exists to remove the usual 10- by 20-cm ellipse of breast skin around the nipple and (2) preservation of the native breast skin dramatically enhances the quality of the reconstruction.

This skin conservation approach appears to be justified in mastectomies when patients are ineligible for lumpectomy radiation. Many of these factors have little to do with a need for wide skin excision (e.g., invasive T1, T2 with an extensive intraductal component, a central tumor that would deform the breast, or multifocality). Favorable conditions for skin-sparing approaches include minimal cancers (T1a, T1b, ductal carcinoma in situ);

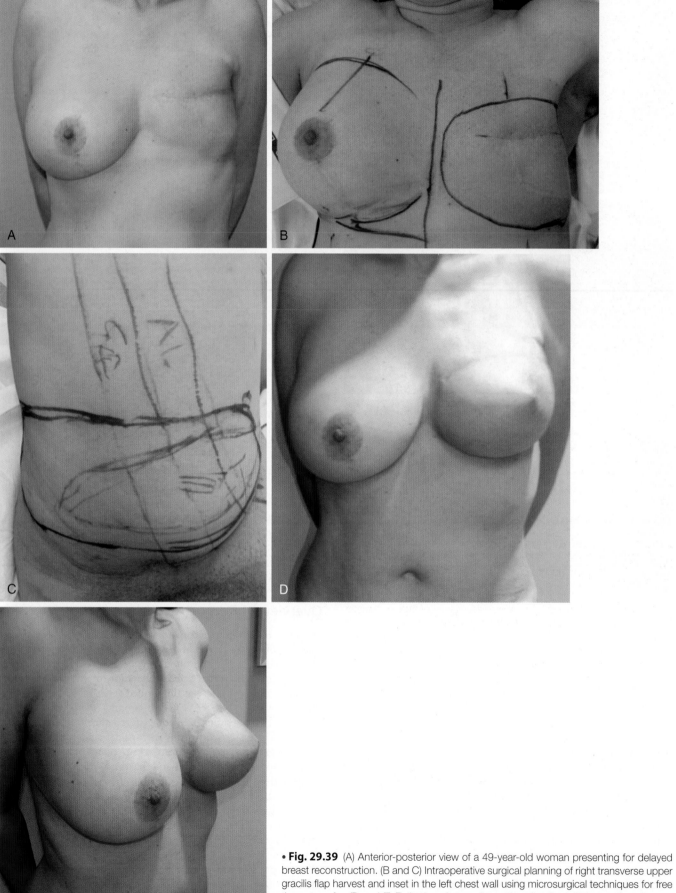

• **Fig. 29.39** (A) Anterior-posterior view of a 49-year-old woman presenting for delayed breast reconstruction. (B and C) Intraoperative surgical planning of right transverse upper gracilis flap harvest and inset in the left chest wall using microsurgical techniques for free tissue transfer. (D and E) Esthetic outcome 6 months after the initial operation demonstrating a larger native breast on the right; patient will undergo right breast reduction for symmetry.

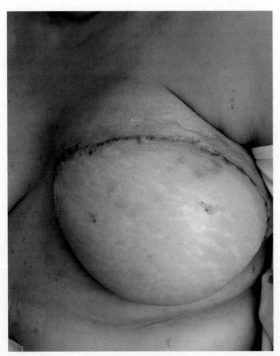

• **Fig. 29.40** A 55-year-old woman on postoperative day 1 after delayed breast reconstruction with free abdominal tissue transfer. Note the "patch" appearance of the abdominal skin on the breast.

diffuse microinvasive or multicentric cancers; benign conditions, such as familial (high-risk) breast cancer or difficult diagnostic breasts; and small breast cancers that are deep in the breast and remote from the overlying skin. Even in large tumors (T2–T4), the expected local recurrences virtually always represent failures together with systemic disease, rather than inadequate locoregional excision. In no immediate reconstructive series has there been any increase in local recurrence that can be related to the autogenous reconstruction.[69–71] A recent Cochrane review of nipple- and areola-sparing mastectomies for the treatment of breast cancer performed a descriptive analyses and meta-analyses of the 11 available nonrandomized comparative studies. Because of the high risk of bias and low quality of such studies, their findings were inconclusive, but no significant difference in local recurrence or OS was seen.[89]

Surgical literature often purports that the purpose of the SSM is to improve "cosmesis." In actuality, SSM provides a major advantage in the quality of every variant of the breast reconstructive procedure, particularly when implant augmentation is planned. Conversely, wide skin excision is the principal requirement for the complex TRAM flap in breast reconstruction; the skin deficit is so extensive that no other reconstruction method would be satisfactory. When limited skin excision has been planned and implemented, simpler variants of reconstruction, such as the autogenous latissimus flap, local flaps, and tissue expanders, can be used because there will be no requirement for surface skin replacement. With increasing evidence that no deleterious outcome results from skin conservation in a broad range (stage presentations) of mastectomy patients, this technique has gained general acceptance as the conventional approach. It can be expected in the future that wide skin excision will have limited indications, such as direct skin invasion or a massive tumor.

Factors Influencing Immediate or Delayed Postmastectomy Reconstruction

The rapid advances in understanding of the fundamental biology of breast cancer in the 20th and early 21st centuries, together with advances in surgical techniques after the advent and application of the vascularized myocutaneous flaps (TRAM and latissimus), have provided viable options for reconstruction after mastectomy. Until recently, few data regarding the influences and attitudes of women who favor the reconstructive procedure were available. The National Cancer Database of the American College of Surgeons evaluated a large sample of women undergoing mastectomy between 1985 and 1990 (n = 155,463) and between 1994 and 1995 (n = 68,348). Reconstruction use and patient and tumor factors in these two time periods were evaluated and compared. The investigators determined that nationally only 3.4% of mastectomy patients of the 1985 to 1990 era selected early or immediate reconstruction; this group size increased to 8.3% in 1994 to 1995. Patient age, income, geographic locale, type of hospital providing treatment, and AJCC tumor stage all influenced the consideration and usage of reconstruction (in univariate analysis). Patients 50 years of age or younger had a 4.3 greater probability for favoring reconstruction than their older patient cohorts (Table 29.3).[90] Of interest, patients with ductal carcinoma in situ were twice as likely as those with invasive carcinoma to favor reconstruction. Thus breast reconstruction is an underused procedure that enhances postmastectomy patient satisfaction and self-esteem.

The principal deterrent for breast reconstruction consideration often follows anecdotal ill-advised consideration of the general oncologic surgeon; previous opinions for an increased probability of failed (and delayed) tumor detection with recurrent disease in the reconstructed breast were not supported by objective data. To answer this essential question, a large analysis of patients (n = 540) undergoing immediate reconstruction after modified radical mastectomy identified 50 patients within this database to have locally advanced breast cancer. Postoperative chemotherapy was given to all patients who underwent immediate reconstruction; radiotherapy was used in 40% of this cohort, depending on tumor/nodal status. At median follow-up of 58.4 months, these patients treated at the University of Texas MD Anderson Cancer Center had no statistically significant differences in local or distant relapse compared with those patients treated with modified radical mastectomy without reconstruction. Furthermore, no differences were evident regarding treatment failure for patients with locally advanced breast cancer who did or did not have immediate breast reconstruction (Table 29.4).[91] Thus immediate reconstruction can be performed with low surgical morbidity and also with acceptable recurrence rates similar to those for patients who did not pursue reconstruction.

In a more recent analysis, Nold and colleagues[92] noted that only 20% to 50% of patients with early-stage disease choose breast conservation procedures. These authors further sought to determine the influences that were most important to select the ablative modified radical mastectomy with or without reconstruction versus breast conservation approaches; both cohorts were eligible for the skin-sparing procedure. Overall, the most influential factor for consideration of a procedure was the "fear of cancer." Women choosing conservation surgery indicated that their surgeon, the (expected) cosmetic result, and psychological issues were more influential in their decision than for those selecting modified radical mastectomy without reconstruction ($p < .02$; Table 29.5).[92] Fear of cancer-related death remained a major factor influencing

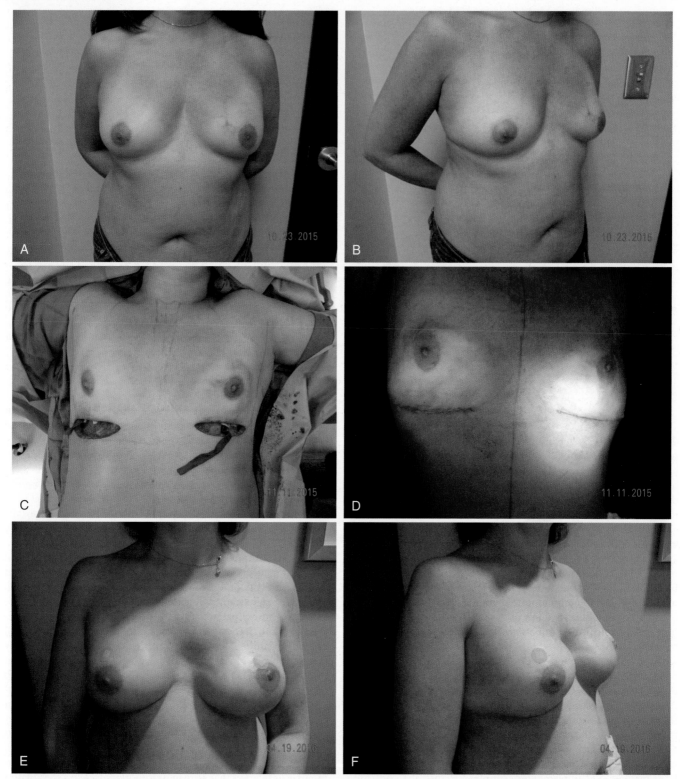

• **Fig. 29.41** (A and B) Anterior-posterior and oblique view of 49-year-old woman presenting for nipple-sparing mastectomy and immediate reconstruction with tissue expanders. (C and D) Intraoperative view of nipple-sparing mastectomy with an inframammary fold incision and immediate view after tissue expander placement. Note the well-preserved skin envelope as demonstrated on (C) as a result of gentle handing during the mastectomy procedure. (E and F) Esthetic outcome 6 months after the initial operation demonstrating completion of expansion process, before final exchange for permanent implant and correction of minor imperfections and asymmetries.

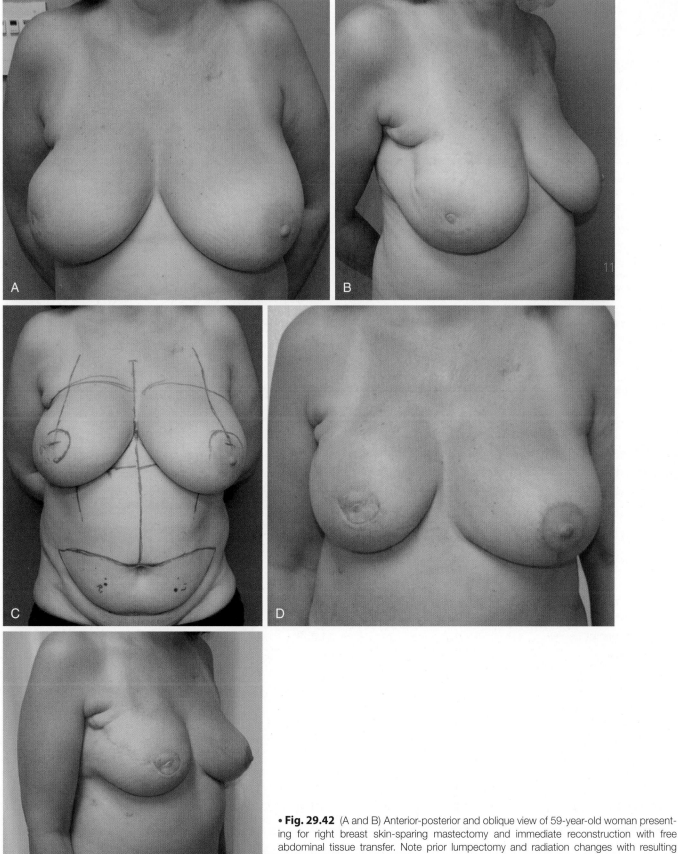

• **Fig. 29.42** (A and B) Anterior-posterior and oblique view of 59-year-old woman presenting for right breast skin-sparing mastectomy and immediate reconstruction with free abdominal tissue transfer. Note prior lumpectomy and radiation changes with resulting asymmetry. (C) demonstrated preoperative planning. (D and E) Show the esthetic outcome 6 months after the initial operation. Please note the abdominal skin was used to replace the nipple-areola complex excised with the mastectomy specimen, which will later be tattooed for color match.

TABLE 29.3 Multivariate Analysis of Factors Influencing the Use of Reconstruction, 1994 to 1995[a]

Variable	Odds Ratio	95% Confidence Interval
Age: ≤50 vs. ≥50 y	4.3	4.2–4.4
PAJCC stage: 0 vs. I–IV	2.1	2.1–2.2
Family income: ≤$40,000 vs. ≥$40,000	2	2–2.1
Ethnicity: non–African American vs. African American	1.6	1.5–1.7
Hospital type: NCI-recognized vs. other	1.4	1.3–1.7
Geographic region: Northeast, Southeast, Mountain, and Pacific vs. Midwest and South	1.3	1.2–1.3

[a]n = 55,728.

NCI, National Cancer Institute; PAJCC, Pathologic American Joint Committee on Cancer.
From Morrow M, Scott SK, Menck HR, et al. Factors influencing the use of breast reconstruction postmastectomy: A National Cancer Database study. J Am Coll Surg. 2001;192:1-8.

TABLE 29.4 Outcome for Locally Advanced Breast Cancer Patients Undergoing Mastectomy With or Without Immediate Breast Reconstruction[a]

Outcome	Immediate Breast Reconstruction (n = 50)	No Reconstruction (n = 72)	p Value
Interval to postoperative chemotherapy (range: number postoperative wound complications percentage)	35 days (5–91)	21 days (8–145)	.05
Major	4/50 (8%)	3/72 (4.2%)	.23
Minor	3/50 (6%)	5/72 (6.9%)	.66
Local recurrence			
Stage IIB	1/23 (4.4%)	2/12 (16.7%)	.22
Stage III	4/27 (14.8%)	7/60 (11.7%)	.70
Distant relapse			
Stage IIB	5/23 (21.7%)	4/12 (33.3%)	.37
Stage III	11/27 (40.7%)	22/60 (36.7%)	.85

[a]Median follow-up of 58.6 months (range 15–116 months).
From Newman LA, Kuerer HM, Hunt KK, et al. Feasibility of immediate breast reconstruction for locally advanced breast cancer. Ann Surg Oncol. 1999;6:671-675.

TABLE 29.5 Responses of Women Undergoing BCS, MRN-R, or MRM-NR Regarding Degree to Which Various Factors Influenced Choice of Surgical Option

Factor[a]	BCS Median (25th, 75th Percentiles)[b]	MRM-R Median (25th, 75th Percentiles)[b]	MRM-NR Median (25th, 75th Percentiles)[b]	p Value
Number	43	14	39	
Family	3 (1, 4)	1.5 (1, 5)	2 (1, 3)	.5989
Primary care physician	1 (1, 3)	1 (1, 1)	1 (1, 2)	.8378
Surgeon	4.5 (3, 5)	3 (1, 4)	2 (1, 5)	.0009
Medical oncologist	1.5 (1, 4)	1 (1, 1)	1 (1, 1)	.0194
Previous (personal) history	1 (1, 2)	1 (1, 1)	1 (1, 1)	.7071
Family history	1 (1, 3)	2.5 (1,5)	1 (1, 3)	.3099
Cosmetic appearance	3 (2, 5)	4 (1, 5)	1 (1, 1)	.0001
Fear of breast cancer	3 (2, 5)	4.5 (4, 5)	5 (3, 5)	.0420
Difficult cancer diagnosis	1.5 (1, 3)	1 (1, 3)	1 (1, 3)	.8581
Concern about radiation	2 (1, 4)	4.5 (1, 5)	3 (1, 5)	.2290
Travel for radiation	1 (1, 1)	1 (1, 1)	1 (1, 1)	.7236
Time for radiation therapy	1 (1, 3)	1 (1, 1)	1 (1, 1)	.7844
Psychological aspects	3 (2, 5)	3 (1, 4)	1 (1, 2)	.0001
Insurance	1 (1, 2)	1 (1, 1)	1 (1, 1)	.1363

BCS, Breast conserving surgery; MRM-NR, modified radical mastectomy without reconstruction; MRN-R, modified radical mastectomy with reconstruction.
[a]Parentheses within rows are used to identify significant treatment differences. Median responses within a row that share the same superscript are not significantly different, and those that have different superscripts are significantly different (p < .05).
[b]Median responses and 25th and 75th percentiles for responses regarding choice of surgical option: 1, did not influence; 2, minimally influenced; 3, influenced; 4, moderately influenced; and 5, greatly influenced decision.
From Nold RJ, Beamer RL, Helmer SD, McBoyle MF. Factors influencing a woman's choice to undergo breast conserving surgery versus modified radical mastectomy. Am J Surg 2000;180:413-418.

women selecting the modified radical without immediate reconstruction. In comparing those with the ablative mastectomy with or without reconstruction, there was a similar fear of cancer-related death; predictably, those who selected reconstruction had greater concern with cosmetic appearance ($p = .0002$). One should emphasize that most local recurrences (>80%) occur near the incision site and the subcutaneous tissue level, easily palpable by physical examination.

A recent meta-analysis by Cochrane database has demonstrated similar outcomes when comparing modified radical, skin-sparing, and nipple-sparing mastectomy. It is important to mention that the quality of data was considered low because of the high probability of selection bias.[93]

In summary, the surgeon's input (opinion) is of paramount concern and importance to the patient considering breast conservation versus an ablative approach with immediate reconstruction. Although proper counseling of the patient regarding equivalent outcomes for recurrence and survival for either ablative procedure is essential, the patient's fear of cancer (relapse and death) may overshadow the surgeon's proper and proactive advice.[94]

Incisions for Axillary Dissection

The advent of SLNB and the early diagnosis of breast cancer (up to 30% of newly diagnosed breast cancers are ductal carcinoma in situ) have had an impact on the application of formal axillary node dissections. Nonetheless, one has to be cognizant of the need for axillary node dissections at the time of the mastectomy or in some instances at a later date. This need for reoperation occurs in as many as 40% of false-negative readings. There are few false-positive results in sentinel node sampling with use of the combined blue dye and isotope mapping techniques. When the former occurs, and permanent pathology of histologically positive nodal disease is present, the surgeon must return to the axilla after breast reconstruction. Cooperation between the oncologic surgeon and the plastic surgeon is essential in these cases, particularly in microvascular free-tissue transfers.[80,95]

Currently, there is some interest in performing the SSM with preservation of the nipple-areola complex. Most data are preliminary, and the technique is applied to selective cases. It should not be used for patients whose tumors are within 2 cm of the nipple-areola complex. Local recurrences under the nipple-areola complex as well as partial or total necrosis of the nipple-areola complex have been observed.[96]

Fig. 29.37 depicts the preferred incision and the optional incisions for axillary dissections performed synchronously with lumpectomy (segmental mastectomy, tylectomy). The surgeon is well advised to complete incisions placed parallel with Langer lines and designed in a curvilinear fashion just caudal to the axillary hairline. These incisions are designed at the time of SLNB and must be enlarged when axillary dissection is indicated for the histologically confirmed positive sentinel node. Preferably, axillary incisions are made separately from incisions of the segmental mastectomy. Optional incisions indicated in Fig. 29.37 obliquely cross Langer lines and are not positioned in axillary skin folds. It is perhaps for this latter reason that delay in primary healing and inferior cosmetic results are obtained. Adequate skin exposure should be provided so that dissection of level I and level II nodes beneath the pectoralis minor is possible without undue traction on the pectoralis major or minor muscles. This principle prevents damage to the medial and lateral (anterior thoracic) pectoral nerves located in the lateral and medial neurovascular bundles, respectively. Incisions placed in a curvilinear transverse, oblique, or vertical fashion all allow adequate access to the axillary vein, the medial border of the pectoralis minor muscle, and the lateral aspect of the latissimus dorsi muscle. This exposure should permit visualization of the long thoracic nerve to the serratus anterior and the thoracodorsal nerve to the latissimus dorsi.

Selected References

26. Madden JL. Modified radical mastectomy. *Surg Gynecol Obstet.* 1965;121:1221.
28. Veronesi U, Cascinelli N, Mariani L, et al. Twenty-year follow-up of a randomized study comparing breast-conserving surgery with radical mastectomy for early breast cancer. *N Engl J Med.* 2002;347:1227-1232.
29. Litiere S, Werutsky G, Fentiman IS, et al. Breast conserving therapy versus mastectomy for stage I-II breast cancer: 20 year follow-up of the EORTC 10801 phase 3 randomized trial. *Lancet Oncol.* 2012;13:412-419.
30. Crago AM, Azu M, Tierney S, et al. Randomized clinical trials in breast cancer. *Surg Oncol Clin N Am.* 2010;19:33-58.
31. Black DM, Hunt KK, Mittendorf EA. Long term outcomes reporting the safety of breast conserving therapy compared to mastectomy: 20-year results of EORTC 10801. *Gland Surg.* 2013;2:120-123.
86. Boneti C, Yuen J, Santiago C, et al. Oncologic safety of nipple skin-sparing or total skin-sparing mastectomies with immediate reconstruction. *J Am Coll Surg.* 2011;212:686-693; discussion 693-5.

A full reference list is available online at ExpertConsult.com.

30

Halsted Radical Mastectomy

KIRBY I. BLAND, V. SUZANNE KLIMBERG, AND EDWARD M. COPELAND III

Historical Aspects for Development of Radical Mastectomy

In 1894 the modern era of breast cancer therapy was transformed when William Stewart Halsted reported the seminal "results of the cure of cancer of the breast." Ten days later the concurrent reports by Willy Meyer of New York indicated that the radical mastectomy followed the evolution of anatomic principles and the advancement of cancer biology of the 19th century. These prior achievements by renowned anatomists, physiologists, and surgeons were the genesis of what were considered "modern" biological and surgical therapies for cancer of the breast. The Halsted radical mastectomy, introduced in 1882 by Halsted at the Roosevelt Hospital in New York City, was popularized and scientifically embraced at the Johns Hopkins Hospital in Baltimore (est. 1889). The operation embodied the concept of routine complete en bloc resection of the breast with the pectoralis major and minor muscles and the regional lymphatics.[1,2] The halstedian approach was largely directed at preventing local or regional recurrences for an oncologic disease considered principally only of locoregional concern. Halsted's synthesis of the techniques of his predecessors in surgery and pathology allowed him to achieve unprecedented local and regional recurrent rates of 6% and 22%, respectively.[1–4] The en bloc technique described by Halsted, although published simultaneously by Meyer,[5] allowed a reduction in the local recurrence rate to 6% from rates of 51% to 82% for renowned European surgeons of the era. Table 30.1 compares the operations available to European surgeons during the era with the accompanying 3-year estimated "cure" rates for breast carcinoma at Johns Hopkins.

Halsted was not the first surgeon to resect the pectoralis major muscle in the course of a radical mastectomy. Wolff[6] documents that in 1570, Barthélemy Cabrol of Montpellier, France, reported the cure of a mammary carcinoma in a 35-year-old woman in whom the pectoralis major muscle was excised and the wound was sprinkled with vitriols.[3] The patient survived 12 years, only to die of cancer of the lower lip. Eminent European surgeons such as Petit, Billroth, Volkmann, and others of the period not infrequently removed portions of the pectoral muscles in resection of various malignancies of the breast.[7] This therapeutic approach violated the principles of en bloc resection of the neoplasm, a dictum espoused by Halsted and Meyer. Joerss[8] attributed the modern operation to Heidenhain. Nonetheless, it was Halsted who advocated *routine* resection of both pectoralis muscles en bloc with breast tissues and all levels (I–III) of axillary nodes. Halsted provided acknowledgments that substantiated the contributions

of other renowned surgeons of this era in formulation and adoption of this procedure.[9]

In its final procedural form, the technique of the radical mastectomy espoused by Halsted embodied the following principles:
- Wide excision of the skin, covering the defect with Thiersch grafts
- Routine removal of both pectoral muscles
- Routine axillary dissection (levels I–III)
- Removal of all tissues en bloc, with wide resection as possible on all sides of the growth
- Routine sacrifice of the long thoracic nerve and the thoracodorsal artery, nerve, and vein

The evolution of the modern radical mastectomy, which began with Cabrol in 1570 and pinnacled with Halsted in 1890,[3] is one of discordant retrogressions. The wide acceptance of the incurability of breast carcinoma, the consequences of sepsis, and the necessity for anesthesia played prominent roles in the delay of the development for surgery of the breast. To attribute the development of the modern operation to a single individual would discredit the remarkable contributions of Halsted's predecessors. The early surgery and pathology pioneers extended the operation because of the clinical observations for the natural history of breast cancer. These leaders of medical science lacked the salient background in biology, pathology, anatomy, pharmacology, and statistics that enabled Halsted to complete the evolution of the radical mastectomy in the late 19th century. Again, the raison d'être of the procedure was local-regional control of disease.

Breast Cancer Treatment in the United States

Trends and Patterns of Care, 1971 to 1984

Fig. 30.1 confirms that most surgeons used the modified radical mastectomy on patients reported in 1971, 1976, 1977, and 1981. In 1972, 48% of patients were reported having had a Halsted-type radical mastectomy, whereas only 3% of patients underwent this procedure in 1981. Trends in the use of radiation therapy and chemotherapy also showed dramatic alterations in application from 1972 through 1981. Trends for the use of radiation therapy in these years are depicted in Fig. 30.2. The proportion of patients at all stages reported to have received irradiation *decreased* substantially as the sole adjuvant therapy in distant disease, from 33% in 1972 to 18% in 1981. However, this trend is most apparent for regional stage disease (45%–21%), in the era. In contrast, the

TABLE 30.1 Chronology of the Mastectomy for Treatment of Breast Cancer With Expectant (Average) 3-Year "Cure Rates"

Type of Operation	Study	Year	No. of Cases	3-Year Cures (%)
Simple mastectomy	Winiwarter (Billroth)[a]	1867–1875		4.7
Average				**4.7**
Complete mastectomy and axillary dissection in most cases	Oldekop[b]	1850–1878	229	11.7
	Dietrich (Lucke)[c]	1872–1890	148	16.2
	Horner[d]	1881–1893	144	19.4
	Poulsen[e]	1870–1888	110	20
	Banks[f]	1877	46	20
	Schmid (Kuster)[g]	1871–1885		21.5
Average				**18.1**
Complete (total) mastectomy, axillary dissection, removal of pectoral fascia and greater or lesser amounts of pectoral muscle	Sprengel (Volkmann)[h]	1874–1878	200	11
	Schmidt[i]	1877–1886	112	18.8
	Rotter[j]		30	20
	Mahler[k]	1887–1897	150	21
	Joerss[l]	1885–1893	98	28.5
Average				**19.9**
Modern radical mastectomy	Halsted[m]	1889–1894	76	45
	Halsted[n]	1907	232	38.3
	Hutchison[o]	1910–1933		39.4
Average				**40.9**

[a]Data from Winiwarter V (Billroth). Beiträge zur statistik d. carcinome. Stuttgart: Gedruckt bei L. Schumacher; 1878.
[b]Data from Oldekop J.[7]
[c]Data from Dietrich G (Lucke). Beitrag zur Statistik des Mammacarcinom. Duch Z F Chir. 1892;33:471.
[d]Data from Horner F. Ueber die Endresultate von 172 operierten Fällen maligner Tumoren der weiblichen Brust. Beitr Z Klin Chir. 1894;12:619.
[e]Data from Poulsen K. Die Geschwülste der Mamma. Arch F Klin Chir. 1891;42:593.
[f]Data from Banks M. A plea for the more free removal of cancerous growths. Liverpool Manchester Surg Rep. 1878;192.
[g]Data from Schmid H (Kuster). Zur statistik der mammacarcinome und deren heilung. Dtsch Z F Chir. 1887;26:139.
[h]Data from Sprengel O (Volkmann). 131 Fälle von Brust-Carcinom. Arch F Klin Chir. 1882;27:805.
[i]Data from Schmidt GB. Die Geschwülste der Brustdrüse. Beitr Z Klin Chir. 1889;4:40.
[j]Data from Rotter J. Günstigere Dauererfolge durch eine verbesserte operative Behandlung der Mammakarzinome. Berl Klin Wochenschr. 1896;33:69.
[k]Data from Mahler F. Ueber die in der Heidelberger Klinik 1887–1897 behandelten Fälle von Carcinoma Mammae. Beitr Z Klin Chir. 1900;26:681.
[l]Data from Joerss K.[8]
[m]Data from Halsted.[1]
[n]Data from Halsted.[2]
[o]Data from Hutchison RG. Radiation therapy in carcinoma of the breast. Surg Gynecol Obstet. 1936;62:653. (Collected figures.)
Modified from Cooper WA. The history of the radical mastectomy. In Hoeber PB, ed. *Annals of Medical History*. Vol. 3. New York: Paul B Hoeber; 1941.

introduction of effective adjuvant and systemic chemotherapy and the emerging principles of pharmacotherapeutics initiated a dramatic increase in the application of chemotherapy. Chemotherapy increased from only 7% of patients treated in 1972 to 22.7% in 1981. This dramatic application of this effective therapy is depicted in Fig. 30.3; this exponential increase in the use of chemotherapy was limited to patients with regional and distant stages of disease. Currently, the use of adjuvant chemotherapy for treatment of localized disease (stages 0 and I) has experienced a renaissance. A discussion of the application of adjuvant chemotherapy and hormonal therapy for breast cancer is provided in Chapters 54 through 57.

The 1982 National Survey by the American College of Surgeons (ACS) evaluated 5-year survival rates by stage, type of treatment, and type of adjuvant therapy. Table 30.2 depicts survival rates for patients initially treated in 1976 by type of operation, with or without adjuvant irradiation, and chemotherapy. Similar survival rates for patients with localized disease were observed for treatment by partial mastectomy alone and by partial mastectomy plus irradiation to the breast, the axilla, or both. In addition, 5-year survival rates for patients treated by the modified radical mastectomy technique were similar to 5-year survival rates for those treated by the Halsted radical mastectomy. Wilson and colleagues[10] noted that survival rates were also similar for those

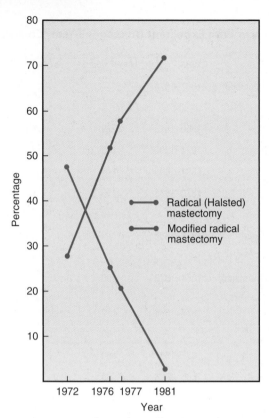

• **Fig. 30.1** Trends in the type of operation performed from 1972 to 1981 in the 1982 National Survey of Carcinoma of the Breast in the United States by the American College of Surgeons. (From Wilson RE, Donegan WL, Mettlin C, et al. The 1982 national survey of carcinoma of the breast in the United States by the American College of Surgeons. *Surg Gynecol Obstet.* 1984;159:309–318.)

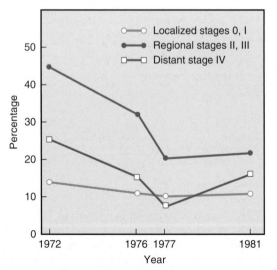

• **Fig. 30.2** Trends in the use of radiotherapy from 1972 to 1981 as reported in the 1982 National Survey of Carcinoma of the Breast in the United States by the American College of Surgeons. (From Wilson RE, Donegan WL, Mettlin C, et al. The 1982 national survey of carcinoma of the breast in the United States by the American College of Surgeons. *Surg Gynecol Obstet.* 1984;159:309-318.)

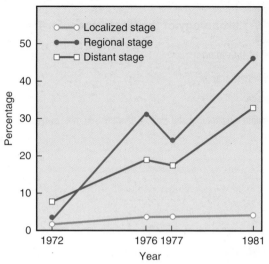

• **Fig. 30.3** Trends in the application of systemic chemotherapy from 1972 to 1981 as reported in the 1982 National Survey of Cancer of the Breast in the United States by the American College of Surgeons. (From Wilson RE, Donegan WL, Mettlin C, et al. The 1982 national survey of carcinoma of the breast in the United States by the American College of Surgeons. *Surg Gynecol Obstet.* 1984;159:309-318.)

who received additional irradiation therapy or chemotherapy with one of the two surgical procedures.

Because the aforementioned publications of short- and long-term surveys are not prospective trials, this bias in treatment selection cannot be eliminated. In addition, follow-up data were limited, and these data represent only the trends in therapeutic approaches. Nonetheless, there has been an important transition in curative surgical procedures used by US surgeons from the Halsted radical to the modified radical mastectomy techniques.[11] This transition was apparent at the time of the 1977 survey reported by Nemoto and associates.[12,13] The 1981 survey[13] confirmed that most patients receiving treatment underwent a modified radical mastectomy rather than a radical mastectomy (77% vs. 3%). This departure from a radical to a less deforming procedure is credited to Sir David Patey and W.H. Dyson[14] of the Middlesex Hospital in London. Patey concluded from scientific study that excision of the pectoralis major muscle was not routinely justified on anatomic or pathologic observations; further, he was able to confirm that complete anatomic nodal clearance of the axilla remained possible, with excision only of the minor muscle. This allowed Patey to coin the term *modified* radical mastectomy after description of the procedure.[15,16]

Thereafter, results of the short-term survey also confirmed an increase in the proportion of patients being treated with partial mastectomy, largely attributed to the seminal contribution of clinical trials conducted by Fisher and coworkers[17,18] in association with the National Surgical Adjuvant Breast and Bowel Project (NSABP). Survival rates of patients treated by the various procedures are not comparable in the absence of more detailed data because of confounding biological and patient-related factors that may affect prognosis.

The 20-year update by Fisher and colleagues[19,20] (2002) confirmed the value of lumpectomy followed by breast irradiation as an appropriate therapy for breast carcinoma—provided that resection margins are clear of neoplasm. Importantly, breast conservation and total mastectomy (which implies radical mastectomy as

TABLE 30.2 Five-Year Survival Rate by Stage, Type of Operation, and Type of Adjuvant Therapy

| | TYPE OF ADJUVANT THERAPY BY STAGE | | | | | | | | |
| | LOCALIZED | | | REGIONAL | | | DISTANT | | |
Type of Operation	None	RT	CT	None	RT	CT	None	RT	CT
Partial Mastectomy									
5-year survival (%)	82.6	83.9	100	64.4	56.9	81	29	9.5	20.4
No. of patients	301	81	7	54	45	8	32	18	37
Total Mastectomy Only									
5-year survival (%)	86.8	81	80.1	60	51.3	55.9	30.2	23.4	19.7
No. of patients	1034	154	37	183	116	32	72	44	43
Total Mastectomy With Low Axillary Dissection									
5-year survival (%)	92.6	88	82.7	75	64.7	74	24.8	19	36.4
No. of patients	540	55	24	242	159	77	15	17	13
Modified Radical Mastectomy									
5-year survival (%)	92.4	89.2	84.3	80.2	72.3	71.6	46.1	29.4	32.4
No. of patients	6537	630	280	2131	1292	1553	85	55	85
Radical (Halsted) Mastectomy									
5-year survival (%)	92.8	89.4	88.7	78	73.1	71.1	52.5	51.4	51.5
No. of patients	3058	335	104	1190	795	640	50	29	37

CT, Chemotherapy; RT, radiation therapy.
Modified from Wilson RE, Donegan WL, Mettlin C, et al. The 1982 national survey of carcinoma of the breast in the United States by the American College of Surgeons. *Surg Gynecol Obstet.* 1984;159:309-318.

an overtreatment) have *equivalent* disease-free, distant disease-free, and overall survival rates (Fig. 30.4). The 20-year analysis (2002) by Veronesi and associates[21] validated the findings of Fisher and the NSABP—long-term survival is *equivalent* for women undergoing breast conservation compared with radical mastectomy (Fig. 30.5) and tumor size (<1 cm vs. >2 cm) of the primary lesions are similar (Fig. 30.6). This European study further confirmed the crude cumulative incidence of *local recurrence* after radical mastectomy and recurrence after breast conservation therapy. Fig. 30.7 indicates that the cumulative incidence of local recurrence was 8.8% with breast conservation versus 2.3% for radical mastectomy at 20 years. No differences were evident between the two groups relative to rates of contralateral disease, second primary cancers, or distant metastases.

The ACS conducted two surveys for the treatment of breast carcinoma in the United States: a long-term survey in 1976 and a short-term survey in 1981.[10] Table 30.3 shows that in the short-term survey, more than twice the percentage of patients were treated by partial mastectomy (7.2%) compared with the long-term survey, which reported that 2.8% of surgeons used this technique in the primary therapy of breast cancer ($p < .0001$). The most significant change in this survey was in the type of operations used for treatment of operable breast cancer. There is an increased use of modified radical mastectomy (55.6% in the long-term survey compared with 78.2% in the short-term survey) and a marked decline in the reported use of the Halsted radical mastectomy (27.5% of patients in the long-term survey compared

with 3.4% in the 1981 data; see Fig. 30.1). For each stage of disease, there was a greater reported use of the modified radical procedure in the more recent short-term survey data compared with that for patients treated 5 years earlier. Interestingly, no significant changes were observed in the other types of surgical procedures between 1976 and 1981.

When treatment modalities were evaluated according to the clinical stage in the ACS survey, 95% of patients were treated in the long- and short-term surveys by surgical treatment alone or in combination with other modalities. Table 30.4 confirms that in the 1976 long-term survey, 60.6% of patients were treated by operation alone, compared with 58.8% in the 1981 short-term analysis. In addition, the use of surgical therapy plus irradiation (with or without chemotherapy) decreased from 19.8% to 16.6%, and the use of chemotherapy (with or without irradiation) with operation increased from 16.4% to 22.7% during this 5-year period. The change was limited to patients with regional and distant disease, and there was no significant change in the use of other treatment modalities between the long- and short-term surveys. For both analyses, 82% to 84% of patients in the localized disease stage were treated with surgery alone. For both surveys, the use of operative therapy as a sole modality decreased with advancing stage of disease, and the proportion of patients treated with surgery alone was similar in both surveys (see Table 30.4). Furthermore, operation plus irradiation was used more often than operation plus chemotherapy in the treatment of patients with cancer diagnosed as localized or regional to adjacent

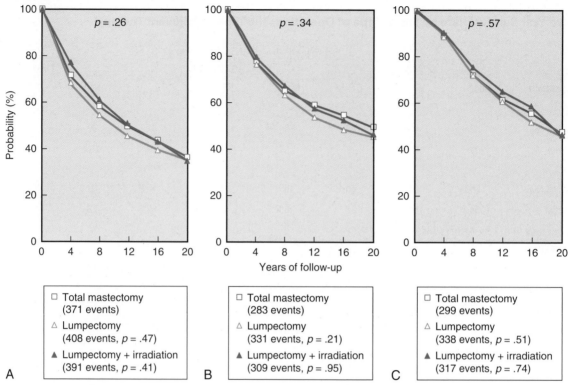

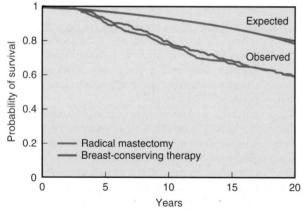

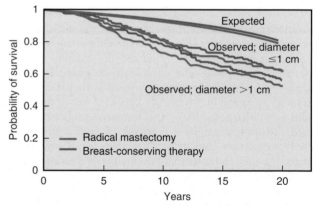

tissue. For the long-term study, operation plus irradiation and operation plus chemotherapy were used equally (24.2% vs. 24.1%) for treatment of patients with axillary node involvement. The short-term study confirmed that operation plus chemotherapy was 3.5 times more likely to be used than operation plus radiation (35% vs. 10.4%) for treatment of patients with positive

axillary nodes. Wilson and colleagues[10] noted that in both surveys, similar proportions of patients with regional disease underwent operation followed by radiation and chemotherapy. For patients with disease in the advanced stage, irradiation, chemotherapy, or hormone therapy, alone or in combination, was used more often (42.1% long term and 38.7% short term).

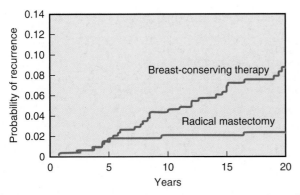

• **Fig. 30.7** Crude cumulative incidence of local recurrences after radical mastectomy and recurrences in the same breast after breast-conserving therapy. (From Veronesi U, Cascinelli N, Mariani L, et al. Twenty-year follow-up of a randomized study comparing breast-conserving surgery with radical mastectomy for early breast cancer. *N Engl J Med.* 2002; 347:1227-1232. Copyright © 2002. Massachusetts Medical Society. All rights reserved.)

Trends and Patterns of Care, 1985 to 2002 National Cancer Database—American College of Surgeons Commission on Cancer

The evolution of less radical approaches for the therapy of breast cancer followed the convincing reports of the past two decades for the efficacy and equivalency for locoregional control with conservative approaches (see Chapter 32). Since 1985, the National Cancer Database (NCDB) of the Commission on Cancer of the ACS tracked therapy trends for breast cancer. These data, illustrated in Tables 30.5 and 30.6, identify the high usage of breast conservation for early-stage disease (T_1, T_2; stage 0) by US Census Region in 1990.[22] The trends and patterns of care by board-certified fellows of the ACS reflect decreasing usage of radical mastectomy in 1985, 1988, and 1990 (1.9%, 1.5%, and 0.6%, respectively). A similar pattern was observed for modified radical mastectomy with 63.2%, 64.8%, and 59.7% of surgeons using the procedure in 1985, 1988, and 1990, respectively (see Table 30.6). The explanation for decreasing use

TABLE 30.3	**Type of Operation and Stage Distribution of Patients With Carcinoma of the Breast**									

	CLINICAL STAGE REGIONAL TO:									
	LOCALIZED		AXILLARY NODES WITH OR WITHOUT ADJACENT TISSUE		ADJACENT TISSUE ONLY		DISTANT		TOTAL	
Operation	n	%	n	%	n	%	n	%	n	%
Long-Term Survey (1976)										
Partial mastectomy	408	3	74	0.8	58	8.1	153	14.3	693	2.8
Total mastectomy only	1261	9.3	203	2.2	178	24.7	278	26	1920	7.8
Total mastectomy with low axillary dissection	632	4.6	509	5.5	35	4.9	98	9.2	1274	5.2
Modified radical mastectomy	7584	55.7	5481	59.1	295	41	361	33.7	13,721	55.6
Radical (Halsted) mastectomy	3571	26.2	2909	31.4	144	20	169	15.8	6793	27.5
Extended radical mastectomy	152	1.1	99	1.1	9	1.2	11	1	271	1.1
TOTAL	13,608	100	9275	100	719	100	1070	100	24,672	100
Short-Term Survey (1981)										
Partial mastectomy	819	8.5	236	3.4	58	12.1	170	22.1	1283	7.2
Total mastectomy only	530	5.5	129	1.9	73	15.2	184	23.9	916	5.2
Total mastectomy with low axillary dissection	511	5.3	340	5	26	5.4	83	10.8	960	5.4
Modified radical mastectomy	7436	77.1	5777	85	302	62.9	312	40.6	13,827	78.2
Radical (Halsted) mastectomy	295	3	272	4	17	3.5	19	2.5	603	3.4
Extended radical mastectomy	57	0.6	41	0.6	4	0.8	1	0.1	103	0.6
TOTAL	9648	100	6795	100	480	100	769	100	17,692	100

From Wilson RE, Donegan WL, Mettlin C, et al. The 1982 national survey of carcinoma of the breast in the United States by the American College of Surgeons. *Surg Gynecol Obstet.* 1984;159:309-318.

TABLE 30.4 Type of Treatment and Stage Distribution of Patients With Carcinoma of the Breast

| | | | CLINICAL STAGE REGIONAL TO: | | | | | | | |
| | LOCALIZED | | AXILLARY NODES WITH OR WITHOUT ADJACENT TISSUE | | ADJACENT TISSUE ONLY | | DISTANT | | TOTAL | |
Operation	n	%	n	%	n	%	n	%	n	%
Long-Term Survey (1976)										
Surgical treatment only	11,592	84.4	3395	35.8	454	53.9	261	14.1	15,702	60.6
Surgical treatment and radiation	1275	9.3	2289	24.2	148	17.6	165	8.9	3877	15
Surgical treatment and chemotherapy	460	3.4	2284	24.1	57	6.8	215	11.6	3016	11.6
Surgical treatment and hormone therapy	75	0.5	132	1.4	12	1.4	103	5.6	322	1.2
Surgical treatment, radiation, and chemotherapy	154	1.1	911	9.6	34	4	142	7.7	1241	4.8
Surgical treatment and others[a]	52	0.4	264	2.8	14	1.7	184	10	514	2
Others[a]	120	0.9	198	2.1	123	14.6	778	42.1	1219	4.7
TOTAL	13,728	100	9473	100	842	100	1848	100	25,891	100
Short-Term Survey (1981)										
Surgical treatment only	8065	82.2	2444	35	285	53.5	140	11.2	10,934	58.8
Surgical treatment and radiation	1035	10.6	731	10.4	94	17.6	56	4.5	1916	10.3
Surgical treatment and chemotherapy	355	3.6	2444	35	44	8.3	209	16.7	3052	16.4
Surgical treatment and hormone therapy	78	0.8	179	2.6	8	1.5	96	7.7	361	1.9
Surgical treatment, radiation, and chemotherapy	88	0.9	857	12.3	37	6.9	181	14.4	1163	6.3
Surgical treatment and others[a]	27	0.3	140	2	12	2.3	87	6.9	266	1.4
Others[a]	162	1.6	192	2.7	53	9.9	485	38.7	892	4.8
TOTAL	9810	100	6987	100	533	100	1254	100	18,584	100

[a]Radiation, chemotherapy, or both, and radiation, hormone therapy, or both.
From Wilson RE, Donegan WL, Mettlin C, et al. The 1982 national survey of carcinoma of the breast in the United States by the American College of Surgeons. *Surg Gynecol Obstet.* 1984;159:309-318.

TABLE 30.5 Percentage of Breast Cancer Cases With Partial (Segmental) Mastectomy by US Census Region, 1990, Stages 0 and I Cases

Region	1985	1988	1990
New England	39.9	44	52.6
Mid-Atlantic	16.4	33.6	48.9
South Atlantic	27.8	27.2	32
East North Central	19.6	25.9	40.7
East South Central	28.3	16.3	17.5
West North Central	14.1	20.1	24.2
West South Central	25.8	20.6	28.8
Mountain	14.5	25	40.1
Pacific	34.1	36	41.3
All regions	25.8	29.8	38.1
No. of cases	5592	12,420	18,641

From Winchester DP. Standards of care in breast cancer diagnosis and treatment. *Surg Oncol Clin North Am.* 1994;3:85.

TABLE 30.6 Percentage of Breast Cancer Cases by Type of Surgery by Year of Diagnosis

Surgery	1985	1988	1990
Radical mastectomy	1.9	1.5	0.6
Modified radical mastectomy	63.2	64.8	59.7
Total mastectomy	3.4	3.8	2.8
Partial (segmental) mastectomy	18.4	22.2	28.4
Subcutaneous mastectomy	0.5	0.5	0.5
Surgery type unknown	3.5	1	1.1
No surgery	7	5.4	4.5
Unknown if surgery done	2.1	0.8	2.4
TOTAL	100	100	100
No. of cases	14,509	26,465	39,869

Modified from Winchester DP. Standards of care in breast cancer diagnosis and treatment. *Surg Oncol Clin North Am.* 1994;3:85.

TABLE 30.7 Changes in Distribution of Patients by Type of Operation by Year of Diagnosis

Type of Operation	PERCENTAGE OF PATIENTS				
	1972 (n = 15,132)	1976 (n = 24,672)	1981 (n = 17,692)	1983 (n = 17,295)	1990 (n = 24,356)
Partial (segmental) mastectomy	3.4	2.8	7.2	13.1	25.4[a]
Total mastectomy, no nodes	11.5	7.8	5.2	4.2	4.1[b]
Total mastectomy, nodes	32.6	55.6	78.2	75.2	65.8[a]
Radical mastectomy	45.3	27.5	3.4	1.7	0.4[a]
Extended radical	1.8	1.1	0.6	0.1	<0.1
None	5.4	5.2	5.4	4.6	4.2[b]

[a]The difference for the rates of these operations for 1985 and 1990 was statistically significant ($p < .0005$). For extended radical mastectomy, $p = .03$.
[b]Denotes $p > .05$ (not statistically significant). Data from 1972, 1976, and 1981 are included for comparison but were not analyzed statistically.
From Osteen RT, Cady B, Chmiel JS, et al. 1991 national survey of carcinoma of the breast by the Commission on Cancer. *J Am Coll Surg*. 1994;178:213-219.

TABLE 30.8 Stage Distribution of Patients by Surgical Procedures[a]

Operation	Median Age (yr)	Stage Unknown (%)	PAJCC STAGE (%)							No. of Patients
			0	I	IIA	IIB	IIIA	IIIB	IV	
< Total, no nodes	69.2	34.6	22.2	4.7	2.5	1.1	0.7	4.8	19.4	3319
< Total, nodes	59.4	6.2	7.9	19.8	11.9	8.2	3.7	3.6	5.7	5095
Subcutaneous	56.5	0.6	2	0.2	0.2	0.3	0.2	0.4	0.6	157
Total, no nodes	71.8	9.6	11	2	2.2	1.3	0.9	7.5	8.5	1519
Total, nodes	63	21.2	52.4	71	81.1	87.6	90.3	75.5	39.5	28,960
Radical	60.8	0.8	0.4	0.5	0.9	1	2.2	3.1	1.8	392
Extended	55	0	0.1	0	0	0	0.2	0.3	0.2	17
Surgery type	62.4	26.1	3.8	1.3	0.9	0.5	1.5	4.4	22.5	1863
No. of patients	—	3980	2484	13,600	10,614	5871	1786	1527	1773	—

[a]Each column represents the percentage of patients with that stage disease who had the operation listed in that row; that is, 22.2% of patients with stage 0 disease were treated by less than total mastectomy without a node dissection.
PAJCC, Pathologic American Joint Committee on Cancer; < Total, less than total mastectomy.
From Osteen RT, Cady B, Chmiel JS, et al. 1991 national survey of carcinoma of the breast by the Commission on Cancer. *J Am Coll Surg*. 1994;178:213-219.

of the radical procedure is found in the shift to the segmental (partial) mastectomy, which represented 28.4% of mastectomies in 1990.[23]

Surgical therapy with breast conservation is being used with increasing frequency; partial (segmental) mastectomy use was 3.4%, 7.2%, and 25.4% in 1972, 1981, and 1990, respectively (Table 30.7). However, modified radical mastectomy remains the most frequently used surgical therapy for breast cancer by those surveyed. The most significant trend in usage was the decrease in radical mastectomy ($p < .0005$); the frequencies in 1972, 1981, and 1990 were 45.3%, 3.4%, and 0.4%, respectively. Since 1972, the radical and extended radical procedures have been virtually replaced by total mastectomy with or without axillary nodal sampling (see Table 30.7).[23]

For the 1990 survey, the criteria on which the surgeon based his or her selection of the operative procedure are depicted in

Tables 30.8 and 30.9. These data illustrate the stage, age distribution (see Table 30.8), and geographic variations (see Table 30.9) that determine the selection process. Radical and extended radical techniques are rarely used except in advanced local disease (stages IIIA or IIIB). Moreover, most US surgeons have replaced the radical procedure with the modified radical (Patey, Auchincloss-Madden) approach.[23,24]

Recent trends for surgical procedures confirmed by the NCDB indicate that patients are being treated in an earlier stage of disease. Bland and colleagues[25] reported the percentage and number of cases by combined American Joint Committee on Cancer (AJCC) stage group and year of diagnosis (Table 30.10) from 1985 to 1995. Convincing are the evolving trends to earlier disease stage (stage 0, I); in contrast, a decrease from 39.2% for stage II disease (1985) to 32.2% (1995) was evident during this decade, with decrease of stage III from 11.6% (1985) to 7.4% in

TABLE 30.9 Frequency of Surgical Procedures by Region

Operation	Canada + US Pass.	New England	Middle Atlantic	South Atlantic	E. North Central	E. South Central	W. North Central	W. South Central	Mountain	Pacific
	REGION (% TREATED BY OPERATION TYPE)									
< Total, no nodes	4.7	13	10.2	6.8	7.4	4.1	5.6	6.1	6	8.2
< Total, nodes	11.8	17.5	13.8	11.6	10.8	6.1	9.9	8.2	11.3	4.9
Subcutaneous	0.9	0.3	0.2	0.3	0.4	0.5	0.4	0.5	0.5	0.5
Total, no nodes	3.3	4.4	4.3	3.7	3.4	3.3	3.6	3.5	3.9	3
Total, nodes	66	58	64.6	72.4	72.2	79	74.5	75.5	72.9	68.3
Radical	5.2	0.7	1	0.9	0.7	2.5	1.2	1.4	1.3	0.4
Extended	—	—	—	0.1	0.1	—	—	—	—	—
Surgery type unknown	8	6	5.8	4.2	5.2	4.5	4.8	4.8	4.2	4.5
No. of patients	212	4137	6782	5287	7836	2213	3288	2886	1946	6958

E, East; *Pass.*, passport; *< Total*, less than total mastectomy; *W*, west.
Osteen RT, Cady B, Chmiel JS, et al: 1991 national survey of carcinoma of the breast by the Commission on Cancer. *J Am Coll Surg.* 1994;178:213-219.

TABLE 30.10 Percentage and Number of Cases by Combined AJCC Stage Group and Year of Diagnosis

PAJCC/CAJCC Stage	1985		1990		1995	
	n	%	n	%	n	%
Stage 0	2249	7.4	8968	11.2	14,790	14.3
Stage I	10,705	35.1	31,797	39.8	43,363	41.9
Stage II	11,959	39.2	27,922	35	33,315	32.2
Stage III	3554	11.6	6832	8.6	7616	7.4
Stage IV	2050	6.7	4299	5.4	4377	4.2
Total	30,517	100	79,818	100	103,461	100
Unknown	12,519		9154		4562	
Cases	43,036		88,972		108,023	

AJCC, American Joint Committee on Cancer; *CAJCC*, Clinical American Joint Committee on Cancer; *PAJCC*, Pathologic American Joint Committee on Cancer.
From Bland KI, Menck HR, Scott-Conner CE, et al. The National Cancer Database 10-year survey of breast carcinoma treatment at hospitals in the United States. *Cancer.* 1998; 83:1262-1273.

1995 in the same interval. These trends are most likely a result of increased use of high-quality mammography screening and patient education. Patient education and increased access to diagnostic clinics have aided early diagnosis and downstaging of this neoplasm.

Table 30.11 reflects the relative survival by combined AJCC stage and treatment from 1985 to 1990. Evident again is the decreasing use of modified radical mastectomy with or without radiotherapy in early-stage diseases (stage 0/I), with essentially no use of the Halsted procedure by US surgeons. Still the most commonly used procedure for stage II/III/IV disease is the modified radical mastectomy with or without radiotherapy.[25] Surgeons are increasingly unlikely to use subcutaneous mastectomy for other than stage 0 disease.[25] The report by Horiguchi and colleagues[26] confirms greater nodal retrieval and positivity in patients undergoing radical procedures than those treated with subcutaneous mastectomy. The local recurrence rate shows a threefold increase in the subcutaneous mastectomy cohort (3.8% vs. 1.3%). No differences were evident in the disease-free or overall survival rates between these two groups.

Figs. 30.8 and 30.9 depict trends of US surgeons, as reported by the NCDB, for choice of operation relative to AJCC stage of disease. A decreasing application of the modified radical or the Halsted procedure is evident for stage 0, I, and II diseases (see Fig. 30.8) with concurrent increased use of breast conservation for those stages (see Fig. 30.9). This 1985 to 1998 NCDB analysis depicts the rare application of the Halsted procedure for any stage disease (Fig. 30.10). This trend has been evident since 1985.

This trend in rate and magnitude of change in application of breast conservation from radical, modified-radical, and total mastectomy is also evident in Canada. The report by Gaudette and coworkers[27] exemplifies the surgeon's decision to decrease mastectomy rates from 62.2% to 37.9% per 100,000 patients between 1981 and 2000. Clearly, transition to less use of the Halsted and less radical (total) mastectomies followed publication of results of the *equivalency* of segmental mastectomy and radiation to the more ablative procedure. The variations in these trends by Canadian surgeons advising patients of survival equivalence of the procedures is evident in Table 30.12.

Trends in Selection of Mastectomy Therapies, 2000 to 2016

The more recent applications of ablative procedures to manage early breast carcinoma (stages 0, I, and II) have continued to

TABLE 30.11 — Relative Survival of Breast Carcinoma Patients by Combined AJCC Stage and Treatment, 1985 to 1990

Stage	Treatment Mastectomy	Radiation Therapy	Systemic Therapy	Entering Patients	0	1	2	3	4	5	6	7	8	9	10	SE
0	Partial, no axillary dissection	No	No	2027	100	100	99	99	99	99	98	98	98	98	98	3
0	Partial, no axillary dissection	Yes	No	638	100	100	100	100	100	100	100	99	99	99	99	6
0	Partial with axillary dissection	Yes/no	Yes/no	876	100	100	99	99	98	99	99	96	93	93	92	4
0	Subcutaneous/total	Yes/no	Yes/no	1086	100	100	100	100	99	99	99	96	94	90	90	4
0	Modified radical	No	No	3451	100	100	100	100	100	100	100	97	97	97	97	2
0	None	Yes/no	Yes/no	479	100	96	93	91	91	91	91	90	92	91	86	6
0	Other treatment			824	100	97	95	93	93	91	90	88	87	87	87	4
0	All treatment			9381	100	100	99	99	99	99	99	96	95	95	95	1
I	Partial, no axillary dissection	No	No	1684	100	97	95	93	90	87	81	75	73	71	66	5
I	Partial, no axillary dissection	Yes	No	1284	100	100	100	99	97	96	94	90	87	86	85	4
I	Partial, no axillary dissection	Yes	Yes	512	100	95	91	88	84	78	76	61	58	58	58	12
I	Partial with axillary dissection	No	No	1242	100	100	98	96	94	94	91	88	86	86	85	4
I	Partial with axillary dissection	Yes	No	5469	100	100	100	100	100	100	99	97	96	96	94	1
I	Partial with axillary dissection	Yes	Yes	2800	100	100	100	100	100	100	100	95	89	86	86	6
I	Modified radical	No	No	14,200	100	100	100	100	100	99	97	93	93	92	92	1
I	Modified radical	No	Yes	5062	100	100	100	99	98	97	95	91	89	87	84	3
I	Other treatment			4899	100	98	96	94	92	90	89	86	84	83	81	2
I	All treatment			37,152	100	100	99	99	98	97	95	92	90	89	88	1
II	Partial with axillary dissection	Yes	Yes	2911	100	100	97	95	92	88	85	81	78	75	72	3
II	Modified radical	No	No	9861	100	99	96	93	89	86	82	78	75	72	71	1
II	Modified radical	No	Yes	11,835	100	100	95	91	87	83	79	72	70	67	65	1
II	Modified radical	Yes	Yes	1780	100	98	91	84	77	71	68	62	58	54	51	3
II	Other treatment			7962	100	96	91	87	82	78	75	69	67	64	62	1
II	All treatment			34,349	100	99	94	91	86	83	79	73	70	68	66	1
III	Modified radical	No	No	1372	100	91	82	74	68	63	60	55	51	50	47	3
III	Modified radical	No	Yes	2702	100	96	83	72	64	58	52	46	45	41	38	2
III	Modified radical	Yes	Yes	1594	100	95	82	70	60	53	48	41	36	35	31	3
III	Other treatment			2844	100	85	70	60	50	44	40	35	32	29	28	2
III	All treatment			8512	100	92	79	68	60	54	50	44	41	38	36	1
IV	Partial, no axillary dissection	Yes/no	Yes/no	882	100	61	40	26	21	14	10	8	5	4	4	2
IV	Partial with axillary dissection	Yes/no	Yes/no	305	100	74	43	33	25	18	17	14	12	12	12	3
IV	Subcutaneous/total	Yes/no	Yes/no	382	100	63	43	31	21	15	12	12	9	8	6	3
IV	Modified radical	No	No	289	100	71	47	40	31	27	26	22	19	16	15	4
IV	Modified radical	No	Yes	681	100	79	54	41	29	22	17	13	12	11	11	2
IV	Modified radical	Yes	Yes	458	100	78	54	41	33	24	19	14	14	12	12	3
IV	No	No	No	352	100	32	21	14	10	9	9	7	7	7	7	2
IV	No	Yes	No	142	100	46	29	21	10	9	6	4	4	4	4	3
IV	No	No	Yes	800	100	56	37	22	14	9	7	4	4	4	4	1

Continued

TABLE 30.11	Relative Survival of Breast Carcinoma Patients by Combined AJCC Stage and Treatment, 1985 to 1990—cont'd															
		Radiation Therapy	Systemic Therapy	Entering Patients	YEARS SURVIVED											
Stage	Treatment Mastectomy				0	1	2	3	4	5	6	7	8	9	10	SE
IV	No	Yes	Yes	508	100	54	35	23	14	8	5	2	1	1	1	1
IV	Other treatment			629	100	76	38	29	20	16	12	10	9	7	6	2
IV	All treatment			5428	100	63	42	30	21	16	12	10	8	7	7	1

AJCC, American Joint Committee on Cancer; *SE*, standard error.

From Bland KI, Menck HR, Scott-Conner CE, et al. The National Cancer Database 10-year survey of breast carcinoma treatment at hospitals in the United States. *Cancer*. 1998;83:1262-1273.

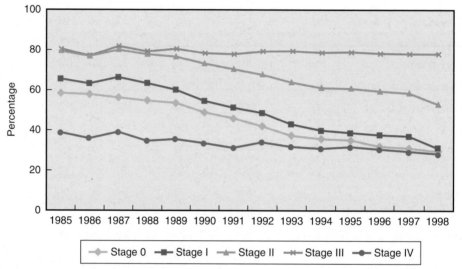

• **Fig. 30.8** Percentage of breast cancers receiving modified or radical mastectomy during initial course of therapy by American Joint Committee on Cancer stage of disease in cases diagnosed between 1985 and 1998, according to National Cancer Database.

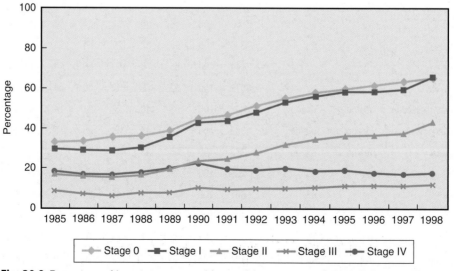

• **Fig. 30.9** Percentage of breast cancers receiving partial mastectomy during initial course of therapy by American Joint Committee on Cancer stage of disease in cases diagnosed between 1985 and 1998, according to National Cancer Database.

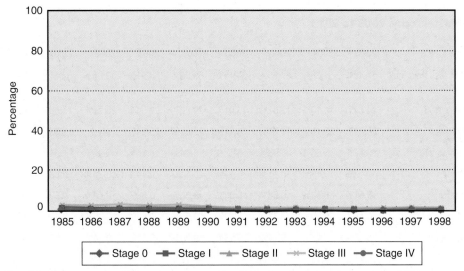

• **Fig. 30.10** Percentage of breast cancers receiving Halsted radical mastectomy during initial course of therapy by American Joint Committee on Cancer stage of disease in cases diagnosed between 1985 and 1998, according to National Cancer Database.

| TABLE 30.12 | Age-Standardized[a] In-Patient Hospital Separation Rates per 100,000 for Breast Cancer Surgery in Canada and Its Provinces, 1981–1984 to 1997–2000 |

	MASTECTOMY					BREAST-CONSERVING SURGERY				
Province	1981–84	1985–88	1989–92	1993–96	1997–2000	1981–84	1985–88	1989–92	1993–96	1997–2000
Canada	61	49.4	46	38.9	38.2	20.4	37.1	43.6	41.7	38.2
BC	69.1	59.7	58.6	47	44.6	12.9	29.1	32.6	38.2	40.1
AB	55.7	50.5	50.4	41.7	46.1	14.8	26.5	35.1	34.1	38.6
SK	70.1	55.7	58	48.9	59.1	10.3	29.1	44.7	37.2	31.9
MB	78.4	65.1	66.9	55.7	48.7	5.5	12.1	17.6	21.9	29.7
ON	61.9	49.6	46.1	37.3	35.1	24.8	44.3	49.3	44.1	34.8
QC	52.5	37.9	28.9	24.8	24.9	26.1	44.4	52.4	49.9	47.3
NB	65.4	58.8	64.3	63.2	53.4	8.3	15	24.7	31.6	36.3
NS	71.2	55.6	54.6	63.2	67.3	14.6	28.3	35.1	33.2	27.9
PE	38.5	71.4	71.2	69.3	75.4	22.2	19.7	27.7	24.5	30
NL	55	56	65	65.9	66.7	6.2	10.8	16.4	15.7	20.4

[a]Rates are age-standardized to the 1991 Canadian population.

AB, Alberta; BC, British Columbia; MB, Manitoba; NB, New Brunswick; NL, Newfoundland; NS, Nova Scotia; PE, Prince Edward Island; ON, Ontario; QC, Quebec; SK, Saskatchewan.

From Gaudette LA, Gao R-N, Spence A, et al. Declining use of mastectomy for invasive breast cancer in Canada, 1981–2000. *Can J Public Health.* 2004;95:336-340.

decline. This trend in reduction in total mastectomy follows the objectives of the American College of Surgeons (ACS), Society of Surgical Oncology, the American Cancer Society, the American Society of Breast Surgeons, and various surgical societies to better educate surgeons. More than 25 years of data note that breast conservation surgery is equivalent to total mastectomy in terms of disease-free and overall survival. Such trends are evident in the cancer statistics of the NCDB at the ACS (Table 30.13).[28] When evaluated cumulatively for stage and type of surgical procedure from 2003 to 2013, the Halsted radical mastectomy comprises 0.05% of total procedures, the majority of which are performed when patient presents with stage II or III disease (Table 30.14)

To date, the halstedian procedure is applied principally to advanced local disease (e.g., chest wall and skin fixation) that did not respond completely to neoadjuvant chemotherapy initiated for purposes of cytoreduction.

Of note, Fig. 30.12 (see later) defines an escalation in use of total (simple) mastectomy NOS (not otherwise specified), 2003 to 2013 from 14.9% to 27%. Increase for use of this procedure is likely a result of increasing application of the total mastectomy with immediate reconstruction for advanced or multicentric disease.

The NCDB of the Commission on Cancer, ACS, documented the diminishing application of both the modified and radical

TABLE 30.13 Trends in Mastectomy, 2003 to 2013[a]	2003	2004	2005	2006	2007	2008	2009	2010	2011	2012	2013
Partial mastectomy, NOS; less than total mastectomy, NOS	57.40%	57.36%	57.55%	57.15%	55.20%	53.91%	53.09%	52.71%	53.33%	52.51%	52.80%
Total (simple) mastectomy, NOS	14.87%	16.13%	17.52%	19.01%	20.90%	22.34%	24.29%	25.56%	26.13%	27.04%	27.38%
Modified radical mastectomy	20.83%	19.18%	17.31%	16.21%	15.87%	15.24%	14%	12.82%	11.28%	10.40%	9.45%
None; no surgery of primary site	5.47%	5.88%	5.98%	6%	6.44%	6.95%	7.02%	7.31%	7.35%	7.79%	7.95%
Subcutaneous mastectomy	0.12%	0.11%	0.11%	0.11%	0.11%	0.14%	0.20%	0.38%	0.55%	0.87%	1.23%
Radical mastectomy, NOS[b]	**0.51%**	**0.53%**	**0.58%**	**0.58%**	**0.55%**	**0.58%**	**0.60%**	**0.50%**	**0.42%**	**0.39%**	**0.37%**
Mastectomy, NOS	0.48%	0.52%	0.57%	0.58%	0.55%	0.55%	0.50%	0.43%	0.61%	0.66%	0.34%
Unknown if surgery performed	0.06%	0.07%	0.14%	0.16%	0.20%	0.12%	0.14%	0.14%	0.15%	0.19%	0.33%
Surgery, NOS	0.21%	0.18%	0.19%	0.17%	0.13%	0.14%	0.14%	0.13%	0.15%	0.11%	0.12%
Local tumor destruction, NOS	0.04%	0.02%	0.02%	0.02%	0.01%	0.01%	0.01%	0.01%	0.01%	0.01%	0.01%
Extended radical mastectomy	0.02%	0.02%	0.03%	0.03%	0.03%	0.03%	0.02%	0.02%	0.02%	0.02%	0.01%

[a]n = 1552 hospitals.
[b]This row is bold because it is the topic of this chapter.
NOS, Not otherwise specified.
From National Cancer Database Commission on Cancer. Trends in Mastectomy 2003 to 2013. *Annual National Cancer Database NCDB Benchmark Report,* February 26, 2016.

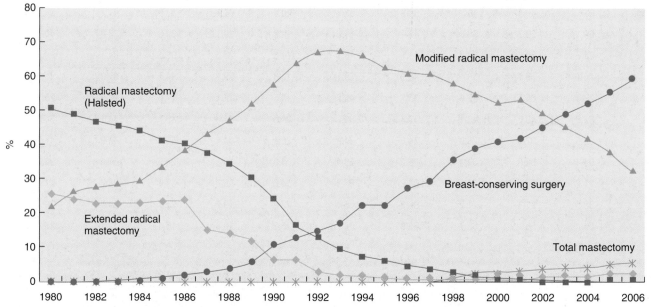

• **Fig. 30.11** Changing trends in surgical procedures for breast cancer in Japan. (From Sonoo H, Noguchi S. Academic Committee of the Japanese Breast Cancer Society. Results of questionnaires concerning breast cancer surgery in Japan 2004-2006. *Breast Cancer.* 2008;15:3-4.)

mastectomies for the surgical therapy of breast carcinoma. This conversion to breast conservation is evident in other countries in North America and Western Europe as well as in Japan.[29] Fig. 30.11 depicts results of the Japanese Breast Cancer Society (JBCS) survey of 1980 to 2006. Japanese surgeons, like their Western colleagues, have made a major alteration of the breast therapy since 1975 from the Halsted radical procedure to the more liberal use of modified radical mastectomy and breast-conserving surgery.

The 2008 publication by Sonoo and Noguchi[30] further reflects the increasing use of breast conservation approaches since 1986; this conservation procedure currently exceeds the use of the modified radical procedure, an event that occurred in Japanese women (see Fig. 30.11) in 2003. Similarly, sentinel lymph node biopsy has rapidly accelerated in use since its introduction in 1996; in 2003 21.5% of Japanese patients with breast cancer underwent sentinel lymph node biopsy.[30,31]

TABLE 30.14 First-Course Surgery by Stage of Breast Cancer Diagnosed, 2003–2013, All Diagnosis Types, All Types of Hospitals in All States[a]

First-Course Surgery		STAGE 0	I	II	III	IV	NA	UNK	TOTALS N	%
1	None; no surgery of primary site	15,274	17,928	20,300	13,897	54,781	163	27,687	150,030	6.82%
		10.20%	11.90%	13.50%	9.30%	36.50%	0.10%	18.50%	100%	
2	Local tumor destruction, NOS	147	100	51	20	22	1	25	366	0.02%
		40.20%	27.30%	13.90%	5.50%	6%	0.30%	6.80%	100%	
3	Partial mastectomy, NOS; less than total mastectomy, NOS	287,033	576,337	252,861	39,667	8557	540	37,079	1,202,074	54.62%
		23.90%	47.90%	21%	3.30%	0.70%	.	3.10%	100%	
4	Subcutaneous mastectomy	2383	3383	2092	421	33	16	166	8494	0.39%
		28.10%	39.80%	24.60%	5%	0.40%	0.20%	2%	100%	
5	Total (simple) mastectomy, NOS	111,690	182,891	136,486	37,984	6073	943	15,832	491,899	22.35%
		22.70%	37.20%	27.70%	7.70%	1.20%	0.20%	3.20%	100%	
6	Modified radical mastectomy	17,049	65,388	117,813	95,549	10,575	299	11,205	317,878	14.44%
		5.40%	20.60%	37.10%	30.10%	3.30%	0.10%	3.50%	100%	
7[b]	**Radical mastectomy, NOS**	**902**	**2307**	**3652**	**3268**	**476**	**54**	**452**	**11,111**	**0.5%**
		8.10%	20.80%	32.90%	29.40%	4.30%	0.50%	4.10%	100%	
8	Extended radical mastectomy	59	112	113	117	32	6	18	457	0.02%
		12.90%	24.50%	24.70%	25.60%	7%	1.30%	3.90%	100%	
9	Mastectomy, NOS	1945	3635	3360	1362	288	24	947	11,561	0.53%
		16.80%	31.40%	29.10%	11.80%	2.50%	0.20%	8.20%	100%	
10	Surgery, NOS	909	720	542	258	207	18	633	3287	0.15%
		27.70%	21.90%	16.50%	7.80%	6.30%	0.50%	19.30%	100%	
11	Unknown if surgery performed	678	652	404	122	284	3	1349	3492	0.16%
		19.40%	18.70%	11.60%	3.50%	8.10%	0.10%	38.60%	100%	
	Total	438,069	853,453	537,674	192,665	81,328	2067	95,393	2,200,649	100%
		19.9%	38.8%	24.4%	8.8%	3.7%	0.1%	4.3%	100%	

[a]n = 1552 hospitals.
[b]This row is bold because it is the topic of this chapter.
NOS, Not otherwise specified.
From National Cancer Database Commission on Cancer. Trends in Mastectomy 2003 to 2013. *Annual National Cancer Database NCDB Benchmark Report,* February 26, 2016.

Contemporary NCDB Bench Reports suggest that in US hospitals there is a *reduction* in the frequency of Halsted mastectomy in the 10-year interval from 0.51% (2003) to 0.37 (2013). The most common overall procedure, partial (segmental) mastectomy, had reduction in frequency from 57.4% (2003) to 52.8% (2013) with simultaneous increase in total (simple) mastectomy, 14.87% (2003) to 27.38% (2013) (see Table 30.13). This observation is likely a result of incorporation of skin-sparing mastectomies with or without myocutaneous flap, or implant and reconstruction. Moreover, the operative choices of patients with breast cancer have trended to procedural selection based on genetic and risk counseling that favors total (simple) mastectomy with or without sentinel node biopsy in these populations. Of great interest is that there has also been a major reduction in the modified

radical mastectomy as first-course operative choice by certified surgeons of the ACS based on NCDB Benchmark Reports. The frequency diminished 11.38% in this 10-year interval (Fig. 30.12)

The cumulative first-course surgery report for all breast cancer diagnoses from 2003 through 2013 (Table 30.15), which includes more than 1500 hospitals in all 50 states and 2.20 million procedures, notes the following frequencies: radical mastectomy 0.5%, partial mastectomy 54.6%, modified radical mastectomy 14.4%, nonsurgical treatment of the primary site 6.8%, and total (simple) mastectomy NOS 22.3%. The reduction in choice of partial mastectomy by breast cancer patients and choice of total breast removal reflects the options given as first-course surgery with the use of reconstructive procedures.[29]

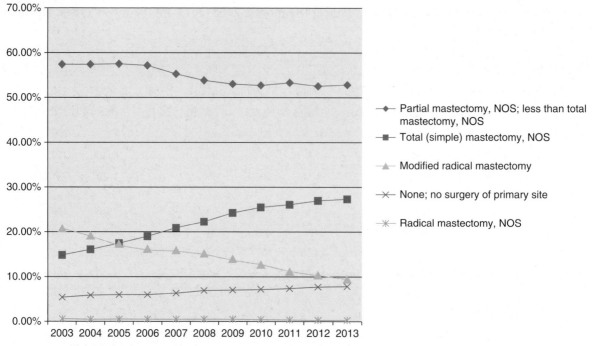

• **Fig. 30.12** Annual National Cancer Database (NCDB) Benchmark Reports showing first-course surgery, all diagnoses, all hospitals, all states (n = 1552 hospitals). Most frequently used surgeries compared with radical mastectomy. *NOS*, Not otherwise specified. (NCDB Commission on Cancer, February 26, 2016.)

TABLE 30.15 First-Course Surgery of Breast Cancer Diagnosed, 2003 to 2013, All Diagnosis Types, All Hospital Types in All States

	First-Course Surgery	n	%
1	None; no surgery of primary site	150,030	6.82
2	Local tumor destruction, NOS	366	0.02
3	Partial mastectomy, NOS; less than total mastectomy, NOS	1,202,074	54.62
4	Subcutaneous mastectomy	8494	0.39
5	Total (simple) mastectomy, NOS	491,899	22.35
6	Modified radical mastectomy	317,878	14.44
7	Radical mastectomy, NOS	11,111	0.5
8	Extended radical mastectomy	457	0.02
9	Mastectomy, NOS	11,561	0.53
10	Surgery, NOS	3287	0.15
11	Unknown if surgery performed	3492	0.16

NOS, Not otherwise specified.
From National Cancer Database Commission on Cancer. Trends in Mastectomy 2003 to 2013. *Annual National Cancer Database NCDB Benchmark Report*, February 26, 2016.

Indications for Use of the Halsted Radical Mastectomy

Modern radiobiology and chemotherapy directed to receptor-specific targeting allows cytoreduction of the primary breast neoplasm, and these less radical (modified radical and partial) mastectomies that are increasingly used in clinics throughout the world. Radical mastectomy is only occasionally necessary to achieve locoregional control of disease in the breast, axilla, and chest wall (<1%). Breast cancer mortality rates before and after the introduction of the Halsted mastectomy attest to the effectiveness of this treatment as the most definitive step in the management of breast cancer.[32] Until the advent of adjuvant chemotherapy with or without monoclonal/receptor specific therapy with modern irradiation, little improvement in survival data for patients with breast cancer was documented. A growing body of data confirms that the extent of the procedure can be lessened while maintaining survival rates equivalent to those of the radical approach for the treatment of breast cancer.[12,13,16–18,33–38]

Retrospective data from the Italian study by Scorpiglione and colleagues[39] in 1995 reaffirms the importance of patient education to allow participation in therapeutic options; efforts to enhance awareness of alternative therapies appropriate for tumor stage should reduce unnecessary radical procedures.[40] The enlightening prospective report by Grilli and associates[41] suggests that the Halsted radical mastectomy was more likely to be inappropriately performed on patients who were less educated and in institutions with low patient volume. Moreover, the 25-year prospective study by Staunton and coworkers[42] at St. Bartholomew's Hospital in London further reaffirms the value of the Patey mastectomy with preservation of the pectoralis major muscle for patients with T_1 and T_2 tumors. The equivalent locoregional control rates of the Patey mastectomy (see Chapter 31) and the Halsted mastectomy account for the diminishing application of the radical procedure internationally.

The major consideration for operations less extensive than the classic Halsted mastectomy is based on tissue preservation to enhance the cosmetic and functional results. Box 30.1 presents the relative indications for use of the Halsted radical mastectomy with advanced locoregional disease.

- Advanced locoregional disease with fixation to pectoralis major muscle (T_2, T_3, T_{4a-c}; stages IIIA, IIIB, IIIC), when refractory to induction chemotherapy and irradiation
- Advanced locoregional disease with skin ulceration (T_{4b}; stage IIIB) unresponsive to radiochemotherapy
- Recurrent advanced, locoregional disease (T_2, T_3, T_4) after partial (segmental) mastectomy with tumor fixation to pectoralis major muscle ("salvage" mastectomy)
- For completion of the radical procedure with locoregional recurrence after modified/segmental mastectomy when tumor invades chest wall and is refractory to cytoinduction chemotherapy
- High-lying advanced peripheral lesions near clavicle/sternum with tumor fixation to muscle (stages IIA, IIB; stages IIIA, IIIB)

[a]All presentations of advanced locoregional disease should receive induction cytotoxic drug therapy, radiotherapy, or both before radical mastectomy. Staging to rule out systemic disease should precede induction therapy.

Of note, major transitions from the halstedian era of breast cancer treatment have resulted from the equivalent locoregional control that is evident with contemporary alternative breast conservation options.[43] However, the increasing application of breast conservation surgery has more recently defined an indication for the Halsted procedure. With local advanced-regional recurrence, after conservation approaches, in the presence or absence of regional disease, the radical mastectomy may be necessary when disease invades the pectoralis major muscle. This aggressive "salvage mastectomy" is necessary for large (bulky) recurrences, especially for posterior lesions that recur with fascial or muscle fixation.

The important study by Korzeniowski and colleagues[44] from the Sklodowska-Curie Institute in Poland has received little recognition. These investigators evaluated 10 years of data for survival and recurrence rates in 1068 patients with breast cancer treated with Halsted radical mastectomy between 1952 and 1980. Univariate and multivariate analyses confirmed the prognostic significance of tumor size, histologic type and grade (Bloom classification), and involvement of axillary nodes. In this large analysis, young age was a significant risk parameter for locoregional disease-free survival. For stage I, T_1 tumors, the prognosis was excellent regardless of histologic grade (80%–90% 10-year disease-free survival); for stage I, T_2 tumors, survival was statistically dependent on histologic grade and type. For stages II and III (node-positive) patients, evidence of increasing numbers of positive nodes and higher histologic grade represented an independent adverse effect on survival and locoregional control. Hathaway and associates[45] and Osborne and Simmons[46] determined that radical surgical therapy and reconstruction are indicated in locally advanced and locally recurrent disease; the procedure was completed with low morbidity and mortality rates and provided excellent local control of disease. Radical surgical procedures may be the only available technique for locoregional control of locally advanced (fixed, ulcerated) disease, especially for patients who have previously received total breast irradiation and multidrug cytotoxic therapy.[47–49]

No indications exist for the extended radical mastectomy with internal mammary node dissection in the contemporary practice of breast surgery. Proponents of the extended procedure suggested

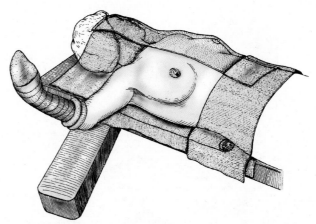

• **Fig. 30.13** Typical position for draping patient for operations of cancer of the right breast. The ipsilateral hemithorax is positioned at the margin of the operative table with a sheet roll that provides slight elevation to the ipsilateral shoulder and hemithorax. This position potentially prevents subluxation and abduction of the shoulder with stretch of the brachial plexus. Draping of the periphery of the breast is inclusive of the supraclavicular fossa and the entire shoulder to allow adequate mobility for adduction of the shoulder and arm across the chest wall. The elbow should be easily flexed and extended without undue tension.

that it has an advantage over the Halsted radical approach, especially for medial quadrant lesions.[50–53]

With the introduction of sentinel node staging in early and advanced disease (see Chapters 41 and 42), the role of axillary node dissection after tumor downstaging with neoadjuvant chemotherapy for advanced disease has been questioned. The analysis by Kuerer and coworkers[54] at the University of Texas MD Anderson Cancer Center confirmed the incomplete accuracy of clinical assessment of the axilla by physical examination combined with ultrasound assessment. Patients being considered for modified radical or Halsted mastectomy with positive findings on preoperative physical or ultrasound examination should receive axillary dissection to enhance locoregional disease control.

Technique of Radical Mastectomy

After induction of general anesthesia, the patient is positioned supine on the operating table with a sheet roll that allows slight elevation of the ipsilateral shoulder and hemithorax. Ideally, the ipsilateral hemithorax should be positioned at the margin of the operating table. The surgeon must be aware of the potential for subsequent subluxation and abduction of the shoulder on the arm board to prevent stretch of the brachial plexus with potential injury by motor denervation of the shoulder and arm. This complication is best avoided by padding the arm board to allow elevation of the forearm and hand in a relaxed position (Fig. 30.13). The operator should confirm that the ipsilateral arm and shoulder have free mobility for adduction across the chest wall; the elbow should be easily flexed and extended without tension.

The involved breast with the ipsilateral neck and hemithorax is "prepped" to the table margin inclusive of the shoulder, axilla, arm, and hand. Towels may be stapled or secured with towel clips to the skin with draping of the shoulder, lower neck, sternum, and upper rectus abdominis musculature within the planned operative field (see Fig. 30.13). We prefer to isolate the hand and forearm with an occlusive Stockinette (DeRoyal Industries, Powell, TN) cotton dressing and secure them with

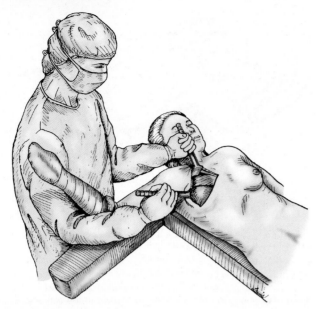

• **Fig. 30.14** Position of the first assistant for right radical mastectomy. The surgical assistant, positioned cephalad to the armboard and shoulder, is able to provide traction, control, and protection of the arm and shoulder. Undue traction of chest wall musculature with potential damage to the brachial plexus can be avoided by ensuring free mobility of the shoulder and elbow that are being controlled by the first assistant.

a Kerlix or Kling (Johnson and Johnson, New Brunswick, NJ) cotton roll that is carefully tied below the elbow. Thereafter sterile sheets isolate the anesthesiologist from the operating site. We prefer to position the first assistant over the shoulder (cephalad to the arm board) on the ipsilateral side of the procedure (Fig. 30.14) so that the muscular retraction with extension and abduction of the arm and shoulder that is necessary for dissection of the axilla can be accomplished without undue stretch on the brachial plexus.

The operation is initiated with the ipsilateral arm in a relaxed, extended position on the padded arm board. Incisions are made according to the guidelines discussed in this chapter and in Chapters 29 and 31. Skin incisions are made with a cold scalpel. Tissue dissection and flap elevation may be completed with electrocautery, cold scalpel, or the neodymium:yttrium aluminum garnet (Nd:YAG) laser scalpel.[55]

Indications for consideration of the Halsted radical mastectomy include larger breast lesions (T_2, T_3, T_4) that have gross involvement (fixation) of the skin and/or the pectoralis major (Fig. 30.15, *inset*) after pretreatment with neoadjuvant chemotherapy. Additional indications that are considered refractory to induction therapy and irradiation include the peripheral (highlying) lesions near the clavicle in patients who are otherwise not candidates for radiation therapy. The skin flaps are designed to encompass wider margins than those for modified radical techniques; this is particularly necessary with incomplete (partial)

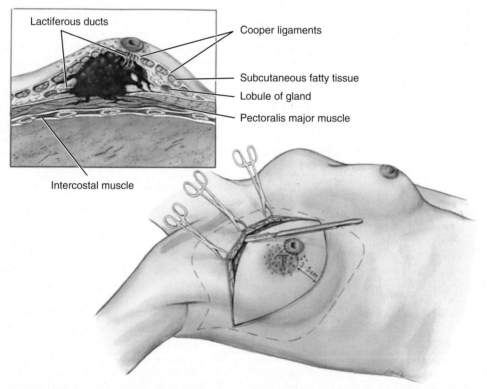

Lactiferous ducts

Cooper ligaments

Subcutaneous fatty tissue

Lobule of gland

Pectoralis major muscle

Intercostal muscle

• **Fig. 30.15** *Inset*, Large breast lesions (T_2, T_3, T_4) may present with gross fixation to the skin and/or pectoralis major musculature. The radical mastectomy is designed to encompass wider skin flaps than the modified technique. The margins designed and developed should encompass normal skin and breast parenchyma 3 to 5 cm from the periphery of the tumor. This wider margin ensures tumor clearance and facilitates skin closure without redundancy of tissue flaps. The design of elevated flaps is inclusive of skin margins at the periphery of the breast on the chest wall. The broken line indicates the limits of the dissection and includes the following: superior, the inferior border of the clavicle at the subclavius muscle; lateral, the anterior margin of the latissimus dorsi muscle; medial, midline of the sternum; and inferior, the inframammary fold with extension of dissection to the cephalic extension of the aponeurosis of the rectus abdominis tendon.

clinicopathologic responses to neoadjuvant therapy. To obtain adequate surgical margins that encompass the primary neoplasm and involved skin, the surgeon may need to elevate skin flaps at the periphery of the breast (see Fig. 30.15). This procedure necessitates an en bloc resection of the breast and the skin overlying the tumor, as well as the pectoralis major and minor muscles, with a complete axillary dissection of level I to III nodes. The limits of the dissection are delineated:

superiorly by the inferior border of the clavicle at the subclavius muscle;
laterally by the anterior margin of the latissimus dorsi muscle;
medially at the midline of the sternum; and
inferiorly at the inframammary fold with extension to the aponeurosis of the rectus abdominis tendon, approximately 2 cm inferior to the caudal extent of the breast.

As described previously, cutaneous flaps should be elevated with a thickness of 7 to 9 mm; however, flap thickness invariably depends on the patient's habitus and lean body mass. The interface for elevation of this flap is the plane deep to the cutaneous vasculature, which can be accentuated with tension on the flaps by towel clips placed in the margins of the incision or by retraction hooks. This technique of retraction is essential to allow exposure of the subcutaneous component of the flap because it overlies the breast parenchyma. Flap elevation may be accomplished with electrocautery or cold scalpel dissection.

Exposure of the superolateral aspect of the wound allows identification of the humeral insertion of the pectoralis major muscle and then continuation of the dissection in a central and superomedial direction with muscular elevation to allow exposure of the pectoralis minor tendinous insertion. The insertion of the pectoralis major on the humerus is transected and rotated medially. The surgeon must be aware of the anatomic position of the cephalic vein and its relationship to the deltopectoral triangle. The dissection begins medially with resection of the pectoralis major at its cranial clavicular attachments. This maneuver allows the surgeon direct access to the axilla; thereafter, the tendinous portion of the pectoralis minor muscle is divided at its insertion on the coracoid process of the scapula (Fig. 30.16). This muscle is likewise elevated from the axilla with careful ligature and division of perforating musculature branches from the thoracoacromial artery and vein. The medial (anterior thoracic) pectoral nerve, which commonly penetrates the pectoralis minor before innervation of the pectoralis major, is ligated and divided at its origin from the medial cord of the brachial plexus. As the surgeon continues the medial resection of the pectoralis major, the lateral (anterior thoracic) pectoral nerve (which originates from the lateral cord and runs in the medial neurovascular bundle) should be identified, ligated, and divided. We prefer to continue the dissection in the superomedial-most aspect of the elevated flap so that the pectoralis major is divided from its medial origin at the costosternal junction of ribs 2, 3, 4, 5, and 6 (Fig. 30.17). The resection of the pectoralis musculature invariably allows the surgeon to encounter multiple perforator vessels (lateral thoracic and anterior intercostal arteries) at its periphery that are end arteries to the pectoralis major and minor. Perforator branches from the intercostal muscles that take origin from the intercostal arteries and veins are also encountered.

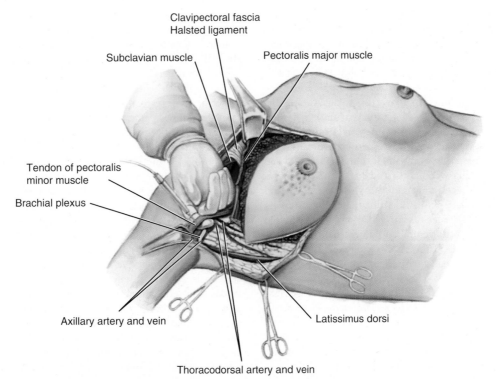

Clavipectoral fascia
Halsted ligament
Subclavian muscle
Pectoralis major muscle
Tendon of pectoralis minor muscle
Brachial plexus
Axillary artery and vein
Latissimus dorsi
Thoracodorsal artery and vein

• **Fig. 30.16** Exposure of the superolateral aspect of the mastectomy wound following division of the humeral insertion of the pectoralis major muscle. The insertion of the pectoralis minor on the coracoid process of the scapula is transected and rotated medially with en bloc dissection of Rotter interpectoral nodes. Technically, the dissection commences on the anterior and ventral aspects of the axillary vein to incorporate levels I to III nodes. Division of the pectoralis major and minor tendons allows the surgeon direct access to the floor of the axilla.

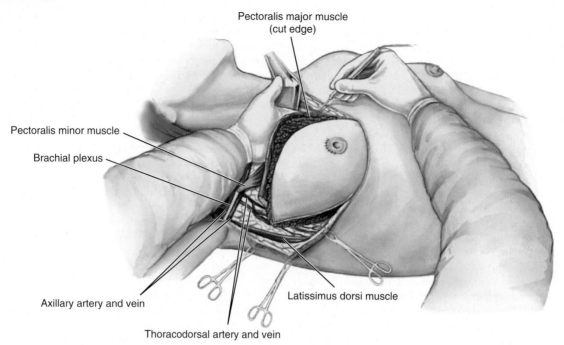

Pectoralis major muscle
(cut edge)

Pectoralis minor muscle

Brachial plexus

Axillary artery and vein

Latissimus dorsi muscle

Thoracodorsal artery and vein

• **Fig. 30.17** Superomedial dissection of the elevated pectoralis minor and pectoralis major muscles en bloc with the breast. The breast parenchyma remains intact with the pectoralis major fascia. Illustrated is the medial extent of the dissection along the costoclavicular margin with division of insertion of the pectoralis major on ribs 2 through 6 and the pectoralis minor on ribs 2 through 5. Multiple perforator branches from the intercostal muscles are encountered at the origin of the intercostal arteries and veins. After superomedial and inferomedial dissection, the axillary contents are fully exposed to allow completion of the Patey axillary dissection of levels I to III nodes.

All divided tributaries should be individually clamped, ligated, and tied with nonabsorbable 2-0 or 3-0 suture. With division of the pectoral muscles and inferomedial traction of the specimen, the axillary contents are fully exposed, and origin of the pectoralis minor on ribs 2 through 5 can be visualized and divided at this level. With this maneuver, the Rotter interpectoral nodes are swept en bloc into the specimen to allow full visualization of the axillary vein to the level of Halsted (costoclavicular) ligament, which is recognized as condensation of the clavipectoral fascia. Level III (apical, subclavicular) nodes can be dissected at this level.

Surgeons typically prefer to work lateral to medial to allow en bloc dissection of the axillary contents (see Chapter 41 for figures that illustrate axillary dissection techniques). The most lateral and ventral aspect of the axillary vein is identified, and the investing deep layer of superficial fascia of the axillary space is incised sharply with the scalpel on its ventral and anterior surface of the vein, with dissection and exposure of all venous tributaries. It is inadvisable to dissect the axilla with electrocautery for fear of thermal damage to the axillary vein and electrostimulation of the cephalad-placed brachial plexus or its motor branches. Because the *medial and lateral (anterior thoracic) pectoral nerves* have previously been sacrificed with elevation of the pectoralis major and minor muscles, the entire extent of dissection along the anterior axillary vein allows ligation and division of venous tributaries coursing inferiorly and anteriorly without fear of neural injury.

All loose areolar tissues at the juncture of the axillary vein with the anterior margin of the latissimus dorsi are swept inferomedially to be inclusive of the lateral (axillary) nodal group (level I). Care is taken to preserve the *thoracodorsal artery and vein,* and the surgeon should be aware of the origin of the *thoracodorsal nerve,* which invariably courses medially to these vascular structures.

This nerve originates from the posterior cord and may run a variable course in the central axillary space upon the teres major as it courses inferolaterally to innervate the latissimus dorsi muscle. As dissection in the axilla commences, the major branch of the *intercostobrachial* nerve, which transverses the axillary spaces at right angles to the latissimus medial to lateral, is identified. This nerve, which is sensory to the medial arm and axilla with fibers from lateral cutaneous branches of the second and third intercostal nerves, is sacrificed without prolonged morbidity.

Typically, the lateral *(axillary) nodal group* level I, is swept anteriorly or posteriorly around the thoracodorsal neurovascular bundle to be incorporated en bloc with the *subscapular group of nodes (level I),* which are medially placed between the thoracodorsal nerve and the lateral chest wall. With dissection of these two nodal groups and the investing areolar tissues, the posterior boundary of the axillary space with exposure of the teres major muscle is evident. Medial dissection with clearing of the ventral surface of the axillary vein allows direct visualization of the subscapularis muscle. Inferior dissection of the external mammary nodes of level I is deferred. Preferably, dissections of the *central nodal group (level II)* and the *apical or subclavicular (level III) nodes* are completed before removal of the external mammary level. We favor this technique with clearing of the superomedial areolar and nodal contents to the costoclavicular (Halsted) ligament. Thereafter the level III group can be labeled with a metallic marker or suture to provide the pathologist precise identification of this nodal group, which may have therapeutic and prognostic value. These two nodal groups are subsequently retracted inferiorly with the partially dissected components of level I groups. Nodal dissection begins with en bloc removal of the external mammary group that is medial and contiguous with the breast. The operator is reminded to dissect from the cephalad to caudad direction parallel with early identification of the *thoracodorsal neurovascular bundle*. This maneuver is important in dissection to prevent neural injury and allows direct access to venous tributaries posterior to the axillary vein. The surgeon then encounters the chest wall, and dissection is continued in a cephalocaudal direction to allow rapid identification of the *long thoracic nerve (respiratory nerve of Bell)* within the investing fascia of the serratus anterior that provides motor innervation to this muscle. After incision of the serratus fascia, this nerve is dissected throughout its course in the medial axillary space from its superiormost origin near the chest wall and brachial plexus to the innervation of the serratus anterior.

On occasion, extranodal extension of metastatic disease with nodal involvement of the external mammary, subscapular, or lateral (axillary) nodal groups of level I initiates tumor fixation and invasion of the thoracodorsal neurovascular bundle. When such pathology is encountered, the surgeon should sacrifice this neurovascular structure at the ventral surface of the axillary vein. Artery and vein should be ligated separately with nonabsorbable 2-0 sutures to avoid subsequent hematoma formation. Relatively little disability is evident with denervation of the latissimus dorsi muscle; however, with sacrifice of the thoracodorsal neurovascular structures, myocutaneous flaps that use the latissimus dorsi must be excluded for reconstruction purposes. Every attempt should be made to preserve the long thoracic nerve for fear of permanent disability with the "winged scapula" and shoulder apraxia that follow denervation of the serratus anterior.

Thereafter the axillary contents anterior and medial to the long thoracic nerve are swept inferomedially with the specimen; the surgeon should ensure that division of the inferiormost boundaries of the axillary contents is deferred until preserved innervations of the long thoracic and thoracodorsal nerves are

visualized. Any point of origin of the pectoralis major muscle from the second through the sixth rib left intact with the medial dissection is divided such that en bloc resection of the pectoralis major is accomplished over the retromammary bursa. The surgeon continues the dissection in this avascular plane to sweep the breast and axillary contents toward the aponeurosis of the rectus abdominis tendon to complete extirpation of the specimen as an en bloc procedure (Fig. 30.18).

The surgeon, assistants, and scrub nurse should reglove (and optionally regown). Clean instruments for flap closure are preferred to avoid the potential for wound implantation of tumor. The wound is then copiously irrigated with saline to evacuate residual tissue and clots. Points of bleeding from intercostal perforators are identified, clamped, and ligated to diminish hematoma and seroma accumulation. Closed-suction catheters (18–20 French) are placed through separate stab-type incisions that enter the inferior margin of the flap at approximately the anterior axillary line (see Fig. 30.18, inset). These Silastic catheters are positioned with the lateral catheter in the axillary space just medial to or on the surface of the latissimus dorsi to provide drainage of the axilla. The second, longer catheter is placed through the anteriormost skin incision superomedially to evacuate serum and blood of the large surface area dissected from the chest wall. The drains are secured at skin level with 3-0 nylon sutures. Suction catheters should not be secured to the chest wall with sutures because of the potential for muscle injury and hemorrhage with removal.

The surgeon should carefully inspect tissues for devascularization that results from the trauma of dissection or tangential incisions, which contribute to subsequent skin necrosis and wound dehiscence. We prefer closure with interrupted 2-0 absorbable synthetic sutures placed in the subcutaneous tissues that purchase the cutis reticularis of the skin without tension. The skin may

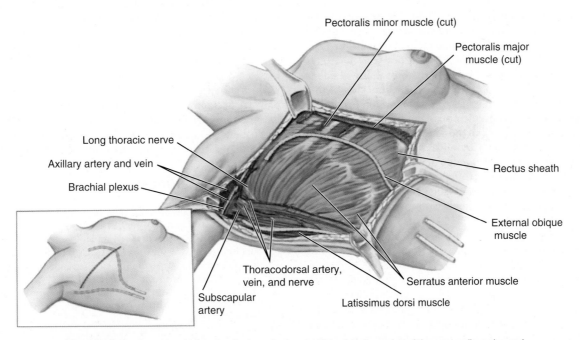

• **Fig. 30.18** The complete Halsted radical mastectomy with residual margins of the pectoralis major and minor muscles. Ideally, preservation of the long thoracic nerve ensures innervation of the serratus anterior. Innervation of the latissimus dorsi muscle is ensured with preservation of the thoracodorsal nerve that accompanies the neurovascular bundle of the posterior axillary space. *Inset,* Position of closed-suction catheters (18–20 French) placed through separate stab wounds that enter the inferior margin of the flap at approximately the anterior axillary lines.

be closed optionally with subcuticular 4-0 synthetic absorbable sutures or stainless steel staples. Steri-Strips are applied across (vertical to) the incision when subcuticular sutures are used in the closure. After irrigation, the closed-suction catheters are connected and maintained on continuous low to moderate suction with large reservoir vacuum bottles. Closure of dead space by suturing of skin flaps to underlying muscle combined with early removal of closed suction drains has been reported by O'Dwyer and colleagues[56] to diminish the incidence of seroma formation. Light, bulky dressings are applied to the entire area of dissection and are taped securely in place, although some surgeons prefer compression dressings over flaps inclusive of the margins of dissection. This practice may initiate central damage to the flap and potential skin necrosis if undue pressure is applied with taping. The dressing should remain intact until the third or fourth postoperative day. Typically wound catheters may be removed when drainage becomes predominantly serous and has decreased to a maximum of 20 to 25 mL during a 24-hour interval. Shoulder exercises are initiated on the day after removal of the drainage catheters.

With development of protracted serosanguineous or serous drainage, the catheters may be shortened and the portable suction device may be secured in the most comfortable position for ambulation. This practice requires the patient to pay strict attention to hygienic care of the catheters and the sites of skin entry and necessitates frequent dressing changes. In addition, the patient should be instructed to temporarily limit the range of motion of the shoulder and arm to augment flap adherence to the chest wall. The physician should periodically inspect the volume and composition of fluid emanating from the catheter and should be aware of the potential for retrograde infection of the axillary space. Interval seroma aspiration may be required. Wound care and complications after mastectomy are comprehensively reviewed in Chapter 34.

Often the defect created with the Halsted mastectomy is too great to allow primary wound closure. The defect may be grafted with split-thickness skin (0.018–0.020 inch) obtained with a dermatome from the anterolateral thigh or buttock (Fig. 30.19). To immobilize the skin graft and enhance the probability of adherence ("graft-take") to the chest wall, the partial-thickness skin is stented with bolsters (see Fig. 30.19) or compression foam mesh that is stapled in position. Catheters are not necessary when perforated skin grafts are applied to the defect. The stents placed over the split-thickness skin grafts are not removed until the fifth or sixth postoperative day, unless undue drainage (serum, blood, or suppuration) from beneath the grafts is evident. This practice increases the probability of graft adherence, which is further enhanced with postoperative shoulder immobilization for large defects.

The more recent application of *temporary* biological dressings or wound vacuum with negative-pressure wound therapy (Vacuum Assisted Closure [KCI, San Antonio, TX]) is a better alternative than skin grafts, especially when concern of pathologic margin positivity of the chest wall require postresection irradiation.

Split thickness grafts have a high failure rate and a quite poor cosmetic result with irradiation postoperatively. The option below of myocutaneous-flaps for reconstruction adds superior coverage to the defect recreated with the Halsted mastectomy.

With biological dressings or Wound VAC suction, which are used more frequently than split thickness skin grafts, patients will be offered *immediate breast reconstruction* with the Halsted mastectomy. This alternative for cosmetic/functional enhancement of

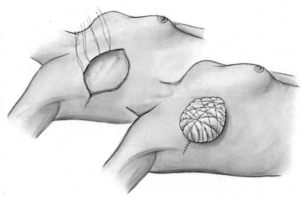

• **Fig. 30.19** *Top,* Large defect that is expectant with creation of large skin flaps inclusive of the periphery of the breast for T_3 and T_4 lesions with fixation to the pectoralis major. Such large defects must be grafted with split-thickness skin (0.018–0.020 inch) that is preferably obtained through a dermatome from skin of the anterior/lateral thigh or buttock. An additional option for closure is the myocutaneous latissimus dorsi flap. *Bottom,* The partial-thickness skin graft held in position with a compression stent created with cotton gauze mesh. These large skin defects do not require catheter drainage. Alternatively, compression foam mesh as the stent may be applied over the split-thickness skin graft. Foam mesh may be stapled in place at the margin of the skin defect.

the patient is being applied more routinely internationally.[57–59] When adverse biological factors are present, the surgeon may defer reconstruction with the temporary coverage just described. However, the Wales prospective trial, conducted by Patel and colleagues[60] over 10 years, suggests that immediate reconstruction is widely applicable and technically feasible without long-term effects on the development of local recurrence or metastatic disease.

The NCDB has also studied factors influencing a patient's decision to submit to breast reconstruction after mastectomy. Morrow and associates[61] considered that reconstruction was an underutilized option in the management of 155,463 women studied between 1985 and 1990 and 68,348 patients evaluated between 1994 and 1995. In these two cohorts, early/immediate reconstruction increased from 3.4% to 8.3%. Influential in the patient's decision for reconstruction are age, income, geographic location, hospital size and type, and tumor stage. Both physician and patient education are essential to properly inform patients of their options, including the risks involved in reconstruction.

Selected References

14. Mannu GS, Bahlerao A. Century of breast surgery from radical to minimal. *Can J Surg.* 2014;57:E147-E148.

19. Fisher B, Anderson S, Bryant J, et al. Twenty-year follow-up of a randomized trial comparing total mastectomy, lumpectomy, and lumpectomy plus irradiation for the treatment of invasive breast cancer. *N Engl J Med.* 2002;347:1233-1241.

20. Rabinovitch R, Kavanagh B. Double helix of breast cancer therapy: intertwining the Halsted and Fisher hypotheses. *J Clin Oncol.* 2009;27:2422-2423.

21. Veronesi U, Cascinelli N, Mariani L, et al. Twenty-year follow-up of a randomized study comparing breast-conserving surgery with radical mastectomy for early breast cancer. *N Engl J Med.* 2002;347:1227-1232.

29. Silverstein MJ. Radical mastectomy to radical conservation (extreme oncoplasty): a revolutionary change. *J Am Coll Surg.* 2016;222:1-9.

A full reference list is available online at ExpertConsult.com.

31

Modified Radical Mastectomy and Simple Mastectomy

KIRBY I. BLAND, HELENA R. CHANG, AND EDWARD M. COPELAND III

Modified Radical Mastectomy

Historical Evolution of the Surgical Technique

The rationale for the Halsted radical mastectomy was largely to achieve local and regional control of the breast cancer. The mastectomy techniques invented by Halsted's predecessors in surgery and pathology allowed him to achieve unprecedented success in obtaining this objective without the availability of irradiation or chemotherapy. The techniques now known as the Halsted radical mastectomy and the modified radical mastectomy are an evolution of these methods, which used varying degrees of breast extirpation and lymphatic dissection (Table 31.1).

In contrast to the Halsted radical mastectomy, the modified radical mastectomy defines a surgery of complete breast removal, with the inclusion of the tumor, overlying skin, and axillary lymphatics, with preservation of the pectoralis major muscle. Preservation of the pectoralis major muscle provides for better cosmesis of the chest wall.

In 1894, Halsted[1] and Meyer[2] independently reported their individual techniques for the successful therapy of breast carcinoma with radical mastectomy. The initial clinical experience by Halsted suggested that the pectoralis major muscle was removed concomitantly with the axillary node dissection. The pectoralis minor muscle was transected only for technical expediency during the axillary dissection and was thereafter reapproximated to close the posterior superior axillary space. Soon after, however, Halsted advocated Meyer's concept of the routine resection of both muscles. This method, once advocated by both Halsted and Meyer, became the state-of-the-art operative procedure for decades in treating cancer of the breast.

However, both American and British surgeons began to develop more conservative procedures. By 1912, Murphy[3] had abandoned the Halsted radical mastectomy in favor of preserving both pectoral muscles. This practice was based on the experiences of Bryant of London, who acknowledged only one case of recurrent breast carcinoma in the pectoral muscles in patients followed over a 40-year clinical review period.[3] Furthermore, the practice by Grace[4] to perform only the simple mastectomy in certain patients went unchallenged until the widely acclaimed reports of the modified radical mastectomy by McWhirter,[5] Patey and Dyson,[6] and Patey[7] in the 1940s. This paradigm shift to focus on surgery with muscle preservation has continued since the 1960s. In 1972, 30% of patients with breast cancer were treated with modified radical

mastectomy and 50% with radical mastectomy. By 1981, only 3% received radical mastectomy, and 73% had modified radical mastectomy. The Consensus Development Conference on the treatment of breast cancer in 1979 stated that the modified radical mastectomy was the standard of treatment for women with stages I and II breast cancer during that period of time.[8,9] Any other local or regional treatment developed thereafter must be compared with results of modified radical mastectomy.[10–17]

Retrospective Studies of the Modified Radical Mastectomy

Multiple retrospective clinical studies were conducted to evaluate the survival outcomes after modified radical mastectomy and are summarized in Table 31.2. These series clearly demonstrated that the rate of survival decreased as the tumor size increased and the lymph node metastases became evident. In these nonrandomized, retrospective studies, there appeared to be no survival benefit obtained by a complete axillary dissection to include level 3 nodes or removal of the pectoralis minor muscle (Patey vs. Auchincloss-Madden techniques). Although a rigorous statistical comparison was not applied, the survival rates at 5 and 10 years after the modified radical mastectomy were clearly affected by the initial stage of the disease (i.e., stage I vs. stage II), and the survival rates deteriorated with longer follow-up.

Further analysis of these series also demonstrated survival rates for operable breast cancer as a function of the status of the axillary lymph nodes at the time of modified radical mastectomy (Table 31.3). Survival was not only inversely related to the presence of a positive lymph node but also decreased proportionate to the number of positive lymph nodes. Similarly, the local and regional recurrence rates after modified radical mastectomy were affected by the stage of disease at the time of treatment (Table 31.4).

Support for limiting the level of lymph node dissection was demonstrated by Madden and colleagues[18] using the Auchincloss technique, which questioned the need to completely dissect the axillary contents. Madden et al. reported a local recurrence rate of 10%.[18] Auchincloss[19] found that the apical nodes (level 3) should be removed if clinically involved because of the high rate of recurrence if these nodes were found to be positive and not subsequently removed. However, if these level 3 nodes were clinically negative, complete axillary dissection was unnecessary because mastectomy with excision of levels 1 and 2 and pectoralis preservation had control and survival rates identical with more

TABLE
31.1 **Historical Development of Modified Radical Mastectomy**

Study	Year	Surgery
Moore[a]	1867	Segmental breast resection, selective axillary dissection
Volkmann[b]	1875	Total breast extirpation, with removal of pectoralis major fascia, preservation of pectoralis major muscle
Gross[c]	1880	Total mastectomy and complete axillary dissection
Banks[d]	1882	Modified radical mastectomy, with pectoralis preservation
Sprengel[e]	1882	Total mastectomy and selective axillary dissection
Kuster[f]	1883	Total mastectomy and routine axillary dissection
Halsted[g]	1894	Radical mastectomy
Meyer[h]	1894	Radical mastectomy
Murphy[i]	1912	Radical mastectomy, modified by pectoralis preservation
McWhirter[j]	1948	Modified radical mastectomy with radiotherapy
Patey[k,l]	1948	Modified radical mastectomy with resection of pectoralis minor
Madden[m,n]	1965	Modified radical mastectomy with pectoralis preservation

[a]Data from Moore CH. On the influence of inadequate operations on the theory of cancer. *R Med Chir Soc Lond.* 1867;1:244.

[b]Data from Volkmann R. Geschwülste der mamma (36 Fälle) Beitrage zur Chirurgie. Leipsig; 1895:310.

[c]Data from Gross SW. *A Practical Treatment of Tumors of The Mammary Gland Embracing Their Histology, Pathology, Diagnosis and Treatment.* New York: Appleton; 1880.

[d]Data from Banks WM. On free removal of mammary cancer with extirpation of the axillary glands as a necessary accompaniment. *BMJ.* 1882;2:1138.

[e]Data from Sprengel.[118]

[f]Data from Küster E. Zur behandlung des brustkrebses verhandlungen der deutschen gesellschaft für Chirurgie. Leipsig; 1883:288.

[g]Data from Halsted.[1]

[h]Data from Meyer.[2]

[i]Data from Murphy.[3]

[j]Data from McWhirter.[5]

[k]Data from Patey and Dyson[6] and Patey.[7]

[l]Data from Madden et al.[18] and Madden.[20]

radical approaches.[18–23] Furthermore, if Rotter nodes were not involved, clearance of these interpectoral nodes was found to be unnecessary.[18,20] Further retrospective studies by Dahl-Iversen and Tobiassen,[24] Handley,[25] Hermann,[26] and Nemoto and Dao[27] confirmed similar survival results between the classic radical mastectomy and the modified radical mastectomy and that these two procedures were equal in the recovery of axillary lymph nodes.

Baker and associates[28] of Johns Hopkins University compared the results of modified radical mastectomy with radical mastectomy in the treatment of operable breast cancer. For 205 patients with stage I cancer, 60 with stage II disease, and 67 with stage III disease (based on the tumor, node, metastasis [TNM] system), there were no statistically significant differences in 5-year survival when the results of the radical mastectomy were compared with those of the modified radical mastectomy. Furthermore, no statistically significant differences in incidence of locoregional recurrence were evident in patients with stages I and II disease when the results of the two surgical procedures were compared. In contrast, individuals with stage III disease treated with modified radical mastectomy had a statistically significant ($p = .002$) higher incidence of local recurrence (chest wall and axilla) compared with patients treated with radical mastectomy. Baker and colleagues[28] concluded that modified radical mastectomy is the treatment of choice in patients with TNM stages I and II disease. For patients with stage III disease, the radical mastectomy provided a greater

probability of locoregional control of disease but did not enhance survival.

Crowe and coworkers[29] reported a 16-year experience of locoregional recurrence in a series of 1392 patients treated for operable breast cancer with modified radical mastectomy. They found that most cases of locoregional recurrence occurred within the first 3 years of treatment. Among patients with locoregional recurrence, distant metastases had developed in 64%. Large size of tumor and positive nodes were associated with rapid, locoregional recurrence. Furthermore, the incidence of developing distant failure was associated with the time of locoregional recurrence. In summary, the size and nodal status of the original cancer, as well as the length of the locoregional disease-free interval, were found to directly affect the likelihood of developing metastasis.

These and other observations support the conclusion that extirpation of the pectoralis major muscle is not essential to provide locoregional control of stages I and II disease (Columbia Clinical Classification A and B). It must be noted that neither procedure was adequate for achieving locoregional control of TNM stage III breast cancer or Columbia Clinical Classification C and D tumors (see Section XV). In properly selected patients with stages I and II disease, these retrospective analyses for the modified radical procedure show survival and control rates comparable to the more radical procedure. Chapters 50 and 51 contain comprehensive

TABLE 31.2 Results of Retrospective Clinical Trials of Patients Treated With Modified Radical Mastectomy Alone[a]

Study	Location/Affiliation	Technique	No. of Patients	Disease Stage	ABSOLUTE SURVIVAL (%)	
					5-yr	10-yr
Handley Thackray, 1969[b]	United Kingdom	Patey	77	I	75	61
			58	II	57	25
Delarue, 1969[c,d]	Toronto	Madden	75	I	61.8	—
			25	II	51.4	—
Madden, 1972[e,f]	New York City	Madden	94	I	81.6	63
				II	32.4	17
Robinson, 1976[g]	Mayo Clinic	Madden	280	I	81	—
				II	54	—
Meyer, 1978[h]	Rockford, Illinois	Madden	175	I–III	74	43
Baker, 1979[d,i]	Johns Hopkins University	Patey	91	I	90	—
			22	II	72	—
			31	III	45	—
Leis, 1980[j,k]	New York Medical College	Patey	397	I	—	72.2
			333	II	—	40.2
Nemoto, 1980[d,l]	American College of Surgeons	Mixed	8906	I	65.1	—
			7832	II	35.1	—
Hermann, 1985[d,m]	Cleveland Clinic	Madden	358	I	73	56
			211	II	55	28

[a]Includes some patients treated with radical mastectomy with equivalent results.
[b]Data from Handley RS, Thackray AC. Conservative radical mastectomy (Patey's operation). *Ann Surg.* 1969;170:880.
[c]Data from Delarue NC, Anderson WD, Starr J. Modified radical mastectomy in the individualized treatment of breast carcinoma. *Surg Gynecol Obstet.* 1969;129:79.
[d]TNM classification.
[e]Data from Madden et al.[18]
[f]Manchester classification.
[g]Data from Robinson et al.[14]
[h]Data from Meyer et al.[43]
[i]Data from Baker et al.[28]
[j]Data from Leis HP Jr. Modified radical mastectomy: definition and role in breast cancer surgery. *Int Surg.* 1980;65:211.
[k]Columbia Clinical Classification.
[l]Data from Nemoto T, Vana J, Bedwani RN, et al. Management and survival of female breast cancer: Results of a national survey by the American College of Surgeons. *Cancer.* 1980;45:2917.
[m]Data from Hermann RE et al.[44]

discussion of local, regional, and systemic complications that may ensue with the modified radical mastectomy.

Prospective Trials for the Modified Radical Mastectomy

During the 1970s, two prospective randomized trials by Turner in Manchester, England, and by Maddox at the University of Alabama, Birmingham, compared the Halsted radical mastectomy with the modified radical mastectomy. The study by Turner and associates[30] consisted of 534 patients with T_1 or T_2 (N_0 or N_1) carcinoma of the breast and demonstrated that after a median follow-up of 5 years, there was no significant difference in disease-free survival, overall survival, or locoregional control rates (Table 31.5).

The study by Maddox and associates[31,32] compared modified radical mastectomy with radical mastectomy in 311 patients with stages I to III breast cancers. Patients with positive lymph nodes

were randomized to receive chemotherapy. Results of this study demonstrated no significant difference in the 5-year disease-free survival rate but did show a significant decrease in local recurrence rates after the radical mastectomy (Table 31.6). A trend toward improved overall survival after radical mastectomy versus modified radical mastectomy was evident after 5 years (84% vs. 76%, respectively) and became more evident after 10 years (74% vs. 65%, respectively; Fig. 31.1). Although there was no significant difference in the overall survival rate between the procedures in patients with smaller cancers, the ultimate survival rate for patients with T_2 or T_3 tumors was significantly better after the radical mastectomy (Fig. 31.2).

Subsequent prospective trials performed in the 1980s and 1990s also observed no significant difference in survival between the Halsted radical mastectomy and the modified radical mastectomy. The study performed by Morimoto at the University of Tokushima, Japan, compared modified radical mastectomy with radical mastectomy in patients with stage II disease who received

TABLE 31.3 Five- and 10-Year Survival Rates as a Function of Axillary Nodal Status After Modified Radical Mastectomy

Study and Year	Clinic or Study Group	No. of Patients	SURVIVAL RATE FOR PATIENTS WITH NEGATIVE NODES		SURVIVAL RATE BY NUMBER OF POSITIVE NODES					
					ANY		1–3		≥4	
			5-yr	10-yr	5-yr	10-yr	5-yr	10-yr	5-yr	10-yr
Handley and Thackray, 1969[a]	United Kingdom	135	75	57	61	25	NA	NA	NA	NA
Madden, 1972[b]	New York City	94	82	63	32	17	NA	NA	NA	NA
Robinson, 1976[c]	Mayo Clinic	339	80[g] (93)		48[g] (55)		61[g] (72)		37[g] (42)	
Nemoto, 1980[d]	American College of Surgeons	24,136	71.8		40.4		63.1–58.8[h]		51.9–22.2[h]	
Hermann, 1985[e]	Cleveland Clinic	564	78	62	55	28	66	41	47	25
Martin, 1986[f]	Mayo Clinic	208	87	74	—	56	NA	NA	NA	NA

NA, Not available.

[a]Data from Handley RS, Thackray AC. Conservative radical mastectomy (Patey's operation). Ann Surg 170:880, 1969.
[b]Data from Madden et al.[18]
[c]Data from Robinson et al.[14]
[d]Data from Nemoto T, Vana J, Bedwani RN, et al. Management and survival of female breast cancer: results of a national survey by the American College of Surgeons. *Cancer.* 1980;45:2917.
[e]Data from Hermann et al.[44]
[f]Data from Martin JK et al. Is modified radical mastectomy really equivalent to radical mastectomy in treatment of carcinoma of the breast? *Cancer.* 1986;57:510.
[g]Determinate survival.
[h]Range inclusive of number of positive nodes.

TABLE 31.4 Local and Regional 5- and 10-Year Recurrence Rates of Various Sites in Retrospective Studies After Modified Radical Mastectomy

Study and Year	Clinic or Study Group	No. of Patients	Disease Stage	SITE (%)	
				Chest Wall Scar or Operative Field	Axilla
Delarue, 1969[a]	Toronto General[g] (Canada)	43	I	0	0
		32	II	12.5	—
		25	III	15	—
Madden, 1972[b]	New York City[h]	94	I–III	10	0
Handley, 1976[c]	United Kingdom[h]	77	A[i]	10	1.8
		58	B	22.6	0.1
		8	C	63.6	9.1
Baker, 1979[d]	Johns Hopkins[g]	91	I	13.2	1.1
		22	II	9.1	4.5
		31	III	22.6	22.6
Leis, 1980[e]	New York Medical College[h]	116	0	0	0
		397	I	5	0.08
		333	II	13.8	0.08
Crowe, 1991[f]	Case Western	917	LN–	6.5	2.7
		475	LN+	9	8.4

LN–, Lymph node negative; *LN+,* Lymph node positive.
Staging is TNM unless otherwise noted.
[a]Data from Delarue NC, Anderson WD, Starr J. Modified radical mastectomy in the individualized treatment of breast carcinoma. *Surg Gynecol Obstet.* 1979;129:79.
[b]Data from Madden et al.[18]
[c]Data from Handley.[25]
[d]Data from Baker et al.[28]
[e]Data from Leis HP Jr. Modified radical mastectomy: definition and role in breast cancer surgery. *Int Surg.* 1980;65:211.
[f]Data from Crowe JP et al.[29]
[g]Five-year recurrence rates.
[h]Ten-year recurrence rates.
[i]Columbia Clinical Classification.

TABLE 31.5 Manchester Trial Results: Overall Survival, Disease-Free Survival, and Local and Distant Disease-Free Survival Rates (%) for Radical and Modified Radical Mastectomy According to Clinical and Pathologic Stage at Entry

	No. of Patients Followed Up	Overall Survival (5-yr)	Disease-Free Local Recurrence (5-yr)[a]	Disease-Free of Distant Metastases (5-yr)[a]	Overall Disease-Free Survival (5-yr)[a]
All Cases					
Radical	278	70	75	63	58
Modified	256	70	79	63	58
Clinical Stage I					
Pathologic Stage I					
Radical	119	80	85	79	69
Modified	108	79	90	79	71
Pathologic Stage II					
Radical	52	57	57	52	39
Modified	49	62	74	62	57
Clinical Stage II					
Pathologic Stage I					
Radical	41	85	91	79	79
Modified	38	78	88	71	70
Pathologic Stage II					
Radical	64	55	59	47	38
Modified	59	55	56	45	30

[a]Figures indicate the percentages of patients not experiencing each event regardless of any other outcome.
From Turner L, Swindell R, Bell WG, et al. Radical versus modified radical mastectomy for breast cancer. *Ann R Coll Surg Engl.* 1981;63:239-243.

TABLE 31.6 University of Alabama Prospective Randomized Trial to Compare the Halsted Radical Mastectomy With the Modified Radical Mastectomy: Local Recurrence Rates of the Two Techniques

	MODIFIED RADICAL MASTECTOMY						HALSTED RADICAL MASTECTOMY					
			LOCAL RECURRENCE						LOCAL RECURRENCE			
			5-YR		10-YR				5-YR		10-YR	
Disease Stage	No. of Patients	%	n	%	n	%	No. of Patients	%	n	%	n	%
I	43	13.8	4	9.3	NA	NA	37	11.9	2	5.4	NA	NA
II	112	36	8	7.1	NA	NA	83	26.7	3	3.6	NA	NA
III	20	6.4	4	20[a]	NA	NA	16	5.1	1	6.3[a]	NA	NA
Total	175	56.2	16	9.1[b]	20	11.4[c]	136	43.7	6	4.4[b]	8	5.8[c]

NA, Not available.
[a]p = nonsignificant.
[b]p = .09.
[c]p = .04.
Modified from Maddox WA, Carpenter JT Jr, Laws HL, et al. A randomized prospective trial of radical (Halstead) mastectomy versus radical modified mastectomy in 311 breast cancer patients. *Ann Surg.* 1983;198:207-212; and Maddox WA, Carpenter JT Jr, Laws HL, et al. Does radical mastectomy still have a place in the treatment of primary operable breast cancer? *Arch Surg.* 1987;122:1317-1320.

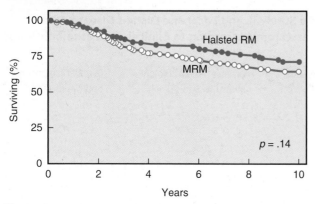

• **Fig. 31.1** Overall survival of patients who underwent radical mastectomy (*RM*; n = 136) and modified radical mastectomy (*MRM*; n = 175) (*p* = .14). (From Maddox WA, Carpenter JT Jr, Laws HT, et al. Does radical mastectomy still have a place in the treatment of primary operable breast cancer? *Arch Surg*. 122:1317-1320. Copyright © 1987, American Medical Association. All rights reserved.)

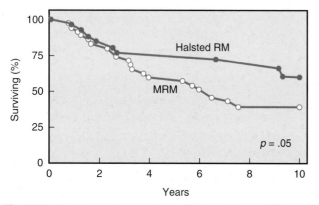

• **Fig. 31.2** Survival curves comparing radical mastectomy (*RM*; n = 25) and modified radical mastectomy (*MRM*; n = 36) for patients with T_2 tumors with clinically positive axillary nodes or T_3 tumors. There was significantly better survival after radical mastectomy (*p* = .05). (From Maddox WA, Carpenter JT Jr, Laws HT, et al. Does radical mastectomy still have a place in the treatment of primary operable breast cancer? *Arch Surg*. 1987;122:1317-1320. Copyright © 1987, American Medical Association. All rights reserved.)

TABLE 31.7	University of Tokushima Prospective Trial to Compare Modified Radical Mastectomy With Extended Radical Mastectomy in Patients With Stage II Disease Treated With Chemotherapy				
Operation	No. of Patients	5-yr DFS	5-yr DFS for Positive Nodes	5-yr OS	5-yr OS for Positive Nodes
MRM	96	87.2	75.6	93.2	84.4
ERM	96	82.7	73.3	92.4	87.8

DFS, Disease-free survival; *ERM*, extended radical mastectomy; *MRM*, modified radical mastectomy; *OS*, overall survival.

Modified from Lerman C, Narod S, Schulman K, et al. BRCA1 testing in families with hereditary breast-ovarian cancer: a prospective study of patient decision making and outcomes. *JAMA*. 275:1885-1892.

local recurrence rate was 5%. Symptomatic lymphedema occurred in 2% of patients, and half of those patients had adjuvant radiation treatment. Given the excellent result in controlling the disease, rapidity in achieving the therapeutic and staging goals, and minimal morbidity, the authors concluded that modified radical mastectomy continued to be a good choice for treating patients with primary operable breast cancer.

Simple Mastectomy

The term *simple mastectomy* is synonymous with *total mastectomy*. This procedure represents further modification of the modified radical mastectomy in that it preserves not only the pectoral muscles but also the axillary lymph nodes. The rationale for this modification is based on the hypothesis that breast cancer is a systemic disease and the outcomes are affected by complex host-tumor interactions. Thus this hypothesis suggests that variations in locoregional therapy are unlikely to substantially affect survival and that biological rather than anatomic factors are responsible for metastatic dissemination.[13,35–42] The regional lymph node may represent an indicator of the existent host-tumor relationship such that a positive lymph node reflects a permitted metastatic development. Accordingly, the simple mastectomy is designed to treat local disease and omit regional nodal dissection because the latter has no influence on survival and risks significant surgical morbidity. Studies comparing the total mastectomy with more radical procedures and examining the role of postoperative radiation therapy are summarized in the following sections.

Retrospective Studies of the Simple Mastectomy

Eight retrospective studies[43–50] comparing simple mastectomy with or without postoperative radiation therapy showed no significant difference in survival after 5 years but indicated a trend toward improved 10-year survival after radiation therapy (Table 31.8). These retrospective studies spanned three decades and used a variety of techniques and surgeons, making rigorous statistical comparison difficult. However, it appears evident that the survival rates achieved with simple mastectomy with or without irradiation are comparable to those obtained with radical mastectomy. The local and regional recurrences were not specifically addressed in these retrospective studies but are extensively addressed in the prospective trials.

postoperative chemotherapy.[33] The results showed no significant difference in 5-year survival, overall survival, or local recurrence between the two groups (Table 31.7). However, nodal metastasis did adversely affect 5-year survival in both groups.

A prospective 25-year follow-up in 193 patients with operable breast cancer who were treated with Patey's modified radical mastectomy was reported by Staunton and associates[34] at St. Bartholomew's Hospital, London. Of those patients, 66% had stage I disease, 24% stage II, and 9% stage III. Of the patients, 42% received hormonal treatment and 9% received chemotherapy. Six percent of patients underwent radiation as part of their initial treatment. The 5-, 10-, and 15-year survival rates for clinical stage I breast cancer ($T_1/T_2 N_0$) were 90%, 79%, and 74%; for stage II ($T_1/T_2 N_1$), 81%, 64%, and 60%; and for stage III ($T_3 N_0/N_1$), 78%, 70%, and 0%, respectively. The 5-, 10-, and 15-year survival rates for patients without nodal metastases by pathologic staging were 95%, 90%, and 84%, respectively, and for patients with positive nodes, 68%, 43%, and 40%, respectively. The isolated

TABLE 31.8 Survival Results of Retrospective Clinical Trials for Simple Mastectomy With or Without Radiotherapy

Study and Year	Clinic or Study Group	No. of Patients	Disease Stage	ABSOLUTE SURVIVAL (%) 5-YR −RT	5-YR +RT	10-YR −RT	10-YR +RT
Williams et al., 1953[50]	St. Bartholomew (United Kingdom)	110	I	77	67	33	40
		45	II	—	35	—	21
Smith and Meyer, 1959[49]	Rockford, Illinois	97	I and II	54	—	32	—
Shimkin et al., 1961[48]	Rockford, Illinois	103	I and II	51	—	31	—
Devitt 1962[46]	Ottawa (Canada)	119	I	—	68	—	45
		30	II	—	56	—	47
Den Besten and Ziffren, 1965[45]	University of Iowa	133	I	55.7	—	—	—
		95	II	33.7	—	—	—
Kyle et al., 1976[47]	Cancer Research Campaign (United Kingdom)	1152	I[a]	78	79	—	—
		1116	II	71	76	—	—
Meyer et al., 1978[43]	Rockford, Illinois	252	I and II	69	—	40	—
Hermann et al., 1985[44]	Cleveland Clinic	355	I	78	—	60	—
		47	II	53	—	37	—

RT, Radiotherapy.
[a]Manchester Staging Classification.

Evolution of Simple Mastectomy With Sentinel Lymph Node Biopsy

In recent years, a sharp increase in performing simple mastectomies and variations of this procedure has been reported across the United States. Many patients who were traditionally treated by breast conserving surgery for early breast cancer or modified radical mastectomy for large primary cancer are now choosing simple mastectomy and sentinel lymph node biopsy. The trend of skipping modified radical mastectomy is no longer limited to those with clinically negative axilla with proven negative sentinel lymph nodes. A similar approach has been extended to patients who have limited metastatic sentinel lymph nodes and those who have pathologically proven metastasis and are converted to node-negative disease by neoadjuvant chemotherapy.

American College of Surgeons Oncology Group (ACOSOG) Z0011 study[51,52] demonstrated that among patients with lumpectomy, limited positive sentinel lymph nodes and postoperative whole breast radiation, there was no difference in overall and disease-free survival rates between groups of patients with and without axillary lymph node dissection. The same approach has been extended into managing patients with mastectomy who had limited metastasis found in the sentinel lymph nodes. Fu and coworkers[53] recently reported that postmastectomy radiation without axillary lymph node dissection was as effective as those with axillary lymph node dissection in patients with mastectomy and limited metastasis in sentinel lymph nodes.

The 2013 ACOSOG Z1071 Alliance study showed that 41% node-positive patients became node negative after neoadjuvant chemotherapy,[54] which further suggested this group of patients traditionally treated by axillary lymph node dissection could now have sentinel lymph node biopsy with simple mastectomy.

Parallel to the increasing use of simple mastectomy in treating invasive breast cancer, a growing use of simple mastectomy is also observed in treating young women with ductal carcinoma in situ (DCIS).[55] It is well known that DCIS is associated with an excellent survival outcome after either breast conserving treatment or mastectomy. For many years, lumpectomy with radiation was preferred by many for treating DCIS. Using National Cancer Database (NCDB), Rutter and coworkers[55] demonstrated a decreased use of mastectomy rates in treating DCIS from 1998 (36%) to 2004 (28%) before rising again through 2011 (33%). Although controversial, some studies also suggested that positive resection margins after mastectomy do not increase chest wall recurrence in women with DCIS.[56,57] If this finding is confirmed, the trend of choosing simple mastectomy by young women with DCIS may continue to grow even if it does not affect the long-term survival.

Prospective Trials for the Simple Mastectomy With and Without Irradiation

The trend toward more conservative surgery led to prospective randomized clinical trials to study simple mastectomy with or without radiation therapy in the treatment of breast cancer. The Groote Schur trial[58] in South Africa compared total mastectomy with radical mastectomy without irradiation in 96 patients with stages I and II breast cancer. This trial was terminated after only 3 years because of the high recurrence rate in the simple mastectomy group. Axillary lymph node and skin flap recurrences were seen in 9.8% and 13.7% of patients, respectively, leading to the conclusion that total mastectomy without irradiation should not be used.

A study by Turnbull and associates[59] evaluated 150 patients with stages I and II breast cancer who underwent simple mastectomy with or without irradiation. This study showed a higher operative field recurrence rate (27.6%) for patients with stages I and II disease who had simple mastectomy alone. Addition of radiation therapy decreased operative field recurrence to 10.8%. Early survival was not affected by radiation therapy.

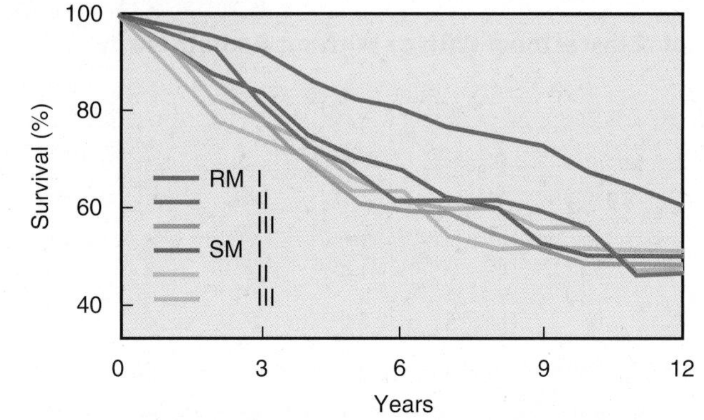

• **Fig. 31.3** Crude survival rates for cases according to international stage of the disease and treatment option. *RM I,* Radical mastectomy for stage I; *SM III,* simple mastectomy plus radiotherapy for stage III, and so forth. (From Langlands AO, Prescott RJ, Hamilton T. A clinical trial in the management of operable cancer of the breast. *Br J Surg.* 2980;67:170-174.)

TABLE 31.9	Edinburgh Royal Infirmary—Cardiff Trial (1967–1973): Axillary Recurrence in Patients With Negative and Nonidentified Nodes Treated by Simple and Radical Mastectomy

	NO. OF PATIENTS	
Treatment	Total	With Axillary Recurrence (%)
Mastectomy alone (simple mastectomy)	64	10 (15.6)
Mastectomy with axillary clearance (radical mastectomy)	66	1 (1.5)

From Forrest AP, Stewart HJ, Roberts MM, Steele RJ. Simple mastectomy and axillary node sampling (pectoral node biopsy) in the management of primary breast cancer. *Ann Surg.* 1982;196:371-378.

TABLE 31.10	Edinburgh Royal Infirmary—Cardiff Trial (1967–1973): Chest Wall Tumor Recurrence[a]

	NO. OF PATIENTS	
Treatment	Total	With Chest Wall Recurrence (%)
Simple mastectomy and axillary radiotherapy	39	10 (25.6)
Radical mastectomy and radical radiotherapy	31	2 (6.5)

[a]Patients had positive nodes at the time of mastectomy.
From Forrest AP, Stewart HJ, Roberts MM, Steele RJ. Simple mastectomy and axillary node sampling (pectoral node biopsy) in the management of primary breast cancer. *Ann Surg.* 1982;196:371-378.

Further studies comparing the simple mastectomy with irradiation versus radical mastectomy demonstrated mixed results. The Copenhagen trial[60] evaluated 666 patients with a 25-year follow-up. This study showed that overall survival rates were identical between study groups at 5 years (60%), 10 years (40%), and 25 years (28%). Recurrence-free survival at 25 years was 58% for radical mastectomy and 45% for simple mastectomy with irradiation in women with stage I disease; however, this was not statistically significant. The 25-year survival rates for patients with and without lymph node metastasis were 20% and 60%, respectively, demonstrating that nodal status has a strong prognostic value for long-term survival.

The Edinburgh trial[61,62] compared simple mastectomy with postoperative radiotherapy to radical mastectomy in 490 patients. In contrast to the Copenhagen study, this trial demonstrated a better, 12-year survival rate in patients with stage I disease in the radical mastectomy group (Fig. 31.3). A significant difference was also seen in the axillary recurrence rate in the simple mastectomy group versus the radical mastectomy group (12% vs. 3%).

As a result of these differences in recurrence rates based on nodal status, more prospective clinical trials have compared the simple mastectomy with lymph node sampling and subsequent radiation therapy versus radical mastectomy and radiation therapy if lymph node involvement was detected. Similar to previous studies, these results show no difference in overall survival between those having simple mastectomy and irradiation versus radical mastectomy; however, recurrence rates tended to be lower with the more radical procedure.

The Edinburgh Royal Infirmary–Cardiff trial[63–65] evaluated 200 patients with T_1 and T_2 disease over a 14-year period. The study compared simple mastectomy and lymph node sampling versus radical mastectomy with irradiation for either group if lymph nodes were involved. The data showed increased axillary recurrence after simple mastectomy versus radical mastectomy (15.6% vs. 1.5%, respectively) if lymph nodes were negative (Table 31.9). Significant chest wall recurrence was seen after simple mastectomy with axillary irradiation versus radical mastectomy with irradiation (25.6% vs. 6.5%, respectively) if lymph nodes were positive (Table 31.10). However, overall survival was identical for both groups (Fig. 31.4). Further analysis of this study

with respect to the recurrence data shows that radiation after total mastectomy without any nodal removal reduced the locoregional recurrences from 41% to 19%, and the recurrences were further reduced to 5% if histologically proven negative nodes were found in the mastectomy specimen (Table 31.11).

To determine whether radiation therapy in patients with histologically proven nodal metastases would be as effective as axillary clearance, Forrest and colleagues[64,65] conducted a randomized trial to study 417 patients who had mastectomy and node sampling or full axillary clearance. Those who had positive nodes by sampling received radiation therapy. Patients with positive nodes received cyclophosphamide, methotrexate, and fluorouracil (CMF) or oophorectomy if they were premenopausal; tamoxifen was given to postmenopausal women and premenopausal women with negative nodes. The incidence of distant metastasis and the 12-year overall survival rate were the same in both groups. Although the radiation reduced chest wall recurrences in node-positive patients compared with patients with axillary clearance, the latter group showed slightly fewer axillary recurrences (3% vs. 5.4%). Adjuvant systemic treatment reduced locoregional recurrences in node-positive women of both groups.

The Manchester Regional Breast Study[66,67] compared simple mastectomy with or without irradiation in stage I patients and radical mastectomy alone in stage II patients. The study consisted of 1020 patients with a 5- to 10-year follow-up and showed that the addition of radiation therapy after simple mastectomy did not affect the survival in patients with stage I disease but reduced the recurrence rate at the chest wall and nodal basin (Table 31.12). There was no significant difference in survival or recurrence for

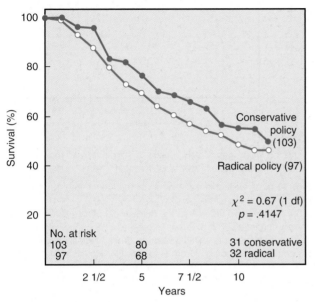

• **Fig. 31.4** Survival of all patients included in the Cardiff trial in April 1981. *df*, Degrees of freedom. (From Forrest AP, Stewart HJ, Roberts MM, Steele RJ. Simple mastectomy and axillary node sampling (pectoral node biopsy) in the management of primary breast cancer. *Ann Surg.* 1982;196:371-378.)

those in the stage II groups treated by either simple mastectomy with radiation or radical mastectomy.

The Cancer Research Campaign Clinical Trial[47,66,68] was another study that evaluated simple mastectomy with or without irradiation. This trial consisted of 2243 patients with a mean follow-up of 11 years. Results showed no difference in overall survival rates (Fig. 31.5). However, there was a significantly higher recurrence rate in the simple mastectomy-only group than the group with simple mastectomy and radiation therapy (Fig. 31.6). The recurrence rate appeared to be proportional to tumor grade, and prophylactic irradiation was proposed to treat patients at high risk for recurrence. Subsequent follow-up of this trial after a 19-year interval reported by Houghton and associates[69] demonstrated that local recurrence was significantly reduced by adding radiation to simple mastectomy. Overall survival rates remained similar between the two treatment groups; however, there were more non–breast cancer deaths observed in the irradiated patients. These non–breast cancer deaths included deaths resulting from cardiac causes and nonbreast malignancies.

The trials of the National Surgical Adjuvant Breast and Bowel Project (NSABP) have played a key role in determining the appropriate surgical course for patients with cancer. Protocol NSABP-B-04 in the 1970s evaluated 1655 patients with an average follow-up of 11 years.[37] The study compared simple mastectomy with and without axillary irradiation versus radical mastectomy and showed no difference in disease-free survival between these groups for patients with clinically negative lymph nodes and no difference in distant and locoregional recurrence-free survival between simple mastectomy with irradiation versus radical mastectomy in patients with clinically positive lymph nodes (Fig. 31.7). However, in those node-negative patients who had

TABLE 31.11	Edinburgh Trial: Locoregional Recurrence According to Whether Nodes Were Identified for Histologic Examination at Mastectomy				
	NO. OF PATIENTS, NODES IDENTIFIED AND HISTOLOGICALLY NEGATIVE		NO. OF PATIENTS, NODES NOT IDENTIFIED		
Treatment	Total	With Recurrence (%)	Total	With Recurrence (%)
Mastectomy alone	114	18 (16)	59	24 (41)
Mastectomy with radiotherapy	112	6 (5)	57	11 (19)

Forrest AP, Stewart HJ, Roberts MM, Steele RJ. Simple mastectomy and axillary node sampling (pectoral node biopsy) in the management of primary breast cancer. *Ann Surg.* 1982;196:371-378.

TABLE 31.12	Manchester Regional Breast Study (1970–1975): Primary Control Related to Clinical Stage and Treatment for Stages I and II Disease							
			PERCENT FREE FROM RECURRENCE					
			CHEST WALL		AXILLA		SUPRACLAVICULAR	
Clinical Stage	Treatment	No. of Patients	5-yr	10-yr	5-yr	10-yr	5-yr	10-yr
I	Simple mastectomy	359	84	80	67	63	89	85
	Simple mastectomy + radiotherapy	354	94	91	84	81	92	89
			p = .0002		*p* = .0001		*p* = .20	
II	Radical mastectomy	148	66	64	76	71	80	77
	Simple mastectomy + radiotherapy	159	77	63	75	72	87	86
			p = .22		*p* = .95		*p* = .15	

From Lythgoe JP, Palmer MK. Manchester regional breast study—5 and 10 year results. *Br J Surg.* 1982;69:693-696.

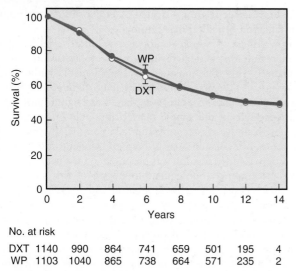

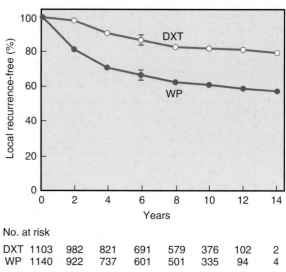

No. at risk

DXT	1140	990	864	741	659	501	195	4
WP	1103	1040	865	738	664	571	235	2

No. at risk

DXT	1103	982	821	691	579	376	102	2
WP	1140	922	737	601	501	335	94	4

• **Fig. 31.5** All evaluable patients: survival in watch policy (*WP*) and radiotherapy groups (*DXT*) ($\chi^2 = 0.02$, $p = .88$, hazard ratio = 1). "No. at risk" represents the number of patients alive at entry and biennially thereafter. This number decreases in the later years because there are fewer patients with relevant trial times. Vertical bars indicate the 95% confidence intervals. (From Berstock DA, Houghton J, Haybittle J, Baum M. The role of radiotherapy after total mastectomy for patients with early breast cancer. *World J Surg.* 1985;9:667-670.)

• **Fig. 31.6** All evaluable patients: local recurrence-free in watch policy (*WP*) and radiotherapy groups (*DXT*) ($\chi^2 = 120.93$, $p < .001$, hazard ratio = 2.69). "No. at risk" represents the number of patients alive at entry and biennially thereafter. This number decreases in the later years because there are fewer patients with relevant trial times. Vertical bars indicate the 95% confidence intervals. (From Berstock DA, Houghton J, Haybittle J, Baum M. The role of radiotherapy following total mastectomy for patients with early breast cancer. *World J Surg.* 1985;9:667-670.)

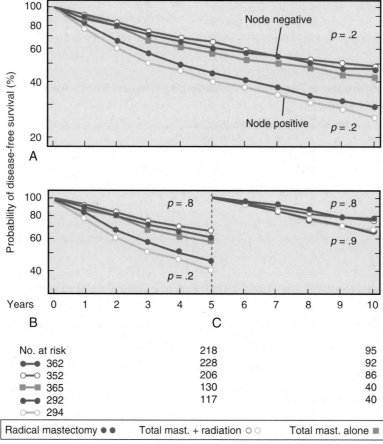

No. at risk

●—●	362	218	95
		228	92
○—○	352	206	86
■—■	365	130	40
●—●	292	117	40
○—○	294		

Radical mastectomy ● ●	Total mast. + radiation ○ ○	Total mast. alone ■

• **Fig. 31.7** Disease-free survival for patients treated with radical mastectomy (*mast.*), total mastectomy plus radiation, or simple mastectomy alone. Survival disease-free through 10 years (A), during the first 5 years (B), and during the second 5 years for patients disease free at the end of the fifth year (C). There were no significant differences among the three groups of patients with clinically negative nodes or between the two groups with clinically positive nodes. (From Fisher B, Redmond C, Fisher ER, et al. Ten-year results of a randomized clinical trial comparing radical mastectomy and total mastectomy with or without radiation. *N Engl J Med.* 1985;312:674-681.)

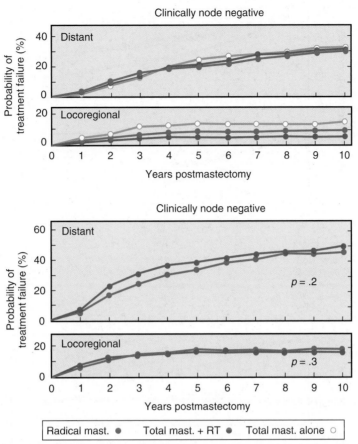

• **Fig. 31.8** Locoregional and distant treatment failures as the first evidence of disease in patients with clinically negative and positive nodes who were treated with radical mastectomy *(mast.),* total mastectomy and radiation, or total mastectomy alone. For node-negative patients, there were no significant differences in distant disease occurring as a first treatment failure among the three groups, whereas locoregional disease was best controlled in the group receiving radiation. For node-positive patients, there was no significant difference in distant or locoregional disease between the two groups. *RT,* Radiation therapy. (From Fisher B, Redmond C, Fisher ER, et al: Ten-year results of a randomized clinical trial comparing radical mastectomy and total mastectomy with or without radiation. *N Engl J Med*. 1985;312:674-681.)

local recurrence, the rate was lowest after simple mastectomy with irradiation (Fig. 31.8). This trial also demonstrated that results after 5 years accurately predicted the outcome at 10 years (Fig. 31.9).

With the advancement in adjuvant systemic treatment coupled with sentinel lymph node biopsy and selective use of radiation, the oncologic safety after simple mastectomy has been significantly improved. Furthermore, several studies also showed that there is no difference in local recurrence between skin-sparing and nonsparing mastectomy[70] and no difference in disease-free survival.[71]

Contralateral Prophylactic Mastectomy

In addition to the noticeable rise of therapeutic mastectomy, an even more dramatic trend is seen in women with unilateral breast cancer to choose contralateral prophylactic mastectomy.[72–74] Although the reasons for this change are unclear, Fu and colleagues[75] reported a retrospective analysis of 373 breast cancer patients treated by mastectomy between 2002 and 2010 in a single institution. Of the 373 patients, 55.5% had bilateral mastectomy and 44.5% had unilateral mastectomy. In this study,

younger age, early-stage breast cancer, family history of breast and/or ovarian breast, personal history of *BRCA* mutation, history of multiple breast biopsies, and preoperative magnetic resonance imaging were found to be associated with bilateral mastectomy compared with the unilateral mastectomy group. Even after excluding those with bilateral breast cancer, the same predictors for choosing contralateral prophylactic mastectomy remained unchanged. Similar association factors with contralateral prophylactic mastectomy have also been reported by others.[76–78] Of the 151 patients with unilateral breast cancer and bilateral mastectomy, 75% had immediate reconstruction. It is clear that the availability of immediate reconstruction and improved esthetic options contribute to the trend of choosing contralateral prophylactic mastectomy in treating women with early breast cancer.

In addition to an overall increase in choosing simple mastectomy (with skin sparing or nipple sparing) with or without sentinel lymph node biopsy for treating breast cancer, a trend of selecting contralateral prophylactic mastectomy has been observed across the United States. Many questions remain unanswered in the practice of contralateral prophylactic mastectomy. The first and foremost question is whether contralateral prophylactic mastectomy reduces a second breast cancer event and improves cancer

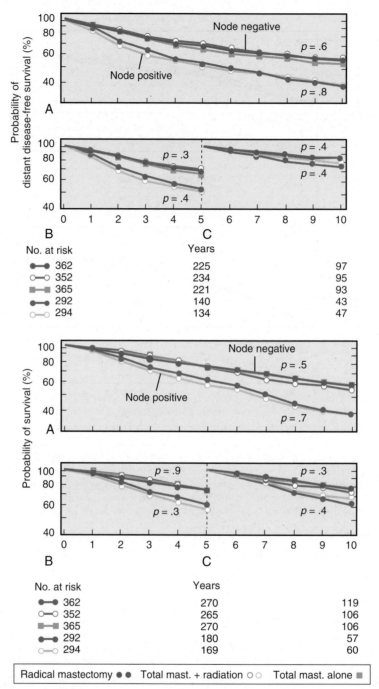

• **Fig. 31.9** Distant disease-free survival and overall survival for patients treated with radical mastectomy *(mast.),* simple mastectomy and radiation, or simple mastectomy alone. *Top panel,* Disease-free survival through 10 years (A), during the first 5 years (B), and during the second 5 years for patients free of distant disease at the end of the fifth year (C). *Bottom panel,* Disease-free survival through 10 years (A), during the first 5 years (B), and during the second 5 years for patients alive at the end of the fifth year (C). There were no significant differences among the three groups of patients with clinically negative nodes or between the two groups with positive nodes. (From Fisher B, Redmond C, Fisher ER, et al. Ten-year results of a randomized clinical trial comparing radical mastectomy and total mastectomy with or without radiation. *N Engl J Med.* 1985;312:674-681.)

specific survival. Kruper and colleagues[79] use SEER—the Surveillance, Epidemiology and End Results database—to compare the outcomes of 26,562 cases of therapeutic mastectomy and contralateral prophylactic mastectomy with 138,826 cases of unilateral therapeutic mastectomy. After propensity score matched analysis, the authors found that contralateral prophylactic mastectomy was associated with better disease-free and overall survival rates in all subset analyses including patients across all stages of disease and across estrogen receptor–positive and –negative breast cancer groups. However, a limitation of the SEER database is that it does not allow removing bias that may affect survival outcomes.[80] Others have reported similar observations, but all had the same limitation in data analysis.[81]

With contralateral prophylactic mastectomy rates continuing to rise and an unclear therapeutic value of the procedure, answers for other associated issues such as complication rates, short- and long-term effects on patient satisfaction, and cost-effectiveness have been scrutinized to better inform patients regarding risks and benefits of this added procedure. Miller and coworkers[82] assessed complication rates associated with contralateral prophylactic mastectomy by comparing 209 cases of contralateral prophylactic mastectomy with 391 cases of unilateral mastectomy in cancer patients performed in a single institution between 2009 and 2012. The authors found that the contralateral mastectomy group was 1.5 times more likely to have any complication and 2.7 times more likely to have a major complication compared with unilateral mastectomy group. Older studies[83,84] also described the risks of surgical complications after bilateral mastectomy with or without reconstruction. A 2015 study reported by Silva and colleagues[85] that compared the complication rates of the two groups showed only a modest difference in postoperative complication rates, however: 8.8% after unilateral mastectomy and 10.1% after bilateral mastectomy for overall complication rate and 4.2% and 4.6%, respectively, for surgical site infection.

In addition to a potential increase in complications because of added contralateral prophylactic mastectomy, concern for delaying adjuvant therapy has been raised. Sharpe and colleagues[86] reported that bilateral mastectomy was associated with a delay to adjuvant chemotherapy; however, in multivariate analysis this association became significant. There is no delay in receiving adjuvant radiation and hormonal therapy.

The added cost for contralateral prophylactic mastectomy is also a concern. According to recent data from a major private health insurer, the average cost of a bilateral mastectomy with reconstruction was $30,500 compared with $18,500 for unilateral mastectomy with reconstruction. A recent report by Edwards and coworkers[87] suggested that in high-risk individuals, bilateral mastectomy is cost-effective compared with subsequent imaging screening based on Medicare reimbursement rates. The reported cost analysis did not include the costs for subsequent cancer diagnosis, treatment, and supportive care.

Beyond the concerns of surgical complications and cost associated with added contralateral prophylactic mastectomy, it is also important to assess the long-term effects of this procedure on women at the levels of body image, sexuality, and overall health. Studies were done to compare bilateral mastectomy with those in the general population, unilateral mastectomy, and breast conserving therapy. Unukovych and colleagues[88] reported that no difference was found in health-related quality of life, including anxiety, depression, and sexuality, before and after contralateral prophylactic mastectomy and between women with contralateral prophylactic mastectomy and those in the general population, although more than half of the patients reported at least one body image issue at 2 years after surgery. When patients with reconstruction after contralateral prophylactic mastectomy and unilateral mastectomy were compared, the former group was associated with higher mean score for breast and outcome satisfaction.[89] Both groups had a similar health-related quality of life (HR-QoL). Sexual dysfunction was observed in both breast conserving therapy and mastectomy groups. However, postoperative sexual dysfunction was more significant in patients after mastectomy. Further subset comparisons between unilateral mastectomy and bilateral

mastectomy with or without reconstruction was not performed in this study.[90]

Although mastectomy with or without reconstruction clearly affects women's body image and sexuality, Rosenberg and associates reported that 80% of patients who chose contralateral prophylactic mastectomy were confident in their decision, and 90% would have made the same decision again.[91] As such, the trend of contralateral prophylactic mastectomy may continue to rise, especially in young women with breast cancer.

Prophylactic Simple Mastectomy in High-Risk Patients

Advances in molecular biology have played a key role in identifying women at increased risk for breast cancer. Although age and family history have been recognized as the important factors in determining risk, the discovery of the *BRCA1* and *BRCA2* gene mutations associated with breast cancer risk has provided an objective means to identify women at high risk for developing breast cancer.[92–96] These women not only carry a significantly increased risk of developing breast cancer but are also more likely to develop it at an early age.[94,97–100] Therefore, identification of these patients by genetic testing is critical if any aggressive measures to reduce the risk of developing breast cancer are to be considered. Currently, the most effective prevention for breast cancer is prophylactic mastectomy. However, prospective data are limited. Guidelines for considering prophylactic mastectomy have been proposed, but there is no absolute indication for this procedure (Box 31.1).[101,102] These guidelines recommend that prophylactic mastectomy may be considered in patients without a history of breast cancer but who are at increased risk of developing breast cancer or who have clinical conditions known to make evaluation of the breasts difficult.[101] Conditions recognized for their increased risk of breast cancer include atypical hyperplasia with a high-risk family history of breast cancer, lobular carcinoma in situ, history of a first-degree relative with premenopausal bilateral breast cancer, and dense breasts that are nodular, which make evaluation exceptionally difficult.

• BOX 31.1 Indications for Prophylactic Total Mastectomy: Society of Surgical Oncology Position Statement (1995)

Patients With No History of Breast Cancer

Atypical hyperplasia
Any history of lobular carcinoma in situ
History of relative with premenopausal breast cancer
Dense, nodular breasts in association with atypical hyperplasia
Family history of premenopausal breast cancer

Patients With Unilateral Breast Cancer

Presence of lobular carcinoma in situ
Large breast that is difficult to evaluate
Diffuse microcalcifications
Risk factors:
    Atypical hyperplasia
    Family history in first-degree relative
    Age <40 years at diagnosis

Modified from Bilimoria M, Morrow M. The woman at increased risk for breast cancer: evaluation and management strategies. CA Cancer J Clin. 1995;45:263–278.

A retrospective study of prophylactic mastectomy in women with a family history of breast cancer was reported by Hartmann and associates[103] at the Mayo Clinic. This study demonstrated a significantly decreased incidence of breast cancer after prophylactic mastectomy after a mean follow-up of 14 years. Only 7 of 639 patients developed breast cancer after prophylactic mastectomy. All who developed breast cancer had a previous subcutaneous or incomplete mastectomy. None of the patients who underwent simple mastectomy developed breast cancer; however, the difference was not statistically significant. A similar retrospective study of 1500 patients by Pennisi and Capozzi[104] showed comparable results but considered only patients undergoing subcutaneous mastectomy.

When genetic testing for inherited breast cancer becomes better understood and more available, many women will be attracted to the idea of risk-reducing mastectomy. Currently, *BRCA1* or *BRCA2* mutations and several other forms of hereditary breast cancer seem to be the only agreed-on indication for prophylactic mastectomy. De Felice and colleagues[105] reported that bilateral prophylactic mastectomy significantly reduced breast cancer incidence in *BRCA1/2* mutation carriers with or without previous salpingo-oophorectomy. Critiques of this study included short median follow-up of 4 years and lack of information on breast cancer–specific and overall survivals of these women.

The results of a prospective trial to examine women with the *BRCA1* or *BRCA2* mutation who underwent prophylactic mastectomy versus regular surveillance were reported by Meijers-Heijboer and associates.[94] The patients who underwent prophylactic mastectomy had no incidence of breast cancer, whereas the surveillance group developed breast cancer at a rate comparable to that of other patients with the same genetic mutation.[94,106] However, mean follow-up in this recent study was only 3 years, and therefore results should be interpreted with caution (Fig. 31.10).

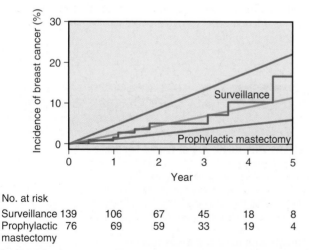

No. at risk

Surveillance 139	106	67	45	18	8
Prophylactic 76	69	59	33	19	4
mastectomy					

• **Fig. 31.10** Actuarial incidence of breast cancer among women with *BRCA1* or *BRCA2* mutation after prophylactic mastectomy or during surveillance. The surveillance group includes data obtained before prophylactic mastectomy in 76 of the 139 women. The green line represents the probability of breast cancer during surveillance and the blue lines the 95% confidence interval. Values were calculated with the use of an exponential model in which the hazard rate was assumed to be constant. (From Meijers-Heijboer H, van Geel B, van Putten WL, et al. Breast cancer after prophylactic bilateral mastectomy in women with a *BRCA 1* or *BRCA 2* mutation. *N Engl J Med.* 2001;345:159-164. Copyright 1999 Massachusetts Medical Society. All rights reserved.)

Although long-term prospective data are not yet available, all these studies indicate that prophylactic simple mastectomy may be considered by high-risk patients to reduce their risk of developing breast cancer. In addition to being advised of available data on risk reduction and the extent of surgery involved, patients should also be advised of the psychosocial aspects of the prophylactic mastectomy and reconstruction before proceeding with this therapy. Patients should be willing to accept the finality of prophylactic mastectomy but also realize that plastic surgeons can provide excellent breast reconstruction to restore body image.

Studies have shown that nipple-sparing mastectomy is safe, feasible, and preferred by most young women who choose to have risk-reducing mastectomy. Indeed, the use of nipple-sparing simple mastectomy has been shown to have increased since the early 2000s.[107–111] In 2015, Yao and associates[112] reported a single-institution experience including 397 nipple-sparing mastectomy procedures in 201 *BRCA1/2* mutation carriers, and 150 of these women underwent nipple-sparing prophylactic mastectomy. Four cases (2.7%) were found to have incidental cancer, and none had nipple-areolar complex (NAC) involvement. Only 1 of the 150 patients with nipple-sparing prophylactic mastectomy developed non-NAC breast cancer with a mean follow-up of 32.6 months. The authors concluded that nipple-sparing prophylactic mastectomy in *BRCA1/2* carriers was safe in risk-reduction setting.

It is reasonable to assume a better cosmetic outcome in most women with nipple-sparing prophylactic mastectomy than those with skin-sparing mastectomy. A 2015 supportive study showed that women with nipple-sparing simple mastectomy had significantly high levels of long-term satisfaction of their body image and sexual well-being compared with skin-sparing mastectomy.[113]

As knowledge in breast cancer risk assessment grows, demonstrating survival advantage and improved cosmetic and psychological outcomes after risk-reducing mastectomy, the trend of young women choosing nipple-sparing mastectomy will continue.

Role of Surgical Excision of Primary Tumor in Patients With Stage IV Disease

Stage IV breast cancer is usually considered incurable, and treatments are largely directed toward palliation. According to the SEER report, approximately 3.5% of women diagnosed with breast cancer in the United States present with metastatic disease at the time of diagnosis.[114] Conventional treatment for metastatic breast cancer is limited to chemotherapy, hormonal therapy, and radiation because the vast majority of these patients do not survive more than 5 years after diagnosis.

The common thought is that patients with widespread cancer are heavily treated and debilitated, and therefore they are not good candidates for major surgery and general anesthesia. Together, the belief of the cancer patients' survival is determined by the metastatic disease and is not affected by the persistence of primary tumor. Thus surgical extirpation of the primary tumor is usually not offered. Surgery is only considered when a symptomatic breast lesion (e.g., bleeding, ulceration, and pain of the primary tumor) exists that cannot be controlled through other means. However, recent literature investigating the role of lumpectomy and mastectomy in patients with metastatic breast cancer suggests that there might be a survival benefit if the primary tumor is removed.

In 2002 Khan and associates published the results of a study that included 16,023 patients with stage IV disease. Approximately 43% of these patients received no operation with or without a combination of other types of treatments, and 57% underwent partial or total mastectomy. Patients who had primary tumor removed with clear margins had a better survival rate than those who did not have surgery. Other factors that were also associated with survival were type of metastasis (bone being the least aggressive), number of metastatic foci, and use of systemic therapy.[115,116]

Another recent study by Babiera and associates, from the MD Anderson Cancer Center, analyzed a similar population of patients who were diagnosed with stage IV disease and had intact primary tumors. The primary end points were death and progression of metastatic disease. All patients were treated with some form of systemic therapy, and 37% (82/224) had surgery. The study showed a trend in favor of the tumor removal but did not detect a statistically significant survival benefit in these patients.[117]

In 2006 Rapiti et al.[119] reported the surgical removal of primary breast cancer in 300 patients with metastatic breast cancer at diagnosis. The data from this study showed a significant survival improvement in patients who had primary tumor removed, particularly when clear margins were obtained. The 5-year breast cancer–specific survival was 27% and 12% for women who had surgical removal of primary tumor with clean margin and women who did not have surgery (*p* = .049), respectively. Similar to what was previously suggested, the benefit was greater in patients with metastases limited to bone.[119]

Another study, using the 1988–2003 SEER program data, analyzed 9734 patients with metastatic breast cancer. Surgery was performed in 47% of the patients, and survival rates were better in women who had surgery for removal of the primary tumor compared with those who did not.[120] Other studies also showed similar results,[121,122] favoring survival improvement by surgery in patients with stage IV disease.

Thus far, the published literature on this topic has all been retrospective in nature, and a major bias of the finding could be that the healthier women with limited tumor metastasis were selected for surgery. Surgical resection, especially with tumor margin clearance, appears to be of some benefit for patients with stage IV breast cancer at time of diagnosis. The benefit seems to be greater in women with limited metastatic disease and favorable response to systemic therapy. Many questions remain unanswered, including timing of surgery, need of axillary dissection, and the role of added radiation therapy in this set of patients.

Modified Radical Mastectomy Technique

The modified radical mastectomy consists of an en bloc resection of the breast, including the nipple-areola complex, the axillary lymphatics, and the overlying skin near the tumor. Several variations of this technique, described by Auchincloss,[19] Handley,[25] and Madden,[20] represent the common technique that preserves the pectoralis major and minor muscles but has incomplete clearance of level 3 axillary nodes. This technique is more likely to preserve the medial pectoral nerve as it penetrates the pectoralis minor muscle. The Patey technique involves removal of the pectoralis minor muscle and complete axillary node dissection.[6,7] Although this technique attempts to spare the medial and lateral pectoral nerves, the more extended nodal removal together with the resection of the pectoralis minor muscle make pectoral nerve preservation difficult to accomplish.

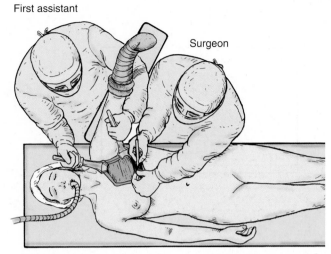

First assistant

Surgeon

• **Fig. 31.11** Position of patient for left modified radical mastectomy at margin of operative table. The first assistant is cephalad to the armboard and shoulder of the patient to allow access to the axillary contents without undue traction on major muscle groups. Depicted is the preferential isolation of the hand and forearm with an occlusive Stockinette cotton dressing secured distal to the elbow. This technique allows free mobility of the elbow, arm, and shoulder to avoid undue stretch of the brachial plexus with muscle retraction.

Anesthesia and Positioning

The patient is positioned supine for induction of general anesthesia. The patient is to be positioned at the edge of the operating table to provide simple access to the operative field without undue traction on the muscle groups and brachial plexus (Fig. 31.11). Further protection of the brachial plexus from shoulder subluxation should be achieved by placing the ipsilateral arm on a padded armboard.

Sterile Skin Preparation

The ipsilateral breast, neck, hemithorax, shoulder, and arm are prepped with the standard povidone-iodine solution or other skin preparation solutions. The preparation should extend well across the midline and include the complete circumferential prep of the ipsilateral shoulder, arm, and hand. The ipsilateral forearm and hand should then be isolated with Stockinette dressing and secured with Kling or Kerlix cotton rolls. Sterile drapes are placed to provide a wide operative field and then secured to the skin. The first assistant is positioned craniad to the shoulder of the ipsilateral breast to provide adequate retraction and arm mobilization without undue traction on the brachial plexus. Once positioning and preparation are complete, adequate mobility of the ipsilateral shoulder and arm should be reassessed before commencing the operation.

Skin Incision and Skin Flap Development

The choice of skin incision and the design of skin flaps are carefully planned with respect to the quadrant in which the primary neoplasm is located so that adequate margins can be ensured and primary closure achieved (Fig. 31.12). In most cases, primary closure is possible unless undue tension or flap devascularization requires extensive margin debridement.

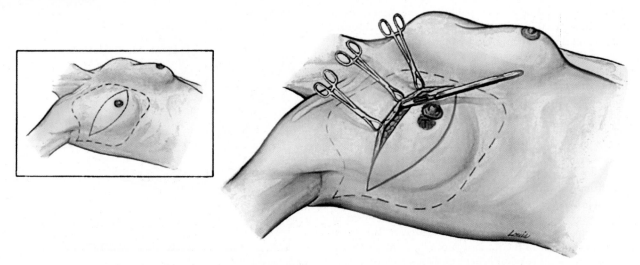

• **Fig. 31.12** *Inset,* Limits of the modified radical mastectomy are delineated laterally by the anterior margin of the latissimus dorsi muscle, medially by the sternal border, superiorly by the subclavius muscle, and inferiorly by the caudal extension of the breast approximately 3 to 4 cm inferior to the inframammary fold. Skin flaps for the modified radical technique are planned with relation to the quadrant in which the primary neoplasm is located. Traditionally, margins are ensured by developing skin edges 3 to 5 cm from the tumor margin. Skin incisions are made perpendicular to the subcutaneous plane. Flap thickness should vary with patient body habitus. Flap tension should be held perpendicular to the chest wall with flap elevation at the plane deep to the cutaneous vasculature, which is accentuated by flap retraction.

The limits of the modified radical mastectomy, regardless of the skin incision used, are delineated laterally by the anterior margin of the latissimus dorsi muscle, medially by the sternal border, superiorly by the subclavius muscle, and inferiorly by the caudal extension of the breast approximately 3 to 4 cm below the inframammary fold.

Skin incisions are made perpendicular to the subcutaneous plane. Retraction hooks or towel clips are placed on the skin margins to provide appropriate elevation and retraction of the skin margin. Retraction should be achieved with constant tension on the periphery of the elevated skin margin at a right angle to the chest wall. The use of "countertraction" against the assistant's traction helps maintain consistent flap thickness and improves visualization within the operative field. Skin flap thickness should vary with patient body habitus but ideally will be 4 to 8 mm. The interface for flap elevation is developed deep to the cutaneous vasculature and should be maintained evenly to provide consistent thickness, which helps avoid devascularization of the tissue planes.

Removal of Breast

Removal of the breast is carried out from superior to inferior with the inclusion of the pectoralis major fascia (Fig. 31.13). The pectoralis major fascia is dissected from the musculature in a plane parallel to the course of the muscle fibers. The operator applies constant inferior traction on the breast and fascia. Multiple perforator vessels will be encountered from the lateral thoracic or anterior intercostal arteries, which supply the pectoralis muscles. These perforators should be identified, clamped, divided, and ligated or clipped.

The breast, inclusive of the skin and elevated pectoralis fascia, should be elevated en bloc. The lateral margin of the mastectomy ends at the anterior margin of the latissimus dorsi muscle. The loose areolar tissue of the lateral axillary space is then elevated after careful identification of the lateral extent of the axillary vein in

its course along the axillary artery and brachial plexus. Dissection craniad to the axillary vein should be avoided because of the risk of damaging the brachial plexus and the infrequent observation of nodal tissue craniad to this vein. However, the axillary vein should be sharply exposed after division of the deep layer of the superficial fascia in the axillary space. All venous tributaries should be divided and ligated. The use of electrocautery should be avoided at this stage because of the risk of thermal damage to the vessel walls and the nearby brachial plexus and motor branches.

Dissection of pectoralis minor begins with proper positioning such that the shoulder of the ipsilateral arm is abducted. The borders of pectoralis minor are delineated and retracted to visualize the insertion of pectoralis minor on the coracoid process, where it can be divided or preserved. Care must be taken to identify and preserve the medial and lateral pectoral nerves because they penetrate the pectoralis minor muscle. These nerves may be sacrificed if pectoralis minor resection is necessary. Resection of pectoralis minor muscle allows for better exposure of level 3 nodes as well as full visualization of the axillary vein along its course beneath this muscle and its entry into the chest wall.

Operative Techniques for Variations of Simple Mastectomy

The surgical techniques for simple mastectomy have evolved over the years. Today most patients opting for mastectomy, whether unilateral or bilateral, choose skin-sparing or nipple-sparing mastectomy when immediate reconstruction is planned unless the skin involvement by cancer is extensive. Although patient preference is an important factor in selecting the type of simple mastectomy, some may not choose nipple-sparing procedure for their cancer treatment, particularly in the presence the following conditions: Paget disease, bloody or clear spontaneous nipple discharge, tumor within 2 cm of nipple, significant ptosis, smoking, and/or

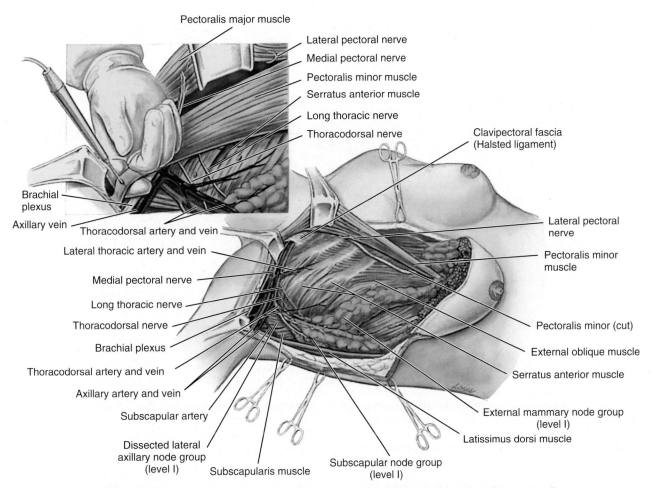

• **Fig. 31.13** *Inset,* Digital protection of the brachial plexus for division of the insertion of the pectoralis minor muscle on the coracoid process. All loose areolar and lymphatic tissues are swept en bloc with the axillary contents. Dissection commences superior to inferior with complete visualization of the anterior and ventral aspects of the axillary vein. Dissection craniad to the axillary vein is not advised, for fear of damage to the brachial plexus and the infrequent observation of gross nodal tissue cephalad to the vein. Investing fascial dissection of the vein is best completed with the cold scalpel following exposure, ligation, and division of all venous tributaries on the anterior and ventral surfaces. Caudal to the vein, loose areolar tissue at the junction of the vein with the anterior margin of latissimus is swept inferomedially inclusive of the lateral (axillary) nodal group (level 1). Care is taken to preserve the neurovascular thoracodorsal artery, vein, and nerve in the deep axillary space. The thoracodorsal nerve is traced to its innervation of the latissimus dorsi muscle laterally. Lateral axillary nodal groups are retracted inferomedially and anterior to this bundle for dissection en bloc with the subscapular (level 1) nodal group. Preferentially, dissection commences superomedially before completion of dissection of the external mammary (level 1) nodal group. Superomedial dissection over the axillary vein allows extirpation of the central nodal group (level 2) and apical (subclavicular; level 3) group. The superomedialmost extent of the dissection is the clavipectoral fascia (Halsted ligament). This level of dissection with the Patey technique allows the surgeon to mark, with metallic clip or suture, the superiormost extent of dissection. All loose areolar tissue just inferior to the apical nodal group is swept off the chest wall, leaving the fascia of the serratus anterior intact. With dissection parallel to the long thoracic nerve (respiratory nerve of Bell), the deep investing serratus fascia is incised. This nerve is closely applied to the investing fascial compartment of the chest wall and must be dissected in its entirety, cephalic to caudal to ensure innervation of the serratus anterior and avoidance of the "winged scapula" disability.

obesity. Surgical delay of complete devascularization of the NAC may improve nipple viability after nipple-sparing mastectomy in women with high-risk conditions such as previous mastopexy or extremely thin patients.[123]

Just as preserving the skin envelope of the breast during mastectomy improves cosmetic outcome, incision placement for mastectomy is also important in the final esthetic appearance. For skin-sparing mastectomy, circumareolar or elliptical incision is the most commonly used approach with different variations of this incision to accommodate other oncologic and body habitus considerations. For nipple-sparing mastectomy, one may choose inframammary fold incision if women have appropriate body habitus, breast size, tumor location, and relationship to the previous incision. Radial or lateral incisions may also be chosen

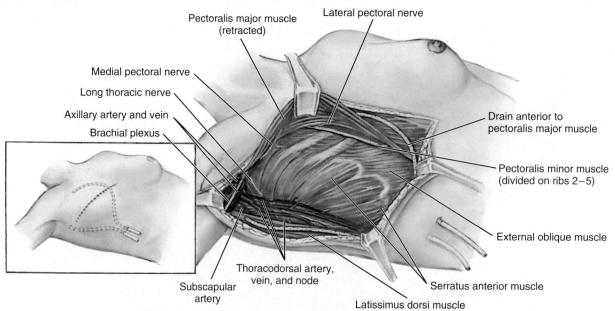

• **Fig. 31.14** The completed Patey axillary dissection variant of the modified radical technique. The dissection is inclusive of the pectoralis minor muscle from origin to insertion on ribs 2 to 5. Both medial and lateral pectoral nerves are preserved to ensure innervation of pectoralis major. With completion of the procedure, remaining portions of this muscle are swept en bloc with the axillary contents to be inclusive of Rotter interpectoral and the retropectoral groups. *Inset,* After copious saline irrigation, closed-suction Silastic catheters (10 French) are positioned via stab incisions placed in the inferior flap at the anterior axillary line. The lateral catheter is placed approximately 2 cm inferior to the axillary vein. The superior, longer catheter placed via the medial stab wound is positioned in the inferomedial aspect of the wound bed anterior to the pectoralis major muscle beneath the skin flap. The wound is closed in two layers with 3-0 absorbable synthetic sutures placed in subcutaneous planes. Undue tension on margins of the flap must be avoided; it may necessitate undermining of tissues to reduce mechanical forces. The skin is closed with subcuticular 4-0 synthetic absorbable or nonabsorbable sutures. After completion of wound closure, both catheters are connected to bulb suction. Light, bulky dressings of gauze are placed over the dissection site and secured in place with occlusive dressings and an Ace bandage.

depending on the other concerns. Preoperative discussion of nipple-sparing mastectomy should include the situations when the NAC needs to be removed after mastectomy for oncologic or other reasons.

Regardless of the type of mastectomy, the anatomic principle of removal of all breast tissue should be adhered to because residual breast tissue can lead to a second breast cancer. It is important to know that not all skin flaps are of equal thickness and that breast tissues interdigitate with subcutaneous fat. One study suggested that most residual breast tissue after skin-sparing mastectomy was detected in the middle circle of the superficial dissection plane and in the outer lower quadrant.[124] Others have suggested that the residual breast tissues could be found in peripheral skin, the inframammary fold, and the NAC.[125–130]

Dissection of Axillary Lymph Nodes

Resection of the axillary nodes is performed en bloc to prevent disruption of lymphatics in the axilla (Fig. 31.14). The dissection begins medially with extirpation of central (level 2) groups and sometimes with apical nodal (level 3) groups. The superomedial-most aspect of the dissection is marked at the costoclavicular ligament to allow the pathologist to examine for extension of nodal disease, which may have subsequent therapeutic and prognostic significance.

Inferolateral retraction of level 2 and 3 nodes, en bloc with level 1 nodal removal, is conducted in a craniad to caudad manner in parallel with the thoracodorsal neurovascular bundle. The loose areolar tissue at the juncture of the axillary vein with the anterior margin of latissimus dorsi is swept inferomedially to include the lateral (axillary) nodal group (part of level 1). Care should be taken to identify and preserve the thoracodorsal neurovascular bundle, which lies deep in the axillary space and is fully invested with loose areolar tissue and nodes of the lateral group. The subscapular nodal group (also level 1) is identified between the thoracodorsal neurovascular bundle and the chest wall. This group is swept away, en bloc, with the attached lateral group. Preservation of the thoracodorsal neurovascular bundle is essential for subsequent breast reconstruction using a myocutaneous flap of latissimus dorsi.

Once the chest wall and medial axillary space are encountered, the long thoracic nerve must be identified and preserved to prevent permanent disability with a winged scapula and shoulder apraxia from denervation of the serratus anterior muscle. The location of this nerve is consistently found applied to the investing fascia of the chest wall and is anterior to the subscapularis muscle. Additional technique includes identification of the serratus anterior and its innervation, the long thoracic nerve, with identification of a consistent venous branch from the thoracodorsal vein that courses medial to the chest wall. This venous branch leads directly to the long thoracic nerve at the juncture of the venous branch with the chest wall. The axillary contents anterior and lateral to this nerve are divided, once again en bloc, with the specimen. Before dividing the inferiormost extent of the axillary contents, the long thoracic and thoracodorsal neurovascular bundles must be visualized and preserved.

Closure

The surgical field is carefully inspected for hemostasis and lymphatic leakage. Points of bleeding or disrupted lymph channels are identified, clamped, and individually ligated. The wound is copiously irrigated with warm saline. The skin margins are carefully inspected for devascularization. Any severely traumatized or devascularized skin edges should be debrided before the closure.

Closed-suction Silastic catheters (10 French) are placed via separate stab incisions that enter the inferior flap near the anterior axillary line. The lateral catheter is placed in the axillary space approximately 2 cm inferior to the axillary vein on the ventral surface of the latissimus dorsi muscle to drain the axilla.

A longer, second catheter is placed into the inferomedial aspect of the wound bed to provide continuous drainage of blood and serum from the space between the skin flaps and chest wall. Both catheters should be secured in place with separate 2-0 nonabsorbable sutures.

The wound is closed in two layers with absorbable 3-0 synthetic suture to approximate subcutaneous tissue and absorbable or nonabsorbable 4-0 synthetic suture to close skin. Steri-Strips are applied perpendicularly to the wound. Suction catheters are connected to bulb suction.

Postoperative Care

The operative dressing should remain intact for 72 hours unless there is concern for flap viability. Suction catheters should remain in place for approximately 1 week until drainage becomes serous and less than 20 to 25 mL over a 24-hour period. Shoulder and arm range-of-motion exercises may be initiated the day after drains are removed.

In the rare cases with protracted serous or serosanguineous drainage, continued suction may be used via the lateralmost (dependent) catheter. Long-term catheter use requires the patient to be instructed in the hygienic care of the catheter and skin wounds as well as frequent dressing changes. Further details regarding protracted wound drainage are provided in Chapter 50 in the discussion of postoperative care after the Halsted radical mastectomy.

Selected References

52. Giuliano AE, Hunt KK, Ballman KV, et al. Axillary dissection vs no axillary dissection in women with invasive breast cancer and sentinel node metastasis: a randomized clinical trial. *JAMA*. 2011;305:569-575.
53. Fu Y, Chung DU, Cao M-A, et al. Is axillary lymph node dissection necessary after sentinel lymph node biopsy in patients with mastectomy and pathological N1 breast cancer? *Ann Surg Oncol*. 2014;21:4109-4123.
75. Fu Y, Zhuang Z, Dewing M, et al. Predictors for contralateral prophylactic mastectomy in breast cancer patients. *Int J Clin Exp Pathol*. 2015;8:3748-3764.
86. Sharpe SM, Liederbach E, Czechura T, et al. Impact of bilateral versus unilateral mastectomy on short term outcomes and adjuvant therapy, 2003–2010: a report from the National Cancer Data Base. *Ann Surg Oncol*. 2014;21:2920-2927.
94. Meijers-Heijboer H, van Geel B, van Putten WL, et al. Breast cancer after prophylactic bilateral mastectomy in women with a BRCA1 or BRCA2 mutation. *N Engl J Med*. 2001;345:159-164.

A full reference list is available online at ExpertConsult.com.

32

Breast Conservation Therapy for Invasive Breast Cancer

AMY E. RIVERE, V. SUZANNE KLIMBERG, AND KIRBY I. BLAND

Breast conservation therapy is the complete removal of breast cancer with a margin of normal tissue surrounding the tumor. This is standardly followed by radiation therapy (RT). The primary goals of breast conservation therapy are to provide a survival equivalent to mastectomy, an acceptable rate of local recurrence, and a cosmetic outcome that is acceptable to the patient.

Historical Perspective

Breast conservation therapy (BCT) for carcinoma was first described in 1924 by Sir Geoffrey Keynes, an English surgeon at St. Bartholomew Hospital in London.[1] Keynes, who used radium seeds as an adjunct to surgery, reported a 5-year survival rate of 77% for women with clinically negative lymph nodes and 36% for those with clinically enlarged lymph nodes (N_1, N_2). In 1939 M. Vera Peters, a radiation oncologist in Toronto, began treating patients who had undergone conservative surgery with radiation.[2–4] By the 1950s and 1960s, breast conservation became increasingly accepted in clinical practice, and in some institutions this therapeutic approach was considered standard. In the early 1970s, several trials were undertaken in an effort to confirm the equivalency of mastectomy and BCT. Six randomized trials[5–17] and two meta-analyses[18,19] conducted in the United States and Europe documented the equivalence of lumpectomy and radiation with mastectomy; this was achieved with a low rate of local recurrence while preserving cosmetic and functional outcome. Four clinical trials now have more than 20 years of follow-up, which further confirm long-term results.[13–16]

At the time of the initial National Surgical Adjuvant Breast and Bowel Project (NSABP) report in 1985 by Fisher and associates,[20] which documented the 5-year equivalence of breast-conserving surgery compared with mastectomy, only 23.9% of stage I breast cancer patients in the United States eligible for breast conservation underwent the procedure. After Dr. Fisher's report, the use of breast conservation increased to 34.6% in the United States for stage I patients according to the Surveillance, Epidemiology, and End Results (SEER) data.[21] In 1990, the National Institutes of Health Consensus Development Conference recommended that breast conservation treatment is an appropriate method of primary therapy for the majority of women with stage I and II breast cancer. Furthermore, it suggested that the procedure is preferable because it provides survival rates equivalent to those of total mastectomy and axillary dissection while preserving the breast.[22] After this landmark recommendation, 53.4% of eligible breast cancer patients in the United States underwent conservative treatment.[21] In an American College of Surgeons Commission on Cancer National Cancer Database (NCDB) study of 16,643 women with stage I or II breast cancer who were treated in 1994, Bland and coworkers[23] confirmed that only 42.6% were treated with a breast-conserving approach. A recent query of the NCDB of stage 0 to II breast cancer included 553,593 patients and showed lumpectomy rates of 66.4%, not significantly changed from 67.7% in 2003. In the group of women who were 45 years old or younger, lumpectomy rates dropped from 61.3% in 2003 to 49.4% in 2010.[24] Most reports indicate that the majority of women who present with breast cancer do not have contraindications to conservative surgery.[24–26] Reasons for underutilization of breast conservation include patient preference, age, and poor prognostic factors. Patient preference is influenced by complex issues regarding access to care, concerns for cancer recurrence, and the impact of surgery on body image and sexuality.[27,28] Medical comorbidity is rarely a major factor in the underutilization of breast-conserving therapy.[26]

Survival

The first and primary goal of breast-conserving surgery is to achieve survival that is equivalent to mastectomy. Six randomized prospective trials comparing breast conservation surgery with mastectomy have been conducted (1972–1989). The specifics of treatment protocols are depicted in Table 32.1. In 2013 van Hezewijk performed a seventh randomized prospective trial evaluating hormonal therapy with a secondary outcome that demonstrated a significantly higher recurrence rate in mastectomy alone but equivalent survival in patients undergoing mastectomy with RT or lumpectomy with RT.[29] No significant differences in overall or disease-free survival rates were evident in any of the trials. The 20-year follow-up has been reported for several of these trials, confirming the long-term survival equivalence.[13–17] Moreover, the Early Breast Cancer Trialists' Collaborative Group performed a meta-analysis, including 3100 patients from seven randomized trials. No difference in 10-year survival was observed (Fig. 32.1).[18] The more recent outcomes data published between 2007 and 2015 have actually demonstrated survival advantage of BCT compared with mastectomy, but most of these studies have been retrospective[30] (Table 32.2).

TABLE 32.1	Prospective Randomized Trials Comparing Breast Conservation With Mastectomy									
							LOCAL RECURRENCE		OVERALL SURVIVAL	
Trial	No. of Cases	Follow-Up (yr)	Tumor Size (cm)	BCT Surgical Margins	RT Boost		BCT (%)	Mx (%)	BCT (%)	Mx (%)
NSABP	1851	20	4	Tumor free	No		14	10	46	47
Milan	701	20	2	—	Yes		9	2	42	41
NCI	247	18	5	Grossly free	Yes		22	6	59	58
EORTC	868	10	5	1-cm gross	Yes		20	12	65	66
Danish	793	20	Any	Grossly free	Yes		NR	NR	58	51
Gustave-Roussy	179	15	2	2-cm gross	Yes		9	14	73	65

BCT, Breast conservation therapy; *EORTC*, European Organization for Research and Treatment of Cancer; *Mx*, mastectomy; *NCI*, National Cancer Institute; *NR*, no response; *NSABP*, National Surgical Adjuvant Breast and Bowel Project; *RT*, radiation therapy.

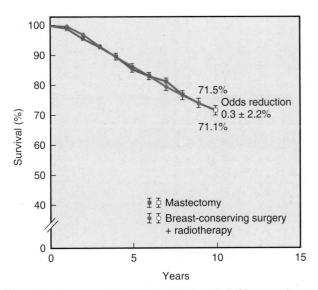

• **Fig. 32.1** Ten-year survival among approximately 3100 women in seven randomized trials comparing mastectomy with breast-conserving surgery plus radiotherapy. Squares represent the women assigned to receive mastectomy, and circles represent those assigned to receive breast-conserving surgery plus radiation therapy. The percentages at the ends of the curves are overall survival rates. (From Early Breast Cancer Trialists' Collaborative Group. Effects of radiotherapy and surgery in early breast cancer: an overview of the randomized trials. *N Engl J Med.* 1995;333: 1454-1455.)

Initiated in the late 1970s, the NSABP B-06 study prospectively randomized 1851 women to receive total mastectomy, lumpectomy, and lumpectomy with radiation. Patients enrolled in this seminal study by Fisher and coworkers[13] had stage I or II breast cancer with tumor diameters that were less than 4 cm. For the lumpectomy candidates, tumors were resected with the intent of removing adequate surrounding tissue that would ensure negative pathologic margins and an acceptable cosmetic outcome. However, approximately 10% of patients in the breast preservation arm had positive margins. Those with positive margins underwent total mastectomy and continued to be followed (Figs. 32.2 and 32.3). Axillary node dissection was performed in all

patients. All patients with positive axillary lymph nodes received adjuvant chemotherapy. Overall cumulative survival at 20-year follow-up was 47% in women treated with mastectomy, 46% in women treated with lumpectomy alone, and 46% in those treated with lumpectomy followed by radiation. The cumulative incidence of death from any cause was 47.7% in women with negative nodes and 63.3% in women with positive nodes[13] (Fig. 32.4).

At 15 years' evaluation, independent prognostic determinants of poor survival were identified from the NSABP B-06 trial. These factors included ipsilateral breast tumor recurrence (IBTR), race, positive nodal status, nuclear grade, histologic type, and patient age. Women younger than 40 years of age and older than 65 years of age had a decreased overall survival compared with women between 40 and 65 years of age.[31] At 20-year follow-up, the IBTR was 39.2% in women who underwent lumpectomy and 14.3% in women who underwent lumpectomy and breast irradiation, but no significant differences in terms of disease-free survival, distant disease–free survival, or overall survival between the three groups.[13]

In a retrospective analysis from the MD Anderson Cancer Center,[32] 1043 women with stage I or II breast carcinoma who were treated with BCT were evaluated with respect to survival. The 5- and 10-year disease-specific survival rates were 94% and 87%, respectively. On multivariate analysis, independent predictors of poor disease-specific (cancer-related) survival included tumor size greater than 2 cm, positive surgical margins, and ipsilateral breast tumor recurrence. Ipsilateral breast tumor recurrence and positive surgical margins have been shown in other studies to be associated with a decreased survival.[31,33,34] These data suggest that aggressive local therapy to minimize ipsilateral breast tumor recurrence is important.

Local Recurrence

The second goal of BCT is to maintain local control with an acceptable rate of local recurrence. Most clinicians agree that a 10-year local recurrence rate of 5% to 10% (<1% per year) is acceptable.[35] Tumor recurrence is defined by most investigators as recurrent tumor at or near the primary site of the index quadrant of therapy. In the randomized and retrospective trials comparing breast conservation with mastectomy, ipsilateral recurrence rates

TABLE 32.2 Studies Comparing Outcomes for Breast Conservation Treatment and Mastectomy

Author/Year	Center/Country	Treatment Period	No. of Pts.	Study Type	Comparison of Survival	Comparison of Local Control	BCT Rate	Results/Comments
Hwang et al. 2013[147]	Duke University, USA	1990–2004	112,154 Stage I, II	Retrospective, California Cancer Registry	HR for OS BCS + RT: 0.72 (0.68–0.76) Mx: 1.0	NR	55%	BCS + RT associated with higher breast cancer specific survival at almost 10-yr follow-up. For every potential confounding factor related to mortality evaluated, women with Mx more likely to die within 3 years.
Agarwal et al. 2014[148]	University of Michigan, USA	1998–2008	132,149 <4 cm <4 LN+	Retrospective, SEER	HR for survival (p <.001) BCS + RT: 1.0 Mx: 1.31 (1.25–1.39) Mx + RT: 1.47 (1.34–1.61)	NR	70%	Patients with BCT improved breast cancer specific survival
Van Hezewijk et al. 2013[29]	Multicenter trial, various countries (TEAM trial)	2001–2006	9231 ER, PR+	Prospective	HR 5-yr OS: (p <.001) BCS + RT: 1.0 Mx: 1.22 (1.02–1.47)	HR for LRR (p = .01) BCS Mx only BCS + RT 1.0 Mx 1.53 (1.10–2.11)	54.1%	Significantly higher LRR in patients with Mx only
Martin et al. 2007[149]	Australian National University	1995–1999	2787	Retrospective	Hazard of death reduced by 55.88%	NR	51.5%	Patients with BCS better survival than mastectomy
Hofvind et al. 2015[150]	Cancer Registry of Norway	2005–2011	9547	Retrospective, Norway Registry	HR of death at 6 yr BCT: 1.0 Mx: 1.7 (1.3–2.4)	NR	61.1%	Women treated with BCT have significantly better breast cancer-specific survival

BCS, Breast-conserving surgery/lumpectomy only; BCT, breast conservation treatment/lumpectomy with radiotherapy; DFS, disease-free survival; ER, estrogen receptor; HR, hazard ratio; LN, lymph node status; LR, local recurrence; Mx, mastectomy; NR, not reported; OS, overall survival; PR, progesterone receptor; Pts, patients; RT, radiotherapy/radiation treatment; SEER, Surveillance Epidemiology and End Results database; TEAM, Tamoxifen Exemestane Adjuvant Multicenter trial.

From Tan MP. Is there an ideal breast conservation rate for the treatment of breast cancer? Ann Surg Oncol. 2016;23:2825-2831. doi: 10.1245/s10434-016-5267-3.

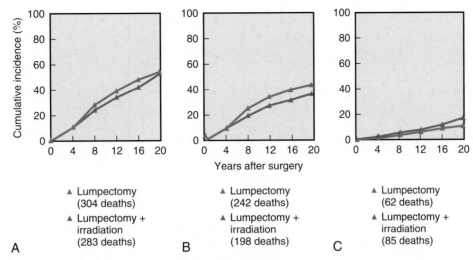

• **Fig. 32.2** Cumulative incidence of death from any cause (A), death after a recurrence or a diagnosis of contralateral breast cancer (B), and death in the absence of a recurrence or contralateral breast cancer (C) in 570 women treated with lumpectomy alone and 567 treated with lumpectomy plus breast irradiation. Data are for women whose specimens had tumor-free margins. (From Fisher B, Anderson S, Bryant J, et al. Twenty-year follow-up of a randomized trial comparing total mastectomy, lumpectomy, and lumpectomy plus radiation for the treatment of invasive breast cancer. *N Engl J Med.* 2002;347: 1233-1241.)

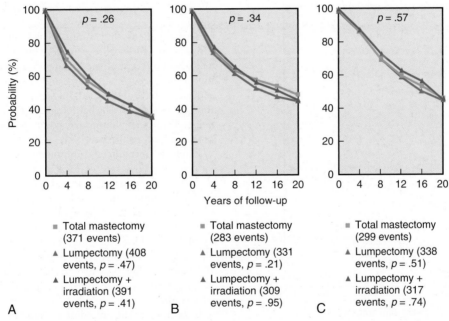

• **Fig. 32.3** Disease-free survival (A), distant disease-free survival (B), and overall survival (C) in 589 women treated with mastectomy, 634 treated with lumpectomy alone, and 628 treated with lumpectomy plus irradiation. In each part, the p values above the curve are for the three-way comparison among the treatment groups, and the p values below the curves are for the two-way comparisons between lumpectomy alone or with irradiation and total mastectomy. (From Fisher B, Anderson S, Bryant J, et al. Twenty-year follow-up of a randomized trial comparing total mastectomy, lumpectomy, and lumpectomy plus irradiation for the treatment of invasive breast cancer. *N Engl J Med.* 2002;347:1233-1241.)

were similar in both groups; local recurrence rates of 5% to 22% have been reported for breast conservation and local recurrence rates of 2% to 14% have been reported for mastectomy[5–17] (see Table 32.1). Modern NSABP protocols of systemic therapy for patients undergoing BCT have demonstrated local recurrence rates of 3% to 6% and 5% to 10% in node-negative and node-positive patients, respectively.[36,37]

In the NSABP B-06 trial, 70% of all ipsilateral breast recurrences occurred within the initial 10 years of therapy (40% in the first 5 years; 30% in the second 5 years)[13] (Fig. 32.5). These data of the NSABP and other institutions demonstrate a persistent risk of local recurrence through 20 years of follow-up.[38–42] In contrast, most local recurrences after mastectomy are evident within the first 36 months.

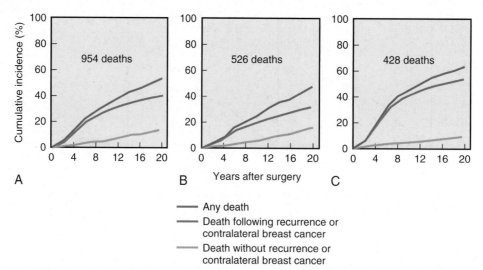

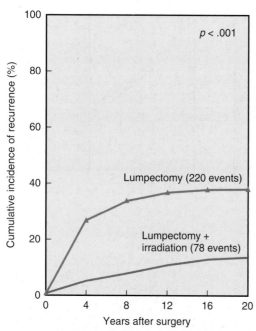

• **Fig. 32.4** Cumulative incidence of death from any cause, death after a recurrence or a diagnosis of contralateral breast cancer, and death in the absence of a recurrence or contralateral breast cancer among all 1851 women (A), 1156 women with negative axillary nodes (B), and 695 women with positive axillary nodes (C). (From Fisher B, Anderson S, Bryant J, et al. Twenty-year follow-up of a randomized trial comparing total mastectomy, lumpectomy, and lumpectomy plus irradiation for the treatment of invasive breast cancer. *N Engl J Med.* 2002;347:1233-1241.)

• **Fig. 32.5** Cumulative incidence of a first recurrence of cancer in the ipsilateral breast during 20 years of follow-up among 570 women treated with lumpectomy alone and 567 treated with lumpectomy plus breast irradiation. The data are for women whose specimens had tumor-free margins. (From Fisher B, Anderson S, Bryant J, et al. Twenty-year follow-up of a randomized trial comparing total mastectomy, lumpectomy, and lumpectomy plus irradiation for the treatment of invasive breast cancer. *N Engl J Med.* 2002;347:1233-1241.)

Risk factors for the development of local recurrence have been evaluated in multiple trials. Paramount in reduction of risk for recurrence in patients undergoing BCT is adequate surgery and the application of RT. Several studies, randomized and retrospective, have confirmed a significantly higher rate of local recurrence

when RT is omitted after breast conservation[6,7,13,43–46] (see Fig. 32.5).

Several patient- and tumor-related issues have been identified as risk factors for local recurrence. Young age is commonly associated with poor pathologic features and typically conveys a higher rate of local recurrence. Kurtz and coworkers[47] and Vrieling and associates[48] have related the increased rate of local recurrence to non–age-related adverse pathologic variables; however, other analyses confirm that young age is an independent risk factor for increased local recurrence.[49–52]

Extensive intraductal component (EIC) has been associated with an increased rate of local recurrence because of a higher likelihood of residual disease and because tumor-free margins are less likely. Tumors are considered to contain an EIC component when more than 25% of the tumor is composed of ductal carcinoma in situ (DCIS), both within the tumor and in the periphery.[53–55] However, a number of studies have confirmed that when negative margins are achieved, as opposed to close or positive margins, the presence of EIC is not associated with an increased rate of local recurrence and does not preclude breast conservation.[56–61]

In addition to the preceding patient- and tumor-related factors, there are treatment-related factors that can decrease the incidence of local recurrence. The addition of adjuvant chemotherapy and hormonal therapy can further decrease the rate of local recurrence. One retrospective study demonstrated a 66% decrease in local recurrence when patients were given adjuvant hormonal therapy.[62] In the NSABP B-13 trial, patients with node-negative, estrogen receptor (ER)–negative disease were randomized to a chemotherapy arm or a no-treatment arm. The 8-year rate of recurrence in the ipsilateral breast was 13.4% in the nontreatment arm but only 2.6% in the chemotherapy arm of the study.[62]

For ionizing RT to be effective in tumor control, the primary tumor must be completely excised with pathologically confirmed negative margins. RT is not delivered as an adjunctive therapy to compensate for inadequate surgery; rather this modality is an adjunct to sterilize the operative field of the index quadrant of therapy. Pathologic margin status is the most important factor associated with ipsilateral breast tumor recurrence. Patients with positive surgical margins may have an associated increased risk of local recurrence (5%–25%).[56,57,63–70] For many years, the recommended margin of tissue surrounding tumor remained in question, but a conference was held in 2014 and, based on a meta-analysis, found that no ink on tumor cells was adequate, and in fact, additional margin distance did not significantly improve ipsilateral breast tumor recurrence or survival.[71] This conference held by the Society of Surgical Oncology (SSO) and American Society for Radiation Oncology (ASTRO), in collaboration with the American Society of Clinical Oncology (ASCO) and the American Society of Breast Surgeons (ASBS).[72–75] Adherence to the consensus recommendation of no ink on tumor provides a means to decrease reexcision rates, improve cosmetic results, and decrease health care costs. It is understood that local recurrence is likely influenced by the interaction of factors and not one factor alone. Wider excision may be necessary with extensive EIC, young age, lack of systemic therapy, or delayed RT to ensure low rates of local recurrence according to Horst and colleagues[72]; however, the SSO/ASTRO consensus reports no decrease in IBTR for young patients, unfavorable tumor biology, lobular cancers, or tumors with EIC when wider margins were taken.[73] The standard treatment of a local recurrence after BCT is mastectomy; however, some have adopted local excision alone for recurrence (e.g., ductal carcinoma in situ or for small invasive tumors), consequently accepting an increased risk of additional recurrence.[35] There are now many studies in support of repeat breast-conserving therapy for IBTR as a safe option in a select group of patients.[76–79] Although there are no prospective trial results comparing breast-conserving surgery with or without RT to mastectomy for IBTR, several retrospective studies have concluded that salvage lumpectomy followed by partial breast irradiation is equal to mastectomy as treatment for IBTR in selected patients—most favorably those >50 years old, those with recurrences (≤2 cm), late recurrences (>48 months), single-site recurrences—and would provide acceptable cosmetic results as suggested by Vila and colleagues.[79] The most commonly used method of partial breast irradiation applied after salvage lumpectomy for IBTR is multicatheter interstitial brachytherapy, but balloon catheter brachytherapy, conformal external beam RT, and intraoperative RT can also be used.[79]

Cosmetic Outcome

An acceptable cosmetic appearance is the third goal of breast conservation surgery. Cosmetic outcome depends principally on the patient's view of the cosmetically acceptable breast; however, many analyses use the radiation oncologist's and/or surgeon's determinants of outcome results (Fig. 32.6). Factors that may affect cosmetic outcome include the volume of tissue removed compared with the breast size and the location of the tumor. Tumors in the medial and inferior breast quadrants, when resected, may result in adverse cosmetic outcome compared with tumors in other quadrants of the breast.[80] In one study of patients' appraisal of cosmetic outcome, 96% of patients found their operated breasts to have an acceptable appearance, and most viewed their operated breasts to have an acceptable ("good") outcome.[81]

In a retrospective review from the Joint Center for Radiation Therapy, the examining physician evaluated the cosmetic outcome. Good or excellent cosmetic outcome was noted in 94% of 655 patients. In this cohort, the extent (volume) of breast tissue resection correlated with the patient's assessment of cosmetic outcome.

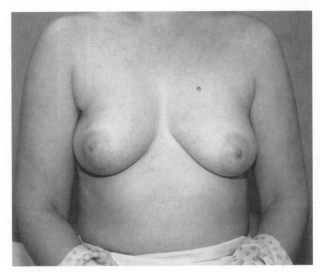

• **Fig. 32.6** Cosmetic results of breast-conserving surgery 5 years after lumpectomy, axillary dissection, and breast irradiation.

When the amount of resected breast tissue was less than 35 cm³, 85% of patients had excellent scores and 96% had good or excellent scores. When the resected breast tissue was larger than 85 cm³, only 51% had excellent scores and 94% had either excellent or good scores.[82] In the study by Cochrane and associates comparing patient satisfaction versus an independent panel assessment of cosmesis, the volume of breast tissue removed was an accurate predictor of cosmesis and patient satisfaction.[80] Other studies examining cosmetic outcome after lumpectomies confirm similar results.[83,84]

A consensus conference, the Collaborative Attempt to Lower Lumpectomy Reoperation Rates (CALLER), was held by the ASBS in 2015 to reduce lumpectomy reoperations and improve cosmetic outcomes. The recommendations reported by Landercaster and colleagues included preoperative imaging with full field digital mammography with ultrasound as needed, minimally invasive breast biopsies for diagnosis, multidisciplinary breast teams, localization techniques for nonpalpable cancers, oncoplastic techniques, specimen orientation of three or more margins, intraoperative surgeon-reviewed specimen radiograph, consideration of shave margins and pathology assessment of margins intraoperatively, compliance with the previously mentioned SSO-ASTRO margin guideline, and routine use of patient reported outcomes specific to breast surgery when feasible.[85]

A randomized controlled trial by Chagpar and colleagues randomized 235 patients intraoperatively who were undergoing partial mastectomy for stage 0 to III breast cancer to have further cavity shave margins or no further margins.[86] The positive specimen margin in both groups was similar before randomization, but the shave group showed a significantly lower positive margin rate than the no shave group (19% and 34%, respectively). In addition, there was a reduction in the rate of reexcision surgery for margin clearance from 21% in the no shave group to 10% in the shave margin group ($p = .02$). Minimizing the need for reexcision to obtain clear margins will be beneficial in terms of cosmetic result after lumpectomy.

Patient Selection

Careful patient selection is essential to ensure a low rate of local recurrence and an acceptable cosmetic outcome. A thorough

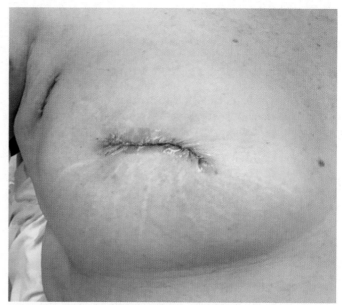

• **Fig. 32.7** Central lumpectomy with excision of the entire nipple-areolar complex for Paget disease of the nipple. This technique can also be used for a tumor that lies just beneath the nipple-areolar complex.

history, physical examination, and mammographic examination are vital in choosing suitable candidates for BCT. Improvement in our understanding of risk factors for local recurrence and improvement in imaging technology have significantly reduced the incidence of local recurrence since the mid-1980s. Patients are not candidates for breast conservation if they have a high probability of recurrence, possess a high probability of complications from RT, have an unacceptably poor cosmetic result, or prefer mastectomy.

Several factors prohibit the use of BCT (Box 32.1). Pregnancy is an absolute contraindication to RT because of radiation scatter and its potential for fetogenesis maturation injury. Although the breast-conserving surgical procedure may be performed during pregnancy, RT should not be delivered in any gestational period. Clearly, the gestational period of greatest fetal risk is the first trimester. Patients with extensive malignant-appearing microcalcifications are not suitable candidates for breast conservation. This mammographic presentation typically suggests diffuse ductal carcinoma in situ. A history of prior therapeutic radiation to the breast region or mediastinum/lung in most circumstances can be prohibitive to conservative surgery with radiation. Finally, patients who have persistently positive margins are unsuitable for breast conservation.[87,88] Two or more primary tumors in separate quadrants (multicentric disease) of the breast may represent a contraindication to breast-conserving surgery. Multifocal (multiple tumors within the same quadrant) disease is typically not a contraindication to breast conservation, if it is possible to perform complete removal of the lesions with negative margins while maintaining a cosmetically acceptable outcome.

Other factors that may contraindicate breast-conserving surgery include a history of collagen vascular disease and a diminutive breast size relative to tumor size. Collagen vascular disease may result in increased toxicity from RT. Neoadjuvant chemotherapy may be offered as an alternative in patients whose primary tumor is too large to undergo breast conservation at initial presentation.[82] Cytoreduction with neoadjuvant chemotherapy does not improve survival but may render some patients who would otherwise have had mastectomy to be candidates for BCT. Family history,[84,87,88] positive lymph nodes, bilateral breast cancer, and lobular histology[89,90] should not exclude patients for breast conservation if otherwise eligible. Paget disease of the breast also should not be excluded from BCT as long as a careful preoperative

imaging assessment of the breast is performed, often including breast magnetic resonance imaging (MRI) due to the frequency of underlying mammographically occult breast cancer as well as multicentricity and multifocality associated with Paget disease. With negative surgical margins and application of adjuvant radiotherapy, a systematic review including 43 studies reported by Helme and colleagues found oncologic outcomes of BCT for Paget to be equivalent to mastectomy.[91] A central lumpectomy with excision of the entire nipple-areolar complex is required for cases of Paget disease of the nipple that qualify for BCT (Fig. 32.7).

Magnetic Resonance Imaging

Several studies have been published indicating that MRI may be a useful adjunct to traditional breast imaging due to its increased sensitivity and specificity compared with traditional breast imaging. MRI has the imaging capability to detect mammographically and clinically occult tumor foci within the ipsilateral breast in approximately 25% of patients with known breast cancer.[92–94] A 2012 European radiologic systematic review and meta-analysis reports MRI detected additional disease in 20% of women on the ipsilateral side and 5.5% in the contralateral breast. In addition, Plana and colleagues reported 12.8% of women with true positive MRI findings converted to a more extensive surgery, most commonly from BCT to bilateral mastectomies.[95] Review of the available literature states clear guidelines for the use of breast MRI in patients with at least a 20% to 25% lifetime risk of the development of breast cancer as a screening tool,[96] but no clear guidelines exist for the use of MRI as a perioperative tool for patients diagnosed with breast cancer.[97] The results of a literature review by Pilewskie and King in 2014 showed little to no statistically significant decrease in IBTR rates, contralateral breast cancer rates, or improvement in survival rates with use of breast MRI. There does appear to be some benefit to MRI for lobular cancers, mammographically occult primary cancers, and measurement of tumor response to neoadjuvant chemotherapy to determine potential for BCT.[97] The role of MRI as a surveillance strategy to follow women post-BCT has not been determined but may have clinical benefit in some high-risk situations and will require additional investigation.[98]

Operative Technique

The goal of breast-conserving surgery is to achieve a low rate of local recurrence while preserving cosmetic outcome. Lumpectomy (segmental mastectomy, partial mastectomy, tylectomy) is the most common form of breast-conserving surgery internationally. Several aspects of technique are emphasized.

Localization

With advances in breast imaging, we have seen an increase in the number of small, nonpalpable breast lesions requiring surgical intervention. A Cochrane review by Chan and colleagues reported that wire-guided localization (WGL) of breast lesions remains the gold standard and in survey results is the predominantly used tool to localize nonpalpable breast lesions for excision.[99] Eleven randomized controlled trials were included with the majority of comparisons of WGL, radioguided occult lesion localization (ROLL), and radioactive iodine (^{125}I) seed localization (RSL). There was no statistically significant difference in terms of successful localization, positive margin rate, and reexcision rate among these options. These are all invasive methods of localization that require an additional procedure before surgery, leading to scheduling conflicts and patient discomfort and inconvenience. Arentz and colleagues reported on their 10-year experience with Hematoma-directed ultrasound-guided (HUG) breast lumpectomy in 2010.[100] They reported a statistically significant decreased positive margin rate on lumpectomies for malignancy using intraoperative ultrasound (IOUS) for HUG compared with performing WGL.[100] A recent review by Volders and colleagues compares the data on IOUS guidance for localization compared with previously mentioned methods. The positive margin rates with IOUS guidance range from 0% to 17% as opposed to the more commonly utilized techniques with rates up to 40% in some studies.[101] In addition, IOUS prevents patients from needing an additional procedure before surgery, thereby alleviating scheduling conflicts and decreasing anxiety and discomfort for the patient.

Incision

An incision corresponding to Langer or Kraissl lines is usually used; although some surgeons prefer radial incisions at the 3, 6, or 9 o'clock positions (Fig. 32.8). In the past, an incision remote from the tumor was inadvisable; however, with the acceptance of oncoplastic techniques, this has become more acceptable. An incision directly over the tumor can always be used, but often can lead to a poor cosmetic result, especially in the upper inner quadrant. Tumors that are very near to the skin surface also typically require an incision directly over the tumor to ensure a negative anterior margin. Today we use a variety of incisions with cosmetic end result in mind, often utilizing a circumareolar incision or in a natural skin fold, where the scar will be somewhat hidden.

Tumor Removal

The tumor is removed so that it is completely surrounded by normal breast parenchyma. The surgeon's objective is to remove

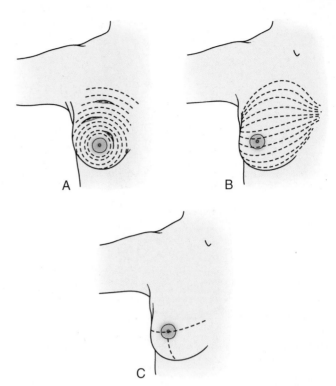

• **Fig. 32.8** Recommended locations of incisions for performing breast conservation. The most cosmetically acceptable scars result from incisions that follow the contour of Langer (A) or Kraissl lines (B). Radial incisions may be preferred for lesions at the 3, 6, or 9 o'clock positions (C).

an amount of tissue adequate to achieve negative specimen margins. An attempted resection amount of 0.5 to 1 cm of grossly normal breast tissue resulted in histologically negative margins in 95% of 239 patients in the experience of Kearney and Morrow.[102] Larger resections may be necessary for invasive ductal carcinomas with EIC and for infiltrating lobular carcinomas; these clinical presentations have convincingly greater probability of pathologic multifocality and multicentricity. Undermining of skin, with thin skin flaps, is strongly discouraged because this technique results in an unfavorable cosmetic result after radiation. Conserving the subcutaneous fat prevents skin retraction and indentation concavity (Fig. 32.9). No special effort is made to include pectoral fascia in the specimen unless the lesion is attached to or approximates this anatomic boundary.

Quadrantectomy

Lumpectomy is the preferred method of breast conservation in North America. Quadrantectomy is an alternative form of breast conservation popularized by Veronesi of the Milan Cancer Center. This technique requires the removal of the neoplasm via a radial incision of T_1 tumors (<2 cm) with a 2- to 3-cm cuff of normal tissue, skin, and pectoralis fascia around the tumor. For tumors located in the upper outer quadrant of the organ, this approach is completed en bloc with the axillary dissection. In the Milan II trial, recurrence was inversely related to the volume of breast tissue resected.[5]

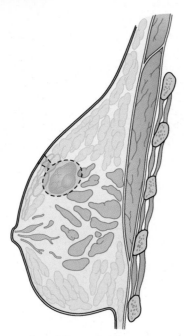

• **Fig. 32.9** Preservation of the underlying adipose and breast tissue prevents an unfavorable cosmetic result.

Oncoplastic Surgery

Oncoplastic breast surgery is an emerging group of procedures that makes it possible for more patients to become candidates for breast conservation; it is covered extensively in Chapter 40. This technique allows patients with larger tumors to preserve the breast with wide excisions and reconstruction of the defect. Without this technique, these patients would either choose a mastectomy or accept an inferior cosmetic outcome.

Oncoplastic surgery can be performed using either volume displacement or volume replacement techniques. Volume displacement techniques allow for reconstruction of the resection defect by transposing tissue from elsewhere in the breast. These techniques can include a batwing mastopexy lumpectomy (Fig. 32.10), radial segmental lumpectomy, donut mastopexy lumpectomy (Fig. 32.11), reduction mastopexy lumpectomy[103,104] (Fig. 32.12), and a round block technique using a periareolar incision especially for inner quadrant lesions. With volume replacement techniques, local tissue such as a latissimus dorsi flap can be used to fill the defect. This may be preferable when volume displacement techniques are unable to provide a satisfactory result with regard to shape and size of the breast, particularly if the patient is unwilling to undergo surgery on the opposite breast. See Chapter 40 for additional details on oncoplastic breast surgery.

Evaluation of Margins

Gross assessment of specimen margins is important to ensure adequate surgical excision of the neoplasm. Minimal manipulation of the lumpectomy specimen during excision allows for optimal margin evaluation by the pathologist. Close or involved margins can be immediately reexcised when determined on gross examination by the surgeon. Intraoperative ultrasound (IOUS) guidance may be used to view the presence of tumor within the specimen ex vivo and perform an ultrasound assessment of margins.[100,101] As previously mentioned, in the ASBS consensus

on reduction of lumpectomy reoperations, intraoperative surgeon-reviewed specimen radiograph was recommended as a tool to decrease positive margin rate and therefore reduce reexcision rate.[85] An additional tool recommended by the consensus is to mark at least three sides of a lumpectomy specimen to indicate the in vivo orientation of the tissue, allowing for margin directed targeting of specific tissue location in cases of required reexcisions.[85] The surgeon may use a variety of techniques to prepare the specimen for pathologic analysis by spatially orienting the specimen in three-dimensional planes. Indelible ink or sutures should be used to indicate the cephalad, caudad, medial, lateral, anterior, and posterior margins to enable the pathologist to properly orient the specimen before sectioning. Some surgeons prefer to perform oriented "shave margins" for each of the biopsy cavity walls. These procedures are completed in the event of close or positive margins so that limited, "margin-directed" reexcision can be performed if necessary. This technique further provides pathologic correlation with the specimen margins. In Chapgar's previously mentioned randomized shave margin trial, the reexcision rate was diminished by half in the group that underwent cavity shave margins.[86] As an alternative, Klimberg and colleagues performed "touch-prep" cytology for intraoperative evaluation of margin status with a sensitivity of 96.39% and specificity of 100%, but the process is time-consuming and expensive.[105] Once gross removal is adequate, intraoperative imaging has been performed, and the specimen is properly oriented with markings, histologic analysis with permanent sectioning of the lesion is performed by the pathologist.

There has been strong evidence that the standard of care is percutaneous diagnostic breast biopsy rather than excisional biopsy due to an increased ability to achieve negative margins at the time of surgery.[85,106–108] With core biopsy directed by ultrasound or stereotactic guidance technology, precision in biopsy is assured. This approach allows the greatest probability of clear histologic margins at first attempt of segmental resection, thus reducing unnecessary reexcisions.

Closure

After meticulous hemostasis of the lumpectomy site has been achieved, the wound is closed. Many surgeons attempt oncoplastic parenchymal reconstruction to close "dead space" of the surgical defect. No drain of any type (open/closed) is placed in the wound. The deep dermis (cutis reticularis) is approximated using an absorbable suture. The skin is then carefully approximated with a continuous monofilament subcuticular suture of absorbable material or Dermabond may be used to seal the incision.

Reexcision

Reexcision for invasive breast cancer should be undertaken for patients with either unknown margins or positive margins defined as ink present on tumor upon pathology review. Reexcision is reported as necessary in 20% to 30% of breast-conserving surgeries,[84,102] but with the SSO/ASTRO consensus guideline of no ink on tumor for reexcisions,[73] the necessary rate of reexcision should decline.[74,75] Pathologically positive margins increase the likelihood that residual cancer will be evident with reexcision. Several studies have demonstrated that on reexcision for positive margins, 40% to 70% of women will have residual disease.[33,57,68,102,109,110] In patients with close margins (<2 mm), reexcision demonstrated residual disease in 22% to 25%.[57,68,110] According to the

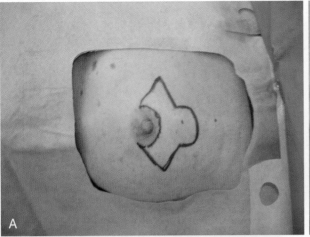

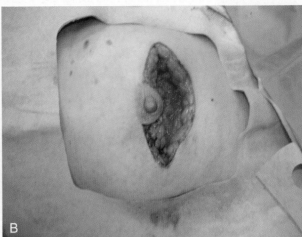

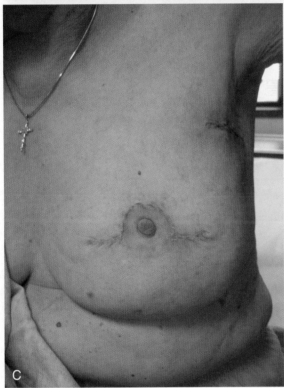

• **Fig. 32.10** Batwing mastopexy lumpectomy for large subareolar breast cancer. (A) Preincision markings after ultrasound localization of the tumor. (B) Intraoperative defect cavity after lumpectomy is performed. (C) The final result is a lift of the breast, often performed bilaterally.

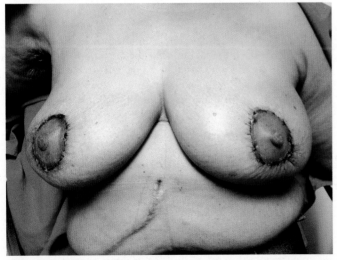

• **Fig. 32.11** Donut mastopexy lumpectomy. A bilateral Benelli lift-type procedure is performed after the lumpectomy specimen is removed from the affected breast.

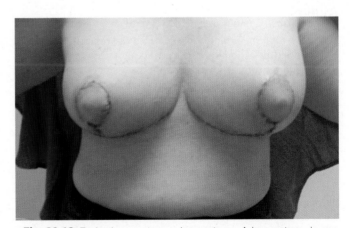

• **Fig. 32.12** Reduction mastopexy lumpectomy. A lumpectomy is performed in the affected breast, followed by bilateral mastopexy to create symmetry.

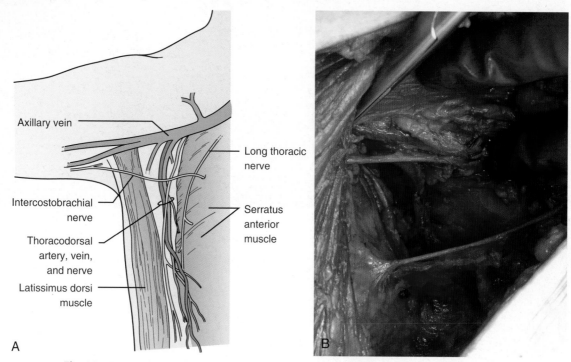

• **Fig. 32.13** The axilla. Schematic drawing labeled with the contents of the axilla (A) and the axilla in vivo after an axillary lymph node dissection has been performed (B).

meta-analysis of 33 studies and 28,162 patients produced from the consensus on specimen margins, positive margins were associated with at least a twofold increase in IBTR compared with patients with negative margins, despite the addition of boost RT, endocrine therapy, or having tumors with favorable biology.[73] In addition, there was no significant benefit to obtaining wider margins on specimens in cases of invasive lobular cancer, patients aged 40 years and younger, or patients with EIC in contrast to the current National Comprehensive Cancer Network and other guidelines that margins less than 1 mm are considered inadequate for ductal carcinoma in situ.[73,111] When a repeat operation is required for patients with initially positive or unknown margins in an attempt to obtain negative margins, the risk of recurrence equates to an initially resected negative margin.[58]

Axilla

Sentinel lymph node biopsy has replaced the necessity for initial axillary node dissection for most patients with breast cancer. Decision regarding surgical therapy of the breast does not influence the decision for axillary surgery. The current standard of care is to reserve axillary node dissection for patients with positive sentinel nodes or for those with contraindication(s) to sentinel lymph node biopsy. The purpose of both axillary dissection and sentinel node biopsy is to stage the patient's disease regarding lymph node involvement with tumor. The therapeutic and survival advantage (or lack thereof) afforded by axillary node dissection is controversial. The specifics of sentinel node biopsy and management of the axilla are extensively discussed elsewhere in this text (see Chapters 41 to 43).

With the exception of high-lying neoplasms of the axillary tail of Spence, the incision used for axillary dissection is separate from that used for removal of the index tumor in the breast. A curvilinear transverse incision is preferred just below the axillary hairline, preferably in a skin fold. For patients with small stature, exposure of the axilla may require a curved, nonradial incision that parallels the latissimus dorsi posteriorly and the pectoralis muscle anteriorly.

Traditional axillary dissection includes nodal groups from axillary levels I and II (Fig. 32.13). The anatomic delineation of this dissection includes the anterior belly of the latissimus dorsi muscle laterally, the axillary vein superiorly, caudal and ventral surfaces of the axillary vein, the medial border of the serratus muscle medially, and the teres major muscle posteriorly. Removal of the pectoralis minor muscle is not advised, except when palpable nodes are evident at level III; this clinical presentation may require a level III dissection. The thoracodorsal nerve and long thoracic nerves to the latissimus dorsi and serratus anterior muscles, respectively, should be identified and preserved. The intercostal-brachial nerve should also be preserved when possible to maintain sensation to the axilla and medial arm. The axillary vein should be visualized on its ventral and caudad surface and preserved because it is dissected beneath the pectoralis minor muscle. These boundaries represent the minimal limits for the dissection. Although the surgical site in the conserved breast is not drained, a closed-suction drain is left in the axilla for 5 to 10 days postoperatively until drainage approximates less than 20 to 30 mL per day.

Radiation Therapy

Radiation and Its Role in Breast Conservation

RT remains a key component in the delivery of breast-conserving therapy. As mentioned previously, the rationale behind its use is to eliminate residual occult microscopic disease in the breast after lumpectomy. Six randomized trials[10,13–17] and two meta-analyses[18,112] have established the role of lumpectomy and RT in accomplishing the goal of locoregional control and organ preservation, as well as providing survival outcomes that are equivalent to those achieved with mastectomy. The largest trial is the NSAPB B-06; its 20-year follow-up continues to demonstrate a statistically significant decrease in local failure and a trend toward improved disease-free survival ($p = .07$) in the group that received RT compared with the group who received lumpectomy alone.[13] Importantly, the lumpectomy plus RT group also continued to demonstrate no difference in survival compared with the mastectomy group, a finding that has been confirmed with equally long follow-up in a second randomized trial from the Milan group,[14] as well as from both the Danish breast-conservation randomized trial[16] and the European Organization for Research and Treatment of Cancer (EORTC).[15]

In 2005, the Early Breast Cancer Trialists' Collaborative Group published a meta-analysis demonstrating an absolute survival benefit at 15 years of follow-up in 7300 patients treated with breast-conserving surgery and RT of 5.4% ($p = .0002$).[112] This translated clinically into the prevention of one disease-related death for every four invasive cancer recurrences prevented by RT. It was the first publication documenting a survival benefit in early-stage breast cancer patients treated with RT. This proportional reduction in mortality from the reduction in locoregional recurrences held true for all women treated with RT, irrespective of age or tumor characteristics, and it was seen in both prior and more recently performed clinical trials (with or without systemic therapy).

Radiation Therapy Versus No Radiation Therapy

Before the demonstration of a proportional survival advantage in early-stage breast cancer patients treated with RT, several groups initiated investigations questioning whether a subset of patients with favorable disease could be identified and treated successfully with lumpectomy alone, thus avoiding RT. The NSABP addressed this question in women with tumors measuring 1 cm or less (T_{1a}, T_{1b}), who were randomized to tamoxifen alone, RT alone, or tamoxifen and RT.[113] The trial was stratified by age (≤ 49 or ≥ 50), with approximately 80% of women entered older than 50 years of age, and 70% of the tumors measuring 5 to 10 mm in size (T_{1b}). The study found a statistically significant reduction in ipsilateral breast tumor recurrences for patients receiving RT versus tamoxifen alone ($p = .008$), as well as a further reduction in ipsilateral breast tumor recurrence when tamoxifen was added to the RT compared with RT alone ($p = .01$). Six additional randomized trials performed in favorable subsets of patients with early-stage disease have also confirmed a decrease in locoregional recurrence with the addition of RT.[44–46,114,115] Table 32.3 illustrates the locoregional recurrence rates for patients prospectively randomized to

TABLE 32.3 Ipsilateral Breast Tumor Recurrences in Patients Treated With Lumpectomy Alone on Randomized Trials

Study	N[A,B] Surgery Alone TAM	RT	TAM+ RT	Systemic Therapy CMF	TAM	Tumor Size (cm)	Nodal Status	Age (yr)	% IBTR Surgery Alone TAM	RT	TAM + RT	Follow-up TAM	RT	TAM + RT
Fisher et al., 2002[113]	334	332	334	—	+ TAM in 2/3 arms	≤1	–	Any	22.8%	11.7%	4.4%	89.2 mo	85.8 mo	86.9 mo
Fisher et al., 2002[113]	334	332	334	—	—	≤1	+/–	Any	16.5%	9.3%	2.8%		8 yr	
Clark et al., 1996[44]	207/421			—	—	≤2	–	≥50	22.4%				10 yr	
Forrest et al., 1996[45]	126	125		ER–	ER +	≤2	+/–[c]	≤70	26.2%	4%			5.7 yr	
Liljegren et al., 1999[115]	197	184		—	—	≤2	–	≤80	24%	8.5%			10 yr	
Renton et al., 1996[46]	210	208		ER–	ER +	≤5	+/–	Any	35%	13%			82 mo	
Holli et al., 2001[114]	71	80		—	—	<2	–	>40	18.1%	7.5%			6.7 yr	
Fyles et al., 2004[116]	383	386		—	+	≤5	–	≥50	17.6%	3.5%			8 yr	
					+	≤2[b]	–	≥50	5.9%	0.4%			5 yr	
Hughes et al, 2004[117]	319	317		—	+	≤2	–	≥70	4%	1%			5 yr	

[a]Patients with one or more positive lymph nodes received systemic therapy with melphalan and fluorouracil.

[b]Subgroup analysis of 611 women with T1 ER-positive lesions.

[c]Premenopausal women with positive nodes were excluded.

CMF, Cyclophosphamide, methotrexate, fluorouracil; *ER*, estrogen receptor; *IBTR*, ipsilateral breast tumor recurrence; *LN*, lymph node; *RT*, radiation therapy; *TAM*, tamoxifen.

nine clinical trials investigating whether surgery alone would provide adequate locoregional control in a "low-risk" subset.

However, two randomized trials have identified a subset of patients aged 60 years and older whose recurrence rates remain acceptably low at 5 years of follow-up.[116,117] In the Hughes trial,[117] women 70 years of age or older with clinical stage I, ER-positive breast cancers were randomized after lumpectomy with negative margins (no tumor at ink) to receive tamoxifen plus RT or tamoxifen alone. Axillary node dissection was allowed but discouraged, and thus the majority of patients (63% in tamoxifen plus RT and 64% in tamoxifen alone) did not have surgical nodal assessment. At 5 years, locoregional control was superior with the addition of the RT arm (LRR of 1% vs. 4%, $p < .001$); however, this low failure rate in the tamoxifen-only arm was thought to be clinically acceptable. This trial (conducted from 1994 to 1999) was updated at San Antonio in 2006 with a median follow-up of 8.2 years and confirmed the initial findings of clinically low rates of recurrence in the tamoxifen-only arm, but the Cancer and Leukemia Group B (CALGB) 9343 trial data was updated in 2013 demonstrating that at 10 years, 98% of patients in the tamoxifen plus RT arm were free from local and regional recurrence compared with only 90% of those receiving tamoxifen alone.[118,119] Survival was found to be equivalent between the groups.

The second trial by Fyles and coworkers randomized 769 women 50 years of age or older with stage T_1 to T_2, N_0, ER-positive breast cancers to lumpectomy and RT plus tamoxifen versus tamoxifen alone.[116] Pathologically negative nodes were required for entry. However, a subset of patients did not undergo surgical axillary staging (17.1% RT plus tamoxifen and 17.5% tamoxifen-only arms) but were N_0 by clinical staging. At 5 years, the rate of relapse in the ipsilateral breast was 7.7% in the tamoxifen versus 0.6% in the RT plus tamoxifen group ($p < .001$), and this increased to 17.6% versus 3.5% at 8 years. Other variables associated with local relapse on univariate analysis included higher pathologic grade, larger tumor size (T_2), negative receptor status, and treatment with tamoxifen alone. A subgroup analysis of 193 women with tumors 1 cm or less in diameter, ER-positive receptors, and 60 years of age or older showed no significant difference in the rate of local relapse (1.2% in the tamoxifen group vs. 0% in the tamoxifen plus RT group, $p = .16$) at 5 years.

Although these trials provide encouraging results for the subset of patients 60 to 70 years of age or older with small (≤2 cm), node-negative, ER-positive tumors, it is important to keep in mind that longer follow-up in other randomized trials has demonstrated higher rates of failure over time, and this risk persists beyond 20 years. As RT has continued to demonstrate a significant reduction in locoregional recurrence in both trials, and because radiation is generally well tolerated, individualized recommendations regarding the need for adjuvant RT should take physiologic age and life expectancy into consideration.

A Cochrane based systematic review included four large multicenter trials with high-quality randomization procedures to evaluate the benefit of RT with BCT for a diagnosis of DCIS.[120] There was a statistically significant reduction in ipsilateral breast recurrence with a hazard ratio of 0.49 (95% confidence interval 0.41–0.58, $p < .00001$). All analyzed subgroups showed benefit from the use of radiotherapy supporting its use for all women undergoing lumpectomy for DCIS.

As an alternative to RT in patients who are at low risk for recurrence and therefore may gain minimal if any benefit from RT, radiofrequency ablation can be considered intraoperatively after lumpectomy. We initially reported on a 100-patient pilot trial with a 5-year disease-free survival of 88% with only two patients having true in-breast recurrences. Three patients had recurrences at the biopsy needle tract, not considered true in-breast recurrences, and two elsewhere recurrences. Excellent or good cosmetic outcome was reported by 92% of patients, and there was a low complication rate of 6%.[121] A 250-patient multicenter trial has been completed and is awaiting trial maturity.[122]

Radiation Therapy Sequencing

The sequencing of radiation and chemotherapy after surgery is beyond the scope of this chapter. However, in patients with negative nodes and small ER-positive tumors who do not require chemotherapy as part of their treatment, radiation may commence after surgery. A retrospective analysis performed at Harvard in the 1980s compared 653 patients with node-negative stage I to II breast cancer who received breast-conserving surgery followed by postoperative radiation at three intervals after surgery: within 4 weeks (n = 283), from 5 to 8 weeks (n = 308), and from 9 to 12 weeks (n = 54).[123] This study confirmed no increase in local recurrences in patients who received radiation within 8 weeks postoperatively. Definitive conclusions were not drawn with regard to the 9- to 12-week group because of accrual of small numbers.

A retrospective analysis from the Netherlands reported the results of treatment with breast-conserving therapy and postoperative radiation for 514 stage I to II cancers and found that the surgery-radiotherapy interval along with T-stage and margin status were independent predictors of recurrence ($p < .05$).[124] Several other retrospective analyses have suggested that there is an increased risk of local recurrence at 5 years when RT is delayed more than 8 weeks after surgery.[125–130] A recent meta-analysis reviewing 10 retrospective studies and 7401 patients has confirmed a 62% increased risk of local recurrence for patients treated with breast-conserving surgery and radiation at an interval of 9 to 12 weeks compared with one of less than 8 weeks.[129] Finally, a SEER analysis, which included 13,907 women 65 years of age and older with stages I to II breast cancer, reviewed factors associated with the time interval between surgery and the initiation of RT and whether delay in treatment influenced survival.[130] The authors noted an association between the delay in initiation of RT (>3 months) and older age, black race, advanced stage, single status, and the presence of excess comorbidities. Although uncommon, these delays were associated with poor survival. In the absence of prospective data, it is safe to recommend that the surgery-radiation interval should not exceed 8 weeks, and the RT should preferably commence within 6 weeks.

Radiation Therapy Technique

Standard technique to deliver whole breast radiation has traditionally consisted of opposed tangent fields applied to the ipsilateral breast and chest wall. Attempts to improve dose homogeneity through the treated tissue historically relied on the application of devices or manipulation of variables that modulate the radiation beam, such as the addition of wedges, use of higher beam energies, or change in beam weighting. More recently, several institutions have investigated the use of intensity modulated RT (IMRT) to achieve superior dose homogeneity and coverage and/or avoidance of normal tissue. Two prospective randomized trials in women with early-stage breast cancer have now demonstrated an improvement in acute and late toxicity in the treated breast with the use of IMRT compared with standard tangents.[131,132] In the Canadian trial, 358 patients were randomized to standard breast RT or IMRT. The IMRT group had a significant improvement in dose distribution, and this translated into a significant reduction in moist skin desquamation (31.2% with IMRT vs. 47.8% with standard treatment, $p = .002$).[132] In the British trial, 306 women with larger breast size were randomized between standard two-dimensional radiotherapy versus three-dimensional IMRT.[131] The primary end point was change in breast appearance scored from serial photographs taken at 1, 2, and 5 years after RT. The group receiving standard RT was 1.7 times more likely to experience a change in breast appearance compared with patients treated with IMRT ($p = .008$). Additional significant improvements in the IMRT group included a reduction in palpable induration in the center of the breast, the pectoral fold, the inframammary fold, and the boost site. There were no reported differences between groups with regard to breast firmness, tenderness, or quality of life.

Although these data with IMRT are encouraging, follow-up is limited, and some authors have raised concerns regarding the risk of second malignancies and the effect of low-dose spillage and its late influence for tissue toxicity, especially in the setting of cardiotoxic drugs.[133,134] Larger trials with longer follow-up and assessment of these end points are necessary to establish this technique as a new standard.

Radiation Dose: The Use of a Tumor Bed Boost

Doses used to boost the tumor bed after whole breast radiation generally range from 10 to 20 Gy and can be delivered with either an appositional electron beam, a conformal photon field arrangement, or through brachytherapy. A recent report from the William Beaumont Hospital reviewed the results for 552 stage I and II breast cancer patients treated with external beam radiation to the whole breast followed by an electron, photon, or interstitial brachytherapy boost. The authors noted no significant difference in either local recurrence rates or cosmetic outcome between the techniques.[135] The issue of using a radiation boost was a subject of controversy for many years, in part because of the comparable results of the NSABP B-06 trial, which did not incorporate a boost, to trials that used this additive therapy. In 1997 a trial published from Lyon, France, randomized 1024 patients with tumors measuring 3 cm or less to receive 50 Gy of radiation to the whole breast followed by either a 10-Gy boost to the tumor bed or no further therapy. The results confirmed a statistically significant decrease in local recurrence at 5 years in the group receiving a boost (3.6%) compared with the group who received no further therapy (4.5%, $p = .044$).[136]

In 2001, the European Organization for Research and Treatment of Cancer prospectively randomized 5318 patients with stage I or II breast cancer and microscopically negative margins on resection to receive 50 Gy of radiation to the whole breast, followed by randomization to either a 16-Gy boost to the tumor bed or no further therapy.[137] Patients with positive nodes received adjuvant systemic therapy, equating to chemotherapy in the premenopausal patients and hormonal therapy in the postmenopausal patients. This study has recently been updated, confirming the local control benefit from the addition of a boost, with a median follow-up period of 10.8 years.[138] The actuarial rate of local recurrence at 10 years was 10.2% for those receiving no further treatment, compared with 6.2% for those receiving a boost ($p < .0001$). Although patients 40 years of age or younger experienced the largest risk reduction from the addition of a boost (23.9% vs. 13.5%, $p = .0014$), the relative risk reduction (41%) was significant in all age groups.

Length of Radiation Treatment

Standard RT generally consists of 45 to 50 Gy delivered daily in 25 to 28 fractions with tangential beams to the breast plus-or-minus surrounding lymphatics, followed by a boost to the tumor bed of 10 to 20 Gy. Three randomized trials investigating shorter treatment intervals and/or alternative fractionation schemes have been reported, and they have demonstrated equivalent local control and cosmetic effects between the shorter (3- to 4.5-week) and standard (5-week) fractionation arms.[139–141] Haviland and colleagues reported an update on 10 years of follow-up using a hypofractionated RT regimen of 40 Gy over 13 to 15 fractions with equal safety and efficacy to the standard 25 fractions.[142]

Several alternatives to whole breast RT have been developed decreasing the radiation field as well as the time course of administration. These come in the form of interstitial catheters, applicator-based brachytherapy, and external beam RT, typically given over the course of 1 week.[119] There are ongoing trials awaiting maturation of data on long-term outcomes of accelerated partial breast irradiation, but at 6.7 years after ASTRO stratified patients into suitable, cautionary, and nonsuitable groups in terms of the use of three-dimensional conformal external beam RT, we find that all three groups had a 1.2% ($P = .99$) or less tumor bed recurrence rate.[119]

In addition, another partial breast treatment method for local therapy consists of a single treatment of intraoperative RT (IORT). The ELLIOT trial compared IORT with electrons to whole breast RT in 1205 patients and concluded that overall survival was equal, but the IBTR was significantly higher in the IORT arm at 11.3% at 5 years in the higher risk group; however, there were fewer patients with skin and pulmonary damage in the IORT group.[143,144] Similarly, the TARGIT-A trial used 50-kV x-rays (IORT) compared with whole breast external beam RT showing a 5-year recurrence rate of 3.3% and 1.3%, respectively ($p = .042$).[145,146] This technique is only available at specific centers due to the high cost of establishing the technology for IORT and its unknown long-term follow-up data.

Selected References

13. Fisher B, Anderson S, Bryant J, et al. Twenty-year follow-up of a randomized trial comparing total mastectomy, lumpectomy, and lumpectomy plus radiation for the treatment of invasive breast cancer. *N Engl J Med*. 2002;347:1233-1241.

71. Houssami N, Macaskill P, Marinovich L, Morrow M. The association of surgical margins and local recurrence in women with early-stage invasive breast cancer treated with breast-conserving therapy: a meta-analysis. *Ann Surg Oncol*. 2014;21:717-730.

85. Landercasper J, Attai D, Atisha D, et al. Toolbox to reduce lumpectomy reoperations and improve cosmetic outcome in breast cancer patients: The American Society of Breast Surgeons Consensus Conference. *Ann Surg Oncol*. 2015;22:3174-3183.

86. Chagpar AB, Killelea BK, Tsangaris TN, et al. A randomized, controlled trial of cavity shave margins in breast cancer. *N Engl J Med*. 2015;373:503-510.

98. Shah C, et al. The role of MRI in the follow-up of women undergoing breast-conserving therapy. *Am J Clin Oncol*. 2016;39:314-319.

100. Arentz C, et al. Ten-year experience with hematoma-directed ultrasound-guided (HUG) breast lumpectomy. *Ann Surg Oncol.* 2010;17:S378-S383.
101. Volders JH, et al. Current status of ultrasound-guided surgery in the treatment of breast cancer. *World J Clin Oncol.* 2016;7:44-53.
111. Gradishar WJ, et al. National Comprehensive Cancer Network Clinical Practice Guidelines in Oncology. Version 2.2016. https://www.nccn.org/professionals/physician_gls/pdf/breast.pdf.
118. Hughes KS, et al. Lumpectomy plus tamoxifen with or without irradiation in women age 70 years or older with early breast cancer: long term follow-up of CALGB 9343. *J Clin Oncol.* 2013;31:2382-2387.

A full reference list is available online at ExpertConsult.com.

33

Breast Reconstruction and Oncoplastic Surgery

ERIC J. WRIGHT, GORDON K. LEE, CRISTIANO BONETI, LUIS O. VASCONEZ, AND JORGE I. DE LA TORRE

Just as the surgical management of breast cancer has evolved, so too has the field of breast surgery. Patient and surgeon expectations are no longer limited to recreating a breast mound but instead to recreate esthetically pleasing, symmetrical breasts, thus improving the quality of life and body image.[1] The number of women undergoing reconstruction continues to increase each year.[2] Breast reconstruction must be accomplished without handicapping any future treatment for the breast cancer and keeping the operation relatively simple, reproducible, and, most important, safe. The surgical changes in the treatment of breast cancer have changed dramatically from the Halsted radical mastectomy to the breast-conserving therapies of today.[3] To perform breast reconstructions or breast reductions, one must know the ideal esthetics of the breasts, the diagnosis, and the surgical reconstructive objectives. This chapter covers breast reconstruction after mastectomies, breast reductions, and oncoplastic breast surgery, an evolving field that combines all available techniques. The surgical description of common reconstructive techniques is described.

Role of Reconstruction in Breast Cancer Treatment

Breast reconstruction is performed to correct anatomic abnormalities, and thus it is always a functional procedure. It is expected that any reconstructive breast procedure will improve appearance after mastectomy or radiation injury. After the passage of a 1998 federal law that ensures coverage from insurance providers for breast reconstruction in the setting of breast cancer treatment, the prevalence of reconstruction continues to increase.

Until the late 1970s and early 1980s, breast reconstructions were mostly performed in delayed fashion after mastectomy. At that time, there were a number of concerns about performing immediate breast reconstruction related to the oncologic safety of reconstruction: the possibility of hiding local recurrences, seeding of the breast tumor throughout the chest or donor site, and interference with adjuvant chemotherapy.[4]

Many studies have subsequently been done to address each concern for immediate breast reconstruction.[5–9] As far as oncologic safety is concerned, most local recurrences occur either in the subcutaneous tissue or along the scar within 3 years after the mastectomy.[10] This is true regardless of whether the patient has undergone breast reconstruction. Multiple studies have confirmed the safety of immediate breast reconstruction, even for patients with advanced disease.[11–13] Consequently, recurrences are easily detected with palpation or inspection. To address the concerns of seeding the donor site, reconstructive surgeons, in cooperation with oncologic surgeons, have adopted two separate surgical fields including all instruments. One study demonstrated that the majority of the patients who underwent immediate reconstruction were able to initiate adjuvant chemotherapy within 6 weeks of mastectomy and reconstruction.[14] A significant percentage of patients who underwent mastectomy without reconstruction had the institution of adjuvant chemotherapy delayed beyond 6 weeks as a result of the persistence of seromas along the axilla or chest skin flap necrosis. The overall complication rates for these two groups of patients were also identical (18%).

Several determining factors are reviewed with the patient before deciding on the type of breast reconstruction. Each of the techniques described in this chapter has advantages and disadvantages. Factors include the type of mastectomy (i.e., nipple- and skin-sparing technique vs. standard modified radical mastectomy), body habitus, opposite breast size and shape, previous abdominal surgery, history of smoking, and of course the overall health of the patient. Equally important is a comprehensive understanding of breast cancer. Patients expected to receive postoperative radiation will have irreversible changes to the chest wall tissues that inevitably alter the final cosmetic result. A discussion with the patient regarding the expected outcomes needs to occur, and in selected cases, delaying the reconstruction process may be the best option for those who want the best result. Finally, the wishes and desire of the patient are considered when determining the best reconstructive plan. The decision of breast reconstruction should involve a multidisciplinary team coordinated with all of the treating specialties.

The reconstructive breast surgeon should be familiar and proficient at performing all reconstructive options. Each patient has her specific goals and challenges, and thus there is no standardized procedure that fits all breast reconstructions. Preoperative

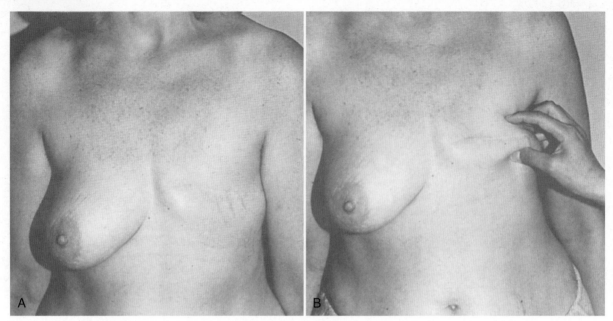

• **Fig. 33.1** (A and B) Ideal low and oblique modified mastectomy closure. The breast skin is slightly redundant, and the inframammary fold is still present.

evaluation and counseling on the reconstruction options and expectations are critical to achieve the desired results.

Definition of the Mastectomy Deformity

Mastectomy

From the standpoint of the reconstructive surgeon, the ideal total mastectomy should preserve the pectoralis major muscle and skin that is not essential to the tumor resection. When this approach is used, the functional considerations of mobility of the shoulder and soft tissue coverage of the ribs are achieved (Fig. 33.1). Extensive skin excision, which results in a tight skin closure, has not been shown to enhance survival, but it does make reconstruction much more difficult. Autogenous flaps are needed after mastectomies with a radical skin excision.

The placement of the incision for a non–nipple- or skin-sparing mastectomy is an important factor that determines the overall outcome. In this regard, the foremost consideration is to place the incision in the appropriate lines of skin tension. It is easy to identify the exact direction of the skin tension lines by pinching the skin to accentuate the wrinkles. Rather than using the standard transverse ellipse, an incision is chosen in the lower or lateral breast, which provides adequate access for any mastectomy. A low and oblique closure is preferred because it is better hidden and offers much better shoulder and chest mobility than a higher incision. The worst choice for a closure in a patient who will eventually have a breast reconstruction is the transverse Patey incision. It is inelastic and unexpandable and results in the least attractive scars (Fig. 33.2). Large-breasted women with grade II to III ptosis can have the skin flap size reduced with a Wise-pattern reduction technique, described later in this chapter. With the continued increase in nipple-sparing mastectomy, several studies have been published regarding the ideal incision location.[15,16] The two commonly advocated locations are the infero-lateral inframammary incision and the vertical infraareolar incision. The decision for the location of the incision for

nipple-sparing mastectomy procedures should be based on the oncologic surgeon's ability to safely perform the mastectomy and the reconstructive surgeon's experience.

Partial Mastectomy/Lumpectomy

The biggest advantage of breast conservation is the preservation of breast sensation. Even though some reconstructed breasts may look as good as natural breasts, we currently do not have reconstruction techniques that can restore nipple sensation. When a complete mastectomy is not performed, the residual defect resulting from the partial mastectomy or lumpectomy can be addressed by several methods. This has created the term *oncoplastic breast surgery*.[17] With this procedure, different pedicles of breast tissue can be elevated to recontour the breast. Various techniques to reconstruct the breast using reduction mammaplasty techniques have been described in the patient undergoing breast conservation therapy and radiation.[18] Larger defects can be filled with autogenous flaps, with or without skin to allow for a natural shape. The favorable nature of the partial mastectomy defect is the reason that a central tumor should never be the sole justification for choosing a complete mastectomy instead of lumpectomy and radiation. When the lumpectomy deforms the breast, and even when it is necessary to remove the nipple, conservation therapy is still a good option.

Reconstructive Surgical Methods

Early on, radical mastectomy was the only treatment for breast cancer. Wide and extreme resections of the breast and skin were performed and allowed to heal in by granulation. This changed after World War II with the greater use on sheet skin grafting, developed in the 1920s. Sheet skin grafting was only used in major centers until the development of the Brown dermatome in the 1950s. By the 1960s, extensive skin flap elevation and primary closure were accepted as safe, having been introduced 20 years earlier.[19] Tube skin grafts were initially used for the most widely

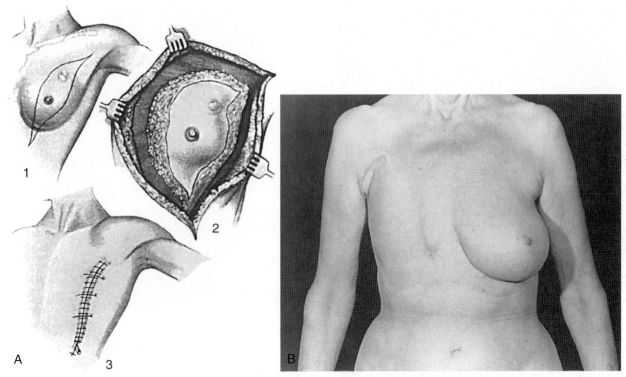

• **Fig. 33.2** (A) Illustration from *Geschickter's Diseases of the Breast* (1943). Note the extent of the proposed skin excision in this simple mastectomy, in which primary closure is obviously a challenge. (B) A 1979 clinical example of this mastectomy with a vertical closure demonstrates the same principles of wide skin excision, performed nearly 40 years later.

accepted tissue reconstruction[20] (Figs. 33.3–33.6) but were arduous and impractical for chest wall reconstruction. Tansini used a latissimus dorsi myocutaneous flap in the early 1900s[21–24] (Fig. 33.7) primarily for wound closure (Figs. 33.8–33.10), and the technique is basically how it is performed today. The slow implementation of the latissimus flap was due in part to the opposition of stalwarts like Halsted who did not think it was safe.[22,25] Tissue reconstruction of chest wall defects after mastectomy became more widely used by the 1970s and in the 1980s when Hartrampf introduced the pedicled abdominal flap.[26]

Early breast implants were made of polyurethane foam, paraffin, or allogenic implants. To avoid some of the severe complications that were reported, silicone gel implants were introduced and popularized by Cronin and Gerow.[27–29]

Tissue Expansion/Implants

The initial experience with prepectoral placement of implants was complicated by capsular fibrosis and capsule formation, erosion of skin, and distortion of the shape of the reconstructed breast. To solve this problem, tissue expanders were introduced in the early 1980s.[30] Expanders allowed extension of the skin as well as the underlying muscle, and implant reconstruction gained acceptance with this advance.[9] After the wound heals, gradual expansion allows for formation of an appropriate size pocket for an implant. With the wide use of skin- and nipple-sparing techniques, expansion of the submuscular pocket is still necessary, even though the skin does not need expansion. The expander fills the void of the extirpated breast so that the overlying spared skin does not wrinkle. Full tissue coverage requires long surgical times.

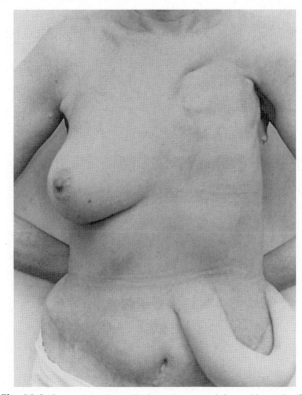

• **Fig. 33.3** Correction of a radical mastectomy defect with a tube flap, created from the abdominal panniculus.

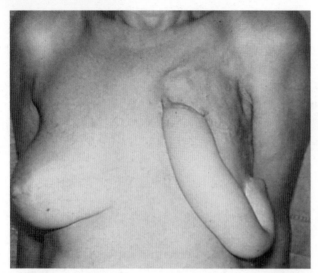

• **Fig. 33.4** Intermediate inset of the tube flap after separation from its abdominal blood supply. This process of "waltzing" a tube-flap from the abdomen to the chest was used by Halsted and Billroth.

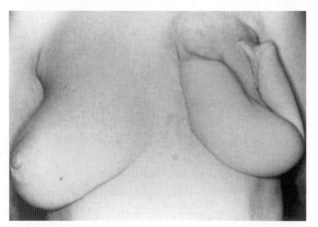

• **Fig. 33.5** Final inset into the sternum before shaping.

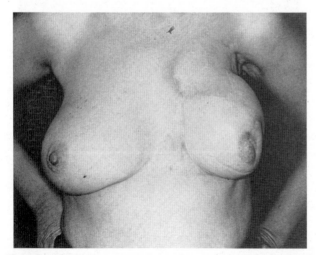

• **Fig. 33.6** The lateral half of the tube flap was then detached laterally and inset into the upper sternum to create the breast shape. This type of reconstruction usually took more than a year to complete, with more than a dozen procedures.

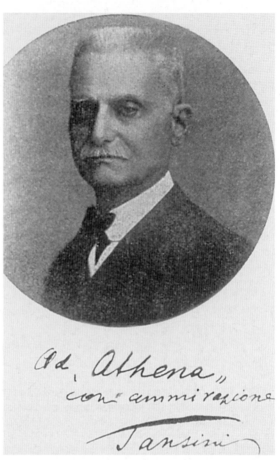

• **Fig. 33.7** Iginio Tansini, the distinguished professor of surgery at the University of Pavia at the turn of the 20th century. The Tansini method of mastectomy used the latissimus dorsi myocutaneous flap to close the radical mastectomy. His primary closure predated sheet skin graft closure by some 20 years. (From Maxwell GP. Iginio Tansini and the origin of the latissimus dorsi musculocutaneous flap. *Plast Reconstr Surg*. 1980;65:686-692.)

Pectoralis coverage with partial sling matrix coverage is expensive but requires less operative time. Explantation rates are generally low and secondary to infection and, more rarely, pain. If expanded too quickly, necrosis of the overlying skin or disruption of the suture line can occur. Despite a complication rate of up to 30%, selected groups have learned to do this well, with acceptable complication rates.[31,32] With the advent of tissue matrix to cover the implant, the patient can undergo direct-to-implant placement.[33,34] Although useful for the avid athlete, the cosmetic result of direct to implant is estimated to be 90% of the submuscular implant because tension on the skin has to be limited. For the right patient, cosmesis can be excellent.

Reconstruction With Acellular Dermal Matrix

In the past, reconstruction with implants placed subcutaneously resulted in numerous complications. The technique evolved to a subpectoral muscle placement with elevation of the serratus muscle or just its fascia to cover the lower and lateral aspect of the submuscular pocket. The concept changed with the introduction of acellular dermal matrix (ADM), used as an inferior sling to cover the lower pole of the implant.[35] The ease of use and availability of ADM makes it an attractive adjunct to this method of

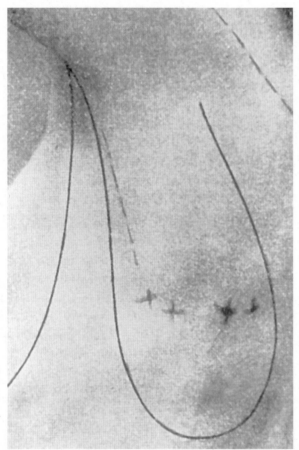

• **Fig. 33.8** Outline of the latissimus myocutaneous flap in the lateral view. Skin was carried on the anterior surface of the latissimus muscle in this proximally based flap. (From Maxwell GP. Iginio Tansini and the origin of the latissimus dorsi musculocutaneous flap. *Plast Reconstr Surg.* 1980;65:686-692.)

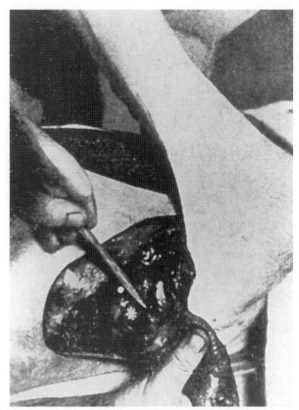

• **Fig. 33.9** Elevation of the latissimus flap with the patient in the supine position. The radical mastectomy defect is seen anteriorly. Note that Professor Tansini is operating without gloves. (From Maxwell GP. Iginio Tansini and the origin of the latissimus dorsi musculocutaneous flap. *Plast Reconstr Surg.* 1980;65:686-692.)

reconstruction, where most of the current reconstructions are subpectoral and sub-ADM over the lower portion of the implant.

The use of ADM has generated its own problems, including prolonged seroma, infection, and increased cost. A modification to the technique is reconstruction with an implant covered circumferentially with ADM and placed in the subcutaneous position.[36]

Surgical Technique for Tissue Expander/Acellular Dermal Matrix

The patient is prepped with new drapes after completion of the mastectomy. The arms have been secured in an extended position, allowing for the patient to be placed in the sitting position during the procedure. The mastectomy skin flaps are assessed for perfusion, and hemostasis is obtained. The pectoralis major muscle is elevated from the lateral border, releasing the inferior attachments from the chest wall up to the sternal attachments. A tissue expander is chosen based on the chest diameter. The lateral border is marked extending over the serratus muscle in accordance with the diameter of the expander. A piece of ADM is then sutured to the inframammary fold medially and to the chest wall laterally following the curvature of the chest. Once the ADM is secured, the tissue expander is placed in the subpectoral/sub-ADM pocket. The pectoralis is then sutured over the superior portion of the ADM. The expander can be inflated to a point where no tension

has been placed on the skin. With nipple-sparing mastectomies, greater expansion allows for more appropriate placement of the nipple, which aids in the postexpansion position. Two drains are placed exiting the pocket in the inferolateral position. The skin edges are trimmed because of the trauma of retraction during the case. A three-layered closure is performed (Figs. 33.11–33.13).

Myocutaneous Flaps

Subpectoral implants are useful when most of the skin of the breast can be saved. However, in the face of the removal of large amounts of skin as in the modified radical mastectomy and radical mastectomy, muscle and skin coverage is needed.

Surgical Technique of the Latissimus Flap

Latissimus dorsi breast reconstruction was reintroduced in the 1970s. Latissimus reconstruction allows for replacement of the shape of the pectoralis muscle and breast and skin. However, the latissimus does not have enough volume to be used by itself for a full breast. Use with an underlying implant was initially good but deteriorated over time.[37] Nevertheless, the latissimus dorsi myocutaneous flap gave the first acceptable results with breast reconstruction after radical mastectomy.

The patient should be marked preoperatively in an upright standing position. The transverse skin island to be used should be no wider than 6 cm and should be fashioned at the approximate level of the bra strap. Depending on the preference of the operating team, the plastic surgeon can harvest the latissimus

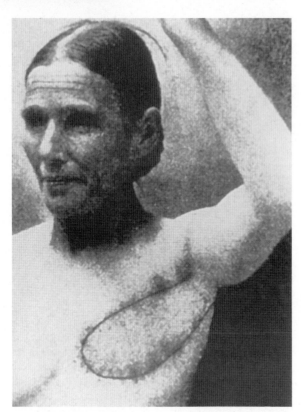

• **Fig. 33.10** Transposed latissimus flap into the left radical mastectomy defect. Instead of taking months to heal the wound, the latissimus flap provided immediate closure. Halsted called this myocutaneous flap procedure "unnecessary and hazardous," even though it was the predominant method of mastectomy closure in Europe at the time. (From Maxwell GP. Iginio Tansini and the origin of the latissimus dorsi musculocutaneous flap. *Plast Reconstr Surg*. 1980;65:686-692.)

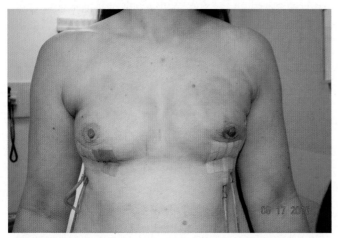

• **Fig. 33.11** The immediate postoperative picture after bilateral nipple-sparing mastectomies with immediate tissue expander placement in a 40-year-old woman.

in the lateral decubitus position, and the flap can be placed in the axilla and closed. The patient can then be repositioned supinely, and oncologic team removes the breast. This minimizes the amount of patient turning on the operating table. Alternatively, the mastectomy can proceed first with subsequent harvest of the latissimus. When axillary node dissection or sentinel lymph node biopsy is to be performed, care should be taken by the

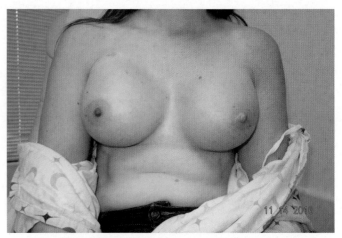

• **Fig. 33.12** Completion of the expansion process.

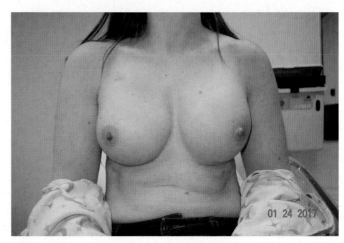

• **Fig. 33.13** Final result after removal of the tissue expanders and placement of the permanent implants.

oncologic team not to damage the blood supply to the flap, the thoracodorsal vessels. After dividing the peripheral origin of the muscle, the skin and underlying muscle are rotated into the breast pocket through a subcutaneous tunnel and sutured to the anterior chest wall. This creates the pocket for an implant. Together with the muscle and subcutaneous fat, the transfer creates the new breast mound.[38] The autogenous latissimus dorsi flap is also the procedure of choice for partial mastectomy defects rather than the more complex TRAM flap. If less than 50% of the breast volume is removed, the autogenous latissimus flap can result in perfect correction for lumpectomy-irradiation failures that require mastectomy.

Irradiated skin is best excised if damage is considerable and should be avoided in areas of skin with telangiectasia, dermal and subcutaneous atrophy, edema, and, in some cases, subcutaneous fibrosis to avoid postoperative skin necrosis, implant extrusion, and wound infection or disruption. At a minimum, the skin flap should be elevated and, if possible, at the submuscular plane. If an implant is used, it must be covered in its entirety with muscle because if the irradiated skin disrupts, the implant will be protected by the muscle layer. There is a greater chance for more severe capsular contracture in postirradiated patients, but the latissimus dorsi myocutaneous flap itself is quite safe and can even be used to cover radiation-exposed implants (Figs. 33.14–33.19).

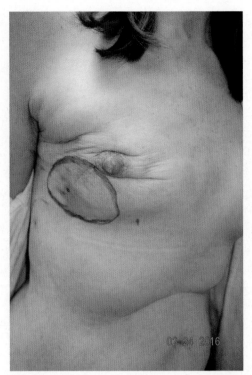

• **Fig. 33.14** History of mastectomy and radiation with soft tissue scarring and radiation skin changes in a 43-year-old woman. Area marked in the circle is planned for excision and replacement with the latissimus muscle flap skin.

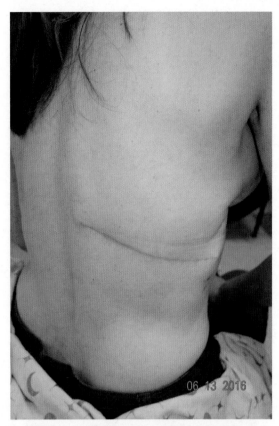

• **Fig. 33.16** Postoperative latissimus donor site scar within the bra line.

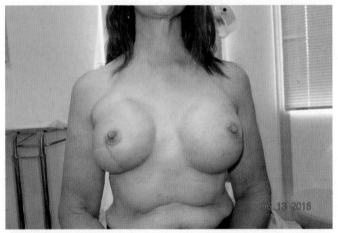

• **Fig. 33.15** Postoperative result after expansion of the latissimus muscle flap and placement of the permanent implant.

Surgical Technique of the Thoracoepigastric Flap

The thoracoepigastric flap is a useful and safe method to add skin and protective coverage to an implant in the most precarious area, the lower pole of the implant. It is a transposition flap, and the secondary defect can usually be closed primarily by advancing the lower abdominal skin with a scar lying close to the inframammary fold.[39] The outlining of the thoracoepigastric flap should be made to extend no further than the midaxillary line, preferably to the anterior axillary line. The flap is outlined at what the surgeon perceives to be the inframammary fold and is elevated at the subfascial levels along the axillary line, superficial to the anterior

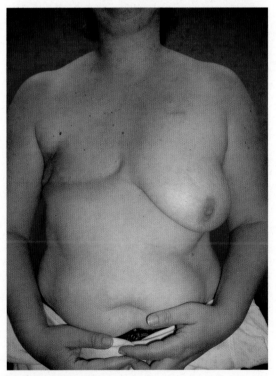

• **Fig. 33.17** History of delayed reconstruction. This 39-year-old woman has a history of radiation. Preoperative picture before a latissimus flap and tissue expander placement.

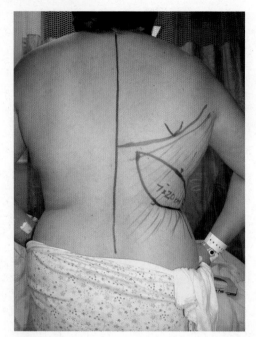

• **Fig. 33.18** Latissimus flap preoperative markings.

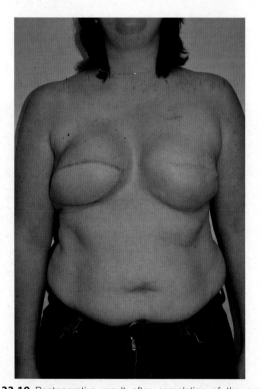

• **Fig. 33.19** Postoperative result after completion of the expansion process and placement of the permanent implant. The latissimus skin component was used to make the inferior pole of the breast after excision of the radiated skin.

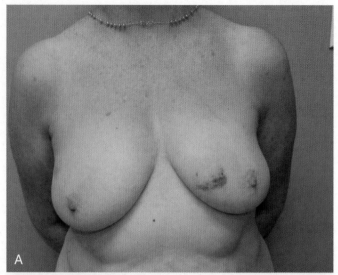

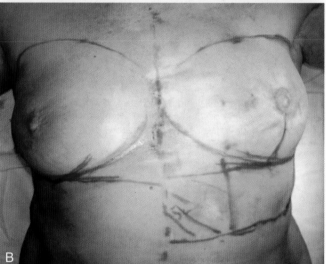

• **Fig. 33.20** (A) A 63-year-old woman undergoing left mastectomy for a stage II breast cancer. (B) Intraoperative markings of the limits of the breast and thoracoepigastric flap design.

rectus sheath. The blood supply of the flap is provided by the perforating vessels from the epigastric arcade, which usually emerge approximately 4 to 5 cm from the midline. At least one of these perforators, or preferably two or three, should be preserved. If necessary to obtain the length of the flap and allow it to reach to the lateral aspect of the defect to be reconstructed, it is preferred that the surgeon back-cuts the flap at the midline of the abdomen, thus preserving the perforators. The medial dissection should stay away from these perforators. The secondary defect is usually closed with minimal or no undermining by advancing the abdominal skin. The flap is effective in providing coverage to the lower portion of the reconstructed breast, which is usually done with an implant. The upper portion of the implant is covered with the pectoralis major muscle, but its coverage is precarious in its lower half (Figs. 33.20–33.22).

Surgical Technique of the Abdominal Transverse Rectus Abdominis Myocutaneous Flap

The era of autogenous myocutaneous flaps began in 1982 with the description by Hartrampf of the pedicled transverse rectus abdominis myocutaneous (TRAM) flap.[40,41] This procedure was the first breast reconstruction using only living tissue, and it achieved the first uniformly good results with any type of mastectomy. The pedicled TRAM is based on the superior epigastric vessels and typically involves dissection of the entire rectus abdominis muscle. The flap is then tunneled through a subcutaneous tunnel to the

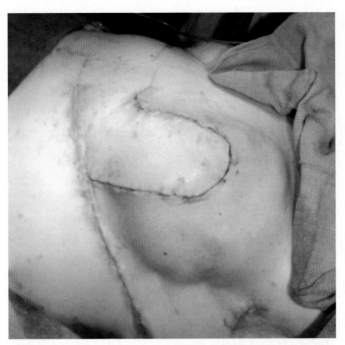

• **Fig. 33.21** Intraoperative view of the flap inset over a silicone implant.

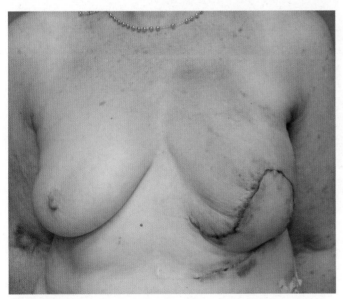

• **Fig. 33.22** Postoperative anterior-posterior view of early postoperative result.

chest. In the 1990s, microvascular transfer of the TRAM flap expanded the indications for the breast reconstruction to high-risk patients who were not acceptable candidates for the pedicle TRAM flap,[42,43] such as patients with diabetes, smokers, obese patients, and those who have had previous radiation. The deep inferior epigastric vessels, with their greater blood supply to the flap, were used for flap perfusion, requiring anastomosis to either the thoracodorsal or internal mammary vessels. However, similar to the pedicled TRAM, the entire rectus abdominis muscle is used for the flap. As the techniques of microsurgery and anatomic knowledge of the abdominal wall perfusion improved, the use of perforator flaps evolved. The deep inferior epigastric vessels branch into medial and lateral rows before entering the rectus muscle. As

the branches travel superiorly, perforating vessels (perforators) branch traveling superiorly to supply the overlying subcutaneous tissue and skin. Dissection of these perforators allowed for the preservation of the surrounding rectus muscle. A muscle-sparing TRAM is performed when a small muscle cuff is taken around the perforating vessels. When all muscle is preserved, it is known as a deep inferior epigastric perforator (DIEP) flap. The DIEP flap has been shown to be a safe option with less abdominal wall morbidity compared with pedicled and free TRAM flaps.

For all of the abdominally based flaps, the lower abdominal skin and subcutaneous tissue, similar to what is discarded for an abdominoplasty, is used to reconstruct the breast. For the muscle-sparing TRAM and DIEP flaps, dissection proceeds laterally to medially until the lateral row perforators are seen. Dissection then proceeds from the medial aspect, identifying the medial row of perforators. Once the perforator options have been determined, a decision is made as to which will be used for flap perfusion. The fascia is incised around the chosen perforators, and intramuscular dissection is performed until the perforator joins the deep inferior epigastric vessels on the underside of the rectus muscle. The medial row perforators are preferred because the innervation to the rectus muscle will be maintained. Once the deep inferior epigastric vessels have been freed, the flap is ready for harvesting. The chest must be prepared with exposure of the internal mammary vessels or thoracodorsal vessels. The internal mammary vessels are more commonly used because of the ability to shape the breast tissue in a more medial position. The third costocartilaginous segment is removed along with the intercostal muscles to expose the internal mammary vessels. Using microsurgical techniques, the vessels of the flap are anastomosed with the chest vessels. The abdominal fascia is closed, followed by skin closure after drain placement. If the flap is performed in an immediate reconstruction, the skin can be deepithelialized, leaving only a small segment to be used for postoperative monitoring. In the delayed setting, the inferior pole of chest skin is removed (Figs. 33.23–33.25).

Other nonabdominally based breast reconstruction options exist. Patients who have had previous abdominal surgeries including abdominoplasty are not candidates for TRAM/DIEP flaps. With these patients, another option is the use of gluteal tissue, known as superior gluteal artery perforator (SGAP) or inferior gluteal artery perforator (IGAP) flaps.

Oncoplastic Surgery

The combination of oncologic treatment with reconstruction principals at the time of resection is called oncoplastic surgery. In breast cancer, it is usually applied to cancers treated with partial mastectomy where the reconstruction is accomplished by mobilizing the remaining breast tissue to restore the natural shape of the breast. It is often accompanied by a contralateral breast reduction for volume symmetry. Several studies have demonstrated the safety of this approach but have also shown that it leads to larger resection volumes.[44,45] To perform an oncologically sound excision and a safe reconstruction, this technique requires extensive knowledge of various breast reduction pedicles. Some defects are more amenable to oncoplastic procedures than others (e.g., inferior and lateral defects) (Figs. 33.26–33.27).

Reconstruction With Fat Grafting

With recent advances in fat grafting techniques and the popularization of fat grafting as a universal filler,[46] select patients may

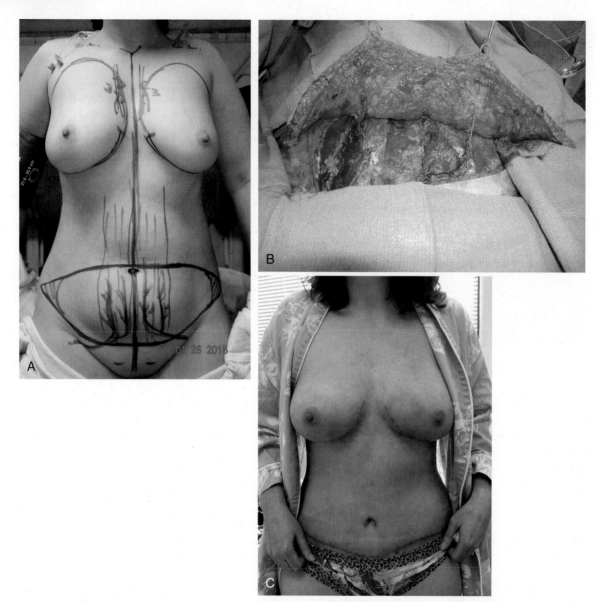

• **Fig. 33.23** (A) Preoperative markings of a deep inferior epigastric perforator flap for immediate bilateral breast reconstruction. The deep inferior epigastric vessels are marked. In addition, the third rib is marked for the planned segmental cartilage resection for access of the internal mammary vessels. (B) Intraoperative photo after flap elevation and perforator dissection. (C) Postoperative results.

undergo reconstruction with autologous fat grafting alone. The ideal method is still evolving, but several theories exist. The work pioneered by Dr. Roger Kouri suggests that the recipient area may require previous suctioning to increase the subcutaneous space and improve neovascularization; other surgeons believe that shearing forces between harvest and grafting play a more significant role in graft take versus reabsorption. The disadvantages of this method of reconstruction include the need for multiple procedures at 3-month intervals, fat necrosis, infection, and inability to obtain symmetry with a large opposite breast.

Opposite Breast Considerations

The most immediate deformity occurring from unilateral breast cancer treatment is asymmetry. Aside from esthetic deformity and the psychological impact it causes, if a significant volume difference exists, the resulting weight imbalance leads to severe back and neck pain. Therefore to treat or prevent such deformity and disability, contralateral breast procedures can be performed to alleviate the symptoms. Currently, there is increased demand for immediate symmetry procedures.

Reduction Mammaplasty

Macromastia is the condition of having abnormally large breasts. Clinically the condition is defined as breast hypertrophy with associated pathologic findings that are the direct or indirect result of excess breast weight, volume, and/or breast malposition. Although breast hypertrophy can result in symptomatic macromastia, because body shapes and sizes vary widely, no universal measurements exist to describe clinically important macromastia. Large breasts can impede physical activities such as exercise, sports, and strenuous work. The inframammary fold can be

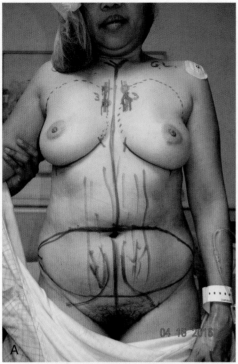

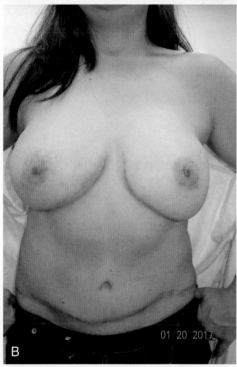

• **Fig. 33.24** (A) Preoperative markings on 45-year-old woman planned for immediate bilateral breast reconstruction after mastectomies with bilateral deep inferior epigastric perforator flaps. The flaps will be deepithelialized beneath the mastectomy skin. (B) Postoperative results.

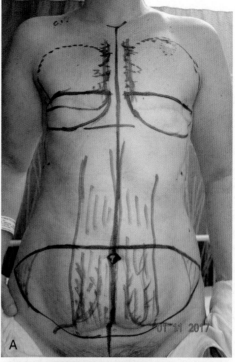

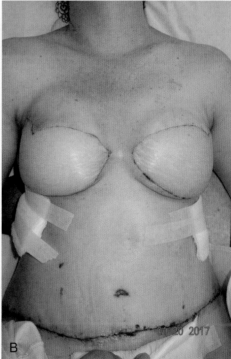

• **Fig. 33.25** (A) Delayed breast reconstruction with bilateral deep inferior epigastric perforator flaps. Inferior pole of the breast skin will be excised and replaced with the abdominal skin to allow for improved breast shape. (B) Early postoperative results.

difficult to reach for many of these patients, making hygiene in this region more arduous. This inframammary skin is at risk for maceration and intertriginous changes and therefore infection.

Although surgical treatment for macromastia has been described for more than 100 years, early techniques involved mastectomy or simple amputation of the breast. Because most of

the essential technical elements of reduction mammaplasty had been developed by the 1930s, further advancement resulted from refinements in skin incision placement, pedicle design, and parenchymal resection patterns.[47] In 1956, Wise expanded this concept, resulting in the inverted T scar.[48] In addition to constructing a classification system for breast ptosis, in 1976 Regnault described

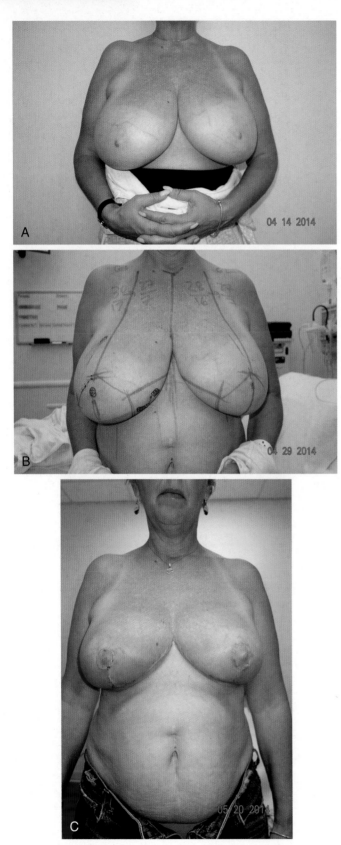

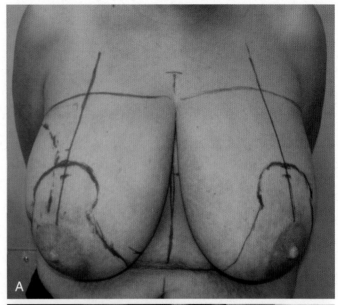

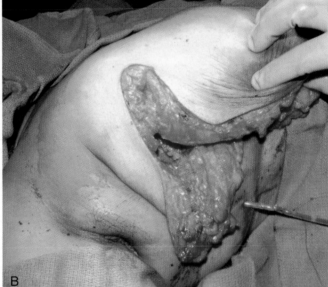

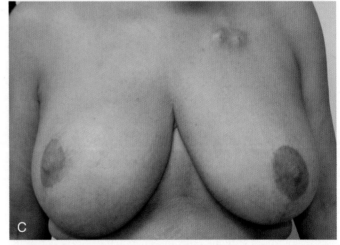

• **Fig. 33.26** (A) Preoperative 60-year-old woman with right breast cancer planned for lumpectomy. (B) Preoperative markings for oncoplastic resection and reconstruction with left reduction for symmetry. (C) Postoperative results.

• **Fig. 33.27** (A) Preoperative markings for oncoplastic resection and reconstruction for treatment of right breast cancer. (B) Intraoperative photo of the skin redraping after specimen removal. (C) Postoperative results.

the B mammaplasty, which limited the inframammary scar to the lateral portion of the breast. The vertical scar approach, first described by Lassus in 1970 and popularized by Lejour in the 1990s, eliminated the entire inframammary scar.[49,50]

Reduction mammaplasty typically involves removal of 400 to 2000 g of breast tissue, as well as a skin-tightening procedure, or mastopexy. Before proceeding with any intervention, mammograms should be ordered according to guidelines established by the National Cancer Institute, the American Cancer Society, and the American College of Radiology, all of which recommend annual (once a year) mammograms for women older than 40 years of age. Preoperative laboratory studies are required as mandated by the patient's age and health. There are various reduction mammaplasty techniques performed. The procedure may be performed in an outpatient or 23-hour stay setting.[51] Preoperative markings are made with the patient in the standing position. Determining the correct height of the nipple position is the key to preserving breast esthetics after reduction. In most patients the nipple should be at or slightly above the inframammary fold. It is important to avoid placing the nipple too high because this is the most difficult esthetic problem to correct. The new location of the nipple is determined by transposing the inframammary fold to the anterior breast surface. The breast should be gently supported to account for elevation of the inframammary fold, and the distance from the sternal notch to the new nipple is usually between 19 and 22 cm. Once the proper nipple location has been ascertained, the remaining skin incisions are marked. In addition, the chest midline, each breast meridian, and the inframammary folds are marked.

The two components of the reduction are the skin closure pattern and the nipple perfusion pedicle. The most common techniques are an inverted-T skin closure with an inferior nipple-areolar pedicle or vertical skin closure with a superior/superomedial nipple-areolar pedicle. Mastopexy corrects the breast ptosis by tightening the skin without removing any breast tissue. Both of these procedures can be performed without adverse effects on palpation or mammographic diagnosis of future breast masses. Reduction mammaplasty may be the only procedure indicated in mastectomy patients who do not want reconstruction. A unilaterally large breast often causes more neck and back pain than bilateral enlargement because of the marked asymmetry in weight. In patients who have breast reconstruction, reduction mammaplasty or mastopexy procedures are essential for symmetry, which is the reason for the reconstruction.[52]

Long-term follow-up is needed to evaluate the esthetic result, scar maturation, symptom relief, and patient satisfaction.[53] After reduction mammaplasty, patients consistently report improvement in physical symptoms.[54] Objective postoperative improvement is documented using photographs and measurements. Subjective symptoms such as headaches, arm pain, and decreased breast pain are partially or completely relieved in more than 90% of patients. One survey of patients indicated that almost 100% of the respondents would either definitely or probably seek the procedure again.[55]

Although patients have a high level of satisfaction with improvement in symptoms and body image, breast reductions have a relatively high rate of complications. Between 42% and 50% of patients had some complications, with 15% considered major and 5% required corrective surgery.[56] Patients who undergo surgery of the breast are prone to the complications that accompany any operation, including anesthetic reactions, pain, infection, bleeding, hematoma, seroma, and pulmonary emboli.

Complications specific to breast reduction fall into one of three major categories: vascular insufficiency, nipple-areola dysfunction, or esthetic deficiency.

Vascular insufficiency can result in loss of either the skin flaps or the nipple. If the skin flaps are affected, it is most commonly at the inferior portion of the vertical limb at its junction with the inframammary incision. This wound breakdown is usually relatively small and can, in most cases, be treated with local wound care. A subclinical decrease in nipple perfusion occurs in a significant number of patients.[57] Partial or complete slough of the nipple is a dramatic but fortunately rare occurrence.[58,59] Necrosis of the nipple can occur as a result of excess skin tension or from pedicle torsion or compression. If identified early, nipple compromise can be addressed by ensuring that the pedicle is not in some way constricted, accomplished by releasing a too tight skin envelope or by converting to a free nipple graft procedure. Fatty necrosis secondary to poor perfusion of the breast adipose tissue can result in focal areas of firm or even calcified tissue, which can be painful and, as indicated earlier, confound cancer surveillance.

Dysfunction of the nipple-areola complex includes both loss of innervation and inability to lactate. Sensory hypesthesia can be partial or complete and may be permanent or temporary. Although objective measurements demonstrate a decrease in sensitivity to pain, pressure, and light touch, subjective reports from patients indicate that in most cases, no sensory deficiency is perceptible within several weeks of surgery. Various techniques offer different rates of sensory changes, with the free nipple graft demonstrating the lowest rate of sensory preservation. In general, sensory innervation is more likely to be maintained if the pectoralis fascia is preserved. There are few studies to evaluate the rate of lactation in postreduction patients.[53] The range of preservation of the ability to breastfeed appears to be greater than 50%; however, in many cases supplementation is required.

Esthetic outcomes can be the most difficult to assess and achieve.[54] Asymmetry is usually present preoperatively, and regardless of the technique used or the experience of the surgeon, it will be present to some degree postoperatively. If the distance between the nipple and the inframammary fold is too long, the breast will "bottom-out," and the glandular tissue will appear ptotic over several months, even if the nipple is at the inframammary fold. Upper pole flatness and lateral fullness can also appear as late undesirable outcomes. Improper positioning of the nipple can lead to the perception that it is too high with respect to the most projecting portion of the breast mound, a problem that is difficult to correct. Alternatively, the nipple may appear to be too low, at a point below the site of maximum breast mound projection. This lower position is esthetically suboptimal but easier to correct than high positioning. Incisions usually heal well, with the inframammary scar typically being the more visible over time. Frequently, the vertical incision becomes nearly imperceptible over time, and this is particularly true in patients with paler skin tones. Complications after breast reduction are most often minor. When needed, surgical revision can typically be performed with the patient under local anesthesia in the office or outpatient setting. Careful preoperative counseling and individualized operative planning can help ensure that the notably high satisfaction levels for reduction mammaplasty are maintained (Fig. 33.28).

Augmentation Mammaplasty

Augmentation of the normal breast is generally discouraged because saline and silicone implants are densely radiolucent,

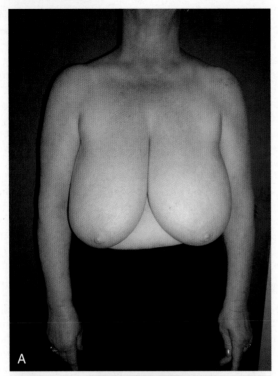

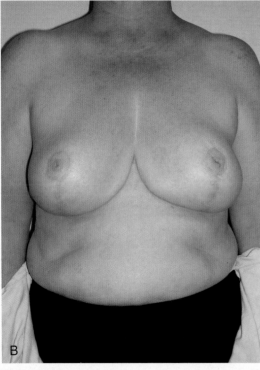

• **Fig. 33.28** (A) Preoperative photo of a 58-year-old woman with symptomatic macromastia. Planned procedure is bilateral reduction mammoplasty with Wise pattern skin resection and inferior pedicle for nipple and areola. (B) Six-month postoperative result.

which obscures mammographic diagnosis of breast cancer. The new triglyceride implant has the same radiodensity of breast tissue, so tiny calcifications can be visualized through the implant. Subpectoral augmentation is generally preferred over prepectoral augmentation, which has a higher incidence of firmness and can interfere with mammographic examination.

Nipple Reconstruction

Nipple-areola reconstruction represents the final part of breast reconstruction. Without the nipple, the breast does not look like a breast. Successful nipple-areola reconstruction restores the shape of the nipple, the shape of the areola, and the color of both entities. The shape of the areola is the foundation for the nipple and is created by a constricted circular closure of the autogenous flap. The nipple is formed by local bilobed or trilobed flaps.[52] The arms of these flaps are wrapped around themselves to form a standing cone. The colors of the nipple and areola are provided by imbedding pigments with a tattoo machine. The color of the nipple is usually darker than that of the areola, which provides additional spatial differentiation. Nipple reconstruction can be performed at the time of an immediate reconstruction, but it is usually performed at a later time, when the shape of the reconstructed breast is definitive. Nipple reconstruction is not without complications. Nipple reconstruction in patients with a history of radiation have complication rates greater than 40%.[55,56] Ultimately, the desire for nipple-areolar reconstruction can be decided by the patient.[57]

Reconstruction Postradiation

When indicated, radiation to the chest wall not only reduces cancer locoregional recurrence but also causes a permanent and irreversible change in shape, skin texture, and elasticity.[58] Discoloration, hair loss, and telangiectasis are common changes that vary in intensity according to the severity of radiation changes. When tissue expanders are used as the method of choice after radiation therapy, these local changes translate into suboptimal esthetic results and a threefold increase in the complication rate.[59] Capsular contracture, implant extrusion, and poor esthetic results occur more frequently after radiation. Therefore radiation therapy is considered a contraindication to the use of tissue expanders. There is also a subset of patients who have previously been treated with lumpectomy and radiation who present for breast reconstruction. Although the complication rate is higher compared with nonirradiated patients, tissue expander reconstruction can still be undertaken with acceptable results.[60]

Autologous breast flaps suffer the effects of radiation as well. Increased rates of flap contracture and fat necrosis occur leading to poor cosmetic outcomes.[61,62] Therefore many believe delayed reconstruction with autologous flaps are indicated in the setting of previous or planned radiation therapy with the benefit of transferring healthy, nonradiated tissue to allow for improved overall outcomes. The disadvantage is the loss of mastectomy skin flaps and the psychological impact of the temporary mastectomy defect for the patient.

Timing of Breast Reconstruction

Breast reconstruction can occur at the time of the mastectomy (immediate reconstruction) or after the mastectomy has been completed (delayed reconstruction). The majority of women prefer to have immediate reconstruction, which alleviates the psychological effects of not having breasts or living with a mastectomy deformity and allows for fewer surgeries and preserving breast skin. Nonetheless, delayed reconstruction is preferred in certain circumstances. Delayed reconstruction can occur weeks to years after mastectomy, usually after completion of all postmastectomy therapies (chemotherapy/radiation). Radiation therapy is known to adversely affect reconstruction outcomes. As mentioned earlier, plastic surgeons may prefer to avoid implants and perform an autologous flap after completion of radiation therapy. Regardless of the timing, there are numerous benefits of undergoing breast reconstruction.[63] Breast reconstruction can be a way to move past the cancer treatment phase, both physically and emotionally, allowing the patient to have improved self-esteem and feel more "normal."

However, surgeons should be concerned about undertaking reconstructions at any time in patients who are poor candidates. It is always a disservice to undertake a complex reconstruction when a patient is still emotionally unstable, has unrealistic expectations, or is in poor health and informed consent cannot be properly obtained.

Conclusions

Contemporary oncology practice guided by clinical trials has directed our understanding of breast cancer treatment to allow new combinations of chemotherapy, reconstruction, and radiation that were not realized a generation ago. Early in the 20th century, the surgeon was alone in taking responsibility for treatment of breast cancer, when the only treatment was the radical mastectomy. Today there is support from several disciplines, and the surgical oncologist should be the leader of this coordinated effort. Helping the patient choose among the numerous reconstructive options requires the efforts and mutual cooperation of both the surgical oncologist and the reconstructive surgeon.

Selected References

13. Park SH, Han W, Yoo TK, et al. Oncologic safety of immediate breast reconstruction for invasive breast cancer patients: a matched case control study. *J Breast Cancer*. 2016;19:68-75.

14. Medina-Franco H, Vasconez LO, Fix RJ, et al. Factors associated with local recurrence after skin-sparing mastectomy and immediate breast reconstruction for invasive breast cancer. *Ann Surg*. 2002;235:814-819.

17. Gurleyik G, Karagulle H, Eris E, Aker F, Ustaalioglu BO. Oncoplastic surgery; volume displacement techniques for breast conserving surgery in patients with breast cancer. *Acta Chir Belg*. 2017; 1-7.

31. Cordeiro PG, McCarthy CM. A single surgeon's 12-year experience with tissue expander/implant breast reconstruction: part II. An analysis of long-term complications, aesthetic outcomes, and patient satisfaction. *Plast Reconstr Surg*. 2006;118:832-839.

34. Colwell AS. Direct-to-implant breast reconstruction. *Gland Surg*. 2012;1:139-141.

A full reference list is available online at ExpertConsult.com.

34

Wound Care and Complications of Mastectomy

STEPHEN R. GROBMYER AND KIRBY I. BLAND

Rehabilitation of the postmastectomy patient produces problems of varying complexity. This chapter reviews commonly used approaches for the care of postmastectomy wounds and addresses the complications encountered in these patients. The goals of postoperative care are to anticipate and prevent adverse events and to accelerate recovery.

Care of the Postmastectomy Wound

The various operative techniques used in the treatment for breast carcinoma are described elsewhere in this text. Complications after any operation can be minimized with thorough preoperative evaluation, meticulous technique, hemostasis, and wound closure. In addition to the standard oncologic evaluation, preoperative evaluation includes assessment of the patient's overall physiologic condition, with particular emphasis on tolerability of anesthesia, uncontrolled diabetes, hypertension, anemia, coagulopathy, or steroid dependency.

Technique at operation and wound closure is an essential part of wound repair. Meticulous hemostasis must be confirmed before closure. Closed-suction drains should be placed into the mastectomy wound site, because most patients will develop a seroma. We prefer closed-suction catheter drainage of the mastectomy wound, commercially available as Blake (Ethicon, Johnson & Johnson Health Care Systems, Piscataway, NJ) or Jackson-Pratt tubing (Baxter Healthcare, Deerfield, IL), and each system should be appropriately placed at operation to allow superomedial and inferolateral positioning to ensure thorough, dependent aspiration. After the wound is closed, the tubing is connected to a closed suction system to ensure removal of all wound contents (e.g., clots, serum). Suction catheter drainage, as a rule, is necessary for 5 to 10 days postoperatively. Earlier removal of the catheters is allowed only when the function of this closed-system technique is compromised. Routinely, catheters are removed only when less than 30 mL of serous or serosanguineous drainage is evident for two consecutive 24-hour intervals.

The skin is closed in two layers using absorbable suture. Thereafter, the skin margins may be covered with strips of surgical tape or wound adhesive. A light, dry gauze dressing is applied to the incision. Pressure dressings over the dissected skin flaps are unnecessary and do not decrease the amount and rate of seroma formation.[1] Postoperatively, the wound is carefully inspected with regard to flap adherence, and the patient is encouraged to resume preoperative activity.

In most circumstances, the breast cancer patient is allowed to begin the gradual resumption of presurgical activities. Younger women usually regain full range of motion of the arm and the shoulder soon after drain removal, whereas some older patients may require intense (supervised) exercise for several months before attaining their former levels of activity. Visits from volunteers of the American Cancer Society or the Visiting Nurse Association are of particular value for psychosocial and physical recovery of the postmastectomy patient.

Complications of Mastectomy

Mastectomy has traditionally been a safe operation with low morbidity and mortality.[2] Although the incidence of postoperative complications is low, physicians should be aware of the morbidity unique to mastectomy and axillary node dissection.

An analysis of National Surgical Quality Improvement Program data recently reported that return to the operating room was the most common morbidity after breast surgery, followed by superficial and deep surgical site infections.[3] Complications can lead to readmissions after mastectomy. A recent report demonstrated a readmission rate of 5.59% after breast surgery with infections being the most common indication for readmission.[4] A detailed review of complications after mastectomy are outlined in the following sections

Lymphedema

Lymphedema affects 6% to 30% of all patients who have had a modified radical mastectomy and is a lifelong risk after the procedure.[5-7] Lymphedema occurs as a consequence of the en bloc ablation of lymphatic routes (nodes and channels) within the field of resection of the primary mammary tumor. The subsequent increase in plasma hydrostatic pressure that results with removal of these conduits may follow the surgical procedure, irradiation, or uncontrolled progression of neoplasm. Injury, capillary disruption, infection, obstruction to lymphatic or venous outflow, hyperthermia, or exercise will accelerate protein leakage into these tissues. The incidence of lymphedema may be significantly reduced by the use of the axillary reverse mapping procedure advocated by Klimberg and colleagues.[8]

Previous attempts to evaluate the degree of arm lymphedema have been classified by Stillwell[9] according to the percentage of volume increase. This methodology has been subsequently investigated and further refined.[10] We grade an increase of less than 10% in arm volume as mild, whereas an increase of greater than 80% is classified as severe

Factors that have been identified as risk factors for the development or progression of lymphedema include the extent of axillary dissection, the use of axillary radiotherapy, pathologic nodal status, infection or injury, and obesity.[11–14] Gilchrist[15] stresses the importance of free and complete active range of motion of the arm and shoulder in the early postoperative period. Traditionally it has been believed and taught that avoidance of excessive sun exposure, injections, infections, or other potentially active or passive injury to the ipsilateral extremity is paramount to prevent lymphedema. Two recent studies, however, have challenged this notion. A study by Ferguson and coworkers[16] involved prospective evaluation of a large cohort of breast cancer patients. Factors associated with lymphedema development include high body mass index, cellulitis, prior axillary node dissection, and regional radiation therapy. These authors found no association between injections in the arm, blood pressure measurements in the arm, air travel, or trauma and lymphedema. This is similar to the findings in the Physical Activity and Lymphedema (PAL) trial, which showed no association between blood draws, blood pressure measurements, and air travel on lymphedema risk.[17] Further study is warranted to further define the optimal balance of lifestyle management, upper extremity precautions, and lymphedema risk.

Furthermore, early recognition of incipient edema by the patient and immediate physical therapy with compression massage often alleviates and augments the prophylaxis of further edema. When lymphedema is severe, the mechanical expression of tissue fluid, with application of an intermittent pneumatic compression device, may be helpful, although a recent small randomized trial has questioned its value compared with conservative measures.[18] The physician may wish to prescribe antibiotics if there is evidence of supervening cellulitis. The arm should be elevated above heart level when the patient is inactive. A more thorough discussion of medical, mechanical, and surgical treatment of chronic lymphedema is provided in Chapter 36.

Wound Infection

Wound infection after mastectomy have been reported to be between 1% and 20%.[19] A large 2012 study from the Mayo Clinic reported infection rate between 2.7% and 8.0% depending on the definition of wound infection used.[20] Infectious complications have been shown to be more common in patients having bilateral mastectomy compared with unilateral mastectomy.[21]

Infection of the mastectomy wound or ipsilateral arm may represent serious morbidity in the postoperative patient and produces an immediate disability that may progress to late extensive tissue dissection that creates thin, devascularized skin flaps. Thereafter, progressive tissue necrosis provides a medium that supports bacterial proliferation with invasive tissue infection. Early debridement of obviously devascularized tissue is an important prophylactic adjunct to prevent progressive invasive infection. When abscess formation does occur, attempts should be made to culture the wound for aerobic and anaerobic organisms, with immediate

Gram stain of identifiable strains to document the bacterial contaminant. The predominant organisms are *Staphylococcus aureus* and *Staphylococcus epidermidis.*[22]

A meta-analysis examining five prospective randomized controlled trials of preoperative prophylactic antibiotics versus placebo demonstrates that prophylactic antibiotics in breast surgery substantially reduce the incidence of postoperative wound infections in breast surgery without any adverse sequelae from the antibiotic administration.[15] We currently use a first-generation cephalosporin before the incision (given intravenously within 30 minutes before the incision) in patients undergoing a mastectomy. Furthermore, it is suggested that reducing postoperative infections is important to prevent delays in adjuvant therapy and reduce cost.[23]

Recent data have suggested that drain antisepsis may have an important role in reducing wound infections after breast surgery. Degnim and colleagues demonstrated that drain bulb irrigation with a dilute sodium hypochlorite solution can significantly reduce bacterial colonization of the drain[24] (Fig. 34.1). Furthermore, in a randomized trial, the technique of drain bulb irrigation combined with the use of chlorhexidine disc dressing was associated with a significant reduction in postoperative infections in breast cancer patients.[25]

Seroma

A seroma is a collection of serous fluid within a surgical cavity that is clinically evident. After a mastectomy, seromas occur in the dead space beneath the elevated skin flaps and represent the most frequent complication of mastectomy, developing in up to 30% of cases.[26,27] With surgical ablation of the breast, the intervening lymphatics and fatty tissues are resected en bloc; thus, the vasculature and lymphatics of the gland are transected. Thereafter, transudation of lymph and the accumulation of blood in the operative field are expected. Furthermore, extensive dissection of the mastectomy flaps results in a large potential dead space beneath the flaps, as does the irregularity of the chest wall, especially in the deep axillary fossa. Continual chest wall respiratory excursions and motion in the shoulder initiate shearing forces that further delay flap adherence and wound repair. Operative technique should minimize lymphatic spillage and transudation of serum to allow rapid adherence of the skin flaps to deep structures without compromise of blood flow to skin flaps or the axilla.

Factors influencing the likelihood of seroma formation include physical activity after surgery, prior history of breast irradiation, obesity, technique at surgery, use of closed-suction drainage, and closure of anatomic dead space; these factors have been examined in many studies. Historically, various techniques for flap fixation and wound drainage have been used to enhance primary wound repair and to minimize seroma accumulation. Two types of external suture fixation have been advocated. In the study by Orr,[28] tension sutures tied over a rubber tubing bolster to fixate the flaps to underlying intercostal muscles and the latissimus dorsi muscle were used. In the report by Keyes and colleagues,[28a] through-and-through flap sutures were tied directly to the skin surface to secure the breast flap to the chest wall. Penrose drains were used to drain excessive accumulation of lymph and blood. Thereafter Larsen and Hugan[29] recommended the application of buried fixation sutures of silk or absorbable material to secure the flaps. These authors secured skin flaps with 30 to 50 subcutaneous cotton sutures and avoided the insertion of any type of drain when possible. Two recent studies[30,31] have reported that quilting sutures are associated with lower rates of seroma formation compared

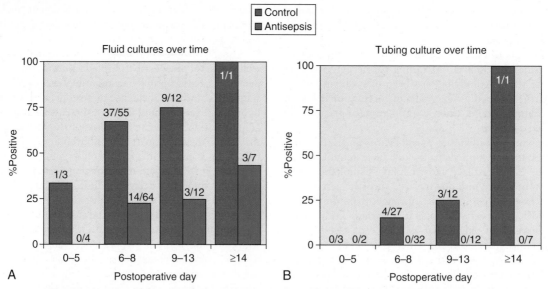

• **Fig. 34.1** (A) Drain fluid cultures from patients with drain bulb irrigation and control patients over time. (B) Drain tubing cultures over time. (From Degnim AC, Scow JS, Hoskin TL, et al. Randomized controlled trial to reduce bacterial colonization of surgical drains after breast and axillary operations. *Ann Surg.* 2013;258:240-247.)

with conventional closure with drains. However, in general, these flap fixation techniques using bolsters, through-and-through sutures from the flap to the underlying chest wall, and quilting sutures have fallen into disfavor because of additional time required to perform these procedures and the emergence of simple and effective suctioning devices.[22]

The use of closed-system suction catheter drainage since the 1990s has greatly facilitated the reduction in protracted serum collections. Removal of serum accumulation was first accomplished by using static drains, such as Paul's tubing, and inserting various soft Penrose drains. Both Paul's tubing and Penrose drains required bulky gauze dressings and multiple dressing changes for the continuous serous soilage expected with wound discharge. In 1947 Murphy[32] proposed continuous closed-suction drainage methods to prevent serum collection beneath extensive flaps. At present, the majority of surgeons use this technique of closed-suction drainage to aspirate excessive collections of serum, lymph, and blood from the mastectomy wound.

In the classic report by Maitland and Mathieson in 1970,[33] 1193 wounds were drained during a 5-year period. Of 153 mastectomies, traditional drainage (i.e., wicks, Penrose) was used in 72, whereas suction drainage was used for the other 81. For operations at various sites, including the genitourinary, alimentary, and biliary tract and soft tissue areas (e.g., breast, thyroid), significant differences were not evident for the two techniques. However, in evaluation of the breast as a subset of the overall analysis, the incidence of wound infection with suction drainage (4.9%) versus traditional drainage (12.50%) was 1.7 times less frequent ($p = .045$). For this subset of the patient population, the authors noted a diminished wound infection rate and increased primary healing with the application of closed-suction drainage techniques.

These results were confirmed by Morris[34] after a controlled clinical trial performed to compare the effectiveness of suction drainage with that of static drainage. For radical mastectomy wounds, this trial established that the rate of wound repair was superior with suction drainage technique. Furthermore, the volume of aspirated drainage was greater with the closed-suction

method, which also afforded a reduction in the infection, tissue necrosis, and wound disruption frequency.

Tadych and Donegan[35] determined the daily wound drainage and total hospital drainage (THD) via a closed-suction system for 49 consecutive patients undergoing a mastectomy to evaluate the frequency of seroma and lymphedema formation. Of this series of patients undergoing modified radical mastectomies and who did not receive irradiation, the THD varied from 227 to 3607 mL and did not correlate with body weight. Ipsilateral edema of the arm directly correlated with THD. Of clinical and practical significance, no patient with less than 20 mL of drainage in the 24 hours before catheter removal developed a seroma.

The extent of surgery also affects seroma formation. A more extensive surgery increases the likelihood of seroma formation in addition to other surgical complications. Aitken and colleagues[36] evaluated 204 consecutive mastectomies (radical and modified radical) in which the techniques used for flap closure and wound management were identical. All potential dead space was obliterated with absorbable sutures that incorporated the pectoralis major, serratus anterior, and latissimus dorsi muscles, as well as the subdermal skin of the axillary flap. Two closed-suction Hemovac drains, one placed in the axillary apex along the lateral part of the chest wall and the other placed over the anterior portion of the chest, were inserted via a separate lower flap stab incision. The average initial volume and total volume of the fluid aspirated from the wounds were similar in both radical and modified radical mastectomy groups (91.1 mL vs. 91.7 mL).

Table 34.1 summarizes the wound complications observed in this series. Postoperative fluid accumulation occurred in 9.31%, with greater frequency in the radical mastectomy group. Infected seroma was identified only in the radical mastectomy group, with an overall frequency of 0.98%. The magnitude of the radical mastectomy procedure perhaps also accounted for the frequency of superficial wound infections, which were more than four times as frequent in this group as in the modified radical mastectomy group. Aitken and Minton[37] identified a decreased incidence of seroma accumulation in these less extensive operations on the

TABLE 34.1 Summary of Wound Complications

	TYPE OF MASTECTOMY			
Complication	Radical (n = 72)	Modified Radical (n = 117)	Simple (n = 15)	Total (n = 204)
Hematoma or seroma	14 (19.44%)	5 (4.27%)	—	19 (9.31%)
Infected seroma	2 (2.78%)	—	—	2 (0.98%)
Superficial wound infection	5 (6.94%)	2 (1.71%)	—	7 (3.43%)

From Aitken DR, Hunsaker R, James AG. Prevention of seromas following mastectomy and axillary dissection. *Surg Gynecol Obstet.* 1984;158:327-330.

TABLE 34.2 Relationship of Dissection Technique, Estimated Blood Loss, and Drain-Related Factors to Postmastectomy Seroma Formation[a]

	Seroma (n = 21)	No Seroma (n = 59)	P[b]
Dissection technique			
Scalpel	5	33	.01
Cautery	16	26	
Estimated blood loss (mL)	90 ± 87	196 ± 165	.006
Drain type[c]			
Blake	4	29	.006
Jackson-Pratt	15	30	
Duration of drains (days)	5 ± 2	6 ± 3	.19
Drainage last day (mL)			
Drain 1	27 ± 47	17 ± 20	.17
Drain 2	22 ± 18	17 ± 13	
Total drainage (mL)			
Drain 1	320 ± 514	213 ± 135	.15
Drain 2	311 ± 493	241 ± 213	.40

[a]Relationships are mean ± standard deviation, except dissection technique and drain type, which are numbers.
[b]P value calculated from the Student t test for continuous variables and chi-square test of homogeneity categorical variables.
[c]Two Hemovac drains were not included in the analysis of risk factors.
From Porter KA, O'Connor S, Rimm E, Lopez M. Electrocautery as a factor in seroma formation following mastectomy. *Am J Surg.* 1998;176:8-11.

breast (simple mastectomy had less incidence than modified radical, which in turn had less incidence than radical mastectomy).

Surgical technique also influences the likelihood of seroma formation. The use of electrocautery increased the rate of seroma formation in one trial in which patients were randomly assigned to dissection of the mastectomy flaps with either scalpel or electrocautery. Seromas developed in 38% of the electrocautery group versus 13% of the scalpel group (p = .01; Table 34.2).[38] Some patient characteristics also affect seroma formation. Three studies indicate that patients with a higher body mass index have an increased rate of seroma formation.[39–41] The incidence of seroma formation also increases with age.[42]

The effect of shoulder mobility restriction in diminishing serous wound discharge after radical mastectomy was evaluated in a randomized prospective clinical trial by Flew.[43] Of 64 consecutive patients nursed in the wards of the Guy's Breast Unit in London, shoulder movement restriction reduced the mean volume of drainage by 40% in those who had immobility for the first 7 postoperative days compared with the group in whom early arm exercises were encouraged. This study confirmed a reduction in drainage duration (days) by 29%. Both the number of patients requiring an operation and the need for multiple aspirations were reduced in the shoulder-restricted group; however, differences were not statistically significant between the two subgroups in duration of hospital stay. Shoulder mobilization did not result in increased shoulder stiffness, although the author confirmed an increased incidence of mild, but transient, lymphedema of the arm when the technique was used. Schultz, Barholm, and Grondal[42] confirmed these findings in their study of 163 patients undergoing modified radical mastectomy (Fig. 34.2). Postoperatively, patients were randomized to physiotherapy on day 1 or day 7. Seromas occurred more frequently in the early mobilization group versus the delayed group. There was no statistically significant difference between the two groups in the late outcome of shoulder function.

However, three studies relate no difference in seroma formation based on delayed or early mobility.[11,44,45] In a prospective randomized trial by Petrek and colleagues,[11] 57 women undergoing modified radical mastectomy or axillary node dissection with breast preservation were randomized to early or delayed mobilization of the ipsilateral arm. Patient characteristics, including type of surgery, were similar in each group. There was no statistically significant difference in seroma formation (Table 34.3). It is the

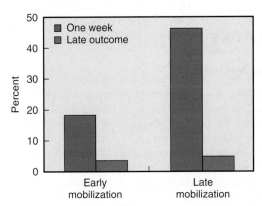

• **Fig. 34.2** Frequency of impaired shoulder mobility after modified radical mastectomy. A significantly higher incidence of impairment occurred after 1 week in the delayed mobilization group (p < .001). There was no significant difference in late outcome. (From Schultz I, Barholm M, Grondal S. Delayed shoulder exercises in reducing seroma frequency after modified radical mastectomy: a prospective randomized study. *Ann Surg Oncol.* 1997;4:293–297.)

practice of the authors to allow arm mobility immediately after surgery but delay a structured exercise routine until after the drains have been removed.

Multiple studies of sclerosing agents; thrombin; and fibrin glue, patches, and sealants in an effort to decrease seroma

TABLE 34.3	Response Variables by Early and Delayed Arm Mobilization Groups[a]		
Variable	Early Group (n = 27)	Delayed Group (n = 30)	P
Inpatient drainage (mL)	558 ± 114 (58–3265)	603 ± 76 (125–2020)	.3498
Inpatient stay (days)[b]	6.9 ± 1.4 (3–36)	6.5 ± 0.6 (2–14)	.2883
Outpatient drainage (mL)	223 ± 100 (0–2080)	117 ± 41 (0–280)	.7133
No. of aspirations	2.6 ± 1.3 (0–34)	2.0 ± 0.5 (0–9)	.2092
Duration (days)	15.0 ± 5.7 (0–150)	13.2 ± 3 (0–58)	.6061
Total drainage (mL)	781 ± 195 (58–5013)	729 ± 102 (125–2777)	.4622

[a]Values represent mean ± SE (range) and P values for the equality of distributions (Mann-Whitney test).
[b]Sample size for the early group is 24, and for the delayed group is 28.
From Petrek J, Peters MM, Nori S, et al. Axillary lymphadenectomy. A prospective, randomized trial of 13 factors influencing drainage, including early or delayed arm mobilization. *Arch Surg.* 1990;125:378-382.

formation after mastectomy have been performed and yielded inconsistent results. A meta-analysis of 11 trials of fibrin glue and sealants to reduce drainage and seroma formation was performed by Carless and Henry.[46] Results indicated that fibrin sealant did not reduce the rate of postoperative seroma, the volume of drainage, or the hospital stay.

Pneumothorax

Pneumothorax, a rare complication, develops when the surgeon perforates the parietal pleura with extended tissue dissection or with attempts at hemostasis for perforators of the intercostal musculature. Pneumothorax is more commonly seen in patients undergoing a radical mastectomy after removal of the pectoralis major musculature.[47] Respiratory distress is recognized in the operative or the immediate postoperative periods, and pneumothorax is confirmed with a chest x-ray study. Immediate therapy with closed thoracostomy drainage of the pleural space is essential as soon as pneumothorax is verified.

Tissue Necrosis

Skin grafting after radical mastectomy, as originally proposed by Halsted,[48] is rarely required in the management of the modern mastectomy wound. Stents applied over split-thickness skin grafts, which are necessary for large tissue defects, should be removed on the fifth or sixth postoperative day. Early and periodic wound care, including debridement with wet-to-dry saline dressings, affords optimal wound management to ensure adequate "take" of the graft application.

A commonly recognized complication of breast surgery is epidermolysis or necrosis of the developed skin flaps or skin margins. Budd and colleagues[49] observed major skin necrosis in 8% of their patients, a rate similar to that found in other series. Bland and associates observed an incidence of 21% for minor and major necrosis of mastectomy skin flaps with associated wound infection.[50,51]

Local debridement is usually unnecessary in minor areas of necrosis (i.e., 2 cm² area). Larger areas of partial or full-thickness skin loss require debridement and, on occasion, the application of split-thickness skin grafts. Rotational composite skin flaps and subcutaneous skin tissue can be used from the lateral chest wall or the contralateral breast to cover the defect.

Hemorrhage

Although not specifically designed to detect bleeding, the use of closed-suction catheter drainage allows early recognition of hemorrhage, an uncommon complication of mastectomy. Hemorrhage is reported as a postoperative complication in 1% to 4% of patients and is manifested by undue swelling of flaps of the operative site and increased bloody drainage.[19] Early recognition of this complication is imperative. Hemorrhage may be treated by aspirating the liquefied hematoma and establishing patency of the suction catheters. The application of a light compression dressing reinforced with Elastoplast tape should diminish the recurrence of this adverse event. Moderate to severe hemorrhage in the immediate postoperative course is rare and is best managed with wound reexploration. Early, severe hemorrhage is most often related to arterial perforators of the thoracoacromial vessels or internal mammary arteries. Direct suture ligation is advisable. Thereafter closed drainage systems are replaced, and tubing patency is ensured before wound closure.

Surgeons hold varying opinions as to the best technique to elevate skin flaps for performance of total mastectomy. Electrocautery, cold scalpel, Shaw hot knife, and, more recently, laser have been used to create skin flaps for modified radical and radical mastectomies. The cold scalpel has the advantage of minimal tissue injury but may present formidable bleeding problems unless used concomitantly with direct suture ligation or electrocoagulation. Excessive bleeding may obscure the operative field with blood, and the extensive dissection may leave the hematologically compromised patient anemic at termination of the procedure. In contrast, electrocoagulation minimizes blood loss.[37,52] However, the experimental studies by Keenan and colleagues[53] suggest that the tissue damage initiated with cautery injury may diminish the host response to infection.

In a prospective nonrandomized study of 60 patients undergoing total mastectomy,[54] no statistical differences for infection rate, operating time, wound discharge, or hospital stay were noted with use of the cold scalpel compared with the electrocautery. These authors determined that use of the electrocautery allowed significantly greater blood loss, estimating that blood loss was 440 mL versus 651 mL for the scalpel and electrocautery, respectively. Kakos and James[52] completed a similar prospective analysis for comparison of blood loss with the electrocautery versus the scalpel in 50 mastectomy patients. Average blood loss in this series was 960 mL in the scalpel group versus 160 mL in the electrocautery group. Of 25 scalpel-group patients, 24 (96%) received transfusions, compared with only 6 of 25 (24%) in the electrocautery group. Wound necrosis was not different in the two groups.

Miller and associates[55] conducted a randomized prospective study to investigate differences in blood loss and postoperative complications in patients undergoing modified radical mastectomy with use of the electrocautery and scalpel. Skin flaps were created with the cold scalpel in 24 patients and with electrocautery in 25 patients. The two groups were similar with respect to age, stage of disease, size of tumor, and body weight. Use of the electrocautery allowed patients to have significantly reduced operative blood loss compared with patients whose skin flaps were created with the cold scalpel (352 vs. 507 mL, respectively; *p* < .05). None of the patients who underwent electrocautery required transfusion. The primary advantage of the electrocautery was the reduction in blood loss; surprisingly, operating time was not significantly shortened with use of the electrocautery technique. These authors acknowledge that the axillary dissection is the time-limiting factor of the procedure, and because of neurologic injury induced with use of electrocoagulation, axillary dissection techniques used by the surgeons were identical in both subgroups. Total postoperative Hemovac drainage and hospital stay were not significantly different between the two groups. Although the number of fever days and wound complications were slightly higher in the electrocoagulation group, this difference was not statistically significant. Miller and associates[55] concluded that use of the electrocautery for the development of skin flaps in the performance of a mastectomy reduces blood loss without incurring a greater incidence of wound complications.

Cautery appears to be the most suitable surgical instrument for tissue plane dissection in the procedure. However, it has the expectant limitation of neurostimulation and heat injury with dissection around motor nerves, such as the brachial plexus, and of motor innervation to muscles of the axillary space, including the medial/lateral pectoral, long thoracic, and thoracodorsal nerves to the pectoralis major, serratus anterior, and latissimus dorsi muscles, respectively. For these reasons, most surgeons use a combination of both techniques.

As indicated by Miller and associates,[56] the known risks of blood transfusions include hepatitis (0.26%–1%), transfusion allergic reactions (1%–19%), and acquisition of human immunodeficiency virus. Each of these transfusion-related complications necessitates constant reexamination of the indications for transfusion, with deliberate attempts to reduce transfusion requirements at mastectomy in the nonanemic patient.

Injury to Neurovascular Structures

Injury to the brachial plexus is also a rare complication of mastectomy.[57] This is most commonly avoided by meticulous (cold scalpel) sharp dissection in and about the neurovascular bundle and through the development of tissue planes that parallel the neurilemma and the wall of the axillary vein to allow en bloc resection of lymphatic structures and fatty tissues.

The sensory innervation of the breast is derived from the lateral and anterior cutaneous branches of the second through the sixth intercostal nerves. The patient usually experiences moderate pain in the operative site, shoulder, and arm in the immediate postoperative period. Because of the necessity of extensive flap development, the patient may note hypesthesia and paresthesia, as well

as occasional "phantom" hyperesthesia in the mastectomy site. Originally described by Ambrois Paré in 1551,[58] phantom breast syndrome is a continued sensory presence of the breast after it has been removed. It is a phantom pain in 17.4% of cases, and in 11.8% of cases it presents as a nonpainful phantom sensation such as itching, nipple sensation, and premenstrual-type breast discomfort.[59] Most symptoms occur within the first postoperative day and remain fairly constant. Preoperative education may help relieve anxiety should symptoms develop.

Hypesthesia of the upper medial arm is a common postmastectomy complaint and results from denervation of one or more of the intercostobrachial nerves traversing the axillary space that are sectioned in the conduct of the axillary dissection. These sensations disappear gradually with wound healing.[60] The patient should be assured that abnormal sensations will usually subside within 3 to 8 months postoperatively. However, normal sensation may never return to the denervated axilla, medial arm, and hemithorax.

Less common are injuries to the thoracodorsal nerve and the long thoracic nerve (respiratory) of Bell. The thoracodorsal, or subscapular, nerve innervates the latissimus dorsi muscle in its course with the thoracodorsal (subscapular) vessels and is commonly sacrificed when lymphatics are discovered to be involved with metastases at axillary dissection. Sacrifice of this nerve results in minimal physical disability; the patient observes weakness of internal rotation and abduction of the shoulder after denervation and paralysis of the latissimus dorsi muscle.

Conversely, injury or transection of the long thoracic nerve of Bell, which innervates the serratus anterior muscle, produces instability and unsightly prominence of the scapula ("winged scapula"). The patient sustaining such an injury will often complain of shoulder pain at rest and with motion for many months after the procedure. All attempts should be made to preserve this nerve, yet its involvement with invasive neoplasm or nodal extension may require that it be sacrificed to ensure adequate en bloc resection.

The lateral and medial pectoral nerves to the pectoralis major muscles and the motor innervation to the pectoralis minor exit the brachial plexus to enter the posterior aspects of these muscles in the proximal axilla. Preservation of the pectoralis major and its function is the objective of the modified radical mastectomy. Thus maintenance of the integrity of the medial and lateral pectoral nerves is paramount to ensure subsequent function of the pectoralis major. Section of the medial pectoral nerve with motor denervation of the pectoralis musculature allows progressive atrophy of these muscle groups with resultant cosmetic and neurologic morbidity.

Deep Venous Thrombosis

Venous thromboembolism (VTE) is a potentially life-threatening complication of surgical procedures requiring general anesthesia. Fortunately, deep venous thrombosis (DVT) and VTE. Reported rates of DVT are between 0.16% and 0.23%.[61,62] These low rates suggest that routine chemical prophylaxis in breast cancer surgery patients is not warranted.[61] Mechanical prophylaxis before the induction of anesthesia and in the postoperative period for hospitalized patients should be used. In those who develop a DVT, the median time to diagnosis is postoperative day 14.[61] Factors that have been reported to be associated with a slightly higher rate of DVT include obesity, inpatient status, venous catheterization, and prolonged operative times (>3 hours).[62] Breast cancer stage has not been found to correlate with DVT risk in breast cancer surgery patients.

Postmastectomy Pain Syndrome

Postmastectomy pain syndrome is chronic pain (>3 months) that is localized to the "anterior or lateral region of the thorax, axillary and/or medial upper arm, causing burning pain, shooting pain, pressure sensation and numbness."[63] It has been reported to occur in up to 47% of patients after breast cancer surgery.[63] Factors associated with postmastectomy pain syndrome include age over 40 years, adjuvant radiation therapy, and axillary lymph node dissection.[64] Interventions including gabapentinoids and antidepressants may have a role in reducing postmastectomy pain.[65] Others have advocated the use of Botox injections in the chest wall musculature at the time of mastectomy to reduce the incidence of postmastectomy pain.[66] There also may be a role for ultrasound-guided trigger point injections for the treatment of postmastectomy pain syndrome.[67,68]

Selected References

11. Petrek JA, Senie RT, Peters M, Rosen PP. Lymphedema in a cohort of breast carcinoma survivors 20 years after diagnosis. *Cancer.* 2001;92:1368-1377.

18. Dayes IS, Whelan TJ, Julian JA, et al. Randomized trial of decongestive lymphatic therapy for the treatment of lymphedema in women with breast cancer. *J Clin Oncol.* 2013;31:3758-3763.

19. Vitug AF, Newman LA. Complications in breast surgery. *Surg Clin North Am.* 2007;87:431-451, x.

23. Olsen MA, Chu-Ongsakul S, Brandt KE, et al. Hospital-associated costs due to surgical site infection after breast surgery. *Arch Surg.* 2008;143:53-60, discussion 1.

61. Andtbacka RH, Babiera G, Singletary SE, et al. Incidence and prevention of venous thromboembolism in patients undergoing breast cancer surgery and treated according to clinical pathways. *Ann Surg.* 2006;243:96-101.

A full reference list is available online at ExpertConsult.com.

35

Quality Measures and Outcomes for Breast Cancer Surgery

JEFFREY LANDERCASPER, CAPRICE C. GREENBERG, AND STEVEN L. CHEN

To say that the first 15 years of the 21st century has seen more emphasis on quality and performance measurement of hospitals and doctors than was seen in the entire 20th century is no exaggeration. Furthermore, payers of care, including the US government, have proposed shifting American medical reimbursement policy to payments that are tied to quality and performance instead of the number of services provided or procedures performed. The Department of Health and Human Service's current target is that 50% of Medicare payments should be tied to quality or value through alternative payment models by 2018.[1] Furthermore, public transparency of performance and what providers of care will be held accountable for will dramatically increase in the coming years. Change is occurring so rapidly that the benefits and risks they pose to patients and providers are not entirely known. Because these shifts are so consequential—and likely irrevocable—it behooves us to understand the opportunities and pitfalls that we face in advance. In this rapidly evolving framework of health care measurement, surgeons and other providers of care must ask themselves whether they are willing to be the stewards of it all. This chapter is a primer for breast surgeons interested in performance measurement and improvement.

Why Measure Quality?

The quality of health care received, including breast cancer care, varies by geography, institution, patient characteristics, and care provider.[2–32c] These variations account for the known disparities and inequities in care. Access to care and quality of care sometimes differ by socioeconomic status, education level, insurance status, and race. Documented quality concerns also include variations in appropriateness of care, with under- and overutilization of services resulting in differences in cost without adding value. The Institute of Medicine (IOM) provides notable examples of quality of care gaps in its seminal publications *To Err Is Human: Crossing the Quality Chasm* and *Delivering High Quality Cancer Care: Charting a New Course for a System in Crisis.*[17,22,24] Such gaps exist along the entire continuum of cancer care, from diagnostic evaluation to survivorship, and include safety issues, unacceptable variability of care, and examples of failure to adopt evidence-based cancer care.[3–10,23] Examples of these gaps include unnecessary diagnostic surgical excisional biopsies instead of needle biopsies and disproportionate numbers of patients undergoing breast-conserving therapy without receiving breast irradiation based on economic

and insurance status. Some variability is evident even within institutions participating in national clinical trials.[4]

There are other reasons to measure quality. Health care spending in the United States is currently rising faster than anywhere else in the world. This spending is not sustainable, nor is it associated with better outcomes. The Commonwealth Fund concludes that when based on cost and outcomes, the United States' overall health care ranking is lower than that of nearly all of the countries of western Europe, New Zealand, and Australia.[11] In a cross-national comparison of health care spending per capita in 11 high-income countries, spending in the United States far exceeded that of the other countries, largely driven by greater use of expensive technologies and notably higher prices. Despite this heavy investment, the United States ranked lower in many measures of population health, such as life expectancy and the prevalence of chronic conditions. An inverse association usually exists between quality and cost of care, so better quality care would be expected to lower costs, which would help to address our health care fiscal crisis.[11,12,33] Increased cost of care is often associated with overutilization or waste of care.[13] These and other observations motivated multiple professional organizations including the American Society of Breast Surgeons (ASBrS) to participate in the American Board of Internal Medicine's Choosing Wisely campaign, a national effort aimed at promoting appropriate care and reducing wasteful care.[13] For example, routine systemic imaging to search for metastatic breast cancer preoperatively, then later during patient follow-up after initial treatment of early-stage breast cancer, is noncompliant with evidence-based guidelines and does not improve patient survival; rather, it increases care costs and leads to unnecessary additional testing and biopsies for false-positive findings.[14]

Lastly, simply developing valid approaches to measure and report quality can have an important impact. Many studies have provided proof of concept that measuring breast cancer care quality and providing peer performance comparison usually correlate with improved care.[15,34]

Who Are the Stakeholders for Quality Measurement?

The stakeholders interested in health care quality include patients and their providers of care, but they also include purchasers, payers, professional organizations, policy makers, patient advocacy groups, and the government.[35] Although all stakeholders desire high-quality care, their perspectives and goals may differ. A historical example of differing stakeholder opinions occurred more than a decade ago when breast cancer patients were offered, then wanted, reconstruction after mastectomy but could not afford it because it was not covered by their insurance plan. From the payer's perspective, reconstruction was costly and characterized as an optional "cosmetic" operation. In contrast, from the provider and patient perspective, reconstruction was of benefit—an attempt to restore normality, both physically and emotionally, after cancer surgery. Resolution of these conflicting arguments did not occur until after federal legislation, the Women's Health and Cancer Rights Act of 1998, mandated reimbursement.[36] This regulatory action resulted from a collaboration between stakeholders that including policy makers.

What Is the American History of Surgical Quality Measurement?

Ernest Codman at Massachusetts General Hospital was one of the first US surgeons to advocate for measurement of surgical outcomes, believing they provided the foundation for improvement.[37,38] Dr. Codman reported the end results of 337 surgical patients treated from 1911 to 1916. He concluded there were 123 errors and 4 "calamities." He advocated for surgeon accountability and transparency, and he recommended development of national patient registries. These were prescient concepts and remain relevant today. Unfortunately most of Dr. Codman's peers disagreed with him. Thus, as a result of his quality advocacy, he was the victim of professional rebukes and social ostracism. There were likely many other surgical leaders interested in quality and outcomes research after the era of Ernest Codman, but few seminal conceptual articles were published on quality measurement during the next half of the century, perhaps reflecting Codman's experience.

In the 1960s, Avedis Donabedian, a health care researcher at the University of Michigan, began refining the concepts of quality measurement, moving away from an unstructured peer-review method, such as traditional morbidity and mortality conferences, toward an objective "outcome-driven process."[39,40] He created a taxonomy of quality measurement based on structure, process, and outcomes of care—later called the *Donabedian Trilogy*—which is still in use today. Since the late 1990s, additional domains of quality to audit have been recommended. These include patient access, patient experience, affordability, population health, safety, effectiveness, and efficiency.[17-20]

Moving beyond concepts and motivated by recognition of disparate care in the Department of Veterans Affairs hospitals, the development of methods to provide hospital-level peer performance comparison for surgical outcomes was accomplished in 1991.[34] Beginning in 1994, Shukri Khuri and others described the system of auditing, peer comparison, and risk-adjusted analytics used by the American College of Surgeons (ACS) and the Department of Veterans Affairs (VA) to report surgical outcomes.[21,32] They provided hospitals with report cards of postoperative morbidity and mortality. In 2004 the VA hospital program evolved into the ACS National Surgical Quality Improvement Program (NSQIP).[34] Other notable surgeon champions of breast cancer quality improvement in recent years include David Winchester, Stephen Edge, Eric Whitacre, and Cary Kaufman. All

provided pioneering work in the development of breast quality measurement by programs such as the Commission on Cancer (CoC),[41] the National Accreditation Program for Breast Centers (NAPBC),[42] the ASBrS Mastery of Breast Surgery Program,[43] and the National Consortium of Breast Centers (NCBC).[44] These programs have been recently summarized.[45] The contemporary strategies to improve patient quality that are endorsed by multiple organizations are listed in Table 35.1.

What Are Quality and Value?

Many organizations have defined quality[17,22,24–26,35,44] (see Table 35.1). The IOM defines health care quality as an iterative process with six aims: safety, effectiveness, timeliness, efficiency, equitability, and patient centeredness.[17]

Value of care has a broader meaning than *quality* of care.[46,47] In addition to quality, cost is considered. Spending on breast cancer care is substantial—not surprising because it is the most commonly diagnosed non–skin cancer in women. Breast cancer expenditures account for the largest share of cancer-related spending.[48] In 2006 Porter and coworkers[46] defined a value metric as "patient health outcomes achieved per health care dollars spent." Others describe it as the simple ratio of quality to cost of care. In his monograph *Discovering the Soul of Service,* Leonard Berry takes a patient-centered approach, defining the value of care as the ratio of quality to burdens, in which burdens can be both financial and human.[49] Using a Surveillance, Epidemiology, and End Results (SEER)-Medicare database, Hassett and colleagues recently explored the relationship between breast cancer care, cost, and outcomes—as measured by adherence to recommended treatments and survival—in 99 geographic regions.[14] Convincingly, they identified significant variability in all. They failed to identify an association between survival and cost of care. Process measures that assessed necessary and unnecessary therapies did not correlate with survival and they found evidence of expenditures for treatments not recommended. Other investigations have also provided evidence of unnecessary expenditures that did not aid survival, suggesting overutilization of some services with no gain.[13] As the United States moves away from a system of fee-for-service and toward value-based reimbursement, many definitions of value are already in use or anticipated. Nearly all have or will have a quality metric in the numerator and a cost metric in the denominator, resulting in the creation of a value metric.

What Are Safety in Surgery and Diagnostic Errors?

Diagnostic errors and *patient safety* are commonly included under the rubric of *quality.* Surgical safety is of great importance for all surgical subspecialties, and safe surgery is necessary for good breast cancer surgical outcomes. Surgical safety checklists and safety improvement methodology have been nicely reviewed elsewhere.[50-53] Direct observation of care may identify root causes of safety issues.[54,55]

Diagnostic errors in medicine are common but underreported, according to a recent comprehensive review.[27] The IOM's updated 2015 definition of *diagnostic error* is "the failure to (a) establish an accurate and timely explanation of the patient's health problem(s) or (b) communicate that explanation to the patient."[27] This definition frames this quality issue from the patient's perspective, recognizing that errors may harm the patient, then parses it;

TABLE 35.1	National Health Care Policy Stakeholder Quality Improvement Objectives	
Organization	**Objective Name**	**Objectives**
Institute of Medicine[a]	Six Aims	• Safe • Effective • Patient centered • Timely • Efficient • Equitable
Institute for Healthcare Improvement[b]	Triple Aim	• Improve the patient experience • Improve population health • Reduce per capita cost
Agency for Healthcare Research and Quality and the National Quality Strategy[c]	Three Aims	• Better care • Healthier communities • More affordable care
	Six Priorities	• Safer care • Person and family partnership in care • Effective communication and coordination of care • Effective prevention and treatment practices • Promoting best practices in communities for health • More affordable health for patients, employers, and governments
	Nine Levers	• Provider measurement and feedback • Public reporting of cost, care, and outcomes • Learning and technical assistance to help organizations • Certification, accreditation, and regulation to meet quality standards • Consumer incentives to adopt healthy behavior • Provider rewards and incentives • Improve health information technology efficiency • Foster innovation and rapid adoption • Workforce development—invest in next generation of health care providers

[a]Committee on Quality of Health Care in America, Institute of Medicine. *Crossing the Quality Chasm: A New Health System for the 21st Century.* Washington, DC: National Academies Press; 2011.
[b]The IHI Triple Aim. Institute for Healthcare Improvement <http://www.ihi.org/engage/initiatives/TripleAim/Pages/default.aspx>.
[c]The National Quality Strategy. Agency for Healthcare Research and Quality <http://www.ahrq.gov/workingforquality>.

accuracy, timeliness, and communication can all be measured, then segregated for audits and tracking. Diagnostic errors have been described as "missed opportunities," either errors of omission (failure to order tests or procedures) or commission (ordering unnecessary tests, such as overutilization of systemic imaging in early-stage breast cancer patients). Relevant examples of diagnostic errors of omission in breast cancer care include delayed diagnoses attributable to misses on screening mammography and failure to recognize imaging-pathology discordance of breast lesions after image-guided needle biopsy that showed benign, indeterminate, or high-risk findings. Multiple reviews and publications have highlighted the reasons for a delayed diagnosis of breast cancer.[56–59]

How Do We Identify a Gap in the Quality of Care?

The World Health Organization identifies gaps in health care quality by recognition of variability of care.[26] Gaps are identified when measurements of actual care do not match achievable care and when variability of performance coexists with evidence that high levels of performance are obtainable.[17,35,60,61] For breast care, searches for variability can be conducted in national databases such as the SEER and the National Cancer Database (NCDB).[62,63] For example, interrogation of the NCDB and the American

Society of Breast Surgeons databases recently identified wide variability of reexcision rates after breast-conserving surgery for cancer, indicating a performance gap.[64–66] Searching for variability has been the primary method for identification of disparities and inequities of care based on socioeconomic status, race, location of care, and other demographic characteristics.

Where Are the Databases for Quality and Clinical Outcomes Research?

Institutions throughout the United States are generating an ever-increasing amount of electronic data. The American Recovery and Reinvestment Act of 2009 included $17 billion in Medicare/Medicaid incentive payments for the adoption of electronic health records (EHRs) starting in 2011, and reductions in Medicare/Medicaid reimbursement for nonadopters beginning in 2015.[67] In addition to the obvious economic implications, this mandate represents an enormous opportunity to evaluate quality and clinical outcomes. The ability to access and analyze these data will markedly improve our ability to study practice patterns, compare the effectiveness of treatment beyond clinical trials, evaluate performance, and provide objective feedback to practitioners. Although significant progress is being made, we currently still rely primarily on the secondary use of administrative data and manual abstraction from cancer registries.

The secondary use of administrative data, the most common data source for such activities, is limited for breast cancer care by the need for accurate pathologic data, such as stage and histology. The abstraction of administrative data from hospital systems (e.g., discharge data) can be available from a variety of sources, such as state hospital associations or private consortiums, such as the University HealthSystem Consortium.[68] Other administrative data exist in the form of insurance claims. Such data are more flexible than discharge data but can be cumbersome to analyze and often represent a biased sample of the population. For example, Medicare claims are often used to evaluate quality and outcomes, but Medicare data come only from patients aged 65 years and older. Thus their utility is limited for cancers that primarily occur in young patients (e.g., testicular cancer) because the biology and treatment of the disease in elderly patients are different from those in younger patients (e.g., breast cancer). Furthermore, claims data cannot be linked to the medical record for more specific information as advances are made (e.g., genomic profiling). These data are, however, extremely well suited to surgical questions. Because they are tied directly to payment, surgical and other procedure codes are reliable and represent a clear, distinct intervention.

Clinical cancer registries exist at the institutional, state, and national levels. State cancer registries vary greatly in terms of the completeness of data. The most common national cancer registries are the SEER and the NCDB of the CoC. The NCDB abstracts data from the more than 1200 CoC-accredited institutions, representing more than 70% of the newly diagnosed cancers in the United States. It is an extremely powerful tool for investigating quality and outcomes that are directly tied to clinical care; however, limitations in the capture of treatment information can limit its application for such measures. It is also important to recognize that the NCDB is not a population-based data set. SEER, on the other hand, now collects data from 18 sites around the United States that were selected to ensure representation of socioeconomic and racial diversity. Because it includes all individuals living in the site, this is a population-based data source, which can be important for generalizability. Another major and well-recognized limitation of cancer registries is the inability to accurately track recurrence. As patients move from one geographic region to another, and even between hospitals within a region, longitudinal outcomes can be difficult to track, and capture of recurrence, in particular, is noted to be unreliable.

Such registries can provide accurate pathologic and other cancer-specific information, but often have less accurate information on treatment, and little to no information on comorbidity. In addition, data elements in cancer registries are manually collected and entered, making it extremely resource-intensive to collect and maintain, resulting in a considerable lag time before data are available for analysis. A number of initiatives have linked cancer-specific variables from registry data to the details of treatment available in administrative data in order to take advantage of both sources. The best example is SEER-Medicare, which links cancer registry data from SEER with Medicare claims data.[69]

Many of the data elements that are lacking in traditional administrative data sources, including cancer-specific variables, are available as unstructured free text in EHRs. To access these data in a cost-efficient manner, automated approaches can be used to extract key measures pertaining to patient, disease, and treatment characteristics. To date, a number of EHR-based initiatives abstract data from multiple institutions and systems to create a virtual data warehouse. Perhaps the most relevant for the quality and outcomes of breast cancer patients is the National Cancer Institute–funded Cancer Research Network,[70] which draws from multiple health maintenance organizations. With the continued expansion of EHRs, a number of new national initiatives aim to increase the availability of these data for the evaluation of clinical effectiveness, quality, and outcomes. The National Patient-Centered Clinical Research Network,[71] a major initiative of the Patient-Centered Outcomes Research Institute, funds the creation of multiple large data warehouses with standardized data structure.

How Do We Measure Quality?

Physician competency may be assessed using a number of methods.[35,45] Hospitals require credentialing, states require licensing, and the American Board of Surgery requires certification. These are mandatory basic levels of surgeon competency. They do not necessarily measure surgeon technical proficiency. The shared goal of these activities is the desire to increase the likelihood that quality care will be provided during a surgeon-patient encounter. After these administrative and regulatory entry thresholds have been achieved, recertification, credentialing, and licensing are most often based on annual Continuing Medical Education credits, essential for maintenance of board certification. Occasionally, peer review by a Department Chair is necessary for renewal of hospital privileges. More recently, direct measurement of postoperative outcomes has been used for some credentialing decisions and by some payers of care for patient steerage decisions. Increasingly, the most common method of assessing care provider performance has been quality measurement and peer comparison.[28,32,34,72–74] These methods provide a potential framework for departure from fee-for-service systems of reimbursement to incentivized pay-for-performance systems.[75,76]

Quality of care is measured by auditing outcomes. From existing patient registries, there is a vast body of information on general and breast surgeon outcomes, especially postoperative morbidity and mortality. Complications are costly and delay patient recovery. However, because the likelihood of death or major morbidity after breast operations is so low compared with more complex general surgical operations, it is of limited use for quality improvement in breast care.[77,78] As a result, breast-focused organizations have endorsed other measures of quality. A common method of measuring breast surgeon quality is to measure their compliance rate with an evidence-based process of care. This seemingly simple evaluation of provider quality has recently been scrutinized. Although guideline compliance is intuitively the best care, a few studies dispute the notion that higher measured compliance rates always identify better surgeon quality and reliably improve patient outcomes. The hypothesis that maximization of guideline adherence is best care may be too simplistic because there can be valid reasons for noncompliance with guidelines, such as patient preferences, limited life expectancy, and comorbidities. Using the patient registry for certified breast centers in Germany, Jacke and colleagues[79] reported on 104 quality indicators that were based on guidelines, categorizing the care decisions of each study patient as either *adherent* or *divergent*. Overall guideline adherence increased and divergence decreased over 8 years, resulting in a twofold increase in quality as measured by the *process of care*. However, a systematic effect of adherence linked to overall survival was not evident, reflecting what the authors termed an "adherence paradox" because increased guideline compliance was not associated with a better outcome.

Procedural volume as a surrogate measure of quality is controversial.[80–84] The controversy stems not only from the use of volume as a measure of competency per se but, rather, its potential use for distribution of care. This use of volume as an accountability measure restricting a surgeon's eligibility to care for a patient needing a specific operation has been proposed and endorsed by some hospital systems.[84] For now, the proponents of using volume for case distribution are focusing on complex gastrointestinal procedures, such as hepatic, pancreatic, and bariatric surgery. Although not yet used for patient steerage in breast care, a direct volume-outcome relationship has been reported.[82] The primary argument for using volume as a measure of quality is that some studies indicate a significant association between higher volume and better outcomes. However, surgeons with lower case volume have demonstrated outcomes comparable to those of high-volume centers.[85] Furthermore, patients often prefer care that is closer to home and to their social support system.

Quality of care can also be measured from the patient's perspective by patient survey. These are termed *patient-reported outcomes* (PROs). They are also called *patient-centered* and *patient experience* quality measures. Multiple patient surveys are available, including those specific to both general or breast surgeons. The surgical care questions embedded in these surveys assess the domains of access, timeliness, and pain control, as well as functional, psychological, sexual, and cosmetic outcomes.[86–93]

What Is a Quality Measure, and Where Do We Find Them?

A quality measure (QM) is a fraction that attempts to quantify quality in a domain of care.[16,35,60,94–105] A QM has a specific numerator, denominator, and inclusion and exclusion criteria. Collectively, these are the *specifications* of a QM. There are multiple measure types, reflecting measurement in different domains of care. Measure types include the Donabedian trilogy of structure, process of care, and outcomes. Newer domains of care for QM development include access, timeliness, patient-centeredness, affordability, efficiency (appropriateness), efficacy (evidence-based), care coordination, cost/resource, and population health.

Structure or *setting* of care reflects the environment in which a care provider practices. For example, a geographic and scheduling model that provides patient navigation and care coordination with all specialty care providers meeting with the newly diagnosed patient at the same time and place would be a structure expected to engender care coordination and high-quality patient-centered care. Another important structural measure that is being developed is the requirement for a survivorship care plan at the completion of treatment. For a breast surgical encounter, examples of operative structure that foster better care are the availability of intraoperative specimen imaging with immediate radiologic interpretation and immediate access to histologic assessment in the operating room during breast-conserving surgery for nonpalpable breast cancers. The measurement of a structural QM is usually dichotomous: it is either present or absent. For example, the structural presence of a tumor board is necessary for NAPBC accreditation.[42]

Process of care measurements usually involve auditing compliance with evidence-based treatments, such as National Comprehensive Cancer Network (NCCN)-recommended care for management of the axilla or adjuvant chemotherapy, endocrine, or radiation treatments within a designated timeframe.[8] For process measures, the difficulty often lies in determining the appropriate denominator based on inclusion and exclusion criteria. For example, the recommendations for chemotherapy include age, histology, receptor status, and tumor size. As previously discussed, such specific characteristics can be challenging to obtain from existing data sources.

An *outcome* QM determines the actual results of care. Key outcomes of cancer treatment—overall survival, disease-free survival, and local regional recurrence—are important to measure but have limited use as a single-surgeon QM due to the attribution issues, as well as to the long length of follow-up required. Cancer recurrence depends on the actions and recommendations of multiple nonsurgeon providers, patient choice, and adherence to treatment, none of which are completely controlled by the surgeon. Other limitations in the use of outcome measures include low case volume and event rates for many breast surgical procedures, limiting the ability to provide stable estimates.

The most common general surgery outcome measures focus on postoperative complications after surgery, such as venous thromboembolism, bleeding, sepsis, organ failure, and surgical site infection. They are limited in their relevance for breast surgeons because they are such infrequent events.[77,78] As a result, efforts to develop more meaningful breast surgeon–specific QMs have occurred (Table 35.2). Surgeon- and breast center–specific QMs are listed in Table 35.3.

TABLE 35.2 Breast Center and Breast Surgeon Quality Measurement Programs in the United States

Organization	Breast Center	Breast Surgeon	Breast Oncologist	Hospital
American Society of Breast Surgeons[a]		✗		
American Society of Clinical Oncologists			✗	
National Consortium for Breast Centers	✗	✗		
National Accreditation Program for Breast Centers	✗			
Commission on Cancer				✗
National Surgical Quality Improvement Program[b]		✗		✗

[a]Only program that allows breast surgeon participation in Centers for Medicare and Medicaid Services incentivized payment programs.
[b]The National Surgical Quality Improvement Program includes measures of breast morbidity and mortality outcomes in its general surgeon reporting.

TABLE 35.3 **Breast-Specific Quality Measures**[a]

	PQRS Measures

American Society of Breast Surgeons	PQRS Measure No. 262: Image Confirmation of Successful Excision of Nonpalpable Image-Localized Breast Lesion
	PQRS Measure No. 263: Preoperative Diagnosis of Breast Cancer by Minimally Invasive Biopsy
	PQRS Measure No. 264: Sentinel Lymph Node Biopsy in Clinical Stage I and II Invasive Breast Cancer
	Non-PQRS (society endorsed) Measures
	Surgeon Assessment for Hereditary Cause of Breast Cancer
	    Surgical Site Infection and Cellulitis after Breast and/or Axilla Surgery
	    Specimen Orientation for Partial Mastectomy or Excisional Breast Biopsy Specimens
	    Unplanned Reoperation Within 30 days After Mastectomy
	    Selection of Prophylactic Antibiotic—First- or Second-Generation Cephalosporin (modified PQRS No. 21)
	    Discontinuation (<24 hours) of Prophylactic Parental Antibiotics (Non-Cardiac Procedures) (modified PQRS No. 22)

National Accreditation Program for Breast Centers and the Commission on Cancer	Radiation therapy after breast-conserving therapy Chemotherapy in hormone receptor–negative patients stage T1c and higher Endocrine therapy in hormone receptor–positive patients stage T1c and higher Core needle biopsy rate for new cancer diagnosis Breast-conserving therapy rate Radiation therapy in mastectomized women with four or more positive nodes
National Consortium for Breast Centers	1. Imaging Timeliness of Care—Time Between Screening Mammogram and Diagnostic Mammogram 2. Mammography Call Back Rate 3. Surgical Timeliness of Care—Time Between Diagnostic Mammogram and Open Surgical Biopsy/Excision (no needle biopsy performed) 4. Imaging Timeliness of Care—Time Between Diagnostic Mammogram and Needle/Core Biopsy 5. Surgical Timeliness of Care—Time Between Needle Biopsy and Initial Breast Cancer Surgery 6. Needle Core Biopsy Rate 7. Pathology Timeliness of Care—Time Between Initial Breast Biopsy (excluding open surgical) and Pathology Results 8. Pathology Timeliness of Care—Time Between Open (incisional/excisional) Initial Breast Biopsy and Pathology Results 9. Pathology Timeliness of Care—Time Between Initial Breast Cancer Surgery and Pathology Results 10. Pathology Report Completeness—Tumor Size 11. Pathology Report Completeness—Margin Analysis 12. Pathology Report Completeness—Margins Identified 13. Pathology Report Completeness—Lymph Node Analysis 14. Pathology Report Completeness—Specimen Sampling Adequacy 15. Five Year Stage Specific Survival Rate 16a. Pathology Report Completeness—ER and PR Receptor Measurement for Invasive Disease 16b. Pathology Report Completeness—ER and PR Receptor Measurement for In Situ Disease 17. Surgical Care—Sentinel Node Biopsy 18. Patient Satisfaction Survey—Use 19. Patient Satisfaction Survey Development 20. Patient Satisfaction Survey Response Rate 21. Patient Satisfaction Survey Measure—Shared Decision Making for Choice of Surgical Option for Breast Surgery 22. Patient Satisfaction Survey Measure—Cosmetic Results Following Breast Reconstruction 23a. Breast Conservation Surgery—Overall Rate (actual patients) 23b. Breast Conservation Surgery—Rate for Eligible Patients (potential eligible patients) 24a. Chemotherapy Use—Rate for Stage II and III ER Negative and PR Negative Breast Cancer (actual) 24b. Chemotherapy Use—Rate for Stage II and III ER Negative and PR Negative Breast Cancer (potential) 25a. Post-Lumpectomy Radiation—Rate for Invasive Breast Cancer (actual) 25b. Post-Lumpectomy Radiation—Rate for Invasive Breast Cancer (potential) 26a. Adjuvant Endocrine Therapy—Rate for Invasive Breast Cancer (actual) 26b. Adjuvant Endocrine Therapy—Rate for Invasive Breast Cancer (potential) 27. Radiation Therapy—Break in Treatment 28. Reconstructive Breast Surgery—Myocutaneous Tissue (Flap) Complication Rate 29. Adjuvant or Neoadjuvant Chemotherapy—Complications Resulting in Inpatient Hospitalization Rate 30. Ambulatory Breast Cancer Surgery—Unplanned Overnight Stay Rate 31. Breast Conservation Surgery—Re-Excision Rate
ASCO Quality Oncology Practice Initiative Measures	N = 62 breast measures[b]

PQRS, Physician Quality Reporting System.

[a]The quality measures listed are simplified descriptions. Full specifications of the measure are accessible through the organizations' websites.

[b]Available at http://www.asco.org/quality-guidelines/summary-current-qopi-measures.

Recent advances in QMs include the development of cross-cutting and composite QMs. *Cross-cutting* is a term describing a single QM expected to be relevant to multiple specialties. Examples include *medication reconciliation post discharge, functional outcome assessment, pain assessment and follow-up,* and *care plan.*[106] Providing a cancer patient with a portable (whether paper or electronic) staging and survivorship document, and updating that document as the patient's circumstances change, is an example of a cross-cutting QM. In this example, the document is iterative, changing over time from diagnosis through treatment, but it remains relevant forever to aid care coordination and communication.

A composite measure summarizes a group of QMs that are related in some way, such as multiple processes of care related to a specific disease condition or to an episode of patient care.[107] In describing one type of use of a composite QM, the Agency for Healthcare Research and Quality (AHRQ) suggests the measure denominator be the sum of processes that constitute a panel of appropriate process measures. With this example, the numerator is the sum of the processes of appropriate care that are actually delivered. Surveys describing PROs in multiple domains of care can also be reported as a single composite number. The survey may calculate separate scores for as many as eight domains of mental and physical health after breast cancer surgery, and then combine all to create a single composite score of 0 to 100, with higher scores representing better health quality.[108] Composite measures can include a functionality allowing different statistical weighting for the individual measures used in the construct of the measure. Composite measures with weighting were better than using individual postoperative complication rates or hospital volume to explain hospital-level variations in quality after bariatric surgery.[109]

The newest measure types under development by the National Quality Forum (NQF) are cost/resource measures.[110] These measures are intended to determine risk-adjusted payments to providers for an episode of care. Initially, the NQF is developing these for medical conditions, such as acute myocardial infarction. Bundled payments for surgical episodes of care are being developed.

The programs and their quality measures available for reporting on the care of patients with breast cancer are listed in Tables 35.2 and 35.3. They have been recently reviewed.[45] Most programs provide peer comparison. In the CoC program, rapid feedback is provided on whether compliance with QMs, such as endocrine therapy for hormone receptor–positive breast cancer patients, was accomplished. This feedback exemplifies one of the first national efforts to link QM reporting to the notion that reporting can improve quality by using time-sensitive prompts. The ASBrS Mastery[SM] is the only program that provides surgeons with the opportunity to participate in Centers for Medicare and Medicaid Services (CMS)-incentivized payment and penalty programs with breast surgeon–specific measures (Table 35.3).[43] An example of the full specifications of one of these measures is provided in Fig. 35.1.

What Are the Quality Reporting Systems in the Public Sector?

The interest in quality measures is complemented by the desire for payers and the public to collect metrics of quality and potentially distribute them. Because there is virtually an unlimited number of programs that occur across the private sector, we focus on the public sector in this chapter.

The Tax Relief and Health Care Act of 2006 created the Physician Quality Reporting Initiative, which CMS implemented as the Physician Quality Reporting System (PQRS). This provided for a bonus payment of as high as 1.5% for participation in data collection. The program was made permanent in 2008 and required that CMS post the names of eligible physicians and group practices, which can currently be found on the Medicare Physician Compare website.[75] In 2010 the Affordable Care Act (ACA) required further changes, most importantly the implementation of a feedback mechanism and an appeals process. It also required the development of penalties that began in 2015. Penalties for nonparticipation in PQRS would be as high as 2% of payments, based on the reporting from 2 years prior (e.g., 2015 penalties would be based on 2013 participation).

In addition to those incentives and penalties, there are potential additional incentives and penalties based on the value modifier (VM), which is intended to measure resource use relative to quality. Based on 2014, providers will be tiered into low-, average-, and high-cost, as well as low-, average-, and high-quality tiers. Those that overperform (e.g., average or high quality for low cost, or high quality for average cost) will be rewarded with additional incentives. A 1% additional bonus is also available for those groups serving high-risk beneficiaries based on average risk scores. The VM dollars at risk will depend on eligible provider group size and year of reporting. In 2016 and 2017, it will range up to a 2% and 4% penalty, respectively, reflecting care in 2014 and 2015. The upper limit of incentivized reward has not been determined at the time of this writing.

The requirements for individual physicians to avoid the PQRS penalty for 2017 (to be performed in 2015) are as follows. Physicians may report data based on paper claims, directly via an EHR, via Registry, or via a Quality Clinical Data Registry (QCDR). Each has slightly different requirements; however, they generally must include reporting of at least nine measures across three or more National Quality Strategy Domains selected from the PQRS Measures list for that year, which in 2016 includes more than 250 measures.[111] In addition, one of those measures must come from the cross-cutting measure list.[106] Although the bulk of the measures apply most closely to primary care–oriented specialties, a number of them have been submitted by the ASBrS and were designed with breast surgeons in mind. Measures that are oncology- or specialist communication–focused may also be appropriate for breast surgeons. Breast surgeons wanting to report breast surgery–specific measures can find more information on the ASBrS website.[43]

Group practices may choose to report together; however, to do so they should register for the Group Practice Reporting Option. Groups do not have a paper claims options, but groups larger than 25 qualify for a Web interface option. In addition, groups reporting together should also plan to work with a CMS-certified vendor to administer the Consumer Assessment of Healthcare Providers and Systems (CAHPS) survey. This is required for groups of more than 100 eligible professionals but can also be utilized for any group larger than two as an option.

Late in 2015, CMS released Quality and Resource Use Reports (QRURs) to all solo practitioners and group practices nationwide based on the 2014 data; however, these data will affect only groups with 10 or more eligible professionals. To avoid the penalty that is based on the VM, groups must have reported successfully on PQRS measures as well, or had at least one member participate

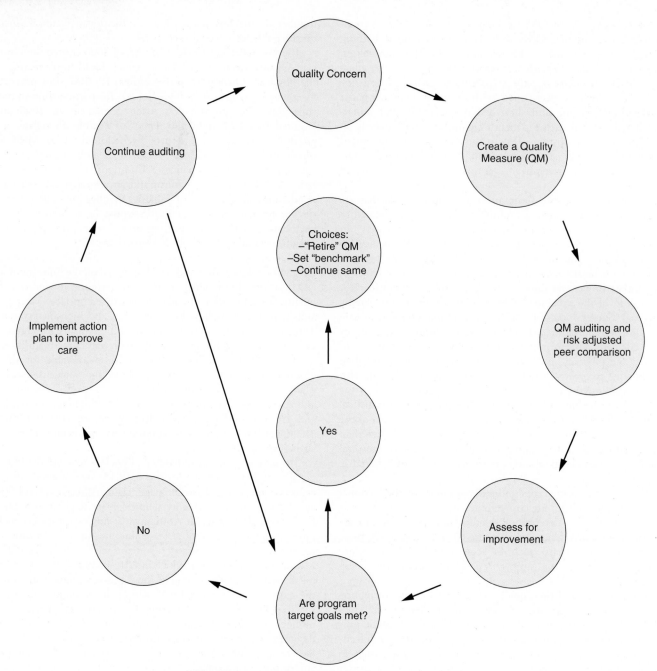

• **Fig. 35.1** The quality improvement plan-do-study-act cycle.

in the Medicare Shared Savings Program. Details can be found on the CMS website for the precise calculation.[76] Quality measures include those utilized through PQRS as well as hospital admissions or chronic conditions for acute diagnoses that may be avoidable and 30-day hospital readmissions. Cost measures are based on the Fee for Service Medicare claims that are attributed to the group. These are calculated both overall and on specific conditions as well. Providers are tiered into high-, average-, and low-cost, calculated based on the standard deviation of the cost scores.

There have been a number of criticisms of the current approach to quality reporting in programs described earlier. First and foremost, the incentive payments have been tied primarily to participation and not achievement of any specific targets. Most of the current measures are focused on the process of care, rather than risk-adjusted outcomes of care. In addition, payments have been an all-or-nothing approach, meaning that for providers who are unable to achieve the reporting threshold, no payments are given at all.

What Is the Future of Public Quality Measurement Reporting?

In 2015, the Medicare Access and CHIP Reauthorization Act (MACRA) was passed, creating two new payment systems—the Merit-Based Incentive Payment System (MIPS) and the Advanced Alternative Payment Models (APMs).[111a] Collectively, these are called the CMS Quality Payment Programs (QPP). Beginning January 1st, 2017, all surgeons needed to participate in one of these two programs to avoid a negative payment adjustment penalty for their billing of Medicare patients.

MIPS incorporated the preexisting PQRS, the Value-Based Payment Modifier Program (VBPMP), and the Medicare Electronic Health Record incentive program into it. MIPS assigns providers a composite performance score (0–100) based on four categories. The score is based on quality (60% weight), improvement activities (15% weight), advancing care information (25% weight), and cost (0% weight in 2017, to be determined 2018 and beyond).[111a,111b] Surgeons choosing the MIPS pathway can "pick their pace" from the following options and payment adjustments in 2017: *no participation* (negative 4%), *submit a minimum amount* of Medicare data such as a single QM or one improvement activity (may avoid a downward adjustment), *partial submission of 90 days* of Medicare data (neutral or small positive adjustment), or *full participation* of 2017 Medicare data (moderate positive adjustment). Although MIPS began with up to 4% payment adjustments, they reach 9% by 2022. From 2020 to 2025, MIPS is the only method for those not participating in an APM to achieve positive updates. Because MIPS is budget-neutral, half of its participants will receive a bonus. The other half will have no adjustment or a negative adjustment.

MIPS allows group instead of individual reporting. By law, surgeons who report with their group cannot report individually, meaning that in most cases, they will not be reporting on specialty-specific QM; rather their performance is rolled into the population-based (e.g., screening mammography compliance), cross-cutting (e.g., medicine reconciliation), or patient reported outcome QMs selected by their group.

There are two types of APMs.[111a] Both aim to shift reimbursement away from volume and toward quality and cost (value). The first is an accountable care organization (ACO). ACOs focus on payments to large organizations, with capitation-based reimbursing for a population of patients over a time interval. They are less relevant to individual surgeons and out of scope for this chapter. The second type of APM is based on a "bundled payment" or an "episode of care" payment model. These arrange for multiple providers to be paid as a group for a service. As currently designed by CMS, APMs are intended to bear more than a nominal financial risk compared to provider risk in MIPS. APM providers bear greater cost burdens for poor patient outcomes. On the other hand, they receive more reward for good patient outcomes achieved at a lower than average cost. Initially, CMS will incentivize APMs by allowing providers to receive a 5% upward payment adjustment simply for participating. Existing APM models can be found on the CMS QPP website.[111a] Newer APM models are under development. Many specify how an APM entity (group of multiple different types of care providers) receives CMS reimbursement for an episode of care. For example, in a breast surgical APM, a fixed dollar reimbursement could be provided by CMS for all the care inputs into the pre-, post- and intra-operative care surrounding a procedure, such as a modified radical mastectomy with immediate reconstruction. These bundled payment APMs will be adjusted for quality of care. After CMS reimbursement, the APM entity parses portions of the fixed reimbursement to the anesthesiologist, breast surgeon, plastic surgeon, and others. The most mature of these models is the comprehensive care for joint replacement (CJR) model.[111c] CMS has stated an ambitious goal of wanting 50% of all Medicare fee-for-service payments to be made via alternative payment models by 2018.[111c]

How Do We Create the Best Quality Measures?

Constructing a perfect measure of provider quality, allowing fair, risk-adjusted differentiation between performance tiers, free of bias, rapidly actionable for improvement, captured without undue burden to busy providers and with face value for every stakeholder is elusive and challenging. As a result, multiple organizations and stakeholders have chosen different pathways and provided different recommendations for QM development and ranking. The NQF provides comprehensive and explicit criteria for desirable attributes.[60] The Institute for Healthcare Improvement[112] and AHRQ are other respected leaders for QM development, naming the preferred principles for QM creation. Endorsement by the NQF—considered the highest level of endorsement—ensures that the QM has met specific and rigorous scientific standards. Public and private payers accept NQF endorsement as a criterion for using a QM in incentivized programs that link compliance with the QM to reimbursement. The NQF measure evaluation criteria include importance, scientific acceptability, feasibility, and a search for competing measures. A comprehensive explanation of how each of these criteria is achieved is accessible on the NQF website. Briefly, a QM's *importance* is determined by whether (1) the measure focus is evidence based and (2) a quality gap (performance variation) is present. *Scientific acceptability* means the measure is reliable (consistent) and valid (credible). Validity means that the measure specifications—numerator, denominator, inclusion, exclusion, and risk adjustment criteria—are exact and evidence based. Importantly, for outcome measures, the NQF emphasizes the evidence-based risk adjustment strategies based on patient factors known to influence the outcome should not initially include factors related to disparities in care. Otherwise, disparities and inequities of care such as race, socioeconomic status, and geography may be missed during initial measurement and peer comparison. *Feasibility* means data capture can occur without undue burden. This is difficult to achieve. Lastly, the NQF recommends review of *related or competing* QMs. After review, the different measure stewards should harmonize, retire, modify, or replace some measures, if possible.

How Do We Rank a List of Many Quality Measures?

Many measures of quality describe best patient care. Because the list is long but resources to audit them are not, how do we choose which to develop into a QM? This challenge has been addressed differently by different organizations.[13] The ACS and the ASBrS have used a modified Delphi appropriateness methodology for ranking.[113,114] The modified Delphi process first has a call for potential candidate measures. After a list is made, an iterative process is used in which each member of a panel assigns a validity score from 1 to 9 for each QM on the master list, where 1 signified *definitely not valid*, 5 signified *uncertain/equivocal validity*, and 9 signified *valid*. After ranking, a panel discussion followed. The process is then repeated after panelists provide evidence and arguments for either increasing or decreasing the importance of the measure. Using the Rand manual methodology for ranking, measure domains with a median score from 7 through 9 are considered valid measures.[113] Other methods have been described to aid the prioritization or ranking of QMs. In a sophisticated approach to development of some of the first NQF-endorsed QMs for breast cancer treatment in 2008, Hassett and colleagues described a quantitative formula for determining both the existence and the magnitude of a quality gap for different types of recommended breast cancer treatments endorsed by the NCCN.[61] With this method, the NCCN database of more than 9000 patients treated by NCI-designated Comprehensive Cancer Centers was used to determine highest and overall concordance rates and number of nonconcordant patients with recommended treatments. This objective information was combined with a qualitative assessment of the importance of each guideline by content experts for ranking.

How Are Quality Measures Used?

Once hard to find, QMs now seem ubiquitous, endorsed by professional organizations and audited in nearly every hospital and clinic. Nearly all medical specialties have developed QMs, and nearly all health systems now have quality departments, champions, or officers who, in nonuniform ways, manage quality data. Increasingly, QMs have been used by public and private payers of care to try to improve appropriateness, quality, and value of care. When measures are used for quality improvement, an audience is engaged to measure performance. The QM becomes a tool to probe for gaps in care. Audits identify the gaps. If any interventions are introduced to improve care, further auditing determines its effectiveness (see Fig. 35.1).

Quality measures are also used for peer performance comparison, quality improvement, surveillance, accountability, and research. *Accountability* means that the QM is used for patient steerage or incentivized performance programs or that it has public transparency. With patient steerage, the results of measurement are used by patients and consumers of care to direct where patients are eligible to seek and receive care. In this case the consumers and purchasers of care can be health plans, industry, private businesses, or the state and federal governments. Incentivized payment programs mean performance is linked to reimbursement to include pay for participation, pay for reporting, penalize for not reporting, pay for above average performance, and penalize for below performance programs. Public transparency is already used by the CMS to display cost, charge, and quality data on its website.[115] If a QM is used for accountability, it should be supported by a high level of evidence. Furthermore, the measure and the care domain being measured should be judged as important by providers, patients, and payer stakeholders. Surveillance measures may have lesser levels of evidence supporting their importance, but there ought to be some belief that tracking performance for the measure will be beneficial.[116]

Examples of breast-specific QMs used by the CoC and the NAPBC for surveillance, quality improvement, and accountability are the breast-conserving therapy rate, the needle biopsy rate for diagnosing new breast cancers, and the rate of receipt of postmastectomy radiation therapy in women with four or more positive nodes, respectively.[116]

Existing and newer proposed uses of QM are for milestones (requisite targets for surgeons in training), hospital credentialing, state licensure, and American Board of Surgery maintenance of certification; QM is also used by employers to discriminate between applicants. To better integrate quality science and the appropriate application of QM into surgical education, the ACS launched the NSQIP Quality In Training Initiative in 2011.[117] This initiative aims to aid surgeons-in-training and their residency directors by providing both a QM curriculum and actual outcomes data to them for the operative cases in which a resident assisted. The goal is for surgical residents to learn the general principles of measurement and improvement and incorporate them in their future practice.

An increasing number of companies and news organizations are using publically available CMS data for public reporting of QM on their industry websites. In doing so, they provide the public with a surgical outcome measurement and sometimes a physician or hospital rating. Their methodologies for rating and ranking are not always transparent and two companies using the same CMS data may have disparate ratings for the same hospital or provider.[118]

How Do We Analyze Quality Data and Provide Fair Peer Comparisons?

Conceptually, the actual capture of surgeon outcome data is straightforward. The analysis is not. The risk adjustment for comparisons and the assignment of attribution for an outcome to an individual surgeon is difficult. The ACS provides information and education regarding stewardship responsibilities and the preferred statistical analysis of patient registries used for quality measurement.[119,120] In NSQIP, participating institutions are provided with risk-adjusted peer performance comparison of standard morbidity and mortality outcomes via transmission of graphic displays of observed-to-expected ratios with confidence intervals. A comprehensive analysis of their methods for risk adjustment for patient and hospital characteristics to improve the fairness of their peer comparisons is out of scope for this chapter, but the ACS and others have described analytic methodologies used for peer comparison, including patient mix, case mix, and shrinkage adjustment strategies, as well as logistic regression, hierarchical modeling, and random variation. Recently in recognition that the overall care of a population of patients may improve naturally over time, a difference-in-differences econometrics methodology has been used to distinguish between quality improvement attributed to a planned intervention or initiative versus the natural drift to better care over time.[34,120–122] Fairness of peer comparison is also enhanced by including specific exceptions and exclusions to the formal specifications of a QM. The ASBrS Mastery[SM] Program provides these adjustments (see Fig. 35.1). An exclusion means a patient has a condition that removes the patient from the compliance denominator for *performance met*. For example, the case of a patient with stage III inflammatory cancer would be excluded from reporting on the QM of percentage of newly diagnosed clinically negative stages I and II breast cancer patients who undergo sentinel lymph node biopsy. Such a case would not be included in the surgeon's reporting or performance rates. An exception for this same QM would be the case of a patient who has a palpable suspicious node discovered intraoperatively (positive for cancer on frozen section) who undergoes full axillary dissection. This case is reported because it meets the denominator criteria, but the surgeon is not penalized because the correct action was taken. The surgeon receives credit for the sentinel lymph node reporting rate but is not penalized for performance.

What Is a Benchmark?

The verb *benchmarking* is used consistently in the health care literature to mean comparison. Comparison of measured results can occur between care providers or between a single institution or individual to an established benchmark. Measuring care, then comparing it—*benchmarking*—is integral to quality improvement. In contrast to benchmarking, the term *benchmark* is used inconsistently with different meanings. A benchmark is a point of comparison (personal communication, February 2, 2015, Alesia D. Hovatter, Health Policy Analyst, Center for Clinical Standards and Quality, Centers for Medicare and Medicaid Services). The different uses of the term *benchmark* and its ambiguity come from all the options for point of comparison.

Historically, benchmarks have been variably defined as highest achievable performance, average (mean) performance, with or without standard deviations, lowest acceptable performance, a quality plausibility threshold, a target goal, a specific decile of performance, or a standard of care. In 2012 the National Healthcare Quality Report and the IOM defined a benchmark as a quantifiable "highest level of performance achieved so far."[29] The European Society of Breast Cancer Specialists' (EUSOMA) recommended lexicon for a benchmark—for an individual QM—is to set both a quality goal and a quality target.[123,124] In 2015 CMS endorsed the ABC™ method for creating a benchmark. This method requires a large database containing patient quality information.[125] A specific formula then takes into account the results from lower volume institutions, so that exemplary results from a few low-volume care providers do not overly inflate the benchmark. Benchmarking and benchmarks are requirements for CMS acceptance of QM programs wanting to participate in government-sponsored incentivized QM programs.

Many developers of measurement programs in the United States provide benchmarking but do not yet name benchmarks. In contrast, EUSOMA was an early adopter and endorser of multiple benchmarks in its breast center cancer QM program.[123] For example, their recommended minimum standard rate of new breast cancer patients receiving a diagnosis by needle biopsy preoperatively is 80%, and their target goal is 90%. Their minimum standard and target goal for proportion of patients receiving a single breast operation is 80% and 90%, respectively, for patients with invasive cancer and 70% and 90%, respectively, for patients with pure ductal carcinoma in situ. The NAPBC and the CoC have also set target goals. The NAPBC recommends that breast centers audit their breast-conserving therapy rate to determine whether they have achieved a 50% rate. In addition, they recommend enrollment of at least 2% of patients into clinical trials. The CoC recently established expected estimated performance rates for multiple breast cancer–related QMs. For CoC-accredited centers due for survey in 2016, the expected performance rate is 90% compliance for the NQF-endorsed QMs of radiation after lumpectomy, radiation after mastectomy in patients with four or more positive nodes, and receipt of hormone therapy in stage I T1c or greater receptor-positive patients. They also recommend that needle biopsy be the diagnostic method in at least 80% of patients receiving a new breast cancer diagnosis.[116]

How Do We Improve Quality?

The goals of all quality improvement programs include reducing variability of care, narrowing the performance curve of care, and moving the median bars of performance in the correct direction. The principles of quality improvement are summarized in Fig. 35.2. Many organizations provide strategies for how to improve quality of care.[34,42,60,96,101,124,126–132] Improvement begins with measurement. QMs are a tool for measuring. With their use,

measurement is more specific and usable for comparisons and assessment of trends. Measurement, that is, peer comparison (with some level of transparency) in industry and health care, may drive improvement without any other specific strategy other than workers' inherent drive to function as well as or better than their peers. This phenomenon has been called the *Hawthorne effect,* named after seminal studies performed in the 1950s at the Hawthorne Works in Cicero, Illinois.[133] In a series of experiments to increase factory line production at the Hawthorne Electric Plant, investigators audited employee output of goods, before and after the workers were informed they were being subjected to auditing. Later, interventions to improve the work environment occurred. Employee output increased above baseline more by the investigators' unplanned intervention (i.e., the notification of auditing) than it did with the planned intervention of workplace environmental enhancement. Subsequent interventions to increase worker reimbursement for better factory output followed, echoing but preceding the development of conceptually similar incentivized models for health care improvement in use today.

Improvement strategies can be broadly classified by approaches that focus on individual care providers or, alternatively, the systems in which they care for patients. Of course, there is much overlap. An example is the improvement in the percentage of newly diagnosed breast cancer patients receiving their diagnosis by needle biopsy in a large multiinstitutional health system in Wisconsin.[134] Variability among care providers and hospitals—all under the governance of a single organization—was recognized by measurement of a specifically defined needle biopsy rate QM. A system-wide quality improvement approach to education, transparency, prospective auditing, targets, and consequences was developed. Quickly, variability was reduced and overall care was improved.[134]

Quality improvement strategies aimed at individual providers often audit measures of personal performance, then provide peer comparison, with or without the establishment of target goals. This has been called a *quality cycle,* and it is the primary methodology of most quality programs (see Fig. 35.2). Additional incentives for performance improvement, such as accountability uses of QM—public transparency, enhanced payments for participation or performance, avoidance of penalties for not participating or poor performance—may be added to these programs. The relative and absolute effectiveness of these added incentives to improve individual surgeon and national aggregate performance is not yet known, but new programs have emerged each year, driven by the continued recognition of the need to reduce variability and costs of care.

Quality improvement tools to improve care also focus on systems of care. The list of these tools is long and filled with abbreviations and acronyms (Table 35.4). Comprehensive reviews of quality improvement strategies are available online and updated annually.[126,135]

Clinical and translational research successes are important but not always sufficient to improve care on a national scale. There is ample documentation of delays in time to adoption of new or better treatments after publications of randomized trials, meta-analyses, and specialty society guidelines. In other words, the publication of evidence-based studies demonstrating better care and the subsequent expert endorsement of them does not always change care quickly.[3–10,13,14,23,28,30,45,136–141] For example, after randomized trials demonstrated that hypofractionated whole breast radiation was equally effective to standard longer, costlier radiation schedules in select patients after breast-conserving surgery, the American Society of Therapeutic Radiation Oncologists

MEASURE TITLE: Unplanned 30 day reoperation after mastectomy
MEASURE DESCRIPTION: Percent of patients undergoing mastectomy who do not require an unplanned secondary breast or axillary operation within 30 days of the initial procedure.
DENOMINATOR: Patients undergoing unilateral or bilateral mastectomy as their initial procedure for breast cancer or prophylaxis.
NUMERATOR: Patients undergoing unilateral or bilateral mastectomy as their initial procedure for breast cancer or prophylaxis who do not require an unplanned secondary breast or axillary operation within 30 days of the initial procedure.
Exclusions (The patient is not in the denominator; i.e., no reporting on this patient):
- Patients undergoing breast-conserving surgery as their initial operation for breast cancer
- Patients undergoing central line reservoir IV access procedures within 30 days after initial mastectomy

Exceptions (The surgeon receives credit for reporting on this patient for this measure but is not penalized if he/she did not meet the performance requirement because there was a valid reason for reoperation not attributed to the quality of the breast surgeon; i.e., the reoperation is attributed to someone else):
- Patients who undergo a planned "cosmetic" procedure in either breast within 30 days after their initial breast operation
- Patients who have a contralateral breast reoperation by the plastic surgeon for a complication in a breast not operated on by the breast surgeon
- Patients with flap ischemia/necrosis (not native skin flap necrosis) who undergo reoperation for debridement of flap or assessment of vascularity or revascularization after a tissue transfer reconstructive operation performed by the plastic surgeon
- Patients with placement of expander or implant who undergo reoperation by plastic surgeon for expander/implant leak or any other prosthetic condition requiring reoperation
- Patients with a false-negative intraoperative sentinel node assessment; i.e., patient underwent immediate intraoperative histologic assessment of SLN with findings of no nodal metastasis but then had postoperative identification of positive SLN necessitating an axillary reoperation

The Measure Query seen by surgeon:

"If this procedure was an initial mastectomy, did this patient have a reoperation for any reason within 30 days?"

The drop-down list seen by breast surgeon:

No
NA – Not an initial mastectomy
NA – Patient underwent lumpectomy as initial operation
Yes – Reop. for central line reservoir placement
Yes – Bleeding requiring exploration
Yes – Surgical site infection
Yes – Postop. ID of positive SLN: no intraop. assessment
Yes – Margin close or positive
Yes – Mastectomy skin necrosis
Yes – Reconstructive flap necrosis
Yes – From plastic surgeon attribution to include transfer of primary care
Yes – From pathologist attribution (Postop. ID of positive SLN: false-negative intraop. SLN)
Yes – Preoperative imaging did not identify lesion in patient undergoing prophylactic mastectomy
Yes – Postop. ID of invasive cancer in DCIS patient with no SLN performed
Yes – Other: Please specify

*American Society of Breast Surgeons Mastery[SM] Program

• **Fig. 35.2** Example of a fully specified quality measure compliant with Centers for Medicare and Medicaid lexicon and ready for reporting by a surgeon in a patient registry. *DCIS*, Ductal carcinoma in situ; *IV*, intravenous; *SLN*, sentinel lymph node. (From the American Society of Breast Surgeons Mastery[SM] Program.)

endorsed their use and included hypofractionated schedules in their Choosing Wisely recommendations. Despite the evidence and expert endorsement, wide variations in adoption persist, with some geographic regions reporting very low use.[6] Rosenberg and coworkers[142] recently performed a claims-based analysis of adoption of seven Choosing Wisely recommendations for patients with common general medical conditions. They identified disappointingly low levels of adoption and concluded that more aggressive strategies would be needed to increase implementation. As a result of many similar observations, active dissemination and implementation policies have been developed (see Table 35.4).

New methods of quality improvement are emerging. As methods for personal improvement, "coaching" and "crowdsourcing" hold promise for surgeons.[143–148] In some studies, coaching, to include video review, assesses surgeon technical proficiency of skills, thereby providing opportunity for technical improvement

based on direct observation. A recent study linked a judged video assessment of technical skills to postoperative outcomes.[145]

Do Quality Measurement and Improvement Programs Work?

Performance improvement initiatives do not always succeed.[142] We only know if a regional or national program is effective by measuring predefined outcomes of program success and investigating whether unintended outcomes occurred as a result of the program.[142,149] More difficult to measure, but still important, is what additional burdens of data entry, whether financial or time, were necessary for providers to participate in a program.

In a recent presentation, Lemeneh Tefera, MD, using the Medicare database, reported that the all-cause hospital readmission rate

TABLE 35.4	Quality Improvement Tools		
Name		**Acronym**	**Reference**
Agency for Healthcare Research and Quality: Comprehensive Unit-based Safety Program		CUSP	http://www.ahrq.gov/professionals/education/curriculum-tools/cusptoolkit/index.html
Agency for Healthcare Research and Quality: D and I strategies		D and I	http://www.ahrq.gov/professionals/systems/hospital/qitoolkit/qiroadmap.html#implementing
Toyota's LEAN and Toyota Production System		Toyota's LEAN and TPS	http://www.ncbi.nlm.nih.gov/pmc/articles/PMC3678835/ and Going Lean in Health Care. IHI Innovation Series white paper. Cambridge, MA: Institute for Healthcare Improvement; 2005.
Plan-Do-Study-Act/Plan-Do-Check-Act		PDSA or PDCA	https://www.deming.org/theman/theories/pdsacycle and https://innovations.ahrq.gov/qualitytools/plan-do-study-act-pdsa-cycle
Institute for Healthcare Improvement: Model for Continuous Quality Improvement		IHI-Model for CQI	http://www.ihi.org/about/Pages/ScienceofImprovement.aspx and http://www.ihi.org/resources/Pages/HowtoImprove/default.aspx
Total Quality Management		TQM	http://www.toyota-global.com/company/history_of_toyota/75years/data/company_information/management_and_finances/management/tqm/change.html
Six Sigma		Six Sigma	http://www.hopkinsmedicine.org/innovation_quality_patient_care/areas_expertise/lean_sigma/about/
National Quality Strategy Levers		NQS 9 Levers[a]	http://www.ahrq.gov/workingforquality/about.htm

[a]See Table 35.1.

in the United States had declined significantly during the 4-year period ending 2014. By dates, this correlated with the implementation of the value-based purchasing and quality improvement programs implemented under the ACA. In addition, Tefera reported an estimated 17% reduction in hospital-acquired conditions, along with $12 billion and 50,000 lives saved.[150] These results suggest success; however, many other efforts to improve quality were ongoing during this same period. It is therefore difficult to determine which specific program(s) was the primary driver of better care.

Separate from state and federal government, multiple professional organizations representing providers of care offer different improvement programs. All contain measures of quality and outcomes and provide peer comparison. These programs differ in their metrics, analytic methods, and risk adjustment. Only a few are breast specific. There is good evidence that many, but not all, of these programs, demonstrate improvement in performance over time.[34,74,121,151–160] Multiple studies demonstrate a correlation between NSQIP participation and improvements in care, cost, and outcomes. For example, Hall and colleagues investigated the NSQIP database for 118 hospitals.[155] They found an association between hospital participation and reductions in complications and death. Both initially "worse-performing" and "well-performing" hospitals improved over time. Eighty-two percent of participating hospitals saw improvement in morbidity, and 66% saw reduction in mortality.[155] Building a business case for quality improvement, it was estimated that each patient having a major surgical complication had an estimated additional cost of at least $11,000.[154] Given the magnitude of reduction of complications associated with NSQIP participation, this translates into millions of dollars of cost savings per hospital per year. Recent investigations of the NSQIP database confirm continuing trends in improvement by participating hospitals each year.[153]

In contradistinction, a recent report interrogating the outcomes and expenditures for more than a million Medicare patients concluded no improvements in quality or cost of care before and after NSQIP hospital participation when using a difference-in-differences analytic approach to account for expected underlying natural drifts to better outcomes by all hospitals during the study time period.[121]

Have the Breast-Specific Quality Measurement Programs Improved Breast Care?

The American Society of Clinical Oncology quality program and the European breast programs have demonstrated performance improvement over time.[140] Brucker and coworkers reported striking improvement in multiple metrics in a German breast center patient registry.[151] From 2003 to 2007, the percentage of patients receiving the diagnosis of breast cancer by needle compared with open biopsy increased from 58% to 88%. EUSOMA results were more modest but still generally support the concept that auditing of QMs and peer comparison in Europe were associated with improvement.[15]

What Are the Risks of Quality Measurement?

There are risks of quality measurement.[35,161] As a consequence of either public transparency or in an attempt to achieve a benchmark, metrics may pressure providers of care to devote inordinate energy to look good. This effort to always be above average may change their normal practice of care. As a result, intentional or not, providers may exclude high-risk patients from audits, report outcomes selectively, or recommend that patients at high risk for poor outcomes forgo a specific procedure. This has been termed *risk aversion.* Hence too much emphasis on individual surgeon metrics could result in a health care quality measurement paradox. For example, the mastectomy rate, a measure of population quality, may worsen, but during this same time period, single-surgeon reexcision lumpectomy rates improve because surgeons may deny higher risk patients the option of breast-conserving surgery. In other words, surgeons change the eligibility criteria they use for an operation as a consequence of programs designed to improve care.[161] Not only might the mastectomy rate increase if reexcision rates are weighted too heavily, but other unintended adverse consequences could emerge as well.[161]

Another risk of performance measurement is the inappropriate assignment of an institution or surgeon to a low-quality tier due to lack of appropriate risk adjustment.[162-165] A notable recent example of this is the measurement of unplanned readmission rates within 30 days after hospital discharge. After years of CMS auditing this measure, Congress enacted the Hospital Readmissions Reduction Program, penalizing hospitals with higher-than-expected readmission rates up to 3% of their total Medicare payments.[166] Readmission rates declined significantly from 19% to 17.8% from 2008 to 2013, viewed as successful accountability use of a readmission rate as a QM.[163] Unfortunately, penalties more often occurred in academic and safety-net hospitals for reasons later found not to be under their control. Barnett and colleagues[164] reported that patients who were sicker, poorer, or less educated and who had fewer social supports were readmitted far more often than other patients. They concluded that hospitals were being penalized based on their underlying patient population, not on their lack of good quality care. Moreover, these patient characteristics were not included in any risk adjustment model before the decision of who to penalize. Thus if statistical confounders are either not known or known but not used during comparisons, then the risk of wrongful assignment of a hospital or surgeon to a low-quality performance decile is real.[162]

What Are the Future Challenges in Quality Measurement?

Despite widespread acceptance of the need to identify and address gaps in the quality of health care, there are challenges. For institutions, these include lack of funding for measurement, lack of provider engagement, lack of a business model to sustain a quality program, and lack of understanding of how to improve, once gaps have been identified. For surgeons, conceptual challenges exist when additional burdens of data entry are required for measurement of their performance. Surgeons are often asked to personally enter quality data into a database to report whether they were compliant with recommended care or to record a postoperative outcome. From the surgeons' perspective, they are inherently dedicated to best care, but extra data entry is a burden. This burden is nearly always unfunded, and providers of care can now be heard describing themselves as *typists* and *abstractors.*

Surgeons and other stakeholders have not yet identified the sweet spot between necessary but burdensome auditing and the surgeons' need to devote the majority of their time to direct patient care. In addition, regulatory oversight is perceived as irritating and heavy-handed by some. During the auditing of health care, surgeons, as well as all other care providers, understand that decisions and actions regarding real patient care do not always fit into the simplistic yes/no response format of a performance measure. Exceptions to meeting the performance requirements of a QM do not uniformly reflect a quality concern, yet few QMs can take all circumstances into account to allow distinction between a real quality concern versus justifiable reason for deviation in meeting performance for a process of care measurement.

Some surgeons have a skeptical view of the worthiness of QM programs in general, questioning their value, accuracy, and ability to accurately adjust for risk before peer comparison. For example, how can you risk adjust for the surgeon's act of selecting patients for surgical procedures?[84] Undoubtedly, this process, which is unique to each surgeon, can be linked to surgical outcomes, but can current risk-adjustment models for patient and tumor characteristics, even if they are state of the art, adequately adjust for all comorbidities in the selection process? The selection process is increasingly a team effort, with specialists in preoperative optimization and prehabilitation assisting in patient selection for surgery. Because selection is linked to outcome, to whom do you now attribute a bad outcome?

Linking an unwanted outcome to a single care provider is challenging. For example, to whom is breast tumor recurrence after breast-conserving therapy 5 years earlier attributed? Should it be attributed to poor surgery, noncompliant radiation or medical oncology treatment, or inadequate shared decision-making regarding choices for adjuvant therapies? Or should it be considered unavoidable owing to aggressive tumor biology or to patient choice to defer treatment? Assigning attribution for a poor outcome or wrong process of care is difficult, especially for composite measures of care. Cancer recurrence and reoperation rates are good examples of results of care that are dependent on multiple processes and specialties.

Another systems challenge is the lack of harmonization of QMs. If performance reporting for a measure reflects the same domain of care but their specifications are different, they must be calculated and reported separately. For example, CMS and NSQIP calculate time at risk for readmission differently: CMS uses 30 days from discharge, and NSQIP uses 30 days from operation. To improve harmonization, the stewards of QM must collaborate to reconcile these differences.

Lastly, there will be challenges in the US government's schedule to implement the Department of Health and Human Service's goals for value-based payments to providers and hospitals. Such a rapid change in the nation's health care structure for reimbursement has never occurred. The targets were for 85% of Medicare fee-for-service payments to be tied to quality or value by 2016, and 30% of Medicare payments to be tied to quality or value through alternative payment models by 2016 (50% by 2018).[1]

Conclusion

Oversight and regulation of surgical care, quality, and outcomes are unlikely to go away anytime soon. The current rate of rise of health care costs for Medicare is not sustainable. Twenty-five percent of privately insured working-age people and 53% of the lower income citizens of the United States find health care unaffordable. This lack of affordability will continue to be a major driver of change.[167] Despite challenges, we must accept ownership of measurement and improvement activities. General and breast surgeons have compelling reasons to advance the science of quality measurement and improvement. Aside from the patients themselves, we remain their strongest advocate for good surgical outcomes. We understand the types of unwanted outcomes that occur after breast surgery and the local resources available to prevent, treat, and monitor them. We also understand the nuances of patient care, the complexity of hospital systems and their operating rooms, and the unique needs of surgical patients. Thus we are best positioned to develop our measurement programs. In its essence, quality care for each patient begins at the local level with individual surgeons. Despite any surgeon's perceived worthiness of the existing quality initiatives, it behooves us to provide practical and scientific advice to quality program developers, then choose some level of participation in a program that fits best with the surgeon's personal notion of the best balance between burdens of reporting and opportunity to improve care at the local or national level. If we do not accept our obligation to improve cost, care, and outcomes, others will do it for us. Excellent resources are available to help providers of care negotiate the quality landscape and succeed.[127,168–170] All maintain a clearinghouse

of quality resources, a blueprint for quality infrastructure, and primers for education—collectively, the catalysts for driving improvement.

Selected References

17. Institute of Medicine. Committee on Quality of Health Care in America. *Crossing the Quality Chasm: A New Health System for the 21st Century.* Washington, DC: National Academy Press; 2001.
20. Berwick DM, Nolan TW, Whittington J. The Triple Aim: care, health, and cost. *Health Aff.* 2008;27:759-769.
168. National Quality Forum. http://www.qualityforum.org/Home .aspx. Accessed 8 December 2015.
169. Agency for Healthcare Research & Quality. http://www.ahrq.gov. Accessed 8 December 2015.
170. Institute for Healthcare Improvement. http://www.ihi.org/Pages/ default.aspx. Accessed 8 December 2015.

A full reference list is available online at ExpertConsult.com.

36

Lymphedema in the Postmastectomy Patient: Pathophysiology, Prevention, and Management

AMY E. RIVERE AND V. SUZANNE KLIMBERG

Lymphedema is the most dreaded complication of breast cancer surgery. It may result in functional, esthetic, and psychological problems, thereby affecting the quality of life of the breast cancer patient. It also predisposes patients to development of infections, decreased functional ability and range of motion, and potential development of malignant lymphangiosarcoma (Stewart-Treves syndrome). It adversely affects quality of life, job performance, and health care costs.

Lymphedema is the result of the functional overload of the lymphatic system in which volume of lymph is greater than the transport capability of the lymphatic channels. The increase in oncotic pressure in the peripheral tissues due to accumulation of macromolecules leads to accumulation of fluid in the interstitial spaces. This protein-rich environment can lead to infection if the integument is broken with minor abrasion or trauma. Lymphedema can begin insidiously at variable periods after axillary treatment. The swelling can range from mild to a seriously disabling enlargement of the arm. Research in this area has been limited because of the variable development over long periods of time and inconsistent subjective versus objective diagnostic definitions of lymphedema. Lymphedema has been viewed as less important than the eradication of cancer and detection of recurrence. There is little in the literature about the prevalence of breast cancer–related lymphedema (BCRL), but Greene and associates estimated that it was 1 in 1000 patients. Incidence of lymphedema has been reported to be somewhere between 0% and 77% in literature (Table 36.1).[1–15] The length of follow-up, type of measurement technique, and definition of lymphedema varies from study to study.

The extent of surgery, patient age, obesity, infection, and adjuvant treatment have been reported to be associated risk factors for the development of lymphedema. The relationship between association of axillary metastases, use of tamoxifen, presence of pre-existing health conditions, tumor size, and time course of the development of lymphedema has not been consistently reported in the literature.

History

In approximately 1622, anatomic dissections by Gasparo Aselli of Italy revealed mesenteric lacteals. In well-fed dogs, these vessels contained a milky white fluid that drained into a large mesenteric node.[16] Later, the French anatomist Jean Pecquet recognized the thoracic duct and its importance in the understanding of the lymphatic system. In 1953 the Scandinavians Rudbeck and Bartholin were the first to use the term lymphatics, but the function of the lymphatics remained a mystery.[16]

In the 18th century, those in William Hunter's School of Anatomy in London studied the anatomy and physiology of the lymphatic system. The work, as summarized by Hunter, showed that "the lymphatic vessels are the absorbing vessels all over the body … and constitute one great and general system."[17] It is probable that Cruickshank (1786), disciple of William Hunter, was the first person to describe in detail the human breast lymphatics in a fresh cadaver of a woman who had died during childbirth.

In 1860 Virchow[18] was one of the first to recognize the importance of the lymphatic system in cancer, believing that lymph nodes acted as a barrier to cancer spread. The radical surgical procedures developed shortly thereafter, including radical mastectomy, radical neck dissection, and abdominal perineal resection, were based on the concept that there was a stepwise progression of cancer spread from the lymph nodes to systemic areas. In fact, Sir Berkeley Moynihan (1865–1936) wrote, "The surgery of malignant disease is not the surgery of organs; it is the anatomy of the lymph node system."[19]

One of the first articles to describe chronic lymphedema as a complication was written by Matas[20] in 1913. Matas stated the following:

> By elephantiasis we mean a progressive histopathologic state or condition which is characterized by a chronic inflammatory fibromatosis or hypertrophy of the hypodermal and dermal connective tissue which is preceded by and associated with lymphatic and venous stasis, and may be caused by any obstruction or mechanical interference with the return flow of the lymphatic and venous currents.[21]

Halsted[21] later expounded on it with his article concerning "elephantiasis chirurgica."

TABLE 36.1	Incidence of Lymphedema						
Reference	Year	Follow-Up (mo)	No. of Patients	Measurement	SLNB	ALND
Schrenk et al.[1]	2000	15	35, 35	Not reported	0	57
Sener et al.[2]	2001	24	303, 117	C >20%	3	17
Swenson et al.[3]	2002	12	169, 78	Survey	9	17
Haid et al.[4]	2002	>36	57, 140	Subjective, CE	4	27
Blanchard et al.[5]	2003	29	894, 164	Subjective	6	34
Schijven et al.[6]	2003	38%, 50% ≤12	180, 213	Subjective	1	7
Ronka et al.[7]	2005	12	43, 40	Subjective	13	77
ALMANAC[8]	2006	12	478, 403	C	5	13
Francis et al.[9]	2006	12	26, 73	Volume	17	47
ACOSOG Z0011[10]	2007	12	445, 446	C >2 cm (20%)	6	11
Swiss Multicenter[11]	2007	31, 30	449, 210	C	4	19
McLaughlin et al.[12]	2008	60	600, 336	C	5	16
NSABP B-32[13]	2010	36	2008, 1975	Volume (≥10%)	8	14
Sagen et al.[14]	2014	30	187, 204	Volume	3	17
Sackey et al.[15]	2014	36	140, 280	Volume	20	45

ALND, Axillary lymph node dissection; *C,* circumference; *CE,* clinical examination; *SLNB,* sentinel lymph node biopsy.

Anatomy

Current understanding of the lymphatic system of the breast is based primarily on the work of Sappey in the 1850s who showed that the upper torso drains from a subareolar plexus to the ipsilateral axilla. In 1903 Poirer and Cuneo summarized the results of Sappey, added their results from fetal studies using Gerota's method of staining lymphatics with oil painting dye and published a comprehensive anatomy book of the lymphatic system.[22] Figs. 36.1 and 36.2 show the Poirer and Cuneo summary of breast drainage and Sappey's findings. A recent study published by anatomist Ian Taylor's group[23] described the anatomy of the breast, and his findings are discordant with the current knowledge of the breast lymphatics. However, Dr. Taylor and colleagues[23] described the lymphatics of the breast by cannulating the lymphatic vessels in cadavers and injecting radiopaque material containing lead oxide, with a repetition of the process until the first lymph node (sentinel node [SLN]) for each collector was reached (Fig. 36.3). The procedure was performed around the entire periphery of the specimen in the subcutaneous plane and around the internal thoracic artery in the vicinity of the perforating branches of the internal thoracic. Blue dye and hydrogen peroxide were used to stain the lymphatic vessels from the nipple and areola. The lymphatic collectors were traced to the first-tier node and color-coded, and all collectors draining to the same first-tier node were given the same color (see Fig. 36.3).

The lymphatics were identified to branch in the peripheral region and then joined to form large collectors that remained

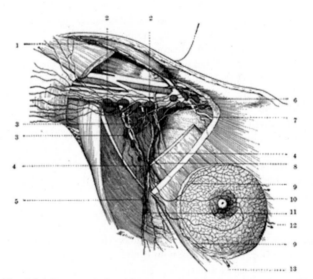

• **Fig. 36.1** Poirer and Cuneo's summary of the breast drainage. This diagram was based on the anatomic and clinical findings of several people, including Sappey. (From Suami H, Pan W-R, Mann GB, Taylor GI. The lymphatic anatomy of the breast and its implications for sentinel lymph node biopsy: a human cadaver study. *Ann Surg Oncol.* 2007;15: 863-871.)

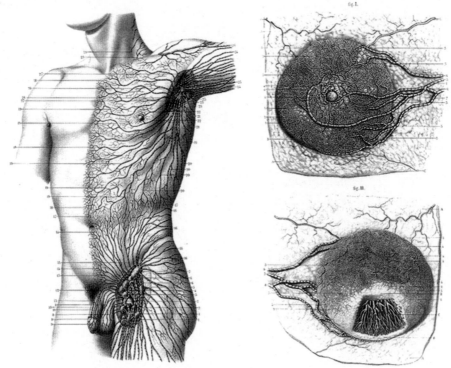

• **Fig. 36.2** Sappey's 1874 drawing of the superficial lymphatics of the upper torso *(left)* and female breast *(right)*. (From Suami H, Pan W-R, Mann GB, Taylor GI. The lymphatic anatomy of the breast and its implications for sentinel lymph node biopsy: a human cadaver study. *Ann Surg Oncol.* 2007;15: 863-871.)

uniform in diameter until they reached the SLN. All superficial lymphatics entered a lymph node in the axilla close to the lateral edge of the pectoralis minor muscle. Lymphatics that passed over or through the breast ended by draining into the same first-tier lymph nodes. Lymphatics in the areolar region were found to be a dense network of lymph capillaries and precollectors in the dermis (Fig. 36.4). In the breast region, most of the lymphatics ran between the dermis and the breast tissue and traversed the breast tissue to reach axillary lymph nodes.[23]

The internal mammary lymphatics were identified along the internal mammary vessels and lymph nodes identified in the intercostals spaces. No connections between collecting lymphatics along the branches of the internal mammary artery and superficial lymphatics were identified; the superficial lymphatics passed laterally toward the axilla.

The observation that the lymphatics pass through the breast tissue or superficial to it is also supported by the studies done by Turner-Warwick,[24,25] who demonstrated a direct pathway from the injection site to the axillary lymph node.

The conclusions were as follows:

• Lymph vessels passing through the breast contribute to breast drainage.
• If the tracer was injected deeply it reached two sets of nodes, as opposed to when it was injected subareolarly or intradermally, where it reached one node only. This difference explains the false-negative rate of sentinel node biopsy because more than one sentinel node can drain the breast.
• Another anatomic explanation for false-negative results after sentinel node biopsy is the variation in the distribution of the perforating lymphatics. The perforating system is

connected to the deep lymphatic vessels. In all quadrants of the breast and especially for deep and medial tumors, cancer can spread via internal mammary lymphatics and intradermal injection does not demonstrate the internal mammary lymphatics.

• No evidence of a centripetal anatomic lymphatic pathway draining the breast tissue toward the subareolar plexus and then toward the sentinel node was identified.
• Accurate lymphatic mapping requires intraparenchymal injection.

Lymph Nodes and Lymphatics Draining the Upper Extremity

Most but not all lymphatics from the upper limb drain into lymph nodes in the axilla.[26] Some can bypass the axilla and drain directly into the subclavian vein. In addition, axillary nodes receive drainage from an extensive area on the adjacent trunk, which includes regions of the upper back and shoulder, the lower neck, the chest, and the upper anterolateral abdominal wall. Axillary nodes also receive drainage from approximately 75% of the mammary gland. The 20 to 30 axillary nodes are generally divided into five groups on the basis of location (Fig. 36.5).

1. Humeral nodes are found posteromedial to the axillary vein above the second intercostal nerve and receive most of the lymphatic drainage from the upper limb.
2. Pectoral nodes occur along the inferior margin of the pectoralis minor muscle along the course of the lateral thoracic vessels and receive drainage from the abdominal wall, the chest, and the mammary gland.

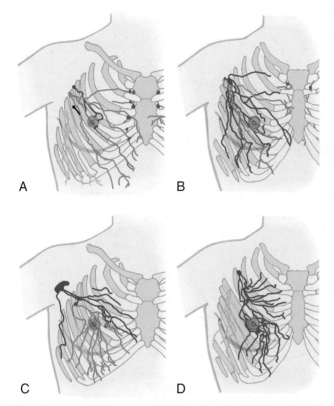

• **Fig. 36.3** (A and C) Male lymphatics. (B and D) Female lymphatics. Tracing distally of lymphatics of both partial upper torsos from each first-tier lymph node color-coded: pectoral nodes (*green, orange, black,* and *yellow*), subclavicular node *(light blue)*, and internal mammary node *(red)*. Lymphatics from nipple and areolar region drain into green colored lymph nodes. Breast lies in the pathway of collecting lymphatics that start peripherally. Although the majority of breast drains into one sentinel node as in (D), every breast area is drained by more than one first-tier node. (Modified from Suami H, Pan W-R, Mann GB, Taylor GI. The lymphatic anatomy of the breast and its implications for sentinel lymph node biopsy: a human cadaver study. *Ann Surg Oncol.* 2007;15:863-871.)

3. Subscapular nodes on the posterior axillary wall in association with the subscapular vessels drain the posterior axillary wall and receive lymphatics from the back, the shoulder, and the neck.
4. Central nodes are embedded in axillary fat and receive lymphatics from humeral, subscapular, and pectoral groups of nodes.
5. Apical nodes are the most superior group of nodes in the axilla and drain all other groups of nodes in the region. In addition, they receive lymphatic vessels that accompany the cephalic vein as well as vessels that drain the superior region of the mammary gland.

Klimberg and colleagues first described the drainage of the arm within the axilla using a technique of axillary reverse mapping (ARM).[27,28] Variations in arm drainage were seen including the traditional teaching of lymphatics from the arm running just beneath the axillary vein either above or below; a sling low in the axilla as much as 3 to 4 cm below the vein; a lateral or medial apron of nodes that could be separated from the underlying axilla proper and then a cord of lymphatics or even a chain of nodes that came across low in the axilla. Our group demonstrated that a majority of the time, these lymphatics could be separated from the lymphatics draining the breast within the axilla as well as major variations of that drainage (Fig. 36.6).[29] Efferent vessels from the apical group converge to form the subclavian trunk, which usually joins the venous system at the junction between the right subclavian vein and the right internal jugular vein in the neck. On the left, the subclavian trunk usually joins the thoracic duct in the base of the neck.

The lymphatics of the upper limb drain directly into a terminal group of lymph nodes in the axilla either directly or passing through a group of lymph nodes. Lymphatics deep to the fascia follow the neurovascular bundles, whereas the superficial lymphatics follow the superficial veins with the exception of the lymphatics of the hand and back of the forearm. Lymphatics from the hand enter the forearm along the cephalic and basilic vein, whereas the deep lymphatics follow the radial, ulnar, interosseous,

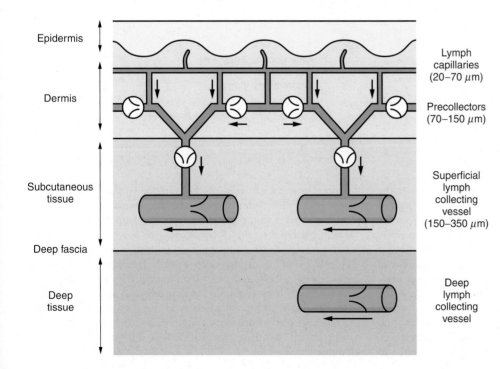

• **Fig. 36.4** Schematic diagram of the relationship between the lymph capillaries, precollectors, and lymph collecting vessels. (Modified from Suami H, Pan W-R, Mann GB, Taylor GI. The lymphatic anatomy of the breast and its implications for sentinel lymph node biopsy: a human cadaver study. *Ann Surg Oncol.* 2007;15:863-871.)

Epidermis

Dermis

Subcutaneous tissue

Deep fascia

Deep tissue

Lymph capillaries (20–70 μm)

Precollectors (70–150 μm)

Superficial lymph collecting vessel (150–350 μm)

Deep lymph collecting vessel

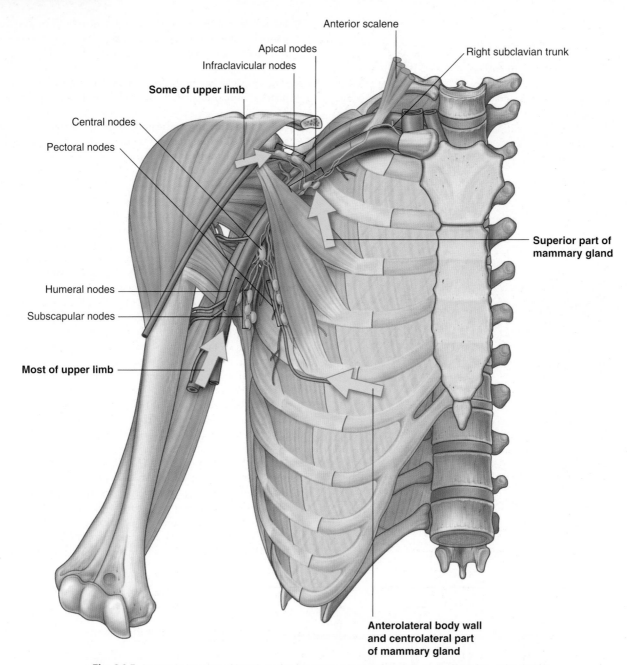

• **Fig. 36.5** Anatomic location of lymph nodes by groups; humeral nodes, pectoral nodes, subscapular nodes, central nodes, and apical nodes. (From Drake R. *Gray's Anatomy for Students*. 13th ed. Philadelphia: Churchill Livingstone; 2005.)

and brachial neurovascular bundles and end at the lateral or the humeral group of lymph nodes. In some patients, lymphatics accompany the axillary vein. The superficial lymphatics are more numerous, and they appear to communicate with the deep vessel lymphatics along their course in the arm.[29] More recent reports by Suami and Taylor[30] did not identify a communication between the superficial and the deep system. They also reported that most lymphatics from the arm drain into one main lymph node in the axillary region, that some lymphatics run along the posterior arm and bypass the main node and enter other smaller nodes, and that there can be interconnections between these nodes (Figs. 36.7 and 36.8). However, a later report published by Suami and

Taylor[31] pointed out that the lymphatics on the limb from the mastectomy side were different compared with the normal arm. They noticed a complete absence of the superficial lymphatic system proximal to the elbow because of blockage of lymphatic channels and identified a circuitous pathway that bypassed these lymphatics to reach the deep system facilitated by backflow through the precollectors and lymph capillaries in the dermis of the forearm. They concluded that previously undetected lymph channels between the superficial and the deep system open due to blockage of the superficial system caused by axillary dissection and reported that these channels may be helpful in prevention of lymphedema.

Pathophysiology

The lymphatic system develops during the embryologic phase as part of the vascular system. The components of the lymphatic fluid include endothelial cells, protein, water, tissue products, and

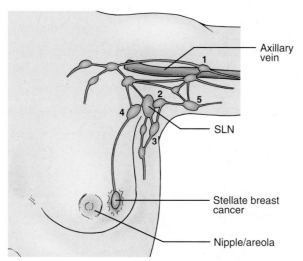

• **Fig. 36.6** Variations in axillary reverse mapping (ARM): anatomic variation in ARM drainage. (1) Traditional teaching of lymphatics from the arm running juxtaposed to the axillary vein either above or below; (2) sling low in the axilla; (3) lateral apron; (4) medial apron (lateral and medial aprons consist of multiple blue nodes); (5) entwined cord of lymphatics or lymph node chain. *SLN*, Sentinel lymph node. (From Boneti C, Korourian S, Bland K, et al. Axillary reverse mapping: mapping and preserving arm lymphatics may be important in preventing lymphedema during sentinel node biopsy. *J Am Coll Surg.* 2009;206:1038-1042.)

other foreign particles. It is believed that the mammalian lymphatic system evolves from the fusion of clefts in the perivenous mesoderm layers.

The lymph capillaries form a network more extensive than that of blood capillaries. In some tissues, such as the skin, gastrointestinal tract, and lung, the lymphatics can be quite extensive. Other organs, such as the bone marrow and brain, do not contain any lymphatics. In the breast, the lymphatics may penetrate the pectoralis fascia when coursing to the axilla. The lymph capillaries, which begin as closed saccules, consist of a single layer of endothelium without gaps. Unlike blood vessels, the lymphatic vessels have an absent or poorly developed basement membrane. This facilitates intercellular movement of plasma proteins and lipids that are too large for venous absorption. Lymphatics reabsorb the fluid exuded by the blood capillaries, but they are also capable of taking up material that is quite large to drain into the collecting lymph vessels.[30] Normally, the pressure in the lymphatic vessels is negative or 0 mm H_2O. After an axillary dissection, intralymphatic pressure becomes positive, and lymphatic flow can be 10 times slower than normal.

The collecting lymph vessels are thin-walled structures with valves every 2 to 3 mm. The smaller collecting vessels have an inner coat of elastic longitudinal fibers and endothelial cells and an outer layer of connective tissue. The larger vessels have an additional middle smooth muscle coat, which aids transport of the fluid. These larger vessels coalesce and travel parallel with the veins to the draining lymph nodes.[30]

In the fetus, the lymph nodes form after the various plexuses develop. Foci of lymphocytes begin to accumulate within a network of lymphatic capillaries and eventually form lymph nodes. The afferent lymphatic enters the outside of the node into the marginal sinus. This structure surrounds the node and has a

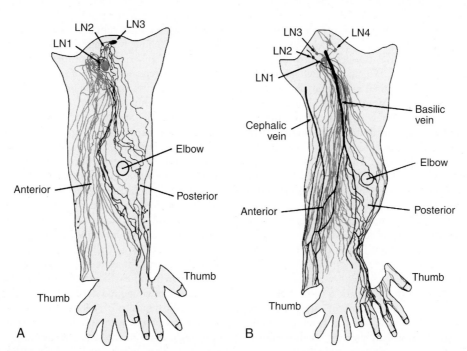

• **Fig. 36.7** (A) Tracing of lymphatics distally from each lymph node and color-coded to define territories. Note that territories of each node do not overlap; orange territory can drain either into LN1 or LN3. Interconnections within each territory are noted. (B) Veins have been injected. Also noted is the dominant territory of LN1 that connects proximally to two other nodes, LN3 and LN4. (Modified from Suami H, Taylor GI. The lymphatic territories of the upper limb: anatomic study and clinical implications. *Plast Reconstr Surg.* 2005;119:1813-1822.)

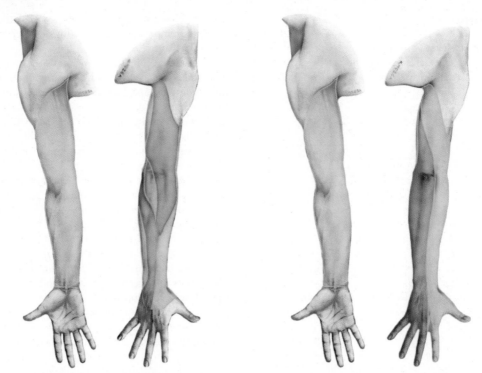

• **Fig. 36.8** Lymphatic territories of each sentinel node colored to match those of Fig. 36.7. (Modified from Suami H, Taylor GI. The lymphatic territories of the upper limb: anatomic study and clinical implications. *Plast Reconstr Surg.* 2005;119:1813-1822.)

delicate retinaculum that will trap particulate material, including metastatic cells. Thus the marginal sinus is the first site for metastases to be found. The efferent lymphatic vessel leaves the hilum of the node.[30]

The normal function of the lymphatics is to return proteins, lipids, and water from the interstitium to the intravascular space. High hydrostatic pressures in arterial capillaries force proteinaceous fluid into the interstitium, resulting in increased interstitial oncotic pressure that draws in additional water that then constitutes the lymph fluid. Before returning to the blood, stream lymph passes through lymph nodes where its composition is altered. Interstitial fluid normally contributes to the nourishment of tissues. Approximately 90% of the fluid returns to the circulation via entry into venous capillaries. The remaining 10% is composed of high-molecular-weight proteins and their oncotically associated water, which is too large to readily pass through venous capillary walls. The lymph then flows into the lymphatic capillaries where pressures are typically low and can accommodate the large size of the proteins and their accompanying water. The lymph fluid then passes through various lymph nodes to join the venous circulation.

When the lymphatic system is altered either as the result of infection, malignancy, or surgery, the lymphatic transport capacity is reduced. This leads to increased production of interstitial fluid that then exceeds the rate of lymphatic return, therefore leading to stagnation of high-molecular-weight proteins in the interstitium. Compared with other forms of edema, this fluid contains high concentration of proteins, whereas other forms of edema are secondary to hypoproteinemia. The high oncotic pressure in the interstitium favors the accumulation of additional water. The accumulation of protein and fluid is a transitory phase lasting 1 to 3 weeks. This then leads to latent phase, which can last from

4 months to 10 years. There may be no clinical signs and symptoms in the latent phase.

Accumulation of interstitial fluid leads to dilatation of the remaining outflow tracts and valvular incompetence that causes reversal of flow from subcutaneous tissues into the dermal plexus. Persistent swelling and stagnant protein eventually lead to fibrosis and provide an excellent culture medium for bacteria to grow, allowing for repeated bouts of cellulitis.

The lymphatic walls undergo fibrosis, and fibrinoid thrombi accumulate within the lumen, obliterating much of the remaining lymph channels. Spontaneous lymphovenous shunts may form. Lymph nodes harden and shrink, losing their normal architecture.

In the interstitium, protein and fluid accumulation initiates a marked inflammatory reaction that leads to increased macrophage activity and destruction of elastic fibers. Fibroblasts migrate into the interstitium and deposit collagen. As a result of this inflammatory reaction, there is a change from the initial pitting edema to the brawny nonpitting edema characteristic of lymphedema. Local immunologic mechanisms are suppressed, predisposing to chronic infections as well as to malignant degeneration of lymphangiosarcoma (Stewart-Treves syndrome).

The skin becomes thickened and gives the typical peau d'orange appearance of congested dermal lymphatics. The epidermis forms thick scaly deposits of keratinized debris; cracks and furrows develop, leading to accumulation of bacteria and leakage of lymph from the surface of the skin. The resulting infection and inflammation further aggravate the edema. The clinical treatment of lymphedema is based on prevention of this vicious cycle.

This entire sequence of events develops in only a small percentage of patients after complete axillary lymph node dissection (ALND) or radiation therapy. The precipitating factors for the development of overt lymphedema are unknown. In patients where the lymphatics accompany the cephalic vein instead of the axillary vein, the incidence of lymphedema formation is reduced because in those cases the lymphatics bypass the axilla. Radiation therapy and repeated bouts of infection may be important factors in the development of lymphedema.

Lymphedema becomes clinically apparent when the compensatory mechanisms are inadequate to combat the requirements of lymphatic flow. The process of lymphatic regeneration may be altered in some patients. Another possible mechanism in lymphedema formation could be alterations in blood flow caused by either venous obstruction or increased arterial flow as a result of reflex sympathetic effects of neurologic injury associated with axillary or breast surgery (postmastectomy syndrome).[32-34]

Etiologic Risk Factors and Incidence

Six contributing factors have been shown to influence the incidence of brachial edema after treatment for breast cancer: radiation therapy, obesity, age, operative site, incision type, and history of infection.[35,36] The increased incidence of post-ALND lymphedema formation in older versus younger women may be caused by the formation of lymphovenous anastomoses in younger women that can bridge the lymph and blood circulation systems but which are closed under normal circumstances. When increased pressure in the lymph system causes the lymphovenous anastomoses to open, this alternate route accomplishes lymph drainage. These lymphovenous anastomoses are much less common in older persons.[37] The occurrence of postoperative wound complications, particularly infection, but also hematoma and/or seroma formation or flap necrosis, was identified as an independent risk factor for the development of lymphedema.[38,39] The presence of axillary metastases and thus the extent of surgery has been found to be associated with increased risk of lymphedema formation by some groups.[40-42]

Adding radiation therapy has been shown to increase the incidence of lymphedema from 20% to 52%.[43,44] The incidence of lymphedema is lessened if transverse rather than oblique incisions are used in the axilla.[35] Others have suggested that the extent of axillary dissection is an important contributing factor. Limiting the axillary dissection to level I and II nodes and preserving the level III nodes and lymphatic collateral channels around the shoulder may decrease the incidence of acute and chronic lymphedema. Larson and colleagues[45] reported that the risk of lymphedema was 37% when full level I through III ALND was carried out, compared with 8% when a level I to II ALND was performed. They also found a correlation between the risk of lymphedema formation and the number of removed lymph nodes; when more than 10 lymph nodes were removed, the risk of edema was 28% versus 9% if 1 to 10 lymph nodes were found in the resected specimen. Petrek and associates[46] have described posttreatment weight gain/obesity as a risk factor for lymphedema formation.

Recent adoption of lymphatic mapping and SLN biopsy (SLNB) for women with invasive breast cancer has minimized the risk of lymphedema while providing accurate staging of the axillary nodal basin. The hypothesis that the histology of the SLNs reflects the histology of the remaining nodes in the basin is well documented. This approach limits the risk of lymphedema mainly to those with positive nodes (see Table 36.1).

Postsurgical BCRL is hypothesized to be caused by disruption of the lymphatics draining the arm. Lymphatics from the arm, back, and breast all drain to the same nodal basin under the arm.

Such lymphatics are indistinguishable in appearance and for the most part in location. Scarring that occurs with surgery, chemotherapy, and radiation may attribute to this mechanical obstruction. However, primary lymphatic flow does vary with the individual patient and genes that may influence lymphedema such as *SOX18*, *CCBE1*, *GJC2*, *GATA2*, *KIF11*, and *VEGFC* making an individual more at risk for lymphedema after surgical disruption of lymphatics.[47]

Incidence

The risk of lymphedema with ALND averages 28% with a range that varies in the literature from 11% to 57% in larger trials.[48] It varies over time depending on type of measurement and extent of surgery, but most lymphedema occurs by 3 years and may continue over a lifetime. The variation in lymphedema rates also reflects the great variability in the technique of axillary node dissection between surgeons, how closely lymphedema is monitored, length of follow-up,[46,48,49] and, questionably, the number of positive lymph nodes,[50] postoperative irradiation,[51] extent of surgery, body habitus, and a number of other patient characteristics.[49,51]

Although the lymphedema rate is much lower with the SLNB, it is still clinically significant. Because so many more patients undergo SLNB, the actual number of patients who get lymphedema due to SLNB approximates the number that will get lymphedema after an ALND. The incidence of lymphedema after SLN mapping averages 6.3% with a range that has been reported to be between 0% and 23%. In the Axillary Lymphatic Mapping Against Nodal Axillary Clearance (ALMANAC) trial, lymphedema was observed in about 5% of breast cancer patients after SLNB.[52] In the prospective international multicenter study organized by the American College of Surgeons Oncology Group (ACOSOG), trial Z0010, upper limb lymphedema (as determined by arm circumference measurements with a difference of 1 cm between arms) was observed in about 7% of patients with breast cancer after SLNB, performed by a wide range of surgeons.[53] The National Surgical Breast and Bowel Project (NSABP-32) trained a cohort of surgeons in SLNB and randomized 5400 patients to SLNB followed by ALND versus SLNB alone demonstrating an 8% risk of BCRL with SLNB.[13] Randomized controlled trials reported that SLNB compared with ALND leads to a significant reduction in postoperative complications (see Table 36.1).

However, the advent of SLNB does not solve the problem of BCRL because just as many women get lymphedema from a negative SLNB as do women from an ALND. Few studies considered incidence, risk factors and treatment costs of BCRL among working-age women after breast cancer treatment, reporting that the BCRL population had significantly higher rehabilitative medical costs ($14,877 to $23,167) with twice as much risk to develop BCRL complications, such as lymphangitis or cellulitis, compared with "BCRL-free" population (odds ratio = 2.02, p = .009).[54,55]

Francis and colleagues[9] described applicability of standardized terminology from Common Terminology Criteria for Adverse Events (CTCAE; Table 36.2) to the incidence of and severity of postoperative acute lymphedema during the first year after SLNB and ALND. According to this report, the incidence of lymphedema was 16.8% after SLNB and 47.1% after ALND. After SLNB, acute lymphedema of severity level I developed in 65% and severity level II in 35%. In the ALND group, severity level II lymphedema reached 60%.

TABLE 36.2 Common Terminology Criteria for Adverse Events, v3.0[a]

Limb	Level I	Level II	Level III	Level IV
Edema	5%–10% interlimb discrepancy in volume or circumference	>10%–30% interlimb discrepancy in volume or circumference	>30% interlimb discrepancy in volume; lymphorrhea; gross deviation from normal anatomic contour; interferes with activities of daily living	Progression to malignancy (i.e., lymphangiosarcoma); amputation indicated; disabling

[a]According to the National Cancer Institute, which has standardized reporting of adverse events in clinical trials.
From Francis WP, Abghari P, Du W, Rymal C, Suna M, Kosir MA. Improving surgical outcomes: standardizing the reporting of incidence and severity of acute lymphedema after sentinel lymph node biopsy and axillary lymph node dissection. *Am J Surg.* 2006;192:636–639.

TABLE 36.3 Lymphedema: Extent of Surgery and Radiation

	Follow-Up (mo)	Measurement	SLNB + WBXRT	ALND + WBRXT	SLNB + WBXRT + RNI	ALND + WBXRT + RNI
ACOSOG Z0011[10] (2007)	12	Arm circumference >2 cm (20%)	6	11		
NSABP B-32[13] (2010)	36	Volume displacement	8	14		
EORTC AMAROS[64] (2014)	60	Arm circumference (10%)		13	5	
NCIC-CTG MA.20[65] (2015)	114	EORTC QLQ-C30		4.5 58% G1 38% G2 4% G3 (10% SLNB)		8.4 25% G1 65% G2 10% G3

ALND, Axillary lymph node dissection; *EORTC AMAROS,* European Organization for Research and Treatment of Cancer after Mapping of the Axilla: Radiotherapy or Surgery; *NCIC-CTG,* National Cancer Institute of Canada Clinical Trials Group; *RNI,* regional lymph node irradiation; *SLNB,* sentinel lymph node biopsy; *WBXRT,* whole breast irradiation.

Lymphedema From Radiation Treatment

Radiation therapy has been found to be an independent risk factor for the development of lymphedema with incidence reported as high as 2% to 5% even without axillary surgery.[56,57] With radiotherapy targeted to the breast, some dose reaches level I and level II nodes, depending on the technique and the anatomy of the patient.[58,59] The exception is in the case of prone positioning where only 13% of level I and none of level II or III receive a radiation dose.[60] Axillary radiation is associated with 2 to 4.5 times greater risk of development of lymphedema and 8 to 10 times greater risk with the combination of radiation and ALND.[61–63] Effect on the development of lymphedema with radiation therapy is also observed with radiation therapy to the breast or chest wall (Table 36.3).[10,13,64,65]

Classification

Lymphedema is classified as primary or secondary and as acute or chronic:

- Primary lymphedema is secondary to congenital abnormalities of the lymphatic system, including lymphatic hypoplasia or dysfunction of the lymphatic valves.
- Secondary lymphedema is a common morbidity from treatment of malignancy, such as treatment of breast cancer patients with axillary surgery or radiation therapy.
- Acute lymphedema typically occurs within 6 months of mastectomy and lasts 3 to 6 months. It is pitting in nature and is usually transient and self-limited and is more pronounced at the end of the day. There is no evidence suggesting increased risk of development of chronic edema.
- Chronic lymphedema is typically present for 3 months and is nonpitting in nature. There are skin changes associated with it, and these patients are prone to cellulitis and ulcer formation.

According to the International Society of Lymphology Staging System, lymphedema also may be described in terms of its stage[66]:

- Stage 0: This stage is also known as latent or subclinical. Swelling is not clinically evident despite impaired lymph transport. It may exist months or years before overt edema occurs.
- Stage I: This stage represents an early accumulation of fluid relatively high in protein content and subsides with limb elevation. Pitting may occur.
- Stage II: Limb elevation alone rarely reduces tissue swelling, and pitting is manifest. Late in stage II, the limb may or may not pit as tissue fibrosis supervenes.
- Stage III: This stage encompasses lymphostatic elephantiasis, where pitting is absent and trophic skin changes such as acanthosis, fat deposits, and warty overgrowths develop.

Within each stage, severity based on limb volume difference can be assessed as minimal (<20% increase), moderate (20%–40% increase), or severe (>40% increase).

Patient History and Measurement of Lymphedema

Symptoms of chronic lymphedema are usually elicited by taking an accurate history of the patient. Patients complain of an overall increase or "fullness" of the extremity, with a corresponding "heaviness" and decreased functional ability. In chronic cases after mastectomy, there may be considerably decreased range of motion and function caused by interstitial fibrosis along the tendinous and ligamentous structures, resulting from increased deposition of protein-rich lymphatic fluids in the tissues. Some recent studies have shown increased arterial inflow[32] and venous outflow[33] to the extremity of the affected side. Svensson and colleagues, using color Doppler ultrasound, noted that the mean percentage of blood flow was 32% higher in the arm on the side of the mastectomy, compared with the contralateral normal arm. If the arm on the side of the mastectomy had lymphedema, then blood flow was 68% higher. This study showed an identifiable increase in arterial flow to treatment-side arms that was worse in those arms already edematous. This was caused by a neurologic deficit with loss of sympathetic vasoconstrictor control. A critical part of the history of patients with acute and chronic lymphedema should include a careful delineation of paresthesias of the hand or forearm, pain and/or numbness of the hand, weakness and dropping articles in the affected hand, coolness of the hand, and variations in pain with the extreme changes in temperature principally cold. Svensson and colleagues noted that more than half of their patients showed evidence of venous outflow obstruction, with venous congestion present in 14% of them.

Diagnosis can be established on the basis of an accurate history and a thorough physical examination. Assessment of the progression of edema is essential in the postoperative care of patients. Several methods have been attempted. Each alone may have its inherent shortcomings, but when used in combination they can give the practitioner an adequate means of following a patient's progression or response to therapy. Photography at preoperative and postoperative visits can be useful in determining the onset and progression of lymphedema. It is important that the photographs be taken at the same focal distance and time of day. Lymphedema is time and activity dependent. Views taken in the morning generally show an overall decreased edema in patients. Therefore afternoon photographs depict a more accurate assessment of a patient's progression and level of disability. Objective techniques used to assess lymphedema include measurement of arm circumferences, ultrasound, water displacement technique, tonometry, optoelectric perometry, bioimpedance, and combined optoelectric perometry, 3D stereophotogrammetry and bioimpedance.[48,67–74] Radiologic studies such as lymphoscintigraphy, magnetic resonance imaging (MRI), and computed tomography (CT) may be necessary in difficult cases.

The National Cancer Institute has standardized reporting of adverse events in clinical trials, called the Common Terminology Criteria for Adverse Events (CTCAE), version 3 (see Table 36.2). Other rating scales described in the literature include the late effects of normal tissues and objective, subjective, and analytic components. Also described is the three-point scale of the American Physical Therapy Association, which grades lymphedema into mild, moderate, and severe.

Circumferential measurements using reference points to bony landmarks may also be a practical and simple way to follow a patient's lymphedema.[68] In severe cases, bony landmarks may be obscured. In postmastectomy patients, the ulnar styloid and the tip of the olecranon are the best landmarks. Differences in circumferential measurement between two opposing limbs are noted at multiple landmarks. These measurements are totaled for each limb and compared. If there is a difference greater than 10 cm, lymphedema exists.[67] The drawbacks to measuring lymphedema

by circumferential measurements include inability to take into account volume differences from left-right dominance, muscle atrophy, fibrous tissue deposition, and weight gain, which may be inaccurately attributed to fluid accumulation. This can be overcome by comparison measurement to the opposite extremity at baseline and follow-up. Additionally, this method is time-consuming, has potential for subjective errors, and measures the overall volume of the limb.

Water displacement is the most accurate method of documenting changes in edema.[74] It is accomplished by measuring the volume of fluid displaced after the affected extremity is placed in a tank of water. Kissin and colleagues[61] found that a water displacement measurement of 15 cm above the epicondyle was the most sensitive index. A value of 200 mL included 96.4% of patients with subjective lymphedema. This would appear to be the best objective criterion with which to judge lymphedema and response to therapy. However, these techniques are time-consuming and are limited to facilities that have the equipment to perform the study. Bioelectrical impedance techniques are the most recent developments for evaluating accumulation of fluid in affected extremities.[69–71]

Tonometry evaluates the resistance of the tissues when compression is applied, giving an estimate of the amount of pressure in the arm depending on the amount of adipose tissue fluid or fibrotic induration. The tonometer does not give an absolute amount of each component; it gives only a relative indication of the amount of each component. The degree of compressibility has been correlated with circumference and therefore with the amount of lymphedema. The electronic tonometer has two plungers: an outer one that is compressed fully when applied to the area being measured and an inner one that moves freely and is located in the center of the inner plunger. The lymphometer is gently pressed into the tissue. When the outer plunger is fully compressed, a beep is heard, during which time the inner plunger is forced into the tissue. The measurement of the inner plunger is locked and read during the beep. A maximum value (measure of hardness of tissues) is obtained if the inner plunger did not move into the tissue at all, and a minimum value (measure of softness of tissues) is obtained if the inner plunger is forced maximally into the tissues. It is important to compare the two sides and the same level in the same person, because tissue tonicity may vary from time to time even in normal individuals. The indurometer is a tool designed to replace the tissue tonometer and measures the resistance to an applied force to quantitate the amount of fibrosis present in the extremity. The two were compared in an international multicenter trial. The tonometer was found to be less variable, but the indurometer was easier to use.[75,76]

In the normal healthy person, the volume of the extracellular subcompartment is approximately 25% of the total volume. Hence methods that measure total limb volume, are thought to inherently suffer from a sensitivity four times less than any technique that measures extracellular volumes directly.[69,70] Lymphedema is not simply an increase in volume but also an alteration of the dermal and subcutaneous tissues accompanying the increase in protein concentration of the extracellular fluid. Such changes alter the resistance of the tissue to compression, and a measure of this resistance can be used to reflect the extent of the changes.

Bioimpedance spectroscopy is a noninvasive technique that directly measures lymph fluid volume. An electrical current is passed through a body segment, and impedance to flow is measured. Impedance to current flow is inversely related to fluid accumulation. The principles behind this technique are that tissues such as fat and bone are insulators, that electrolyte fluid conducts electricity, that low-frequency currents selectively pass through the extracellular fluid compartments, and that high-frequency currents pass through both extra- and intracellular compartments. The fact that lymphedema is an addition to the extracellular fluid compartment indicates that multiple frequency bioimpedance analysis is an accurate measure of lymph fluid impedance. Reduced impedance values in a measured extremity are considered indicative of lymphedema. Although this technique provides valuable information complementary to volume measurements, it is information about changes associated with lymphedema after the initial stages and as such may not be useful in the early diagnosis of the condition. Cornish and associates studied 102 female patients, 20 of who developed lymphedema in the 24 months after breast cancer surgery.[77] In each of these 20 cases, using bioimpedance predicted onset of lymphedema up to 10 months before the condition could be clinically diagnosed, thus allowing the early institution of preventative measures. This small study claimed a 100% sensitivity of bioimpedance, demonstrating a vast improvement on the currently used circumferential technique, which proved to have a sensitivity of only 5% for the purposes of early detection.[77] ImpediMed's L-Dex U400 is a noninvasive bioimpedance spectroscopy (BIS) tool to assess the extracellular fluid differences between the arms by measuring resistance to electrical current flow. At very low frequencies, the current travels predominantly through the extracellular fluid compartment of limbs. The L-Dex U400 device uses an "impedance ratio" methodology to assess unilateral lymphedema of the arm. The resistance at 0 kHz (theoretical) in the affected/at-risk arm is compared with the resistance at 0 kHz (theoretical) in the unaffected arm as represented by the following ratio: unaffected/affected or at risk. By this method the unaffected arm acts as an internal and subject specific control with high sensitivity allowing for subclinical detection compared with traditional techniques. BIS uses standardized cutoffs and has been shown to have excellent interobserver variability. Measurements are made by attaching electrodes to the patient's skin. The current is imperceptible to patients and would be equivalent to that received by holding an AA battery. Once both arms are measured the device calculates an L-Dex value. Abnormal L-Dex values include those outside the normal range (± 10 L-Dex units) and a change of greater than 10 from baseline. This measurement is not quantitative.

Extracellular fluid volume measurement by MRI[78] or CT[79] have also been used to determine the cross-sectional composition of the limb at small increments along the limb length and are accurate but time-consuming and expensive.

A recent multicenter trial compared multifrequency bioimpedance electrical analysis with perometry arm measurement for the early detection and intervention of lymphedema. The primary end point was an arm volume increase of 10% or more compared with the contralateral arm by perometer at 2 and 5 years after axillary node clearance. Of 964 patients, 612 had minimum 6-month data compared with 1-month baseline. Thirty-one patients by perometry and 53 by BIS were deemed to have lymphedema. There was moderate correlation between the two methods, but the authors concluded arm volume measurements remain gold standard.[80]

To date, no studies have been reported that identified a subset of patients at risk of developing postmastectomy lymphedema by means of a preoperative lymphoscintigram.

Nonoperative Management of Lymphedema

The initial treatment of chronic secondary lymphedema should be managed through nonsurgical measures. Adequate patient education with respect to activity levels and infection prophylaxis plays an important role in patients' long-term care. Physical therapy, in conjunction with compression garments or sequential-gradient compression-type pumps, is used in the care of patients with chronic lymphedema. A multidisciplinary and multimodal approach to the treatment of chronic lymphedema has been shown to reduce overall limb volume by at least half in 72% of patients treated.[81,82] Patients may have paresthesias of the hand or forearm, pain and/or numbness of the hand, weakness in the affected hand, coolness of the hand, and variations in pain with the extreme changes in temperature, principally cold. If any of these symptoms are elicited, stellate ganglion block may rapidly alleviate the symptoms and greatly reverse the amount of lymphedema when present.[83] Many patients mistake such pain for lymphedema. We have had great success at our institution using trigger point injections of the scapulothoracic bursae for chronic pain after surgery including that of the chest wall and pain radiating down the arm.[84] Infection prophylaxis is an important component in the care of patients with chronic extremity lymphedema who are prone to repeated infections, because accumulation of protein-rich fluid creates a rich culture medium for bacterial growth. The more lymphedematous the tissues, the more susceptible they are to infections. Infection itself increases the risk of lymphedema by 50%. Simple injuries may lead to generalized infections, lymphangitis, and cellulitis, which can cause further lymphatic destruction and blockage of remaining channels.[22] Extensive patient education in skin care, such as the immediate care of any open wound and proper nail care, is a simple but important necessity in lymphedema treatment. Ample evidence in the literature suggests that the more severe the lymphedema, the greater the risk of cellulitis and extremity infection. Each subsequent episode of infection increases the risk of bacteremia and systemic toxicity to the patient and worsens the lymphedematous condition in the extremity.

Extremity elevation (periodic elevation of the affected extremity) is the simplest form of self-care that a patient can do to reduce chronic lymphedema. The patient should be instructed on proper height and elevation of the affected extremity for the most satisfactory results. Nighttime elevation of the extremity has been shown to have the most dramatic effect.

Diuretics are of minimal aid in the treatment of chronic lymphedema resulting from oncologic surgery or metastatic spread of the disease. This type of therapy should be reserved for early treatment of primary lymphedema patients, although its effects are transient at best.

Massage can be an effective therapy in the long-term treatment of a chronic lymphedematous extremity. However, lack of experienced personnel limits the availability of this treatment. This has led to a plethora of devices that massage through mechanical or compressional means.[85] These sequential compression machines provide a pumping-like action to the extremity and were developed to improve the lymph and venous circulation in the lymphedematous limb. The pneumatic massage device includes a sleeve and an air control unit; the sleeve envelops the limb and consists of five pneumatic cuffs, and the air control unit supplies compressed air into the sleeve. A method of undulatory massage is used to improve lymph flow. This method involves sequential inflation and deflation of the cuffs. The first cuff is inflated first to a pressure of 80 mm Hg, followed by the second cuff, and the first cuff is not deflated until the third cuff is inflated to prevent the lymph from flowing backward. During this process, the blood flow waves are recorded using a Doppler flowmeter. A 2014 review evaluating 287 lymphedema patients included in seven randomized controlled trials showed that intermittent pneumatic compression therapy could alleviate lymphedema, but there was no significant difference compared with standard management.[85]

Results were difficult to interpret because of the variability in methods, and further randomized trials are needed to determine true effectiveness of the treatment. It was noted in Brown's analysis of the Prescription and Adherence to Lymphedema self-care (PAL) trial that compliance was poor in terms of compression pump use, finding that 42% of women admitted to less than 25% adherence to compression pump use, perhaps because of the effect of treatment on quality of life.[86]

A randomized controlled trial published in 2015 by Uzkeser and colleagues[87] divided 31 postmastectomy lymphedema patients into two groups; group I (n = 15) without intermittent pneumatic compression therapy and group II (n = 16) with intermittent pneumatic compression therapy. This study used ultrasonography for evaluation of dermal thickness as a part of the assessment for lymphedema changes in combination with arm volume, circumference, and pain measurements. Both groups received complex decongestive physical therapy with skin care, manual lymphatic drainage, compression bandages and exercises, and were treated five times per week for 3 weeks. Both groups showed significant limb volume reduction, but there was no significant advantage to the pneumatic compression group.

Complete Decongestive Physiotherapy

Complete or complex decongestive physiotherapy or therapy (CDP/T) is a noninvasive therapy that is considered the standard of care. CDP/T, first described in the late 1800s, has been further improved by Földi.[88] Physiologically, because of communication of the lymphatic vessels between various body regions, CDP can help shunt fluid out of the compromised extremity. CDP can be performed in a hospital setting or during home-based physical therapy.

Physical therapy is offered in two phases. Phase I lasts for 4 weeks and comprises four segments. The first is skin care, which improves and maintains the normal skin integrity while decreasing the risks of infection. The second segment involves manual lymphatic drainage. This is a daily therapy designed to remove excess lymphatic fluid and open collateral lymphatics, allowing the nonsurgical or unaffected regions to aid the compromised regions in draining excess lymphatic fluid. The third segment deals with compression bandaging to maintain and increase compartment pressure and prevent retrograde flow of lymphatic fluid. The fourth segment involves specialized physical therapy exercises followed by lymphatic massage. Massage therapy is based on first emptying the lymphatics of the trunk. The Földi technique[88] of massage is then applied to areas adjacent to the compromised extremity. The therapist concentrates on the central portions of the limb, gradually working toward the distal portion of the extremity. This forces the excess lymphatic fluids into watershed regions of the body, which allows the fluid access to the unaffected lymphatic collateral circulation. This therapy is delivered by specialists certified by the Lymphology Association of North America.

Phase II consists of applying low resistance short-stretch compressive bandages. They are applied in multiple layers and are

designed to enhance lymphatic pumping. More commonly, at home patients will use specially measured compression garments because they are easier to apply by the patient themselves. The use of elastic sleeve therapy alone has been shown to decrease limb girth by 15%.[36] Maintaining the overall benefits from CDP depends largely on whether patients continue their exercises and have intermittent CDP. Studies from Australia have shown that these techniques reduce extremity size by 65%.[89] However, they require skilled personnel and a strong daily commitment to complete.

A recent meta-analysis of 10 randomized controlled trials (RCTs) of manual lymphatic drainage alone was not effective in preventing postoperative lymphedema.[90] However, a systematic review of 26 studies of CDP that includes manual lymphatic drainage and 9 RCTs demonstrated decreased limb volume and improved quality of life with CDP.[91] On average, limb reductions of up to 50% can be achieved. However, three small randomized trials comparing CDP versus compression garments[92–94] showed no significant difference in extremity volume reduction (ranged from 23% to 46%) in 4 to 6 weeks of therapy. Dayes and associates continued to follow patients for a year, and this lack of difference was maintained, as well as a lack of differences in quality of life and arm function. Although this has brought controversy to the efficacy of CDP, it is effective.[94] Whatever method is chosen needs to be one that the patient can comply with on a daily basis to be effective.

Exercise

Although not all forms of exercise are beneficial to patients with extremity edema, those that increase circulation in the affected extremity are recommended. These include swimming, biking, and isometric exercises. Medical management should involve a multidisciplinary approach in the patient's long-term care. This includes patient education, instruction in home physical therapy exercises, maintenance of normal range of motion and strength in the affected extremity, and preservation of existing motion. The overall treatment plan may include education and instruction in elevation of the affected extremity; skin care precautions; massage techniques; pumping exercises; and appropriate active-assisted, active, and resistive exercises. A physical therapist can train the patient in fitting and using compression garments and in monitoring the use of sequential-gradient compression-type pumps. Therapy used in conjunction with garments and pumps as well as patient education, skin maintenance, and eradication of bacterial and fungal skin infections can reduce extremity girth and lymphatic volume.

There has been persistent reluctance to allow women at risk for the development of lymphedema participate in upper extremity weight training activities, but there is more recent evidence that there is no adverse effect of weight training, and it may in fact improve range of motion, strength, and even quality of life.[95]

With obesity rates in cancer survivors on the rise, the National Comprehensive Cancer Network (NCCN) has embarked on a campaign to encourage healthy lifestyle, including exercise, in survivors.[96] A systematic review of the literature looked at 11 studies involving 1091 women either with or at risk for the development of BCRL. Low- to moderate-intensity weight training was used with a slow progression and under supervision, resulting in significantly improved upper extremity strength (standardized mean difference [SMD] 0.93, 95% confidence interval [CI] 0.73–1.12), with no increase in arm volume (SMD –0.09, 95% CI

–0.23 to 0.05) or incidence of breast cancer–related lymphedema (relative risk 0.77, 95% CI 0.52–1.15). The overall effect of weight training on lymphedema favored improvement in severity and incidence of breast cancer–related lymphedema, but this did not reach statistical significance.[95] Cormie and colleagues randomly assigned 62 women with breast cancer–related lymphedema (discrepancy in arm volume >5%) to high-load resistance exercise (n = 22) or low-load resistance exercise (n = 21) or usual care (n = 19).[97] After 3 months of participation, no lymphedema adverse events or exacerbations had occurred in any of the three groups, and there was a significant improvement in muscle strength, muscle endurance, and quality-of-life/physical functioning in the two exercise groups compared with the usual care group. An additional systematic review and meta-analysis is also in line with these studies and even provides data supporting progressive resistance training in breast cancer as a tool for risk reduction of breast cancer–related lymphedema versus control conditions (odds ratio = 0.53, 95% CI 0.31–0.90; I^2 = 0%).[98] There was improvement in muscle strength without increase in limb volume, and when the two studies that evaluated patients undergoing active adjuvant treatment were excluded, there was also a significant improvement in health-related quality of life. With the current data, the NCCN is in support of women with lymphedema participating in supervised exercise programs while wearing a compression sleeve starting with low weights and low repetitions with gradual increases.[96] Pusic and associates completed a systematic review of quality-of-life outcomes in breast cancer survivors and found that exercise and complete decongestive therapy were associated with improved overall quality of life.[99]

Hyperbaric Oxygen

The pathologic correlates of the response to hyperbaric oxygen in irradiated tissues have been studied in animals and include neovascularization, organization, and marked reductions in fibrous tissue.[100]

Nonrandomized trials have suggested that there might be a therapeutic effect of hyperbaric oxygen on arm lymphedema.[101] Gothard and colleagues followed with a phase III trial of 58 patients with moderate lymphedema per arm volume. They performed patient self-assessments with the UK SF-36 Health Survey Questionnaire. There was no significant difference between the treatment and control in median volume of the arm or questionnaire results after 12 months of treatment.[102]

Benzopyrones

Few drugs are being studied for treatment of chronic lymphedema.[103] Benzopyrones are appropriate for the treatment of lymphedema because they cause proteolysis and phagocytosis of macrophages, improve lymph flow, and promote regulation of tissue osmolarity.[104] This decreases the overall volume of high-protein concentrate edema by stimulating proteolysis.[105] These agents directly increase the number of macrophages at the site of high-protein lymphedema, which increases the normal proteolysis by the cells.[106] By increasing proteolysis and the number of macrophages, excess plasma protein is removed and overall edema decreases. Coumarin (Venalot), a benzopyrene, breaks down large protein molecules, facilitating absorption of the proteins into the vascular system at the level of the capillaries. Pentoxifylline (Trental) has been used in ameliorating postradiation fibrosis and may be used in refractory cases of lymphedema associated with radiation fibrosis to ameliorate the swelling and fibrosis. A recent Cochrane review found 15 randomized controlled trials testing the benzopyrones oxerutins (Paroven), coumarin, Venastat (horse chestnut seed), Cyclo 3 Fort (combined *Ruscus aculeatus*, hesperidin methylchalcone, and ascorbic acid), or Daflon (combination Diosmin and Hesperiden) or a combination versus placebo.[107] The authors deemed is was not possible to draw conclusions about the effectiveness of benzopyrones in lymphedema treatment due to the poor quality of the trials. The trial by Loprinzi and associates was the best of the trials and found no effectiveness of coumarin over placebo and reported one case of hepatotoxicity.[108]

Prevention of Lymphedema

Sentinel Lymph Node

Clearly the biggest effect on BCRL has been the development and proof of concept for SLN biopsy, which is covered nicely in Chapter 42. The major definitive RCT to show that SLNB significantly reduces the risk of lymphedema over ALND is the NSABP B-32.[54,109] The NSABP B-32 trial was a multicenter trial of 5611 women with invasive breast cancer randomized to receive immediate ALND or SLND only if the SN was negative. The primary aim of the study was overall and disease-free survival. Secondary aims were to determine long-term control of regional disease, compare morbidity, and determine the risk of systemic recurrence in patients who have pathologically node-negative lesions. The NSABP B-32 study collected data on surgical and pathologic accuracy, technical success, and variations of success by technique used in a broad general population of surgeons. The SLN was identified in level I and II of the axilla in 98.6% of cases. The overall accuracy was 97.1%, with a false-negative rate of 9.8%. After mean follow-up of 95.6 months, overall survival, disease-free survival, and regional control were equivalent between treatment arms, demonstrating that when the SLN is negative, SLNB without ALND is safe and appropriate surgical management in clinically node negative patients.[110] In terms of lymphedema, the trial showed significant arm volume differences at 36 months between the SLNB group (8%) and the ALND group (14%) by volume displacement.

The Medical Research Council of the United Kingdom completed the ALMANAC trial, which was a phase III multicenter randomized trial including 15 centers that performed a two-armed prospective trial randomizing patients to SLNB followed by ALND or the SLNB alone. If the SLN was negative, no further surgery was performed; if the SLN was positive, ALND or axillary irradiation completed the treatment. The primary end points were axillary morbidity, health economics, and quality of life. The results showed overall improved quality of life in the SLNB group (*p* < .003).[8] Similar to B-32, lymphedema was 5% after SLNB versus 13% for ALND at 1 year. The Sentinella/GIVOM trial as well as many others have demonstrated that the single biggest impact on reducing lymphedema of the upper extremity for staging the axilla has been less surgery in the form of SLNB.[111]

Nonoperative Management of the Axilla

As reduction of BCRL is minimized with less surgery, many have investigated replacing surgery with radiation therapy when the SLNB was positive. In 1998 Greco and associates randomized 381 patients with positive axilla to ALND versus radiation of the axilla. With 26-month follow-up they had equivalent oncological results.[112] Similarly Veronesi and associates reported a larger trial with 63-month follow-up.[113] Galper and associates from the Joint Center for Radiation Therapy also studied 292 patients with positive SLNs with ALND (n = 292) versus axillary radiation (n = 126) and again found similar results with only 2 axillary recurrences in the radiation group versus none in the ALND group.[114] This set the stage for the AMAROS trial (After Mapping of the Axilla: Radiotherapy or Surgery Trial), which is a prospective randomized phase III noninferiority trial randomized 1425 women with clinical T1-2N0 invasive breast cancer with a positive SLN to axillary radiation versus ALND.[64] Axillary recurrence was low in both arms (0.43% in the ALND vs. 1.19% in the axillary radiation arm) and no differences in disease-free and overall survival. Lymphedema was significantly higher in the ALND arm (23%) compared with the axillary radiation arm (11%) at 5 years ($p < .0001$). Further follow-up of the radiation arm will determine whether the morbidity remains low.[64]

The SOUND (Sentinel node vs. Observation after axillary UltrasouND) trial is an ongoing prospective randomized trial of SLNB versus no axillary staging of clinical negative axilla by ultrasound.[115] The Quick-DASH assessment was used and includes 11 items to measure physical function and symptoms in persons with any or multiple musculoskeletal disorders of the upper limb. In the preliminary report of the first 180 patients recruited there was significant higher morbidity in the SLNB group versus the nonoperative arm.

Axillary Reverse Mapping and Reanatomosis

Axillary Reverse Mapping

Axillary reverse mapping (ARM) was first described by Klimberg and colleagues in 2007 and describes the variation in anatomy of the lymphatic drainage from the arm within the axilla (see Fig. 36.6).[27,28,116,117] It involves mapping the drainage of the arm with blue dye as well as mapping the drainage of the breast with split mapping and decreases the likelihood of disruption of lymphatics and subsequent lymphedema. Technetium sulfur colloid is injected in the subareolar plexus, and blue dye is injected subcutaneously in the ipsilateral upper extremity (split mapping). Tummel and associates recently published the follow-up data on 654 patients with an overall lymphedema rate of 2.5% identifying a lymphedema rate of <1% in the SLNB group and 6% in the ALND group. There was crossover (where the ARM node was identified as the SLN) in 3.8% of patients. It is our practice now to reanastomose or reapproximate the afferent and efferent limbs of any crossover node because they are SLNs and should be removed. Axillary recurrence rates in this prospective phase II trial were 0.2% for SLNB and 1.4% for ALND. Studies that have reported high ARM node positivity have not used split mapping and have not performed the procedure as described. Simply mapping the lymphatics from the arm does not elucidate which ones have co-drainage pathways from the breast. This study also makes clear that the technique of the SLNB does matter and the surgeon should take care to reapproximate cut lymphatics. In the only prospective randomized trial, Yue and colleagues randomized patients undergoing a modified radical mastectomy to ARM or no ARM. In the control group, the lymphedema rate at 20 months was 6% versus that of the ARM group (33%; $p < .001$).[117a]

LYMPHA (Lymphedema Microsurgical Preventive Healing Approach)

Boccardo and associates have championed the idea of LYmphedema microsurgical Preventive Healing (LYMPHA), which entails performing a lymphatic-venous anastomoses at the time of ALND. To date they have reported 74 patients with only 3 developing lymphedema after ALND with 8- to 12-month short-term follow-up.[118] The procedure requires microscopic expertise. Our data with ARM would suggest that a simple approximation of lymphatics may also suffice and does not require this expertise.[116]

Operative Management of Lymphedema

Surgical treatment should be instituted for patients for whom previous medical modalities have failed or for those who have had long-term complications. The earliest form of surgical intervention dates back to Lisfranc in 1841 and mostly consisted of excision of the swollen tissue.

In the past century, a number of surgical treatment plans were attempted on the basis of reconstruction of lymphatic channels. Initial trials were attempted by Handley in 1908 and involved the burying of silk and other synthetic materials in the soft tissues to mimic lymphatic channels. High rates of infection, extrusion of the suture, and very limited transient improvement caused this technique to be abandoned. Emmanuel Kondoleon (1879–1939) devised the Kondoleon operation for elephantiasis of the lower extremity in which long, elliptical incisions on the lateral aspect of the extremity were made, starting from the iliac crest and ending above the external malleolus. Subcutaneous tissue and fascia were excised corresponding to the skin incision. Heavy, continuous catgut was used to close the incision, and a tightly applied wrap was used over the extremity during the postoperative period.

Another approach involves removing subcutaneous fat and placing a dermal flap within the muscle to encourage superficial-to-deep lymphatic anastomoses.

Modern procedures can be divided into excisional procedures, tissue transfer, liposuction, and lymphovenous shunts.

Excisional Procedures

Patients who have massive lymphedema with overlying skin breakdown may benefit from the Charles procedure, which has mainly been used for lower extremity lymphedema. In this technique, skin and subcutaneous tissue are removed to the level of the underlying fascia and the extremity is covered with split-thickness skin grafts. Although the cosmetic appearance of the limb is not favorable, this procedure allows an incapacitated patient to return to normal activity. A moderate hospital stay is required, and wound-healing problems can occur in the skin-grafted areas. The risk/benefit evaluation is favorable because these patients are homebound or bedridden if left untreated, but it is a procedure of last resort. In a prospective study of 11 patients with upper extremity BCRL, Salgado and associates developed a one-stage procedure that enabled a radical reduction of lymphedematous tissue with preservation of the perforator vascular supply to skin.[119] The authors achieved significant circumference reduction above and below the elbow but not at the wrist and hand. Complications were minimal in this group.

Tissue Transfer for Refractory Lymphedema

The anecdotal observations of some patients having some benefit in the reduction of lymphedema with reconstructive procedures of the breast by rotational flaps to the area of the chest wall and axillary area have been noted. Theoretically, the flaps may bring alternative lymphatic drainage to the area of lymphatic congestion. Patients with long-standing lymphedema develop hypertrophy of the adipose tissues, which causes refractoriness to conservative measures. Surgical techniques such as bridging procedures, total excision with skin grafting, reduction, and microsurgical reconstruction involving lymphovenous shunts or transplantation of lymph vessels have been used for treatment of refractory lymphedema. None of these methods have yielded satisfactory or long-lasting results. Microsurgical procedures that involve creating anastomosis between dilated lymph channels or lymph collectors and the venous system have been performed with marginal results in the 30% to 40% range, equivalent to a placebo effect. These procedures required wearing a compression garment after surgery and did not result in complete reduction of arm swelling because the hypertrophied adipose tissue remained unchanged. Tissue transfer procedures are becoming popular, with plastic surgeons harvesting groin nodes and reimplanting them in the axilla or hand. By all accounts, reported studies are small with five prospective (n = 10–21)[120–123] and four retrospective studies[124–127] (n = 9–24) and numerous case reports. Follow-up time has been from 6 to 96 months. Volume reduction has been reported in all but two studies and has ranged from a reduction of 22% to 81%. Patient selection and surgeon expertise are the key to achieving good results.[128]

Liposuction

Patients with late-stage or long-standing lymphedema do not respond to conservative measures such as manual lymph drainage and pressure therapy. Brorson and Ohli[129] did a study on 11 patients with nonpitting postmastectomy edema. They measured the arm volume in patients with lymphedema by plethysmography and then subjected them to liposuction; arm volumes were measured. A complete reduction of the excess arm volumes was achieved in 6 months. Analysis of the aspirate showed 93% adipose tissue. Volume-rendered CT, which was also used to analyze the arm volumes, estimated the amount of excess adipose tissue in the lymphedematous arm to be 81%. The increased adipose hypertrophy may be from a physiologic imbalance of blood and lymphatic flow resulting in impaired macrophage clearance of lipids.[130] Others feel that the fat cell is an endocrine organ in and of itself and is perturbed when cytokine-activated inflammation occurs.[131,132] Recent research shows a direct relationship between lymph flow and adipose deposition.[133]

Liposuction for lymphedema was first performed in 1987 at the Department of Plastic and Reconstructive Surgery, Malmö University, Sweden.[134] The treatment was performed under general anesthesia using the "dry technique," which involves an injection of either local anesthetic or epinephrine and 15- to 20 3-mm-long incisions. Liposuction was done circumferentially from hand to shoulder, and hypertrophied fat was removed through cannulas connected to a vacuum pump. The treated portion of the arm is compressed by bandages to control bleeding and postoperative edema. Incisions are left open to allow drainage. A compression garment is then applied. Postoperatively, the arm is elevated during the hospital stay usually for 3 to 4 days. The patient alternates between two standard compression sleeves during the first two postoperative weeks, which is followed by controlled compression therapy for a 12-month period. Controlled compression therapy involves using custom-made garments after measuring the arm at each visit. A prerequisite to maintain the effects of liposuction in patients with chronic lymphedema is the continuous use of compression garments that are remeasured yearly. Liposuction does not cause any further disruption of lymphatics and decreases the incidence of erysipelas. This results from the removal of proteinaceous fluid and adipose tissue and increased blood flow to the tissues. There have been no recurrences reported in this study on 15 years of follow-up.[134]

There are four other prospective studies of 11 to 37 patients using liposuction to reduce lymphedema of the upper extremity.[135–137] All but one demonstrated 103% to 123% volume reduction in the involved arm. Qi and associates demonstrated an 18% reduction.[136]

Lymphovenous Shunts

An alternative microsurgical technique described by Campisi and colleagues[138,139] involves performing interposition autologous lymphatic-venous-lymphatic anastomoses. This procedure represents an alternative to direct lymphatic-venous shunts and is based on the abundance of large-caliber venous tributaries. The lymphatic collectors can be placed at both ends of the venous graft sites. The lymphatic-venous-lymphatic anastomoses consist of inserting suitably large and lengthy autologous venous grafts between lymphatic collectors above and below the site of obstruction to the lymphatic flow (Figs. 36.9 and 36.10).

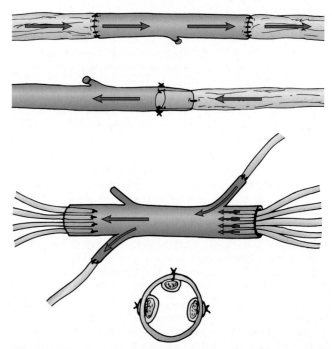

• **Fig. 36.9** A schematic drawing of the derivative multiple lymphatic venous anastomoses and the reconstructive multiple lymphatic venous lymphatic anastomoses technique with the interposition of an autologous vein graft between lymphatics above and below the obstacle to the lymph flow. (From Campisi CC, Ryan M, Boccardo F, Campisi C. A single-site technique of multiple lymphatic-venous anastomoses for the treatment of peripheral lymphedema: long-term clinical outcome. *J Reconstr Microsurg.* 2016;32:42–49.)

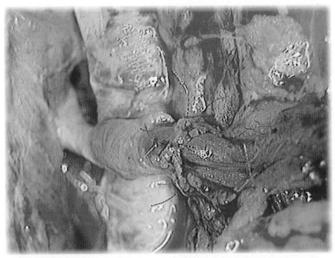

• **Fig. 36.10** Multiple lymphatic venous anastomoses: the passage of blue lymph into the vein branch, as seen under the operating microscope, verifies the patency of the anastomosis. (From Campisi CC, Ryan M, Boccardo F, Campisi C. A single-site technique of multiple lymphatic-venous anastomoses for the treatment of peripheral lymphedema: long-term clinical outcome. *J Reconstr Microsurg.* 2016;32:42–49.)

Contraindications to this procedure include lymph node hyperplasia or aplasia and extensive obliteration of superficial and deep lymphatic collectors.

Campisi and associates have the most experience with this technique and have reported their results in a retrospective manner with reportedly good results for the treatment of early-stage lymphedema.[138,139] However, for later, advanced, and chronic stages, this therapeutic option is not suitable. Seven prospective studies of upper extremity lymphedema in 10 to 100 patients with 12 to 109 months of follow-up have demonstrated 2% to 50% decrease in limb volume.[140–146] However, a recent study suggested that the net effect of lymphatic venous anastomosis was minor and that the main reduction in lymphedema was due to the application of complete decongestive therapy.[147] Larger prospective trials are needed to determine utility.

Postmastectomy Pain Syndrome

Postmastectomy pain syndrome is a recognized complication of breast surgery and is found in about 20% of women after mastectomy. Often patients confuse such pain with the possible onset of lymphedema. It is defined as a chronic (continuing for 3 or more months) neuropathic pain affecting the axilla, medial arm, breast, and chest wall after breast cancer surgery. Risk factors for persistent postmastectomy pain syndrome include young age and obesity. The relationship between postmastectomy pain syndrome and radiation therapy, chemotherapy, and tamoxifen is difficult to establish. The symptoms are distressing and may be difficult to treat. In a carefully performed cross-sectional study by Beyaz and associates, the prevalence was 36% and significantly more frequent after mastectomy.[148] Typically, such patients are treated with gabapentin, and antiseizure medications have limited benefit for such pain syndromes. We have reported that we think most of this syndrome is due to shoulder bursitis probably from positioning for surgery. As such we have had great success with trigger point injections in the scapulothoracic bursa (upper and lower shoulder blade). The bursitis injection consists of a mixture of

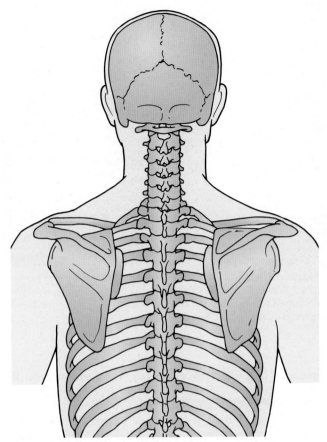

• **Fig. 36.11** Representing the anatomic location of the scapulothoracic bursa where a trigger point injection for postmastectomy syndrome would be given. (From Kaufmann T, Chu F, Kaufman R. Postmastectomy lymphangiosarcoma (Stewart-Treves syndrome): report of two long-term survivals. *Br J Radiol.* 1991;64:857.)

short-acting local anesthetic (4.5 cc of lidocaine 1%), a long-acting local anesthetic (4.5 cc of bupivacaine 0.5%), and a corticosteroid (40 mg of methylprednisolone) injected under the shoulder blade (Fig. 36.11).[84] The success rate was 83.5% with complete relief of pain and another 12.6% with significant improvement with only four patients (3.9%) not responding. A pectoral block can be added for such patients.[149] All patients should follow with heat to the affected shoulder blade and analgesics to decrease inflammation. The injection can be repeated as necessary, but this is rarely needed.

Lymphangiosarcoma: a Rare but Fatal Complication of Long-Standing Lymphedema

A rare complication of chronic extremity lymphedema is the development of lymphangiosarcoma. This tumor is a rare form of soft tissue neoplasm. In 1906 Lowenstein[150] first commented on this condition with respect to posttraumatic chronic lymphedema of the upper extremity. In 1948 Stewart and Treves were the first to associate the condition with postmastectomy edema.[151,152] The incidence ranges from 0.07% to 0.45%.[153] Histologically, the tumor consists of vascular cavities lined with spindle-shaped

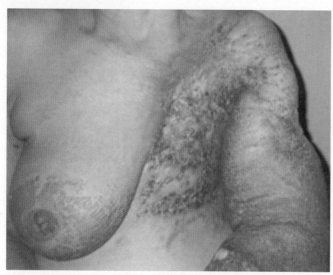

• **Fig. 36.12** Angiosarcoma of the arm extending onto the chest wall. (From O'Donnell TF Jr. The management of primary lymphedema. In: Ernst CB, Stanley JC, eds. *Current Therapy in Vascular Surgery*. 2nd ed. Philadelphia: BC Decker; 1991.)

endothelial cells with large nuclei and prominent nucleoli. The median time between mastectomy and development of this tumor is 10 years.[154] The primary lesion tends to form multiple satellites that may spread further or enlarge and ulcerate. Involvement of the underlying muscle is a late finding and is rare (Fig. 36.12).[155] Metastasis usually occurs early in the disease and is generally to the lungs.[156] Development can be divided into three phases: prolonged lymphedema, angiomatosis, and angiosarcoma.[157] Treatment includes local excision, wide excision, amputation, radiation therapy, chemotherapy, and combination therapy. Median survival of patients is 19 months after diagnosis.[154] The disease has a predictable course with rapid progression and a fatal outcome.[158]

Summary

Postmastectomy patients and their caregivers are often faced with the problematic management of upper extremity chronic lymphedema. Until recent years, this condition was neglected because of poor understanding of the cause and abnormal physiology behind the condition. Consequently, most patients were completely untreated or undertreated. This resulted in a lifelong struggle for many patients, with a condition that eventually led to crippling disability. In the past, patients were told that this condition was something that they had to live with.

An accurate knowledge of the physiology and pathophysiology of lymphedema is necessary to understand the rationale of treatment techniques available. An accurate assessment of the degree of impairment should be established before initiating either

short- or long-term care. Although surgical intervention and treatment have been tried in the past and are much improved, the standard of care now is conservative medical management. The basis of conservative therapy is reduction of existing edema while controlling formation of new edema. Observation techniques, including photography, circumferential measurement, and water displacement, may be used in the long-term monitoring of lymphedema.

The best chance for patients is primary prevention of lymphedema. Newer, minimally invasive surgical techniques in the initial treatment and diagnosis of breast cancer, such as SLNB, may decrease the overall number of node dissections being completed. This in turn will decrease the number of patients subjected to the threat of lymphedema. The addition of procedures such as ARM can help delineate the drainage of the arm so the lymphatics can be protected and, if necessary, reapproximated at the time of surgery.

A multidisciplinary approach is needed to maximize available treatment regimens. Surgeons, nurses, and physical and occupational therapists play active roles in the care of chronic lymphedema patients. Appropriate patient education and instruction in self-care are paramount in the long-term care of patients, because repeated infections worsen lymphedema. Patient education should include instruction in exercise, activities to avoid, extremity elevation, and infection prophylaxis.[159] A realistic approach to the long-term care of this condition coupled with therapeutic and emotional support can ensure a productive and less debilitating lifestyle to patients with chronic extremity lymphedema.

Acknowledgment

We gratefully acknowledge the contributions of Paramjeet Kaur, Christopher A. Puleo, and Charles E. Cox, who authored this chapter in previous editions.

Selected References

84. Boneti C, Arentz C, Klimberg VS. Scapulothoracic bursitis as a significant cause of breast and chest wall pain: underrecognized and un dertreated. *Ann Surg Oncol.* 2010;17(suppl 3):321-324.

96. Denlinger CS, Ligibel JA, Are M, et al. Survivorship: healthy lifestyles, version 2.2014. *J Natl Compr Canc Netw.* 2014;12: 1222-1237.

115. Gentilini O, Botteri E, Dadda P, et al. Physical function of the upper limb after breast cancer surgery. Results from the SOUND (Sentinel node vs. Observation after axillary Ultra-souND) trial. *Eur J Surg Oncol.* 2016;42:685-689.

116. Tummel E, Ochoa D, Korourian S, et al. Does axillary reverse mapping prevent lymphedema after lymphadenectomy? *Ann Surg.* 2017;265:987-992.

139. Campisi CC, Ryan M, Boccardo F, Campisi C. A single-site technique of multiple lymphatic-venous anastomoses for the treatment of peripheral lymphedema: long-term clinical outcome. *J Reconstr Microsurg.* 2016;32:42-49.

A full reference list is available online at ExpertConsult.com.

37

Assessment and Designation of Breast Cancer Stage

LEIGH NEUMAYER AND REBECCA K. VISCUSI

Staging: Past, Present, and Future

Staging plays an integral role in the management of breast cancer. Classifying patients by stage places them in prognostic groupings based on the best current available evidence gained from observation studies or clinical trials. The role of the surgical oncologist both past and present has been to acquire the pathologic tissues required to accurately diagnose, measure, and determine nodal staging of patients' tumors. The major disciplines of surgery, medical oncology, and radiation oncology use current breast cancer staging classifications for determining the extent of disease, predicting overall survival, and providing guidance for therapy. Furthermore, epidemiologists and public health researchers rely on uniform breast cancer staging methods to evaluate trends in breast cancer incidence, screening programs, treatment outcomes, and risk factors worldwide. Finally, staging also plays an integral part in advances in breast cancer research and in the application of basic science to clinical science (translational research).

In the past, the cancer staging system was quite simplistic. Neoplasms were staged on the basis of clinical evaluation alone as operable or inoperable and classified as local, regional, or metastatic. However, there were limitations in accurately predicting the outcome in patients, and therefore the importance of deriving a more sophisticated staging system had been realized. Clinical staging is largely based on simple physical measurements such as size of the tumor or extent of anatomic spread of the disease to regional lymph nodes and distant organ sites at the time of diagnosis. These measurements are static and permit only limited evaluation of an ever-changing, heterogenous neoplasm that often has been in existence for years before the initiation of the staging process. Furthermore, advancements in breast cancer research and the development of new therapies have led to more treatment options (e.g., systemic chemotherapy, hormonal and other novel biologic therapies); however, the impact of treatment on long-term prognosis is not incorporated. Even today, the classification schemas for staging patients are limited by the inability to accurately assess the biological behavior of tumors and only minimal levels of molecular data are available.

Current staging schematics use a combination of clinical and pathologic factors, which are both useful in providing prognostic information. Clinical parameters historically have been used to predict survival because of the simplicity in obtaining the data.

The clinical system may serve to guide initial therapy based on all available preoperative data that include history, physical and laboratory examinations, and biopsy material. However, tumors are now detected at very early stages, before they become clinically evident; as a result, histopathologic staging based on the primary tumor and local/regional lymph nodes has proved to be more accurate in predicting survival. The pathologic system, because of its ability to precisely define the histology and the extent of disease, is more accurate for grouping of patients with similar prognoses and for planning subsequent therapies.

Future staging systems will likely include new technologies and in-depth molecular, genetic, and pathologic analysis of the tissue specimens. The introduction of the sentinel lymph node (SLN) technique has allowed more accurate staging with much less morbidity to the patient compared with a complete axillary node dissection. With improvements in the sensitivity of detection methods, including histopathologic assays and molecular techniques, microscopic and submicroscopic tumor metastases can be detected. The recent expansion of genetic knowledge associated with the Human Genome Project has provided a large number of molecular tools that may prove valuable in the evaluation of tumor progression and overall survival. Molecular staging using reverse transcriptase polymerase chain reaction (RT-PCR), microarray analysis, and proteomics to identify unique gene and protein expression profiles may allow the detection of occult cancer before it becomes clinically evident and may provide more accurate information to help determine prognosis and survival with minimal morbidity to the patient. Finally, more accurate molecular staging may allow ablative rather than extirpative procedures and molecular-directed systemic therapies to be used. The increasing use of molecular staging and assessment of tumor response could potentially affect future staging systems by including biological markers to pretreatment clinical stage and posttreatment pathologic staging.

Clinical, Pathologic, and Biological Markers and Factors in Determining Prognosis

Central to any staging system are identifiable objective tumor and host characteristics that are prognostic of tumor progression. A number of clinical and pathologic factors have been identified that

| TABLE 37.1 | Prognostic Factors in Breast Cancer |

Clinical Histopathologic Factors	Biologic Factors
Age	Angiogenesis (VEGF)
Tumor size	Proliferation (MIB-1/Ki67/mitotic index)
Tumor location	Growth factor receptor (EGFR/HER2/neu)
Tumor histology	Cell cycle regulators (*p53/c-myc/*cyclins)
Tumor grade	Proteases (uPA/PAI-1/cathepsin D)
Hormone receptor status	Bone marrow micrometastasis
Vascular invasion	Circulating tumor cells
Lymph node status	Molecular subtype
Distant metastasis	Multiparameter gene expression analysis (MammaPrint/Oncotype Dx)

EGFR, Epidermal growth factor receptor; *HER2*, human epidermal growth factor receptor 2; *MIB-1*, methylation inhibited binding protein-1; *VEGF*, vascular endothelial growth factor.
Modified from Bundred NJ. Prognostic and predictive factors in breast cancer. *Cancer Treat Rev.* 2001;27:137-142.

may predict the long-term outcome in patients with breast cancer. Generally accepted prognostic factors include age, tumor size, lymph node status, histologic tumor type and grade, mitotic rate, hormone receptor status, and human epidermal growth factor receptor 2 (HER2/neu) status. A number of other biological factors have also been studied and provide information regarding the potential for aggressive behavior of tumors (Table 37.1).

Prognostic factors are important for forecasting outcomes in individual patients and can be used to help refine treatment choices. A prognostic factor is capable of providing information on clinical outcome at the time of diagnosis, independent of therapy. Such factors are usually indicators of growth, invasion, and metastatic potential. Nodal status is the most important parameter used to define risk category in early breast cancer and is considered a "pure" prognostic factor; that is, nodal status does not affect response to systemic therapy. On the other hand, a predictive factor is capable of providing information on the likelihood of response to a given therapeutic modality. Such markers are either within the target of the treatment or serve as modulators related to expression and/or function of the target. Estrogen receptor status is a predictive factor because it indicates the likelihood of response to endocrine therapy, but its role as an independent prognostic factor is controversial. In contrast, expression of the HER2/neu oncogenes may not only be an important prognostic factor in at least some subsets of patients with breast cancer; it may also provide some indication of the likelihood of response to certain chemotherapeutic agents. Therefore the HER2/neu oncogene has a dual role as prognostic and predictive factor.

Traditionally the dogma has been that prognostic factors help physicians determine which patients with breast cancer need adjuvant therapy, whereas predictive factors indicate which adjuvant therapy is most appropriate. The most important benefit of prognostic classification may be to help physicians identify patients in whom adjuvant therapy could be avoided, thus preventing treatment-related side effects. In theory, the identification, validation, and application of suitable predictive and prognostic factors

helps ensure that only those patients likely to benefit will receive a given treatment.

Clinical Factors

Clinical staging is based on physical examination and information gathered from various imaging modalities. A thorough physical examination should consist of inspection and palpation of all of the breast tissue, the skin overlying the breasts, and the regional lymph nodes (axillary, infraclavicular, supraclavicular, and cervical). Important characteristics to note are the tumor size, whether there is extension into the chest wall, involvement of the overlying skin (e.g., erythema, induration, or edema), and presence of lymphadenopathy. Mobility of the involved regional lymph nodes is also important to note as a prognosticating indicator, with fixed nodes with extracapsular extension having a worse prognosis.

Imaging modalities such as mammogram, ultrasound, and contrast-enhanced magnetic resonance imaging (MRI) are available and useful as an adjuvant to the physical examination. The US Food and Drug Administration first approved the use of digital mammography in 2000 and further approved three-dimensional tomosynthesis in 2011. Although the data are still somewhat limited regarding tomosynthesis, a recent retrospective analysis performed by Friedewald and coworkers that included almost 460,000 patients demonstrated its use was associated with an increase in the overall cancer detection rate with concurrent decrease in the recall rate.[1]

In regard to MRI usage, there is sufficient evidence supporting use of MRI for screening purposes in women with a known genetic mutation as well as women with a lifetime risk of developing breast cancer greater than 20%[2]; however, its use in women with a known breast malignancy is more controversial. MRI is being used with increasing frequency in an effort to assess extent of disease in the affected breast, evaluate for presence of multifocal and multicentric disease, and detection of cancer in the contralateral breast. Opponents of this trend argue that the increased sensitivity of MRI leads to more false-positive results, further necessitating unnecessary biopsies and larger surgeries. In a meta-analysis performed by Houssami and colleagues, additional disease was detected on MRI in the affected breast in 16% of cases with only a 66% positive predictive value.[3] Likewise, the Comparative Effectiveness of MR Imaging in Breast Cancer (COMICE) trial is a prospective randomized study that was designed to investigate the clinical efficacy of preoperative MRI in women with breast cancer. When comparing MRI findings with histopathology, they noted 38% of patients in whom mastectomy was felt to be necessary based on MRI findings would have been candidates for breast conservation based on histology.[4]

Primary Tumor Characteristics

Tumor Size

Tumor size is one of the most important prognostic markers of invasive breast cancer. It is defined as the maximal size of the invasive component of the primary tumor on pathologic examination. Clinical evaluation of tumor size has been included in many staging systems as an independent predictor of survival.[5-7] The potential for metastasis increases in a linear relationship with the size of the primary tumor (Fig. 37.1).[5] Furthermore, there is a distinct relationship between increasing tumor size and the probability of axillary nodal metastasis.[8] These investigators demonstrated that tumors must reach 3.1 to 4 cm in diameter to generate axillary metastasis in 50% of patients (Table 37.2). Fisher[9] has likewise shown that tumor size correlates with disease-free survival at 10 years, even when controlled for nodal metastases (Fig. 37.2). Tumor size is particularly useful as a prognostic tool in patients with no involvement of regional lymph nodes and may alter adjuvant treatment options. For instance, patients with small tumors (<1 cm) who have lymph node–negative disease have an excellent overall prognosis. A study from the Surveillance, Epidemiology, and End Results (SEER) Program demonstrated that the 10-year breast cancer–specific mortality in this group of patients is only 4%, whereas their overall mortality is 24%.[10] Thus, patients with small tumors with lymph node–negative disease have a five-fold higher risk of dying from causes other than breast cancer. It is also true, however, that patients with small tumors can have metastasis to the axillary lymph nodes, and conversely, more than one-third of patients with tumors greater than 6 cm in palpable diameter have negative lymph nodes, thus demonstrating the limited predictiveness of tumor size alone.[11]

Tumor Location

Tumor site is generally not included as a prognostic factor to identify patients at higher risk of relapse. However, tumor location

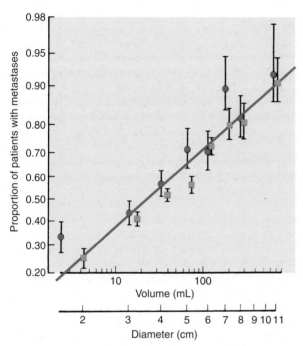

• **Fig. 37.1** A linear relationship exists between tumor size (volume or diameter) and potential for metastases. (From Koscielny S, Tubiana M, Lê MG, et al. Breast cancer: relationship between the size of the primary tumor and the probability of metastatic dissemination. *Br J Cancer.* 1984;49:709.)

TABLE 37.2	Relationship Between Tumor Size and Axillary Metastases	
Tumor Diameter (cm)	No. of Patients	Axillary Node Positive (%)
0.1–0.5	147	28.6
0.6–1	960	24.7
1.1–2	4044	34.1
2.1–3	3546	42.1
3.1–4	1917	50.1
4.1–5	1135	56.5
>5	1232	64.5

Modified from Nemoto T, Vana J, Bedwani RN, et al. Management and survival of female breast cancer: results of a national survey by the American College of Surgeons. *Cancer.* 1980;45:2917-2924.

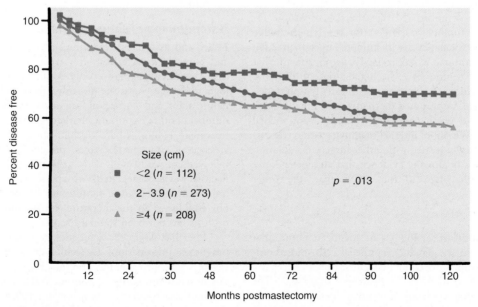

• **Fig. 37.2** Primary tumor size correlates with disease-free survival in patients undergoing curative surgery. (From Fisher ER. Prognostic and therapeutic significance of pathologic features of breast cancer. *NCI Monogr.* 1986;1:29.)

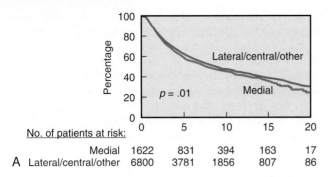

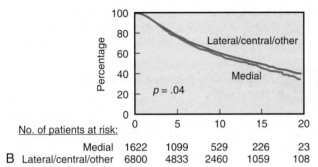

• **Fig. 37.3** (A) Disease-free survival and (B) overall survival according to predominant site of primary tumor. (From Colleoni M, Zahrieh D, Gelber RD, et al. Site of primary tumor has a prognostic role in operable breast cancer: the international breast cancer study group experience. *J Clin Oncol.* 2005;23:1390.)

has a significant prognostic utility, especially for axillary lymph node–negative patients. Several investigators from single institutions and data obtained from SEER have found that medial and central locations of tumor are associated with a 29% to 46% increase risk of developing systemic relapse and 20% to 46% increase risk of breast cancer–related death compared with the lateral location.[11–14] A study from the International Breast Cancer Study Group that included more than 8000 patients confirmed these results but also demonstrated that the risk of relapse for patients with medial tumors was largest for the lymph node–negative patients and for patients with tumors larger than 2 cm (Fig. 37.3).[15] Furthermore, a recent study demonstrated that lower inner quadrant tumors have the highest risk of mortality compared with other locations in women with early lymph node–negative breast cancer.[16] A proposed mechanism for the increased risk of metastases and death from breast cancer from medial tumors is occult involvement of internal mammary nodes (IMNs) that are not systematically treated with either surgery or radiation therapy. In fact, there is growing evidence that the lower inner quadrant drains more often to the IMNs than the other quadrants.[17,18]

Tumor Histology

The great majority of breast carcinomas are adenocarcinomas that derive from the mammary glandular epithelial cells, most commonly cells from terminal ductal lobular units. Breast cancer is a heterogenous disease with up to 21 histologic subtypes.[19] The most common type was classified as invasive ductal carcinoma, not otherwise specified (NOS); however, the nomenclature was recently changed by the World Health Organization (WHO) in 2012 to invasive carcinoma of no special type (NST).

Approximately 25% of invasive breast cancers are classified as special types of breast cancer and show distinctive growth patterns, cytologic features, clinical presentation, and behavior.[20] Next to inflammatory carcinoma, which is the most aggressive form of primary breast cancer with a 5-year survival rate of approximately 50%,[21] pleomorphic lobular, metaplastic, and micropapillary carcinomas carry a poor prognosis. Tubular, cribriform, mucinous, papillary, medullary, and adenoid cystic subtypes have more favorable prognoses.[19]

Tumor Grade

Histologic grading is a strong predictor of overall and disease-free survival in patients with invasive breast cancer; it is felt to be equivalent to lymph node status based on a number of independent studies.[22] Nuclear grading is the cytologic assessment of tumor cells and it is applied to all invasive and in situ carcinoma of the breast. The WHO endorses a histologic grading system based on criteria established by Bloom and Richardson and Elston and Ellis, known as the Nottingham Grading System.[23,24] This grading system incorporates three cytoplasmic and nuclear characteristics including extent of nuclear pleomorphism, degree of tubule formation, and number of mitotic features.[22] Hensen and colleagues performed a SEER review of 22,616 cases of breast cancer and calculated 5-year survival rates based on grade alone. Survival at 5 years was estimated to be 93% for grade 1, 82% for grade 2, and 65% for grade 3. In addition, when evaluating grade and stage together, they noted that women with stage II disease and grade 1 tumors had the same survival rates as women with stage I disease and grade 3 tumors, suggesting that incorporating grade into current staging systems could help more accurately predict outcome.[25]

Similarly, Fisher and colleagues[26] examined histologic grade in relationship to 5-year treatment failures and found that there is a significant correlation between these two factors in patients with absent nodal metastases or with four or more positive lymph nodes. Furthermore poor histologic grade is a significant predictor of pathologic complete response (26%) compared with good histologic grade (14%) in the setting of neoadjuvant chemotherapy.[27,28]

Histopathologic Features of Tumor

Fisher and associates[29] examined the relationship of pathologic and clinical characteristics to 5-year survival in 1000 patients treated with radical mastectomy. Although they found that pathologic nodal status was the most dominant influence on treatment failure rates and corresponding survival, they also identified a number of other important predictors of short-term (<24 months) treatment failure. Characteristics such as perineural invasion, absence of sinus histiocytosis, presence of glycogen, and skin involvement correlated with poor long-term survival. Tumor necrosis was also associated with a poor clinical outcome. However, independent prognostic significance of this histologic feature is not established in the literature. Furthermore, quantification of necrosis has not been standardized.

Other histologic characteristics have also been found to bear prognostic information. These include lymphovascular invasion, elastosis, glycogen staining, and the presence or absence of numerous host inflammatory responses. Evaluation of lymphovascular invasion is particularly important in small lesions without nodal involvement because it can identify patients with high risk of recurrence. In addition, it has also been found to have a strong association with breast cancer–specific survival and distant disease free survival.[30] On the contrary, presence of tumor-infiltrating lymphocytes has been associated with improved overall survival and distant disease-free survival, especially in triple-negative breast cancers.[31]

Estrogen and Progesterone Receptors

Both estrogen receptors (ER) and progesterone receptors (PR) are essential prognostic indicators in patients with breast cancer, and more importantly, they are highly predictive of benefit from endocrine therapy in both the adjuvant and metastatic settings. Knight and colleagues[31a] and Osborne and McGuire[32] have shown that ER status affects survival, independent of axillary nodal status with ER positivity generally correlating with a better prognosis. Similarly, another study has demonstrated longer survivorship for PR-positive patients than for PR-negative patients.[33] Receptor status has also been shown to be predictive of response in patients receiving chemotherapy. In the neoadjuvant setting, several studies have confirmed that ER-negative tumors are more likely to decrease in size in response to chemotherapy.[28,34,35] However, although ER-negative tumors are more likely to achieve pathologic complete response with neoadjuvant chemotherapy, affected patients have less favorable 5-year overall and progression-free survival rates compared with those with ER-positive disease. One proposed explanation for this finding was the beneficial effect of postoperative hormonal therapy available to patients with ER-positive tumors, which could supersede the significance of achieving pathologic complete response in this setting.[35]

HER2/neu Expression

HER2/neu-positive phenotype accounts for about 15% of patients. Amplification or overexpression of HER2/neu has been found to portend a poor prognosis, correlating with other factors associated with poor prognosis such as tumor grade, size, nodal status, and hormone receptor status.[36] Furthermore, it is also considered a predictive factor in that it predicts response to targeted therapy.

Tumor Growth Rate and Proliferation

Anatomic methods for staging breast cancer have withstood the test of time and remain the gold standard; however, these methods often provide only a static or instantaneous view of what is actually occurring at the molecular and cellular levels. Attempts at measuring dynamic characteristics (clinical and pathologic) have also been predictive of tumor progression. Clinical measurements of flux of tumor volume over time and pathologic determinations of cell kinetics have both been useful. Most of breast cancer prognostic factors are directly or indirectly related to proliferation, and increased proliferation correlates strongly with poor prognosis, irrespective of the methodology used to assess proliferation. Measurements of tumor doubling time, although not clinically practical, have been shown to correlate with prognosis. Multiple studies have demonstrated a wide range of doubling times, not only between patients but also within the same patient over time.[37–39] This heterogeneity is typical of breast cancer. Evaluation of tumor cell kinetics through growth fraction estimates has been used for the assessment of proliferation rate and its relation to prognosis.[40] The growth fraction can be assessed by immunohistochemistry (IHC) of proliferation-associated antigens, such as ki67, cyclin A, cyclin D, cyclin E, p27, p21, thymidine kinase (TK), topoisomerase IIα, proliferating cell nuclear antigen (PCNA), geminin, or minichromosome maintenance (McM) proteins. Of these, ki67 has extensively been studied alone or with MIB1, which is an

antibody that reacts against ki67. There is a good correlation between ki67 and MIB1 staining,[41] and a pronounced decrease in the ki67/MIB1 labeling index is associated with a good response to preoperative treatment with chemotherapy or tamoxifen.[42–44] In a recent review by Luporsi and coworkers, ki67 was found to be significantly associated with disease-free survival with seven randomized controlled trials and two meta-analyses in multivariate analysis. In addition, in the neoadjuvant setting, an elevated ki67 was associated with a higher likelihood of complete pathologic response.[45]

Flow cytometry has recently been used to estimate cellular kinetics and to detect the presence of aneuploidy. Flow cytometry permits rapid, single-cell analysis of DNA content per cell, enabling the determination of the fraction of cells within the S phase and the ploidy levels within tumor cell proliferation. However, despite extensive literature on flow cytometry, the results obtained by this method are still not widely used in everyday practice, because there is high intratumor heterogeneity of the S-phase fraction and multiple methodologies to determine S-phase fraction by flow cytometry.[46,47] In general, a high S-phase fraction is associated with a higher risk of metastatic recurrence in lymph node–negative patients. Furthermore, it has been suggested that flow cytometry also influences the response to chemotherapy in neoadjuvant, adjuvant, and metastatic settings.[48–57]

Other methods used to assess the growth fraction are the incorporation techniques with tritium-labeled thymidine (3H-TdR) and bromodeoxyuridine (BrdU), which theoretically provide the gold standard of cellular proliferation.[58,59] These methods are more sensitive than standard histologic tests that enumerate the relative number of mitoses and have demonstrated some promise in their ability to identify aggressive, rapidly growing tumors. With tritiated thymidine, tumor cells are sampled from the specimen and then incubated with 3H-TdR, which is taken up by cells in the DNA synthetic or S phase. Measuring 3H-TdR uptake then permits the estimation of the percentage of cells in the S phase (thymidine labeling index). Many studies have shown that a high thymidine labeling index is associated with poor prognosis in lymph node–positive and –negative patients with breast cancer,[60–62] and patients with a high index benefit from adjuvant chemotherapy.[63] However, incorporation techniques can be tedious and time-consuming, and they are impractical for routine use; this hampers their worldwide application, despite the very good prognostic value of the thymidine labeling index. This index does, however, correlate with histologic characteristics such as tumor grade and may be important in the staging of lymph node–negative patients.[63]

One the most powerful, practical, and well-reproduced indicators of proliferation and prognosis is the mitotic activity index (MAI).[64–66] As mentioned previously, MAI is part of the histologic grade system and represents by far the most important contributor to the prognostic value of histologic grade. The proliferation factor MAI is one of the strongest prognostic factors in patients younger than 71 years with lymph node–negative invasive breast cancer, without adjuvant systemic treatment and with long-term follow-up.[67] Moreover, patients with rapidly proliferating tumors significantly benefit from adjuvant systemic therapy, in contrast to those with low proliferation.[68] Recently, Baak and colleagues[67] demonstrated that among women with small, low-grade, lymph node–negative invasive breast cancer who usually do not receive systemic therapy, MAI ($\geq 10/1.6$ mm^2) was able to identify accurately those patients at high risk of distant metastatic disease or death. The 10-year overall survival rates for MAI less than 10

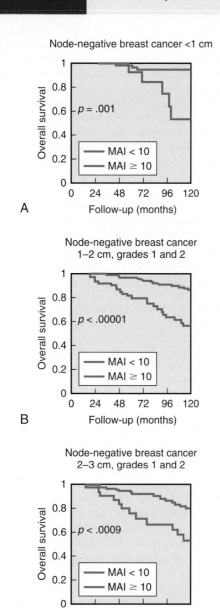

A

Node-negative breast cancer <1 cm

B

Node-negative breast cancer
1–2 cm, grades 1 and 2

C

Node-negative breast cancer
2–3 cm, grades 1 and 2

• **Fig. 37.4** Overall survival associated with mitotic activity index *(MAI)* in patients with tumors less than 1 cm diameter (all grades) (A), 1 to 2 cm (grades 1 + 2) (B), and 2 to 3 cm (grades 1 + 2) (C). (From Baak JP, van Diest PJ, Janssen EA, et al. Proliferation accurately identifies the high-risk patients among small, low-grade, lymph node-negative invasive breast cancers. *Ann Oncol.* 2008;19:649–654.)

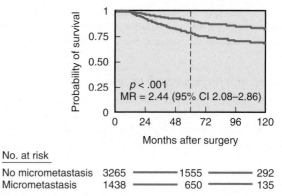

No. at risk			
No micrometastasis	3265	1555	292
Micrometastasis	1438	650	135

• **Fig. 37.5** Breast cancer–specific survival according to the presence or absence of bone marrow micrometastasis. *CI,* Confidence interval; *MR,* mortality rate. (From Braun S, Vogl FD, Naume B, et al. A pooled analysis of bone marrow micrometastasis in breast cancer. *N Engl J Med.* 2005;353:793. Copyright © 2005 Massachusetts Medical Society. All rights reserved.)

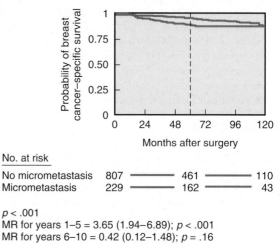

No. at risk			
No micrometastasis	807	461	110
Micrometastasis	229	162	43

$p < .001$
MR for years 1–5 = 3.65 (1.94–6.89); $p < .001$
MR for years 6–10 = 0.42 (0.12–1.48); $p = .16$

• **Fig. 37.6** Breast cancer–specific survival in low-risk patients with no adjuvant systemic therapy, according to the presence or absence of bone marrow micrometastasis. *MR,* Mortality rate. (From Braun S, Vogl FD, Naume B, et al. A pooled analysis of bone marrow micrometastasis in breast cancer. *N Engl J Med.* 2005;353:793. Copyright © 2005 Massachusetts Medical Society. All rights reserved.)

versus 10 or higher in women with tumor diameter less than 1 cm were 94% and 67%, respectively (Fig. 37.4). The authors concluded that these high-risk patients identified by MAI should be considered for adjuvant systemic therapy.

Biological Markers

With the development of monoclonal antibody technology, antibodies specific for breast cancer have been developed. These antibodies can be used to detect microscopic disease not easily seen on routine histopathology by using immunoperoxidase technology and radioimmunoassay. They may be useful in accurately staging the anatomic extent of axillary disease and distant disease

such as tumor infiltration of bone marrow.[69] The presence of isolated tumor cells in the bone marrow of women with early-stage breast cancer may be an independent marker of disease recurrence and shortened survival.[70] However, controversy exists regarding the independent influence of occult metastatic cells on prognosis. Braun and colleagues[71] performed a pooled analysis involving more than 4700 patients from several prospective studies and revealed that bone marrow micrometastases did predict an independent poor outcome (Fig. 37.5). Compared with women without bone marrow micrometastases, patients with bone marrow disease had larger tumors, tumors with a higher histologic grade, more frequent lymph node metastases, and more hormone receptor–negative tumors. Furthermore, in a subgroup analysis of low-risk patients with tumors less than 2 cm and without lymph node metastases who did not receive chemotherapy, the difference in distant disease-free survival between those patients who had micrometastases versus those who did not was very small (Fig. 37.6). These data suggest that the presence of bone marrow micrometastases may often reflect other prognostic factors already discerned from the primary tumor characteristics and lymph node status. The American College of Surgeons Oncology Group (ACOSOG) Z10 study is a prospective observational study whose primary objective was to investigate the association between survival and disease-free survival in women with early-stage breast cancer (T_{1-2}) and detected metastases within SLNs and bone marrow specimens using IHC. Of the specimens noted to be negative on hematoxylin and eosin (H&E) stain that were further evaluated with IHC, 10.5% of SLNs and 3% of bone marrow aspirates were found to be positive for tumor. Importantly, no difference in overall survival or disease-free survival was seen in women with H&E-negative, IHC-positive SLNs. However, there was a significant association between decreased overall survival and occult bone marrow metastases with no significant difference in disease-free survival. The authors concluded that although presence of occult bone marrow metastases may help identify high-risk women, the incidence was too low to recommend routine bone marrow aspiration in women with early-stage breast cancer.[72]

Similar to detection of disseminated tumor cells in bone marrow, novel methods that measure circulating tumor cells (CTCs) in the peripheral blood have also been developed.[73–75] Currently, there is only one US Food and Drug Administration–approved test, the CellSearch assay (Veridex, Warren, NJ). This assay is based on the enumeration of epithelial cells, which are separated from the blood by antibody-coated magnetic beads and identified with the use of fluorescently labeled antibodies against cytokeratin and with fluorescent nuclear stain. Several studies have confirmed that the presence of CTCs is associated with a poor outcome in patients with metastatic disease.[76–78] Cristofanilli and associates[79] measured CTCs before systemic treatment in patients with metastatic disease and found that levels of CTCs equal to or higher than 5 per mL of whole blood were the most significant predictors of progression-free and overall survival. Furthermore, these CTC levels after the first course of hormone therapy or chemotherapy predicted no treatment response. A recent Southwestern Oncology Group (SWOG) study further confirmed the poor prognostic significance of CTCs in metastatic breast cancer patients; however, they failed to find a survival benefit of early change to an alternate systemic therapy.[80] Although measuring CTCs shows promise, it still faces a number of challenges in terms of identification and full understanding of clinical significance,[81] and their use in diagnosis, treatment management, or staging is currently not recommended.[47]

Tumor markers, such as CA15-3, CA27-29, and carcinoembryonic antigen (CEA), are not very sensitive or specific for breast cancer and are not recommended for screening, diagnosis, or staging.[47] Cathepsin D, a lysosomal proteolytic enzyme with a critical role in protein catabolism and tissue remodeling,[82] has been used as a marker of invasion and poor prognosis in breast cancer.[82,83] However, the magnitude in predicting outcome is relatively small, and routine clinical use of this marker is also not recommended.[47] Other novel biologic markers recently found to be associated with prognosis are the urokinase plasminogen activator (uPA) and the plasminogen activator inhibitor (PAI-1), which are part of the plasminogen activating system. Several studies have suggested that overexpression of uPA and/or PAI-1 are strongly associated with poor prognosis in lymph node–negative cancer, and when these two factors are combined, they are associated with a two- to eightfold higher risk of recurrence and death.[84,85] Furthermore, Janicke and coworkers[86] found in a prospective randomized trial that low or high levels of uPA and/or PAI-1 can

help stratify who will benefit from adjuvant chemotherapy in patients with lymph node–negative breast cancer. In their study, for all women treated without systemic chemotherapy, the 3-year recurrence rate was significantly lower for those with low expression of uPA and PAI-1 (6.7% vs. 14.7%). The independent prognostic value of high levels of uPA and/or PAI-1 was confirmed in a pooled analysis involving 8377 breast cancer patients by the European Organization of Research and Treatment of Cancer-Receptor and Biomarker Group.[87] In both lymph node–positive and lymph node–negative patients, higher levels of uPA and/or PAI-1 were independently associated with poor relapse-free and overall survival (Fig. 37.7). Currently, uPA and/or PAI-1 measured by enzyme-linked immunosorbent assay has been recommended for the determination of prognosis in patients with newly

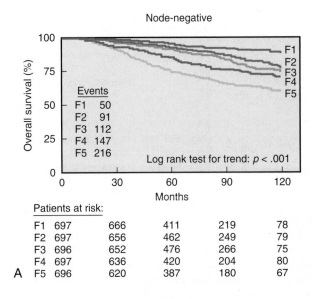

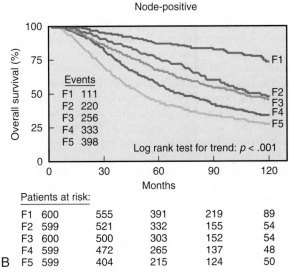

• **Fig. 37.7** Overall survival as a function of categorized prognostic scores of urokinase-type plasminogen activator (uPA) and its inhibitor (PAI-1) in lymph node–negative (A) and lymph node–positive (B) breast cancer patients. Prognostic scores were divided in five groups (F1–F5) with the use of their 20th, 40th, 60th, and 80th percentiles. (From Look MP, van Putten WL, Duffy MJ, et al. Pooled analysis of prognostic impact of urokinase-type plasminogen activator and its inhibitor PAI-1 in 8377 breast cancer patients. *J Natl Cancer Inst.* 2002;94:116.)

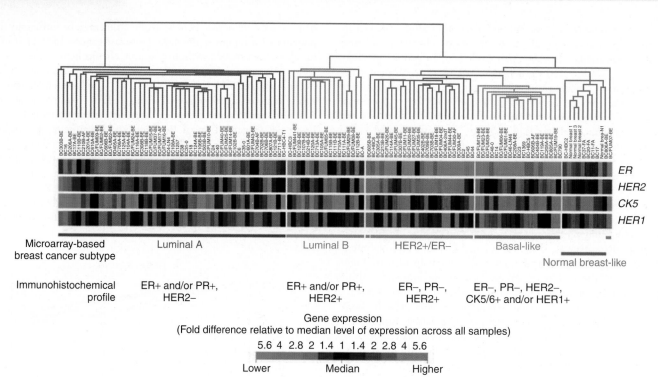

• **Fig. 37.8** Microarray-based breast cancer subtypes and their immunohistochemical profile. *ER,* Estrogen receptor; *PR,* progesterone receptor. (From Carey LA, Perou CM, Livasy CA, et al. Race, breast cancer subtypes, and survival in the Carolina Breast Cancer Study. *JAMA.* 2006;295:2492.)

diagnosed, lymph node–negative breast cancer by the American Society of Clinical Oncology.[47] However, despite comprehensive validation, they are infrequently used clinically.[88] Possible explanations include the large amount of tissue needed for the assay originally, the requirement of fresh or freshly frozen tissue, and the availability and convenience of other multiparameter assays, such as MammaPrint and Oncotype Dx.[47]

Oncogenes may be related to the complex phenomenon of human breast cancer initiation and progression through the process of gene amplification, mutation, chromosomal breakage, or insertion of retroviral promoters near oncogenes.[89] Although studies of individual oncogenes and tumor suppressor genes may prove fruitful in identifying poor patient prognosis, simultaneous analysis of expression of multiple genes in individual tumors is a new approach to breast cancer classification and has shown promise in providing greater accuracy in predicting outcomes and in aiding selection of therapies for individual patients. Using RNA expression array technology, initially four and then after further refinement, five breast cancer molecular subtypes were identified and validated in both clinically and ethnically diverse patient populations.[90–93] These five subtypes include basal-like, HER2/neu-overexpressing, luminal A, luminal B, and normal breastlike (Fig. 37.8). These subtypes have been compared with clinical outcomes; luminal-type cancers tend to have the most favorable long-term survival, whereas the basal-like and HER2/neu-overexpressing are most sensitive to chemotherapy but have the worst prognosis overall (Fig. 37.9).[91,94,95]

The true prognostic or predictive value of the molecular classes is unknown because there is a strong correlation between molecular class and conventional histopathologic prognostic factors. For example, Pusztai and colleagues[96] found that all luminal-type cancers were ER positive, and 63% of these were also low or

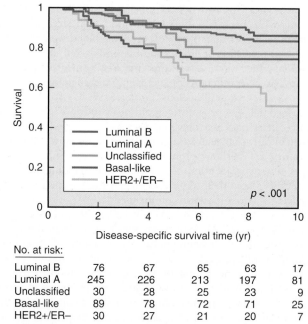

No. at risk:

Luminal B	76	67	65	63	17
Luminal A	245	226	213	197	81
Unclassified	30	28	25	23	9
Basal-like	89	78	72	71	25
HER2+/ER–	30	27	21	20	7

• **Fig. 37.9** Survival of patients with breast cancer according to molecular subtype. *ER,* Estrogen receptor. (From Carey LA, Perou CM, Livasy CA, et al. Race, breast cancer subtypes, and survival in the Carolina Breast Cancer Study. *JAMA.* 2006;295:2492.)

intermediate histologic grade. This contrasted with their finding that 95% of basal-like cancers were ER negative, and 91% were high histologic grade. Furthermore, the majority of basal-like cancers are characterized by the absence of ER receptor, PR receptor, and HER2/neu expression, and they are also associated with p53 gene mutations and a high proliferation rate.[97] Because of these characteristics, basal-like cancer is usually referred to as *triple-negative* breast cancer in daily practice. However, although the terms tend to be used interchangeably, they are not completely synonymous, because a small proportion of basal-like cancers do express hormone receptors or HER2/neu. Several studies have confirmed that triple-negative breast cancers are characterized by an aggressive clinical history, an earlier age of onset, and *BRCA1*-related breast cancer.[97,98] Recently, Bauer and colleagues[99] found that the relative survival for women with triple-negative breast cancer was poorer than for women with other types of breast cancer, with 77% of women surviving 5 years after diagnosis, compared with 93%. Finally, several studies have confirmed that African American women and Hispanic women were found to have a higher incidence of triple-negative phenotype.[94,99] These recent results might explain biologic disparities in long-term survival of breast cancer associated with race.

Molecular profiling has also been used to stratify patients with early breast cancer into prognostic groups, and information gained by these methods may outperform standard clinical and pathologic prognostic features. Several multiparameter assays that do not overlap have been developed and include the Rotterdam signature,[100] the Breast Cancer Gene Expression Ratio,[101] Mamma-Print,[102] and Oncotype Dx,[103] but only the last two are currently commercially available. For instance, MammaPrint (Agendia BV, Amsterdam, the Netherlands), is a 70-gene signature (largely consisting of genes regulating proliferation, invasion, metastasis, stromal integrity, and angiogenesis) used to stratify patients into a prognostic group using DNA microarrays originally in fresh frozen tissue.[102] This was designed by comparing gene expression in lymph node–negative patients, younger than 53 years of age with T_1 or T_2 breast cancers who developed metastases within 5 years of diagnosis, compared with a matched group that did not develop metastasis. At 10 years, van de Vijver and colleagues[104] demonstrated that both overall survival (95% vs. 55%) and distant metastasis-free survival (85% vs. 51%) were significantly greater in those classified as having a good prognosis according to their gene expression profile alone. The estimated hazard ratio for distant metastases by signature was 5.1 ($p < .001$) and remained significant when adjusted for lymph node status. This signature has since been validated with an independent data set, can now be performed using formalin fixed paraffin embedded tissue, and is currently being utilized in prospective, randomized trial titled Microarray In Node Negative Disease May Avoid Chemotherapy (MINDACT).[105,106] The hypothesis of the trial is that molecular profiling can lead to improved risk assessment thereby reducing the number of patients receiving adjuvant systemic therapy without compromising long-term outcome. Results of the pilot phase including the first 800 patients was published and showed that, compared with Adjuvant! Online, use of MammaPrint resulted in a potential 8.25% reduction in chemotherapy use. Results of long-term outcome are still pending.[107]

On the other hand, Oncotype Dx (Genomic Health Inc., Redwood City, CA) is a 21-gene real-time RT-PCR assay on formalin-fixed, paraffin-embedded tissue, with 15 cancer-related genes and six reference genes, that is currently being studied to help predict the chance of recurrence in patients with lymph node–negative, ER-positive breast cancer. The assay calculates a recurrence score, which stratifies patients into low, intermediate, and high risk of recurrence.[108,109] Paik and colleagues evaluated this assay among women treated with tamoxifen in the National Surgical Adjuvant Breast and Bowel Project (NSABP) B-14 trial.

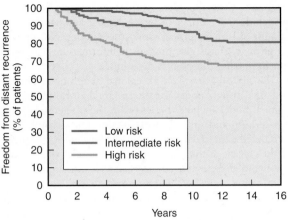

No. at risk:

Low risk	338	328	313	298	276	258	231	170	38
Intermediate risk	149	139	128	116	104	96	80	66	16
High risk	181	154	137	119	105	91	83	63	13

• **Fig. 37.10** Likelihood of distant recurrence according to recurrence score categories of a 21-gene prognostic signature (Oncotype Dx). (From Paik S, Shak S, Tang G, et al. A multigene assay to predict recurrence of tamoxifen-treated, node-negative breast cancer. *N Engl J Med.* 2004;351;2817. Copyright © 2004 Massachusetts Medical Society. All rights reserved.)

Kaplan-Meier estimates of 10-year disease recurrence rate in the three groups were 6.8%, 14.3%, and 30.5% (Fig. 37.10), respectively, and there was also a significant relationship between recurrence score and overall survival.[109] Currently this assay is being studied in a clinical trial (Trial Assigning IndividuaLized Options for Treatment [TAILORx]), evaluating the role of chemotherapy in lymph node–negative patients. Patients deemed to be high risk are given chemotherapy and hormone therapy, patients in the intermediate group are randomized to hormonal therapy alone or combination chemotherapy plus hormonal therapy, and patients in the low-risk group are treated with hormone therapy alone.[110] The initial results of the lowest risk group (scores of 0–10) were recently published. At 5 years the rate of freedom of recurrence from breast cancer at a distant site in these 1626 women assigned to receive endocrine therapy alone was 99.3% and the overall survival was 98.0%.[110] As more results from this trial enrolling more than 10,000 women emerge, the utility of the Oncotype Dx will continue to evolve.

Lymph Node Status

In the late 19th century, Halsted[111] described how breast cancer spreads systematically from the primary breast tissue to the ipsilateral axilla and is finally disseminated into the systemic circulation. The presence of axillary nodal metastasis was considered a poorer prognostic factor compared with improvement in survival with a more radical operation. However, this theory has been challenged over the years when it became evident that more extensive mastectomies proved to have survival benefit equal to that of less extensive, breast conserving operations.[112,113] Furthermore, up to 30% of patients with lymph node–negative disease eventually develop recurrent metastatic disease.[114] However, once the diagnosis of breast cancer has been established, the lymph node status remains the most powerful predictor for long-term survival.[115] Over the years, lymph node staging has been refined to include the number of lymph nodes, and more recently, the amount of tumor burden within these nodes. Not only does the lymph node status give prognostic information, it is also important in making therapeutic decisions.

The clinical assessment of regional lymph nodes must include ipsilateral axillary nodes and interpectoral, or Rotter, nodes. Other regional nodes include the IMNs in the intercostal spaces along the sternum and supraclavicular nodes. For a lymph node to be considered supraclavicular, it must be located in a triangle bound by the clavicle at the base, the internal jugular vein medially, and omohyoid muscle and tendon laterally and superiorly. Physical examination, however, is notoriously inaccurate in preoperative assessment of the presence of lymph node metastasis. In fact, microscopic evidence of tumor can be demonstrated in one-third of patients in the absence of palpable axillary lymph nodes. Clinical examination has a false-positive rate for detection of axillary metastases ranging from 25% to 31%. False-negative rates range from 27% to 33%.[115,116]

Axillary Nodal Disease

Results of a national survey by the American College of Surgeons (ACS) involving 20,547 women with breast cancer clearly demonstrated a strong linear association between the number of histologically involved axillary nodes and 5-year survival (Fig. 37.11).[8] Furthermore, in a 10-year clinical trial, Fisher, Fisher, and Redmond,[117] reporting for the NSABP, found that patients with negative axillary lymph nodes had 5- and 10-year survival rates of 78% and 65%, respectively. Similarly, the number of positive nodes correlated with the 5- and 10-year treatment failures. No positive nodes was associated with a 20% treatment failure rate at 10 years, whereas more than four positive nodes was associated with a 71% treatment failure rate. Not only is axillary lymph node metastasis a time-dependent variable, but it also seems to be a marker for a more aggressive tumor phenotype. Jatoi and associates[118] have shown that patients with four or more involved lymph nodes at the time of initial diagnosis have a significantly worse outcome after their first recurrence (Fig. 37.12).

Although axillary nodal status is an important prognostic indicator, its therapeutic role is more to clear the axilla of gross disease. Historically, there was a push to perform extensive axillary dissections to obtain accurate prognostic information. Certainly, complete dissection of all three levels of lymph nodes (Patey dissection) not only provided the maximum amount of prognostic information but also cleared the axilla of gross disease and was thought

to obviate the need for axillary irradiation. Before the advent of SLN techniques, several studies addressed the extent of axillary dissection and determined that, in certain cases, a level 1 dissection could be predictive of the actual involvement of the remaining nodal basin. Boova and colleagues[119] examined the contents of 200 consecutive mastectomy and total axillary dissection specimens. The average number of lymph nodes recovered from each level was 14 at level 1, 11 at level 2, and 8 at level 3. Of the patients, 40% had axillary metastases, with half of these involving only level 1 (Table 37.3). Interestingly, seven patients (3.5% of all patients and 8.7% of those with lymph node metastases) had positive nodes at level 2 and/or 3 without positive nodes at level 1 (skip metastasis). These authors concluded that level 1 dissections could be accurate predictors of the status of the entire axillary lymph node basin, assuming that an adequate number of lymph nodes has been sampled. Fisher and coworkers[120] also suggested that dissection of levels 1 and 2 is more than adequate in most cases to accurately predict prognosis. The current standard

TABLE 37.3	Patterns of Axillary Nodal Involvement: Levels 1, 2, and 3
Nodal Status	**No. of Patients (%)**
All levels negative	120 (60)
Level 1 positive	39 (19.5)
Levels 1 and 2 positive	19 (9.5)
Levels 1, 2, and 3 positive	11 (5.5)
Levels 1 and 3 positive	4 (2)
Level 2 positive[a]	5 (2.5)
Level 3 positive[a]	1 (0.5)
Levels 2 and 3 positive[a]	1 (0.5)

[a]Skip metastasis group.

Modified from Boova RS, Bonanni R, Rosato FE. Patterns of axillary nodal involvement in breast cancer. Predictability of level one dissection. *Ann Surg.* 1982;196:642-664.

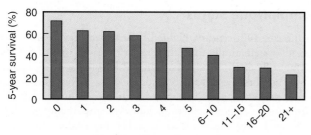

• **Fig. 37.11** Survival of breast cancer according to number of histologically involved axillary lymph nodes. (From Nemoto T, Vana J, Bedwani RN, et al. Management and survival of female breast cancer: results of a national survey by the American College of Surgeons. *Cancer.* 1980; 45:2917.)

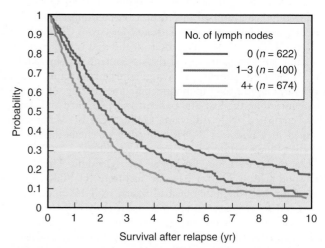

• **Fig. 37.12** Survival after first relapse by number of positive axillary lymph nodes. (From Jatoi I, Hilsenbeck SG, Clark GM, Osborne CK. Significance of axillary lymph node metastasis in primary breast cancer. *J Clin Oncol.* 1999;17:2334.)

of care for a complete axillary lymph node dissection includes both level 1 and level 2 lymph nodes with procurement of at least 10 lymph nodes.

Sentinel Lymph Node Mapping

The introduction of SLN mapping technology has challenged the classic approach to breast cancer staging that involves routine axillary lymph node dissection. The SLN concept supports the notion that breast cancer cells spread in an orderly fashion via direct lymphatic communication from the primary tumor to the SLN. Therefore the SLN is most likely to be the first site of metastasis within the lymph node basin. Currently, SLN mapping for breast cancer has become the primary means for accurately assessing nodal metastasis. On average, one to three SLNs may be found within an axillary basin. A number of large, single, and multiinstitutional trials have now demonstrated the accurate predictability of the SLN technique in staging the axilla in breast cancer patients by using various injection techniques with technetium sulfur colloid, isosulfan blue, or a combination of both agents.[121–124] The optimal technique for most is a combination of blue dye and technetium sulfur colloid. A SLN identification rate of more than 95% is the rule, with accuracy rates exceeding 95% and a false-negative rate of approximately 2%. A well-trained multidisciplinary team must be systematically assembled to ensure the success of the procedure. Long-term follow-up is needed to define the true false-negative rate—that is, to identify axillary recurrences in patients with breast cancer with negative SLNs and no complete axillary dissections. Initial studies suggest that this risk is less than 1% (0.2%–0.3%).[125,126]

In addition, the accuracy of the SLN mapping technique is enhanced by the ability to improve on the histologic examination of the lymph node when 1 to 3 lymph nodes, as opposed to 15 to 20 lymph nodes, in a complete node dissection are submitted for a more detailed examination. Routine histologic examination with serial step sectioning and H&E staining is performed to identify tumor deposits within the lymph node. Furthermore, IHC, with cytokeratin assays, shows an increased rate of detection of occult micrometastatic disease, further improving the accuracy of the technique.[127] Cote and colleagues[128] noted that occult nodal metastases were detected in 7% of patients with H&E sections and in 20% with IHC. Other investigators have also shown the increase in detection of occult micrometastatic disease in patients who were determined to be lymph node–negative based on routine histologic methods.[129,130] In a study by Schreiber and associates,[131] up to 9.4% of the patients were upstaged with the addition of IHC and serial sectioning. However, to date the clinical significance of identifying micrometastatic and submicrometastatic disease as a prognostic variable is controversial. A population-based analysis by Chen and coworkers[132] evaluated 209,720 patients with invasive breast cancer without distant metastases and no more than three axillary nodes using the SEER registries. Overall, patients with micrometastases no larger than 2 mm had a significant worse 5-year survival (86%) than patients without nodal metastases (90%) and better than patients with macrometastases in no more than three nodes (82%; Fig. 37.13). Cox and coworkers noted that 16% of patients with micrometastasis (>0.2 mm and <2 mm) and 9% of patients with isolated tumor cells or small-cell clusters not greater than 0.2 mm by IHC on SLN biopsy will have additional positive non-SLN if an axillary lymph node dissection is performed.[133] As stated previously, ACOSOG Z10 showed that of the specimens noted to be negative on H&E stain that were further evaluated with IHC, 10.5% of

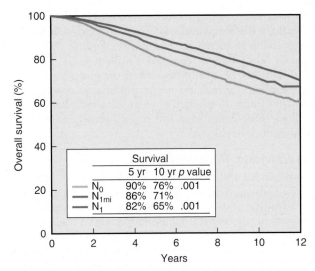

• **Fig. 37.13** Prognostic significance of lymph node micrometastases in breast cancer. (From Chen SL, Hoehne FM, Giuliano AE. The prognostic significance of micrometastases in breast cancer: a Surveillance, Epidemiology, and End Results population-based analysis. *Ann Surg Oncol.* 2007;14;3378.)

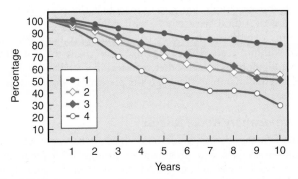

• **Fig. 37.14** Ten-year overall survival in patients without lymph node metastases (1), with axillary lymph node metastases only (2), with internal mammary node metastases (3), and with both groups involved (4). (From Veronesi U, Cascinelli N, Greco M, et al. Prognosis of breast cancer patients after mastectomy and dissection of internal mammary nodes. *Ann Surg.* 1985;202:702.)

SLNs were found to be positive for tumor with no difference in overall survival or disease-free survival compared with women with IHC negative SLNs.

Internal Mammary Nodal Disease

The status of the IMNs has been a point of controversy since the time of Halsted in the 1890s. Prospective randomized trials have failed to demonstrate a benefit in survival for women who had complete IMN dissections (extended radical mastectomy) while incurring significant operative morbidity. However, other studies have shown a prognostic significance of metastasis to the IMNs.[134–137] Veronesi and associates[138] reported 10-year overall survival rates according to IMN disease and/or axillary lymph node disease among patients who had extended radical mastectomy (Fig. 37.14). The study clearly demonstrated a marked difference in overall survival between patients without any nodal disease (80%) and patients with only IMN disease and only axillary lymph node disease, with an overall survival of 53% and

55%, respectively. Furthermore, the presence of both IMN disease and axillary lymph node disease was associated with the worst outcome with an overall survival of 30%. Positive IMNs can be found in up to 10% of cases when axillary nodes are negative and in as many as 26% of cases when the primary tumor location is medial.[139] Lymphatic mapping techniques may lead to the ability to identify IMNs with improved accuracy; however, there is still appreciable morbidity. The surgical management of IMNs remains controversial.

Supraclavicular Nodal Disease

Historically, supraclavicular lymph nodes involved with tumor indicated advanced disease and were associated with a poor prognosis. Positive supraclavicular lymph nodes were considered to have survival rates similar to those with distant spread rather than of regional nodal disease.[140,141] More recent studies suggest that the outcomes of patients with these tumors are comparable to those of patients with locally advanced disease rather than distant metastatic disease.[142]

Currently, routine scalene lymph node biopsies are not indicated. In the prechemotherapy era, scalene lymph node biopsy was performed to determine operability of breast cancer patients with advanced local disease but without evidence of distant metastases. It was noted by Papaioannou and Urban,[143] however, that when scalene lymph nodes were pathologically positive, despite the use of radical mastectomy with adjuvant radiotherapy, no patients were disease free after 1 year, and more than 50% were dead within 3 years. These data once again suggested that metastasis to lymph node beds other than regional (axillary, clavicular, and internal mammary) suggests the presence of distant systemic disease.

Intramammary Nodal Disease

Intramammary lymph nodes (intraMLNs) have received little attention as potential prognostic indicators for patients with breast carcinoma and are largely overlooked by radiologists, pathologists, and surgeons. Recently interest for intraMLNs as a marker of disease severity has increased with the introduction of SLN biopsy and lymphatic mapping because detection of intraMLNs is likely to occur more frequently by preoperative lymphoscintigraphy and intraoperative gamma probe scanning of the breast. By definition, intraMLNs are surrounded by breast parenchyma, a feature that distinguishes them from low axillary lymph nodes. Histopathologic studies of breast specimens containing intraMLNs have revealed that these lymph nodes may be present in any quadrant of the breast and can yield a variety of pathologic findings, including metastatic carcinoma in the ipsilateral breast.

The prevalence of intraMLNs has been reported to range between 1% and 28%.[144,145] Egan and McSweeney[144] were the first to address the prognostic significance of intraMLN in breast cancer. They found that in stage I disease, positive intraMLNs were associated with a poor prognosis (10-year survival rate, 79%); however, intraMLNs were not found to be associated with poorer prognosis in stage II disease. Because of this, patients with breast carcinoma accompanied by intraMLN metastases are traditionally considered to have stage II disease, even in the absence of axillary lymph node involvement. Recently Shen and colleagues[146] evaluated 130 patients with intraMLNs. IntraMLN metastases were found in 28% of all cases, and isolated intraMLN metastases were documented in 5% of all cases. The presence of intraMLN metastases was associated with poorer 5-year overall

survival compared with non-intraMLN involvement (64% vs. 88%). Furthermore, intraMLN was found to be a significant independent predictor of survival in patients with axillary lymph node involvement as well as among those without axillary involvement. Similar results have reported that intraMLN metastases is a marker of disease severity and that the presence of metastatic disease in an intraMLN is associated with a high rate of axillary nodal involvement.[147]

Pathologic Assessment of Lymph Nodes

Molecular staging using techniques such as RT-PCR is allowing the detection of one tumor cell in the background of a million. Adoption of these technologies has raised the likelihood of finding micrometastases. Furthermore, accurate molecular analysis of all or part of the SLN offers the potential to reduce false-negative findings significantly and overcome limitations that occur with standard methods of intraoperative SLN analysis. Currently, intraoperative SLN analysis methods such as imprint cytology (touch preparation) and frozen section suffer from poor and variable sensitivity and a lack of standardization.[148,149] Compared with final pathology results, the reported sensitivity of frozen section SLN analysis varies from 58% to 87%.[150] Imprint cytology has similar limitations in sensitivity.[151] Recently, Backus and colleagues[152] were able to identify an optimal two-gene expression marker set (mammaglobin, cytokeratin 19) for detection of clinically actionable metastasis in breast SLNs using microarray methods. Furthermore, they developed a rapid RT-PCR assay (GeneSearch Breast Lymph Node [BLN] Assay; Veridex, Warren, NJ) using these two markers; it generates a result in less than 30 minutes. The authors assessed the utility of RT-PCR assay in SLNs of 254 breast cancer patients, reporting a sensitivity of 90% and specificity of 94%. Blumencranz and associates[153] recently validated this RT-PCR assay in a prospective study at 11 clinical sites. The assay detected 98% of metastases larger than 2 mm and 88% of metastases larger than 0.2 mm. Micrometastases were less frequently detected (57%), and assay-positive results in nodes found to be negative by histology were rare (4%). The authors concluded that the use of the BLN assay overcomes conventional histologic sampling errors and can reduce the need for second surgeries to complete the axillary dissection on SLN-positive patients. Similar results have been reported by other authors who used this commercially available assay, and prospective trials are under way to further characterize its utility in daily practice.[154] Other indices that portend an unfavorable prognosis for breast cancer relate to the presence of gross rather than microscopic disease in the lymph nodes and/or the presence of extranodal disease.[155,156]

Evolution of Staging Systems

Early staging systems for breast cancer were based on the feasibility of operative intervention. Most tumors were classified as either operable or inoperable; however, this grouping did not offer any significant prognostic information. In 1905 the German physician Steinthal[157] recommended three classifications for patients with breast cancer: (1) tumors not larger than "a plum" and clinically not associated with skin or axillary lymph node involvement, (2) large tumors adherent to the skin with palpable enlarged axillary lymph nodes, and (3) large tumors diffusely involving the breast with skin, deep muscle, and supraclavicular lymph node involvement. This classification was based on clinical factors that were perceived as important in predicting prognosis. Early on, it was clear that surgeons had identified some of the most ominous

TABLE 37.4	Manchester System
Stage I	The tumor is confined to the breast. Involvement of the skin may be present, provided the area is small in relation to the size of the breast
Stage II	The tumor is confined to the breast and associated lymph nodes are present in the axilla
Stage III	The tumor extends beyond the breast as demonstrated by the following: a. Skin invasion or fixation of a large area in relation to the size of the breast or skin ulceration b. Tumor fixation to the underlying muscle or fascia; mobile axillary nodes
Stage IV	The tumor extends beyond the breast as shown by the following: a. Fixation or matting of the axillary nodes b. Fixation of tumor to chest wall c. Deposits in supraclavicular nodes or in the opposite breast d. Satellite nodules or distant metastases

Modified from Patterson R. *The Treatment of Malignant Disease by Radium and X-Rays.* London: Edward Arnold; 1948.

TABLE 37.5	Portmann Classification
Stage I	
–	Skin—not involved
+	Tumor—localized to breast, mobile
–	Metastases—none
Stage II	
–	Skin±not involved
+	Tumor—localized to breast, mobile
+	Metastases—few axillary lymph nodes involved in microscopic evaluation; no other metastases
Stage III	
–	Skin—edematous; brawny red induration and inflammation not obviously caused by infection; extensive ulceration; multiple secondary nodules
++	Tumor—diffusely infiltrating breast; fixation of tumor or breast to chest wall; edema of breast; secondary tumors
++	Metastases—many axillary lymph nodes involved or fixed; no clinical or roentgenologic evidence of distant metastases
Stage IV	
+/–	Skin—involved or not involved
+/++	Tumor—localized or diffuse
+++	Metastases—axillary and supraclavicular lymph nodes extensively involved; clinical or roentgenologic evidence of more distant metastases

Modified from Portmann UV. Clinical and pathological criteria as a basis for classifying cases of primary breast cancer. *Cleve Clin Q.* 1943;10:41-47.

prognostic indicators for breast cancer. It is also interesting to note the inclusion of primary tumor size in this primitive staging scheme. An unpopular but insightful system was proposed by Lee and Stubenbord[158] in 1928. Their system included an index of the rate of tumor growth. This method was the first to attempt assessment of the biology of individual tumors and their potential for progression.

In 1940 the four-stage Manchester classification was introduced (Table 37.4).[159] It permitted staging based solely on clinical criteria, including the extent of local involvement by the primary tumor, the presence and mobility of palpable enlarged axillary lymph nodes, and the presence of distant metastases. Neither pathologic information nor tumor size was included in this system. In 1943 Portmann[160] described a staging system that incorporated clinical, pathologic, and roentgenographic characteristics of breast cancers and evaluated each lesion based on three categories: skin involvement, the location and mobility of the primary tumor, and the extent of local and distant metastases (Table 37.5). Haagensen and Stout[161] evaluated 568 patients with breast cancer who were treated with radical mastectomy. In 1943 they published the following criteria of inoperability, which were based on the clinical characteristics of patients who were clearly incurable by aggressive surgery alone:

- Extensive edema of the skin overlying the breast or edema of the arm
- Satellite nodules of the breast or parasternal tumor nodules
- Inflammatory carcinoma
- Supraclavicular or distant metastases
- Two or more of the five "grave signs" of locally advanced cancer:
  1. Breast skin edema
  2. Breast skin ulceration
  3. Tumor fixation to chest wall
  4. Axillary lymph node fixation to skin or deep tissues
  5. Enlarged axillary lymph nodes larger than 2.5 cm in diameter

Haagensen and Stout also advocated the use of biopsy material in the determination of inoperability. Their proposed "triple biopsy" included sampling the primary tumor, apical axillary nodes, and IMNs as part of the pretreatment evaluation. This represented the first attempt at including pathologic data in the staging process.

Although largely derived from Haagensen and Stout's criteria of inoperability, the Columbia Clinical Classification (CCC) ignored the use of tumor size and any biopsy material or other pathologic data. It has, however, been successfully used to separate groups of patients with distinctly different survival rates.[162] Staging was determined on the basis of physical examination and other roentgenographic information in an attempt to simplify and streamline the staging process. Four stages were defined (Table 37.6). Stages A and B were both used to describe operable cancers, but stage B referred to palpably enlarged, unfixed axillary lymph nodes (presumed to represent regional metastases). Based on the five "grave signs" listed previously, stage C defined a group of patients with cancers that were locally advanced. In stage D, the tumors were considered inoperable as defined by the "criteria of inoperability." Patients with stages A and B disease were treated with radical mastectomy, whereas those with stages C and D disease underwent radiation therapy.

TABLE 37.6	Columbia Clinical Classification
Stage A	No skin involvement or fixation of the tumor to the chest wall. Axillary nodes are not palpable.
Stage B	No skin involvement or fixation of the tumor to the chest wall. Clinically palpable nodes, but <2.5 cm in transverse diameter and not fixed to overlying skin or deeper structures of the axilla.
Stage C	Any one of the five grave signs of advanced breast carcinoma: 1. Limited edema of the skin involving less than one-third of the skin over the breast 2. Skin ulceration 3. Fixation of the tumor to the chest wall 4. Massive involvement of axillary lymph nodes measuring >2.5 cm in transverse diameter 5. Fixation of the axillary nodes to overlying skin or deeper structures of the axilla
Stage D	Any patient with signs of advanced breast carcinoma: 1. A combination of any two or more of the five grave signs listed under stage C 2. Extensive edema of the skin (involving more than one-third of the skin over the breast) 3. Satellite skin nodules 4. The inflammatory type of carcinoma 5. Clinically involved supraclavicular lymph nodes 6. Internal mammary metastases as evidenced by a parasternal tumor 7. Edema of the arm 8. Distant metastases

Modified from Haagensen CD, Cooley E, Kennedy CS, et al. Treatment of early mammary carcinoma: a Cooperative International Study. *Ann Surg.* 1964;157:157-179.

Despite initial acceptance, the CCC has since been replaced by the current TNM system, which incorporates both clinical and pathologic features. This system was adopted for many reasons, including its initial simplicity, clinical applicability, and universal utility. Moreover, it is clear that since the 1990s, because of the widespread use of screening mammography and public education, breast cancers are being detected earlier, with fewer delays in diagnosis. This has necessarily shifted the contemporary population of patients being evaluated to earlier stages at diagnosis. In turn, the need for elaborate classification schemes based on generally advanced clinical criteria has become obsolete. At present, patients need to be stratified into groups based on subtler, less advanced characteristics of disease progression. This is necessary not only because many women now have small or nonpalpable tumors but also because not all small tumors have the same biological behavior (e.g., growth, metastases).

The TNM system, developed in France by Pierre Denoix[163] in the 1940s, represented an attempt to classify cancer based on the major morphologic attributes of malignant tumors thought to influence prognosis: size of the primary tumor (T), presence and extent of regional lymph node involvement (N), and presence of distant metastases (M). In 1958 the International Union Against Cancer (UICC) described the first recommendations for the staging of breast cancer based on the TNM system.[164] Subsequently, the American Joint Committee on Cancer (AJCC) published a breast cancer staging schematic based on the TNM system in its first cancer staging manual in 1977.[165] Since then, the AJCC's proposals have undergone somewhat parallel and confluent evolutionary changes to those of the UICC; in 1987, for the first time, a truly universal staging system was developed, and differences between them were eliminated. The current UICC and AJCC staging systems for breast cancer are now identical. This alliance permits collaboration in multiinstitutional trials on an international level.

The TNM system was originally conceived to be a simple system that would classify patients into various groups, each with a different survival rate and prognosis. There were binary choices for each evaluable patient and tumor characteristic. For instance, T$_0$ represented the absence of tumor; T$_1$ represented the presence of tumor. Similarly, N$_0$/M$_0$ and N$_1$/M$_1$ represented the absence or presence of regional or distant metastatic disease, respectively. Any patient could be rapidly classified into one of eight possible groups that could then be stratified into any number of stages based on observed survival frequencies. Such a classification system would have been simple, logical, and easy to commit to memory for future use. Although the TNM system was originally simple in design, modifications were necessary to improve prognostic power and stage definition. A large number of clinical and pathologic prognostic indicators have been identified since the inception of the TNM system (see the section on clinical and pathologic correlates with prognosis). The TNM system is the only system to date that has successfully incorporated many of these factors. For this reason, despite the observation that this method of staging for breast cancer has become more complicated, it is also highly practical and adaptable. It provides more prognostic information and better stratifies patients for the purpose of guiding therapy than do other systems that are based largely on clinical criteria alone.

The more precisely the clinician is able to define specific groups of patients who should undergo equivalent therapeutic regimens, the greater the probability that medical scientists should be able to reduce the number of patients with aggressive disease who are undertreated and those with limited disease who are overtreated. As more and more prognostic indices are identified and successful therapeutic modalities discovered, changes within the TNM classification will be required to encompass these advancements; for this reason, binary choices have become quaternary (N$_0$, N$_1$, N$_2$, N$_3$) or greater (T$_0$, T$_{is}$, T$_1$, T$_2$, T$_3$, T$_4$). Further delineation within each subcategory has also been added.

Current Staging System

Currently, the most popular staging system is the TNM system, based on the AJCC, sponsored by the American Cancer Society (ACS) and the American College of Surgeons. The AJCC staging system was extensively modified in 2002 leading to the updated sixth edition, representing the culmination of many years of evolution of the AJCC and ACS. The seventh edition was subsequently published in 2010, and the eighth edition published in late 2016 for implementation in early 2018.[166] Major changes between the sixth and seventh edition are highlighted in this section. Despite these unified efforts, however, the current system will certainly undergo future changes. The best staging system should be flexible and continue to evolve with new prognostic data.

The current staging system requires microscopic confirmation and histologic typing of the tumor before attempting any stage classification. Any patient with documented breast cancer may then be staged by clinical (clinical or preoperative, designated by a "c" prefix) or pathologic criteria (pathologic or postoperative, designated by a "p" prefix). The clinical-diagnostic staging process requires a complete physical examination, with determination of the extent of ipsilateral and contralateral neoplastic involvement of skin, breast tissue, regional and distant lymph nodes, and underlying muscles. Imaging modalities such as mammogram, ultrasound, and breast MRI are useful as an adjuvant to the physical examination. According to the AJCC, imaging findings must be collected within 4 months of diagnosis to be incorporated as a staging element.[166] Relevant imaging findings may include tumor size, presence or absence of regional lymph node disease, extension into the underlying chest wall, or presence of distant metastasis. Laboratory examinations, as well as further imaging may be indicated in certain patients to evaluate for distant spread. Current National Comprehensive Cancer Network (NCCN) guidelines recommend baseline laboratory testing (complete blood count, platelet count, liver function tests, and alkaline phosphatase) for all patients with invasive breast cancer. For stages I–IIB, the recommendation is for symptom-directed additional staging (bone scan, computed tomography [CT] scan of chest and/or abdomen and pelvis). Bone scans might be done in the setting of bone pain or elevated alkaline phosphatase. Likewise, abdominal CT and/or chest CT should be considered with the presence of abdominal or pulmonary complaints or abnormal laboratory values. The role of positron emission tomography (PET) in the initial staging evaluation of breast cancer is uncertain. For patients with stage IIIA or IIIB, one should consider chest/abdomen/pelvis CT and possibly a bone scan as the risk of distant metastases is increased in these patients. Per NCCN guidelines, PET is currently not indicated in stage I or II and is considered an optional way of staging patients with more advanced disease.

The pathologic classification involves all the data used in clinical staging; however, this more definitive staging system can be implemented only after the resection of the primary tumor and regional lymph nodes. It requires that no macroscopic tumor be present at the margins of resection. Should tumor be present at the margins on gross examination of the resected specimen, the code T_x is applied, indicating that the pathologic stage cannot yet be determined. Some pathologic examination of the axillary lymph nodes (SLN biopsy or axillary lymph node dissection) is also required. The current TNM staging system based on the seventh edition of the AJCC staging manual is summarized in the following sections.

Specific Stages

T Stage (Tumor Size)

Clinical tumor stage is the size of the tumor (reported in centimeters) based on the physical examination and various imaging modalities (e.g., mammogram, ultrasound, MRI; Table 37.7). The pathologic T stage is based on the tumor size on the final pathologic specimen measuring only the invasive component. New to the seventh edition is the specific recommendation that, for small tumors that can be submitted in one paraffin block, the most accurate determination of pathologic stage is the microscopic measurement. However, for a large tumor that requires multiple blocks, the gross measurement is preferred. Furthermore, in

TABLE 37.7 AJCC Primary Tumor (T) Classification for Breast Cancer

Tx	Primary tumor cannot be assessed
T0	No evidence of primary tumor
Tis	Carcinoma in situ
Tis (DCIS)	DCIS
Tis (LCIS)	LCIS
Tis (Paget)	Paget disease of the nipple *not* associated with invasive carcinoma in situ (DCIS and/or LCIS) in the underlying breast parenchyma. Carcinomas in the breast parenchyma associated with Paget disease are categorized based on the size and characteristics of the parenchymal disease, although the presence of Paget disease should be noted.
T1	Tumor ≤20 mm in greatest dimension
T1mic	Microinvasion ≤1 mm in greatest dimension
T1a	Tumor >1 mm but ≤5 mm in greatest dimension
T1b	Tumor >5 mm but ≤10 mm in greatest dimension
T1c	Tumor >10 mm but ≤20 mm in greatest dimension
T2	Tumor > 20 mm but ≤50 mm in greatest dimension
T3	Tumor > 50 mm in greatest dimension
T4	Tumor of any size with direct extension to chest wall and/or to the skin (ulceration or skin nodules). *Note:* invasion of the dermis alone does not qualify as T4
T4a	Extension to the chest wall, not including only pectoralis muscle adherence/invasion
T4b	Ulceration and/or ipsilateral satellite nodules and/or edema (including peau d'orange) of the skin, which do not meet criteria for inflammatory carcinoma
T4c	Both T4a and T4b
T4d	Inflammatory carcinoma (see "Rules for Classification")

AJCC, American Joint Commission on Cancer; *DCIS,* ductal carcinoma in situ; *LCIS,* lobular carcinoma in situ.
From Edge SB, Byrd DR, Compton CC, Fritz AG, Greene FL. *AJCC Cancer Staging Manual.* 7th ed. New York: Springer; 2010:360.

patients with small tumors who have undergone diagnostic core needle biopsy, especially vacuum-assisted sampling, measuring residual tumor at time of surgery may lead to understaging. However, simply adding maximum dimensions of the invasive cancer seen within the biopsy specimen may lead to overestimation. In this scenario, a combination of imaging and gross and microscopic histologic findings should be used to determine final tumor size.

Special circumstances include multicentric or multifocal disease and use of neoadjuvant therapy. For multiple synchronous ipsilateral primary carcinomas, the largest tumor is used for the T classification and the physician should document that there are multiple primaries with their corresponding sizes and characteristics. Bilateral synchronous breast cancers are staged separately as separate primaries. For patients undergoing neoadjuvant therapy, a pretreatment pathologic size is not possible to ascertain. Pretreatment staging should be based on clinical considerations. Posttreatment size is designated ypT and should be determined by using a combination of gross and microscopic disease. In instances where residual disease consists of multiple tumor foci, the final size is determined by the largest contiguous focus of invasive cancer.

The T$_{is}$ classification includes ductal carcinoma in situ, lobular carcinoma in situ, or Paget disease of the nipple with no invasive tumor, designated as T$_{is}$ (DCIS), T$_{is}$ (LCIS), and T$_{is}$ (Paget), respectively. The authors' acknowledged that the terms *ductal intraepithelial neoplasia* (DIN) and *lobular intraepithelial neoplasia* (LIN) have been proposed but are currently not widely accepted. They further clarified that only DIN lesions containing DCIS or LCIS should be classified as T$_{is}$ (DCIS) or T$_{is}$ (LCIS). Paget disease of the nipple with an associated invasive or noninvasive tumor is classified based on the malignant component. The T$_{is}$ (Paget) designation should only be used if no underlying malignancy is present. Although there is controversy regarding LCIS, whether this is merely a marker for increased risk of developing breast cancer or a precursor of invasive lobular carcinoma, LCIS is currently reported as a malignancy in this staging system. A further addition to the seventh edition includes the recommendation that size of noninvasive cancer be listed. Although size will not change T stage, it may influence further management.

T$_1$ is designated for tumors that are 2 cm or smaller and subclassified as T$_{1mic}$, T$_{1a}$, T$_{1b}$, and T$_{1c}$. Microinvasive breast cancer is defined as a focus of tumor less than or equal to 0.1 cm in greatest dimension. When there are multiple foci of microinvasion, the T designation is based on the largest of the foci and not the additive sum of these. T$_2$ tumors are between 2 and 5 cm, and T$_3$ tumors are larger than 5 cm. Tumors with direct invasion into the chest wall or skin are designated as T$_4$ tumors, with subclassification based on edema, extension to chest wall, skin ulceration, peau d'orange, or inflammation. Of note, chest wall extension does not include invasion into the pectoralis major alone. Inflammatory cancer is classified as T$_{4d}$ and remains a clinical diagnosis characterized by erythema of the skin that involves a third of the breast. A biopsy showing tumor emboli within dermal lymphatic is confirmatory but not necessary to make the diagnosis, and care should be taken to differentiate from local advanced cancer involving the skin or dermal lymphatic invasion without clinical signs of inflammatory cancer.

N Stage

Clinical nodal staging is based on physical examination or imaging studies, including CT scans, MRI, and ultrasound but excluding lymphoscintigraphy (Table 37.8). If the regional lymph nodes cannot be assessed clinically (previously removed or not removed for pathologic examination), they are designated cN$_X$. If no regional nodes are involved with tumor, it is designated as cN$_0$. Categorization of clinical regional lymph node involvement is based on whether the lymph nodes are mobile (cN$_1$) or fixed (cN$_{2a}$) and evidence of involvement of the ipsilateral infraclavicular lymph nodes (cN$_{3a}$) or ipsilateral supraclavicular lymph nodes (cN$_{3b}$). Metastasis to ipsilateral supraclavicular lymph node disease was considered to have a prognosis similar to that for patients with distant disease; however, the overall survival is better and was changed to stage N$_{3c}$ in the revised 2002 AJCC staging system. Designation of ipsilateral IMN disease is dependent on involvement of other nodal basins. Metastasis within ipsilateral IMN without other nodal disease is designated

TABLE 37.8	AJCC Clinical Regional Lymph Nodes (N) Classification for Breast Cancer
N$_X$	Regional lymph nodes cannot be assessed (e.g., previously removed)
N$_0$	No regional lymph node metastases
N$_1$	Metastases in movable ipsilateral level I, II axillary lymph node(s)
N$_2$	Metastases in ipsilateral level I, II axillary lymph nodes that are clinically fixed or matted, or in clinically detected[a] ipsilateral internal mammary nodes in the *absence* of clinically evident axillary lymph node metastases
N$_{2a}$	Metastases in ipsilateral level I, II axillary lymph nodes fixed to one another (matted) or to other structures
N$_{2b}$	Metastases only in clinically detected[a] ipsilateral internal mammary nodes and in the *absence* of clinically evident axillary level I, II lymph node metastases
N$_3$	Metastases in ipsilateral infraclavicular (level III axillary) lymph node(s) with or without level I, II axillary lymph node involvement; or in clinically detected[a] ipsilateral internal mammary lymph node(s) with clinically evident level I, II axillary lymph node metastases; or metastases in ipsilateral supraclavicular lymph node(s) with or without axillary or internal mammary lymph node involvement
N$_{3a}$	Metastases in ipsilateral infraclavicular lymph node(s)
N$_{3b}$	Metastases in ipsilateral internal mammary node(s) and axillary lymph node(s)
N$_{3c}$	Metastases in ipsilateral supraclavicular lymph node(s)

AJCC, American Joint Commission on Cancer.

[a]*Clinically detected* is defined as detected by imaging studies (excluding lymphoscintigraphy) or by clinical examination and having characteristics highly suspicious for malignancy or a presumed pathologic macrometastasis based on fine-needle aspiration biopsy with cytologic examination. Confirmation of clinically detected metastatic disease by fine-needle aspiration without excision biopsy is designated with an (f) suffix, for example, cN3a(f). Excisional biopsy of a lymph node or biopsy of a sentinel node, in the absence of assignment of a pT, is classified as a clinical N, for example, cN$_1$. Information regarding the confirmation of the nodal status will be designated in site-specific factors as clinical, fine-needle aspiration, core biopsy, or sentinel lymph node biopsy. Pathologic classificaiton (pN) is used for excision or sentinel lymph node biopsy only in conjunction with a pathologic T assignment.

From Edge SB, Byrd DR, Compton CC, Fritz AG, Greene FL. *AJCC Cancer Staging Manual.* 7th ed. New York: Springer; 2010:360.

as cN$_{2b}$ and cN$_{3b}$ when in conjunction with other areas of nodal disease.

SLN biopsy techniques have dramatically changed the pathologic staging of patients with breast cancer. Patients are now being diagnosed with earlier tumor stages with the detection of microscopic and submicroscopic metastatic tumor deposits. This was reflected and incorporated into the revised 2002 AJCC pathologic staging system for the first time. This revised system also incorporated the assessment of microscopic disease based on IHC and molecular techniques (RT-PCR).

Pathologic staging of the lymph nodes is based on biopsies taken from SLN excision or complete axillary lymph node dissections (Table 37.9). The largest dimension of confluent or contiguous tumor cells is used to determine the size of metastatic disease. When multiple tumor deposits are seen, the size of disease is

TABLE 37.9	AJCC Pathologic Regional Lymph Nodes (pN) Classification for Breast Cancer[a]
pN_X	Regional lymph nodes cannot be assessed (e.g., previously removed, or not removed for pathologic study)
pN_0	No regional lymph node metastasis histologically
	Note: Isolated tumor cell clusters (ITC) are defined as small clusters of cells not greater than 0.2 mm, or single tumor cells, or a cluster of fewer than 200 cells in a single histologic cross section. ITCs may be detected by routine histology or by IHC methods. Nodes containing only ITCs are excluded from the total positive node count for purposes of N classification but should be included in the total number of nodes evaluated.
$pN_0(i-)$	No regional lymph node metastases histologically; negative IHC
$pN_0(i+)$	Malignant cells in regional lymph node(s) no greater than 0.2 mm (detected by H&E or IHC including ITC)
$pN_0(mol-)$	No regional lymph node metastasis histologically; negative molecular findings (RT-PCR)
$pN_0(mol+)$	Positive molecular findings (RT-PCR), but no regional lymph node metastases detected by histology or IHC
pN_1	Micrometastases; or metastases in 1–3 axillary lymph nodes; and/or in internal mammary nodes with metastases detected by sentinel lymph node biopsy but not clinically detected (RT-PCR)[b]
pN_{1mi}	Micrometastases (greater than 0.2 mm and more than 200 cells, but none greater than 2 mm)
pN_{1a}	Metastases in 1–3 axillary lymph nodes, at least one metastasis greater than 2.0 mm
pN_{1b}	Metastases in internal mammary nodes with micrometastases detected by sentinel lymph node dissection but not clinically detected[b]
pN_{1c}	Metastases in 1–3 axillary lymph nodes and in internal mammary lymph nodes with micrometastases detected by sentinel lymph node dissection but not clinically detected[b]
pN_2	Metastases in 4–9 axillary lymph nodes; or in clinically detected[c] internal mammary lymph nodes in the *absence* of axillary lymph node metastases
pN_{2a}	Metastasis in 4–9 axillary lymph nodes (at least one tumor deposit greater than 2.0 mm)
pN_{2b}	Metastases in clinically detected[d] internal mammary lymph nodes in the *absence* of axillary lymph node metastases
pN_3	Metastases in 10 or more axillary lymph nodes, or in infraclavicular (level III axillary) lymph nodes, or in clinically detected[d] ipsilateral internal mammary lymph nodes in the *presence* of one or more positive level I, II axillary lymph nodes; or in more than three axillary lymph nodesand in internal mammary lymph nodes with micrometastases or macrometastases detected by sentinel lymph node biopsy but not clinically detected[c]; or in ipsilateral supraclavicular lymph nodes
pN_{3a}	Metastases in 10 or more axillary lymph nodes (at least one tumor deposit greater than 2.0 mm) or metastases to the infraclavicular (level III axillary) lymph nodes
pN_{3b}	Metastases in clinically detected[d] ipsilateral internal mammary lymph nodes in the *presence* of one or more positive axillary lymph nodes; or in more than three axillary lymph nodes and in internal mammary lymph nodes with micrometastases or macrometastases detected by sentinel lymph node biopsy but not clinically detected[c]
pN_{3c}	Metastasis in ipsilateral supraclavicular lymph nodes

AJCC, American Joint Commission on Cancer; *H&E*, hematoxylin and eosin; *IHC*, immunohistochemical; *RT-PCR*, reverse transcriptase polymerase chain reaction.

[a]Classification is based on axillary lymph node dissection with or without sentinel lymph node biopsy. Classification based solely on sentinel lymph node biopsy without subsequent axillary lymph node dissection is designated (sn) for "sentinel node," for example, $pN_0(sn)$.

[b]RT-PCR.

[c]*Not clinically detected* is defined as not detected by imaging studies (excluding lymphoscintigraphy) or not detected by clinical examination.

[d]*Clinically detected* is defined as detected by imaging studies (excluding lymphoscintigraphy) or by clinical examination and having characteristics highly suspicious for malignancy or a presumed pathologic macrometastases based on fine-needle aspiration biopsy with cytologic examination.

From Edge SB, Byrd DR, Compton CC, Fritz AG, Greene FL. *AJCC Cancer Staging Manual.* 7th ed. New York: Springer; 2010:360.

classified based on the largest deposit. If the regional nodes cannot be assessed pathologically (previously removed or not removed for pathologic examination), they are designated pN_X. If no regional lymph nodes are involved with tumor, it is designated as pN_0. Further subclassification of pN_0 allows the distinction between the identification of microscopic cells based on IHC or molecular techniques (RT-PCR). Isolated tumor cells are defined as single tumor cells or small clusters not greater than 0.2 mm, usually detected with IHC or molecular methods but that may be verified on H&E stains. Isolated tumor cells usually show no evidence of metastatic activity and are designated $pN_{0(i+)}$. Pathologic node positivity is based on the number of lymph nodes involved. pN_1 is divided into four categories, including pN_{1mic} (micrometases >0.2 mm and/or 200 cells but <2 mm), pN_{1a} (metastases in 1–3 positive nodes), pN_{1b} (histologically confirmed IMN metastases in the absence of SLN disease), and pN_{1c} (histologically confirmed IMN disease in the presence of SLN disease). Additionally, pN_2 is also divided into two categories including pN_{2a} (metastases in

<table>
<tr><td colspan="2">TABLE 37.10 AJCC Distant Metastasis (M) Classification for Breast Cancer</td></tr>
</table>

M_x	No clinical or radiographic evidence of distant metastases
$cM_0(i+)$	No clinical or radiographic evidence of distant metastases, but deposits of molecularly or microscopically detected tumor cells in circulating blood, bone marrow, or other nonregional nodal tissue that are no larger than 0.2 mm in a patient without symptoms or signs of metastases
M_1	Distant detectable metastases as determined by classic clinical and radiographic means and/or histologically proven larger than 0.2 mm

AJCC, American Joint Commission on Cancer.
From Edge SB, Byrd DR, Compton CC, Fritz AG, Greene FL. *AJCC Cancer Staging Manual.* 7th ed. New York: Springer; 2010:360.

4–9 positive nodes) and pN_{2b} (radiographically or clinically IMN disease in the absence of SLN disease). pN_3 includes pN_{3a} (metastases in 10 or more axillary nodes or ipsilateral infraclavicular lymph nodes), pN_{3b} (radiographically or clinically confirmed IMN disease in the presence of SLN disease or histologically confirmed IMN disease with 3 or more positive axillary nodes), and pN_{3c} (metastases in ipsilateral supraclavicular lymph nodes). In the previous AJCC 1997 staging system, the designation of pathologically fixed, matted nodes were separate categories. In the revised AJCC 2002 staging system and continued into the 2009 system, there is not a distinction for fixed or matted lymph nodes.

M Stage

Distant metastatic disease is designated as M_1 disease (Table 37.10). Evidence of metastatic disease may be based on clinical history and physical examination, with or without the assistance of various imaging modalities and biochemical markers. When feasible to obtain, pathologic confirmation is recommended. New to the 2009 AJCC staging system is the $M_0(i+)$ category that includes presence of circulating tumor cells, disseminated tumor cells within the bone marrow, and micrometastases <0.2 mm incidentally found within other organ tissue. In the absence of other radiographic or clinical evidence of distant disease, this category does not change the overall stage but may portend an unfavorable prognosis.

Stage Groupings

There are five stage groupings (0, I, II, III, and IV) in the new TNM staging system, all of which include subdivisions (Table 37.11). Stage 0 (T_{is} N_0 M_0) refers to preinvasive cancers (carcinoma in situ) that have not penetrated the basement membrane of the duct or lobule. There are no regional or distant metastases associated with this stage at initial diagnosis and these tumors have an excellent prognosis. In the 2009 AJCC staging system, stage I has been further subdivided into stage IA (T_1 or T_{1mic} N_0 M_0) and stage IB (T_0 or T_1, N_{1mi}, M_0). Stage IIA (T_0 N_1 M_0, T_1 or T_{1mic} N_1 M_0, T_2 N_0 M_0) and stage IIB (T_2 N_1 M_0, T_3 N_0 M_0) are reserved for cases with regional lymph node metastases or cancers bigger than 5 cm and carry a worse prognosis. Stage IIIA (T_0 N_2 M_0, T_1 N_2 M_0, T_2 N_2 M_0, T_3 N_1 M_0, T_3 N_2 M_0), stage IIIB (T_4 N_0 M_0, T_4 N_1 M_0, T_4 N_2 M_0), and stage IIIC (any T N_3 M_0) refer to larger tumors that are locally advanced and thus have

<table>
<tr><td colspan="2">TABLE 37.11 AJCC Stage Grouping and Histopathologic Grading System Classification for Breast Cancer</td></tr>
</table>

Stage Grouping

Stage 0	T_{is} N_0 M_0
Stage IA	$T_1{}^a$ N_0 M_0
Stage IB	T_0 N_{1mi} M_0 T_1 N_{1mi} M_0
Stage IIA	T_0 $N_1{}^b$ M_0 $T1^a$ $N_1{}^b$ M_0 T_2 N_0 M_0
Stage IIB	T_2 N_1 M_0 T_3 N_0 M_0
Stage IIIA	T_0 N_2 M_0 $T1^a$ N_2 M_0 T_2 N_2 M_0 T_3 N_1 M_0 T_3 N_2 M_0
Stage IIIB	T_4 N_0 M_0 T_4 N_1 M_0 T_4 N_2 M_0
Stage IIIC	Any T N_3 M_0
Stage IV	Any T N M_1

Histologic Grade

G_x	Grade cannot be assessed
G_1	Low combined histologic grade (favorable)
G_2	Intermediate combined histologic grade (moderate favorable)
G_3	High combined histologic grade (unfavorable)

^{a}T_1 includes T_{1mic}.
^{b}T_0 and T_1 tumors with nodal micrometastases only are excluded from stage IIA and are classified stage 1B.

Note. M_0 includes $M_0(i+)$. The designation pM_0 is not valid; any M_0 should be clinical. If a patient presents with M_1 before neoadjuvant systemic therapy, the stage is considered stage IV and remains stage IV regardless of response to neoadjuvant therapy. Stage designation may be changed if postsurgical imaging studies are carried out within 4 months of diagnosis in the absence of disease progression and provided that the patient has not received neoadjuvant therapy. Postneoadjuvant therapy is designated with "yc" or "yp" prefix. Of note, no stage group is assigned if there is a complete pathologic response (CR) to neoadjuvant therapy, for example, $ypT_0ypN_0cM_0$.
From Edge SB, Byrd DR, Compton CC, Fritz AG, Greene FL. *AJCC Cancer Staging Manual.* 7th ed. New York: Springer; 2010:360.

an unfavorable prognosis. Stage IV (any T any N M_1) refers to distant systemic spread of disease with a significantly poor survival (Fig. 37.15).

Histopathlogic Grade

The AJCC-recommended histologic grading system is based on the Nottingham combined histologic grade (see Table 37.11).[23] The grade "G" of the tumor is designated based on the morphologic features of the primary tumor (tubule formation, nuclear pleomorphism, and mitotic count) by assigning a value of 1 to 3 (1, favorable; 3, unfavorable). The scores are added together for each feature. Grade 1 tumors have a combined score of 3 to 5 points; grade 2, 6 to 7 points; and grade 3, 8 to 9 points.

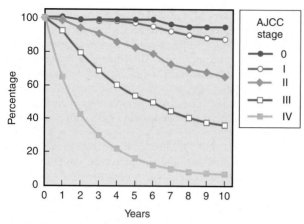

• **Fig. 37.15** The relative survival for breast cancer patients according to the American Joint Committee on Cancer (AJCC) stage group. (From Bland KI, Menck HR, Scott-Conner CE, et al. The National Cancer Database 10-year survey of breast carcinoma treatment at hospitals in the United States. *Cancer.* 1998;86:1262.)

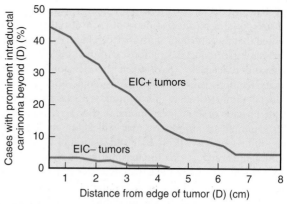

• **Fig. 37.16** Frequency distribution of prominent intraductal carcinoma at various distances from the edge of the primary tumor. *EIC,* Extensive intraductal component. (From Holland R, Connolly JL, Gelman R, et al. The presence of an extensive intraductal component (EIC) following a limited excision correlates with prominent residual disease in the remainder of the breast. *J Clin Oncol.* 1990;8:113.)

Extent and Multicentricity of In Situ and Invasive Carcinoma

The terms *multicentricity* and *multifocality* have been used for decades to indicate seeming or real multiplicity of cancer within an individual breast. The terms have no intrinsically different meanings but have recently been interpreted as follows: *multicentricity* indicates multiple but independent sites of origin usually in a separate duct system or relatively remote from one another; *multifocality* indicates multiple foci of the same tumor, relatively close to each other, usually in the same quadrant. Multicentricity has been considered an important factor when planning breast conserving surgery. However, many cases that would have previously been deemed multicentric in the past are now recognized as multiple lesions within a breast segment that result from spread of intraductal carcinoma within the three-dimensional duct system. Although multicentricity is important in planning surgical therapy, its true prevalence is much less than originally estimated. Indeed, extent of disease, in situ or invasive, is a concept that has essentially replaced that of multifocality and multicentricity, particularly in the planning of surgical therapy.

The prevalence of true multicentricity is difficult to estimate from the literature. Studies conducted in the mid-20th century showed rates of multicentric lesions ranging from 13% to 35%. The implications of these additional lesions are still not fully understood.

In 1994 Faverly, with Holland and associates,[167] applied three-dimensional imaging to study the distribution of intraductal carcinoma as constrained by the anatomy of the breast duct system. Since then, Ohtake and associates[168] and Mai and colleagues[169] have used computer-generated reconstructions of the mammary duct system in three dimensions to study the pattern of distribution of intraductal and invasive carcinoma in relation to the duct system. They discovered that apparent multicentricity is often the result of intraductal spread of the tumor. This finding has highlighted the problem of formulating a useful definition of multicentricity based on distance or quadrant.

Other studies have added the elements of time and biology (natural history) by observing the evaluation (or lack of it) of clinical disease in the living breast after partial mastectomy. The results of breast conserving surgery show that recurrent disease most often occurs locally, within the spatial constraints that the geometry of the duct system places on the spread of in situ carcinoma. Simply put, more than 90% of local recurrences of breast carcinoma in many women treated with breast conserving surgery are in the immediate vicinity of the primary tumor.[170] This implies that the extensiveness of in situ carcinoma within a duct system and margin status are the more relevant issues for predicting outcome in most cases.[171,172]

A perfect definition of multicentricity referable to all settings is essentially impractical because of the difficulties inherent in visualizing the three-dimensional microanatomy of the breast. Distinguishing independently originating breast carcinomas from multiple foci of invasion resulting from intramammary spread of carcinoma along ducts is difficult. Therefore multicentricity as a descriptor is necessarily arbitrary and becomes a function of the method used for detection. Consider here the anatomy of the breast. The breast is a branching gland with 15 to 20 collecting (lactiferous) ducts exiting at the nipple. Each of these ductal systems or lobes subserves hundreds of lobular units, which are collections of acinar elements.[173] In a three-dimensional reconstruction based on one patient, Ohtake and colleagues[174] noted that only 2 of the duct systems actually communicated with one another, and the remaining 14 were anatomically independent. Although the ductal systems are not grossly definable anatomic units separated by septa, only immediately adjacent radiating ductal systems overlap (Fig. 37.16), with limited opportunity for communication.[173] Quadrants represent an attempt to divide the breast into independent duct systems; however, the boundaries are drawn arbitrarily, and true duct systems may overlap into an adjacent quadrant at the periphery.

Given this anatomy, apparent multicentricity resulting from spread along a single duct system would be expected to appear in a radial distribution from nipple to periphery. This radial distribution, combined with the irregular branching system of duct systems that exists in three-dimensions, explains the fact that a single intraductal breast cancer may appear as separate foci in the two-dimensional slides routinely used for diagnosis. Mai and colleagues,[169] who performed computer-assisted three-dimensional reconstruction of intraductal and invasive mammary carcinoma (lobular carcinoma was excluded) from 30 mastectomy specimens, found that intraductal carcinoma presented with radial distribution corresponding to the geometry of each ductal system. They also noted that multiple foci of invasive carcinoma were connected by intervening intraductal carcinoma within a single duct system. Ohtake and colleagues[174] have taken the viewpoint that multicentricity requires demonstration of histologic noncontinuity of intraductal tumor through the mammary ductal tree. Of note, there are no cases of lobular carcinoma in their series. As stringent as this requirement appears, it may still allow an overestimate of true multicentricity. Both Mai and associates[169] and Faverly and colleagues[167] report that discontinuities of intraductal tumor within a single mammary duct tree, detected at a subgross level, are not uncommon. Studies indicate that the phenomenon of "pagetoid spread" of intraductal carcinoma[175] may lead to apparent discontinuities in intraductal tumor that originate from the same "index" carcinoma.

Studies using molecular biology to differentiate independent sources for multicentric carcinoma also support the concept of a single index case that spreads through the duct system.[176–178] As such, the true definition of multicentric should require demonstration of independent molecular events that result in the local occurrence of carcinoma in independent duct systems. This definition would require three-dimensional reconstruction of the duct systems along with molecular profiling studies, procedures that are not a part of routine processing of breast specimens. Therefore multicentricity is likely to remain arbitrarily defined. Extent of disease is more amenable to measurement in routine pathologic examination of specimens. Given that the prevalence of true multicentricity is overestimated, extent of disease may be more relevant in the majority of cases when planning breast conserving surgical therapy.

Biological Studies

Evaluation of multicentric tumors using subcellular and molecular technologies has expanded current understanding of the true biological nature of multicentric tumors and may allow more precise definitions of multicentric and extensive. Two hypotheses, excluding intramammary metastases, have been introduced to explain the etiology of multicentric disease. One of these suggests that the multiple sites develop by intraductal spread, which may appear discontinuous at the subgross level, from an "index" case. The other hypothesis supports the concept of a genetic alteration that occurs during development and distributes extensively or locally in the breast depending on the stage of development at which it occurs. This first hit predisposes the affected region, and a second, localized genetic event results in carcinoma.[179] If the latter hypothesis is correct, there will be a combination of shared and distinct molecular events that define the separate foci of carcinoma.

Noguchi and associates,[177] in a study of 30 patients with invasive mammary carcinoma (ductal), demonstrated that clonality within a tumor could be established by measuring the restriction fragment length polymorphism (RFLP) of the tumor using the X-linked phosphoglycerate kinase gene (*PGK*). They then evaluated individual foci of invasive mammary carcinoma (ductal) in each of three women with two, three, and four separate ipsilateral lesions. They found that the separate foci exhibited the identical RFLP for each patient, strong evidence that seemingly independent foci of cancer are likely to be related.

A study applying cytogenetic analysis[178] to multicentric tumors ("macroscopically distinct," 5–15 mm apart) also supports the hypothesis of intraductal spread of tumor as the major mechanism for apparent multifocality. However, the presence of cytogenetically unrelated clones within a single focus suggests that breast cancer may in fact be polyclonal. Thus diverging molecular evolution of a single focus may make it difficult to differentiate between independent "index" cases and evolution of tumor that has spread from a single "index" case. In fact, molecular evolution may in part explain histologic heterogeneity in DCIS within independent duct systems.

Fujii and colleagues[176] studied invasive tumors for allelic losses at seven chromosomal loci and compared the alterations in these tumors with those present in DCIS within the same breast. A high degree of concordance of specific losses between the in situ and invasive lesions supports the concept of multifocal rather than truly multicentric carcinoma. A variable degree of heterogeneity in allelic losses at one or more loci in 8 of the 20 cases examined is again attributed to some degree of clonal divergence in the evolution of breast cancer.

Early protein-based immunocytochemical techniques,[180] certainly the least reliable of these methodologies, generated conflicting results in a study of 24 cases of "separate" tumors. More recently a study of morphology combined with IHC for ER, PR, HER2/neu, and ki67 in 32 patients who had undergone modified radical mastectomy supported the hypothesis that multicentric mammary carcinoma results from intraductal spread.[181] As noted earlier, all but one (97%) of the patients in that study had identical histology in the separate tumor foci.

Associated Factors

Numerous authors have proposed various factors to be associated with increased risk of multicentricity, defined by occurrence in multiple quadrants or within a minimum distance. The problem with interpreting these studies is the inherently arbitrary definition of multicentricity in standard pathology reports. As described earlier, many of the lesions called multicentric are likely multifocal manifestations of DCIS or multiple foci of invasion with intervening intraductal carcinoma. The presence of a lesion in the nipple or subareolar area is perhaps the most clearly and consistently demonstrated factor for multicentricity.[181,182] Mai and coworkers[169] discovered that DCIS exhibited a pyramidal shape, "fanning out" from the nipple to the posterior of the breast. As described earlier, it is possible that the convergence of the duct systems at the nipple explains the seemingly increased multicentricity in the subareolar tissue.

Studies looking for a relationship between multicentricity and tumor size,[171,182–190] patient age,[182,186,188,190] family history,[188,191] or nodal status[182,187–190,192–194] have generated mixed results. Lagios, Westdahl, and Rose[184] found an association of multicentricity with tubular carcinoma. Among other factors studied and shown to have no relationship to receptor status are height, weight, parity,[195] specific breast or quadrant involved, amount of necrosis,[183] nuclear grade, expression of the adhesion molecule CD44v6,[196] preexisting or concurrent benign breast disease,[182,190] and bilaterality.[190]

Clinical Follow-Up Studies

The primary relevance of multicentric disease is essentially for patients who desire or undergo breast conserving therapy. Middleton and coworkers,[181] who studied multicentricity in patients who had undergone mastectomies, found no difference in disease-free survival for women with apparently multicentric versus unicentric invasive carcinoma. In their earlier study, 75% of the cases were invasive mammary carcinoma, and 25% had infiltrating lobular carcinoma. The authors were unable to determine whether the equivalence in survival rates was a result of the type of treatment the women received.

Studies using extensive three-dimensional reconstruction suggest that multicentricity of carcinoma, either DCIS or an invasive (not lobular) carcinoma associated with DCIS, defined as independent sources of tumor located in separate duct systems, is actually an unlikely event, whereas multifocality of either invasive or in situ carcinoma is not uncommon. Given the near-complete independence of the ductal systems, breast conserving surgery may be adequate therapy when disease is localized and, if based on a segmental anatomy, may also be adequate when extensive or invasive or multifocal DCIS is present. The latter may also present with foci of invasive carcinoma, but these will originate within the same duct system nearly 90% of the time.

As such, the phenomenon of extensive intraductal carcinoma with multifocal invasive or in situ tumor is the more commonly encountered issue than true multicentricity when planning surgical therapy for a patient with breast carcinoma. The collaborative study between medical schools at Nijmegen and Harvard represents one of the early comprehensive studies to address an EIC as a clinically relevant factor in the study of breast carcinoma.[197] The definition of an EIC for this study was similar to that in a previous study by Schnitt and associates[198] and consisted of two criteria: (1) DCIS was present prominently (≥25%) within the infiltrating tumor, and (2) DCIS was present clearly extending beyond the infiltrating margin of the tumor. Mastectomy specimens from 214 patients were studied with a three-dimensional reconstructive technique; the study design was predicated on a practical clinical question: can the findings in an excisional biopsy predict residual tumor within the remaining breast? Excisional biopsies with extensive in situ carcinoma were in fact far more likely (74% vs. 42%) to be associated with residual carcinoma, primarily in situ disease, in the mastectomy specimen. The EIC-positive patients were also more likely to have additional foci of invasive carcinoma within the breast at the time of mastectomy. However, this difference was small and reached statistical significance only within the immediate vicinity of the primary tumor (within 2 cm of the margin of the primary tumor). The major difference, then, between the EIC-positive and EIC-negative tumors was in the extent of the in situ disease of ductal type within the remainder of the breast (Fig. 37.17).[171] Intralymphatic channel tumor involvement was not different between the two tumor types.

The Holland study on the predictive capability of EIC produced results compatible with other studies on this phenomenon.[199–201] It has been confirmed in studies from Amsterdam[202,203] and London.[204] Other earlier studies did not support the predictive usefulness of EIC with regard to local treatment failure. This disparity may be explained by the fact that one of these studies used a large resection[205] and the other required histologic documentation of tumor-free margins.[206]

The more recent studies with three-dimensional reconstruction by Ohtake and coworkers[174] along with Mai and coworkers,[169] described earlier in this chapter, also support the concept of extensive intraductal carcinoma as an important factor in determining the effectiveness of breast conserving therapy. However, this does not necessarily imply that breast conserving therapy will not be successful. Mai and coworkers attribute the success of segmental

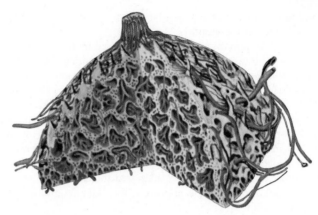

• **Fig. 37.17** Proposed anatomy of the breast with partial lobar oriented ductal system. However, recent studies have shown that the human ductal system is more complex than simple radiating anatomy. Although anastomoses between ductal systems may not occur, individual ductal systems may overlap with each other with respect to the area of the breast they serve much like venous drainage networks. One ductal system may not be confined to a single breast quadrant. (Redrawn from Love SM, Barsky SH. Anatomy of the nipple and breast ducts revisited. *Cancer.* 2004;101:1947.)

resection in treating breast carcinoma to the high prevalence of DCIS restricted to a single duct system. They go even further and suggest that failures using segmental resection for small carcinomas may in part be related to the pyramidal shape of the distribution of the DCIS. Supportive of this hypotheses is a small study of mastectomy specimens obtained after local failure following lumpectomy, which found that recurrences were located in the same quadrant as the primary lesion and were present radial to the initial tumor (either closer to the nipple or toward the axilla).[207] Mai and coworkers also suggest involvement of the nipple and lack of recognition of an EIC associated with a small, palpable invasive lesion as possible causes for failures in segmental resections.

Clinical Implications of Multicentricity

A number of prospective, randomized clinical trials have demonstrated equivalent survival for in situ and invasive breast cancers treated with mastectomy or breast conservation.[207–209] Therefore, the current standard of care for the management of both invasive and in situ breast cancers is a breast conserving approach. One of the major contraindications to a breast conserving approach is the presence of multicentric disease.[210] In addition, the presence of an EIC coexistent with an invasive breast carcinoma predicts an increased risk of local failure with a breast conserving approach. Two large European randomized trials (the Breast Cancer Cooperative Group of the European Organisation for Research and Treatment of Cancer [EORTC] and the Danish Breast Cancer Cooperative Group [DBCG]) compared breast conserving therapy and mastectomy in stages I and II breast cancer. In their analysis, Voogd and colleagues reported that the risk of local recurrence after breast conserving therapy for women with infiltrating ductal carcinomas with EIC was 2.52 times higher than that in those without EIC. The 10-year actuarial rates were 21% and 9%, respectively.[211] Therefore it is critical to accurately assess the extent of disease so that the appropriate surgical intervention can be planned. The consideration of partial breast irradiation only amplifies the importance of accurately determining whether multicentric disease is present.

Another important clinical question raised by the presence of multicentric invasive breast cancer is the appropriate method for nodal assessment. SLN biopsy has become the standard of care for evaluating the nodal status in patients with clinically node-negative breast cancer. The presence of multicentric disease was initially thought to be a contraindication to the performance of SLN biopsy because of concerns that these tumors might involve more than one dominant lymphatic drainage pattern. This might result in inaccurate nodal staging and high false-negative rates.[212,213] A number of investigators have addressed this issue and demonstrated that the technique appears to be valid in multicentric disease as well.[214–217]

In conclusion, the definition of multicentricity is still somewhat controversial, and although its presence (at least tumors in more than one quadrant) is considered a contraindication to breast conservation surgery, the true clinical implications of multicentricity are as controversial as its definition. On the other hand, extent of disease appears to be of more importance and has implications as far as risk of local recurrence.

Acknowledgment

We gratefully acknowledge the contributions of Alfredo Santillan, John Kiluk, and Charles Cox, who authored this chapter in previous editions.

Selected References

1. Friedewald SM, Rafferty EA, Rose SL, et al. Breast cancer screening using tomosynthesis in combination with digital mammography. *JAMA*. 2014;311:2499-2507.

22. Rakha EA. Breast cancer prognostic classification in the molecular era: the role of histological grade. *Breast Cancer Res*. 2010;12:207.

34. Jeruss JS, Mittendorf EA, Tucker SL, et al. Combined use of clinical and pathologic staging variables to define outcomes for breast cancer patients treated with neoadjuvant therapy. *J Clin Oncol*. 2008;26:246-252.

45. Luporsi E, André F, Spyratos F, et al. Ki-67: level of evidence and methodological considerations for its role in the clinical management of breast cancer: analytical and critical review. *Breast Cancer Res Treat*. 2012;132:895-915.

81. Castlea J, Shakera H, Morrisa K, et al. The significance of circulating tumour cells in breast cancer: a review. *Breast*. 2014;23:552-560.

109. Paik S, Shak S, Tang G, et al. A multigene assay to predict recurrence of tamoxifen-treated, node-negative breast cancer. *N Engl J Med*. 2004;351:2817-2826.

137. Veronesi U, Marubini E, Mariani L, et al. The dissection of internal mammary nodes does not improve the survival of breast cancer patients. 30-year results of a randomised trial. *Eur J Cancer*. 1999;35:1320-1325.

210. Morrow M, Harris JR. Practice guidelines for breast conservation therapy in the management of invasive breast cancer. *J Am Coll Surg*. 2007;205:362-376.

A full reference list is available online at ExpertConsult.com.

38

Lobular Carcinoma in Situ of the Breast

KRISTINE E. CALHOUN AND BENJAMIN O. ANDERSON

Lobular neoplasia is the overarching nomenclature used to describe the spectrum of proliferative but noninfiltrative changes seen within the lobular units of the breast. Lobular neoplastic lesions include atypical lobular hyperplasia (ALH) and lobular carcinoma in situ (LCIS), each of which is associated with an increased risk of developing a subsequent invasive breast cancer (IBC).[1,2] Pathologically, lobular neoplasia is diagnosed when the acini of the terminal duct lobular units are filled and distended by small, uniform, loosely cohesive cells.[3] The distinction between ALH and LCIS has historically been based on the degree of histologic change observed by the pathologist. At the cellular and proteinomic levels, ALH and LCIS have striking similarities to invasive lobular cancers (ILC) with most staining positive for estrogen receptors (ERs), having low proliferative index rates, and being ErbB2 (HER2/neu) negative.[3]

Although recognized since the 1940s as a unique histopathologic finding, controversy remains regarding both the clinical significance and overall invasive malignant potential of LCIS. LCIS is a marker for the development of invasive carcinoma, but the location for that subsequent cancer is not confined to the site at which LCIS was found. Actually, LCIS is a significant breast cancer risk factor for subsequent cancer in both breasts and with either ductal or lobular histology. Analogous to ductal carcinoma in situ (DCIS) and invasive ductal carcinoma, genetic evidence suggests that LCIS can be a nonobligatory precursor of ILC. However, the frequency with which malignant progression from LCIS to ILC actually occurs remains an area of vigorous debate. From a diagnostic perspective, management dilemmas continue as to whether LCIS requires surgical excision when it is seen on percutaneous needle sampling or if there are cases in which no further workup beyond needle biopsy is required. At the opposite extreme, there is debate if some LCIS cases should be removed with negative surgical margins after open surgical biopsy for therapeutic purposes, which then begs the question of whether radiation therapy should be offered to these potentially more aggressive cases. Although treatment strategies have evolved from routine mastectomy to surveillance since LCIS was first described,[4] some in the medical community continue to question whether more aggressive intervention should occur in selected LCIS cases.

The purposes of this chapter are to define the historical background that led to our current understanding of LCIS biology, delineate histopathologic features of classic and "pleomorphic" LCIS, discuss the clinical presentation and natural history of LCIS, examine the evidence for and against routine surgical excision after the diagnosis of LCIS on image-guided sampling, review the role for chemoprevention in LCIS management, and discuss the role of surgical prophylaxis for LCIS in the small subgroup of patients for whom it may be appropriate.

Historical Background

LCIS as a Premalignant Lesion

Lobular neoplasia was initially described in 1941 when Foote and Stewart published their classic report of LCIS.[4] At that time, LCIS was generally seen in conjunction with ILC, as illustrated in Godwin's 1952 case report in which he describes it as a premalignant lesion.[5] Because LCIS was believed to be an obligate precursor to invasive cancer, mastectomy was initially recommended as an appropriate therapeutic procedure after its histologic diagnosis on breast biopsy, and this remained the standard of care for the next 40 years. Today we recognize the selection bias from that period before mammographic screening when all breast cancers were diagnosed as clinically detected findings such as palpable masses. In today's era of mammographic imaging and needle biopsy, we are now able to examine lobular neoplasia in isolation and recognize that early reports greatly exaggerated its malignant potential (Table 38.1).[4–11]

LCIS as a Risk Factor for Invasive Breast Cancer and Lobular Neoplasia

In the late 1970s the dominant belief that LCIS required therapeutic mastectomy was questioned when Haagensen at Columbia and Rosen at Memorial Sloan-Kettering both independently began to advocate for less drastic management.[9,12] In Haagensen's series, 211 women with pure LCIS underwent excision alone and were followed for evidence of development of subsequent IBC. Of the women, 10% developed an ipsilateral breast cancer, and 9% were subsequently diagnosed with a contralateral invasive tumor.[9] When occurring in the same breast, the invasive cancers were not always found at the original LCIS biopsy site. Haagensen argued that LCIS is better described as a risk factor than a preinvasive cancer because longitudinal series show IBC of either ductal or lobular histology developing in either breast with similar frequency. As a risk marker for cancer, bilateral mastectomy was felt to be overly aggressive and largely unnecessary in the setting of LCIS.

To dissuade surgeons from managing LCIS as a malignant lesion warranting mastectomy, Haagensen and colleagues recommended reclassifying LCIS as *lobular neoplasia*, thus eliminating the word *carcinoma* from the name and removing any distinction between ALH and LCIS.[9] They reasoned that avoiding

TABLE 38.1	Evolution of Lobular Carcinoma in Situ (LCIS)	
1865	Cornil[6]	Described intraepithelial breast carcinoma in lobules
1919	Ewing[7]	Published photomicrographs of LCIS
1931	Cheatle and Cutler[8]	Challenged whether malignant-appearing cells confined to lobules/ducts were "precancerous"
1941	Foote and Stewart[4]	Coined term *lobular carcinoma* in situ
1950s		LCIS generally seen together with invasive cancer, assumed to be premalignant hazard
1952	Godwin[5]	Suggested that LCIS evolves into ILC; recommended mastectomy for treatment
1978	Haagensen et al.[9]	Defined *lobular neoplasia* (ALH and LCIS) as fundamentally benign
1980s		LCIS shifts to being identified as a risk factor for invasive cancer
1996	Frost et al.[10]	Describes pleomorphic LCIS
2000	Middleton et al.[11]	Proposes relationship between pleomorphic LCIS and pleomorphic ILC

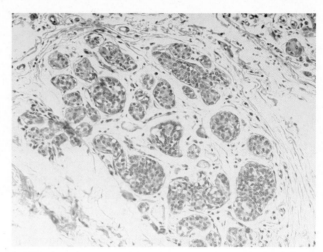

• **Fig. 38.1** Histologic spectrum of classic lobular carcinoma in situ. Low-grade monotonous appearing nuclei with scant cytoplasm—so-called type A cells.

mastectomy was appropriate because of both the low incidence of subsequent breast cancer observed and the nearly equal hazard of contralateral breast cancer, which would be left unaddressed by a unilateral mastectomy. In a 21-year follow-up study of Haagensen and colleagues' original patients, among the 99 patients available for follow-up, 24% developed either DCIS or IBC, far lower than the rates that would be expected with an obligate precursor malignant lesion.[13] Observation in place of mastectomy was gradually accepted as adequate management for lobular neoplasia, leading ultimately in the 1990s to the abandonment of routine mastectomy after an LCIS diagnosis.

Continued Definition of LCIS as a Unique Stage 0 Preinvasive "Cancer"

Despite a growing body of supportive evidence, there still exists some resistance to the hypothesis that lobular neoplasia represents a single pathologic entity of limited malignant potential. Several large professional entities, including the Surveillance, Epidemiology, and End Results (SEER) Program, the National Surgical Adjuvant Breast and Bowel Program (NSABP) and the American Joint Commission on Cancer, have continued to classify LCIS as a Stage 0 lesion at this time, although significant discussion regarding whether this should be the case is underway and this designation may change. Despite this classification, there is agreement that observation rather than mastectomy is now the preferred course of treatment when lobular neoplasia is diagnosed.

LCIS similarly continues to be included in the National Comprehensive Cancer Network (NCCN) Breast Cancer Guidelines, although specific cancer management is not recommended if the classic form of LCIS alone is identified at biopsy.[14] Inclusion in cancer guideline documents is unfortunate because it can perpetuate concern among women diagnosed with LCIS and stimulate fear that they too have breast cancer, when they fundamentally do not.

LCIS Histopathology

Morphologic Features of LCIS

The histologic distinction between lobular and ductal neoplastic processes was initially based on location in the ductal-lobular system and differences in cytologic characteristics. In their original 1941 description, Foote and Stewart described LCIS as a proliferation of small, uniform, discohesive cells filling and often distending the acinar units within a lobule.[4] In this classic form of LCIS, the nuclei are round, have indistinct nucleoli, uniform chromatin and a distinctly monotonous, low-grade appearance with minimal mitotic activity (Fig. 38.1). The lobular-based proliferation of LCIS is typically solid, without the architectural lumen formation typical of cribriform pattern DCIS. Lobular proliferations that fill and distend at least 50% of the acini in a lobule are classified as LCIS, whereas involvement of less than 50% of the acini is considered ALH (Fig. 38.2). Because this definition of lobular distention can be subjective and the 50% threshold is somewhat arbitrary, some pathologists prefer the all-encompassing term *lobular neoplasia,* whereas others favor the separate terminology, arguing that it remains clinically useful because LCIS conveys a higher IBC risk than does ALH. Page and colleagues estimated that ALH conveys a four- to fivefold increased invasive cancer risk, whereas LCIS conveys a full nine-fold increased risk in the absence of endocrine suppression.[15]

LCIS frequently extends beyond the lobules to involve the ductal system. This pattern of spread has a Pagetoid appearance, meaning that the neoplastic cells infiltrate from the lobule down into the adjacent duct, separating the basement membrane from the overlying epithelium, displacing and often attenuating the normal ductal epithelial layer (Fig. 38.3). As with other etiologies,

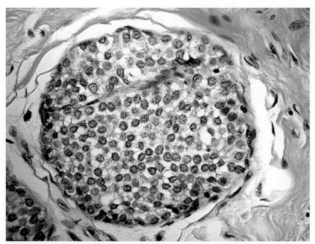

• **Fig. 38.2** Lobular carcinoma in situ. This acinus is completely filled with loosely cohesive, small round cells with hyperchromatic nuclei. The cells are evenly spaced and markedly distend the acinar space. (400×.)

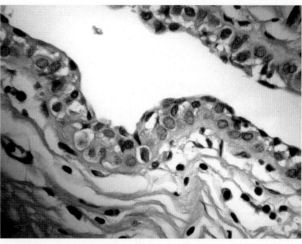

• **Fig. 38.4** Loss of epithelial cadherin (E-cadherin) expression supports the lobular phenotype of the process. Thin, attenuated E-cadherin positive normal ductal cells are still present.

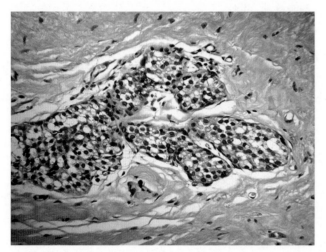

• **Fig. 38.3** Pagetoid extension of lobular carcinoma in situ up a duct.

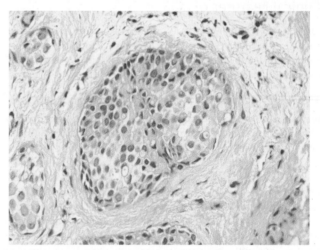

• **Fig. 38.5** Pleomorphic lobular carcinoma in situ has high-grade nuclei and is often associated with comedo-type necrosis, closely mimicking high-grade comedo ductal carcinoma in situ.

there can be significant variation in the degree and extent to which LCIS involves the breast. Uncommonly, classic LCIS will appear especially florid, with markedly distended lobules and foci of necrosis. These cases can be difficult to distinguish from DCIS, which more classically contains this type of central necrosis.[16] Expression of the cell adhesion molecule E-cadherin (E-cadherin) is typically lost in LCIS and retained in DCIS, making the use of immunohistochemistry staining for this marker useful in this differential (Fig. 38.4).[17–19]

Pleomorphic LCIS

There have been multiple descriptions of LCIS showing an in situ lobular pattern of growth similar to the classic LCIS form (see Fig. 38.1) but a high-grade, pleomorphic cytology that more resembles the aggressive phenotype of high-grade DCIS.[9,11,20-23] Such lesions have been variably called *pleomorphic LCIS* (Fig. 38.5). In contrast to the monomorphic cells of classic LCIS, pleomorphic LCIS cells have marked nuclear atypia, demonstrate variation in size and have frequent to abundant mitotic activity. The pleomorphic form of LCIS more frequently contains central comedo necrosis, making its appearance strikingly similar to

comedo-type high-grade DCIS. In the past, pleomorphic LCIS was commonly diagnosed as high-grade DCIS by pathologists who were concerned that the high-grade cytology represented an aggressive in situ process that should be managed as such. A molecular factor that distinguishes lobular from ductal pathology is the expression of E-cadherin, a cellular adherence protein that is present in ductal pathology but is absent in lobular disease. The development of an immunohistochemical test for E-cadherin helped standardize pathology interpretation and is now a standard discriminating test when the in situ morphology is unclear or ambiguous. Histologic clues to this diagnosis include finding a discohesive appearance within a solid, high-grade in situ lesion, the presence of intracytoplasmic lumens or the coexistence of classic LCIS. E-cadherin staining is often required for confirmation that the cells are lobular in origin. It has been speculated that pleomorphic LCIS may have an increased likelihood of being associated with ILC and, in particular, its pleomorphic subtype that is among invasive cancers known to be more biologically aggressive.[11,17,19-20,23]

Immunohistologic Features and Molecular Genetics of LCIS

Most often, classic LCIS is strongly positive for ER expression and, in keeping with its low-grade biology, rarely demonstrates HER2 overexpression or p53 alterations.[24,25] This behavior contrasts with pleomorphic LCIS, which typically has lower levels of ER expression and can be positive for HER2 overexpression or contain p53 alterations, factors that all suggest a more aggressive behavior at the cellular level.[11,23] Molecular analysis of pleomorphic LCIS suggests that although it is highly likely to contain some of the same molecular alterations seen in classic LCIS (such as 1q gains and 16q losses), it frequently has accumulated additional alterations that are more typical of high-grade ductal carcinomas.[26,27]

Clinical Presentation, Natural History, and Biologic Significance of LCIS

Clinical Features of LCIS

LCIS typically presents as an asymptomatic, occult lesion incidentally discovered during histologic workup for another clinical or radiographic indication. Only rarely will LCIS present as a discrete lesion seen either by mammogram or ultrasound.[28] It is even less common for lobular neoplasia to present as a clinically palpable mass. Most instances of LCIS are incidentally discovered on breast biopsy conducted for another reason. Although fewer than 5% of breast biopsies performed for benign conditions ultimately yield a diagnosis of LCIS, it is hypothesized that the true incidence may be much higher in the general female population because a large number of women with lobular neoplasia remain undiagnosed as they have no other indication for breast biopsy.[3,29]

LCIS is commonly widespread in the breast, with patterns that are multifocal, multicentric, and/or bilateral. Early publications detailed its multifocal nature,[4,30] noting that when patients underwent mastectomy after surgical biopsy showing LCIS, the breast specimen commonly had residual disease in areas outside the biopsy cavity, with a diffuse speckled, microscopic distribution through multiple lobules of a given region. Rosen and colleagues observed that LCIS was commonly multicentric, being present in multiple quadrants of the breast in 24 of 50 (48%) mastectomy specimens.[31] Beute and colleagues found that among 119 patients diagnosed with LCIS between 1974 and 1987 in their institution, 82 had both breasts sampled either by mirror-image biopsy or contralateral mastectomy. Of these, LCIS was found to be bilateral in half (41/82) of the patients.[32]

Risk of Subsequent Invasive Carcinoma After LCIS Diagnosis

Women diagnosed with LCIS are typically quoted to have an 8- to 10-fold increased lifetime risk for developing breast cancer in both the ipsilateral and the contralateral breast.[14] The absolute risk of breast cancer after LCIS is 20% to 25% after 20 years.[33] Mathematical modeling suggests that during the first 15 years after biopsy, women with LCIS have 10.8 times the risk of breast cancer development compared with women of comparable age who lack proliferative disease findings on breast biopsy.[15] A more recent publication from Memorial Sloan Kettering Cancer Center examining 29 years of clinical surveillance reported a 15.8% rate of

TABLE 38.2	Selected Long-Term Follow-up Studies of Patients With Lobular Carcinoma in Situ
Haagensen, 1986[35]	
Mean follow-up, years	14.7
Ipsilateral cancer	11%
Contralateral cancer	27/258 (10%)
Anderson, 1974[36]	
Mean follow-up, years	15
Ipsilateral cancer	20%
Contralateral cancer	17%
Wheeler et al., 1974[37]	
Mean follow-up, years	15.7
Ipsilateral cancer	4%
Contralateral cancer	15%
Page et al., 1991[15]	
Mean follow-up, years	19
Ipsilateral cancer	15%
Contralateral cancer	10%
Rosen et al., 1978[12]	
Mean follow-up, years	24
Ipsilateral cancer	22%
Contralateral cancer	20%
King et al., 2015[34]	
Mean follow-up, years	29
Ipsilateral cancer	10%
Contralateral cancer	5%

subsequent breast cancer development among 1060 women diagnosed previously with LCIS.[34] The majority of the cancers were ipsilateral (63%), with 25% contralateral and 12% bilateral with both ductal and lobular invasive histology. Chemoprevention was the only factor found on multivariate analysis to influence breast cancer risk, substantially decreasing it.[34] On average, they found a 2% annual incidence of breast cancer development in the setting of a prior diagnosis of LCIS.

In general, the risks of cancer in the ipsilateral and the contralateral breast are approximately equal, as shown in multiple longitudinal studies of patients diagnosed with LCIS by surgical biopsy (Table 38.2).[12,15,34–37] These studies illustrate the primary reason that LCIS is not typically treated surgically with lumpectomy: the only logical operation would be a bilateral mastectomy, which would be unnecessary approximately 80% of the time. It is possible that some subgroups of LCIS may exhibit a more aggressive unilateral biology and preinvasive behavior. The extent of LCIS (few lobules vs. extensive disease) and subtyping based on classic versus pleomorphic histopathology has not always been a standard part of pathology reports. As a result, retrospective analysis of population-based data is challenging, and additional prospective data are necessary to answer this question. Rendi and colleagues attempted to provide more clarity on whether the amount of LCIS seen at core needle sampling had any correlation with the risk of identifying subsequent invasive disease. In their study of 106 patients with pure lobular neoplasia diagnosed on core sampling, they found that among the 33 patients with pure LCIS, the upgrade rate at excision for malignancy was 4.4% and only occurred when extensive (more than four foci) of LCIS was present initially.[38] Such findings have allowed the NCCN screening and diagnosis panel to suggest that for individuals with classic LCIS on core sampling where the finding is concordant with breast imaging findings, surveillance alone is sufficient and surgical excision may not be necessary for definitive diagnosis.[39]

Female Steroid Hormones and LCIS

Changing Incidence Rates of LCIS and the Influence or Exogenous Hormones on Lobular Carcinogenesis

The incidence rates of ILC increased steadily from 1977 to 1999, whereas the incidence rates of IDC increased at a similar rate until 1987 and then leveled off until 1999.[40,41] Since 1999, however, rates of both ILC and IDC have declined by approximately 4% per year.[42] LCIS incidence rates increased in parallel with ILC rates from 1977 to 1999, although rates of LCIS held steady from 1999 to 2006, despite a decline in ILC during that same time period. On the basis of available SEER data from the United States, LCIS rates are highest among women aged 50 to 69 years, but although diagnosis of LCIS increased up until 2006 for women aged 30 to 49 and aged 70 years or older, rates fell after 2002 among women 50 to 69 years of age. In contrast, ILC rates remain highest among women 70 years of age or older, with declines in ILC cases since 2002 among both 50- to 69-year-old women and those aged 70 years and older. ILC rates among women 30 to 49 years of age have increased slowly over the past 30 years but remain much lower than the rates seen among women 50 years of age and older.

Rising rates of all lobular pathology through 2002, as well as their subsequent fall, may be related to changing patterns of combined estrogen and progestin menopausal hormone therapy (CHT) use. Although it is established that CHT use increases breast cancer risk,[4,5] almost all studies that have reported on associations between CHT and risk of ILC versus IDC indicate that this association varies by histologic type.[9,12,13] In these studies, CHT use is associated with 2.0- to 3.9-fold increases in ILC risk, but has much less of an impact on IDC risk. The publication of the Women's Health Initiative randomized trial results of CHT use in 2002, which demonstrated that the risks of long-term CHT use (for >5 years) outweighed its benefits, resulted in a dramatic decline in the use of CHT among women worldwide. It has been hypothesized that abrupt cessation in CHT use is at least partially responsible for the decline in total breast cancer rates after 2002 observed in the United States and may account for the drop in ILC and LCIS incidence rates since 2002 primarily among women most likely to be CHT users, those 50 to 69 years of age. Despite this reasonable hypothesis, others have argued that saturation of screening, and not a decrease in CHT use, may be a greater contributor to the decline in overall breast malignancy rates demonstrated since 2002.[42] Interestingly,

a more recent SEER database study suggests that the rate of LCIS increased from 2.00 in 100,000 patients in 2000 to 2.75 in 100,000 patients in 2009.[43]

In general, lobules become atrophic and tend to disappear after menopause unless the patient is taking hormone therapy. Despite this finding, Wellings and colleagues reported that some human mammary lobules persist after menopause and certain atypical lobules are morphologically similar to preneoplastic alveolar nodules that occur in strains of mice with a propensity for developing mammary carcinoma.[44] They suggest that these persistent atypical mammary lobules could be precancerous in human beings. These findings might help explain why ILC rates are highest among women 70 years of age and older.

Not all cases of LCIS are diagnosed in the postmenopausal setting. A recent publication by McEvoy and colleagues identified 58 women with atypical breast lesions, including eight with pure LCIS, diagnosed under age 35 years. At median follow-up of 86 months, seven of the cohort had developed breast cancer, with four among those initially found to have LCIS, two whose initial lesion was ALH and one whose initial lesion was atypical ductal hyperplasia (ADH). There were four ipsilateral cancers, including three initially diagnosed with LCIS and three contralateral cancers ultimately identified at a mean age of 41 years. These authors concluded that young women with atypical lesions were at a strikingly high risk of developing breast cancer and advocated for close clinical surveillance and follow-up.[45]

Endocrine Chemoprevention for LCIS

Chemoprevention of Invasive Breast Cancer

On the basis of the finding that LCIS signifies an increased risk of ipsilateral and contralateral breast cancer development, devising a systemic chemoprevention strategy makes biological sense in this patient population. Unfortunately, the literature from randomized trials directly addressing breast cancer risk reduction among patients with LCIS is limited. Tamoxifen is a selective ER modulator (SERM) with both agonist and antagonist properties commonly used in the treatment of both early-stage and metastatic breast cancer. Tamoxifen has also been shown to decrease the risk of contralateral breast cancer[46] in women receiving treatment in the adjuvant setting, and thus was chosen for evaluation in the prevention setting. Historically, four large randomized clinical trials evaluated the use of tamoxifen for breast cancer risk reduction. Two of these trials showed a statistically significant reduction in the incidence of IBC among women treated with 5 years of tamoxifen compared with those that received placebo.[47,48] In the NSABP P-01 prevention trial, there was a 49% reduction in the incidence of IBC ($p < .00001$), whereas the International Breast Cancer Intervention Study (IBIS-I) showed a 27% reduction in risk among individuals taking the drug ($p = .004$). Two additional trials reported smaller, nonsignificant decreases in breast cancer risk among tamoxifen-treated women,[49,50] whereas a meta-analysis that combined results from all four trials showed a 34% to 38% reduction in breast cancer risk.[51]

Only the NSABP P-01 trial specifically evaluated a subset of participants with LCIS. This trial enrolled 13,388 women at increased risk of breast cancer by virtue of an elevated Gail model score (5-year risk ≥1.66% of developing breast cancer), age greater than 60 years, or a past history of biopsy-proven LCIS or ADH. Participants in this trial were randomized to tamoxifen (20 mg daily) versus placebo, for a planned duration of 5 years. Six percent of study participants had a history of LCIS, and an additional 9.1% of enrollees had a history of atypia. As noted earlier, a 49% reduction in breast cancer incidence was seen overall in this study. The relative risk of breast cancer was 0.44 (95% confidence interval [CI] 0.16–1.06) among women with a history of LCIS and 0.14 (95% CI 0.03–0.47) among women with a history of atypia. Importantly, no reduction was seen in the risk of ER-negative breast cancer, nor was a difference in overall survival noted between the two study arms. On the basis of the NSABP P-01 trial results, the US Food and Drug Administration (FDA) approved tamoxifen for breast cancer prevention.

Raloxifene is another SERM that has a slightly different side effect profile than its cousin, tamoxifen. In initial studies testing its efficacy for treating and preventing postmenopausal osteoporosis, patients taking raloxifene were also noted to have a reduced incidence of breast cancer.[52,53] This led to the Study of Tamoxifen and Raloxifene (STAR) trial, a head-to-head comparison of raloxifene to tamoxifen for breast cancer chemoprevention, in which the two agents were shown to be equivalent in terms of reducing the risk of IBC in postmenopausal women.[54] Slightly more than 9% of study participants had a history of LCIS. Overall, breast cancer events were similar in women with LCIS compared with that of the entire study population and did not differ by treatment arm. Interestingly, the number of noninvasive breast cancers was lower among tamoxifen-treated women (30 vs. 44 women cases of DCIS; 21 vs. 29 cases of LCIS). It is important to note that although the NSABP P-01 trial included both pre- and postmenopausal women, only postmenopausal women were eligible for the STAR trial. Thus although the STAR trial resulted in FDA approval for raloxifene for the indication of breast cancer risk reduction in postmenopausal women, tamoxifen remains the only FDA-approved agent for breast cancer chemoprevention in premenopausal women.[55]

Aromatase Inhibitors for Chemoprevention

In clinical trials in the adjuvant treatment setting, aromatase inhibitors have been shown to be superior to tamoxifen in terms of their effect on contralateral breast cancer,[56] leading to interest in investigating these agents in the prevention setting. Two placebo-controlled clinical trials examining the efficacy of aromatase inhibitors for prevention of breast cancer in postmenopausal women have now been published. The IBIS-II study enrolled postmenopausal women aged 40 to 70 at increased risk of breast cancer, including women with a history of LCIS, atypical hyperplasia (AH), or surgically treated DCIS, and randomized participants to anastrozole versus placebo for a period of 5 years.[57] There were a total of 154 (8%) patients with LCIS/AH in the treatment arm, plus 190 (10%) with LCIS/AH in the placebo arm. Overall, there was a significant decrease in the number of breast cancers identified in the anastrozole group, and although it did not reach statistical significance, women with LCIS/AH and without prior hormone replacement therapy (HRT) exposure in the anastrozole had an increased benefit and greater risk reduction than others in the study.[57] These results were similar to the MAP.3 study, which enrolled postmenopausal women at least 35 years of age and at increased risk of breast cancer based on either the Gail Model or a previous history of LCIS, AH, or DCIS.[58] Women with atypia/LCIS accounted for 11% of the overall study participants. Study participants were randomized to either 5 years of exemestane (Aromasin) or placebo and stratified based on Gail score and current aspirin use. At 3 years follow-up, of

4560 patients enrolled, 11 cancers had developed in the treatment group and 32 in the placebo arm, and the superiority of exemestane to placebo was seen in all subgroups, including those with LCIS.[58] The American Society of Clinical Oncology in 2013 updated their guidelines on chemoprevention for breast cancer, recommending tamoxifen for premenopausal women, as well as raloxifene or exemestane for use in postmenopausal females.[59] (The IBIS-II trial results were published after this guideline update.)

Finally, the safety of using combined HRT (CHRT) in women with a history of LCIS is currently unknown. Indirect evidence of a potential relationship between CHRT and lobular carcinoma, as well as the potential for increased breast density and reduced mammographic sensitivity, argue against using CHRT in this population.

Surgical Intervention for LCIS

Surgical Excisional Biopsy Showing LCIS

Historical data indicate that lobular neoplasia is found in 0.5% to 4% of excisional biopsies and 1.5% of core needle breast biopsies. Typically, additional invasive intervention is not indicated when LCIS is diagnosed by surgical excision, even when the lesion is seen at the surgical margin. Because LCIS generally does not itself require surgical treatment, surgical biopsy showing LCIS should not itself demand further intervention because surgical margins are not clinically relevant. Unlike surgical treatment for DCIS or invasive cancer, it is not necessary to surgically remove more breast tissue simply because the tissue that was excised had LCIS at the edge of the excision specimen. This conclusion is supported by a 2004 study of 40 patients with invasive cancer and associated lobular neoplasia. Although 14 of the patients had either close (<2 mm) or frankly positive margins for lobular neoplasia, none suffered local recurrence in the breast after a median of 67 months' follow-up.[60] Such results suggest that observation can safely replace excision when margins show LCIS involvement.

Core Needle Samples Showing LCIS

Percutaneous core needle biopsy is the sampling method now typically used for the primary evaluation of suspicious breast findings. Although the benefits of tissue sampling with this technique are established, needle biopsy has an inherent potential risk of sampling error or underestimation of malignancy due to collecting smaller specimens than are obtained at surgery. The likelihood of such underestimation has been extensively studied for ADH at core needle biopsy. Surgical excision is recommended in this setting because approximately 20% of ADH cases have been shown to have coexistent in situ or invasive malignancy identified at subsequent excisional biopsy.

It remains more controversial whether surgical excision is also required when LCIS is the most severe histopathology result identified by core needle biopsy sampling. Evidence-based management recommendations have been challenging due to the relatively infrequent occurrence of pure LCIS at percutaneous biopsy. LCIS has been reported to comprise from 0.2% to 1.2% of core biopsy results,[61–63] and thus most studies have included only small numbers of patients. Generalization of study results has been problematic because a variety of biopsy devices and needle gauges have been used. There is little question that excision is indicated when LCIS is present and this result is discordant relative to the clinical or imaging finding, or when it is found along with other high-risk lesions, such as a radial scar or ADH, which are themselves indications for surgical biopsy.[62] Although the number of cases in each study is small, historical results suggested rates of underestimation of malignancy for LCIS were comparable to those seen with ADH. In a multisite investigation of cases with LCIS as the most severe core needle sampling histopathology, Lechner and associates found 34% (20/58) were associated with malignancy at surgical excision,[61] whereas Shin and Rosen reported upgrade rates of 21% (3/14) in this setting.[64] Mahoney and colleagues hypothesized that excision might not be necessary when LCIS was found using larger caliber 11-gauge vacuum-assisted breast biopsy, but their study still demonstrated malignancy in 33% (4/12) cases.[63]

More recently, a multicenter investigation from Italy found that the rate of upstage to malignancy after excision when LCIS was found during image guided sampling was 18%.[65] Their entire cohort included women with pure LCIS, as well as LCIS associated with other high-risk lesions, but among the small subset of individuals with pure LCIS, a 20.3% upstage rate was identified. Rendi and colleagues also found a high risk of upstage to cancer when extensive (more than four) foci of LCIS were seen on core sampling.[38] In contrast, another study of 87 cases of lobular neoplasia found an upgrade rate of only 3.4% and only when the imaging Breast Imaging Reporting and Data System (BI-RADS) score was 4 or higher, when there was concurrent ADH, or in the setting of a breast cancer history in either breast.[66] These authors challenged the need for routine surgical excision and instead proposed that clinical and radiographic surveillance is appropriate when the core needle sampling finding of lobular neoplasia, including classic LCIS, is concordant with imaging and the patient has no prior or current cancer history. A similarly low 3% rate of upgrade to malignancy was also recently reported for a multicenter, prospective trial of 77 patients with pure lobular neoplasia on core biopsy.[67] These authors also endorsed observation, not excision, for patients with pure LN on core biopsy and concordant imaging findings.

On the basis of the results of these and other small studies and on the clinical experience of their expert panel, the NCCN breast cancer diagnosis and screening guidelines have progressively softened their recommendation that surgical excision for all cases of LCIS found at core needle biopsy is required. Guidelines as of 2016 state that excision for classic LCIS should be performed if pathology and imaging findings are discordant or when LCIS is found in conjunction with ADH, whereas observation alone is now allowed for classic LCIS that is concordant with imaging findings.[39] The NCCN guidelines do acknowledge in a footnote that multifocal/extensive LCIS associated with more than four terminal ductal lobular units (TDLU) may be associated with an increased risk of invasive disease being found at excision for classic LCIS, in keeping with the Rendi and colleagues article, but do not specifically state that these cases require excision. It seems reasonable, and is within the NCCN guidelines, to recommend excision for classic LCIS seen on core biopsy when there are discordant pathology and imaging findings, when the lesion is associated with additional atypical findings (ALH, ADH, FEA, etc.), when the lesion is extensive and/or involves more than four TDLUs, and when the classic LCIS is associated with a mass on imaging. In the setting of pleomorphic LCIS, the NCCN recommends management along the breast cancer treatment pathway.[39]

The Use of Breast Magnetic Resonance Imaging for Lobular Neoplasia

Although the use of bilateral breast magnetic resonance imaging (MRI) among women at high risk for the development of breast cancer has been investigated, no current recommendations address the use of screening MRI among those with lobular neoplasia. American Cancer Society guidelines updated in 2015 support annual MRI screening for limited groups of individuals, such as women with known BRCA mutation carriers, those with high-risk conditions such as Li-Fraumeni syndrome and Cowden disease, individuals exposed to chest radiation between the ages of 10 and 30, and those with a calculated lifetime breast cancer risk greater than 20% to 25% based on family history.[68] The American Cancer Society found insufficient evidence to recommend routine annual MRI for women diagnosed with LCIS, ALH, or ADH in the absence of other high-risk conditions, citing a lack of data due to a paucity of studies specifically addressing women with these risk factors, whereas the most recent NCCN cancer screening guidelines state that MRI for patients with a history of LCIS or ADH/ALH can be considered.[39]

Some studies have specifically looked at the role of MRI in the setting of lobular neoplasia. One from Memorial Sloan-Kettering Cancer Center reported results when MRI was used as a screening tool for women with biopsy-proven ADH and/or LCIS, but not ALH. MRI led to an increased number of biopsies among the 182 individuals (135 with LCIS) who submitted to the screening versus the 196 who declined. The addition of surveillance breast MRI led to detection of otherwise occult malignancy in 4% (5 of 135) of women with LCIS undergoing this test. Of note, when a new cancer was subsequently diagnosed, individuals in the MRI cohort were found to have earlier stage lesions than those followed with conventional imaging.[69] In addition, Sung and associates investigated the use of MRI in 220 women with a history of LCIS. During their study period, 17 cancers were detected, 12 with MRI alone and 5 with mammography alone. They concluded that MRI is a useful adjunct to traditional mammogram in patients with prior findings of LCIS and resulted in a 4.5% incremental breast cancer detection rate.[70] A more recent study from Ehasani and colleagues evaluated 282 high-risk women with MRI, including 40 with a history of LCIS and/or AH. They reported a breast cancer detection rate of 4.6% during the study period, with 10 of 13 found by MRI, and 2 of those among women with LCIS, suggesting again that MRI may be a useful adjunct to traditional clinical examination and mammography in these high-risk patients.[71]

Breast Conservation in Patients Who Have LCIS Coincident With Invasive Cancer

In general, the presence of LCIS in conjunction with an invasive malignancy is not a contraindication for breast conserving surgery. Although studies have some mixed results, the majority of reports have failed to demonstrate an increased risk of ipsilateral breast cancer recurrence after breast conservation for invasive cancer coincident with LCIS.[72,73] Abner and colleagues from Harvard's Joint Center for Radiation Therapy found that the 8-year local recurrence rate was 13% among the 119 patients with associated LCIS adjacent to the tumor compared with 12% for the 1062 patients without associated LCIS (p = not significant).[73] The extent of LCIS did not appear to affect the risk of recurrence. Two additional publications continue to support these findings. Pierce and colleagues identified 64 individuals treated with lumpectomy who had LCIS and an invasive lesion present. Local control rates when LCIS was present were excellent and equal to those seen in women without evidence of LCIS, even if the lobular neoplasia was multifocal and/or involved the surgical margin.[74] In addition, Morrow and colleagues failed to find a correlation between LCIS either in the surgical specimen or the resection margin and local failure in an analysis of 2894 women treated with breast conserving therapy over a 27-year period.[75]

In contrast to these favorable reports, some authors have instead suggested that patients with IBC and coincident LCIS (IBC + LCIS) may be at increased risk for ipsilateral breast tumor recurrence, with some citing the presence of LCIS as an independent risk factor for local failure after breast conserving therapy.[76–78] Despite these conflicting data, our institution does not routinely offer reexcision to individuals solely based on the presence of LCIS at a surgical margin, even if the specimen is a lumpectomy for invasive cancer.

Controversy remains about what to do when the involved margin reveals the pleomorphic LCIS. Limited data suggest that individuals with pleomorphic LCIS may have poorer outcomes than those with the classic subtype. It is possible that pleomorphic LCIS, like DCIS, should be excised with negative surgical margins. The historic data regarding outcomes of patients with pleomorphic LCIS were worrisome. In 1991 Page and colleagues described cancer risk implications among different patterns of the LCIS spectrum.[15] Thirty-nine patients with a diagnosis of isolated LCIS underwent surgical biopsy, not mastectomy, and were followed for an average of 19 years. The absolute risk of invasive cancer was 17% at 15 years. The histologic pattern of 10 invasive carcinomas developing in 9 patients was predominantly of the lobular type, with 3 pure and 4 variant types representing 70% of the developed carcinomas. Three of those women with IBC died at an average interval of 5.3 years. All 3 women had a histologic pattern of pleomorphic ILC.[15] In general, pleomorphic ILC with associated LCIS appears to portend a poorer outcome when the sparse data in the literature are examined. In a 1992 report from Italy, the authors described 10 cases of pleomorphic ILC, 6 of which included LCIS.[79] Six of 10 patients died within 42 months of diagnosis. Three other patients developed recurrence or distant metastases at short intervals. The authors concluded that pleomorphic ILC is a highly lethal variant of invasive carcinoma.

In 1992, Weidner and Semple compared the clinical course of 25 cases of classic ILC with 16 cases of pleomorphic ILC.[80] Survival until recurrence was significantly worse in the patients with pleomorphic ILC. Patients with positive nodes and pleomorphic histology were 30 times more likely to experience breast cancer recurrence than patients with the classic ILC histology. A more recent article by Bentz and colleagues evaluated 12 patients with pleomorphic ILC, 11 of whom had long-term clinical follow-up.[20] Of the 12 cases, 7 had coexisting pleomorphic LCIS. Nine patients developed fatal metastatic disease, with a median survival of 2.1 years. Middleton and colleagues from the National Cancer Institute identified 38 cases of pleomorphic ILC.[11] Pleomorphic LCIS was associated with pleomorphic ILC in 45% of cases. Of the 19 patients available for follow-up, 7 had no evidence of disease at last examination (range 1–15 years), 3 were alive with disease (range 2–14 years), and 9 were dead of disease (range 2 months to 9 years). Six patients had subsequent diagnoses of tumor in the contralateral breast. Their analysis showed that pleomorphic ILC tends to appear in older postmenopausal women who present with locally advanced disease.

These findings suggest that pleomorphic ILC may be as aggressive as most forms of IDC and that pleomorphic LCIS could be a harbinger for that aggressive underlying biology. This part of the spectrum of LCIS may warrant different management than classic LCIS. Although large case series are lacking due to the rarity of pure pleomorphic LCIS, two recent studies have shed additional light on pleomorphic LCIS as an entity. Flanagan and colleagues looked at 23 cases of pure pleomorphic LCIS diagnosed over a 15-year period.[81] These authors found that of 21 patients undergoing surgery for a core biopsy finding of pleomorphic LCIS, 33% had a subsequent diagnosis of invasive cancer and 19% had DCIS identified. In addition, 48% of the cases revealed extensive, multifocal pleomorphic LCIS and 71% were found to have a close or positive surgical margin. When negative margin resection was attempted, mastectomy was the usual outcome. Interestingly, they identified no ipsilateral breast cancer recurrences, even when close or positive margins persisted and suggested that negative margin resection for pleomorphic LCIS may not always be necessary.[81]

Another publication, however, found a 19.4% (n = 6) local recurrence rate among 47 women diagnosed with pleomorphic LCIS. In this study, two of the local recurrences occurred in women with positive pleomorphic LCIS margins, with the other four recurrences happening despite negative surgical margins. More surprising was the finding that 7 women with positive pleomorphic LCIS margins had not suffered from a recurrence at the time of publication.[82] A clear consensus regarding pleomorphic LCIS margin management fails to exist and each patient should be discussed individually.

Is There a Defined Role for Surgical Prophylaxis With LCIS?

In general, LCIS is no longer believed to be a pathologic entity that mandates surgery. Although the risk of developing invasive cancer with LCIS is elevated above the general population, most women with this diagnosis will not develop IBC within their natural lifetimes. Of those women who do get breast cancer, the relative risk appears to be similar for both breasts. Thus, if one were to perform surgery for LCIS, the only logical operation would be bilateral total mastectomy. One of the most important changes in the surgical management of lobular neoplasia, therefore, has been the abandonment of routine mastectomy after a diagnosis of LCIS, a change supported by data from the NSABP, which suggested that LCIS could be safely treated conservatively and that mastectomy was not required for oncologic control.[83]

Although such surgery is felt to be excessive for the majority of individuals with LCIS, there may be circumstances in which bilateral mastectomy is a reasonable consideration. Bilateral prophylactic mastectomy (with or without reconstruction), regardless of the reason why it is performed, confers greater than a 90% risk reduction against the development of subsequent breast cancer.[84] If a patient is otherwise a reasonable candidate for prophylactic surgery, such as an individual from a high-risk family in which genetic testing is noninformative or those with a known genetic mutation, and if that woman is then found to have LCIS, she might have heightened consideration for such a procedure. Any use of prophylactic surgery for breast cancer risk reduction must be highly individualized and warrants considerable introspection before a definitive decision is made. Counseling for both medical and psychological issues is mandatory, as is ample time to make an appropriate personal decision. We generally recommend referral to our high-risk clinic for a thorough discussion of nonsurgical options, including more rigorous surveillance and chemoprevention.

Conclusions

LCIS, which is defined as involvement of more than 50% of the affected acini of the lobule, exists as two main subtypes, classic and pleomorphic. Since the initial description of LCIS in the 1940s, our understanding of the lesion has changed dramatically and continues to evolve. Historically, LCIS was felt to be a direct precursor to invasive malignancy. With time, LCIS instead came to be thought of instead as a marker for the development of malignancy in either breast. Aggressive surgical resection mandating bilateral mastectomy was replaced with programs of surveillance involving clinical and radiographic examinations. By combining epidemiologic evidence arguing that LCIS confers increased bilateral risk of developing invasive cancer with current molecular evidence that supports lobular neoplasia as a precursor lesion, a model encompassing both concepts has emerged. Although lobular neoplasia may be a precursor to some invasive carcinomas with its frequent multifocal and bilateral distribution and relatively low lifetime risk of evolving into an invasive carcinoma, this biologic entity can be treated as a "risk indicator" lesion without complete surgical resection. Future challenges will determine whether there are high-risk subtypes of LCIS, such as the pleomorphic form, that may behave as high-risk precursor lesions requiring surgical or hormonal-based therapeutic interventions.

LCIS is usually discovered incidentally during biopsy for another clinical or radiographic indication. LCIS incidence appears to be influenced by the use of exogenous hormones, with diagnoses decreasing concurrent with decreasing CHT use since 2002, with a slight increase between 2002 and 2009. When LCIS is identified, the lifetime risk of an invasive cancer is thought to be 8 to 10 times that seen among women who lack such a diagnosis. The risk of invasive cancer development can be decreased by the use of a chemopreventive antihormonal endocrine agent, such as tamoxifen, raloxifene, or an aromatase inhibitor. Tamoxifen is approved for both pre- and postmenopausal women with lobular neoplasia, whereas raloxifene is approved only for those who are postmenopausal.

When LCIS is diagnosed on a core needle biopsy, current guidelines recommend consideration of diagnostic surgical excisional sampling for discordant pathology/imaging findings, with extensive LCIS, and when the lesion is associated with other atypical findings, core biopsy is used to eliminate the possibility of a missed malignancy. Observation alone without excision is being offered to an increasing number of individuals with classic LCIS on core sampling that is deemed concordant with imaging findings. Aggressive surgical resection of all LCIS disease to achieve a negative surgical margin, even at the time of lumpectomy for a concurrent invasive tumor, is not advocated because LCIS is often multicentric, multifocal, and bilateral. Such clinical presentations make bilateral mastectomy the only way to ensure removal of all of the LCIS present, an approach that is therapeutically aggressive (and unnecessary) for this high-risk factor, unless there are other compelling and confounding breast cancer risk factors present. Finally, the biological behavior of pleomorphic LCIS remains controversial in terms of long-term outcomes and risk of invasive cancer development.

Selected References

34. King TA, Pilewskie M, Muhsen S, et al. Lobular carcinoma in situ: a 29-year longitudinal experience evaluating clinicopathologic features and breast cancer risk. *J Clin Oncol.* 2015;33:3945-3952.

38. Rendi MH, Dintzis SM, Lehman CD, et al. Lobular in-situ neoplasia on breast core needle biopsy: imaging indication and pathologic extent can identify which patients require excisional biopsy. *Ann Surg Oncol.* 2012;19:914-921.

55. Visvanathan K, et al. American Society of Clinical Oncology clinical practice guideline update on the use of pharmacologic interventions including tamoxifen, raloxifene, and aromatase inhibition for breast cancer risk reduction. *J Clin Oncol.* 2009;27:3235-3258.

67. Nakhlis F, Gilmore L, Gelman R, et al. Incidence of adjacent synchronous invasive carcinoma and/or ductal carcinoma in situ in patients with lobular neoplasia on core biopsy: results from a prospective multi-institutional registry (TBCRC 020). *Ann Surg Oncol.* 2016;23:722-728.

81. Flanagan MR, Rendi MH, Calhoun KE, et al. Pleomorphic lobular carcinoma in situ: radiologic-pathologic features and clinical management. *Ann Surg Oncol.* 2015;22:4263-4269.

A full reference list is available online at ExpertConsult.com.

39

Ductal Carcinoma in Situ of the Breast

MELINDA S. EPSTEIN, MICHAEL D. LAGIOS, AND MELVIN J. SILVERSTEIN

Ductal carcinoma in situ (DCIS) of the breast is a heterogeneous group of lesions with diverse malignant potential and a range of treatment options. Before the 1980s, DCIS was not uniformly accepted as a fully noninvasive disease[1] and only represented 1% of all breast biopsies.[2] In patients diagnosed with DCIS, the disease commonly presented with a palpable mass, bloody nipple discharge, or Paget disease and was usually extensive, exceeding 50 mm.[3,4] DCIS now accounts for approximately 25% of newly diagnosed breast cancers[2] and is the most rapidly growing subgroup in the breast cancer family of disease with more than 60,000 new cases diagnosed in the United States during 2016.[5,6] Most new cases of DCIS are small, nonpalpable, and identified mammographically.

It is now well appreciated that DCIS is a stage in the neoplastic continuum in which the majority of biological alterations required for the development of invasive breast cancer are already present,[7] including but not limited to, proliferation, evading growth suppression, resisting cell death, replicative immortality, inducing angiogenesis, and activating invasion and metastasis.[8] Although DCIS is a precursor lesion for most invasive breast tumors, not all DCIS lesions have sufficient time or the genetic alterations required for progression to invasive disease.[9–11]

Contemporary therapies for DCIS range from simple excision to various forms of wider excision (i.e., segmental resection, quadrant resection, oncoplastic resection), all of which may or may not be followed by radiation therapy. When breast preservation is not feasible, total mastectomy is performed, often skin and/or nipple-areola-sparing and frequently with immediate reconstruction. Sentinel node biopsy is not necessary for most patients with DCIS. It should be considered only for those with palpable DCIS, tumors exceeding 50 mm, and lesions thought to be suspicious for invasion. It should also be considered if mastectomy is being performed.

Because DCIS is a group of heterogeneous lesions[12,13] and patients have a wide range of personal needs that must be considered during treatment selection, no single approach will be appropriate for all forms of the disease or for all patients.

Current treatment decisions are based on a variety of measurable prognostic factors, including tumor extent, margin width, nuclear grade, age, and the presence of comedonecrosis. Physician experience and physician bias also play a role. Unfortunately, randomized clinical trials have often failed to record these prognostic factors, thus making it impossible to validate them. Furthermore, if information on prognostic factors were collected during a trial, it was often done with inconsistent standards, making it impossible to confirm their significance. In part, such deficiencies were due to the methods of tissue examination used during the trials. Indeed, early pathologic standards favored limited sampling, resulting in the inability to determine the size (extent), margin involvement, and presence of microinvasion or larger areas of invasion. For example, in the Memorial Sloan Kettering Cancer Center nomogram[14] DCIS size was excluded entirely because the data were not collected during the period of accrual. Similarly, in 2006 Wong and colleagues[15] sought to compare low-risk versus high-risk DCIS based on pooled data from hospitals in Boston, Massachusetts. Unfortunately, the hospitals involved in the trial could not agree on consistent standards to determine tumor size, margin width, or grade.

Even randomized trials that did collect prognostic factor information using consistent standards were often unable to validate them. Indeed, randomized trials that focused on the benefits of irradiation and tamoxifen, such as the National Surgical Adjuvant Breast and Bowel Project (NSABP) B-17,[16] NSABP B-24,[17,18] UK/ANZ DCIS,[19] European Organization of Research and Treatment of Cancer (EORTC) 10854,[20] and SweDCIS[21] were unable to establish the validity of prognostic factors when analyzed retrospectively. Tumor size and margin status could often not be accurately assessed in the NSABP B-17[16] trial slides and specimen x-rays were frequently hard to locate after 5 to 10 years of follow-up. Similarly, in the EORTC 10854[20] trial only 22% of the DCIS had a measurable size and 10% of the entered cases in the trial were not classified as DCIS on later central review. Regardless of the inability of these trials to validate the use of radiation and tamoxifen in DCIS patients to prevent local recurrences, there are thousands of women who today are routinely recommended to undergo radiation therapy and at least 5 years of tamoxifen for small, low-grade, widely excised DCIS for a benefit limited to 4 in 100 patients.

The recognition of prognostic factors that influence ipsilateral breast recurrence in DCIS (i.e., tumor extent, margin width, nuclear grade, age, and the presence of comedonecrosis) evolved not out of randomized trials, but out of early prospective follow-up studies.[4,22–26] These prospective studies fortuitously used serial sequential tissue examination and mammographic concordance, techniques later strongly endorsed by the College of American Pathologists[27] and shown to permit a more accurate and reproducible determination of DCIS extent in comparison with older methods.[28] By requiring complete examination of the resection for DCIS, there was a reduced chance of overlooking microinvasive foci, inadequate margins and the full extent of the disease process. Moreover, there was a better opportunity to establish concordance with the imaging.

The Changing Nature of Ductal Carcinoma in Situ

There have been dramatic changes in the past 20 years that have affected the diagnosis and treatment of patients diagnosed with DCIS. Before mammography was common, DCIS was rare, representing less than 1% of all diagnosed breast cancers.[2] Today DCIS is common, representing 25% of all newly diagnosed cases and as much as 30% to 50% of cases of breast cancers diagnosed by mammography.[13,23,29–31]

Previously, most patients with DCIS presented with clinical symptoms such as a palpable breast mass, bloody nipple discharge, or Paget disease.[3,4] Today most DCIS lesions are nonpalpable and generally detected by imaging alone.

Until approximately 25 years ago, the treatment for patients with DCIS was mastectomy. Today almost 75% of newly diagnosed patients with DCIS are treated with breast preservation.[32] In the past, when mastectomy was common, reconstruction was uncommon; if it was performed, it was generally done as a delayed procedure. Today reconstruction for patients with DCIS treated by mastectomy is common and is regularly done immediately at the time of mastectomy. In the past, when a mastectomy was performed, large amounts of skin and the nipple were discarded. Today, it is considered perfectly safe to perform a skin-sparing mastectomy for DCIS and, in most instances, nipple-areola–sparing mastectomy.

In the past, there was little confusion. All breast cancers were essentially considered the same, and mastectomy was the only treatment. Today all breast cancers are recognized as different, and there is a range of acceptable treatments for each lesion. These changes were brought about by a number of factors, most importantly increased mammographic surveillance and the acceptance of breast conservation therapy for invasive breast cancer.

The widespread use of mammography changed the way DCIS was detected. In addition, it changed the nature of the disease detected by allowing us to enter the neoplastic continuum at an earlier time with a much smaller size than seen by Ashikari and colleagues.[33] It is interesting to note the impact that mammography had on The Breast Center in Van Nuys, California, in terms of the number of DCIS cases diagnosed and the manner in which they were diagnosed.[34]

From 1979 to 1981, the Van Nuys group treated an average of five DCIS patients per year. Only two lesions (13%) were nonpalpable and detected by mammography. In other words, 13 patients (87%) presented with clinically apparent disease, detected by the old-fashioned methods of observation and palpation. Beginning in 1982, when new state-of-the-art mammography units and a full-time experienced radiologist were added, the number of new DCIS cases dramatically increased to more than 50 per year, most nonpalpable.

The total of 1855 DCIS patients discussed in this chapter were accrued at the Van Nuys Breast Center from 1979 to 1998, the University of Southern California/Norris (USC/Norris) Comprehensive Cancer Center (NCCN)from 1998 to 2008, and at Hoag Memorial Hospital Presbyterian from 2008 to through 2015. Analysis of all 1855 patients through 2015 shows that 1655 DCIS lesions (89%) were nonpalpable. If we look at only those diagnosed during the past 8 years at Hoag, as screening mammography has improved, 95% were nonpalpable.

Another factor that has had a significant impact on how we currently think about DCIS was the acceptance of breast conservation therapy (lumpectomy, axillary node dissection, and radiation therapy) for patients with invasive breast cancer. Until 1981, the treatment for most patients with any form of breast cancer was mostly mastectomy. However, since that time, numerous prospective randomized trials have shown an equivalent survival rate for patients with invasive cancer treated with breast conservation therapy or mastectomy.[35–40] It made little sense to continue treating less aggressive DCIS with mastectomy while treating more aggressive invasive breast cancer with breast preservation. Moreover, current data suggest that many patients with DCIS can be successfully treated with breast preservation, with or without radiation therapy.[41–43] This chapter discusses how easily accessible data may aid in the complex treatment selection process.

Pathology

Classification

Although there is no universally accepted histopathologic classification, most pathologists have traditionally divided DCIS into five major architectural subtypes (papillary, micropapillary, cribriform, solid, and comedo), often comparing the first four (noncomedo) with comedo.[23,44,45] Comedo DCIS is frequently associated with high nuclear grade,[23,44,45] aneuploidy,[46] a higher proliferation rate,[47] HER2/neu gene amplification or protein overexpression,[48–52] and aggressive clinical behavior.[22,53–55] Noncomedo lesions tend to be just the opposite.

However, architectural classification alone is not adequate to segregate patients into high- and low-risk categories. There is no uniform agreement among pathologists of exactly how much comedo DCIS must be present to consider the lesion a comedo DCIS. Furthermore, in our series of patients, approximately 75% of DCIS lesions had significant amounts of two or more architectural subtypes, making division by a predominant architectural subtype problematic. Although, it is clear that lesions exhibiting a predominant high-grade comedo DCIS pattern are generally more aggressive and more likely to recur if treated conservatively than low-grade noncomedo lesions, architectural subtyping alone is insufficient to precisely segregate patients by risk of recurrence. Azzopardi and colleagues[56] recognized this in 1979.

Nuclear grade is a better biological predictor of cancer behavior than architecture and therefore has emerged as a key histopathologic factor for identifying aggressive tumors.[4,22,25,55,57,58] Thus, to more accurately stratify patients by risk of recurrence, current classifications have focused on both necrosis and nuclear grade. As a result, in 1995 the Van Nuys group introduced a new pathologic DCIS classification,[59] the Van Nuys Classification, based on high nuclear grade and the presence or absence of comedo-type necrosis.

The Van Nuys group selected high nuclear grade as one of the factors in their classification because there was general agreement that patients with high nuclear grade lesions recur at a higher rate and in a shorter time period after breast conservation than patients with low nuclear grade lesions.[4,22,55] Comedo-type necrosis was also chosen because its presence also suggests a poorer prognosis[60,61] and it is easy to recognize.[62] Douglas-Jones and colleagues[63] have shown that the Van Nuys system is the most reproducible of the available classifications.

The details of the Van Nuys Classification System can be found in Fig. 39.1. There is neither a minimum nor a specific amount of high nuclear grade DCIS nor a minimum amount of comedo-type necrosis required in this classification. Furthermore, the subtleties

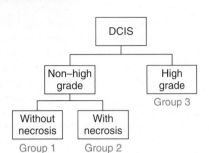

• **Fig. 39.1** The original Van Nuys ductal carcinoma in situ *(DCIS)* classification system. DCIS patients are separated in high nuclear grade (grade 3) and non–high nuclear grade (grades 1 and 2). Non–high nuclear grade cases are then separated by the presence or absence of necrosis. Lesions in group 3 (high nuclear grade) may or may not show necrosis.

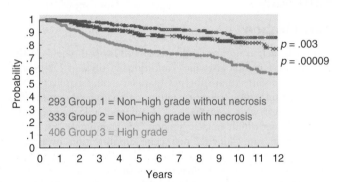

• **Fig. 39.2** Probability of local recurrence-free survival for 1148 breast conservation patients using Van Nuys ductal carcinoma in situ pathologic classification. Comparison of group 2 or group 3 versus group 1.

of the intermediate-grade lesion, essential in other systems, are not important in the Van Nuys classification; only nuclear grade III cells (large, pleomorphic cells with prominent nucleoli and coarse clumped chromatin)[22,59,60] need be recognized.

The Van Nuys classification is useful because it divides DCIS patients into three biological groups with different risks of local recurrence after breast conservation therapy (Fig. 39.2). When combined with tumor size, age, and margin status, the Van Nuys Classification is an integral part of the USC/Van Nuys Prognostic Index (USC/VNPI), a system that will be discussed in detail.

Progression to Invasive Breast Cancer

Which DCIS lesions will become invasive, and when will that happen? These are the most important questions in the DCIS field today. Currently, there is intense molecular biological study regarding the progression of genetic changes in normal breast epithelium to DCIS and then to invasive breast cancer. It is now appreciated that DCIS is a stage in the neoplastic continuum in which the majority of genetic and epigenetic changes required for the development of invasive breast cancer are already present,[7] including but not limited to proliferation, evading growth suppression, resisting cell death, replicative immortality, inducing angiogenesis, and activating invasion and metastasis.[8]

Immunohistochemical and Molecular Phenotypes in DCIS

It has been recognized for some time that there is a substantial concordance between the nuclear grade of DCIS and its associated invasive carcinoma, such that low-grade DCIS lesions, regardless of the classification scheme used, are largely associated with lower-grade invasive carcinomas, whereas high-grade DCIS tumors are associated with higher-grade invasive carcinomas. Similarly, the frequency of specific biomarkers in DCIS varies with the grade of the lesion. Estrogen and progesterone receptors are usually expressed in low-grade DCIS but less so in high-grade lesions. In contrast, HER2/neu overexpression and elevated proliferative markers such as ki67 are more often observed in high-grade DCIS and less often in low-grade lesions. More recently, surrogate molecular phenotypes defined by immunohistochemistry have been used to identify DCIS phenotypes corresponding to luminal A, luminal B, HER2, and triple-negative/basal phenotypes in invasive breast cancer. Luminal A and B DCIS phenotypes are more frequent in the low to intermediate nuclear grade lesions, whereas HER2, triple-negative/basal phenotypes are more common among high-grade DCIS.[64,65]

Microinvasion

The incidence of microinvasion was difficult to quantitate until 1997 because there was no formal or universally accepted definition of what constituted microinvasion. The first official definition of what is now classified as pT1mic disease was published in the 5th edition of the *Manual for Cancer Staging* read as follows: "Microinvasion is the extension of cancer cells beyond the basement membrane into adjacent tissues with no focus more than 1 mm in greatest dimension. When there are multiple foci of microinvasion the size of only the largest focus is used to classify the microinvasion (do not use the sum of the diameters of all individual foci). The presence of multiple foci of microinvasion should be noted, as it is with multiple larger invasive carcinomas."[66]

If even the smallest amount of invasive disease is found upon excision or mastectomy in the presence of a large DCIS, the lesion should not be classified as DCIS but as invasive cancer. In concordance with the TNM staging system, if the invasive foci is 1 mm or smaller, the tumor should be defined as a T1mic with an extensive intraductal component (EIC).

Foci of microinvasion that consist of single cells have been shown to have no impact on patient outcome whereas foci comprising cohesive groups of cells have been found to be associated with an increased rate of distant recurrence and death.[67] In contrast to the number of cells within a focus of microinvasion, the number of microinvasive foci in a lesion have a small impact on breast cancer mortality; patients with multiple foci have a comparable outcome to patients with a single focus of microinvasion, 5.8% versus 1%.[67]

Multicentricity and Multifocality of Ductal Carcinoma in Situ

Multicentricity is generally defined as DCIS in a quadrant other than the quadrant in which the original DCIS (index quadrant) was diagnosed. There must be normal breast tissue separating the two foci. Because the definition of multicentricity differs between investigators, the reported incidence of multicentricity also varies. Reported rates vary from 0% to 78%,[68–71] averaging about 30%, have been reported. Twenty-five years ago, the 30% average rate of multicentricity was used by surgeons as a rationale for mastectomy in patients with DCIS.

In 1990, Holland and colleagues[72] investigated the rate of multicentricity in 82 mastectomy specimens by preparing whole-organ sections every 5 mm, a variation of Egan's subgrossing technique.[73] Each section was radiographed, and paraffin blocks were made from every radiographically suspicious spot. In addition, an average of 25 blocks were taken from the quadrant containing the index cancer; random samples were taken from all other quadrants, the central subareolar area, and the nipple. The microscopic extension of each lesion was verified on the radiographs. The resulting data demonstrated that most DCIS lesions were larger than expected (50% were greater than 50 mm), involved more than one quadrant by continuous extension (23%), but, most importantly, were unicentric (98.8%). Only 1 of 82 mastectomy specimens (1.2%) had multicentric distribution with separate lesions in a different quadrant separated by normal tissue. This study suggested that complete excision of a DCIS lesion was possible due to unicentricity but might be extremely difficult due to larger than expected size. In an update, Holland reported whole-organ studies in 119 patients, 118 of whom had unicentric disease.[74] This information, when combined with the fact that most local recurrences are at or near the original DCIS, suggests that the problem of multicentricity is not important in the DCIS treatment decision-making process.

Multifocality is defined as separate foci of DCIS within the same ductal system. Studies of both Holland and colleagues[72,74] and Noguchi and colleagues[75] suggest that a great deal of multifocality may be artifactual, resulting from examining a three-dimensional entity in two dimensions on a glass slide. It would be analogous to saying that the branches of a tree were not connected if the branches were cut through one plane, placed separately on a slide, and viewed in cross section.[76] Multifocality may be due to small gaps of DCIS or skip areas within ducts as described by Faverly and colleagues[77] and is more easily recognized when a serial sequential tissue processing technique as opposed to random sampling is employed.

Detection and Diagnosis

The importance of quality mammography in the identification of DCIS cannot be overemphasized. Currently, more than 90% of patients with DCIS present with a nonpalpable lesion detected by mammography. The most common mammographic finding is microcalcification, frequently clustered and generally without an associated soft tissue abnormality.[78] More than 80% of DCIS patients exhibit microcalcifications on preoperative mammography, the patterns of which may be focal, diffuse, or ductal, with variable size and shape.[78] Patients with comedo DCIS tend to have "casting calcifications" that are linear, branching, and bizarre and are almost pathognomonic for comedo DCIS[78] (Fig. 39.3). However, when noncomedo lesions are calcified, they tend to have fine granular powdery calcifications or crushed stone–like calcifications (Fig. 39.4). It is important to note that some DCIS lesions, even with prominent comedonecrosis, fail to exhibit mammographic microcalcifications; among others, microcalcifications are seen only intermittently. Indeed, 32% of noncomedo lesions in our series did not have mammographic calcifications, making the DCIS more difficult to find and the patients more difficult to follow, if treated conservatively.

A major problem confronting surgeons relates to the fact that calcifications do not always map out the entire DCIS lesion, particularly those of the noncomedo type. Even if all the calcifications are removed, noncalcified DCIS may be left behind. Conversely, the majority of the calcifications may suggest a lesion larger than the true DCIS lesion. However, calcifications more

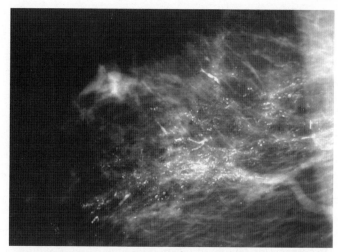

• **Fig. 39.3** Mediolateral mammography in a 43-year-old woman that shows irregular branching calcifications. Histopathology showed high-grade comedo ductal carcinoma in situ, Van Nuys group 3.

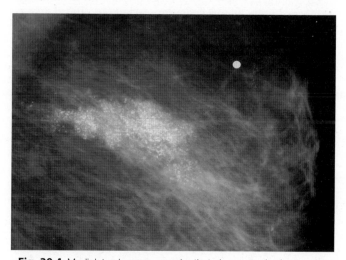

• **Fig. 39.4** Mediolateral mammography that shows crushed stone–type calcifications.

accurately approximate the size of high-grade and/or comedo lesions than low-grade and/or noncomedo lesions.[79]

If a patient's mammogram shows any abnormality (i.e., calcifications, architectural distortion, nonpalpable mass), additional radiologic workup needs to be performed. This should include compression and magnification views. Ultrasonography should also be performed on all suspicious calcifications to rule out the presence of a mass that can be biopsied with ultrasound guidance. In addition, magnetic resonance imaging (MRI) has become increasingly popular and is often used to map out the size and shape of biopsy-proven DCIS lesions or invasive breast cancers and to rule out other foci of multifocal, multicentric or contralateral cancer. MRI has the advantage of detecting DCIS that has not undergone calcification.

Biopsy Techniques

If radiologic workup shows an occult lesion that requires biopsy, there are multiple approaches: fine-needle aspiration biopsy (FNAB), core biopsy (i.e., stereotactic, ultrasound guided, MRI guided), and directed surgical biopsy using guide wires or radioactive localization. FNAB is generally of little help for nonpalpable DCIS. Although with FNAB it is possible to obtain cancer cells, there is no architecture. So although cytopathologists can identify the presence of malignant cells, they cannot determine whether the lesion is invasive.

Stereotactic core biopsy became available in the early 1990s and is now widely used. Dedicated digital tables and add-on upright units make this a precise procedure. Large-gauge vacuum-assisted needles are the tools of choice for diagnosing DCIS using these techniques. Ultrasound-guided core biopsy also became popular in the 1990s but is of less value for DCIS because most DCIS lesions do not present with a mass that can be visualized by ultrasound. Nonetheless, all suspicious microcalcifications should be evaluated by ultrasound because a mass will be found in 5% to 15%[29] of patients. Proper pathologic examination of a large-gauge core biopsy for microcalcification requires confirmation of the microcalcification in the core as well as at least serial levels to adequately sample the tissue. Radiographic-pathologic correlation is required to confirm concordance.

Open surgical biopsy should only be used if the lesion cannot be biopsied using minimally invasive techniques. This should be a rare event with current image-guided biopsy techniques and occurs in less than 5% of cases.[29,80] If excision using needle localization is performed, whether for diagnosis or treatment, intraoperative specimen radiography and correlation with the preoperative mammogram is mandatory.[81,82] Margins should be inked or dyed and specimens should be serially sectioned and, if necessary, a second x-ray of the slices should be obtained. The tissue sections should be arranged and processed in sequence. Pathologic reporting should include a determination of nuclear grade, an assessment of the presence or absence of necrosis, the measured extent of the lesion (calculated on the basis of the slices prepared), and measurement of all margins, in particular, the closest margin.[27,82,83] The major architectural subtypes should also be included in the diagnosis.[84] If the patient is motivated for breast conservation, a multiple wire–directed oncoplastic excision can be planned. This will give the patient her best chance at two opposing goals: clear margins and good cosmesis.[85]

Treatment

For most patients with DCIS, there is no single correct treatment. There will generally be a choice. The choices, although seemingly simple, are not. As the choices increase and become more complicated, frustration increases for both the patient and physician.[86,87]

Treatment End Points for Patients With Ductal Carcinoma in Situ

When evaluating the results of treatment for patients with breast cancer, a variety of end points must be considered. Important end points include local recurrence (both invasive and DCIS), regional recurrence (such as the axilla), distant recurrence, breast cancer–specific survival, overall survival, and quality of life. No study to date has shown a significant difference in distant disease-free or breast cancer–specific survival in patients with pure DCIS, regardless of any treatment.[88] In our series of 1855 patients with DCIS, the breast cancer–specific mortality rate is 0.7% at 10 years. Numerous other DCIS series[89–94] also confirm an extremely low mortality rate with DCIS. Consequently, local recurrence has become the most commonly used and important end point when evaluating treatment for patients with DCIS.

Forty to fifty percent of local recurrences after treatment for DCIS are invasive. Approximately 10% to 20% of DCIS patients who develop local invasive recurrences develop distant metastases and die of breast cancer.[95,96] Long term, this translates into a mortality rate of approximately 0.5% for patients treated with mastectomy, 1% to 2% for conservatively treated patients who receive radiation therapy, and 2% to 3% for patients treated with excision alone.

It is clearly important to prevent local recurrences in patients treated for DCIS. They are demoralizing. They often lead to mastectomy and if they are invasive, they upstage the patient and are a threat to life. However, protecting DCIS patients from local recurrence must be balanced against potential detrimental effects of the treatments given.

Treatment Options

Mastectomy

Mastectomy is, by far, the most effective treatment available for DCIS if the goal is simply to prevent local recurrence. Most mastectomy series reveal local recurrence rates of approximately 1% with mortality rates close to zero.[97] In our series of 576 DCIS patients treated with mastectomy, none of whom received radiation therapy or tamoxifen, we have had 13 local recurrences (9 invasive and 4 DCIS). One of the patients with an invasive local recurrence developed metastatic disease. In addition, two other patients developed metastatic breast cancer without developing a local recurrence. The absolute rate of distant recurrence was 0.5%.

However, mastectomy is an aggressive form of treatment for patients with DCIS. It clearly provides a local recurrence benefit but only a theoretical survival benefit. As well, during an era where breast conservation is increasingly used for treatment of invasive breast carcinoma, it is difficult to justify mastectomy, particularly for otherwise healthy women with screen-detected DCIS. Mastectomy is indicated only in cases of true multicentricity or when a unicentric DCIS lesion is too large to excise with clear margins and an acceptable cosmetic result. In our opinion, no DCIS lesion in too large to excise if the breast is large enough to accommodate an oncoplastic reduction with a good cosmetic result.

Initially it was thought that DCIS was not part of the spectrum of disease related to breast cancer–associated genes *BRCA1* and *BRCA2*. However, an association between DCIS and these genes is now recognized.[98,99] Genetic positivity for *BRCA1* or *BRCA2* is not an absolute contraindication to breast preservation, although many patients who test positive for a deleterious mutation and who develop DCIS seriously consider bilateral mastectomy and salpingo-oophorectomy.

Breast Conservation

Breast conservation for DCIS can take the form of excision alone or excision plus radiation therapy. The most recently available Surveillance Epidemiology and End Results (SEER) data reveal that 70% of patients with DCIS are treated with breast conservation,[100,101] nearly equally divided between with and without radiation therapy.

Clinical trials have shown that local excision plus radiation therapy in patients with negative margins provides excellent rates of local control.[18,89,92–94,102–104] Some cases of DCIS may not recur or progress to invasive carcinoma when treated by excision alone.[22,88,105–109] Although we know that this may be true for many cases of DCIS, it is not true for all cases. Because we are currently unable to determine which DCIS lesions will progress to invasive disease and, if they do, over what period of time, the use of radiation therapy for high-risk DCIS patients should be considered.

Are We Overtreating Ductal Carcinoma in Situ?

Until 2008 the standard treatment for DCIS, recommended by NCCN guidelines, was mastectomy or lumpectomy plus radiation therapy. In 2008, the NCCN modified its recommendations and suggested that selected low-risk DCIS patients could be treated with excision alone.[110] The definition of who was low risk and who could be treated with excision alone was not defined and therefore left to clinical judgment.

During 2015 the media saw numerous lay articles focusing on the issue of whether DCIS was being overtreated.[111,112] These articles questioned whether excision alone for DCIS was overtreatment.

To address the issue of possible overtreatment, the Low-Risk DCIS (LORIS) Trial[113,114] was undertaken in the United Kingdom. This trial randomized screen-detected, favorable, low- and intermediate-grade DCIS to standard surgical treatment versus active monitoring (surveillance) (needle biopsy alone with no additional treatment and yearly mammography surveillance).[113,114] Each group of patients will be followed for 10 years with a yearly mammogram, and the end point will be invasive recurrence.

Given that it will take at minimum of 10 years to gather meaningful results from the LORIS trial, we queried our database for a cohort of patients that could be considered similar to the LORIS Trial's active monitoring group. We compared them with patients treated using a standard surgical approach.[115] Because NCCN guidelines[110] state that DCIS with surgical margins less than 1 mm are inadequate, we used that definition as a surrogate for the LORIS surveillance arm. In contrast, we considered DCIS patients with surgical margin widths 1 mm or greater as adequately treated and as a surrogate for standard treatment. The patients were subdivided by low nuclear grade versus high.

The 10-year local recurrence probabilities were statistically significant (<0.001) for low grade versus high grade and for narrow margins less than 1 mm versus wide margins 1 mm or greater. When the two factors were combined, excision alone with margins 1 mm or greater yielded a local recurrence rate at 10 years of 13% for low-grade DCIS and 36% for high-grade DCIS ($P < .001$). For patients who had inadequate margins of less than 1 mm, excision alone yielded a 10-year local recurrence rate of 51% for low-grade and 67% for high-grade lesions. These data show that margins less than 1 mm lead to local recurrence rates of greater than 50% at 10 years and are inadequate. These data suggest that needle biopsy alone, regardless of grade, will lead to extremely high recurrence rates, half of which will be invasive.

Intraoperative Radiation Therapy for Ductal Carcinoma in Situ

Whole breast radiation therapy (WBRT) is often recommended for women treated for DCIS after breast conserving surgery (BCS) because several prospective randomized trials have demonstrated a 50% to 60% reduction in ipsilateral breast cancer recurrence for DCIS patients treated with WBRT.[19,116–119] Local failure in a patient that has received WBRT usually leads to a recommendation for mastectomy, as reirradiation is associated with extremely high levels of toxicity to the breast.[120] As a result, recent advances in radiation therapy have focused on replacing traditional WBRT

with shorter hypofractionated regimens or accelerated partial breast irradiation (APBI).

Intraoperative radiation therapy (IORT) is an APBI approach in which all radiation is delivered directly to the lumpectomy site during surgery. Because 60% to 75% of DCIS patients treated with BCS recur at or near the original tumor site,[121–123] limiting the radiation dose to the tumor bed during lumpectomy allows radiation to be delivered in a single dose to the region where recurrence would most likely happen, eliminating compliance issues,[124] reducing radiation exposure to normal tissues, and reducing radiation-induced toxicity. The simplicity of IORT makes this technique extremely appealing for patients with either invasive or noninvasive breast carcinoma.

The rationale for using IORT in women diagnosed with pure DCIS is supported by the TARGIT-A trial, a prospective randomized IORT-APBI trial that examined the equivalence of IORT compared with standard WBRT treatment for patients with early-stage invasive breast cancer.[125–127] Half of the patients enrolled in the TARGIT-A trial were found to have concurrent early-stage invasive cancer and DCIS upon pathologic examination.[125,126] Yet regardless of the presence of a DCIS component, equivalent local recurrence rates were observed among patients treated with WBRT and IORT.[125–127] Thus data from TARGIT-A demonstrates that IORT is capable of preventing recurrences in both DCIS and early-stage invasive breast carcinomas.

Since publication of the TARGIT-A trial, additional studies have documented the efficacy of APBI in patients with DCIS. In 2011 an update on the American Society for Breast Surgery MammoSite Registry Trial was published, examining a subset of 194 patients with DCIS as the primary pathology.[128] The local recurrence rate for DCIS patients treated with APBI was 3.4%, comparing favorably with the 5-year recurrence rate of 7.5% for WBRT patients reported in the NSABP B-17 trial.[129] In addition, publications from William Beaumont Hospital and Bryn Mawr Hospital studies support the findings of the MammoSite Registry Trial, concluding that that APBI as part of BCS for pure DCIS is associated with excellent local control and survival rates.[130,131] Other studies treating DCIS patients with IORT reached similar conclusions.[132,133] Taking these, and other, studies into account there is no reason to conclude that IORT would be less effective in treating DCIS patients than WBRT. Indeed, DCIS is now included as an acceptable histology by the American Brachytherapy Society and American Society for Breast Surgery.[134,135]

In summary, IORT is a promising new treatment modality that greatly simplifies the delivery of postexcision radiation therapy in patients diagnosed with DCIS. The efficacy of IORT for the treatment of DCIS has been confirmed in numerous trials. IORT makes breast conservation possible for women that could not tolerate or would not be available for 3 to 6 weeks of conventional whole breast radiation therapy.

Reasons to Consider Excision Alone

There clearly are patients with DCIS who require mastectomy. They generally have lesions too large to remove with a cosmetically acceptable result. In addition, some patients are simply more comfortable with mastectomy. However, the majority of patients, more than 70%, are good candidates for breast conservation, and half of these can probably be treated with excision alone, if adequate margins are obtained. Here are a number of reasons to consider excision alone for selected patients with DCIS.

Common Use. Excision alone is already common in spite of the randomized trial data that suggest that all conservatively treated patients benefit from radiation therapy. SEER Data reflect that excision alone is being used as complete treatment for DCIS in 35% of all DCIS patients. American doctors and patients have embraced the concept of excision alone for DCIS.

Anatomic. Evaluation of mastectomy specimens using the serial subgross tissue processing technique reveals that most DCIS is unicentric (involves a single breast segment and is radial in its distribution).[4,58,72,74,77,136] Using the same technique and evaluating patients with 25 mm or less of disease provided additional support that the majority of image detected DCIS can be adequately excised.[4,22] This means that in many cases, it is possible to excise the entire lesion with a segment or quadrant resection, possibly curing the patient without additional therapy. Holland and Faverly have shown that if 10-mm margins are achieved in all directions, the likelihood of residual DCIS is less than 10%.[77]

Biological. DCIS is a heterogeneous group of diseases with different architectures, different nuclear grades, and unpredictable malignant potentials. Some nonaggressive DCIS lesions carry a low potential, about 1% per year, of developing into an invasive tumor.[76,88,105,137–139] This is only slightly more than lobular carcinoma in situ, a lesion that is routinely treated with careful clinical follow-up.

Pathology Errors. The differences between atypical ductal hyperplasia and low-grade DCIS may be subtle. It is not uncommon for atypical ductal hyperplasia to be classified as DCIS. Such patients treated with excision and radiation therapy are indeed "cured of potential DCIS" but incur significant risks of morbidities.

Prospective Randomized Data. Prospective randomized DCIS trials show no difference in breast cancer–specific survival or overall survival, regardless of treatment after excision with or without breast irradiation.[89,92–94,104]

Radiotherapy May Cause Harm. Numerous studies have shown that WBRT for breast cancer may increase mortality from both lung cancer and cardiovascular disease.[140–144] As well, radiation fibrosis due to therapy may change the texture of the breast and skin, making mammographic follow-up more difficult and can result in delayed diagnosis if there is a local recurrence. Because there is no proof that breast irradiation for patients with DCIS improves survival and there is proof that radiation therapy may cause harm, it makes perfect sense to spare patients from this potentially dangerous treatment whenever possible.

Socioeconomic. Radiation therapy is expensive and time consuming (as much at $40,000 and taking 3–7 weeks).

Increased Risk. Some studies show that there are more invasive recurrences in irradiated patients than nonirradiated patients.[15,108] In our own series, 44% of excision only patients that recurred did so with invasive disease whereas 55% of irradiated patients who recurred, recurred with invasive cancer ($P < .01$). In our series, the median time to recurrence after excision alone was 40 months, whereas after excision and irradiation it was 78 months ($P < .01$). All subsets of DCIS show substantial delays in recurrence after irradiation—less in high grade and longest in low grade—and this delay can alter the perceived benefit of irradiation.[145]

Only One Time. If radiation therapy is given for the initial DCIS, it cannot be given again, at a later time, even if there is a small invasive recurrence. In general, we prefer to withhold radiation in DCIS patients initially and only give it to the few that ultimately recur with invasive disease. The use of radiation therapy with its accompanying skin and vascular changes make

skin-sparing mastectomy, if needed in the future, more difficult to perform.

Improved Patient Selection. The gold standard for local recurrence rates in irradiated patients is a 16% at 12 years as established by the NSABP B-17 trial.[18,89,102,118] A subsequent update showed a 19.8% local recurrence rate in the irradiated arm of B-17 at 15 years.[118] However, by using tools such as the USC/VNPI, it is now possible to select patients that recur at a rate of 8% or less at 12 years without radiation therapy (USC/VNPI scores 4–6).

NCCN Guidelines. Finally, within the 2008 NCCN guidelines, excision without radiation therapy has been added as an acceptable treatment for selected DCIS patients with low risk of recurrence.[110]

Prospective Randomized Ductal Carcinoma in Situ Trials

The NSABP B-06 protocol is the only prospective randomized trial that has compared mastectomy with breast conservation for patients with DCIS, albeit inadvertently.[70,129] Although this study investigated invasive disease, during central slide review a subgroup of 78 patients was confirmed to have pure DCIS without any evidence of invasion.[70] There were three treatment arms: total mastectomy, excision plus radiation therapy, and excision alone. Axillary nodes were removed regardless of the treatment assignment. After 83 months of follow-up, the percent of patients with local recurrences were zero for mastectomy, 7% for excision plus radiation therapy, and 43% for excision alone.[146] Despite these large differences in local recurrence, there was no difference among the three treatment groups in breast cancer-specific survival.

Numerous prospective randomized trials have demonstrated a significant reduction in local recurrence for DCIS patients treated with radiation therapy compared with excision alone: the NSABP (protocol B-17)[102]; the European Organization for Research and Treatment of Cancer (EORTC) protocol 10853[104]; the United Kingdom, Australia, New Zealand DCIS Trial (UK/ANZ Trial)[92]; and the Swedish Trial.[94] However, none of these trials has reported a survival benefit.[18,19,89,92,93,102–104,118,147–149]

In the NSABP B-17 Trial, more than 800 patients with DCIS excised with clear surgical margins were randomized into two groups: excision alone versus excision plus radiation therapy. The main end point was local recurrence, invasive or noninvasive. The definition of a clear margin was nontransection of the DCIS. The results of NSABP B-17 were updated in 1995,[148] 1998,[103] 1999,[18] 2001,[89] and 2011.[118] After 15 years of follow-up, there was a statistically significant, 50% decrease of both invasive and noninvasive local recurrences in patients treated with radiation therapy compared with those treated with excision alone (19.8% and 35%, respectively).[118] There was no difference in distant disease-free or overall survival in either arm. These data led the NSABP to continue recommending postoperative radiation therapy for all patients with DCIS who chose to save their breasts. Clearly, this recommendation was based on the decreased local recurrence rates rather than survival advantages.

Results from the EORTC 10853 trial, designed almost identically to the NSABP B-17 trial, were published in 2000[104,147] and updated in 2006.[149] After 10 years of follow-up, 15% of patients treated with excision plus radiation therapy had recurred locally compared with 26% of patients treated with excision alone.[149] As in the NSABP B-17 Trial, there was no difference in distant disease-free or overall survival in either arm of the EORTC Trial. Although in the initial report there was a statistically significant increase in contralateral breast cancer in patients who were randomized to receive radiation therapy, this was not observed when the data were updated.

The UK/ANZ Trial was published in 2003[19] and updated in 2011.[92] In this trial, 1694 patients that had been excised with clear margins (nontransection of DCIS) were randomized to receive radiotherapy (yes or no) and/or to tamoxifen versus placebo. This yielded four subgroups: excision alone, excision plus radiation therapy, excision plus tamoxifen, and excision plus radiation therapy plus tamoxifen. With a median follow-up of 12.7 years, those who received radiation therapy demonstrated a statistically significant decrease in ipsilateral breast tumor recurrence, similar in magnitude to the NSABP B-17 and EORTC trials. As with the NSABP and the EORTC, there was no difference in survival, regardless of treatment, in any arm of the UK DCIS trial.

The Swedish DCIS Trial[94] randomized 1067 patients into two groups: excision alone versus excision plus radiation therapy. In contrast to the trials discussed earlier, microscopically clear margins were not mandatory. Indeed, 22% of patients had microscopically unknown or involved margins. The cumulative incidence of local recurrence at 10 years was 21.6% for excision only and 10.3% for excision plus radiation therapy with an overall hazard ration of 0.33 ($P < .0001$).[94] There were 15 distant metastases and breast cancer related deaths in the excision only arm and 18 in the excision plus radiation therapy (P = nonsignificant).[94,150] As in the NSABP B-17, EORTC, and UK/ANZ trials, women treated with radiotherapy in the Swedish DCIS trial exhibited lower recurrence rates.[94] However, the trial found no evidence in the relative risk of invasive and noninvasive recurrences and no difference in distant disease-free or overall survival in either arm.[94]

In 2007 Viani and colleagues[93] published a meta-analysis of the four prospective randomized DCIS trials comparing excision alone with excision plus radiation therapy. Pooled data on 3665 patients revealed a 60% reduction of both invasive and DCIS recurrences ($P < .00001$) with the addition of radiation therapy. There was, however, no decrease in distant metastases in those who received radiation therapy, nor was there any survival benefit. Patients with high-grade lesions and involved margins received the most benefit from radiation therapy.

In 2010, the Early Breast Cancer Trialists Collaborative Group (EBCTCG)[151] published an overview of the four randomized DCIS trials, reaching very similar conclusions to Viani and colleagues.[93] The EBCTCG reaffirmed a lower local recurrence rate in all subgroups of patients who received adjuvant radiation therapy but no significant effect on breast cancer or all-cause mortality.[151]

Tamoxifen for Ductal Carcinoma in Situ

Tamoxifen is now considered a standard adjuvant agent for local control in DCIS patients undergoing breast conservation with or without irradiation. This viewpoint is largely due to the initial results of NSABP B-24[18] and the UK/ANZ Trial,[92] both which claimed a small but significant benefit for ipsilateral local control and contralateral chemoprevention.

Results of the NSABP B-24 trial[18] were first published in 1999 and updated in 2011.[19,118] In the B-24 protocol, more than 1800 DCIS patients were treated with excision and radiation therapy,

and then randomized to receive either tamoxifen or placebo. After 15 years of follow-up, 16.6% of patients treated with placebo had recurred locally, whereas only 13.2% of those treated with tamoxifen had recurred.[118] The difference, although small, was statistically significant for invasive local recurrences but not for DCIS recurrences.

Similar to the results of the NSABP B-24 trial, the UK/ANZ Trial also demonstrated that tamoxifen significantly reduced the incidence of ipsilateral DCIS recurrences but not invasive recurrences.[92] The scale of risk reduction was comparable to those observed in the NSABP B-24 trial. Moreover, tamoxifen provided no additional benefit in those who were irradiated.[92]

However, in 2012 when Allred and colleagues reexamined the rates of ipsilateral recurrences in a subset of 732 patients from NSABP B-24 trial, p values for the differences between tamoxifen versus placebo fell short of statistical significance.[17] Similarly, when Cuzick and colleagues provided an update of the UK trial in 2011,[19] there was no significant difference in either ipsilateral or contralateral events between patients with or without tamoxifen therapy. These findings are exactly opposite those seen in the NSABP B-24 trial.[18] Of interest, upon reanalysis, patients that did not receive radiation showed significant differences in contralateral events related to tamoxifen. Because only the ipsilateral breast undergoes radiation therapy, it is unclear why contralateral events are suppressed by tamoxifen in the nonirradiated group, but not in the irradiated group.

Based on the results of these clinical trials, Warrick and Allred[152] concluded that tamoxifen is probably overused and advocate more selective use of the drug. They particularly note that a major benefit would be seen in patients with estrogen-positive disease who are premenopausal with extensive high-grade disease and/or narrow margins. On the whole, the clinical benefit of tamoxifen intervention based on the randomized trials is meager at best.

Determination of HER2/neu Status and Potential Benefit of Neoadjuvant Trastuzumab

The HER2/neu gene is amplified or overexpressed in approximately 25% to 30% of invasive breast carcinomas.[153] It is now standard of care to treat HER2/neu-positive invasive breast cancers greater than 10 mm with the monoclonal antibody trastuzumab (Herceptin). Indeed, this therapy has had a major impact on relapse in patients with HER2/neu-positive invasive breast cancers. Although approximately 40% of DCIS lesions also exhibit amplification and/or overexpression of HER2/neu,[50,52,154,155] there is a lack of evidence that HER2/neu-positive DCIS will respond to trastuzumab therapy in a manner equivalent to invasive disease.

In 2012, Von Minckwitz and colleagues[156] examined the effect of chemotherapy plus trastuzumab on HER2/neu-positive DCIS adjacent to HER2/neu-positive invasive breast cancer. Treatment reduced the volume of adjacent DCIS suggesting the possibility of a therapeutic impact of chemotherapy plus trastuzumab on the HER2/neu-positive in situ component.

In contrast, in 2011 Kuerer and colleagues[157] described the results of a pilot study in which patients with large areas of HER-2/neu-positive DCIS (mean 5.2 cm) received a single dose of trastuzumab with follow-up surgical excision and reevaluation 14 to 28 days post therapy. No overt histologic response to the biological therapy was recorded; there was no alteration in ki67 or cleaved caspase.[157] However, pretreatment increased antibody-dependent cell-mediated cytotoxicity.[157]

Predicting Local Recurrence in Conservatively Treated Patients With DCIS

There are now sufficient, readily available data that can aid clinicians in differentiating patients who significantly benefit from radiation therapy after excision from those who do not. These same data can identify patients who are better served by mastectomy because recurrence rates with breast conservation even with the addition of radiation therapy are unacceptably high.

Our research[4,22,26,57,59,139,158] and the research of others[55,60,106,107,148,159] has shown that various combinations of nuclear grade, the presence of comedo-type necrosis, tumor size, margin width, and age are all important factors that can be used to predict the probability of local recurrence in conservatively treated DCIS patients.

Treatment Selection for Patients With DCIS of the Breast Using the University of Southern California/Van Nuys Prognostic Index

In 2008 the NCCN included excision alone as an acceptable treatment alternative for patients with DCIS, validating an actual practice in the United States in which almost 50% of conservatively treated patients do not receive postexcisional breast irradiation.[110] However, the NCCN did not define the subset of patients in which excision without radiation therapy was appropriate.[110] Researchers have attempted to accomplish this for years but with only marginal success. Multivariate analysis has shown that six factors are independent predictors of local recurrence in patients with DCIS treated with breast conservation: treatment (radiation therapy yields a lower local recurrence rate than excision alone), age (older age is better), size (smaller size is better), nuclear grade (lower grade is better), margin width (wider margins are better), comedonecrosis (no necrosis is better).[160–162]

In 1995, the Van Nuys Classification was developed that used a combination of nuclear grade and necrosis to predict local recurrence.[59] In 1996, the Van Nuys Prognostic Index added size and margin width to the numerical algorithm[25] and in 2002, the USC/VNPI added age at diagnosis to the algorithm.[158,162] These studies collected all pathologic features in a prospective fashion but treatment (excision alone vs. excision plus radiation therapy) was not randomized.

The USC/VNPI was devised by combining four statistically significant independent prognostic factors for local tumor recurrence (tumor size, margin width, age, and pathologic classification (determined by nuclear grade and the presence or absence of comedo-type necrosis). Each of the four prognostic predictors was scored 1, 2, or 3, where 1 is the most favorable and 3 the least favorable. Table 39.1 details this scoring system. The individual scores for each of the four prognostic factors were added together to give an overall score ranging from a low of 4 (least likely to recur) to a high of 12 (most likely to recur). Prior published recommendations were excision alone for those who score 4, 5, or 6; excision plus radiation therapy for those who score 7, 8, or 9; and mastectomy for those who scored 10, 11, or 12.[4,7]

In this chapter, we use the USC/VNPI to analyze local recurrence rates and to update treatment recommendations in a large

TABLE 39.1 The USC/VNPI Scoring System^a

Score	Size	Margin	VN Class	Age
1	≤15 mm	≥10 mm	Grade 1–2 without necrosis	>60
2	16–40	1–9	Grade 1–2 without necrosis	40–60
3	>40	<1	Grade 3	<40

^{a}A score of 1 (best) to 3 (worst) is given for each of four factors (size, margin width, pathologic classification, and age). The individual scores are totaled to give an overall USC/VNPI Score ranging from 4 (best) to 12 (worst).

USC/VNPI, University of Southern California/Van Nuys Prognostic Index.

series of patients with pure DCIS for whom all histopathologic factors were collected within a prospective database. When originally published in 1996, the Van Nuys Prognostic Index was based on 333 patients.[25] With five times as many patients accrued since originally described, sufficient numbers of patients currently exist for analysis by individual score rather than groups of scores.

From 1979 through 2015, 1855 patients with pure DCIS were treated. No patients with invasive cancer, no matter how small the invasive focus, were included; 576 patients were treated with mastectomy, 424 with excision and standard radiation therapy, 131 with excision and intraoperative radiation therapy (IORT), and 724 with excision alone.

No patient received any form of chemotherapy. Endocrine therapy was used at the discretion of the medical oncologist. Treatment was not randomized. Patient preference, after full disclosure and discussion of available data, was the major factor in the treatment decision-making process.

Every effort was made to excise all lesions completely and to examine microscopically all excised tissue. Localization by bracketing wires, intraoperative radiography of the specimen, and correlation with the preoperative mammogram were performed in every case. The specimen was oriented and margins were marked with ink or colored dye.

IORT is a new and experimental form of therapy. Although we have accrued 131 patients to a prospective IORT database, the median follow-up for this subgroup in only 24 months. Therefore they have not been included in any analyses in this chapter.

Pathologic Evaluation

The resected tissue was sectioned sequentially into uniform slices. The entire resection was embedded in sequence. Pathologic evaluation included determination of the histologic subtype, nuclear grade, the presence or absence of comedo-type necrosis, the maximal extent of the lesion, and margin width.

The size of small lesions was determined by direct measurement of stained slides. The size of larger lesions was determined by a combination of direct measurement and calculation according to three-dimensional reconstruction with a sequential series of slides. This approach is now the recommended protocol of the College of American Pathologists and is an absolute prerequisite for the determination of a USC/VNPI score.[27,82]

Margin width was determined by direct measurement or ocular micrometry. The smallest single distance between the edge of the tumor and an inked line delineating the margin of normal tissue was reported. Margins in patients who underwent reexcision and in whom no additional DCIS was found were reported as being equivalent to 10 mm in width.

Pathologic classification was determined by dividing tumors into three groups by using the Van Nuys DCIS Classification: grade 1 = low or intermediate nuclear grade without necrosis; grade 2 = low or intermediate nuclear grade with necrosis; and grade 3 = high nuclear grade with or without necrosis. Necrosis was not quantified but classified as present or absent. Nuclear grade was determined by the highest nuclear grade present, not by average grade.

Any ipsilateral breast event, regardless of location, was included in analyses called "all local recurrences." However, a subgroup of local recurrences were scored as "true local recurrences" if they were at or near the primary tumor, within the same quadrant as the primary tumor or within 5 cm of the primary tumor.

Statistical Analysis

Time to local recurrence, calculated as the time from date of diagnosis to the date of local recurrence, was used as the end point. Any ipsilateral breast event, regardless of quadrant, was counted as a local recurrence. The quadrant of recurrence was also recorded, making it possible to analyze all local recurrences and same quadrant local recurrences. Data from patients who did not have a local recurrence were censored at the date of last follow-up. Kaplan-Meier plots were used to estimate the probability of remaining free of local recurrence at 12 years. The statistical significance between survival curves was determined by the log-rank test.

In previous papers, patients were grouped by USC/VNPI scores of 4, 5, and 6, scores of 7, 8, and 9, and scores of 10, 11, and 12.[4,7] In this study, all analyses were done by individual scores from 4 to 12. The goal was to define the parameters necessary to allow a local recurrence rate of less than 20% at 12 years for each individual score. Less than 20% local recurrence rate at 12 years was an arbitrary choice but seemed reasonable on the basis of previously reported prospective randomized data; for example, the NSABP-B17 data at 12 years showed a 16% local recurrence rate with irradiation and a 32% recurrence rate without irradiation.[89,118]

Local recurrence rates, regardless of treatment were so low for all patients who scored 4, 5, or 6 (<8% for all scores) that they were grouped together in the final analysis. Local recurrence rates, regardless of treatment, were so high for patients who scored 10, 11, or 12 (greater than 40% for all scores) that they were also grouped together in the final analysis. Patients who scored 7, 8, or 9 are shown by individual score.

Results

After removing 131 patients treated with excision plus IORT, there were 1724 patients to be analyzed, 576 treated with mastectomy, 424 treated with excision plus standard radiation therapy, and 724 patients treated with excision alone.

Among 556 patients treated by mastectomy, there were 13 local recurrences, 9 of which were invasive. The Kaplan-Meier probability of local recurrence at 12 years after mastectomy for DCIS was 4%. Eleven (85%) local recurrences after mastectomy occurred in patients who scored 10 to 12 using the USC/VNPI. There were 2 local recurrences after mastectomy in patients who scored 7 to 9 and none in patients who scored 4 to 6.[163]

Among 424 patients treated with excision plus radiation, there were 79 local recurrences, 43 of which were invasive. The Kaplan-Meier probability of any local recurrence at 12-years after excision plus radiation therapy for DCIS was 24%. When same quadrant

local recurrence is used as the end point, there were 58 true local recurrences after excision plus radiation therapy. The Kaplan-Meier probability of true local recurrence at 12-years after excision plus radiation therapy for DCIS was 19%. Twenty-one local recurrences (27%) were in quadrants different from the index lesion and considered to likely represent new primaries.

Among 724 patients treated with excision alone, there were 130 local recurrences, 54 (42%) of which were invasive. The Kaplan-Meier probability of any local recurrence at 12 years after excision alone for DCIS was 31%. When true local recurrence is used as the end point, there were 118 true local recurrences after excision plus radiation therapy. The Kaplan-Meier probability of true local recurrence at 12 years after excision alone for DCIS was 29%. Twelve local recurrences (9%) were in quadrants different from the index lesion and considered to most likely represent new primaries.

The average follow-up was 88 months for all patients, 105 months for patients who received radiation therapy, 79 months for patients treated with excision alone, and 84 months for patients treated with mastectomy.

Thirteen patients treated with breast conservation developed metastatic breast cancer after a local invasive recurrence, 11 of whom died from breast cancer. Eighty patients died from causes not related to breast cancer. The 12-year Kaplan-Meier probability of dying from breast cancer among all 1724 patients with DCIS was 0.8%. A meta-analysis of four prospective randomized DCIS trials by Viani and colleagues[93] revealed that the probability of dying from breast cancer after treatment for DCIS was extremely low and statistically identical regardless of treatment.

Fig. 39.5 shows 392 patients with scores of 4, 5, or 6 analyzed by treatment (excision alone vs. excision plus radiation therapy). The local recurrence rate at 12 years for all patients who received radiation therapy was 3.5%. As all local recurrences after radiation therapy were in different quadrants, the true local recurrence rate should be considered 0%. For those treated with excision alone, the all local recurrence rate was 7.5% (P = nonsignificant). The same quadrant or true local recurrence rate was 6.7%. When analyzed by individual score, those who scored 4, 5, or 6, regardless of treatment, had a local recurrence rate less than 8% at 10 years and hence were grouped together.

Fig. 39.6 shows 638 breast conservation patients who scored 7, 8, or 9. Neither treatment curve meets the less than 20% local recurrence guideline at 12 years. Therefore each score (7, 8, and 9) was analyzed individually by various margin widths (1, 2, 3, 5, and 10 mm), with and without radiation therapy.

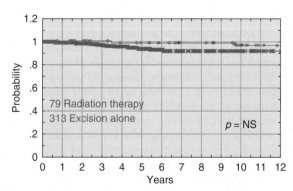

• **Fig. 39.5** Local recurrence-free survival for 392 patients with University of Southern California/Van Nuys Prognostic Index (USC/VNPI) scores of 4, 5, or 6 analyzed by treatment: 79 excision plus radiation therapy (blue) versus 313 excision alone (red). NS = no significant difference.

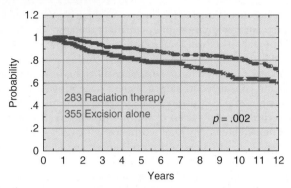

• **Fig. 39.6** Local recurrence-free survival for 638 patients with University of Southern California/Van Nuys Prognostic Index (USC/VNPI) scores of 7, 8, or 9 analyzed by treatment: 283 excision plus radiation therapy (blue) versus 355 excision alone (red) (p = .002).

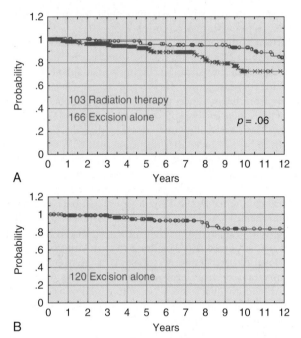

• **Fig. 39.7** (A) Local recurrence-free survival for 269 patients with University of Southern California/Van Nuys Prognostic Index (USC/VNPI) scores of 7 analyzed by treatment: 103 excision plus radiation therapy (blue) versus 166 excision alone (red) (p = .06). (B) Local recurrence-free survival for 120 patients with USC/VNPI scores of 7 and margin width of 3 mm or more treated by excision alone.

Fig. 39.7A shows 269 patients who scored 7. The local recurrence rate at 12 years for those who scored 7 and received radiation therapy was 16% but for those treated with excision alone, it was 28%. The next step was to analyze various margin widths for patients who scored 7 and were treated with excision alone to find the margin width necessary to lower the local recurrence rate to less than 28% at 12-years.

Fig. 39.7B shows 120 patients who scored 7, were treated with excision alone, and who had margin widths of 3 mm or more. This subgroup had a local recurrence rate of 16% at 10 years, meeting the requirement.

This process was repeated for patients who scored 8 to 12. The minimum treatment necessary to achieve a local recurrence rate less than 20% at 10 years is detailed in Table 39.2. Regardless of margin width, no patient who scored 10, 11, or 12 could achieve

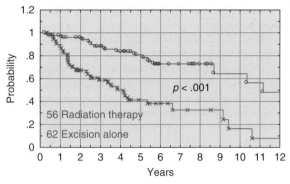

• **Fig. 39.8** Local recurrence-free survival for 118 patients with University of Southern California/Van Nuys Prognostic Index (USC/VNPI) scores of 10, 11, or 12 analyzed by treatment: 62 excision plus radiation therapy (red) versus 56 excision alone (blue) (p < .001).

TABLE 39.2	Minimum Treatment Recommendations to Achieve a Local Recurrence Rate Less Than 20% at 12 Years Using the USC/VNPI Scoring System	
USC/VNPI	**Treatment**	**12-Year Recurrence**
4, 5, or 6	Excision alone	<8%
7, Margins ≥3 mm	Excision alone	16%
7, Margins <3 mm	Radiation	19%
8, Margins ≥3 mm	Radiation	11%
8, Margins <3 mm	Mastectomy	0%
9, Margins ≥3 mm	Radiation	17%
9, Margins <3 mm	Mastectomy	0%
10, 11, or 12	Mastectomy	8%

USC/VNPI, University of Southern California/Van Nuys Prognostic Index.

a local recurrence rate less than 40% with radiation therapy, and it was necessary to recommend mastectomy for the entire group. Fig. 39.8 shows 118 breast conservation patients who scored 10, 11, or 12.

Discussion of Using USC/VNPI to Select Treatment

Radiation therapy after excision for DCIS has routinely been shown to decrease the local recurrence rate by approximately 50% in multiple prospective randomized trials.[21,89,104,118,164] Despite this, no trial has demonstrated difference in breast cancer specific survival, regardless of the treatment used.[93] Because no treatment is associated with an increase in survival, whenever possible we should strive for the lowest amount of treatment that yields an acceptable local recurrence rate.

With five times as many patients as originally published, the USC/VNPI can be more finely tuned to aid in the treatment decision-making process. To achieve a local recurrence rate of less than 20% at 10 years, our data support excision alone for patients scoring 4, 5, or 6 and patients who score 7 but have margin widths 3 mm or greater.

Excision plus radiation therapy achieves the less than 20% local recurrence requirement at 10 years for patients who score 7 and have margins less than 3 mm, patients who score 8 and have margins 3 mm or greater, and for patients who score 9 and have margins 5 mm or greater.

Mastectomy is required for patients who score 8 and have margins less than 3 mm, who score 9 and have margins less than 5 mm and for all patients who score 10, 11, or 12 to keep the local recurrence rate less than 20% at 10 years.

If the closest margin width is less than 10 mm and the patient is amenable to reexcision, the USC/VNPI can theoretically be lowered by 1 to 2 points. Margin width is the only variable under surgical control. Neither grade nor size can be reduced by reexcision.

The pattern of local recurrence in patients treated with excision alone and excision plus radiation therapy is different and merits comment. Ninety-one percent of local recurrences in patients treated with excision alone occurred within the same quadrant as the index lesion compared with only 73% in patients treated with excision plus radiation therapy ($P < .001$). Fifty-four of 130 (42%) of local recurrences were invasive in patients treated with excision alone whereas 43 of 79 (54%) of local recurrences were invasive in patients treated with excision plus radiation therapy ($P < .01$). The median time to local recurrence after excision alone was 39 months, whereas after excision plus radiation therapy, it was 66 months ($P < .01$). Radiation therapy has a profound impact on the nature, location, and timing of local recurrence in patients with DCIS.

The choice of less than 20% local recurrence rate at 10 years was somewhat arbitrary, although the NSABP reported 19.6% at 15 years for patients treated with excision and radiation therapy.[118] If one were to elect 10% or 15% as the maximum allowable recurrence rate, the recommendations would change to include more mastectomies, more radiation therapy, and less excision alone. If one were to accept 25% or even 30% as the maximum allowable recurrence rate, the recommendations would change to include more excision alone, more radiation therapy, and fewer mastectomies.

Using the USC/VNPI for Patients Undergoing Mastectomy

Patients with DCIS who are treated with mastectomy seldom recur locally or with metastatic disease. We questioned whether the USC/VNPI could predict these infrequent events.[163] In our series 576 patients with pure DCIS were treated with mastectomy. Average follow-up was 86 months. 16 patients developed recurrences: 2 metastatic without local recurrence, 1 metastatic with a preceding local recurrence, and 13 local recurrences without metastatic disease. Eleven of 16 (69%) recurrences were invasive; five (31%) were DCIS. Fifteen of 16 (94%) patients who recurred had multifocal disease; 10/16 (63%) had multicentric disease. Using the USC/VNPI, patients scoring 4 to 9 were compared with those scored 10 to 12 in Table 39.3 and Fig. 39.9.

DCIS patients scoring 10 to 12 using the USC/VNPI were significantly ($P < .001$) more likely to develop recurrence after mastectomy than patients scoring 4 to 9. At particularly high risk were young patients with large high-grade tumors and close or involved mastectomy margins. These data should be used when counseling a patient who is considering postmastectomy radiation therapy.

Oncotype DX Breast DCIS Score

Which conservatively treated DCIS patients will develop local recurrences, and will the recurrence be invasive? Recently, a

TABLE 39.3 Using the USC/VNPI for Mastectomy			
USC/VNPI Score	4–9	10–12	P Value
N	303	273	
Average age	55	47	<.01
Average nuclear grade	2.07	11	<.01
Local recurrence only	2	11	<.01
Local recurrence then metastatic	0	1	NS
Metastatic only	0	2	NS
No. invasive recurrences	2	9	<.01
Probability recurrence at 12 years	1.2%	8%	<.01

NS, Nonsignificant difference; *USC/VNPI*, University of Southern California/Van Nuys Prognostic Index.

Five hundred seventy-six patients who underwent mastectomy were assigned USC/VNPI scores and divided into those who scored 4 to 9 versus those who scored 10 to 12. The groups are compared in the table.

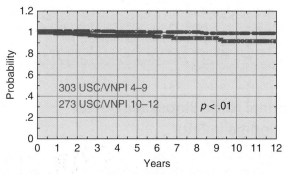

• **Fig. 39.9** Local recurrence-free survival for 576 mastectomy patients grouped by University of Southern California/Van Nuys Prognostic Index (USC/VNPI). 303 mastectomy patients who scored 4 to 9 (blue) versus 273 patients who score 10 to 12 (red) ($p < .01$).

multigene expression assay called Oncotype DX Breast for DCIS (Genomic Health, Redwood City, California) was developed in an effort to shed light on these two questions that physicians have been asking for decades.[165] The assay evaluates the expression level of seven prognostic genes normalized to the expression of five reference genes to calculate the DCIS score (ranging from 1 to 100) and is completely independent of the clinicopathologic features of a tumor.[165] Similar to the USC/VNPI, the Oncotype DX Breast DCIS score is intended to help select low-risk DCIS patients that do not require radiation therapy.

The Oncotype DX Breast DCIS assay was validated by Solin and colleagues using tissue samples of patients enrolled in the Eastern Cooperative Oncology Group (ECOG) E5194 study, a nonrandomized, prospective, multicenter study designed to compare the treatment of DCIS using surgical excision with or without radiation therapy.[165,166] When test DCIS scores were divided into low-risk (DCIS score <39), intermediate-risk (DCIS score 39–54), and high-risk (DCIS score ≥55) groups,[167] the overall local recurrence rates were found to be 10.6%, 26.7%, and 29.5% respectively at 10 years.[165] At 10 years, the invasive local recurrence rates for the 3 groups were 3.7%, 12.3%, and 19.2%, respectively.[165] These data have been supported in a Canadian population-based validation study.[167] Thus both study authors concluded that the Oncotype DX Breast DCIS test predicts the risk of both local and invasive local recurrences and provides physicians with data that complements traditional clinical and pathologic data.

However, the majority of physicians that order this test do not appreciate the limitation of these validated results. First, only very low-risk DCIS patients were enrolled in the ECOG E5194 study. The ECOG E5194 study was restricted to patients with tumor margins ≥ 3 mm. Permissible size was also restricted, with low- or intermediate-grade DCIS ≤ 25 mm and high grade ≤ 10 mm in size. Therefore the Oncotype DX Breast DCIS score is only applicable that meet these criteria. Second, although the results of the population-based study by Rakovitch and colleagues support the overall conclusions of the ECOG E5194 study, it also draws attention to the inability of the DCIS score to differentiate intermediate- and high-risk DCIS.[167] Specifically, in situ tumors with intermediate and high Oncotype DX Breast DCIS scores exhibited similar recurrence risks (33% and 27.8%, respectively).[167] Third, because the assay does not account for predictive factors such as age, margin width, extent of disease, and necrosis it is unlikely to be accurate for the majority of patients. Finally, the cost of the test is excessive, currently costing each patient approximately $4000 out of pocket.

There may come a time when there is an affordable genetic test that can accurately predict the likelihood of both local recurrence and local invasive recurrence in the majority of DCIS patients. However, this will not be a test that does not take into account proven predictive factors.

Sentinel Node Biopsy for Ductal Carcinoma in Situ

Although axillary lymph node dissection for DCIS patients has been abandoned for more than 20 years,[168–170] we do perform sentinel node biopsy on selected DCIS patients. We perform it for all patients with DCIS who are undergoing a mastectomy. In addition, we perform sentinel node biopsy if there is any suspicion on breast imaging or core biopsy pathology that there may be an invasive component. We also perform a sentinel node biopsy for palpable DCIS.

Summary

DCIS is now a relatively common disease, and its frequency is increasing. Most DCIS detected today will be nonpalpable and will be detected by mammographic calcifications. It is not uncommon for DCIS to be larger than expected by mammography, to involve more than one quadrant of the breast, and to be unicentric but multifocal in its distribution. Not all microscopic DCIS will progress to clinical cancer, but if a patient has DCIS and is not treated, she is more likely to develop an ipsilateral invasive breast cancer than is a woman without DCIS.

The initial breast biopsy should be a percutaneous image-guided core biopsy. After establishment of the diagnosis, the patient should be counseled. Preoperative evaluation should include digital mammography with magnification views and ultrasonography. MRI is liked by some, shunned by others. We obtain an MRI on every patient diagnosed with any form of breast cancer. If she is motivated for breast conservation, the surgeon, plastic surgeon, and radiologist should plan the procedure together carefully, using multiple wires to map out the extent of the lesion.

The first attempt at excision is the best chance to get a complete excision with a good cosmetic result. Reexcision often yields a poor cosmetic result and the overall plan should be to avoid reexcision whenever possible.

High-grade comedo DCIS is more aggressive and malignant in its histologic appearance and is more likely to be associated with a subsequent invasive cancer than the lower-grade noncomedo subtypes. Comedo DCIS treated conservatively is also more likely to recur locally than noncomedo DCIS. However, separation of DCIS into two groups by architecture is an oversimplification and does not reflect the biological potential of the lesion as well as stratification by nuclear grade and comedo-type necrosis.

The USC/VNPI uses five independent predictors to predict the probability of local recurrence after conservative treatment for DCIS: tumor size, margin width, nuclear grade, age, and the presence or absence of comedo-type necrosis. In combination, they can be used as an aid to identifying subgroups of patients with different recurrence potentials. For example, patients who score 4, 5, or 6 using the USC/VNPI have extremely low probabilities of local recurrence after excision alone. If size cannot be accurately determined, margin width by itself can be used as a surrogate for the USC/VNPI, although it is not as precise and is associated with an increased risk of local recurrence.

Oncoplastic surgery combines sound surgical oncologic principles with plastic surgical techniques. Coordination of the two surgical disciplines may help to avoid poor cosmetic results after wide excision and may increase the number of women who can be treated with BCS by allowing larger breast excisions with more acceptable cosmetic results. Oncoplastic surgery requires cooperation and coordination of surgical oncology, radiology, and pathology. Oncoplastic resection is a therapeutic procedure, not a breast biopsy, and is performed on patients with a proven diagnosis of breast cancer. New oncoplastic techniques that allow for more extensive excisions can be used to achieve both acceptable cosmesis and widely clear margins, reducing the need for radiation therapy in many cases of DCIS.[171]

When considering the entire population of patients with DCIS without subset analyses, prospective randomized trials have shown that postexcisional radiation therapy can reduce the relative risk of local recurrence by about 50% for conservatively treated patients. However, in some low-risk DCIS patients, the costs may outweigh the potential benefits. Despite a relative 50% reduction in the probability of local recurrence, the absolute reduction may be only a few percent. Moreover the local recurrence rate at 15 years for NSABP B-17's irradiated arm is 20%.[118] Although local recurrence is extremely important, breast cancer–specific survival is the most important end point for all patients with breast cancer, including patients with DCIS, and no DCIS trial has ever shown a survival benefit for radiation therapy compared with excision alone.

In recent years, an increasing number of selected patients with DCIS have been treated with excision alone. Excision alone has now become an acceptable form of treatment for selected patients since the 2008 NCCN Guidelines.[110] The decision to use excision alone as treatment for DCIS should only be made if the patient has been fully informed and has participated in the treatment decision-making process.

Selected References

4. Lagios M, Westdahl P, Margolin F, Rose M. Duct Carcinoma in situ: relationship of extent of noninvasive disease to the frequency

of occult invasion, multicentricity, lymph node metastases, and short-term treatment failures. *Cancer.* 1982;50:1309-1314.

25. Silverstein MJ, Poller D, Craig P, et al. A prognostic index for ductal carcinoma in situ of the breast. *Cancer.* 1996;77: 2267-2274.

26. Silverstein MJ, Lagios M, Groshen S, et al. The influence of margin width on local control in patients with ductal carcinoma in situ (DCIS) of the breast. *N Engl J Med.* 1999;340:1455-1461.

118. Wapnir I, Dignam J, Fisher B, et al. Long-term outcomes of invasive ipsilateral breast tumor recurrences after lumpectomy in NSABP B-17 and B-24 randomized clinical trials for DCIS. *J Natl Cancer Inst.* 2011;103:478-488.

151. Early Breast Cancer Trialists Collaborative Group. Overview of the randomized trials of radiotherapy in ductal carcinoma in situ of the breast. *J Natl Cancer Inst Monogr.* 2010;41:162-177.

A full reference list is available online at ExpertConsult.com.

40

The New Paradigm: Oncoplastic Breast Conservation Surgery

COLLEEN M. O'KELLY PRIDDY, NIRAV B. SAVALIA, AND MELVIN J. SILVERSTEIN

The adoption of breast conserving therapy as an acceptable alternative to mastectomy opened the door to a wide and varied range of partial breast reconstruction techniques. The term *oncoplastic breast surgery*, as suggested by Werner Audretsch in 1993,[1] describes the concept of local tissue rearrangement that would allow for wide resection of tumors while preserving or improving breast cosmesis. Although the term has been used more broadly to include nipple- and skin-sparing mastectomies with immediate reconstruction, this chapter focuses on immediate or delayed partial breast reconstruction with volume-displacing or volume-replacing techniques after wide excision of the primary lesion. In other words, oncoplastic breast conservation. A contralateral mammaplasty or mastopexy is generally required for symmetry due to the loss of volume from removal of the index cancer.

Traditionally, surgical oncologists are trained to remove the cancer at all costs, with little emphasis placed on the importance of the cosmetic result. Many women have simple excisions and appear to have a reasonable cosmetic outcome in the early postoperative period, but the early results are sometimes misleading. The addition of scarring, resolution of the seroma, and radiotherapy ultimately reveals the true esthetic outcome many months or even years later.

Oncoplastic breast conservation surgery is a new paradigm combining sound oncologic principles with plastic surgery techniques, allowing for wide excision of tumors with minimized risk of involved margins and simultaneous prevention of the deformities commonly associated with simple excisions and postradiotherapy fibrosis.[2] It requires a philosophy that the appearance and function of the breast after tumor excision is important; the patient will live with this result for the rest of her life. The goals of oncoplastic breast surgery include complete removal of the lesion with negative margins, a good to excellent cosmetic result, and the definitive procedure at a single operation. Over the past 30 years we have developed a comprehensive multidisciplinary oncoplastic approach for the surgical treatment of breast cancer.[3-6] This requires an approach that includes coordination with the surgical oncologist, radiologist, plastic surgeon, medical oncologist, pathologist, radiation oncologist, and genetic counselor. As improved breast imaging and neoadjuvant chemotherapy allow a larger number of women to be considered for breast conservation, the combination of oncologic and plastic surgery disciplines also increases the number of women who may be treated with breast conserving surgery by allowing larger

excisions with more acceptable cosmetic results.[7] These techniques are applicable to patients with both noninvasive (ductal carcinoma in situ [DCIS]) and invasive breast cancers. Furthermore, now that excision without radiation therapy is an accepted treatment for patients with biologically favorable DCIS, widely clear margins are of even greater importance than previously appreciated.[8,9]

An important goal in caring for a woman with breast cancer is to go to the operating room once and perform a definitive procedure that does not require reoperation. The first attempt to remove a cancer is critical, offering the best chance to remove the entire lesion in a single piece, evaluate its true extent and margin status, and to achieve the best possible cosmetic result. The concept of a one-stage operation is important in the psychological and emotional recovery of a cancer patient.[10] Fewer procedures allow the patient to quickly move on with her life, to the next phase of treatment, if necessary. With this in mind, it is of highest importance to thoroughly stage the cancer preoperatively and carefully plan the operation. This is accomplished by reviewing the patient's full diagnosis, stage, pathology, imaging, risk of recurrence, and risk of developing cancer in the contralateral breast. Whenever possible, the initial breast biopsy should be performed using a minimally invasive percutaneous technique.[11] This usually provides ample tissue for diagnosis and biomarker analysis and should be possible in more than 98% of cases.[12] Preoperative knowledge of tumor biology can sometimes be exploited by using neoadjuvant systemic therapy, which will often downstage a tumor and convert the definitive operation from mastectomy to breast preservation.

General Considerations

Leading the Oncoplastic Team

Of utmost importance is a dedicated team approach. At our facility, the oncologic breast surgeon assumes the role of "leader" to guide the team and ensure excellent communication among all team members. During the first visit we generate a "flight plan" that summarizes the diagnosis, includes photos of the patient's chest and relevant imaging, and lists the plan of action leading up to and including the planned operation (Fig. 40.1). The flight plan is given to the patient, distributed to all team members, and updated and revised, if necessary, as the patient moves through the consultation process.

Diagnosis: RIGHT Grade II ductal carcinoma in situ,
ER/PR Positive, 12:00 position, spanning 27 mm on MRI.
12 mm on manno. 5 cm from nipple

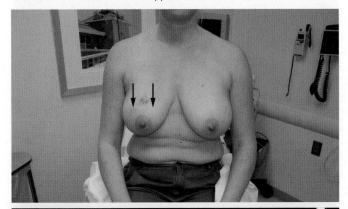

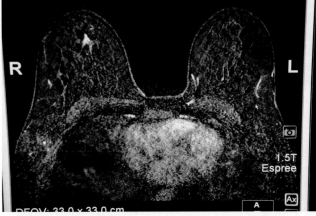

1. RIGHT wire guided segmental resection using split reduction
2. LEFT mastopexy for symmetry
3. Plastic surgical consultation with Dr. Davalia 949-759-0980
4. IORT consultation
5. Genetic counseling

• **Fig. 40.1** Example flight plan.

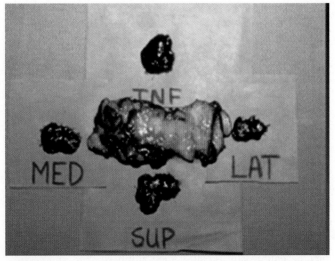

• **Fig. 40.2** The main specimen has been excised with four additional pieces representing the new margins. These additional specimens are clearly smaller than the true margins. Therefore the surgeon cannot be truly certain that the margins are negative. Removal of a single large specimen allows improved confidence in the margin status.

Rationale for Oncoplastic Breast Surgery

The primary goal of breast conservation is to achieve local control with adequate margins while maintaining breast cosmesis.[13] Unfortunately, as many as 36% of simple excisions fail to achieve adequate margins in a single operation, leading to reexcision, worsening cosmesis, and conversions to mastectomy.[14] The benefits of breast conservation compared with mastectomy are preservation of a sense of wholeness, retaining normal breast sensation, and limited morbidity from device-based or autologous reconstruction. The benefits are even greater when adjuvant radiotherapy must be added to postmastectomy reconstruction.[15]

A few of the factors implicated in poor cosmetic results after breast conservation are age greater than 60, tumors larger than 2 cm, small breast size, reexcision for inadequate margins, improper scar orientation, breast tissue resection greater than 100 cm^3 independent of breast size, breast ptosis, tumors located in the central, medial, or lower quadrants, and radiation dose inhomogeneity.[16–20] The common theme among all these limitations is that the removal of tissue without proper reshaping of the breast allows scarring and postradiation fibrosis to reveal an unreconstructed cavity, imbalance in breast tissue distribution, and

distortion of the nipple-areola complex (NAC). These limiting factors are largely overcome when an oncoplastic reconstruction is performed. Oncoplastic breast conservation allows rebalancing of the breast. The breast is reconstructed with either a volume displacing or volume replacing technique. This ability to maintain breast balance while reducing breast volume expands the pool of patients who could be considered candidates for breast conservation. This is of particular benefit to the patient with advanced disease who would need adjuvant radiotherapy regardless of mastectomy. These techniques are referred to as extreme oncoplasty or radical breast conservation and are discussed later in this chapter.[21,22]

Currently, because many as 40% to 50% of new breast cancer cases are discovered by modern state-of-the-art imaging.[11] Intraoperatively they are often grossly both nonpalpable and not visible to the surgeon's eye. Under these circumstances, the surgeon essentially operates blindly. Multiple hooked wires can help define the extent of the lesion and guide surgical excision.[23] Using bracketing wires or other newer forms of localization, the surgeon can usually excise the entire lesion within a single piece of tissue, sometimes including overlying skin as well as prepectoral fascia as the anterior and posterior margins. The tissue should be precisely oriented for the pathologist. Intraoperative two-view specimen radiography is extremely useful in localizing the lesion within the specimen, estimating margin distance, and ensuring complete removal.

If the specimen is removed in multiple pieces, rather than a single piece, accurate size and margin assessment may be compromised. Fig. 40.2 shows an excision specimen with four additional pieces that represent the new margins, but clearly the additional specimens do not encompass the full margin, leading to uncertainty about complete excision.

Reconstructive Goals

A common misconception is that the goal of breast reconstruction is to create the "perfect breast." In actuality, the goal should be to achieve an outcome that best suits the *patient's* goals for treatment and desires for final breast appearance. The patient's esthetic goals are often tempered by the complexity of many of the most modern and technically state-of-the-art reconstructive methods. In the same vein, the default reconstructive goal should not be to simply maintain the patient's current appearance. With this in mind, the reconstructive plan can be formulated only after analysis of the tumor size and location, the preoperative breast shape, size, and degree of ptosis, and understanding the patient's oncologic needs and reconstructive desires. The ideal is to minimize the amount of surgery, donor sites, recovery periods, risk of complications, and failure rates, while maximizing the desired esthetic and oncologic outcome.

Many reconstructive options exist, ranging from a simple tissue rearrangement to complex microvascular tissue flap reconstruction. Each step toward a more complex procedure must be carefully weighed against the patient's expectation of results and assessment of the risk to benefit ratio. Reconstructive surgeons may be tempted to use all of their advanced skills and create a complex surgical plan with multiple operations. However, the patient may be satisfied with the reasonable breast shape and symmetry achieved with a simpler course. The decision must be an amalgam of what is oncologically necessary and the simplest reconstructive plan that achieves the patient's goal. Our goal has always been to go to the operating room once, completing the oncologic and reconstructive portions of the case in a single procedure, if possible. The decision to use volume displacement techniques (in other words, to use existing breast volume to reconstruct the defect, versus volume replacement techniques that use regional or distant tissue flaps of varying complexity) depends on the reconstructive needs. Volume displacement techniques offer the simplest solution when there is adequate native breast tissue and the patient accepts a smaller reconstructed breast as well as the need for contralateral surgery to correct asymmetry. Volume replacement allows maintenance of the preoperative breast size but often requires longer operative time, longer recovery, and has associated donor-site morbidity. Our practice is devoted primarily to volume displacement reconstruction and defers to mastectomy only when this is not feasible. In other words, mastectomy (although sometimes appropriate and necessary) is our last choice and never our default option.

To help patients understand the value of oncoplastic breast conservation, they must be educated about their options and the rationale for patient selection and merits of simple excision versus oncoplastic breast conservation. For surgeons, the ability to predict the postlumpectomy deformity leads to understanding the importance of patient selection.

Women with smaller breasts (A/B cup) and minimal ptosis can be challenging. Simple excisions of small tumors are often believed to have little esthetic effect. This is often true when the tumor is in the upper or upper outer breast and a layered glandular repair is performed. However, even the smallest tumor can result in a postlumpectomy deformity if excised from the lower pole of the breast. Postoperative scarring will deform the lower pole and retraction will displace the NAC inferiorly, resulting in the classic "bird's beak" deformity (Fig. 40.3). This can be avoided by recentralizing the NAC over the reshaped breast mound immediately after the resection. With larger tumors, a prediction about the size of the defect will determine eligibility for breast conservation. If the predicted remaining breast is deemed adequate for reconstruction with glandular rearrangement, then oncoplastic breast surgery can be planned. However, if these predictions are inaccurate, then a post lumpectomy deformity will result. In retrospect, these

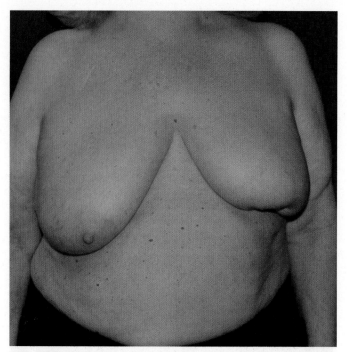

• **Fig. 40.3** "Bird's beak" deformity after excision of a lower pole tumor from the left breast.

patients may have been better managed with volume replacement techniques or with skin- or nipple-sparing mastectomy. These missteps can only be avoided with experience, and the novice oncoplastic surgeon should be wary.

Women with larger breasts (C/D cup and beyond) and ptosis will benefit from oncoplastic breast surgery both oncologically and esthetically. An oncoplastic approach will allow a larger excision with higher probability of obtaining adequate margins as well as correction of breast ptosis and macromastia. Furthermore, the correction of macromastia yields the benefit of better adjuvant radiotherapy dose homogeneity with resultant long-term maintenance of cosmesis.[24]

Preoperative Planning

Preoperative planning requires discussion among, at a minimum, the oncologic surgeon and the radiologist. Usually a plastic surgeon, medical oncologist, radiation oncologist, and others should be included as well. All of the preoperative tests must be carefully evaluated and integrated with information about the pathologic subtype, size and extent of the lesion, size of the breast, lesion position within the breast, patient wishes, among other concerns. Other particular concerns include invasive lobular cancers that may be larger than expected based on initial imaging, extensive in situ components with similar risk for underestimation on imaging, patient desire for symmetry, and timing of the symmetrizing procedure.

Various options for the timing of oncoplastic breast surgery have been suggested.[25,26]

• **Immediate:** Definitive oncoplastic breast surgery at the time of tumor resection. This is a single-stage approach that has the advantage of using surgically naive tissue for reconstruction but may require repeat operations if margins are not clear and may necessitate mastectomy if the proper margins cannot be identified at reexcision.

- **Delayed-immediate:** Delay of oncoplastic breast surgery until final pathologic margins are confirmed to be clear, usually one to 3 weeks later and before the delivery of radiotherapy. This is a staged approach that has the advantage of definitively clearing the margins before committing to oncoplastic breast surgery but the downside of requiring multiple operations.
- **Delayed:** No oncoplastic breast surgery until after completion of adjuvant systemic and radiation therapy, usually 1 to 2 years later. This has the advantage of minimizing the potential delay of initiation of adjuvant therapy from wound-healing complications, but has the highest complication rates and least favorable esthetic outcomes.

In our practice, we have evaluated our postoperative margin status after initial surgery, specifically comparing simple elliptical excisions and Wise-pattern mammaplasty excisions. For tumors spanning 50 mm or more, the elliptical excision group (n = 250) had negative margins (defined as no ink on tumor[27] in 88% of cases. The oncoplastic reduction group (n = 300) had negative margins in 97% of cases. For tumors spanning more than 50 mm in the extreme oncoplastic group (n = 125), the negative margin rate was 87%.[22] As such, we feel justified in routinely performing immediate oncoplastic breast conservation in virtually all patients who are candidates for breast conservation. Even for tumors larger than 50 mm, the positive margin rate is similar to that of simple excisions with margin shaving.[14] In the case of positive margins, early reexcision before scarring has obliterated the dissected planes allows re-creation of the excisional defect for more accurate reexcision. When conversion to mastectomy is indicated, it is of benefit for the macromastia patient to have had the preliminary skin reduction and NAC repositioning. This patient who, before this failed oncoplastic breast conservation, may not have been a good candidate for NAC-sparing mastectomy may now successfully have the procedure after allowing 1 to 2 months of healing for revascularization of the NAC.

The skin overlying the tumor does not always need to be removed as a rule. However, when skin is not removed the anterior margin may be close or involved. We always measure skin-to-tumor distance using all three imaging modalities (mammography, ultrasound, and magnetic resonance imaging). If the skin-to-tumor distance is less than 10 mm, we remove the overlying skin. For patients with DCIS in whom we do not plan to irradiate postoperatively, we generally remove the overlying skin to ensure a negative anterior margin.

It is expected that oncoplastic resection of the index tumor will result in asymmetry. Given that breast asymmetry after breast conservation is known to affect psychosocial functioning and quality of life, the value of contralateral symmetry surgery is not debated.[28] The ideal timing for surgery of the contralateral breast would be after the index breast has been treated and adjuvant radiotherapy has been delivered. It is well accepted that the index breast will respond to radiotherapy with a variable degree of volume loss, fibrosis, and loss of elasticity. At a second operation the contralateral breast can be reduced and lifted for symmetry after these postradiotherapy changes have stabilized. Although ideal symmetry can be achieved in this staged approach, the index breast may continue to slowly shrink for years due to ongoing radiation injury.

When presented with the option of having two separate operations over the span of 1 to 2 years versus having both operations performed in the same setting, albeit with somewhat less accurate symmetry, it is rare that a patient prefers a staged approach. Virtually all are willing to accept the lesser symmetry from a single-stage approach when educated about the long-term effects of radiation therapy. With that in mind, a small fraction of our patients do return 3 to 4 years after surgery to have a secondary procedure for the contralateral breast to maintain symmetry.

Surgical Considerations

On the day of surgery, the patient undergoes wire localization (we do this the afternoon before surgery if the operation is scheduled as a first-start case) and sentinel node mapping by the radiologist. Just before surgery, generally in the preoperative holding area, she is marked in the upright position and counseled one final time. In the operating room, she is positioned on the operating table with her arms secured to the arm boards at 90 degrees. This allows for the head of the bed to be raised 45 to 90 degrees during the operation to assess symmetry. Assuming a bilateral procedure is planned, a two-team approach is used. While the oncologic surgeon is resecting the tumor from the index breast, the plastic surgeon is performing the contralateral breast symmetry procedure. After the tumor has been resected, the index breast is reconstructed, thus minimizing any increase in operative time. Drains are generally not required for these operations. At the conclusion of the procedure, the patient's breasts are wrapped in a compressive dressing for 24 to 48 hours to minimize seroma, ecchymosis, and hematoma.

With the range of oncoplastic approaches, precise and thorough communication between the plastic surgeon and oncologic surgeon is crucial. Proper preoperative planning, combined with knowledge of the blood supply of the breast, will usually allow preservation of a robust pedicle for the NAC and minimize necrosis.

Oncoplastic Techniques

Simple Glandular Flap Techniques

Glandular rearrangement can range from basic undermining and closure of a defect to tissue rearrangement with glandular flaps. The basic technique is to achieve closure of the parenchymal defect independent of the skin. An incision is made for access, often within the periareolar border, but can be anywhere on the breast. Through this incision, skin flaps are elevated (akin to mastectomy flaps) to expose the involved region of the breast. Once the excision is complete the adjacent parenchyma is freed from the underlying chest wall fascia. At this point, if primary closure of the defect is possible without deforming the breast, then it is performed with interrupted sutures. If primary closure is not possible, then the parenchyma can be further freed both from the overlying skin and underlying fascia. Care must be taken to preserve an adequate blood supply. This technique should be avoided in a predominantly fatty breast to avoid fat necrosis. The mobilized flaps of glandular tissue from both sides of the defect can then be rotated or advanced into the defect and sutured into place. Any dimpling of the overlying skin should be conservatively undermined before skin closure (Fig. 40.4).

Crescent, Hemibatwing, and Batwing Techniques

For lesions in the upper hemisphere (generally in the 08:00–04:00 positions going clockwise), crescent, batwing, or hemibatwing excisions may be used. These excisions lift the NAC, and a

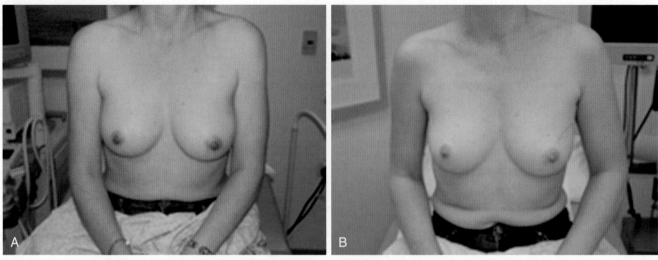

• **Fig. 40.4** Radial ellipse technique: preoperative (A) and 6-month postoperative (B) photos. A 2-cm left upper outer quadrant cancer was removed using a radial elliptical incision.

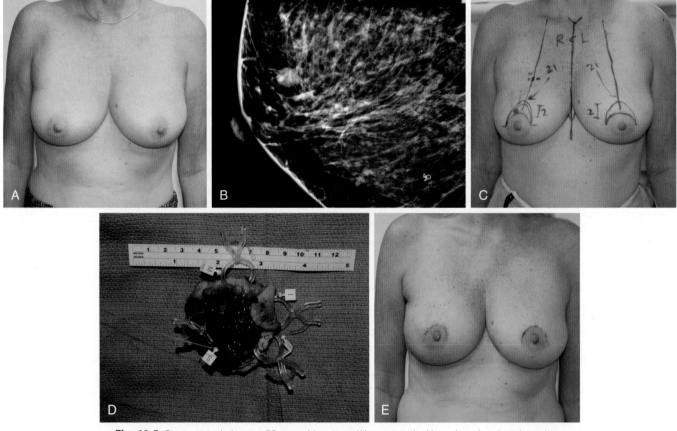

• **Fig. 40.5** Crescent technique: a 56-year-old woman (A) presented with an invasive ductal carcinoma of the right breast spanning 7 mm on mammogram at the 12:00 border of the areola (B). A crescent mastopexy (C) allowed excision of a 44-g specimen including the skin margin (D). A contralateral crescent mastopexy provided symmetry (E). Final pathology revealed a 1.1-cm invasive cancer and 5 cm of ductal carcinoma in situ with all negative margins.

contralateral crescent is often done simultaneously for symmetry. Generally, crescents are only appropriate for breasts with minimal or grade I ptosis that do not require reshaping. We typically limit movement of the NAC to a maximum of 2 cm. The upper hemisphere of the areola is meticulously marked, and an analogous second crescent is marked no more than 2 cm higher. The skin within the crescent is excised and access to the breast is gained. Once again, skin flaps are elevated to expose the breast gland, and the resection is performed. Glandular advancement of the lower pole parenchyma and overlying NAC is performed, and the parenchymal defect is repaired. The incision is then easily closed in layers, resulting in a minor correction of ptosis (Fig. 40.5).

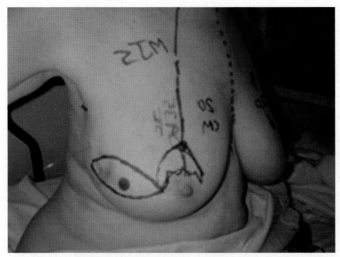

• **Fig. 40.6** Hemibatwing technique: preoperative marking for a hemiba-twing excision, which is a combination of a supraareolar crescent and a radial ellipse.

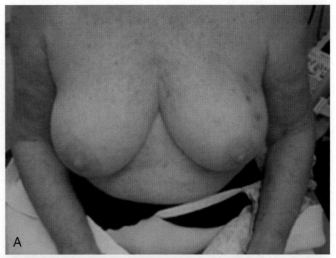

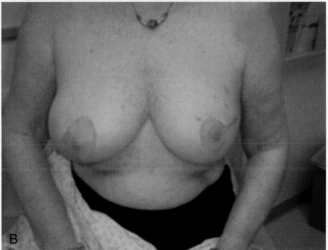

• **Fig. 40.7** Hemibatwing technique: (A) preoperative and (B) 1-month postoperative photos. A lateral invasive ductal carcinoma in the 02:00 position of the left breast was excised with a hemibatwing. A crescent mastopexy was done for symmetry on the right breast.

The batwing technique is essentially a crescent mastopexy with two wings on either side of it.[3] It allows a more aggressive mastopexy to be performed without the need for raising skin flaps or creation of pedicles for the NAC. This method is ideal for an upper pole tumor where a wide area of tissue is involved or in a previously irradiated breast where minimal tissue undermining is critical to avoiding necrosis. This procedure preserves the nipple on an extremely broad inferior pedicle.

A hemibatwing is a combination of a radial elliptical excision and a crescent excision (Fig. 40.6). This achieves dual goals: lifting the NAC while excising a radial segment of the breast. It can be combined with a crescent mastopexy of the contralateral breast for symmetry (Fig. 40.7).

A clamshell technique is also possible, combining two mirror-image batwings with the NAC in between (Fig. 40.8). The center point of these two batwings will determine the final NAC position. The benefit of this technique over a simple batwing is that it allows a larger area of tissue to be excised from an entire hemisphere of the breast. Enough tissue is spared within the clamshell pattern to allow it to be de-epithelialized and advanced into the excavated hemisphere. As with the batwing, this procedure is ideal for patients in whom minimal tissue undermining is important. We commonly use the clamshell pattern in previously irradiated patients who develop a new or recurrent cancer and desire another attempt at breast conservation. In addition, this technique allows for breast conservation in patients with multicentric disease with or without skin involvement.

Vertical Mammaplasty, Inframammary Excision, and Central Excision Techniques

The vertical mammaplasty excision removes a triangular-shaped piece of tissue from the lower breast hemisphere. It is ideal for patients with tumors in the 05:00 to 07:00 position who do not want the NAC elevated as it would be with a standard reduction (Fig. 40.9). It leaves an inverted T-shaped scar. A classic vertical mammaplasty relies on liposuction for additional contouring[29]; this is used judiciously or not at all in oncoplastic reconstruction to minimize the potential for seeding of tumor cells. The incision for the inframammary approach is placed just slightly above the inframammary sulcus. In the upright position, this scar is hidden. This incision is an excellent choice for lesions in the posterior inferior position of the breast. It does not remove any skin and generally does not change the size or shape of the breast. Lesions in the upper hemisphere can be reached using this incision.

When the NAC is involved by tumor, the central excision of breast tissue is incorporated into an inverted T mammaplasty that allows for reshaping and immediate NAC reconstruction. This technique takes advantage of breast ptosis to advance an inferiorly based island of tissue into the central defect. It is also feasible to reconstruct a NAC on this island of tissue, which can be tattooed later to complete the reconstruction (Fig. 40.10). Alternatively, the Grisotti technique can be used for smaller defects.[30] It relies on rotation-advancement of a laterally based tissue island with minimal reshaping of the remainder of the breast.

Round Block Mastopexy (Benelli) and Reduction Mammaplasty Techniques

After 30 years of using a range of oncoplastic approaches, it has become clear to us that the best and most consistent results are

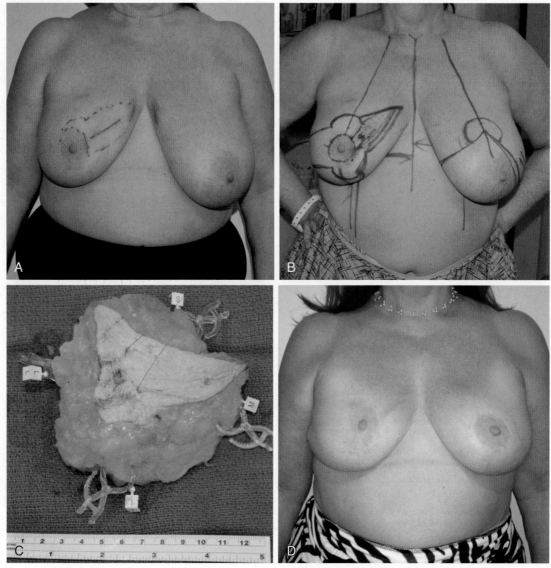

• **Fig. 40.8** Clamshell technique: a 60-year-old woman (A) presented with a recurrent ductal carcinoma in situ (DCIS) of the upper inner quadrant of the right breast (treated previously with three excisions and radiation therapy). She had been offered mastectomy and autologous flap reconstruction at an outside institution but declined. Instead, she chose an excision with a clamshell-type reconstruction and contra-lateral breast reduction for symmetry (B). Final specimen weighed 175 g (C) and contained 2.9 cm of DCIS with negative margins. (D) shows the final postoperative result.

obtained using a round block (Benelli) excision in women with smaller breasts and grade I ptosis and with a reduction mamma-plasty in women with medium to large breasts and grade II or III ptosis. An elliptical or triangular extension can be added to either of these approaches, in which case they are called split-Benelli or split-reduction.[31,32]

The round block (Benelli) mastopexy gives excellent results for lesions in small to medium breasts with mild to moderate ptosis (Fig. 40.11).[33] This technique allows 360-degree access to the breast, and the final scar is limited to the circumareolar border. The inner circle is drawn to the desired NAC diameter within the baseline areola. The outer circle is drawn eccentrically, with its center point higher than the current nipple position, allowing elevation of the NAC upon closure. Conversely, if no upward movement of the NAC is desired, the two circles can be drawn concentrically. The diameter of the outer circle should not exceed twice the diameter of the inner circle. The skin within these circles

is deepithelialized, and the dermis incised 5 mm inside the outer ring, and access to the breast is gained. The skin flaps can be raised circumferentially down to the chest wall, thus retaining the NAC on a central pedicle. Once the entire gland is exposed in this manner, a pie-shaped wedge of tissue can be resected easily from any location in the breast and the defect closed with minimal undermining off the chest wall. The skin is then redraped and the incision closed with a permanent pursestring closure around the areola. The result is a rounder, lifted breast. Any scalloping or wrinkles that develop after final closure due to size discrepancy between the length of the inner and outer circles will flatten out over the course of a few months.

The workhorse of oncoplastic surgery at our facility is the Wise pattern mammaplasty.[34] This powerful technique owes its versatil-ity to several key features. First, it allows the use of virtually any pedicle for the NAC (superior, lateral, medial, inferior, central, and bipedicle; we generally prefer a superior or medial pedicle).

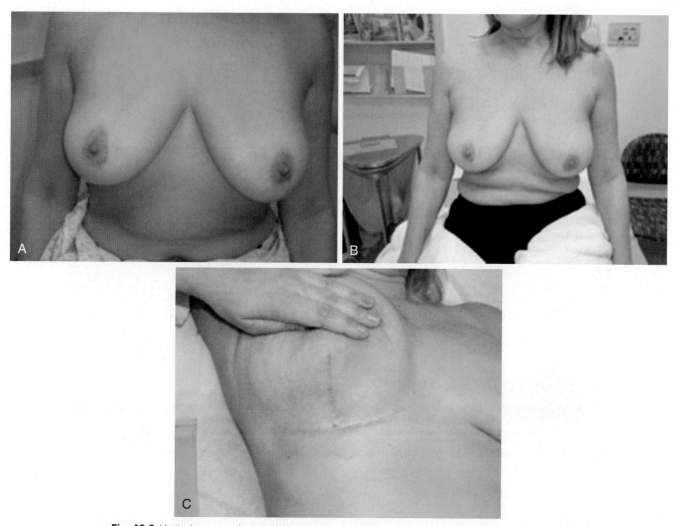

• **Fig. 40.9** Vertical mammaplasty technique: preoperative (A) and 2-year postoperative (B) photos. This patient underwent excision of a 2-cm invasive cancer in the 06:00 position of the right breast using a triangle excision. This was chosen because she did not want any change in appearance after surgery. A reduction excision was suggested, but she declined. (C) The incision appears as an inverted T.

Second, significant tissue rearrangement can be performed with multiple secondary pedicles independent of the NAC. Finally, the wide skin resection allows the most aggressive correction of ptosis. These factors combine to allow exposure to the entire breast, the ability to widely resect tissue from any quadrant, and the opportunity to significantly reduce overall breast volume to aid radiation dose homogeneity.

The Wise pattern mammaplasty requires the creation of three triangles: vertical, medial, and lateral. The inferior borders of all three triangles are incorporated into the inframammary fold incision, limiting the scars to the circumareolar border, the vertical midline of the breast, and the inframammary crease (Fig. 40.12). Tumors located in the inferior pole can be easily incorporated in the incision, with the overlying skin, through a standard Wise pattern. The vertical pillars are then plicated and the NAC inset into the keyhole. If the NAC cannot be saved, a nipple can be re-created immediately or as a delayed procedure. This technique allows the lower pole and central tumors to be easily excised along with the overlying skin to avoid a close or positive anterior margin.

When the tumors are located in areas that do not naturally fall within a standard Wise pattern, two options exist. The first is to perform a standard Wise pattern technique and to tunnel under skin flaps to reach the distant tumor. This is acceptable if the tumor is deep and the anterior margin is not felt to be of concern. However, for most cases when the tumor is located outside the Wise pattern, our preferred alternative is to excise the tumor with the anterior skin margin. For tumors located in the upper outer or upper inner quadrants, the Wise pattern may be reconfigured to include the tumor with the overlying skin, in a split reduction.

When the NAC is involved by tumor, the central excision of breast tissue is incorporated into an inverted T mammaplasty that allows for reshaping and immediate NAC reconstruction. This technique takes advantage of breast ptosis to advance an inferiorly based island of tissue into the central defect. It is also feasible to reconstruct a NAC on this island of tissue that can later be tattooed to complete the reconstruction. Alternatively, the Grisotti technique can be used for smaller defects.[30] This relies on rotation advancement of a laterally based tissue island with minimal reshaping of the remainder of the breast.

In a split reduction, the lateral or medial triangle of the Wise pattern is not positioned at the base of the breast but advanced

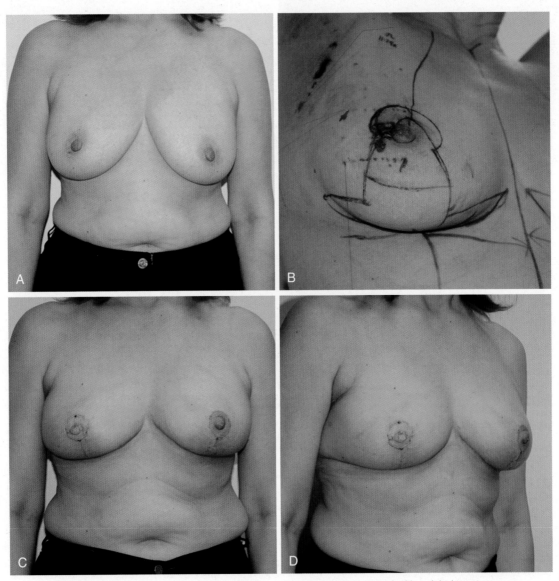

• **Fig. 40.10** Central excision technique: a 60-year-old woman (A) presented with a right breast cancer involving the nipple-areolar complex (NAC). She underwent neoadjuvant chemotherapy followed by a central reduction with excision of the NAC via an inverted-T reduction pattern reconstruction and NAC reconstruction on an inferiorly based parenchymal segment (B). The left breast was reduced with a standard Wise pattern technique for symmetry (C and D).

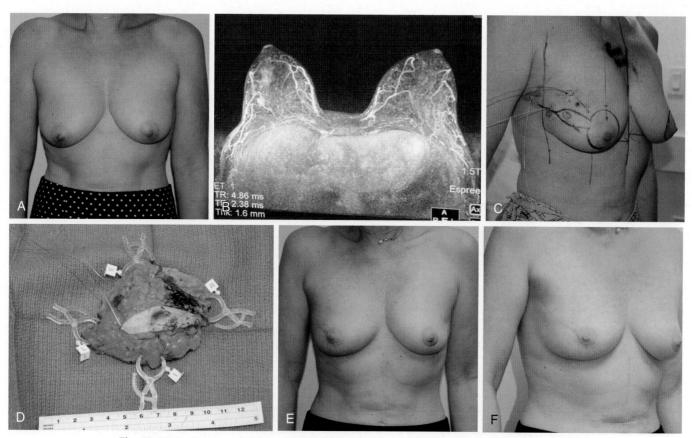

• **Fig. 40.11** Circumareolar/Benelli technique: a 47-year-old woman (A) presented with an invasive cancer of the right breast at the 10:00 position spanning 25 mm on magnetic resonance imaging (B). After neoadjuvant chemotherapy, a circumareolar/Benelli approach (C) with lateral skin ellipse over the tumor allowed excision of a 75-g specimen (D); final pathology revealed a 1.4-cm invasive ductal carcinoma with negative margins and 3/10 positive axillary lymph nodes. (E and F) Postoperative appearance.

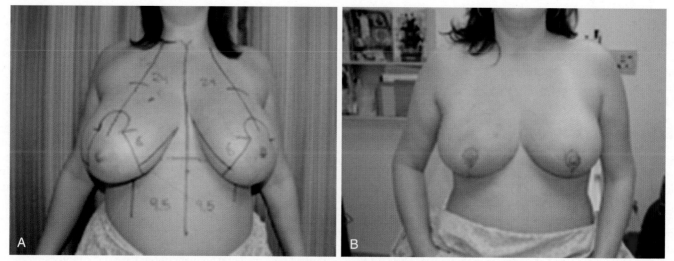

• **Fig. 40.12** Wise-pattern reduction mammaplasty technique: preoperative (A) and 1-week postoperative (B) photos. A 12-mm tumor was removed from the lower inner quadrant of the right breast using a standard Wise pattern reduction.

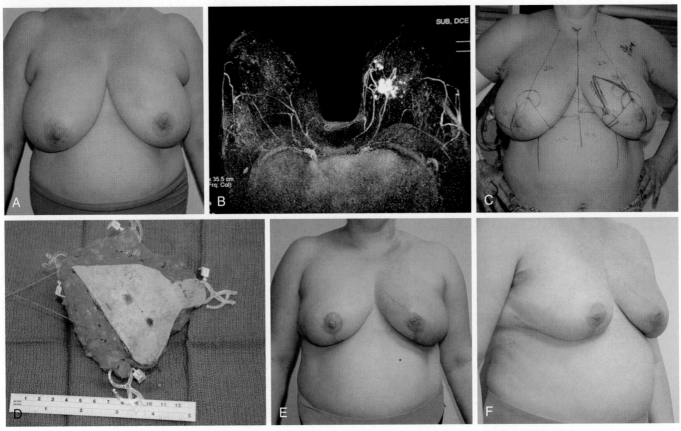

• **Fig. 40.13** Split reduction technique: a 43-year-old woman (A) presented with a multifocal left breast cancer with ductal carcinoma in situ component in the upper inner breast. There were approximately 20 lesions spanning 74 mm by 72 mm on magnetic resonance imaging (B). After neoadjuvant chemotherapy, she underwent a split reduction of the left breast and contralateral Wise pattern reduction for symmetry (C). The specimen weight was 266 g from the upper inner breast (D) and revealed a 9.5-cm span of multifocal invasive tumors with negative margins. The postoperative photos (E and F) demonstrate the final outcome after adjuvant radiation therapy to the left breast.

cephalad to a position directly overlying the tumor (Figs. 40.13 through 40.15). The medial or lateral vertical limb of the inverted T is split on the side of the tumor excision to accommodate the higher position of the medial or lateral triangle. When the tumor is located in the 12:00 position, the split occurs at the apex of the keyhole rather than along the vertical limbs of the pattern.

Extreme Oncoplasty

In 2008, we wondered how far we could push the oncoplastic envelope. We had been performing oncoplastic resections for unifocal stage I and II disease for years. We also encountered many patients with larger or multifocal/multicentric tumors who seemed technically amenable to oncoplastic resection, but there were no prospective randomized data to support breast conservation for these patients. We always believed that the relationship between the size of the breast and the span of the tumor was key: a large breast with a large tumor could tolerate a large resection. So we began our "Extreme Oncoplasty Program" to provide second opinions for patients who wanted to save their breast but had been told that they needed a mastectomy.

Extreme oncoplasty is a breast conserving operation using oncoplastic techniques for a patient who, in most physicians' opinions, requires a mastectomy. Due to the nature of these lesions, most of these patients will also need postmastectomy radiation therapy. Extreme oncoplasty can be considered, if the breast is large enough to support it, for patients with tumors larger than 50 mm, multifocal or multicentric lesions, extensive DCIS or an extensive intraductal component greater than 50 mm, a previously irradiated breast with a new or recurrent cancer within that breast, and locally advanced breast cancers with a limited or partial imaging response to neoadjuvant chemotherapy (Fig. 40.16).[35] Patients such as these have generally not been considered acceptable candidates for breast conservation because the prospective randomized trials on which breast conservation is based only allowed inclusion of unifocal tumors up to 5 cm in extent. There are no prospective randomized data for larger, multifocal, or multicentric lesions, and there are not likely to be any. But what is the difference between a 48-mm cancer that qualifies and a 52-mm cancer that does not? When breast conservation is performed for a patient who turns out to have a 55- or 60-mm cancer on final pathology, most of us will irradiate that breast if the margins are negative and not convert to a mastectomy just because of a size larger than 50 mm. It is important to recognize that we are doing this without the support of any Level I evidence.

The most important reason to consider extreme oncoplasty is that breast conservation yields a better quality of life compared with the combination of mastectomy, reconstruction, and

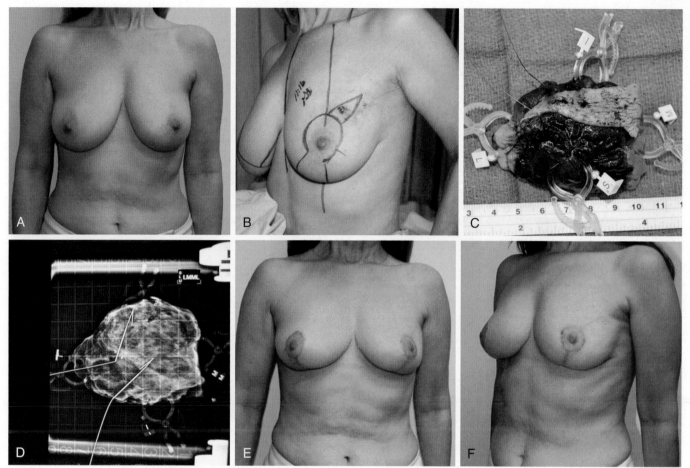

• **Fig. 40.14** Split reduction technique: a 53-year-old woman (A) presented with an invasive lobular carcinoma of the left upper outer breast spanning 2 cm on magnetic resonance imaging. A split reduction pattern was used for the left breast (B), and standard Wise pattern reduction was performed on the right for symmetry. A 62-g specimen was excised (C and D) and revealed a 6-cm invasive lobular carcinoma on final pathology with negative margins. It is likely that this tumor would have required reexcision or conversion to mastectomy with traditional methods of breast conservation. (E and F) Postoperative appearance.

radiation therapy, and survival is likely the same.[36] Consider the quality of life with the combination of mastectomy, reconstruction, and radiation therapy. For most patients, a retropectoral expander will be placed at the time of mastectomy. This causes significant pain. There are drains, a foreign body, the potential for infection, and the additional time required for expansion, all of which can have a significant impact on the patient's life. The final reconstruction requires another operation: the expander to implant exchange or perhaps an autologous flap. If an autologous flap is used it is a longer procedure, with additional operative risks and donor site morbidity. There may be additional operations to adjust the breast and nipple as well as tattoos for the areola. Then there is the opposite breast to consider; many patients will consider prophylactic mastectomy and reconstruction or a reduction for symmetry. The mastectomy or mastectomies will almost always leave insensate breast(s). The final cosmetic result can range from poor to excellent, but our experience in looking at more than 1000 reconstructed patients tells us that fewer than 40% would be rated as excellent by us.

After a mastectomy with reconstruction, most of these high-risk patients need radiation therapy.[37] Currently patients with tumors greater than 5 cm, four or more positive nodes, and

sometimes 1 to 3 positive nodes receive radiation therapy.[38,39] Additionally, patients with extensive lymphovascular invasion get radiation therapy, as will patients with close or involved margins after mastectomy. In other words, radiation therapy will be recommended for many patients after mastectomy and certainly for nearly all patients who qualify for extreme oncoplasty. If the patient is going to be given radiation therapy regardless of surgical approach, we generally prefer to save her breast with an acceptable cosmetic result, if it is technically possible and oncologically sound.

Radiation therapy is not friendly to postmastectomy reconstruction.[40] There is a risk of capsular contracture if an implant-based reconstruction is used, or breast shrinkage if autologous tissue is used. Radiation therapy is inconvenient from the patient's perspective, expensive, causes some morbidity, and may interfere with the timing of chemotherapy. Because no mastectomy removes 100% of the breast, if radiation therapy is not given the remaining 5% to 10% of the overall breast tissue and dermal lymphatics are not treated, which may contribute to an increased local recurrence rate.

Compare this to oncoplastic breast conservation with a simultaneous contralateral reduction for symmetry: a single operation,

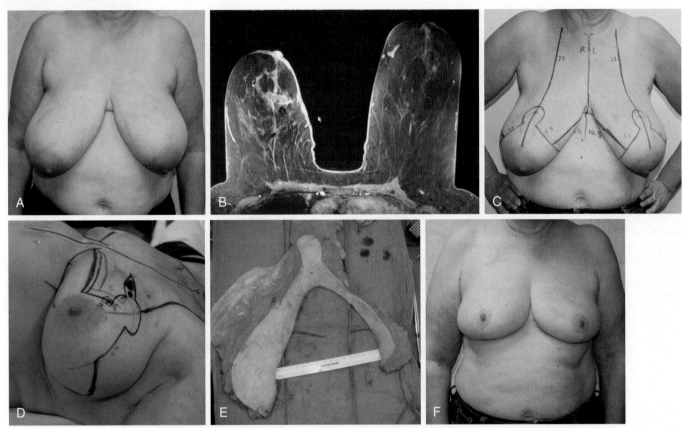

• **Fig. 40.15** Split reduction technique: a 56-year-old woman (A) presented with a left breast invasive carcinoma and ductal carcinoma in situ of the upper inner quadrant, spanning 19 mm on mammography. (B) Preoperative magnetic resonance imaging. She underwent a split reduction excision of the tumor (C and D) with negative margins (E). In addition, the index breast was significantly reduced, and a contralateral Wise pattern reduction was performed for symmetry. The final results (F) are shown 1 year after adjuvant radiotherapy to the left breast.

no drains, and better esthetics both immediately and later. There is less pain, less expense, a shorter hospital stay (this is often an outpatient procedure), no foreign body, and no donor site morbidity. The breasts are more functional and sensate. All of this results in better body image and a happier patient.[41] Most importantly, breast conservation with a reduction allows the patient to forget that she had breast cancer—not right away, but at some point in the future. In 6 months or a year, the patient will be getting dressed, and she has two normal reduced breasts. They look good, they are nearly always sensate, and she feels like she is just a normal woman. She will be reminded of breast cancer only when she sees it on television or it is time for an appointment with her doctor. If she had a mastectomy, even with an excellent reconstruction, she will be reminded of her cancer on a daily basis for the rest of her life.

We have followed our extreme oncoplasty patients very carefully.[21] The extreme cases, on average, have cancers about three times the size of our standard oncoplastic cases. The extreme specimens weighed about 70 grams more. No ink on tumor was achieved only 86% of the time during the first excision due to the larger size of the extreme tumors; 12% of patients underwent reexcision, and 5% ultimately underwent mastectomy. The local recurrence rate for the extreme cases is slightly but not significantly higher (1.5% vs. 1.2% over a mean follow-up of 24 months), as would be expected for patients with larger cancers.

There are no long-term recurrence or survival data at this point for extreme patients. There was overwhelming patient satisfaction with the oncoplastic program as measured by a patient satisfaction survey.

Summary

The techniques discussed here are our most commonly used methods of oncoplastic breast surgery. The premise of our general techniques is discussed, but each operation must be individualized for the patient at hand. Many patients present to us seeking breast conservation after having been told elsewhere that it would be technically challenging or impossible. A large number of these women have been spared mastectomies by using the carefully selected and designed techniques described. The importance of individualization of these techniques cannot be overstated: we frequently make intraoperative adjustments to the preoperative markings to modify the skin envelope, modify the NAC pedicle if necessary, and often use secondary and tertiary parenchymal pedicles to reconstruct defects. The ability to maintain flexibility is important, and communication between disciplines is critical.

Oncoplastic surgery combines sound oncologic surgical principles with plastic surgical techniques. Coordination of these two disciplines helps avoid poor cosmetic results after wide excision and increases the number of women who can be treated with

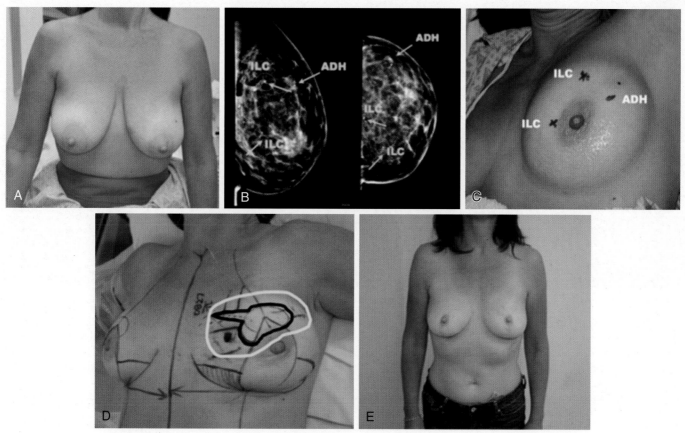

• Fig. 40.16 Extreme oncoplasty: a 48-year-old woman (A) presented with two foci of invasive lobular carcinoma *(ILC)* and an additional focus of atypical ductal hyperplasia *(ADH)* (B and C). The disease spanned nearly half her left breast and was in multiple quadrants. She underwent a wire-localized extreme split reduction excision (D); the black line indicates the skin that was removed and the yellow line the total tissue removed. Final pathology revealed two foci of ILC spanning 42 mm. With the ADH, the total disease spanned 81 mm. All margins were negative. The final results (E) are shown 2.5 years after adjuvant radiotherapy to the breast.

breast conserving surgery by allowing larger breast excisions with more acceptable cosmetic results. Oncoplastic surgery requires cooperation and communication of a large multidisciplinary team. New oncoplastic techniques that allow more extensive excisions can be used to achieve both acceptable cosmesis and widely negative margins, reducing the need for radiation therapy in many cases of DCIS. Extreme oncoplasty is a breast conserving operation using oncoplastic techniques for a patient who, in most physicians' opinions, requires a mastectomy. Because of the size and extent of these lesions, most of these patients will also need postmastectomy radiation therapy. Extreme oncoplasty can be considered, if the breast is large enough to support it, for patients with tumors larger than 50 mm, multifocal or multicentric lesions, extensive DCIS or extensive intraductal component greater than 50 mm, previously irradiated breasts with a new or recurrent ipsilateral cancer, and large locally advanced breast cancer with a partial or complete imaging response to neoadjuvant chemotherapy. Oncoplastic breast surgery and extreme oncoplasty are win-win approaches, allowing removal of the cancer with wide margins while often achieving better cosmesis than before surgery. They both require a philosophy that the appearance, function, and sensation of the breast after cancer surgery are important.

Selected References

3. Anderson BO, Masetti R, Silverstein MJ. Oncoplastic approaches to partial mastectomy: an overview of volume-displacement techniques. *Lancet Oncol.* 2005;6:145-157.

6. Savalia NB, Silverstein MJ. Oncoplastic breast reconstruction: patient selection and surgical techniques. *J Surg Oncol.* 2016;113: 875-882.

20. Waljee JF, Hu ES, Newman LA, Alderman AK. Predictors of breast asymmetry after breast-conserving operation for breast cancer. *J Am Coll Surg.* 2008;206:274-280.

22. Silverstein MJ. Radical Mastectomy to Radical Conservation (Extreme Oncoplasty): A Revolutionary Change. *J Am Coll Surg.* 2015.

25. Kronowitz SJ, Kuerer HM, Buchholz TA, Valero V, Hunt KK. A management algorithm and practical oncoplastic surgical techniques for repairing partial mastectomy defects. *Plast Reconstr Surg.* 2008;122:1631-1647.

28. Waljee JF, Hu ES, Ubel PA, et al. Effect of esthetic outcome after breast-conserving surgery on psychosocial functioning and quality of life. *J Clin Oncol.* 2008;26:3331-3337.

35. Silverstein M, Savalia N, Khan S, Ryan J. Extreme oncoplasty: breast conservation for patients who need mastectomy. *Breast J.* 2015;21:52-59.

A full reference list is available online at ExpertConsult.com.

41

Therapeutic Value of Axillary Node Dissection and Selective Management of the Axilla in Small Breast Cancers

RAQUEL PRATI, HELENA R. CHANG, AND MAUREEN A. CHUNG

Controversy has long existed regarding the biological implications and surgical treatment of regional lymph node metastasis in invasive breast cancer. Several factors have resulted in a renewed evaluation of axillary node dissection. First is the continuing biologic controversy that axillary lymph node metastases are "indicators but not governors" of outcome in breast cancer.[1] Indeed in all human cancers with few exceptions, this biological concept has been proved repeatedly,[2-6] and in most studies addressing this issue, lymph node metastases have proved to be indicators only.[7] Another factor that has led to resurgence of interest in the role of axillary node dissection is the downward trend in tumor size secondary to mammographic screening and the resulting decrease in proportion of patients with lymph node metastasis. Use of primary tumor characteristics and genomic patterns to aid in decisions to administer systemic chemotherapy, the failure of high-dose therapy with bone marrow support, and the increasing indications for systemic adjuvant therapy in most cases have also challenged the need for axillary node dissection. Finally, with the advent of sentinel lymph node biopsy and its widespread application,[8] the need for complete axillary evaluation has been questioned. This chapter summarizes the role of the lymphatic system in breast cancer and factors that have led to the decreased need for surgical axillary evaluation. Alternatives to axillary lymph node dissection, including axillary observation only in patients with small tumors, treatment of the axilla with tangential whole breast radiotherapy fields or axillary radiotherapy, lymph node evaluation by four- and five-node sampling, sentinel node biopsy, and the use of ultrasound to stage the axilla are also discussed. The continuing controversy surrounding the potential value of axillary dissection in breast cancer patients is explored.

Lymphatic Function and Nodal Metastases

A brief analysis of anatomy, physiology, biological function, and metastatic specificity of the lymphatic system adds to our understanding of lymph node metastasis and its impact on survival. The lymphatic system was first described by Asselius in Pavia in 1622.[9] It was not until 1863, however, that the relationship between the lymphatic system and lymph nodes was made by His.[10] The lymphatic system serves four purposes:

1. Return of interstitial fluids and proteins to the blood and the conduction of absorbed fats of the intestinal tract to the vascular system by way of intestinal lacteals and the thoracic duct
2. Exposure of foreign antigens to lymph node lymphocytes for generation of acquired specific immunity
3. Production and dissemination of antigen-specific T lymphocytes
4. Production and maturation of plasma cells that produce antigen-specific antibodies

Lymphatic fluid contents can either pass through the lymph node or bypass the lymph node entirely to enter the hematogenous system. The predominant pattern is for lymph to flow through the afferent lymphatic channels to the lymph node for maximum exposure of foreign antigens to lymphocytes. Because lymph fluid can either pass through the lymph node or bypass the lymph node directly into the hematogenous system, it is not surprising that studies show that metastatic cancer cells arriving at the lymph node by afferent lymphatic channels may transit through or bypass the lymph node entirely through lymphatic channels or lymphatic venous anastomoses.[11,12] Metastatic cancer cells that drain directly into the lymph node may lodge and remain without progressive growth (this may be exemplified by isolated tumor cells), be destroyed by physiologic processes that occur in the lymph node, or lodge and grow in the lymph node and become metastases. The presence of metastatic cancer cells in the lymph node is therefore only an indication of the ability of the cancer cell to metastasize from the primary tumor site and not necessarily proof of later nodal metastatic growth. As clinical trials show, many patients with lymph node metastases may harbor systemic cells or micrometastases; however, significant proportions of patients develop systemic disease without any evidence of lymph node metastases. In these patients, it is conceivable that the metastatic cancer cell bypassed the lymph node and entered the hematogenous system directly or transited the node without residual evidence of its presence. Another major subgroup of patients has lymph node metastases but never develops systemic disease. The number of lymph node metastases is the major factor in this statistical relationship to later systemic metastatic disease; patients with only one-node metastases have an excellent prognosis, whereas those with more than 10-node metastases have a very poor prognosis.

The advent of sentinel lymph node biopsy has furthered our knowledge of the lymphatic system of the breast. Sentinel lymphadenectomy has proven that drainage of lymph from the breast is orderly through one or two initial draining nodes, or sentinel lymph nodes.[13] These sentinel lymph nodes tend to be close to the breast. Injection of blue dye or radioactive tracer in the breast parenchyma around the primary tumor, in the overlying skin, or around the nipple all drain to the same sentinel lymph nodes.[14,15] These studies have shown that the breast lymphatic drainage is orderly, and thus the distribution of lymph, metastatic cells, and nodal metastases are not random events but rather highly structured, defined, and sequentially based on the anatomy and physiology of the lymphatic system.

There are five models of when and how tumors develop metastasis[16] (Fig. 41.1). In clonal selection, metastasis develops as the final step in a multistep process. The Halstedian view of breast cancer follows this model. In parallel evolution, metastasis occurs early in tumor progression and is independent of the primary tumor. This model is in agreement with the Fisherian model of breast cancer. Tumor cells develop metastasis at varying rates in the dynamic heterogeneity model. In clonal dominance, clonal cells with the most metastatic potential outgrow other tumor cells to dominate the primary tumor mass and metastatic deposits. The stem cell model suggests that only the stem cells have the capacity to metastasize. Regardless of the model, a cancer cell has to detach from the primary tumor mass (loss of cell-to-cell adhesion), invade the blood and lymphatic vasculature, extravasate into parenchymal tissue, and colonize that tissue.

Extensive research work is being conducted on the specificity of the interaction between metastatic cancer cell and recipient organ. Cancer cells, selected by sequential harvesting of specific organ site metastasis and reinjected intravenously into animal models, display an inability to lodge or grow in organs other than the source from which they were obtained.[17] It has been shown that metastatic subclones with different gene expression profiles developed metastases in different organs despite being derived from the same breast cancer cell line.[18] Brodt and colleagues[19] demonstrated lymph node specificity of human lymphatic metastatic cells grown in nude mice and provide further evidence for organ specificity of lymph node metastases. This distinct organ-specific metastatic behavior has been eloquently proven by animal studies in which individual cells from the effusion of a breast cancer patient differed in their ability to metastasize to the bone, lung, or adrenal organs.[20] These observations provide evidence for Paget's "seed and soil theory."[21] Unknown as yet are the exact physiologic mechanisms that permit or prevent lodging and progressive growth of organ-specific metastatic cells, but they may be related to cytokine function, electrical charge, structural aspects of the metastatic cell surface, or other tissue features in the receptor organ.[22–24] Metastatic cancer cells have to be able not only to detach from the primary organ and invade the lymphatic system but also to attach to the lymphatic metastatic site via specific interaction between cell and endothelial or lymph node structural element receptors. Once attachment has occurred, these cancer cells have to evade possible immune system rejection and produce angiogenic factors that are essential for growth. These cells that lodge and grow in lymph nodes may have no ability to lodge and grow in other organs or other organ endothelial cells.

Patients can harbor metastases in different organs such as the lymph node, liver, or bone. What is unclear is whether some of these metastases are directly derived from the primary tumor

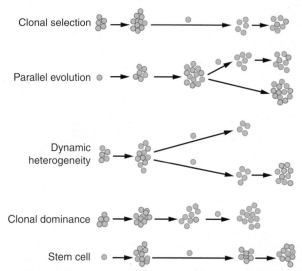

• **Fig. 41.1** Models of the metastatic process. Five models have been proposed for metastatic development. (Redrawn with permission from Talmadge JE. Clonal selection of metastasis within the life history of a tumor. *Cancer Res.* 2007;67:11471-11475.)

(synchronous seeding) or if some of the metastatic deposits metastasized to other organs (metachronous seeding). The current concept of lymph nodes as indicators, not governors, of survival would support synchronous seeding.[1] Overwhelming data from randomized trials do support this concept. However, the recent overview of outcomes after radiotherapy for breast cancer does suggest a survival benefit in those patients who received radiotherapy and had better locoregional control. If metachronous seeding can occur, axillary clearance of lymph nodes that harbored metastatic disease should result in better outcome. These differing concepts of seeding are further complicated by self-seeding in which disseminated tumor cells can return to the primary tumor site and grow.[25]

Most breast cancers drain to the axilla irrespective of the quadrant location for the primary index lesion. Tumors located in the inner quadrants of the breast have the greatest likelihood of draining to the internal mammary nodes[26] (Fig. 41.2). However, even in these patients, the primary tumor also drains to the axilla.[27] The few patients with metastasis to the internal mammary nodes are more likely to have larger tumors, more aggressive disease, and multiple positive axillary lymph nodes.[28] Indeed, in a recent analysis of 6000 breast cancer patients, the incidence of internal mammary lymph node recurrence was 0.1%, with almost of all these patients also having systemic recurrence.[29]

Bone marrow micrometastasis in breast cancer patients in the absence of lymph node involvement supports the concept of direct hematogenous spread. Braun and associates[30] reported that one-third of node-negative breast cancer patients have bone marrow micrometastasis and that their presence increased relapse. Combined data from nine studies involving 4703 breast cancer patients suggested that the presence of bone marrow micrometastasis was a significant prognostic factor for both overall and breast cancer–specific survival.[31] Presence of micrometastasis increased twofold the likelihood of disease recurrence and dying of breast cancer and was a significant prognostic factor after controlling for tumor size, lymph node involvement, tumor grade, and hormone receptor status.

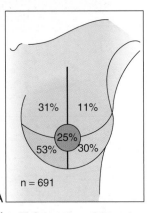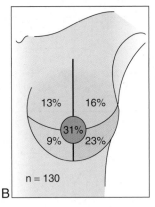

• **Fig. 41.2** Location of the primary tumor in patients with a positive internal mammary chain sentinel node. Breast cancers located in the lateral quadrants can drain to the internal mammary nodes. (A) Most breast cancers that drain to the internal mammary nodes are located in the medial aspect of the breast. (B) Most patients with positive internal mammary nodes, however, will have a lesion in the lateral aspect of the breast. (Redrawn with permission from Estourgie SH, Tanis, PJ, Nieweg, OE, et al. Should the hunt for internal mammary chain sentinel nodes begin? An evaluation of 150 patients. *Ann Surg Oncol.* 2005;10: 935-941.)

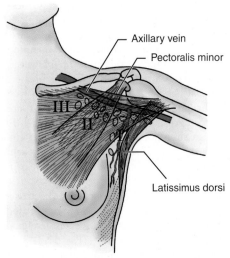

• **Fig. 41.3** Anatomy of the axilla. The axillary triangle is defined by the axillary vein, the latissimus dorsi muscle, and the chest wall. The level I lymph nodes are inferior and lateral to the pectoralis minor, the level II lymph nodes are behind the pectoralis minor and below the axillary vein, and the level III lymph nodes are medial to the pectoralis minor and below the axillary vein.

Axillary Anatomy and Evaluation

The axillary space is defined by the axillary vein superiorly, the serratus anterior medially, and the latissimus dorsi laterally. The pectoralis muscles are anterior to the medial portion of the axilla. The pectoralis minor is used to divide the axilla into three levels: level I nodes are lateral to the pectoralis minor, level II nodes are behind the pectoralis minor, and level III nodes are medial to the pectoralis minor (Fig. 41.3). The interpectoral (Rotter) nodes are found between the pectoralis major and minor muscles along the lateral pectoral nerve.

There has been considerable debate regarding appropriate extent of axillary node dissection. A complete axillary dissection removes all three levels of lymph nodes, whereas a partial axillary dissection may refer to the removal of level I and II nodes or only level I nodes. Most axillary metastases involve either level I or II nodes. Indeed, sentinel node mapping has shown that low level I lymph nodes are frequently a site of metastatic disease. Veronesi and coworkers reported that the likelihood of "skip metastases" (i.e., involvement of level III nodes in the absence of level I and II involvement) was less than 1%.[32] Similarly, Rosen and colleagues studied 429 patients with axillary node metastases and found isolated disease in level III in only 0.2% of the specimens.[33] Sentinel node mapping has shown that the breast can bypass level I nodes to drain into level II nodes. It is not surprising that the reported rate of skip metastases to level II nodes is as high as 25%.[34] Contemporary axillary dissection in breast cancer refers to the removal of level I and II lymph nodes.

The axilla can be evaluated by clinical examination, noninvasive imaging, minimally invasive surgery, and axillary clearance. Axillary node dissection is considered the gold standard, and it is the modality to which all methods are compared. Clinical examination of the axilla is not an accurate method to evaluate the axilla. Sentinel lymphadenectomy has proved that axillary metastases can be present in more than 30% of patients with a clinically negative axilla. Alternatively, about 25% of patients with axillary adenopathy have no metastatic disease. This is especially valid if the patient has had a recent intervention in the breast.

Axillary lymph nodes can often be seen on mammograms. They are not clinically suspicious unless they are greater than 2 cm in size or have loss of the fatty hilum. Ultrasound is the best noninvasive method to assess lymph nodes. Lymph nodes that are less than 1 cm in size and have a centrally located hilum are most likely benign. Conversely, lymph nodes that are large and have a thick, eccentric hilum are suspicious for metastatic disease. Sonographic diagnosis of lymph nodes will be accurate in approximately 70% of cases. Accuracy of axillary ultrasound can be improved when coupled with fine-needle aspiration cytology (FNAC). FNAC of axillary lymph nodes is very sensitive, and the false-negative rate is less than 1%.[35-37] Several centers have shown that proceeding directly to axillary node dissection based on a positive FNAC is cost-effective and spares up to 40% of patients the intermediate step of a sentinel node biopsy.[38,39] Patients with negative FNAC proceed to sentinel node biopsy because of the known sampling error, especially in patients with micrometastasis.

The likelihood of nodal involvement correlates directly with increasing tumor size.[40] Although the exact numbers varied, in general, the likelihood of nodal involvement with a T$_{1a}$ tumor was 5% to 10%, with T$_{1b}$ 10% to 20%, and with T$_{1c}$ greater than 20%.[41] However, these percentages were based on conventional axillary node dissections, often on registry data with their inherent discrepancies. The advent of sentinel lymphadenectomy has resulted in intense histologic examination of lymph nodes and an increased detection of smaller-sized metastasis and upstaging. The incidence of positive lymph nodes based on tumor size and detected by sentinel lymphadenectomy is depicted in Table 41.1. Because most breast cancer patients with clinically negative axilla are treated with sentinel lymphadenectomy, results based on this surgical approach and method of lymph node evaluation are included. The likelihood of lymph node metastases in T$_{1a}$

TABLE 41.1 Incidence of Lymph Node Metastases Based on Tumor Size in Breast Cancer Patients Undergoing Sentinel Lymphadenectomy[a]

Series	No.	Evaluation	T_{1mic}	T_{1a}	T_{1b}	T_{1c}	T_2
Memorial Sloan Kettering Cancer Center[b]		Overall includes IHC	11%	14%	22%	36%	58%
		Serial section	5%	10%	18%	32%	53%
		H&E alone	2%	5%	13%	25%	45%
University of California, Davis[c]	577	NS	—	15%		31%	56%
European Working Group[d]	2929	Overall includes IHC	6.5%	10%		16% T < 1.5	—
Mayo Clinic[e]	77	Overall includes IHC	7.8%	—	—	—	—
Mayo Clinic, University of Pennsylvania[f]	222	Overall includes IHC	—	4%	20%	24%	49%
University of Istanbul[g]	400	Overall includes IHC	—	18%	24%	33%	52%

H&E, Hematoxylin and eosin staining; *IHC*, immunohistochemistry; *NS*, not significant; *T*, tumor size (T_{1a}, T ≤ 0.5 cm; T_{1b}, 0.5 < T ≤ 1 cm; T_{1c}, 1 < T ≤ 2 cm; T_2, 2 < T ≤ 5 cm).
[a]Immunohistochemistry has resulted in an increased detection of nodal disease.
[b]Data from Bevilacqua.[44]
[c]Data from Vanderveen KA, Schneider PD, Khatri VP, et al. Upstaging and improved survival of early breast cancer patients after implementation of sentinel node biopsy for axillary staging. *Ann Surg Oncol.* 2005;13:1450-1456.
[d]Data from Cserni G, Bianchi S, Vezzosi V, et al. Sentinel lymph node biopsy in staging small up to 15 mm breast carcinomas. Results from a European multiinstitutional study. *Pathol Oncol Res.* 2007;13:5-14.
[e]Data from Gray RJ, Mulheron B, Pockaj BA, et al. The optimal management of the axillae of patients with microinvasive breast cancer in the sentinel lymph node era. *Am J Surg.* 2007;194:845-848, discussion 848–849.
[f]Data from Reynolds C, Mick R, Donohue JH, et al. Sentinel lymph node biopsy with metastasis: can axillary dissection be avoided in some patients with breast cancer? J Clin Oncol. 1999;17:1720-1726.
[g]Data from Ozmen et al.[70]

cancers is 10% to 18%. Higher rates are encountered if immunohistochemistry is used to evaluate the lymph nodes. Lymph node metastases are observed in up to 24% of patients with T_{1b} tumors and approximately one third of patients with T_{1c} cancers. Similar to T_{1a} cancers, a higher incidence of lymph node metastases is seen when immunohistochemistry is used to evaluate the lymph node. Approximately 50% of patients with T_2 tumors have nodal involvement. It is clear that intense histologic evaluation of sentinel lymph nodes has resulted in increased identification of nodal metastasis, especially isolated tumor cells and micrometastasis.[42] It has been shown that in countries that have adopted sentinel lymphadenectomy in the management of patients with early breast cancer, lymph node metastasis has increased 13%.[43] For example, intense histologic analysis of sentinel lymph nodes has resulted in an increased detection of metastases in microinvasive breast cancer from 2% to almost 10%.[44] Most of the metastases identified in these patients are micrometastases or isolated tumor cells, and the clinical significance of these small tumor deposits is debated. In addition to tumor size, prognostic factors associated with increased incidence of lymph node metastasis include tumor grade, age, hormone receptor status, and presence of lymphovascular invasion. The special subtypes of ductal carcinoma such as colloid, papillary, and tubular have been reported to have a low likelihood of lymph node metastasis. For example, in a meta-analysis of pure tubular carcinomas, positive nodes were seen in 7% of patients and none in patients with tumors less than 1 cm.[45] However, the advent of sentinel lymphadenectomy has also increased nodal positivity. Leikola and coworkers reported that almost 30% of patients with tubular carcinomas had a positive sentinel lymph node, including tumors less than 1 cm. The average size of the metastasis was small (0.17 mm), and in most patients only the sentinel lymph node was positive for disease.[46]

Surgical techniques for evaluating the axilla include sentinel lymphadenectomy, limited axillary clearance, and axillary node dissection. For many decades, axillary node dissection was an important tool in the management of breast cancer because of its ability to determine the number of positive nodes involved with disease and because it had a low rate of regional recurrence. Axillary recurrence after a level I and II dissection is less than 3%.[47] However, axillary node dissection has significant morbidity, including lymphedema, paresthesias, and nerve damage. The widespread application of mammographic screening and smaller tumor size at presentation has resulted in approximately only 25% of women having nodal disease at the time of presentation.[47a] An axillary node dissection in node-negative women provides no therapeutic benefit other than prognostic information, and the advent of sentinel lymphadenectomy to stage the axilla has relegated axillary node dissection to the treatment of patients with known positive nodes. Despite the complications associated with axillary node dissection, it remains the gold standard for surgical evaluation of the axilla in breast cancer patients with large tumors (>T2) and/or with known axillary node metastatic disease.

Sentinel lymphadenectomy is a minimally invasive technique that can stage the axilla in breast cancer patients. Since its initial description in 1994,[13] sentinel lymphadenectomy has been rapidly incorporated into clinical practice. The advantage of sentinel lymphadenectomy is that patients who have no nodal metastases can avoid a formal axillary node dissection. The ability to detect at least one sentinel lymph node is in the high 90th percentile.[48] In most patients, only two sentinel lymph nodes are removed, and therefore a disadvantage is that those patients who have positive sentinel lymph nodes may need to have a completion axillary node dissection to determine the number of positive nodes. An international consensus conference agreed that sentinel node biopsy was a suitable replacement for axillary node dissection in early breast cancers.[49]

The early studies of sentinel lymphadenectomy reported false-negative rates in patients who had immediate completion axillary node dissections. The false-negative rate, defined as node-positive patients with negative sentinel lymph nodes divided by all patients with positive axillary lymph nodes, ranged from 9.6%[50] to 11.4%[51] in early studies. The excellent results obtained with this technique led to early abandonment of a completion axillary node dissection in patients with negative sentinel lymph nodes. There have been multiple institutional studies that have reported outcomes of patients with negative sentinel lymph nodes who did not have a formal axillary node dissection. Clinical axillary recurrence rates from single institutions in patients with negative sentinel node biopsy alone are negligible and less than 1.5%.[52–56] A similar low axillary recurrence of 0.6% was reported by the Swedish Multicenter Cohort Study of 3534 patients after 3 years of follow-up.[57] In the European Institute of Oncology randomized trial of sentinel lymphadenectomy and axillary node dissection, patients with negative sentinel lymph nodes did not have completion axillary node dissection. There have been 2 axillary recurrences out of 167 patients with a negative sentinel lymph node who did not have completion axillary dissection after a median follow-up of 102 months.[50,58]

Patients undergoing sentinel lymphadenectomy alone have less morbidity compared with those who have a completion axillary node dissection. The European Institute of Oncology study randomized 516 patients to sentinel node biopsy followed by immediate axillary node dissection or axillary node dissection only if the sentinel lymph node was positive for metastatic disease.[50] Besides the results previously mentioned, less morbidity, as measured by axillary pain, paresthesias, arm mobility, and arm swelling was observed in the sentinel node group. The Axillary Lymphatic Mapping Against Nodal Axillary Clearance (ALMANAC) trial randomized patients with operable breast cancer to sentinel lymphadenectomy or axillary node dissection. The primary outcome measures were arm and shoulder morbidity and quality of life. Patients randomized to sentinel lymphadenectomy had a decreased risk of lymphedema and sensory loss and perceived better quality of life than those undergoing axillary dissection.[59] National Surgical Adjuvant Breast and Bowel Project (NSABP) B-32 randomized patients to sentinel node biopsy followed by immediate axillary node dissection or sentinel lymphadenectomy without formal axillary dissection if the sentinel lymph nodes were negative. The primary end points of this trial were survival, regional control, and morbidity. This trial randomized 5611 patients between 1999 and 2004. Findings demonstrated overall survival, disease-free survival, and regional control to be similar between groups with mean time on study for SLN negative patients of 95.6 months.[60,61] The American College of Surgeons Oncology Group (ACOSOG) Z0011 randomized patients with a positive sentinel lymph node to observation or completion axillary node dissection; women in the latter group had more wound infections, seromas, and paresthesias.[62] Women in the completion axillary node dissection arm were more likely to have lymphedema. An Italian trial (Sentinella-GIVOM)[63] and a UK trial (Cambridge/East Anglia)[64] are designed in a similar manner to NSABP B-32. Both of these studies have reported arm morbidity and better quality of life in patients randomized to the sentinel lymphadenectomy arm alone. In summary, sentinel lymphadenectomy is a minimally invasive surgical technique that can accurately stage the axilla in breast cancer patients with less morbidity than a level I/II axillary node dissection.

Sentinel lymphadenectomy can provide information about whether breast cancer patients have nodal disease, but because there is limited sampling of nodes, it cannot be used to determine the number of positive lymph nodes. There has been much debate about the need for a completion axillary node dissection in patients with a sentinel lymph node positive for metastatic disease.[65] Total number of positive nodes is important prognostic information because an increasing number of positive nodes correlates with decreased survival. Furthermore, additional positive axillary lymph nodes may influence decisions regarding adjuvant treatment. However, as discussed earlier, axillary node metastases are indicators, and not governors, of survival, and therefore the therapeutic benefit of further surgery may be minimal. Most patients with a positive sentinel lymph node have no further axillary disease,[51] and there is clearly no benefit to removing negative axillary lymph nodes. Delayed axillary dissection is also associated with increased operative time.[66] Furthermore, adjuvant chemotherapy is seldom altered by information gathered from the completion axillary dissection.[42]

These arguments have resulted in discussions of whether patients with a positive sentinel lymph node need to have a completion axillary node dissection and methods to predict which patients will have a positive non–sentinel lymph node. Patients with positive sentinel lymph nodes but no residual nodal disease would derive little benefit from a completion axillary node dissection. Size of metastasis is most predictive of likelihood of non–sentinel node metastasis. Micrometastases are defined as having a size of more than 0.2 mm but not greater than 2 mm. Isolated tumor clusters are not greater than 0.2 mm, have no evidence of proliferation or stromal reaction, and are located in lymphatic sinuses.[67] As shown in Table 41.2, about 50% of patients with metastatic deposits greater than 2 mm (macrometastases) have residual disease identified on completion axillary node dissection. However, patients with micrometastases, especially isolated tumor clusters, are less likely to have further positive sentinel lymph nodes after completion axillary dissection. An exception is the series from University of Helsinki in which 26% of patients with a sentinel lymph node micrometastasis had tumor deposits in non–sentinel lymph nodes. Immunohistochemical analysis of non–sentinel lymph nodes may partially explain the high rate of non–sentinel lymph node involvement in the Helsinki series.[68] In addition to size of metastasis, tumor features may be used to predict patients likely to have non–sentinel lymph node metastases. Patients with a macrometastasis, lymphovascular invasion in the primary tumor, extranodal extension, or a high ratio of involved to noninvolved sentinel lymph nodes are more likely to metastasize to non–sentinel lymph nodes.[69–71] Patients with a solitary positive sentinel lymph node accompanied by additional negative sentinel lymph nodes are unlikely to have residual disease.[72]

These risk factors are difficult to apply to the individual patient who may be unsure if she should proceed to a completion axillary dissection. Nomograms have been designed to assist physicians and patients in this decision-making process. The first computerized model for prediction of positive non–sentinel lymph nodes in patients with a positive sentinel lymph node was reported from the Memorial Sloan Kettering Cancer Center (MSKCC).[73] This nomogram was created using the data from 702 patients who had had a sentinel lymphadenectomy followed by completion axillary dissection. Factors used in calculating risk in this nomogram

TABLE 41.2   Likelihood of non-SLN Metastasis After Axillary Node Dissection in Patients With a Positive SLN[a]

Size of Metastasis	Series	No.	Incidence of non-SLN Metastasis (%)
Macrometastasis	John Wayne Cancer Institute[b]	101	63
	European Institute of Oncology[c]	794	50
	Rush-Presbyterian-St. Luke's-Roosevelt[d]	63	46
	University of Texas MD Anderson Cancer Center[e]	92	48
	University of Ferrara[f]	38	43
	Netherlands Cancer Institute[g]		
	Mayo Clinic/University of Pennsylvania[h]	24	80
	Istanbul University[i]	130	56
Micrometastasis	John Wayne Cancer Institute[b]	93	26
	European Institute of Oncology[c]	318	21
	Rush-Presbyterian-St. Luke's-Roosevelt[d]	30	20
	Netherlands Cancer Institute[e]	106	19
	Mayo Clinic/University of Pennsylvania[f]	36	25
Micrometastasis and isolated tumor cluster	Mayo Clinic[j]	28	7
	University of Ferrara[f]	58	14
	Istanbul University[i]	18	11
	Helsinki University[k]	84	26
	Univ. of Texas MD Anderson Cancer Center[e]	30	17
Isolated tumor cluster	John Wayne Cancer Institute[l]	61	5
	Rush-Presbyterian-St. Luke's-Roosevelt[d]	31	19
	European Institute of Oncology[c]	116	15

SLN, Sentinel lymph node.

[a]Patients with SLN containing micrometastases and isolated tumor clusters are less likely to have residual disease after completion axillary node dissection.

[b]Data from Turner RR, Chu KU, Qi K, et al. Pathologic features associated with nonsentinel lymph node metastases in patients with metastatic breast carcinoma in a sentinel lymph node. *Cancer.* 2000;89:574-581.

[c]Data from Viale G, Maiorano E, Pruneri G, et al. Predicting the risk for additional axillary metastases in patients with breast carcinoma and positive sentinel lymph node biopsy. *Ann Surg.* 2005;241:319-325.

[d]Data from Menes TS, Tartter PI, Mizrachi H, et al. Breast cancer patients with pN0i + and pN1mi sentinel nodes have high rate of nonsentinel node metastases. *J Am Coll Surg.* 2005;200:323-327.

[e]Data from Hwang et al.[80]

[f]Data from Carcoforo P, Maestroni U, Querzoli P, et al. Primary breast cancer features can predict additional lymph node involvement in patients with sentinel node micrometastases. *World J Surg.* 2006;30:1653-1657.

[g]Data from van Rijk et al.[42]

[h]Data from Reynolds C, Mick R, Donohue JH, et al. Sentinel lymph node biopsy with metastasis: Can axillary dissection be avoided in some patients with breast cancer? *J Clin Oncol.* 1999;17:1720-1726.

[i]Data from Ozmen et al.[70]

[j]Data from Gray RJ, Pockaj BA, Conley CR. Sentinel lymph node metastases detected by immunohistochemistry only do not mandate complete axillary lymph node dissection in breast cancer. *Ann Surg Oncol.* 2004;11:1056-1060. [k]Data from Leidenius et al.[68]

[l]Data from Calhoun KE, Hansen NM, Turner RR, Giuliano AE. Nonsentinel node metastases in breast cancer patients with isolated tumor cells in the sentinel node: implications for completion axillary node dissection. *Am J Surg.* 2005;190:588-591.

included tumor size, histology and grade, lymphovascular invasion, multifocality, hormone receptor status, method used to analyze the sentinel lymph nodes, and the number of positive and negative sentinel lymph nodes. The model was subsequently applied to 371 patients. The MSKCC nomogram has been validated by several centers.[74–77] Although it has been shown to be a good predictive tool, limitations include overestimation of risk in patients with sentinel lymph node that contain micrometastasis only,[75] differences in pathologic examination of the node,[76] and volume of metastasis and presence of extracapsular extension.[77] The MSKCC nomogram has been shown to be more accurate than clinical judgment in predicting likelihood of non–sentinel lymph node metastasis and need for completion axillary node dissection.[78] Although the MSKCC nomogram has been validated by other institutions, caution should be used when applied to patients who have a preoperative axillary ultrasound showing a normal-appearing sentinel lymph node and a positive sentinel

lymph node. In this group of patients, the MSKCC nomogram may overestimate the risk of non–sentinel lymph node metastasis.[79]

A mathematical scoring system using clinical and pathologic factors to predict likelihood of metastases in non–sentinel lymph nodes has been developed at the MD Anderson Cancer Center.[80] This algorithm was based on 131 breast cancer patients who had a positive sentinel node and underwent completion axillary dissection. Factors predictive of a positive non–sentinel node were a primary tumor greater than 2 cm, presence of a macrometastasis (i.e., metastatic deposit >2 mm), and lymphovascular invasion. Patients with a score of 4 all had further axillary metastases after completion axillary dissection.

A drawback of the MSKCC nomogram is that size of metastasis is not included in the model.[81] The presence of immunohistochemistry metastasis is used as a surrogate for micrometastasis. Although the MD Anderson model does include size of metastasis as a factor, only four variables are used in their mathematical algorithm. The ability of both of these models has been compared, and in a retrospective series of 186 sentinel lymph node–positive patients, the MSKCC was found to be more useful in individualizing surgical management of the axilla in sentinel lymph node–positive patients.[82] These models may be helpful in counseling patients who are unlikely to have non–sentinel lymph node metastasis or who are poor surgical candidates. The S classification of sentinel lymph nodes may be used to predict non–sentinel lymph node metastasis in patients with a positive sentinel lymph node. This classification system was initially described in patients with malignant melanoma and measures the maximum distance between tumor cells and the interior margin of the respective lymph node capsule for each positive sentinel lymph node.[83] The S classification system used depth of invasion as a surrogate for size of metastasis. SI is defined as subscapular tumor cells no deeper than 0.3 mm, SIII has tumor cells deeper than 1 mm below the capsule, and SII has a depth between SI and SIII. In a recently published study of 36 patients with a positive sentinel lymph node, there were no non–sentinel lymph nodes positive for metastasis in patients classified as SI, whereas 61% of patients with SIII had non–sentinel lymph nodes positive for metastasis.[84] A study by the same group retrospectively looked into the capability of predicting presence of metastases and overall survival in a population of 236 patients with a positive sentinel node followed by axillary lymph node dissection. This study concluded that this system allowed adequate prediction of the likelihood of the involvement of non-SLN and with a good OS prognosis with a mean follow-up of 65 months.[85] Although encouraging, the S classification of sentinel lymph nodes would still need to be validated in a larger cohort of breast cancer patients. In summary, it is difficult to accurately predict which patients with a positive sentinel lymph node will have residual disease after completion axillary node dissection. Patients with immunohistochemistry-positive sentinel lymph nodes or who fit ACOSOG Z0011 trial population profile do not need to undergo completion axillary node dissection.[86,87] Within this group, caution should be reserved for patients with T$_3$ and T$_4$ tumors because these are the patients most likely to have non–sentinel lymph node involvement.

It has been argued that axillary clearance is not needed in patients with positive sentinel lymph nodes because tangential fields from breast radiotherapy cover the axilla. Studies have looked at whether tangential breast radiotherapy fields overlap in breast cancer patients treated with breast conservation. Initial studies were difficult to interpret because the extent of the axilla was difficult to define using plain films. The advent of sentinel lymphadenectomy allowed marking of the sentinel lymph node with a clip. Radiotherapy fields in relation to this clip could be determined and the radiation dose to the clip calculated. In a small study of 36 women, the clip marking the sentinel lymph node fell within the tangential breast radiotherapy fields 94% of the time with a radiation dose greater than 4400 cGy in 50% of the patients.[88] A larger study of 106 patients confirmed that the sentinel lymph node clip was within the tangential fields used for breast radiotherapy but surprisingly was not covered by standard axillary radiation fields.[89] These results suggest that residual axillary disease within the axilla would be treated in patients undergoing breast radiotherapy and therefore that completion axillary dissection may not be necessary in patients with a positive sentinel node.

Two large randomized studies were designed to address the need for completion axillary dissection in breast cancer patients with a positive sentinel lymph node. The ACOSOG Z0011 study randomized breast cancer patients with a positive sentinel lymph node to completion axillary dissection or observation.[93] Patients in the observation arm did not have radiotherapy fields altered to include the axilla. Decisions regarding adjuvant systemic chemotherapy were based on primary tumor characteristics. This study randomized 891 patients with 446 patients undergoing lumpectomy and radiation for T1 or T2 tumors and clinically negative axilla. At a median follow-up of 6.3 years, there were no differences in local recurrence or regional recurrence in the two comparison groups, suggesting that sentinel lymph node procedure without axillary node dissection offers adequate regional control in patients with up to 2 positive sentinel lymph node.[87] The European Organization for Research and Treatment of Cancer 10981 to 22023 After Mapping of the Axilla: Radiotherapy or Surgery (AMAROS) trial was designed to compare regional control in patients with a positive sentinel lymph node randomized to delayed axillary dissection or axillary radiotherapy.[94] This intergroup noninferiority phase III study addressed whether axillary radiation therapy provides equivalent regional control with fewer side effects compared with further axillary node dissection in cases where the sentinel lymph node is positive. Patients with tumors up to 5 cm and clinically negative axillary lymph nodes were eligible. The type of breast treatment was either breast conservation followed by whole breast radiation or mastectomy followed or not by chest wall radiation. Primary end point for patients with a positive sentinel lymph node was axillary recurrence in 5 years with secondary measured outcomes including recurrence-free, disease-free, and overall survival; shoulder mobility; lymphedema; and quality of life. A total of 4823 patients were enrolled from 2001 to 2010, with 4806 of them being eligible for randomization to either receive axillary node dissection or axillary radiotherapy.[95,96] A positive sentinel lymph node was found in 1425 patients with 244 of them assigned to receive axillary node dissection and 681 axillary radiotherapy (intention-to-treat patient population). With 6.1 years of median follow-up it was seen that the 5-year axillary recurrence was 0.43% and 1.19% respectively, a difference without statistical significance, whereas lymphedema in the ipsilateral arm was significantly more frequently seen in the axillary dissection arm at 1, 3, and 5 years. Ipsilateral arm range of motion and quality of life were not significantly different between groups.[96]

Although a level I and II dissection has been part of treatment practice worldwide, many surgeons in the United Kingdom have preferentially used four-node sampling for many decades.[97] Four-node sampling involves removal of palpable lymph nodes by surgical exposure beginning at the axillary tail until four axillary lymph nodes have been identified.[98] Chetty and colleagues[99] reported the Edinburgh Breast Unit experience with this technique in their prospective study of 466 patients randomized to level III axillary dissection or four-node sampling and axillary radiotherapy or, in the latter half of the trial, observation only of patients with negative nodes. There was no statistical difference in the proportion of women with positive lymph nodes or in the regional nodal recurrence rate between the two arms. Long-term regional control was excellent, with relapse rates of 5% at 10 years with no detriment in survival.[100] A similar prospective study of four-node sampling in 237 women demonstrated that this surgical approach to the axilla accurately predicted axillary status in 98% of patients.[101] These results should not be surprising because in a comparative study of four-node sampling and sentinel lymph node biopsy, the sentinel lymph node was contained within the four nodes sampled 80% of the time.[102]

Five-node biopsy has also been suggested as an alternative to axillary clearance in women with breast cancer. This technique involves removal of five lymph nodes with dissection beginning at the axillary tail. The accuracy of five-node sampling to evaluate nodal status has been reported[103] in a prospective trial of 415 breast cancer patients. The sensitivity of five-node biopsy was 97.3% (95% confidence interval 97.1%–97.5%), with a negative predictive value of 98.5% (95% confidence interval 98.4%–98.6%). The accuracy of five-node sampling was similar for cancers detected clinically or mammographically (97.9% and 95.8%, respectively). There were four false-negative cases in this study, resulting in an overall false-negative rate of 1%. If only patients with a positive lymph node were included in the denominator, the false-negative rate was 2.7% (4/149). The sensitivity of sampling only four nodes was negligibly lower than that reported for five-node biopsy (96%). This study concluded that five-node sampling was an accurate test for staging the axilla in breast cancer. Because all patients in this study had an axillary node dissection after five-node sampling, the morbidity of this surgical technique could not be evaluated.

Axillary Radiotherapy

Axillary radiotherapy is an alternative to surgical dissection. Axillary surgical dissection provides nodal information and excellent regional control. However, the increasing use of tumor features to guide systemic therapy recommendations makes nodal information less important. Patients enrolled in the NSABP B-04 trial had their axilla treated in three possible manners: observation alone, axillary node dissection, and axillary radiotherapy. The low regional recurrence rate with no diminution in survival in the arm randomized to axillary radiotherapy has prompted the use of axillary radiotherapy in the management of breast cancer patients. Other studies have reported their results on axillary radiotherapy for regional control in women with breast cancer. Overall, excellent regional control has been achieved with axillary radiotherapy with no decrease in survival (Table 41.3).

The longest follow-up comparing axillary dissection to axillary radiotherapy has been reported from the Institut Curie in France.[104] This study randomized 658 women with breast cancers less than 3 cm in size and clinically negative axilla to axillary dissection or axillary radiation. All patients had breast conserving therapy, and adjuvant systemic therapy was directed by treating physician. The mean age of all patients at randomization was 52 and 50.6 years for patients randomized to axillary surgery or radiotherapy, respectively. There was no significant difference in overall survival, disease-free survival, metastases, or local recurrences between the groups after a median follow-up of 15 years. The likelihood of axillary recurrence was 1% in the group having axillary clearance compared with 3% in the group treated with axillary radiotherapy. The authors concluded that axillary radiotherapy had a higher, albeit quite low, rate of axillary recurrence compared with surgical dissection with no difference in survival. Ten-year follow-up has been reported from three other studies. The University of Medicine and Dentistry of New Jersey (UMDNJ)/Yale series consists of results obtained in approximately 2000 women treated at these institutions. Most patients in this series had an axillary node dissection. There was excellent regional control regardless of axillary treatment in this study. The Danish and Japanese series were prospective studies. There were slightly more nodal recurrences in women treated with axillary radiotherapy in the Japanese series (axillary radiotherapy: 4.6%; axillary node dissection: 1.3%). There was no reported difference in regional control in the Danish series; however, women randomized to axillary radiotherapy also received tamoxifen.

TABLE 41.3 **Comparison of Axillary Node Dissection and Axillary Radiotherapy in Breast Cancer Patients[a]**

Study	Time Period	No.	Follow-Up (Years)	Treatment	Regional Recurrence (%)	Survival
Danish Study[a,b]	1991–2000	180	10	BCS, TAM, AxRT	1.1	10 years: 80%
	T_{1-2}	340		BCS, AND	1.5	10 years: 75%
Japanese Study[a,c]	1983–2002	80	10	BCS, AND	1.3	T_1: 95% T_2: 93%
	T_{1-2}	1134		BCS, AxRT	4.6	T_1: 93% T_2: 90%
Univ. of Medicine and Dentistry of New Jersey/Yale[d]	1973–2003	590	10	BCS, AxRT	3	—
		1330		BCS, AND	2	—
Italian+[e]	1995–1998	221	5	BCS, AxRT	0.5	95%
	T < 1.2 cm	214		BCS	1.4	97%
Institut Curie[f]	1982–1987	658	15	BCS, AND	1	74%
	T < 3 cm			BCS, AxRT	3	76%

AND, Axillary node dissection; *AxRT*, axillary radiotherapy; *BCS*, breast conservation surgery; T_1, tumors ≤2 cm; T_2, >2 but ≤5 cm; *TAM*, tamoxifen.

[a]Axillary radiotherapy results in good regional control of the axilla in breast cancer patients with no decrease in overall survival.

[b]Data from Spruit PH, Siesling S, Elferink MA, et al. Regional radiotherapy versus an axillary lymph node dissection after lumpectomy: A safe alternative for an axillary lymph node dissection in a clinically uninvolved axilla in breast cancer. A case control study with 10 years follow up. Radiat Oncol 2007;2:40.

[c]Data from Fujimoto N, Amemiya A, Kondo M, et al. Treatment of breast carcinoma in patients with clinically negative axillary lymph nodes using radiotherapy versus axillary dissection. Cancer 2004;101:2155-2163.

[d]Data from Pejavar et al.[92]

[e]Data from Veronesi et al.[121]

[f]Data from Ahlgren et al.[103]

The AMAROS trial included and randomized 1425 patients with a positive sentinel lymph node (pathologic staging) to receive axillary radiation or axillary lymph node dissection. These women had T1–2 primary breast cancer and originally clinically negative axilla. At a median follow-up of 6.1 years, there was a relatively low number of recurrence events. There was no significant difference in the 5-year axillary recurrence rates between the two groups, both being very low (0.43 and 1.19% for axillary lymph node dissection and RT-only groups, respectively). Disease-free survival was also similar; overall survival was not statistically different between the 2 groups. The only and significant difference between the groups was the higher incidence of lymphedema in the axillary lymph node dissection group at 1, 3, and 5 years.[96]

Therapeutic Role of Axillary Node Dissection

There are two explanations for why more extensive axillary surgery may influence survival. Extent of axillary node dissection may have an impact on survival because of better staging of patients. A Surveillance, Epidemiology, and End Results (SEER) database report of 257,157 breast cancer patients published in 2005 found that the total number of lymph nodes removed predicted survival.[105] Specifically, women who had more than four lymph nodes removed did substantially better than those who had fewer lymph nodes surgically excised. A similar study of 464 stage I breast cancer patients concluded that excision of less than 10 axillary lymph nodes was associated with a decrease in survival.[106] To determine whether some of the favorable outcome associated with greater number of nodes excised resulted from better selection of patients for adjuvant systemic therapy, Weir and colleagues evaluated extent of axillary dissection in patients who did not receive systemic therapy.[107] Their study included 2278 women treated for breast cancer from 1989 to 1993 in British Columbia, Canada. More recurrences and a worse overall survival were noted in patients who had fewer axillary lymph nodes excised and who had not received systemic therapy. This association between number of axillary lymph nodes and outcome disappeared in those who received systemic therapy, underlining the benefit of systemic therapy in treatment of micrometastatic disease. A study that contradicts the belief that extent of axillary node dissection influences survival because of better staging was reported by Camp and associates. In this small study of 290 node-negative breast cancers treated from 1982 to 1993, patients who had more than 20 lymph nodes removed had a worse 5-year survival (85%) compared with those with a lesser dissection (96%).[108] This study has been criticized because of its small sample size. Indeed, a larger study of 2229 patients treated during the same time period reported that neither 5-year nor long-term survival was influenced by the number of lymph nodes removed during dissection.[109] It is feasible that the association between increased survival and number of axillary lymph nodes excised may be less remarkable with the advent of sentinel lymphadenectomy, directed excision of lymph nodes, and the increased histologic evaluation of excised lymph nodes. The ratio of positive lymph nodes to total lymph nodes may be an important issue in axillary evaluation in patients with node-positive breast cancer. Indeed, the number of lymph nodes excised should be irrelevant if the lymph nodes are truly negative for metastatic disease. Van der Wal and coworkers[110] retrospectively evaluated 453 stage I and II breast cancers and examined total number of lymph nodes excised and the ratio of number of positive lymph nodes to total number excised. They found a significantly better 10-year survival in node-negative patients who

had more than 14 lymph nodes excised (89% and 79% for those with >14 lymph nodes and those with <14 lymph nodes excised, respectively). For node-positive patients, the total number of lymph nodes excised and the ratio of positive lymph nodes to total number of lymph nodes excised were significant risk factors for poor survival outcome. The association of poor outcome with this ratio supports the hypothesis that more extensive axillary surgery provides better staging information and selection of patients for adjuvant therapy.

Alternatively, excision of lymph nodes harboring microscopic foci of disease may improve survival. There are surprisingly few data that address the issue of whether cancer cells that have metastasized to the lymph node can metastasize. If breast cancer cells in the lymph node can metastasize, then there should be a survival advantage to axillary clearance. Conversely, if only primary tumor cells can metastasize, then treatment of lymph node metastases should have no impact on survival. Results from the NSABP B-04 trial are often used to support the concept that "lymph nodes are predictors but not governors of survival." However, there are two reasons the results of the NSABP B-04 may not be applicable today. During the period that the NSABP B-04 was conducted and until recently, 50% of breast cancer patients presented with nodal disease.[111] These patients were at significant risk for systemic disease, and an axillary node dissection may not have provided much benefit. However, with contemporary breast cancer screening with annual mammography, tumor size has decreased, and the likelihood of nodal metastasis at the time of presentation is approximately 25%.[112] The main drawback of the B-04 trial was the number of patients randomized to each arm. This study had a power of only 70% and 40% to detect survival differences of 7% and 5%, respectively.

Results from three randomized trials support the therapeutic value of axillary control. The Stockholm radiotherapy trial randomized 960 premenopausal patients to preoperative or postoperative radiotherapy or no radiotherapy after modified radical mastectomy. Radiotherapy produced a fivefold decrease in local recurrence risk and in node-positive women, postoperative radiotherapy decreased the risk of distant metastases. This trial suggested that local recurrence was a predictive factor for secondary systemic disease.[113] The Danish Breast Cancer Cooperative Group randomized 3000 high-risk breast cancer patients who had undergone mastectomy and axillary clearance to postmastectomy radiotherapy or observation.[114] Patients were deemed high risk because of large tumor size or skin or muscle invasion (T$_3$ or T$_4$ tumors) and/or positive axillary lymph nodes. Postmastectomy radiotherapy involved axillary, supraclavicular, and internal mammary lymph nodes. The locoregional recurrence rate was 14% in those patients receiving postmastectomy radiotherapy compared with 49% in those who did not receive it.[115] Most of the locoregional recurrences involved the chest wall. This study has been criticized because the axillary node dissection was inadequate, with only a median of seven nodes were removed. Furthermore, combination Cytoxan, methotrexate, fluorouracil (CMF) or tamoxifen was used for premenopausal and postmenopausal women, respectively; these therapies would be considered inadequate by contemporary guidelines.

The British Columbia randomized radiation trial was designed to determine the impact of postmastectomy radiation on survival in node-positive premenopausal women who received adjuvant CMF chemotherapy.[116] The study was conducted from 1979 to 1986 and included 318 women. All women had a modified radical mastectomy in which a median of 11 nodes was removed followed by CMF chemotherapy. The arm randomized to post-mastectomy radiation had significantly less locoregional recurrence and better breast cancer–specific survival and overall survival after 20 years of follow-up.[117] Eighteen percent of the patients assigned to chemotherapy alone had an isolated locoregional recurrence compared with 7% assigned to chemotherapy and radiation. The 20-year breast cancer–specific and overall survival were 38% and 37% in the group that received chemotherapy alone and 53% and 47% for the group assigned to chemotherapy and radiation. The improved outcome was independent of number of positive nodes. The results of both the Danish and British Columbia trials suggested that locoregional control secondary to adequate treatment of the axilla improved survival and had a therapeutic value.

Pooling of results with meta-analysis is one way to overcome the difficulty of small sample size. The potential therapeutic value of axillary node dissection and regional control has been raised by the results published from the Early Breast Cancer Trialists' Collaborative Group (EBCTG).[118] This review summarizes results available from 42,000 women in 78 randomized trials. If axillary node dissection has no therapeutic benefit, there should be no difference in survival in node-positive women undergoing mastectomy treated with or without postmastectomy radiotherapy. Fig. 41.4 summarizes the results on local recurrence and breast cancer mortality in women treated with mastectomy and axillary clearance with or without postmastectomy radiation. The results from 36 trials of patients treated with mastectomy and axillary clearance or axillary sampling randomized to radiotherapy or no radiotherapy were included for analysis. There was no difference in mortality in women with node-negative disease treated with or without postmastectomy radiation. However, there was significantly worse survival in node-positive women who did not receive postmastectomy radiotherapy with an absolute difference in survival of 5.4%. Patients with more than four positive nodes benefited the most from postmastectomy radiotherapy. The beneficial effect of radiotherapy of local and regional recurrences was independent of age.

Selective Management of Axilla

Even though the morbidity of sentinel lymphadenectomy is much lower than that of axillary node dissection, complications are not negligible. Considerable research has been conducted in trying to identify a group of breast cancer patients in whom the likelihood of nodal metastasis is so low that axillary evaluation can be omitted. The incidence of nodal metastases increases with tumor size and the extent of pathologic examination of the lymph node. Because more women now are diagnosed with small breast cancers, is it possible to identify a subset with a negligible incidence of prognostically significant lymph node metastases greater than 2 mm in diameter? If it were possible to identify a subset of women with excellent prognosis based on size and lack of nodal macrometastases, the need for surgical axillary evaluation could be obviated. Before widespread mammographic screening, few women had small breast cancers (T_{1a} and T_{1b}). The incidence of nodal metastases was derived from registry or population-based large databases as summarized in Table 41.4.[41] As shown in this table, the incidence of nodal metastases for T_{1a} breast cancers (invasive breast cancers ≤ 5 mm) was more than 10%. Initial evaluation of this data would suggest that one is not able to identify a subset of women in whom the incidence of nodal metastases is very low. However, Whitten and colleagues[119] found

that more than 50% of women identified as having T_{1a} breast cancers in registry data had misclassification of the T_{1a} size on actual pathologic review of the cancers and actually had larger breast cancers. Data from individual institutions that have performed a pathologic review of their T_{1a} breast cancers report an overall incidence of nodal metastasis less than 5%. As shown in Table 41.5, adverse prognostic factors may include high nuclear grade, lymphovascular invasion, age younger than 35 years at diagnosis, and breast cancers diagnosed by clinical examination. Even when these prognostic factors are included, the incidence of nodal metastases in T_{1a} breast cancers is less than 5% (4.9%). However, nodal metastases in these studies were based on axillary node dissections, and the advent of sentinel lymphadenectomy has resulted in an increased incidence of nodal metastases, particularly micrometastases.

Although the incidence of nodal metastases has increased for each tumor size classification, there are some groups for whom the likelihood is still low. Attempts have been made to develop nomograms that can predict nodal involvement in the era of sentinel lymphadenectomy. Kaufman and associates have described an axillary treatment scale, Kaufman axillary treatment scale (KATS) based on tumor size, patient age, and tumor grade.[120] Patients are rated 1 to 4 for tumor size, 1 to 3 for age, and 1 to 2 for tumor grade. When applied to a SEER database, KATS scores of 3 and 4 identified patients with an average node-positive rate of 4.4%. Although it could be argued that patients with low KATS scores may not need axillary dissection, patients in this database had conventional axillary surgery and not sentinel lymphadenectomy.

A nomogram to predict a positive sentinel node in breast cancer patients was developed using patients treated at MSKCC in New York.[44] The initial nomogram was modeled using data collected from 4608 breast cancer patients and validated in a subsequent 3037 patients. Factors associated with a positive sentinel node were age, tumor size, tumor type, lymphovascular invasion, tumor location, multifocality, and hormone receptor status. The nomogram is based on "points," with the number of points predicting probability of sentinel lymph node metastasis (Fig. 41.5). Although this nomogram is useful in counseling patients, the authors state that this model is imperfect, with an area under the curve of 0.754, and should only be used as an estimate of risk.

Data reported from clinical trials support that some patients do not need axillary evaluation. Most trials included older women and replaced axillary evaluation with tamoxifen. Overall, axillary observation in older women with small breast cancers has resulted in few axillary recurrences and good survival. The Italian trial was a large multicenter randomized control trial in breast cancer patients older than 45 years of age with tumors less than 1.2 cm and clinically negative axillae[121] comparing axillary radiotherapy with observation. With a median follow-up of 63 months, there have been more regional recurrences in those women who received no further treatment to the axilla after breast conserving treatment (1.4%) compared with those who received axillary radiotherapy (0.5%). However, there was no difference in disease-free survival between the groups. The International Breast Cancer Study Group (IBCSG) and the Italian equivalent of the National Cancer Institute used tamoxifen as a surrogate for axillary dissection in older women. The IBCSG and the Italian Istituto Nazionale dei Tumori (NCI) randomized women older than 60 or 65 years of age, respectively, to tamoxifen with and without axillary node dissection in patients undergoing breast conserving surgery. The overall

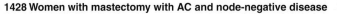

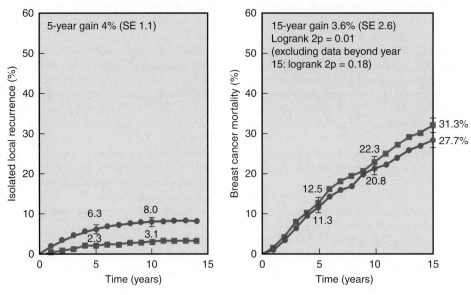

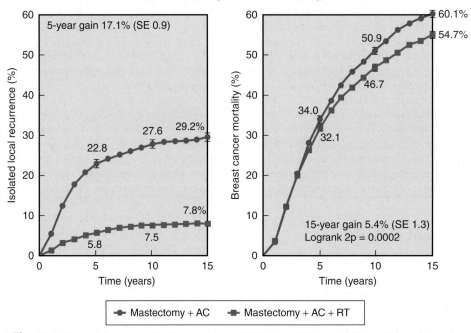

• **Fig. 41.4** Therapeutic value of axillary clearance (AC) and radiotherapy (RT) in node-positive breast cancer: Results from Early Breast Cancer Collaborative Trialists Group. Patients with node-positive breast cancer treated with AC and axillary RT had fewer recurrences and a better overall survival. *SE,* Standard error. (From Clarke M, Collins R, Darby S, et al: Effects of radiotherapy and of differences in the extent of surgery for early breast cancer on local recurrence and 15-year survival: an overview of the randomised trials. Lancet 2005;366:2087-2106.)

survival was equivalent in both arms for both studies, but the Italian NCI study reported more regional recurrences in women not receiving axillary node dissection. These studies confirm the results of the NSABP B-04 of no decrease in survival in women who do not have removal of axillary lymph nodes (Table 41.6). Another Italian study by Martelli and colleagues designed to assess the safety of omitting axillary lymph node dissection in elderly patients without palpable axillary lymph nodes failed to show significant difference in breast cancer mortality between the groups with and without axillary dissection after a median follow-up of 15 years. This study included 671 patients of 70 years of age and older treated between 1987 and 1992 with 172 receiving and 499 not receiving axillary lymph node dissection and all of whom received tamoxifen for at least 2 years. In patients with pT1a breast cancer, axillary relapse was 5.8% in the no-dissection group and 3.7% in the dissection group.[122]

The prognostic and therapeutic role of surgical evaluation of the axilla remains controversial. Presence of nodal metastases is an important prognostic factor in breast cancer patients and is used to guide recommendations for systemic therapy. Sentinel lymphadenectomy is a minimally invasive surgical technique that has resulted in an increased detection of nodal metastases. It can accurately predict which breast cancer patients have nodal disease, but its role as the only surgical intervention in node-positive patients is being evaluated. Newer studies are challenging the statement that "lymph node metastases are predictors and not governors of outcome" in this era of early breast cancer detection.

Targeted Axillary Lymph Node Dissection

Sentinel lymph node biopsy has been historically discouraged for patients who undergo neoadjuvant chemotherapy due to a concern of a higher false negative (FN) rate in this patient population. This was the original recommendation by the guideline for sentinel lymph node biopsy in breast cancer published by ASCO in 2005.[123] Now this recommendation is being modified and may be offered before or after neoadjuvant chemotherapy, although the outcome for patients who were node positive and become negative after the systemic treatment has not been extensively studied.[124]

The ACOSOG Z1071 (Alliance) trial was designed to evaluate accuracy of sentinel lymph node biopsy after chemotherapy in T0–4 N1–2 M0 breast cancer patients. The overall FN rate of sentinel lymph node biopsy in this group was 12.6% and varied significantly depending on whether single (20.3%) or dual (10.8%) tracer was used. The number of sentinel lymph nodes removed also influenced the FN rate with the lowest rate of 9.1% seen in patients who had three or more lymph nodes removed, but as high as 31% when only one was removed.[125] The SN FNAC study from Canada also aimed to study the accuracy of sentinel lymph node biopsy in patients with biopsy proven positive node (T0–3, N1–2) before neoadjuvant chemotherapy. An FN rate of 8.4% was reported, considering that IHC use was mandatory in this study and all sizes of nodal metastasis were included in the positive lymph node category. A higher FN rate of 13.3% was

TABLE 41.4 Nodal Positivity in T_{Ia} Breast Cancer From Tumor Registries

Series	Time Period	No. of T_{Ia} Cancers	Lymph Node Positive (%)
SEER	1988–1993	12,950	9.6
Rhode Island Tumor Registry/Bay State	1984–1995	230	11.3
British Columbia Cancer Agency, Canada	1989–1992	196	13.3
Oklahoma College of Medicine	1965–1989	74	12.2
Kitakyushu Medical Center, Japan	1970–1996	17	18
New York Presbyterian, Cornell University	1990–1996	199	16

SEER, Surveillance, Epidemiology, and End Results.
Modified from Chung MA, Wazer D, Cady B. Contemporary management of breast cancer. *Obstet Gynecol Clin North Am.* 2002;29:173-188.

TABLE 41.5 Nodal Positivity in T_{Ia} Breast Cancer for Single-Institution Reports

Series	Time Period	n	Lymph Node Positive (%)	Adverse Prognostic Factors
Mallinckrodt/St. Luke's	1969–1988	29	0 (0)	—
Joint Center for Radiation Therapy/Harvard Medical School	1968–1986	10	1 (10)	—
Memorial Sloan Kettering Cancer Center, New York	1989–1991	60	6 (10)	High nuclear grade, LVI
Mt. Sinai Medical Center, Miami, Florida	1990–1997	24	0 (0)	High nuclear grade
Breast Center, Van Nuys, California	1979–1995	92	4 (4)	LVI, high nuclear grade, palpable lesion
Loyola Medical Center, Illinois	1989–1996	23	1 (4.3)	High nuclear grade, LVI
Presbyterian Hospital, Carolinas Medical Center, North Carolina	1987–1994	82	3 (4)	—
Rush-Presbyterian–St. Luke's Medical Center	1987–1992	21	1 (5)	—
St. Joseph Hospital, Colorado	1987–1994	74	3 (4.5)	High nuclear grade
John Wayne Cancer Institute	1988–1994	20	2 (10)	—
Mount Sinai Medical Center, New York	1993–1998	105	8 (8)	Age <40 and LVI
Virginia Mason Hospital, Washington	1977–1987	34	1 (3)	—
Centro per lo Studio e la Prevenziona Oncologica of Florence	1970–1992	31	0 (0)	—
Total	—	605	30 (4.9)	

LVI, Lymphovascular invasion.
Modified from Chung MA, Wazer D, Cady B. Contemporary management of breast cancer. *Obstet Gynecol Clin North Am.* 2002;29:173-188.

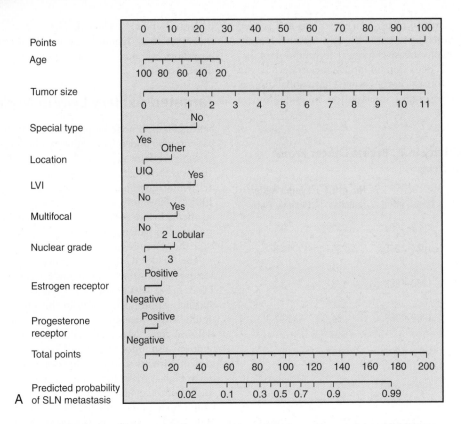

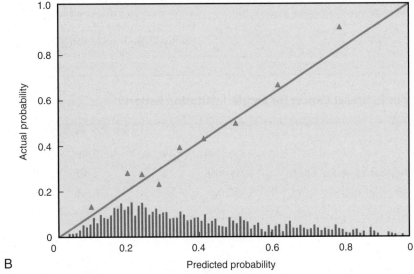

• **Fig. 41.5** Schematic diagram of Memorial Sloan Kettering Cancer Center nomogram that predicts likelihood of nodal metastases in breast cancer patients. *LVI,* Lymphovascular invasion; *SLN,* sentinel lymph node; *UIQ,* upper inner quadrant. (From Bevilacqua JL, Kattan MW, Fey JV, et al. Doctor, what are my chances of having a positive sentinel node? A validated nomogram for risk estimation. *J Clin Oncol.* 2007;25:3670-3679.)

seen if isolated tumor cells and micrometastatic disease were considered negative lymph nodes. Similarly to the ACOSOG Z1071, the use of dual tracer improved the accuracy of the sentinel lymph node biopsy.[126] Another prospective study, the SENTINA study, revealed that patients who were cN+ and converted into ycN0 (no baseline axillary node biopsy or FNA was done in these patients) had a FN rate of 14.2% by the sentinel lymph node biopsy procedure and an 80.1% identification rate. Similar to the

ACOSOG Z1071, FN rates decreased if a higher number of lymph nodes were removed and dual tracer was used for sentinel lymph node mapping.[127]

A more recently developed technique, targeted axillary lymph node dissection, may significantly lower the FN rates of SLNB in this subset of patients. The procedure is offered to patients with a positive node before neoadjuvant chemotherapy. It consists of removing the known metastatic lymph node at the time

TABLE 41.6   Outcome in Breast Cancer Patients Treated With Observation Only (With or Without Tamoxifen)

Study	Time	No	Treatment	Regional Recurrence	Overall Survival
Italian+[a]	1995–1998	221	BCS, AxRT	0.5%	95%
	T <1.2 cm	214	BCS,	1.4%	97%
International Breast Cancer Study Group Trial 10–93[b]	1993–2002	234	BCS, AND, TAM	—	6 y: 67%
	Age >60 y	239	BCS, TAM	—	6 y: 66%
National Cancer Institute, Italy[c]	1996–2000	110	BCS, TAM	1.8%	BCS: 96%
	Age 65–80 y T <2 cm	109	BCS, AND, TAM	0%	BCS: 96%

AND, Axillary node dissection; *AxRT,* axillary radiotherapy; *BCS,* breast conserving surgery; *T,* tumor size; *TAM,* tamoxifen.

[a]Data from Veronesi et al.[121]

[b]Data from International Breast Cancer Study Group; Rudenstam CM, Zahrieh D, Forbes JF, et al. Randomized trial comparing axillary clearance versus no axillary clearance in older patients with breast cancer: first results of International Breast Cancer Study Group Trial 10-93. *J Clin Oncol.* 2006;24:337-344.

[c]Data from Martelli G, Boracci P, De Palo M, et al. A randomized trial comparing axillary dissection to no axillary dissection in older patients with T1N0 breast cancer: results after 5 years of follow-up. *Ann Surg.* 2005;242:1-6, discussion 7-9.

of removing tracer detected sentinel lymph nodes. This has been studied by Caudle and associates at the MD Anderson, where the originally clipped positive node was localized with an I[125] seed under the ultrasound and sentinel nodes were mapped with the injection of radioisotope and/or blue dye. Dual tracer injection was not mandatory. FN rate was 10.1% in patients who underwent conventional sentinel lymph node biopsy followed by axillary lymph node dissection compared with 2% when targeted axillary dissection was followed by axillary lymph node dissection. They also reported an FN rate of 4.2% when only the clipped lymph node alone was removed.[128] A recent analysis of ACOSOG Z1071 (Alliance) patients who had a clip placed during the core needle biopsy of the node showed an FN rate of 6.8% when the clipped node was removed during the sentinel lymph node biopsy.[129] These studies demonstrated that axillary staging in patients who received preoperative chemotherapy was possible by a more limited procedure to reduce morbidity associated with axillary evaluation. It is noteworthy that there has been no large study to define long-term outcomes in patients with conversion to negative axilla by neoadjuvant chemotherapy when axillary lymph node dissection is not performed.

Selected References

87. Giuliano AE, McCall L, Beitsch P, et al. Locoregional recurrence after sentinel lymph node dissection with or without axillary dis-section in patients with sentinel lymph node metastasis. *Ann Surg.* 2010;252(3):426-433.

96. Donker M, van Tienhoven G, Straver ME, et al. Radiotherapy or surgery of the axilla after a positive sentinel node in breast cancer (EORTC 10981-22023 AMAROS): a randomized, multicenter, open-label, phase 3 non-inferiority trial. *Lancet Oncol.* 2014;15:1303-1310.

118. Clarke M, Collins R, Darby S, et al. Effects of radiotherapy and of differences in the extent of surgery for early breast cancer on local recurrence and 15-year survival: an overview of the randomised trials. *Lancet.* 2005;366:2087-2106.

124. Lyman GH, Temin S, Edge S, et al. Sentinel lymph node biopsy for patients with early-stage breast cancer: American Society of Clinical Oncology clinical practice guideline update. *J Clin Oncol.* 2014;32:1365-1383.

126. Boileau JF, Poirier B, Basik M, et al. Sentinel node biopsy after neoadjuvant chemotherapy in biopsy-proven node-positive breast cancer: the SN FNAC study. *J Clin Oncol.* 2015;33:258-264.

129. Boughey JC, Ballman KV, Le-Petross HT, et al. Identification and resection of clipped node decreases the false-negative rate of sentinel lymph node surgery in patients presenting with node-positive breast cancer (T0-T4, N1-N2) who receive neoadjuvant chemotherapy. Results from ACOSOG Z1071 (Alliance). *Ann Surg.* 2016;263:802-807.

A full reference list is available online at ExpertConsult.com.

42

Lymphatic Mapping and Sentinel Lymphadenectomy for Breast Cancer

ALICE CHUNG AND ARMANDO E. GIULIANO

Intraoperative lymphatic mapping and sentinel lymph node dissection (SLND) has replaced axillary lymph node dissection (ALND) as a minimally invasive and highly accurate staging procedure for early invasive breast cancer.[1] The status of the axillary lymph nodes is an important prognostic indicator for overall survival in breast cancer. It is the presence or absence of lymph node metastases, the number of tumor positive nodes, and the size of the primary tumor that determine the pathologic stage.[2] The prognostic information derived from ALND has been sufficiently crucial such that clinically uninvolved lymph nodes have been removed for staging with no therapeutic benefit. The therapeutic role of ALND and selective management of the axilla for minimally invasive breast cancer are addressed in Chapter 41.

History of Sentinel Node Concept in Breast Cancer

Surgeons, radiologists, and pathologists have had a long-standing interest in the draining lymphatics of malignant disease. Tumors have unique lymphatic drainage patterns (e.g., Virchow node for gastric cancer, Delphian node for thyroid cancer). The urologist Ramon Cabanas coined the term *sentinel node* (SLN) as a specific group of lymph nodes associated with the superficial epigastric vein for penile carcinoma.[3] Preoperative lymphangiograms were used to direct the anatomic dissection to resect this specific lymph node center. In his series, a positive lymph node center was identified in 15 patients, and complete inguino-femoro-iliac dissection demonstrated no additional positive nodes in 80% (12 of 15). Penile carcinoma was staged with preoperative lymphangiograms to identify the specific nodal center at risk for metastases, and bilateral biopsy of the SN center with inguino-femoro-iliac dissection was performed only when tumor cells were discovered in the SN center. On the basis of these results, when the sentinel nodal center was negative, no further nodal dissection was indicated.[3]

The SN concept is founded on the principle that the afferent lymphatic channel draining a primary tumor courses to the first, "sentinel," lymph node in that specific regional lymphatic basin (Fig. 42.1). Morton and colleagues at the John Wayne Cancer Institute (JWCI) first tested the sentinel node hypothesis in an animal model and then validated it in patients with melanoma.[4]

Investigators next asked if this minimally invasive technique could be applied to staging of breast cancer.[5,6] Radiographic imaging to stage the axilla had been attempted to identify nodal metastases in breast cancer, but no predictable preoperative technique had emerged with sufficient sensitivity and specificity to replace formal ALND.[7,8] Interestingly, Kett and Lukacs had reported that the first regional lymph node, the "Sorgius node," could be identified in breast cancer using direct mammalymphography.[7] Contrast material, Lipiodol Ultra-Fluide, was injected into a lymphatic collecting channel that had been visualized after intradermal injection of patent blue violet into the areola.[7] Benign lymph nodes could be distinguished from malignant nodes by the pattern of distribution of contrast material in the node. This technique did not attain general acceptance for diagnosing malignant nodes in breast disease. It was labor-intensive, time-consuming, and required serial roentgenography preoperatively for at least 24 hours. In addition, an ALND had to be performed regardless of the preoperative imaging studies to isolate the suspected lymph nodes. Postoperative roentgenograms of the excised axillary nodes were necessary to distinguish nodes that contained metastatic deposits from those that did not. Simplification of the technique with indirect lymphography was attempted but still required multiple projections of the axilla taken at regular intervals followed by surgery 24 to 48 hours later. The correlation of pathologically positive nodes with radiographically opacified nodes was poor, and the technique was abandoned.[8]

Armed with this historical information and the success of intraoperative lymphatic mapping for melanoma, three technical approaches for SN identification in breast cancer evolved: dye-directed lymphatic mapping, isotope-based radiolocalization, and the combination of vital dye and isotope techniques.[5,6,9–12]

Evolution of Dye-Directed Sentinel Lymphadenectomy for Breast Cancer

In October 1991, the feasibility of lymphatic mapping and sentinel lymphadenectomy in breast cancer was investigated in the hope of developing a more accurate staging procedure with less morbidity than ALND.[5] Several hypotheses for SLND in breast cancer were proposed and tested in a prospective manner.[5,11,13–15] The discoveries made by answering each hypothesis have brought us to the current acceptance of observation of the axilla in SN-negative patients. Although these studies established a technique and showed the

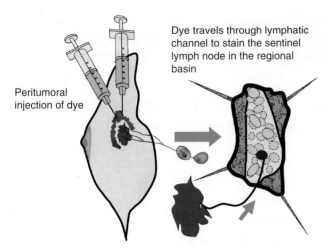

Peritumoral injection of dye

Dye travels through lymphatic channel to stain the sentinel lymph node in the regional basin

• **Fig. 42.1** Schematic diagram of blue dye transit from primary breast tumor to sentinel node.

TABLE 42.1	Comparison of Axillary Staging by Standard ALND and SLND	
	ALND (n = 134)	SLND (n = 162)
Median number of excised axillary nodes/basin (range)	19 (8–40)	21 (6–46)
Median number of positive axillary nodes/basin (range)	1 (1–27)	2 (1–33)
Number of patients with axillary metastasis	39 (29.1%)	68 (42%)[a]
≤2 mm by H&E	4 (3%)	15 (9.2%)[b]
≤2 mm by H&E or IHC	4 (3%)	26 (16%)[c]
≤2 mm by IHC	0	11 (6.8%)

ALND, Axillary lymph node dissection; *H&E,* hematoxylin and eosin; *IHC,* immunohistochemistry; *SLND,* sentinel lymph node dissection.
[a]*p* < .03.
[b]*p* < .004.
[c]*p* < .0005.
Modified from Giuliano AE, Dale PS, Turner RR, et al. Improved axillary staging of breast cancer with sentinel lymphadenectomy. *Ann Surg.* 1995;222:394-401.

feasibility of SLND, new questions emerged from these initial studies that were the basis of national clinical trials and rigorous scientific research (see later discussion).

In the absence of any prior experience with intraoperative lymphatic mapping for breast cancer, a learning period was required to define the technical aspects of the procedure. Several factors were identified that determined its ultimate success. These included patient selection, injection method, dissection technique, and histopathologic evaluation of the SN.

Surgical Feasibility

Could an SN be identified intraoperatively in breast cancer? In 1991, there was no established protocol for intraoperative lymphatic mapping for breast cancer. The purpose of this first pilot study was to establish a method of intraoperative lymphatic mapping and SLND in breast cancer and to determine the feasibility, safety, and accuracy of the procedure for early-stage breast cancer.[5] To accomplish this, intraoperative lymphatic mapping and SLND were followed by a completion level I, II, and some III ALND in all patients with invasive breast cancer, even those with advanced tumors and grossly involved nodes who we now know are not candidates for the procedure. The technical variables that were evaluated included the quantity of isosulfan blue dye (0.5–10 mL), the appropriate site of injection (tumor vs. parenchyma vs. biopsy site), and time interval from injection to axillary incision (1–60 minutes) required for successful identification of the SN.

There were two phases to this study: the early phase (I), or the technical development period, and the second phase (II), a refinement of a technique. During phase I, the ability to identify the SN was 58.6% with an accuracy of 94.3%. As the technical variables were refined and the method evolved in phase II, the identification rate was 78% with 100% accuracy. The probability of excising a tumor-bearing SN was significantly greater with SLND (61.9%) than with random axillary node sampling (17.5%; *p* < .0001).

This study must be put into the proper context of the time in which it was reported. It was a pilot study to determine whether the SN concept could be applied to breast cancer in the absence of any established criteria or guidelines. The ability to find the SN was lower than hoped for and disheartening, but the observation that, when discovered, it truly reflected the status of the axilla was exciting. This was sufficient to persist in further investigation.

Histopathologic Staging

To improve accuracy, a modification of the technique was discovered by evaluating the causes for a false-negative node in the pilot study. Of the five false-negative SNs, four could have been identified by intraoperative frozen section analysis or by postoperative immunohistochemistry (IHC). The second study considered whether focused histopathologic evaluation of the SN with serial section and IHC could improve the SN identification rate and reduce the false-negative rate.[13]

ALND alone was compared with SLND followed by completion ALND. In the SLND group, the SN was evaluated by frozen section hematoxylin and eosin (H&E) and permanent sections with H&E and IHC, whereas the non-SNs were evaluated by H&E alone. Axillary metastases were identified in 29.1% of the ALND group and 42% of the SLND group (*p* < .03). The difference resulted from the increased sensitivity in the detection of micrometastases by H&E and IHC in the SLND group versus the ALND group (16% vs. 3%, respectively; Table 42.1).

This study demonstrated that frozen section diagnosis, multiple levels of SN analysis, and IHC increased the accuracy of axillary staging. Micrometastases were easier to identify in the SN with multiple levels and IHC, although the clinical significance of IHC-detected micrometastases has not been shown to affect survival. This topic is discussed further later in this chapter and more extensively in Chapter 43.

Prospective Validation

The two initial studies established the methodology, feasibility, safety, and histopathologic processing of the SN. ALND still remained the established method of staging for the treatment of breast cancer in 1994. For an alternative approach to be considered, the new technique required prospective and systematic validation.[11] From July 1994 to October 1995, 107 patients with

TABLE 42.2	Sentinel Node Identification Rate and Detection of Sentinel Node Metastases by Size of Metastasis	
Variable		**No. of Patients**
SLND procedures		107
Detecting sentinel node		100 (93.5%)
Tumor-involved axillae		42
Sentinel node positive		42
With macrometastases		23
With micrometastases		19
Detected by H&E		10
Detected by IHC		9

H&E, Hematoxylin and eosin; *IHC,* immunohistochemistry; *SLND,* sentinel lymph node dissection.
Modified from Giuliano AE, Jones RC, Brennan M, Statman R: Sentinel lymphadenectomy in breast cancer. J Clin Oncol 1997;15:2345-2350.

TABLE 42.3 Relationship of Primary Tumor Size and Status of Sentinel Node

Primary Tumor Size	No. of Patients	SENTINEL NODE POSITIVE		SENTINEL NODE NEGATIVE	
		n	%	n	%
T_1	64	22	34.4	42	65.6
T_{1a}	4	1	25	3	75
T_{1b}	18	8	44.4	10	55.6
T_{1c}	42	13	31	29	69
T_2	34	18	52.9	16	47.1
T_3	2	2	100	0	0
All	100	42	42	58	58

Modified from Giuliano AE, Jones RC, Brennan M, Statman R. Sentinel lymphadenectomy in breast cancer. *J Clin Oncol.* 1997;15:2345-2350.

TABLE 42.4 Confirmation of the Sentinel Node Hypothesis Using IHC to Detect Metastasis in Nonsentinel Nodes When the Sentinel Node Is Tumor Free

	H&E	IHC	IHC Conversion Rate (%)	P Value
Lymph node evaluation				
Tumor in sentinel lymph node	0/157	10/157	6.4	<.0001
Tumor in nonsentinel lymph node	0/1087	1/1087	0.1	
Patient evaluation				
Patient with sentinel node metastases	0/70	10/70	14.3	<.0001
Patient with sentinel lymph node metastases only	0/60	1/60	1.7	

H&E, Hematoxylin and eosin; *IHC,* immunohistochemistry.
Modified from Turner RR, Ollila DW, Krasne DL, Giuliano AE. Histopathologic validation of the sentinel lymph node hypothesis for breast carcinoma. Ann Surg. 1997;226:271-278.

TABLE 42.5 Final Tumor Status of Sentinel and Nonsentinel Lymph Nodes

Tumor Status	No. of Patients (%)
Lymph node positive	59 (57.3)
Lymph node negative	44 (42.7)
Sentinel node positive only	25 (24.3)
Sentinel node and nonsentinel node positive	18 (17.5)
Nonsentinel node positive only	1 (1)
Total	103 (100)

Modified from Turner RR, Ollila DW, Krasne DL, Giuliano AE. Histopathologic validation of the sentinel lymph node hypothesis for breast carcinoma. Ann Surg. 1997;226:271-278.

potentially curable breast cancer underwent SLND with the mature method. The SN was identified in 93.5%, and 66.7% of those with a tumor-positive SN had no other tumor-bearing axillary lymph nodes (Table 42.2). The status of the axilla relative to the tumor size is shown in Table 42.3.

There were no false-negatives, with a specificity and sensitivity of 100%. Axillary staging with SLND was validated for this defined patient population using strict technical guidelines for identification and evaluation of the SN. Since then a number of prospective clinical trials have confirmed the feasibility of intraoperative lymphatic mapping, its accuracy, and its oncologic safety in clinically node-negative breast cancer.

Complete Nonsentinel Node Staging and Proof of Principle

The SN hypothesis was not immediately accepted but challenged as an artifact of increased SN histopathologic processing and not a reflection of the status of the axilla. This challenge led to the initiation of the pivotal study of lymphatic mapping in breast cancer and proof of principle that the SN is the first regional node draining the primary tumor.[15]

Complete histopathologic evaluation of SNs and non-SNs was performed with serial sectioning, H&E, and IHC in all cases of H&E-negative SNs. H&E staining identified a tumor-bearing SN in 32% of patients, and IHC upstaged an additional 14.3% (Table 42.4). In 60 patients whose SNs were negative by H&E and IHC, 1087 non-SNs were examined at two levels by IHC. Only one additional tumor-positive node was identified. The SN was sufficient for staging and therapy in 57.3% of patients because they had no additional nodal disease (Table 42.5).

This study provided evidence that the SN is the first draining lymph node from the primary tumor and is not an artifact of histopathologic evaluation. The SN hypothesis was validated and has been confirmed by independent investigators.[16–18]

TABLE 42.6	Sentinel Node Histopathology in Clinical Trial of Patients With a Tumor-Free Sentinel Node	
	No. of Patients/ Total Patients	Percent of Patients
Sentinel node identified	124/125	99.2
Sentinel node negative	67/124	54
Sentinel node positive	57/124	46
>2 mm	26/57	45.6
≤2 mm	31/57	54.4
H&E identified	9/31	29
IHC identified	22/31	71

H&E, Hematoxylin and eosin; *IHC,* immunohistochemistry.
From Giuliano AE, Haigh PI, Brennan MB, et al. Prospective observational study of sentinel lymphadenectomy without further axillary dissection in patients with sentinel node-negative breast cancer. J Clin Oncol. 2000;18:2553-2559.

Prospective Study of Sentinel Lymphadenectomy Alone for a Tumor-Free Sentinel Node

Standardization of the SLND technique, validation with completion ALND, and complete histopathologic assessment of the SN and non-SNs confirmed the accuracy and prognostic value of SLND. The natural segue in the incorporation of SLND was the study to determine whether ALND could be avoided when the SN was negative. The purpose of the next study was to determine the complication rate and the local recurrence rate in women who had a tumor-free SN who did not undergo ALND.[14] This was the first study to eliminate ALND in SN-negative patients.

Women with tumors of 4 cm or less underwent SLND for staging as the only axillary treatment if the SN contained no tumor cells. Completion ALND was performed when the SN contained metastatic cells. Patients did not receive axillary irradiation. SLND identification rate was 99% (Table 42.6). Complications occurred in 20 patients (35%) undergoing ALND after SLND, but in only two patients (3%) undergoing SLND alone (*p* = .001). The complications in both groups were minimal, primarily wound seromas. There were no locoregional recurrences at 39 months. Subsequent studies support these findings.[19] The axillary recurrence rates are under 1% in the majority of large studies.[20]

SLND can eliminate the need for ALND in patients who have negative SNs, because removal of negative axillary lymph nodes does not alter disease outcome. The role of SLND alone for SN-negative breast cancer patients has been investigated in large national and international trials (see later discussion).

Identification of the Sentinel Node in Breast Cancer by Radiolocalization

During the 1970s and 1980s, radiocolloid lymphoscintigraphy was shown to be a versatile and simpler technique than mammalymphography, but the prognostic value of axillary lymphoscintigraphy alone was insufficient to avoid axillary dissection for staging. In the early 1990s, experimentation with radiolocalization of the SN on the skin surface that could direct surgical removal with a gamma detection probe was initiated in an animal model.[21] Gamma probe–guided SN identification had some theoretical advantages: the location of the SN could be identified, surgery could be confined to a small area in a nodal basin, the SN could be distinguished from non-SNs by quantitative counts, and extraaxillary SNs could be detected.

In 1993, Krag and coworkers reported a pilot study in 22 patients that established intraoperative radiolocalization of an SN in breast cancer. Unfiltered technetium-99m–labeled (^{99m}Tc) human sulfur colloid (0.5 mCi suspended in 0.5 mL saline) was injected in a 180-degree arc oriented toward the axilla, successfully identified a radioactive node in 82%, and reflected the status of the axilla in all these cases.

Identification of the Sentinel Node With Preoperative Lymphoscintigraphy and Intraoperative Radioguided Surgery

In 1997 Veronesi and colleagues reported a large series of patients who had subdermal injection of ^{99m}Tc-human colloidal albumin, preoperative lymphoscintigraphy, and intraoperative gamma probe detection of the SN.[12] The SN was identified in 98% of cases and accurately predicted the status of the axilla in 97.5%. In the large majority of early-stage breast cancer patients, the combination of preoperative lymphoscintigraphy with intraoperative radiolocalization could locate an SN in the axilla with a high degree of accuracy.[12]

Combined Technique of Vital Dye and Radioisotope

The group from the Moffitt Cancer Center adapted the discoveries made from blue dye lymphatic mapping and isotope radiolocalization and reported on the combined technique in 62 women.[10] The authors predicted that the ability to identify the SN by combined technique would be greater. In fact, in their hands, the SN was localized successfully in 92% of patients. A hot spot could be identified on the skin of the axilla and therefore limit the axillary exploration, minimizing tissue disruption. Radiocolloid identified more SNs, but in no case did a "hot" nonblue node contain micrometastatic disease.[10] No skip metastases were identified in this small series.

Global Experience With Sentinel Lymphadenectomy in Breast Cancer

From these lead studies, blue dye alone, radioisotope alone with or without preoperative lymphoscintigraphy, or combined dye and nuclide,[5,6,10,12] investigators from many large academic centers and smaller community hospitals in the United States and throughout the world rapidly experimented with variations on the techniques.[22] These studies demonstrate a high accuracy rate and a low false-negative rate (Table 42.7).[5,6,10–12,23–63] The value of the technique is inherent to the successful identification of the correct SN that reflects the status of the axilla.

Definition of the Sentinel Node

Morton first defined the SN as the first lymph node that receives afferent lymphatic drainage from the primary tumor.[4] As the

TABLE 42.7 Sentinel Lymph Node Identification and Success Rate

Author	Year	No. of Patients	Success (%)	Sensitivity (%)	NPV (%)	False Negative (%)	Accuracy (%)
Vital Dye Technique							
Guiliano[5]	1994	174	66	88	94	4.3	96
Guiliano[11]	1997	107	94	100	100	0	100
Guenther[23]	1997	145	71	90	96	9.6	97
Dale[25]	1998	21	66	100	100	0	100
Koller[29]	1998	98	98	96	94	5.8	97
Flett[30]	1998	68	82	83	93	17	95
Morgan[41]	1999	44	73	83	91	16.7	94
Imoto[42]	1999	88	74	86	89	13.7	94
Kern[44]	1999	40	98	100	100	0	100
Morrow[45]	1999	50[a]	88	95	—	—	96
Ilum[55]	2000	161	60	86	87	14.3	93
Motomura[60]	2001	93[b]	84	81	93	19	95
Radioisotope Technique							
Krag[6]	1993	22	82	100	100	0	100
Veronesi[12]	1997	163	98	95	95	4.7	98
Pijpers[24]	1997	37	81	100	100	0	100
Krag[28]	1998	157	93	95	98	4.9	98
Krag[26]	1998	443	93	89	96	11.4	97
Crossin[32]	1998	50	84	88	98	12.5	98
Borgstein[33]	1998	130	94	98	98	2.2	98
Offodile[34]	1998	41	98	100	100	0	100
Snider[37]	1998	80	88	93	98	7	99
Rubio[38]	1998	55	96	88	95	11.8	96
Veronesi[39]	1999	376[c]	99	93	94	6.7	97
Miner[31]	1999	57	97	92	98	7.7	98
Feldman[40]	1999	75	93	81	92	19	94
Moffat[47]	1999	70	89	90	96	10	97
Zurrida[51]	2000	376	99	93	94	6.7	97
Fraile[54]	2000	132	96	96	97	4	98
Rink[55]	2000	123	94	92	96	7.7	97
Mariani[58]	2000	197[d]	97	86	92	13.7	95
Combined Technique							
Albertini[10]	1996	62	92	100	100	0	100
Barnwell[35]	1998	42	90	100	100	0	100
O'Hea[36]	1998	59	93	85	92	15	95
Kollias[43]	1999	117	81	94	97	6.5	98
Morrow[45]	1999	42[e]	86	97	—	—	96
van der Ent[46]	1999	70	100	96	98	3.7	99

TABLE 42.7   **Sentinel Lymph Node Identification and Success Rate—cont'd**

Author	Year	No. of Patients	Success (%)	Sensitivity (%)	NPV (%)	False Negative (%)	Accuracy (%)
Hill[48]	1999	104[f]	93	89	91	10.6	95
Mariani[58]	2000	197[d]	97	86	92	13.7	95
Doting[52]	2000	136	93	95	96	5.1	98
Imoto[53]	2000	59	93	92	94	8	96
McMasters[63]	2000	562	90	94	98	5.8	98
Smillie[59]	2001	106	84	95	96	6	98
Motomura[60]	2001	138[g]	95	100	100	0	100
Frisell[63]	2001	75	92	89	93	11	96
Tafra[62]	2001	529	87	87	95	13	96

Sensitivity = (true positive)/(true positive + false negative).
Negative predictive value (NPV) = (true negative)/(true negative + false negative).
False negative = (false negative)/(true positive + false negative).
Accuracy = (true positive + true negative)/(total number of patients).
[a]Blue dye arm only.
[b]Indigocyanine green arm only.
[c]Includes subgroup of 54 patients who had patent blue dye and isotope.
[d]Analysis of 197 of 284 cases with axillary lymph node dissection.
[e]Blue dye and radioisotope arm.
[f]Subgroup of 104 of 500 cases with axillary lymph node dissection.
[g]Combine indigocyanine green and isotope arm.

techniques have varied to include radioisotope, dye, or a combination, the definition of the SN has become more complex. Operational definitions of the SN have evolved from technology.[64] These include the first blue node, the hottest node, the suspicious palpable node, and the node to which a blue lymphatic tracks. Problems are encountered when the SN is defined by technique. Radioactive lymph nodes are detected by lymphoscintigraphy and gamma detection probes. Lymphoscintigrams can visualize primary and secondary echelon nodes as well as nonaxillary sites.[64] The brightest nodes, however, may be bright because of the distance from the gamma counter, not because they are the first to receive metastases. Likewise, the gamma detection probe finds the hottest node that may be the node to which open lymphatic channels have been diverted rather than the less radioactive SN because tumor has occluded the lymphatics and obliterated the nodal tissue. The physiologic principle described by Morton, however, has not changed and governs the SN concept. The definition of the SN in breast carcinoma is the first node or nodes to which lymph drainage and metastasis occurs from the primary tumor.[65] The SN is usually an axillary node, but it can in rare cases be found in nonaxillary locations.[65] The breast is a parenchymal organ that has the potential to drain to multiple nodal basins. Do breast parenchymal, subcutaneous, dermal, and/or periareolar lymphatics flow to the same axillary nodes that govern lymphatic drainage?[66] When blue dye was injected intraparenchymally in the same quadrant as the primary tumor or in a discordant quadrant from the tumor and radioisotope was injected intradermally over the tumor, the SN was blue and hot in 93.9% of cases with concordant quadrant injections and 92.5% in discordant quadrant injections. In another study, peritumoral blue dye and subareolar isotope resulted in 97% blue nodes that were 98% concordant for blue-hot nodes.[67] These studies confirm the SN concept and suggest that there may be a primary nodal drainage pattern from the breast and that this most likely can be identified by a variety of techniques.

Multicenter Lymphatic Mapping Trials

The first multicenter trial was initiated in 1995 to evaluate the ability of surgeons with varied experience in SLND to identify and to accurately stage the axilla using the radioisotope technique.[26] Eleven surgeons entered 443 patients into the study. The SN was identified using a gamma detection probe. A completion level I and II ALND was performed in all cases. A level III dissection was performed for suspicious nodes. Failure to identify a hot spot before excision of the SN was associated with a previous excisional biopsy, age 50 years or older, and medial tumor location. The SN was identified in 88.6% of cases. The accuracy was 96.8%, the negative predictive value was 95.7%, and the sensitivity was 89%. The false-negative rate ranged from 0% to 28.6%. All 13 false-negative SNs occurred with medial hemisphere tumors. The SN was located in a region outside the axilla in 8% of cases. Variations in success were attributed to both surgeon experience and patient characteristics.[26]

This study was followed by the 42-center Department of Defense Multicenter Trial of Breast Lymphatic Mapping, which required surgeons to participate in a 2-day course using an intraparenchymal injection of blue dye and radioisotope. Patients were randomized to SLND alone if the SN was negative or SLND followed by ALND.[61] Preoperative lymphoscintigraphy was performed in 84% of cases and demonstrated at least one SN in 66%. The nodal drainage pattern was to the axilla in 99.9%, axilla only in 78%, internal mammary in 14%, internal mammary only in 2%, and other sites in 5%. The success rate for identifying the

SN was 92% at the Moffitt Cancer Center, 91.4% at other university centers, and 85.2% in community/regional centers. The SN was positive in 32% of patients, and the only site of metastases in 63%. Skip metastases were identified for a false-negative rate of 4%. There were no axillary recurrences in the SLND-alone group at 16 months. This multicenter trial demonstrated successful mapping, a low skip metastasis rate, and a reliable performance rate for both university and nonuniversity institutions, thus confirming not only the accuracy of SLND but its widespread feasibility.

In another multicenter trial, surgeons from academic institutions and the private sector attended a formal lymphatic mapping course with hands-on experience in a training laboratory facility first.[62] The surgeons achieved a 90% identification rate and a 4.3% false-negative rate when they had performed more than 30 cases. Multivariate analysis demonstrated the poorest success rate in older patients (≥50 years) and by inexperienced surgeons (≤10 cases). Identification was not affected by type of prior surgery (fine-needle aspiration, core biopsy, excision), filtered or unfiltered ^{99m}Tc, time from injection to surgery, tumor size, or tumor location. The false-negative rate was worse for central lesions ($p < .02$).

In one of the largest multicenter studies evaluating the optimal SLND technique, 99 surgeons enrolled in the University of Louisville Breast Cancer Sentinel Lymph Node Study and performed SLND in 806 patients.[63] The surgeons were provided flexibility in choosing the technique. Each case was evaluated for patient and tumor characteristics, identification rate, false-negative rate, and technique used. There was no difference in SN identification for dye alone or dye plus isotope (86% vs. 90%, respectively). The false-negative rate was significantly lower with the dual agents (11.8% vs. 5.8%, $p < .05$). The isotope-dye combination resulted in more SNs removed (2.1 vs. 1.5, $p < .0001$). In this large study, the optimal technique with the lowest false-negative rate was dual-agent SLND. With this technique the false-negative rate is low enough to be considered a suitable alternative to ALND in routine surgical practice.

The prospective Swedish Multicenter Cohort Study in 3354 patients from 26 hospitals treated by 131 surgeons demonstrated a negative SN in 2246 cases, and no further ALND was performed.[69] Peritumoral, subcutaneous, or intracutaneous injection of radioisotope was followed with lymphoscintigraphy. SNs were identified intraoperatively with a handheld gamma detection probe. At 37 months, nodal failure was 1.2%. The overall survival was 91.6%, and the disease-free survival was 92.1%.

Clinical, Pathologic, and Technical Aspects of Sentinel Lymphadenectomy

Patient Selection Criteria

Guidelines for successful SN identification require appropriate patient selection, defined tumor characteristics, and technical validation.[19] A variety of factors may interfere with the accuracy of this procedure and decrease the chance of correctly identifying the SN (Table 42.8).[70] The technique can be used effectively in all age groups, in both males and females, with breast conservation surgery (BCS) or mastectomy, at the time of primary excision or reexcision, in bilateral breast cancer, after long-interval reduction mammoplasty, and with breast implants. American Society of Clinical Oncology (ASCO) guidelines are shown in Table 42.9.[19]

TABLE 42.8	Factors Associated With Failure to Identify the Sentinel Node			
Factor	Fraction Failed SN	Percent Failed SN	Chi-Square	P Value
Body Mass Index (kg/m²)			22.2687	.0001
<18.5	0/74	0		
18.5–24.9	9/1881	0.5		
25–29.9	25/1562	1.6		
30–49.9	29/1406	2.1		
≥50	2/41	4.9		
Age (yr)			20.5185	.0004
≤39	1/330	0.3		
40–49	8/1171	0.7		
50–59	18/1668	1.1		
60–69	21/1253	1.7		
≥70	23/845	2.7		
Pathologic Tumor Stage			1.6780	.4322
T_1	58/3947	1.5		
T_2	12/1063	1.1		
T_3	0/68	0		
Final Nodal Status			2.6198	.1055
Negative	59/3981	1.5		
Positive	11/1251	0.9		
Biopsy Type			0.3915	.5315
Excisional	21/1606	1.3		
Nonexcisional	45/2921	1.5		
Histology			1.3555	.5078
Ductal	60/4324	1.4		
Lobular	7/435	1.6		
Other	4/495	0.8		
Tumor Location			3.8406	.1466
Medial	21/1069	2		
Central	15/1167	1.3		
Lateral	35/3008	1.2		
Final Number of Positive Nodes			4.5380	0.4748
0	56/4060	1.4		
1	6/325	1.8		
2	0/132	0		
3	1/86	1.2		
4	0/38	0		
≥5	4/154	2.6		

SN, Sentinel lymph node.

From Posther K, McCall LM, Blumencranz PW, et al. Sentinel node skills verification and surgeon performance data from a multicenter clinical trial for early-stage breast cancer. *Ann Surg.* 2005;242:593-602.

TABLE 42.9 Recommendations and Levels of Evidence for Sentinel Lymph Node Dissection Based on Updated 2014 Guidelines by the American Society of Clinical Oncology		
Clinical Circumstance	Recommendation for Use of Sentinel Node Biopsy	Level of Evidence[a]
T_1 or T_2 tumors	Acceptable	Good
T_3 or T_4 tumors	Not recommended	Insufficient
Multicentric tumors	Acceptable	Intermediate
Inflammatory breast cancer	Not recommended	Insufficient
DCIS with mastectomy	Acceptable	Limited; Informal Consensus
DCIS without mastectomy	Not recommended except for large DCIS (>5 cm) on core biopsy or with suspected or proven microinvasion	Insufficient
Suspicious, palpable axillary nodes	Not recommended	Good
Older age	Acceptable	Intermediate
Obesity	Acceptable	Intermediate
Male breast cancer	Acceptable	Limited
Pregnancy	Not recommended	Insufficient
Evaluation of internal mammary lymph nodes	Acceptable	Limited
Prior diagnostic or excisional breast biopsy	Acceptable	Intermediate
Prior axillary surgery	Acceptable	Intermediate
Prior nononcologic breast surgery (reduction or augmentation mammoplasty, breast reconstruction)	Acceptable	Intermediate
After preoperative systemic therapy	Acceptable	Intermediate
Before preoperative systemic therapy	Acceptable	Intermediate

DCIS, ductal carcinoma in situ.

[a]Levels of evidence:

- Good: multiple studies of sentinel lymph node dissection (SLND) test performance based on findings on completion of axillary lymph node dissection (ALND).
- Intermediate: moderate confidence that the available evidence reflects the true magnitude and direction of the net effect. Further research is unlikely to alter the direction of the net effect; however, it might alter the magnitude of the net effect.
- Limited: few studies of SLND test performance based on findings on completion of ALND or multiple studies of mapping success without test performance assessed.
- Insufficient: on studies of SLND test performance based on findings on completion of ALND and few if any studies of mapping success
- Informal Consensus: the available evidence was deemed insufficient to inform a recommendation to guide clinical practice. The recommendation is considered the best current guidance for practice, based on informal consensus of the expert panel.

From Lyman G, Giuliano AE, Somerfield M, et al. American Society of Clinical Oncology Guideline recommendations for sentinel lymph node biopsy in early-stage breast cancer. *J Clin Oncol*. 2005;23:7703-7720, and Lyman GH, Temin S, Edge SB, et al. Sentinel lymph node biopsy for patients with early-stage breast cancer: American Society of Clinical Oncology clinical practice guideline update. *J Clin Oncol*. 2014;32:1365-1383.

Age

Sentinel lymphadenectomy has been used to stage the axilla in individuals spanning all decades.[5] The identification of the SN, however, has been less successful in older patients.[70] The failed ID rate is 0.3% for women 39 years of age or younger and 2.7% for those 70 years of age or older.[70] The results from the National Surgical Adjuvant Breast and Bowel Project (NSABP) B-32 trial show a statistically significant, but not clinically relevant, difference in identification rates by 49 years of age or less versus 50 years of age or more, whereas a recent study shows similar identification rates.[71,72] A combination of vital dye and isotope improves identification in older patients.[60,73]

SLND is an option for axillary staging of the older patient. The role of ALND for elderly patients has been questioned because it has significant morbidity.[71,74] SLND provides prognostic information about axillary status with little or no morbidity and changes local and/or systemic treatment in 14% of cases.[74] In another study, SN status was associated with significantly different rates of systemic therapy in women 70 years of age or older.[71] Hormonal therapy was used in 86.9% of women with a positive SN versus 54.3% with a negative SN, and chemotherapy was used in 24% and 2.8%, respectively. The difference in use of systemic therapy for SN-positive patients occurred with tumors smaller than 1 cm and between 1 and 2 cm but not with tumors larger than 2 cm.

Gender

Although male breast cancer accounts for less than 1% of breast cancer cases, the use of SLND has been studied in both male and female patients.[75,76] Conventional surgical management of male breast cancer has been modified radical mastectomy, but more men are diagnosed with node-negative disease and can avoid ALND.[77] Combined data from a number of series show a 96% identification rate, with 45% of patients having a positive node, and in 56% of those cases the SN is the only positive node.[72] SLND is a less invasive staging procedure that is applicable to men with breast cancer who have a clinically negative axilla.[77]

Body Habitus

Failure to identify the SN is correlated with an increased mean body mass index (BMI).[70] There is a progressive increase in failure rate as BMI increases above 26.[70] The JWCI experience also finds SN identification to be more challenging in the obese patient, and the combined vital dye and radioisotope technique may be considered for these patients.

Pregnancy and Lactation

The safety of SLND with radioisotope in pregnancy has been studied by Pandit-Taskar and colleagues at the Memorial Sloan-Kettering Cancer Center (MSKCC).[78] Retrospective data from nonpregnant women with breast cancer and SN biopsy were used in a phantom model calculation of the radiation-absorbed dose of ^{99m}Tc-sulfur colloid after a single intradermal dose of 0.1 mCi on the morning of surgery or 0.5 mCi on the afternoon before surgery. The highest estimated dose received by the fetus was with the 2-day protocol, measured at 0.014 mGy and is less than the National Council on Radiation Protection and Measurements limit to the pregnant woman.[78] Three other theoretical studies reach similar conclusions.[79–81] Although radiolabeled technetium is probably safe in pregnancy, clinicians are reluctant to use it, and the ASCO guidelines do not recommend it.[19,82] Use of isosulfan blue dye is contraindicated because there are no data in human pregnancy regarding whether fetal harm can result from intrauterine dye exposure, and it is classified by the US Food and Drug Administration as a category C drug in pregnancy. One small series of 25 pregnant patients reported use of methylene blue in 7 patients without any complications.[83]

Previous Breast or Axillary Surgery

Previous breast reduction surgery, surgical implants, extensive injuries, burns, previous reconstructive surgery to the breast or axilla, surgery for hidradenitis, or congenital lymphatic problems may have an effect on the feasibility of the procedure with insufficient evidence to recommend it.[19]

Application of the technique to recurrent disease, especially after SLND, has been shown to be feasible,[84,85] although some question its value.[86–88] Success of reoperative axillary surgery has been shown to be inversely related to the number of nodes removed initially and has been due in part to lymphoscintigraphy, which may identify sites of nonaxillary drainage.[88] Preoperative lymphoscintigraphy shows variable drainage pathways and slower migration of radiocolloid but can be performed successfully in patients with ipsilateral breast tumor recurrence.[86] Ugras and coworkers found that rates of axillary failure, nonaxillary failure, distant recurrence and death did not differ between clinically node-negative patients with local recurrence who had axillary restaging (n = 47; 57%) versus those who did not (n = 36; 43%).[89] The use of adjuvant therapy was similar between groups and the authors suggest that because randomized trials support the use of systemic therapy for all patients with invasive local recurrence, axillary staging may not be necessary in clinically node-negative patients.

Previous Excision

Previous excision was considered a contraindication in some of the earlier SLND studies.[10,12,33,39,40] It was hypothesized that when the breast lymphatics are transected, the drainage pattern would not be reliable. Haigh and associates demonstrated that there were no statistically significant differences for SN identification rate or accuracy by biopsy method (fine-needle aspiration, core biopsy or excision), excision volume, time from initial biopsy to SLND, tumor size, and tumor location by univariate and multivariate analysis.[90] In another study, 2206 patients were enrolled, and there was no statistically significant difference between SN identification rate or false-negative rate between those patients who had needle biopsy or excisional biopsy.[91] Similar findings are observed in the European Institute of Oncology, where more than 50% of the patients present for definitive treatment after an excisional biopsy and have an SLND with 99% identification rate and axillary failure of 0.7%.[92]

Tumor Features

Type of Carcinoma

Invasive Carcinoma. Axillary staging is essential for management of invasive carcinoma. The largest proportion of cases in published series of SLND for breast cancer have been performed for invasive ductal carcinoma (82.3%), followed by invasive lobular carcinoma (8.3%) and other subtypes (9.4%).[70] A contraindication to SLND after neoadjuvant chemotherapy is inflammatory breast cancer.[93]

Ductal Carcinoma In Situ and Ductal Carcinoma In Situ With Microinvasion. Ductal carcinoma in situ (DCIS), by definition, cannot give rise to axillary metastases; however, sampling error at the primary site, ipsilateral nodal recurrence, as well as distant metastatic disease can be identified in a small percentage of cases.[94–96] The incidence of lymph node metastases in small reported series has a wide range of variability—from 0% to 22% (Table 42.10).[97] The largest series of patients with pure DCIS shows the presence of SN metastases in 1.4% of cases and does not support the routine use of SLND in DCIS.[95] The critical issue with DCIS is the risk of microinvasion and as a consequence the risk of metastasis. Ipsilateral nodal recurrence is a surrogate marker for axillary involvement at the time of diagnosis. In the NSABP B-17, the ipsilateral nodal recurrence was 0.83 per 1000 patient-years, and in B-24, it was 0.36 per 1000 patient-years.[94] Given this low rate of metastases, we do not recommend SLND for DCIS.

DCIS with microinvasion does carry a real incidence of metastatic potential, and SN biopsy is recommended.[98] However, if there is no evidence of microinvasion, guidelines published by ASCO[82] and the National Comprehensive Cancer Network[99] do not recommend axillary staging in women undergoing BCS. If invasive cancer is discovered at the time of lumpectomy, SLND can be performed at a later time. SLND may be appropriate when mastectomy is performed in patients with DCIS with risk of invasion.[98] Risk factors for invasion include a palpable mass, mammographic mass, histology suspicious for microinvasion, or extensive disease (>5 cm).

Identification of an SN with tumor cells will upstage DCIS from stage 0 to stage IB and may lead to chemotherapy recommendations. The clinical relevance of positive SNs in DCIS and also in DCIS with microinvasion is unknown. Before offering SLND to the individual with a diagnosis of DCIS, the impact of the results must be considered. Identification of a positive SN presents a therapeutic quandary to the patient and the treating team.[100] This is an area that needs further investigation. SLND for DCIS is recommended for mastectomy patients.[19] In those patients who are undergoing BCS, SLND may be considered for

| TABLE 42.10 | Percentage of Lymph Node Metastasis With DCIS and DCISM | | | | | | |

First Author	Year	DCIS			DCISM		
		%	n	mm	%	n	mm
van la Parra	2007	4.4	2	1	50	3	2
Veronesi	2005	1.8	9	5			
Mittendorf	2005	22	9	4			
Camp	2005	3.3	1	1	15.4	2	
Farkas	2004	0	0				
Rahusen	2003	0	0				
Lara	2003	13	13	13			
Kelly	2003	2	3	3			
Intra	2003				9.7	4	2
Intra	2003	3.1	7	5			
Cserni	2002	10	1	1			
Cox	2001	13	26		20	3	
Pendas	2000	5.7	5				
Klauber-DeMore	2000	12	9	7	10	3	2
Zavotsky	1999				14.3	2	

DCIS, Ductal carcinoma in situ; *DCISM,* ductal carcinoma in situ with microinvasion; *mm,* micrometastases; *n,* number of positive sentinel nodes.
From van la Parra RFD, Ernst MF, Barneveld PC, et al. The value of sentinel lymph node biopsy in ductal carcinoma in situ (DCIS) and DCIS with microinvasion of the breast. *Eur J Surg Oncol.* 2008;34:631-635.

patients who present with a mass, have suspected microinvasion, or are found to have extensive DCIS because these may be found to be invasive on excision.[19] These patients may prefer SLND at the time of surgical resection to avoid a second operation.

Feasibility of Sentinel Lymph Node Dissection for Palpable Versus Nonpalpable Tumors

SLND for nonpalpable tumors has been approached with different options. The lesion can be injected with stereotactic guidance, with mammographic localization before wire placement, or with ultrasound guidance.[37] An approach to nonpalpable lesions that requires SN resection is radioguided occult lesion localization (ROLL) together with SN biopsy (SNOLL), which has been shown to be an accurate and safe technique for localizing nonpalpable breast tumors.[101] Radioisotope is injected directly into the lesion under ultrasound or mammographic guidance, and a second dose is injected peritumorally or subdermally for SN biopsy. A systematic review identified seven studies of SNOLL in 983 patients with nonpalpable breast cancer. Overall complete tumor resection rates ranged from 82% to 91% with successful SN identification rates ranging from 88% to 100%.[102]

Multifocal or Multicentric Disease

Multifocality and multicentricity have been relative contraindications to SLND but are currently acceptable.[19] A multiinstitutional validation study in 130 patients undergoing SLND followed by ALND in 125 of the patients with multicentric cancer demonstrated a 91.5% identification rate and a 4% false-negative rate.[103] There are a number of case reports, retrospective and prospective studies, and multicenter trials using a variety of methods to perform SLND with an identification rate of 85.7% to 100%, a false-negative rate of 0% to 33.3%, and an accuracy of 77.8% to 100% (Table 42.11).[104]

| TABLE 42.11 | Sentinel Lymph Node Biopsy in Multifocal-Multicentric Breast Tumors Published in the Literature, 1999–2006 | | | | | | |

Author	Year	Study	No. of Patients	Mapping Technique	ID (%)	FN (%)	ACC (%)
Mertz	1999	Prospective	16	A*	98	0	100
Schrenk	2001	Prospective	19	A^blue ± A*	100	0	100
Kim	2002	Case reports	5	1ID* + T^blue	100	nv	nv
Fernandez	2002	Multicenter trial	53	T*+blue or ID*+blue or A*+blue	98	0	100
Ozmen	2002	Prospective	21 (males/females)	T^blue	85.7	33.3	77.8
Kumar	2003	Retrospective	59 (48 AD)	T^blue + 1–2ID*	93.5	0	100
Tousimis	2003	Retrospective	70	T*+blue	95.9	8	96
Kumar	2004	Retrospective	10 (8 AD)	T* or A*+blue	100	0	100
Goyal	2004	Multicenter trial	75 (AD or S)	T*+blue	94.6	8.8	95.8
Knauer	2006	Multicenter trial	150 (125 AD)	ns (* or/+blue)	ns	4.1	97.4
Ferrari	2006	Prospective	31	2ID* or A*	100	7.1	96.8

A, Areolar injection of radioisotope (A*) or blue dye (A^blue); *AD,* Axillary dissection; *ID,* intradermal injection of radioisotope (ID*) or blue dye (ID^blue) over one (1ID) or two (2ID) neoplastic foci; *ns,* nonspecified; *S,* lymph node sampling; *T,* peritumoral injection of radioisotope (T*) or blue dye (T^blue).
From Ferrari A, Dionigi P, Rovera F, et al. Multifocality and multicentricity are not contraindications for sentinel lymph node biopsy in breast cancer surgery. *World J Surg.* 2006;4:79.

Palpable Axillary Lymph Nodes

The role of SLND for patients with clinically suspicious axillary nodes is somewhat problematic. Patients with clinically suspicious lymph nodes have been excluded from the majority of published series. Clinical examination is the oldest and simplest method to evaluate regional lymphatics, but its accuracy is limited. Many patients have undergone core biopsy or excisional biopsy and have inflammatory hyperplasia of lymph nodes that are free of tumor and would be denied the advantage of a minimally invasive SLND. The correlation of clinical examination followed by ALND or SLND shows that the risk of lymph node metastasis is 40.4% if the clinical assessment is negative, 61.5% if the lymph nodes are palpable but not suspicious, and 84.4% if clinically suspicious and is considered of little value.[105] Clinical examination is subject to false-positive results in 53% of patients with moderately suspicious nodes and 23% of those with highly suspicious nodes.[106] If preoperative evaluation with imaging studies or tissue sampling does not clearly identify metastatic disease, SLND should be considered as an option in staging of the axilla. There is no reason to exclude these patients from SLND on the condition that the clinically suspicious node is resected and analyzed.

Applications of Sentinel Lymphadenectomy

Sentinel Lymphadenectomy and Operative Procedure

SLND can be performed successfully with BCS, mastectomy, or nipple- or skin-sparing mastectomy.[91,107] The technique can be used for synchronous bilateral lesions equally effectively as for unilateral disease. When immediate reconstruction is planned, staged SN biopsy before mastectomy facilitates surgical planning to avoid the complications of discovering a tumor-positive SN after reconstruction, especially when autologous tissue is used.[108,109] Ipsilateral new primary tumor is no longer a contraindication in selected cases.[88] The incidence of occult invasive carcinoma in prophylactic mastectomy is approximately 5% to 10%.[110,111] In a meta-analysis of 14 studies of 2708 patients who had prophylactic mastectomy and SLND, the frequency of occult invasive cancer was 1.8%, and the rate of positive SNs was 1.2%.[112] This rate is lower than the incidence of allergic reactions that may occur with isosulfan blue dye (reported to be as high as 2.7%)[113,114] and therefore does not justify using the dye for lymphatic mapping in this setting. To avoid the need to stage the axilla after prophylactic mastectomy, especially in conjunction with immediate reconstruction, SLND can be performed with prophylactic mastectomy.[111] Boughey and colleagues conducted a decision analytical model that predicted that 73 SLNDs are required to prevent one axillary dissection.[115] They calculated the probability of complications per breast cancer detected was ninefold greater with routine use of SLND over performing ALND only when occult invasive cancer is discovered after mastectomy. On the basis of these findings, the authors did not recommend SLND with prophylactic mastectomy. The use of magnetic resonance imaging in addition to SLND raises costs and misses most occult malignancies, and it is not recommended for prophylactic mastectomy because of the low rate of invasive carcinoma and the absence of nodal disease in those cases.[110] There is currently no evidence to support SLND in prophylactic mastectomy.

Preoperative Chemotherapy

Preoperative chemotherapy has been successfully incorporated into the breast cancer treatment algorithm for smaller breast cancers that are less likely to have tumor-positive lymph nodes. It can clear the axilla of microscopic nodal disease in a fraction of patients with positive axillary nodes.[116] Preoperative chemotherapy results in pathologic nodal downstaging and no adverse outcome in the axilla.[117] The proportion of patients with negative nodes increases as tumor response to preoperative chemotherapy improves. Although chemotherapy has the potential to sterilize nodal disease, it is uncertain what the degree of conversion may be.[118] For this reason, the timing of SLND in relationship to preoperative chemotherapy, is controversial. A number of studies suggest the feasibility of performing SLND after preoperative chemotherapy in clinically node-negative patients (Table 42.12).[119] Meta-analysis shows a pooled identification rate of 90% and an

TABLE 42.12	Sentinel Lymph Node Biopsy Identification Rates After Preoperative Chemotherapy in Patients With Breast Cancer		
Reference	**Year**	**No. of Patients in Whom SLND Attempted**	**No. of Patients in Whom SN Identified**	**Identification Rate (%)[a]**
Nason et al.	2000	15	13	87 (62–96)
Fernandez et al.	2001	40	34	85 (71–93)
Tafra et al.	2001	29	27	93 (78–98)
Brady	2002	14	13	93 (68–99)
Stearns et al.	2002	26	23	88 (71–96)
Piato et al.	2003	42	41	98 (87–100)
Balch et al.	2003	32	31	97 (84–99)
Haid et al.	2003	45	42	93 (82–98)
Mamounas	2003	428	363	85 (81–88)
Schwartz & Meltzer	2003	21	21	100 (84–100)
Reitsamer et al.	2003	30	26	87 (70–95)
Aihara et al.	2004	20	17	85 (63–95)
Shimazu et al.	2004	47	44	94 (83–98)
Hauschild et al.	2004	29	29	100 (88–100)
Patel et al.	2004	42	40	95 (84–99)
Kang et al.	2004	54	39	72 (59–83)
Tio et al.	2004	89	83	93 (86–97)
Lang et al.	2004	52	50	96 (87–99)
Shen et al.	2004	70	65	93 (84–97)
Kinoshita et al.	2004	46	42	91 (79–97)
Bonardi et al.	2004	102	99	97 (92–99)
Pooled data		1273	1142	90 (88–91)

[a]Values in parentheses are 95% confidence intervals.
SLND, Sentinel lymph node dissection; *SN*, sentinel lymph node.
From Xing Y, Foy M, Cox DD, et al. Meta-analysis of sentinel lymph node biopsy after preoperative chemotherapy in patients with breast cancer. *Br J Surg.* 2006;93:539-546.

overall accuracy of 94% with a sensitivity of 88% and a negative predictive value of 90%.[119] The major advantage of performing SLND after preoperative chemotherapy is that some patients who have axillary nodes downstaged by chemotherapy can be spared the morbidity of ALND. ASCO guidelines published in 2014 state that in clinically node-negative patients undergoing preoperative chemotherapy, SLND may be offered before or after chemotherapy and that completion ALND is recommended when nodal disease is discovered after neoadjuvant chemotherapy.[82] When patients present with node-positive disease but are downstaged by neoadjuvant chemotherapy to clinically node-negative disease, the use of SLND after preoperative chemotherapy remains controversial. This clinical scenario has been addressed by three prospective trials—the SENTINA (n = 592 patients),[120] American College of Surgeons Oncology Group (ACOSOG) Z1071 (n = 663),[121] and SN FNAC (n = 153)[122]—in which SLND was followed by ALND. The SN identification rate in the respective trials were reported to be 80.1%, 92.9%, and 87.6%; the overall false-negative rates were 14.2%, 12.6%, and 13.3%, respectively. The predetermined acceptable false-negative rate in the ACOSOG Z1071 and SN FNAC trials was less than 10%. The reported false-negative rates clearly exceeded this number, although additional analyses identified certain subsets where the false-negative rate was lower than 10%. In the SENTINA and ACOSOG Z1071 trials, the false-negative rate was improved by use of dual agent lymphatic mapping and removal of more SNs. In the SN FNAC trial, the false-negative rate was reduced to 8.4% by use of IHC to evaluate for nodal metastases and designation of presence of isolated tumor cells as node-positive disease, and the authors argue that consideration of any size metastases identified by IHC as node-positive would potentially enable 30% of patients to avoid ALND. The results of this trial were reported as an unplanned interim analysis before meeting the goal accrual of 300 patients due to slow accrual as well as publication of the ACOSOG Z0171 results. On the basis of the data from these trials, the ASCO 2014 guidelines state that SLND may be offered but that the procedure is less accurate in this subset of patients. The recommendation is considered by ASCO to be of moderate strength based on intermediate quality evidence. Despite this statement, it is important to understand that there has been no clinical trial that has provided substantial evidence to support omission of axillary dissection in this setting.

Management of the Internal Mammary Lymph Sentinel Node

The prognostic value of the internal mammary nodal status is high, particularly when both axillary and internal mammary nodes are either negative with improved survival or positive leading to a significantly decreased survival.[123] Lymphoscintigraphy or gamma detection probe can identify drainage patterns and stratify individuals into those who may benefit from staging the internal mammary lymph node (IMLN) by SLND.[124] This may be one advantage of lymphatic mapping with radioisotope compared with blue dye. Presence of IMLN metastases is strongly associated with axillary nodal metastases, and the incidence of IMLN involvement is approximately 3%.[125] The role of SLND for an IMLN is still undergoing evaluation and may be of importance for patients with negative axillary nodes and small tumors who would not normally receive adjuvant chemotherapy.[126]

The surgical approach to IMLNs has been much simplified by lymphoscintigraphy and gamma probe detection. The procedure can now be performed through a small incision at the lateral sternal margin.[125] The pectoral muscle fibers are separated, and the intercostal muscles are divided for 3 to 4 cm, avoiding pleural injury. The perivasal adipose tissue is separated, and the gamma probe is inserted. The node is identified and resected. The fibers of the pectoralis are reapproximated. One hundred and forty-two patients underwent the procedure at the European Institute of Oncology in Milan and MSKCC with no complications.[125]

IMLN lymphatic drainage was demonstrated in 22% of patients in one study with 24% of them demonstrating metastases.[127] Management was changed as a result of these findings. Radiation fields were extended in 85% of these patients and additional systemic therapy was given in 30%. In another study of 72 patients who had IMLN biopsy, 10 patients (14%) had metastases identified by IMLN biopsy. Radiation therapy to the IM nodes was added to the adjuvant radiation protocol in all 10 patients, and adjuvant chemotherapy was added to one patient who had a negative axilla.[128] The authors found that IMLN involvement was significantly correlated with worse overall survival. Routine SN biopsy of IMLN is not standard practice, but it does warrant further investigation to determine appropriateness of the procedure and identification of patient populations who may benefit.[126]

Predictors of Sentinel Node Metastases

Tumor Size and Risk of Sentinel Node Metastases

Tumor size is a predictor of nodal metastases. Is there a size so small that SLND can be omitted or too great where SLND is not practical? Surgeons have attempted to define a subgroup of patients at a low enough risk of nodal metastasis in whom axillary dissection may be omitted. The incidence of nodal metastases is the lowest for T_1 tumors. It is in this group that investigators have tried to define the risk more accurately. Giuliano and coworkers studied incidence of nodal involvement in T1 tumors and demonstrated H&E nodal metastasis in 10% of T_{1a} lesions, 13% of T_{1b}, and 30% of T_{1c}.[129] When SNs were examined by IHC staining, 15% of patients with either T_{1a} or T_{1b} lesions had evidence of tumor cells in the SN. These data suggest that the risk of axillary metastases is sufficiently high to warrant axillary staging for T_{1a} and T_{1b} lesions. Tumor size is a predictor of SN positivity—that is, the larger the tumor, the greater the likelihood of detecting a positive SN. The frequency of SN positivity by method of analysis is shown in Fig. 42.2.[130]

Although the risk of axillary metastases is too high to omit staging for T_{1a} and T_{1b} lesions, the role of SLND at the other end of the spectrum, for large tumors (≥5 cm), is controversial. Large size has been considered an exclusion criterion because of insufficient evidence.[19] Several studies have looked at lymphatic mapping for larger tumors and found high identification rates and accuracy.[131–138] In 41 patients with a mean tumor size of 7.12 cm and a clinically negative axilla, 73% of patients had a tumor-positive SN.[138] There was one false-negative SN for an incidence of 3% and an overall positive axillary status of 76%. Three patients had micrometastases with no additional positive nodes. The significant predictors of non-SN positivity were SN macrometastases and tumor size greater than 7 cm. The SN reflected the status of the axilla in 98% of cases and could have prevented axillary surgery in a quarter of the cases. A second series of 103 patients from the University of Pennsylvania and the Mayo Clinic with tumors that were T_2 or larger demonstrated a 99% accuracy for axillary staging.[137] This study confirmed that the presence of macrometastases predicted non-SN metastases, although 37.5% of their patients with micrometastases had additional non-SNs that

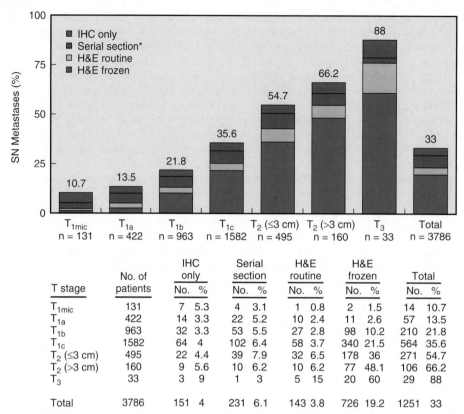

T stage	No. of patients	IHC only		Serial section		H&E routine		H&E frozen		Total	
		No.	%	No.	%	No.	%	No.	%	No.	%
T$_{1mic}$	131	7	5.3	4	3.1	1	0.8	2	1.5	14	10.7
T$_{1a}$	422	14	3.3	22	5.2	10	2.4	11	2.6	57	13.5
T$_{1b}$	963	32	3.3	53	5.5	27	2.8	98	10.2	210	21.8
T$_{1c}$	1582	64	4	102	6.4	58	3.7	340	21.5	564	35.6
T$_2$ (≤3 cm)	495	22	4.4	39	7.9	32	6.5	178	36	271	54.7
T$_2$ (>3 cm)	160	9	5.6	10	6.2	10	6.2	77	48.1	106	66.2
T$_3$	33	3	9	1	3	5	15	20	60	29	88
Total	3786	151	4	231	6.1	143	3.8	726	19.2	1251	33

• **Fig. 42.2** Frequency of sentinel lymph node *(SN)* metastasis by T stage and method of detection of metastases in modeling group. The table provides the precise patient numbers and percentages represented graphically in the figure. *Includes SN metastases found on serial sections by hematoxylin and eosin *(H&E)* or H&E as a result of immunohistochemistry *(IHC)*. (From Bevilacqua JL, Kattan MW, Fey JV, et al. Doctor, what are my chances of having a positive sentinel node? A validated nomogram for risk estimation. *J Clin Oncol.* 2007;25:3670-3677.)

were positive. SN staging can be performed in patients with large tumors before initiation of preoperative chemotherapy as discussed previously. Canavese compared SLND in 64 cases of locally advanced breast cancer to SLND in a historical control group of early-stage tumors and found comparable SN identification (93.8%), false-negative (5.1%), and overall accuracy (96.7%) rates.[139] Given the paucity of data in this patient population, ASCO 2014 guidelines state that there is insufficient evidence to support SLND in patients with T3 to T4 tumors who will undergo primary surgery.

Number of Sentinel Nodes Removed

The mean number of SNs removed varies among large institutional series (Table 42.13).[140] Some investigators have asked whether there is an improvement in SN identification and accuracy with the number of SNs removed.[141,142] In the University of Louisville Breast Cancer Sentinel Lymph Node Study, there was a 90% identification rate with an 8.3% false-negative rate in a total of 1436 patients undergoing SLND.[141] Fifty-eight percent of the patients had multiple SNs removed. The false-negative rate was 14.3% when a single SN was removed compared with 4.3% when multiple SNs were removed (*p* < .0004). Logistic regression analysis revealed that the use of blue dye alone was an independent factor for a single SN (*p* < .0001). The ability to identify multiple SNs, when they can be demonstrated, enhanced the identification rate and the accuracy. In one study, the first two SNs removed predicted the status of the axilla in 98% of cases.[143] The mean

number of SNs removed in another study was 2.5 with a 98% accuracy when less than three SNs were resected and 100% with four, recommending termination of further node removal to reduce morbidity and cost.[140] In another study, the first three nodes removed predicted the status of the axilla in 98% of cases, but 4% had a positive SN detected in four to eight additional sites.[142] These authors concluded that there is no upper limit to the number of SNs that are at risk for metastases and that all blue and/or hot nodes should be removed. They predicted that removal of additional nodes would not have an adverse effect. However, it is likely that complications, especially lymphedema, are related to the number of lymph nodes removed. Chagpar and coworkers report a higher false-negative rate when SN biopsy is limited to the removal of only three SNs (10.3%) compared with an overall rate of 7.7% when all SNs were removed.[144]

Significance of Micrometastases

SLND for breast cancer has improved staging of the axilla compared with routine ALND.[13] However, a dilemma has evolved from focused histopathologic assessment of the SN with IHC.[145] This topic is covered more extensively in Chapter 66. SN evaluation with IHC can upstage SN-negative patients.[13] The International (Ludwig) Breast Cancer Study Group used serial subsectioning and H&E staining of axillary lymph nodes to identify metastases.[146] Nine percent of the patients had micrometastases and a statistically significant reduction in survival. The current standard pathologic evaluation of the SN is by multiple

TABLE 42.13 Studies Examining How Many Nodes Needed to Be Removed Before Identifying All Positive Sentinel Lymph Nodes

Institution	No. of Positive Sentinel Lymph Nodes	One Node (%)	Two Nodes (%)	Three Nodes (%)	Four Nodes (%)	Five Nodes (%)	Six to Eight Nodes (%)
MD Anderson Cancer Center/Duke	278 (11%)	79	96	99	100	N/A	N/A
University of Michigan	132 (18%)	66	86	98	100	N/A	N/A
Mayo Clinic	103 (22%)	87	95	98	100	N/A	N/A
Beaumont Hospital	172 (24%)	76.6	91	97	98.8	99.4	100
Ludwig Boltzmann	105 (40%)	91.4	99	100	N/A	N/A	N/A
Virginia Mason	129 (24%)	65	98.4	99.2	100	N/A	N/A
Memorial Sloan-Kettering Cancer Center	241 (15%)	75.3	92.9	98	99.1	99.6	100
Wagga Wagga (Australia)	33 (29%)	88	97	100	N/A	N/A	N/A
University of South Florida	128 (27%)	89	98.4	99.2	100	N/A	N/A
Ohio State University	104 (29%)	83	97	98	99	100	N/A

From Zakaria S, Degnim AC, Kleer CG, et al. Sentinel lymph node biopsy for breast cancer: how many nodes are enough? *J Surg Oncol.* 2007;96:554-559. Reprinted with permission of John Wiley & Sons, Inc.

subsectioning and dedicated screening.[147–149] This approach would have identified some of the metastatic tumor deposits in the Ludwig Study. A reevaluation of the Ludwig V study confirmed a statistically significant difference in disease-free survival when micrometastases were detected by H&E ($p = .001$) but not by IHC ($p = .09$).[150]

The clinical significance of micrometastases was evaluated prospectively by the ACOSOG Z0010 and NSABP-B32 trials. The ACOSOG Z0010 trial was a prospective multicenter trial designed to evaluate occult disease in the bone marrow and SN of women with clinical T1–2N0M0 invasive breast cancer treated with lumpectomy and SLND.[151] Blinded analysis of the SN by IHC and bone marrow by immunocytochemistry was performed in a central laboratory on the 3904 SNs that were histologically negative by H&E. Adjuvant treatment recommendations were made on the basis of H&E examination of the axillary nodes. Clinicians were blinded to the results. Among 5184 patients with SN, 1239 (23.9%) had metastases identified by routine H&E. IHC detected an additional 350 (10.5%) with SN metastases. SN metastases detected by IHC did not have a significant impact on 5-year overall survival. Bone marrow micrometastases were identified in 105 of 3491 (3.0%) of cases examined and bone marrow IHC positivity was significantly associated with worse overall survival. The authors concluded that SN metastases identified only by IHC likely have no clinical significance, and the incidence of bone marrow micrometastases is too low to justify routine bone marrow aspirations in this population. Occult metastases were also investigated by the NSABP-B32 trial subset analysis, where 3887 tissue blocks from histologically negative SN were reexamined with serial sectioning and IHC.[152] Occult metastases were identified in 15.9% with no difference in overall survival between those with occult metastases and those without occult metastases (94.6% and 95.8%, respectively). The authors concluded that the difference in overall survival, although statistically significant, was so small that there is no added clinical benefit to performing additional sectioning and IHC of H&E negative SN.

Isolated tumor cells in the SN should be distinguished from micrometastases.[153] The 7th edition of the American Joint Committee on Cancer (AJCC) TNM staging system in breast cancer has altered the definition of stage 1 breast cancer to reflect the findings on the prognostic significance of micrometastases. Stage IA includes T1 tumors that are pathologically node negative by H&E and IHC. Stage IB includes T1 tumors with micrometastases in the lymph nodes (N1mic). The American Society of Breast Surgeons released a position statement on SN micrometastases in August 2011, stating that SN micrometastases detected only by IHC are clinically insignificant and that routine use of IHC staining of SNs is unnecessary and should be limited to selective use at the discretion of the pathologist. IHC is of value to detect metastases from infiltrating lobular carcinoma, which may be difficult to detect with H&E.

Management of the Axilla When the Sentinel Node Is H&E Positive

When the SN contains metastases, the standard recommendation for patient management has traditionally been ALND. The ACOSOG Z0011 trial challenged this doctrine and revolutionized the surgical management of SN-positive axillary nodes in early breast cancer. The trial was a prospective phase III noninferiority trial that randomized 891 patients with clinical T1 or T2N0M0 breast cancer with a tumor-positive SN to completion ALND or observation of the axilla. All patients were treated with lumpectomy and whole breast radiation.[154,155] At median follow-up of 6.3 years, there was no difference between the two treatment arms with respect to local-regional recurrence (3.1% with ALND and 1.6% with SLND alone), overall survival (91.8% with ALND vs. 92.5% with SLND alone), and disease-free survival (82.2% with ALND and 83.9% with SLND alone). These findings, although initially met with controversy, have led to significant reduction in ALND in the appropriately selected patient with a positive SN. Patients with a positive SN who are considered suitable for observation of the axilla include those with clinically node-negative T1–2 tumors that have fewer than three positive SNs treated with lumpectomy, SLND, whole breast radiation, and systemic therapy, without evidence of significant extranodal extension.

Radiation Treatment of the Axilla

Radiation of the axilla has been investigated in patients who have not undergone ALND, and it may be an option for patients who have a positive SN after SLND. A randomized trial of ALND versus radiation of the axilla in breast conservative management in 381 patients revealed one axillary recurrence in each arm at a median follow-up of 26 months.[156] In a randomized trial comparing no axillary treatment with axillary radiotherapy, there were three regional failures (expected: 43) in the no-treatment arm and one (expected: 10) in the radiotherapy arm at 63 months follow-up.[157]

The Joint Center for Radiation Therapy has investigated the role of axillary radiation when a limited number of positive nodes have been resected.[158] They studied 292 patients with stage I and II breast cancer who had axillary irradiation without ALND and 126 who had limited axillary surgery (five or fewer lymph nodes removed) and axillary irradiation. Regional nodal failure was detected in 6 of 418 (1.4%) patients at 8 years. Four had simultaneous local and distant disease, and two had isolated axillary failure. The regional failures occurred in 3 of 218 patients who had axillary irradiation without ALND (1 supraclavicular and 2 axillary) and in 3 of 42 patients (1 infraclavicular and 2 axillary) who had pathologically involved limited axillary dissection. There were no axillary recurrences in the 84 patients who had limited axillary surgery with pathologically negative nodes and axillary irradiation. This limited study suggests that axillary radiation may offer an alternative to ALND for SN-positive patients. The Joint Center has designed a protocol to determine the efficacy of axillary irradiation after a positive SN and to identify subgroups that may benefit from axillary irradiation.[158] The After Mapping of the Axilla: Radiotherapy or Surgery Trial (AMAROS) prospective randomized phase III noninferiority trial randomized 1425 women with clinical T1–2N0 invasive breast cancer with a positive SN to axillary radiation versus ALND.[159] With a median follow-up of 6.1 years, there was a low number of axillary recurrences in both arms (0.43% [95% confidence interval 0–0.92] in the ALND arm and 1.19% [0.31–2.08] in the axillary radiation arm) and no differences in disease-free and overall survival. There was significantly higher rate of lymphedema in the ALND arm (23%) compared with the axillary radiation arm (11%) at 5 years ($P <$ .0001). The data from this study suggest that axillary radiation provides comparable local control to ALND in clinically node-negative SN-positive patients with lower rates of lymphedema.

Technical Considerations

General Technical Considerations

The opportunity to save a patient from ALND or to improve staging through SLND depends on accurate identification of the SN. This accuracy is a combination of correct localization and complete histopathologic evaluation. The rate of nonlocalization depends on the method of detection and the experience of the institution (see Table 42.7).[5,6,10–12,23–63] Examples of SLND techniques with dye, isotope, or combined dye and isotope are discussed in the following sections.[9] Identification rates by technique are shown in Table 42.14.[22] Differences in the ability to find the

SN include variations in methodology: type of vital dye and/or radioisotope, timing of surgery after dye or isotope injection, site of injection (peritumoral, subdermal, intradermal, subareolar), and filtered versus unfiltered isotope.[9,22] Risk factors associated with unsuccessful lymphatic mapping include surgeon inexperience, medial hemisphere lesions, extensive axillary tumor burden, and extranodal extension of metastases.[160] Other studies report failure to identify the SN because of multifocal or multicentric tumors, previous excision, large biopsy cavity, skip lesions, and micrometastases, as discussed previously. The most important factor for successful SN identification remains the surgeon and his or her team's experience with any given technique.

Lymphatic Mapping With Vital Dye

Selection of Optimal Dye for Intraoperative Lymphatic Mapping

The selection of an appropriate vital dye is critical for a successful procedure. The optimal dye for lymphatic mapping has been studied in an animal model.[161] Three different dyes were investigated: cyalume, a fluorescent dye; methylene blue, a water-soluble dye; and isosulfan blue, a dye with selective avidity for the lymphatics. Cyalume readily identified the lymphatics but also stained the surrounding interstitial tissue creating a high background. Methylene blue proved to be unsatisfactory in the animal model because of poor uptake by the lymphatics. The success rate of methylene blue with radioisotope is reported to be equivalent to isosulfan blue with isotope.[162,163] Isosulfan blue is conjugated to albumin, taken up by the lymphatics readily, and retained in the lymphatics and SN without leak into extralymphatic tissues.[164] The more concentrated compound available outside of the United States is Patent Blue V, which has similar functional characteristics. Indigocarmine has been used successfully in Japan. It has a higher intralymphatic retention with a high degree of success.[42,53] Indigocyanine green has also been used successfully.[60] Evan's blue dye has been used for successful identification of axillary and internal mammary SNs.[165]

Complications of Dye Injection

The safety and efficacy of isosulfan blue dye was first studied in a rat model and then investigated in 11 volunteers and 543 patients in the 1980s.[166] Up to 15 mg of a 1% solution injected into the extremity resulted in a 97.4% success rate to identify the lymphatic vessels, with no adverse reactions and minimal allergic reactions in patients (≤1%). Isolated case reports of adverse reactions with blue dye including allergic urticaria and anaphylaxis have been reported, but this rate is extremely low.[167] Data from the NSABP B-32 trial shows 0.4% grade 1 and 2 allergic reactions and 0.2% grade 3 and 4 with no deaths.[63] The data from ACOSOG Z0010 trial show 0.1% anaphylaxis with isosulfan blue alone or in combination with radiocolloid, axillary wound complications in 1%, axillary seroma in 7.1%, and axillary hematoma in 1.4%.[168] Hives covering the trunk and upper extremities, not associated with hypotension, resolve within 24 to 48 hours after administration of methylprednisolone and diphenhydramine.[167] Management of hypotensive anaphylaxis includes discontinuation of anesthetic agents; administration of fluids; and administration of epinephrine, diphenhydramine hydrochloride, and corticosteroids.[167] Intraoperative plasma histamine levels may be elevated at the time of reaction.[167] Postoperative skin testing to isosulfan blue may be a useful test.[167] The anaphylactic reaction seems to be an immunoglobulin E reaction and may occur as long as 30 minutes

TABLE 42.14 Characteristics of Studies Included in Systematic Review

Study	No. Completing Study	Percentage of Positive Lymph Nodes	Proportion Mapped Successfully	Technique[a]	PROPORTIONS Total Positive Lymph Nodes	Total Positive SNs
Olson et al., 2000	223	43.14	0.91	2	0.43	0.41
Cox, 2000	484	72.48	1	2	0.72	0.72
Noguchi et al., 2000	674	41.39	0.99	2	0.41	0.37
Tafra et al., 2001	48	30.04	—	2	0.30	0.26
Krag et al., 1998	443	28.15	0.93	2	0.28	0.25
Veronesi et al., 1999	376	48.52	0.99	2	0.49	0.45
Winchester et al., 2000	72	72.22	0.75	1	0.72	0.65
Laurisen et al., 2000	80	55.13	0.98	2	0.55	0.55
Bobin et al., 2000	243	37.78	0.93	2	0.38	0.35
de Kanter et al., 2000	199	34.39	0.92	2	0.34	0.32
Canavese et al., 2001	212	37.38	0.97	2	0.37	0.35
Giuliano et al., 1997	172	36.84	0.66	0	0.37	0.32
Ilum et al., 2000	159	50.52	0.61	0	0.51	0.43
Krag et al., 1998	157	50	0.76	2	0.50	0.48
Bembenek et al., 1999	146	46.23	0.81	1	0.46	0.42
Doting et al., 2000	136	46.83	0.93	2	0.47	0.44
Morrow et al., 1999	139	20.09	0.79	2	0.29	0.25
Fraile et al., 2000	132	39.37	0.96	1	0.39	0.38
Borgstein et al., 1997	104	43.27	1	1	0.43	0.42
Nos et al., 1999	122	30.89	0.88	0	0.31	0.28
Cserni et al., 2000	122	74.34	0.93	2	0.74	0.67
Nwariaku et al., 1998	119	28.13	0.81	2	0.28	0.27
Kollias et al., 1999	117	32.63	0.82	2	0.33	0.31
Giuliano et al., 1994	107	42	0.93	0	0.42	0.42
Reynolds et al., 1999	95	44.52	—	0	0.45	0.41
Molland et al., 2000	86	50	1	0	0.50	0.48
Bobin et al., 1999	100	46.99	0.83	0	0.47	0.45
Koller et al., 1998	98	53.13	0.98	0	0.53	0.50
Jaderborg et al., 1999	79	31.25	0.81	2	0.31	0.30
Sandrucci and Mussa, 1998	84	43.84	0.87	1	0.44	0.41
Roumen et al., 1997	83	40.35	0.69	1	0.40	0.39
Nason et al., 2000	82	46.97	0.80	2	0.47	0.39
Snider et al., 1998	80	20	0.88	1	0.20	0.19
Folscher et al., 1997	79	53.13	0.41	0	0.53	0.38
van der Ent et al., 1999	70	38.57	1	2	0.39	0.37
Mertz et al., 1999	79	42.11	0.97	1	0.42	0.41
Vaggelli et al., 2000	76	49.25	0.95	1	0.49	0.49

Continued

TABLE 42.14 Characteristics of Studies Included in Systematic Review—cont'd

Study	No. Completing Study	Percentage of Positive Lymph Nodes	Proportion Mapped Successfully	Technique[a]	PROPORTIONS Total Positive Lymph Nodes	Total Positive SNs
Rodier et al., 2000	73	50	0.84	0	0.50	0.46
Moffat et al., 1999	70	35.48	0.89	1	0.35	0.32
Noguchi et al., 1999	72	46.03	0.86	2	0.46	0.40
Flett et al., 1998	68	37.50	0.82	0	0.38	0.32
Martin et al., 2000	758	32.59	0.89	2	0.33	0.31
Gucciardo et al., 2000	50	41.86	0.86	1	0.42	0.30
Altinoyollar et al., 2000	60	44.89	0.82	0	0.45	0.39
O'Hea et al., 1998	59	41.82	0.93	2	0.42	0.36
Chatterjee et al., 1998	60	35.59	0.97	2	0.36	0.34
Clark et al., 1999	55	40.38	0.95	2	0.40	0.38
Breslin et al., 2000	51	58.14	0.84	2	0.58	0.51
Crossin et al., 1998	50	17.39	0.84	1	0.17	0.15
Mechella et al., 2000	48	35.71	0.88	1	0.36	0.31
Galli et al., 2000	46	34.09	0.96	1	0.34	0.27
Morgan et al., 1999	44	37.50	0.73	0	0.38	0.31
Langer et al., 2000	44	53.66	0.93	2	0.54	0.51
Barnwell et al., 1998	42	39.47	0.90	2	0.39	0.39
Liu et al., 2000	41	51.28	0.93	2	0.51	0.49
Offodile et al., 1998	41	45.00	0.98	1	0.45	0.45
Hsieh et al., 2000	41	39.02	1	1	0.39	0.34
Ratanawichitrasin et al., 1998	40	25.71	0.88	0	0.26	0.20
Delaloye et al., 2000	40	30.77	0.98	2	0.31	0.31
Kern, 1999	40	38.46	0.98	0	0.38	0.38
Horgan et al., 1998	38	50	0.92	0	0.50	0.42
Kowolik et al., 2000	37	27.27	0.89	2	0.27	0.24
Berclaz et al., 1998	34	33.33	0.97	2	—	—
Borgstein et al., 1997	25	56	1	2	0.56	0.56
Kapteijn et al., 1998	30	38.46	0.87	0	0.38	0.38
Schneebaum et al., 1998	30	32.14	0.93	2	0.32	0.25
Canavese et al., 2000	55	35.80	1	0	0.36	0.30
Forner et al., 2000	21	38.10	1	2	0.38	0.33
Schrenk and Wayand, 2001	19	52.63	1	2	0.53	0.53

SN, Sentinel lymph node.

[a]0, blue dye alone; 1, radiocolloid alone; 2, both blue dye and radiocolloid.

From Kim T, Giuliano AE, Lyman GH. Lymphatic mapping and sentinel lymph node biopsy in early-stage breast carcinoma. *Cancer.* 2005;106:4-16, and Van Zee KJ, Manasseh DM, Bevilacqua JLB, et al. A nomogram for predicting the likelihood of additional nodal metastases in breast cancer patients with a positive sentinel node biopsy. *Ann Surg Oncol.* 2003;10:1140-1151.

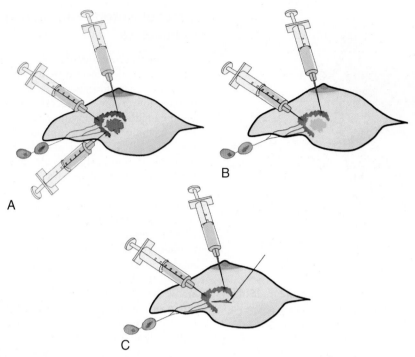

• **Fig. 42.3** Injection technique for lymphatic mapping and sentinel lymphadenectomy. Dye is injected into the parenchyma on the axillary side of the tumor when the tumor is palpable (A). If the tumor has been previously removed, dye is injected into the wall of the biopsy cavity on the axillary side (B). If the tumor is nonpalpable, the tumor is triangulated on the mammogram and the guidewire is used to localize the region of the tumor for peritumoral injection along the axillary side (C).

to 1 hour after injection.[169] Intraoperatively, isosulfan blue can affect pulse oximetry.[170,171] Although this is a pseudo-desaturation with PaO_2 remaining normal, surgeons and anesthesiologists must investigate the clinical situation and the potential causes of desaturation.[170] Relatively minor problems include transient staining of the epidermis that can take several weeks to several months to fade completely. There is a transient change in color of the urine and stool to a greenish hue. Although these are temporary events, unless patients are forewarned about what to expect, this can cause a great deal of unnecessary distress.

In contrast to isosulfan blue, methylene blue has not been associated with anaphylactic reaction.[167] Local reactions of skin erythema, superficial ulceration, or necrosis have been reported with intradermal injections. Partial skin loss usually responds to topical Silvadene therapy, with no need for surgical debridement.[167] Methylene blue should not be injected intradermally or subdermally because of risk of skin ulceration.[172]

Anesthetic Considerations

Sentinel lymphadenectomy is usually an outpatient procedure. Axillary exploration can be performed under general anesthesia, conscious sedation with local, or local anesthesia alone.[173] SLND under local anesthesia requires expert surgeons, quick and precise surgery, and minimal use of electrocautery. Local anesthesia may not be appropriate for some patients.

Vital Dye Injection Technique

After adequate anesthesia, the patient is positioned at the edge of the operating room table with the arm extended at 90 degrees and prepped free. Five milliliters of 1% isosulfan blue is injected peritumorally or around the biopsy cavity in an arc toward the

axilla.[13,162] Successful SN identification has been reported when isosulfan dye is injected into sites other than breast parenchyma: subdermal, intradermal, intradermal periareolar, and subareolar.[9] For palpable lesions, dye is injected into the breast parenchyma around the axillary side of the tumor. For mammographically or ultrasonographically detected lesions, dye is injected adjacent to the localization needles or with the use of ultrasound guidance. For tumors previously removed by excisional biopsy, dye is injected into the wall of the biopsy cavity on the axillary side but not into the cavity itself (Fig. 42.3). Dye injected into biopsy cavities or directly into the tumor does not gain access to the afferent lymphatics and therefore will not identify the sentinel node.

The average interval between dye injection and axillary incision is 5 minutes. The time can be modified for individual patients, such as in older patients or in those with a higher BMI. In the latter case, more time is required for dye to opacify the lymphatics. Dye transit time from primary to axilla is related to the location of the tumor, with shorter transit times for lesions in the axillary tail and longer ones for those in the lower inner quadrant. Typically 3 to 4 minutes and 7 to 10 minutes should be allowed for dye to travel, respectively, from lesions in these locations. This time delay often seems endless for the surgeon; therefore, strict monitoring of time is recommended. Disregard of this simple fact may contribute to the difficulties that some have had with the dye-directed technique. Improved blue node identification has been reported with breast or three-stage lymphatic massage.[174,175]

Dissection Technique

SLND is typically performed during mastectomy or partial mastectomy. A 2- to 3-cm transverse incision is made 1 cm below the

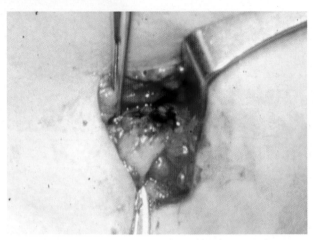

• **Fig. 42.4** Lymphatic channel leading to sentinel node.

hair-bearing area of the axilla slightly anterior to the midaxillary line, preferably in a skin crease for improved cosmesis. Skin flaps are not developed for this procedure. The clavipectoral fascia is identified and incised. The arm is abducted to bring the axillary content outward into the operative field. Gentle blunt dissection is initiated at the margin of the pectoralis major in the zone containing the pectoral nodes, the most likely region to contain the SN. If no blue lymphatic is identified, attention is redirected to the known zones of nodal clustering (e.g., external mammary, central subscapular, subclavicular) in levels I and II. The SN is located in level I in 83% of cases, level II in 15.6%, and level III in 0.5%.[72] The blue lymphatic trunk is followed to the SN and traced proximally and distally to locate other blue nodes (Fig. 42.4). Omission of this step can result in missing a more proximal or distal blue node and can be another reason for a false-negative SN. After removal of the SN, the axillary space is gently explored and palpated for suspicious, palpable nodes. These are removed and identified as suspicious. Disregard for palpable nodes has been the cause of false-negative SNs in several series. After all SNs are identified, they are sent for pathologic evaluation.

Radiolocalization and Lymphatic Mapping With Isotopes

Radiopharmaceutical

The optimal radioactive tracer for SN identification should have properties that permit rapid migration from the site of injection to the draining lymphatics.[176] The agent must identify the SN and retain its activity long enough to allow identification in the operating room. The biokinetics of radioactive particulate flow and absorption depend on particle size.[177] The most commonly used agents for SLND are colloidal radioisotopes that are transported through the lymphatics and phagocytized by macrophages in the SN. A variety of agents have been used: ^{99m}Tc-sulfur colloid, ^{99m}Tc-human serum albumin, ^{99m}Tc-antimony sulfur colloid, ^{99m}Tc-dextran, and ^{99m}Tc-tin.[9] ^{99m}Tc-tilmanocept is a novel receptor binding molecular agent approved by the US Food and Drug Administration in 2014 for lymphatic mapping in solid tumors that has advantages over the other radiocolloids, including rapid injection site clearance, high retention in the sentinel node, and low distal node accumulation.[178]

Effect of Isotope Filtration on Dose and Volume of Injectate

The desirable properties of an ideal radiocolloid for SLND include rapid reabsorption from injection site, reasonable migration time to permit identification and surgical scheduling, high degree of retention, a low second echelon pass-through rate, low cost, minimal radiation exposure, ease of preparation, consistency, and reproducibility of the technique.[28] The SN retains larger particle sizes better. Filtered colloids are more uniform in size and move more rapidly through the reticuloendothelial system into the intravascular space. Investigators who have used unfiltered[26,31,36–38,40,47–50] or filtered isotopes[10,26,27,35,37,43,45,48,59,179] have achieved similar success rates for identification and accuracy. The size of particles in filtered ^{99m}Tc-sulfur colloid is less than 10 nm, whereas unfiltered particles average a size of 305 to 340 nm.[180] The unfiltered radioisotope results in poorer quality gamma camera images because of the low uptake of large particles and is more suitable for the intraoperative gamma detection probe than preoperative lymphoscintigraphy.[181] Other investigators have used isotopes with smaller particulate size: ^{99m}Tc-human serum albumin is less than 4 nm, ^{99m}Tc-dextran less than 4 nm, and ^{99m}Tc-antimony sulfur colloid 15 to 50 nm.[180] Tilmanocept has an average diameter of 7 nm.[178] To counterbalance the more rapid penetration of the lymphatics by filtered compounds and compounds with smaller particles, a larger dose is usually administered.[180] Doses of less than 0.5 mCi,[6,10,27,36,48] 1 mCi,[26,31,32,35,37,38,40,45,47,50] or greater than 1 mCi[46] have been used.

Transport through the lymphatic channels is dependent on the anatomy and physiology of the lymphatic channel.[182] Lymph flow depends on a delicate balance between intraluminal pressure and interstitial pressure. Just as particle size has an effect on rate of lymphatic migration and nodal retention, volume of injection has an effect on flow.[182] Some argue that small volumes are better because they do not disturb the homeostatic fluid balance. Others argue that large volumes increase interstitial pressure, which leads to greater lymphatic reabsorption and flow. The volumes of injection have varied from the small volume (0.5 mL) studied initially[6] to larger volumes (8 mL) more recently.[40,47,181] Tanis and associates suggest that high volumes may increase transmural pressure and improve flow, but this is at the cost of lymphatic channel expansion and anchoring filament stretch leading to increased diffusion.[182] Krag and coworkers, on the other hand, suggest that the increased volume leads to improved microcirculation, the opening of the leaflets of the vascular endothelium to permit fast flow rates, and entrance of large particles, which are retained in the first echelon nodes.[181] One point to consider is that larger volumes lead to a greater zone of diffusion. This larger area of radioactivity, especially in the upper outer quadrant, can cause difficulty for radiolocalization of the SN.[182] Lymph flow is complex and affected by patient characteristics such as state of hydration, physical exercise, and medications, as well as breast massage, isotope characteristics, volume of injectate, and particulate size.[182] Despite variations in technique, successful lymphatic mapping can be achieved with experience at individual investigator institutions, both academic and community hospitals.[61]

Injection Site

When Krag and colleagues[6] described SLND with a gamma detection probe, the isotope was injected peritumorally. Other investigators have examined the role of subdermal, intradermal, or subareolar/periareolar injection.[9,12,39,48,50,55,57,58,183–185] A prospective randomized trial comparing intradermal, intraparenchymal, and subareolar injection routes for SLND demonstrated a significantly greater rate of localization, more rapid transit by lymphoscintigraphy, and shorter time to surgery with the intradermal injection.[184] Internal mammary nodes are rarely visualized with intradermal injection.[183,184] In another randomized multicentric trial comparing periareolar and peritumoral injection of radiotracer and blue dye, both locations resulted in a 99.1% detection rate and a high concordance rate.[183] Subareolar injection offers some advantages over peritumoral injection (e.g., nonvisualization of nonpalpable tumors, increased distance of radioactivity from the axilla for upper outer quadrant lesions, good choice for multicentric disease).[186] An important aspect of lymphatic mapping is that each investigator must follow rigorous adherence to a defined method, data collection, and analysis.

Timing of Injection, Lymphoscintigraphy, Intraoperative Gamma-Probe Detection

The technical variations for radioisotope-directed SLND also affect detection of a radioactive node by lymphoscintigraphy or by gamma-detection probe (Fig. 42.5). In a prospective trial to evaluate the feasibility of using lymphoscintigraphy in conjunction with gamma probe detection for SN identification, 89% of the patients demonstrated focal accumulations of isotope.[33] The scintigraphic failure rates were greater in patients with previous excision, 36% versus 4% ($p < .005$). Failure to visualize SN occurred with large injection site overlap and a large breast hematoma. In another study, failure to visualize an SN was associated with peritumoral injection, patient age greater than 60 years, and upper outer quadrant tumor location.[187] A single radioactive focus was identified in 77%, two foci in 21%, and three foci in 2.6%.[33] The distribution of these foci was not affected by the location of the tumor. The primary flow was toward the axilla. Examination of variations in pattern and intensity as a function of time demonstrate no significant differences between early and late lymphoscintigrams.[33,188] A small number of patients (3.4%) do not demonstrate a radioactive focus until late, and those (5.1%) who do not have clearly visible foci even after overnight exposure also have low SN counts at the time of surgery.[33] The mean transit time to first localization with dynamic imaging varied with intradermal (8 ± 14 minutes), intraparenchymal (53 ± 49 minutes), and subareolar (22 ± 29 minutes) injection sites.[184] Aberrant drainage patterns have been demonstrated by lymphoscintigraphy and gamma probe detection, especially to the IMLN. Preoperative lymphoscintigraphy demonstrates the highest rate of internal mammary node drainage with intraparenchymal injection (11%), followed by periareolar (2%) injection, and the lowest was for intradermal injection (1%).[184] The management of this small subgroup of patients is quite controversial and discussed subsequently.

Surgical Technique for Radioguided Sentinel Lymphadenectomy

The surgical approach to SLND for a hot node varies slightly from the method of dye-directed surgery.[6,26–28,181] Radioactivity at the primary tumor site is identified with the gamma detection probe. The breast is swept in concentric circles the size of the detection probe to define the zone of diffusion and identify any hot spots. The goal of the intraoperative gamma detection probe is to survey

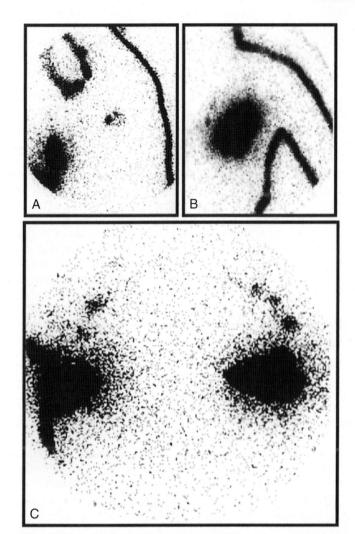

• **Fig. 42.5** Preoperative lymphoscintigraphy. (A) A left anterior oblique view of a sentinel node. (B) Drainage to the internal mammary lymph node in a patient with a previous axillary sentinel lymph node dissection. (C) Bilateral lymphoscintigraphy in a patient with bilateral breast cancers.

all common breast nodal drainage sites for activity: breast, axilla, infraclavicular, supraclavicular, and internal mammary nodal basins. A major difficulty has been the definition of the SN or radioactive node. A hot spot is defined as any location with a cumulative 10-second count greater than 25.[6,31,40] Other authors use different criteria for an SN such as audible counts, the hottest node, a 10:1 ratio of SN to background, or a fourfold reduction in counts after the SN is removed.[12,27,33,36,39,46,48] At times the node with the highest counts is not the SN. Some have suggested that the absolute count is not as critical as the ratio of the hottest node to the background because there are variations in uptake of radioactivity.[189] When a hot spot is identified, the probe is angled to identify the point of maximum intensity. This defines the line of sight and angle of dissection. A small, 3- to 4-cm incision is made over the hot spot. The soft tissues are divided and the gamma detection probe is inserted to reestablish the line of sight. This sequence is repeated and readjusted until the SN is identified by maximum counts. The radioactive SN is resected. The surface of the SN is checked for point of maximum intensity of counts per second. This location can be marked with a suture for the pathologist. It is usually the location of the metastatic focus. Verification that this is truly the SN is done by an ex vivo count of the SN and in vivo background count. Remaining radioactive SNs are removed until the background is less than one-tenth the counts of the hottest node.

Hottest Node

Lymph nodes with the highest radioactive uptake usually contain the largest relative volume of metastasis.[33] Obstruction of the lymphatics by tumor metastases changes the pattern of flow. Increased immunologic competency of the SN may be reflected by higher uptake of isotope.[33] Lymph nodes with hyperplasia or fatty degeneration may demonstrate slow uptake or reduced activity.[33] A positive SN is the hottest node in 74% to 77% of cases, but if only the hottest node would have been removed, 23% to 26% of the positive SNs could be missed.[62,190] Complete replacement of the SN by tumor may result in minimal or no uptake. All suspicious palpable nodes must be removed at the time of SLND.

Pearls to Remember for the Combined Technique

Lymphatic mapping with a combination of blue dye and isotope combines the features of these two modalities (Fig. 42.6). Following are some "pearls" to remember:

- Vigorously shake the colloid before injection to disperse clumps of particles.
- Realize that although radiolocalization works with same-day or second-day isotope injections, the optimal time from radioisotope injection to surgery varies by site of injection.
- Inject each agent separately (comixing causes precipitation of both detectors).

- Operate in a bloodless field, and have good retraction.
- Clip nonblue hot lymphatic channels, and maintain the probe's line of sight.
- Do not cut the blue lymphatic.[155] The blue lymphatic should remain intact as a map to the SN.

Histopathologic Evaluation

The histopathologic assessment of axillary lymph nodes has traditionally consisted of bivalving the node and evaluating it with H&E stain. The limited number of SNs removed, usually one to three, has permitted more exhaustive and sophisticated techniques to be instituted. This has led to some controversy in the pathologic management of the SN. Some investigators recommend intraoperative frozen section analysis and permanent section evaluation with both H&E and IHC.

The American College of Pathologists has established guidelines for SN processing,[147] as has the European Working Group for Breast Screening Pathology.[148] SNs can be processed in the operating room or be studied by permanent H&E stain. The American College of Pathologists recommends that the SN be bivalved along the longitudinal axis and sectioned into 1.5- to 2-mm slices. Intraoperative examination can be performed by frozen section or imprint cytology. The SN is then submitted in formalin for histologic assessment with H&E staining. It is recommended that each block be sectioned at three levels. If metastases are identified (Fig. 42.7), macrometastases, micrometastases, IHC, or reverse transcriptase-polymerase chain reaction (RT-PCR) metastases should be described according to the new AJCC guidelines.[2,191]

Intraoperative frozen section analysis of the SN has some drawbacks, including accuracy of diagnosis, cost of the procedure, and potentially increased operative time.[192] A number of studies have

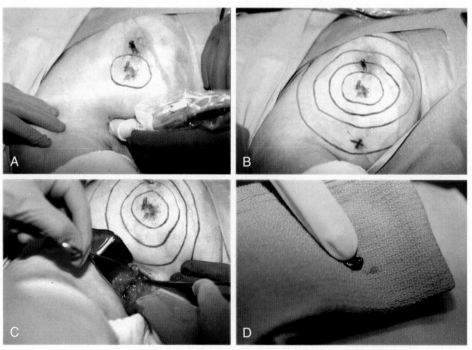

• **Fig. 42.6** Combined blue dye and radioguided sentinel lymph node dissection. (A) The location of the axillary hot spot is determined. (B) Isobars of decaying radioactivity are demonstrated. (C) A blue lymphatic is identified that courses to the blue and radioactive sentinel node. (D) The presence of radioactivity in the resected node is confirmed with the gamma detection probe.

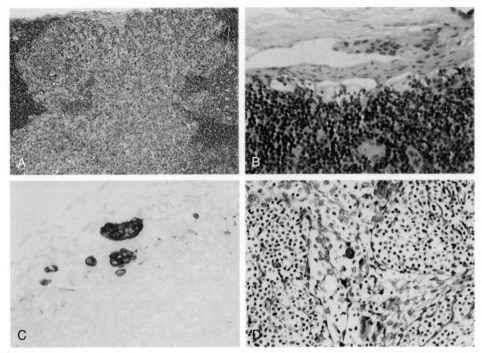

• **Fig. 42.7** Histopathology images of sentinel node metastases. (A) Hematoxylin and eosin (H&E)-positive macrometastasis. (B) H&E micrometastasis. (C) Cluster of immunohistochemistry (IHC)-positive cells. (D) Single IHC-positive cell.

demonstrated a frozen section false-negative rate that ranges from a low of 5.5% as reported by Veronesi and colleagues,[39] who performed exhaustive complete intraoperative frozen section and IHC analysis of the SN, to a high of 54%.[193] The sensitivity of frozen section to identify SN metastases is tumor-size dependent.[192,194] Frozen section can identify macrometastases with greater sensitivity than micrometastases.[192,194] A false-positive SN was identified in one study.[194] Imprint cytology is an alternative method to detect a tumor-positive SN in the operating room that some authors have found to be sensitive, whereas others find it less reliable.[149,195] Frozen section can identify axillary metastasis in the SN if ALND is planned at the same operation, in which case the patients undergo standard level I and II axillary dissection.[196] The ACOSOG Z0011 trial demonstrated that a positive SN in select patients undergoing BCS is not always an indication for completion ALND, and thus frozen section analysis of SN in patients undergoing lumpectomy is not warranted. However, ALND is still recommended in SN-positive patients undergoing mastectomy, and frozen section may have utility in sparing mastectomy patients from a second operation for ALND if nodal metastases are identified at the time of the mastectomy. If axillary metastases are not identified with frozen section, no further axillary surgery needs to be performed if permanent sections are concordant.[13] A negative SN is further evaluated at the previous two H&E levels with IHC. The cytokeratin IHC staining is performed using the MAK-6 antibody cocktail to low- and intermediate-molecular-weight cytokeratin. More extensive evaluation with seven additional levels for IHC did not increase the incidence of IHC-positive SNs. The role of IHC for SN is controversial, and this issue is discussed later in this chapter.

A portion of the lymph node can also be processed for multiple marker reverse transcriptase polymerase chain reaction (RT-PCR) analysis and has comparable sensitivity to histopathologic evaluation of the entire SN.[197] The sensitivity is 98.1% for metastases greater than 2 mm, 94.7% for metastases greater than 1 mm, and 77.8% for metastases greater than 0.2 mm. The results were obtained in 40 minutes intraoperatively. A quantitative RT-PCR assay has been developed using 43 potential markers.[198] A validation set using four markers individually or in combination was compared with histologic analysis. The results demonstrated 97.8% accuracy for a two-marker assay and could be performed in less than 35 minutes intraoperatively. RT-PCR evaluation of the SN has the potential to provide an automated standardized analysis of SN and could prove to be more cost-effective and practical than the current standard evaluation of SN. However, molecular analysis of SN is unlikely to be of clinical relevance in view of recently reported results of the ACOSOG Z0010 and NSABP-B32 trials on micrometastases.

False-Negative Sentinel Nodes

Investigators have attempted to characterize the causes of false-negative SNs. Explanation for false-negative rates may have to do with injection methodology; lymphatic physiology; aberrant lymphatic patterns; tumor-replaced nodes that are either not blue or have a lower radioactivity count than adjacent second echelon nodes to which lymphatic flow is unimpeded by tumor occlusion; and surgeon, nuclear medicine, and pathologist experience. The false-negative rate ranges from 0% to 29.4% in single-institution studies (average, 8.4% across studies; median, 7%).[22] The European Institute of Oncology single-institution, randomized prospective trial reports a false-negative rate of 8.8%.[199] The data from the multiinstitutional, randomized prospective NSABP B-32 trial reports a false-negative rate of 9.8% and an overall accuracy of 97.1%.[72] Differences in tumor location (medial and lateral tumors higher than central), type of diagnostic biopsy (excision/incisional biopsy higher than fine-needle aspiration or core needle biopsy) and number of SNs removed (1 > 2 > 3 > 4

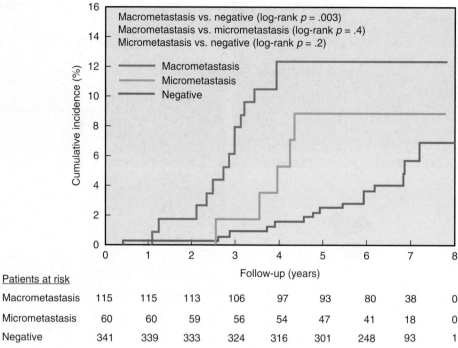

• **Fig. 42.8** Breast cancer–related events in the combined axillary lymph node dissection group and sentinel lymph node dissection group according to the status of the sentinel node. (From Veronesi U, Paganelli G, Viale G, et al. Sentinel-lymph-node biopsy as a staging procedure in breast cancer: Update of a randomised controlled study. *Lancet Oncol.* 2006;7:983-990.)

> 5) affected the false-negative rate. The Sentinella/GIVOM academic and small community hospital multiinstitutional trial has found a much higher false-negative rate (16.7%).[200] The participants in this trial were required to have performed at least 15 cases with no false-negative SNs, but no formal instruction was required.

Predictors of Nonsentinel Node Metastases

During recent decades, the size of primary tumors has decreased, and the incidence of axillary metastases has decreased correspondingly. In a meta-analysis, the SN is the only positive node in 47% of patients from large centers.[22] The randomized prospective NSABP B-32 trial found that in patients with a positive SN who had an ALND, 61.4% contained metastases in the SN only.[72] Omission of ALND when an SN is negative has been generally accepted as a reliable method of axillary staging with low regional recurrence rates, and the question of whether all patients with a positive SN require ALND, which was addressed in the ACOSOG Z0011 trial will be discussed later in this chapter..

Predictors of non-SN metastases have been identified in individual centers.[201] Non-SN metastases can be identified by H&E or by the more sensitive method, IHC, in 14.7% of nonsentinel nodes when the SN is positive.[202] According to multivariate analysis, tumor size, size of SN metastasis, extranodal hilar tumor invasion, and peritumoral lymphovascular invasion are independent variables predictive of non-SN metastases.[202] Tumor size greater than 5 cm was associated with a non-SN metastasis in 78.6% of patients. If the SN metastasis was greater than 2 mm, non-SN metastasis occurred in 62.4%.[202] Similar findings have been reported by Rahusen and colleagues, who demonstrated that patients with only one positive SN or micrometastasis less than 1 mm had significantly less non-SN involvement (40% vs. 78%)

than patients with macrometastases (27% vs. 49%).[203] In a multiinstitutional study, non-SN metastases were related to size of SN metastasis, primary tumor size, and lymphovascular invasion.[204] These studies identify small tumor size, SN micrometastasis, and absence of lymphovascular invasion as predictors of the SN as the only positive node.

The MSKCC group has developed a nomogram that is a tool to help estimate the risk of additional nodal disease when the SN is positive (Fig. 42.8).[201] The nomogram uses pathologic size, tumor type, nuclear grade, lymphovascular invasion, multifocality, estrogen receptor (ER) status, histopathologic method used to detect a positive SN, and number of negative SNs to predict the likelihood of additional positive non-SNs. The nomogram was established using retrospective data and was evaluated in a prospective manner at MSKCC and found to have improved prediction capability. The nomogram has been tested by several other groups with fair to good reliability, but at the same time its clinical usefulness has been questioned.[205] In addition, the relevance of these prediction tools has diminished as the role of ALND continues to evolve, as ALND for SN-positive patients decreases, and as tumor biology becomes the more important factor in determining therapy.

Morbidity of Sentinel Lymphadenectomy

Axillary dissection is associated with lymphedema, paresthesias, infections, and decreased range of motion.[14] Lymphatic mapping and sentinel lymphadenectomy result in much less morbidity than complete axillary dissection.[14,199] There is elimination of an axillary drain, less patient discomfort, and decreased incidence of lymphedema or neurovascular injury.[206] In the randomized Milan trial, axillary pain, numbness, paresthesias, and arm swelling

TABLE 42.15 Lymphedema in ALND Versus SLND

Study	SLND (No.)	ALND (No.)	Lymphedema SLND (%)	Lymphedema ALND (%)
Schrenk	35	35	0	17
Haid	57	140	4	27
Swenson	169	78	4	14
Blanchard	683	91	6	34
Schijven	180	213	1	7
Ronka	43	40	13	77
Leidenius	92	47	5	28
Mansel	515	516	5	13

ALND, Axillary lymph node dissection; *SLND*, sentinel lymph node dissection.
From Thompson M, Korourian S, Henry-Tillman R, et al. Axillary reverse mapping (ARM): a new concept to identify and enhance lymphatic preservation. *Ann Surg Oncol.* 2007;14:1890-1895.

persisted to a significantly greater extent in the ALND than the SLND group.[199] Surgical complications were statistically greater in the SLND plus ALND arm than in the SLND-only arm of the ACOSOG Z0011 trial, as well as wound infections ($p < .016$), seromas ($p < .0001$), paresthesias ($p < .0001$), and subjective lymphedema at 1 year ($p < .0001$).[207] Overall quality of life and arm functioning scores were better in the SLND group in the Axillary Lymphatic Mapping Against Nodal Axillary Clearance (ALMANAC) trial.[208] The risk of lymphedema after SLND ranges between 0% and 13% compared with 7% to 77% for ALND (Table 42.15).[209] The incision is smaller, and there is less pain, less limitation of motion, and fewer neurologic sequelae.

Variations in arm lymphatics contribute to the risk of developing lymphedema. A concept toward preventing arm lymphedema that was introduced in 2007 is axillary reverse mapping (ARM).[209,210] This technique uses 2.5 to 5 mL of isosulfan blue injected intradermally or subcutaneously in the tissue of the upper inner arm to map the lymphatics draining the arm. This procedure allowed preservation of the lymphatics draining the arm in all but one case. A recent systemic review identified eight prospective trials of ARM in 1142 patients undergoing axillary surgery for breast cancer.[211] Lymphedema rates were reported to range from 0% to 6% in ARM-assisted SLND procedures and 5.9% to 24% in ARM-assisted ALND procedures. Crossover nodes between the breast and arm lymphatics were identified in 0% to 10% of cases with 0% to 20% of nodes containing metastatic disease. Preservation of these crossover nodes raises concern that metastases in these nodes could be retained when using the ARM technique. Survival and recurrence data with extended follow-up on this technique are not available; therefore, the oncologic safety of the procedure remains unknown.

Learning Curve

Guidelines

As SLND is now the standard means for staging the axilla in clinically node-negative breast cancer, appropriate training and quality control are essential. The accuracy of SLND depends on the experience of the surgeon, pathologist, and nuclear medicine physician. How do surgeons acquire the skills, how many cases are sufficient for the surgeon to feel confident that the false-negative rate will be low, and how frequently should the surgeon be performing these cases to remain proficient?[206] What are the best methods of SLND to produce the highest identification rate and the lowest false-negative rate?

When new technology is introduced into practice, guidelines are established and should be adhered to by the medical community.[212] Cox and colleagues established a training program in which 16 surgeons performed lymphatic mapping in 2255 patients. The technique was combined isotope and blue dye. Each surgeon was trained in a 2-day course.

The American Society of Breast Surgeons has recommended a greater than 95% identification rate with a false-negative rate of 5% to 10% or less and suggests that axillary recurrence rates in SN-negative patients should not exceed 1%.[82] Surgeons must have completed an American Board of Medical Specialties–approved surgical residency program and have attained or be eligible for board certification by the American Board of Surgery. Training in the technique of SLND is part of the curriculum in all accredited surgical training programs.

Prospective Randomized Clinical Trials

NSABP B-32

The NSABP B-32 multiinstitutional study randomized 5611 women with invasive breast cancer to receive immediate ALND or SLND only if the SN was negative.[72] The aims of the study were to determine long-term control of regional disease, compare the effect of these two treatment arms on disease-free and overall survival, compare morbidity, and determine the risk of systemic recurrence in patients who have pathologically node-negative lesions. The NSABP B-32 study collected data on surgical and pathologic accuracy, technical success, and variations of success by technique used in a broad general population of surgeons. SNs were removed in 97.2% of cases. The SN was identified in level I and II of the axilla in 98.6% of cases. The overall accuracy was 97.1%, with a false-negative rate of 9.8%. Allergic reactions to blue dye occurred in 0.7% of cases. After mean follow-up of 95.6 months, overall survival, disease-free survival and regional control were equivalent between treatment arms, demonstrating that when the SN is negative, SLND without ALND is safe and appropriate surgical management in clinically node-negative patients.[213]

The European Institute of Oncology randomized controlled study is modeled on the NSABP B-32 protocol.[199] Women with tumors less than 2 cm were randomized to SLND only if the SN was tumor-free or to SLND followed by ALND. In the ALND group, 32% had a positive SN, and 8 of 174 SN-negative patients had a false-negative node. In the SLND-only group, the SN was positive in 36% with one axillary failure (expected: 8) at a median follow-up of 79 months. Breast cancer–related events by size of SN metastasis are shown in Fig. 42.9.[199] The overall survival was 96.4% in the ALND group and 98.4% in the SLND-only group.[199] The interpretation of this trial is that only SLND for SN-negative cancer decreases morbidity and cost with a lower than expected axillary failure rate. The Sentinella/GIVOM trial involved a similar randomization but found a false-negative rate of 16.7%.[200] Despite this high false-negative rate, there was only one axillary failure in the SLND-only group at 55.6 months. The

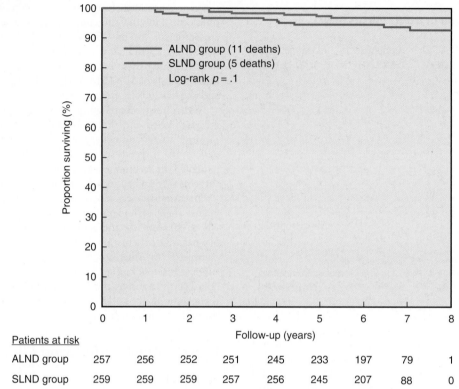

• **Fig. 42.9** Randomized European Institute of Oncology Trial for sentinel node–negative patients comparing sentinel lymph node dissection *(SLND)* alone to SLND followed by axillary lymph node dissection *(ALND)*. The graph shows overall survival in the ALND group versus the SLND group. (From Veronesi U, Paganelli G, Viale G, et al. Sentinel-lymph-node biopsy as a staging procedure in breast cancer: update of a randomised controlled study. *Lancet Oncol.* 2006;7:983-966.)

overall survival was 95.5% in the ALND group and 94.8% in the SLND-only group.

ACOSOG Z0010

The ACOSOG Z0010 trial is a prospective nonrandomized study in patients with stage I or II clinically node-negative breast cancer treated with breast conservation, SLND, and bilateral bone marrow aspiration. If the SN was negative, no further ALND was undertaken. The SN was evaluated by H&E only. Further analysis of metastatic potential was determined by blinded evaluation of the SN and bone marrow by IHC analysis. The objectives of this study were to determine the prevalence and significance of IHC-positive micrometastases in lymph nodes, bone marrow, or both in stage I and IIA breast cancer and determine risk of local recurrence. The basis for this protocol was that the prognostic assessment of the axilla has historically been determined on the basis of H&E staining, and this has dictated the design of established adjuvant treatment. A secondary objective was to determine the morbidity of SLND. The surgical complication rate was low among a wide range of surgeons.[168] Anaphylaxis occurred in 0.1%, seroma in 7.1%, and wound infection in 1.4%. Younger age was associated with a higher incidence of paresthesias and increased BMI with lymphedema. As mentioned previously in this chapter, the authors found that IHC-detected SN metastases did not appear to have an impact on overall survival, and the incidence of bone marrow IHC positivity was too low to justify routine bone marrow aspiration.[151]

The enormous amount of literature on the technique of SLND, the surgical learning curve and outcome of only SLND for SN-negative patients suggest that there is probably no role for further randomization of women to full ALND in the absence of SN metastases. Regional lymph node metastasis can be accurately identified by SLND. It is these patients, if any, who are likely to benefit from ALND. If a benefit can be achieved from ALND, it will not be in node-negative women.

ACOSOG Z0011

The ACOSOG Z0011 trial randomized women with clinical T1–2N$_0$M$_0$ breast cancer who have breast conservation and SLND and a positive SN to ALND or no ALND. Both arms received whole-breast radiotherapy. The primary end point of the study was overall survival. Secondary end points included comparison of surgical morbidities associated with SLND plus ALND versus SLND alone and disease-free survival. Adverse surgical effects were reported in 70% of the SLND plus ALND group.[207] Patients in the ALND group had significantly more infections, seromas, paresthesias, and erythema of the drain site.

The basis of this trial was that the SN is the only positive node in a large number of cases, breast irradiation treats the lower axilla, and chemotherapy is recommended based on status of the axilla, not on the number of positive nodes.[214] In addition, tumor biology dictates outcome more than the operation performed. Axillary staging with sentinel lymphadenectomy has demonstrated the SN to be the only site of metastases in an average of

47% of nodal dissections from large high-volume breast centers.[22] A large percentage of women are completely staged by removal of the SN alone and may achieve regional control with no further treatment. In addition, prior randomized trials have shown no effect on survival with ALND.[215–219]

The standard treatment for breast conservation includes irradiation of the breast to reduce local recurrence rates. The radiation fields for the breast extend into the axilla through opposing tangential fields. Veronesi has shown that there is an orderly spread of breast cancer to the axilla that follows a predictable pattern.[220] The invasion of level II or III without level I metastases occurred in only 1.3% of cases. The sentinel lymph node has been identified in level I in 62.8% of the cases.[5] Similar findings have been reported by the Moffat group,[47] who identified the SN in level I in 83% of the cases. Tangential breast irradiation after breast-conserving surgery overlaps the level I axillary nodes.[221] No isolated regional nodal failures were identified in patients with early-stage breast cancer with clinically negative axillary lymph nodes treated with two-field tangential breast irradiation alone, without ALND or third nodal field radiation.[221] Opposing tangential fields used to irradiate the breast after BCS may ablate residual low axillary metastases. The results of this trial as previously mentioned showed that there was no significant difference in overall or disease-free survival between the two arms.[154,155] Despite the fact that as many as 27% of patients treated with ALND had additional involved nodes, presumably patients treated with SLND alone had a similar number of involved nodes left in place.

Traditionally, ALND has been performed to identify patients with pathologically uninvolved nodes who would not benefit from adjuvant chemotherapy and those with positive lymph nodes who would be given chemotherapy. Today administration of chemotherapy is often based on the size of the primary tumor, its biological characteristics, and patient-specific risk. Randomized clinical trials support the role of adjuvant systemic therapy irrespective of the nodal status if the primary tumor has adverse features.[222] Therefore, many breast cancer patients with unfavorable primary tumor characteristics receive chemotherapy independent of axillary lymph node status and may not need to have an ALND performed to determine therapy.

Reporting of the results of this trial was initially met with controversy because many feared that patients would be placed at undue risk by leaving potential axillary nodal disease untreated.

However, there has been a large body of evidence with long-term follow-up, even before the Z0011 trial, supporting the notion that axillary treatment in the form of ALND or axillary radiation does not significantly affect survival (Table 42.16).[157,217–219,223–225] Table 42.17 lists a number of studies demonstrating negligible rates of axillary recurrence with follow-up time ranging from 25 to 42 months in patients with positive SNs that did not have ALND. The results of the Z0011 trial confirm these findings.

Concern also arose that the trial was only applicable to older patients with estrogen responsive tumors containing limited disease burden, and that younger patients with higher risk tumors were underrepresented in Z0011. However, several investigators have studied the applicability of the Z0011 trial to various patient populations. Chung and coworkers evaluated whether the Z0011 trial eligibility criteria applied to 186 SN-positive patients with young age at diagnosis (<50), ER-negative tumors, or HER2-positive tumors and found that 84% of clinically node-negative patients met the eligibility criteria for the trial and could have

TABLE 42.16 Randomized Trials in Addition to Z0011 Demonstrating No Significant Effect of Axillary Treatment on Survival

Study	N	Treatment Arms	F/U (yr)	Survival Difference
NSABP-B04[219]	1159	RM/TM/TM + RT	25	NS
Cancer Research Campaign[217]	2243	TM/TM + RT	18	NS
Manchester[218]	1022	TM/TM + RT	34	NS
Martelli[223]	671	ALND/No ALND	15	NS
Louis-Sylvestre[224]	658	ALND/AxRT	15	NS
Veronesi[157]	435	No AxTx/AxRT	5	NS
Galimberti[225]	934	ALND/No ALND	5	NS

ALND, Axillary dissection; *AxRT,* axillary radiation; *AxTx,* axillary treatment; *F/U,* Follow-up; NS, not significant; *NSABP,* National Surgical Adjuvant Breast and Bowel Project; *RM,* radical mastectomy; *RT,* radiation therapy; *TM,* total mastectomy.

TABLE 42.17 Studies Demonstrating Axillary Recurrences After a Tumor-Positive Sentinel Lymph Node Biopsy and No Axillary Lymph Node Dissection

Author	Year	No. of Patients	Recurrences	Interval to Recurrence (months)	Median Follow-Up (months)
Guenther	2003	46	0	—	32
Fant	2003	31	0	—	30
Naik	2004	210	3	11,19,46	25
Langer	2005	27	0	—	42
Jeruss	2005	73	0	—	27
Hwang	2007	196	0	—	30

From Rutgers EJT. Sentinel node biopsy: interpretation and management of patients with immunohistochemistry-positive sentinel nodes and those with micrometastases. *J Clin Oncol.* 2008;26:689-702.

been spared ALND.[226] Yi and colleagues evaluated the applicability of the Z0011 trial results to their population of 488 patients with clinical T1-2N0 breast cancer and one or two positive SNs treated with breast conserving therapy.[227] They found that 75% of patients were eligible for the trial and could have avoided ALND. The most common reason for Z0011 ineligibility in their study was presence of three or more positive SNs. Only 12.5% of patients in this study had ER-negative tumors, and the authors did not report data on HER2-positivity. Dengel and colleagues[228] conducted a prospective series of consecutive patients with a positive SN treated with breast conserving therapy. They found that 84% of their patients qualified for the Z0011 trial. These studies demonstrate that the Z0011 trial applies to the large majority of patients with SN-positive breast cancer, including those with higher risk tumor features.

Although initially met with controversy, this trial has now proven to be a landmark trial that changed the standard of care in the surgical management of the axilla for SN-positive patients. We currently await the results of the 10-year follow-up, which will be reported in the near future.

ALMANAC

The Medical Research Council of the United Kingdom funded a two-phase study: the ALMANAC trial.[229] Phase I was a learning phase in which 15 centers performed 40 SLND procedures followed by completion ALND. A 90% success rate and a false-negative rate of less than 5% were required for entry into phase II. Phase II was a two-armed prospective trial that randomized patients into SLND followed by ALND or the SLND alone. If the SN was negative, no further surgery was performed; if the SN was positive, ALND or axillary irradiation completed the treatment. The primary end points were axillary morbidity, health economics, and quality of life. The results showed overall improved quality of life in the SLND group ($p < .003$).[208] The presence of lymphedema was 5% versus 13% at 1 year for SLND versus ALND, respectively. Drain use, length of hospital stay, and time to return to normal activities of daily living were shorter for the SLND group. SLND was associated with reduced morbidity and improved quality of life and should be considered the treatment of choice for clinically node-negative early-stage breast cancer patients.[208]

AMAROS Trial

The European Organization of Research and Treatment of Cancer funded the After Mapping of the Axilla: Radiotherapy or Surgery Trial (AMAROS). This was a prospective randomized phase III noninferiority trial comparing axillary irradiation to ALND for a positive SN; it included 1425 women with clinical T1–2N0 invasive breast cancer with a positive SN randomized to axillary radiation versus ALND.[159] After median follow-up of 6.1 years, the 5-year axillary recurrence rate in the ALND arm was 0.43% (95% confidence interval 0–0.92) and 1.19% (0.31–2.08) in the axillary radiation arm. The planned noninferiority test was underpowered due to the low number of events. The one-sided 95% confidence interval for the underpowered noninferiority test on the hazard ratio was 0 to 5.27 with a noninferiority margin of 2. There were no differences between the two groups with respect to disease-free and overall survival, but the rate of lymphedema was significantly higher in the ALND arm (23%) compared with the axillary radiation arm (11%) at 5 years ($p < .0001$). The authors concluded that axillary radiation offers SN-positive patients similar rates of local control to ALND with less morbidity.

Summary

Lymphatic mapping with vital dyes or radioisotope is accurate and safe. Sentinel lymphadenectomy with focused histopathologic evaluation of the SN improves axillary staging. The procedure can be performed on an outpatient basis, has less morbidity and fewer complications, and is more cost-effective than routine axillary dissection. SLND is now the standard procedure for patients with clinically node-negative breast cancer. ALND in many appropriately selected SN-positive patients has been abandoned. The current national trials will continue to clarify the role of ALND and axillary radiation in SN-positive patients as the importance of tumor biology and genomics in determining prognosis and therapy continues to increase.

Selected References

72. Krag DN, Anderson SJ, Julian TB, et al. Technical outcomes of sentinel-lymph-node resection and conventional axillary-lymph-node dissection in patients with clinically node-negative breast cancer: results from the NSABP B-32 randomised phase III trial. *Lancet Oncol.* 2007;8:881-888.

151. Giuliano AE, Hawes D, Ballman KV, et al. Association of occult metastases in sentinel lymph nodes and bone marrow with survival among women with early-stage invasive breast cancer. *JAMA.* 2011;306:385-393.

155. Giuliano AE, Hunt KK, Ballman KV, et al. Axillary dissection vs no axillary dissection in women with invasive breast cancer and sentinel node metastasis: a randomized clinical trial. *JAMA.* 2011;305:569-575.

159. Donker M, van Tienhoven G, Straver ME, et al. Radiotherapy or surgery of the axilla after a positive sentinel node in breast cancer (EORTC 10981-22023 AMAROS): a randomised, multicentre, open-label, phase 3 non-inferiority trial. *Lancet Oncol.* 2014;15:1303-1310.

229. Clarke D, Khonji N, Mansel R. Sentinel node biopsy in breast cancer: ALMANAC trial. *World J Surg.* 2001;25:819-822.

A full reference list is available online at ExpertConsult.com.

43

Detection and Significance of Axillary Lymph Node Micrometastases

MELISSA PILEWSKIE AND HIRAM S. CODY III

Since the days of Halsted, breast cancer has been viewed as a disease that begins locally and is subject to a predictable, orderly, and sequential process of spread, first to regional lymph nodes and then to systemic sites.[1] From the 1970s, Fisher[2] has popularized the alternative hypothesis that most breast cancers are systemic from the outset and that outcome is governed more by the presence of occult systemic metastases than by variations in local treatment. In the Halstedian model, the most aggressive local treatment should be the most curative, and in the "Fisherian" model, greater emphasis is placed on systemic treatment. In fact, neither model by itself can encompass the broad range of clinical behaviors familiar to any physician who treats breast cancer. This broad range has given rise to the most recent paradigm, the *spectrum hypothesis,*[3] which suggests that the optimal treatment of each cancer must be tailored to its unique (and perhaps separate) propensities for local progression and for systemic metastasis.

In determining where a given breast cancer lies on the spectrum of potential outcomes, axillary lymph node (ALN) status has been, to date, the single best prognostic factor. Despite this, the outcome for good-prognosis breast cancer is not uniformly favorable, and as many as 30% of ALN-negative patients die of distant metastases despite adequate local therapy. It is logical to suspect that more intensive surveillance for subclinical regional or systemic disease might have uncovered this metastatic potential, and for patients with breast cancer, this search has focused on three sites: the ALN,[4] the bone marrow,[5] and the peripheral blood.[6] This chapter focuses on the identification, significance, and surgical management of occult metastases in the ALN.

Definition and Classification of Axillary Lymph Node Micrometastases

The concept of occult ALN metastasis in breast cancer was first articulated in 1948 by Saphir and Amromin.[7] In radical mastectomy specimens previously found to be ALN negative on routine single-section pathologic examination, they retrospectively performed serial sections (SS), taking an average of 332 sections per paraffin block. They identified ALN metastases in 33% (10/30) of cases and recommended that SS of the ALN in breast cancer should become routine.

The term *micrometastasis* was first used in 1971 by Huvos and colleagues,[8] who suggested a distinction between ALN *macrometastasis* (tumor foci ≥2 mm in diameter) and *micrometastasis* (<2 mm in diameter). This distinction was carried forward to the 1997 (5th) edition of the American Joint Committee on Cancer (AJCC) Staging Manual,[9] in which micrometastases less than or equal to 2 mm were categorized as pN1a disease and regarded as prognostically equivalent to pN0 (node-negative) disease. The AJCC has more recently further subcategorized nodal micrometastases into those less than or equal to 0.2 mm (pN0(i+) or "isolated tumor cells" [ITCs]) and 0.2 to 2 mm (pN1mi or "micrometastases") in the 2002 (6th) edition,[10] and 2010 (7th) edition.[11] Nodal metastases greater than 2 mm in diameter are categorized as pN1 or "macrometastases."

Prognostic Significance of Axillary Lymph Node Micrometastases: Retrospective Data

A large body of retrospective data assessing the prognostic significance of micrometastases fits into two categories: (1) studies in which patients classified initially as ALN positive are stratified by size of ALN metastasis and (2) studies in which patients classified initially as ALN negative are found on further study to be ALN positive.

Classification by Size of Axillary Lymph Node Metastasis

Three early studies from Memorial Sloan Kettering Cancer Center found (1) comparable overall survival at 8 years for patients with ALN micrometastases (<2 mm) versus negative ALN[8]; (2) better overall survival at 14 years for those with micrometastases rather than macrometastases[12]; and (3) worse disease-free survival (DFS) at 12 years for those with *single* micrometastasis or *single* macrometastasis than node-negative disease.[13] In parallel, a contemporaneous report from the National Surgical Adjuvant Breast and Bowel Project (NSABP) B-04 trial[14] demonstrates worse 4-year DFS for patients with axillary micrometastases and macrometastases compared with patients with negative nodes. A subsequent report from Cox and colleagues[15] reaches the same conclusion, finding significantly worse overall survival and DFS for patients with pN1mi versus pN0 disease. Conversely, in a multiinstitutional French retrospective review comprising 8001 patients treated between 1999 and 2008, Houvenaeghel and colleagues found no significant difference in recurrence-free survival or overall survival in patients with nodal micrometastases (either pN0(i+) or pN1mi) compared with pN0 patients.[16]

TABLE 43.1 Frequency and Prognostic Significance of Occult Axillary Metastases in Retrospective Studies of More Than 100 Patients Initially Staged as Node Negative by Varying Histopathology Techniques[a]

Method Author (Year)	No. of Patients	Converted to Node-Positive (%)	Follow-Up (yr)	Disease-Free Survival	Overall Survival
Serial Sections					
Wilkinson (1982)	525	17	15	NS	NS
Ludwig (1990)	921	9	5	$p = .003$	$p = .002$
Neville (1991)	921	9	6	$p = .0008$	$p = .0009$
Cote (1999)	736	7	12	$p = .001$	$p = .0005$
IHC					
Trojani (1987)	122	11	10	$p < 0.003$	$p = .02$
de Mascarel (1992)	129	10	10	$p = .01$	$p = .007$
Hainsworth (1993)	343	12	6.5	$p < .05$	NS
Cote (1999)	736	20	12	$p = .09$	NS
Umekita (2002)	148	14	8	$p = .0009$	$p = .0001$
Reed (2004)	385	12	25	NS	NS
Serial Sections + IHC					
McGuckin (1996)	208	25	5	$p = .007$	$p = .02$
Nasser (1993)	159	31	11	$p = .04$	$p = .07$
Millis (2002)	477	13	19	—	NS
Cummings (2002)	203	25	10	$p = .016$	—
Kahn (2006)	214	14	8	NS	NS
Tan (2008)	368	23	18	$p < .001$	$p = .02$

DFS, Disease-free survival; *IHC*, immunohistochemistry; *NS*, not specified.
[a]Among studies with more than 100 patients.

Classification by Frequency of Occult Axillary Lymph Node Metastases

Dowlatshahi and colleagues[17] reviewed in detail 31 studies (1948–1996) that attempted to define the frequency and significance of occult metastases found on further analysis of ALN originally classified as negative. All are retrospective, span different time periods, and comprise different patient populations. Many contain fewer than 100 patients and lack the statistical power to detect small but significant differences in outcome. All use various combinations of SS and/or immunohistochemistry (IHC) staining for cytokeratins. Despite these caveats, some strong overall trends emerge:

- Occult micrometastases are found consistently among patients who are ALN negative by routine examination. All studies but one identify ALN micrometastases in 7% to 42% of patients initially staged as ALN negative.
- Occult micrometastases may be prognostically significant. Six of the seven studies with more than 100 patients demonstrate significantly worse overall survival and/or DFS for patients with micrometastases compared with those with negative ALN.
- The yield of IHC-detected micrometastases is greater for lobular than for duct carcinomas. All of the studies that

distinguish between duct and lobular tumor type demonstrate IHC micrometastases 2 to 10 times more frequently with invasive lobular than with invasive duct cancers.

Table 43.1[18–32] summarizes series with more than 100 patients, including (1) eight published before 1997, (2) the second Ludwig study (1999),[19] and (3) six more recent studies (2002–2008) of similar methodology.[20,23,25,28,29,31] Of the six recent studies, half find ALN micrometastases to be prognostically significant and half do not. A more recent (2004–2011) Surveillance, Epidemiology, and End Results study of 93,070 patients who were pN0 by routine H&E reports the results of IHC cytokeratin staining; 5% were converted to pN0(i+) and 7% converted to pN1mi. In a multivariate model controlling for demographic and tumor characteristics, compared with pN0 patients, overall survival was significantly worse for pN1mi (hazard ratio [HR] 1.399, $p < .0001$) but not for pN0(i+) disease (HR 1.071, $P = .33$).[33]

The Ludwig Studies of Axillary Lymph Node Micrometastases

The Ludwig Trial V was designed to test the effect of a single dose of perioperative combination chemotherapy, and it reported 5-year results for ALN-positive[34] and ALN-negative patients in 1988 and

1989, respectively.[35] The authors then examined the lymph node tissue blocks from 921 of the 1275 patients originally staged as pN0[18] using a meticulous SS methodology and central pathologic review. Occult ALN metastases were found in 9% of patients; at 5 years, both overall survival and DFS were significantly worse.

In 1999 Cote and colleagues[19] reported 10-year results for 736 of the original 921 patients, adding IHC (a single section from a single level, stained with the anticytokeratin antibodies AE-1 and CAM 5.2) to the previous SS methodology (two H&E stained sections from each of six levels). Single-section IHC detected micrometastases far more often than SS/H&E (20% vs. 7%), particularly in patients with invasive lobular carcinomas (39% vs. 3%). Although 10-year DFS and overall survival were worse for SS/H&E-detected micrometastases, by 23% and 18%, and for IHC-detected micrometastases, by 8% and 5%, respectively, this margin was significant only for H&E-detected disease. Grouped by menopausal status, both H&E- and IHC-detected micrometastases were highly significant in postmenopausal but not in premenopausal women.

Logistical Hurdles in the Detection of Axillary Lymph Node Micrometastases

Although the preceding results present heterogenous outcomes for patients with micrometastasis, the authors of the first Ludwig study[18] in 1991 present a persuasive case for their conclusion that SS analysis of "negative" ALN should "be considered as part of the routine pathology examination"; few pathology departments then or since have had the resources to do so. The Ludwig investigators examined an average of 12 tissue blocks per patient, and 12 H&E-stained slides per block, in 921 patients to identify occult metastases in 83 individuals, or nearly 1600 slides to identify one additional node-positive patient. The earlier Wilkinson SS study[32] had a strikingly similar yield, examining 1449 slides to identify a single positive ALN. On the basis of these formidable logistics, the pathologic examination of axillary lymph node dissection (ALND) specimens with a single H&E-stained section per node has remained standard care at most institutions worldwide.

The advent of sentinel lymph node (SLN) biopsy has changed this practice. Pioneered in its modern form by Morton and colleagues[36] and first reported for breast cancer by Alex (1993)[37] and Giuliano and colleagues (1994),[38] SLN biopsy has largely replaced ALND for breast cancer staging at many centers in the United States and worldwide. Sixty-nine observational studies[39] and seven randomized trials[40–46] of SLN biopsy validated by a "backup" ALND confirm that SLN biopsy is feasible, accurate, and safe for patients with stage I to IIIa invasive breast cancer, with less postoperative morbidity than that of ALND.[42] Most importantly, SLN biopsy is a targeted examination of an average of two to three nodes (those most likely to contain metastases) versus the 15 to 20 removed in a standard ALND. SLN biopsy therefore makes enhanced pathologic analysis by SS and IHC logistically feasible and allows the identification of a group of patients whose risk of systemic relapse might otherwise go unrecognized.

Role of Enhanced Pathology in Sentinel Lymph Node Biopsy

Enhanced pathologic techniques using SS and IHC staining have played at least four roles in the evolution of SLN biopsy for breast cancer: (1) improved staging of the axilla; (2) validation of the SLN hypothesis; (3) reduction in the rate of false-negative SLN; and (4) the prediction of non-SLN metastases in patients with positive SLN.

Improved Axillary Lymph Node Staging

Giuliano and colleagues[47] first documented the improved sensitivity of IHC analysis in SLN specimens; comparing patients having SLN biopsy (analyzed both by H&E and IHC) plus completion ALND (analyzed by H&E) with those having conventional ALND (analyzed by H&E), positive ALNs were significantly more frequent in the group having enhanced pathology (42% vs 29%), as was the proportion of micrometastases among the ALN-positive patients (38% vs 10%). A number of subsequent studies have confirmed these findings, which are quite consistent with the data in Table 43.1; the yield of positive SLN biopsy is increased 10% to 20% by the addition of IHC to conventional H&E analysis.

Validation of the Sentinel Lymph Node Hypothesis

Two elegant studies have used both SS and IHC to validate the SLN hypothesis. Turner and colleagues[48] prove that a negative SLN is highly predictive of a negative axilla: in 60 patients who had SLN biopsy followed by a completion ALND and whose SLNs proved negative both on H&E and IHC, all of the remaining ALNs were also analyzed by both H&E and IHC, and only one of 1087 nonsentinel nodes, less than 0.1%, contained a metastasis. Conversely, Weaver and colleagues[49] show that the SLN is the node likeliest to be positive; among 431 patients in a multicenter validation trial of SLN biopsy, they found that nodal metastases were far more frequent in the SLN than in non-SLNs (16% vs. 4%). They further demonstrated that occult nodal metastases identified by SS and IHC (in patients initially staged as node negative) were also far more likely to involve the SLN than the non-SLNs (4% vs. 0.35%).

Reduction in the Rate of False-Negative Sentinel Lymph Node Biopsy

The false-negative rate of SLN biopsy (the proportion of node-positive cases in which the SLN is negative) should be as small as possible, ideally 5% or less. Although there is no consensus regarding the optimal method for pathologic examination of SLNs, it is quite clear that the use of IHC increases the sensitivity of SLN biopsy, thereby decreasing the false-negative rate. Liberman[4] has compared the results of 26 SLN validation trials that used H&E staining with seven trials that used IHC and demonstrates increased sensitivity (92% vs 97%) and a decreased false-negative rate (8% vs 3%) for the latter method.

Risk of Nonsentinel Lymph Node Metastasis in Micrometastatic Sentinel Lymph Node–Positive Patients

With the advent of SLN biopsy, it was logical to ask whether ALND should be mandatory for all SLN positive patients, especially those with micrometastases. In a meta-analysis of 25 studies, Cserni and colleagues[50] found that non-SLNs were positive in 20% of patients with SLN micrometastases and in only 9% of those whose SLNs were positive only on IHC. Two other meta-analyses found that in women with pN0(i+) or pN1mi disease, non-SLN metastases were present in 12% to 20% of patients. Other variables (such as larger tumor size or lymphovascular invasion [LVI]) also increase the risk of non-SLN metastases. Van Zee and associates[51] have developed and prospectively validated a multivariate nomogram that estimates the risk of non-SLN metastasis using nine variables, one of which is method of SLN metastasis detection (IHC, SS, or routine H&E); the others are frozen section, tumor size, tumor type/grade, number of positive SLNs, number of negative SLNs, LVI, multifocality, and estrogen receptor status. This tool has been validated by independent data sets worldwide[52–55] and has allowed a growing number of SLN positive patients in our own practice to avoid ALND altogether.[56]

Prognostic Significance of IHC-Detected Micrometastases: Prospective Studies

The retrospective studies cited in Table 43.1 are insufficient to prove that occult ALN metastases, whether detected by SS or IHC methods, are prognostically significant. In a retrospective study from Memorial Sloan Kettering Cancer Center, the authors used their current pathologic protocol for the examination of SLNs to reassess the axillary tissue blocks of 368 patients initially staged as pN0 between 1976 and 1978, and have reported 20-year results.[29] All patients had mastectomy/ALND, none had systemic adjuvant therapy, and the ALNs were reexamined by SS and IHC. Of 368 patients, 83 (23%) were converted to node-positive; compared with patients who remained pN0, the prognosis of those with pN0(i+) was worse and the prognosis of those with pN1mi was substantially worse. This study is valuable as a historic baseline but is of less relevance in an era of earlier diagnosis and widespread adjuvant systemic therapy. We now have two landmark prospective trials that address the prognostic significance of IHC-detected micrometastases in present-day patients.

American College of Surgeons Oncology Group Z0010 Trial

The American College of Surgeons Oncology Group (ACOSOG) Z0010 trial enrolled 5210 patients (1999–2003) with cT1–2N0 disease in a prospective observational design.[57] All patients had breast-conserving surgery, and all systemic therapy decisions were based on SLN status as determined by H&E stains. The H&E negative SLNs were then evaluated with IHC stains, and 10.5% were converted to node positive. At 5 years, overall survival and DFS did not significantly differ between those who were IHC negative and IHC positive (Fig. 43.1, Table 43.2). In Z0010, 83% of patients received chemotherapy and 68% hormonal therapy.

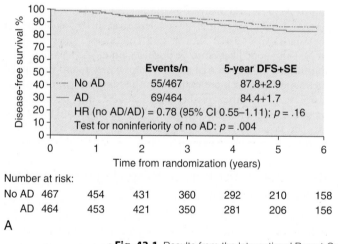

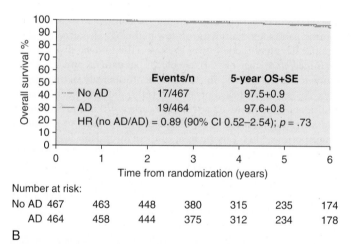

Number at risk:

No AD	467	454	431	360	292	210	158
AD	464	453	421	350	281	206	156

A

Number at risk:

No AD	467	463	448	380	315	235	174
AD	464	458	444	375	312	234	178

B

• **Fig. 43.1** Results from the International Breast Cancer Study Group trial. (A) DFS and (B) OS (n = 931) among women undergoing ALND versus SLNB alone for the management of axillary nodal micrometastases. *AD,* Axillary lymph node dissection; *DFS,* disease-free survival; *OS,* overall survival; *SLNB,* sentinel lymph node biopsy. (From Galimberti V, Cole BF, Zurrida S, et al. Axillary dissection versus no axillary dissection in patients with sentinel-node micrometastases (IBCSG 23-01): a phase 3 randomised controlled trial. *Lancet Oncol* 2013;14:297-305.)

TABLE 43.2 Survival Outcomes Between Women With and Without Occult Nodal Metastases Detected by IHC in the NSABP B-32 and ACOSOG Z0010 Trials

Study (Year)	SLN H&E Negative	Occult Metastases by IHC	5-YEAR DFS			5-YEAR OS		
			IHC Negative	IHC Positive	*P* value	IHC Negative	IHC Positive	*P* value
NSABP B-32 (2011)	3268	15.9%	89.2%	86.4%	.02	95.8%	94.6%	.03
ACOSOG Z0010 (2011)	3326	10.5%	92.2%	90.4%	NS	95.7%	95.1%	NS

ACOSOG, American College of Surgeons Oncology Group; *DFS,* disease-free survival; *H&E,* hematoxylin and eosin; *IHC,* immunohistochemistry; *NS,* not specified; *NSABP,* National Surgical Adjuvant Breast and Bowel Project; *OS,* overall survival; *SLN,* sentinel lymph node.

| TABLE 43.3 | Recurrence and Survival Outcomes Between Women With Sentinel Lymph Node Micrometastases Managed With SLNB Alone Compared With Completion ALND | | | | | | | | | |

			REGIONAL RECURRENCE		ANY DISEASE RECURRENCE[a]			DEATHS		
	Total N	Additional Positive Nodes in ALND	SLNB Alone	ALND	SLNB Alone	ALND	P value	SLNB Alone	ALND	P value
AATRM 048/13/2000 (2013)	233	15/112 (13%)	1.7%	0.9%	2.5%	1%	NS	0	0.9%	—
IBCSG 23–01 (2013)	931	59/464 (13%)	1%	0.2%	8.1%	9.7%	NS	4%	4%	NS

ALND, Axillary lymph node dissection; *IBCSG,* International Breast Cancer Study Group; *NS,* not specified; *SLNB,* sentinel lymph node biopsy.
[a]Including any local, regional, or distant recurrence, excludes contralateral breast cancer.

National Surgical Adjuvant Breast and Bowel Project B-32 Trial

The NSABP B-32 trial compared SLN biopsy alone with SLN biopsy plus ALND among 3989 SLN negative patients in a prospective randomized design and found no differences in overall survival or DFS; a false-negative rate of 10% in the ALND arm did not adversely affect outcome for patients who had SLN biopsy alone. SLNs were examined by H&E, with IHC allowed only for confirmation, and treatment decisions (as in ACOSOG Z0010) were based on SLN status as determined by H&E. Their axillary tissue blocks were then sent for central review, additional serial sections, and IHC staining. Occult SLN metastases were found in 15.9% of patients (11.1% pN0(i+), 4.4% pN1mi, and 0.4% pN1), and, compared with those whose SLNs remained negative, 5-year DFS and overall survival were worse by small but statistically significant margins (89% vs. 86%, *p* = .02; and 96% vs. 95%, *p* = .03, respectively; Table 43.2).[58] In B-32, 90% of patients received systemic therapy (40% chemotherapy and 68% hormonal).

Both ACOSOG Z0010 and NSABP B-32 clearly demonstrate that the presence of IHC-detected SLN metastases is of little, if any, prognostic significance among breast cancer patients treated according to current guidelines for systemic adjuvant therapy. The differences in DFS and overall survival found by NSABP B-32 are statistically significant, but one must question whether they are clinically significant. Because the overwhelming majority of patients in both trials had already received systemic adjuvant therapy in the absence of IHC status, it is inconceivable that the information gained from IHC could have appreciably changed outcomes, and, in our view, routine use of IHC stains for SLN examination is no longer needed. Current National Comprehensive Cancer Network guidelines note that SLN involvement is defined by multilevel nodal sectioning with H&E alone, and routine IHC is not recommended.[59]

Surgery for SLN Micrometastases: A Shifting Paradigm

Many publications, virtually all retrospective, address the role of ALND in patients with SLN micrometastases and suggest that ALND, in general, is not required. This is confirmed by clear trends in patterns of care. A review from the National Cancer Database shows that between 1998 and 2005, a growing proportion of women with SLN micrometastases did not undergo

ALND, increasing from 25% to 45% (*p* < .001).[60] The same study, subject to the limitations of uncontrolled comparisons, shows no difference between SLN-only (802 patients) and SLN-ALND (2357 patients) in axillary local recurrence (0.4% vs. 0.2%) and 5-year relative survival (99% vs. 98%).

We now have two randomized trials that address this issue. The International Breast Cancer Study Group (IBCSG) 23-01 trial[61] recruited 934 women (2001–2010) from 27 institutions; all had a primary breast cancer 5 cm or less with SLN micrometastases and were randomized to no further surgery (SLN biopsy alone) versus completion ALND. Additional positive nodes were found in 13% of the ALND arm, but at 5 years median follow-up, there were no significant differences in DFS or overall survival, and the rate of axillary local recurrence in both arms was less than 1% (Table 43.3).

The Spanish Multicenter Clinical Trial AATRM 048/13/2000[62] accrued 233 women (2001–2008) with tumor size less than 3.5 cm and an SLN micrometastses and compared no further surgery with ALND. At a median follow-up of 5.2 years, there were only four events, including two axillary recurrences in the SLN-only arm and one axillary soft tissue recurrence after ALND. DFS was 98% and did not differ between groups (Fig. 43.2, see also Table 43.3).

Unresolved Controversies

Are Immunohistochemistry-Positive Cells Metastases or Displacement Artifacts?

In an era when preoperative diagnosis by core needle biopsy is routine, some nodal "metastases" may be artifactual. Rosser[63] suggests that IHC-detected "micrometastases" are not metastases at all but rather the passive transport to the SLN of tumor cells and epithelial debris dislodged by manipulation of the breast. In a small series, Carter and associates[64] found subcapsular epithelial cells associated with macrophages, foreign-body giant cells, and blood cells, suggesting postbiopsy traumatic displacement rather than biologic metastasis. Bleiweiss[65] reported 25 cases in which benign epithelial cells were found in the SLNs of patients with proven breast cancers, 88% of these concordant with benign intraductal papillomas that had presumably been dislodged by a biopsy procedure. Finally, Moore and coworkers[66] reviewed 4016 cases of SLN biopsy to determine whether prior manipulation of the tumor site was related to the frequency of SLN metastasis. Comparing patients who had no biopsy, fine-needle aspiration, core biopsy, or surgical biopsy, IHC positive SLNs were found in

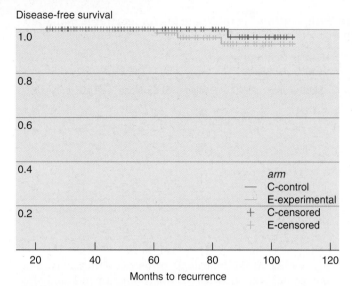

Disease-free survival

• **Fig. 43.2** Results from the Multicenter Clinical Trial AATRM 048/13/2000; disease-free survival (n = 233) among women undergoing axillary lymph node dissection versus sentinel lymph node biopsy alone for the management of axillary nodal micrometastases. (From Solá M, Alberro JA, Fraile M, et al. Complete axillary lymph node dissection versus clinical follow-up in breast cancer patients with sentinel node micrometastasis: final results from the multicenter clinical trial AATRM 048/13/2000. *Ann Surg Oncol.* 2013;20:120-127.)

1%, 3%, 3.8%, and 4.6% of cases, respectively (*p* = .002). In contrast, the frequency of H&E positive SLNs was unrelated to method of biopsy. Although some proportion of SLN metastases may be artifactual, there is at present no reliable way for pathologists to distinguish passive and active spread, and decisions regarding systemic therapy in this setting must be individualized.

Can Pathologic Evaluation of SLNs Be Standardized?

Although the role of IHC staining is in decline, there is, to date, no standardized method for the pathologic evaluation of SLNs, either intraoperatively or on permanent sections, and institutional protocols vary widely.[67] Pathologists disagree in the classification of nodal metastases as pN0(i+) and pN1mi disease.[68] Lymph node metastases comprise a heterogeneous collection of pathologic findings, and it may be overly simplistic to categorize them on the basis of size alone, as is done in the current AJCC staging system.[11] Turner and colleagues[69] have demonstrated that specialized training programs using a more specific set of histologic criteria for lymph node staging can improve the rate of agreement between pathologists; posttraining, they observed increased rates of agreement for all cases (from 72% to 96%), for lobular

carcinoma (from 55% to 100%), and for isolated tumor cells (from 68% to 98%). The challenge, still unmet, is to develop standardized protocols for SLN processing and interpretation that are simple, reproducible, cost-effective, and clinically relevant.

Conclusions and Future Directions

SLN biopsy has largely replaced ALND as the procedure of choice for ALN staging. We now have definitive prospective studies, ACOSOG Z0010 and NSABP B-32, showing that routine use of IHC is no longer justified, and two randomized trials showing that for many patients with SLN micrometastases, ALND is no longer needed. Next-generation trials will probably compare SLN biopsy to no axillary staging for early-stage breast cancer.

Looking ahead, we have entered an exciting era in which gene expression profiling promises more accurate prognostication[70–72] and better prediction of response to therapy[73] than conventional histopathology, challenging the primacy of axillary node status. First-generation clinical trials testing this hypothesis, such as the European Organization of Research and Treatment of Cancer (EORTC) 10041 Microarray in Node-Negative Disease May Avoid Chemotherapy (MINDACT),[74] Trial Assigning IndividuaLized Options for Treatment (Rx) (TAILORx),[75] and RxPonder[76] are underway, and others are certain to follow. In the shorter term, these technologies will be integrated into practice alongside lymph node staging and other standard methods, allowing further refinement in our ability to prognosticate and predict. In the longer term, we must ask whether genomic technologies will identify new therapeutic targets, leading to more effective systemic therapies, eventually rendering lymph node staging obsolete.

Selected References

50. Cserni G, Gregori D, Merletti F, et al. Meta-analysis of non-sentinel node metastases associated with micrometastatic sentinel nodes in breast cancer. *Br J Surg.* 2004;91:1245-1252.
57. Giuliano AE, Hawes D, Ballman KV, et al. Association of occult metastases in sentinel lymph nodes and bone marrow with survival among women with early-stage invasive breast cancer. *JAMA.* 2011;306:385-393.
58. Weaver DL, Ashikaga T, Krag DN, et al. Effect of occult metastases on survival in node-negative breast cancer. *N Engl J Med.* 2011;364:412-421.
61. Galimberti V, Cole BF, Zurrida S, et al. Axillary dissection versus no axillary dissection in patients with sentinel-node micrometastases (IBCSG 23-01): a phase 3 randomised controlled trial. *Lancet Oncol.* 2013;14:297-305.
62. Sola M, Alberro JA, Fraile M, et al. Complete axillary lymph node dissection versus clinical follow-up in breast cancer patients with sentinel node micrometastasis: final results from the multicenter clinical trial AATRM 048/13/2000. *Ann Surg Oncol.* 2013;20:120-127.

A full reference list is available online at ExpertConsult.com.

44

Intraoperative Evaluation of Surgical Margins in Breast Conserving Therapy

STEPHEN R. GROBMYER, STEPHANIE A. VALENTE, AND EDWARD M. COPELAND III

Breast conserving therapy (BCT) is the preferred treatment approach for most patients with early-stage breast cancer. The combination of complete resection of the primary lesion with tumor-free margins and radiotherapy provides excellent local tumor control. There exists a balance between the extent of lumpectomy performed to achieve tumor-free margins and the resultant cosmesis of the breast. Because pathologic margin status is an important prognostic factor for local failure after segmental resection of in situ or invasive breast carcinoma, pathologic examination of margin status plays a key role in BCT. The inability to obtain clear margins at the time of partial mastectomy for malignancy remains a significant clinical problem. Intraoperative evaluation of margin status may permit immediate reexcision of involved margins, minimizing the need for secondary operative procedures. Unfortunately, at present, all methods used to evaluate margin status intraoperatively have some technical or practical limitations. The technique of margin evaluation varies significantly between institutions because it is unclear which approach is most accurate and cost effective. This chapter reviews data regarding the prognostic significance of margin status, describes the techniques currently used for intraoperative evaluation of margins, and compares the relative benefits and limitations of each approach.

The 1990 National Institutes of Health Consensus Conference on Breast Cancer stated that breast conservation surgery followed by radiation therapy is the preferred method of treatment for stage I and II breast cancer.[1] This recommendation was made after several large, randomized clinical trials found that women with early-stage breast cancer treated with BCT had long-term survival rates equivalent to those treated with mastectomy.[2–9] These studies report local failure rates of 5% to 15% at 5 to 12 years after wide excision and radiation therapy.

Women with isolated local recurrence are usually treated with salvage mastectomy, and 64% to 92% of them remain disease free at 5 years.[10–12] Although local failure is relatively uncommon, it represents a failure of breast conservation and should be prevented when possible.[2,7,13] This concern has led to the investigation of the risk factors for local recurrence after BCT.

Local recurrence after BCT may be the result of inappropriate patient selection, inadequate operative technique or radiation therapy, or inherent biological characteristics of the tumor. Margin status, tumor size, axillary lymph node status, tumor grade, hormone receptor status, patient age, lymphovascular invasion, presence of extensive intraductal carcinoma, and not receiving chemotherapy or hormonal treatment have been identified as prognostic factors for local recurrence.[13–17] Historically, numerous studies have found that surgical margin status is an important predictor of local recurrence after wide excision of invasive breast cancer (Table 44.1).[4,5,17–50] Singletary[51] performed a meta-analysis of these studies and found that 30 of the 34 studies show a significantly higher local recurrence rate after "margin-positive" resection compared with those with negative margins. Furthermore, when these studies were grouped according to how the negative margin was defined (i.e., not defined, >1 mm, >2 mm), the differences in local recurrence rates between positive and negative margins were highly significant for each group.[51] On the basis of these collective data, it is now generally agreed that a margin-negative resection is required for optimal local tumor control.

Many early studies of BCT considered gross tumor excision to be adequate, regardless of the extent of microscopic margin involvement.[2,6] More recently, attention has focused on the adequacy of microscopic margin status for patients undergoing BCT. A recent consensus panel of the Society of Surgical Oncology and The Society for American Radiation Oncology has recommended that the use of "no ink on tumor" should be the standard for a safe margin in patients with stages I and II invasive breast cancer undergoing BCT in the context of modern multidisciplinary therapy.[52]

Surgical margin status is also an important determinant of local tumor control in ductal carcinoma in situ (DCIS). However, there is no consensus about what constitutes an adequate margin in patients with DCIS undergoing BCT. Silverstein and associates[53] found margin width to be the most important prognostic factor for local recurrence after excision of DCIS. They stratified patients into three risk groups based on margin width: a high-risk group with margins 1 mm or smaller, an intermediate-risk group with margins 2 to 9 mm, and a low-risk group with margins 10 mm or larger. Their studies indicated that if appropriate adjuvant therapy is used, women with margins 1 mm or larger have low (12%) local recurrence rates at 8 years.[53] Several other investigators[54,55] have confirmed these findings, and they are also supported by a meta-analysis by Boyages and coworkers.[56] A recent large retrospective analysis of 2996 patients with DCIS demonstrated that a wider margin width was associated with improved local control in patients not receiving adjuvant radiation therapy but not in those receiving adjuvant radiation therapy.[57]

When inadequate surgical margins are obtained at the time of first operation, the required second operative procedure produces

TABLE 44.1 Margin Status and Local Recurrence After Breast Conserving Therapy

Study	Definition	Follow-Up (yr)	LOCAL RECURRENCE (%) Negative Margin	Positive Margin
Anscher et al.[17]	ND[a]	3.5	1.5	9
Burke et al.[21]		5	2	15
Clarke et al.[22]		10	4	10
Cooke et al.[23]		4.2	3	13
Fourquet et al.[25]		8.6	8	29
Heimann et al.[29]		5	2	11
Leborgne et al.[32]		6.3	9	6
Mansfield et al.[33]		10	8	16
Pezner et al.[38]		4	0	14
Pierce et al.[39]		5	3	10
Ryoo et al.[42]		8	5	13
Slotman et al.[45]		5.7	3	10
van Dongen et al.[5]		8	9	20
Veronesi et al.[4]		6.6	9	17
Assersohn et al.[18]	>1 mm	4.8	0	3
Gage et al.[27]		9.1	3	9/28[b]
Park et al.[36]		10.6	7	14/27[c]
Recht et al.[41]		4.8	3	22
Schnitt et al.[44]		5	0	21
Dewar et al.[24]	>2 mm	10	6	14
Freedman et al.[26]		6.3	7	12
Hallahan et al.[28]		3	5	9
Kini et al.[31]		10	6	17
Markiewicz et al.[34]		6	10	4
Obedian et al.[35]		10	2	18
Peterson et al.[37]		6.1	8	10
Solin et al.[47]		5	3	0
Smitt et al.[46]		10	2	22
Touboul et al.[49]		7	6	8
Wazer et al.[50]		7.2	4	16
Pittinger et al.[40]	>3 mm	4.5	3	25
Horiguchi et al.[30]	>5 mm	3.9	1	11
Schmidt-Ullrich et al.[43]		5	0	0
Bartelinke et al.[19]	Micro[d]	6	2	9
Borger et al.[20]	Micro[d]	5.5	2	16
Spivack et al.[48]	Micro[e]	4	4	18

[a]Negative margin not defined.
[b]Nine percent with focally positive margin; 28% with greater than focally positive margin.
[c]Fourteen percent with focally positive margin; 27% with greater than focally positive margin.
[d]Negative margin defined as more than one microscopic field.
[e]Negative margin defined as no microscopic foci of tumor at inked margins.
Modified from Singletary SE. Surgical margins in patients with early-stage breast cancer treated with breast conservation therapy. *Am J Surg.* 2002;184:383-393.[51]

additional physical discomfort and emotional distress for patients and increases the cost of treating their disease. Furthermore, reexcision is associated with a less desirable cosmetic result[58] and may delay initiation of adjuvant therapy. This has prompted extensive interest and research in the field of intraoperative analysis of the margins to reduce the need for reexcision of involved margins.

All methods used for intraoperative evaluation of margin status have some technical or practical limitations. For example, segmental resection specimens have a large surface area and are often irregular, making it difficult for the pathologist and surgeon to determine the "true" margin, even if orientation and inking methods are used. Any technique used to evaluate margin status in the operating room must be relatively simple, rapid, reproducible, and inexpensive for it to be practical and cost-effective.

Frequency of Margin-Positive Partial Mastectomy

Margin-positive mastectomy remains a significant clinical problem. Rates of margin-positive mastectomy range greatly in reported series and vary between 12% and 68%.[59-62] A recent large analysis of 2206 women undergoing partial mastectomy demonstrated significant variation in rates of margin positive lumpectomy related to the surgeon and institution where procedures were performed.[63] Some have suggested that certain histologic subtypes, such as invasive lobular carcinoma, are associated with higher rates of margin positivity after partial mastectomy.[64] Other factors that have been associated with having margin-positive partial mastectomy include larger tumor size, extensive intraductal component, younger patient age, lymphovascular invasion, and axillary nodal metastases.[31,61,65] Patients with these features may benefit from more aggressive intraoperative strategies to obtain clear margins.

Pathologic Assessment of Margin Status and Specimen Handling

Optimal margin assessment is predicated on proper specimen handling because improper handling can introduce artifacts that greatly limit sensitivity of margin analysis. The importance of specimen handling has been recently highlighted by the Consensus Conference on Nonpalpable Image-Detected Breast Cancers.[66] Surgical specimens should be oriented by the surgeon for proper pathologic processing.[66] When specimen radiography is performed, substantial compression should be avoided because it can fracture the specimen and create false (artifactual) margins after inking.[66] Inking of the six sides of the specimen is performed by either the surgeon at the time of surgery or the pathologist before gross inspection.

Gross Intraoperative Inspection of Tumor Margins

Serial sectioning techniques have been the cheapest, most popular, and most widely used methods to evaluate margins. Most studies correlating local recurrence rates to surgical margin status used serial sectioning procedures of some type, although there is significant variability in the technique and extent of margin evaluation between studies.

Gross intraoperative specimen margin inspection involves careful handling and orientation of the specimen for the pathologist. Serial sectioning is performed intraoperatively after margin-directed inking of the specimen. The relationship of the tumor to gross margins is analyzed, and additional margins are excised at the time of surgery based on the findings. The results of recent studies using gross intraoperative analysis of tumor margins after partial mastectomy have been variable. Balch and associates[67] studied 254 patients in whom gross intraoperative analysis of margins was performed. These authors found that this technique does not reflect true margin status in 25% of women, and the authors concluded that gross inspection alone is not ideal for intraoperative margin assessment. Cabioglu and coworkers recently studied 264 patients undergoing partial mastectomy.[68] These authors combined gross specimen inspection with selective frozen section analysis and specimen radiography. They found that this aggressive approach reduced the incidence of margin-positive partial mastectomy by approximately 50% and demonstrated excellent rates of local control.

Cavity Shave Margin Technique

The cavity shave margin technique is also currently used by many surgeons for margin analysis. This technique samples the tumor bed by shaving samples from the walls of the excision cavity. The use of cavity margins has been well studied and is advocated by some groups.[69-72] When the cavity margin technique is used, after the lumpectomy specimen is removed, separate specimen shave biopsies of the sides of cavity margin are performed and these specimens are oriented, inked and sent for permanent sectioning. The permanent hematoxylin and eosin (H&E) stains of the cavity margins are analyzed to determine the "final" or "true" margin status. Distance from tumor (if present) to ink on the cavity margin is used by some to determine adequacy of final margin. For some groups, cavity margins are interpreted as either positive or negative depending on the presence or absence of tumor in the cavity margin specimen.[69,71] This particular technique has been associated with reduced rates of margin-positive resection and very low rates of ipsilateral recurrence after adjuvant therapy. Huston and colleagues[72] and Cao and associates[70] have both reported a reduction in margin-positive resection rates with the use of the "cavity margin" technique without intraoperative frozen section. A randomized controlled trial of cavity shave margins in patients having lumpectomy for stage 0 to III breast cancer demonstrated a 50% reduction in the rates of margin positive lumpectomy and the subsequent need for reexcision without an associated increase in complication rates or a worse cosmesis[73] (Table 44.2). It is noteworthy that the margin positive excision rate in the control group (lumpectomy with no cavity margins) of this randomized trial was high—34%—which limits somewhat the significance of the conclusions.

TABLE 44.2	Effect of Lumpectomy Cavity Shave Margin: Results of a Randomized Trial[73]		
Treatment	Total No. of Patients	No. of Positive Margins	Margin + Rate
Shave margin	119	23	19%
No shave margin	116	39	34%

TABLE 44.3	Value of Lumpectomy Cavity Shave Margin-Frozen Section: University of Florida Experience[71]	
No. of operations		97
Sensitivity		58.1%
Specificity		100%
Positive predictive value		100%
Negative predictive value		75%
Accuracy		82%

Frozen Section Analysis

Frozen section analysis (FSA) is a commonly used technique for the intraoperative assessment of margin status. In the past, FSA was primarily used for the diagnosis of palpable breast lesions undergoing excisional biopsy, where it has demonstrated accuracy rates of 96% to 98% for both invasive and in situ lesions.[74–76] With the emergence of fine-needle aspiration cytology and image-guided core biopsy as alternatives to excisional biopsy, the role of FSA has shifted primarily to intraoperative margin assessment. Frozen section is commonly used with the "shaved margin" technique. Using this technique, Weber and coworkers[77] performed FSA in 166 patients and reported the sensitivity and specificity of FSA to be 91% and 100%, respectively. Reported work from the University of Florida also suggests that the use of frozen sections of cavity margins is an effective strategy for improving outcomes after partial mastectomy for breast cancer[71] (Table 44.3). Boughey and colleagues[78] compared rates of reoperation in their institution, which routinely uses frozen section of margins to rates of reoperation reported through the National Surgical Quality Improvement Program (NSQIP). Patients having a lumpectomy for cancer in their institution with intraoperative frozen section analysis of margins had a significantly lower rate of reexcision compared with NSQIP patients (3.6% vs. 13.2%).[78]

Financial costs associated with performance of intraoperative FSA are offset by savings associated with reduced rates of required reoperation to clear margins. Importantly, this technique is associated with high rates of local control and low rates of ipsilateral tumor recurrence (1.9% at 5.6 years of follow-up).[69] Another recent study by Olson and associates[79] similarly supports the value of intraoperative frozen section of "cavity margins." Performance of intraoperative FSA can be technically challenging, resource-intensive, and consume valuable operative time, which has limited its utilization.[80] In inexperienced hands, it may be technically difficult to freeze adipose tissue, and tissue artifacts may result from freezing.

Intraoperative Cytologic Evaluation by Touch Preparation

Cytologic examination with touch prep has emerged as a technique for evaluating margin status during resection of breast malignancies. The technique was initially described in the early 20th century[81,82] and has been referred to as imprint cytology and scrape cytology in addition to touch prep. This approach has gained popularity recently because of reports of margin-positive rates of up to 50% with gross evaluation of the tumor specimen[83]

as well as the previously described limitations of frozen section. Proponents of touch prep claim that in the hands of an experienced cytopathologist, it may even be more accurate than permanent section because it samples the entire surface area of the resected specimen.[84]

Intraoperative analysis of margins by touch prep is a relatively rapid and simple procedure.[84] The excised tumor specimen is pressed onto a glass slide on all six of its surfaces (superior, inferior, medial, lateral, anterior, and posterior), with the hypothesis that tumor cells will adhere to the slide to a greater degree than fat. The slide is fixed in methanol, stained with H&E, and analyzed by a cytopathologist. In experienced hands, this process reportedly takes 2 to 15 minutes to complete.[84–87]

Several studies have compared the accuracy of touch prep with gross evaluation and serial sectioning. Cox and coworkers[85] were the first to report the use of touch prep for intraoperative evaluation of margin status in 1991. In a study of 114 patients undergoing partial mastectomy for breast malignancies, touch prep was 97% accurate at determining margin status.[85] The same group subsequently published a series of 114 segmental resections for DCIS and 701 resections for invasive carcinoma and reported local recurrence rates of 6% and 3% at 4 and 3.5 years of median follow-up, respectively.[88,89] This group has also reported that use of intraoperative imprint cytology is associated with lower rates of ipsilateral tumor recurrence rates compared with conventional margin analysis.[90] Klimberg and colleagues[84] also found touch prep to have an exceptionally high diagnostic accuracy of 100% in a group of 83 women undergoing partial mastectomy for breast malignancy.

Other studies have shown less promising results with intraoperative touch prep. Saarela and colleagues[91] reported a much poorer correlation with gross evaluation and serial sectioning. In their study of 53 partial mastectomies with adequate touch prep cytology, the false-negative rate was 63%, the false-positive rate was 11%, and sensitivity was only 38%. This low diagnostic accuracy led them to conclude that intraoperative touch prep was of no value. However, their institutional experience with the technique is considerably less than that of others who have reported better correlation with permanent section. This suggests that their results may be explained primarily by a lack of experience with the technique. A study by Creager and associates[92] reported a false-negative rate of 20% in the community hospital setting. This group concluded that touch prep is a useful technique for intraoperative evaluation of margin status, but they were unable to achieve accuracy approaching that reported at high-volume centers.[84,85] The variable results obtained at different institutions explain why there continues to be debate regarding the utility of touch prep for intraoperative evaluation of margin status.

Several studies have compared the diagnostic accuracy of touch prep with that of frozen section.[85–87] These reports suggest that the two techniques are roughly equivalent, with touch prep having a slightly higher propensity for false-positive results (Table 44.4). More recent data do not include comparison between touch prep and frozen section due to institutional biases that have developed for one technique over the other. Enhanced touch prep that involves staining fresh tissue with specific antibodies may have a role in the future in further improving intraoperative touch prep analysis of margins.[93]

Intraoperative Ultrasound

Ultrasonography has been used in breast surgery in an attempt to improve rates of margin-free resection of nonpalpable lesions.

Image-guided wire localization has traditionally been used to direct excision of nonpalpable breast lesions. Initially, intraoperative ultrasound (IOUS) was described as an alternative to wire-guided excision.[94] IOUS can replace the need for a standard wire or radioactive seed placement localization technique in some cases and is more convenient for the patient. IOUS use for tumor localization, however, has been expanded to include intraoperative assessment of margin status.[95–100] It was hypothesized that IOUS would increase margin-negative resection rates, increase margin width, decrease the volume of breast tissue excised, and improve esthetic outcome compared with wire-guided excision of nonpalpable lesions.[95,97,98,100] It has also been proposed that IOUS could achieve similar results during excision of palpable breast malignancies.[96]

Several trials have evaluated margin status after IOUS-guided excision of nonpalpable breast malignancies (Table 44.5).[95,96,98,100] These studies report margin-positive excision rates of 0% to 18% with IOUS-guided excision.[95,97,98,100] This is quite favorable compared with the 47% to 60% margin-positive rate historically reported in studies of wire-guided excision.[101,102] The studies with matched historical controls were quite small, and none were able to demonstrate a statistically significant difference in margin-positive lumpectomy rates. A trend toward greater margin width was seen in ultrasound-guided resection compared with previous reports of wire-guided excision, but this was not statistically significant.[95,100] Several studies suggest a difference in the volume of breast tissue excised, but this has not been correlated with esthetic outcome.[95,97,100]

A study has evaluated the utility of IOUS as a technique to guide excision of palpable lesions.[96] This prospective study randomized women with T_1 and T_2 invasive carcinomas to IOUS-guided lumpectomy or standard BCT. The tumor volume excised between the two groups was similar, and of the IOUS patients, 3.5% of IOUS-guided lumpectomies had a positive margin, whereas 29% of BCT patients had involved margins. The operative time, costs, and patient impression of cosmetic results were not statistically different between the groups.[96] Several other studies[103,104] have similarly shown superiority of ultrasound-guided excision to wire-localized excision in terms of lower rates of margin-positive excision and lower volumes of resection. These studies support the use of IOUS as a technique to help reduce rates of margin-positive partial mastectomy.

Klimberg and coworkers[105] have recently described the continuous ultrasound-guided breast excision (CUBE) technique and reported negative final margins in 12 consecutive patients in whom this novel technique was used.

Intraoperative Specimen Radiography

Intraoperative specimen imaging is another approach that has been advocated for reducing rates of margin-positive partial mastectomy and is commonly used. Several authors have documented[106,107] a significant reduction in the rate of partial mastectomy with the use of two-view specimen mammography to guide decisions regarding intraoperative reexcision of margins. After surgical resection of the specimen, the orientated specimen is then either transported to radiology where a mammography machine is used to take an x-ray of the specimen or a cabinet x-ray machine in the operating room is used to x-ray the specimen. The specimen is radiographed and then flipped 90 degrees and x-rayed again such that all six margins can be visualized. The surgeon and radiologist are both able to see the specimen radiograph, and additional margin tissue can be taken at that time if needed. The pathologists can also reference the specimen radiograph when preparing the specimen for permanent sectioning.

Other Approaches and Emerging Technology for Margin Analysis

Intraoperative imaging with magnetic resonance imaging has recently been explored and has been demonstrated to be feasible and safe in a small phase I clinical trial,[108] although expense and

TABLE 44.4	Comparison of the Accuracy of Touch Prep and Frozen Section Analysis for the Intraoperative Evaluation of Margin Status				
		TOUCH PREP		FROZEN SECTION	
Study	n	False Positive	False Negative	False Positive	False Negative
Tribe[87]	311	0.7	5.2	0	1.6
Esteban et al.[86]	140	1	2	1.1	0.7
Cox et al.[85]	111	2.7	0	0	4.5

TABLE 44.5	Intraoperative Ultrasound for the Evaluation of Margin Status						
Study	Type	n	Lesion Size (cm)	Volume (cm³)	Percent Margin Positive	Distance to Margin (mm)	Operating Room Time (min)
Rahusen et al.[98]	Prospective	19	1.2	—	11	—	—
Paramo et al.[97]	Prospective	15	1.1	30	0	—	53
Harlow et al.[95]	Retrospective	65	1.1	97.2	4.8	8±6	—
Snider et al.[100]	Retrospective	22	1.1	62.6/81.1	18	6.6±2.8	—
Tummel et al.[105a]	Prospective	12	—	—	0	—	—

aContinuous ultrasound-guided breast excision (CUBE) technique.

limited access to technology will likely limit the further development of this technology. Two recent clinical trials have used optical coherence tomography for the intraoperative assessment of lumpectomy cavity margins.[109,110] Both trials suggest that the use of such technology may have a role in reducing the rates of margin positive lumpectomy.

Multiple other imaging technologies and techniques are currently under development that may have a role in the future in the assessment of intraoperative margin status. Technologies currently under development for this application include Raman spectroscopy,[111] radiofrequency spectroscopy,[112] radioguided intraoperative margin evaluation,[113] and photoacoustic tomography.[114]

Summary and Conclusions

Margin status correlates with the risk of local recurrence after partial mastectomy for breast malignancies. Historically, a significant portion of patients undergoing partial mastectomy for malignancy required reexcision to obtain clear margins. These reexcisions are associated with increased cost, patient anxiety, and possibly a delay in the initiation of adjuvant therapy. As a result, development of accurate, expeditious, and reproducible techniques for intraoperative evaluation of margin status is of great clinical importance. The historical standard technique for determining margin status is en bloc excision with gross evaluation of margins, serial sectioning, and routine histopathologic evaluation. Because this approach is associated with margin-positive rates of 25% to 50% or more and increased resources and operative time, other techniques for intraoperative evaluation of margin status have been devised and should strongly be considered. These include the use of specimen radiograph, frozen section, touch prep, cavity shave margins, or IOUS. When applied by experienced surgeons and pathologists, each technique has been reported to result in margin-positive rates lower than those obtained with gross evaluation and serial sectioning alone. Each approach has significant practical and theoretical limitations, and there are no compelling data to indicate that one is superior to another. At present, we believe experienced surgeons

and pathologists can use many of these techniques effectively. Use of these technologies within an institution may best be performed in the context of a system to track outcomes to optimize quality and value of care. At present, choice of technique should be geared toward the expertise available in a given practice setting. Further research is needed to determine the most accurate, cost-effective, and widely applicable approach in general clinical practice.

Selected References

51. Singletary SE. Surgical margins in patients with early-stage breast cancer treated with breast conservation therapy. *Am J Surg.* 2002;184:383-393.
52. Moran MS, Schnitt SJ, Giuliano AE, et al. Society of Surgical Oncology-American Society for Radiation Oncology consensus guideline on margins for breast-conserving surgery with whole-breast irradiation in stages I and II invasive breast cancer. *Ann Surg Oncol.* 2014;21:704-716.
53. Silverstein MJ, Lagios MD, Groshen S, et al. The influence of margin width on local control of ductal carcinoma in situ of the breast. *N Engl J Med.* 1999;340:1455-1461.
57. Van Zee KJ, Subhedar P, Olcese C, Patil S, Morrow M. Relationship between margin width and recurrence of ductal carcinoma in situ: analysis of 2996 women treated with breast-conserving surgery for 30 years. *Ann Surg.* 2015;262:623-631.
69. Camp ER, McAuliffe PF, Gilroy JS, et al. Minimizing local recurrence after breast conserving therapy using intraoperative shaved margins to determine pathologic tumor clearance. *J Am Coll Surg.* 2005;201:855-861.
71. Cendan JC, Coco D, Copeland EM 3rd. Accuracy of intraoperative frozen-section analysis of breast cancer lumpectomy-bed margins. *J Am Coll Surg.* 2005;201:194-198.
73. Chagpar AB, Killelea BK, Tsangaris TN, et al. A randomized, controlled trial of cavity shave margins in breast cancer. *N Engl J Med.* 2015;373:503-510.
84. Klimberg VS, Westbrook KC, Korourian S. Use of touch preps for diagnosis and evaluation of surgical margins in breast cancer. *Ann Surg Oncol.* 1998;5:220-226.

A full reference list is available online at ExpertConsult.com.

45

Surgical Management of Early Breast Cancer

RAQUEL PRATI, KIRBY I. BLAND, AND V. SUZANNE KLIMBERG

It is imperative that *early breast cancer* be defined before surgical treatment is discussed. The National Cancer Institute defines early breast cancer as breast cancer that has not spread beyond the breast or the axillary lymph nodes. This includes ductal carcinoma in situ and stage I, stage IIA, stage IIB, and stage IIIA breast cancers. (www.cancer.gov). However, others have defined early breast cancer as noninvasive and invasive breast cancers smaller than 20 mm.[1] For the purposes of this chapter, *early invasive breast cancer* is defined as invasive breast cancers up to 20 mm in size. The surgical management of lobular or ductal in situ cancers is discussed elsewhere.

The approach to surgical treatment of breast cancer has changed dramatically over the past century and in particular the past few decades. The halstedian view of local growth with lymphatic predominance dictated extensive surgeries to treat breast cancer. This philosophy was challenged by the Fisherian thesis[2] that breast cancer was systemic in origin and therefore details and extent of surgical treatment for the primary cancer and the regional lymph nodes did not govern survival. This hypothesis of breast cancer growth has now been replaced by the spectrum biological theory described by Hellman.[3] The spectrum model of breast cancer emphasizes that not all breast cancers behave alike and the importance of progressive tumor growth with increasing likelihood for metastasis with tumor size. According to the spectrum hypothesis, there are some breast cancers that metastasize early in their development. These are the patients who, despite participation in a breast cancer screening program and having small breast cancers, die of metastatic disease. At the other end of the spectrum, there are some breast cancers that, despite large size, never develop metastatic disease. These are the small subset of patients with large breast primaries who do well with aggressive local treatment alone. However, the vast majority of breast cancers fall in the middle. Initially, these tumors are localized within the breast. With time, these tumors progressively increase in size and become more likely to develop metastatic disease. These patients derive the most benefit from breast cancer screening programs. Because the vast majority of patients fall within this category of size influencing likelihood of metastasis, it is not surprising that small breast cancers have the best prognosis.

Screening for breast cancer with mammograms has resulted in a dramatic change in breast cancer presentation and mortality. Although there continues to be some debate regarding benefit of breast cancer screening using mammograms,[4] overall there is consensus that mammographic screening results in a decrease in breast cancer mortality of approximately 20% in women 40 to 74 years of age who have been invited to participate in screening.[5] The benefits of mammographic screening are best exemplified by results from the Swedish mammographic trials. In these trials, the rate of breast cancer mortality in patients invited to participate in mammographic screening was compared with the rate in those who were not. Overall, there was a reduction of breast cancer mortality of 44% in the seven Swedish counties exposed to mammographic screening.[6] The use of mammography for breast cancer screening and benefits of particular guidelines have been a matter of much debate for decades, especially since the US Preventive Services Task Force (USPSTF) and the American Cancer Society (ACS) were published in the late 2000s for average-risk women. USPSTF recommends biennial screening mammography starting age 50 until age 74 with individualized recommendations based on personal risk for women in their 40s. The ACS recommends annual mammography for women starting at age 45 until age 54, continuing with biennial study as long as overall life expectancy is of 10 years or longer. This is valid for average risk women, meaning a lower than 15% lifetime risk of breast cancer.[7-9]

The resultant implementation of mammograms to screen for breast cancer has altered breast cancer presentation. The state of Rhode Island is an example of a population that is well screened for breast cancer because screening is universally covered, and the effect on breast cancer presentation, treatment, and outcome over a long time period has been reported.[10] Approximately 80% of Rhode Island women participate in breast cancer screening, which is defined as having had a mammogram within the previous 2 years.[11] The Rhode Island Cancer Registry data regarding invasive breast cancer presentation and mortality in 17,522 female residents diagnosed between 1987 and 2008, inclusive, were analyzed for demographic and pathologic factors. Data were analyzed by four time periods: 1987 to 1992, 1993 to 1998, 1999 to 2003, and 2004 to 2008. Statistically significant improvements occurred over the four successive time periods, in mean cancer size (23.7, 20.9, 19.6, and 19.3 mm, $p < .0001$), pathologic grade (grade I: 12, 15, 19, and 17%; grade III 57, 41, 36, and 35%, $p < .0001$), breast conserving surgery (38, 56, 67, and 71 %, $p < 0.0001$) and mortality (37.3, 31.4, 25.1, and 22.6 per 100,000/year, $p < 0.0001$).These results confirm that breast cancer screening within a population results in smaller invasive breast cancers and greater proportion of lower-grade lesions. Detection of smaller tumors by mammography increased the rate of breast conservation surgery from less than 30% before 1990 to more than 70% in most recent years in Rhode Island.

The vast majority of early breast cancers are detected by screening mammograms. Mammographic features of malignancy include a satellite or oval mass, with or without microcalcifications, and microcalcifications that can be clustered, pleomorphic, or "casting" in appearance. Breast cancer biology and prognosis may be influenced by mammographic appearance. Tabar and colleagues evaluated mammographic tumor appearance with breast cancer outcome in patients from the Swedish Breast Cancer Screening Trials.[12] They reported that breast cancers could be classified into five categories based on mammographic features: stellate mass without calcifications, oval mass without calcifications, powdery calcifications with or without a mass, crushed stonelike calcifications with or without a mass, and casting-type calcifications. Casting-type microcalcifications were identified in only 7% of patients, but these patients were three times more likely to have lymph node involvement.[12,13] It has also been reported that patients who present with casting-type microcalcifications were more likely to have poor prognostic features such as positive axillary lymph nodes, hormone receptor negativity, and HER2/neu amplification, as well as a worse outcome independent of tumor size.[14]

Preoperative Evaluation

Preoperative needle biopsy and breast imaging should be performed before breast cancer surgical treatment. Despite clinical suspicion of a malignancy, either by clinical examination or imaging test, it is important that a preoperative biopsy be obtained. Masses can be biopsied by fine-needle aspiration or core needle biopsy. Core needle biopsy is preferable because information on invasion, hormone receptor status, tumor grade, and, in some cases, lymphovascular invasion can be evaluated and is considered the standard of care and a quality measure for breast cancer treatment.[15] Core needle biopsies can be guided by palpation for palpable masses or by stereotactic or sonographic guidance for mammographic or ultrasound abnormalities, respectively. In contemporary management, upward of 85% of breast cancers should be diagnosed preoperatively. A cancer diagnosis before initial surgical treatment leads to more definitive local excision, a greater proportion with negative tumor margins, and thus a decreased need for reexcision, and the ability to evaluate the axilla simultaneously.[16] Patients can also be appropriately counseled before surgery regarding choices such as breast conservation versus mastectomy and neoadjuvant therapy, if appropriate.

However, there are some instances in which a preoperative cancer diagnosis may not be feasible. A stereotactic biopsy for suspicious or indeterminate microcalcifications may not be technically feasible because of proximity to the skin or chest wall. These patients should proceed directly to needle localization and excision. Additionally, approximately 25% of patients with a preoperative needle biopsy may be upstaged to malignancy after surgical excision. A radiologic diagnosis of radial scar mandates surgical excision because of the difficulty in differentiating a radial scar from a low-grade lesion on core needle biopsy. Finally, patients with clotting abnormalities should probably proceed directly to surgery instead of a preoperative needle biopsy.

Although many patients are diagnosed based on imaging abnormalities, there are still a few patients who present with a palpable mass. All patients with breast cancer should have, at minimum, a mammogram. A mammogram permits evaluation of the breast for disease outside the affected quadrant and may provide an estimate of tumor size. Disease outside the affected quadrant precludes the use of breast conservation and may be helpful in planning surgical treatment.

The role of magnetic resonance imaging (MRI) in the patient newly diagnosed with breast cancer is still being debated.[17] Preoperative breast MRI may be used to evaluate the ipsilateral or contralateral breast. Additional tumor can be identified in the ipsilateral breast in 13% to 31%[18–27] of patients resulting in a wider excision in 3% to 14% or conversion to mastectomy in up to 25%.[23,26–28] These results have suggested that candidates for breast conservation surgery should have a preoperative breast MRI. However, it is unclear whether the occult disease identified on breast MRI is clinically important and would not be adequately treated with whole breast radiotherapy. Long-term local recurrence for patients treated with breast conservation is approximately 10%, which is significantly lower than the rate of additional tumor identified on breast MRI. A small retrospective study reported a higher local recurrence rate of 6.8% in women who had conventional imaging compared with 1.2% in those who had received a preoperative MRI ($p < .01$).[29] However, these rates of local recurrence are quite low and different from the series reported by Solin and colleagues where preoperative MRI at the time of diagnosis was not associated with any improvement in outcome.[30] There are even fewer data regarding the role of breast MRI to detect occult disease in the contralateral breast. As demonstrated by Wang and colleagues, the detection of synchronous contralateral breast cancer seems to be increased by the use of preoperative MRI. In this Surveillance, Epidemiology, and End Results (SEER)-Medicare database study, this observation was not offset by a similar decrease of subsequent contralateral cancer occurrence among older women with stages I and II breast cancer, leading to the authors' conclusion that breast MRI might lead to overdiagnosis.[31] The largest study addressing this issue comes from the American College of Radiology Imaging Network,[32] in which occult contralateral disease was identified in 3.1% of participants. The mean diameter of the invasive tumors was 1 cm and was not influenced by menopausal status, dense breast tissue, or tumor histology. A previously published meta-analysis, including 18 studies on MRI and detection of contralateral breast cancer, also shows that there is an increase in detection of contralateral breast cancer without clear evidence of benefit because this could be leading to overdiagnosis.[33] At present, there is no convincing evidence to suggest that the use of preoperative MRI improves local control in women, but it may permit better definition of extent of disease and decrease the need for reexcision to obtain negative surgical margins. In the Choosing Wisely Initiate of the American Society of Breast Surgeons, one of the five tests or interventions that physicians and patients should question is the routine ordering of MRI.[34,35] In an individual person data meta-analysis preoperative MRI for staging the cancerous breast did not reduce the risk of local or distant recurrence.[35] MRI is especially useful when occult breast cancer presents via axillary lymphadenopathy or in those with *BRCA* mutations, but there is no evidence that it lessens reexcision rate, local recurrence, or mortality. In addition, MRI adds to false-positive biopsy rate, extra procedures, and costs, and often delays surgery or ends with increased patient anxiety and questionably a higher mastectomy rate.

Surgical Options for Early Breast Cancer

Surgical management of early breast cancers can be divided into breast conservation surgery or mastectomy and axillary sampling.

TABLE 45.1   Randomized Clinical Trials of Mastectomy Compared With Breast Conservation Surgery for Invasive Breast Cancer

Study	No. of Patients	Time Period	Tumor Size (cm)	Follow-up	Surgery	Local Recurrence Rate	Breast Cancer Survival	Overall Survival
"QUART": Milan Cancer Institute[a]	701	1973–1980	T ≤ 2	20 y	QUART	9%	73.9%	58.3%
					Radical mastectomy	2%	75.7%	58.8%
NSABP B-06[b]	2163	1976–1984	T ≤ 4	69% >20 y	L + AND	40%	64.4	46%
					L + RT + AND	14%	63.3	46%
					MRM	10%	63	47%
NCI[c]	247	1979–1987	T ≤ 5	10 y	L + RT + AND	18	ns	77
					MRM	4	ns	75
Gustave-Roussy[d]	179	1972–1980	T ≤ 2	15 y	L + AND	9%	73%	
					MRM	14%		65%
EORTC[e]	868	1980–1986		10 y	L + AND	20%	65%	
					MRM	12%		66%
Danish Cancer Group[f]	904	1983–1989		6 y	L + AND	3%	79%	
					MRM	4%		82%

AND, Axillary node dissection; *EORTC,* European Organization for Research and Treatment of Cancer; *L,* lumpectomy; *MRM,* modified radical mastectomy; *NCI,* National Cancer Institute; *NSABP,* National Surgical Adjuvant Breast and Bowel Project; *QUART,* quadrantectomy, axillary node dissection, and radiotherapy; *T,* tumor size.

[a]Data from Veronesi U, Cascinelli N, Mariani L, et al. Twenty-year follow-up of a randomized study comparing breast-conserving surgery with radical mastectomy for early breast cancer. *N Engl J Med.* 2002;347:1227-1232.

[b]Data from Fisher B, Anderson S, Bryant J, et al. Twenty-year follow-up of a randomized trial comparing total mastectomy, lumpectomy, and lumpectomy plus irradiation for the treatment of invasive breast cancer. *N Engl J Med.* 2002;347:1233-1241.

[c]Data from Poggi MM, Danforth DN, Sciuto LC, et al. Eighteen-year results in the treatment of early breast carcinoma with mastectomy versus breast conservation therapy: The National Cancer Institute Randomized Trial. *Cancer.* 2003;98:697-702.

[d]Data from Arriagada R, Le MG, Rochard F, Contesso G. Conservative treatment versus mastectomy in early breast cancer: Patterns of failure with 15 years of follow-up data. Institute Gustave-Roussy Breast Cancer Group. *J Clin Oncol.* 1996;14:1558-1564.

[e]Data from van Dongen JA, Voogd AC, Fentiman IS, et al. Long-term results of a randomized trial comparing breast-conserving therapy with mastectomy: European Organization for Research and Treatment of Cancer 10801 trial. *J Natl Cancer Inst.* 2000;92:1143-1150.

[f]Data from Blichert-Toft M, Rose C, Andersen JA, et al. Danish randomized trial comparing breast conservation therapy with mastectomy: six years of life-table analysis. Danish Breast Cancer Cooperative Group. *J Natl Cancer Inst Monogr.* 1992;(11):19-25.

Breast conservation surgery includes radiotherapy. Practice guidelines for breast conservation therapy in patients with invasive breast cancer have been published and provide a good review.[36] There have been six randomized trials addressing the outcome of breast cancer patients treated with breast conservation surgery or mastectomy, and a full discussion is contained in Chapter 50. As summarized in Table 45.1, there is no difference in overall survival whether mastectomy or breast conservation is selected. In most of the trials, there was no significant difference in local recurrence in the treated breast compared with chest wall recurrences after mastectomy, and for the most part, these local breast recurrences can be addressed with mastectomy. Although patient choice may dictate surgical treatment, there are some patients for whom a mastectomy should be recommended. Contraindications for breast conserving therapy for breast cancer include prior history of whole breast radiotherapy, active collagen vascular disease precluding radiotherapy, inability to obtain tumor-free margins despite multiple surgical excisions, first and second trimester of pregnancy, cancers originating in two separate quadrants, and diffuse microcalcifications occupying more than one quadrant. These patients are best served with mastectomy. Histology, location of tumor, patient age, and tumor size (except relative to breast size) are not contraindications to breast conserving therapy.

Determination if a patient is a candidate for breast conservation should begin with the initial history and physical examination.[36] Although a significant family history for breast cancer does not preclude breast conservation, these patients are at significant risk for contralateral breast cancers and may opt for genetic testing. Prior history of therapeutic radiotherapy involving the breast region excludes the use of additional radiotherapy, and these patients are best served by mastectomy. This might be questioned in the scenario where a patient received accelerated partial breast radiation and the breast cancer is diagnosed in a different breast area. A few studies, like the one published by GEC-ESTRO Breast Cancer Working Group in 2013, suggest that in a selected population of patients with ipsilateral breast tumor recurrence, a technique of accelerated partial breast radiation could be considered in patients previously treated with lumpectomy and radiation. In this particular study, multicatheter radiation has been used with excellent/good cosmetic results in 85% of the patients. Overall survival rate is equivalent to those patients submitted to mastectomy at the time of recurrence.[37] The presence of breast implants, possibility of pregnancy, and symptoms of metastatic disease should all be included in the patient history. Physical examination is focused on evaluating the breast and regional lymphatics. Tumor size, if the lesion is palpable, is important, and ratio of tumor size to breast volume and the presence of multiple tumors should be noted. Fixation of the tumor to the skin should be evaluated. Evidence of a locally advanced cancer such as skin edema and ulceration and erythema excludes these patients from breast conservation. Because patient preference is important, the option of breast conservation or mastectomy with or without reconstruction should be discussed even if the patient is an excellent candidate for breast conservation.

Breast Conservation Surgery

The vast majority of patients with early breast cancer are candidates for breast conserving therapy. Indeed, the rate of breast conservation in well-screened populations approaches 80%. The objective of breast conservation surgery for breast cancer is to excise the primary tumor to negative surgical margins while maintaining a cosmetically acceptable breast. Surgical removal of the primary breast cancer while preserving the breast has been called partial mastectomy, wide local excision, lumpectomy, segmental mastectomy, and tumorectomy. All imply surgical removal of the tumor with a grossly negative margin. Quadrantectomy implies excising a quarter of the breast and is more extensive. A quadrantectomy is more likely to result in negative surgical margins but may compromise cosmesis. As breast cancers have decreased in size, the ability to surgically excise breast cancers with a good cosmetic result has increased.

Preoperative localization is required in nonpalpable breast cancers and those that are difficult to palpate. Most nonpalpable breast cancers are localized with a guidewire (needle localization) in the mammography suite immediately before surgery. If needle localization is used, a specimen radiograph is obtained in the operating room to verify that the abnormality and the localizing clip has been included within the excised tissue (Fig. 45.1). When specimen radiography is performed, two views, including an orthogonal one, is the standard. The mammographic abnormality can be localized for the pathologist either with a needle or images of the specimen performed in a grid. Although guidewire localization is most widely used for nonpalpable lesions it is difficult and painful for the patient often accompanied by vasovagal events. New approaches to localize the lesion have been described, including marking the breast cancer with a hematoma. In this technique, intraoperative ultrasound is used to localize the hematoma and guide excision.[38] Hematoma-directed ultrasound guidance (HUG) compared with needle localization breast biopsy for excision of nonpalpable lesions has been described over a 10-year period in 455 patients. Margin positivity was significantly lower for HUG (24%) compared with needle localization breast biopsy (47%) (p = .045).[39]

Another technique to guide localization of nonpalpable tumors is cryo-assisted excision. This technique uses intraoperative cryoablation to create an ice ball around the primary tumor followed by ultrasound guidance during surgical excision.[40] In a prospective randomized trial of cryo-assisted and guidewire needle localization, there was no difference in margin positivity (28% for cryo-assisted localization and 31% for guidewire localization).[41] A major disadvantage of this approach is that freezing artifact of the primary tumor may result in difficulties with histologic examination.[42]

Another technique with increasing data in the literature is radioactive iodine seed localization, which uses an iodine-125 seed for localization of nonpalpable lesions or previously clipped lesions that have disappeared on imaging due to complete

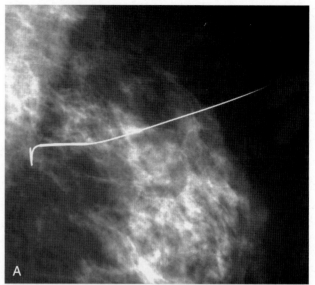

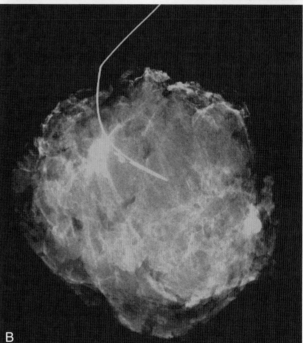

• **Fig. 45.1** Nonpalpable breast cancers should be localized by a guidewire preoperatively and the excised specimen imaged to verify that the lesion has been excised. (A) Mammogram with preoperative needle localization. (B) Specimen radiograph of the excised breast tissue with a clip marking the abnormality.

response to neoadjuvant chemotherapy. This has been seen as equivalent to the needle localization in noninferiority studies and meta-analysis.[43–45]

A pilot study has been published recently describing implantation of infrared-activated, electromagnetic wave-reflective device for localization of nonpalpable breast lesions.[46] The reflector was implanted up to 7 days before the procedure with mammography or ultrasound guidance. Of the 50 patients studied, all had the reflector and lesion successfully removed suggesting a viable alternative to standard wire localization.

Some of the disadvantages of the wire localization compared with the localization of nonpalpable lesions with radioactive

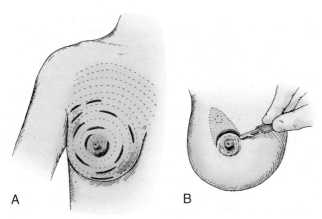

• **Fig. 45.2** (A) Surgical incisions should be placed along Langer lines. (B) Incisions close to the areola border are preferable as they can be masked by the areola border and easily included in a mastectomy, if one is later required.

iodine seed and the electromagnetic wave reflective device include work-flow limitations because the wire needs to be placed on the day of surgery, potentially delaying surgical start times and preventing these procedures to be the first ones of the day. The HUG procedure does not have this disadvantage but must usually be performed within 5 weeks of the biopsy. Possible wire migration during patient transportation is also another disadvantage, potentially misguiding the surgeon on the optimal targeted tissue removal.

Surgical incision placement in breast conserving surgery is important for optimizing cosmetic results. Surgical incisions should be placed to optimize cosmetic results but should not compromise surgery if a mastectomy is needed. Incisions should be placed along Langer or Kraissl lines (lines of tension) because this decreases keloid formation and optimizes cosmesis. On the breast, these incisions are usually circular and are illustrated in Fig. 45.2. Exceptions to this rule are lesions Located in the lower hemisphere of the breast up to and including nine and three o'clock lesion are best addressed with radial incisions. Curvilinear incisions are recommended if only breast tissue is being excised. A radial incision is recommended in the inferior breast if skin is to be included within the excision. When taking skin, a parallelogram is advised compared with an ellipse. In this scenario, the radial incision minimizes ptosis of the nipple. Incisions are best placed as close to the nipple-areola complex as possible because this incision can be easily included if a mastectomy is warranted.

A periareolar incision to remove the breast primary has gained popularity in recent years. This incision permits access to all quadrants of the breast, can be easily accommodated if a mastectomy is needed in the future, and has an excellent cosmetic outcome because the incision is often masked by the areolar border.[47] This incision works well if the lesion is sufficiently deep to the skin such that a 1-cm skin flap can be made. Thinner skin flaps may result in denting of the skin. It is imperative that the biopsy site be clearly marked with clips or a fiducial marker if this incision if used so that radiotherapy planning is not jeopardized. Procedures such as this, the round block technique, and others are termed *oncoplastic* and are covered in Chapter 40.

The decision to include skin depends on tumor location. Mammograms and, in particular, ultrasounds can help estimate the distance between the lesion and subcutaneous tissue. If the lesion is superficial, skin should be included within the excision. Excision

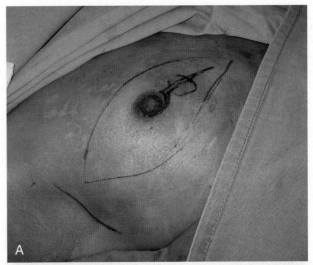

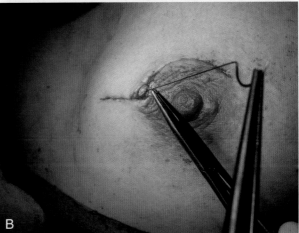

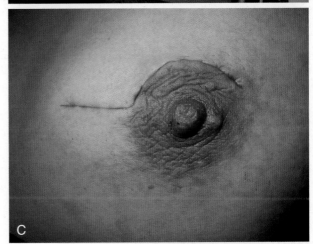

• **Fig. 45.3** A boomerang incision around the areola is recommended for superficial lesions close to the areola that require skin excision. Skin is included with the incision, and placement of a boomerang does not compromise vascular supply to the nipple. (A) Drawing of the skin incision. (B and C) Skin closure. (From Tan MP. The boomerang incision for periareolar breast malignancies. *Am J Surg.* 2007;194:690-693.)

of skin is not required for lesions more than 1 cm deep to the subcutaneous tissue. Superficial lesions close to the areola border that require excision of skin are best approached using a boomerang incision (Fig. 45.3).[48] These lesions can sometimes be challenging; inappropriate technique can lead to nipple devascularization and deviation. A boomerang incision is a combination of a radial incision over the superficial lesion and a boomerang around the areola. This type of incision has been shown to produce excellent cosmetic results, does not compromise margin status, and can be easily included in a mastectomy incision, if needed later. Large batwing incisions are usually reserved for oncoplastic procedures and are addressed elsewhere.[49]

There has been some debate as to whether the needle biopsy site has to be excised at the time of definitive surgery. Although seeding of the biopsy tract has been reported to be as high as 32%,[50] recurrence at the core needle biopsy site is much lower, at approximately 1% when radiation is used. Furthermore, in a retrospective review of 530 patients with stage I and II breast cancer treated with breast conservation surgery and radiotherapy, there was no difference in local recurrence after a median follow-up of more than 70 months if the patients had a preoperative needle biopsy.[51] It is feasible that the tumor deposits identified by washings are not clinically viable or are easily treated with postoperative radiotherapy. Indeed, a local recurrence rate at the needle biopsy site of up to 27% has been reported for patients treated with mastectomy.[52] Therefore, it is recommended that biopsy sites be excised in breast cancer patients treated with mastectomy or partial mastectomy who do not receive postoperative radiotherapy.

The breast lesion should be excised as one specimen; morcellation of the excised tissue should be avoided. Excision as a single specimen is extremely important for tumor size determination and margin assessment. Excision with a knife is recommended because in some instances, cautery artifact at the margin may interfere with determination of margin status. Sharp smooth incisions should be used along the margins; multiple small nicks at the margin may make it difficult to determine whether a margin is involved with tumor. Once the breast tissue is removed, it should be immediately oriented, preferably with colored inks (Fig. 45.4). The use of six colored inks has been shown to decrease the volume of tissue excised if a margin is found to be positive because it is possible to identify the margin involved and avoid who bed reexcision.[53] Examination and then specimen imaging (ultrasound and/or mammography) should confirm removal of the lesion, all of the calcifications and the clip. In addition, many surgeons perform shaved margins of the cavity after tumorectomy. Chagpar and colleagues recently published the results of a randomized trial of 235 patients undergoing partial mastectomy for breast cancer with and without shaved margins.[54] Patients undergoing shave margins had a significantly lower rate of positive margins than those in the no-shave group (19% vs. 34%, $p = .01$), as well as a lower rate of second surgery for margin clearance (10% vs. 21%, $p = .02$).

Meticulous hemostasis should be obtained after surgical excision. Although most postoperative breast hematomas do not require surgical intervention, they are painful, may increase infection, and may delay initiation of postoperative breast radiotherapy. Hematoma formation may obscure postoperative changes, resulting in unnecessary biopsy to preclude recurrent disease. Before breast closure, four clips or a fiducial marker should be placed to localize the biopsy site. These clips aid in radiotherapy planning and mark the area for future mammography. However, clips should not be placed in the biopsy site if accelerated radiotherapy by a balloon catheter is planned because these clips can puncture the balloon.

It is debatable if the biopsy site should be reapproximated before skin closure. Closure of the biopsy site may lead to a worse breast cosmesis. Conversely, leaving the biopsy site in place encourages seroma formation and potentially better cosmesis.[55] Newer techniques that close the deep and superficial layers have also been advocated.[56] These newer techniques include alignment of the parenchyma at right angles to the incision and reapproximation of the deep and superficial suture lines without closure of the central biopsy site. A recent report confirms that leaving the biopsy site in place does achieve a better cosmetic result. However, in this study, it was more difficult to differentiate between postoperative changes and recurrence.[57] Drains in the breast should be avoided, and the skin should be reapproximated using a subcuticular technique. Staples should be avoided on the skin.

The objective of breast conservation surgery is to excise the tumor to negative surgical margins (tumor-free margin or negative margin) with acceptable breast cosmesis. There was much controversy regarding the definition as to what constitutes a negative surgical margin for excision of breast cancer.[58] The definition used by the National Surgical Adjuvant Breast and Bowel Project was no tumor cells at the transected margin. Others have used 2 to 5 mm as the cutoff for a tumor-free margin, whereas others have focused on the extent of margin involvement.[59] Approximately half of the patients with a positive margin have residual disease at mastectomy, with higher rate of residual disease in those patients with multiple close margins.[60] If feasible and needed, multiple reexcisions do not affect local recurrence if a negative surgical margin is ultimately obtained.[61] In 2014, the Society of Surgical Oncology and the American Society for Radiation Oncology issued a consensus guideline on margins for patient undergoing lumpectomy and whole breast radiation for stages I and II invasive breast cancer, which has also been endorsed by the American Society of Clinical Oncology.[62,63] The panel of experts used a study level meta-analysis of margin width and ipsilateral breast tumor recurrence (IBTR) of 33 studies including a total of 28,162 patients. There was no clear evidence that wider margins than "no ink on tumor" reduce IBTR for patients with stage I and II disease receiving whole breast radiation. It has been stated in the study that this guideline should not be applied to patients with pure ductal carcinoma in situ (DCIS), those who received preoperative chemotherapy, or those who receive accelerated partial breast radiation or no radiation at all after breast conservation.

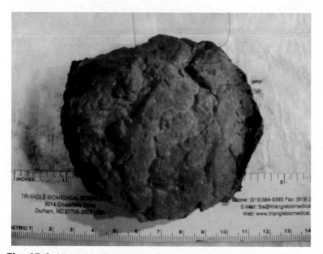

• **Fig. 45.4** All excised breast specimens should be oriented. The use of six colored inks permits easy reexcision if a margin is positive for tumor cells.

• **Box 45.1** **Standards for Breast Conservation for Patients With Early Breast Cancer**

Mammography (2)
1. All patients should have preoperative mammography.
2. Size of the mammographic abnormality should be included in the report.

Labeling of the Surgical Specimen (3)
1. Laterality of the specimen
2. Involved breast quadrant
3. Orientation of the specimen

Pathology Report (10)
1. Microscopic confirmation of disease
2. Tumor size
3. Histologic type
4. Histologic grade
5. Presence or absence of lymphatic and blood vessel invasion
6. Macroscopic margin status
7. Microscopic margin status
8. Estrogen receptor status
9. Progesterone receptor status
10. Presence of in situ disease

Radiotherapy (6)
1. Radiotherapy administered after breast conservation surgery
2. Documentation of dosimeter or dose distribution
3. Planning on a dedicated simulator
4. Treatment 5 days per week
5. Dose planning with use of tissue compensators
6. Avoidance of breast bolus to minimize skin toxicity

Systemic Therapy (1)
1. Systemic therapy for patients with positive nodes

Modified from Winchester DP, Cox JD. Standards for breast-conservation treatment. CA Cancer J Clin. 1992;42:134-162. This material is reproduced with permission of Wiley-Liss, Inc., a subsidiary of John Wiley & Sons, Inc.

In 1992, the American College of Surgeons, the American College of Radiology, the College of American Pathologists, and the Society of Surgical Oncology published guidelines for breast conserving therapy that included 22 standards.[64] Box 45.1 summarizes these standards.[64] Although most of the guidelines related to pathology report content, three of the standards were related to the surgical specimen. These standards included labeling the breast involved (laterality), noting the affected quadrant, and orienting the breast specimen. In a follow-up study in 2002,[65] there was excellent compliance with information regarding laterality. Approximately two-thirds of breast specimens were oriented. However, only about one-fifth of surgeons noted the affected quadrant. This has recently been updated with the development of and publication of the National Accreditation Program for Breast Centers Standards Manual (Box 45.2).[66] This accreditation process for a center has 29 standards that includes standards involving center leadership and the utilization of an interdisciplinary breast cancer conference, clinical management, research, community outreach, professional education, and quality improvement. In particular relation to surgical care is the surgical correlation with imaging/concordance; preoperative planning after needle biopsy; offering lumpectomy or mastectomy with or without reconstruction; lymph node surgery, including sentinel lymph node biopsy, initial surgical correlation, and treatment planning;

as well as medical and radiation oncology consultation, education, support, rehabilitation, and survivorship programs.

Mastectomy

Early breast cancers can also be treated with a mastectomy. Multiple randomized trials have shown that there is no difference in overall breast cancer survival whether breast conservation or mastectomy is performed. Mastectomy, however, does result in fewer breast recurrences. A benefit of mastectomy is that for most women, postmastectomy radiation is not needed. The technical aspects of mastectomy are discussed in detail in Chapter 31. In general, mastectomy implies the removal of breast and overlying skin and includes the nipple-areola complex. The mastectomy incision should incorporate the previous biopsy scar. The preferred mastectomy incision uses a modified Orr incision that is slightly oblique from the transverse line and cephalad toward the axilla (Fig. 45.5). This incision removes the nipple-areola complex, allows access to the axilla, and provides an acceptable cosmetic result. This type of mastectomy should be used if no plastic reconstruction of the breast is planned because it minimizes skin on the chest wall, which can become irritated by wearing breast prosthesis. Patients can have either immediate or delayed reconstruction of the breast with this type of mastectomy. The breast should be oriented with sutures after removal and the posterior margin inked. If the primary breast lesion is not clinically palpable, a radiograph of the excised breast can be performed to aid in pathologic evaluation.

A variant of the classic mastectomy is the skin-sparing mastectomy. This operation is best used if plastic surgical reconstruction of the breast is planned. A skin-sparing mastectomy includes removal of the breast parenchyma with minimal removal of the overlying skin. Underlying pectoralis fascia is included with the excised breast specimen. The remaining native breast skin and inframammary fold provide for excellent cosmetic results when the breast is reconstructed with either autologous tissue or an implant. A skin-sparing mastectomy is usually performed through a circular incision around the areola with a hockey-stick extension if needed (Fig. 45.6). The nipple-areola complex is usually included with a skin-sparing mastectomy.

Variants of the skin-sparing mastectomy include nipple skin-sparing mastectomy, which has been advocated by some as being cosmetically superior to a skin-sparing mastectomy. However, a nipple-sparing mastectomy does leave some ductal tissue beneath the nipple, which some have suggested may lead to increase nipple areolar recurrence.[67] However, a meta-analysis and review of the literature published in 2015 included 20 studies and a total of 2207 patients who underwent nipple-sparing mastectomy for breast cancer treatment, with majority of them being stage I or II. This study suggested likely absence of adverse oncological events when nipple-sparing mastectomies were performed. This is particularly true in carefully selected patients with early-stage breast cancer, with the authors recognizing the limitations of this being a meta-analysis of observational studies in the setting of an outcome that is unlikely to be evaluated in a randomized clinical trial setting.[68]

Axillary Evaluation

The most important prognostic feature of an early breast cancer is nodal involvement. Nodal involvement suggests that the primary tumor has the capability to spread systemically. The

---

• BOX 45.2 **National Accreditation Program for Breast Centers Standards Manual 2014**

1. Imaging
   a. Screening mammography (digital or analog)
   b. Diagnostic mammography (additional views beyond screening mammography and workup of a clinical abnormality)
   c. Ultrasound
   d. Breast MRI
2. Needle Biopsy
   a. Needle biopsy—palpation-guided
   b. Image guided—stereotactic
   c. Image guided—ultrasound
   d. Image guided—MRI
3. Pathology
   a. Report completeness/CAP protocols
   b. Radiology-pathology correlation
   c. Prognostic and predictive indicators
   d. Gene Studies (if available)
4. Interdisciplinary Conference
   a. History and findings
   b. Imaging studies
   c. Pathology
   d. Pre- and posttreatment interdisciplinary discussion
5. Patient Navigation
   a. Facilitates navigation through system for the patient
6. Genetic Evaluation and Management
   a. Genetic risk assessment
   b. Genetic counseling
   c. Genetic testing
7. Surgical Care
   a. Surgical correlation with imaging/concordance
   b. Preoperative planning after biopsy for surgical care
   c. Breast surgery: lumpectomy or mastectomy
   d. Lymph node surgery: sentinel node/axillary dissection
   e. Post initial surgical correlation/treatment planning
8. Plastic Surgery Consultation/Treatment
   a. Tissue expander/implants
   b. TRAM/latissimus dorsi
   c. DIEP flap/free flaps (if available)
9. Nursing
   a. Nurses with specialized knowledge and skills in diseases of the breast

10. Medical Oncology Consultation/Treatment
    a. Hormone therapy
    b. Chemotherapy
    c. Biologics
    d. Chemoprevention
11. Radiation Oncology Consultation/Treatment
    a. Whole breast irradiation with or without boost
    b. Regional nodal irradiation
    c. Partial breast irradiation treatment or protocols
    d. Palliative radiation for bone or systemic metastasis
    e. Stereotactic radiation for isolated or limited brain metastasis
12. Data Management
    a. Data collection and submission
13. Research
    a. Cooperative trials
    b. Institutional original research (not part of national trials)
    c. Industry sponsored trials
14. Education, Support, and Rehabilitation
    a. Education along continuum of care (pretreatment, during, posttreatment)
    b. Psychosocial support: i. individual support; ii. family support; iii. support groups
    c. Symptom management
    d. Physical therapy (for example, lymphedema risk reduction practices, and management, shoulder ROM)
15. Outreach and Education
    a. Community at-large education (including low-income/medically underserved)
    b. Patient education
    c. Physician education
16. Quality Improvement
    a. Continuous quality improvement through annual studies
17. Survivorship Program
    a. Follow-up surveillance
    b. Rehabilitation
    c. Health promotion/risk reduction

CAP, *College of American Pathologists;* DIEP, *deep inferior epigastric perforator;* MRI, *magnetic resonance imaging;* ROM, *range of motion;* TRAM, *transverse rectus abdominis myocutaneous (flap).*

---

likelihood of spread to the axillary lymph nodes increases with primary tumor size. Approximately 25% of breast cancer patients have positive lymph nodes at the time of diagnosis. Clinical evaluation of the axilla is notoriously inaccurate and should not be used as the primary method to stage the axilla in most patients. Surgical evaluation of the axilla is usually used for patients with breast cancer. Surgical evaluation includes sentinel lymphadenectomy, axillary node dissection, and the more recently described targeted axillary dissection.

Sentinel lymphadenectomy is a minimally invasive surgical technique that is used to stage the axilla. This surgical approach can be used to determine which patients have nodal disease and which do not. Because on average only two lymph nodes are removed, sentinel lymphadenectomy cannot accurately indicate the number of lymph nodes involved with tumor. Sentinel lymphadenectomy should be used in patients with a clinically negative axilla, a situation most frequently encountered in patients with early breast cancer.

Although the original description of sentinel lymphadenectomy used only one tracer, most centers today use a combination

of dyes. The most frequent combination used is radioactive protein (technetium sulfur colloid) and blue dye (Fig. 45.7). The radioactive protein can be filtered or unfiltered. Blue dyes used include isosulfan blue, methylene blue, or patent blue dye. If radioactive protein is used, it is usually injected 2 hours before surgery or up to the day before for early-morning cases. The blue dye is usually injected in the operating room followed by breast massage for approximately 5 minutes. The tracers can be injected in the tissue around the primary tumor, in the skin overlying the primary tumor or the periareolar area.

Sentinel lymphadenectomy commences with a transverse incision in the low axilla, two to three finger-breadths below the axillary apex. The sentinel lymph nodes are encountered after incision of the clavipectoral fascia. All hot (radioactive), warm, and/or blue nodes are considered sentinel lymph nodes. If radioactive protein is used, a background less than 10% of the hottest node is considered "cold." After all sentinel lymph nodes are removed, the axilla is palpated to ensure that there are no firm nodes. All firm nodes should be removed; they may represent lymph nodes that the dye cannot drain to because of complete nodal replacement with tumor. The clavipectoral fascia should be reapproximated during closure to avoid a bulging seroma in the axilla. Patients undergoing a mastectomy can still have axillary evaluation with sentinel lymphadenectomy. A separate axillary incision is not required. Placement of a drain after sentinel lymphadenectomy is usually not required unless accompanied by a mastectomy.

Sentinel lymphadenectomy is the preferred surgical approach in women with early breast cancer. Until the introduction of sentinel lymphadenectomy, axillary node dissection was the

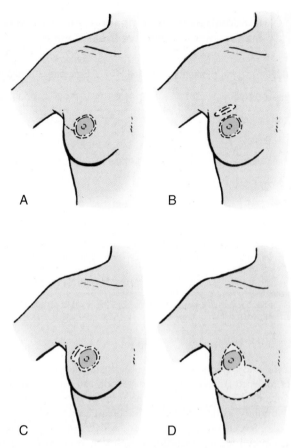

A   B

C   D

• **Fig. 45.6** Skin-sparing mastectomy incisions. The objective of a skin-sparing mastectomy incision is to optimize cosmetic results by leaving the skin envelope without jeopardizing breast cancer treatment. The classic incision is shown in (A) and consists of a circular incision around the areola with a hockey-stick extension. (B–D) depict variations of the classical incision. It is important to note that previously placed incisions to excise the cancer should be removed along the nipple and areola. (From Carlson GW. Trends in autologous breast reconstruction. In: Robb GL, Miller MJ, eds. *Seminars in Plastic Surgery*. New York: Thieme; 2004:79-87.)

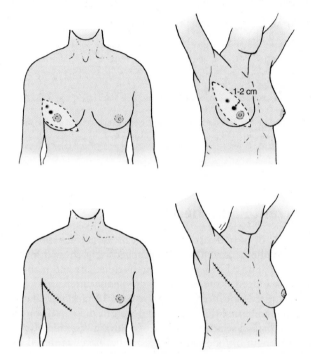

• **Fig. 45.5** Classic mastectomy incision. The classic mastectomy incision, also known as the Orr incision, is obliquely placed along the chest wall and includes skin and the nipple-areola complex. This incision permits easy access to the axilla.

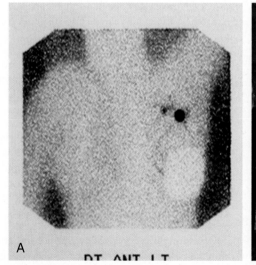

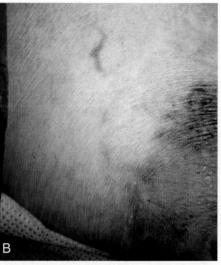

• **Fig. 45.7** Use of blue dye and technetium sulfur colloid to identify the sentinel lymph node. The sentinel lymph node can be identified after injection of radioactive protein and blue dye. (A) Lymphoscintigram after injection of technetium sulfur colloid in the skin overlying the breast cancer. (B) Periareola injection of blue dye and the blue-stained lymphatic channels.

TABLE 45.2	Randomized Trials Comparing Breast Conservation Surgery With and Without Radiotherapy in the Management of Invasive Breast Cancer							
Study	No. of Patients	Time Period	Tumor Size (cm)	Follow-up	Surgery	Local Recurrence Rate (%)	Breast Cancer Survival (%)	Overall Survival (%)
Uppsala–Orebro	381	1981–1988	T ≤ 2	109 mo	BCS, RT, AND	9	88	78
Breast Cancer					BCS, AND	24	90	78
Study Group[a]								
Ontario Clinical	837	1984–1989	T ≤ 4	7.6 y	BCS, AND	35	81	76
Oncology Group[b]					BCS, RT, AND	11	84	79
Finnish Trial[c]	152		T ≤ 2	6.7 y	BCS, AND	18	99	—
					BCS, RT, AND	8	98	—

AND, Axillary node dissection; *BCS*, breast conserving surgery; *RT*, whole breast radiotherapy; *T*, tumor size in centimeters.

[a]Data from Liljegren G, Holmberg L, Bergh J, et al. Ten-year results after sector resection with or without postoperative radiotherapy for stage I breast cancer: a randomized trial. *J Clin Oncol.* 1999;17:2326-2333.

[b]Data from Clark RM, Whelan T, Levine M, et al. Randomized clinical trial of breast irradiation following lumpectomy and axillary dissection for node-negative breast cancer: an update. Ontario Clinical Oncology Group. *J Natl Cancer Inst.* 1996;88:1659-1664.

[c]Data from Holli K, Saaristo R, Isola J, et al. Lumpectomy with or without postoperative radiotherapy for breast cancer with favorable prognostic features: results of a randomized study. *Br J Cancer.* 2001;84:164-169.

operation most frequently used to evaluate the axilla in breast cancer patients. An axillary node dissection can provide information on nodal involvement and the number of nodes involved. Contemporary axillary dissection in breast cancer refers to the removal of level I and II lymph nodes. Axillary node dissection has significant morbidity, including lymphedema, paresthesias, and nerve damage, and an axillary node dissection in node-negative women provides no therapeutic benefit other than prognostic information. Axillary dissection is usually reserved for patients with positive sentinel lymph nodes, those with grossly positive nodes, and those with early breast cancer who cannot have a sentinel lymph node biopsy. In 2010 Giuliano and colleagues reported the American College of Surgeons Oncology Group (ACOSOG) Z0011 trial.[69] They reported equivalent local recurrence and survival in patients with two or more positive nodes on sentinel node biopsy and whole breast radiation therapy with or without full axillary node dissection. Nondissection of the axilla with positive nodes is considered a viable choice equal to axillary node dissection. Of note is that a majority of these patients did receive radiation to the axilla. Also objective lymphedema was not different between the sentinel and axillary lymph node dissection groups in Z0011. This study and its ramification are described in detail in Chapter 42.

Targeted axillary dissection has been more recently described and includes the performance of sentinel lymphadenectomy in combination with the localization and removal of a clipped and biopsy-proven positive lymph node(s) in patients who have undergone neoadjuvant chemotherapy. The goal is to allow a more selective removal of nodes in an attempt to prevent axillary node dissection and its possible associated morbidities. A prospective study has revealed a false-negative rate of 2% compared with approximately 10% when sentinel lymphadenectomy was performed alone. Sample size limited the statistical comparison, but research is ongoing.[70] The Alliance trial has also suggested that the evaluation of the positive clipped lymph node should be considered when performing sentinel lymphadenectomy in post-neoadjuvant chemotherapy patients allowing for significant reduction of false negative rates in this group.[71]

Adjuvant Radiotherapy

Treatment of early breast cancer with breast conservation usually involves radiotherapy. This is comprehensively covered in Chapters 47, 50, and 51. There has been much debate and many trials that have addressed the need for radiotherapy after breast conservation surgery for cancer. There have been 14 randomized clinical trials that addressed this issue. The details of these trials vary with regard to patient selection, the use of adjuvant systemic treatment, and the length of follow-up. Three studies have compared breast conserving surgery with and without radiotherapy: the Uppsala-Orebro, Ontario, and Finnish studies (Table 45.2). These studies collectively showed that breast radiotherapy decreased local recurrence approximately 70% but that there was no difference in overall survival. A meta-analysis of all trials of breast conserving surgery with and without radiotherapy reported that there was a threefold increased risk of local recurrence if radiotherapy was omitted.[72] The meta-analysis also suggested that there was a small survival benefit with breast radiotherapy.

It is feasible that radiotherapy may be omitted or replaced by tamoxifen in a select group of early breast cancers. Several studies have evaluated replacement of radiotherapy with tamoxifen (Table 45.3). Although the local recurrence rate with breast conservation surgery and tamoxifen was less than 10% for most of the studies, this number was higher than that reported with breast radiotherapy. The Milan trial was a prospective trial of elderly patients in which tamoxifen replaced breast radiotherapy.[73] In this study of 354 elderly women, recurrences occurred in 8% of patients treated with breast conservation surgery and tamoxifen. These results suggested that radiotherapy is superior to tamoxifen in decreasing local breast recurrence for patients treated with breast conservation.

The randomized trials allowed the comparison of radiotherapy and no radiotherapy for breast cancers in general but did not permit discrimination between different breast cancers. Breast cancer is a heterogenous disease, and some cancers are more likely to recur after breast conservation treatment. Breast cancers with a higher rate of local recurrence after breast conservation include

TABLE 45.3 Local Recurrence and Survival in Women With Invasive Breast Cancer Treated With Tamoxifen and/or Radiotherapy

Series	No. of Patients	Treatment/Inclusion	IBTR %	Outcome
NCI, Milan[a]	354	BCS, TAM, no RT, no AND	15 y: 8.3	15-y BCS: 23%
		Above with T₁ only	15 y: 7.3	
CALGB[b]	636	BCS, RT	4	5-y OS: 86%
		BCS, RT, TAM	1	5-y OS: 87%
Canadian trial[c]	769	BCS, TAM	5 y: 8	5-y OS: 92%
		BCS, RT, TAM	5 y: 1	5-y OS: 92%
NSABP-21[d]	1009	TAM	13.5	94%
		RT	6.9	94%
		TAM + RT	2.7	93.4%
Scottish trial[e]	585	BCS, TAM	28	93%
		BCS, TAM, RT	6	93%
St. George (United Kingdom)[f]	418	BCS, TAM	35	
		BCS, TAM, RT	13	

AND, Axillary node dissection; *BCS,* breast conserving surgery; *CALGB,* Cancer and Leukemia Group B; *IBTR,* ipsilateral breast tumor recurrence; *NCI,* National Cancer Institute; *NSABP,* National Surgical Adjuvant Breast and Bowel Project; *OS,* overall survival; *RT,* whole-breast radiotherapy; *TAM,* tamoxifen.

[a]Data from Martelli G, Miceli R, Costa A, et al. Elderly breast cancer patients treated by conservative surgery alone plus adjuvant tamoxifen: fifteen-year results of a prospective study. *Cancer.* 2007;112:481-488.

[b]Data from Hughes KS, Schnaper LA, Berry D, et al. Lumpectomy plus tamoxifen with or without irradiation in women 70 years of age or older with early breast cancer. *N Engl J Med.* 2004;351:971-977.

[c]Data from Fyles AW, McCready DR, Manchul LA, et al. Tamoxifen with or without breast irradiation in women 50 years of age or older with early breast cancer. *N Engl J Med.* 2004;351:963-970.

[d]Data from Fisher B, Bryant J, Dignam JJ, et al. Tamoxifen, radiation therapy, or both for prevention of ipsilateral breast tumor recurrence after lumpectomy in women with invasive breast cancers of one centimeter or less. *J Clin Oncol.* 2002;20:4141-4149.

[e]Data from Forrest AP, Stewart HJ, Everington D, et al. Randomised controlled trial of conservation therapy for breast cancer: 6-year analysis of the Scottish trial. Scottish Cancer Trials Breast Group. *Lancet.* 1996;348:708-713.

[f]Data from Renton SC, Gazet JC, Ford HT, et al. The importance of the resection margin in conservative surgery for breast cancer. *Eur J Surg Oncol.* 1996;22:17-22.

TABLE 45.4 Risk Factors Associated With an Increased Likelihood of Local Recurrence in Breast Cancer Patients Treated With Breast Conservation Surgery and Radiotherapy

Prognostic Factor	Relative Risk of Local Recurrence[a]
Age <45 y	4.09
Age <50 y	1.2–2
Mammogram suggestive of multicentricity	2.3
Diffuse microcalcifications	3.8
Presence of extensive intraductal component	2.2–9
Presence of comedocarcinoma	3.5
Histology (lobular vs. ductal)	2.8
Positive surgical margin	2.6–16.7
Tumor size (>2 cm)	2
Positive lymph nodes	2.5
p53 overexpression	9.28

[a]Relative risk expressed as a multiple if prognostic factor is absent or age is >65.
From Bland KI, Daly JM, Karakousis CP, eds. *Surgical Oncology, Contemporary Principles and Practice.* New York: McGraw-Hill, 2001:966.

Outcome After Surgical Management of Breast Cancer

Outcome after the surgical management of early breast cancer is based on tumor size and lymph node involvement. The largest population-based series of patients with small breast cancers is derived from the SEER registry. In this study of more than 50,000 patients with breast cancers less than 1 cm, the 10-year breast cancer–specific survival was 96%. Similar survival rates of more than 20 years have been reported from the Swedish Breast Cancer Screening Trials. In general, women with breast cancers less than 1 cm have greater than 90% long-term survival. Although women with tumors greater than 1 cm still have an excellent outcome, it is comparatively worse than those with smaller tumors. These data suggest that, within the spectrum hypothesis, 1 cm is the cutoff where the likelihood of lymph node metastases begins to increase. Table 45.5 summarizes the series that have reported outcome of patients with early breast cancers published since the late 1990s.

The vast majority of early breast cancer patients can be surgically treated with breast conservation surgery with radiotherapy. There are several special circumstances that need to be discussed. These circumstances include management of the elderly patient, preoperative diagnosis of a radial scar, patients with breast cancers of lobular histology, and patients with a strong family history of breast cancer.

Management of the Elderly Patient

The two biggest risk factors for breast cancer are increasing age and being female, and therefore it is not surprising that the incidence of breast cancer is greatest in older women. Issues related to breast cancer management in elderly patients have been

those that occur in young patients (age <40 years),[74] have a high tumor grade,[75] lymphovascular invasion,[76] tumor cells at the margin,[77] and invasive cancers with an extensive intraductal component.[76] Table 45.4 summarizes risk factors for local recurrence after breast conservation surgery. Computerized web-based tools have been developed to assist patients and physicians regarding an individual patient's risk of recurrence. One such tool is ipsilateral breast tumor recurrence (IBTR!; www.tufts-nemc.org/ibtr/). IBTR! uses data from randomized trials and institutional reports to estimate a woman's 10-year risk of local recurrence based on age, margin status, lymphovascular invasion, tumor size, tumor, and use of adjuvant chemotherapy and antiestrogens and to calculate the additional benefit, if any, of breast radiotherapy.[78]

TABLE 45.5   Outcome of Women Diagnosed With Early Breast Cancer

Series	Time Period	No. of Patients	Overall Survival	Breast Cancer Survival
SEER[a]	1998–2001	51,246	Overall 10 y: 75.9% T$_{1a}$N$_0$ 10 y: 78.6% T$_{1b}$N$_0$ 10 y: 75.0%	10 y: 96% 10 y: 96% 10 y: 96%
NCCH, Japan[b]	1967–1995	1699 T$_{1a}$: 38 T$_{1b}$: 26 T$_{1c}$: 1405	10 y: 91.9% 20 y: 70.7% 10 y: 86.8% 20 y: 76.7% 10 y: 83.9% 20 y: 70.1%	
NCI, Italy[c]	1997–2001	425 T$_{1mic}$: 24 T$_{1a}$: 76 T$_{1b}$: 325	DFS 4 y: 100% 4 y: 97.0% 4 y: 97.6%	
Swedish Two County[d]	1977–2001	714 T$_{1a}$,T$_{1b}$: 300 T$_{1c}$: 414		24 y: 94% 24 y: 96% 24 y: 93%
MSKCC[e]	1989–1991	T$_{1a}$,T$_{1b}$: 290	Overall 6 y: 91% DFSS 6 y: 92%	
Finland[f]	1945–1984	T$_{1a}$, T$_{1b}$:80 T$_{1c}$: 130		20 y: 92% 20 y: 75%
British Columbia[g]	1989–1991	T$_{1a}$,T$_{1b}$: 430 T$_{1c}$: 57	10-y DFSS: 82% 10-y DFSS: 75%	10 y: 92% 10 y: 90%
Netherlands[h]	1999–2005	T$_{1a}$: 2398 T$_{1b}$: 9599 T$_{1c}$: 29114	Overall 5-y: 93% Overall 5-y: 93% Overall 5-y: 88%	5 y[i]: 99% 5 y[i]: 100% 5 y[i]: 96%
	2006–2012	T$_{1a}$: 3846 T$_{1b}$: 12213 T$_{1c}$: 34163	Overall 5-yr: 95% Overall 5-y: 95% Overall 5-y: 91%	5 y[i]: 100% 5 y[i]: 101% 5 y[i]: 98%

Breast cancer survival in women diagnosed with early disease. Only studies published within the past 10 years are included.

DFS, Disease-free survival; *DFSS,* disease-free specific survival; *MSKCC,* Memorial Sloan Kettering Cancer Center; *NCCH,* National Cancer Center Hospital; *NCI,* National Cancer Institute; *SEER,* Surveillance, Epidemiology, and End Results.

[a]Data from Hanrahan EO, Gonzalez-Angulo AM, Giordano SH, et al. Overall survival and cause-specific mortality of patients with stage T1a,bN0M0 breast carcinoma. *J Clin Oncol.* 2007;25:4952-4960.

[b]Data from Ichizawa N, Fukutomi T, Iwamoto E, Akashi-Tanaka S. Long-term results of T1a, T1b and T1c invasive breast carcinomas in Japanese women: validation of the UICC T1 subgroup classification. *Jpn J Clin Oncol.* 2002;32:108-109.

[c]Data from Colleoni M, Rotmensz N, Peruzzotti G, et al. Minimal and small size invasive breast cancer with no axillary lymph node involvement: the need for tailored adjuvant therapies. *Ann Oncol.* 2004;15:1633-1639.

[d]Data from Tabar L, Chen HHT, Yen MFA, et al. Mammographic tumor features can predict long-term outcomes reliably in women with 1–14-mm invasive breast carcinoma. *Cancer.* 2004;101:1745-1759.

[e]Data from Mann GB, Port ER, Rizza C, et al. Six-year follow-up of patients with microinvasive, T1a, and T1b breast carcinoma. *Ann Surg Oncol.* 1999;6:591-598.

[f]Data from Joensuu H, Pylkkanen L, Toikkanen S. Late mortality from pT1N0M0 breast carcinoma. *Cancer.* 1999;85:2183-2189.

[g]Data from Chia SK, Speers CH, Bryce CJ, et al. Ten-year outcomes in a population-based cohort of node-negative, lymphatic, and vascular invasion-negative early breast cancers without adjuvant systemic therapies. *J Clin Oncol.* 2004;22:1630-1637.

[h]Data from Saadatmand S, Bretveld R, Siesling S, et al. Influence of tumor stage at breast cancer detection on survival in modern times: population based study in 173797 patients. *BMJ.* 2015;351:h4901.

[i]Observed survival divided by expected survival of corresponding general population matched by sex, age, and year of diagnosis.

reviewed.[79] Although many geriatric patients with breast cancer die of other causes, age alone should not be a barrier to treatment. Breast cancer screening with mammography has been shown to decrease mortality. Although few women older than 70 years of age were included in the screening trials, it is likely that older women also benefit from screening mammography. However, the benefits of screening need to be weighed against comorbidities. The American Geriatrics Society recommends that screening mammography be continued until the woman has a life expectancy that is less than 4 years (www.americangeriatrics.org). The ACS recommends annual mammography for women starting at age 45 until age of 54, continuing with biennial study as long as overall life expectancy is of 10 years or longer.

Breast conservation surgery plus radiotherapy or mastectomy is the recommended treatment for women with breast cancer, irrespective of age. There have been several trials comparing surgery plus or minus tamoxifen to tamoxifen alone for elderly patients (Table 45.6). It is generally agreed that tamoxifen alone

TABLE 45.6	Effect of Omitting Surgery on Overall Survival and Local Recurrence in Elderly Women With Breast Cancer			
No. of Patients	Follow-up (mo)	Treatment	Overall Survival (%)	Local Recurrence (%)
164	120	Tamoxifen	39	57
		Surgery	27[a]	9[b]
135	24	Tamoxifen	85	44
		Surgery	74.6[a]	24.6[c]
200	72	Tamoxifen	67	56
		Surgery	72[a]	44[a]
474	80	Tamoxifen	38.7	47.2
		Surgery and tamoxifen	45.6[a]	11[b]
171	41	Tamoxifen	68	27
		Surgery	72[a]	6[b]
455	151	Tamoxifen	28.8	50
		Surgery and tamoxifen	37.7[b]	16[b]

Surgery excision is superior to tamoxifen alone in elderly patients with breast cancer who are medically fit.
[a]No significant difference between tamoxifen versus surgery and tamoxifen or surgery alone.
[b]Significant difference between tamoxifen versus surgery and tamoxifen or surgery alone.
[c]Significance not reported.
From Wildiers H, Biganzoli L, Fracheboud J, et al. Management of breast cancer in elderly individuals: recommendations of the International Society of Geriatric Oncology. Lancet. 207;8:1101-1115.

is inferior to surgery with or without tamoxifen for local control in the medically fit elderly patient.[80] It is unclear whether surgery improves overall survival. In summary, age alone should not be used to guide surgical treatment of the elderly patient.

A continuing area of controversy is whether elderly patients treated with breast conservation need radiotherapy. Older patients often have significant morbidities, and they are more likely to die of diseases other than their breast cancer. Furthermore, breast cancers in older women may be less aggressive and more indolent than those diagnosed in younger counterparts. The Canadian series included 769 women older than 50 years of age and randomized them to breast conserving therapy, tamoxifen, and/or radiotherapy. Despite a similar 5-year survival of 92%, the local recurrence was 8% in those treated with tamoxifen alone; this was eightfold higher than those treated with radiotherapy and tamoxifen.[81] The Cancer and Leukemia Group B (CALGB) conducted a similar randomized trial but included only women older than 70 years of age.[82] In this study of 636 women with T1NoMo estrogen receptor–positive breast cancer treated with lumpectomy, the ipsilateral breast tumor recurrence after 5 years was 4% in those women who had surgery and tamoxifen compared with 1% in those who received radiotherapy in addition to surgery and tamoxifen. However, with the recently reported median follow-up of 12.6 years recurrence with radiation was 2% and with tamoxifen only 10%.[83]

Invasive Lobular Breast Cancer

Invasive lobular breast cancer is characterized by Indian filing of cells and is often not associated with a mass. Because of difficulty in its diagnosis, invasive lobular breast cancers tend to be larger than invasive breast cancers at diagnosis. Large population studies have shown that invasive lobular breast cancer can be treated with breast conservation surgery with a similar recurrence rate to that of invasive ductal cancers.[84] Hence, the histologic diagnosis of an invasive lobular carcinoma does not preclude breast conservation

surgery. Contemporary management of invasive lobular carcinoma does not mandate lobular carcinoma in situ (LCIS)-negative margins. Some studies have reported a significantly higher incidence of invasive lobular carcinoma after a diagnosis of LCIS[85] and demonstrated that the recurrence rate of invasive lobular carcinoma was higher when associated with LCIS (15% vs. 6%).[86] Only a few previous studies have evaluated the impact of LCIS at the surgical margin and recurrence of invasive disease. Abner and colleagues[87] demonstrated no difference in recurrence rates in patients with LCIS-positive and LCIS-negative surgical margins (15% and 12%, respectively), whereas Sasson and associates[86] reported a significant increase in recurrence with LCIS-positive margins (29%) compared with those patients with LCIS-negative margins (6%).

Family History of Breast Cancer

Family history of breast cancer is not a contraindication for breast conservation because the rate of local recurrence in patients with first- and second-degree relatives with breast cancer is not significantly higher compared with women with no family histories. However, testing for genetic mutations BRCA1 and BRCA2 can identify those patients who are at a significant risk of metachronous breast cancers. Overall, there is no difference in survival in patients who are BRCA1 and BRCA2 positive compared with those who are negative.[88,89] However, the rate of contralateral breast cancer was sixfold higher in BRCA mutation carriers versus controls (39% vs. 7%).[90]

One of the issues often raised with newly diagnosed breast cancer patients is the timing of genetic testing relative to surgical intervention.[91] BRCA testing in the United States currently takes 3 weeks to complete, and this waiting period may not be acceptable to some patients. If the patient has decided that she would proceed with breast conservation if negative, one approach that can be used is to proceed with breast conservation surgery while waiting for BRCA test results. Radiotherapy is not initiated until

BRCA results are available. If the patient is *BRCA* negative, she can then proceed to radiotherapy. If she is *BRCA* positive, the patient can proceed to mastectomy if she so desires.

Minimally Invasive Ablative Therapies

Emerging treatments for breast cancer include the use of ablative therapies.[92] The most common ablative therapies for breast cancer are radiofrequency ablation and cryoablation. Other less common ablative techniques include microwave ablation, interstitial laser therapy (ILT), and high-intensity focused ultrasound (HIFU) ablation. These ablative therapies can be guided by ultrasound, stereotactic methods, or MRI. The marked benefit of these ablative approaches is that they can be performed in the office or ambulatory setting with minimal anesthesia and in the future may obviate the need for a surgical incision. To date, all percutaneous ablative approaches have been followed by surgical resection to document pathologic destruction of all viable tissue. However, as data accumulate regarding optimal patient and tumor selection and appropriate use of these techniques, surgical resection of the ablated cancer may not be required.

Radiofrequency Ablation

In radiofrequency ablation (RFA), an electrode is placed percutaneously under radiologic guidance, typically ultrasonography or MRI. The same radiologic method is then used to monitor the thermotherapy during the procedure. The electrode delivers an alternating current that generates ionic agitation, causing friction and thus localized heat production in the targeted tumor. Once target temperatures, which range from 45°C to 50°C, are reached, protein denaturation and coagulative necrosis occur[93] (Fig. 45.8).

RFA has been used to ablate tumors of many histologic types in the liver, lungs, and kidneys. Its complication rate is low, with a mortality rate of less than 0.8% and a morbidity rate of 5% to 10%.[94] This is being further studied in breast cancer through multiple phase II trials.[95–111] All have enrolled fewer than 100 patients, relied on ultrasonographic guidance, and, in general, confirmed that RFA can satisfactorily necrose breast tumors (Table 45.7). Noguchi and colleagues[99] reported the results of 10

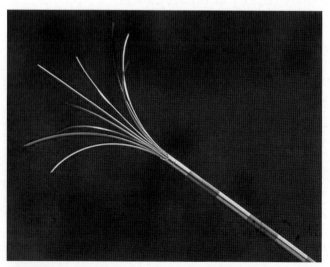

• **Fig. 45.8** Typical radiofrequency ablation probe. (Courtesy AngioDynamics, Inc.)

patients with biopsy-proven invasive (7) or noninvasive breast cancers (3) that were treated with RFA before surgical resection. The average tumor size was 1.1 cm, and no tumor was larger than 2 cm. Maximum ablation temperatures of 95°C were reached in all patients and maintained for 15 minutes. After treatment, seven patients underwent wide local excision, and three patients received total mastectomies. Seven patients underwent sentinel lymph node biopsy, and three underwent complete lymph node dissections. No lymph nodes were positive for metastatic disease. No complications of RFA were noted. Histologic evaluation of the resected specimens showed that on hematoxylin and eosin (H&E)–stained sections, marked changes were observed in less than one third of cancer cells in 9 of 10 patients. Tumor cells ranged from necrotic to normal-appearing. However, when examining nicotinamide adenine dinucleotide–stained sections to assess for tumor viability, the authors found no viable tumor in any of the radiofrequency-ablated regions in all of the treated tumors. This implies that the necrosis zone could be underestimated if assessed by standard histopathologic analysis with H&E staining alone. Others have reported less than 100% complete ablation (see Table 45.7). Klimberg and colleagues described a different concept of percutaneous excision followed by percutaneous ablation using the HUG technique.[108] Using this technique in a phase II trial, 15 patients received radiofrequency ablation, and all showed 100% ablation and negative margins on whole mount pathology of the ablation site. With large vacuum-assisted devices, this seems like a good option. On the basis of these studies, others have reported low morbidity and recurrence in small trials with percutaneous ablation alone without resection with or without radiation and follow-up of patients with periodic fine-needle aspiration or biopsy.[101,112–116] Oura and colleagues reported the largest trial of 52 patients treated with RFA with only one burn. They were followed with FNA biopsy. At 15-month follow-up, they reported only one detected recurrence.[113]

Although most studies have attempted to assess whether RFA is a potential replacement for lumpectomy in breast conserving therapy, one group of researchers has proposed a new use for RFA in the treatment of early-stage breast cancer.[117,118] Klimberg and coworkers proposed that excision followed by intracavitary hyperthermia with RFA (eRFA) could decrease the need for reexcision of inadequate margins, leading to improved cosmesis and a decreased risk of local recurrence without the need for radiation. Two groups of patients were evaluated in their initial study. In the first group, patients underwent prophylactic mastectomy. Ex vivo, the mastectomy specimen was used to simulate a 1 × 1-cm lumpectomy, and the resulting cavity was then subjected to RFA. Pathologic evaluation showed that RFA was associated with a consistent radial ablation diameter, and proliferating cell nuclear antigen staining confirmed 100% nonviable tissue within the ablation zones. The second group of patients underwent lumpectomy and intraoperative eRFA for the treatment of T$_1$ or T$_2$ breast cancers. The average tumor size in this patient population was 1.6 cm. If intraoperative margins were tumor-positive after eRFA, the patient underwent immediate reresection. Ten patients had close (eight patients with 1-mm margins, one patient with a 2-mm margin) or positive (one patient) margins on the final pathologic evaluation. None of these patients underwent reexcision. Seventeen patients with positive nodes underwent post-eRFA radiotherapy, and two others had undergone preoperative radiotherapy. At a median follow-up of 24 months, no patients showed evidence of local recurrence. Two patients had ipsilateral regional recurrences. Long-term results of a single institution

TABLE 45.7 Clinical Trials on Radiofrequency Ablation and Breast Cancer

Authors	Year	n	Tumor Size/Stage	Treatment	Time (min)	IHC Analysis	Complete Ablation (%)	Complications
Izzo et al.	2001	26	T1–T2	LeVeen US-guided RFA (margin >5 mm)	15 × 2	NADH	96	Skin burn (1)
Burak et al.	2002	10	≤2 cm	Radiotherapeutics RFA → surgery after 1–3 wk	30 × 2	CK 8/18 IHC	96	Skin burn (= 1)
Hayashi et al.	2003	22	<3 cm	SB RFA → surgery after 1–2 wk in outpatient setting	15	NADH	19/22	Wound infection (4) Skin necrosis (1)
Fornage et al.	2004	21	≤2 cm	Intraoperative RFA 70 Starbust (SB) & SBXL	15	NADH	100	None
Noguchi et al.	2006	10	≤2 cm	StarBurst RFA → surgery	18	NADH	100	None
Earashi et al.	2007	17	<3 cm	StarBurst	18	NADH	100	None
Khatri et al.	2007	15	≤1.5 cm	Cool-Tip	21 × 22	NADH	100	Skin puckering n = 2
Medina-Franco et al.	2008	25	<4 cm	Elektrotom	11 × 3	NADH	76	Skin burn n = 3
Manenti et al.	2009	34	≤2 cm	RFA → surgery after 4 weeks			33/34	
Imoto et al.	2009	30	≤2 cm	LeVeen	18 × 2	NADH	92	Skin burn n = 2 Muscle burn n = 7
Wiksell et al.	2010	31	<1.6 cm	?	10	H&E only	84	Skin burn n = 1 Muscle burn n = 2 Pneumothorax n = 1
Kinoshita et al.	2010	49	≤3 cm	Cool Tip	9 × 2	NADH	76	Skin Burn n = 2 Muscle burn n = 3
Ohtani et al.	2011	41	<2 cm	Cool Tip	?	H&E only	88	Skin burn n = 1
Klimberg et al.	2011	15	≤1.5 cm	StarBurst XL RFA → surgery	15	PCNA	100	MRI not predictive
Vilar et al.	2012	14	<3 cm	LeVeen RFA → surgery (after 4 wk)	?	H&E only	100	MRI not predictive in 50%
Schassburger et al.	2014	18	<16	NeoDynamics	10	H&E & CK 8 IHC	100	Performed under local anesthesia

H&E, Hematoxylin and eosin; *NADH,* nicotinamide adenine dinucleotide; *PCNA,* proliferating cell nuclear antigen; *RFA,* radiofrequency ablation; *SBXL,* StarBurst XL.

phase II pilot trial of ablation after breast lumpectomy added to extend intraoperative margins (ABLATE I) 100 patients were accrued.[118] Patients with ER + ductal or invasive cancer greater than 3 cm were eligible for the trial. During the study mean follow-up period of 62 months ± 24 months (68-month median follow-up) in patients not treated with radiation therapy, there were two in-site tumor recurrences treated with aromatase inhibitor, three biopsy entrance site recurrences treated with excision and radiation therapy to conserve the breast, and two recurrences elsewhere and 1 contralateral recurrence; all three were treated with mastectomy. The ABLATE II multicenter prospective phase II trial has just closed to accrual (250 patients) and has reported no recurrences on interim analysis at 16 months. This concept will need further follow-up to be offered as an alternative to those who can't or won't take radiation therapy. Previous studies of RFA shed light on several important aspects of the procedure that will prove invaluable as this technique is refined. Tissue acquisition before ablation is essential for tumor confirmation

and tumor marker analysis, optimal ablation occurs most reproducibly in tumors smaller than 2 cm, and tumors treated with RFA must be at least 1 cm away from the skin to minimize the risk of burning local noncancerous tissue. Finally, although ultrasound is convenient and can be performed as an outpatient clinic procedure, it does not accurately measure tumor volume, and thus use of this imaging modality alone may increase the risk of residual (untreated) cancer and local recurrence. This limitation may be addressed by the availability of MRI-compatible RFA probes and the increased use of MRI for initial screening assessment, for probe placement, and for real-time procedure monitoring.

Cryoablation

During cryoablation, a cryoprobe is radiologically guided into the center of the targeted lesion. Cooling gas (argon, nitrogen, or liquid nitrogen) flows into the probe tip and causes a local freezing phenomenon. Usually two or three freeze-thaw cycles in one setting are used in an attempt to eradicate the tumor.

Cryoablation attacks tumor cells in two ways. First, direct cell injury occurs when cells closest to the cryoprobe quickly form intracellular ice, which shears cell membranes. Farther from the cryoprobe, tumor cells are frozen more slowly. Ice forms extracellularly, creating a hypertonic extracellular environment. Osmotic shifts drive water out of the cells, causing dehydration and cell membrane damage. During the thawing cycle, water rushes back into the cells secondary to the relative hypotonicity of the extracellular environment; this results in intracellular edema and lysis (Figs. 45.9 and 45.10).

The second effect of cryoablation is vascular in nature: The initial freeze causes vasoconstriction and a relative decrease in blood flow with anoxia and damages the capillary endothelium, which leads to leakage, thrombosis, and target-tissue anoxia. As blood vessels thaw, a compensatory vasodilation with resultant hyperperfusion, which has been theorized to lead to free radical formation, further exacerbates endothelial damage over several days.[119]

Pfleiderer and associates published a pilot study of 15 patients with T$_1$ or T$_2$ breast cancer who underwent cryoablation.[119] The mean tumor size was 2.2 cm (range, 0.9–4 cm). Sixteen tumors (one patient had multifocal disease) were treated with two freeze-thaw cycles with a minimum freeze cycle temperature of −146°C. Tumors were surgically resected 5 days after cryoablation. Five tumors were smaller than 1.5 cm and showed no remaining invasive carcinoma. Two of these tumors showed DCIS adjacent to the cryoablated lesion. Eleven tumors were 1.6 cm or larger; all showed remnants of invasive carcinoma with subtotal necrosis on H&E-stained sections. In a larger trial, Pfleiderer and coworkers published a larger trial that consisted of 30 patients with tumors 1.5 cm or smaller. Twenty-nine of 30 patients successfully underwent cryoablation. A histologic review of all postresection tumor specimens revealed no viable tumor within the cryoablated lesion. However, remnant DCIS was found beyond the margins of the cryolesions in 5 of 29 patients. Significant complications included one instance of arterial hemorrhaging after cryoprobe removal (attributed to trauma during initial placement of the probe), and a seroma that required no intervention before resection of the primary tumor.[120]

Sabel and colleagues published a multicenter, phase I trial in which 27 of 29 patients with confirmed T$_1$ breast cancers underwent ultrasonographic-guided cryoablation with two freeze-thaw cycles. Continuous ultrasonography was performed during the procedure to analyze the ice ball around the cryoprobe. Surgical resection was performed 1 to 4 weeks after cryoablation. The average tumor size was 1.2 cm. Postresection histologic evaluation revealed no viable invasive cancer in 84% of patients. DCIS was found adjacent to the treatment zone in four patients and was believed to represent multifocal disease in two patients. The likelihood of complete ablation correlated with tumor size, with all tumors smaller than 1 cm completely ablated and 63% of tumors

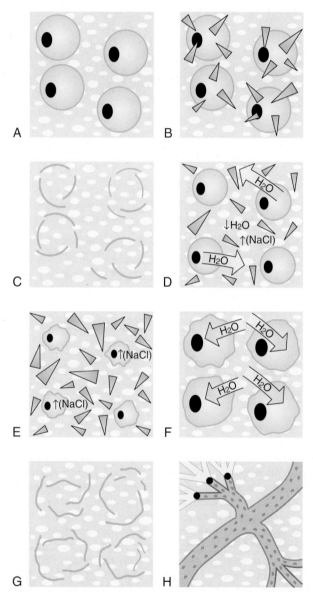

• **Fig. 45.9** Mechanism of cryoablation. (A) Cells in equilibrium. (B) Intracellular ice formation close to cryoprobe. (C) Shearing of cell membranes secondary to extreme cooling. (D) Farther away from the cryoprobe, movement of intracellular water toward the hypertonic extracellular environment. (E) Flaccid cells. (F) Rush of water back into thawing cells. (G) Cytolysis. (H) Capillary endothelial damage creating delayed thrombosis and local hypoxia (3–5 days). (Modified from Kaufman CS, Littrup PJ, Freman-Gibb LA, et al. Office-based cryoablation of breast fibroadenomas: 12-month followup. *J Am Coll Surg.* 2004;198:914-923.)

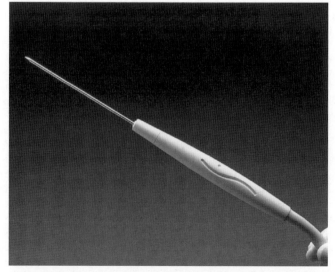

• **Fig. 45.10** Typical cryoablation probe. (Courtesy of Sanarus Medical.)

smaller than 1.5 cm completely ablated. Nodal assessment at the time of surgery revealed that 4 of 25 patients had tumor-positive sentinel lymph nodes, showing that the cryoablation had no effect on subsequent sentinel lymph node analysis.[121] Morin and associates published a phase I study of 25 patients with T_1 or T_2 breast tumors treated with cryoablation. In this study, the safety, efficacy, and predictability of MRI-guided cryosurgery were assessed. Mammography, ultrasonography, scintimammography, and MRI were performed before cryoablation and 1 month after cryoablation, before surgical resection of the ablated tumor. Thirteen cases were declared technically totally complete. Among these cases, no viable tumor cells remained in the surgically resected specimen. This study concluded that the combination of the interventional radiologist's periprocedural radiologic assessment and scintimammographic findings enabled a 96% accurate prediction of histopathologic results.[122]

Most recently the Alliance Cooperative group has reported a large phase II trial exploring cryoablation in the percutaneous treatment of invasive cancers in a multicenter setting.[123] A total of 19 centers contributed 99 patients, of which 86 patients (87 breast cancers) with invasive ductal carcinoma less than 2 cm with less than 25% intraductal component and tumor enhancement on MRI were evaluable for data analysis. Final pathology demonstrated successful ablation in 66 of 87 (75.9%) cancers. The negative predictive value of MRI was 81.2% (90% confidence interval 71.4–88.8). There are certain limitations to cryoablation, not the least of which is that no study today has shown complete ablation to date. Total ultrasound reflection occurs at the ice interface; consequently, no structure is visible beyond the ice ball. Therefore the ice ball's exact dimensions remain unknown when ultrasonography is used for monitoring; however, this drawback may be avoided by using MRI instead of ultrasonography. Another shortcoming of cryoablation is that the ice ball persists for up to 1 month or more postprocedurally, which obscures physical examination and radiology interpretations. No large-scale trials have been performed to test the efficacy of cryoablation for the treatment of early-stage breast cancer. The ACSOG has proposed a phase II trial to determine the rate of complete tumor ablation in breast cancer patients treated with cryoablation. Secondary objectives of this trial include evaluating the negative predictive value of MRI in the postablation setting to determine residual invasive ductal carcinoma or DCIS.

Interstitial Laser Therapy

During interstitial laser therapy (ILT), a percutaneous optical fiber is used to deliver laser light to a targeted tumor. Radiologic guidance is used to place the 16- to 18-gauge probe that contains the optic fiber. The interaction between the laser photons and the tumor results in the absorption, diffusion, and refraction of laser light into the targeted tissue area. The near-infrared photons are absorbed and transformed into heat, causing protein denaturation and coagulative necrosis.[124] Temperatures are monitored with thermal sensors attached to the treatment probe, which allows for measurements of core temperatures during the procedure.[125] MRI thermal mapping, a form of noninvasive real-time monitoring, is additionally available because the optical fibers used in ILT are MRI-compatible.

Few case reports[126,127] of ILT are found in the literature. Harries and coworkers reported a case series of 44 patients with primary breast cancer treated with an 805-nm diode laser placed percutaneously and monitored by ultrasonography or computed tomography before surgical resection. The patients were followed for 2 to 26 months. Three patients had the ILT procedures terminated early because of pain. There were no histologic signs of laser-induced damage within the resected tumors in four patients. One patient had a small hematoma as a result of the procedure. The authors concluded that ultrasonography could not accurately assess laser-induced tissue damage.[128]

Akimov and colleagues reported a case series of 35 patients with primary breast cancer treated with an Nd:YAG 1064-nm pulse-wave laser. Twenty-eight patients underwent laser ablation followed by surgical resection within 1 to 11 days, and seven patients underwent laser therapy alone. The 28 patients who underwent laser ablation and surgical resection had a mean tumor size of 3 cm (range 1–6 cm). Follow-up ranged from 5 to 33 months. Three-year survival was extrapolated to be 92% in the postmenopausal population and 27% in the premenopausal population. In the seven patients who underwent laser ablation without resection, tumor size ranged from 2.5 to 4 cm. Local control was achieved in five of these seven patients. Complications included gaseous rupture of one tumor and skin burns in four patients.[129]

Dowlatshahi and associates reported the largest case series of ILT. The group published findings on 54 patients with T_1 breast cancer treated with an 805-nm laser. Fifty patients had invasive carcinoma, and four had in situ disease. The average tumor size was 1.3 cm (range 0.5–2.3 cm). The average laser energy given was 5900 J (range 2500–14,000 J), the average diameter of necrosis seen was 1.7 cm (range 1–3.2 cm), and the maximum peripheral temperature achieved was 60°C. Forty-eight patients underwent surgical resection after ILT. Complete tumor ablation was seen in 70% of patients. Residual disease was attributed to several factors, including inadequate laser energy (during the learning phase), involuntary motion in an overly sedated patient, technical failures such as malfunctioning thermal probes and fluid pumps, suboptimal target visualization secondary to a post–needle biopsy hematoma and excessive fluid inflation, and large (>2 cm) tumor size. Tumors were not surgically resected in two patients. These tumors were monitored for 6 to 24 months and eventually developed into oil cysts that were percutaneously drained. Acellular debris was present within the cysts.[130]

Van Esser and colleagues reported on 14 patients with small invasive breast carcinomas (mean of 17 mm) that underwent ultrasound-guided laser with a mean treatment time of 21 minutes (range 15–30 minutes). The tumor was completely ablated in seven (50%) of the patients. One patient had a skin burn, and one had a localized pneumothorax.[131] Most recently Haralddottir and colleagues examined and found favorable immune responses in 24 patients with breast cancer with a follow-up time of 116 (range = 91–136) months.[132]

The benefits of ILT include laser fibers that are MRI-compatible and high tissue temperatures that can be achieved extremely quickly but with limited size compared with RFA. Klimberg and colleagues found that laser ILT was much more unpredictable than RFA.[108] However, with its limited target field, ILT requires precise targeting and multiple applications. Additionally, no randomized controlled trials have confirmed the safety and efficacy of ILT for early-stage breast cancer.

Microwave Ablation

In microwave ablation, two microwave phased array waveguide applicators compress the breast. Microwaves applied to the living

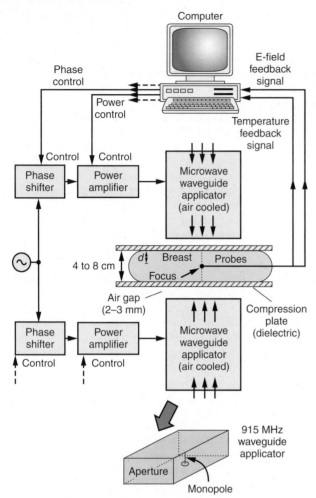

• **Fig. 45.11** Diagram for a dual-channel adaptive microwave phased array thermotherapy system for treating breast cancer. The high water content of breast carcinoma cells means that these cells heat more rapidly than the normal surrounding breast tissue exposed to the microwave field. (Modified from Gardner RA, Vargas HI, Block JB, et al. Focused microwave phased array thermotherapy for primary breast cancer. *Ann Surg Oncol*. 2002;9:326-332.)

phased array therapy were applied to early-stage breast cancers in an attempt to identify the minimal thermal dose required to safely but completely necrose tumor cells. Twenty-five patients with an average tumor size of 1.8 cm underwent 80- to 120-cumulative equivalent minute (CEM) thermal doses relative to 43°C. Escalating doses were applied in cohorts of five patients each. The procedure was terminated early in one patient because of pain. Of the remaining 24 patients, 23 received tumoricidal temperatures (>43°C). Four patients with inaccurate tumor temperature readings and two patients who received suboptimal thermal doses were excluded from the efficacy analysis. Of the remaining 19 patients, 8 patients received CEM thermal doses of 158.9 to 206 minutes; this cohort had a mean 84% (range 60%–100%) tumor necrosis as assessed by H&E staining. Nine patients received a thermal dose of 107.8 to 147.8 minutes. Six of these nine patients displayed a mean 40% (range 25%–95%) tumor necrosis. Two patients received a thermal dose of 82.8 to 97.2 minutes. One of these two patients showed 50% tumor necrosis. From this study, it could be concluded that 140 CEM predicted 50% tumor response and that 210 CEM predicted 100% tumor response. A 50% tumor response was predicted at peak temperatures of 47.4° C, and 100% tumor response was predicted at 49.7°C. Complications reported in the last cohort of study included severe pain in one patient, pain in seven patients, brief skin erythema in four patients, breast or areolar edema in five patients, and skin burns in two patients.[134] This was followed by a randomized institutional trial of preoperative microwave treatment of invasive cancer. Zero of 34 (0%) patients had positive tumor margins, whereas positive margins occurred in 4 of 41 (9.8%) patients receiving BCS alone (*p* = .13). In a randomized study for patients with large tumors, based on ultrasound measurements, the median tumor volume reduction was 88.4% (n = 14) for patients receiving FMT and neoadjuvant chemotherapy, compared with 58.8% (n = 10) reduction in the neoadjuvant chemotherapy-alone arm (*p* = .048).[135] Zhou and colleagues described an ablate-and-resect study of ultrasound-guided microwave coagulation of small breast cancers. Complete tumor coagulation in 95% of cases (36 of 38).[136] However, complications included thermal injuries to the skin and pectoralis major muscle.

High-Intensity Focused Ultrasound Ablation

HIFU ablation is a noninvasive procedure in which a piezoelectric transducer generates focused ultrasound beams that penetrate soft tissue and focus on the targeted tumor. The absorbed energy in the tissue is converted into heat as it propagates through the tumor, leading to peak temperatures of 55°C to 90°C and resultant protein denaturation and coagulative necrosis within seconds. HIFU is the only technique that does not require a probe placement.[137,138] Early attempts at using HIFU ablation were hampered by an inability to accurately define the volumetric dimensions of the targeted tumor mass and the natural variations in tissue densities that caused the mass, which made it difficult to predict not only the shape, size, and location of the tumor but also the amount of ultrasound energy required to reach it. However, advances in imaging technology have made it possible now to accurately identify tumors and their volumetric dimensions. This increased anatomic resolution has led to renewed interest in HIFU. Ultrasonography or MRI can be used to guide the HIFU procedure.

The best studied HIFU ablation technique is magnetic resonance guided focused ultrasound (MRgFUS) ablation. Before

tissue produce dielectric heat by stimulating agitation between water molecules within the tissue; this leads to frictional heating and coagulative necrosis. When applied to cancer cells, microwaves heat the cancer cells with high water contents but not cells with lower water contents such as normal breast adipose and glandular tissue cells (Fig. 45.11).

Gardner and coworkers described a pilot study in which 10 women with breast cancers 0.9 to 4 cm in diameter underwent microwave ablation followed by mastectomy within 27 days. For these patients, the mean tumor equivalent thermal dose was 51.7 minutes (range 24.5–100 minutes), the mean peak tumor temperature was 44.9°C (range 43.3–47.7), and the mean treatment time was 34.7 minutes (range 12–40 minutes). Six patients showed 29% to 60% tumor reduction as assessed by ultrasonography. On histology, four patients showed significant ischemic tumor necrosis (40%–60% of total tumor volume), and six patients showed some degree of tumor apoptosis (82%–97%).[133]

Vargas and colleagues reported a prospective, multicenter phase II trial in which escalating doses of focused microwave

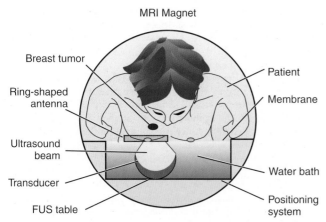

• **Fig. 45.12** Illustration of magnetic resonance imaging *(MRI)*-guided focused ultrasonography ablation system for breast cancer. Transducer-focused ultrasound *(FUS)* beams increase the temperature inside the breast tumor, resulting in coagulative necrosis at the focal point. (Modified from Gianfelice D, Khiat A, Amara M, et al. MR imaging-guided focused US ablation of breast cancer: histopathologic assessment of effectiveness—initial experience. *Radiology.* 2003;227:849-855. © Radiologic Society of North America.)

MRgFUS ablation, the patient is placed in a prone position, and MRI in three planes is used to identify the location and dimensions of the targeted lesion. During the HIFU ablation, the patient's breast is placed in a ring-shaped MRI surface coil, and degassed water is placed between the breast and the ultrasound transducer to enhance acoustic coupling. Patients are usually treated with intravenous analgesics and mild sedatives before the procedure to alleviate pain, anxiety, and claustrophobia, as well as to minimize movement. MRI is used to map temperature changes in real time while the tumor is ablated (Fig. 45.12).

In a feasibility study of MRgFUS ablation of breast fibroadenomas,[139] Hynynen and associates found that temperature alterations inversely affect T_1 tumors' relaxation times, which can be seen on T1-weighted images, and that temperature alterations also affect proton magnetic resonance frequency, which can be seen on phase-shift images. Postprocedure, contrast-enhanced MRI can be used to identify perfused and nonperfused ablated tissue.[140] In the study, 8 of 11 tumors ablated with MRgFUS showed a partial or complete response on postresection pathologic specimen evaluation. The study confirmed the use of temperature-sensitive, phase-difference-based MRI to monitor MRgFUS ablation in real time and the use of T1-weighted postprocedure images to determine response to treatment.

Focused ultrasound can also be performed under ultrasound guidance. Using ultrasonography for guidance, Wu and coworkers enrolled 48 patients, of whom 23 underwent HIFU ablation before modified radical mastectomy. The average tumor size was 3.1 cm (range, 2–4.7 cm). Histopathologic analysis of the resected specimens showed complete tumor necrosis as well as necrosis of the surrounding normal tissue in all patients treated with HIFU.[141] The initial feasibility studies were followed by a series of small phase I and phase II trials of MRgFUS ablation, all with fewer than 30 patients.[141-143] Most recently, Furusawa and colleagues published a study of 21 breast cancer patients treated with MRgFUS ablation, with nodal assessment by sentinel lymph node biopsy or complete dissection without surgical resection of the primary tumor. Follow-up was performed every 3 months with MRI and ultrasonography. Patients had an average tumor size of 1.5 cm and an average follow-up of 14 months. Recurrence occurred in only 1 patient, who had a pure mucinous carcinoma that recurred at 10 months.[144] Complications included breast edema, which usually resolved within 7 to 10 days after the procedure, and pain. Also, intermittent skin burns attributed to technical miscalculations, some requiring resection during postablation surgery, were noted, which have been attributed to technical miscalculations during MRgFUS. The main advantage of MRgFUS ablation is that it is completely noninvasive. Unlike RFA, cryoablation, or laser ablation, MRgFUS ablation does not require an incision for intratumoral probe placement. The technique can also deliver focused energy to the targeted tissue with an accuracy within 1 mm. Additionally, temperature changes are monitored within the tissue in real time, allowing the operator to easily achieve the desired thermal effect within the tissue.[145]

The main disadvantage is the long treatment times (35–150 minutes). Although MRI is more sensitive than either mammography or ultrasonography in assessing invasive cancer, it cannot routinely identify lesions smaller than 5 mm. Additionally, MRI has 80% to 95% sensitivity in detecting invasive breast cancer but it has only 70% to 75% sensitivity in detecting DCIS.[146] MRgFUS can be used to ablate small, focused areas of tissue. Although this is an advantage to targeting only tumor cells, it requires complex treatment planning with multiple overlapping ablation zones.

Irreversible Electroporation

Irreversible electroporation (IRE) is an ablation strategy based on the principle of electroporation in which electric pulses are used to create nanoscale defects in the cell membrane and induce permeability. Thermotherapy techniques destroy both cancerous and normal tissue. In contrast, IRE affects only the cell membrane, leaving intact the extracellular matrix, including ducts, collagen and elastin, and vessels and nerves.[147] In an orthotopic human breast cancer animal model Neal and colleagues have shown the potential of this modality.[148,149] Although this new technique sounds promising, a possible hurdle is the amount of pain associated with it.

Percutaneous or transcutaneous ablation has many issues to answer before becoming a mainstream treatment but when improvements in imaging become a reality so will ablation of breast cancer.

Summary

The advent of screening mammography and its widespread application has resulted in more patients being diagnosed with small invasive breast cancers. Most of these early breast cancer patients can be treated with breast conservation surgery and sentinel lymphadenectomy followed by radiotherapy. Preoperative planning includes a tissue diagnosis of cancer before proceeding to surgery and assessment of whether the patient can receive radiotherapy. Surgical incisions used in breast conservation surgery should be placed such as to maximize cosmesis but not compromise a mastectomy, if one is needed. Surgeons should play an active role in inking the margins and assessing margin status intraoperatively. Shaved margins aid in obtaining negative margins. Sentinel lymphadenectomy for axillary evaluation has become the primary tool in axillary evaluation in patients with early breast cancers. Percutaneous ablation has been shown to adequately treat primary and metastatic disease in multiple organs, including the liver, kidneys, lungs, brain, and prostate. Questions regarding its applicability to breast cancer treatment have arisen over the past 2 decades. Although no large, randomized trials have been performed to assess the feasibility of replacing lumpectomy with percutaneous ablation in breast conserving therapy for early-stage breast cancer, a growing body of literature supports the safety and efficacy of percutaneous ablation and stresses the importance of undertaking such a trial.

Selected References

15. Clifford EJ, De Vol EB, Pockaj BA, Wilke LG, Boughey JC. Early results from a novel quality outcomes program: the American Society of Breast Surgeons' Mastery of Breast Surgery. *Ann Surg Oncol.* 2010;17(suppl 3):233-241.
39. Arentz C, Baxter K, Boneti C, et al. Ten-year experience with hematoma-directed ultrasound-guided (HUG) breast lumpectomy. *Ann Surg Oncol.* 2010;17(suppl 3):378-383.
49. Landercasper J, Attai D, Atisha D, et al. Toolbox to reduce lumpectomy reoperations and improve cosmetic outcome in breast cancer patients: The American Society of Breast Surgeons Consensus Conference. *Ann Surg Oncol.* 2015;22:3174-3183.
54. Chagpar AB, Killelea BK, Tsangaris TN, et al. A randomized, controlled trial of cavity shave margins in breast cancer. *New Engl J Med.* 2015;373:503-510.
63. Buchholz TA, Somerfield MR, Griggs JJ, et al. Margins for breast-conserving surgery with whole-breast irradiation in stage I and II invasive breast cancer: American Society of Clinical Oncology endorsement of the Society of Surgical Oncology-American Society for Radiation Oncology consensus guideline. *J Clin Oncol.* 2014;32:1502-1506.
66. NAPBC Standard Manual 2014 Edition. <https://www.facs.org/~/media/files/quality%20programs/napbc/2014%20napbc%20standards%20manual.ashx>; 2014. Accessed 5 April 2016.
98. Fornage BD, Sneige N, Ross MI, et al. Small (≤2-cm) breast cancer treated with US-guided radiofrequency ablation: feasibility study. *Radiology.* 2004;231:215-224.
108. Klimberg VS, Boneti C, Adkins LL, et al. Feasibility of percutaneous excision followed by ablation for local control in breast cancer. *Ann Surg Oncol.* 2011;18:3079-3087.

A full reference list is available online at ExpertConsult.com.

46

Biological Basis of Radiotherapy of the Breast

SUZANNE EVANS, MELISSA YOUNG, SUSAN HIGGINS, AND MEENA S. MORAN

Radiotherapy Techniques: Introduction

Radiation therapy (RT) is one of the major therapeutic modalities used in the management of early-stage breast cancer and offers significant reductions in local-regional relapse after breast conserving surgery for most patients, as well as a potential for reducing breast cancer–specific mortality risk in selected subgroups. Breast conservation therapy (B), defined as local excision of the primary tumor followed by RT, is considered a standard management option for women with early-stage disease, based on multiple randomized prospective trials of invasive and noninvasive cancers with long-term follow-up.[1,2] In the setting of invasive cancers, RT has been shown to reduce in-breast recurrences by a relative risk reduction of approximately two-thirds and also confers a small, but statistically significant, long-term survival benefit when delivered after breast conserving surgery.[2] Similarly, RT has been demonstrated to reduce both invasive and noninvasive in-breast recurrences by approximately 50% in all subgroups across the wide spectrum of ductal carcinoma in situ (DCIS) subtypes, although the pooled data from meta-analysis fail to show a similar survival benefit with radiation for DCIS.[1] In these early randomized trials that established the integral role of radiation as a component of B, the majority of patients received conventionally fractionated, whole breast radiation therapy (WBRT), delivered to doses of 45 to 50 Gy in 1.8- to 2.0-Gy fractions, over a 5- to 6-week period. Recent technological advancements have resulted in improvements in the therapeutic ratio of RT by minimizing radiation exposure to normal tissue (such as heart, lung, and unaffected breast) while maintaining tumor control and, in some cases, allow for more accelerated treatment delivery in selected patients, with options such as accelerated partial breast irradiation (APBI) and hypofractionated WBRT (hWBRT). This chapter reviews basic rationale and radiobiology of RT and describes modern methods and techniques currently used early-stage breast cancer.

Radiation Therapy Modalities: External Beam Versus Brachytherapy

There are two major, yet very different, modalities for the delivery of RT: (1) external-beam RT (EBRT), in which radiation is generated outside the body and delivers high-energy photon or electron x-ray beams to the intended target (whole breast, lumpectomy cavity, etc.), and (2) brachytherapy, in which radioactive sources are placed inside of the patient in close proximity to the tumor and typically emit radiation of lower energy intended to treat only the volume of tissue in the immediate vicinity to the source. Brachytherapy is the less common delivery technique that mandates dedicated equipment, sources, room shielding, and specific expertise for handling and delivery; EBRT is more widespread and most commonly delivered using cobalt machines or linear accelerators (LINACS). Cobalt machines deliver photon energies of 1.2 and 1.3 MV and have the ability to adequately penetrate and treat most tumors sites that are not located deep within tissue. Several major disadvantages that limit the use of cobalt machines in clinical practice include a larger penumbra (less precisely defined beam edge), inability to deliver adequate doses to deeper tissues, and exposure to radiation to therapy staff from radioactivity from the active Co-60 source. Many of the original RT phase III trials that initially established the benefits of RT used cobalt machines and subjected the patients randomized to radiation in these trials with inadvertent radiation exposure to normal tissues such as heart, lung, and contralateral breast. With long-term follow-up, there is a large body of data demonstrating the subsequent and significant consequences of older delivery techniques including higher risks of second malignancy (in lung and contralateral breast) and, in cases of left breast treatment, development of cardiovascular disease and cardiac-related deaths.[3] Hence, cobalt machines across North America and Europe have mostly been replaced by LINACS in the past 25 years. Unlike Cobalt machines, LINACS do not continuously emit radioactivity so personnel exposure concerns are minimized. Furthermore, additional benefits include, but are not limited to, a wide range of beam energies extending from 4- to 6-MV photons (typically used for breast cancer) to 18 to 20 MV (sometimes used in larger breasted patients but more typically used for deep tumor sites such as those within the abdomen or pelvis). LINACs also offer a range of therapeutic electron beams, which are less penetrating and can be used in combination with photons. Contemporary LINACS also offer automated multileaf collimation, intensity-modulation capabilities, on-board imaging, and other technological advances all designed to deliver a more precise, conformal dose of radiation.

Alternatively, brachytherapy has been used to deliver an additional RT "boost" to the lumpectomy cavity after WBRT, for accelerated partial breast techniques (APBI, discussed later in the chapter), and for previously radiated patients who require retreatment to limited areas such as in the instance of chest wall recurrences. Brachytherapy can be delivered in conjunction with EBRT or alone but is generally not used to implant larger volumes or deeply situated tumor sites such as regional lymph nodes. The brachytherapy procedure typically requires the placement of radioactive sources into temporary catheter(s), which are placed in close proximity to the tumor or tumor bed. Iridium-192 (Ir^{192}) is the most commonly used source, has a half-life of 74.2 days, and emits an average photon energy of 0.38 MV, which allows for feasible shielding against radiation exposure for personnel. Modifications to the rate and distribution of RT into the surrounding tissues can be achieved by varying the type of implant catheters, the number of sources, and their placement. Hence, brachytherapy can be delivered as either "low-dose rate" (LDR) or "high-dose rate" (HDR) (see the ABPI section).

The beam characteristics of electron EBRT, high-energy photon EBRT, and brachytherapy (lower-energy) are important for understanding their application in breast cancer treatment. Generally, the higher the photon energy, the greater the penetration to deeper depths, but the lower RT dose to the skin surface. Electron beams travel a finite depth in tissue, therefore are useful for the RT "boost" dose, where an "en-face" electron field typically delivers RT to a limited area surrounding the lumpectomy cavity after WBRT, or for treatment of the chest wall or internal mammary nodes (for which more superficial treatment is advantageous to reduce exposure to underlying heart and lung). Electron beams similarly increase the depth of penetration with increasing energy; however, unlike photons, surface dose increases with increasing electron energy. The use of various photon or electron beam energies allows for tailoring the radiation dose distribution to the individual patient's anatomy. Alternatively, the low-energy photons emitted from brachytherapy sources (Ir^{192}) do not penetrate tissues deeply and hence only deliver RT to a limited area surrounding the source.

Radiobiological Considerations

The rationale for using conventional fractionation (small daily fractions of 1.8–2.0 Gy per day to a total dose of 45–50 Gy) is based on theoretic radiobiological modeling of the relative sensitivity of normal tissue compared with cancer cells to changes in daily fraction size. Historically, normal tissue, relative to most tumor types, was considered to be more sensitive to fraction size. Thus smaller daily fractions have traditionally been used with the rationale that larger daily fractions theoretically increased the risk of damage to normal cells relative to tumor kill, resulting in a higher potential for late-reacting (normal) tissue complications.[4] Breast cancers, like most other tumors, were presumed to have low sensitivity to changes in fraction size relative to normal tissue. More recently, it was established that for breast cancer explicitly, the sensitivity to fraction size is similar to that of surrounding normal tissue, based on radiobiologic calculations of cell survival curves of breast cancer cells relative to normal breast tissue.[5] For example, for most tumor subtypes, delivering a 2-Gy fraction would result in more tumor kill compared with normal tissue kill, but if fraction size is increased to 4 Gy, normal cell kill becomes increasingly greater than tumor cell kill, resulting in a decrease in the therapeutic ratio (increasing toxicity relative to tumor cell

kill). Unique to breast cancer, however, the cell survival curves of breast tumor cells relative to normal breast tissue are similar, suggesting similar sensitivity to changes in fractionation. Therefore, if increasing the fraction size has minimal effect on the therapeutic ratio in breast cancer, there may be little or no therapeutic advantage to using smaller daily fraction sizes in breast cancer.[4] In fact, these radiobiological estimations are clinically supported by several phase III trials, which randomized patients to conventional fractionation compared with various hWBRT regimens, and suggest similar tumor control and noninferiority in late tissue complications and cosmesis.[5-7] As such, hWBRT is now more routinely incorporated into clinical practice in selected subsets of patients, and has decreased the treatment delivery of EBRT from typically 5+ weeks to 3+ weeks. The vast majority of patients on these trials were treated to the intact breast (not postmastectomy), did not receive regional-nodal radiation or prior chemotherapy, and had invasive cancers, but the indications for appropriate patient populations for hWBRT are evolving.

Anatomic Considerations for Radiation Delivery

As the field of radiation oncology has moved toward more conformal techniques for delivering uniform doses of radiation throughout the breast and chest wall, reconstructed breast or chest wall and nodal target delineation is critical for accurate treatment delivery and better sparing of normal tissue. Significant interobserver variations in target delineation in breast cancer radiotherapy planning have been previously reported.[8-10] Notably, the Radiation Therapy Oncology Group (RTOG) evaluated interobserver variability of target and normal structure delineation of nine radiation oncologists specializing in breast radiotherapy and found as little as 10% overlap, with standard deviations up to 60% in volume variation, for contouring of regional nodes and anatomic structures across this group of breast experts.[11] To promote standardization of target volumes and improve quality, the RTOG created a breast contouring guidelines with accompanying atlas. The consensus guidelines are summarized in Tables 46.1 and 46.2.[12] Using predetermined anatomic definitions, an averaged contour was generated from this cohort of experts and confirmed using consensus software tools.[13] These standards of volume definition should allow for future studies pertinent to radiation therapy techniques and/or treatment volumes to be more consistently report and improve upon reproducibility and generalizability.

External-Beam Techniques and Considerations

Standard Treatment Field Setup

The majority of patients who receive external beam radiotherapy to the intact breast are treated using tangential photon fields. Initially the patient undergoes a "simulation," a procedure to obtain anatomic information that allows the design of the treatment fields. This can be done using a conventional x-ray simulator, which has the same geometry as the treatment machine but provides diagnostic-quality fluoroscopy and x-ray films, or, more recently, with a computed tomography (CT) simulator, which provides axial slices and more anatomic information to

TABLE 46.1   Anatomic Boundaries of Breast and Chest Wall Contours for Radiotherapy Planning

	Cranial	Caudal	Anterior	Posterior	Lateral	Medial
Breast	Clinical reference + second rib insertion	Clinical reference + loss of CT-apparent breast	Skin	Excludes pectoralis muscles, chest wall muscles, ribs	Clinical reference + mid axillary line typically, excludes latissimus dorsi muscle	Sternal-rib junction
Breast + chest wall	Same	Same	Same	Includes pectoralis muscles, chest wall muscles, ribs	Same	Same
Chest wall	Caudal border of the clavicle head	Clinical reference + loss of CT-apparent contralateral breast	Skin	Rib-pleural interface (includes pectoralis muscles, chest wall muscles, ribs)	Clinical reference/mid axillary line typically, excludes latissimus dorsi muscle	Sternal-rib junction

CT, Computed tomography.
Modified from the RTOG Breast Cancer Contouring Atlas. <http://www.rtog.org/CoreLab/ContouringAtlases /BreastCancerAtlas.aspx>. Accessed January 19, 2016.

TABLE 46.2   Anatomic Boundaries of Lymph Node Contours for Radiotherapy Planning

	Cranial	Caudal	Anterior	Posterior	Lateral	Medial
Supraclavicular	Caudal to cricoid cartilage	Junction of brachiocephalic-axillary veins/caudal edge of clavicle head	Sternocleidomastoid (SCM) muscle	Anterior aspect of the scalene muscle	Cranial: lateral edge of SCM muscle Caudal: junction of first rib-clavicle	Excludes thyroid and trachea
Axilla Level I	Axillary vessels cross lateral edge of pectoralis minor	Pectoralis major muscle insert into ribs	Plane defined by anterior surface of pectoralis major and latissimus dorsi muscle	Anterior surface of subscapularis muscle	Medial border of latissimus dorsi muscle	Lateral border of pectoralis minor muscle
Axilla Level II	Axillary vessels cross medial edge of pectoralis minor muscle	Axillary vessels cross lateral edge of pectoralis minor	Anterior surface of pectoralis minor muscle	Ribs and intercostal muscles	Lateral border of pectoralis minor muscle	Medial border of pectoralis minor muscle
Axilla Level III	Pectoralis minor muscle insert on cricoid	Axillary vessels cross medial edge of pectoralis minor	Posterior surface of pectoralis major muscle	Ribs and intercostal muscles	Medial border of pectoralis minor muscle	Thoracic inlet
Internal mammary	Superior aspect of the medial first rib	Cranial aspect of the fourth rib	Encompass the internal mammary/thoracic vessels	Encompass the internal mammary/thoracic vessels	Encompass the internal mammary/thoracic vessels	Encompass the internal mammary/thoracic vessels

SCM, Sternocleidomastoid.
Modified from the RTOG Breast Cancer Contouring Atlas. <http://www.rtog.org/CoreLab/ContouringAtlases/BreastCancerAtlas.aspx>. Accessed January 19, 2016.

individualize dose distribution of the radiation beams. In either case, the patient is placed in the treatment position, typically supine with her arms positioned over her head to move the arm out of the radiation field and reduce the skin fold in the inframammary region. The typical borders of the chest wall/ breast radiation fields are superiorly the inferior clavicular head; inferiorly 2 to 3 cm below the inframammary fold; medially the midsternum; and laterally 2 cm beyond palpable breast tissue (often at the anterior border of the latissimus dorsi muscle). At the time of "simulation," adhesive wires can be placed to encompass the clinical breast volume, as well as to highlight the lumpectomy scar, which are useful to visualize and delineate the clinical breast volume on the imaging with either fluoroscopy or CT images. These images are ultimately used to generate a radiation treatment plan customized for each individual patient's anatomy.

Two-Dimensional Versus Three-Dimensional Conformal Versus Intensity-Modulated Radiation Therapy

Historically, breast radiotherapy treatment planning consisted of two-dimensional planning, which consisted of fluoroscopic simulation to establish treatment fields. The radiation beams were arranged tangentially to limit the exposure to underlying heart, lung, and contralateral breast, but the dose calculations were based on treatment planning using only a single plane in the middle of the breast (central axis). However, given the variations in the contour of breast tissue from its superior to inferior extent, there was significant heterogeneity of the dose distribution across the treatment plan, leading to "hot spots" and or "cold spots" that were not accounted for (i.e., distribution of dose within the breast will be greatest in the thinnest portions of the breast leading to "hot spots" and vice versa). In the modern era of radiotherapy, the use of CT scanners has allowed for three-dimensional (3D) planning to replace earlier two-dimensional (2D)-based planning methods and better define target volumes across the entire breast volume (not just at the central axis) and more precisely avoid organs at risk. Increasingly sophisticated algorithms use 3D information to conform the dose distribution, to the target and provide more homogenous doses of radiation treatment.

Several methods are available to deliver a more homogeneous dose to the breast/chest wall volume. MLC takes advantage of the small computer-controlled motorized small metallic leaves in the head of the machine, which essentially function as automated mini blocks to deliver a more conformal dose by shaping the radiation beam edges. Furthermore, "wedges," are often used, which are wedge-shaped pieces of metal used to attenuate the beam depending on the slope and thickness of the breast or chest wall to achieve a more uniform distribution of the radiation dose by attenuating the dose delivered the breast/chest wall to better match its contour. When electron beams are used, such as for internal mammary nodal treatment or lumpectomy "boost dose," physical blocks are placed in the path of beam in the machine head to deliver a more conformal electron beam dose. Three-dimensional treatment techniques make use of subfields within the larger fields (field in field) to decrease the "hotspots," achieved using the MLCs described earlier. Dose inhomogeneity is associated with worse skin toxicity,[14] breast pain,[15] and poorer long-term cosmesis[16]; therefore these methods are routinely used to improve radiation dose homogeneity. Unlike 2D treatment planning, 3D planning requires evaluation of the dose distribution over the entire breast, not just at the central axis. The field-in-field techniques can be forward or inverse planned, and use "subfields" that block segments of tissue that would otherwise be receiving higher doses (Fig. 46.1). Modifications to the weighting of these subfields and mixing of photon energies can optimize dose homogeneity.

Inverse-planned IMRT (most commonly with coplanar beams) makes use of computerized software that generates the treatment plan and radiation beam specifications using a priority-based algorithm that takes the defined clinical volume relative to prioritized

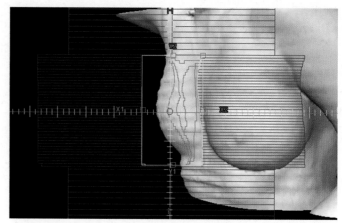

• **Fig. 46.1** A "beam's-eye view" of breast treatment. The open field is outlined in yellow, and the brown outlines are indicative of areas that are blocked during a portion of the treatment to improve dose homogeneity.

dose constraints for normal tissues into consideration. Although inverse-planned IMRT requires less time for planning and can provide excellent homogeneity and normal tissue sparing, particularly for anatomically challenging cases, disadvantages include more radiation monitor units (MU) for treatment and more low-dose radiation exposure to larger volumes of normal tissue, with concerns regarding potential long-term toxicity such as secondary malignancies.[17] Furthermore, IMRT requires longer daily treatment time and increases health care costs and therefore is reserved at our institution for select cases where acceptable dose constraints cannot otherwise be met using 3D conformal RT (3D-CRT) methods.[18,19] Caution should be exercised when considering rotational IMRT techniques or fixed-gantry IMRT techniques using multiple angles and noncoplanar beams, because such methods can increase dose to normal tissue structures.[20] Although standards for homogeneity have yet to be consistently adopted, the RTOG 1005 protocol specifies a maximal hot spot in the breast planning target volume to no more than 115% prescribed dose and aims for no more than 5% of the breast planning target volume to receive more than 110% prescribed dose[21]; Guidelines of the Danish Breast Cancer Cooperative Group describe recommendation for dose distributions ranging from 95% to 107%.[22]

Patient Positioning

The traditional positioning for breast cancer treatment has been supine with arms up over the head, but recent advances in immobilization allow for various other positioning techniques. The prone breast board requires the patient to lay prone on the board with the affected breast hanging down within a "cut-out" section of the board. The prone position is advantageous in selected patients to elongate the breast, produce a more uniform shape to improve dose inhomogeneity,[23] and avoid dose to underlying heart and lung. Its use is limited in that it cannot be used for patients needing regional nodal radiation due to interruption of the beams by the board and treatment table (see "Prone Technique for Cardiac Avoidance" later in the chapter). Lastly, the prone board may not be ideal for patients with lumpectomy cavities that are medial or those close to the chest wall because this position may not adequately allow for treatment of the breast/chest wall volume and may be better treated in the supine position. Patients with bilateral breast cancer are also best treated in the supine position.

Image-Guided Radiation Therapy (IGRT)

Variation in the day-to-day set up can lead to underdosing of the target or overdosing to organs at risk, especially if field edges are adjacent to critical targets and the volume being treated is very conformal to the tumor volume. Furthermore, in patients where the light field of the radiation beam cannot be directly visualized on the skin, such as is the case with some prone breast boards, the accuracy of positioning using standard methods may be difficult to verify in the treatment room. Several image-guided positioning verification techniques may be employed in these settings. These include standard portal imaging, which uses the (megavoltage) treatment beam to obtain an image of the treatment field in relation surrounding soft tissue and bony anatomy that is compared with digitally reconstructed images derived from the treatment planning CT scan. Orthogonal kilovoltage imaging can be obtained to use bony anatomy to confirm setup of the patient in the room and is sometimes used for IMRT or partial breast radiotherapy when exact localization is more critical. Lastly, surface imaging makes use of camera-based imaging to produce a 3D rendering of the patient in real time and can be used to confirm interfractional positioning and intrafractional movement.

Boost Treatment Planning

After whole breast radiation, an additional dose may be delivered to the lumpectomy bed and is often referred to as "boost" treatment. Depending on the depth or location of the lumpectomy cavity, either photon or electron beams may be used. Electron beams are often used in situations in which targets are more shallow in the body and have the advantage of less penetration, and thus the potential for better sparing of surrounding normal tissue (e.g., lung, heart, breast tissue outside of the boost target). Alternatively, for deeper cavities where the electron beams may not provide adequate dose distribution or for centers without electrons, photon beams may be used to deliver the boost.

The lumpectomy cavity can be a challenge to delineate. Radiation oncologists typically rely on the treatment planning CT scan to identify surgical clips in the tumor bed and postsurgical changes including seromas and surgical scar tissue. Delineation of the anterior, posterior, superior, inferior, medial, and lateral aspects of the tumor bed by the surgeon at the time of lumpectomy is the most reliable method for boost cavity delineation, particularly when full thickness closure of the lumpectomy is performed (Fig. 46.2). When superficial closures are performed, the cavity is often easier to delineate; however, boost volumes may be larger as seroma accumulation can be more prominent. Presurgical mammograms and other breast imaging are also sometimes used to determine the location of the tumor bed for boost delineation.

Typically, once the lumpectomy cavity is delineated, a margin of 1 to 2 cm is placed around this region to define the "boost volume."[24,25] In the European Organization of Research and Treatment of Cancer boost trial[26] electrons, photons and brachytherapy boosts were permitted, although treatment planning was primarily performed two-dimensionally. Currently, 3D boost delineation is encouraged because surgical techniques have evolved such that the lumpectomy scar and cavity are not always proximate.

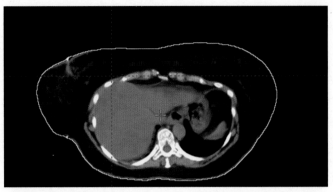

• **Fig. 46.2** An example of a full-thickness closure of a lumpectomy cavity without surgical clips. Although the general surgical area can be estimated, the exact borders of the cavity are indistinct.

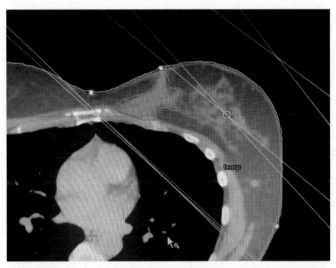

• **Fig. 46.3** A very medial lumpectomy cavity, which makes a heart block difficult. In this case, deep inspiration breath hold technique was used to separate the heart from the lumpectomy cavity.

Cardiac Avoidance in Breast Radiotherapy Planning

The modern radiation oncologist must carefully consider cardiac dose in treatment planning for breast cancer. Darby and coworkers[27] have demonstrated a linear relationship between cardiac dose and cardiac outcome. Current technological advancements that allow for minimizing cardiac dose include heart blocking, enhanced patient positioning and verification, active breathing modalities, accelerated partial breast treatment, altered fractionation, 3D or fixed gantry intensity-modulated radiation therapy (IMRT) treatment planning, and protons.

The Role of the Surgeon

To achieve cardiac avoidance, there needs to be good collaboration between the surgeon and the radiation oncologist. Cardiac avoidance often can involve some interplay between breast coverage and cardiac avoidance (Fig. 46.3). As such, it is absolutely essential that the surgical bed is well visualized (see previous section "Boost Treatment Planning").

Heart Blocks

Individualization of the treatment field with a heart block may be appropriate, in the setting of a readily identifiable lumpectomy cavity. Before placing a heart block, the radiation oncologist should review preoperative imaging to understand the relationship of the tumor to the chest wall. This is particularly important in the setting of oncoplastic reduction or any situation in which the lumpectomy cavity is ambiguous, to avoid placing the heart block in a location that formerly harbored tumor. The use of a heart block typically only reduces the previously targeted breast tissue by 2.8% and has been demonstrated not to compromise local control.[28] In appropriately selected patients, heart blocks offer a simple technique to decrease cardiac volume while maintaining local control.

Patient Positioning

Appropriate patient positioning and immobilization allows for better geometry and treatment angles in women treated for breast cancer, and is a commonly used method to alter distribution of breast tissue and critical normal tissue structures. The use of adequate immobilization has allowed for improved treatment conformality and has advanced the ability of radiation oncologists to achieve adequate normal tissue avoidance.

Supine Breast Board

The use of the breast board promotes the forward movement of the tissues of the breast, which allows for less inclusion of tissues deep to the chest wall.[29] Improvements in position have been shown to reduce the mean cardiac dose in comparison to treatment with flat positioning and collimation.[30]

Prone Breast Board

In a review of women simulated with both prone and supine positioning, prone positioning decreased the volume of heart in the field for 85% of the patients.[31] Women of all breast volumes had a reduction in cardiac volume with the greatest effect noted in larger breast volumes.[31] The radiation oncologist may wish to review a preoperative magnetic resonance imaging scan, if performed, before simulating prone as a minority of women will have their heart fall anteriorly with prone positioning. Although this technique requires experience with the prone board for daily positioning and reproducibility, once mastered, it provides an alternative method for decreasing cardiac dose.

Deep Inspiration Breathing Techniques

Deep inspiration breath hold (DIBH) involves gating both the radiation beam and patient breathing to deliver the radiation only when the heart is most advantageously placed within the chest. DIBH takes advantage of the inferior and posterior displacement of the heart caused by deep inspiration (Fig. 46.4). A CT-based study found the heart is entirely removed from the field in nearly half of the patients, and the use of DIBH results in an 80% reduction in cardiac volumes overall.[32] With either inspiratory gating or DIBH, the median heart volume receiving >50% of the dose has been shown to decrease from 19% to 3%.[33] Hence, the use of gating or DIBH has significantly decreased the cardiac volume and toxicity in the modern era, and is a major advancement in our technology for treating breast cancer patients.

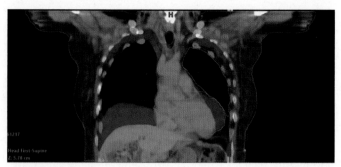

• **Fig. 46.4** The free breathing scan (heart outlined in pink) is blended with the deep inspiration breath-hold scan. Note the inferior and posterior displacement of the heart with this technique.

Accelerated Partial Breast Irradiation

APBI is another means of cardiac avoidance in carefully selected women. For appropriately selected early-stage breast cancer patients, as dictated by national guidelines,[34] APBI is used to treat substantially less normal breast and hence, significantly reduces the dose to the heart (see the later section, "Accelerated Partial Breast Irradiation," and "Radiation Modalities" earlier in the chapter). Data from National Surgical Adjuvant Breast and Bowel Project B-39 protocol demonstrated that for patients with poor cardiac anatomy, 3D-CRT APBI resulted in an 84% reduction in the mean cardiac dose in comparison with WBRT.[34] Regardless of the modality of APBI, the decrease in treated volume offers marked cardiac avoidance, although long-term outcomes of local control from phase III trials have yet to be reported.

Hypofractionation

hWBRT has been demonstrated to be equivalent in terms of tumor control and normal tissue toxicity (see "Radiobiological Considerations and hWBRT" earlier in the chapter).[7] It has been demonstrated that the most the commonly adopted regimens 40 Gy in 15 fractions from the START B Trial[6] and 42.5 Gy in 16 fractions from the Ontario Trial[7] are estimated to deliver less dose to the heart compared with standard fractionation schedules of 50 Gy delivered in 25 fractions, based on radiobiological models that adjusted for fraction size.[35] To further clinically support this, the 10-year update of the START data did not show any increase in cardiac events with hWBRT.

3D Planning

Advances in computerized treatment planning allow for more efficient plan optimization. Several iterations of treatment plans with various energies, mixed energies, beam angles, MLC positioning, and field-in-field arrangements can be developed to decrease the dose to the heart.

Protons

Proton therapy shows great promise in reducing cardiac dose. Lin and colleagues compared DIBH photon IMRT with proton therapy, and the mean cardiac dose could be reduced from DIBH IMRT at 1.6 Gy to as low as 0.009 Gy with proton therapy.[36] However, an added incremental benefit of diminishing cardiac doses to ultra low-dose levels (<2 Gy) has not been demonstrated,[2] so it remains unclear whether the clinical benefit of protons is justifiable given their expense.

Accelerated Partial Breast Irradiation

APBI techniques were developed with the goal of decreasing the overall treatment time associated with standard whole breast radiotherapy. The rationale for treatment of a select portion of the breast, as opposed to the whole breast, comes from data collected in both retrospective and prospective studies showing that the majority of local recurrences occur in close proximity to the tumor bed. Ipsilateral breast tumor recurrences (IBTR) in areas other than the tumor bed are extremely rare and represent only 3% to 4% of all IBTR cases.[37] On the basis of these concepts, APBI techniques were designed to treat a select portion of the breast, usually the lumpectomy cavity plus a margin of approximately 1 to 2 cm, over the course of 1 week. APBI treatment techniques include methods that use external beam photons (3D conformal EBRT), methods that use brachytherapy (such as interstitial or balloon-based brachytherapy), and techniques that deliver photons or electrons to the tumor bed intraoperatively (IORT).

Techniques for Delivery of APBI

External Beam/3D Conformal Radiation Therapy

Methods that use EBRT APBI are delivered after breast conserving surgery, employing multiple external beam fields to target the tumor bed (with margin) while sparing organs at risk, including the thyroid, opposite breast, heart, and lungs. Major advantages of using 3D-CRT include the familiarity of linear accelerators for most radiation oncologists (hence, no special expertise or dedicated equipment required), the noninvasive delivery approach, and the availability of the pathology results of the surgical specimen (including the margin status, size of the tumor, lymph node status, and information regarding focality of the tumor) before treatment, allowing for proper patient selection. Treatment is usually delivered over the course of 5 days/1 week, using 10 fractions that are delivered twice a day, with at least 6 hours between treatments.[38] The total dose ranges from 35 to 38.5 Gy.[38,39] Similar to WBRT planning, a CT is performed with the patient typically in the supine position and should encompass both breasts and normal tissue structures, beginning at or above the mandible and extending below the inframammary fold to include the entire lung. Of note, the delineation of target volumes begins with defining and contouring the excision cavity, and thus it is essential that the excision cavity can be clearly identified on the CT scan. With regard to beam arrangement, a typical 3D-CRT plan uses 4 to 5 noncoplanar beams to meet the dose constraints to normal tissue structures such as heart and lung. Classically, two of the beams are positioned as standard tangents, and the other two to three beams are noncoplanar. In general, none of the beams are directed at the critical normal structures (heart, lung, contralateral breast).

Brachytherapy

In general, there are three categories of brachytherapy techniques for the treatment of breast cancer: interstitial brachytherapy, which uses catheters and individual strands of LDR radiation sources (usually Ir[192] wire) or, alternatively, an HDR source, to encompass the target; balloon brachytherapy, which uses a balloon device to deliver dose to the target; and intraoperative radiation therapy, which uses a device to deliver dose to the tumor bed during surgery.

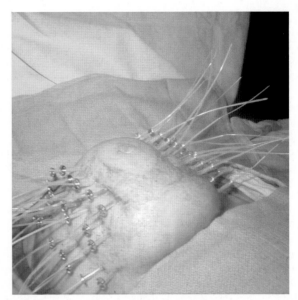

• **Fig. 46.5** A skin rendering of a typical interstitial implant, showing the large number of insertion sites used with protruding catheters. Each insertion site leaves a small scar, which can be cosmetically displeasing to some women.

Interstitial Brachytherapy. Interstitial brachytherapy (IBT) is the oldest of the APBI techniques[40–43] and has the most mature data regarding efficacy and toxicity. However, significant disadvantages of IBT include the relatively complex technique associated with a steep learning curve that requires a high level of expertise and dedicated resources and equipment that are not readily available in all radiation therapy departments. Furthermore, its invasive delivery method with its inherent risk of infection requires the catheters be placed into the lumpectomy bed and left protruding from the skin for at least 1 week after insertion, which some patients may find unpleasant and inconvenient (Fig. 46.5). The number and arrangement of catheters needed for treatment are determined before the procedure. The volume and extent of the cavity are delineated by imaging, which is used to generate a treatment plan using a dedicated brachytherapy treatment planning software. As discussed earlier, brachytherapy can be delivered using either LDR or HDR delivery methods (see "Radiation Modalities"). For LDR procedures, the patient is typically hospitalized in a shielded room for the duration of treatment. As with other LDR brachytherapy procedures, the appropriate radiation safety procedures must be used to minimize exposure to personnel, including the nursing staff. HDR therapy is delivered with a high activity source (most commonly Ir[192]), using a remote afterloading device in a dedicated suite that is specifically shielded for radiation delivery using the given source.

Intracavitary Brachytherapy Balloon-Based Brachytherapy. Like interstitial brachytherapy, intracavitary brachytherapy is an invasive procedure and potentially carries with it the risk of infection. However, compared with interstitial techniques, intracavitary techniques require less expertise and are, from a technical standpoint, more straightforward. Several types of single lumen and multiple lumen balloon catheters are currently commercially available for intracavitary breast brachytherapy. The device can be placed at the time of surgery into an open cavity, inserted after the lumpectomy into the cavity using ultrasound guidance or placed into the closed cavity as a second surgical procedure through the lumpectomy incision site.[44] Placement of the device after surgery allows for evaluation of the final pathologic results of the definitive surgery before insertion of the device, avoiding the risk of aborting the treatment if pathology reveals contraindications to a partial breast approach (e.g., positive margins or positive lymph nodes).[45] Once the treatment device is in place, the patient undergoes a CT can to evaluate the integrity and placement of the balloon. Specifically, the balloon symmetry, integrity of the catheter, the distance of the balloon from the skin, and conformance of the balloon to the cavity are assessed. It is important to confirm that there are no significant pockets of air or fluid between the device and the breast tissue[46] and to ensure the distance of the balloon to the skin is ≥7 mm because this metric has been correlated with a lower incidence of radiation dermatitis, fat necrosis, and skin fibrosis.[44] Once treatment planning is completed, treatment is delivered in the HDR suite using a remote after loading device. Treatment is delivered twice a day, with at least 6 hours between fractions. Each treatment takes approximately 20 minutes. After the last fraction is delivered, the balloon is deflated, and the catheter is removed.

Intraoperative Photon/Electron Radiotherapy. IORT uses a device to deliver radiation therapy to the lumpectomy cavity at the time of surgery. Although the major advantage to IORT is the convenience of receiving the entire course of radiation in a single fraction, problematic issues with this delivery method abound. They include the inability to review final pathology before treatment delivery, inability to accurately verify the doses and volumes of tissue treated, and the risk of the patient requiring a course of standard WBRT in addition to IORT if adverse pathologic features are present.[47] Several portable devices are currently available for IORT. One device delivers low-energy photons (50 kV) using a spherical applicator (diameter 1.5–5.0 cm) that is placed in the region of the tumor bed in direct contact with the breast tissue, delivering 20 Gy at the surface and approximately 5 Gy at a depth of 1 cm over 20 to 45 minutes.[47] Alternatively, a portable linear accelerator is available to deliver electron beams with energies of 6 to 9 MeV to the tumor bed using the applicator tube which is collimated to various diameters (4–8 cm). Before treatment, a lead shield is placed on the pectoralis fascia to protect the lung.[48]

The efficacy and safety of IORT has not been established and requires additional data and longer follow-up.

Conclusions

RT is commonly used in early-stage breast cancer treatment but must be delivered carefully to minimize the risks to critical adjacent structures such as the heart and lung. Technological advances in RT have provided us with various methods for decreasing heart and lung doses, diminishing overall treatment time, and decreasing acute and long-term toxicity with more homogenous dose distributions. These technological advances in RT continue to evolve with even faster and more novel delivery techniques intended to further tailor the treatment to patients' anatomy, improving patient convenience, and ultimately increasing the therapeutic ratio.

Selected References

1. Early Breast Cancer Trialists' Collaborative G, Correa C, McGale P, et al. Overview of the randomized trials of radiotherapy in ductal carcinoma in situ of the breast. *J Natl Cancer Inst Monogr.* 2010;2010:162-177.
2. Early Breast Cancer Trialists' Collaborative G, Darby S, McGale P, et al. Effect of radiotherapy after breast-conserving surgery on 10-year recurrence and 15-year breast cancer death: meta-analysis of individual patient data for 10,801 women in 17 randomised trials. *Lancet.* 2011;378:1707-1716.
3. Clarke M, Collins R, Darby S, et al. Effects of radiotherapy and of differences in the extent of surgery for early breast cancer on local recurrence and 15-year survival: an overview of the randomised trials. *Lancet.* 2005;366:2087-2106.
4. Rowe BMM. Accelerated partial breast irradiation and hypofractionated whole breast radiation. *US Oncol Hematol.* 2011;7:31-37.
5. Group ST, Bentzen SM, Agrawal RK, et al. The UK Standardisation of Breast Radiotherapy (START) Trial A of radiotherapy hypofractionation for treatment of early breast cancer: a randomised trial. *Lancet Oncol.* 2008;9:331-341.

A full reference list is available online at ExpertConsult.com.

47

Radiotherapy and Ductal Carcinoma in Situ

SUSAN A. MCCLOSKEY AND JULIA WHITE

The incidence of ductal carcinoma in situ (DCIS) has risen sharply over the past 2 decades as a result of widespread adoption of screening mammography comprising nearly one in three new breast cancers diagnosed each year.[1] As a result, breast cancer specialists and their patients are faced daily with weighing the multiple treatment options available for DCIS. The local regional treatment patterns for DCIS from 1991 to 2010 in a recent Surveillance, Epidemiology, and End Results (SEER) analysis demonstrated that 69.5% underwent breast conserving surgery and 43% were treated with radiotherapy after breast conserving surgery or lumpectomy.[2] DCIS treated with lumpectomy alone has a distinctive recurrence pattern within the ipsilateral breast characterized by half the events recurring as DCIS and the other half recurring as invasive breast cancer. When breast radiotherapy is used after lumpectomy the primary goals of treatment are prevention of any in-breast recurrence, particularly invasive breast cancer recurrence, and avoidance of mastectomy.

This chapter reviews the current evidence available to guide radiation therapy–specific decision-making after breast conserving surgery and mastectomy for pure DCIS, discusses radiation therapy delivery details, and explores patterns of failure and results of salvage therapy.

Randomized Trials Demonstrate Efficacy of Radiotherapy for Treatment of DCIS

The efficacy of radiotherapy at reducing in-breast recurrence after lumpectomy for DCIS has been demonstrated in five phase III prospective randomized trials (Table 47.1). The first four of these to be conducted—the National Surgical Adjuvant Breast and Bowel Project (NSABP) B-17 trial, the European Organization for Research and Treatment of Cancer (EORTC) 10853 trial, the United Kingdom Coordinating Committee on Cancer Research (UKCCCR) DCIS trial, and the Swedish multicenter (SweDCIS) trial)—now have 15 to 17.5 years follow-up.[3–6] The first trial to be opened was the NSABP B-17 clinical trial, which enrolled 818 women from 1985 through 1990 who had undergone lumpectomy for DCIS with microscopically clear margins and were randomized postoperatively to observation versus whole breast radiotherapy. The most recent analysis done after 17.25 years median follow-up demonstrates a sustained benefit of breast radiotherapy with a 52% reduction in the risk of invasive ipsilateral breast cancer recurrence (hazard ratio [HR] 0.48 95%

confidence interval [CI] 0.33–0.69, $p < .001$) and a 47% relative reduction in the risk of DCIS ipsilateral in-breast recurrence (HR 0.53, 95% CI 0.35–0.8, $p < .001$) compared with those randomized to lumpectomy alone.[3]

The EORTC 10853 trial enrolled 1010 women postlumpectomy with DCIS ≤5 cm in size randomizing cases to observation versus breast radiotherapy over a similar time period (1986–1996). In comparison to NSABP B-17, microscopically clear resection margins were not stipulated for eligibility in this trial, and fewer cases were mammography detected (Table 47.2). However, 15-year outcomes from the EORTC 10853 trial are similar to the NSABP B-17 trial demonstrating a sustained 47% relative reduction in ipsilateral local recurrence and approximately equal reduction in DCIS and invasive cancer recurrences.[4]

The Swedish Breast Cancer group enrolled 1067 women from 1987 to 1999 who had been invited to participate in a mammography screening program and had undergone lumpectomy for DCIS occupying a quadrant or less of the breast. Microscopically clear surgical margins were not required, but a specimen radiograph was done for 97%. At a mean of 8 years of follow-up, a 60% reduction in local recurrence (corresponding relative risk of 0.40; 95% CI 0.30–0.54) was seen with the addition of radiotherapy with similar reductions in risk for ipsilateral invasive and DCIS recurrences.[7] Extended follow-up on this trial was attained by using the unique Swedish national registration number to link the trial database to the Swedish Cancer Registry. With a median follow-up of 17.5 years, 20-year outcomes were reported. In contrast to the other trials, a somewhat smaller overall relative risk reduction of 37.5% was reported in the radiotherapy arm. The cumulative incidence of recurrence was 32.0% in the observed arm (95% CI 28.0–36.0) and 20.0% in the radiotherapy arm (95% CI 16.0–24.0). A much larger relative risk reduction of 67% was seen for DCIS compared with 13.0% for invasive breast cancer recurrence.[6]

The UK/ANZ DCIS Trial accrued 1701 women with DCIS detected in the National Breast Screening Program who had undergone lumpectomy with cancer-free surgical margins between 1990 and 1998. The trial used a 2 × 2 factorial design to assess radiotherapy, tamoxifen, or both in patients with completely excised DCIS. Patients could elect either to enter into the four-way randomization or into one of two separate two-way randomizations. Among the various randomization schemes, 1030 patients were randomized to radiotherapy or observation after lumpectomy. A 68% relative risk reduction and 12.3% absolute

TABLE 47.1 In-Breast Recurrence in Five Phase III Randomized Control Trials Evaluating Radiotherapy for DCIS

Trial	No. of Patients Analyzed	Median Follow-Up (y)	% IPSILATERAL BREAST CANCER RECURRENCE					
			LUMPECTOMY			LUMPECTOMY + RT		
			All	Invasive	DCIS	All	Invasive	DCIS
NSABP B-17[3]	813	17.25	35[a]	19.6	15.4	19.8	10.7	9.1
EORTC 10853[4]	1010	15.7	30[b]	15	15	17	9.5	7.5
UK ANZ[5]	1030	12.7	19.4[c]	9.1	10.3	7.1	3.3	3.8
SweDCIS[6]	1046	17.5	32[d]	—	—	20		
RTOG 9804[9]	629	7.2	7.2[e]	3	4.2	0.8	0.4	0.4

DCIS, Ductal carcinoma in situ; *RT,* radiation therapy; —, data not available in the reference.
[a]Fifteen-year cumulative incidence.
[b]Actuarial 15 years.
[c]Ten-year cumulative incidence.
[d]Ten-year actuarial, 20-year cumulative incidence.
[e]Seven-year cumulative incidence.

TABLE 47.2 Patient and Treatment Variables in the Phase III Randomized Control Trials Evaluating Radiotherapy Effect Postlumepctomy for Ductal Carcinoma in Situ

Trial	Years Accrued	Mammo. Detected (%)	Tamoxifen (%)	Size, Mean	Negative Surgical Margin (%)	High Grade (%)	Comedo-necrosis (%)
NSABP B-17[3]	1985–90	80.5	0	87% <10 mm[65]	100 (82[65])	47[65]	46[65]
EORTC 10853[4]	1986–96	71	0	20 mm	79	38	39
UK ANZ[5]	1990–98	91	53	78% <2 cm[66]	100	75[66]	90[66]
SweDCIS[6]	1987–99	78.7	3	56% <15 mm	80	42[67]	63[67]
RTOG 9804[9]	1999–06	100	62	5 mm	100	0	—

Mammo., Mammogram; —, data point not available in the citation.

risk reduction in ipsilateral cancer recurrences were reported at 10 years (12.7 year median follow-up) with 19.4% recurrences in the observed arm versus 7.1% with radiotherapy (HR 0.32, 95% CI 0.22–0.47, $p < .0001$).[5]

These four trials were included in a meta-analysis by the Early Breast Cancer Trialists' Collaborative Group (EBCTCG) that included 3729 women with a median follow-up of 8.9 years. Radiotherapy approximately halved the rate of ipsilateral breast events (rate ratio 0.46, standard error [SE] 0.05, $2p < .00001$) with no evidence of heterogeneity between the trials in the proportional reduction. Radiotherapy resulted in a larger proportional reduction in the rate of ipsilateral breast recurrence for women more than 50 years of age compared with younger women (rate ratios: age <50 years 0.69, SE 0.12; ≥50 years 0.38, SE 0.06, $2p = .0004$ for the difference between these proportional reductions). The proportional reduction in recurrence by radiotherapy did not differ significantly according to any other clinical or pathologic factor. There was no significant difference in the meta-analysis for breast cancer or overall mortality between treatment arms. There were 50 of 1878 (2.7%) breast cancer deaths for the radiotherapy groups and 44 of 1851 (2.3%) for observation post-lumpectomy. Importantly, there was no significant difference in heart disease deaths in those irradiated versus observed.[8]

The four randomized trials just reviewed were accrued during an era when DCIS was still clinically detected in some, often larger in size, frequently higher grade with significant comedo necrosis and without consistent attention to completeness of excision by negative surgical margins (see Table 47.2). On closer examination, the rise in DCIS incidence seen in the SEER analysis is related to more detection of "noncomedo" DCIS versus higher-risk "comedo" histology that has been relatively stable in incidence.[2] This led to the fifth phase III randomized trial, the Radiation Therapy Oncology Group (RTOG) 9804 trial in "good-risk" DCIS to evaluate whether radiotherapy benefits those who undergo lumpectomy for DCIS with good risk features, that is, mammographically detected, low- or intermediate-grade DCIS, 2.5 cm or less in size, with 3 mm or greater surgical margins. The study did not meet accrual goal and was closed early with 636 enrolled of a planned 1790. The population accrued was uniformly mammography detected, surgical margins consistently negative, with smaller lesion size on average without high nuclear grade compared with the prior phase III trials (see Table 47.2). Roughly two-thirds were treated with tamoxifen. With a median follow-up was 7.17 years, there were 19 in-breast recurrences in the observation arm versus two in the radiotherapy arm. The cumulative incidence of recurrence was 6.7% (95% CI 3.2%–9.6%) in the observation arm versus 0.9% (95% CI 0.0%–2.2%) in the RT arm (HR 0.11; 95% CI 0.03–0.47; p < .001).[9]

Results With Excision Alone in Selected Patients

The majority of women with DCIS are now diagnosed with small, nonpalpable lesions that are detected by mammography. With improved diagnostic, surgical, and pathologic techniques and a better understanding of which factors can affect local recurrence, many investigators have proposed that excision alone may be adequate treatment for DCIS in select women. There have been a series of studies exploring omission in select subsets.

Silverstein and colleagues published results for a nonrandomized series of 706 patients treated in Van Nuys, California, or at the University of Southern California (USC) in Los Angeles (426 by excision alone and 280 by excision and radiotherapy), which showed that the addition of radiotherapy did not decrease the overall rate of local recurrence (17.5% and 16.4% in the two groups, respectively). The authors found that tumor size, margin width, grade, and patient age were independent predictors of local recurrence. They combined these parameters to create the "USC/Van Nuys Prognostic Index."[10] They suggested that patients with intermediate and high scores benefit from the addition of radiotherapy, whereas patients with low scores could be adequately treated with breast conserving surgery alone. Of great importance, the surgical specimens of patients included in this series underwent complete serial sectioning at 2- to 3-mm intervals. Sections were then arranged and processed in sequence. Unfortunately, this kind of painstaking analysis is not available at most treatment centers. Several recent publications that have attempted to validate the USC/Van Nuys Prognostic Index or earlier Van Nuys Prognostic Index have not demonstrated that the score accurately predicts the risk of local recurrence.[11–14]

Two prospective single-arm trials have been conducted in recent years in the United States to test the hypothesis that excision with wide surgical margins may be adequate treatment for patients with small, low-grade lesions. One of these was conducted at the teaching hospitals affiliated with the Harvard Medical School from 1995 to 2002. Eligibility criteria included maximum size of 25 mm, predominant histology nuclear grade 1 or 2, final margins of 10 mm or more or no tumor on reexcision, and no suspicious calcifications on postoperative mammograms. After 158 patients were enrolled, the study was stopped early after a high number of local recurrences were observed. At a median follow-up of 40 months, 13 patients developed an ipsilateral recurrence, for a 5-year actuarial rate of local recurrence of 12%. The authors concluded that radiotherapy could not be safely omitted, even in the population of patients considered to be at lowest risk of recurrence.[15] Updated study results were recently published. With a minimum follow-up of 8 years and a median of 11 years, the 10-year cumulative incidence of local recurrence was 15.6 % indicating substantial and ongoing risk of local recurrence even among women with favorable DCIS undergoing excision alone.[16]

Eastern Cooperative Oncology Group (ECOG) conducted a prospective phase II trial, E5194, of wide local excision alone without radiotherapy for treatment of DCIS. There were two study arms: low- or intermediate-grade DCIS 2.5 cm or less in size and high-grade DCIS 1 cm or less in size. In the low/intermediate-grade arm, 561 women were enrolled, with a median age of 60 and median DCIS size of 6 mm. Thirty-one percent received tamoxifen. In the high-grade arm, 104 women were enrolled before early termination, with a median age of 58 and median DCIS size of 7 mm. Twenty-four percent received tamoxifen. With a median follow-up of 12.3 years, 12-year ipsilateral breast events were 14.4% in the low/intermediate-grade arm and 24.6% in the high-grade arm.[17]

ECOG/ACRIN E5194 and RTOG 9804 suggest that for low- or intermediate-grade DCIS spanning less than 2.5 cm with greater than 3-mm surgical margins, in-breast recurrence rates steadily increase with time but may be acceptably low to justify omission of radiation.

Factors Associated With Local Recurrence

Clinical Factors

Patients presenting with a physical finding (nipple discharge or bleeding, or a palpable mass) have often been found to have a higher rate of local recurrence when treated with breast conserving surgery and radiotherapy than those presenting with only a mammographic abnormality.[4] The poorer prognosis associated with clinical detection may be confounded by young age. Women aged less than 40 to 50 years are less likely to receive regular mammogram screening as their older counterparts. Investigators from MD Anderson Cancer Center found in their large single institutional series of 2037 patients with DCIS, 56.1% of those under 40 years presented with clinical, rather than radiologic, signs of breast cancer, compared with 14% of those over age 40 (p = .001).[18]

Patient Factors

Young age at diagnosis (variously defined as younger than 35, 40, 45, or 50 years) has consistently been associated with higher rates of ipsilateral local failure.[19–23] For example, in the EORTC 10853 randomized trial, women 40 years of age or younger who received radiotherapy had a 10-year local recurrence rate of 34%, compared with 19% for older women.[4] Similar statistically significant differences in local failure in relation to age were demonstrated in two large multiinstitutional retrospective case control studies.[24,25]

In the SweDCIS trial and UK/ANZ trial older women had a proportionally greater benefit from the addition of breast radiotherapy compared with younger women.[5,6] This is further reflected in the EBCTCG meta-analysis where radiotherapy resulted in a larger proportional reduction in the rate of ipsilateral breast recurrence for women aged more than 50 years than for younger women. When the meta-analysis was subdivided into five groups according to age (<40, 40–49, 50–59, 60–69, ≥70), the trend in the proportional reduction in ipsilateral breast recurrence with increasing age was significant (p = .02). The difference between the proportional reduction in recurrence by radiotherapy in younger and older women did not appear to be accounted for by differences in histologic grade or comedonecrosis or by differences in nuclear grade or architecture.[8]

This increased risk of local failure may be related to younger patients having more extensive disease or higher-grade DCIS at presentation, however the recently published Memorial Sloan Kettering Cancer Center experience indicated that recurrence risk decreased with age even after multivariable adjustment for clinicopathologic factors.[20]

Pathologic Factors

Histologic subtype, presence of comedo necrosis, nuclear grade, span/size, biomarkers, and margin status of DCIS have been associated with the risk of local recurrence with or without radiotherapy. NSABP B-17 found the pathologic factors of tumor size >1 cm, presence of comedonecrosis, and margin positivity to significantly affect in-breast recurrence risk.[3] EORTC 10853 found solid or cribriform subtype and positive margins to significantly predict for local recurrence.[4] High grade and large size were found to affect recurrence risk in UK/ANZ[5] and high grade and necrosis were predictive of recurrence in the SweDCIS trial.[6]

In the high-grade arm of the ECOG E5194 observation trial, among 104 women enrolled with a median DCIS size of 7 mm, 12-year ipsilateral breast event rate was 24.6% (vs 14.4% in the low/intermediate-grade arm). The only other variable associated with in-breast recurrence besides trial cohort was DCIS size.[17]

Certain biological markers have also been found to predict local recurrence in DCIS after breast conserving surgery and radiotherapy. Estrogen receptor (ER) negativity, progesterone receptor (PR) negativity, and HER2/neu gene amplification have all been individually associated with an increased risk of local recurrence. In addition, p21-positive DCIS has been found to have a higher risk of recurrence, which is independent of ER, PR, and HER2/neu expression.[26–29]

In most studies with long-term follow-up available, margin status has been associated with the risk of recurrence in patients treated with breast conserving surgery without or with radiotherapy.[3,4,30–32] Investigators at Memorial Sloan Kettering Cancer Center recently examined the impact of margin width on local recurrence among 1374 women treated with excision alone versus 1588 women treated with excision followed by radiation. Among those receiving radiation, 10-year local recurrence rates of 12% and 10% were seen for those with margins of 2 mm or less and greater than 1 cm, respectively. Among those treated with excision alone, 10-year local recurrence rates of 27% and 16% were noted for those with margins of 2 mm or less and greater than 1 cm, respectively. Multivariate analysis indicated that margin width was not a significant predictor of recurrence among women receiving radiation but was highly predictive of recurrence among those undergoing excision alone.[33]

Although margin status is predictive of in-breast recurrence, there remains no consensus as to what the minimum tumor-free margin width should be or whether patients with close or positive margins can be safely treated with breast conserving surgery and radiotherapy. In November 2015, the Society of Surgical Oncology, American Society of Radiation Oncology, and American Society of Clinical Oncology cosponsored a consensus panel on DCIS margins, and we anxiously await publication of the results to inform optimal margins for pure DCIS after excision.

Interestingly, investigators at MD Anderson Cancer Center recently explored rates of residual disease in shaved margins with respect to margin status on main lumpectomy specimen. Rates of residual disease in separately submitted shave margins were 88%, 52%, and 13% in women with positive, less than 2-mm, and greater than 2-mm margins, respectively, indicating that residual disease can be significant, even among women with negative margins.[34]

Imaging Factors

The lack of a postoperative preradiation therapy mammogram to rule out residual calcifications has been correlated with local recurrence. This step was recommended in a 1998 joint statement of the American College of Radiology, the Society of Surgical Oncology, the American College of Surgeons, and the College of American Pathologists.[35] However, Grann and colleagues from Saint Barnabas Medical Center in Livingston, New Jersey, examined findings for 61 patients with DCIS or early invasive cancer who presented with mammographic calcifications and had postoperative mammograms. There were residual calcifications in none of seven patients with close margins (<2 mm) and only 1 of 54 patients with more widely uninvolved margins. Hence, the value of routinely obtaining postoperative mammograms is uncertain.[36]

Tools to Predict Risk

Nomograms have been developed to aid in estimating risk of recurrence after excision alone for DCIS. Investigators from Memorial Sloan Kettering Cancer Center, in an attempt to better provide individualized risk estimates for women with DCIS, combined 10 clinical, pathologic, and treatment factors from 1681 patients into a nomogram that estimates risk of IBTR at 5 and 10 years after breast conserving surgery. Median follow-up was 5.6 years, with 294 women followed for at least 10 years. Internal validation with bootstrap resampling was performed (C-index 0.704; bootstrap validated 0.688). The model separated the population into octiles of 10-year local recurrence risk ranging from approximately 5% to 35%.[37] The model is available as an online tool, where the user can enter the values of all variables and the result is given as a probability of local recurrence at 5 or 10 years (http://nomograms.mskcc.org/Breast/DuctalCarcinomaInSituRecurrencePage.aspx). This nomogram can be particularly helpful in counseling women regarding the anticipated benefits of adjuvant therapy to guide decision-making.

A multigene expression assay, termed Oncotype DCIS, has also been developed to personalize recurrence risk for informed decision making. The Oncotype DCIS score provides an estimate of 10-year risk of any in-breast recurrence (DCIS or invasive) and invasive recurrence among women undergoing breast conserving surgery alone. There have been two validation studies performed, one using data from the ECOG/ACRIN E5194 study and a second using data from the Ontario population-based DCIS cohort. Both validation studies indicated that the Oncotype DCIS score independently predicts and quantifies recurrence risk.[38,39]

Tamoxifen and Radiotherapy

Two prospective, randomized trials have evaluated the role of tamoxifen in women with DCIS treated with breast conserving surgery and radiotherapy (Table 47.3). The NSABP B-24 trial randomized 1798 women treated with lumpectomy and radiotherapy to receive 5 years of tamoxifen or placebo. After a median follow-up of 163 months, the 15-year rate of local recurrence was 16.6% in the placebo group and 13.2% in the tamoxifen group. The absolute reduction was significant for invasive (9% vs. 6.6%) but not for in situ (7.6% vs. 6.7%) recurrence. The rate of contralateral breast cancer was reduced from 8.1% to 4.9% by tamoxifen (p = .023). Overall survival was similar in both arms.[3]

TABLE 47.3   Randomized Trials of Radiotherapy and Tamoxifen in Ductal Carcinoma in Situ

Trial	No. of Patients	Follow-Up (y)	Histology of Recurrence	LOCAL RECURRENCE (%)			NEW CONTRALATERAL PRIMARY (%)		
				No TAM	TAM	P Value	No TAM	TAM	P Value
NSABP B-24[3]	1798	13.6 median	DCIS	7.6	6.7	0.33	2.8	1.6	
			Invasive	9	6.6	0.025	5.3	3.3	
			All	16.6	13.2		8.1	4.9	0.023
UKCCCR[a5]	1576	4.38 median	DCIS	10	7	0.08	NR	NR	NR
			Invasive	4	6	0.23	2	1	0.30
			All	15	13	0.42	3	1	0.07

NR, Not reported; *NSABP*, National Surgical Adjuvant Breast and Bowel Project; *TAM*, tamoxifen; *UKCCCR*, United Kingdom Coordinating Committee on Cancer Research.
[a]Results given include patients who both did and did not receive radiation therapy.

In contrast, the UKCCCR trial did not demonstrate a significant reduction in the risk of ipsilateral breast failure from tamoxifen in the trial as a whole (see Table 47.3) or separately for the 1053 patients treated with excision without radiotherapy (18% crude local failure rate in the placebo arm compared with 17% for the tamoxifen arm) or the 523 patients receiving radiotherapy (6% in both arms).[5] However, only 54% of patients participated in the full 2 × 2 randomization, whereas the others chose whether to take tamoxifen or radiotherapy and were then randomly assigned to the use of the other modality. This design introduces potential bias, and hence it makes interpretation of the results challenging.

There are few data on the role of tamoxifen in DCIS in relation to the tumor's hormone receptor status. Allred and coworkers retrospectively examined the impact of tamoxifen by receptor status among 734 women in NASBP B-24 in whom hormone receptor status was evaluated. Tamoxifen resulted in significant reduction in subsequent breast cancer at 10 years among patients with ER-positive DCIS, whereas women with ER-negative DCIS receiving tamoxifen did not benefit.[40]

NSABP B-35 randomized 3104 postmenopausal women with hormone receptor–positive DCIS after lumpectomy and radiation to tamoxifen or anastrazole for 5 years. With a median follow-up of 9 years, anastrazole resulted in a significant decrease in breast cancer–free interval events versus tamoxifen. The difference was exerted specifically through significant reductions in invasive recurrence and the significant effect was observed only in women under age 60.[41]

Radiation Treatment Techniques

The impact of radiation dose on the risk of local recurrence is uncertain. Several series have found no substantial differences in outcome for the dose range of 50 to 60 Gy, suggesting that a tumor bed dose of 50 Gy may be adequate after lumpectomy with negative margins[42–44] Importantly, the four randomized trials of DCIS after surgical excision used 50 Gy with no tumor bed boost. However, a recent multiinstitutional retrospective analysis from the European Rare Cancer Network found that with a median follow-up of 72 months, patients 45 years of age or younger treated to 50 Gy had a local relapse rate of 28% compared with 14% for patients who received 60 Gy, including that given by a boost to the tumor bed ($p < .0001$).[45]

To address potential overtreatment of DCIS, efforts have been made not only to identify women in whom radiation can be omitted but also to investigate more convenient forms of radiation delivery for those who are advised or elect to receive radiation. Randomized data have emerged to support hypofractionated whole breast radiation and partial breast irradiation among select women with favorable risk invasive breast cancer. Although randomized data are lacking to definitively support alternative fractionation schemes for pure DCIS, several retrospective analyses have been published suggesting excellent outcomes with hypofractionated whole breast radiation and partial breast irradiation for women with DCIS.[46–58] On the basis of emerging data, revision of the American Society for Radiation Oncology consensus statement on partial breast irradiation was recently proposed to include low- or intermediate-grade DCIS, 2.5 cm or less in size, with surgical margins of 3 mm or greater in the acceptable category.

Patterns of Recurrence and Results of Salvage Treatment

Most local recurrences after breast conserving surgery and radiotherapy for DCIS occur in the vicinity of the original tumor site, and approximately 50% are invasive.[3–6,59] Greenberg and coworkers used data from the National Comprehensive Cancer Network Oncology Outcomes Database and from the Cancer Research Network DCIS study to characterize type and treatment of local recurrence after an initial diagnosis of DCIS. Just under 50% of recurrences were invasive, 8.5% experienced a node positive recurrence, and approximately 40% underwent mastectomy at the time of recurrence. Patients who received radiation were significantly less likely to undergo repeat breast conserving surgery than those who did not receive radiation. Among women undergoing reconstruction for recurrence, a greater percentage underwent expander/implant reconstruction who had not received radiation. Surgical complications after surgery for recurrence were significantly more common among women who had received radiation at the time of initial DCIS diagnosis.[60]

The 15-year update of EORTC 10853 reported breast cancer specific survival to be significantly influenced by an invasive recurrence with hazard of dying five times higher compared with patients who did not experience a local recurrence.[4] NSABP B-17 similarly reported significant impact on breast cancer mortality risk among women experiencing an invasive recurrence with a hazard ratio of 7.06 and 10-year probability of breast cancer death 10.4%.[3] In both trials, DCIS recurrence did not affect breast cancer mortality.

Radiation Therapy After Mastectomy

Several recent retrospective analyses have been published assessing postmastectomy recurrence risk in an attempt to identify a subset of women for whom postmastectomy radiation may be beneficial. The studies have failed to identify a high-risk subset. Childs and colleagues retrospectively analyzed 142 women who underwent mastectomy and did not receive postmastectomy radiation. With a median follow-up of 7.6 years, crude rates of chest wall recurrence were 4.8%, 4.3%, and 0% among women with positive, close, and negative margins, respectively.[61] Similarly, Owen and colleagues from British Columbia retrospectively reviewed outcomes according to margin status and other high-risk features among 637 women undergoing mastectomy and no radiation for pure DCIS. With a median follow-up of 12 years, locoregional recurrence (LRR) was 1%. The highest LRR was among women age 40 or younger at 7.5%. No conglomerate of risk factors was found to predict LRR exceeding 15%, and thus the authors concluded that routine use of postmastectomy radiation is not justified.[62]

The MD Anderson group retrospectively analyzed outcomes among 810 women after mastectomy with pure DCIS. With a median follow-up of 6.3 years, among 803 who did not receive postmastectomy radiation, the 10-year LRR rate was 5% for margins 1 mm or less, 3.6 % for margins 1.1 to 2.9 mm, and 0.7 % for margins 3 mm or greater. The MD Anderson series included only five women with positive surgical margins, thus limiting analysis in the positive margin subset.[63] Finally, the largest study published to date retrospectively evaluated outcomes among 1546 women in Ontario who underwent mastectomy for pure DCIS. With a median follow-up of 10.1 years, the investigators were unable to identify a subset of patients with high rate of chest-wall recurrence. Chest-wall recurrence among women age 40 and younger, high-grade DCIS, and positive surgical margins were 5.2%, 3%, and 3%, respectively.[64] Taken together, these retrospective analyses would suggest that postmastectomy radiation is not justifiable for the majority of women with pure DCIS after mastectomy.

Conclusions

Multiple retrospective studies and prospective randomized trials have clearly established the long-term efficacy of breast conserving surgery and radiotherapy in the management of patients with DCIS. Radiation therapy has not been demonstrated to affect breast cancer–specific survival, and thus a careful weighing of risks and benefits must be performed to inform decision-making. Beyond anticipated risk reduction, which has been better honed in recent years via predictive tools and prospective trial data, one must also consider competing risks, radiation risk, patient preference, and salvage options. This era of patient-centered, value-based health care mandates careful consideration of the aforementioned factors to reach a personalized decision for each patient regarding adjuvant radiation therapy.

Selected References

3. Wapnir IL, Dignam JJ, Fisher B, et al. Long-term outcomes of invasive ipsilateral breast tumor recurrences after lumpectomy in NSABP B-17 and B-24 randomized clinical trials for DCIS. *J Natl Cancer Inst.* 2011;103:478-488.
4. Donker M, Litière S, Werutsky G, et al. Breast-conserving treatment with or without radiotherapy in ductal carcinoma in situ: 15-year recurrence rates and outcome after a recurrence, from the EORTC 10853 randomized phase III trial. *J Clin Oncol.* 2013;31: 4054-4059.
5. Cuzick J, Sestak I, Pinder SE, et al. Effect of tamoxifen and radiotherapy in women with locally excised ductal carcinoma in situ: long-term results from the UK/ANZ DCIS trial. *Lancet Oncol.* 2011;12:21-29.
6. Wärnberg F, Garmo H, Emdin S, et al. Effect of radiotherapy after breast-conserving surgery for ductal carcinoma in situ: 20 years follow-up in the randomized SweDCIS Trial. *J Clin Oncol.* 2014;32:3613-3618.
9. McCormick B, Winter K, Hudis C, et al. RTOG 9804: a prospective randomized trial for good-risk ductal carcinoma in situ comparing radiotherapy with observation. *J Clin Oncol.* 2015;33: 709-715.

A full reference list is available online at ExpertConsult.com.

48

Radiotherapy and Regional Nodes

OREN CAHLON AND BERYL MCCORMICK

The importance of regional lymph nodes in breast cancer and their appropriate treatment has undergone dramatic changes in a relatively short period. Although oncologists once considered them the gold standard for prognosis for a patient and prediction of who may benefit from systemic therapy, they have now turned to tumor markers, breast cancer intrinsic subtypes, and the "score" from several available tumor gene sets, such as such as the Oncotype Score (Genomic Health), the Mammoprint, and others. As well, the century-old Halsted concept of the regional lymph nodes as the "next step" toward spread of the cancer from the breast to the nodes and ultimately to distant sites has been replaced with other models, resulting in a marked change in the nodal surgery recommended for a woman with a new breast cancer diagnosis.

These concept changes have had a major influence on the role of radiotherapy (RT) in the management of breast cancer, in addition to the changes in surgical approach. As is clear from recent studies, these new paradigms are applicable to both women who choose breast conservation surgery and those who choose mastectomy. This chapter focuses on recent studies in patients with early-stage breast cancer and the interpretation of the results for radiation treatment planning after breast conservation surgery.

Studies conducted in the 1980s demonstrated the benefit of RT to the chest wall and lymph nodes in women with positive lymph nodes who had a mastectomy followed by systemic chemotherapy and were randomized to receive or not receive postmastectomy RT. These studies demonstrated both a marked reduction in local-regional recurrence and a small but statistically improved survival for those assigned to receive RT.[1–3] Those studies were criticized, however, especially in the United States, for the quite high locoregional recurrence rate in the women who received only surgery as local treatment.

Two new trials, the National Cancer Institute of Canada Clinical Trials Group (NCIC-CTG) MA20 trial[4] and the European Organisation for Research and Treatment of Cancer (EORTC) trial,[5] were conceived to reevaluate the role of nodal RT in women with earlier-stage breast cancer (high-risk node-negative and 1–3 positive nodes), in both patients opting for breast-conservation surgery and those who had a mastectomy.

For women with locally advanced breast cancer (stage III; T3/T4 N1 and T1–4 N2–3), it is generally agreed that the regional lymph nodes should be irradiated, regardless of the type of surgery the patients undergo. This is based primarily on the benefit demonstrated in the randomized postmastectomy radiotherapy (PMRT) trials, which included comprehensive nodal irradiation.[1–3] The primary debate in the patients with stage III disease is whether the internal mammary node (IMN) chain requires coverage.[6] The

debate over the IMN chain is centered around the fact that isolated IMN recurrences in practice are quite rare and that IMN coverage is technically challenging, often increasing unwanted exposure to the heart, lung, and contralateral breast. This topic is discussed briefly in this chapter and also addressed in the chapter on PMRT.

Patient Selection

The debate over the need for nodal coverage in patients undergoing breast conservation with earlier-stage disease (mostly stage II) remains unanswered and is the focus of this chapter. We will consider two distinct groups of patients when considering those who have one to three axillary positive nodes: (1) one to three positive axillary sentinel nodes without completion dissection and (2) one to three positive axillary nodes with completion axillary dissection.

Positive Sentinel Node Without a Completion Axillary Dissection

An important group of patients is those who are clinically node negative and have a positive sentinel node biopsy with minimal disease burden in the axilla. The American College of Surgeons Oncology Group (ACOSOG) Z0011 study was conceived at a time when sentinel node dissection (SLND) was accepted as treatment for women with a negative sentinel node result, but those with a positive sentinel node were routinely undergoing a follow-up full axillary dissection (ALND).[7] This prospective randomized trial was designed to compare completion axillary dissection to no further surgery in women undergoing breast conservation surgery with clinical T1 or T2 N0 M0 breast cancers found to have one or two positive sentinel nodes. Patients with three or more involved sentinel nodes were excluded from the study, as were those "with matted nodes or gross extranodal disease." Approximately 40% of patients in this trial had micrometastases. The primary end point was survival, and the secondary end point was locoregional recurrence. Adjuvant systemic therapy was determined by the treating physician, and whole breast radiation was required, specifically without the use of a "third field" over the supraclavicular region. The originally planned accrual was 1900 patients, but the trial was closed in 2004 with 891 patients randomized, due to "lower than expected accrual and event rates." Published results at a median follow-up time of 6.3 years showed no difference in survival, and no difference in locoregional recurrence between those women randomized to completion ALND and those who received only the sentinel node procedure. The study conclusion was "SLND without ALND can offer excellent regional control and may be reasonable management for selected patients with early-stage breast cancer treated with breast conserving therapy and adjuvant systemic therapy. "

But controversy over this study surfaced soon after the practice-changing surgical results were published, with implications for consideration of postlumpectomy radiation field design.[8] One observation centered on the possibility that some radiation from the tangent breast fields was in fact treating the Level I–II region of the axilla. Was the use of "high tangents" more common in patients who were randomized in the study to the SLND arm only? To address these issues, completed case report forms from the Z 0011 study were reviewed in detail, and more detailed radiation field design information was requested, in a follow-up study by Jagsi and colleagues.[8] Surprisingly, 15% of all women in the study were treated with a third field over the supraclavicular nodes, and from the smaller subset of patients for whom details of radiation field design were known, about half of those with breast tangent fields only had "high tangents," defined as a superior field edge with 2 cm or less from the humeral head, including more of the axilla nodal region. No significant differences in radiation field design were noted between the two Z0011 treatment arms, but the findings of this study confirmed the hypothesis that some of the patients in the study had more nodal irradiation than the Z0011 study design had intended.

The International Breast Cancer Study Group (IBCSG) 23-01 trial had a design similar to the Z0011 trial but included only women with micrometastatic nodal disease and T1-T2 tumors.[9] Additional axillary disease was identified in 13% of patients who had a completion dissection (vs. the 27% in Z0011). This study showed added morbidity with completion dissection and no benefit in terms of disease control, providing additional evidence that ALND is not needed for women with T1–T2 tumors and micrometastases.

For some patients, axillary treatment is still deemed useful. For patients with more than two positive sentinel nodes, axillary treatment is needed. In addition, treatment is recommended for those with high-risk features based on tumor size, type, grade, vascular invasion, and extracapsular extension of cancer in the sentinel nodes. The risk of additional axillary disease can be estimated with the use of a nomogram,[10] which takes these risk factors into account. Several retrospective studies showed that in well-selected, low-risk women, axillary radiation can offer excellent axillary control.[11,12] In 2001, EORTC initiated the 10981-22023 AMAROS trial, a randomized, multicenter, open-label, phase III noninferiority trial in patients with T1–T2 primary, unifocal, invasive breast cancer, with no palpable lymphadenopathy.[13] Patients with tumors of up to 5 cm diameter were eligible. Radiation included the breast/chest wall, axilla, and supraclavicular (with only 10% of patients receiving IMN irradiation). Patients were randomly assigned before any surgery to axillary dissection or axillary radiation if they had a positive sentinel node biopsy. Of the 4806 patients randomized, 30% had positive sentinel nodes. A median of two sentinel nodes were removed and a median of one sentinel node was positive. Approximately 60% of patients had a macrometastasis, and 40% had a micrometastasis or isolated tumor cells. In the axillary dissection arm, 33% of patients had additional axillary metastases. Five-year axillary recurrence was 0.43% (95% confidence interval [CI] 0.00–0.92) after axillary lymph node dissection versus 1.19% (0.31–2.08) after axillary RT. Axillary dissection more than doubled the rate of clinical lymphedema at 5 years (11% vs. 23%). Thus this study

concluded that if further axillary treatment is needed in clinically node-negative, sentinel-node–positive patients, axillary RT could be chosen instead of axillary lymph node dissection because it provides comparable axillary control and less morbidity. Although the National Surgical Adjuvant Breast and Bowel Project B04 trial was conducted many years ago, before sentinel node biopsies and routine use of systemic therapy, that study also showed that, for clinically node-negative women, axillary RT and axillary dissection offer similar rates of long-term axillary control.[14]

Positive Sentinel Node and Completion Axillary Dissection With a Total of One to Three Positive Nodes

For patients who have a sentinel node and completion dissection with one to three positive nodes, there are a number of historical trials, several recent publications, and a few large retrospective series to help guide management. The original rationale for regional node irradiation (RNI) in women with one to three nodes came from the data from the randomized PMRT trials.[1–3] These trials included all node-positive women, including those with one to three nodes. They found a locoregional control, disease-free survival, and overall survival benefit for the entire patient population. However, several large series from Eastern Cooperative Oncology Group trials conducted in the United States in which radiation was not used after mastectomy for women with one to three nodes showed that the locoregional failure rate was much lower than was reported in the randomized trials.[15–17] This led to a number of subset analyses for patients with one to three nodes only, and these analyses continued to show a benefit for this subset of patients.[18,19] However, the subset analysis had the same limitations as the original trials, which were criticized for outdated chemotherapy and inadequate axillary dissections with only an average of eight nodes removed at the time of dissection. The Early Breast Cancer Trialists' Collaborative Group (EBCTG) meta-analysis specifically showed a benefit for women with even just a single positive node.[19] This corroborates prior data showing that the relationship with the most impact may be between a reduction in locoregional recurrence and decreased breast cancer morality in women with a smaller burden of nodal metastases. Women with one to three positive lymph nodes likely have a lower competing risk of distant metastases than those with four or more positive lymph nodes; therefore, a reduction in locoregional recurrence due to locoregional therapies can result in a relatively greater impact on cancer-specific survival.[18,19]

In an effort to better identify criteria for RNI in women with one to three nodes, a number of large retrospective trials from British Columbia and the MD Anderson Cancer Center identified risk factors that place patients at increased risk for locoregional recurrence. MD Anderson had several publications in the early 2000s on a cohort of 1031 women treated with mastectomy and Adriamycin-based chemotherapy without radiation.[20–22] The goal of these studies was to identify risk factors after mastectomy to better select women for PMRT/RNI. These studies identified close or positive margins, microscopic invasion of the nipple, pectoral fascial involvement, presence of lymphovascular space invasion, and gross multicentric disease (>20% nodal involvement, tumors >4 cm, extranodal extension >2 mm) as risk factors for locoregional recurrence. A similar study was published by Truong and colleagues based on 821 treated in British Colombia with mastectomy and systemic therapy but no radiation.[23] They found greater than 25% positive nodal ratio, estrogen receptor (ER) negativity, medial tumor location, and age less than 45 years to be risk factors. On the basis of these factors, clinicians can better estimate the risk of recurrence and potentially avoid overtreating patients at low risk for recurrence.

A randomized study from the Intergroup was launched in 2000 to better characterize the benefit of PMRT in women with T1–T2 lesions and one to three nodes. This study was designed to randomize women, after mastectomy, axillary dissection, and chemotherapy, to PMRT to the chest wall and regional nodes (supraclavicular/axillary apex and IMN chain) but closed due to poor accrual. It is unlikely that this study will be attempted again, and Level I evidence for this particular group of women will not be available.

More modern series from Memorial Sloan Kettering Cancer Center (MSKCC) and MD Anderson have shown that it is possible to identify patients at low risk for locoregional recurrence after mastectomy and chemotherapy.[24,25] Moo and coworkers from MSKCC studied a group of 1087 women with T1/T2 tumors and one to three positive nodes treated at MSKCC from 1995 to 2006. Of this group, 924 did not receive PMRT and 163 received PMRT. Patients who received PMRT were younger, had larger tumors, higher grade, lymphovascular invasion, extranodal extension, and a greater number of nodes. The 5-year rate of locoregional recurrence was equally low in these two groups of patients: 3.2% for RT versus 4.3% for no RT. This suggests that the vast majority of women with one to three nodes do not require PMRT, and those with higher-risk features can have their risk effectively reduced with radiation. This study should not be used to justify that PMRT is not needed in women with one to three nodes. Rather, it supports the selective use of PMRT/RNI in women with risk factors identified in the original MD Anderson and British Columbia papers.

In 2015, three large national trials looking specifically at the question of RNI in lower-risk patients were reported. The data from these trials have lent more support for the use of RNI in women with one to three nodes, although there is still clearly controversy. Given that both also support the use of IMN irradiation (even in relatively low-risk patients), this will likely further the increasing trend of IMN irradiation in the United States. In 2006 a patterns-of-care study showed that IMN irradiation was relatively rare for women with less than 4 nodes.[26] A more recent survey (unpublished Radiotherapy Comparative Effectiveness Consortium [RADCOMP] survey, 2015) showed that there has likely been some more adoption of IMN irradiation in the United States over the past decade.

The NCIC-CTG MA 20 randomized high-risk, node-negative or node-positive breast cancer patients who underwent breast-conservation surgery to whole breast irradiation or whole breast irradiation and regional lymph node irradiation, which included the internal mammary nodes in the first three intercostal spaces, the supraclavicular, and high axillary lymph nodes.[4] High-risk patients were defined as having a 5-cm or larger breast primary or a 2-cm or larger primary with fewer than 10 lymph nodes removed and one of the following higher-risk features: ER-negative, grade III disease, or lymphovascular invasion. Median patient age was 53 years old, and 85% of patients had one to three positive lymph nodes. The primary tumor was larger than 2 cm in 48% of patients, and 43% of patients had grade III disease. Fifty percent of patients had only a single positive node and 75% of patients had ER-positive disease. Nearly all patients received adjuvant chemotherapy (91%), and the majority received adjuvant

endocrine therapy (77%). This trial failed to show a survival benefit, although it did show benefits in locoregional control (95.2% vs. 92.2%), disease-free survival (82% vs. 77%), and distant disease-free survival (86.3% vs. 82.4%). In a prespecified subgroup analysis, patients with ER-negative disease in the nodal irradiation group had a higher 10-year rate of overall survival than did patients in the control group (81.3% vs. 73.9%), a difference that approached statistical significance (hazard ratio 0.69; 95% CI 0.47–1.00; $p = .05$).

Ten-year results from the EORTC 22922 trial were also published in the *New England Journal of Medicine* in 2015 and demonstrated similar results.[5] This trial found that the use of an internal mammary and medial supraclavicular field resulted in a statistical reduction in regional recurrence (4.2% vs. 2.7%) and distant recurrence (19.6% vs. 15.9%), and a trend toward improved overall survival (82.3% vs. 80.7%, respectively; $p = 06$). Eligible patients had pathologically positive axillary lymph nodes or were node negative with central or medial tumors. Median patient age was 54 years. Sixty percent had pT1 tumors, 45% of patients were N0 and an additional 55% had one to three positive nodes, and 74% of patients had ER-positive disease. More than 90% of patients in each study group underwent partial or total axillary lymph node dissection, and the majority of patients received systemic therapy. Although details regarding lymphovascular invasion, extranodal extension, and tumor grade are not available, this seems to be a relatively low-risk patient population to demonstrate a benefit of IMN RT. In the United States, it is relatively rare to offer node-negative patients with small tumors IMN RT. Thus it could be extrapolated that if a group of higher-risk women were included, with higher rates of IMN involvement, the absolute benefit of RT would be greater with a similar relative-risk reduction.

The Danish Breast Cancer Group (DBCG) published a large population-based study demonstrating a survival benefit for IMN RT versus no IMN RT.[27] Although this study was not randomized, its unique design was able to account for biases. In 2003 a decision was made to abandon IMN RT for all left-sided women based on a concern over cardiotoxicity risks of IMN RT and anthracycline use, but to continue to treat all node-positive patients with right-sided breast cancer with IMN RT. Thus although this was not a randomized trial, the unique study design had a naturally random allocation of patients to IMN RT or not. Between 2003 and 2007 3089 patients were treated as part of this study, with 1492 allocated to receive IMN RT based on right-sided disease and 1597 allocated to no IMN RT based on left-sided disease. The patient characteristics were nearly identical between the two groups, as would be expected from a randomized trial. In this study, 60% of patients had one to three positive nodes, 40% were medially located, 42% had T1 tumors, 29% were grade 3, and 20% were ER negative. IMN RT reduced 8-year breast cancer mortality from 23.4% to 20.9%, and overall survival was improved from 72.2% to 75.9% with IMN RT. Subset analysis showed that the benefit was greatest for patients with medially located tumors and four or more positive nodes, with the smallest benefit for women with one to three positive nodes and laterally located tumors. Based on surgical data, it would be expected that patients with medial tumors and larger axillary burden are at greatest risk for IMN involvement.[28]

Although the aforementioned trials have shed significant light on the role of RNI in women with intermediate-risk disease, the community is struggling with the different conclusions reached regarding the need to treat the regional nodes in women with one to three positive lymph nodes, when comparing the Z0011 study to the MA 20 and EORTC trials discussed earlier. However, entry criteria and patient characteristics for these three studies were not identical. The Z0011 study was limited to women with T1–T2 lesions, and the majority, 70%, had T1 breast cancers. In comparison, the EORTC and MA 20 trials allowed up to T3 lesions, with the proportion of T1 cancers in the MA 20 trial about 50%, and in the EORTC trial about 60%. Also, 83% of Z0011 patients were ER positive, an important favorable prognosis marker, compared with only 75% in MA 20. Adjuvant therapy was used in a greater proportion of the Z0011 patients, 96% to 97%, compared with 85% in the other two trials. So in part, the different conclusions can be explained by the Z0011 patients having both a more favorable breast cancer, and a higher likelihood of receiving adjuvant therapy, a treatment recognized to contribute to local and regional control, than MA 20 and EORTC patients.

Accepting the Z0011 surgical conclusions, what should be considered when designing the breast radiation fields? For those women with breast cancer characteristics similar to the more favorable women in the Z0011 study, namely those with T1 lesions, which are ER positive, with involvement of only one axillary lymph node, and who will also be receiving appropriate systemic treatment, the intended breast tangent fields in the Z0011 study should yield the same excellent local-regional control as was demonstrated in the Z0011 study. However, because approximately 50% of patients received high tangents and nearly 20% received a third supraclavicular field, it is possible that it was primarily the 40% of patients with micrometastatic disease who only received breast radiation.

For patients with larger tumors, those with very extensive replacement of the involved sentinel nodes or with extranodal extension, and those with high-grade or estrogen-negative tumors, deliberate inclusion of the lymph nodes at level I–II is a radiation technique to consider because those patients will be at higher risk. Factors such as oncotype score, intrinsic subtype, lymphovascular invasion in the tumor specimen, young age, and ability to tolerate appropriate systemic therapy can also guide the radiation oncologist to design appropriate regional nodal radiation fields in addition to breast radiation. Once a decision is made to treat the nodes, technique is driven by the decisions to include only the level I–II nodes, which can usually be included in the "high-tangent" breast fields, and to include as well the supraclavicular regions and possibly the internal mammary nodes. The techniques discussed in the MA 20 and EORTC section of this chapter are appropriate when more extensive nodal coverage is planned; key to this is contouring the nodes to be included in the patient's treatment plan.

In summary, the Z0011, AMAROS, MA 20, and EORTC trials did not address exactly the same patient populations, and were designed to ask quite different treatment questions. Thus patients with a limited number of positive axillary nodes after breast conserving surgery should be considered in the context of these trials and treated in a way that is consistent with the trial that is most representative of their disease characteristics.

The Z0011 and IBCSG clearly demonstrated that some patients, especially those with micrometastatic disease undergoing breast conservation therapy, do not require axillary surgery or radiation. For patients with slightly higher-risk disease, AMAROS and the modified Z0011 RT fields showed that axillary radiation can safely replace axillary dissection in many patients with one to two positive sentinel nodes and T1–T2 tumors. For patients who still undergo a complete axillary dissection and have one to three positive nodes, the MA 20, EORTC, and DBCG trials established that RNI including IMN RT will improve outcomes for some patients with one to three nodes and T1/T2 tumors, although these studies did not clearly answer which patients need IMN RT and which do not. However, based on the consistency of these results, it is clear that IMN RT can improve breast cancer and overall survival in some patients, and it is important not to undertreat women who can benefit from this. Several recent editorials have shown that there is still significant uncertainty on how to manage the axilla for intermediate-risk patients.[29,30]

Radiotherapy Techniques for Regional Nodes

For many years, two-dimensional planning was used to treat nodal fields based on bony landmarks. Even with the advent of computed tomography–based three-dimensional (3D) planning, many clinicians have continued to use traditional field borders for breast cancer patients. Today 3D-conformal radiation therapy is the most commonly used technique. Many radiation oncologists are now contouring nodal areas at risk (clinical target volumes [CTVs]) for individualized treatment planning but will still often use traditional field borders. The Radiation Therapy Oncology Group (RTOG) atlas was developed to help standardize contouring in the 3D era and many follow this as a general guideline for contouring nodal regions at risk.[31] Similar contouring atlases have been developed by other groups as well and, although they are very similar, there are some subtle differences, reflecting some discrepancies in physician contouring for breast cancer.[32,33] More recently, several groups have reported on patterns of nodal failures.[34–37] On this basis, some of these groups have advocated more generous nodal contours to better cover the posterolateral supraclavicular fossa and possibly even extending the superior border of the supraclavicular field to the cricoid cartilage. However, whether all patients need such generous nodal coverage or whether this should be risk-adapted remains unanswered.[38]

Coverage of the IMN chain with 3D conformal radiation can be achieved with a number of different techniques. Several publications have studies the optimal beam arrangement to maximize target coverage and minimize dose to the surrounding normal structures (lung, heart, contralateral breast).[39–41] As expected, these studies show that there is usually a trade-off between coverage and organ-at-risk doses: techniques with better target coverage typically result in higher organ-at-risk doses. The most commonly used techniques are wide tangent beams or a separate medial electron strip. Intensity-modulated RT/volumetric modulated arc therapy (IMRT/VMAT) are becoming increasingly used for IMN coverage. Most recently, proton therapy has been identified as a particularly good technique for IMN coverage.[42–47] Most physicians choose to cover the first three intercostal spaces for patients receiving prophylactic regional node irradiation (without clinical IMN involvement).[48] For patients with clinical IMN involvement or for primary lesions located in the lower inner quadrant, the first four to five intercostal spaces are usually covered. The lower intercostal spaces are usually more challenging to cover with wide tangents because they often extend down to the level of the heart, and it is difficult to exclude the heart from the tangent fields.

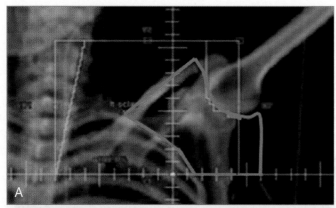

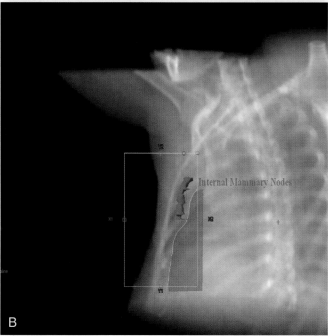

• **Fig. 48.1** (A) Digitally reconstructed radiograph (DRR) demonstrating classic supraclavicular and posterior axillary fields. (B) DRR showing partially wide tangents showing coverage of the upper internal mammary node chain. (From Moran MS, Haffty BG. Radiation techniques and toxicities for locally advanced breast cancer. *Sem Rad Onc.* 2009;19: 244-255.)

3D Conformal Radiation

3D conformal radiation typically uses a 3-, 4-, or 5-field approach to treating the breast/chest wall and nodes, depending on nodal volumes being treated (Figs. 48.1 and 48.2). A classic three-field approach used tangent fields to treat the chest wall/breast and supraclavicular fossa and axillary apex. The supraclavicular field was historically prescribed to a depth of 3 cm, but more recently a prescription depth has been chosen to adequately deliver dose to the designated supraclavicular contour. To cover the more posterolateral portion of the axilla and supraclavicular fossa, a posterior axillary boost can be added as a fourth field to add coverage to the area that is too deep to be reached by the anteriorly angled supraclavicular field. For patients who do not require coverage of the full axilla and more posterolateral portion of the supraclavicular, a fourth field is not needed. A five-field technique uses a medial electron field to cover the IMN chain (matching the shallow tangent fields) and added the aforementioned four

fields (Fig. 48.3). The advantage of the wide-tangent technique is its simplicity. It is achieved by pulling the posterior border of the tangent field posteriorly to encompass the parasternal IMN contour in the first three to five intercostal spaces. A wide tangent field will significantly increase the portion of the lung in the tangent field. Because tangent fields do not have any dose falloff within the field, wide tangents not only increase the low-dose lung exposure (V5–V10), but also the higher-dose lung exposure (V20–V50). In addition, there will often be exposure to the contralateral breast. The medial electron field is a more complicated technique and requires more sophisticated treating planning to properly match the electron field to the shallow tangent field. This technique often gives lower-lung exposure because the electrons have a relatively steep dose falloff and can often give lower heart doses (depending on cardiac anatomy) because the shallow tangents are usually lateral to the cardiac silhouette. The IMN field and tangent field are typically matched on the skin, and this results in an area of chest wall being underdosed, often described as a "cold triangle," and a hot spot in the medial edge of the tangent field because of bowing out of the low-electron isodose levels. In addition, because the electrons are often prescribed to the 90% isodose line, the skin dose is a bit higher in the electron field compared with the breast/chest wall field, increasing acute dermatitis and the potential for permanent skin changes.

A recent publication from MD Anderson showed that, using 3D-conformal radiation with classic fields and techniques, the nodal fields recommended by the RTOG atlas are not entirely covered.[49] Thus although 3D conformal radiation is commonly used and a very good technique for many patients, it has limitations that must be assessed on a case-by-case basis.

Multifield IMRT

Multifield IMRT and VMAT are modern radiation techniques that are now used for select breast cancer patients requiring comprehensive nodal irradiation. Multifield IMRT allows for improved high-dose conformality but at the cost of increased lower-dose exposure (Fig. 48.4). Standard 3D conformal fields result in compromised coverage of target structures. This is probably a reasonable trade-off to lower normal tissue exposure in lower-risk patients. The most common areas that are not completely covered with 3D fields are the IMN chain, posterolateral supraclavicular, and medial and lateral edges of the breast/chest wall. The concave shape of the target volume that includes the medial chest wall/breast/IMN nodes medially and the lateral breast/axilla laterally is well suited for multifield IMRT. It is difficult to sculpt the high isodose lines around this with traditional fields. Studies comparing this technique to 3D-conformal RT show that IMRT/VMAT typically reduce the high-dose exposure to the organs at risk but increase the low-dose exposure due to the "low-dose bath" associated with a multifield technique. For example, the ipsilateral lung V20, V30, V40, and V50 are typically lower with IMRT but the V10 and V5 are higher. Advantages of this technique include the improved homogeneity, obviating the need for matching fields (which create hot and cold spots), faster treatment delivery with VMAT, and high-dose conformality.

Several institutions have completed clinical trials with IMRT for patients requiring comprehensive nodal RT. To our knowledge, there are no published reports of clinical results of IMRT for comprehensive nodal irradiation. Ho reported encouraging early results of a single-arm, phase II protocol from MSKCC in 2013,[50] and longer-term follow-up should be forthcoming.

Proton Therapy

Because of the favorable depth dose characteristics with the Bragg peak, proton-beam therapy allows for more precise dose delivery with maximal sparing of normal tissues (Fig. 48.5). Six dosimetric studies have demonstrated that proton therapy offers optimal target coverage while minimizing heterogeneity and reducing normal tissue exposure.[42–45] Three publications on early clinical results of proton therapy for patients receiving comprehensive nodal irradiation have demonstrated favorable acute toxicity and dosimetry.[44–47] The potential advantages of proton therapy are greatest for patients who require IMN coverage. For patients who do not require IMN coverage, there is typically less need for proton therapy, although there are still some cases with unfavorable cardiac anatomy that can benefit from proton therapy.

Text continued on p. 687

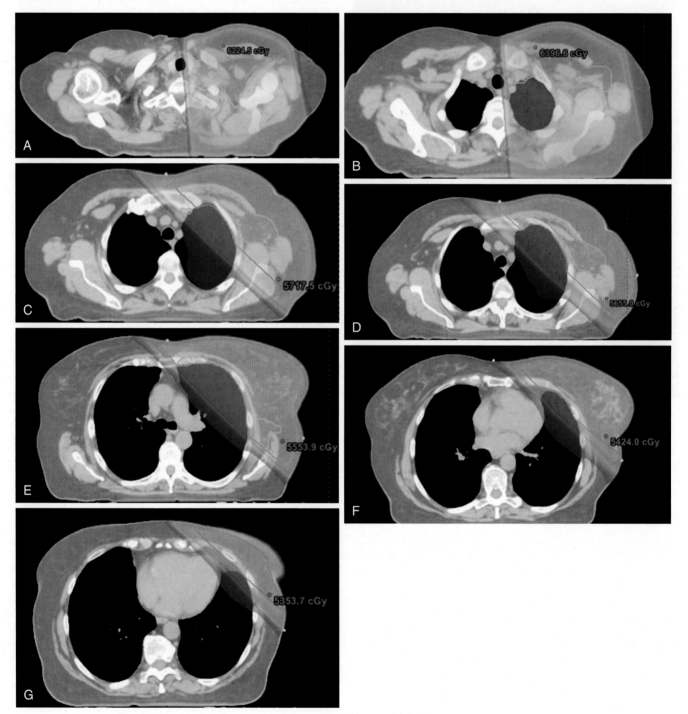

• **Fig. 48.2** Colorwash dose distribution in a patient with stage II left-sided breast cancer receiving postoperative radiotherapy to the left chest wall and regional nodes with a four-field, partially wide tangent technique. (A–G). Axial colorwashes.

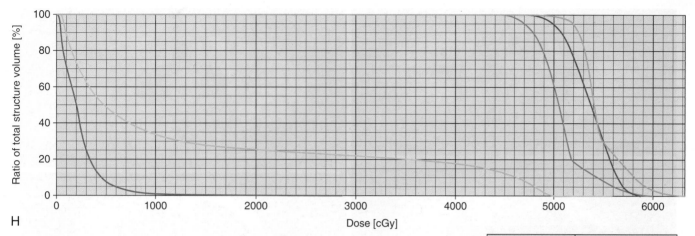

DVH line	Structure
	Heart
	IMN
	SCV
	Axillary nodes

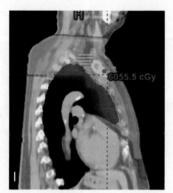

• **Fig. 48.2, cont'd** (H) Dose-volume histogram *(DVH)*. (I) Sagittal colorwash. *IMN,* Internal mammary node; *SCV,* supraclavicular.

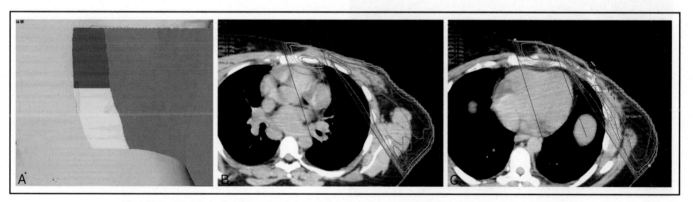

• **Fig. 48.3** (A–C) Skin rendering showing five-field technique with electron strip matched to shallow tangents and axial isodose lines. (From Oh JL, Buchholz TA. Internal mammary node radiation: a proposed technique to spare cardiac toxicity. *J Clin Oncol.* 2009;27:e172-3; author reply, e174.)

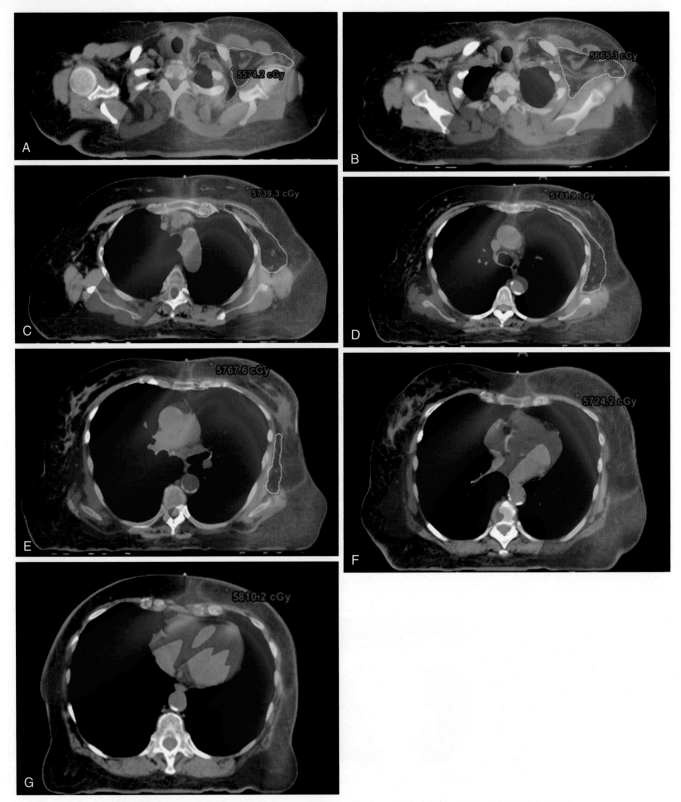

• **Fig. 48.4** Colorwash dose distribution in a patient with stage II left-sided breast cancer receiving post-operative radiotherapy to the left breast and regional nodes with volumetric arc therapy plan and deep inspiration breast hold. (A–E) Axial colorwash. (F) Sagittal colorwash. (G) Dose-volume histogram.

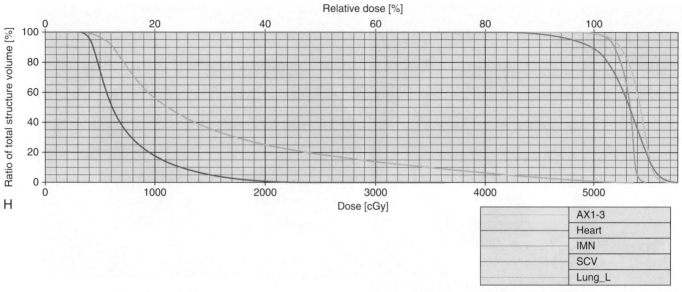

	AX1-3
	Heart
	IMN
	SCV
	Lung_L

• **Fig. 48.4, cont'd** (H) Dose-volume histogram. *IMN*, Internal mammary node; *L*, left; *SCV*, supraclavicular.

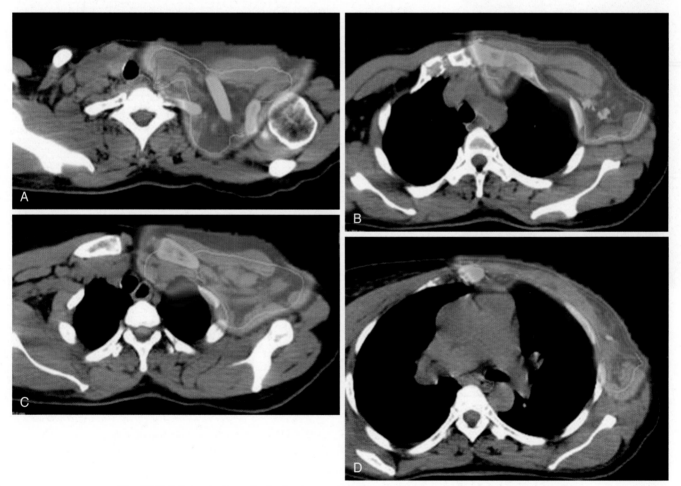

• **Fig. 48.5** Colorwash dose distribution in a patient with stage II left-sided breast cancer receiving postmastectomy radiotherapy to the left chest wall and regional nodes with uniform scanning proton therapy. (A–F) Axial colorwash. *Continued*

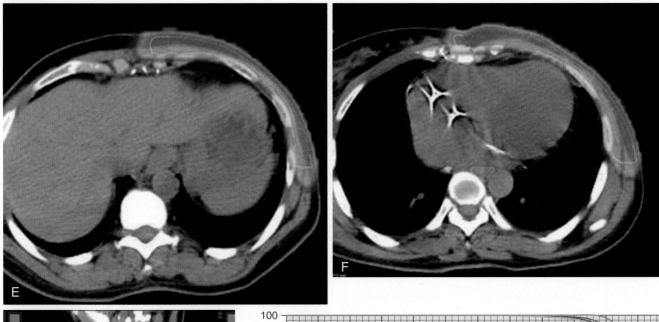

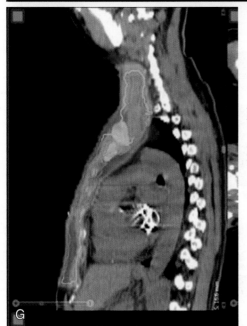

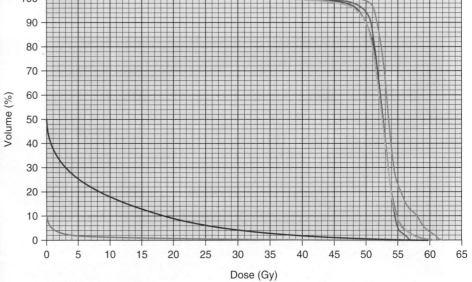

Structures	Min dose (Gy)	Max dose (Gy)	Mean dose (Gy)	Total volume (cc)	Volume at [2.56] Gy
—— PTV50.4-skin	16.33	62.28	52.52	776.55	776.55 cc/100.00%
—— CTV-SCV-50.4	23.27	57.63	52.56	68.75	68.75 cc/100.00%
—— LUNG_L	0	58.2	5.01	1001.97	312.48 cc/31.19%
—— CTV-CW-50.4	1.21	60.74	52.26	483.37	483.37 cc/100.00%
—— CTV-IMN-50.4	46.51	62.27	54.07	8.93	8.93 cc/100.00%
—— HEART	0	50.94	0.38	857.56	23.26 cc/2.71%

☐ White Background

• **Fig. 48.5, cont'd** (G) Sagittal colorwash. (H) Dose-volume histogram. *CTV,* Clinical target volume; *IMN,* internal mammary node; *L,* left; *PTV,* planning target volume; *SCV,* supraclavicular.

The encouraging early clinical results of proton therapy for breast cancer have aided in the development of the RADCOMP trial, a pragmatic randomized control trial of protons versus photons for breast cancer patients requiring comprehensive nodal irradiation including IMN coverage, with the primary end point of reduction in cardiac events at 10 years, which was activated in 2016.[51] The trial will include left- and right-sided cases, breast conservation and mastectomy, and adjuvant and neoadjuvant chemotherapy. The primary eligibility for the trial is the physician intention of IMN irradiation. A biobank and radiorepository are being set up for correlative studies to identify potential biomarkers of late toxicity and to define dosimetric parameters associated with cardiac events, respectively.

Selected References

4. Whelan T, Olivotto I, Chapman J, et al. Regional node irradiation in early stage breast cancer. *N Engl J Med.* 2015;373:307-316.

5. Poortmans PM, Struikmans H, Kirkove C, et al. Internal mammary and medial supraclavicular irradiation in breast cancer. *N Engl J Med.* 2015;373:317-327.

8. Jagsi R, Chadha M, Moni J, et al. Radiation field design in the ACOSOG Z0011 (Alliance) Trial. *J Clin Oncol.* 2014;32:3600-3606.

13. Donker M, van Tienhoven G, Straver M, et al. Radiotherapy or surgery of the axilla after a positive sentinel node in breast cancer (EORTC 10981-22023 AMAROS): a randomized, multicenter, open-label, phase 3 non-inferiority trial. *Lancet Oncol.* 2014;15:1303-1310.

20. Early Breast Cancer Trialists' Collaborative Group. Effect of radiotherapy after mastectomy and axillary surgery on 10-year recurrence and 20-year breast cancer mortality: meta-analysis of individual patient data for 8135 women in 22 randomised trials. *Lancet.* 2014;383:2127-2135.

A full reference list is available online at ExpertConsult.com.

49

Postmastectomy Radiotherapy

PRASANNA ALLURI AND RESHMA JAGSI

Postmastectomy radiotherapy (PMRT) is an integral component of the multimodal treatment of invasive breast cancer in patients with sufficient risk of harboring a reservoir of locoregional disease despite mastectomy and systemic therapy. Microscopic residual disease in the chest wall and/or regional lymph nodes, if left untreated, may seed or reseed distant metastases after initial clearance of distant disease by highly effective contemporary systemic therapies. In addition, occult disease may also serve as a source of locoregional recurrence, which is often highly morbid to the patient in the postmastectomy setting. Therefore, the goal of PMRT is to eliminate residual occult locoregional disease and reduce the risk of both locoregional and distant recurrences.

This chapter focuses on the role of PMRT in the treatment of patients with invasive breast cancer and the evidence regarding the impact of PMRT on locoregional control and overall survival. It begins by reviewing the evidence from randomized trials, followed by a discussion of how best to generalize from these trials and select patients appropriately for treatment, especially among those with N1 and N0 disease, for whom treatment is more controversial. It then turns to special considerations, including axillary management postmastectomy in patients with limited volume node-positive disease treated without axillary node dissection, the role of PMRT in patients who were treated with neoadjuvant chemotherapy, implications of differences in tumor biologic subtype, and the optimal integration of PMRT and breast reconstruction.

Randomized Trials of Postmastectomy Radiotherapy

Although even early randomized trials of PMRT consistently revealed considerable reduction in the risk of locoregional recurrence, initial studies did not demonstrate an improvement in overall survival.[1–3] This is likely due to treatment-related toxicity caused by antiquated radiation techniques such as the classic anterior "hockey stick" photon field, which exposed large volumes of the heart to substantial doses of radiation, resulting in cardiac deaths that offset the salutary effects of PMRT on breast cancer control.[4]

Conclusive evidence for a substantial survival benefit from PMRT was eventually demonstrated in randomized trials from Denmark and British Columbia, initiated in the early 1980s, with landmark publications in the late 1990s. In the British Columbia trial, 318 pathologically node-positive premenopausal patients were randomized to cyclophosphamide, methotrexate,

and fluorouracil (CMF) chemotherapy alone or chemotherapy and PMRT to the chest wall and the regional lymph nodes after modified radical mastectomy with axillary node dissection.[5,6] This study demonstrated both a significant reduction in locoregional failure (from 28% to 10%) and improvement in overall survival (from 37% to 47% at 20 years, $p = .03$) with addition of PMRT. These findings were consistent with the larger Danish 82b trial, which randomized 1708 premenopausal women with high-risk breast cancer (defined as axillary node involvement, tumor size greater than 5 cm, or invasion of the skin or pectoral fascia) to CMF chemotherapy alone or chemotherapy and PMRT after total mastectomy and axillary dissection.[7] This trial also demonstrated both a reduction in locoregional failure (from 32% to 9%) and an improvement in overall survival (from 45% to 54% at 10 years, $p = .001$). The Danish 82c trial, which evaluated the benefits of PMRT in postmenopausal women, randomized 1375 patients younger than 70 years of age with high-risk breast cancer to PMRT and tamoxifen versus tamoxifen alone, after total mastectomy and axillary dissection.[8] This study also demonstrated that PMRT reduced locoregional failure (from 35% to 8%) and improved overall survival (from 36% to 45% at 10 years, $p = .03$). Together the findings from these studies paved the way for a change in paradigm in favor of PMRT in patients with substantial risk of locoregional recurrence after surgery and initial systemic therapy.

Controversies Surrounding Application of Randomized Trial Data in N1 Disease

Some concerns remain, however, regarding the applicability of the findings of these studies to patients who have undergone more comprehensive clearance of axillary levels I and II, which is often the case for patients treated in the United States. The median number of lymph nodes removed in the Danish study (only seven) was lower than what one would expect from a standard axillary dissection of levels I and II performed in the United States. This could have contributed to increased incidence of locoregional failures and amplified the benefit of PMRT; it could also have led to understaging of patients treated on these trials. Of note, locoregional recurrence rates after mastectomy alone in patients with one to three positive lymph nodes were much lower in retrospective American studies of patients treated without PMRT than those noted in the patients treated without radiotherapy in the Danish and British Columbia studies. Analyses of patients treated on Eastern Cooperative Oncology Group[9] and National Surgical Adjuvant Breast and Bowel Project (NSABP)[10] trials suggested a rate of only 13%; other studies, including series from MD

Anderson[11] and the International Breast Cancer Study Group (IBCSG),[12] also demonstrated similar findings. Therefore consensus guidelines developed soon after the landmark publications from these trials did not recommend for or against PMRT for patients with one to three positive lymph nodes,[13] and practice patterns studies showed divided opinion regarding the adoption of PMRT in the United States.[14] The ambiguity remained unresolved after the premature closure in 2003 due to accrual failure of a SWOG/Intergroup randomized control trial designed to assess role of PMRT in patients in the United States with one to three positive lymph nodes.

To address the concerns related to limited axillary dissection, the Danish studies were reanalyzed after pooling the data from both the 82b and 82c studies and including only those patients with 8 or more lymph nodes removed (n = 1152).[15] Remarkably, even though the rates of locoregional failures were lower among patients with one to three involved lymph nodes than those with four or more involved lymph nodes, the same absolute magnitude of survival benefit was observed among these two groups of patients. This was important because a landmark analysis of the Oxford Early Breast Cancer Trialists' Collaborative Group (EBCTCG) comprehensive meta-analysis had suggested that there might be a consistent ratio between prevention of locoregional recurrence and improvement in survival, with one life saved at 15 years for every four locoregional recurrences prevented at 5 years.[16]

More specifically, although initial meta-analyses had raised concerns that any benefits of PMRT were more than offset by cardiac and other toxicity, the 2005 publication reflected the maturation of the large Danish trials and demonstrated a benefit. That study analyzed data from 8340 women with node-positive disease who, after mastectomy and axillary clearance, were randomized to PMRT or no further treatment on trials initiated through 1995. PMRT reduced 5-year local recurrence risk from 22.8% to 5.8%, 15-year breast cancer mortality risk from 60.1% to 54.7% (5.4% absolute risk reduction, $2p = .0002$) and overall mortality from 64.2% to 59.8% (4.4% absolute risk reduction, $2p = .0009$). Yet because this meta-analysis was itself strongly influenced by the inclusion of the large number of patients from the Danish trials, the concerns about inadequate axillary surgery that hampered the interpretation of those trials also extended to this iteration of the meta-analysis.

To address the uncertainty regarding the benefit of PMRT in patients treated with mastectomy and adequate axillary dissection, the EBCTCG more recently performed an updated meta-analysis of 22 trials initiated before 2000 consisting of individual data for 8135 women randomly allocated to adjuvant radiotherapy to the chest wall and regional lymph nodes (supraclavicular or axillary fossa or both, and internal mammary nodes) after mastectomy and axillary surgery versus the same surgery alone.[17] Patients were classified as having axillary dissection (defined as removal of axillary lymph nodes in at least levels I and II or, if this information was not available, removal of at least 10 nodes) or axillary sampling (when less extensive axillary surgery was performed). Among women with axillary dissection and no involved nodes (n = 700), PMRT did not have significant impact on locoregional recurrence, overall recurrence, or breast cancer–specific mortality. Unsurprisingly, for women with four or more involved nodes on axillary dissection, PMRT reduced both locoregional recurrence (from 32.1% to 13.0% at 10 years, $2p = .00001$) and overall recurrence (from 75.1% to 66.3% at 10 years, $2p = .003$), as well as breast cancer–specific mortality (from 80.0% to 70.7% at 20

years, $2p = .04$). More notably, among 1314 women with axillary dissection and one to three involved nodes, for whom the benefit of PMRT had previously not been clearly established, radiotherapy was again observed to reduce locoregional recurrence (from 21% to 4.3% at 10 years, $2p = .00001$), overall recurrence (from 45.5% to 33.8% at 10 years, $2p = .00009$), and breast cancer–specific mortality (from 49.4% to 41.5% at 20 years, $2p = .01$). The vast majority (1133 of 1314) of patients in this group received systemic therapy (CMF or tamoxifen), but the proportional reductions in overall recurrence rates and breast cancer–specific mortality rates did not differ based on whether systemic therapy was given. Furthermore, within the group of 1133 women who had one to three involved nodes on axillary dissection, who received systemic therapy, and for whom additional information regarding the number of positive nodes was available (n = 683), the proportional reduction in locoregional recurrence rate or breast cancer–specific mortality rate did not differ significantly based on whether one, two, or three nodes were involved. Overall, PMRT appeared to prevent one breast cancer death at 20 years for every 1.5 recurrences avoided at 10 years.[17]

These findings have together provided significant impetus for use of PMRT in patients with one to three involved nodes after mastectomy and axillary dissection. For instance, the current National Comprehensive Cancer Network guidelines recommend strongly considering radiation therapy to "chest wall + infraclavicular region, supraclavicular area, internal mammary nodes, and any part of the axillary bed at risk" in this group of patients.[18] Nonetheless, some degree of controversy continues regarding the use of PMRT for patients with one to three involved nodes because the absolute risk of locoregional failure is likely lower with the advent of more effective systemic regimens such as anthracycline-based contemporary chemotherapy regimens, longer courses of endocrine therapy with aromatase inhibitors, and particularly the introduction of targeted agents such as trastuzumab, which were not routinely available in earlier eras. Furthermore, with more screening-detected cancers and surgical and pathologic advances that allow detection of small amounts of nodal involvement, the risk of locoregional recurrence is likely to be even lower among contemporary patients, who have been "upstaged" by more sensitive nodal assessment procedures.[19] Particularly in patients with favorable biology, risks may be considerably lower in the modern era than the 20% documented in the most recent EBCTCG meta-analysis.[17]

Indeed, in an analysis of estrogen receptor (ER)-positive patients enrolled in the NSABP B-28 trial who underwent mastectomy and did not receive PMRT, the 10-year cumulative incidence of locoregional recurrence was less than 10% for those with N1 disease, even among patients with high recurrence score on 21-gene assay.[20] An MD Anderson study presented a retrospective analysis of locoregional recurrence rates in two cohorts of patients with T1–2N1 breast cancer treated with mastectomy and adjuvant chemotherapy, with 19% of patients treated in an early era (1978–1997) and 25% of patients treated in a more recent era (2000–2007) having received PMRT. It revealed that the risk among patients treated in the earlier cohort without PMRT was 9.5% at 5 years and 14.5% at 15 years versus 3.4% at 5 years and 6.1% at 15 years among those who received PMRT; in the later cohort, the 5-year risks were only 2.8% without PMRT and 4.2% with PMRT, leading the authors to conclude that modern treatment advances and the selected use of PMRT for those with high-risk features has allowed for the identification of a cohort at very low risk for LRR in the absence of PMRT.[21] Still, although the lower absolute rates of locoregional recurrence in the absence of PMRT in some of these patient groups suggest that they may not benefit substantially from treatment, it is important to note recent findings from the MA20[22] and EORTC 22922-10925[23] studies that suggest that in some patients with early-stage breast cancer, an important benefit in overall disease control can be attained from comprehensive radiotherapy, even though the risk of regional recurrence itself is not high. There may not be a straightforward ratio between the prevention of locoregional recurrence and the potential for survival benefit.

Special Considerations

Patients With Node-Positive Disease and Undissected Axillae After Sentinel Lymph Node Biopsy

The near universal adoption of sentinel lymph node biopsy as the preferred approach for staging the axilla in recent years has further complicated the management of patients by identifying more patients with limited nodal involvement, including micrometastases and isolated tumor cells. These patients were unlikely to have been included on the randomized trials of PMRT because those patients were treated before sentinel node biopsy techniques made the detection of lower burden axillary nodal metastases more common.

Several recent studies have raised the question of whether select patients with low-volume nodal burden treated in an era of modern systemic therapy require any directed axillary treatment, including subsequent axillary dissection or directed axillary radiation.[19] The IBCSG 23-01 trial randomized patients with primary tumors of 5 cm or less, who on sentinel lymph node biopsy had one or more micrometastatic (defined as less than or equal to 2 mm) sentinel lymph nodes without extracapsular extension, to axillary dissection or no further surgery.[24] The study revealed extremely low axillary recurrence rates and did not show any statistically significant differences in disease-free survival between the two groups (5-year disease-free survival 87.8% in the no axillary dissection group and 84.4% in the axillary dissection group, $p = .16$). However, only 9% of patients in this study underwent a mastectomy, so it is somewhat difficult to draw strong conclusions about the omission of both axillary dissection and PMRT in patients with micrometastatic disease.

The EORTC 10981-22023 AMAROS trial showed no statistically significant difference in axillary recurrence in patients with clinically negative axillae, T1–T2 primary breast cancers, and a positive sentinel lymph node who were randomized to axillary dissection versus axillary radiotherapy.[25] This may increase referral of patients with positive sentinel lymph nodes and no further axillary surgery to radiation oncologists, who must then face complex management decisions in mastectomy patients with incomplete axillary staging information.

Postmastectomy Radiotherapy in Node-Negative Breast Cancer

The use of PMRT in node-negative breast cancer patients is a particularly controversial area. Although the Danish trials included patients with T3–T4 node-negative disease and demonstrated a benefit, recent retrospective pooled analyses, including of five NSABP trials, have suggested that the risk of isolated locoregional failures as a first event in T3N0 patients may be lower (7.1%) than previously expected with omission of radiotherapy after mastectomy.[26] Therefore, many radiation oncologists do not routinely recommend adjuvant radiotherapy in all T3N0 breast cancer patients after mastectomy. Instead a personalized treatment decision based on a number of risk factors such as tumor size, receipt of an inadequate axillary dissection, close or positive margins and the presence of lymphovascular invasion is often warranted.

This is supported by the findings of other studies in node-negative patients with smaller primary tumors, which have suggested that consideration of these other risk factors may predict for locoregional recurrence in the absence of RT.[27–29] In one large retrospective analysis of 1505 T1–2N0 breast cancer patients treated between 1989 to 1999 with mastectomy with clear margins but no adjuvant radiotherapy, histologic grade, lymphovascular invasion, T stage and systemic therapy use were significant predictive factors for locoregional recurrence.[28] For instance, patients with grade 3 disease and concomitant lymphovascular invasion had a locoregional recurrence risk of 21.2% at 10 years. Other retrospective studies have identified tumor size greater than 2 cm, margin less than 2 mm, premenopausal status, lymphovascular invasion, patient age, and nonreceipt of systemic therapy as significant risk factors for locoregional recurrence.[12,27,29] The 10-year risk of rates of locoregional recurrence ranged from 1.2% for node-negative women with no risk factors to 40.6% for women with three risk factors treated in these historical series.[29] These results suggest that the risk of locoregional failure may be substantial in a subset of node-negative patients when PMRT is omitted. However, in the setting of more modern systemic therapy and recognition of the importance of tumor biology, the true risks remain uncertain. Margin status, in particular, has been the subject of recent observational studies, which have suggested that not all patients with close or even positive margins require radiation therapy.[30,31] In sum, the decision regarding PMRT in node-negative patients, particularly those with smaller primary tumors, must be made after comprehensive consideration of the many factors identified in these studies to provide individualized risk assessment for each patient.

Postmastectomy Radiotherapy in Patients Treated With Neoadjuvant Chemotherapy

Although there is considerable evidence from randomized clinical trials evaluating the benefits of PMRT in patients with node-positive breast cancer, none of the patients treated in these trials received preoperative (neoadjuvant) chemotherapy. It has been unclear how best to apply the evidence from the historical PMRT trials to patients treated in the neoadjuvant setting. Therefore retrospective analyses have been undertaken to better guide patient selection in that setting.

Much of the initial information regarding the locoregional outcomes of patients treated with neoadjuvant chemotherapy came from the MD Anderson Cancer Center. Retrospective analyses suggested that patients with locally advanced disease on clinical presentation had a substantial risk of locoregional recurrence in the absence of radiation, even if they had a pathologic complete response to the chemotherapy, with much lower rates when PMRT was administered (33% vs. 3%).[32] However, among the small number of patients with clinical stage I and II disease who achieved a pathologic complete response, there were no locoregional failures at all even in the absence of PMRT.[33]

These findings were further supported by an analysis of patterns of failure after doxorubicin/cyclophosphamide-based neoadjuvant chemotherapy and mastectomy in patients enrolled in the large NSABP B18 and B27 trials (in whom PMRT was prohibited). This analysis revealed that 10-year locoregional recurrence rates in patients with a complete pathologic response in both the nodes and breast were less than 10%, regardless of the tumor size or whether the axilla was clinically positive or negative.[34] On the other hand, patients with pathologically positive nodes after neoadjuvant chemotherapy had more substantial risk of locoregional recurrence after mastectomy without radiotherapy.

More recently, the CTNeoBC investigators combined the pathologic complete response evaluation with information with tumor biology to optimize locoregional management decision in patients receiving neoadjuvant chemotherapy.[35] Their analysis included more than 13,000 patients enrolled in 12 trials of neoadjuvant chemotherapy and most patients received anthracycline and/or taxane-based regimens, with a few trials including trastuzumab. All patients with hormone receptor–positive tumors were supposed to receive at least 5 years of endocrine therapy. Radiotherapy was not administered in a randomized fashion and criteria for administration differed across the studies.

The pathologic complete response was evaluated based on three definitions:

1. absence of invasive cancer and in situ disease in both the breast and nodes (ypT0 ypN0),
2. absence of invasive cancer in the breast and nodes irrespective of the presence of in situ disease in the breast (ypT0/is ypN0), and
3. absence of invasive cancer in the breast irrespective of in situ disease in the breast or disease in the nodes (ypT0/is)

The study has shown that more aggressive subtypes had higher rates of complete pathologic response: 50.3% in HER2-positive, hormone receptor–negative tumors treated with trastuzumab; 33.6% for triple-negative tumors; and 7.5% for hormone receptor–positive, HER2-negative grade 1/2 tumors.[35] Patients with HER2 positive, hormone receptor–negative tumors and triple-negative tumors had the strongest association between pathologic complete response (CR) and long-term outcomes. Triple-negative patients with a pathologic CR had a low 5-year locoregional recurrence of 6.2% after mastectomy, but recurrence risk was significantly elevated at 22.1% when residual nodal disease was present. Similarly, HER2-positive, hormone receptor–negative patients who had mastectomy after neoadjuvant chemotherapy and had complete pathologic CR had a locoregional recurrence risk of only 4.1%, whereas it was 24% with residual nodal disease. Although treatments were not uniform across the patient populations, these data suggest that information regarding breast cancer subtypes and differences in pathologic response to neoadjuvant chemotherapy may be used to design clinical trials to address omission of PMRT in patients with low risk of locoregional recurrence and dose intensification in patients with high risk of locoregional failure. In fact, the NSABP B-51/Radiation Therapy Oncology Group (RTOG) 1304 trial, which opened in August 2013, is evaluating whether omission of PMRT may be acceptable in patients with T1–3N1 disease based on palpation or imaging (ultrasound, computed tomography, magnetic resonance imaging, or positron emission tomography) and pathologic confirmation of axillary involvement without a sentinel node biopsy, who achieve complete pathologic response in the axilla after neoadjuvant chemotherapy.[36]

Tumor Biology Considerations

The importance of tumor biology extends beyond the neoadjuvant setting. In more recent years, it has become widely appreciated that the intrinsic biologic subtype of breast cancer has important prognostic and possibly predictive implications, not only for systemic outcomes but also locoregional control. To assess whether breast cancer subgroups based on the expression of ER, progesterone receptor (PR), and HER2 had any effect on response to PMRT in high-risk patients, Overgaard and coworkers analyzed data from 1000 of the 3083 high-risk breast cancer patients in the pooled Danish 82b and 82c trials randomly assigned to the PMRT group.[37] They constructed the following four subgroups for statistical analysis (Rec+ = ER+ and/or PR+; Rec− = ER− and PR−):

1. Rec+/HER2−
2. Rec+/HER2+
3. Rec−/HER2− (triple negative)
4. Rec−/HER2+

The authors noted significantly improved overall survival after PMRT among Rec+/HER2− patients but not in triple-negative and Rec−/HER2+ patients. Furthermore, significantly diminished improvement in locoregional recurrence control after PMRT was observed when comparisons were made between ER−/PR− tumors versus ER+/PR+ tumors and between triple-negative and Rec−/HER2+ versus Rec+/HER2− tumors. However, the interpretation of these findings has been challenging, given substantial changes in systemic therapy (particularly the introduction of HER2-targeted therapies) since the time of those trials.

Several groups have considered gene expression profiling to identify subsets of patients who may benefit from PMRT.[38,39] In one study, DNA microarrays from 94 breast cancer patients who underwent mastectomy between 1990 and 2001 without PMRT were used to develop two sets of gene expression profiles (one with 258 genes and another with 34 genes) that were independently prognostic, along with ER status, for local control on multivariable analysis.[38] In another study, gene expression profiling was performed in a training set of tumor tissue from 191 patients in the Danish Breast Cancer Cooperative Group 82bc cohort, and a weighted gene expression index (DBCG-RT index) was developed and validated in 112 additional patients.[39] The DBCG-RT profile was able to stratify patients into high and low locoregional risk groups. Furthermore, PMRT reduced locoregional recurrence in the high-risk group but no additional benefit with PMRT was found in the low-risk group. The DBCG-RT profile also identified a subset of triple-negative patients with high risk of locoregional failure who derived significant benefit from PMRT.

Other studies have also investigated the locoregional risk after mastectomy in triple-negative breast cancer specifically.[40] In a large population-based cohort study from Alberta, locoregional recurrence in T1–T2N0 triple-negative breast cancer patients after mastectomy was found to be 10% at a median follow-up of 7.2 years.[41] A multicenter randomized control trial from China demonstrated substantial benefit for PMRT in node-negative triple-negative breast cancer patients.[42] However, because of an unexpectedly large benefit with PMRT noted in this trial and concerns about possible differences in treatments or pathologic assessments, PMRT has not been routinely adopted in this group of patients.

On the other hand, it is possible that some patients with more favorable biology may not require PMRT even when nodes are involved. As noted earlier, in an analysis of ER-positive patients enrolled in the NSABP B-28 trial who underwent mastectomy for N1 disease and did not receive PMRT, the risk of locoregional recurrence was low and ranged from 2.4% to 6.0%.[20] In a study demonstrating the significance of intrinsic subtypes of breast cancer in predicting the risk of locoregional relapse, a six-marker immunohistochemical panel was applied to tissue microarrays to determine intrinsic molecular subtype of tumors from 2985 patients.[43] This study revealed that basal, luminal B, luminal-HER2, and HER2-enriched subtypes were associated with increased risk of locoregional recurrence on multivariable analysis. These findings suggest that the inherent biology of the tumors may provide independent prognostic and predictive information regarding the benefit of PMRT and may warrant validation in a prospective study.[44]

Postmastectomy Radiotherapy and Reconstructive Surgery

With increased access to and receipt of reconstructive surgery after mastectomy,[45] it has become particularly important to determine the best approach to integrate these two treatments. Reconstruction can be achieved with implant-based[46] or autologous tissue-based approaches,[47] and there are several approaches possible for the sequencing of surgery and adjuvant therapy. The acute side effects of radiotherapy on the chest wall and reconstructed breast are inflammatory in nature and include soft tissue edema, skin erythema, and, in some cases, dry or moist desquamation in the treated area of the skin. Late toxicities of radiotherapy can include skin changes, vascular compromise, and soft tissue fibrosis. In the context of breast reconstruction, these effects can lead to increased risk of complications and adverse cosmetic outcomes requiring repeated surgical interventions. Studies have shown that PMRT increases the rate of complications in both autologous and implant reconstruction, including the risk of infection, implant removal, fat necrosis, and capsular fibrosis.[48,49] A recent systematic review of surgical outcomes after autologous and prosthetic reconstruction in 5347 patients showed that PMRT was associated with significantly higher weighted incidence of complications, including reoperation, total complications, and reconstruction failure in patients undergoing prosthetic reconstruction, compared with autologous reconstruction.[50] The type of reconstruction and receipt of radiotherapy also appear to have significant impact on patient-reported quality of life and satisfaction with cosmetic outcomes.[51] Given that immediate reconstruction can affect radiation treatment planning[52] and even possibly recurrence rates,[53] early consultation with a radiation oncologist and a comprehensive discussion of the implications of PMRT on reconstruction with the patient are warranted in all patients considering mastectomy with breast reconstruction.

Conclusions

In summary, PMRT is strongly indicated in patients with locally advanced breast cancer, including those with four or more positive lymph nodes, but it should also be strongly considered in many patients with earlier-stage disease. Individualized risk assessment is necessary to help patients make treatment decisions that are right for them. Recent changes in practice patterns with near universal adoption of sentinel lymph node biopsies for axillary staging, decreasing utilization of axillary lymph node dissection even after discovery of positive sentinel lymph node(s), increasing utilization of neoadjuvant systemic therapy approaches, and growing appreciation of the critical importance of tumor biology in addition to extent of disease add to the complexity of these decisions. Thus the role of PMRT, especially in intermediate-risk patients, continues to evolve. However, considerable evidence does exist to help patients and providers engage in thoughtful discussions about anticipated risks and benefits to come to an appropriately tailored treatment decision that reflects both the best available data and the patient's considered values and preferences.

Selected References

5. Ragaz J, Jackson SM, Le N, et al. Adjuvant radiotherapy and chemotherapy in node-positive premenopausal women with breast cancer. *N Engl J Med.* 1997;337:956-962.
7. Overgaard M, Hansen PS, Overgaard J, et al. Postoperative radiotherapy in high-risk premenopausal women with breast cancer who receive adjuvant chemotherapy. Danish Breast Cancer Cooperative Group 82b Trial. *N Engl J Med.* 1997;337:949-955.
8. Overgaard M, Jensen MB, Overgaard J, et al. Postoperative radiotherapy in high-risk postmenopausal breast-cancer patients given adjuvant tamoxifen: Danish Breast Cancer Cooperative Group DBCG 82c randomised trial. *Lancet.* 1999;353:1641-1648.
10. Taghian A, Jeong JH, Mamounas E, et al. Patterns of locoregional failure in patients with operable breast cancer treated by mastectomy and adjuvant chemotherapy with or without tamoxifen and without radiotherapy: results from five National Surgical Adjuvant Breast and Bowel Project randomized clinical trials. *J Clin Oncol.* 2004;22:4247-4254.
15. Overgaard M, Nielsen HM, Overgaard J. Is the benefit of postmastectomy irradiation limited to patients with four or more positive nodes, as recommended in international consensus reports? A subgroup analysis of the DBCG 82 b&c randomized trials. *Radiother Oncol.* 2007;82:247-253.
16. Clarke M, Collins R, Darby S, et al. Effects of radiotherapy and of differences in the extent of surgery for early breast cancer on local recurrence and 15-year survival: an overview of the randomised trials. *Lancet.* 2005;366:2087-2106.
17. McGale P, Taylor C, Correa C, et al. Effect of radiotherapy after mastectomy and axillary surgery on 10-year recurrence and 20-year breast cancer mortality: meta-analysis of individual patient data for 8135 women in 22 randomised trials. *Lancet.* 2014;383:2127-2135.
26. Taghian AG, Jeong JH, Mamounas EP, et al. Low locoregional recurrence rate among node-negative breast cancer patients with tumors 5 cm or larger treated by mastectomy, with or without adjuvant systemic therapy and without radiotherapy: results from five national surgical adjuvant breast and bowel project randomized clinical trials. *J Clin Oncol.* 2006;24:3927-3932.
37. Kyndi M, Sørensen FB, Knudsen H, et al. Estrogen receptor, progesterone receptor, HER-2, and response to postmastectomy radiotherapy in high-risk breast cancer: the Danish Breast Cancer Cooperative Group. *J Clin Oncol.* 2008;26:1419-1426.
41. Abdulkarim BS, Cuartero J, Hanson J, et al. Increased risk of locoregional recurrence for women with T1-2N0 triple-negative breast cancer treated with modified radical mastectomy without adjuvant radiation therapy compared with breast-conserving therapy. *J Clin Oncol.* 2011;29:2852-2858.

A full reference list is available online at ExpertConsult.com.

50

Breast Conserving Therapy for Invasive Breast Cancers

GARY M. FREEDMAN

reast conservation has been a standard alternative to mastectomy for most patients with early-stage 0 to II breast cancer for decades. The purpose of breast conserving surgery (BCS) is the removal of all gross disease, and as much microscopic disease as possible, from the breast while maintaining a good cosmetic result. Residual microscopic disease may then be treated with postoperative radiation therapy (RT), which has been traditionally directed to the entire preserved breast tissue. This combination of BCS and whole breast radiation therapy (WBRT) has been successful in matching the long-term survival as mastectomy. With modern patient selection and multimodality treatment, BCS and WBRT also will result in equally low rates of local recurrence in the preserved breast compared with the chest wall or reconstructed breast after mastectomy.

This chapter examines patient selection, outcomes, and methods of BCS and WBRT for patients with invasive breast cancer and clinically early-stage I and II disease. Additional sections discuss advances in shortening treatment length for RT by hypofractionation, integration of WBRT with systemic therapy, the management of a local recurrence after WBRT, and when BCS alone without RT may be safely offered to selected patients.

Randomized Trials Comparing Breast Conserving Surgery and Radiation Therapy With Mastectomy

Randomized prospective clinical trials have confirmed that BCS and WBRT are associated with equal long-term survival as mastectomy for patients with stage I-II invasive breast cancer (Table 50.1).[1-6] Meta-analyses of these trials have also confirmed equal distant disease-free survival and overall survival.[7,8] The equivalence of these two options has been acknowledged by the wide oncology community, since at least 1990 to the present, in published consensus statements by the National Institute of Health, the National Comprehensive Cancer Center Network, and the American College of Radiology.[9-11] As a measure of quality clinical practice, the National Accreditation Program for Breast Centers of the American College of Surgeons sets a standard of 50% of eligible patients with early stage to be treated with breast conservation.[12]

The risk of a local recurrence in the breast, or ipsilateral breast tumor recurrence (IBTR), in these randomized trials is much higher than generally observed in more modern series. A risk of IBTR of 15% to 20% after BCS and WBRT in a population of stage I and II patients would be unacceptable today. These studies were conducted between the years 1972 and 1987 and do not represent modern patient selection and multimodality (surgery, systemic therapy) treatment. Many factors may account for the high local recurrence in these trials: suboptimal preoperative imaging compared with modern mammography and ultrasound that may have understaged extensive or multicentric breast cancers; less effective surgical-pathologic correlation to imaging findings, particularly for the nonpalpable mass in an era before modern localization procedures; less effective or underutilized systemic therapy compared with modern systemic and targeted therapies; and inclusion of women who may have been at higher risk for new primaries (not distinguishable from local recurrences in most cases) in the preserved breast due to lack of BRCA mutation testing in that era. The surgical techniques and pathologic margin assessment used for BCS in that era also may be largely responsible for the high IBTR rates in those early experiences. A tumorectomy or wide excision was used in most of these randomized trials, except the Milan that used quadrantectomy, but only the National Surgical Adjuvant Breast and Bowel Project (NSABP) B-06 trial required a negative resection margin. The trials with the highest IBTR rates, the National Cancer Institute (NCI) and the European Organisation for Research and Treatment of Cancer (EORTC), permitted patients with tumors of up to 5 cm (compared with upper size limits of 2–4 cm in the other four trials), and allowed gross tumor resection without microscopic margin assessment. For example, in the BCS and WBRT arm of the EORTC trial, 48% of all patients had microscopically positive margins. It is currently recommended that BCS specimens should be oriented for the pathologist to identify the specific margins, and each designated margin evaluated for involvement and closest distance to invasive carcinoma or ductal carcinoma in situ (DCIS).[13]

These randomized prospective trials show that BCS and WBRT that result in comparable rates of local control as mastectomy will yield comparable overall survival for patients with early-stage breast cancer, not that local control is unimportant. The Early Breast Cancer Trialists' Collaborative Group meta-analysis of randomized trials in the setting of BCS has shown that, as differences in local control rates between two treatments increase, differences in survival may eventually become apparent.[8] Therefore, the goal of BCS and WBRT should be to more closely match or equal the rates of local recurrence of mastectomy—a goal that is now

TABLE 50.1	Overall Survival and Local Recurrence in Six Prospective Randomized Trials in Stage I–II Breast Cancer Comparing Breast Conserving Surgery and Whole Breast Radiation Therapy to Mastectomy Between 1972 and 1989						

			OVERALL SURVIVAL (%)		LOCAL RECURRENCE (%)		
Trial	Years	No.	Mastectomy	BCS + RT	Mastectomy	BCS + RT	Interval Reported
NCI	1979–87	237	44	38	1	22	25 years
Milan	1973–80	701	59	58	2	9	20 years
NSABP	1976–84	1217	47	46	10[a]	14	20 years
EORTC	1980–86	868	45	39	12[b]	20[b]	20 years
Danish	1983–89	793	51	58	21[a]	13[a]	20 years
IGR	1972–79	179	65	73	18	13	15 years

[a]Crude result.
[b]Local-regional recurrence rates 10 years.
BCS + RT, Breast conserving surgery and radiation therapy; EORTC, European Organization for Research and Treatment of Cancer; IGR, Institut Gustave-Roussy; NCI, National Cancer Institute (United States); NSABP, National Surgical Adjuvant Breast and Bowel Project.

TABLE 50.2	Ipsilateral Breast Tumor Recurrence in Prospective Phase III Trials in Stage I–II Breast Cancer That Included Breast Conserving Surgery and Whole Breast Radiation Therapy Beginning After 1990				

Trial	Years	N	IBTR (%)	Years at IBTR	Reference
ACOSOG Z0011	1999–2004	891	2–3	5	16
PRIME II	2003–2009	658	1	5	216
PMH/BCCA	1992–2000	386	4	8	214
OCOG	1993–1996	1234	6	10	14
CALBG 9343	1994–1999	317	2	10	215
START A	1999–2002	2236	6	10	15
START B	1999–2002	2215	4	10	115
MA.20	2000–2007	1832	4	10	17

ACOSOG, American College of Surgeons Oncology Group; CALGB, Cancer and Leukemia Group B; OCOG, Ontario Clinical Oncology Group; PMH/BCCA, Princess Margaret Hospital / British Columbia Cancer Agency; START, Standardisation of Breast Radiotherapy.

Patient Selection for Breast Conserving Surgery and Radiation

The rates of IBTR in prospective phase III trials that included in one of the study arms patients treated with BCS and WBRT from a more modern era after 1990 are much lower since the era of the prospective randomized trials comparing to BCS and WBRT to mastectomy from 1972–1989 (Table 50.2).[14–17] The rates of IBTR of 1% to 3% at 5 years and 2% to 6% at 10 years are now comparable to those achieved by mastectomy for similarly staged patients.

The excellent rates of local control with BCS and WBRT are achieved by means of careful patient selection for BCS, pathologic evaluation, radiation, and systemic therapy. Many factors influence the risk of IBTR, and some of the most important clinical and pathologic factors are closely interrelated and cannot be examined in isolation. For example, young patients (35–40 years old or less at diagnosis) have been reported in older series to have a high rate for IBTR. Yet this age group is also more likely than older women to have an extensive intraductal component (EIC) and close or positive resection margins[18] and also more likely to have been treated with undiagnosed *BRCA* mutation resulting in an apparent higher IBTR rate. In other cases, treatment-related factors, such as extent of surgery or use of systemic therapy, may mitigate the adverse impact of one or more negative prognostic factors. Yet patients whose expected risk of IBTR is very high may still be best served by mastectomy so as not to compromise patient survival. Patient selection for WBRT should also take into account the perceived likelihood of complications from radiation and of an acceptable cosmetic outcome of the preserved breast.

Clinical Factors

There are relatively few clinical patient-related or tumor-related factors that would preclude BCS and WBRT. Young patient age is not alone a contraindication and the risk of IBTR has been markedly reduced in the modern era to low and acceptable levels, comparable in tumor control and survival to mastectomy. Many clinical features or aspects of tumor biology that are associated with an increased risk for IBTR in young women may be more effectively mitigated by optimal patient selection and surgical and systemic therapies. For patients with initial tumor size greater than 5 cm, selected patients with a good response to neoadjuvant chemotherapy may still be candidates for BCS and WBRT. True gross multicentric disease, or diffuse malignant-associated calcifications that cannot be removed, remain indications for mastectomy in most cases. However, multifocal breast cancer within a same

possible with modern multimodality patient selection and treatment.

quadrant/region of the breast can be treated with BCS if done through a single incision with an acceptable cosmetic result to the patient. Similarly, patients with a subareolar tumor location requiring sacrifice of the nipple-areolar complex, or women with small breast size and a large visible volume defect from surgery, may still prefer breast conservation over mastectomy when the subsequent cosmetic appearance is still acceptable to them despite significant asymmetry. Other contraindications to breast conservation with radiation therapy include a history of collagen vascular disease (scleroderma or active lupus with skin involvement, but not rheumatoid arthritis), prior chest wall irradiation, or pregnancy because of the concern for an increased risk of serious complications or severe late radiation effects in the patient or fetus.[19–21]

Patient Age

Age younger than 35 to 40 years old has been associated with an increased risk of IBTR after BCS and WBRT compared with older patients.[22–24] In a meta-analysis of randomized trials comparing BCS with or without WBRT, the risk for any first recurrence (local and distant) by age in node-negative women was 5.9% per year for age younger than 40 years, 2.7% per year for age 40 to 49 years, and 1% to 1.9% per year for 50 years and older.[8] There was also an increased recurrence risk in node-positive women younger than 40 years and a higher breast cancer mortality for women younger than 40 years, compared with older women. However, this does not mean that mastectomy should be the preferred treatment in this age group. The risk for local-regional recurrence (with or without simultaneous distant metastases) is also significantly higher after mastectomy in young women.[25] Mortality is also not reduced in young women with mastectomy compared with BCS and WBRT.[24] For example, a population-based study of 9285 women in Denmark showed that women younger than 35 years treated with BCS and WBRT had a greater risk of IBTR than women ages 45 to 49 years (15% vs. 3%) or women age 50 years or older, but death rates compared with mastectomy groups were the same for each age cohort.[26] In a large population-based study from Canada of 965 women aged 20 to 39, 616 patients had BCS and WBRT and 349 had mastectomy. There were no significant differences in 15-year local-regional recurrence, distant metastases, or survival outcomes between the two groups.[27]

The increased IBTR rates in young women are likely due at least in part to their higher likelihood of having more adverse tumor features than older women. Some of these adverse features are classical pathologic features such as high histologic grade, positive or close resection margins, or a more extensive local tumor burden on reexcisions. This increased risk for IBTR in young women seems to be partly or mostly mitigated when correcting for these adverse prognostic factors by greater surgical attention or modern systemic therapy. For example, a recursive partitioning analysis of more than 900 patients treated with BCS and WBRT found age, margin status, and EIC among the strongest predictors for IBTR, with age the most important.[28] However, when considering women aged 35 years or younger, the risk of IBTR at 10 years was only 3% for patients with negative margins (>2 mm) and EIC-negative tumors compared with 34% when margins were close or positive. Similarly, in a study examining outcome in patients age 40 years or younger in the southern Netherlands, van der Leest and colleagues observed that the risk of IBTR at 10 years was 41% in patients who had an incomplete excision, compared with 16% for those with a

complete excision (*p* = .005), and 22% for patients not receiving systemic therapy, compared with 11% with systemic therapy (*p* = .002).[29]

In more recent studies, the worse prognosis for young women has been attributed to a higher incidence of adverse tumor biology in tumor subtyping and gene expression profiling rather than classical pathologic features.[30] For example, in one study young patients with adverse receptor profiles (luminal B, triple-negative, and HER2 positive) had a higher risk for IBTR that was not observed in young patients with a more favorable luminal A pattern.[31] In a multiinstitutional study of 1434 patients treated with BCS and WBRT, young patient age remained significant with tumor subtyping on multivariate analysis for IBTR but none of the other classical pathologic factors such as grade or margins.[32] However, although statistically significant, the elevated risk for IBTR in the youngest cohort ages 23 to 46 years was 5% compared with less than 2% for older cohorts, a much lower difference and of marginal clinical significance particularly compared with historical studies of age cohorts that did not correct for tumor subtype.[33] In another study of 1058 patients treated with BCS and WBRT, where breast cancer subtype was included in the analysis with other clinical and pathologic traditional risk factors, age less than 40 years was not a significant predictor for IBTR at 10 years (90% vs. 94%, *p* = .08).[34]

Tumor Size

In standard practice, BCS has been limited to patients with tumors approximately 4 to 5 cm so that a resection to negative margins can be achieved with a good cosmetic result. Patients with tumors larger than 5 cm may be able to have BCS with an acceptable cosmetic result in the setting of a large breast size.[35,36] However most women with a large tumor size greater than 5 cm or tumors less than 5 cm with a large size to breast ratio are best considered for neoadjuvant chemotherapy for tumor downstaging before BCS. Patients who respond well to neoadjuvant chemotherapy may become better candidates for BCS and WBRT with acceptable cosmetic results.

The NSABP B-18 trial randomly assigned patients to receive either neoadjuvant or adjuvant chemotherapy.[37] BCS and WBRT were performed for 33% of patients presenting with clinical T3 tumors who were assigned to have neoadjuvant chemotherapy, compared with only 9% of those randomized to immediate surgery followed by chemotherapy. IBTR rates for all patients undergoing BCS and WBRT in the neoadjuvant and adjuvant arms were 11% and 8%, respectively, which difference was not statistically significant. However, the IBTR rate was higher (16%) for patients who needed to have chemotherapy to become eligible for BCS and WBRT, compared with those initially felt to be candidates for BCS before chemotherapy (10%). In an updated report of pooled data of 1890 patients treated with BCS + WBRT in the neoadjuvant therapy trials NSABP B-18 and B-27, the 10-year cumulative incidence of IBTR was 8.1%.[38] In the multivariate Cox proportional hazards model, clinical tumor size was not a significant independent predictor of IBTR. Significant factors for IBTR were age, clinical nodal status, and pathologic nodal status/pathologic breast tumor response to neoadjuvant chemotherapy. In a randomized trial performed by the EORTC, 23% of patients originally felt to require mastectomy were treated with BCS after neoadjuvant chemotherapy; but there was no significant difference in local recurrence rates between the neoadjuvant and adjuvant chemotherapy arms.[39] Other studies have also shown favorable results with BCS and

WBRT. Fifty-two of 84 women with tumors larger than 5 cm responded to neoadjuvant chemotherapy sufficiently to become 3 cm or smaller and were treated with quadrantectomy and WBRT at the National Cancer Institute in Milan, with a 4% rate of IBTR at 8 years.[40] A study conducted by Chen and colleagues at the MD Anderson Cancer Center reported a 5-year IBTR rate of 8% in 110 patients with initial T3–T4 tumors treated by neoadjuvant chemotherapy, BCS, and WBRT.[41] However, careful clinical and pathologic correlation of tumor stage before and after chemotherapy is needed with this approach. For example, marking the tumor location by a clip before neoadjuvant therapy is recommended to localize the area if there is a good response and ensure negative margins.

Gross Multifocal/Multicentric Disease

The presence of clinically or radiologically detected multifocal disease (defined as having two or more tumors in the same quadrant) or multicentric disease (two or more tumors in separate quadrants) has generally been considered a contraindication to breast conservation therapy. Older studies of such patients have reported elevated IBTR rates of 20% to 40%.[42–45] However, other reports have had more favorable outcomes in highly selected patients with multiple lesions. Hartsell and coworkers observed a 4% risk of IBTR for patients with two gross pathologic tumors that were EIC negative and resected with negative margins.[46] Cho and colleagues reported no local recurrences after breast conserving therapy in 15 patients, 9 of whom had multiple lesions detected preoperatively and 6 of whom had such disease detected only by the gross pathology examination.[47] Oh and coworkers found a 6% IBTR rate at 5 years among 20 patients presenting with clinically multifocal disease who were treated with neoadjuvant chemotherapy, BCS, and radiation.[48] Okumura and colleagues reported only one local recurrence in 34 patients treated with BCS for macroscopically multiple tumors detected either before (26) or during (8) surgery.[49] Of note, 20 of the 34 tumors were demonstrated to be microscopically contiguous. Yerushalmi and coworkers reported results for 300 patients with multifocal or multicentric stage I or II breast cancer aged 50 to 69, EIC negative, and with small tumor size.[50] These women treated by BCS + WBRT had an IBTR at 10 years of 5.5%, which was similar to that of separate cohorts of unifocal breast cancer treated by breast conservation or patients with one or more tumors treated by mastectomy.

Genetic Factors

A known genetic mutation in *BRCA* predisposing to breast cancer development is a relative but not absolute contraindication to breast conservation. In a series of 87 women with known *BRCA1* or *BRCA2* mutations, Robsen and colleagues reported a relatively high risk for IBTR (14% at 10 years and 23% at 15 years).[51] However, Pierce and colleagues reported the results of a multiinstitutional case control study which included 160 known *BRCA1-2* mutation carriers and 445 sporadic breast cancer control patients.[52] There was no significant difference in the 15-year risk of IBTR between the *BRCA1-2* patients and the controls (24% vs. 17%). Of note, the risk of IBTR (and contralateral breast cancers) was reduced substantially among those *BRCA1-2* patients who underwent bilateral oophorectomy or who received tamoxifen, compared with those who did not have such additional treatment. Many of the local "recurrences" in patients with *BRCA1-2* mutations may be attributable to the development of new primary tumors, rather than a relapse of the

original cancer. Sixty percent of IBTRs in patients with *BRCA1* or *2* mutations were located in a different quadrant than the index lesion, compared with 29% for control patients. In another report, Pierce and coworkers compared breast conservation to mastectomy in 655 women with known *BRCA1* or *2* mutation.[53] The local recurrence rate at 15 years was 23.5% versus 5.5% ($p <$ .0001), respectively. However, there were no significant observed differences in the incidence of contralateral breast cancer (>40%) or overall survival. Again, in this series most of the apparent IBTR were considered to be most likely new primaries in the preserved breast. There is other indirect evidence that most IBTR in these patients are actually new primaries. Turner and colleagues found that 8 of 52 patients (15%) with IBTR after breast conserving therapy retrospectively were found to have *BRCA1* or *BRCA2* mutations.[54] The mean time to IBTR in these women was 8.7 years, compared with 4.3 years for their overall population. Also, the patterns of relapse histology (compared with the first tumor) and location in the breast were different for the *BRCA* mutation carriers than for other patients, suggesting the majority of these IBTRs were actually new primaries arising later in the preserved breast tissue.

Thus breast conservation therapy is a reasonable option for women at high genetic risk who do not choose to have bilateral mastectomy. Their rates of IBTR, or what may be new primaries in the preserved breast, appear to be reduced to acceptable levels by risk reduction strategies. Closer screening than usual that includes annual magnetic resonance imaging in addition to mammogram is warranted after treatment for the *BRCA*-associated breast cancer patient who chooses breast conservation.

Race

Race is not an independent factor for IBTR after BCS plus RT after controlling for other prognostic factors in most studies.[22,28,55] However, other studies have found a higher risk for IBTR in black women compared with white women.[56,57] The strong link between race and triple-receptor-negative (estrogen receptor [ER], progesterone receptor [PR], and HER2 negative) tumor subtype makes older retrospective studies that do not account for both in their analyses now outdated. It is known that black women have more common presentation with higher stage breast cancer and lower survival and that this is attributed in large part to a higher incidence of triple-negative breast cancer.[58,59] Among 704 women all classified as triple-receptor-negative breast cancer subtype, Perez and coworkers found that black women had the same local recurrence rate as nonblack women (3.0% vs. 5.3%, $p = $ .15).[60] Black women in their study did have a higher stage at presentation and higher incidence of regional nodal recurrence.

Pathologic Factors

Margin status and breast cancer tumor subtype approximated by receptor expression are the two main pathologic factors that have a significant impact on the observed rates of IBTR after BCS and WBRT in modern series. Of these, only positive margin status has the potential to preclude BCS in some cases. There is an extensive list of other pathologic features of early-stage breast cancer that have been studied in mostly retrospective analyses for an effect on IBTR, including major ones of histologic grade, nuclear grade, presence of an EIC, lymphovascular invasion, axillary nodal positivity, and extranodal tumor extension. These other factors have minimal to no effect on IBTR once multivariate analyses that include margins and tumor subtype are taken into account, so should not significantly affect patient selection for BCS and WBRT.

Margin Status

A "positive" margin is generally defined as the microscopic presence of tumor cells at an inked edge when radial margin processing, or "breadloafing," is performed, or the presence of any tumor cells in "shaved" margin specimens. In most series of BCS and WBRT, the risk of IBTR is two to three times greater in the presence of a positive margin compared with a negative margin.[61–73] A negative margin in many studies can be considered one that is without tumor cells at the ink, or simply not positive. This has been the subject of a major consensus statement (discussed subsequently) that will likely increase its more widespread acceptance in clinical practice. However, other studies have tried to make a distinction between patients with varying degrees of negative margins: a "close" margin (defined variously as cancer cells within distances of 1 mm[63,74] or 2 mm[61,62,66,67,75,76]) or a "negative" (wider than 2 mm) margin. Retrospective series of BCS and WBRT with margins that are close less than 1 to 2 mm have been associated with much greater heterogeneity in outcomes, with an increased risk of IBTR in some studies[61,66,67,76–78] but not others.[62,63,74,79–81] For example, Obedian and coworkers found that patients with close or negative margins both had a 10-year IBTR rate of 2%.[62] In another series, Park and colleagues reported the same crude rate of IBTR (7%) at 8 years in patients with either close (≥1 mm) or negative margins.[63] However, in a prospective trial from the same institution, women with close margins randomized to receive chemotherapy before RT had a crude local failure rate of 32%, compared with 4% in patients receiving RT before chemotherapy.[78] Patients with margins wider than 2 mm have more uniformly across studies had a very low risk of IBTR within 10 years after BCS and WBRT.[61,66,67,76,77,80]

The effect of nonnegative margins on IBTR has not been uniform in retrospective studies but associated with heterogeneity based on other clinical and pathologic characteristics. Patient age has been shown in many studies to influence the outcome of involves margins. For example, in a recursive partitioning analysis, Freedman and coworkers showed that close or positive margins were more significant for young patients than for patients older than age 55.[28] Leong and colleagues found that the risk of IBTR in patients with a positive margin was 11% for women age 51 years or older, 21% for women ages 35 to 50 years, and 50% for women age 34 years or younger.[69] Jobsen and colleagues reported that for women 40 years old or younger the 5-year local recurrence rate was 37% when margins were positive and 8.4% when they were negative.[65] Other studies have shown that the number of positive margins[72] and extensive (compared with focal) extent of margin positivity may affect the risk for IBTR several-fold.[63,70,72] For example, Park and coworkers reported an 8-year risk of IBTR of 27% in patients with extensively positive margins, compared with 14% for patients with focally positive margins (involvement that could be encompassed within three or fewer low-power microscopic fields); the risk was 13% for patients with uninvolved margins.[63] The IBTR rate with positive margins was reported to be substantially more than two to three times higher than negative margins in cases of invasive lobular carcinoma or an EIC.[71,82] Systemic chemotherapy has been reported to reduce the impact of a positive margin in some studies[63,66] but not others.[61] In the same study by Park and colleagues, patients with focally positive margins who received systemic therapy had an IBTR rate of 7%

at 8 years, compared with 18% of patients who did not have systemic therapy; however, for patients with extensive margin involvement, systemic therapy had little effect (26% and 29% IBTR rates, respectively).[63] Length of follow-up may be important, with 10-year follow-up needed to observe differences between close and negative margins in some series.[61,68,70,83] For example, Freedman and coworkers found no significant difference in the 5-year cumulative incidence of IBTR for patients with a close or negative margin, but by 10 years a significant difference in IBTR rates was apparent (14% vs. 7%, respectively).[61] Such latency periods of 10 years or more in seeing the rates of IBTR with close margins diverge from those of negative margins has also been shown in other series.[68,70,83] Some have practiced a policy of escalating doses for close or positive margins in an attempt to reduce the perceived higher risk for IBTR, although this did not significantly improve local control in the largest prospective randomized trial (discussed later).[84]

This heterogeneity of results regarding the association between margin status and local recurrence may be explained in part by the relatively loose relationship between margins and the extent of residual disease in the breast after surgery. It is this degree of tumor burden that is likely the determining factor for local control. Most of the preceding studies do not report the recurrence risk based on the histology of the tumor, the type of tumor involving the margin, the number of involved resection margins, or the anatomic location of the involved margins. The width of a resection margin can be limited to the surgeon by tumor location and anatomy—for example, a posterior margin at the posterior fascia or deep muscle of the chest wall, or an anterior margin just below but not involving the skin. These situations may not have the same risk for residual disease at the margin as cases where the margin is bordering on breast tissue. Margin location at an anatomic boundary such as the pectoralis muscle is a common reason for not reexcising a margin before radiation.[85] There is a wide variation in the incidence of having residual disease in patients undergoing reexcision (20%–60%),[18,86,87] which seems to reflect the variability in these other cofactors with margins. Schnitt and colleagues noted residual carcinoma in 88% of specimens identified to have an EIC, compared with 48% of specimens of patients without an EIC in the primary excision ($p = .002$).[86] Mai and coworkers studied serially sectioned lumpectomy specimens and found a relation between having extensive DCIS in the specimen, the incidence of margin involvement, and the risk of more extensive margin involvement.[88] Wazer and coworkers found that the simultaneous presence of an EIC and young age (45 years or younger) were more important than initial margin involvement for predicting the presence of tumor on reexcision.[18] Smitt and colleagues also reported that reexcision findings were related to patient age and the presence of an EIC.[66] Only 11% of patients without an EIC who had close margins had tumor found in the reexcision specimen; this rate was only 10% in patients older than over 65 years. Chism and coworkers found that the risk of having a positive reexcision varied from 15% for patients with T1–T2 tumors with close margins, negative nodes, and no EIC to 83% for those with positive margins, EIC, and positive nodes.[89] Goldstein and colleagues found that increasing amounts of carcinoma near the margin, from the presence of minimal disease to more extensive volume, in addition to the margin width itself, was predictive of IBTR.[68]

Houssami and coworkers conducted a meta-analysis of IBTR after BCS and WBRT, and the relation to final microscopic margin status and the threshold distance for a negative margin.[90]

Thirty-three studies met entry criteria for the analysis that included 32,363 patients and margin data on 28,162 patients. The studies were almost all retrospective and treated patients during 1979–2001. The median prevalence of local recurrence was only 5.3% across the 33 studies. The odds ratio in 33 studies for local recurrence was 1.96 for positive or close versus negative margins. In a subgroup of 19 studies with more specific available data on margin width, the odds ratio was 1.74 for close versus negative, and 2.44 for positive versus negative margins ($p < .001$). However, additional analyses showed that local recurrence did not significantly vary with margin distance of 1, 2, or 5 mm compared with a margin definition of no tumor on ink. In the adjusted model, the odds of local recurrence were associated with margin status ($p < .001$) but not with margin distance ($p = .12$), and there was no statistical evidence that the odds of local recurrence decreased as the distance for negative margins increased ($p = .21$ for trend).

The Society of Surgical Oncology (SSO) and American Society for Radiation Oncology ASTRO) convened a multidisciplinary panel to develop a consensus statement regarding margins for BCS and WBRT.[91] This panel also included representatives of the College of American Pathologists, American Society of Breast Surgeons, American Society of Clinical Oncology, and a patient advocate. The statement was based in large on the meta-analysis by Houssami and colleagues[90] that served as the primary evidence base, with additional topic-specific literature reviews conducted by participants for questions not addressed in the meta-analysis. The statement concerns stage I–II invasive breast cancer treated by BCS and WBRT, and did not include cases of pure DCIS, neoadjuvant chemotherapy, or accelerated partial breast irradiation. Major recommendations of the consensus statement were that positive margins, defined as ink on invasive cancer or DCIS, are associated with a twofold increase in IBTR. Negative margins (no ink on tumor) optimize IBTR, but wider margin widths do not significantly lower this risk; the routine practice to obtain wider negative margin widths than ink on tumor is not indicated. It should be noted that this consensus was not a call for an end to all reexcisions in selected clinical cases based on clinical judgment. There was little data available for the meta-analysis to compare margins of no tumor on ink versus 1 mm or greater. However, the consensus opinion was that (1) given the absence of significance to the meta-analysis of margin widths greater than 1 mm, (2) the baseline very low risk for IBTR in the meta-analysis as a whole of approximately 5%, and (3) other improvements in patient selection and systemic therapy since the years of the studies, it is reasonable to assume that any benefit to wider margins not detectable by the power of the meta-analysis would not be clinically significant or greater than 1% to 2%. Other recommendations by the consensus group made based on secondary data from prospective randomized trials and retrospective studies included that there was no indication that a wider margin width than no ink on tumor was routinely needed for young patient age, EIC, lobular histology, whole breast hypofractionation (daily fraction size >2 Gy), or unfavorable biologic subtypes of invasive cancer.

Table 50.3 summarizes the consensus recommendations of several major organizations for the use of reexcision in the setting of nonnegative margins after BCS before WBRT.[10,91–94] In summary, it is preferable to have a negative margin (no tumor on ink) before radiation to minimize the subsequent risk of IBTR. However, some patients with focal margin involvement are still reasonable candidates for BCS and WBRT, and others may benefit from a reexcision to obtain a wider margin before WBRT, depending on the presence of other risk factors such as age, histology, the location and extent of these margins, and the use of adjuvant systemic therapy.

Tumor Subtyping

Gene expression profiling by use of microarrays is a technique that allows the simultaneous study of expression of tens of thousands of genes to looks for patterns that correlate with clinical end points.

TABLE 50.3 Recommendations for the Use of Reexcision for Nonnegative Margins After Breast Conserving Surgery and Before Whole Breast Radiation for Early-Stage Invasive Breast Cancer

	Invasive Breast Cancer	Reference
American College of Radiology	• A reexcision should be performed for an involved margin. • Wider margins may be more important in select patients (young, estrogen receptor negative, or extensive intraductal component).	92
American Society of Breast Surgeons	• Margin ≥1 mm usually adequate • Consider reexcision for focally positive or <1-mm margins on a case-by-case basis. • Reexcision usually needed for a positive margin.	93
American Society of Clinical Oncology	• Endorses adoption of the SSO/ASTRO Guideline—but flexibility in the application of the guideline is needed in some areas. • Heightened emphasis needed on the importance of postlumpectomy mammography for cases involving microcalcifications.	94
National Comprehensive Cancer Network	• A positive margin should generally undergo further surgery. • Exceptions may be made for selected cases of focally positive margin and absence of extensive intraductal component.	10
Society of Surgical Oncology/American Society for Radiation Oncology	• A positive margin should be defined as no tumor on ink. • Negative margins are optimal for local control in most situations. • Wider margins than no tumor on ink are not routine indications for further surgery.	91

ASTRO, American Society for Radiation Oncology; *SOS,* Society of Surgical Oncology.

This technique has been used in patients with early-stage invasive breast cancer, and gene expression in many studies has been predictive for risk of distant metastases and mortality.[95–97] Many studies have examined the use of gene expression profiles and their prognostic effect for local recurrence with varying degrees of success, and none are currently ready for clinical use in patient selection for BCS and WBRT.[98–101] Mamounas and coworkers[102] examined the 21-gene recurrence score assay Oncotype DX (Genomic Health, Redwood City, CA) that had been successful in predicting distant recurrence for an association with local recurrence. The recurrence score was available from 390 patients with ER-positive and node-negative invasive breast cancer treated on prospective randomized trials by the NSABP with BCS and WBRT. The local-regional recurrence rates were 6.8%, 10.8%, and 14.6% for low, intermediate, and high recurrence scores, respectively ($p = .043$). However, there was a larger variation in IBTR by age with women younger than 50 years (approximately 12%–28% by recurrence score) compared with 50 or older (<5% for all recurrence scores).

Without a validated clinical-use assay to identify these tumors prospectively, these different classes of tumors can be roughly distinguished more easily in clinical practice by expression of currently standard ER, PR, and HER2 receptor testing. Luminal A and B subtypes are associated with positive ER. ER-negative tumors are divided into those positive for HER2, or those of "basal-like" expression associated with low to absent ER, PR, and HER2 receptor expression (or triple-receptor negative).[103] There is an incomplete correlation between basal-like tumors and these receptor expression profiles: from 15% to 45% of basal-like tumors express at least one of these markers, and only 85% of triple-receptor-negative tumors are basal-like by expression arrays.[104] In a multiinstitutional study of breast cancer subtype in 1223 women treated by BCS and WBRT, Hattangadi-Gluth and colleagues reported the 5-year IBTR was 0.2% for luminal A, 1.2% for luminal B, 4.4% for triple negative, and 9% for HER2 positive ($p < .0001$) that was significant on multivariate analysis.[105] Arvold and colleagues reported that HER2 positive (and hormone receptor negative) and triple negative subtypes were associated with increased IBTR.[26] Univariate analysis of individual receptor expression HER2/neu overexpression[106] is not associated with an increased risk of IBTR. Patients with ER-negative tumors had an increased risk of IBTR in some[107] but not all studies.[74,108,109] Triple-negative receptor pattern was significantly associated with local recurrence in some studies[110] but not others.[111–113]

In summary, breast cancer subtyping may be associated with differences in IBTR after BCS and WBRT. However, a less favorable tumor subtype, such as triple-negative or HER2 positive, should not influence patient selection for breast conservation. Two studies have specifically compared patients with T1–2N0 triple negative breast cancer subtype treated with BCS and WBRT to mastectomy and found no significant difference in local-regional recurrence, distant metastases, or survival.[114,115]

Other Pathologic Factors

An EIC is defined as the simultaneous presence of intraductal carcinoma which comprises a prominent portion of the area of the primary mass (generally 25% or more) and of intraductal carcinoma clearly extending beyond the infiltrating margin of the tumor or present in sections of grossly normal adjacent breast tissue. Predominantly noninvasive tumors, with only focal areas of invasion, are also included in this category. The presence of an EIC-positive tumor has been associated with an increased risk of

IBTR after breast conserving therapy, although its effect is minimized by increasing the extent of surgery and obtaining negative margins.[45,61,63,69,70,116,117] Patients with positive axillary nodes do not have an increased risk of IBTR compared with patients with negative nodes; indeed, in many earlier studies, their risk of IBTR was generally lower than that of patients with negative nodes, due to the common use of adjuvant systemic therapy for node-positive but not node-negative patients.[45,116–119] Extracapsular nodal extension[120,121] is not associated with an increased risk of IBTR. High histologic grade has also had a variable association with the risk of IBTR after BCS and WBRT, with an increased risk reported by some series[64,122] but not others.[45,109,123] Similarly, lymphovascular invasion has been associated with a relatively increased risk of IBTR in many[74,109,117,122,124] but not all series.[45,64,119] Local recurrence rates are similar for patients with invasive lobular and invasive ductal carcinoma so not a factor in patient selection.[125,126] Provided margins are negative for invasive disease, the presence of LCIS has also not been associated with an overall increased risk of IBTR.[127,128]

Treatment Factors

Surgery

The extent of BCS may have an impact on IBTR. In the Milan experience, the risk of IBTR was lower in patients undergoing quadrantectomy than tumorectomy,[116] but the cosmetic results of such wide resections tend to be worse than for patients treated with smaller excisions. Therefore more extensive resection beyond that needed to obtain a negative surgical margin is not necessary.

A reexcision may have therapeutic benefit in converting patients with positive margins to negative margins. Patients achieving a negative margin after reexcision have the same risk of IBTR at 10 years as patients with a negative margin obtained after a single excision.[129] However, a negative reexcision does not have therapeutic value. In the study by Chism and colleagues, the 10-year risk of IBTR with close or positive margins not undergoing reexcision was 5%, the same as for women undergoing a reexcision that contained no residual disease.[89] However, perhaps reflecting the higher tumor burden in these patients, the rate of IBTR was 9% in women with residual disease ($p = .038$). Neuschatz and colleagues also found that the risk of IBTR at 12 years was the same for those with no residual tumor on a reexcision as for those patients with initial margin widths of 2 to 5 mm.[67] A reexcision for those patients with initially positive margins, or multiple or extensive close margins, may have more of a diagnostic role to detect patients with a very extensive local tumor burden that suggests mastectomy may be a better option than breast conserving therapy. In patients recommended to have a reexcision before WBRT, a directed reexcision of only the initially involved margins can be employed to reduce volume loss and help to preserve an acceptable cosmetic result.

Radiation Boost

The addition of a radiation therapy "boost," or an extra dose delivered to the excision site after whole-breast irradiation, has been associated with a decreased risk for IBTR compared with giving whole-breast RT alone in randomized trials.[33,130,131] In the EORTC trial, IBTR in the boost and no-boost arms were 12% and 16% at 20 years, respectively. The reduction was statistically significant and proportionally independent of age, but was in magnitude greatest in absolute terms for women age 40 years or younger who had the largest baseline risk of IBTR. However, the EORTC trial did not assess margin status in relation to the in situ component, only invasive breast cancer, and neither trial recorded the exact tumor-free margin width, which may have been quite narrow in some cases. Patients with close or positive margins may also benefit from increased doses given to the tumor bed, which have been reported to decrease the risk of IBTR some series[79,81] but not others.[67,70,74] In the randomized trial by the EORTC of boost versus no boost, for a subgroup of patients available for central pathology review, the risk of IBTR for positive margins was 11.1% compared with 9.4% for negative margins.[132] For patients with microscopic positive margins, a higher boost of 26 Gy was associated with a nonsignificant trend to lower local recurrence compared with 10 Gy (10.8% vs. 17.5%, $p > .1$).[84]

Use of a concurrent boost is a promising method of maintaining a shorter radiation schedule of whole breast hypofractionation, but also gaining the local control benefit of a lumpectomy cavity boost.[133–135] Phase III trials studying hypofractionated WBI with a concurrent boost over 3 weeks, including Radiation Therapy Oncology Group 1005 and IMPORT (Intensity Modulation and Partial Organ) High trial in the United Kingdom, if successful may make this approach more widely accepted for use.

Adjuvant Systemic Therapy

The risk of IBTR is lower in patients treated with adjuvant systemic chemotherapy.[116–118,136] However, adjuvant systemic therapy may delay the time to develop IBTR but not reduce its long-term risk for patients at high risk of local recurrence, such as those with positive margins. Freedman et al found no significant decrease in the IBTR rate at either 5 or 10 years resulting from the use of systemic therapy in patients with negative margins; for patients with positive margins, the use of systemic therapy was associated with a lower rate of IBTR at 5 years, but it did not significantly decrease the 10-year cumulative incidence of IBTR.[61] Adjuvant tamoxifen has also been associated with a decrease in the rate of IBTR.[28,109,119,137,138]

Patient Selection Factors for Hypofractionated Whole Breast Irradiation

Hypofractionation is the use of larger than conventional 2-Gy fraction size and generally means a course of radiation delivered in a fewer number of fractions in a shorter period of time than conventional fractionation. There have been four prospective randomized phase III clinical trials of whole breast hypofractionated radiation (H-WBRT) conducted in the United Kingdom and Canada that have long-term 10-year results (see Table 50.2). These studies were paramount in establishing H-WBRT as a standard of practice and alternative to conventional fractionation worldwide.

The Ontario Clinical Oncology Group (OCOG) trial randomized patients to 42.5 Gy in 16 fractions over 22 days versus 50 Gy in 25 fractions over 35 days.[14,139] Eligibility factors included invasive breast cancer 5 cm or less, pathologically node negative, and negative resection margins (defined as no tumor on ink). Exclusion factors included clinical T4 tumors, multicentric disease, and a breast size too large for satisfactory radiation therapy such as a maximum width and the posterior border of tangential fields greater than 25 cm (large chest wall separation). Chemotherapy was permitted before radiation. There was no regional nodal or

boost radiation. These two radiation schedules were associated with equivalent 10-year IBTR of 6.2% and 6.7%, respectively. H-WBRT was not inferior to conventional fractionation in terms of breast cancer mortality, death from other causes, or overall survival. The late cosmetic appearance was considered good or excellent in approximately 70% of women in both groups. There were similarly no reported differences in 10-year skin and subcutaneous tissue complications.

The Royal Marsden Hospital and Gloucestershire Oncology Center (RMH/GOC), or Standardization of Breast Radiotherapy (START) pilot trial, was a three-arm trial that used 39 Gy or 42.9 Gy in 13 fractions, compared with 50 Gy in 25 fractions, while maintaining the same 5-week treatment length in all arms.[140,141] Eligibility was T1–3, N0-1, age less than 75 years, invasive breast cancer, and BCS with a macroscopic negative margin. Chemotherapy was permitted before or during radiation. A breast boost and regional node irradiation were allowed. The IBTR at 10 years was 12.1% for 50 Gy, 14.8% for 39 Gy, and 9.6% for 42.9 Gy, the differences between 39 and 42.9 Gy being statistically significant ($p = .027$). The most hypofractionated trial arm had a statistically significant change in breast appearance out to 10 years after radiation. There was a statistically significant observed change in breast appearance up to 10 years after radiation more often in the patients receiving 42.9 Gy compared with 39 Gy and 50 Gy (42.3% vs. 27.4% and 35.4%, respectively), but the number with a marked difference remained relatively low in all three arms (10.1%, 3.4%, and 5.6%, respectively). The differences did not reach significance for 39 Gy compared with 50 Gy. The dose for this arm was modified down for the subsequent START A trial.

From this pilot study, the UK Standardisation of Breast Radiotherapy (START) trials A and B were developed.[15,142,143] Trial A compared 50 Gy in 25 fractions, 41.6 Gy in 13 fractions, or 39 Gy in 13 fractions all kept at a duration of 5 weeks (by using every-other-day scheduling in the hypofractionated arms). This was similar to the pilot study described earlier, except for a reduction in dose from 42.9 to 41.6 Gy because of the observed increase in late effects. Trial B compared 50 Gy in 25 fractions over 5 weeks versus 40 Gy in 15 fractions over 3 weeks, a schedule commonly used in the United Kingdom at that time and that was more similar to the Canadian randomized trial. Eligibility included T1–3a, N0-1, invasive breast cancer, and BCS or mastectomy with a margin greater than 1 mm. Chemotherapy, regional node irradiation and boost radiation were all permitted. A sequential boost was permitted on these START trials. There were no differences in 10-year IBTR between the hypofractionation arms and standard fractionation. The local-regional recurrence rates for START A were not significantly different between arms (7.4%, 6.3%, and 8.8%, respectively) or for START B (5.5% and 4.3%, respectively). Rates of breast cancer-specific, disease-free and overall survival were also the same. The late effects of breast appearance, breast edema or hardness, or skin changes were generally equal or better with whole breast hypofractionation, and there were no significant differences in late effects of rib fracture, lung fibrosis, ischemic heart disease or brachial plexopathy.

As a response to the publication of phase III data with 5- to 10-year results, ASTRO convened a task force of experts to make consensus recommendations on the use of H-WBRT in early-stage breast cancer.[144] There was consensus that H-WBRT resulted in equivalent results as conventional fractionation, but for a relatively narrow definition of patients meeting the criteria on the randomized trials and accrued in large numbers on those trials. This was women 50 or older, T1-2, N0, BCS, no systemic chemotherapy, radiation to the breast only, and radiation dose heterogeneity of ±7%. There was no consensus for or against high-grade tumors. There was consensus against H-WBRT for patients not included in the trials, such as DCIS, or underrepresented on the trials such as age less than 50 or needing regional node irradiation. The task force concluded that there were "few data to define the indications for and toxicity of a tumor bed boost" in patients treated with H-WBRT. For patients treated with H-WBRT without a boost as was used on the OCOG trial, 42.5 Gy in 16 fractions was recommended. Lastly, optimization of dose homogeneity was recommended, with a strong recommendation for three-dimensional dose compensation and exclusion of the heart from the primary treatment fields with H-WBRT.

In 2012 ASTRO selected H-WBRT for their first out of five recommendations for the Choosing Wisely campaign, an initiative to foster conversations between patients and physicians about treatments that may be overused, unnecessary or potentially harmful.[145] The recommendation made was "Don't initiate whole-breast radiation therapy as a part of breast conservation therapy in women age ≥50 with early-stage invasive breast cancer without considering shorter treatment schedules." H-WBRT was selected for this campaign due to the high prevalence of radiation for early-stage breast cancer in clinical practice, the potential convenience to patients, the reduced cost of care, the strength of the medical evidence and the previously published ASTRO consensus guideline. The text of the recommendation makes note that physicians could discuss with patients that H-WBRT is appropriate for selected women (but does not go into further detail about selection factors). Physicians could also make it known to their patients that there is relatively shorter 10-year follow-up data compared with longer results of 20 years or more for conventional WBI fractionation.

Current patient selection for H-WBRT should be broadly applicable to most women with early-stage breast cancer after BCS. Since the ASTRO consensus, there has been additional large phase III data and other high-quality evidence with long-term. Age less than 50 should not be used as a sole reason to exclude patients from H-WBRT. The OCOG trial reported no significant difference in local control by age 50 and older versus less than 50 and that age less than 50 years had an odds ratio of 1.64 (95% confidence interval [CI] 1.26–21.5, $p < .001$) compared with 50 and older for having a good or excellent cosmetic result.[14] A meta-analysis of the long-term START pilot, A and B trials also found no significant difference in 10-year local control for ages less than 40, 40 to 49, or 50 and older.[15] The analysis of moderate to marked physician-assessed normal tissue effects on the breast (shrinkage, edema, induration or telangiectasia) was also either not significantly different or actually favored hypofractionation by age in the subgroup analysis. Although there were some initial concerns raised about high-grade and H-WBRT, the randomized trials have shown no difference in the local-regional relapse by grade.[15,146] Left breast cancer was not specifically excluded from the randomized clinical trials of H-WBRT. The START A and B trials specifically did not show an increase in cardiac events for left-sided patients at 10 years with hypofractionation compared with conventional fractionation.[15] The ASTRO task force recommended for H-WBRT exclusion of the heart from the treatment field using basic three-dimensional treatment planning—a good recommendation for any fractionation.[144] Field in field 3D

conformal (forward planning) or intensity modulated radiation therapy (inverse planning), prone position, and deep inspiration breath holding are all standard measures today that may be employed today to reduce cardiac dose.[147–151] From 11% to 36% of patients in the four major studies of H-WBRT had systemic chemotherapy. A meta-analysis of the long-term RMH/GOC, START A and B trials showed no difference in the local-regional relapse by use of chemotherapy.[15] Subgroup analysis of the OCOG trial showed no difference in local control, or association with a good or excellent cosmetic result, between H-WBRT and conventional fractionation for use of systemic therapy in general (chemo and/or endocrine therapy). The sequential administration of chemotherapy before or after radiation should not be a contraindication to delivering H-WBRT. Because of the possible increased soft tissue and cosmetic effects and lack of data in the setting of H-WBRT, concurrent administration of chemotherapy is not recommended. Given the severe nature of the potential complications, the poor response to treatment of plexopathy, and the potential for very late onset, regional node irradiation is currently recommended only with conventional fractionation.

The OCOG trial specifically excluded patients with a breast "deemed too large to permit satisfactory radiation therapy (i.e., the maximum width of breast tissue > 25 cm)."[139] The UK START A and B trials did not specifically exclude patients for a large breast size, but also placed a limitation on the dose inhomogeneity allowed on the central axis during radiation planning of 5% of the prescribed dose (±5%).[142,143] The dose inhomogeneity and hot spots need to be restricted even more with H-WBRT than with conventional fractionation to minimize risks for complications due to the steep late effects curve associated with equivalent tissue effects from altered dose fractionation. Keeping the dose homogeneity within 105% to 110% should keep the isoeffective dose for late effects comparable between 2- and 3-Gy fraction sizes.[152] There have been significant advances in radiation planning that have been able to improve dose homogeneity and reduce complications. Today 3D planning by computed tomography simulator and either field in field 3D conformal (forward planning) or intensity modulated radiation therapy (inverse planning) can reduce dose inhomogeneity and reduce complications such as edema or negative cosmetic effects on the breast.[153–158] In addition to these measures, even a large chest wall separation >25 cm that was used as exclusion in the OCOG trial in the past may be mitigated by differences in patient positionings, such as prone, that can reduce the central axis separation and dose inhomogeneity of large-breasted women.[159–161]

Timing of Radiation Therapy in Relation to Surgery and Systemic Therapy

Radiation therapy is given after BCS, as the appropriateness of breast conserving therapy depends on knowing the pathologic tumor size and final resection margin status. The optimal interval for starting radiation after surgery is unknown. In general, at least 4 to 6 weeks are given to allow wound healing. Delays of starting RT of up to 8 weeks after surgery are not associated with an increased risk of IBTR compared with starting within 4 weeks.[162] A systematic review of 8 retrospective studies involving 6303 patients found that patients who started radiation longer than 8 weeks after surgery had an IBTR rate of 9.1%, compared with 5.8% for patients starting sooner (odds ratio 1.62; 95% CI 1.21–2.16).[163] Therefore, in general it is advisable to begin radiation within 8 weeks of surgery in patients not receiving chemotherapy.

For patients receiving chemotherapy, radiation can be delayed until after its completion. A prospective study of women with stage I or II breast cancer randomized patients to receive a 12-week course of adjuvant chemotherapy before or after radiation.[78] There were no statistically significant differences in time to failure, overall sites of first failure (local or distant), or overall survival between patients treated with early or late radiation. Retrospective studies have either shown a modest increase in IBTR with delay to radiation after chemotherapy[163] or no difference in IBTR with delay of radiation.[164,165] Sequential administration of chemotherapy and radiation is preferable to concurrent treatment because it preserves the efficacy of both adjuvant therapies and minimizes the risk of toxicity and interference of one adjuvant therapy with the other. A randomized trial comparing concurrent to sequential administration of radiation therapy and cyclophosphamide, methotrexate, and fluorouracil (CMF) for patients with negative margins showed no differences in 5-year local control, recurrence-free, or overall survival rates.[166] Potential disadvantages of giving concurrent therapy are also increased incidences of radiation dermatitis or other toxicities.[167,168] Although some studies have shown acceptable toxicity with concurrent radiation and CMF regimens,[168,169] this may not be true of modern dose-dense regimens currently in use today.

Endocrine therapy may be given concurrently or after radiation therapy without effect on local control or survival.[170–172]

Characteristics and Management of Local Failure After Breast Conserving Surgery and Radiation Therapy

Current recommendations for surveillance of patients after breast conservation therapy include monthly patient self-examination, examination by a physician every 4 to 6 months for 5 years, and then yearly, and mammography 6 months after radiation and then yearly.[10] More than 80% of cases of IBTR are detected by mammography and have a median size of 1 to 2 cm.[45,117,173–176] The median interval to the detection of local recurrence is 4 to 6 years.[98,177–180] The time to recurrence appears to be delayed by the use of systemic therapy.[55] More than 80% to 90% of breast recurrences are invasive.[176,177,181–184] Approximately 75% of patients with IBTR will present with isolated (breast-only) recurrence, 5% to 15% will have simultaneous regional recurrence (most commonly axillary), and 5% to 15% will present with simultaneous distant metastases.[45,183–185]

Local recurrences are found in the same quadrant as the original primary tumor in approximately 50% to 90% of cases.[45,61,64,117,177,178,182,183,185–187] With longer follow-up, the proportion of recurrences in other quadrants increases.[177,188] In classification of an IBTR, it is not usually possible to distinguish between a failure to destroy residual tumor cells from the original cancer and those due to the later development of a new primary cancer. An IBTR is commonly considered as a "true recurrence" of the original tumor based on combinations of similar histology, within the same quadrant, and/or occurrence within 5 years of the original primary.[117,180,188–191] Gujral and coworkers classified 79% of IBTR as local recurrence at a median follow-up of 10 years based on location and histology.[191] In a novel study that compared loss of heterozygosity between the original primary and the IBTR, Vicini and colleagues determined that 76% were

clonally related and 24% were different.[192] Consistent with the clinical definition relating time interval to likelihood of being a new primary, the proportion of IBTRs that were clonally related was 93% at 5 years, 67% at 10 years, and 33% at 15 years.

Most studies indicate that a shorter time to the development of local recurrence (particularly within 2–3 years of initial treatment) is a negative prognostic factor, which indicates an aggressive tumor biology with a higher incidence of subsequent distant metastatic disease.[45,107,117,124,176–178,184,186,193–196] Smaller initial tumor size,[107,193,197] initially negative axillary nodes,[176,181,187] positive ER status,[107] and absence of lymphovascular invasion[176] or skin involvement[175,176,181,186,193,198] are favorable prognostic factors. The size of the recurrence has not been a prognostic factor in most series,[175,177,181,185,187,193,198] although it has been in some.[176,181] Patients with recurrences that are pure DCIS or only focally invasive have the highest rates of salvage with mastectomy, with long-term breast cancer–specific survival rates greater than 90%.[177,181,184,185,195]

Mastectomy is generally considered the standard treatment for patients with a clinically isolated IBTR,[10,199] resulting in local control rates of approximately 85% to 95%.[176,177,182–185,198] Exploration of the axilla or axillary dissection shows pathologic nodal involvement in 13% to 58% of patients.[124,177,184,189,200] Although it seems reasonable to give systemic treatment to patients at substantial risk of distant failure after mastectomy based upon its efficacy in the adjuvant setting, studies of patients in this setting have not uniformly confirmed its value.[177,193] A randomized trial of chemotherapy for isolated locoregional recurrence of breast cancer (CALOR) assigned 85 patients to chemotherapy and 77 to no chemotherapy.[201] The 5-year disease-free survival was 69% with chemotherapy and 57% without chemotherapy ($p = .046$). Subgroup analysis showed the benefit limited to ER-negative patients.

Approximately 70% of IBTR may be candidates for salvage BCS. Alpert and colleagues found that only 66% of patients treated by salvage mastectomy would have been potential candidates for further BCS based on tumor size less than 3 cm, 3 or fewer positive axillary nodes, the absence of lymphovascular or skin extension, and concordance of physical examination and mammography findings.[183] Li and colleagues found that 71% of IBTR were favorable based on as unifocal DCIS or T1 2 cm or less, without skin involvement, and a more than 2-year interval from initial treatment.[173] Clinical stage of IBTR predicted for pathologic stage: 95% of patients with clinical T1 IBTR had pathologic T1 disease at salvage mastectomy ($p < .0001$). Results in patients undergoing second BCS as salvage surgery have been mixed with the incidence of a second local failure after wide excision in other published series ranges from 18% to 48%.[176,177,181,200] More stringent patient selection, such as using this approach only for patients with very small recurrences or those with negative margins (or both) might perhaps increase second local control rates.[183]

The experience of second BCS and further RT in selected patients having an IBTR after WBRT shows there is an 11% to 36% risk for second local recurrence. Kurtz and coworkers treated 11 of 50 patients who had recurrences away from the original tumor bed with additional radiation after wide excision.[200] Second local failures occurred in 36% of the patients treated with further irradiation, compared with 31% of those treated with wide local excision alone. Deutsch and colleagues reported on a series of 39 women treated for IBTR by repeat BCS and 50-Gy electron beam reirradiation.[202] The subsequent breast second IBTR rate was 23%, although there were no reported serious sequelae from the

TABLE 50.4 Overall Survival and Local Recurrence Rates in Prospective Randomized Trials of Patients With Stage I–II Breast Cancer Comparing BSC Alone to Breast Conserving Surgery and RT

Trial	Years	Tumor No.	Tamoxifen Size (cm)	% IBTR (%)	BCS	BCS + RT	Follow-up
NSABP B-06 [2]	1976–1984	1137	≤4	0	39.2	14.3	20 y
Uppsala-Örebro[210]	1981–1988	381	≤2	0	24	8.5	10 y
British[213]	1981–1990	400	≤5	If ER+	50	29	20 y
Ontario[211]	1984–1989	837	≤4	0	35	11	8 y median
Scottish[212]	1985–1991	585	≤4	73	24.5	5.8	6 y
Milan[208]	1987–1989	567	≤2.5	12	35	7	10 y
NSABP B-21[138]	1989–1998	673	≤1	All	16.5	2.8	8 y
		336	≤1		0	—	9.3 y
GBCSG[217]	1991–1998	173	≤2	0	34[a]	10[a]	10 y median
		174	≤2	All	8[a]	7[a]	
Canadian[214]	1992–2000	769	≤5	All	12.2	4.1	8 y
CALGB[215]	1995–1999	636	≤2	All	10	2	10 y
ABCCSG[218]	1996–2004	869	<3	All	5.1	0.4	5 y
PRIME II[216]	2003–2009	658	<3	All	4.1	1.3	5 y

[a]Crude result.

ABCCSG, Austrian Breast and Colorectal Cancer Study Group; *BCS*, breast conserving surgery; *BCS + RT*, breast conserving surgery and radiation; *CALGB*, Cancer and Leukemia Group B; *GBSG*, German Breast Cancer Study Group; *NSABP*, National Surgical Adjuvant Breast and Bowel Project.

additional radiation. Hannoun-Levi and coworkers also reported a 23% second local recurrence rate at 5 years in 69 patients with IBTR who were treated by a second BCS and interstitial brachytherapy.[203] Chadha and colleagues treated 15 patients with second BCS and brachytherapy and had a IBTR rate of 11%.[204] In three other series of second BCS and brachytherapy, the second local recurrence rates were 21% to 26%.[181,205,206] Common among these series was the relatively low risk for serious complications from reirradiation. The Radiation Therapy Oncology Group studied prospectively a regimen of salvage BCS and 3D conformal external beam APBI in a favorable subset of patients. Patient selection included IBTR 3 cm or less in size, without imaging evidence of multicentricity, and an interval to recurrence of greater than 1 year. The study has shown feasibility and low acute and 1-year toxicity without second local recurrences.[207]

Breast-Conserving Surgery Without Radiation Therapy

The rationale for giving postoperative WBRT is to treat potential areas of microscopic residual disease left anywhere in the breast after BCS, which may act as a source of local recurrence. However, considerable research has been conducted to determine whether radiation is necessary for all patients after BCS. The prospective randomized studies conducted over the past decades have failed to demonstrate any subgroup of patients, even with very favorable clinical and pathologic selection factors, who do not receive a benefit from radiation in reduction of IBTR. However, the results of trials with careful patient selection have shown a subgroup of

women for whom the statistically significant reduction in IBTR by WBRT may not be clinically significant to them or associated with an increase in overall survival.

In general, the omission of WBRT after BCS is associated with a clinically and statistically significant decrease in breast cancer mortality. The greatest difference was observed in node-positive patients in the Milan quadrantectomy trial: the 10-year overall survival rate was 82% with RT, compared with 62% without it.[208] However, a pooled analysis of published results from 15 prospective randomized trials including 9422 women found the relative risk of mortality was 1.086 (95% confidence interval 1.003–1.175), or an 8.6% excess risk of mortality, if RT was omitted.[209] The Early Breast Cancer Trialists' Collaborative Group metaanalysis of randomized trials included more than 10,800 patients treated on 17 phase III trials of BCS with or without WBRT.[8] The 10-year risk of any locoregional or distant first recurrence was reduced from 35% to 19% ($p < .00001$) and reduced the 15-year risk of breast cancer death from 25% to 21% ($p = .00005$).

There have been numerous prospective randomized trials of BCS with or without WBRT for patients with stage I or II breast cancer (Table 50.4).[2,138,208,210–218] Factors that have been variously associated with an intermediate to high risk of IBTR in patients treated without RT include larger tumor size, younger age, the presence of an EIC, positive axillary nodes, lymphovascular invasion, and invasive lobular histology.[118,208,210–213] Patients with an EIC had a 10-year risk of IBTR of 70% in one study even after quadrantectomy.[208] In the same study, the risk of IBTR without radiation for patients age 65 years or younger was four-fold higher than the risk with RT, with the highest incidence in patients 45 or younger. A subgroup at very low risk of IBTR that did not benefit from radiation could not be identified in the Ontario study; the risk of IBTR was greater than 20% in those with age 50 or older with tumors smaller than 2 cm, patients age 50 years or older with tumors that had nuclear grade 1 to 2, or patients of any age with tumors 1 cm or smaller.[211] In the NSABP B-21 trial, which included only patients with tumors 1 cm or smaller, the risk of IBTR was 16.5% with tamoxifen, 9.3% with radiation, and 2.8% with both modalities.[138] A negative margin of no tumor on ink was used in most randomized prospective trials of BCS without radiation.[2,138,214,215] It is not known whether a wider surgical margin in these cases would further reduce the risk for IBTR when radiation is omitted. The Joint Center for Radiation Therapy conducted a prospective study of BCS alone in a group with the following eligibility criteria: T1 tumor size; unicentric; ductal, mucinous, or tubular carcinomas; no EIC; no lymphovascular invasion; pathologically negative axillary nodes.[219] In addition, there was a requirement for microscopic resection margins of 1 cm or wider or no tumor on reexcision. Even in this group of patients selected for very favorable characteristics, the IBTR rate was 23% after a median follow-up of 7.2 years.

These trials have not been able to demonstrate a clinically definable subgroup that does not have a lower IBTR with radiation. However, these trials have suggested some parameters that might define subgroups of women who may be appropriate candidates for BCS without WBRT because the risk of IBTR is acceptably low and not associated with a survival detriment. The studies outlined in Table 50.4 show a general improvement in results in later years by means of selection criteria for smaller tumor size, ER positivity and use of endocrine therapy, negative margins, and older women. A large randomized trial by the Cancer and Leukemia Group B was conducted of postoperative tamoxifen with or without radiation in 636 women age 70 years or older with T1 tumors that were ER positive with clinically or pathologically negative axillary nodes.[215] The locoregional recurrence at 10 years was 10% in 319 treated with tamoxifen and 2% in 317 treated with tamoxifen and WBRT ($p < .001$). There were no statistically significant differences in distant metastases, death from breast cancer or overall survival. In a Canadian trial, 769 patients age 50 or older with T1 or T2 node-negative breast cancer were randomized to receive tamoxifen alone or tamoxifen and radiation.[214] The median age was 68 years. The 8-year rates of IBTR were 4.1% and 12.2% with and without radiation, respectively ($p < .0001$). There were also no statistically significant differences in distant metastases or survival. The PRIME II trial[216] selected patients felt likely to be low-risk for IBTR without radiation based on age 65 or older, hormone receptor-positive, axillary node-negative, T1–T2 up to 3 cm at the longest dimension, negative margins 1 mm or larger, and grade 3 tumor histology or lymphovascular invasion, but not both. The 5-year IBTR was 4% with BCS and endocrine therapy alone versus 1% with BCS, endocrine therapy and WBRT ($p = .0002$) without differences in survival. The importance of endocrine therapy was shown in the German Breast Study Group trial, where the crude risk of local recurrence at 10 years was 7% to 10% in patients treated either with BCS and WBRT, BCS and tamoxifen, or BCS and both, but was 34% in those treated with BCS alone.[220]

There have been some promising results using tumor genomic expression or intrinsic breast cancer subtyping. Liu and colleagues[221] conducted a retrospective subgroup analysis on 501 of 769 available blocks from the larger Canadian prospective trial that had shown a significant benefit to WBRT after BCS and tamoxifen.[214] They conducted intrinsic subtyping by using immunohistochemical analysis of biomarkers ER, PR, HER2, cytokeratin 5/6, epidermal growth factor receptor, and ki67 to divide patients into luminal A, luminal B, or high-risk subtype. Luminal subtypes seemed to derive less benefit from WBRT (luminal A hazard ratio [HR] 0.40; luminal B HR 0.51) than high-risk subtypes (HR 0.13) that did not reach statistical significance. In an exploratory analysis of women with clinical low-risk (age older than 60 years, T1, grade 1 or 2) luminal A tumors, the 10-year IBTR was 1.3% with tamoxifen versus 5.0% with tamoxifen plus WBRT ($p = .42$). A prospective, single-arm clinical trial of BCS and endocrine therapy (tamoxifen or aromatase inhibitor) for 5 years has been open since 2013 to women with luminal A cancer and age 55 years or older, pT1N0, grade 1 to 2, margins 1 mm or greater, absence of lobular cancers, extensive intraductal component and lymphovascular invasion sponsored by the Ontario Clinical Oncology Group. Another prospective, single-arm clinical trial (IDEA) of BCS and endocrine therapy for 5 years is enrolling women aged 50 to 69 with hormone-sensitive, HER2-negative tumors with a low-risk genomic expression test (Oncotype-DX, GenomicHealth, Redwood City, CA). A third trial (PRECISION) that opened in 2016 is enrolling women 50 to 75 years of age after BCS to omit radiation based on a favorable result of a gene signature assay test (Prosigna, NanoString Technologies, Seattle, WA).

In summary, the optimal patient selection criteria for BCS without WBRT is generally patients aged 65 to 70 years or older or with a reduced life expectancy, with an ER-positive tumor and willing and able to take endocrine therapy for 5 years, tumor size 2 cm or smaller, negative axillary nodes and resection margins. Future patient selection based on ongoing clinical trials may depend more on biologic factors of genomic expression and tumor subtyping rather than traditional clinical and pathologic factors. In low-risk patients, the 5- to 10-year risk of IBTR may be acceptably low to them compared with BCS and WBRT. Although the risk for IBTR may be modestly higher without WBRT, for most women, these IBTRs will be picked up at an early stage by careful follow-up and treatable by salvage BCS with or without RT without detriment in overall survival. Even in favorable low-risk women, for those who want the very lowest risk for IBTR or who do not tolerate endocrine therapy within 6 months of BCS, WBRT is still recommended.

Conclusions

The combination of BCS and WBRT is an effective alternative to mastectomy for the majority of women with early-stage invasive breast cancer, with equal rates of local-regional control and survival. Clinical experience and long-term follow-up of patients have led to improved understanding of clinical and pathologic factors that are important in selecting good candidates for breast-conservation therapy. Together with improvements in surgical techniques and the increased use of adjuvant systemic therapy, this greater understanding has helped to minimize the risk of local recurrence. Hypofractionation that reduces length of treatment to 3 to 4 weeks is now an acceptable option for most women requiring WBRT after BCS, although some women based on young age, regional node treatment or dose homogeneity are suitable for conventional fractionation. Patients who have an IBTR can usually be cured by salvage mastectomy, which is the preferred treatment for most women, but there are promising results in studies of further attempts at BCS and additional RT. Although the majority of women will benefit from postoperative WBRT, with a large reduction in the risk of local recurrence, there may be a subgroup of women for whom this benefit is small and clinically acceptable to them. Women of advanced age or substantial comorbidities, who have small tumors excised with wide margins and are treated with endocrine therapy, will have minimal risks of local-recurrence recurrence or breast cancer mortality with the omission of RT. However, for the majority of women, the use of WBRT after BCS has been associated with a significant improvement in breast cancer mortality and overall survival.

Selected References

8. Early Breast Cancer Trialists' Collaborative G, Darby S, McGale P, et al. Effect of radiotherapy after breast-conserving surgery on 10-year recurrence and 15-year breast cancer death: meta-analysis of individual patient data for 10,801 women in 17 randomised trials. *Lancet*. 2011;378:1707-1716.

14. Whelan TJ, Pignol J-P, Levine MN, et al. Long-term results of hypofractionated radiation therapy for breast cancer. *N Engl J Med*. 2010;362:513-520.

33. Bartelink H, Maingon P, Poortmans P, et al. Whole-breast irradiation with or without a boost for patients treated with breast-conserving surgery for early breast cancer: 20-year follow-up of a randomised phase 3 trial. *Lancet Oncol*. 2015;16:47-56.

91. Moran MS, Schnitt SJ, Giuliano AE, et al. Society of Surgical Oncology-American Society for Radiation Oncology consensus guideline on margins for breast-conserving surgery with whole-breast irradiation in stages I and II invasive breast cancer. *J Clin Oncol*. 2014;32:1507-1515.

215. Hughes KS, Schnaper LA, Bellon JR, et al. Lumpectomy plus tamoxifen with or without irradiation in women age 70 years or older with early breast cancer: long-term follow-up of CALGB 9343. *J Clin Oncol*. 2013;31:2382-2387.

A full reference list is available online at ExpertConsult.com.

51

Partial Breast Irradiation: Accelerated and Intraoperative

CHIRAG SHAH, ELEANOR E. HARRIS, DENNIS HOLMES, AND FRANK A. VICINI

With more than 20 years of follow-up, multiple randomized studies have demonstrated equivalent outcomes between mastectomy and breast conserving therapy.[1–3] Furthermore, multiple studies have demonstrated an increase in local recurrence with the omission of radiation therapy after breast conserving surgery (BCS), and a meta-analysis has demonstrated an improvement in breast cancer mortality with the addition of radiation therapy to BCS.[4–6] As part of the randomized trials, radiation therapy primarily consisted of whole breast irradiation (WBI) using two-dimensional techniques. Over the past several decades, WBI has evolved and with modern radiation delivered using three-dimensional (3D) techniques that allow for improved target coverage and sparing of the heart and other organs at risk.[7] The duration of WBI is typically 3 to $6\frac{1}{2}$ weeks, often including a tumor bed boost, which can make compliance difficult for some patients. Multiple studies have documented that up to 15% to 20% of patients forgo adjuvant radiation therapy, and another subset of patients forgo breast conservation altogether due to an inability to receive adjuvant radiation therapy.[8–11] Although recent studies have documented the clinical efficacy and toxicity profile of hypofractionated WBI, reducing the treatment duration to 3 weeks, many patients continue to seek alternatives that shorten the duration of radiation therapy.[12,13] Partial breast irradiation represents a variety of techniques that allows for adjuvant radiation therapy to be delivered in 1 week or less (Fig. 51.1).

The rationale for WBI is the assumption of the potential for microscopic disease beyond the lumpectomy cavity. However, patterns of failure for patients undergoing breast conservation do not validate this hypothesis because the majority of ipsilateral breast tumor recurrences (IBTRs) occur within close proximity to the lumpectomy cavity, "true recurrences," with lower rates of failures elsewhere in the breast.[14,15] Furthermore, multiple studies have confirmed that the incidence of metachronous new primaries is not altered by the delivery of WBI.[16–18] Finally, pathologic specimen evaluation has documented that in patients undergoing BCS with negative margins that residual disease is most likely located within 1 to 2 cm of the surgical cavity.[19,20] Taken together, these data support the concept of partial breast irradiation, treating the breast tissue in the periphery of the lumpectomy cavity rather than the whole breast in selected patients. This chapter focuses on partial breast irradiation techniques, including accelerated partial breast irradiation (APBI) and intraoperative radiation therapy (IORT).

Accelerated Partial Breast Irradiation

APBI can be delivered using several techniques and fractionation schemes with the most common techniques being interstitial brachytherapy, applicator-based brachytherapy, and external-beam techniques (Fig. 51.2). Interstitial brachytherapy represents the original APBI technique with the longest follow-up to date, followed by development of single lumen applicators and subsequently multilumen applicators and external-beam techniques.

Interstitial Accelerated Partial Breast Irradiation

The interstitial brachytherapy technique had traditionally been used for boost after WBI before the introduction of electron beams on linear accelerators and thus was the first technique used for APBI as monotherapy.[3] A prospective Hungarian trial (1996–1998) with 12-year follow-up used the high-dose-rate (HDR) interstitial multicatheter technique as monotherapy for APBI and demonstrated a 9.3% rate of IBTR in a series of 45 patients with early-stage disease (tumor <2 cm, negative margins, negative nodes [N1mi allowed], low-grade). Toxicity rates were low with a 2% rate of grade 3 fibrosis and a 2% rate of fat necrosis, with 78% of patients having excellent/good cosmesis.[21] This prompted a randomized trial comparing partial breast irradiation (PBI) and WBI in women with early-stage breast cancer (T1N0-1mi, grade 1–2, nonlobular histology, negative margins). Radiation on the partial breast arm was delivered with interstitial brachytherapy (HDR: 7 × 5.2 Gy) or electrons (50 Gy/25 fractions). At 10 years, no difference in the rate of local recurrence was noted (5.9% PBI vs. 5.1% WBI) with no difference in disease-free, cancer-specific, or overall survival noted as well. PBI was associated with improved cosmetic outcomes (81% vs. 63% excellent/good cosmesis).[22] Similarly, a matched pair analysis (matched for age, size, nodal status, estrogen receptor status, hormonal therapy) from William Beaumont Hospital comparing 199 patients receiving interstitial APBI with 199 patients receiving WBI found no difference in 12-year outcomes including local recurrence (3.8% WBI vs. 5.0% APBI), which was confirmed by a second matched pair analysis from Washington University (3.8% WBI vs. 3.0% APBI).[23,24] These outcomes were recently validated by the Groupe Européen de Curiethérapie-European Society for Therapeutic Radiology and Oncology trial; this multiinstitutional phase III noninferiority trial randomized 1184 patients to interstitial APBI with HDR/pulsed-dose-rate (PDR)

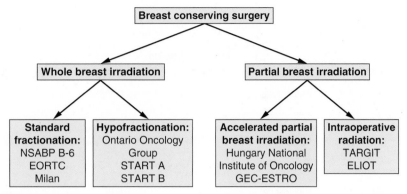

• **Fig. 51.1** Adjuvant radiation therapy options after breast conserving surgery. *EORTC,* European Organization of Research and Treatment of Cancer; *GEC-ESTRO,* Groupe Européen de Curiethérapie -European Society for Therapeutic Radiology and Oncology; *NSABP,* National Surgical Adjuvant Breast and Bowel Project; *START,* UK Standardisation of Breast Radiotherapy.

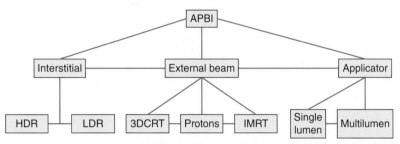

• **Fig. 51.2** Accelerated partial breast irradiation *(APBI)* treatment techniques. *HDR,* High-dose rate; *IMRT,* intensity modulated radiation therapy; *LDR,* low-dose rate; *3D-CRT,* three-dimensional conformal radiation therapy.

implants or WBI with a boost after BCS. Five-year outcomes demonstrated no difference in local recurrence with interstitial brachytherapy (0.9% WBI vs. 1.4% APBI), along with no difference in survival. With respect to toxicity, APBI was associated with a reduction in breast pain and a trend for reduced late grade 2 to 3 skin toxicity (5.7% APBI vs. 3.2% WBI).[25]

Radiation Therapy Oncology Group (RTOG) 9517 was a Phase II trial evaluating interstitial brachytherapy with both low-dose-rate (LDR; n = 33, 45 Gy in 3.5–5 days) and HDR (n = 66, 34 Gy in 10 fractions twice daily) multicatheter implants. Five-year local recurrence rates of 3% and 6% were noted for the HDR and LDR cohorts respectively. With regard to toxicity, 13% developed grade 3 skin toxicity with 66% to 68% rates of excellent/good cosmesis.[26,27] These findings have been confirmed by other single-institution prospective studies as well as retrospective studies that have documented low rates of recurrence and toxicity with high rates of excellent/good cosmetic outcomes that remained stable over time. With respect to dose and fractionation, the majority of studies have used 34 Gy/10 fractions twice daily or 32 Gy/8 fractions twice daily, whereas the Hungarian randomized study used 36.4 Gy/7 fractions twice daily. In cases in which LDR is used, 45 to 50 Gy over 3 to 5 days has commonly been administered. A summary of selected multicatheter interstitial APBI studies are presented in Table 51.1.[28–34]

Applicator Accelerated Partial Breast Irradiation

Interstitial brachytherapy represented a technique that allowed for the delivery of APBI with excellent clinical outcomes. However, due to the technical complexity associated with inserting the catheters, it has been limited to a small number of centers.

However, with the introduction of single-entry applicators whose insertion is less technically demanding, brachytherapy-based APBI became more widely available for patients and is used at a growing number of centers. The initial clinical studies, after US Food and Drug Administration approval in 2002, were performed using the single-lumen MammoSite (Hologic, Bedford, MA) applicator. Benitez and colleagues published results from the initial study of 43 patients with no local recurrences at 5 years and 83% excellent/good cosmesis. Toxicity rates were low including a 9.3% rate of infection and 12% symptomatic seroma rate. Importantly, a skin spacing target of 7 mm was identified to reduce skin toxicity, such as telangiectasias, and improve cosmetic outcomes.[35] The success of this study led to the prospective American Society of Breast Surgeons (ASBS) MammoSite Registry, which enrolled 1449 patients from 2002 to 2004. With a median follow-up of 63 months, the 5-year IBTR rate was 3.8% and excellent/good cosmesis was seen in more than 90% of cases. Toxicity outcomes showed a 9.6% rate of infection, 2.5% rate of fat necrosis, and 13% rate of symptomatic seromas.[36,37] Similar results have been seen by multiple prospective, multiinstitutional, and single-institution studies.[38–45]

Although the initial applicator studies used a single lumen device, advances in design allowed for the development of multilumen applicators providing for more dosimetric degrees of freedom. Multiple dosimetric studies have been performed demonstrating improvements in target coverage as well as reduction in dose to the chest wall, normal breast tissue, and skin, even in cases with limited skin distance.[45–48] Mature data beyond 5 years are limited with this technique, but initial studies have demonstrated low rates of toxicity and excellent clinical outcomes.[38,44,45,49] A multiinstitutional series with 3-year outcomes

TABLE 51.1 Interstitial APBI Studies

Trial/Institution	Patients (n)	Study Type	Median Follow-Up (months)	Technique	Outcomes
GEC-ESTRO	1184	Randomized	78	HDR/PDR	No difference in 5-year local recurrence (0.9% vs. 1.4%); APBI reduced breast pain
National Institute of Oncology Hungary	128 PBI (88 HDR)	Randomized	124	HDR/ electrons	No difference in 10-year local recurrence (5.9% vs. 5.1%); excellent/good cosmesis
William Beaumont Hospital	199	Matched Pair	127	HDR	No difference in 12-year local recurrences (3.8% vs. 5.0%)
Washington University	202	Matched Pair	60	HDR	No difference in 5-year local control (97% vs. 96.2%); excellent/good cosmesis 95%, 10.1% rate of symptomatic fat necrosis
National Institute of Oncology Hungary	45	Prospective	133	HDR	12-year local recurrence 9.3%; excellent/good cosmesis 78%, 2.2% grade 3 fibrosis, 2.2% fat necrosis requiring surgery
RTOG 9517	99	Prospective	73	HDR (66)/ LDR (33)	5-year local recurrence 3% HDR/6% LDR; excellent/ good cosmesis 66%, 13% grade 3 toxicity
Harvard University	50	Prospective	134	LDR	12-year local recurrence 15%; excellent/good cosmesis 67%, 9%/13% grade 3/4 toxicity, 54% moderate/ severe fibrosis, 35% fat necrosis
Multi-Institutional (Germany/Austria)	274	Prospective	63	PDR (175)/ HDR (99)	5-year local recurrence 2%; excellent/good cosmesis 90%, 0.4%/2.2% grade 3 + fibrosis/telangiectasia
Ochsner Clinic	50	Prospective	75	LDR/HDR	Local recurrence 2%; 8% grade 3 or 4 toxicity; comparable outcomes, toxicity, cosmesis compared with WBI cohort
Tufts/Brown University	75	Retrospective	73	HDR	Excellent/good cosmesis 91%
University of Wisconsin	247	Retrospective	48.5	HDR	Local recurrence 2%; Excellent/good cosmesis 93%,
Virginia Commonwealth University;	44	Retrospective	42	LDR (11)/HDR (31)	Local recurrence 0%; excellent/good cosmesis 80% LDR/90% HDR
Orebro University	50	Retrospective	86	PDR	7-year local recurrence 4%; excellent/good cosmesis 56%, 12% fat necrosis

APBI, Accelerated partial breast irradiation; *GEC-ESTRO,* Groupe Européen de Curiethérapie-European Society for Therapeutic Radiology and Oncology; *HDR,* high-dose rate; *LDR,* low-dose rate; *PBI,* partial breast irradiation; *PDR,* pulsed-dose rate; *WBI,* whole breast irradiation.

found the local recurrence rate to be 2.2% in a series of 342 patients, with a 4.4% rate of persistent seromas and 8.5% rate of infection. Excellent/good cosmesis was noted in 88% of patients with these findings substantiated by additional studies.[38] Table 51.2 presents a summary of selected applicator APBI studies.

Two observational studies evaluated brachytherapy based APBI compared with WBI and found higher rates of mastectomy as well as higher rates of toxicity (infectious and noninfectious).[50,51] The limitations of these studies include the design of the study (observational), missing data in the databases used especially regarding use of radiation, short follow-up, failure to control for relevant patient and disease characteristics as well as lack of information for evaluating the reason for the difference in mastectomy rates, and use of billing codes rather than medical records, all of which makes their findings hypothesis generating in light of mature phase III data failing to corroborate their findings.[52,53] With the continued evolution of brachytherapy APBI to include multilumen applicators, it is expected that toxicity rates will continue to decline. The most common dose and fractionation scheme is 34 Gy/10 fractions twice daily; however, shorter courses (e.g., 28 Gy/4 fractions twice daily) are being investigated.

External-Beam Accelerated Partial Breast Irradiation

APBI delivered with external-beam techniques is an appealing option for many patients because it eliminates the need for another procedure after surgery. Although older series have evaluated this technique, with the advent of computed tomography simulation, 3D planning, and image guidance, external-beam APBI can be delivered in multiple techniques with greater accuracy of target volume delineation and treatment delivery.[54,55] Several institutional studies have suggested increased toxicity or poorer cosmesis with 3D conformal radiation therapy (CRT) APBI external-beam techniques, potentially related to larger volumes of normal breast irradiated or specific techniques utilized. However, publication of two randomized trials evaluating external-beam APBI has provided level I data regarding the technique and support the continued study and utilization of the technique.[56,57]

TABLE 51.2 Applicator APBI Studies

Trial/Institution	Patients (n)	Study Type	Follow-Up (months)	Technique	Outcomes
MammoSite Initial Study	43	Prospective	65	Single Lumen	5-year local recurrence 0%; excellent/good cosmesis 83%, 12% symptomatic seromas, 9% infections
ASBS MammoSite Registry	1449	Prospective registry	63	Single Lumen	5-year local recurrence 3.8%; excellent/good cosmesis 91%, 13% symptomatic seroma, 2.5% fat necrosis, 10% infections
Contura Phase 4	342	Prospective registry	36	Multi-Lumen	3-year local recurrence 2.2%; excellent/good cosmesis 88%, 4.4% symptomatic seroma, 8.5% infection
Multi-Institutional (Germany)	23	Prospective	20	Single Lumen	39% serious seroma, 26% telangiectasia, 56% hyperpigmentation
Multi-Institutional (United States)	483	Retrospective	24	Single Lumen	2-year local recurrence 1.2%; excellent/good cosmesis 91%, 9% infections, reduced infection with closed-cavity technique
William Beaumont Hospital	80	Retrospective	22	Single Lumen	3-year local recurrence 2.9%; excellent/good cosmesis 88%, at 3 years, 10% symptomatic seromas, 11% infections, 9% fat necrosis, 88% excellent/good cosmesis
Rush University Medical Center	70	Retrospective	26.1	Single Lumen	Local recurrence 5.7%
Medical University of South Carolina	111	Retrospective	46	Single Lumen	4-year IBTR 5%; excellent/good cosmesis 90%
The Breast Center, Georgia	46	Retrospective	36	Multi Lumen	Local recurrence 2%; excellent/good cosmesis 97%, 4.3% persistent seroma, 2.2% telangiectasia
University of California–San Diego	100	Retrospective	21	Strut Applicator	Recurrence rate 1%; 1.9% symptomatic seroma, 1.9% fat necrosis

APBI, Accelerated partial breast irradiation; *IBTR*, ipsilateral breast tumor recurrence.

The 3D-CRT technique was developed at William Beaumont Hospital with initial dosimetric studies and outcomes demonstrating its feasibility.[58] A 5-year update (205 patients) from the institution demonstrated no recurrences and reasonable rates of chronic toxicity with a 7.5%/7.6% rates of fibrosis/telangiectasias and 81% of patients having excellent/good cosmesis.[59] Similar results were noted in several studies including a subset analysis of National Surgical Adjuvant Breast and Bowel Project (NSABP) B-39, which demonstrated low rates of fibrosis (grade 2 < 12%, grade 3 < 3%, grade 4/5 0%), and an analysis of 100 patients treated with external-beam radiation therapy APBI at New York University using the prone technique, which demonstrated an 89% rate of excellent/good cosmesis at 5 years.[60–62] Also, a small randomized trial from Spain demonstrated no recurrences at 5 years with improved acute toxicity with 3D-CRT APBI.[63] However, other single-institution studies raised concerns regarding toxicity (fibrosis) and poor cosmetic outcomes. Findings from the University of Michigan (which used intensity modulated radiation therapy [IMRT] and active breathing control) and Tufts series were confirmed in part by long-term follow-up of RTOG 0319, a phase II trial that demonstrated deterioration of cosmetic outcomes from 82% excellent/good cosmesis at 1 year to 64% at 5 years with a 5.8% rate of grade 3 toxicity.[64–66] The RAPID trial randomized women after BCS to external-beam APBI (3D-CRT) or WBI (standard/hypofractionated). The trial accrued more than 2100 women, and with median follow-up of 3 years, APBI was found to have higher rates of grade 1 and 2 toxicity (telangiectasias, induration, breast pain, fat necrosis) with no difference in the rates of grade 3 toxicity (1.4% vs. 0%). Cosmetic outcomes were inferior with 3D-CRT APBI.[56] An alternative to 3D-CRT APBI is to use IMRT; initial outcomes from this technique were promising with a phase II study of 136 patients from Lei and colleagues demonstrating a 4-year IBTR rate of 0.7% with 88% to 91% excellent/good cosmesis and low rates of toxicity noted.[67] A randomized study from Florence compared IMRT APBI with WBI delivered with IMRT (standard fractionation); at 5 years, no difference in rates of local recurrence were noted and acute toxicity was improved with APBI (0% vs. 6.5%), as was excellent/good cosmesis (95.1% vs. 89.6%).[57] The dose and fractionation most commonly used is 38.5 Gy/10 fractions BID; however, recent data have demonstrated excellent clinical and toxicity outcomes with 30 Gy/5 fractions every other day. Similarly, an abstract of the IMPORT-LOW trial demonstrated that with 5.8 years of follow-up that once daily fractionation (40 Gy/15 fractions) to the partial breast was noninferior to WBI or WBI with a simultaneous integrated boost (0.5% vs. 1.1% vs. 0.2%) with respect to recurrences as well as toxicity.[68] Table 51.3 provides a summary of selected external-beam APBI series.

Proton therapy represents an alternative external-beam technique compared with 3D-CRT and IMRT (Table 51.4). This technique has undergone continued refinement because of initial concerns regarding toxicity; a study from Massachusetts General Hospital demonstrated 79% of patients having moderate to severe skin color changes at 3 to 4 weeks after treatment and 22% moderate to severe moist desquamation at 6 to 8 weeks.[69] A subsequent update from MGH compared outcomes of 19 patients treated with protons (32 Gy/8 fractions BID) with 79 treated with photons or mixed photons/electrons. With 7-year follow-up, proton therapy was associated with worse cosmesis (62% vs. 94% excellent/good, *p* = .03) as well as higher rates of skin toxicity including telangiectasias, pigmentation changes but no difference in the rates of breast pain, edema, fibrosis, fat necrosis, rib

fracture, or skin desquamation. Also, although not statistically significant there was a higher rate of local recurrence noted (11% vs. 4%).[70] An update of the Loma Linda proton experience (40 Gy/10 fractions daily) was recently published with 5-year outcomes; 100 patients were enrolled with a 3% IBTR and no grade 3 or higher acute skin toxicity. Patient and physician assessed cosmesis was 90% excellent/good cosmesis with no change noted over time.[71] Chang and colleagues reported outcomes of a phase II trial including 30 patients treated with protons (30 CGE/6 fractions daily). With a median follow-up of 59 months, no recurrences had been identified with 69% excellent/good cosmesis at 3 years. Breast retraction was noted to increase during follow-up across all patients.[72]

Expert Consensus Statements

At this time, multiple societies have released evidence-based consensus statements to assist clinicians treating patients off-protocol with APBI (Table 51.5).[73–76] These guidelines are predominantly based on clinical and pathologic features as well as expert/consensus opinion. One of the most commonly used groupings is the American Society of Radiation Oncology (ASTRO) consensus guideline. Published in 2009 and based on the randomized trials and prospective studies available at that time, it recommended three categories (suitable, cautionary and unsuitable) for the selection of patients for APBI off-protocol. Limited data have validated these groupings with multiple studies demonstrating a failure of consensus groupings to stratify by risk of local recurrence. An analysis of the ASBS MammoSite Registry evaluated the risk of local recurrence by ASTRO consensus groupings; at 5 years, no difference in the rate of IBTR was noted by grouping (2.6% vs. 5.4% vs. 5.3%, *p* = .19) with the only factor associated with IBTR being estrogen receptor negativity.[77] These findings have been reproduced by several studies showing no significant relationship between the ASTRO categories and the risk of IBTR.[78–81] However, after the publication of the ASTRO consensus statement, the SEER database has revealed an increase in the number of suitable and decrease in the number of unsuitable patients undergoing brachytherapy-based APBI, demonstrating that clinicians are responding to these guidelines.[82] In light of increasing data on APBI, other statements have been released including those from the ABS, although data validating these guidelines are limited at this time.[74] An update of the ASTRO guidelines is expected in 2017 with preliminary guidelines available for public review.[83]

Future Directions

In the near future, mature results from several randomized trials comparing APBI and WBI are expected and will look to confirm the five randomized studies and prospective institutional data to date that have documented no significant difference in local recurrence outcomes with APBI and WBI. Furthermore, as APBI continues to evolve as a treatment technique, future directions look to reduce the duration of therapy further and use new techniques to reduce the risk of toxicity. With regard to duration, studies are underway evaluating APBI delivered with applicators in 2 days or less. Wilkinson et al. presented outcomes from a prospective study at William Beaumont Hospital where 45 patients received APBI (28 Gy/4 fractions twice daily) using single-lumen applicators. At 4 years, no grade 3 or greater toxicities were noted. Grade 1 to 2 fat necrosis and seromas were observed in 18% and 42% of

TABLE 51.3 Modern External Beam APBI Studies

Trial/Institution	Patients (n)	Study Type	Follow-Up (months)	Technique	Outcomes
RAPID	2135	Randomized	36	3D-CRT	Increased adverse cosmesis with APBI (26% vs. 18%, per patients), increase grade 1–2 toxicity with 3D-CRT
University of Florence	520	Randomized	60	APBI	No difference in local recurrence or survival; improved cosmesis with IMRT APBI (95.1% vs. 89.6%) and reduced rates of acute toxicity
IMPORT LOW	2018	Randomized	68	3D-CRT	No difference in local recurrence: 1.1% WBI vs. 0.2% (WBI with simultaneous boost to cavity) vs. 0.5% PBI
Hospital de la Esperanza	102	Randomized	60	3D-CRT	No local recurrences, APBI lower acute toxicity, no difference chronic toxicity
NSABP B-39/RTOG 0413	1367	Randomized	41	3D-CRT	Grade 2 fibrosis 12%, grade 3 3%
RTOG 0319	52	Prospective	63	3D-CRT	Local recurrence 6%; excellent/good cosmesis 82% year 1/64% year 3, 5.8% grade 3 toxicity
University of Michigan	34	Prospective	60	IMRT	Local recurrence 3%; excellent/good cosmesis 73%, 3.3% grade 2 fibrosis,
New York University	100	Prospective	64	3D-CRT-prone	Local recurrence 1%; excellent/good cosmesis 89%, grade 3 toxicity 2%
Rocky Mountain	136	Prospective	53.1	IMRT	Ipsilateral failure 0.7%; excellent/good cosmesis 88%, 3.6% telangiectasia, 1.4% rib fracture
Canadian Multi-Institutional Trial	104/87 with 3-year + follow-up	Prospective	36 (minimum)	3D-CRT	One local recurrence; excellent/good cosmesis 82%, 1 grade 3 toxicity
Tufts University	80	Retrospective	32	3D-CRT	Excellent/good cosmesis 81%, 7.5% grade 3/4 fibrosis, 11% fat necrosis
William Beaumont Hospital	192	Retrospective	56	3D-CRT	Local recurrence 0%; excellent/good cosmesis 81%, 7.5% grade 3 fibrosis, 7.6% telangiectasias

APBI, Accelerated partial breast irradiation; *IMPORT LOW*, Intensity Modulated and Partial Organ Radiotherapy Low Risk; *IMRT*, intensity modulated radiation therapy; *NSABP*, National Surgical Adjuvant Breast and Bowel Project; *PBI*, partial breast irradiation; *RAPID*, Randomized Trial of Accelerated Partial Breast Irradiation; *RTOG*, Radiation Therapy Oncology Group; *3D-CRT*, three-dimensional conformal radiation therapy; *WBI*, whole breast irradiation.

TABLE 51.4 APBI Proton Studies

Institution	Patients (n)	Follow-Up (months)	Outcomes
Massachusetts General Hospital	19	82.5	7-year local recurrence 11%; 62% excellent/good cosmesis, increased late skin toxicity compared with photons
Loma Linda University Medical Center	100	60	5-year local recurrence 3%; 90% excellent/good cosmesis
Seoul National University	30	59	5-year local recurrence 0%; 69% excellent/good cosmesis

APBI, Accelerated partial breast irradiation.

TABLE 51.5 **Summary of Evidence Based Guidelines**

	Suitable	Cautionary	Unsuitable
ASTRO	Age ≥60 *BRCA* negative Tumor size <2 cm Invasive ductal Negative margins No LVSI ER positive Unicentric pN0 (i +/−) No neoadjuvant therapy	Age 50–59 Tumor size 2.1–3.0 cm DCIS, ILC Close margins (<2 mm) Limited/focal LVSI ER negative	Age <50 *BRCA* positive Tumor >3 cm, T3/4 Positive margins Extensive LVSI Multicentric pN1–3 Neoadjuvant therapy No nodal surgery
	Acceptable Criteria		
ABS	Age ≥50, tumor size ≤3 cm, all invasive subtypes and DCIS, ER positive/negative, negative margins, No LVSI, pN0		
	Low-Risk	**Intermediate-Risk**	**High-Risk**
GEC-ESTRO	Age >50 Tumor size ≤3 cm Negative margins No LVSI Unifocal/unicentric Invasive ductal pN0 No neoadjuvant therapy	Age 40–50 Tumor size ≤3 cm Close margins (<2 mm) Multifocal DCIS pN1mi, pN1a	Age <40 Tumor size >3 cm Positive margins Multifocal/multicentric pNx, pN2a Neoadjuvant therapy
	Selection Criteria		
ASBS	Age ≥45, invasive carcinoma/DCIS, tumor size ≤3 cm, negative margins, sentinel node negative		

ABS, American Brachytherapy Society; *ASBS,* American Society of Breast Surgeons; *DCIS,* ductal carcinoma in situ; *ER,* estrogen receptor; *ILC,* invasive lobular carcinoma; *LVSI,* lymphovascular space invasion.

patients, respectively, but 3 patients did develop rib fractures. Excellent/good cosmesis was reported in 98% of patients. No patients developed local recurrences.[84] Currently, the TRIUMPH trial is enrolling patients and evaluating clinical outcomes and toxicity with a 2-day fractionation schedule using multilumen applicators.[85]

Multiple techniques have been developed to further reduce the toxicities associated with APBI. With respect to brachytherapy, although it has been several years since the introduction of multilumen and strut applicators, only now are data emerging to document the reduction in toxicities compared with single-lumen applicators.[38] With regard to external-beam irradiation, as noted earlier, incorporation of IMRT has demonstrated promising results with a randomized trial demonstrating improvement in toxicity compared with WBI.[57]

Finally, with a growing impetus to evaluate not only the efficacy and toxicity but also the cost-effectiveness, studies continue to be performed evaluating the cost-effectiveness of APBI compared with WBI. Assessment of the cost-effectiveness of radiotherapy approaches should consider cost of capital (equipment, infrastructure modifications), reimbursable treatment-related costs, expenses related to management of recurrences and toxicities, and the economic impact of diminished quality of life and loss of work productivity. Shah and colleagues performed a cost analysis and found that APBI techniques were cost-effective compared with WBI when incorporating costs of recurrence and nonmedical costs.[86] On the basis of outcomes data for IORT from the TARGIT-A and ELIOT trials, a second study from the group concluded that all APBI techniques and WBI were cost-effective

compared with IORT, in part due to higher rates of recurrence with IORT, despite a reduction in absolute cost.[87] However, a second analysis from Alvarado et al. that included Markov modeling did find IORT cost-effective compared with WBI at 10 years.[88] However, this study used low rates of local recurrence inconsistent with current data (3% with IORT and 2.4% with WBI at 10 years compared with 3.3% and 4.4% seen at 5 years from TARGIT and ELIOT) and assumed IORT patients could undergo salvage breast conservation, whereas WBI patients could not with the standard of care remaining salvage mastectomy.

Intraoperative Radiation Therapy

IORT represents an alternative partial breast technique that is typically delivered at the time of lumpectomy but may also be performed after lumpectomy in a second procedure.[89] Potential biological advantages of IORT include limited tumor cell repopulation, a vascularized and oxygenated tumor bed, reduction in cytokine production, and, when using 50-kV photons, a higher relative biologic effectiveness (RBE) factor.[90,91] Potential technical advantages of IORT include reduction in patient setup variability, minimization of dose to organs at risk and patient convenience potentially leading to increased utilization of breast conserving therapy, especially for patients with limited access to radiotherapy facilities.[92] Limitations of the technique include unknown final pathology status (when delivered at time of initial surgery), need for remedial WBI in a cohort of patients, concerns regarding dose at 1 cm with 50-kV techniques, a lack of image guidance techniques consistently used, a lack of dosimetry, limited

TABLE 51.6	**IORT Techniques**				
	Novac 7/Liac	**Mobetron**	**Intrabeam**	**Axxent**	**H.A.M.**
Energy level	High	High	Low	Low	High
Energy type	Electrons	6- to 12-MeV electrons	50-kV photons	50-kV photons	Iridium[192]
Use in standard OR	Yes	Yes	Yes	Yes	No
Application	Various	Various	Breast, skin, and limited other	Breast, skin, and limited other	Various
Setup time (min)	20	20	10–15	20	30–40
Treatment time (min)	3–5	3–5	20–50	20	Up to 40
Cavity shape	Various	Various	Various	Various	Various
Cost (US$) (controller)	>$1M	>$1M	$450K	$250K	$200–300K
Adjustable dose depth	Yes, up to 4 cm	Yes, up to 4 cm	No	No (possible)	Yes, up to 2 cm
Internal shield required	Yes	Generally Yes	No	No	Yes
Incision width	Wide	Wide	Various	Various	Various
Disposable source	No	No	No	Yes	Yes
Disposable applicator	No	No	Yes	Yes	No
Applicator type	Collimator	Collimator	Intracavitary	Intracavitary	Intracavitary

follow-up, and data demonstrating higher rates of recurrences compared with WBI.

IORT is typically delivered using one of two techniques: (1) 20 Gy with a 50-kV x-ray source or (2) 21 Gy with 3- to 12-MeV electrons.[6,93,94] With regard to the 50-kV technique, this is founded on data supporting an increased RBE with decreasing photon energy and the potential for increased RBE with depth due to decreasing energy.[95–97] However, traditional APBI techniques typically provide 34 to 38.5 Gy (in 10 fractions) to 1 cm beyond the cavity compared with 5 Gy at 1 cm with 50-kV x-rays, although the 5 Gy is delivered in a single fraction, which limits radiobiologic comparisons, though concerns exist as to whether the dose is adequate.[98] The Intrabeam Photon Radiosurgery System (Carl Zeiss Meditec, Oberkochen, Germany), uses low-energy x-rays and, based on studies by Vaidya, the physical dose prescription for targeted intra-operative radiotherapy (TARGIT) is 20 Gy administered to the surgical margin, yielding a dose of 5 to 6 Gy at a depth of 1 cm due to steep dose attenuation in breast tissue.[99] Treatment time varies from 20 to 50 minutes based on applicator diameter, with longer treatment times generally required for larger applicators. The Axxent Electronic Brachytherapy System (iCAD, Sunnyvale, CA) is a mobile electronic radiotherapy device that delivers low-energy x-rays as well and uses a dose of 20 Gy at the margin with a treatment time of 8 to 17 minutes depending on applicator diameter.

With the ELIOT technique, 21 Gy is delivered using 3- to 12-MeV electrons and can be delivered with the Light Intraoperative Accelerator (LIAC) (Sardina, Italy), NOVAC 7 (Hitesys, Aprilia, Italy), or Mobetron (IntraOp Medical, Santa Clara, CA) systems.[100,101] The prescription dose of 21 Gy used in the ELIOT method was selected on the basis of a dose-escalation study that confirmed acceptable acute and late toxicity after 21 Gy administered in a single fraction.[102] For both techniques, international standards have also been established for the implementation and maintenance of an IORT program.[100,103]

Another technique is the Mobile High Dose Rate (HDR)-IORT method that uses the Harris-Anderson-Mick (H.A.M.) Breast Applicator (Mick Radio-Nuclear Instruments, Mount Vernon, NY) as a means of delivering high-dose radiotherapy in a shielded operating room.[104] The Memorial Sloan Kettering protocol administers a physical dose of 20 Gy to a depth of 2 cm from the lateral margins and 0.5 cm from the deep margin to the 90% isodose line. IORT delivery time is up to 40 minutes. Table 51.6 provides a summary of IORT techniques.

Randomized Studies

Two large randomized trials have been performed comparing IORT with WBI. TARGIT-A was a randomized, noninferiority trial comparing IORT (50-kV, 20 Gy) with WBI (40–56 Gy with or without boost); 3451 women over the age of 45 with unifocal invasive ductal carcinoma undergoing wide local excision were enrolled. Two cohorts of IORT patients existed in this trial, the prepathology group (two-thirds of patients) who underwent TARGIT at the time of lumpectomy and the postpathology group (one-third of patients) who underwent TARGIT after lumpectomy by reopening the wound. Receipt of WBI for the IORT patients was risk-adapted (e.g., surgical margins <1 mm, extensive ductal carcinoma in situ, infiltrating lobular carcinoma, positive lymph nodes) with 15.2% of all IORT patients receiving supplementary WBI (21.6% prepathology, 3.6% postpathology). With respect to patient characteristics, 40% of patients were 65 or older (2% <45), 15% had grade 3 tumors, 10% were estrogen receptor negative, and 19% were node positive. With a median follow-up of only 29 months, TARGIT was found to have a statistically higher rate of local recurrences (3.3% vs. 1.3%, $p = .04$), within the statistical noninferiority allowance of 2.5%; TARGIT was associated with a nonsignificant increase in local recurrence (2.1% vs. 1.1%, $p = .31$) in the prepathology group, whereas an increase in local recurrence exceeding the 2.5% threshold was noted for the postpathology group (5.4% vs. 1.7%, $p = .07$), which may be due to delays in TARGIT delivery. Given these results, the authors caution against using IORT as a second procedure after the lumpectomy. No difference in axillary recurrences, breast cancer mortality, or overall survival was noted. Rates of grade 3 or 4 skin toxicity were increased with WBI compared with IORT though the number of events remained low (13/1731 vs. 4/1720).[86] Publication of the updated data has elicited debate with competing viewpoints and concern raised regarding the increased rates of local recurrence as well as the statistical methodology of the trial and its design as well as its short follow-up.[105,106]

A second randomized equivalence trial utilizing the ELIOT technique compared IORT to WBI (50 Gy/25 fractions with 10 Gy boost) enrolling 1305 patients. Eligibility included otherwise unselected women age 48 to 75 years old with tumors less than 2.5 cm. No additional WBI was given to the IORT group, with IORT delivered to a dose of 21 Gy using 6 to 9 MeV electrons. With a median follow-up of 5.8 years, IORT was associated with an increase in ipsilateral breast tumor recurrences (4.4% vs. 0.4%, $p < .0001$) with no difference in survival noted (96.8% vs. 96.9%).[86] Five-year rates of IBTR exceeded 10% for patients with tumors >2 cm, four or more positive nodes, grade 3 disease, estrogen receptor–negative tumors, and triple-negative tumors. Higher rates of axillary failure were also noted with IORT (1.0% vs. 0.3%, $p = .03$). IORT was associated with a reduction in overall skin side effects with reductions in erythema, dryness, hyperpigmentation, and pruritis and an increase in fat necrosis. No difference was noted in fibrosis, retraction, pain, or burning between the two arms.[93] It should be noted that large numbers of patients on the trial would not be eligible for PBI in the United States based on current APBI consensus statements. One criticism of the clinical trials evaluating IORT is the lack of longer-term (e.g., 10-year) follow-up compared with WBI, although ELIOT published results with a median follow-up of 5.8 years. Furthermore, it is important to recognize that the initial 5 years of follow-up of other breast conserving therapy trials provides valuable insights into the local recurrence pattern that is likely to be observed with longer follow-up. The Oxford meta-analysis confirmed that two-thirds of all recurrences at 10 years were seen within the first 5 years after treatment.[6] However, as a comparison, it should be noted that none of the five randomized APBI trials found an increase in local recurrence at 5 years compared with WBI, whereas both IORT trials have the potential for greater increases in the TARGIT trial with a median follow-up of only 29 months when presenting the 5-year outcomes. Also, it is interesting to note that rates of local recurrence have started to rise in the IORT studies with further follow-up with questions emerging as to the stability of local control with the technique and the local control benefit of IORT compared with endocrine therapy alone.[107]

Additional Studies

Multiple prospective, single institution, and retrospective analyses have evaluated IORT. The Montpelier Phase II study enrolled 42 patients between 2004 and 2007 with patients receiving 21 Gy via electrons. With 6 years of follow-up, a 9.5% local failure rate was noted with no grade 3 toxicities and 85.7% excellent/good

cosmesis. On post-treatment mammogram, 71% of patients demonstrated fat necrosis with 40% having a palpable mass in the area.[108] Similarly, a prospective study from Italy enrolled 81 patients and demonstrated the feasibility of the technique with low rates of complications noted.[109] A phase II study from Saudi Arabia enrolled 45 patients to receive IORT (20 Gy, 50 kV) with WBI given for tumors greater than 3 cm, lymphovascular space invasion, multifocal disease, extensive intraductal component, and positive nodes. Thirty-six percent of patients required EBRT and 12 developed fat necrosis.[110] Multiple single institution and retrospective series have been published recently, demonstrating the feasibility of multiple IORT techniques, although long-term follow-up with respect to clinical outcomes and toxicity remain limited.[111–114]

Boost

Multiple studies have evaluated IORT when used as a boost to escalate dose to the tumor bed while limiting dose to the skin and organs at risk. A prospective trial from Australia enrolled 55 patients to receive a 5-Gy IORT boost via a 50-kV x-rays followed by WBI. With a median follow-up of 3.3 years, no locoregional recurrences were noted, with 53% and 15% of patients reporting grade 2 and 3 fibrosis, respectively.[115] These findings were confirmed by an analysis of 1109 patients receiving a median of 10-Gy IORT boost delivered via electrons. With 6-year follow-up, a local recurrence rate of 0.8% was noted.[116] Vaidya et al. examined the efficacy of the TARGIT method for delivery of a tumor bed boost (20 Gy) in a case-controlled study of 299 unselected patients scheduled to receive 45 to 50 Gy WBI. At median follow-up of 60.5 months, the 5-year actuarial locoregional recurrence rate of the TARGIT boost was 1.7%.[117] These results, along with several retrospective series, support the use of IORT as a boost because it provides excellent rates of local control and potentially reduces the duration of radiation therapy by eliminating the need for an external beam boost.[118–121]

Future Directions

At this time, multiple studies are underway evaluating IORT and attempting to identify groups of patients who do not have higher rates of recurrences with IORT compared with WBI due to the higher rates of recurrences seen in the TARGIT-A and ELIOT trials. The TARGIT-US Registry trial is currently accruing patients to provide long-term outcomes with IORT. Several single-institution trials are underway as well, and new IORT techniques are being evaluated. APBI and IORT techniques are being studied together with some studies using APBI applicators to deliver single-fraction radiation therapy at the time of surgery and intraoperative computed tomography being evaluated to assist with image guidance.[122] There is interest in longer-term follow-up from the existing randomized trials, as well as further studies to define the optimal selection criteria for IORT alone or when used as a boost, its use in low-risk DCIS or for limited in-breast recurrence.

The array of PBI techniques in general presents an opportunity to study and refine patient selection for each of the available techniques, given that both clinical and technical considerations present limitations for each. The era of PBI has represented a paradigm shift in the treatment of early-stage breast cancer, similar to that of the introduction of breast conserving therapy as an alternative to mastectomy. PBI in particular offers the promise to personalize and optimize local therapy based on evolving eligibility criteria, and future studies will focus on these questions. At this time, there are clear guidelines for the utilization of APBI and five randomized trials comparing APBI to WBI demonstrating no difference in local control; however, in contrast, there are a lack of evidence-based guidelines for IORT, and the Level I evidence available demonstrates higher rates of local recurrence compared with WBI. Such guidelines are needed for IORT as they can help shape appropriate patient selection as APBI guidelines were not created to include IORT. Updated ASTRO partial breast guidelines available for comment include IORT and state that patients should be counseled of increased rates of IBTR with IORT compared with WBI and that outside of clinical trial that IORT is not encouraged due to short follow-up.[83] In light of such recommendations and the data available, the role of IORT remains unclear because, unlike APBI, it has not been found to be comparable to WBI and, further, there are limited data demonstrating its efficacy compared with endocrine therapy alone.

Conclusions

Partial breast irradiation encompasses accelerated partial breast irradiation (APBI) and intraoperative radiation therapy (IORT). At this time, mature data from six randomized trials comparing APBI and WBI demonstrate no difference in outcomes and low rates of toxicity, making APBI a standard treatment option after BCS for appropriately selected patients. IORT, a form of partial breast irradiation different from APBI, offers the potential of a single treatment delivered at the time of surgery. However, off-protocol, IORT is not encouraged with local recurrence rates being higher (although the clinical significance of this is unknown) compared with WBI (while the five randomized APBI trials have not), limited long-term follow-up, and current expert consensus recommending use only on clinical trial. Future studies will evaluate innovations in APBI and shortening dose/fractionation schedules and with respect to IORT provide further data to clarify rates of local recurrence with the technique compared with standard radiotherapy options and help identify appropriate patient selection criteria.

Selected References

21. Polgar C, Major T, Fodor J, et al. Accelerated partial breast irradiation using high-dose-rate interstitial brachytherapy: 12-year update of a prospective clinical study. *Radiother Oncol.* 2010;94:274-279.

22. Polgar C, Fodor J, Major T, et al. Breast-conserving therapy with partial or whole breast irradiation: ten-year results of the Budapest randomized trial. *Radiother Oncol.* 2013;108:197-202.

23. Shah C, Antonucci JV, Wilkinson JB, et al. Twelve-year clinical outcomes and patterns of failure with accelerated partial breast irradiation versus whole-breast irradiation: results of a matched-pair analysis. *Radiother Oncol.* 2011;100:210-214.

25. Strnad V, Ott OJ, Hildebrandt G, et al. 5-year results of accelerated partial breast irradiation using sole interstitial multicatheter brachytherapy versus whole-breast irradiation with boost after breast-conserving surgery for low-risk invasive and in-situ carcinoma of the female breast: a randomised phase 3, non-inferiority trial. *Lancet.* 2016;387:229-238.

36. Shah C, Badiyan S, Ben Wilkinson J, et al. Treatment efficacy with accelerated partial breast irradiation (APBI): final analysis of the American Society of Breast Surgeons MammoSite breast brachytherapy trial. *Ann Surg Oncol.* 2013;20:3279-3285.

56. Olivotto IA, Whelan TJ, Parpia S, et al. Interim cosmetic and toxicity results from RAPID: a randomized trial of accelerated partial breast irradiation using three-dimensional conformal external beam radiation therapy. *J Clin Oncol.* 2013;31:4038-4045.

57. Livi L, Meattini I, Marrazzo L, et al. Accelerated partial breast irradiation using intensity-modulated radiotherapy versus whole breast irradiation: 5-year survival analysis of a phase 3 randomised controlled trial. *Eur J Cancer.* 2015;51:451-463.

68. Coles C, Agrawal R, Ah-See ML, et al. Partial breast radiotherapy for women with early breast cancer: First results of local recurrence data for IMPORT LOW (CRUK/O6/003). Presented at the 10th European Breast Cancer Conference; March 9–11, 2016; Amsterdam, The Netherlands.

89. Vaidya JS, Wenz F, Bulsara M, et al. Risk-adapted targeted intraoperative radiotherapy versus whole-breast radiotherapy for breast cancer: 5-year results for local control and overall survival from the TARGIT-A randomised trial. *Lancet.* 2014;383:603-613.

A full reference list is available online at ExpertConsult.com.

52

Radiation Complications and Their Management

GARY M. FREEDMAN

This chapter discusses the potential complications associated with the use of radiotherapy. These may occur in the weeks during or after radiation or decades after treatment. Improvements in radiation have fortunately led to a decrease in the incidence of many of these complications in patients treated today compared with those treated in the past with outdated techniques and equipment.

Such possible complications, from most to least common, include fatigue; myelosuppression; radiation dermatitis; alterations in the cosmetic appearance of the breast and local soft tissue symptoms; long-term chest wall or soft tissue complications, including rib fractures and brachial plexopathy; pulmonary effects; cardiac complications; and radiation-related second malignancies. (The effects of irradiation on the risks of arm edema and complications after breast reconstructive surgery are discussed in other chapters.) The risk of complications in patients with collagen vascular disease is also discussed.

Fatigue and Myelosuppression

Fatigue is a common side effect in women treated for breast cancer in general and also specifically in association with radiation. Baseline assessments of fatigue in breast cancer patients even before radiation show that approximately 30% or more report fatigue, that is, even higher in patients receiving chemotherapy in addition to radiation.[1,2] Fatigue generally increases during radiation to plateau at weeks 4 and 5 but is usually mild and resolves or returns to pretreatment baseline within a few months of completing treatment.[3–7] Radiation-related fatigue is associated with decreased quality of life in some studies.[4,7] However, in a randomized trial of breast conserving surgery with or without radiation, radiation was associated with increased levels of fatigue but not global differences in quality of life.[8] Fatigue remains common in 40% to 50% of women at end of radiation and even 1 year after completion of treatment.[1] In one longitudinal study of breast cancer survivors, persistent fatigue was reported in approximately 20% of women up to 5 to 10 years from treatment.[9] Fatigue is more common after chemotherapy and radiation compared with either treatment alone.

In managing the patient with fatigue, it is important to rule out other potential causes such as anemia, cardiovascular disease, depression, or hypothyroidism. There is no specific medical treatment for radiation-related fatigue. In a randomized double-blind clinical trial of vitamins or placebo during radiation for breast cancer, there was no improvement in radiation-related fatigue.[10] Physical activity including aerobic and resistance exercise has been associated with reductions in patient-reported fatigue after radiation in randomized trials.[11,12] In a randomized trial, patients assigned to up to three 60-minute classes of yoga or stretching exercises per week during their 6 weeks of radiation had improved fatigue at the end of treatment and 1 to 3 months after treatment compared with patients assigned to usual care (and offered these interventions after radiation).[2] Activity in the structure of a regular community-based exercise program for 6 months beginning during or within 3 months of treatment was shown to reduce even long-term fatigue in participants.[13] However, two comprehensive reviews and meta-analysis of randomized and nonrandomized controlled trials have not shown statistically significant improvements in fatigue or health-related quality of life with physical exercise compared with controls.[14,15] Acupuncture has been associated with improvements in cancer-related fatigue in patients with breast cancer in one prospective randomized trial.[16]

Myelosuppression is also very common during and for a few months after radiation, with the greatest effect on circulating lymphocytes and least effect on platelets and hemoglobin levels.[5] Breast irradiation directly treats a very small volume of total body bone marrow of the chest wall. Because myelosuppression is rarely of clinical significance, blood counts do not need to be routinely checked. Hematologic toxicities appear to be slightly greater in patients treated with chemotherapy after radiation therapy, compared with when chemotherapy is given before radiation.[17] In randomized trials of concurrent versus sequential chemotherapy and radiation, anemia[18] or febrile neuropenia[19] were more frequent with concurrent therapy. For patients receiving concurrent chemotherapy, special attention should be given to signs of infection (local or systemic) or leukopenia. However, the incidence of these problems is low with concurrent radiation and cyclphosphamide-methotrexate-5-fluorouracil (CMF) chemotherapy.[20–22] There is limited experience with radiation and concurrent other systemic chemotherapy, but in one trial the incidence of grade 3 to 4 neutropenia was much higher with concurrent radiation and paclitaxel but not felt to be different than expected from paclitaxel alone.[23]

Radiation Dermatitis and Infections

Acute radiation dermatitis includes a clinical spectrum of signs and symptoms that usually develop slowly during the course of weeks, generally escalating as treatment progresses. These usually become most severe in the last week of radiation or 1 to 2 weeks after completion. Radiation dermatitis begins with generalized dryness and itching of the skin. This will commonly progress to erythema or hyperpigmentation, which may be asymptomatic or mildly painful. This erythema can be confused with acute inflammation of the breast that can also occur in the first weeks of treatment. Often a pruritic papular rash (folliculitis) may occur in the upper inner portion of the chest wall where there is overlap with previously sun-exposed regions of the neck and chest. Desquamation may progress to a moist, weeping reaction due to breakdown of the skin integrity; the latter is particularly likely to be found in the inframammary fold and toward the axillary tail. Patients with such moist desquamation may also have substantial breast discomfort or pain and swelling. Moist desquamation is associated with a reduced global quality of life.[24,25] Rarely, the most severe cases may progress to full thickness skin ulceration and bleeding. The time course of recovery is generally weeks for immediate erythema or desquamation, whereas months may be required for the resolution of hyperpigmentation and swelling.

Acute dermatitis is usually scored by the National Cancer Institute's Common Terminology Criteria for Adverse Events (CTCAE).[26] Grade 1 dermatitis is faint erythema or dry desquamation; grade 2 is moderate to brisk erythema; patchy moist desquamation, mostly confined to skin folds and creases; moderate edema; grade 3 is moist desquamation other than skin folds and creases; bleeding induced by minor trauma or abrasion; grade 4 is skin necrosis or ulceration of full-thickness dermis; spontaneous bleeding from involved site. The incidence of acute radiation dermatitis with breast conserving surgery and modern radiation is approximately 3% grade 0, 35% grade 1, 60% grade 2, and 2% grade 3.[27,28] The definitions used in CTCAE for dermatitis include adjectives such as *mild, moderate,* or *mostly* so are subjective and may allow substantial interobserver variation. Furthermore, each grade encompasses substantial variability in the severity of symptoms experienced by patients. For example, a small 1-cm nonpainful area of moist desquamation in the inframammary fold is scored as grade 2, as would be a 10-cm painful area requiring wound care or a treatment break. Fig. 52.1 shows examples of acute radiation skin toxicity.

Radiation dermatitis is most directly related to increased dose inhomogeneity, which itself is a function of increasing breast size or chest wall diameter.[25,29,30] For this reason, moist desquamation is more common in women with large breasts than those with small breasts.[24,31] Intensity modulated radiation therapy (IMRT) has been associated with a decrease in the rates and severity of acute dermatitis, compared with conventional two-dimensionally compensated "wedged" tangential-field irradiation.[25,31–33] For example, the Sunnybrook Health Sciences Centre and British Columbia Cancer Agency—Vancouver Island Centre in Canada conducted a prospective randomized trial of standard tangential whole breast radiation versus IMRT.[25] The dosimetric characteristics and dose homogeneity of the radiation plans were significantly improved for the patients randomized to IMRT, with a reduction in the median clinically significant maximum dose within the breast tissue (105% vs. 110%) and the volume receiving greater than 105% of the prescribed dose (7.7% vs. 16.9%). Patients randomized to IMRT were less likely to develop acute moist desquamation (31.2% vs. 47.8%), particularly desquamation occurring in the inframammary fold. Improved methods of 3D conformal radiation are able to improve dose homogeneity using forward-based planning and "field-in-field" techniques

compared with simple two-dimensional (2D) wedged tangents. This may make comparisons of acute dermatitis between three-dimensional (3D) conformal tangents (forward planning) and IMRT (inverse planning) less distinguishable compared with the older studies of IMRT compared with 2D tangents.[28] Prone positioning may reduce toxicity previously seen in larger-breasted women by reducing skin folds or decreasing chest wall separation.[34] Whole breast hypofractionation that is now standard for many postlumpectomy patients has been associated with decreased acute radiation skin toxicity compared with conventional fractionation.[35,36]

Randomized controlled trials of topical skin care products used with the goal of mitigating radiation dermatitis in breast cancer patients compared with an aqueous-type cream placebo have been mostly negative or of minimal clinical significance. These include studies of Biafine (Ortho-McNeil Pharmaceuticals, Raritan, NJ), hyaluronic acid, steroids, oil-based emulsions, calendula, glycerine, or miscellaneous natural ingredients.[24,37–42] For example, in one study of mometasone furoate, there were modest reduced average dermatitis scores but the average erythema was only faint or dull for placebo.[38] However, up to 1 in 10 women may have avoided or at least had reduced moist desquamation. These trials are often of limited value because of their small numbers, dermatitis scoring systems used, or radiation techniques. In addition, these agents nearly uniformly have no clear mechanism for reducing radiation dermatitis, so new agents with novel biologic rationale are needed.

The treatment of radiation dermatitis depends on its severity. There are substantial variations from one center to another in the preferred approaches and products used. Grade 1 to 2 dermatitis can be treated first with any number of water-soluble skin moisturizers such as MediChoice (Owens & Minor, Richmond, VA), Lotion Soft (STERIS, St. Louis, MO), or Eucerin (Beiersdorf, Hamburg). As symptoms of dryness, skin pain, or areas of dry peeling increase, petroleum-based emollients such as Aquaphor (Beiersdorf, Hamburg) can be used as needed. However, they should not be used immediately before treatment to prevent bolus effects and increased skin dose. Steroid creams may reduce mediators of inflammation in the skin that are responsible for radiation dermatitis. Therefore a weak-strength cream such as hydrocortisone 1% in most cases will reduce papular eruptions and minor itching of the skin. Over-the-counter strength lidocaine jelly can be used alone or mixed with Aquaphor for temporary relief of skin pain as well. Moist desquamation of the skin is managed by nonstick dressings, aluminium acetate solution in water (Domeboros, Moberg Pharma North America, Cedar Knolls, NJ) or silver sulfadiazine cream (Silvadene, King Pharmaceuticals, Bristol, TN). Prophylactic oral or topical antibiotics are not needed for moist desquamation.

Infections of the breast include fungal superinfections, particularly in the inframammary folds of large-breasted women or as a complication of moist desquamation. These may occur from overuse of antibiotics. Topical antifungal creams are applied for 10 to 14 days, with oral agents reserved for refractory cases. By the end of radiation, the presence of erythema and edema and skin pain can make detection of infection more difficult. Bacterial infections are associated with a marked change or sudden onset in skin color or pain, compared with the usual gradual onset from radiation dermatitis week to week. The pain or redness may appear out of proportion to the expected appearance when present earlier in a course of treatment. The incidence of developing cellulitis or breast abscess during or within 1 year of breast radiation

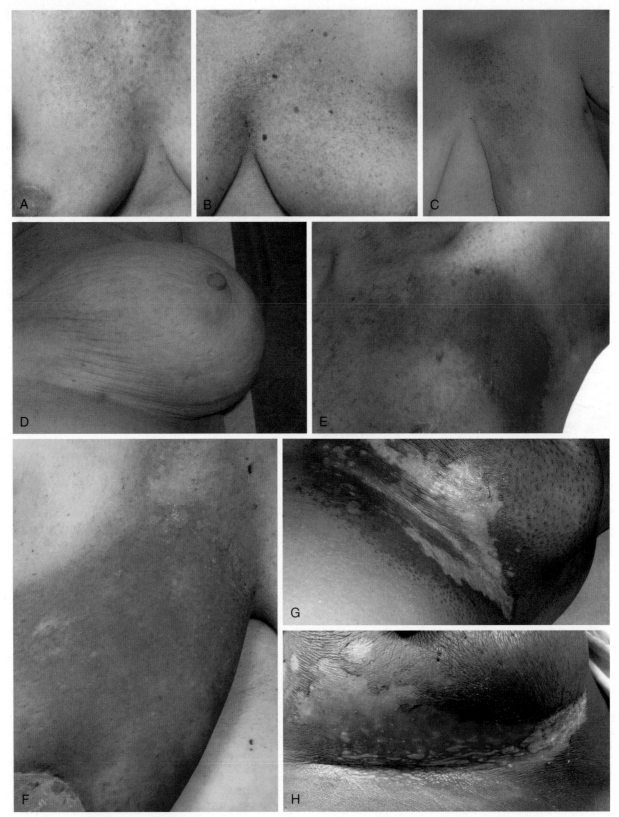

• **Fig. 52.1** Acute radiation dermatitis. The incidence of acute radiation dermatitis with breast conserving surgery and radiation is approximately 3% grade 0, 35% grade 1, 60% grade 2, and 2% grade 3. (A and B) Examples of grade 1 faint or mild maculopapular dermatitis. (C) A case of moderate grade 2 maculo-papular dermatitis. (D) Grade 2 moderate edema of the breast. (E and F) Examples of grade 2 moderate to severe erythema. (G and H) Examples of grade 2 moist desquamation within skin folds.

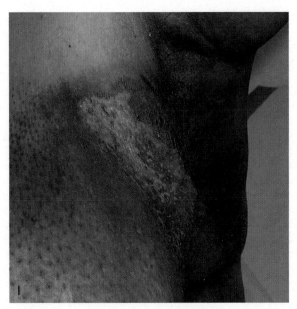

• **Fig. 52.1, cont'd** (I) Grade 3 moist desquamation not confined within a skin fold.

is 1% to 8%.[43–45] In one study, delayed cellulitis continued to occur up to 5 years after treatment, with a cumulative rate of 9%.[44] Cephalexin or ciprofloxacin are used for 10 to 14 days in cases of suspected bacterial infection. For infections refractory to antibiotics, an ultrasound may be needed to rule out an abscess that requires incision and drainage.

Cosmesis and Breast-Related Symptoms

Potential long-term effects of radiation to the breast include breast pain, edema, fibrosis, induration, and hyperpigmentation or telangiectasias of the skin. Alone or combined these can have negative effects on the overall cosmetic result. Approximately 70% to 90% of women have a good or excellent cosmetic result after breast conserving surgery and radiation (Table 52.1).[46–62] Traditional scoring of breast cosmesis has been a simple scale of poor, fair, good, or excellent, with excellent representing no apparent effects of the radiation.[63] It is also important to assess cosmesis at baseline before radiation, in an attempt to distinguish what effects on cosmesis may be due to surgical changes rather than subsequent radiation changes. For example, changes in breast size can be immediate due to volume loss or delayed within months of surgery due to decrease in postsurgical edema or size of a seroma. The European Organisation for Research and Treatment of Cancer developed an objective scoring system that evaluates the treated breast for overall cosmesis and more specific differences in factors including size, shape, symmetry, color, and position of the nipple.[64] Patient-reported cosmetic results often are better than physician-reported or other objective measurements.[54] For example, in one large prospective randomized study, patients reported approximately 94% good or excellent cosmesis compared with only 75% by a five-person panel evaluating their images at 5 years after surgery.[62] The Breast Cancer Treatment Outcome Scale (BCTOS) is a 22-item patient-reported measure of perceived esthetic cosmetic status, functional status and breast-specific pain that has demonstrated validity.[65]

Common symptoms after breast radiation include mild breast discomfort, sensitivity to touch, or shooting pains of the breast that come and go rapidly and unexpectedly. These will generally

TABLE 52.1	Percentage of Women With Good or Excellent Cosmetic Results After Breast Conserving Surgery and Radiation		
Study First Author	Year	N	Good/Excellent (%)
Delouche[46]	1987	410	77
Boyages[47]	1988	121	75
Dewar[48]	1988	592	92
Abner[49]	1991	170	90
Taylor[50]	1995	458	87
Fowble[51]	1996	471	90
Wazer[52]	1997	509	85
Fung[53]	1997	55	85
Romestaing[54]	1997	1024	85
Grills[55]	2003	1178	93
Vass[56]	2005	142	75
Haffty[57]	2006	52	77
Harsolia[58]	2007	172	98
Whelan[59]	2010	451	70
Murphy[60]	2011	2567	95
Hill-Kayser[61]	2012	354	71
Hau[62]	2012	385	74

improve over time. In a randomized prospective clinical trial performed at Princess Margaret Hospital in Toronto, breast pain and quality of life were studied in women treated with breast conserving surgery and tamoxifen with or without radiation.[66] There was no significant difference between the arms in quality-of-life scores for physical function, pain, or breast symptoms within 12 months of treatment. In both treatment arms, the breast-reported symptoms and pain decreased over time, suggesting that the predominant factor causing them was surgery. Serious breast pain requiring medication occurs in approximately 1% of women. Initial management includes nonsteriodal antiinflammatory medication. More severe and persistent symptoms of the breast or chest wall may be treated with trials of medication such as low-dose nortriptyline, venlafaxine, or gabapentin.

Breast edema presents as heaviness, pain, or enlargement of the breast. Signs of edema include a global increase in breast size, skin thickening, or peau d'orange without other inflammatory signs. Delayed drainage from the nipple and areola may cause a distended appearance when moving from sitting to supine position. Risk factors for breast edema are large breast size, axillary node dissection, and upper extremity lymphedema. Mild breast edema may be managed by wearing a sports bra that applies passive hydrostatic pressure to the breast. Moderate to severe cases of edema may be referred to physical therapy for therapeutic massage.

Skin telangiectasias occur in 10% to 30% of women treated with postoperative radiation, and is associated with use of cobalt therapy, a breast boost, or concurrent chemotherapy.[56,67-69] Telangiectasias commonly develop within electron boost fields or skin folds (Fig. 52.2). The time course to their appearance is usually 1 to 2 years, but they may continue to evolve for many years after. Management of asymptomatic telangiectasis is observation, whereas symptomatic telangiectasis causing an unsightly appearance may be treated by sclerotherapy, pulsed dye laser, or electrodessication.[70-72]

The risk of late radiation negative cosmetic effects are most related to total dose, use of a boost, dose per fraction, and dose homogeneity. In a large prospective randomized trial of dose escalation comparing 50-Gy whole breast to 50 Gy plus a 16-Gy tumor bed boost, use of the radiation boost was associated with an increased risk for severe fibrosis (1.8% in the no boost group vs. 5.2% in the boost group; $p < .0001$).[73] In a different randomized trial of 50 Gy plus or minus a 10-Gy boost, a boost was associated with no difference in patient- or physician-reported cosmetic results.[54] However, in a third randomized trial comparing 50 Gy in 25 fractions to 45 Gy in 25 fractions plus a 16-Gy

boost, the physician and objective measurement of good or excellent cosmesis was approximately 80% with boost compared with 70% without boost.[62] This suggests that the beneficial effects of reducing the whole breast dose were greater than the potential negative effects of adding the boost.

A worse long-term cosmetic outcome and complication rate has been reported with doses greater than 50 Gy to the whole breast or daily dose per fraction of 2.5 Gy or higher.[50,74,75] However, in modern studies of whole breast hypofractionation, use of a daily dose higher than 2.5 Gy may no longer be associated with a negative cosmetic results and may actually have improved cosmetic outcomes when combined with sufficient reduction in the whole breast total dose. The Ontario Clinical Oncology Group trial randomized patients to 42.5 Gy in 16 fractions versus 50 Gy in 25 fractions without a tumor bed boost.[59] The late cosmetic appearance was considered good or excellent in approximately 70% of women in both groups. There were similarly no reported differences in 10-year skin and subcutaneous tissue complications. The UK Standardisation of Breast Radiotherapy (START) trials consisted of two separate studies of whole breast irradiation and hypofractionation that allowed a boost.[76] Trial A compared 50 Gy in 25 fractions, 41.6 Gy in 13 fractions, or 39 Gy in 13 fractions in 5 weeks. Trial B compared 50 Gy in 25 fractions over 5 weeks versus 40 Gy in 15 fractions over 3 weeks. The late effects of breast appearance, breast edema or hardness, or skin changes were generally equal or better with whole breast hypofractionation. There was also no significant effect of the boost in these randomized studies. However, in another study of 312 women returning questionnaires for patient-reported outcomes, a boost after whole breast hypofractionation was associated with a modest increase in pain or negative cosmetic results compared with no boost.[77] However, this was of minimal clinical significance with patients reporting only slightly worse cosmetic assessments on the BCTOS (2.3 vs. 2.1, $p = .02$) with use of the boost.

Measures to improve dose homogeneity may reduce the incidence of these complications. Modern computed tomography–based planning by either field in field or forward planned 3D conformal or inverse planned IMRT can reduce dose inhomogeneity and complications such as edema or negative cosmetic effects on the breast.[58,60,78-83] In a trial conducted at the Royal Marsden Hospital in England, 306 women were randomized to receive whole breast radiation after breast conserving surgery using IMRT or conventional two-dimensional tangential radiation therapy.[32] There was improved dose homogeneity with IMRT, with 19% of the IMRT plans showing dose inhomogeneity of greater than or equal to 105% compared with 92% of the conventional plans. Photographic analysis 5 years after treatment showed that there was a change in breast appearance in 58% of patients randomized to conventional treatment, compared with 40% of those randomized to IMRT ($p = .008$). There was a significant relation between the presence of regions of the breast receiving greater than 105% of the dose and any change in breast appearance. Fewer patients treated with IMRT had clinically palpable induration of the breast tissue as well. In the Cambridge Breast IMRT trial, 1145 trial patients were analyzed and 815 with a high predetermined level of dose inhomogeneity were randomized to standard wedged tangential radiation or replanned with a simple intensity modulation technique.[84] The overall 5-year rates of moderate to good cosmesis were 88% with IMRT and 78% with controls and was significant on multivariate analysis. There was also a significantly lower incidence of skin telangiectasias with IMRT.

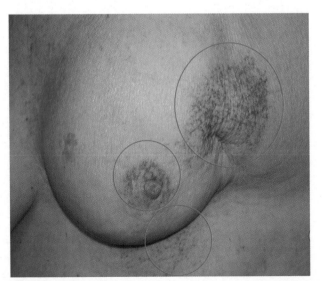

• **Fig. 52.2** Benign radiation-related telangiectasias of the skin in a patient treated with postlumpectomy breast radiation.

Concurrent chemotherapy has been associated with increased rates of breast fibrosis, telangiectasia, hyperpigmentation, breast atrophy, and a worse cosmetic result.[49,69] A group at the former Joint Center for Radiation Therapy of Harvard Medical School reported that 47% of patients treated with chemotherapy had an excellent cosmetic result, compared with 71% of those treated with radiation alone, with good results in 36% and 19%, respectively.[49] This effect was seen predominantly in those patients receiving concurrent radiation and chemotherapy, rather than sequential treatment. However, a study by the University of Pennsylvania did not see a decrease in cosmetic outcomes in relation to the use of chemotherapy, its timing with radiation, or the type of chemotherapy used.[85] However, these studies used predominately CMF, and the results may not be applicable to patients treated with the anthracycline- and taxane-based regimens now in use.

BRCA mutation has not been associated with increased late radiation breast complications.[86,87] An increase in late effects has been reported in patients with a heterozygous mutation of the gene for ataxia telangiectasia (ATM) in many but not all studies.[88–91] Ho and coworkers[92] reported the increase in late grade 2 to 4 subcutaneous side effects was observed in particular association with a 5557 G/A polymorphism of the ATM gene. There are no data on the effects of radiation complications by other breast cancer–associated incidence genes, but more data may be anticipated with the increase in clinical use of commercially available multigene panels for testing newly diagnosed breast cancer patients.

Rib Fracture

Rib fracture was associated with old series of radiation, particularly with the use of orthovoltage radiation due to its giving a higher relative dose to bone than does modern megavoltage radiation. The incidence of rib fracture after breast conserving surgery and radiation in the 1980s and 1990s was reduced to approximately 1% to 2% or less.[51,53,93–95] In the UK START trial, enrolling from 1999 to 2002, the 1% to 2% of reported cases within 10 years included many with history of trauma or metastases.[76] The confirmed cases after imaging and further investigations was 0.3% or less. Rib pain may not always be associated with abnormalities on imaging. Symptomatic rib fractures related to history of breast radiation may be treated with standard measures of pain medication and incentive spirometry. Recovery is usually within 6 to 8 weeks.

Brachial Plexopathy

Brachial plexopathy occurs in approximately 1% of patients. This complication is almost exclusively limited to patients treated with regional nodal irradiation.[96–99] Patients commonly present with pain radiating down the extremity, numbness or weakness, and progressive loss of motor strength of the extremity. Such symptoms may appear years or even decades after treatment.[75] The main differential diagnosis is tumor recurrence in the axillary apical nodes, and magnetic resonance imaging is the best study in distinguishing between these two causes. There is no standard treatment for brachial plexopathy. In one study, five cases of plexopathy were transient and resolved without treatment.[99] A randomized double-blind phase II study of hyperbaric oxygen in these patients failed to demonstrate significant improvement in neurophysiologic tests up to 1 year after treatment.[100]

Pulmonary Complications

Radiation therapy given to the whole breast using tangential beam arrangements will treat approximately 5% to 20% of the ipsilateral lung.[101] Das and colleagues developed a model to estimate the irradiated volume for patients not undergoing three-dimensional CT planning: for each millimeter of central lung distance in a tangential radiation portal, the proportion of irradiated lung was 0.6% on the left side and 0.5% on the right side.[102] In a randomized comparison of supine versus prone positioning, the prone position was associated with significantly lower lung volume in the treatment fields.[103] The need for regional node radiation needs to be carefully weighed against the added risks for toxicity. Adding a supraclavicular or full axillary field will increase the irradiated volume by an average of 7% to 12%.[101,102] The use of IMRT delivered through standard tangential beam arrangements will modestly reduce the volume of irradiated ipsilateral lung. However, some techniques of IMRT through multiple-gantry angles or moving arcs will actually increase low-dose irradiation of the lung, compared with conventional tangential radiation.

The most common complication from pulmonary irradiation is asymptomatic pulmonary scarring, which occurs most commonly in the apical portion of the lung from supraclavicular irradiation (Fig. 52.3). Changes in pulmonary function such as forced vital capacity (FVC), forced expiratory volume in 1 second (FEV_1), and carbon monoxide diffusing capacity (DLCO) have been reported in patients undergoing pulmonary function studies before and after radiation.[101,104,105] Studies differ on how likely such changes resolve. Kimsey and colleagues studied 34 women who underwent tangential breast irradiation with or without regional node irradiation and reported transient 5% to 10% decreases in spirometry parameters that returned to baseline by 2 years.[101] In a study by Jaén and colleagues, pulmonary function studies showed transient modest reductions in FVC, FEV_1, and ventilation that returned to or exceeded baseline.[106] However, reductions in perfusion and DLCO persisted long term and only partially recovered. In a long-term study of pulmonary function after breast radiation, Erven and colleagues studied pulmonary function tests up to 10 years after treatment.[107] An early reduction in vital capacity and forced expiratory volume at 3 to 6 months recovered nearly to baseline by 12 months, but total lung capacity and diffusion capacity of carbon monoxide did not. Small mean

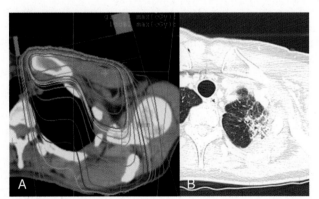

• **Fig. 52.3** Asymptomatic apical pulmonary scarring from supraclavicular irradiation. (A) Isodose distributions showing dose to the lung from an anterior oblique supraclavicular field. (B) Resulting pulmonary fibrosis within 6 months of treatment.

TABLE 52.2	Incidence of Radiation-Related Pneumonitis			
Study First Author	**Year**	**N**	**Pneumonitis (%)**	**Comments**
Fowble[51]	1996	491	0.3	
Zissiadis[108]	1997	438	3	
Fung[53]	1997	55	3.6	Bilateral RT
Pierce[95]	1997	429	<1	
Galper[99]	2000	292	1.2	
Lind[109]	2002	613	0.9	Local RT only
			4.1	Locoregional node RT
Grills[55]	2003	1178	0.3	Breast only
		164	0.6	Breast and regional node RT
Bellon[20]	2004	112	<1	Concurrent CMF
Taghian[110]	2005	41	15	Paclitaxel, regional node RT
		1286	1	
Haffty[57]	2006	109	0	Concurrent chemotherapy
Burstein[23]	2006	40	18	Concurrent paclitaxel
Blom Goldman[116]	2014	89	6 (1[a])	
Whelan[112]	2015	927	0.2[a]	No IMN radiation
		893	1.2[a]	IMN radiation
Choi[111]	2016	366	3.3 (0[a])	No IMN radiation
		356	6.5 (2.5[a])	IMN radiation

CMF, Cyclophosphamide, methotrexate, and 5-fluorouracil; *IMN,* internal mammary nodes; *RT,* radiation therapy.
[a]Grade 2 pneumonitis.

reductions of 5% to 10% from baseline preradiation were observed when rechecked 8 to 10 years after RT.

The incidence of radiation pneumonitis after breast conserving surgery and radiation is shown in Table 52.2.[20,23,51,53,55,57,95,99,108–112] Radiation pneumonitis may present as a triad of dry cough, dyspnea, and low-grade fever. The usual onset of development is within 3 to 9 months of radiation. However, a shorter interval to symptoms within 6 weeks is possible, particularly in patients treated with concurrent paclitaxel.[109,113,114] Imaging studies should indicate an area of pulmonary inflammation that is confined to the radiation field. Pneumonitis will respond to treatment with steroids and is only life-threatening if unrecognized and treated with successive attempts at antibiotic treatment.[98] The risk of pneumonitis is substantially higher when the internal mammary or supraclavicular nodes are treated in addition to the breast or chest wall, compared with treatment of the breast or chest wall alone.[109,112] In a randomized trial reported by Choi and colleagues, 3.6% of patients had grade 1 (asymptomatic or mild symptoms [dry cough], slight radiographic appearances) and 1.2% grade 2

(moderate symptomatic fibrosis or pneumonitis [severe cough], low-grade fever, patch radiographic appearances).[111] All cases of grade 2 were in patients treated to the internal mammary nodes (IMN). Objective measures of predicting pneumonitis by quantitative lung volume measurement is less certain. In the study by Choi and colleagues, IMN radiation was associated with higher lung doses and volumes treated, but there was no correlation with clinically significant grade 2 versus grade 1 pneumonitis. In the study by Kimsey, there were 2 cases of pneumonitis out of 8 patients in whom more than 10% of the lung volume was irradiated, compared with none out of 21 patients with less than 10% irradiated.[101] Lind and colleagues examined 128 patients treated to the breast or chest wall and regional lymph nodes.[115] The mean V20, or volume of lung receiving a dose of 20 Gy or higher, was 27%. The V20 was the most important predictor of pneumonitis on multivariate analysis. In the groups subsequent prospective study of 89 women, where the V20 was kept less than 30% during radiation planning, there were 4 cases of mild and 1 case of moderate pneumonitis.[116]

The incidence of radiation pneumonitis is generally greater in patients treated with concurrent chemotherapy (see Table 52.2). Rates of up to 30% to 50% have been observed in patients treated with high-dose chemotherapy and regional node irradiation.[23,109,110,117,118] However, only 1 in 112 women developed pneumonitis in a trial of concurrent CMF and reduced-dose radiation given to the breast without regional node irradiation.[20]

Bronchiolitis obliterans organizing pneumonia (BOOP) is a rare syndrome of nonproductive cough, fever, and dyspnea with often bilateral pulmonary infiltrates. This distribution outside of radiation fields distinguishes BOOP from radiation pneumonitis. The incidence in studies from Japan has been approximately 1.5 to 2.0%.[119–121] BOOP has not been described in studies reporting complications of breast conserving surgery and radiation from the United States, Canada, and Europe. This may be due to lack of recognition of the syndrome as being distinct from radiation pneumonitis, or perhaps due to a unique risk factor increasing the risk of BOOP in the Japanese population. There are no known patient- or treatment-related risk factors.

Cardiac Complications

The individual prospective randomized trials comparing breast conserving surgery to mastectomy, or breast conserving surgery with or without radiation, did not observe statistically significant differences in nonbreast cancer mortality with radiation.[122–127] However, these studies may not have had sufficient statistical power to detect small differences in cardiac effects. A large meta-analysis of 17 randomized trials of radiotherapy versus no radiotherapy after breast conserving surgery from 1976 to 1999 showed a 3.8% reduction in breast cancer deaths, but only a 3% reduction in death from any cause.[128] This difference may be attributed in large part to increased late effects of radiation on the heart. There was an even greater difference of death from nonbreast cancer causes in postmastectomy randomized trials due to the greater use of regional node, specifically internal mammary node, radiation in postmastectomy trials.

Taylor and colleagues conducted a study of heart and coronary doses given using different radiation techniques prevalent between studies of the 1950s to 1990s.[129] The mean dose to the left anterior descending artery was greater than the mean whole heart dose for all techniques. In general, older radiation techniques that included orthovoltage energies, internal mammary treatment particularly

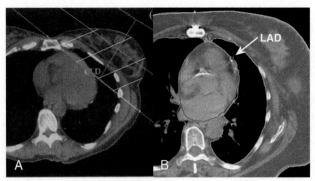

• **Fig. 52.4** Correlation between irradiated heart volume and coronary artery dose. (A) Illustration of the volume of heart *(red)* included in a tangential irradiation portal *(yellow)* sparing most of the whole heart volume. (B) Location of the left anterior descending *(LAD)* on the anterior surface of the heart.

with photon fields, or deep tangential fields were associated with greater heart doses. However, there was large variation due to differences in patient position and anatomy, so that individualized three-dimensional treatment planning of each case is essential. In a retrospective review of 2168 women treated for breast cancer from 1958 to 2001, heart dose was estimated from idealized phantom measurements.[130] They found that the mean heart dose correlated with excess relative risk of coronary events by 7.4% per 1 Gy. In that study period, the mean heart dose was estimated to be 6.6 Gy for women with tumors in the left breast. In a systematic review of 149 studies published during 2003 to 2013, the mean heart dose from left-sided breast radiation therapy was 5.4 Gy.[131] The lowest mean heart doses were from tangential radiation with breathing control (1.3 Gy) or proton radiation (0.5 Gy), and the highest inclusion of internal mammary lymph nodes (8 Gy).

Analysis of whole-heart mean doses alone may be misleading, because conventional tangential fields may still give significant doses to the critical structures of the anterior surface of the heart, including the left ventricular myocardium and coronary arteries (Fig. 52.4).[132,133] Das and colleagues found that more than 80% of patients with left-sided breast cancer had less than 3% of the heart within the fields.[102] Borger and colleagues did not find a correlation between the development of cardiovascular disease and amount of heart in radiation simulation films.[134] But left-sided radiation to even apparently small volumes of the left ventricle has been shown to cause early perfusion deficits in the distribution of the left anterior descending coronary artery.[135] These deficits may persist. In a study from the University of Pennsylvania, after a median follow-up time of 12 years, stress test abnormalities were seen in 59% of patients treated with left-sided radiation therapy, compared with 8% of patients with right-sided lesions.[136] Radiation has been specifically linked to the observance of coronary stenosis in distributions consistent with the radiation fields and cardiac vessel anatomy.[137]

The risk of radiation-related cardiac mortality has generally decreased over time.[138] One study using the Surveillance Epidemiology and End Results (SEER) database from 1973 to 1992 reported an excess rate of fatal myocardial infarction of 1% to 2% (relative risk 1.17; 95% confidence interval 1.01–1.36) over the course of 8 to 18 years from treatment for patients receiving left-sided versus right-sided adjuvant radiation.[139] In contrast, studies limited to patients treated with postlumpectomy radiation have

not generally found differences in cardiac mortality between left- and right-sided irradiation.[134,140–143] However, some of these studies have shown an increase in the number of nonfatal cardiac events associated with left breast irradiation. In a study of patients treated in the Netherlands between 1980 to 1993, there was a relative risk of cardiovascular disease of 1.57 (95% confidence interval 0.83–3.0) after left-sided radiation even when correcting for other potential risk factors such as age, diabetes mellitus, and a preexisting history of cardiovascular disease.[134] A study from the University of Pennsylvania showed that 10% of patients treated to the right breast had developed coronary artery disease by 20 years after treatment, compared with 25% of patients with left-sided cancers.[142] The highest risk for coronary disease was in patients with left-sided radiation and hypertension. A group at the University of Michigan studied patients treated from 1984 to 2000 and observed a cumulative incidence of myocardial infarction/coronary artery disease requiring intervention of 2.7% at 10 years.[144] Left-sided radiotherapy was significantly associated with myocardial infarction, but not all coronary artery disease requiring interventions, suggesting a background incidence in this population not directly caused by the radiation itself. As in other studies, the risk was also related to age and other risk factors. In the UK START trials, after patients with preexisting heart disease at enrollment were excluded, the incidence of confirmed ischemic heart disease for left-sided radiation treated 1999 to 2002 was 0.4% at 10 years.[76]

Achieving as low a cardiac dose as reasonably possible is justified to minimize the long-term risk of cardiac effects. This may be even more important with the increasing use of cardiotoxic chemotherapy regimens, such as dose-dense doxorubicin, taxanes, and trastuzumab. The 3D conformal tangents with forward planning with custom blocking or predefined segments can decrease the heart dose and normal tissue complication probability for late cardiac toxicity compared with using simple wedged tangents.[145–147] Prone positioning may help reduce heart dose in many but not all cases of left-sided breast cancer.[148] In a prospective study of 200 left-sided patients simulated both supine and prone, prone position was associated with an 85% reduction of in-field heart volumes compared with supine.[103] However, a benefit was seen in 85% of patients to prone positioning for the heart volume in the radiation field, but for 15% supine position was better. There can be significant variation in patient anatomy so that there are overlapping ranges of heart dose for IMRT versus 3D, and IMRT may be superior to 3D in heart dose for some patients but not all.[145] IMRT has been reported to reduce dose to heart compared with 3D in most[149–151] but not all studies.[152] Inverse planned IMRT has been shown to improve high doses received by the lung and heart for patients requiring internal mammary node irradiation compared with partly wide tangents or mixed beam plans.[150] However, the trade-off is that the addition of nontangential beams to IMRT increases the low-dose radiation to the heart and V5 dose.[153–157] Mean heart dose can be significantly reduced with respiratory control compared with free-breathing radiation.[151,158–163] Proton radiation therapy may have dosimetric advantages compared with photons due to the property of the positively charged proton depositing the bulk of its energy in tissue in a finite range, or Bragg peak, with essentially no residual radiation beyond this depth. Dosimetric studies have demonstrated very low cardiac dose with proton therapy in the postmastectomy radiotherapy setting even with regional node treatment.[164–167] Proton therapy may reduce risk for cardiac toxicity of radiation compared with photon radiation by reducing not only mean heart dose but also dose to the critical coronary artery structures on the heart's surface.[168] In one study, a scanning proton technique for left-sided irradiation was associated with lower minimum, maximum, and dose to 0.2 cc of the left anterior descending coronary artery than the best possible photon beam radiation technique (IMRT with deep inspiration breath hold).[169] The RADCOMP breast proton versus photon study (clinicaltrials.gov identifier NCT02603341) is being conducted on the hypothesis that proton therapy for locally advanced breast cancer reduces major cardiovascular events, is noninferior in cancer control, and improves health-related quality of life compared with photon therapy.

In addition, diagnosing and treating other risk factors, such as hypertension, diabetes, smoking, and hyperlipidemia, may be important in minimizing complications in patients treated with left-sided radiation.

Second Malignancies

The prospective randomized trials comparing breast conserving surgery and radiation to mastectomy or breast conserving surgery with or without radiation, have shown no statistically significant increases in the risk of contralateral breast cancer or nonbreast cancer malignancy with long-term follow-up.[122,124,126,170–173] However, this is a relatively common event in the breast cancer survivor. In one study from Fox Chase Cancer Center, the risk of second malignancy after breast conserving surgery and radiation was 16% at 10 years, of which approximately half were contralateral breast cancers. Patients aged 35 years or younger and those patients with a strong family history were at a higher relative risk of developing contralateral breast cancer.[174] Many could have been associated with *BRCA* or other germline mutation that would be diagnosed with more widespread availability of genetic testing today. For example, in a study of known *BRCA* mutation carriers treated with breast conservation, ipsilateral breast cancer events reached more than 20% at 15 years, but most were considered new primaries rather than failure to control the primary tumor in the breast.[175] In another study, the risk of second malignancies after breast conserving surgery and was 17.5% at 15 years, no different than for a cohort of patients treated during a similar time period with mastectomy without radiation.[176] Galper and colleagues reported that 8% of 1884 patients developed a second nonbreast malignancy.[177] This represented a 1% increase over expected incidence from the SEER database, which was observed more than 5 years after treatment. These were predominantly lung and ovarian cancers and occurred mainly in women younger than 50 years old at initial diagnosis. Kirova and colleagues studied 16,705 patients, of whom 13,472 received radiation.[178] The only two second malignancies with an increased relative risk at 10 years (compared with nonirradiated patients) were sarcomas (relative risk 7.46) and lung cancer (relative risk 3.09). Another study of 194,789 women from the SEER database treated from 1973 to 1993 found no increased risk of thyroid cancer in irradiated women compared with nonradiated controls and incidence rates similar to the female general population.[179]

The risk of lung cancer has modestly increased in some studies related to the use of older radiation techniques and regional node irradiation. The National Surgical Adjuvant Breast and Bowel Project studied the risk of lung cancer in women treated on prospective randomized trials of postlumpectomy and postmastectomy radiation.[180] There was no increased risk of ipsilateral lung cancer in patients treated to the breast alone with a mean follow-up of 19 years. However, for patients treated with comprehensive regional node irradiation after mastectomy, the cumulative incidence of ipsilateral lung carcinomas at 25 years was 1.5%, which was statistically increased compared with nonirradiated patients. In some studies, the risk of subsequent lung cancer in women with breast cancer was associated with smoking.[176,181] For example, a study using the Connecticut tumor registry, patients treated with radiation before 1980 had an increased risk of ipsilateral lung cancer more than 10 years after treatment, with a relative risk of 2.8, but the effect was greatest in smokers (relative risk 32.7).[182]

There have been reports of sarcomas appearing within radiation fields, usually 10 years or more after treatment, which may or may not be associated with the radiation. The risk is on the order of 1 patient in 200 to 500 or less.[97,174,176,178] Yap and colleagues studied 274,572 cases of breast cancer in the SEER database from 1973 to 1997.[183] The 15-year cumulative incidence of sarcoma was 3.2 per 1000 irradiated patients, compared with 2.3 per 1000 unirradiated patients at 15 years. The majority were angiosarcomas, with respective incidences of 0.9 and 0.1 per 1000 patients. The incidence of angiosarcoma after breast radiotherapy in other studies has been reported to be 0.004% to 0.18%.[177,184] Management is non–skin sparing mastectomy. These tumors are highly aggressive, with local recurrence rates in 50% to 75% and high association with distant metastatic disease.[185,186] Adjuvant reirradiation has been promising for improving local control with relatively low rates of complications.[187,188] Atypical vascular lesions of the skin are rare and generally appear smaller and at an earlier interval as angiosarcoma.[189,190] These should be widely excised because of their possible progression to angiosarcoma in a few case reports.

Complications in Patients With Collagen Vascular Disease

There is controversy regarding whether breast radiation therapy is contraindicated in patients with certain rheumatologic diseases. Such illnesses are rare, hence experience is limited in the specific breast cancer subpopulation. Early retrospective case reports first called attention to a possible connection between collagen vascular disease and radiation complications. Fleck and colleagues reported on five women treated with breast conserving surgery and radiation who had collagen vascular diseases.[191] The only patient with scleroderma experienced telangiectasias, skin necrosis, rib fractures, and interstitial pulmonary fibrosis. One patient with systemic lupus developed soft tissue necrosis and brachial plexopathy. Varga and colleagues reported four patients with systemic sclerosis who had radiation and exaggerated cutaneous and internal fibrotic reactions.[192] One patient with breast cancer had radiation of only 20 Gy to the chest wall and supraclavicular nodes and had complications within 3 months of fibrosis of the skin and chest wall, contractures, and arm swelling. Severe localized skin thickening and fibrosis was also reported in other small case reports.[193,194] Robertson and coworkers reported that one patient with scleroderma developed breast edema, fibrosis, retraction and rib fractures and another patient with rheumatoid arthritis had severe breast swelling, erythema, fibrosis, pain, and retraction that required palliative mastectomy.[195]

In other larger studies, the incidence of complications with collagen vascular disease and radiation has been lower than in isolated case reports but still potentially severe in the cases of scleroderma. The number of cases treated for breast cancer is often small. Ross and coworkers found no significant increased risk for radiation complications in 61 patients, even in 4 patients with scleroderma, but Phan and coworkers found an increase in risk for 2 patients with scleroderma in a series of 38 patients.[196,197] Morris and colleagues reported 16 patients with radiation with history of scleroderma and only 4 of 16 had severe late effects.[198] Three were patients radiated to the pelvis. A patient with scleroderma radiated to the breast (not regional nodes) had painful scar tissue and a cool arm years after treatment. Gold reported on 20 patients with scleroderma who were treated with radiation.[199] Three of the 20 had severe side effects during or shortly after treatment, and 3 had severe (grade 3 or higher) late side effects. Only 1 of these 20 was a patient with breast cancer treated to the chest wall and supraclavicular region who had acute grade 2 and no grade 3 late toxicity within 1 year. In a series of 21 patients with lupus and radiation, in which there was moderate toxicity overall, the 1 patient with breast cancer in the series did not experience grade 3 or higher toxicity.[200] Lin and colleagues reported 86 courses of radiation in 73 patients with collagen vascular diseases and compared them with matched controls without collagen vascular disease.[201] There was no difference in acute toxicity, but an increased incidence of any late toxicity was observed; however, severe late toxicity was most linked to pelvic radiation. Eight patients had breast cancer and 2 (25%) had grade 3 acute toxicity of skin desquamation, and late toxicity was grade 0 in 5 patients, grade 1 in 1 patient, and grade 2 in 2 patients.

In the largest breast cancer–specific series, Chen and coworkers[202] found that there was no significant difference in acute or chronic complication rates for 36 patients with collagen vascular disease treated with breast conserving surgery and radiation for early-stage breast cancer compared with matched controls, except for patients with scleroderma. Two of 4 such patients had severe acute toxicity, and 3 of 4 had late complications (fibrosis, necrosis, or ulceration requiring palliative mastectomy, or skin telangiectasias) including a case of temporary cord paralysis associated with regional neck and internal mammary node irradiation. There was no increased incidence of toxicity with rheumatoid arthritis, lupus, or other cases of less common collagen vascular disorders.

In summary, only scleroderma appears to be an absolute contraindication to radiation. Patients with active lupus should be approached with caution, and a past history of lupus, discoid lupus, or rheumatoid arthritis does not appear to be associated with a higher risk of radiation complications.

Conclusions

Radiation therapy for breast cancer is well tolerated and associated with a low risk of serious complications. The majority of women have good or excellent cosmetic results and a low incidence of long-term pain, fibrosis, or chest wall complications. The incidence of complications to the lung and heart has been steadily decreasing with improvements in radiation technique, more selective use of regional node irradiation, and decreased use of concurrent chemotherapy and radiation. Second malignancy is a rare but potentially serious effect of radiation seen in long-term survivors, but for the newly diagnosed patient with breast cancer, the risk is minimal compared with the potential benefits of radiation.

Selected References

35. Shaitelman SF, Schlembach PJ, Arzu I, et al. Acute and short-term toxic effects of conventionally fractionated vs hypofractionated whole-breast irradiation: a randomized clinical trial. *JAMA Oncol.* 2015;1:931-941.

76. Haviland JS, Owen JR, Dewar JA, et al. The UK Standardisation of Breast Radiotherapy (START) trials of radiotherapy hypofractionation for treatment of early breast cancer: 10-year follow-up results of two randomised controlled trials. *Lancet Oncol.* 2013;14:1086-1094.

103. Formenti SC, DeWyngaert JK, Jozsef G, et al. Prone vs supine positioning for breast cancer radiotherapy. *JAMA.* 2012;308:861-863.

130. Darby SC, Ewertz M, McGale P, et al. Risk of ischemic heart disease in women after radiotherapy for breast cancer. *N Engl J Med.* 2013;368:987-998.

137. Nilsson G, Holmberg L, Garmo H, et al. Distribution of coronary artery stenosis after radiation for breast cancer. *J Clin Oncol.* 2012;30:380-386.

A full reference list is available online at ExpertConsult.com.

53

Radiation Therapy for Locally Advanced Breast Cancer: Historical Review to Current Approach

KILIAN E. SALERNO AND MICHAEL D. MIX

Patients presenting with locally advanced breast cancer (LABC) are at significant risk for locoregional recurrence and distant metastatic disease. Optimal treatment paradigms have changed over time and now include multimodality therapy with systemic therapy, resection, and radiation. Sequence of treatments depends on extent of disease at presentation and degree of resectability at presentation. The role of neoadjuvant chemotherapy is expanding, particularly in patients with triple-negative, HER2-positive, clinically node-positive disease, and in those with unresectable disease. Combination chemotherapeutic regimens are used and most often delivered in a dose-dense fashion. Most often, modified radiation mastectomy is used for surgical management of LABC. Some select noninflammatory breast cancer (IBC) patients with good response to neoadjuvant chemotherapy (NAC) and limited disease extent may be considered for BCS. The role of axillary staging other than axillary lymph node dissection using sentinel node biopsy, especially after NAC, is evolving and under investigation. Locoregional radiotherapy targets the areas at risk: the chest (or breast) and regional nodes. Optimal outcomes require multidisciplinary coordination and delivery of care. Increasingly, treatments will be response adapted and tailored for each patient based on individual risk for recurrence and tumor biology.

This chapter describes the evolution of therapy for LABC. Optimal management requires coordinated multidisciplinary care. Current treatment paradigms for LABC include use of NAC, resection, usually with mastectomy and axillary lymph node dissection, and adjuvant radiation to the chest wall or breast and regional nodes.

Definition

An exact definition of LABC varies among sources and as the stage groupings and TNM definitions have changed in more recent editions of the American Joint Committee on Cancer (AJCC) staging manual.[1,2] Generally, patients with LABC have stage III disease at presentation with large primary breast cancers (cT3, >5 cm) and involved regional nodes; breast cancers with involvement of the skin and/or chest wall, satellite nodules, breast edema, or a combination thereof (cT4a, cT4b, and cT4c), clinical

presentation of IBC (cT4d), or advanced regional nodal disease with either bulky, fixed, matted nodes, presence of infraclavicular, supraclavicular, or internal mammary nodal disease (cN2 and cN3). IBC is a clinical diagnosis on the basis of erythema and/or edema involving a third or more of the skin of the breast with rapid onset (Fig. 53.1).

Some have included stage IIB large node-negative breast cancers (cT3N0) in this grouping. Others have used descriptors such as "fixed" or "skin involvement," but these do not always coincide with staging definitions of skin ulceration or chest wall invasion. Others have included patients spanning IIB to III disease, including node positivity in general because treatment approaches are similar, particularly with expanded use of neoadjuvant therapy.[3]

Stage grouping for LABC has changed over time. Under the seventh edition AJCC, LABC patients would be stage III patients. In previous staging editions, LABC would include both stage III and select stage IV disease (supraclavicular nodal involvement without distant metastases). Supraclavicular nodes were recategorized as N3 disease and no longer M1, and infraclavicular nodes were added to the nodal stage groupings. Additionally, the clinical definition of inflammatory carcinoma is reiterated.

Within LABC, there is significant variability in extent of disease, treatment pathways, and outcomes. Historically and practically, LABC has been divided into operable and inoperable disease. This is reflected in treatment algorithms within the National Comprehensive Cancer Network (NCCN) Breast Cancer Guidelines.[4] Although in the NCCN Guidelines, the term "LABC" is specified on the inoperable pathway, stage III breast cancers are included on pathways for either upfront resection or neoadjuvant chemotherapy followed by resection.

Incidence

Incidence of LABC varies based on the definition used. In 2015 to 2016, there were approximately 250,000 new cases of breast cancer diagnosed and 41,000 deaths in the United States. Over the past 30 years, mortality due to breast cancer has declined significantly (36% from 1989 to 2012). This is primarily a result of early detection due to mammographic screening and

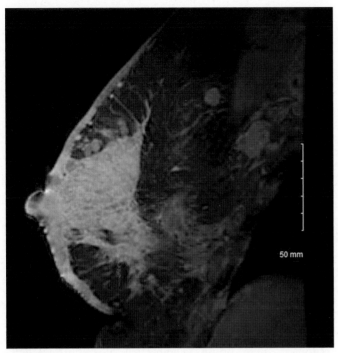

• **Fig. 53.1** Locally advanced breast carcinoma. Breast magnetic resonance imaging scan of sagittal view of a patient with inflammatory breast carcinoma demonstrating diffuse skin thickening, edema, mass-like enhancement throughout the breast, apparent pectoralis muscle invasion, and adenopathy within the axilla and subpectoral regions.

optimizing outcomes in these aggressive cancers as patients are at high risk for local, regional, and distant recurrence. Early involvement of all care providers is crucial and should be maintained throughout the treatment course.

In the past, operable LABC was primarily treated with modified radical mastectomy followed by chemotherapy and postmastectomy radiation. Treatment options have evolved and now increasingly include the use of NAC followed by surgery (mastectomy and breast conserving surgery [BCS] in selected cases), with nodal assessment (axillary dissection with ongoing investigation of sentinel node biopsy) and adjuvant radiation to the chest wall/breast and regional lymphatics.

For patients with inoperable disease at presentation, treatment involves NAC followed by surgery if rendered resectable and adjuvant radiation. For those patients with persistent unresectable disease after chemotherapy, considerations include modification of systemic therapy and/or use of radiation for locoregional control with reassessment for resectability.

Criteria for inoperability were first described by Drs. Haagensen and Stout and included extensive skin edema, chest wall fixation, skin satellite nodules, parasternal deposits, fixed axillary nodes, and arm lymphedema at presentation, but not nipple retraction or skin dimpling itself.[8] In the presence of these cardinal signs, use of radical mastectomy did not lead to permanent cure, and locoregional recurrence (LRR) exceeded 50% at 5 years. These observations led to a transition from radical surgery first to radiation as primary local treatment, then inclusion of systemic therapy, and now combined modality treatment.

Rationale for Use of Systemic Therapy

The rationale for use of systemic therapy includes improvement in overall survival and reduction in recurrence. The Early Breast Cancer Trialists' Collaborative Group (EBCTCG) meta-analysis of systemic therapy trials revealed a significant improvement in survival with use of polychemotherapy and endocrine therapy as well as the influence of age on outcome.[9] The meta-analysis is limited by absence of taxanes or HER2 directed therapies. Anthracycline-based polychemotherapy reduced the annual breast cancer death rate by 38% for those under age 50; 20% for women aged 50 to 69; and for those who were estrogen receptor (ER) positive, 5 years of tamoxifen reduced the annual breast cancer death rate by 31%.

Rationale for use of NAC had traditionally been to render unresectable disease operable. Studies investigating NAC have shown improvement in downstaging, resectability, and conversion from mastectomy to opportunity for breast conservation, without improvement in overall survival compared with adjuvant delivery, however.

A recent meta-analysis of NAC for LABC demonstrated benefit to dose-dense administration over standard schedule dosing for anthracyclines with or without taxanes with increased pathologic complete response (pCR) and overall response (OR) rates (13.5% vs. 9.2% for pCR and 52.5% vs. 45.3% OR).[10] The meta-analysis is limited by number of studies included (six studies), lack of data on ER or HER2 receptor status, and absence of HER2-directed therapies.

In vivo assessment of response to NAC permits potential cross-over to other therapies, including change in systemic therapy, proceeding to surgery directly if resectable, and use of radiation therapy (RT). Use of response has increasingly been incorporated into current clinical trial design and correlative studies.

education.[5] Fortunately, the rates of LABC have similarly declined. LABC remains a global problem, however, with patients frequently presenting with advanced disease.

In 2011, there were approximately 16,000 T3 breast cancers and 70,000 node-positive cancers. Inflammatory carcinomas account for 4000 cases annually.[5] A Surveillance, Epidemiology, and End Results (SEER) report on incidence of LABC and IBC between 1988 and 2000 showed an increased incidence rate (per 100,000 woman years) of IBC from 2 to 2.5, whereas LABC incidence rate decreased from 2.5 to 2.[6]

Outcomes

Historically, patients with LABC have had poor outcomes; 5-year survival rates were 25% to 45% with use of local therapy only (mastectomy, radiation, or both). Per National Cancer Database (NCDB) data from 2001 to 2002, 5-year survival was 66.7% for stage IIIA, 41% for IIIB, and 49.3% for IIIC disease. For those with regional disease at diagnosis in the United States between 2005 and 2011, 5-year relative survival rates were approximately 85% with use of systemic therapy, resection, and radiation. Using the SEER registry, median survival of IBC was 2.9 years versus 6.4 years for other LABC.[6] From a prospective clinical trial of multimodality therapy, 15-year survival was 50% for stage IIIA patients, 23% for stage IIIB patients, and 20% for IBC,[7] demonstrating that there are long-term survivors of LABC and IBC.

General Treatment Paradigms

Treatment paradigms for LABC generally include trimodality therapy. Multidisciplinary coordinated care is integral for

At present, use of NAC has expanded to include patients with lesser disease burden but in whom systemic therapy is indicated and thus given preoperatively versus adjuvantly. This is a particularly common approach in those with select intrinsic subtypes, triple-negative and HER2-positive cancers, and in those with node-positive disease.

Rationale for Postmastectomy Radiation

Original postmastectomy radiation therapy (PMRT) trials demonstrated significant improvements in locoregional control (LRC) and overall survival (OS) with use of PMRT in women with large, node-positive, or otherwise high-risk breast cancers.[11–13] In the Danish 82b of premenopausal women treated with cyclophosphamide, methotrexate, and 5-flurouracil (CMF), LRR was 9% with PMRT versus 32% without ($p < .001$), with improvement in 10-year OS (54% with PMRT vs. 45% in those with CMF alone; $p < .001$). For postmenopausal women treated with tamoxifen on the 82c trial, LRR was 8% with PMRT versus 35% without ($p < .001$), also with improvement in 10-year OS (45% with PMRT vs. 36% in those with tamoxifen alone; $p = .03$). For premenopausal women treated with CMF on the British Columbia trial, use of PMRT was associated with improved LRC (10% vs. 26%; $p = .002$) and 20-year OS (47% with PMRT vs. 37% no PMRT; $p = .03$).

The role for PMRT is covered in Chapter 49.

Meta-analyses investigating the role of PMRT have been conducted to address the role of locoregional radiation in improving outcomes for breast cancer. Whelan and associates evaluated 18 trials and 6300 patients with node-positive disease treated with modified radical mastectomy and systemic therapies. Patients included had stage II or III disease. The use of PMRT reduced any recurrence, odds ratio 0.69 (95% confidence interval [CI] 0.58–0.83); local recurrence odds ratio 0.25 (95% CI 0.19–0.34); and mortality, odds ratio 0.83 (95% CI 0.74–0.94).[14]

The EBCTCG recently published an updated meta-analysis of the effects of PMRT on 10-year recurrence and 20-year survival.[15] The 22 trials included in the analysis were conducted between 1964 and 1986 and included 8135 women. In node-negative women, no effect of RT was seen. In 1314 women with 1 to 3 nodes positive, RT reduced LRR ($2p < .00001$), overall recurrence (relative risk [RR] 0.68, 95% CI 0.57–0.80, $2p = .00006$), and breast cancer mortality (RR 0.80 95% CI 0.67–0.95, $2p = .01$). The same effect was seen in the subgroup of 1133 women treated with systemic therapy. For the 1772 women with four or more lymph nodes involved, RT had similar effects with improvement in LRR ($2p < .00001$), overall recurrence (RR 0.79, 95% CI 0.69–0.90, $2p = .0003$), and reduction in breast cancer mortality (RR 0.87, 95% CI 0.77–0.99, $2p = .04$).

Some have questioned the applicability of the results from these studies to current patients who receive systemic therapies known to be more effective, prolonged endocrine therapy, often have earlier detection, have a greater number of lymph nodes routinely evaluated with axillary lymph node dissections, and receive modern RT techniques. However, at this time, radiation after mastectomy is recommended for patients who present with LABC.

Locoregional Recurrence Rates Without PMRT

Studies of mastectomy with systemic therapy and no PMRT can be used to evaluate LRR risks and patterns of failure in the absence of RT. In the Danish 82b/c trials with 18 years of follow-up, LRR was 49% with the chest wall being the most common first site of recurrence.[16] In the British Columbia trial, 20-year LRR was 21% for women with one to three nodes positive and 41% for four or more involved nodes.[11] Data from the MD Anderson Cancer Center reports and the Eastern Cooperative Oncology Group (ECOG), National Surgical Adjuvant Breast and Bowel Project (NSABP), and International Breast Cancer Study Group trials have been published that include 10-year rates of LRR without PMRT (Table 53.1).[17–20]

Patterns of recurrence in these series were similar to those from the PMRT trials with local recurrence at the chest wall being most common, followed by the supraclavicular fossa, axillary apex, or infraclavicular region. Failure in the dissected axilla is uncommon, and internal mammary nodal recurrence is rare.[18–21]

Guideline Statements for PMRT and LABC

Given the results of the PMRT trials and risks for LRR without RT in high-risk patients, an American Society of Clinical

---

TABLE 53.1 Risk for Locoregional Recurrence After Mastectomy and Systemic Therapy Without Radiation

| Trial | No. of Patients | LOCOREGIONAL RECURRENCE RISK (%) | | Follow-Up (y) |
		1–3 LNs+	≥4 LNs+	
MDACC (Katz et al.[17])	1–3 LNs+ 466 ≥4 LNs+ 419	10	4–9 LNs 21 ≥10 LNs 22	10
ECOG (Recht et al.[18])	1–3 LNs+ 1018 ≥4 LNs+ 998	13	29	10
NSABP (Taghian et al.[19])	1–3 LNs+ 2957 ≥4 LNs+ 2784	13	4–9 LNs 24 ≥10 LNs 32	10
IBCSG (Wallgren et al.[20])	1–3 LNs+ 2404 ≥4 LNs+ 1673	13–25	4–9 LNs 26–35 ≥10 LNs 26–48	10

ECOG, Eastern Cooperative Oncology Group; *IBCSG,* International Breast Cancer Study Group; *LNs,* lymph nodes; *MDACC,* MD Anderson Cancer Center; *NSABP,* National Surgical Adjuvant Breast and Bowel Project.

Oncology consensus guideline recommended PMRT for patients with four or more nodes positive and those with T3 or stage III disease.[22] For patients presenting with LABC, PMRT was recommended. At that time, the authors acknowledged that there was limited randomized data for T3 and operable stage III LABC and for PMRT in the setting of NAC.

Cancer Care Ontario guideline recommendations on locoregional therapy of LABC attempt to address current treatment questions.[3] In general, mastectomy is recommended as the standard of care for patients with LABC, with BCS to be used on a selective basis and not for patients with inflammatory carcinoma. PMRT is recommended for patients with LABC and includes treatment of the chest wall or breast and regional nodal basins. After NAC, adjuvant radiation is recommended for LABC patients, even those with complete pathologic response. Axillary dissection is recommended for nodal staging in LABC because data regarding use of sentinel lymph node biopsy in this setting are limited. Options provided for subsequent management in the setting of progression or lack of response to initial NAC include crossover to a new systemic therapy regimen, immediate surgery if feasible, or radiation with multidisciplinary input and care coordination.

The American College of Radiology convened an expert panel to review the literature for treatment of LABC and updated their Appropriateness Criteria in 2016.[23] The authors highlight the importance of coordinated multimodality care using chemotherapy, surgery, and radiation for optimal outcomes and appropriate initial staging imaging to define extent of disease and subsequent response to NAC. They too acknowledge that few randomized trials specifically address the role of radiation in this setting but recommend RT after mastectomy for most patients, although optimal targets, volumes, and techniques have not been defined. They additionally note that breast conservation may be employed selectively in noninflammatory LABC patients with good response to NAC. Data on breast reconstruction options and RT related toxicities are presented as well.

Studies for LABC

There are limited studies specifically addressing LABC. The available data for radiation in the setting of LABC and with use of NAC are reviewed. Original studies of LABC mostly included patients with operable disease and included use of one modality, then progressed to combinations of treatment modalities and sequence. Subsequent or current trials include few or any LABC patients; in many trials, LABC is an exclusion criterion.

RT Alone for Operable LABC

Recognizing the significant risks for recurrence and death in patients with LABC treated with mastectomy alone, an alternative approach was to use radical radiation in this setting. Use of high-dose irradiation alone in LABC patients treated from 1960 to 1972 demonstrated potential for local control rates greater than 70% but was associated with increased late complications, including fibrosis.[24] In a series of 137 patients with nonmetastatic LABC treated with radiation alone, 90% initial clinical response, 5-year local control of 54%, distant DFS of 28%, and overall survival of 30% were seen.[25] Node-negative disease, use of excisional biopsy, dose of greater than 60 Gy, and use of systemic therapy were associated with improved local control. A follow-up publication of 192 patients with T3–4 or N2–3 disease (some of whom had

excisional biopsy and with greater use of systemic therapy) demonstrated improvement in survival (41% at 5 years and 23% at 10 years).[26] Crude local control was nearly 80% and influenced by dose of greater than 60 Gy delivered.

Neoadjuvant Chemotherapy Followed by Either Resection or Radiation

The Cancer and Leukemia Group B (CALGB) investigated the addition of NAC to primary local therapy, either resection or radiation.[27] This original trial of upfront systemic therapy in stage III breast cancers included patients with cT3N1–2 or cT4N0–2 LABC. Patients were treated with chemotherapy for three cycles (cyclophosphamide, doxorubicin, 5-fluorouracil, vincristine, and prednisone), then reassessed for operability and randomized to either mastectomy or radiation, followed by adjuvant chemotherapy. There were 87 patients evaluable for resection versus radiation with no significant differences noted by local therapy (approximately 50% of patients relapsed, half were local), and there was no survival difference. Radiation was delivered to the breast and regional nodes (supraclavicular, axillary, and internal mammary nodes) to 50 Gy with boost to residual disease (22 Gy to breast and 15–20 Gy to axillary nodes). The study did demonstrate improvement in disease control with systemic therapy in addition to local therapy alone. The median disease control was 2 to 2.5 years. Pre- or perimenopausal status or those presenting with inflammatory disease had worse outcomes.

Resection Followed by Systemic Therapy and Either Observation or Radiation

The addition of RT to resection and systemic therapy was evaluated by the ECOG trialists.[28] Inclusion criteria were those with operable noninflammatory LABC: T4 disease, T3N1–2 or muscle involvement, or T1–2 disease fixed to muscle or with N2 disease. Patients had upfront mastectomy followed by six cycles of systemic therapy with cyclophosphamide, doxorubicin, 5-fluorouracil, tamoxifen, and fluoxymesterone. Those without distant disease were randomized to either observation or radiation. Radiation was delivered to the chest wall and regional nodes to a total dose of 46 to 50 Gy. Patterns of failure differed by treatment regimen. Use of RT was associated with a reduction in LRR (24%–15%) with increased rate of distant relapses (50% vs. 35%), although no difference in time to relapse or overall survival was seen. Patients who developed recurrence after observation were treated with radiation for local control.

Neoadjuvant Systemic Therapy and Radiation for LABC

The French evaluated the potential for upfront systemic therapy and radiation in noninflammatory LABC patients.[29] On this trial, 120 patients received four cycles of anthracycline-based chemotherapy followed by preoperative radiation consisting of 45 Gy to the breast and nodal regions. Patients then received additional local therapy (resection or radiation) and further chemotherapy. The option for subsequent local therapy was response stratified. Those with larger amounts of residual disease proceeded to modified radical mastectomy (MRM), whereas those with less than

3-cm residual disease underwent wide local excision and axillary lymph node dissection, and those with clinical complete response received a radiation boost without resection. The 10-year local failure rates were 4% with MRM, 23% with wide local excision + RT, and 13% with RT alone. Factors associated with DFS included clinical stage, nodal stage, and tumor response. This trial and preceding data from use of radiation alone defined a role for potential preoperative RT in downstaging and local control in LABC unresponsive to NAC.

Inoperable LABC

Patients with inoperable LABC at presentation and resistance to chemotherapy are a rare subset of patients who present a significant treatment challenge. A total of 38 such patients were identified from five institutional trials of NAC (4.4% of patients enrolled).[30] These patients had T3, stage III, or stage IV (isolated supraclavicular involvement and no distant metastatic disease), remained inoperable after upfront anthracycline-based therapy, and then received radiation to the breast and lymph nodes (median dose 45–50 Gy with 10-Gy boost). After RT, 84% were able to proceed to mastectomy, and those treated with all three modalities had improved local control and DFS. Although limited in numbers, the response rates to NAC and RT were informative: 18% clinical response to NAC and additional 26% with RT, and nodal response of 23% with NAC and additional 58% with RT. As in other similar trials of LABC, advanced nodal stage was associated with worse outcomes than primary disease extent. In this cohort, patients expected to have extremely poor outcomes, but OS was 46% at 5 years and 20% at 10 years; distant disease–free survival was 32% at 5 years and 19% at 10 years, demonstrating for the importance of intensive multimodality therapy in the setting of poor upfront response.

Inflammatory Breast Carcinoma

IBC is a subset of LABC associated with high rates of LRR, distant metastases, and poor survival outcomes.[6,7] Historically, patients treated with radical resection developed rapid occurrence of chest wall disease and radical radiation resulted in limited long-term local control and poor survival.[31] The addition of systemic therapy to local treatments improved outcomes. A review of IBC patients treated with doxorubicin-based systemic therapy and radiation from 1974 to 1993 showed response to neoadjuvant therapy influenced risk for local recurrence and those who also received mastectomy had lower rates of local failure.[32]

Current treatment for IBC includes NAC, MRM, and PMRT. A retrospective review of 256 IBC patients treated at a single institution between 1977 to 2004 showed that patients who received all three treatment modalities had improved outcomes versus those who did not (5-year LRC 84% vs. 51%, distant metastasis–free survival 47% vs. 20%, and OS 51% vs. 25%, p < .0001).[33] Factors associated with LRC included response to chemotherapy, surgical margin status, number of lymph nodes involved, and use of taxanes. In patients with limited response to systemic therapy, nonnegative margins, and young age, dose escalation from 60 to 66 Gy given twice-daily improved local control.[33,34] PMRT fractionation and dose evolved over time, shifting from once daily to twice daily treatments, and increase in total dose. This accelerated hyperfractionated course of PMRT with dose escalation to 66 Gy was associated with improvement in LRC, DFS, and OS and was delivered as 51 Gy to the chest wall and regional nodes with a 15-Gy chest wall boost in 1.5-Gy fractions given twice-daily.[33,34] Others have reported local control rates of 87% with once daily treatment and use of skin bolus after taxane-based NAC and mastectomy.[35] There is not a single optimal locoregional radiation treatment approach for IBC, although use of acceleration, bolus, and/or dose escalation should be considered, particularly in patients with poor response to NAC.

Role for PMRT After NAC and Mastectomy

The role for PMRT after NAC was evaluated with a retrospective review of patients treated on six institutional trials of NAC followed by mastectomy from 1974 to 2000.[36] Patients who received PMRT were compared with those who did not. Despite group imbalances (with more advanced patients in the RT group), irradiated patients had improved locoregional control and cause-specific survival. Ten-year actuarial and isolated rates of LRR were lower with use of PMRT (11% vs. 22%, p = .0001 and 8% vs. 20%, p = .0002). Rates of LRR and cancer-specific survival according to clinicopathologic features are summarized in Table 53.2. Radiation reduced LRR in patients with cT3–4 tumors, stage IIB or greater disease, residual tumor size greater than 2 cm, and ypN2–3 disease. Cancer-specific survival was improved with RT for patients with stage IIIB or greater disease, cT4 tumors, and ypN2–3 disease. Additionally, the benefit of PMRT was seen in patients with clinically advanced stage III/IV disease who had pCR at mastectomy (10-year LRR 3% with RT vs. 33% no RT, p = .006).

This initial finding of PMRT benefit, even after pCR, led to subsequent evaluation of LRR in patients with pCR after NAC.[37] Of 106 patients with noninflammatory carcinomas with pCR at mastectomy, 10-year LRR for stage III patients was 33% without PMRT vs. 7% with PMRT (p = .04). For those stage I–II patients with pCR, no LR recurrences were seen at 10 years.

Potential Option for BCS After NAC for LABC

There are no randomized trials of BCS versus mastectomy for patients with LABC. Much of the data for use of BCS in select LABC patients after NAC comes from institutional and retrospective reports. Patient selection usually excludes patients with IBC.

In patients with LABC at presentation, response to NAC and then mastectomy and axillary lymph node dissection were evaluated to predict who might have been candidates for BCS based on clinical and pathologic features.[38] Initial criteria for consideration of BCS were complete resolution of skin edema and small residual tumor (<5 cm) without multicentricity or lymphovascular space invasion. These BCS guidelines were eventually adapted to include resolution of skin or chest wall involvement, lack of multicentricity or extensive microcalcifications, tumor greater than 5 cm, and no contraindications to RT. When applying these guidelines to patients receiving NAC followed by BCS, including 38% who had stage III disease, low rates of recurrence were seen with 5-year ipsilateral breast tumor recurrence (IBTR)-free and LRR-free survival rates of 95% and 91%, respectively. Higher rates of IBTR were observed with cN2–3 disease, residual tumor greater than 2 cm, multifocal residual disease, and presence of lymphovascular space invasion.[39]

The preceding risk factors associated with LRR with BCT versus mastectomy after NAC were evaluated to devise a prognostic index score that was subsequently validated.[40,41] Each factor was scored with one point: cN2–3 disease, LVSI, pathologic residual tumor greater than 2 cm, and multifocal residual disease. Risk for 10-year

TABLE 53.2	Ten-Year Rates of Locoregional Recurrence and Cause-Specific Survival by Clinicopathologic Features From the Mdacc Experience					
	10-YEAR LRR (%)			10-YEAR CSS (%)		
	No RT	PMRT	p Value	No RT	PMRT	p Value
Combined clinical stage						
I–II				73	71	.482
IIIA				64	70	.742
≥IIIB				22	44	.002
≥IIB	26	10	<.0001			
Clinical T stage						
T1	0	8	.535	80	92	.550
T2	10	7	.408	56	66	.977
T3	22	8	.002	71	69	.878
T4	46	15	<.0001	24	45	.007
Clinical N stage						
N0	23	10	.014	65	62	.749
N1	14	9	.062	66	64	.818
N2–3	40	12	<.0001	27	49	.024
Pathologic tumor size (cm)						
0–2	13	8	.051	64	69	.168
2.1–5	31	14	.002	49	53	.887
≥5.1	52	13	.001	25	37	.577
Pathologic nodal stage (No. of LNs+)						
0	11	4	.010	67	81	.271
1–3	13	11	.636	70	56	.179
≥4	59	16	<.0001	18	44	.005

CSS, Cause-specific survival; LNs, lymph nodes; LRR, locoregional recurrence; MDACC, MD Anderson Cancer Center; PMRT, postmastectomy radiation; RT, radiation therapy.

Modified from Huang EH, Tucker SL, Strom EA, et al. Postmastectomy radiation improves local-regional control and survival for selected patients with locally advanced breast cancer treated with neoadjuvant chemotherapy and mastectomy. J Clin Oncol 22:4691-4699, 2004.

LRR was low for patients with score of 0 to 1, lower for mastectomy than BCT with score of 2 (12% vs. 28%, p = .28), and significantly lower with use of mastectomy versus BCT for presence of three to four risk factors (19% vs. 61%, p = .009).

Locoregional Recurrence Risk on NSABP Trials of NAC and Implications for RT

On the NSABP B-18 and B-27 trials, there was no difference in DFS or OS if chemotherapy was given neoadjuvantly or adjuvantly, nor with the addition of docetaxel to doxorubicin and cyclophosphamide. Addition of preoperative docetaxel increased the rates of pCR (26% vs. 13.7%, p < .0001) and pCR was associated with improved outcomes.[42,43] pCR was defined as absence of

invasive tumor in the breast. Patients receiving preoperative therapy, especially those with larger tumors at presentation (>5 cm), were able to achieve downstaging and receive more BCS without a significantly increased rate of in-breast recurrence.[44]

A combined analysis was performed to evaluate 10-year LRR rates after NAC in the absence of RT.[45] The proportion of patients enrolled with cT3 disease varied between 13% to 29% and cN1 27% to 30% on these trials. Patients with T4 or N2 disease were not eligible. Patients received radiation to the breast if they had BCS without nodal irradiation; PMRT was not delivered for those treated with mastectomy. Results from patients treated with BCT were stratified by age and compared by clinically node negative versus positive. For those receiving mastectomy (and no PMRT), results were reported by tumor stage (≤5 cm vs. >5 cm) and by nodal status. Multivariate analysis of predictors for 10-year LRR is summarized in Table 53.3. Rates for LRR were reported by degree of pathologic response seen and pCR rates in the breast and lymph nodes. Recurrence rates were further reported by the number of positive lymph nodes (1–3 vs. ≥4) with risk of LRR increasing with increasing number of residual positive lymph nodes. Importantly, this combined analysis shows that the risk for LRR is significant for most patients with any residual nodal disease following NAC (Figs. 53.2–53.4).

These data can be helpful in trying to predict risk for LRR and thus potential benefit from adjuvant radiation in the setting of NAC. Predictors of LRR include age, clinical tumor and nodal status, and pathologic response in the breast and axillary lymph nodes. For patients with LABC, however, adjuvant radiation to the chest wall/breast and regional nodes is recommended regardless of response to NAC. Current clinical trials are open evaluating locoregional therapies on the basis of nodal response to NAC and are discussed later.

Other Prognostic Factors and Future Directions

Although the NSABP reports pCR as absence of invasive tumor in breast, there are differing definitions of pCR including no residual invasive or in situ disease in the breast and nodes, no invasive disease in the breast or nodes (in situ disease allowed); no invasive disease in the breast with either node-negative or positive disease. With such variability in definition, the prognostic value of achieving pCR differs significantly. The various definitions of pCR and impact of intrinsic tumor subtype on prognosis were compared in an analysis of patients treated on seven NAC trials.[46] The authors suggest that pCR defined as complete absence of disease (invasive and in situ) in the breast and nodes is associated with better discrimination of outcomes and that residual disease in any location should not be considered pCR. These data demonstrate that the prognostic import of pCR differs on the basis of intrinsic subtype.[46] pCR was prognostic for luminal B/HER2-negative, HER2-positive (nonluminal), and triple-negative breast cancers, and not prognostic for luminal A or luminal B/HER2-positive cancers.

An analysis by subtype of patients treated on the Danish PMRT trials showed improved outcomes in patients with hormone receptor–positive disease or HER2-negative disease versus not.[47] This is informative of the influence of intrinsic tumor subtype on locoregional control and outcomes is limited, however, because the systemic therapies used differ significantly from currently used agents.

TABLE 53.3 Multivariable Analysis of Predictors of 10-Year Locoregional Recurrence After Neoadjuvant Chemotherapy Without Radiation From the Combined Analysis of NSABP B-18 and B-27

Variable	No. of Patients	LRR Events	HR	95% CI	p Value
Combined data set	2961				
Age ≥50 vs. <50 y			0.78	0.63–0.98	.03
Clinical tumor size >5 vs. ≤5 cm			1.51	1.19–1.91	<.001
Clinical nodal status cN+ vs. cN–			1.61	1.28–2.02	<.001
Breast/nodal pathologic status					<.001
ypN–/no breast pCR vs. ypN–/breast pCR			1.55	1.01–2.39	
ypN+ vs. ypN–/breast pCR			2.71	1.79–4.09	
Patients treated with mastectomy	1071	131			
Clinical tumor size >5 vs. ≤5 cm			1.58	1.12–2.23	.0095
Clinical nodal status cN+ vs. cN–			1.53	1.08–2.18	.017
Breast/nodal pathologic status					<.001
ypN–/no breast pCR vs. ypN– breast pCR			2.21	0.77–6.30	
ypN+ vs. ypN–/breast pCR			4.48	1.64–12.21	
Patients treated with WLE + RT	1890	189			
Age ≥50 vs. <50 y			0.71	0.53–0.96	.025
Clinical nodal status cN+ vs. cN–			1.70	1.26–2.31	<.001
Breast/nodal pathologic status					<.001
ypN–/no breast pCR vs. ypN–/breast pCR			1.44	0.90–2.33	
ypN+ vs. ypN–/breast pCR			2.25	1.14–3.59	

CI, Confidence interval; *cN,* clinical node; *HR,* hazard ratio; *LRR,* locoregional recurrence; *NSABP,* National Surgical Adjuvant Breast and Bowel Project; *pCR,* pathologic complete response; *WLE + RT,* wide local excision and radiation; *ypN,* pathologic nodal response to neoadjuvant chemotherapy.

Data from Mamounas EP, Anderson SJ, Dignam JJ, et al. Predictors of locoregional recurrence after neoadjuvant chemotherapy: results from combined analysis of National Surgical Adjuvant Breast and Bowel Project B-18 and B-27. *J Clin Oncol* 2012;30:3960-3966.

In the future, it may be possible to further stratify risk for LRR (and hence subsequent expected benefit of adjuvant radiation) on the basis of gene expression profiling. Of patients from the Danish 82b/c trials for whom tissue was available, gene expression analysis was performed to assess risk for LRR without PMRT.[48] Genes were identified to stratify patients into high- and low-risk groups. LRR risk at 20 years was 57% in the high-risk group and 8% in the low-risk group ($p < .0001$). Use of PMRT significantly lowered the risk for LRR in the high-risk group (57% vs. 12% at 20 years, $p < .001$).

Studies of concurrent chemotherapy and radiation have yielded mixed results. In a trial of LABC patients treated with preoperative radiation to 45 Gy to breast and nodes and concurrent paclitaxel, response rates greater than 90% were seen with tolerable toxicities.[49] Subsequent follow-up results demonstrate pathologic response was associated with improved DFS and OS.[50] This is in contrast to another study using concurrent chemoradiation with paclitaxel in which significant and dose-limiting pulmonary toxicity was observed 25% of patients.[51] Use of concurrent chemoradiation remains an area of investigation.

Ongoing studies are evaluating the role of locoregional therapies including axillary surgery and radiation in clinically node-positive patients receiving NAC.

For cT1–3N1M0 patients who convert to node-negative disease (ypN0), the NRG Oncology group is evaluating the role for regional nodal irradiation on the NSABP B51/Radiation

Therapy Oncology Group 1304 trial. Patients treated with mastectomy are randomized to either postmastectomy chest wall and regional nodal irradiation or no radiation. Those treated with lumpectomy receive breast radiation and are randomized to regional nodal irradiation or not. Axillary management allows for either axillary lymph node dissection or sentinel node biopsy.

For patients staged cT1–3N1M0 who have persistent node-positive disease (ypN+ on sentinel node biopsy) after NAC, the Alliance for Clinical Trials in Oncology group is evaluating the role of further axillary surgery versus axillary RT on the A011202 trial. Randomization is to either axillary lymph node dissection plus nodal irradiation excluding the dissected axilla or no further axillary surgery and full axillary nodal irradiation.

The forthcoming results of these studies will be informative and may be applicable to select LABC patients; however, those with more advanced disease at presentation are excluded.

Locoregional Radiation Targets and Techniques for LABC

For LABC, treatment targets include the chest wall or breast and regional lymph nodes; the areas at risk for locoregional recurrence.

In the Danish 82b and 82c and the British Columbia postmastectomy trials, treatment volumes included the chest wall and

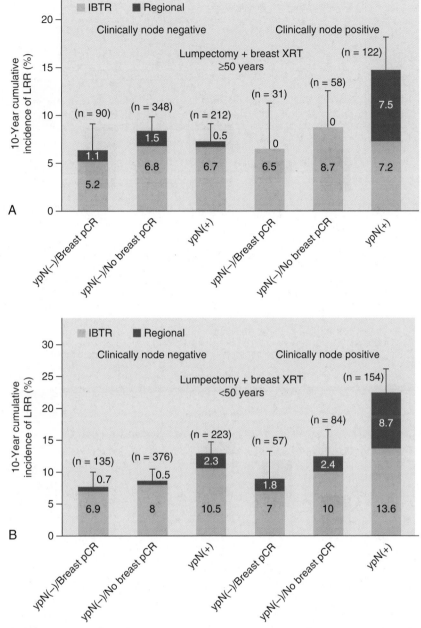

• **Fig. 53.2** Ten-year cumulative incidence of locoregional recurrence *(LRR)* in patients (A) age ≥50 years treated with lumpectomy plus breast external radiotherapy *(XRT)* and (B) younger than age 50 years treated with lumpectomy plus breast XRT. *IBTR,* Ipsilateral breast tumor recurrence; *pCR,* pathologic complete response (after neoadjuvant chemotherapy); *ypN,* pathologic nodal status (after neoadjuvant chemotherapy). (From Mamounas EP, Anderson SJ, Dignam JJ, et al. Predictors of locoregional recurrence after neoadjuvant chemotherapy: results from combined analysis of National Surgical Adjuvant Breast and Bowel Project B-18 and B-27. *J Clin Oncol* 2012;30:3960-3966.)

supraclavicular, axillary, and internal mammary nodal regions.[11–13] In the EBCTCG analysis of radiotherapy after mastectomy and axillary surgery, of the 22 trials with data available, all included RT to the chest wall and supraclavicular and/or axillary fossa, and the IMNs were treated in 20 of 22 trials.[15]

In the contemporary studies of regional nodal irradiation in early-stage breast cancers, treatment volumes include the chest wall or breast; the supraclavicular, axillary, and internal mammary lymph nodes (MA-20 study); or the medial supraclavicular and internal mammary lymph nodes (EORTC 22922 trial).[52,53]

Given the high risk for locoregional relapse in LABC, it is recommended that multimodality therapy with systemic therapy, resection, and comprehensive radiation be delivered. This includes radiation of the chest wall or breast and the supraclavicular, infraclavicular, internal mammary nodal regions, and any portion of the axilla at risk. Areas of initial disease involvement at presentation need to be considered in radiation treatment planning, especially areas not addressed surgically (i.e., supraclavicular, infraclavicular, and/or internal mammary nodal disease). Areas of unresected disease should be considered for boost, and boost is

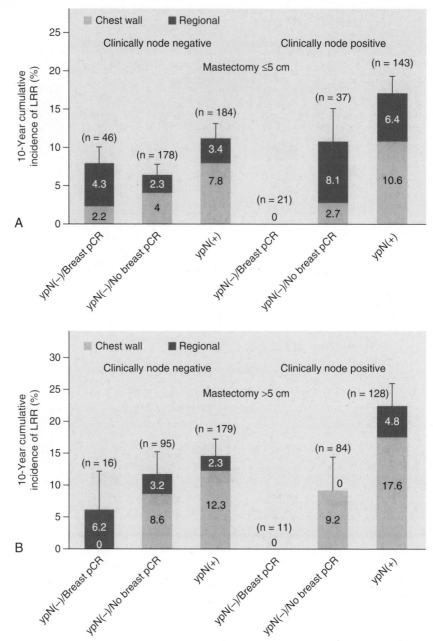

• **Fig. 53.3** Ten-year cumulative incidence of locoregional recurrence *(LRR)* in patients with (A) tumors 5 cm or smaller treated with mastectomy and (B) tumors 5 cm or greater treated with mastectomy. *pCR,* Pathologic complete response (after neoadjuvant chemotherapy); *ypN,* pathologic nodal status (after neoadjuvant chemotherapy). (From Mamounas EP, Anderson SJ, Dignam JJ, et al. Predictors of locoregional recurrence after neoadjuvant chemotherapy: results from combined analysis of National Surgical Adjuvant Breast and Bowel Project B-18 and B-27. *J Clin Oncol* 2012;30:3960-3966.)

recommended for persistent residual disease. The mastectomy incision is often boosted as well.[54–56]

Details of postmastectomy treatment techniques and field design are described in Chapter 49 and regional nodal irradiation in Chapter 48. Radiation treatment associated toxicities are discussed in Chapter 52.

Conclusion

Patients presenting with LABC are at significant risk for locoregional recurrence and distant metastatic disease. Optimal treatment paradigms have changed over time and now include multimodality therapy with systemic therapy, resection, and radiation. Sequence of treatments depends on extent of disease at presentation and degree of resectability at presentation. The role of neoadjuvant chemotherapy is expanding, particularly in patients with triple-negative, HER2-positive, clinically node-positive disease and in those with unresectable disease. Combination chemotherapeutic regimens are used and most often delivered in a dose-dense fashion. Most often, modified radiation mastectomy is used for surgical management of LABC. Some select noninflammatory breast cancer patients with good response to

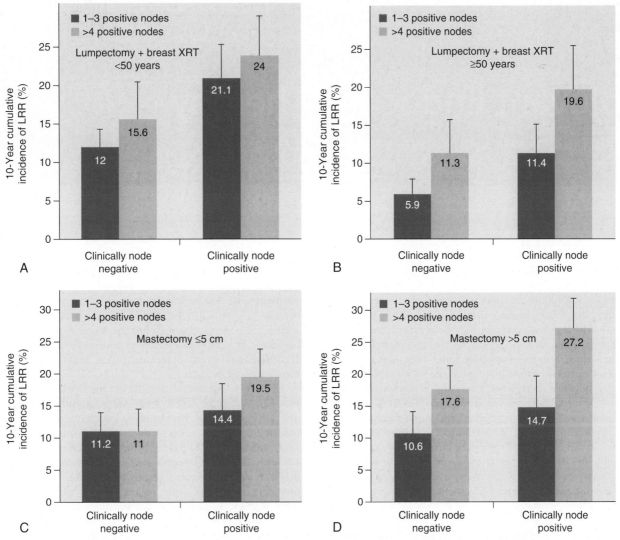

• **Fig. 53.4** Ten-year cumulative incidence of locoregional recurrence *(LRR)* in pathologically node-positive patients (A) age 50 years or younger treated with lumpectomy plus breast external radiotherapy (XRT) according to number of positive nodes; (B) age 50 years or older treated with lumpectomy plus breast XRT according to number of positive nodes; (C) with tumors 5 cm or smaller treated with mastectomy according to number of positive nodes; (D) with tumors 5 cm or greater treated with mastectomy according to number of positive nodes. (From Mamounas EP, Anderson SJ, Dignam JJ, et al. Predictors of locoregional recurrence after neoadjuvant chemotherapy: results from combined analysis of National Surgical Adjuvant Breast and Bowel Project B-18 and B-27. *J Clin Oncol* 2012;30:3960-3966.)

NAC and limited disease extent may be considered for BCS. The role of axillary staging other than axillary lymph node dissection, using sentinel node biopsy, especially after NAC, is evolving and under investigation. Locoregional radiotherapy targets the areas at risk: the chest (or breast) and regional nodes. Optimal outcomes require multidisciplinary coordination and delivery of care. Increasingly, treatments will be response adapted and tailored for each patient based on individual risk for recurrence and tumor biology.

Selected References

3. Cancer Care Ontario Guidelines. Locoregional therapy of locally advanced breast cancer (LABC); 2014. http://www.cancercare.on.ca/common/pages/UserFile.aspx?fileId=334821. Accessed 20 July 2016.

23. American College of Radiology. Appropriateness criteria: locally advanced breast cancer; 2016. acsearch.acr.org/docs/69346/Narrative. Accessed 20 July 2016.

36. Huang EH, Tucker SL, Strom EA, et al. Postmastectomy radiation improves local-regional control and survival for selected patients with locally advanced breast cancer treated with neoadjuvant chemotherapy and mastectomy. *J Clin Oncol.* 2004;22:4691-4699.

37. McGuire SE, Gonzalez-Angulo AM, Huang EH, et al. Postmastectomy radiation improves the outcome of patients with locally advanced breast cancer who achieve a pathologic complete response to neoadjuvant chemotherapy. *Int J Radiat Oncol Biol Phys.* 2007;68:1004-1009.

45. Mamounas EP, Anderson SJ, Dignam JJ, et al. Predictors of locoregional recurrence after neoadjuvant chemotherapy: results from combined analysis of National Surgical Adjuvant Breast and Bowel Project B-18 and B-27. *J Clin Oncol.* 2012;30:3960-3966.

A full reference list is available online at ExpertConsult.com.

54

Adjuvant Endocrine Therapy

KAREN LISA SMITH AND VERED STEARNS

The use of endocrine therapy for breast cancer dates back to the early 1900s when favorable results were reported for the management of inoperable advanced breast cancer with surgical techniques for removing sources of estrogen.[1–3] With the subsequent understanding that breast cancer is a systemic disease in which micrometastases may be present from the time of diagnosis, evaluation of endocrine therapy moved into the adjuvant setting. Studies of oophorectomy after mastectomy for early breast cancer were first reported in the 1950s–1960s.[4] Since then, oral endocrine therapies and nonsurgical methods of ovarian ablation (OA) have been developed and a series of trials evaluating these agents have resulted in adjuvant endocrine therapy becoming a key component of the treatment of early-stage breast cancer.[5–7] In this chapter, we review the current approach to adjuvant endocrine therapy for early-stage invasive breast cancer and ductal carcinoma in situ (DCIS). We also review key trials leading to the development of current treatments and review toxicities and unanswered questions.

Rationale for Adjuvant Endocrine Therapy

Adjuvant endocrine therapy for early-stage invasive breast cancer is given with curative intent. Meta-analyses performed by the Early Breast Cancer Trialists' Collaborative Group (EBCTCG) evaluating individual patient-level data from multiple clinical trials since 1985 have consistently demonstrated that adjuvant endocrine therapy reduces the risk of locoregional recurrence, distant recurrence, contralateral new primary breast cancer, and mortality.[5,6] The benefits of adjuvant endocrine therapy are substantial, with recurrence rates almost halved and mortality rates reduced by approximately one-third.[6] Benefits are long-lasting, with a carryover benefit continuing up to 5 years beyond the conclusion of therapy.[6,8]

In the setting of DCIS, adjuvant endocrine therapy can be considered with the aim of reducing the risk of an in-breast recurrence and for contralateral chemoprevention. However, endocrine therapy has no effect on the risk of distant metastases or mortality after DCIS.[9–12]

Who Is a Candidate for Adjuvant Endocrine Therapy?

The observation that endocrine manipulation can be therapeutic for breast cancer predates the discovery of the estrogen receptor (ER) and progesterone receptor (PR) in breast tumors in the 1970s.[13,14] It has since been established that the benefit from adjuvant endocrine therapy is limited to hormone receptor–positive breast cancer, making hormonal therapy the first "targeted therapy."[6] Approximately 75% of invasive breast cancers are ER and/or PR positive, although breast cancers in young women are less likely to be hormone receptor positive.[15,16] Evaluation of ER and PR status by immunohistochemical assay is required for all breast cancers.[17]

ER status (positive or negative) is the single most important factor predictive of benefit from adjuvant endocrine therapy.[6,11] The strength of ER expression is predictive of the degree of benefit from adjuvant endocrine therapy, with stronger expression associated with greater benefit.[6,18] Current guidelines use 1% expression on immunohistochemical assay as the cutoff to define hormone receptor positivity; however, guidelines grant providers discretion with regard to use of adjuvant endocrine therapy in patients whose breast cancers are only weakly hormone receptor positive (defined as 1%–10%) while endorsing it for those whose breast cancers have stronger expression.[17] Data also suggest greater benefit from adjuvant endocrine therapy in patients whose tumors express both steroid hormone receptors (ER and PR positive) than only one receptor.[19] Controversy exists regarding the relative importance of PR expression in predicting benefit from adjuvant endocrine therapy. Analyses from the EBCTCG suggest that, given ER status, PR status does not predict benefit from adjuvant endocrine therapy.[6] However, ER-negative/PR-positive breast cancer is rare, and because PR is an estrogen-regulated gene, there has been debate about whether ER-negative/PR-positive breast cancer is a true entity.[20,21] Given this uncertainty, adjuvant endocrine therapy is recommended for patients whose breast cancers express both ER and PR and for those whose breast cancers express only one steroid hormone receptor.[17]

Evolving data suggest that factors besides hormone receptor status may affect the degree of benefit from adjuvant endocrine therapy. For example, expression of human epidermal growth factor receptor 2 (HER2) is associated with endocrine resistance. In addition, activation of downstream signaling, such as the PI3Kinase/AKT/mTOR pathway, may be associated with endocrine resistance.[22] Recent trials in the metastatic setting combining endocrine therapy with targeted therapies with the intent of overcoming endocrine resistance have yielded favorable results, and efforts to assess these approaches are ongoing in the adjuvant setting.[23–26]

TABLE 54.1	Current Therapeutic Options for Adjuvant Endocrine Therapy			
Selective Estrogen Receptor Modulators	**Aromatase Inhibitors**	**Ovarian Ablation**	**Ovarian Function Suppression**
Tamoxifen 20 mg oral daily	Anastrozole 1 mg oral daily	Oophorectomy	Goserelin 3.6 mg subcutaneous every 28 days
	Letrozole 2.5 mg oral daily	Ovarian irradiation	Triptorelin 3.75 mg intramuscular every 28 days
	Exemestane 25 mg oral daily		Leuprolide 3.75 mg intramuscular every 28 days

Adjuvant Endocrine Therapy: Mechanism of Action

The binding of estrogen to the ER results in a series of downstream steps that modulate transcription of genes responsible for cellular function, tumor growth, invasion, angiogenesis, and survival. Endocrine therapy either antagonizes the ER or causes estrogen deprivation.[22] Types of endocrine therapy used in the adjuvant setting include selective ER modulators (SERMs), aromatase inhibitors (AIs), OA, and ovarian function suppression (OFS) (Table 54.1).

Selective Estrogen Receptor Modulators

Tamoxifen, a nonsteroidal oral SERM that competes for estrogen binding sites in target tissues including the breast, is the only SERM approved for the adjuvant treatment of breast cancer. Notably, its effects on target genes and tissues are mixed, with antagonistic effects in the breast but agonistic effects on other tissues such as the uterus and bone.[27]

Aromatase Inhibitors

Conversion of adrenal androgens to estrogen by peripheral tissues is the primary source of estrogen in postmenopausal women. AIs block aromatase, the enzyme that converts adrenal androgens to estrogen.[22] Currently available AIs are the third-generation reversible nonsteroidal inhibitors anastrozole and letrozole and the irreversible steroidal inactivator exemestane.[7] AI monotherapy is not effective in premenopausal women because it does not block production of estrogen in the ovaries.[28]

Ovarian Ablation and Ovarian Function Suppression

The ovaries are the primary site of estrogen production in premenopausal women. Ovarian estrogen production can be blocked by OA or by OFS. OA is permanent and is accomplished by oophorectomy or ovarian irradiation. OFS is typically reversible and is accomplished with gonadotropin-releasing hormone (GnRH) agonists, also called luteinizing hormone releasing hormone (LHRH) agonists.[29] When GnRH agonists are used, monthly injections are preferred because ovarian suppression may be inadequate with less frequent injections.[30]

Approaches to Adjuvant Endocrine Therapy for Invasive Early-Stage Breast Cancer

Beginning in the 1980s, the EBCTCG meta-analyses established 5 years of tamoxifen as a standard adjuvant therapy for early-stage invasive breast cancer.[6,31] Although 5 years of tamoxifen remains an option, multiple recent clinical trials have evaluated strategies to improve on the outcomes achieved with 5 years of tamoxifen. In general, strategies that have been evaluated include longer durations of therapy, sequential use of tamoxifen and AIs, AI monotherapy, and the use of OA or OFS. With the expanding data, adjuvant endocrine therapy decisions are increasingly complex and differ by menopausal status.

Evaluating Menopausal Status

Assessment of menopausal status is required for selection of adjuvant endocrine therapy. If postmenopausal status cannot be confirmed, women should be managed as premenopausal. Women can be considered postmenopausal if they meet any of the following criteria: (1) prior oophorectomy; (2) age 60 years or older or (3) under age 60 without a hysterectomy and amenorrheic for at least 12 months in the absence of chemotherapy, SERM therapy, or OFS, with follicle stimulating hormone (FSH) and estradiol concentrations in the postmenopausal range; or (4) under age 60 years with a previous hysterectomy in the absence of chemotherapy, SERM therapy, or OFS, with FSH and estradiol concentrations in the postmenopausal range. It is not possible to determine menopausal status in women who have been treated with OFS. Determining menopausal status after chemotherapy is difficult because amenorrhea may not be a reliable indicator of ovarian function. In this scenario, serial documentation of FSH and estradiol concentrations in the postmenopausal range is required.[32]

Options for Postmenopausal Women With Invasive Early-Stage Breast Cancer

Options for postmenopausal women include monotherapy with tamoxifen or AI for 5 years, tamoxifen for 10 years, AI for 10 years, or sequential therapy for 5 to 10 years.

Tamoxifen Monotherapy for 5 Years: The Historical Standard

In their most recent update, with a median follow-up of 13 years, the EBCTCG investigators demonstrated that approximately 5 years of tamoxifen compared with control was associated with a 39% reduction in the 10-year probability of recurrence of ER-positive early-stage breast cancer (rate ratio 0.61, $p < .00001$). The risk of recurrence was reduced during years 0 to 4 and 5 to 9, but not in years 10 to 14 of follow-up, suggesting a 5-year carry-over effect. Tamoxifen was also associated with a 38% reduction in the risk of contralateral breast cancer compared with control (rate ratio 0.62, $p = .00001$). In addition, tamoxifen monotherapy for approximately 5 years reduced breast cancer mortality by 30% (rate ratio 0.70, $p < .00001$). Mortality benefits from tamoxifen monotherapy for approximately 5 years persist through 15 years of follow-up (Table 54.2). Tamoxifen for 5 years was beneficial regardless of receipt of chemotherapy, nodal status, age at diagnosis, or tumor size. Of note, many of the trials included in the meta-analysis did not require hormone receptor positivity for entry. However, the only factor noted to be predictive of benefit from tamoxifen in the EBCTCG meta-analysis was ER status, and adjuvant tamoxifen is only recommended in the setting of hormone receptor–positive early-stage breast cancer.[5,6]

Data regarding menopausal status are not available in the EBCTCG meta-analysis. However, women of all ages benefited from tamoxifen with slightly higher proportional risk reductions observed in older women.[6] Although tamoxifen monotherapy for 5 years is now rarely used in postmenopausal women, the EBCTCG meta-analysis established a standard therapy to which newer approaches have been compared.

Tamoxifen Monotherapy for 10 Years

The optimal duration of adjuvant tamoxifen therapy is uncertain. The EBCTCG meta-analysis confirmed that 5 years is superior to a shorter duration.[5] However, because up to half of breast cancer recurrences occur after the completion of 5 years of adjuvant tamoxifen, trials have evaluated an extended course of adjuvant tamoxifen (Table 54.3).[6,8,33–37] Initial studies did not demonstrate a benefit for prolonged treatment, but these were limited by small size, short follow-up, and the inclusion of ER-negative participants.[33,34,37] More recently, two larger trials with lengthy follow-up have demonstrated superiority of a 10-year course compared with

5 years. The international Adjuvant Tamoxifen: Longer Against Shorter (ATLAS) trial and its UK counterpart, the Adjuvant Tamoxifen: To Offer More? (aTTom) trial, together aimed to randomize more than 20,000 women who had completed 5 years of adjuvant tamoxifen to an additional 5 years of tamoxifen or to discontinuation of therapy. Both trials allowed enrollment of women regardless of the tumor's ER status, but efficacy analyses for the ATLAS trial are limited to the ER-positive subset and, in the case of the aTTom trial, it is estimated that 80% of the ER-unknown participants were likely ER positive.[8,36] The ATLAS trial demonstrated reduced risk of breast cancer recurrence with extended therapy, with cumulative risks of recurrence during years 5 to 14 of 21.4% in women taking extended therapy compared with 25.1% in controls. In addition, extended therapy was associated with reduced breast cancer mortality in the ATLAS trial with cumulative breast cancer mortality risk during years 5 to 14 of 12.2% in women randomized to extended therapy compared with 15% in controls. The greatest effect of the longer course of tamoxifen on breast cancer mortality in the ATLAS trial occurred in the second decade after diagnosis, consistent with the known carryover effect of tamoxifen.[8] Preliminary findings of the aTTom trial are consistent with those of the ATLAS trial, with late reductions in recurrence and breast cancer mortality with extended therapy (Table 54.4).[36]

Eighty-nine percent of the ER-positive participants in both arms of the ATLAS trial were postmenopausal, and the hazard ratio for recurrence was similar in pre- and postmenopausal study participants, although it did not achieve statistical significance in the premenopausal subset, likely due to small sample size.[8] Data regarding menopausal status of the participants in the aTTom trial have not been reported. Although tamoxifen monotherapy is rarely used for postmenopausal women in this era, data from these trials indicate that tamoxifen monotherapy for 10 years may be considered in postmenopausal women, especially if AI therapy is contraindicated.

Aromatase Inhibitor Therapy for 5 Years

To date, the strategy of treatment with a 5-year course of adjuvant AI therapy compared with tamoxifen for 5 years has been evaluated in three major trials (Fig. 54.1).[38–43] The Arimidex,

| TABLE 54.2 | Absolute Reductions in the Risk of Breast Cancer Recurrence and Mortality at 5, 10, and 15 Years From Diagnosis for Approximately 5 Years of Tamoxifen Compared With Control |

Absolute Reduction in Risk	5 Years	10 Years	15 Years
Breast Cancer Recurrence	12.4%	14.2%	13.2%
Breast Cancer Mortality	3.3%	6.2%	9.2%

Data from the Early Breast Cancer Trialists' Collaborative Group meta-analysis.[6]

| TABLE 54.3 | Trials Evaluating Extended Tamoxifen Therapy for Early-Stage Invasive Breast Cancer |

Trial	ER Status of Study Participants	Sample Size (N)	Reduction in Recurrence With Extended Tamoxifen (Yes/No)	Survival Benefit With Extended Tamoxifen (Yes/No)
Eastern Cooperative Oncology Group[33]	Any ER status	193	No difference for entire study population but longer time to relapse in ER-positive subset	No
Scottish Adjuvant Tamoxifen Trial[35,37]	Any ER status	342	No	No
NSABP B-14[34]	ER positive	1172	Yes: improved disease-free survival with extended tamoxifen	No
ATLAS[8]	Any ER status	12,894 (6846 ER positive)	Yes	Yes
aTTom[36]	ER unknown or ER positive	6953 (2755 ER positive)	Yes	Yes

ATLAS, Adjuvant Tamoxifen: Longer Against Shorter; *aTTom*, Adjuvant Tamoxifen: To Offer More?; *ER*, estrogen receptor; *NSABP*, National Surgical Adjuvant Breast and Bowel Project.

TABLE 54.4	Rate Ratios for Recurrence and Breast Cancer Mortality in the ATLAS and aTTom Trials Demonstrating Delayed Benefit of 10 Years of Tamoxifen Compared With 5 Years of Tamoxifen for Early-Stage Breast Cancer			
Years Since Initiation of Tamoxifen Therapy	**RECURRENCE RATE RATIO (95% CI)**		**BREAST CANCER MORTALITY RATE RATIO (95% CI)**	
	ATLAS[a]	aTTom	ATLAS[a]	aTTom
5–9	0.90 (0.70–1.02)	Years 5–6: 0.99 (0.86–1.15) Years 7–9: 0.84 (0.73–0.95)	0.97 (0.79–1.18)	1.03 (0.84–1.27)
10+	0.75 (0.62–0.90)	0.75 (0.66–0.86)	0.71 (0.58–0.88)	0.77 (0.75–0.97)

[a]Analyses for ATLAS are limited to the ER-positive subset.

ATLAS, Adjuvant Tamoxifen: Longer Against Shorter; *aTTom*, Adjuvant Tamoxifen: To Offer More?; *CI*, confidence interval.

Data from the ATLAS and aTTom trials.[8,36]

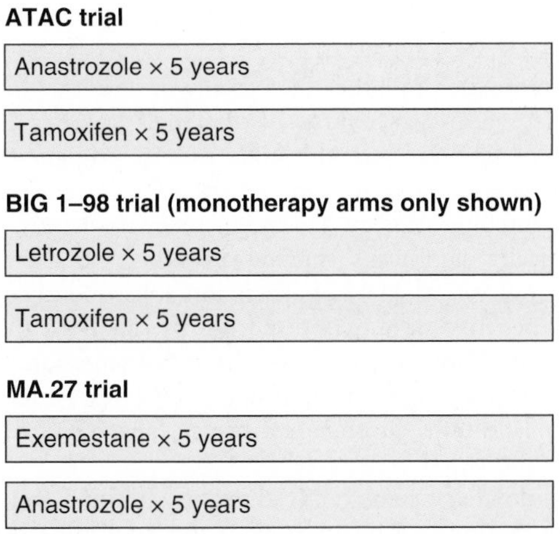

ATAC trial

Anastrozole × 5 years

Tamoxifen × 5 years

BIG 1–98 trial (monotherapy arms only shown)

Letrozole × 5 years

Tamoxifen × 5 years

MA.27 trial

Exemestane × 5 years

Anastrozole × 5 years

• **Fig. 54.1** Design of trials evaluating adjuvant aromatase inhibitor therapy for 5 years for the treatment of invasive early-stage hormone receptor–positive breast cancer. *ATAC*, Arimidex, tamoxifen, alone or in combination; *BIG 1-98*, Breast International Group 1-98; *MA.27*, National Cancer Institute of Canada Trial.

Tamoxifen, Alone or in Combination (ATAC) trial investigators compared 5 years of tamoxifen with 5 years of anastrozole in 6241 postmenopausal women. After a median follow-up of 120 months, the ATAC trial met its primary disease-free survival (DFS) end point favoring anastrozole; however, the benefit was limited to the predefined subgroup of women with hormone receptor–positive breast cancer, which comprised 84% of the trial participants. Among these women, there were statistically significant improvements in DFS, time to recurrence, time to distant recurrence, and the risk of contralateral breast cancer. The reduction in the risk of recurrence with anastrozole compared with tamoxifen was greatest in the first 2 years of treatment but was sustained over time, suggesting a carryover effect for anastrozole also. Despite these benefits, there was no difference in overall survival (OS) between the arms of the ATAC trial.[38–40]

The Breast International Group 1-98 (BIG 1-98) trial investigators evaluated several adjuvant endocrine therapy treatment strategies in 8010 postmenopausal women with hormone receptor–positive early-stage breast cancer. When it initially opened, women were randomly assigned to either 5 years of tamoxifen or 5 years of letrozole therapy. The study was later expanded to include two additional arms to evaluate switching strategies (letrozole for 2

years followed by tamoxifen for 3 years and tamoxifen for 2 years followed by letrozole for 3 years) with the aim of comparing these new arms to letrozole monotherapy.[42] After an initial efficacy report in 2005 demonstrated superiority of letrozole monotherapy over tamoxifen monotherapy, the trial was amended to allow patients randomized to tamoxifen monotherapy to cross over to letrozole, an option which was taken by 25% of such women.[42,43] After a median follow-up of 8.7 years, improved outcomes for letrozole monotherapy were observed for the primary end point, DFS, and for secondary end points including OS, distant recurrence–free interval and breast cancer–free interval. The benefits of letrozole monotherapy over tamoxifen monotherapy were present in both node-positive and node-negative patients (Table 54.5).[43] Results of the comparisons of the switching approaches to letrozole monotherapy are described subsequently.

The National Cancer Institute of Canada (NCIC) MA.27 trial investigators compared 5 years of exemestane monotherapy to 5 years of anastrozole monotherapy in 7576 postmenopausal women with hormone receptor–positive early-stage breast cancer with a primary end point of 5-year event-free survival (EFS). The trial was designed after preclinical evidence suggested that exemestane, a steroidal irreversible suicide inactivator of aromatase, may have greater efficacy than the reversible nonsteroidal AIs. However, after a median follow-up of 4.1 years, there was no difference in the 4-year EFS rate, OS, or disease-specific survival.[41]

Sequential Therapy With Tamoxifen and an Aromatase Inhibitor (or Vice Versa) for 5 Years Total

Switching approaches (tamoxifen followed by an AI or vice versa) for 5 years total have been evaluated in multiple clinical trials to date (Fig. 54.2).[42–51] As described earlier, after initially randomizing women to either 5 years of tamoxifen or 5 years of letrozole, the BIG 1–98 trial expanded to include two additional arms evaluating switching strategies (letrozole for 2 years followed by tamoxifen for 3 years and tamoxifen for 2 years followed by letrozole for 3 years) with the aim of comparing these arms to the letrozole monotherapy arm. After 8.1 years median follow-up, the sequential approaches were not associated with a lower risk of recurrence than letrozole monotherapy, and there were no differences in OS, distant recurrence–free survival, and breast cancer–free interval.[43]

The Intergroup Exemestane Study (IES) investigators randomized 4724 postmenopausal women with early-stage ER-positive or ER-unknown breast cancer who had completed 2 to 3 years of

TABLE 54.5	Recurrence, Survival, and Contralateral Breast Cancer Outcomes in Trials of 5 Years of Adjuvant Aromatase Inhibitor Therapy Compared With 5 Years of Adjuvant Tamoxifen Therapy		
Trial	Recurrence (95% CI, *p*)	Survival (95% CI, *p*)	Contralateral Breast Cancer (95% CI, *p*)
ATAC[a,39]	HR for DFS 0.86 (0.78–0.95, .003) *Favors anastrozole*	HR for OS 0.95 (0.84–1.06, .4) *No difference between tamoxifen and anastrozole*	HR for contralateral breast cancer 0.62 (0.45–0.85, .003) *Favors anastrozole*
BIG 1-98[b,43]	HR for DFS[c] 0.82 (0.74–0.92, .0002) *Favors letrozole*	HR for OS 0.79 (0.69–0.90, .0006) *Favors letrozole*	Not reported[c]

[a]Results presented are limited to the ER-positive subset of participants.
[b]Results presented are for the comparison of letrozole monotherapy to tamoxifen monotherapy.
[c]DFS end point in Breast International Group (BIG) 1-98 included invasive breast cancer relapse, second primary breast, or nonbreast cancer or death without previous cancer event. Separate HR for contralateral breast cancer in BIG 1-98 not reported.
CI, Confidence interval; *DFS,* disease-free survival; *HR,* hazard ratio; *OS,* overall survival.

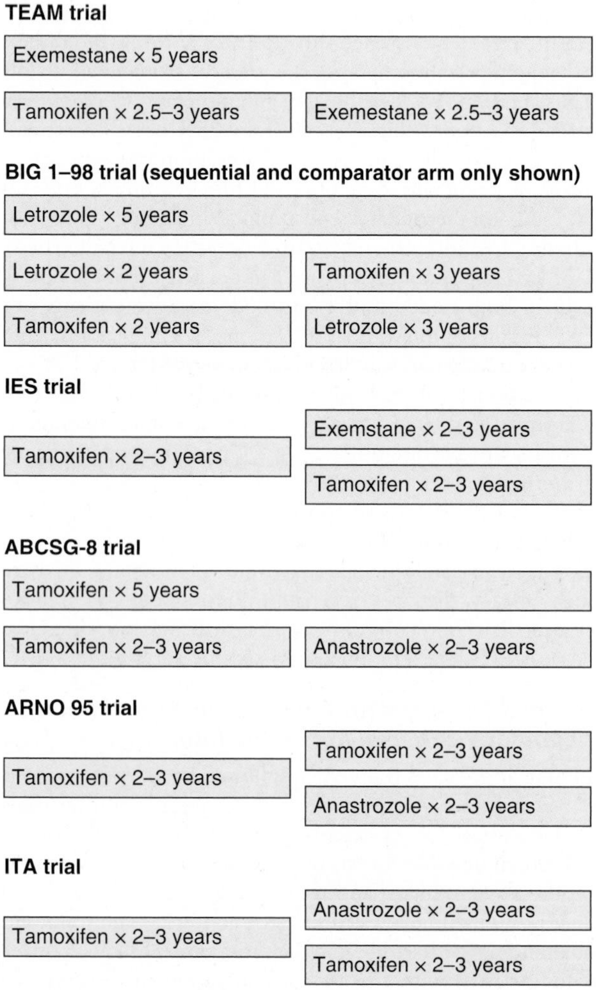

TEAM trial

Exemestane × 5 years	
Tamoxifen × 2.5–3 years	Exemestane × 2.5–3 years

BIG 1–98 trial (sequential and comparator arm only shown)

Letrozole × 5 years	
Letrozole × 2 years	Tamoxifen × 3 years
Tamoxifen × 2 years	Letrozole × 3 years

IES trial

	Exemstane × 2–3 years
Tamoxifen × 2–3 years	Tamoxifen × 2–3 years

ABCSG-8 trial

Tamoxifen × 5 years	
Tamoxifen × 2–3 years	Anastrozole × 2–3 years

ARNO 95 trial

	Tamoxifen × 2–3 years
Tamoxifen × 2–3 years	Anastrozole × 2–3 years

ITA trial

	Anastrozole × 2–3 years
Tamoxifen × 2–3 years	Tamoxifen × 2–3 years

• **Fig. 54.2** Design of trials evaluating switching approaches of tamoxifen and aromatase inhibitors for 5 years total for the treatment of invasive early-stage hormone receptor-positive breast cancer. *ARNO,* Arimidex-Nolvadex Trial 95; *ABCSG,* Austrian Breast and Colorectal Cancer Study Group; *BIG 1-98,* Breast International Group 1-98; *IES,* Intergroup Exemestane Study; *ITA,* Italian Tamoxifen Anastrozole; *TEAM,* Tamoxifen Exemestane Adjuvant Multinational.

adjuvant tamoxifen to either exemestane or continued tamoxifen to complete a 5-year course of therapy.[44,45] After a median follow-up of 55.7 months, the study met its primary end point, DFS, with a 24% reduction in the risk of recurrence associated with the switching strategy. On intent-to-treat analysis, there was no statistically significant survival advantage to the switching strategy. However, when 122 participants subsequently confirmed to be ER negative were excluded from the analysis, there was a modest survival advantage for switching to exemestane, with the divergence in risk appearing approximately 2 years after randomization. In addition, contralateral breast cancer was reduced by 43% with the switching strategy.[45]

The Tamoxifen Exemestane Adjuvant Multinational (TEAM) trial was a randomized phase 3 open-label trial initially designed to compare 5 years of tamoxifen monotherapy with 5 years of exemestane monotherapy in postmenopausal women with early-stage breast cancer. However, when data demonstrating superiority of tamoxifen followed by exemestane compared with tamoxifen alone became available from the IES, the TEAM study design was modified to compare 5 years of exemestane to 2.5 to 3 years of tamoxifen followed by exemestane to complete a 5-year course of therapy. Results reported to date include the intent-to-treat analysis of 4868 women who received tamoxifen followed by exemestane and 4898 women who received exemestane monotherapy with a median 5-year follow-up. Similar to the BIG 1–98 trial, there was no significant difference in outcomes for the two arms, and no subgroups benefited from the AI monotherapy approach compared with the sequential approach.[48]

The Italian Tamoxifen Anastrozole (ITA) trial investigators randomized 448 postmenopausal women who had completed 2 to 3 years of adjuvant tamoxifen for early-stage node-positive ER-positive breast cancer to continue tamoxifen or to switch to anastrozole to complete 5 years of therapy. Although the ITA trial closed early after the release of the ATAC trial results, it demonstrated an improvement in relapse-free survival associated with switching to anastrozole. An OS advantage was not demonstrated, although the study was not powered to detect a survival difference.[47]

The Arimidex-Nolvadex (ARNO) trial 95 and the Austrian Breast and Colorectal Cancer Study Group (ABCSG) trial 8 both compared tamoxifen monotherapy for 5 years to tamoxifen for 2 to 3 years followed by anastrozole to complete 5 years of therapy.

Each enrolled postmenopausal women with hormone receptor–positive early-stage invasive breast cancer who did not receive chemotherapy. Randomization for the ABCSG 8 trial occurred at baseline, whereas randomization for the ARNO 95 trial occurred within 2 years of initiation of tamoxifen. An initial preplanned combined analysis of these two trials demonstrated a 40% improvement in EFS with the sequential approach, with this improvement largely driven by reduction in distant metastases with anastrozole.[50] After a median follow-up of 30.1 months, intent-to-treat analysis of the ARNO 95 trial revealed improved DFS and OS associated with the switch to anastrozole.[49] In contrast, final results of the ABCSG 8 trial did not reveal significant improvements in recurrence-free survival or OS after 60 months median follow-up. Of note, 18% of participants randomized to tamoxifen monotherapy crossed over to receive anastrozole, which may have masked a benefit of switching. Analysis performed to compensate for selective crossover suggested that switching to anastrozole reduced recurrence by 24% (Table 54.6).[51]

TABLE 54.6 Recurrence and Survival Outcomes in Trials Evaluating Switching Approaches of Tamoxifen and Aromatase Inhibitors for 5 Years Total

Trial	Recurrence (95% CI, *p*)	Survival (95% CI, *p*)
BIG 1-98: comparison of letrozole × 2 years followed by tamoxifen × 3 years and letrozole × 5 years[43]	HR for DFS 1.06 (0.91–1.23, .48) *No difference between arms*	HR for OS 0.97 (0.80–1.19, .79) *No difference between arms*
BIG 1-98: comparison of tamoxifen × 2 years followed by letrozole × 3 years and letrozole × 5 years[43]	HR for DFS 1.07 (0.92–1.25, .36) *No difference between arms*	HR for OS 1.10 (0.90–1.33, .36) *No difference between arms*
IES[45]	HR for DFS 0.76 (0.66–0.88, .0001) *Favors tamoxifen followed by exemestane*	Intent-to-treat analysis: HR for OS 0.85 (0.71–1.02, .08) After exclusion of 122 participants subsequently confirmed to be ER-negative: HR for OS 0.83 (0.69–1.00, .05) *Favors tamoxifen followed by exemestane*
TEAM[48]	HR for DFS 0.97 (0.88–1.08, .60). *No difference between arms*	HR for OS 1.00 (0.89–1.14, >.99) *No difference between arms*
ITA[47]	HR for RFS 0.64 (0.52–0.97, .023) *Favors tamoxifen followed by anastrozole*	HR for OS 0.79 (0.52–1.21, .3) *No difference between arms*
ARNO 95[49]	HR for DFS 0.66 (0.44–1.00, .049) *Favors switching to anastrozole*	HR for OS 0.53 (0.28–0.99, .045) *Favors switching to anastrozole*
ABCSG-8[51]	Intent-to-treat analysis: HR for RFS 0.80 (0.63–1.01, .06) *No difference between arms* Censored analysis to compensate for selective crossover: HR for RFS 0.76 (0.60–0.97, *p* not reported) *Favors switching to anastrozole*	HR for OS 0.87 (0.65–1.16, .34) *No difference between arms*

ARNO, Arimidex-Nolvadex trial 95; *ABCSG*, Austrian Breast and Colorectal Cancer Study Group; *BIG*, Breast International Group; *CI*, confidence interval; *DFS*, disease-free survival; *HR*, hazard ratio; *IES*, Intergroup Exemestane Study; *ITA*, Italian Tamoxifen Anastrozole; *OS*, overall survival; *RFS*, recurrence-free survival; *TEAM*, Tamoxifen Exemestane Adjuvant Multinational.

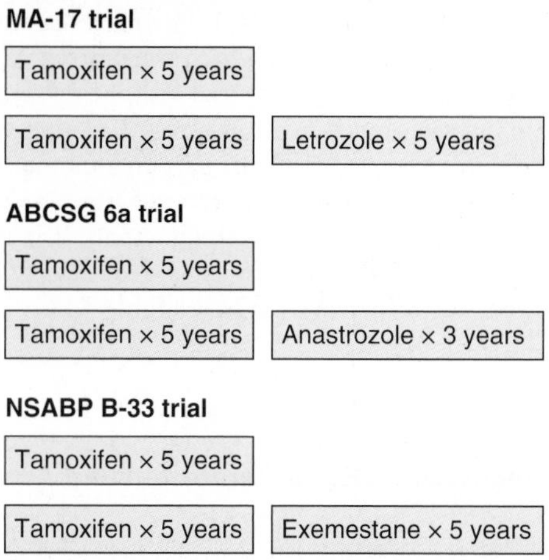

MA-17 trial

| Tamoxifen × 5 years | |
| Tamoxifen × 5 years | Letrozole × 5 years |

ABCSG 6a trial

| Tamoxifen × 5 years | |
| Tamoxifen × 5 years | Anastrozole × 3 years |

NSABP B-33 trial

| Tamoxifen × 5 years | |
| Tamoxifen × 5 years | Exemestane × 5 years |

• **Fig. 54.3** Design of trials evaluating tamoxifen for 5 years followed by an aromatase inhibitor for up to 10 years total for the treatment of invasive early-stage hormone receptor–positive breast cancer. *ABCSG,* Austrian Breast and Colorectal Cancer Study Group; *MA.17,* National Cancer Institute of Canada trial; *NSABP,* National Surgical Adjuvant Breast and Bowel Project.

Tamoxifen for 5 Years Followed by an Aromatase Inhibitor for Up to 10 Years Total

Concerns regarding the risk of late recurrence, the uncertain efficacy of prolonged tamoxifen therapy before the ATLAS and aTTom findings, and emerging data demonstrating the benefits of adjuvant AIs led to the evaluation of extended therapy with AIs after 5 years of tamoxifen therapy in three clinical trials (Fig. 54.3).[52–55] The NCIC MA.17 study was a phase III trial that randomized 5187 postmenopausal women with early-stage hormone receptor-positive breast cancer who had completed approximately 5 years of adjuvant tamoxifen to either placebo or letrozole therapy for 5 years. The study was unblinded after the first interim analysis, and women in the placebo arm were offered the opportunity to cross over to letrozole, an option that approximately two-thirds pursued.[52] Despite extensive crossover, which may dilute findings, this study revealed a 42% improvement in DFS and a 40% improvement in distant DFS with extended adjuvant therapy. There was no effect on OS in the population as a whole, but preplanned subset analysis indicated improved survival in the node-positive subgroup with extended therapy.[53]

Two additional smaller studies have also evaluated the role of extended adjuvant AI therapy in patients who completed 5 years of adjuvant tamoxifen for early-stage breast cancer. The ABCSG 6a study was a continuation of the ABCSG 6 study that compared a 5-year course of tamoxifen to tamoxifen plus aminoglutethimide, an early AI that is no longer in use, demonstrating no advantage to the combination.[56] Postmenopausal women with early-stage hormone receptor–positive breast cancer who completed the ABCSG 6 study were randomized to an additional 3 years of adjuvant anastrozole or to no further adjuvant therapy. After a median follow-up of 62.3 months, intent-to-treat analysis revealed a 38% reduction in the risk of recurrence and a 47% reduction in the risk of distant recurrence with extended anastrozole therapy. Despite these findings, there was no survival advantage associated with extended anastrozole therapy in the ABCG6a study.[54] The National Surgical Adjuvant Breast and Bowel Project (NSABP) B-33 trial investigators randomized 1598 postmenopausal women who had completed approximately 5 years of

TABLE 54.7 Recurrence and Survival Outcomes in Trials Evaluating Switching Approaches of Tamoxifen and Aromatase Inhibitors for Up to 10 Years

Trial	Recurrence (95% CI, *p*)	Survival (95% CI, *p*)
MA.17[53]	HR for DFS 0.58 (0.45–0.76, <.001) *Favors extended letrozole*	HR for OS 0.82 (1.57–1.19, .3) *No difference between arms* Preplanned subset analysis limited to node-positive participants: HR for OS 0.61 (0.38–0.98, .04) *Favors extended letrozole*
ABCSG-6a[54]	HR for RFS 0.62 (0.40–0.96, .031), *Favors extended anastrozole*	HR for OS 0.89 (0.59–1.34, .57) *No difference between arms*
NSABP B-33[55]	HR for DFS 0.68 (95% CI not reported, .07) *Trend in favor of exemestane*	HR for OS not reported Too few deaths in either arm to draw conclusions *No difference between arms*

ABCSG, Austrian Breast and Colorectal Cancer Study Group; *CI,* confidence interval; *DFS,* disease-free survival; *HR,* hazard ratio; *NSABP,* National Surgical Adjuvant Breast and Bowel Project; *OS,* overall survival; *RFS,* recurrence-free survival.

adjuvant tamoxifen for early-stage hormone receptor–positive breast cancer to exemestane or to placebo for 5 years. After the results of the MA.17 trial were reported, the NSABP B-33 trial closed early with approximately half the intended enrollment, and the study was unblinded so that participants in the placebo arm could be offered the opportunity to cross over to exemestane, an option pursued by almost half. Intent-to-treat analysis after 30 months of median follow-up revealed a nonsignificant trend toward improved DFS for the participants originally randomized to exemestane but no difference in survival. These findings are difficult to interpret because they are likely diluted due to extensive crossover and are limited by inadequate power (Table 54.7).[55]

Aromatase Inhibitor for Longer Than 5 Years

The benefits observed with extended adjuvant therapy in trials such as ATLAS, aTTom, and MA.17, along with the favorable findings for adjuvant regimens including AIs compared with 5 years of tamoxifen monotherapy, raise the question of whether more than 5 years of adjuvant AI therapy is beneficial. Multiple ongoing trials aim to answer this question by evaluating different approaches to extended adjuvant AI therapy.[57] First results of one such trial, MA.17R, were recently published. In this phase III, double-blind, placebo-controlled trial, the investigators randomized 1918 postmenopausal women with a history of hormone receptor–positive early-stage breast cancer who were disease-free after 4.5 to 6 years of adjuvant AI therapy to letrozole or placebo for an additional 5 years. Notably, many participants had also received tamoxifen before AI therapy. The primary end point of the MA.17R trial was DFS, which included local or distant recurrence in addition to new contralateral primary breast cancer. Study findings favored extended letrozole with improved 5-year DFS (95% for letrozole compared with 91% for placebo), although much of this difference was attributable to a reduction in new contralateral primary breast cancer. As expected, bone toxicity was greater in the letrozole arm than placebo; however, participants reported favorable quality of life (QOL) with extended AI therapy. To date, survival data are not mature.[58]

Selecting an Adjuvant Endocrine Therapy Regimen for Postmenopausal Women With Early-Stage Invasive Hormone Receptor–Positive Breast Cancer

Given the numerous trials and approaches to adjuvant endocrine therapy that have been evaluated for postmenopausal women with invasive early-stage hormone receptor–positive breast cancer, selecting the "optimal" regimen can be challenging. Interpretation of the findings and cross-trial comparisons are challenging because of the different patient populations, trial designs, and end points. However, a pattern of reduced risk of recurrence with the use of AI monotherapy or sequential therapy (tamoxifen followed by AI or vice versa) compared with tamoxifen monotherapy is seen in most of the trials. This treatment effect with AI therapy appears quickly, with reduced risk of recurrence noted within approximately 2 to 3 years of initiation of AI therapy. However, data from individual trials regarding the effects of AI therapy on breast cancer mortality are less consistent, with some studies demonstrating a survival benefit and others not. Reasons for this are not certain but may be explained by the fact that many of the studies included predominantly low-risk participants and that tamoxifen therapy itself is quite effective; thus identifying a survival difference would require a very large study and long follow-up.

The EBCTCG investigators recently reported an updated meta-analysis of nine trials evaluating 5 years of adjuvant endocrine therapy with AIs or tamoxifen using individual patient-level data from 31,920 postmenopausal women with ER-positive invasive early-stage breast cancer. Although this analysis does not evaluate extended adjuvant endocrine therapy, it is helpful for the purposes of synthesizing the studies evaluating 5-year approaches and provides some clarity regarding whether adjuvant AI therapy has a survival benefit compared with adjuvant tamoxifen therapy. The key finding from this meta-analysis is that AIs are associated with approximately 30% lower risk of breast cancer recurrence compared with tamoxifen during the period of time when the treatments differ (rate ratio 0.70, 95% confidence interval 0.64–0.77) but not afterward. Furthermore, AI monotherapy for 5 years is associated with a 14% reduction in 10-year breast cancer mortality compared with tamoxifen monotherapy, supporting the notion that AIs, like tamoxifen, have a carryover benefit (rate ratio 0.86, 95% confidence interval 0.81–0.99). In addition, this meta-analysis suggests that the benefit of AI therapy is independent of stage, grade, PR status, and HER2 status and that the third-generation AIs have similar efficacy.[7]

It is important to note that the benefits of AIs compared with tamoxifen are relative risk reductions. Although the proportional benefit of an AI compared with tamoxifen is the same regardless of tumor factors, the absolute benefit differs based on the absolute risk.[7] Understanding the absolute level of risk, the expected benefits of each approach, and the side effect profile can guide clinicians in selecting regimens for individual patients. At this time,

there is no best adjuvant endocrine therapy regimen for postmenopausal women, although guidelines suggest inclusion of an AI in the regimen in the absence of contraindications.[59] Criteria for selection of patients in whom to consider extended adjuvant AI therapy have not yet been determined; however, it is reasonable to discuss this option in patients in whom AI therapy is well tolerated, especially in those with a higher risk of recurrence and in whom bone mineral density is favorable.

Options for Premenopausal Women With Invasive Early-Stage Breast Cancer

Recent data have led to rapid changes in the management of premenopausal women with invasive hormone receptor–positive early breast cancer. Accurate assessment of menopausal status is of utmost importance as AI monotherapy is ineffective in women with ovarian function. Current options for premenopausal women include tamoxifen for 5 to 10 years, tamoxifen followed by an AI (if menopause is achieved), and OFS or OA with tamoxifen or an AI.

Tamoxifen Monotherapy for 5 Years

As noted earlier, the EBCTCG meta-analysis revealed a 39% reduction in recurrence and a 30% reduction in mortality with 5 years of tamoxifen. Data regarding menopausal status were not reported, but benefits for tamoxifen were observed for women of all ages including younger than 45 and 45 to 54 years.[6] As is the case for older women, the EBCTCG meta-analysis established 5 years of tamoxifen as a historical standard for premenopausal women.

Tamoxifen Monotherapy for 10 Years

As discussed earlier, the ATLAS and aTTom trials compared 5 and 10 years of tamoxifen, demonstrating reduced recurrence and breast cancer mortality with extended therapy.[8,36] Only 11% of the ATLAS study participants were premenopausal, and although confidence intervals were wide, subgroup analysis favored extended therapy in the premenopausal group.[8] Data regarding menopausal status of the aTTOm trial participants has not been reported. Despite the inclusion of few premenopausal study participants, these trials are particularly relevant to premenopausal women for whom AI monotherapy is not an option.

Tamoxifen for 5 Years Followed by an Aromatase Inhibitor for 5 Years

Also as described earlier, the MA.17 trial evaluated 5 years of letrozole after 5 years of tamoxifen. Participants were required to be postmenopausal at study entry, but women who were premenopausal at diagnosis and who became postmenopausal after chemotherapy during tamoxifen therapy were eligible. The DFS benefit for extended letrozole therapy was greater in women who were premenopausal at diagnosis (hazard ratio 0.26) than in those who were postmenopausal at diagnosis (hazard ratio 0.67).[60]

Ovarian Ablation or Ovarian Function Suppression Plus Tamoxifen or an Aromatase Inhibitor

For many years, the indication for OA or OFS in adjuvant therapy for premenopausal women with early-stage invasive breast cancer was uncertain. The rationale for considering OA or OFS includes the fact that adjuvant chemotherapy trials have demonstrated improved outcomes in young women who develop chemotherapy-induced amenorrhea (CIA), suggesting that part of the benefit of chemotherapy may be explained by its suppression of ovarian function and that inducing amenorrhea in women who do not experience CIA may be of some benefit.[61,62] In addition, the collective data described earlier support the superiority of AI therapy over tamoxifen in postmenopausal women with invasive early-stage hormone receptor–positive breast cancer, and this option is only available to premenopausal women in the setting of OA or OFS.

Analysis of OFS or OA in the EBCTCG 2005 update revealed a 4.3% reduction in the 15-year risk of recurrence and a 3.2% reduction in the 15-year risk of breast cancer mortality with the use of OFS or OA. However, the effects of OFS or OA were smaller in trials in which women also received chemotherapy, potentially because chemotherapy could have induced menopause. In addition, hormone receptor status was not documented in all of the trials included in this meta-analysis, potentially confounding the results.[5] The LHRH-Agonists in Early Breast Cancer Overview Group performed a meta-analysis of LHRH agonists in 16 trials including 9022 hormone receptor–positive premenopausal women with early-stage breast cancer. Overall, this meta-analysis demonstrated a greater benefit with OFS than that observed in the EBCTCG meta-analysis with a 12.7% reduction in the risk of recurrence and a 15.1% reduction in the risk of death after recurrence among women who received LHRH agonists in addition to tamoxifen, chemotherapy, or both, but not among those who received LHRH agonists alone. A definite benefit for the addition of LHRH agonist therapy to tamoxifen alone was not confirmed in this meta-analysis because it was not clear how much of the benefit of the combination was attributable to the tamoxifen component, and not all studies included a comparator arm treated with tamoxifen alone. LHRH agonist–based therapy was observed to be approximately equally effective to chemotherapy in this meta-analysis, although the trials included used older chemotherapy regimens. A particular benefit was observed for the use of LHRH agonists after chemotherapy in women younger than age 40 in this meta-analysis, supporting the use of OFS in women less likely to develop CIA.[63] Based on the results of the older studies included in the EBCTCG and LHRH agonists in Early Breast Cancer Overview Group meta-analyses, the role for OFS or OA was unclear, and for many years, it was not routinely recommended as a component of adjuvant endocrine therapy.[30] However, four modern trials have begun to clarify the scenarios in which OFS or OA may improve outcomes (Fig. 54.4).

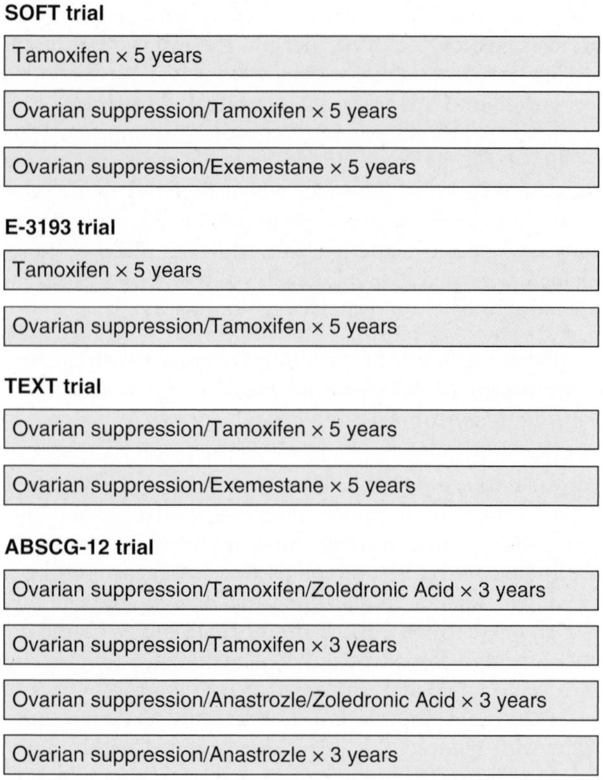

The phase III Suppression of Ovarian Function Trial (SOFT) randomized 3066 premenopausal women with early-stage invasive hormone receptor–positive breast cancer to one of three adjuvant hormonal therapy regimens, each given for 5 years: tamoxifen, tamoxifen plus ovarian suppression, or exemestane plus ovarian suppression. Ovarian suppression could be accomplished by triptorelin, oophorectomy, or ovarian irradiation. Women were stratified by whether they received prior chemotherapy, with documentation of an estradiol concentration in the premenopausal range within 8 months of completion of chemotherapy required for eligibility. The initial analytic plan was to assess DFS, the primary end point, across the three arms using three pairwise comparisons; however, the study enrolled an older and lower risk population than expected and recurrence rates were lower than anticipated, thus the primary analysis was modified to assess whether tamoxifen plus ovarian suppression was superior to tamoxifen alone. After a median follow-up of 67 months, 5-year DFS did not differ between tamoxifen and tamoxifen plus ovarian

SOFT trial

Tamoxifen × 5 years

Ovarian suppression/Tamoxifen × 5 years

Ovarian suppression/Exemestane × 5 years

E-3193 trial

Tamoxifen × 5 years

Ovarian suppression/Tamoxifen × 5 years

TEXT trial

Ovarian suppression/Tamoxifen × 5 years

Ovarian suppression/Exemestane × 5 years

ABSCG-12 trial

Ovarian suppression/Tamoxifen/Zoledronic Acid × 3 years

Ovarian suppression/Tamoxifen × 3 years

Ovarian suppression/Anastrozle/Zoledronic Acid × 3 years

Ovarian suppression/Anastrozle × 3 years

• **Fig. 54.4** Design of trials evaluating ovarian ablation or ovarian function suppression for the treatment of invasive early-stage hormone receptor-positive breast cancer. *ABCSG,* Austrian Breast and Colorectal Cancer Study Group; *E-3193,* Eastern Cooperative Oncology Group Trial; *SOFT,* Suppression of Ovarian Function Trial; *TEXT,* Tamoxifen and Exemestane Trial.

suppression (unadjusted hazard ratio 0.83, 95% confidence interval 0.66–1.04, $p = .10$) (Table 54.8). Notably, outcomes were excellent among the 949 participants who did not receive chemotherapy, with more than 95% of such women in each study arm free from breast cancer at 5 years. In contrast, outcomes were less favorable among the 1084 women who received chemotherapy, a group that was generally younger and more likely to have adverse clinicopathologic features. In this group, 5-year rates of freedom from breast cancer were lower with ovarian suppression, suggesting benefit from ovarian suppression in premenopausal women deemed to be at sufficient risk to warrant adjuvant chemotherapy and who remain premenopausal afterward (Table 54.9). In particular, ovarian suppression was associated with improved rates of freedom from breast cancer among women under age 35, 94% of whom received chemotherapy. In this subgroup, the rate of freedom from breast cancer at 5 years was 67.7% for tamoxifen alone, 78.9% for tamoxifen plus ovarian suppression and 83.4% for exemestane plus ovarian suppression. At this time, survival data from the SOFT trial are not mature, and it remains to be seen whether the differences in recurrence associated with ovarian suppression in the subgroups that benefited translate into a survival benefit.[64]

The Eastern Cooperative Oncology Group (ECOG) investigators have also conducted a trial evaluating the role of ovarian suppression in addition to tamoxifen. E-3193 was a randomized phase III trial comparing 5 years of tamoxifen to 5 years of tamoxifen plus ovarian suppression in a low-risk population of node-negative premenopausal women with hormone receptor-positive

TABLE 54.8   Disease-Free Survival by Arm for Primary Comparisons in Key Trials Evaluating Adjuvant Ovarian Suppression in Premenopausal Women With Hormone Receptor–Positive Invasive Early-Stage Breast Cancer

Trial, N		Tamoxifen	Tamoxifen/Ovarian Suppression	AI/Ovarian Suppression
SOFT[64] N = 3066		84.7%	86.6%	
TEXT/SOFT[66] N = 4690			87.3%[a]	91.1%[a]
E-3193[64] N = 345		87.9%	89.7%	
ABCSG-12[68] N = 1803	With zoledronic acid Without zoledronic acid		88.4% 85.6%	86.9% 83.4%

[a]Indicates statistically significant difference in DFS for comparison of treatment arms.
ABCSG, Austrian Breast and Colorectal Cancer Study Group; *AI*, aromatase inhibitor; *DFS*, disease-free survival; *E-3193*, Eastern Cooperative Oncology Group trial; *SOFT*, Suppression of Ovarian Function Trial; *TEXT*, Tamoxifen and Exemestane Trial.

TABLE 54.9   Five-Year Rates of Freedom From Breast Cancer Stratified by Receipt of Chemotherapy in the SOFT Trial[64]

Endocrine Therapy Arm	Chemotherapy N = 949	No Chemotherapy N = 2033
Tamoxifen	78%	95.8%
Ovarian suppression/ tamoxifen	82.5%	95.1%
Ovarian suppression/ exemestane	85.7%	97.1%

SOFT, Suppression of Ovarian Function Trial.

invasive breast cancer who did not receive chemotherapy. Ovarian suppression could be accomplished by LHRH analog, oophorectomy, or ovarian irradiation. Although the target enrolment was 1600, the trial closed early with only 345 participants due to poor accrual. After a median follow-up of 9.9 years, there was no difference in DFS and OS, the primary end points, between the two arms, a finding likely related to inadequate power and the low-risk population (see Table 54.8). However, the power was adequate for analysis of secondary end points that included patient-reported outcomes (PRO) regarding the effect of OFS on health-related QOL, menopausal symptoms, and sexual function, which are described subsequently.[65]

The Tamoxifen and Exemestane Trial (TEXT) randomized 2672 premenopausal women with hormone receptor–positive early-stage breast cancer to adjuvant OFS plus either tamoxifen or exemestane for 5 years. For the 60% of participants who received chemotherapy, OFS was initiated concurrently with chemotherapy. Women randomized to OFS were allowed to undergo permanent OA after at least 6 months of triptorelin. The initial plan was to compare DFS between the two arms of TEXT; however, as was the case with SOFT, the TEXT study population had lower risk features than anticipated, and the DFS rate was better than expected. The SOFT and TEXT protocols were amended designating a combined analysis of data from both trials as the primary analysis of ovarian suppression plus exemestane compared with

ovarian suppression plus tamoxifen. After a median follow-up of 68 months, the combined TEXT/SOFT analysis including data from 4690 participants revealed improved DFS in the exemestane arm (hazard ratio 0.72, 95% confidence interval 0.60–0.85, $p <$ .001) (see Table 54.8). Benefits of exemestane with ovarian suppression were observed regardless of receipt of chemotherapy, although the absolute risk reduction was greater in those who received chemotherapy. To date, no survival difference has been observed between the two arms, although survival data are not yet mature; however, the trend suggests ovarian suppression plus exemestane may be associated with inferior survival, an unexpected finding that requires confirmation and further follow-up (hazard ratio 1.14, 95% confidence interval 0.86–1.51, $p =$ .37).[66]

OFS with either tamoxifen or an AI was also compared in the ABCSG-12 trial, which randomized 1803 premenopausal women with hormone receptor–positive early-stage invasive breast in a two-by-two factorial disease to 3 years of goserelin with tamoxifen or anastrozole, with or without zoledronic acid. Adjuvant chemotherapy was not allowed, but 5% of the participants underwent neoadjuvant chemotherapy before enrolling.[67,68] Although benefit was observed for the addition of zoledronic acid, the final analysis with regard to endocrine therapy, with a median follow-up of 94.4 months, showed no difference in the primary end point, DFS, between the tamoxifen and anastrozole arms (hazard ratio 1.13, 95% confidence interval 0.88–1.45, $p =$ .335) (see Table 54.8). The reason these findings differ from those of the SOFT/TEXT analysis is not certain but may reflect the small sample size or the relatively low-risk population in the ABCSG-12 trial.[69] It is also possible that the 3-year regimens evaluated in this trial were insufficient and that a difference between the two arms would have been observed with longer therapy. It is doubtful that the difference in findings can be explained by differing efficacy between anastrozole and exemestane.[41] As was suggested in the combined SOFT/TEXT analysis, OS in the AI arm in the ABCSG-12 trial was inferior (hazard ratio for death 1.63, 95% confidence interval 1.05–2.52, $p =$ .03), a finding that requires confirmation.[68]

Selecting an Adjuvant Endocrine Therapy Regimen for Premenopausal Women With Early-Stage Invasive Hormone Receptor–Positive Breast Cancer

As is the case with postmenopausal women, selection of an adjuvant endocrine therapy regimen for premenopausal women with early-stage breast cancer is challenging. One must balance efficacy, risk of recurrence, and toxicity to select the optimal regimen for each patient. Unfortunately, validated biomarkers to identify which patients may benefit the most from each regimen are not currently available. However, evidence from the recent trials evaluating ovarian suppression can be used to guide clinical decisions. These trials demonstrate that although outcomes in premenopausal women with breast cancer are often considered to be unfavorable and adjuvant chemotherapy is often used in this population, properly selected premenopausal women without high-risk features can achieve favorable outcomes with adjuvant endocrine therapy alone.[64,66,68] In addition, the recent data suggest that OFS or OA is unlikely to be of significant benefit in low-risk patients whose disease characteristics do not warrant chemotherapy.[64] Thus a risk-stratified approach for the selection of patients in whom OFS or OA is offered makes sense, with consideration of this approach in those in whom chemotherapy is appropriate, those who are very young or those who have other high-risk features (Fig. 54.5). Such an approach has been recently endorsed in updated American Society of Clinical Oncology guidelines.[70]

Many unanswered questions remain regarding adjuvant endocrine therapy for premenopausal women. For women who receive OFS, the optimal duration is not yet certain, although 3 to 5 years is reasonable.[64,66,68] Furthermore, the optimal endocrine therapy backbone with which to pair ovarian suppression—tamoxifen or an AI—is not certain. Data from the combined SOFT/TEXT analysis suggest improved DFS with AI therapy, a finding that is consistent with studies evaluating AIs in the postmenopausal

setting.[39,43,66] In the ABCSG-12 trial, an advantage for AI therapy over tamoxifen in the setting of ovarian suppression was not observed. Moreover, the potential for a negative effect on survival with the use of an AI plus OFS or ovarian ablation has been raised.[66,68] The reason for a potential adverse survival effect with AI therapy in the setting of ovarian suppression is unclear, although it has been hypothesized that adjuvant AI therapy may predispose to resistance, making subsequent therapy more challenging.[68] It is hoped that further follow-up regarding survival data in the SOFT/TEXT combined will hopefully clarify this issue. At the present, it is not known how the 3- to 5-year regimens including ovarian suppression compare to 10 years of tamoxifen or to 5 years of tamoxifen followed by 5 years of an AI. The optimal time to initiate OFS, especially in women who receive adjuvant chemotherapy, is also uncertain. Additionally, it is not known whether OFS with a LHRH analog is equivalent to OA achieved by oophorectomy or irradiation. However, concern has been raised about possible inadequate suppression of ovarian function with LHRH analogs.[71] At this time, some consider evaluating estradiol concentrations serially in women receiving OFS,[32] although appropriate management in cases in which suppression is inadequate is not clear.

Fertility Considerations in Premenopausal Women With Early-Stage Invasive Breast Cancer Undergoing Adjuvant Endocrine Therapy

Chemotherapy is gonadotoxic and can result in amenorrhea, premature menopause, and infertility.[72] Adjuvant endocrine therapy itself does not impair fertility; however, fertility declines naturally

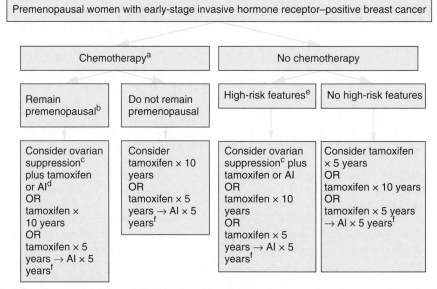

• **Fig. 54.5** Proposed risk-based algorithm to guide selection of premenopausal women with early-stage invasive hormone receptor–positive breast cancer for ovarian suppression or ablation.
[a]Receive chemotherapy or risk sufficient to recommend chemotherapy.
[b]Based on resumption of menses or estradiol level in premenopausal range.
[c]Ovarian suppression can be accomplished by luteinizing hormone releasing hormone analog, oophorectomy, or ovarian irradiation.
[d]Particular benefit noted for ovarian suppression among women younger than 35 in the Suppression of Ovarian Function Trial, 94% of whom received chemotherapy.[60]
[e]Established criteria to define high-risk features are not available. Reasonable considerations include young age, node positive, large tumor, high grade, lymphovascular invasion, and high recurrence score on 21-gene assay.
[f]AI monotherapy can only be considered in women who have become postmenopausal. *AI,* Aromatase inhibitor.

with age during the course of adjuvant endocrine therapy. Data suggest that pregnancy after breast cancer is not associated with higher risk of cancer recurrence,[73] but there are no current data to demonstrate safety of interruption of adjuvant endocrine therapy to achieve pregnancy. Providers must address fertility goals before initiating adjuvant endocrine treatment with the intent of incorporating these goals into treatment plans. In addition, ensuring premenopausal women who do not undergo ovarian suppression use reliable nonhormonal contraception to avoid pregnancy during adjuvant endocrine therapy is required,[74] especially as tamoxifen can induce ovulation. For women who intend to become pregnant after tamoxifen therapy, a washout period of 2 months is recommended.[75]

Timing of Initiation of Adjuvant Endocrine Therapy

For women who do not receive other adjuvant therapy, adjuvant endocrine therapy is typically initiated approximately 4 weeks after surgery. For women who receive adjuvant chemotherapy, adjuvant endocrine therapy is typically initiated after chemotherapy. Although findings have not been consistent, some data suggest a trend toward less favorable outcomes with concurrent administration of chemotherapy and endocrine therapy.[76] Endocrine therapy can be initiated concurrently with or after radiation therapy.[77]

Moving Beyond Hormone Receptor Status: Biomarkers to Guide Therapeutic Decisions in Women With Invasive Early-Stage Hormone Receptor–Positive Breast Cancer

Biomarkers can be prognostic and/or predictive. Prognostic factors provide information about outcomes independent of treatment whereas predictive factors suggest benefit from specific therapies. As discussed earlier, ER is the most important factor predictive of benefit from adjuvant endocrine therapy.[6] In addition, ER and PR provide prognostic information in women with early-stage invasive breast cancer with stronger hormone receptor positivity associated with more favorable outcomes.[78] Established clinical factors such as tumor size, lymph node status, grade, and age also provide prognostic information in women with hormone receptor–positive breast cancer.[32] Additional biomarkers, such as molecular profiles, have emerged in recent years. Key biomarkers and the setting(s) in which they may provide information relevant to the care of women with hormone receptor–positive invasive early-stage breast cancer are reviewed next.

Estimating the Risk of Recurrence in Women Treated With Adjuvant Endocrine Therapy

In clinical practice, it is useful to provide individualized assessment of the risk of recurrence to help guide decisions regarding adjuvant systemic therapy. Validated computer-based models such as Adjuvant! Online can be used to assess the risk of recurrence and mortality in women treated with various adjuvant therapy regimens, including endocrine therapy.[79,80] In addition, several molecular profiles provide prognostic information in women treated with adjuvant endocrine therapy for early-stage hormone

receptor–positive breast cancer.[81] The best validated at this time is the 21-gene Oncotype Dx Recurrence Score (RS), which categorizes hormone receptor–positive invasive early-stage breast cancers into low-, intermediate-, and high-risk groups. The RS estimates the risk of distant recurrence at 10 years with 5 years of adjuvant endocrine therapy and is predictive of benefit from adjuvant chemotherapy.[82–85] Recent data from the Trial Assigning Individualized Options for Treatment (TAILORx) prospectively confirmed excellent outcomes in node-negative individuals with very low RS treated with adjuvant endocrine therapy alone.[86] Trials evaluating the predictive ability of Mammaprint, a 70-gene profile, and of the RS in a node-positive population are ongoing.[81]

Determining the Duration of Therapy: Biomarkers for Late Recurrence

Hormone receptor–positive breast cancer can recur many years after diagnosis.[5,87,88] As noted earlier, extended adjuvant endocrine therapy reduces the risk of recurrence; however, such treatment may involve extended treatment-associated toxicities.[8,36,52,53] Ideally, a tool to identify individuals who are disease free after 5 years of adjuvant therapy, face high risk for late recurrence, and can benefit from extended adjuvant therapy would guide patient selection for extended therapy. To date, several tools have been developed that can identify individuals at risk for late relapse. For example, the breast cancer index (BCI) assay, a gene expression–based signature, identifies patients with hormone receptor–positive node-negative early-stage breast cancer at risk for both early (within 5 years) and late recurrence (>5 years).[89,90] Similarly, one of the implications of the PAM50 risk of recurrence (ROR) score, based on a 46-gene subset of the PAM50 genes plus tumor size, and of the EndoPredict gene expression signature is that both may identify patients at risk for late recurrence.[91,92] Recent data also suggest that higher ER mRNA expression on the Oncotype Dx test may be a prognostic factor to identify women at increased risk of late recurrence.[93] However, although prognostic, there are only limited data currently supporting the use of these biomarkers for predicting benefit of extended adjuvant endocrine therapy. Furthermore, given the ongoing risk of late recurrence and the carryover effect of adjuvant endocrine therapy, data regarding risks of recurrence beyond 10 years are required to better identify those at risk for late recurrence and those who may benefit from extended therapy.

Determining the Type of Endocrine Therapy: Biomarkers Suggestive of Benefit From Tamoxifen or Aromatase Inhibitor Therapy

Several clinicopathologic features may inform preferential benefit from tamoxifen or AI therapy in different scenarios. For example, improved outcomes were observed with letrozole compared with tamoxifen in women with invasive lobular carcinoma or with invasive ductal carcinoma characterized by high proliferative characteristics.[94] In contrast, some studies have suggested reduced efficacy of AI therapy in women with elevated body mass index (BMI), a finding with biological rationale based on levels of aromatase in peripheral fat.[95–99] Although thought-provoking, data are not yet sufficient to recommend using histology, degree of proliferation, or BMI to guide the decision of whether to prescribe tamoxifen or an AI.[59]

Tamoxifen is a prodrug, with its effects mediated primarily by its metabolites 4-hydroxy-tamoxifen and endoxifen. The degree of tamoxifen metabolism varies based on each individual's cytochrome P450 (CYP2D6) alleles. However, the degree of CYP2D6 metabolism in an individual has not been confirmed to predict benefit from tamoxifen, and CYP2D6 testing is not recommended.[32,100-102] Despite this, coprescription of tamoxifen and medications that inhibit CYP2D6 function should be avoided if possible. Commonly used medications in women with breast cancer that have CYP2D6 inhibitory activity include the antidepressants paroxetine, fluoxetine, and bupropion.[32,103]

Approaches to Adjuvant Endocrine Therapy for Ductal Carcinoma in Situ

The prognosis for women with DCIS is excellent, with minimal risk of distant metastases or mortality. However, women with DCIS are at risk for ipsilateral breast cancer recurrence after breast conservation and for contralateral new primary breast cancers and adjuvant endocrine therapy may prevent these outcomes. The results of key trials evaluating adjuvant endocrine therapy for DCIS are described subsequently (Fig. 54.6).[9,10,12,104]

The NSABP B-24 study investigators randomized 1799 women with DCIS who had undergone breast conserving surgery and radiation to either tamoxifen or placebo for 5 years. Compared with placebo, tamoxifen reduced the risk of invasive ipsilateral breast tumor recurrence (IBTR) by 32% (hazard ratio 0.68, 95% confidence interval 0.49–0.95, $p = .025$) and the rate of contralateral new breast cancers by 32% (hazard ratio 0.68, 95% confidence interval 0.48–0.95, $p = .023$). Tamoxifen also reduced the risk of recurrent DCIS in the ipsilateral breast, although this was not statistically significant (hazard ratio 0.84, 95% confidence interval 0.60–1.19, $p = .33$). Younger women, those who presented with a palpable abnormality, and those with positive surgical margins had higher risk of invasive and noninvasive ipsilateral

breast tumor recurrence, although the prognostic effect of positive margins was less among those who received tamoxifen. In addition, the presence of comedonecrosis was associated with high risk of recurrent ipsilateral DCIS. Notably, the risk of distant metastases in the absence of a prior invasive recurrence was low in both arms, and tamoxifen receipt did not influence mortality. However, mortality was increased among women who developed a subsequent invasive ipsilateral recurrence (hazard ratio 1.75, 95% confidence interval 1.45–2.96, $p < .001$).[10]

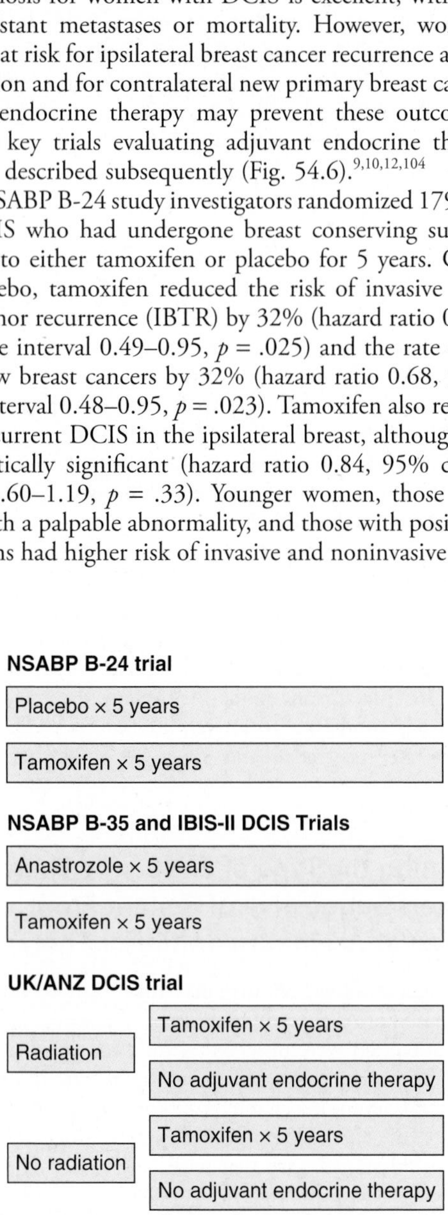

Of note, hormone receptor–positivity was not required for participation in B-24. Approximately 70% of DCIS cases are hormone receptor positive. Subsequent to the publication of B-24, the investigators assessed ER and PR on a subset of the study participants (N = 902) and determined that the benefits of tamoxifen were limited to the hormone receptor–positive group. Similar to findings in invasive breast cancer, the addition of PR to ER status did not add to prediction of benefit from adjuvant tamoxifen. Among the ER-positive group, tamoxifen was associated with a statistically significant reduction in the risk of any breast cancer event (hazard ratio 0.58, 95% confidence interval 0.415–0.81, $p = .0015$), any invasive breast cancer (hazard ratio 0.53, 95% confidence interval 0.34–0.82, $p = .005$) and any contralateral breast cancer (hazard ratio 0.5, 95% confidence interval 0.28–0.88, $p = .02$). Aside from tamoxifen, the only factor associated with breast cancer recurrence was age, with greater risk of recurrence in participants under 50 years at study entry.[11]

The UK/ANZ DCIS trial randomized 1694 women with DCIS who had undergone breast conserving surgery with negative margins to radiation, tamoxifen or both in a 2 × 2 factorial design. The majority of the study participants were 50 to 64 years old, with only a small fraction of younger women. Hormone receptor positivity was not required for eligibility. After a median follow-up of 12.7 years, tamoxifen reduced the 10-year risk of new breast events from 24.6% to 18.1% (hazard ratio 0.71, 95% confidence interval 0.58–0.88, $p = .002$). However, the ipsilateral benefit of tamoxifen was limited to reducing the risk of future DCIS (hazard ratio 0.70, 95% confidence interval 0.51–0.86, $p = .03$) because tamoxifen did not reduce the risk of future ipsilateral invasive breast cancer (hazard ratio 0.95, 95% confidence interval 0.66–1.38, $p = .79$). It is not clear why the UK/ANZ and B-24 findings differ with regard to the effect of tamoxifen on future ipsilateral invasive breast cancer, although it may be partly explained by the younger age distribution in the B-24 study compared with the UK/ANZ study. Overall, tamoxifen reduced the 10-year risk of future contralateral breast cancer events from 4.2% to 1.9% in the UK/ANZ study (hazard ratio 0.44, 95% confidence interval 0.25–0.77, $p = .005$), a similar degree of risk reduction as in the B-24 study. Tamoxifen did not influence mortality in the UK/ANZ trial.[12]

Adjuvant AI therapy has also been investigated for chemoprevention in postmenopausal hormone receptor–positive women with DCIS. Findings from the NSABP B-35 study, a phase III trial that randomized 3104 women to anastrozole or tamoxifen for 5 years after completion of breast conserving therapy, were recently presented. After a median follow-up of 6.8 years, anastrozole was associated with a 27% reduction in the risk of any future breast cancer event, with 93.5% of participants in the anastrozole arm and 89.2% of participants in the tamoxifen arm estimated to be free of breast cancer at 10 years. However, the benefits of anastrozole compared with tamoxifen were limited to women under age 60, and OS was excellent in both groups.[9] In

NSABP B-24 trial

Placebo × 5 years
Tamoxifen × 5 years

NSABP B-35 and IBIS-II DCIS Trials

Anastrozole × 5 years
Tamoxifen × 5 years

UK/ANZ DCIS trial

Radiation	Tamoxifen × 5 years
	No adjuvant endocrine therapy
No radiation	Tamoxifen × 5 years
	No adjuvant endocrine therapy

• **Fig. 54.6** Design of trials evaluating adjuvant endocrine therapy for ductal carcinoma in situ (DCIS). *IBIS*, International Breast Cancer Intervention Studies; *NSABP*, National Surgical Adjuvant Breast and Bowel Project; *UK/ANZ*, United Kingdom/Australia and New Zealand.

contrast, in the similarly designed International Breast Cancer Intervention Studies (IBIS)-II DCIS trial (n = 2980), anastrozole was noninferior to tamoxifen, but superiority of the AI was not demonstrated.[104] The explanation for the difference in findings between the NSABP B-35 and IBIS-II DCIS trials is not certain, although the lack of superiority of anastrozole in the IBIS-II DCIS trial may be due to inadequate power in the setting of low event rates.[104] Regardless, one can safely conclude that either tamoxifen or anastrozole is a reasonable option for postmenopausal women with ER-positive DCIS.

Common Side Effects of Adjuvant Endocrine Therapy

Although there is overlap, the side effects associated with the different types of endocrine therapy differ. Common side effects and approaches to management are discussed next.

Menopausal Symptoms

Hot flashes and sweats are reported in approximately 40% to 60% of women receiving AIs or tamoxifen, with studies suggesting more frequent hot flashes with tamoxifen.[40–42,45,48,51,53,105,106] The frequency of hot flashes appears to be similar with the different AI.[41] In premenopausal women, the addition of ovarian suppression to tamoxifen is associated with substantially more hot flashes and sweats; however, hot flashes are rarely severe.[64,65] Hot flashes are also common with ovarian suppression plus AI therapy, although less frequent than with ovarian suppression plus tamoxifen. Similarly, rates of sweats are higher with tamoxifen plus ovarian suppression than with AI plus ovarian suppression.[66,107] Hot flashes improve over time during the course of adjuvant ovarian suppression, although not to baseline.[64,66,107] Of note, data regarding rates and trends in hot flash severity over time are not available for extended tamoxifen therapy. Hot flashes are difficult to manage; pharmacologic agents, behavioral interventions, and acupuncture, among other approaches are used, with selective serotonin or reuptake inhibitors (SSRIs) or serotonin norepinephrine reuptake inhibitors (SNRIs) particularly effective.[108–110]

Vaginal dryness is also a commonly reported menopausal symptom during adjuvant endocrine therapy. Among postmenopausal participants of trials evaluating tamoxifen and AIs, vaginal dryness was reported more frequently with AI therapy.[48,104,106,111] Not surprisingly, ovarian suppression in premenopausal women is associated with high rates of vaginal dryness, and it is particularly common in those treated with concurrent AI therapy.[64,66,107] Tamoxifen is also associated with vaginal discharge in up to approximately 15% of women.[40,105,111] The first approach to managing vaginal dryness due to adjuvant endocrine therapy is often use of nonhormonal vaginal moisturizers and lubricants.[112,113] For women in whom this is unsuccessful, intravaginal estrogen may be considered, although there are concerns about systemic absorption and its potential effect on cancer recurrence, especially with concurrent AI therapy.[114,115]

Sexual Dysfunction

Loss of libido is reported by approximately 30% to 45% of women receiving adjuvant endocrine therapy. Among postmenopausal women, loss of libido is slightly more commonly associated with AI therapy than with tamoxifen therapy.[105,111] Not unexpectedly, the addition of ovarian suppression to tamoxifen therapy in premenopausal women is more strongly associated with loss of libido than tamoxifen alone.[64,65] Furthermore, paralleling the experience of postmenopausal women, loss of libido is more frequently experienced by premenopausal women receiving ovarian suppression plus AI therapy than by those receiving ovarian suppression plus tamoxifen therapy.[66,107] AI therapy is also associated with dyspareunia in 15% to 20% of postmenopausal women.[111] Similarly, exemestane in combination with ovarian suppression is associated with dyspareunia in approximately one third of premenopausal women.[66] Premenopausal women receiving exemestane plus ovarian suppression report more difficulty becoming sexually aroused than those receiving tamoxifen plus ovarian suppression.[107] Sexual functioning is worst in the first 2 years of adjuvant endocrine therapy and improves over time.[65]

Sexual dysfunction in women receiving adjuvant endocrine therapy is likely underidentified and undertreated. Inquiry into sexual health should be routine, and symptoms should be addressed.[113] Because vaginal dryness can contribute to sexual dysfunction, this should be managed as described earlier. Data also suggest that pelvic floor rehabilitation may help with sexual dysfunction and that topical lidocaine may alleviate dyspareunia.[113,116]

Uterine Disorders

In contrast to its antagonist effect on breast tissue, tamoxifen acts as an agonist to the ER in the endometrium, which can predispose to endometrial hyperplasia, endometrial atypia, and, rarely, endometrial cancer.[6,8,40,42,45,48,51,104,105] Studies evaluating tamoxifen and AIs in postmenopausal women have consistently demonstrated higher rates of postmenopausal vaginal bleeding among women treated with tamoxifen.[40,42,45,48,105] However, the incidence of endometrial cancer among women treated with up to 5 years of tamoxifen is only 1.2% at 10 years, approximately three times the incidence in women treated with AIs.[7,40] The risk of endometrial cancer is 74% higher in women treated with 10 years of tamoxifen compared with women treated with 5 years of tamoxifen, although the absolute risks remain small.[8,36] Studies have consistently demonstrated that the risk of endometrial cancer associated with tamoxifen increases with age, with virtually no risk before age 45.[6–8,36] Notably, the risk of death due to endometrial cancer in women treated with adjuvant endocrine therapy is extremely low.[8,36,40] Screening for uterine cancer in women receiving tamoxifen is not recommended, but prompt evaluation of abnormal vaginal symptoms is required.[117]

Thromboembolism

Tamoxifen is associated with a small risk of thromboembolism. However, reported rates rarely exceed 3%, and this risk is primarily limited to women older than 55 years.[6,40,42,45,48,49,64,66,104] The risk of mortality due to pulmonary embolism is only 0.2% even with 10 years of tamoxifen therapy.[8]

Cardiovascular Disorders

Initial studies suggested a negative effect of AI therapy on cardiovascular health, but this has not been confirmed. Overall, tamoxifen appears to have a favorable effect on lipid profiles, whereas AI therapy appears to have a neutral or negative effect.[118,42,45,119] Some studies have reported a higher incidence of myocardial infarction, heart failure, or other cardiac events in women receiving an AI compared with tamoxifen monotherapy, but others have not. Overall, a longer duration of AI therapy is associated with higher odds of cardiovascular disease.[38,42,45,48,53,120] A meta-analysis of seven randomized trials suggested a 34% higher risk of cardiac events in trials of third-generation AIs compared with tamoxifen; however, the absolute increase in risk was only 0.57%, and the number needed to harm was more than 180.[121] Despite these findings, the risk of death due to cardiovascular cause does not appear to be higher with AI therapy than tamoxifen therapy in postmenopausal women.[53]

Some studies have also suggested slightly higher rates of hypertension in postmenopausal women in association with AI therapy compared with tamoxifen.[45,48,104] Among premenopausal women, ovarian suppression is associated with hypertension in up to 23% of women.[64] Reported rates of stroke and transient ischemic attack in association with adjuvant endocrine therapy are low, although some studies suggest a slight increase with tamoxifen.[6,40]

Mood Disturbances

Mood disturbances are common in women receiving endocrine therapy for early-stage breast cancer. Approximately 10% to 20% of postmenopausal women treated in trials evaluating AIs and tamoxifen experienced depression, with no significant difference in the likelihood of depression according to endocrine therapy type.[40,45,48] Depression is even more frequent in premenopausal women undergoing adjuvant endocrine therapy, with approximately half of the participants in the SOFT and TEXT trials reporting depression, although depression was typically of low grade.[64,66] Given the frequency of depression, providers must screen patients and initiate therapy as appropriate.[113] Standard treatments may be used, although antidepressants that are strong inhibitors of CYP2D6 should be avoided in patients receiving tamoxifen.[32,103]

Bone and Joint Pain

Approximately one-third of postmenopausal women treated with AIs experience arthralgias or myalgias which are usually described as symmetric stiffness or achiness.[40,42,48,51] Tamoxifen is also associated with bone and joint pain although less frequently.[40,45,104,106] Musculoskeletal symptoms are particularly common among premenopausal women receiving ovarian suppression.[64,66,107]

The mechanism behind arthralgias associated with endocrine therapy is uncertain. Often women who do not tolerate one AI due to joint pain can rotate to another with better tolerance.[122,123] The optimal approach to managing AI-associated arthralgias is uncertain, and multiple approaches have been tried including analgesics, antiinflammatory agents, exercise, and vitamin D repletion, among others.[123,124] Up to approximately 20% of women discontinue AI therapy due to muscle and joint pain.[125]

Loss of Bone Mineral Density, Osteoporosis, and Fractures

AI therapy in postmenopausal women is associated with a rapid loss of bone mineral density (BMD) within the first 6 to 12 months of treatment.[126–128] However, this stabilizes and tends to improve after completion of therapy.[127,129] There is no difference in the degree of loss of BMD between the steroidal and nonsteroidal AI.[130] Despite the loss of BMD, osteoporosis is only reported in 5% to 10% of postmenopausal women in trials evaluating AIs and tamoxifen therapy.[45,48,53] Importantly, women who initiate adjuvant AI therapy with normal BMD are unlikely to develop osteoporosis during treatment.[126,127]

Premenopausal women undergoing adjuvant endocrine therapy also face a substantial risk of osteoporosis. Although protective against loss of BMD in postmenopausal women, approximately 10% of premenopausal women treated with tamoxifen monotherapy develop osteoporosis.[64] The addition of ovarian suppression to tamoxifen is associated with osteoporosis in almost one-quarter of premenopausal women, and almost 40% of those treated with ovarian suppression plus an AI develop osteoporosis.[64,66]

The frequency of fracture in association with adjuvant endocrine therapy is difficult to measure and reported rates have varied across trials. Overall, AI therapy is more strongly associated with fracture than tamoxifen with the absolute increase in fracture risk with AI therapy greatest in older women.[7,38,42,45,48,51,53,66,126] The increase in fracture risk associated with AI therapy resolves after completion of therapy.[38,127]

Management of osteopenia and osteoporosis in women receiving adjuvant endocrine therapy is an area of controversy. Guidelines recommend monitoring with dual energy x-ray absorptiometry scans during therapy, although it is not clear that T-scores are the best predictor for fractures[131,132] Women should be assessed for other fracture risk factors such as tobacco use, low BMI, personal or family history of fragility fracture, and/or steroid use.[132] Bisphosphonates and denosumab can improve BMD in women receiving adjuvant endocrine therapy, although to date, only denosumab has been associated with a reduction in fractures.[131,133] Intriguing data also suggest that bone-targeted therapies may be associated with improved breast cancer outcomes in postmenopausal women receiving adjuvant endocrine therapy.[131] At this time, clear criteria for selection of individuals in whom bisphosphonates or denosumab should be considered for the purposes of improving bone health and for the identification of individuals in whom avoiding AI therapy due to concerns about BMD should be considered are not certain.

Quality of Life

Despite the many side effects, women taking adjuvant endocrine therapy enjoy relatively good QOL. However, data are conflicting regarding whether QOL declines during adjuvant endocrine therapy.[105,107] Overall, QOL appears to be similar for women treated with AIs and tamoxifen, even among premenopausal women concurrently receiving ovarian suppression, although specific side effects differ.[55,104–107,111] Whether ovarian suppression is associated with a decline in QOL is controversial; however, any decline in QOL improves with time.[65]

Adherence to Adjuvant Endocrine Therapy

Despite the substantial benefits associated with adjuvant endocrine therapy, rates of discontinuation and nonadherence are high, with women younger than 40 most likely to discontinue therapy.[134] Unfortunately, early discontinuation and nonadherence to adjuvant endocrine therapy are associated with a higher risk of mortality.[135]

Conclusion

Treatment options for adjuvant endocrine therapy have rapidly expanded since the early 2000s. This growing menu of options has improved outcomes compared with the historical standard of 5 years of tamoxifen monotherapy. However, selection of the optimal therapy for each individual patient has become increasing complex. Patients and providers must carefully weigh the underlying risk of cancer recurrence, the expected benefit from the adjuvant endocrine regimen(s) under consideration and the expected therapeutic toxicities all within the context of underlying health conditions and individual preferences. The future promises to bring further evolution as results from ongoing trials evaluating biomarkers and the combination of endocrine therapy and targeted therapies become available with the aims of improving outcomes, better identifying candidates for specific therapies, and overcoming endocrine resistance.[25,26,81]

Selected References

5. Effects of chemotherapy and hormonal therapy for early breast cancer on recurrence and 15-year survival: an overview of the randomised trials. *Lancet.* 2005;365:1687-1717.
6. Davies C, Godwin J, Gray R, et al. Relevance of breast cancer hormone receptors and other factors to the efficacy of adjuvant tamoxifen: patient-level meta-analysis of randomised trials. *Lancet.* 2011;378:771-784.
7. Dowsett M, Forbes JF, Bradley R, et al. Aromatase inhibitors versus tamoxifen in early breast cancer: patient-level meta-analysis of the randomised trials. *Lancet.* 2015;386:1341-1352.
70. Burstein HJ, Lacchetti C, Anderson H, et al. Adjuvant endocrine therapy for women with hormone receptor-positive breast cancer: American Society of Clinical Oncology Clinical Practice Guideline Update on Ovarian Suppression. *J Clin Oncol.* 2016;34: 1689-1701.
99. Dowsett M, Cuzick J, Ingle J, et al. Meta-analysis of breast cancer outcomes in adjuvant trials of aromatase inhibitors versus tamoxifen. *J Clin Oncol.* 2010;28:509-518.

A full reference list is available online at ExpertConsult.com.

55

Adjuvant and Neoadjuvant Systemic Therapies for Early-Stage Breast Cancer

CESAR A. SANTA-MARIA AND WILLIAM J. GRADISHAR

Although surgery is the cornerstone therapy for early-stage breast cancer, adjuvant systemic therapy can improve relapse rates through eradication of micrometastatic disease. First reported in the 1970s, adjuvant chemotherapy for breast cancer can decrease the risk of distant metastasis and improve survival of patients initially diagnosed with early-stage disease.[1] Although initial adjuvant studies included only the use of nontargeted cytotoxic chemotherapy, a deeper understanding of breast cancer biology has led to several agents designed to target specific molecular aberrancies. The identification of the estrogen receptor (ER) and human epidermal growth factor receptor 2-neu (HER2), mechanistic understanding, and subsequent translational investigation has been one of the most important advances in all of oncology, ushering in the targeted era of cancer therapy.

The journey of optimizing systemic adjuvant therapy has been dynamic, challenging traditional theorems of oncology, with successes and failures along the way, and further research is still needed. The "more is better" approach to cancer therapy that dominated oncologic strategies since the 1960s and 1970s has been investigated in the development of adjuvant strategies, yet although this led to the incorporation of highly effective cytotoxic therapy such as anthracyclines and taxanes into modern regimens, it also led to the use of highly toxic approaches including bone marrow transplantation that were not beneficial. Lessons derived from these early studies have helped form novel research approaches using more specific populations, powerful biomarkers, and targeted therapies.

Guidance in a Changing Landscape: St. Gallen and the National Comprehensive Cancer Network

Adjuvant and neoadjuvant therapies are constantly changing as new research leads to more potent strategies. The most recognized set of guidelines that influence physicians all around the world comes from the National Comprehensive Cancer Network (NCCN).[2] A total of 26 experts from centers in the United States publish guidelines every year based on data from clinical trials. These treatment guidelines provide guidance for the management of the different subtypes and stages of breast cancers based on currently available research, which can help physicians formulate treatment recommendations.

Every few years, experts in the field of oncology gather in St. Gallen, Switzerland, and provide guidelines based on available evidence for the therapy of early-stage breast cancer. In the most recent publication, stemming from the 2013 St. Gallen conference, experts identified key areas where research is needed such as in patients with aggressive phenotype ER-positive breast cancers or those that lack ER and HER2, the so-called triple-negative breast cancers (TNBC).[3] Duration and role of combination targeted therapies were also discussed, as well as recommended follow-up for patients with early-stage breast cancer.

Biology Defining Therapy: Breast Cancer Subtypes

Breast cancer is a heterogeneous disease comprising of several molecular subtypes, which are commonly extrapolated into clinical subtypes based on receptor status such as the ER or HER2.[4,5] Subtypes of breast cancer can be defined using gene expression microarrays, which cluster analysis can identify as basal-like, Erb-B2-positive, normal breast–like, and luminal epithelial categories. Luminal subtypes are most commonly associated with the ER and progesterone receptor (PR) for which hormonal therapies are an integral component of adjuvant therapy; however, not all ER-positive tumors respond well to hormone therapy.[6] Molecularly, luminal subtypes can be categorized as luminal A or B, and phenotypically behave as distinct entities. In this regard, Luminal B tumors tend to have higher histologic grade, ki67, and an increased risk of relapse compared with luminal A tumors.[7,8] Clinical considerations with more aggressive phenotype ER-positive disease include the incorporation of cytotoxic chemotherapy, and hormone therapies are typically used as well; more research is needed to develop more effective therapies for this subtype. The Erb-B2-positive subtype correlates most closely with HER2 positive tumors. HER2 was first described in the 1980s and can be found to be overexpressed in 25% to 30% of breast cancers. Although historically HER2 was a marker that predicted inferior outcomes, the development of anti-HER2 agents has made this subtype among the most treatable and prognosis has significantly improved.[9,10] Patients with TNBC most commonly correlate with basal subtypes. These cancers tend to have aggressive pathologic features, and treatment is typically limited to cytotoxic agents.[11]

Adjuvant Chemotherapy

Cytotoxic chemotherapy agents were the first adjuvant drugs developed for patients with early-stage breast cancers. They remain an important therapy for all subtypes of breast cancer; however, in HER2-positive subtypes, the addition of anti-HER2 therapies to chemotherapy is a critical component of treatment; this is described later in the chapter. Patients with ER-positive disease may benefit from adjuvant chemotherapy, although numerous factors are considered when deciding chemotherapy, these are discussed later in this chapter as well. For patients with TNBC adjuvant chemotherapy is of particular importance, as these tumors tend to have a higher risk of recurrence, and cytotoxic chemotherapy is currently the only systemic adjuvant option these patients have.

First-Generation Regimens

Nitrogen mustards and antifolates were found to have anticancer effects during the mid-twentieth century, paving the way for powerful combination regimens in numerous disease settings.[12,13] In 1976 the first successful adjuvant regimen for early-stage breast cancer was published, demonstrating that treatment with cyclophosphamide, methotrexate, and 5-fluorouracil (CMF) after surgery in patients with lymph node–positive disease could improve long-term survival.[1] The CMF regimen would serve as a gold standard to which other adjuvant regimens would be added or compared with for decades to come.

Introduction of Anthracyclines

Anthracyclines were developed as an anticancer antibiotic derived from *Streptomyces* bacterium that have several mechanisms of action, including intercalation of DNA and RNA inhibiting synthesis, and inhibition of topoisomerase II, which interferes with DNA supercoiling and relaxation.[14] Initially found to be active against pediatric malignancies, anthracyclines were first tested in breast cancer in the metastatic setting where they were found to have anticancer activity.[15] The National Surgical Adjuvant Breast and Bowel Project (NSABP) B-15 and B-16 studies investigated the regimen of adriamycin and cyclophosphamide (AC) in node-positive breast cancer and found that it was equivalent to CMF but better tolerated.[16,17] A large meta-analysis by the Early Breast Cancer Trialists' Collaborative Group (EBCTCG) confirmed that four doses of AC was at least equivalent to CMF (relative risk [RR] 0.98, standard error [SE] 0.05, $2p = .67$).[18]

In efforts to improve the CMF regimen, methotrexate was substituted for an anthracycline, leading to the development of the 5-fluorouracil, adriamycin, and cyclophosphamide (FAC) and 5-fluorouracil, epirubicin, cyclophosphamide (FEC) regimens. The Grupo Español de Investigación en Cancer de Mama (GEICAM; Spanish Breast Cancer Research Group) compared FAC with CMF and found that in node-negative disease 5-year disease-free survival (DFS) was 75% versus 67% favoring FAC ($p = .0378$).[19] The National Cancer Institute of Canada Clinical Trials Group (NCIC CTG) similarly performed a comparison of FEC versus CMF and found that 5-year relapse-free survival (RFS) rates were 63% compared with 53%, favoring FEC ($p = .009$) with an overall survival (OS) advantage as well (77% vs. 70%, $p = .03$, chemotherapy, respectively).[20] The importance of anthracyclines in the adjuvant setting was also highlighted in the National Epirubicin Adjuvant Trial (NEAT) and the BR9601 trial

by the Scottish Cancer Trials Breast Group (SCTBG). In these studies, patients with early-stage breast cancer were randomized to epirubicin or no-epirubicin before CMF, and both 5-year RFS and OS were improved in the epirubicin group (76% vs. 69%, and 82% vs. 75%, $p < .001$ for all comparisons, respectively).[21] The aforementioned meta-analysis by the EBCTCG also found that patients receiving anthracycline doses greater than four cycles of AC (i.e., FEC or FAC) had breast cancer mortality rates superior to CMF (RR = 0.78, SE 0.06, $2p = .0004$).[18]

Addition of Taxanes to Anthracycline-Based Chemotherapy

Derived from plants of the genus *Taxus,* taxanes are a class of anticancer drugs developed in the 1970s that work by disrupting microtubule function.[22] Paclitaxel and docetaxel were initially evaluated in metastatic breast cancer and found to be an effective option for anthracycline-resistant patients.[23,24] Based on their activity in the metastatic setting, numerous studies have been conducted to assess the efficacy of adding taxanes to adjuvant.

The addition of paclitaxel to AC was evaluated in the Cancer and Leukemia Group B (CALGB) 9344 trial.[25] In this trial, 3121 patients with axillary node-positive breast cancer were initially randomized to compared three doses of adriamycin (60 mg/m², 75 mg/m², and 90 mg/m²) as part of the standard AC regimen and then randomized to four cycles of paclitaxel (175 mg/m² every 3 weeks) versus no further therapy. There was no difference in outcome based on the different AC regimens, but there was a significant improvement both in RFS (hazard ratio [HR] 0.83, $p = .0023$) and in OS (HR 0.82, $p = .0064$) with the addition of paclitaxel.

A weekly schedule of paclitaxel was investigated in the GEICAM 9906 study, which included a total of 1248 patients with axillary node–positive early-stage breast cancer.[2] Patients were randomized into one of two treatment arms: (1) FEC90 (5-fluorouracil 600 mg/m², epirubicin 90 mg/m², cyclophosphamide 600 mg/m²) every 3 weeks for a total of six cycles, (2) or FEC90 every 3 weeks for four cycles followed by paclitaxel 100 mg/m² every week for eight cycles. After a median of 46 months, there was a significant difference in DFS (85% vs. 79%, HR 0.63, $p = .0008$) in favor of the taxane arm; however, there was no significant difference in OS (95% vs. 92%, HR 0.74, $p = .137$).

A similar benefit was seen when adding docetaxel to anthracycline-based therapy. In the Protocole Adjuvant dans le Cancer du Sein (PACS; French Adjuvant Study Group) 01 trial, 1999 women with node-positive breast cancer were randomized to receive six cycles of FEC100 (5-fluorouracil 500 mg/m², epirubicin 100 mg/m², cyclophosphamide 500 mg/m²) or three cycles of FEC100 followed by three cycles of docetaxel 100 mg/m².[26] At 5 years, DFS was 78% in the taxane-containing arm compared with 73% in the nontaxane arm (HR 0.82, $p = .012$), and OS also significantly favored the taxane-containing arm (91% vs. 87%, HR 0.73, $p = .017$).

The Eastern Cooperative Oncology Group (ECOG) E1199 trial was a four-arm study designed to assess whether docetaxel was better than paclitaxel and whether weekly versus every-3-week administration was better.[27] AC was administered initially for four cycles every 3 weeks. Subsequently patients were randomized to one of four arms: (1) paclitaxel 175 mg/m² every 3 weeks for four cycles (control group); (2) paclitaxel 80 mg/m² every week for 12 doses; (3) docetaxel 100 mg/m² every 3 weeks for four cycles; and

(4) docetaxel 35 mg/m^2 every week for 12 doses. The odds ratio (OR) for DFS was 1.27 (95% confidence interval [CI] 1.03–1.57) in the weekly paclitaxel arm (p = .006) and 1.23 (95% CI 1.00–1.52) in the every-3-week docetaxel arm (p = .02) compared with the control group; however, only the weekly paclitaxel group had an OS benefit (OR = 1.32, 95% CI 1.02–1.72, p = .01). Exploratory analysis demonstrated that benefit was seen primarily in HER2-negative patients irrespective of ER status.

In contrast, retrospective studies suggest that patients with ER-positive disease are likely to derive lesser benefit from taxanes. A retrospective analysis in a subgroup of patients who participated in the Intergroup 9344 trial found that patients with HER2-positive tumors benefited from paclitaxel regardless of their hormone receptor status. However, in HER2-negative patients, paclitaxel only benefited the hormone receptor–negative patients.[28] Furthermore, data from the CALGB analyzed retrospectively showed that chemotherapy was of little or no benefit in lymph node–positive and hormone receptor–positive patients.[29]

A meta-analysis of 13 trials including 22,903 patients identified was performed to assess survival benefits of the addition of a taxane to an anthracycline-containing regimen.[30] The pooled analysis demonstrated improved DFS (HR 0.83, 95% CI 0.79–0.87, p < .00001) and OS (HR 0.85, 95% CI 0.79–0.91, p < .00001) with the addition of taxanes, with an absolute improvement of 5% in DFS and 3% in OS. The investigators also found that the benefit from taxanes was significant for both ER-positive and ER-negative patients and was independent of whether paclitaxel or docetaxel was used. There was no benefit seen whether taxanes were given concurrently with anthracyclines or sequentially.

In summary, addition of taxanes after anthracycline-based therapy can improve survival in patients with early-stage breast cancer, particularly those with high-risk features such as lymph node involvement. Most data suggest that benefit independent of ER status and that weekly paclitaxel is the most effective taxane regimen.

Dose Density

Chemotherapy works by first-order kinetics (half -life), meaning that a chemotherapy drug will kill a constant proportion of tumor cells, rather than constant numbers.[31] Human cancer cells grow by nonexponential Gompertzian kinetics, which means tumors have an initial rapid growth curve which levels off as they outgrow nutrients and blood supply. Because cells are more sensitive to chemotherapy during the rapid growth phase, more frequent (dose-dense) administration of cytotoxic agents rather than increased doses was hypothesized to kill more cancer cells.[32]

To test this hypothesis, the CALGB performed a study of 2005 women with axillary node–positive breast cancer who were randomly assigned to receive one of the following regimens: (1) sequential doxorubicin, paclitaxel, and cyclophosphamide administered every 3 weeks; (2) the same sequence administered every 2 weeks with filgrastim; (3) AC followed by paclitaxel administered every 3 weeks; or (4) AC followed by paclitaxel administered every 2 weeks with filgrastim.[33] At a median follow-up of 36 months, there was a statistically significant improvement on DFS for the dose-dense regimens (every 2 weeks) compared with the every 3-week regimen (4-year DFS 82% vs. 75%, respectively, RR = 0.74, p = .01). OS was also improved in the dose-dense arms but did not reach statistical significance (3-year OS 92% vs. 90%, respectively, RR = 0.69, p = .013). There was no difference

between sequential and concurrent arms. Notably, both ER-positive and ER-negative patients benefited from dose density, but this was particularly noted in the ER-negative subgroup (19% vs. 32% in ER-positive vs. ER-negative group, respectively, in terms of relative reduction in hazard). Toxicity was comparably between arms, although severe neutropenia was less frequent in patients who received the dose-dense regimens.

To confirm findings, a meta-analysis assessing dose density was performed.[34] Patients treated with dose-dense regimens had better DFS (HR = 0.83, 95% CI 0.73–0.94, p = .005) and OS (HR = 0.84, 95% CI 0.72–0.98, p = .03). Benefit was only seen in ER-negative (HR = 0.71, 95% CI 0.56–0.89) and not ER-positive disease (HR = 0.92, 95% CI 0.75–1.12). Again, dose density was not associated with an increase in treatment related events.

Although dose density has been accepted as a standard of care in patients with TNBC, controversy still exists in ER-positive disease. This likely stems from the biological fact that most ER-positive tumors tend to be more indolent in nature (i.e., luminal A–like); however, special consideration should be made when treating patients with aggressive phenotype ER-positive disease because these tend to be more chemoresponsive (i.e., luminal B–like).[6]

Non–Anthracycline-Containing Regimens

Anthracyclines can have potent anticancer effects, but they can have significant long-term toxicity. A dreaded consequence of use of adjuvant anthracyclines for breast cancer is the risk of bone marrow neoplasms. The overall rate of marrow neoplasms has been found to be as high as 0.46 per 1000 person-years in patients treated with adjuvant chemotherapy.[35] Anthracyclines are also associated with cardiotoxicity, which can be acute or chronic. Acute cardiotoxicity is rare, reported in approximately 3.2% of patients treated with anthracyclines, and may include arrhythmias, acute congestive heart failure, myocarditis, and myocardial infarction.[36] Chronic cardiotoxicity can occur subclinically (OR = 6.25, 95% CI 2.58–15.13) or be clinically significant (OR = 5.43, 95% CI 2.34–12.62) most frequently manifesting as an irreversible heart failure.[37] To test whether nonanthracycline regimens could be as effective as anthracycline-based regimens US Oncology performed an adjuvant trial in women with stage I to III breast cancer patients who were randomized to either doxorubicin at 60 mg/m^2 and cyclophosphamide at 600 mg/m^2 given every 3 weeks for four cycles (AC) and docetaxel at 75 mg/m^2 and cyclophosphamide at 600 mg/m^2 given every 3 weeks for four cycles (TC). With a median follow-up of 7 years, the DFS rate was significantly superior for TC compared with AC (81% vs. 75%, respectively; HR = 0.74; 95% CI 0.56–0.98, p = .033), and OS were the same (87% vs. 82%, respectively; HR = 0.69, 95% CI 0.50–0.97, p = .032).[38] Both regimens were well tolerated, with TC having a higher incidence of febrile neutropenia and AC having three long-term fatal toxicities (one patient with heart failure and two with marrow events). From the results of this trial, TC emerges as a valuable regimen in the adjuvant treatment of breast cancer and may replace AC as a "standard of care" for women who are not considered eligible or appropriate for a combination of an anthracycline and taxane. For high-risk disease in which patients are eligible for anthracycline-based therapy, combination anthracycline and taxane-based therapy is preferred. Currently, a phase III study is comparing TC with combination anthracycline and taxane-based therapy (clinicaltrials.gov identifier NCT00493870).

Bone Marrow Transplant

The rationale behind the use of high-dose chemotherapy (HDC) necessitating stem cell support is based on the fact that because some chemotherapy could kill some cancer cells, more chemotherapy should kill more cancer cells and thus increase the cure rate. The dose-limiting event of chemotherapy was thought to be myelotoxicity; therefore harvesting the bone marrow before treatment with HDC and reinfusing it after treatment is complete was thought to allow for safe administration of HDC. Investigation of this strategy, however, was impaired by the political and social climate of the times as well as one of the largest scandals in medical research history, resulting in the needless overtreatment of thousands of patients with breast cancer and delays in obtaining definitive data.

In the early 1980s the identification of human immunodeficiency virus (HIV) and acquired immunodeficiency syndrome (AIDS) spurred the development of anti-HIV medications and put into question the ethics of drug development when there are patients with serious or life-threatening diseases. This led the US Food and Drug Administration (FDA) to develop measures of providing such patients new treatments as early as possible. Breast cancer advocates had likewise formed powerful groups and were at the forefront of these issues.[39] Despite a review of HDC with autologous stem cell transplant (ASCT) in breast cancer published in 1992, which stated that although responses were impressive, there were insufficient data to conclude whether this was superior to or worse than conventional dose chemotherapy, this procedure became increasingly popular outside of clinical trials.[40] Furthermore, at the 1992 American Society of Clinical Oncology (ASCO) Annual Meeting, a randomized control trial from South Africa was presented demonstrating significant response rates and improvements in survival.[41] These circumstances delayed accrual of patients to definitive phase III studies. It was not until the 1999 ASCO Annual Meeting that studies demonstrating that HDC with ASCT offered no benefit compared with standard adjuvant regimens were finally presented. The Philadelphia Bone Marrow Transplant Group found that bone marrow transplant did not improve survival in patients with metastatic breast cancer.[42] Furthermore, results from the CALBG 9082, Southwestern Oncology Group (SWOG) 9114, and NCIC MA-13 studies did not demonstrate a benefit in high-risk early-stage breast cancer.[43] In addition, the highly publicized research misconduct found after an audit in the trials presented by the South African group at the 1992 ASCO meeting demonstrated why there had been discordant results. Thus after almost 2 decades and thousands of women being needlessly transplanted, this practice finally came to an end.

Despite the harm and controversy surrounding HDC with bone marrow transplantation, there are valuable lessons to be learned. The most important is the crucial importance of level of evidence when prescribing a therapy; evidence-based medicine is a standard of care in all of medicine, and especially in oncology. Exposure to toxic medications in the absence of known benefit should be considered with extreme caution and preference given to enrollment into clinical trials. In addition, although mechanisms to grant early approval of promising medications are important, there must be a strategy to complete definitive studies. A case in point is the antivascular endothelial growth factor receptor (VEGF) inhibitor, bevacizumab, in metastatic breast cancer. Although initial early-phase studies showed promise, which led to accelerated approval, the definitive studies were able to be conducted, and when results showed no benefit, approval was repealed.[44]

ER-Positive Disease

Hormone receptor–positive breast cancers use estrogen to develop and grow. Antiestrogen therapies were the first targeted therapy developed in any cancer, but not all breast cancers responded to these treatments.[45] It was not until the development of a powerful predictive biomarker, the ER, that studies could be designed testing optimal treatment strategy in the adjuvant setting.[46] Despite the importance of antiendocrine therapy, however, some patients benefit from additional systemic therapy with cytotoxic chemotherapy. Identifying who is likely to benefit from chemotherapy is a crucial decision to make in patients with early-stage ER-positive disease.

Considering Chemotherapy

As previously discussed, chemotherapy works best on cells that are rapidly dividing rather than those that have a slower growth curve. This basic biological principle helps guide the benefits patients may, or may not, derive from chemotherapy. Standard pathologic examination can frequently lend clues. Patients with more aggressive appearing tumors (i.e., high grade) or that have high proliferation indices (high ki67) generally tend to respond better to chemotherapy than those that are low grade with low ki67.[8] Numerous gene expression assays have been developed and studied to help both define clinical behavior and benefit from adjuvant chemotherapy.

Genomic Profiling for Risk Stratification

The Predictor Analysis of Microarray 50 (PAM50) assay is a 50-gene test designed to characterize the intrinsic subtype of a tumor and can help distinguish between luminal A– and B–like tumors.[47] It is performed using quantitative reverse-transcriptase polymerase chain reaction (RT-PCR) on a formalin-fixed paraffin-embedded (FFPE) tissue sample, and a risk of recurrence (ROR) score is generated that stratifies patients into a low, medium, or high score is also computed. This has been validated retrospectively in the Adjuvant Tamoxifen or Anastrozole (ATAC) trial and in the Austrian Breast Cancer Study Group (ABCSG)-8 trial, where ROR scores could identify those at higher risk of recurrence.[48,49]

The Onco*type* DX test is the most validated genomic assay to prognosticate patients with ER-positive disease and help guide the decision to recommend chemotherapy. After RNA extraction from FFPE tissue, primers and probes for 21 specific genes are used to quantitate RNA expression by RT-PCR. The expression of each gene is measured in triplicate and then normalized relative to a set of five reference genes (*ACT* [the gene encoding β-actin], *GAPDH, GUS, RPLPO,* and *TFRC*). A recurrence score (RS) is then calculated, giving a score from 0 to 100. The initial validation studies were performed on patients with node-negative, ER-positive breast cancer in the NSABP B-20 study where patients were randomized to tamoxifen versus tamoxifen with CMF.[50] Of the 2363 patients enrolled, 651 were assessed based on tissue availability (227 treated with tamoxifen, and 424 treated with tamoxifen plus chemotherapy). In this retrospective study, patients with a recurrence score of 31 or greater had a significant benefit from chemotherapy (RR = 0.26, 95% CI 0.13–0.53) compared with patients with a RS less than 18 who did not benefit from chemotherapy (RR = 1.31, 95% CI 0.46–3.78). The Trial Assigning Individualized Options for Treatment (TAILORx) study was designed to prospectively validate the RS in women with hormone receptor–positive node-negative breast cancer. Patients with a score from 0 to 10 were assigned to receive endocrine therapy, and patients with a score of 26 or higher were assigned to receive chemotherapy in addition to endocrine therapy. Those with intermediate scores (11–25) were randomized to receive endocrine therapy alone or in combination with chemotherapy. Results for those with a score of 0 to 10 have been published and confirmed that these patients have an invasive DFS of 93.8% (95% CI 92.4–94.9), and OS of 98% (95% CI 97.1–98.6). The Rx for Positive Node, Endocrine Responsive Breast Cancer (RxPONDER) study is investigating the RS in patients with hormone receptor–positive, node-positive disease, where those with a RS 25 or less are randomized to receive endocrine therapy alone or in combination with chemotherapy (clinicaltrials.gov identifier NCT01272037). In summary, Onco*type* Dx testing may be considered in patients with hormone receptor–positive, node-negative patients to help determine the potential benefit of chemotherapy but is still considered investigational in node-positive disease.

MammaPrint is a 70-gene expression assay that includes a comprehensive assessment of genes integral to oncogenesis, including apoptosis evasion, self-sufficiency in growth signals, insensitivity to antigrowth signals, limitless replication, tissue invasion and metastasis, and angiogenesis.[50a] The MINDACT trial was a large prospective clinical trial enrolling 6693 patients with early stage breast cancer randomizing patients with clinically high-risk disease but low MammaPrint scores to adjuvant chemotherapy versus no chemotherapy.[50b] Notably, the chemotherapy used was anthracycline-based or docetaxel with capecitabine; third-generation regimens including both anthracycline and taxanes were not used. Investigators identified 1128 evaluable patients with high clinical risk and low MammaPrint scores. DFS at 5 years in those who received chemotherapy was 95.9% (95% CI 94–97.2) versus 94.7% (95% CI 92.5–96.2) in those who did not receive chemotherapy, which was not a statistically significant difference (HR = 0.78, 95% CI 0.5–1.21, p = .27). A key strength of this study was that it couched molecular risk stratification in clinical risk. Important limitations, however, include the fact that a heterogenous patient population was selected, including patients with HER2-positive disease (9.5%) and TNBC (9.6%). While this detracts some of the predefined statistical power in regard to the ER-positive group, there is insufficient power to make any conclusions regarding the HER2-positive and TNBC group. The study included both lymph node–negative and lymph node–positive patients. While the lymph node–positive group is not adequately powered for, it is also important to consider the chemotherapy regimens used. Patients received either anthracycline- or taxanes-based regimens, and data exists suggesting that, in node-positive disease combination, third-generation regimens (i.e., including both anthracycline and taxanes) are not noninferior to second-generation regimens. Therefore MammaPrint is also an option for patients with ER-positive, node-negative breast cancer, particularly if they are at high clinical risk and wish to avoid chemotherapy.

When to Consider Chemotherapy for ER-Positive Disease

In essence, what genomic biomarkers are attempting to characterize is disease biology, which is the ultimate driver as to whether a patient's tumor is likely to benefit from adjuvant chemotherapy. Although these genomic assays are sophisticated methods of assessing disease biology, other markers are part of routine pathologic workup that can assess biology as well. In a time when health

economics and cost-effectiveness are considerations, these markers should be considered when formulating patient treatment plans, particularly when results would not change management. Numerous studies have found that ki67, HER2, and hormone receptor status can approximate luminal A versus B phenotypes.[51] Although histologic grade or ki67 alone have significant variability between different laboratories and as single variables do not reliably predict RS; simple models using these markers together can predict RS with high fidelity.[52,53] Indeed, these routine markers can be integrated into a formula and result in score called the immunohistochemical 4 (IHC4) score.[54] In the Arimidex, Tamoxifen, Alone or in Combination (ATAC) trial, IHC4 scores were found to offer similar prognostic information then the Oncotype Dx RS.[54] The Optimal Personalized Treatment of Early Breast Cancer Using Multiparameter Analysis (OPTIMA) study is investigating how some of these markers compare with one another, and results are awaited.[55]

In the meantime, oncologists must personalize care when considering chemotherapy for ER-positive disease. Biological factors must be balanced with clinical factors, including anatomic stage and patient factors such as comorbidities and performances status. Although the standard of care for node-positive disease includes the addition of adjuvant chemotherapy, studies such as RxPONDER may help identify patients where chemotherapy is not beneficial, thus sparing them of undue toxicity. The use of genomics to assess biology is important but should be put into context of other pathologic markers and how additional data would influence therapy.

Tamoxifen

The selective ER modulator tamoxifen is a cornerstone therapy for patients with ER-positive breast cancer who are either premenopausal or postmenopausal and not a candidate for an aromatase inhibitor (AI). The effects of 5 years of adjuvant tamoxifen is potent; at 15 years, it decreases the risk of recurrence from 46.1% to 33.0% (log-rank $2p$ < .00001) and decreases breast cancer mortality from 32.7% to 23.6% (log-rank $2p$ < .00001).[46] Numerous studies have investigated the use of tamoxifen beyond 5 years including the Scottish Adjuvant Tamoxifen Trial (SATT), NSABP-14, and the joint ECOG E4181 and E5181 analysis, which failed to consistently demonstrate a DFS or OS benefit.[56–58] These studies were generally small, and ER status was either negative or unknown in many patients. For more than 2 decades, 5 years of adjuvant tamoxifen was considered a standard of care until two large studies found 10 years was superior. The Adjuvant Tamoxifen: Longer Against Shorter (ATLAS) trial enrolled 6846 patients with ER-positive disease who were treated with 10 versus 5 years of tamoxifen.[59] Ten versus 5 years of treatment resulted in a significant reduction in recurrence (18% vs. 20.8% respectively, RR = 0.84, 95% CI 0.76–0.94), breast cancer mortality (9.7% vs. 11.5%, respectively, p = .01), and improvements in OS (18.6 vs. 21.1%, respectively, p = .01). The Adjuvant Tamoxifen: To Offer More? (aTTom) trial reported that 2755 women with ER-positive breast cancer allocated to 5 versus 10 years of tamoxifen had a similar benefit.[60] The aTTom study found that compared with 5 years, 10 years of tamoxifen resulted in a significant reduction in recurrence (16.7 vs. 19.3%, RR = 0.85, 95% CI 0.76–0.95) and a trend toward improved breast cancer mortality. Notably, in both the ATLAS and aTTom trials benefit of extended tamoxifen occurred almost 10 years after initiating treatment, suggesting that these therapies have a carryover effect in terms of disease recurrence. Furthermore, these were studies with generalized eligibility criteria and included patients from stage I to III tumors, subset analysis did not identify a specific group that benefited more, thus the results are considered to be applicable to a diverse patient population. Although the risk of pulmonary embolism is present while patients are on tamoxifen, this risk ends upon cessation of therapy; this was not the case for the risk of endometrial cancer, which persisted even after therapy ended. The ATLAS study did not demonstrate an increase in pulmonary embolism or endometrial cancer-associated deaths; however, the aTTom trial did demonstrate a small increased risk of endometrial cancer–associated death (RR 1.83, 95% CI 1.09–3.09). Limitations of these extended tamoxifen studies include the fact that most patients were postmenopausal, where AIs have become the standard of care; furthermore, how this regimen compares with others, such an AI after tamoxifen or the addition of ovarian suppression is not addressed.

Aromatase Inhibitors

As their name implies, AIs inhibit aromatase and prevent the peripheral conversion of androgens to estrogens. Two main subclasses of AIs have been approved: steroidal (i.e., exemestane) and nonsteroidal (i.e., anastrozole and letrozole). Numerous studies have pitted 5 years of tamoxifen versus 5 years of AIs, and a meta-analysis conducted by the EBCTCG involving postmenopausal women with early-stage ER-positive breast cancer found that AIs reduced recurrence particularly in the first year (RR = 0.64, 95% CI 0.52–0.78) and years 2 to 4 (RR = 0.8, 95% CI 0.68–0.93) and had lower 10-year breast cancer mortality (RR = 0.85, 95% CI 0.75–0.96).[61] Thus for women who are postmenopausal and have hormone receptor–positive breast cancer, AIs have emerged as the adjuvant endocrine treatment of choice.

Postmenopausal women who are initially treated with tamoxifen derive benefit if they switch to an AI. The Intergroup Exemestane Study found that exemestane versus tamoxifen after 2 to 3 years of tamoxifen for a total of 5 years of endocrine therapy led to improvements in recurrence or death (HR = 0.76, 95% CI 0.66–0.88, p = .0001).[62] The Italian Tamoxifen Arimidex trial, found similar benefits of the switch method compared with 5 years of tamoxifen.[63] Completing an additional 5 years of an AI after 2 to 3 years of tamoxifen has also been found to be beneficial. The aforementioned EBCTCG meta-analysis found that this strategy reduced recurrence during years 2 through 4 (RR = 0.56, 95% CI 0.46–0.67), as well as breast cancer mortality (RR = 0.84, 95% CI 0.72–0.96).[61] The importance of adding adjuvant AIs can further be seen in the NCIC CTG MA.17 trial, in which patients were randomized 5 years of letrozole versus placebo after completing 5 years of tamoxifen.[64] After a median follow-up of 30 months, those treated with letrozole had improved DFS either locally or contralaterally (HR = 0.58, 95% CI 0.45–0.76, p < .001) or in terms of distant metastasis (HR = 0.60, 95% CI 0.43–0.84, p = .002), although no OS benefit was seen.

The question as to whether 10 years of AI therapy is better than 5 years is being evaluated in the MA.17 extension trial (clinicaltrials.gov identifier NCT00754845) and NSABP B-42 (clinicaltrials.gov identifier NCT00382070). Although the current standard of care is 5 years of adjuvant AI in early-stage breast cancer, patients with particularly high-risk disease can be considered for extended therapy; however, providers must weigh the lack of data and potential long-term toxicity of AI therapy, including to bone health and cardiovascular risks.

Ovarian Suppression

Chemotherapy-induced amenorrhea has been associated with improved outcomes in patients with early-stage breast cancer.[65,66] Indeed, an EBCTCG meta-analysis demonstrated improved recurrence rates ($2p < .00001$) and breast cancer mortality ($2p = .004$) in patients receiving ovarian suppression compared with no ovarian suppression.[67] However, a later meta-analysis by the EBCTCG found that the addition of ovarian suppression to tamoxifen did not improve recurrence rates (HR = 0.85, 95% CI 0.67–1.09) nor mortality (HR = 0.84, 95% CI 0.59–1.19) but in fact increased grade III toxicities, such as menopausal symptoms and sexual dysfunction.[68] To demonstrate the efficacy of ovarian suppression, the Suppression of Ovarian Function Trial (SOFT) and Tamoxifen and Exemestane Trial (TEXT) were performed. A joint analysis investigating exemestane with ovarian suppression compared with tamoxifen with ovarian suppression demonstrated improved 5-year DFS (91.1% vs. 87.3%, respectively, HR = 0.72, 95% CI 0.60–0.86, p = .0002).[69] These data unfortunately did not have a comparator arm without ovarian suppression. It was not until the SOFT study was presented and published a few months later that the benefit of adding ovarian suppression to tamoxifen was evaluated, and it did not provide benefit for the entire treated population (DFS HR = 0.83, 95% CI 0.66–1.04, p = .1).[70] The study was also stratified by those who received versus did not receive chemotherapy, and secondary objectives investigated freedom from breast cancer (FFBC) rates in tamoxifen, versus tamoxifen with ovarian suppression, versus AI with ovarian suppression. Adding ovarian suppression to tamoxifen did not improve FFBC in the entire cohort (HR = 081, 95% CI 0.63–1.03) nor in patients treated with chemotherapy (HR = 0.78, 95% CI 0.6–1.02); however, patients receiving 5 years of AI with ovarian suppression did experience improved FFBC compared with tamoxifen alone in the entire cohort (HR = 0.64, 95% CI 0.49–0.83) and in those receiving chemotherapy (HR = 0.65, 95% CI 0.49–0.87). In an unplanned subset analysis in patients less than 35 years of age (n = 350, 11% of total cohort), the majority of whom were treated with chemotherapy, suggested that the addition of ovarian suppression to either tamoxifen or an AI improved FFBC compared with 5 years of tamoxifen. Importantly, the addition of ovarian suppression was associated with more side effects including those of estrogen deprivation, and the long-term effects on cardiovascular and bone health remain unknown.

Optimal Endocrine Therapy for Pre- and Postmenopausal Women

Navigating through data on various adjuvant endocrine therapy approaches can be challenging, and it is important to weigh the benefit and toxicity of therapy to each individual patient. For patients who are premenopausal and have ER-positive breast cancer, the standard of care remains tamoxifen, which may be prescribed for up to 10 years. Premenopausal patients with high-risk disease requiring chemotherapy may be considered for ovarian suppression therapy with an AI. The benefit of adding ovarian suppression to tamoxifen has only been demonstrated in a small subset analysis of patients less than 35 years of age.[70] For patients who are premenopausal but become postmenopausal during the first 5 years of tamoxifen, additional therapy with up to 5 years of an AI should be considered. For patients who are postmenopausal, the standard of care currently remains 5 years of adjuvant

AI therapy. Based on the experience with extended tamoxifen, providers may consider extended AI therapy in high-risk patients understanding the lack of data and known long-term toxicities of AIs on bone and cardiovascular health.

Bisphosphonates in ER-Positive Breast Cancer

Bisphosphonates inhibit bone resorption due to osteoclasts and can increase bone density. They are approved for numerous indications, including osteoporosis, osteitis deformans, hypercalcemia of malignancy, and decreasing fractures in patients with bone metastasis. In addition, preclinical data suggest that they may prevent tumor cell adhesion to bones, induce tumor apoptosis, antagonize growth factors, and have antiangiogenic effects.[70a–70d]

Numerous studies have been conducted using various adjuvant bisphosphonates in early breast cancer. The AZURE study was a large phase 3 study investigating zoledronic acid in high-risk early breast cancer, and while the overall analysis did not show a difference in DFS (HR = 0.94, 95% CI 0.82–1.06, p = .3), it did show reduced risk of bone metastasis at any time (HR = 0.84, 95% CI 0.68–0.97, p = .02), especially in those who were postmenopausal (HR = 0.77, 95% CI 0.63–0.96).[70e] Other studies have also shown survival benefit in patients receiving various bisphosphonates, and although not all met their primary endpoint, many found benefit in subset analysis focusing on postmenopausal patients.[70f–70i] To help clarify some of the discordance, a large patient-level meta-analysis was conducted by the EBCTCG involving 18,766 women.[70j] The meta-analysis included studies using various bisphosphonates, schedules, and duration. Furthermore, studies had varied adjuvant chemotherapy and endocrine regimens. Although overall reduction in recurrence was not significant (RR = 0.94, 95% CI 0.87–1.01, 2p = .08), distant recurrence was improved (RR = 0.91, 95% CI 0.83–0.99, 2p = .03), particularly bone recurrence (RR = 0.83, 95% CI 0.73–0.94, 2p = .004). The benefit was seen only in postmenopausal women; premenopausal women did not derive benefit. While this meta-analysis is the highest level data available to support use of bisphosphonates, the heterogeneity across studies and use of bisphosphonate limit the interpretability.

The benefits of bisphosphonates on bone health, however, are clear. Estrogen is an important hormone in maintenance of bone density, and after menopause many women will have decrements in bone density. Aromatase inhibitors in particular are known to decrease bone density and can indeed increase the risk of fracture. Bisphosphonates are known to improve bone density and decrease fractures in patients with early breast cancer.[70j] Patients undergoing therapy with aromatase inhibitors should undergo bone density screening routinely and be treated with bisphosphonates as indicated.

Thus, while the benefits of bisphosphonates on recurrence and survival in breast cancer are not entirely clear, the added benefits of bone health have led some societies to issue recommendations to either consider or frankly recommend these agents, although the optimal scheduling and duration of therapy is unknown.[70k,70l]

HER2-Positive Disease

HER2 was first described in the 1980s, and found to be amplified or overexpressed in 25% to 30% of breast cancers. HER2-positive breast cancers historically were among the most aggressive

with poorest prognosis; however, the incorporation of anti-HER2 therapies has vastly improved outcomes. Through translational research, a monoclonal antibody, trastuzumab, was developed to target HER2, and clinical studies demonstrated significant clinical benefit when combined with chemotherapy, first in the metastatic setting and then as adjuvant therapy for early-stage breast cancer.[9,10]

Trastuzumab

Trastuzumab is a monoclonal antibody targeting HER2 and HER4 and was the first anti-HER2 therapy approved for use in patients with HER2-positive breast cancer. The landmark trial of adjuvant trastuzumab for early-stage breast cancer was performed by the Breast Cancer International Research Group (BCIRG), which investigated the addition of trastuzumab to adjuvant chemotherapy.[10] The regimens investigated were standard AC followed by docetaxel; AC followed by docetaxel and trastuzumab (AC/TH); and docetaxel, carboplatin, and trastuzumab (TCH). The original report with a median follow-up of 65 months demonstrated that 5-year DFS for AC/docetaxel was 75%, which was significantly lower compared with 84% in the AC/TH arm (HR = 0.64, p < .001) and 81% in the TCH arm (HR = 0.75, p = .04); OS was also superior in the AC/TH and TCH arms (87% vs. 92% and 91%, respectively, p = .04 for both AC/TH and TCH). Although not powered to assess differences between AC/TH and TCH, the study found there was no significant differences in DFS and OS between these two arms, albeit there was a nonsignificant trend suggesting AC/TH was superior). The final results presented at the 2015 San Antonio Breast Cancer Symposium (SABCS) found that a median of 10.3 years follow-up, there are persistent improvements in DFS and OS in the trastuzumab-based arms but that DFS HRs for AC/TH and TCH are closer than those observed in the 5-year analysis (AC/TH HR = 0.70, 95% CI 0.60–0.83, p < .001; TCH HR = 0.76, 95% CI 0.65–0.90, p < .001).[71] Notably, TCH has significantly lower rates of cardiomyopathy than AC/TH (0.4% vs. 2%, respectively, p = .0005). A large meta-analysis including 11991 patients confirmed the DFS and OS benefits of adding trastuzumab to adjuvant chemotherapy in early-stage breast cancer (HR 0.60, 95% CI 0.50–0.71, p < .0001) and HR = 0.66, 95% CI 0.57–0.77, p < .00001, respectively).[72] The OS of trastuzumab is noted when giving concurrently with chemotherapy (HR = 0.64, 95% CI 0.53–0.76) versus sequentially (HR = 0.85, 95% CI 0.43–1.67). These results demonstrate that TCH is likely as potent as AC/TH and has lower rates of cardiotoxicity, making this a preferred regimen (Fig. 55.1).

Duration of Therapy

The aforementioned meta-analysis also demonstrated that trastuzumab for less than 6 months did not provide OS benefit (HR = 0.55, 95% CI 0.27–1.11). Indeed, the Protocol for Herceptin as Adjuvant therapy with Reduced Exposure (PHARE) trial, which compared 6 versus 12 months of adjuvant trastuzumab, found that 6 months was not noninferior to 12 months of therapy (DFS 91 versus 94%, respectively, HR 1.28, 95% CI 1.05–1.56).[73] The Herceptin Adjuvant (HERA) trial investigated if a longer duration of trastuzumab improved DFS.[74] Compared with 12 months of adjuvant trastuzumab, 24 months of therapy did not improve DFS (HR = 0.99, 95% CI 0.85–1.14) nor OS (HR = 1.05, 95% CI 0.86–1.28) but did increase cardiotoxicity (7.2% decrease in left ventricular ejection fraction in the 2-year group, compared

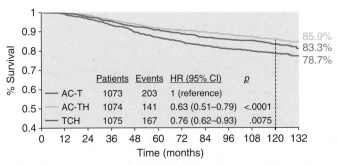

• **Fig. 55.1** Breast Cancer International Research Group 006 overall survival. *AC,* Adriamycin and cyclophosphamide; *AC-TH,* AC followed by paclitaxel and trastuzumab; *CI,* confidence interval; *HR,* hazard ratio; *TCH,* docetaxel, carboplatin, and trastuzumab. (Data from Slamon D, et al. Presented at the 2015 San Antonio Breast Cancer Symposium; December 8–12, 2015; San Antonio, Texas; Abstract S5-04.)

with 4.1% in the 1-year group, *p* < .0001). These data demonstrate the importance of adjuvant trastuzumab and that optimal duration of therapy is 1 year (see Fig. 55.1). Other trials are addressing shorter durations of trastuzumab of therapy compared with the standard 1 year.

Deescalation of Therapy: Small HER2-Positive Tumors

Although smaller tumors (i.e., <1 cm) typically have very good prognosis, data suggest that those that are HER2-positive have higher recurrence rates than those who are HER2-negative.[75,76] Adjuvant studies investigating trastuzumab typically have included predominantly larger and/or node positive tumors, and thus the benefit of anti-HER2 for smaller tumors is not clearly defined.[72]

A patient-level meta-analysis was conducted including patients with HER2-positive tumors less than 2 cm with or without positive nodes across five randomized trials including the Herceptin Adjuvant (HERA), North Central Cancer Treatment Group (NCCTG) N9831, NSABP B-31, French Federation of Cancer Centers Sarcoma Group Protocole Adjuvant dans le Cancer du Sien (FNCLCC-PACS) 04, and Finland Herceptin (FinHER) trials. At 8 years of follow-up, the addition of trastuzumab in both in ER-positive and ER-negative cohorts was associated with improved recurrence rates (24.3% vs. 17.3%, *p* < .001 in ER positive; 33.4% vs. 24%, *p* < .0001 in ER negative) and OS (11.6% vs. 7.8%, *p* = .005 in ER positive; 21.2% vs. 12.4%, *p* = .0001 in ER negative).[77] Although these numbers notably include patients with node-positive disease, this demonstrates the importance of adjuvant trastuzumab. In subset analysis, those with ER-positive disease with one or no nodes, the addition of trastuzumab improved recurrence rates from 12.7% to 19.4% (DFS gain 6.7%, *p* = .005), but no OS (absolute gain of 2.1%, *p* = .12). These data suggest that there may be populations of patients who may be suitable candidates assessing deescalation of therapy strategies.

To explore this strategy, a single arm study investigating the combination of adjuvant paclitaxel with trastuzumab in HER2-positive tumors less than 3 cm with no lymph node macrometastasis was performed. After a median follow-up of 4 years, the 3-year rate of survival free from invasive disease was 98.7% (95% CI 97.6–99.8). This regimen was very well tolerated with only 3.2% (95% CI 1.7–5.4) of patients developing grade III neuropathy and 0.5% (95% CI 0.1–1.8) developing symptomatic congestive heart failure.[78] Although these data are not definitive given the single-arm design and short follow-up, they demonstrate that

patients treated with this regimen may do exceptionally well (see Fig. 55.1).

Several studies are now in progress to assess deescalation strategies. The ATEMPT trial (NCT01853748) is investigating trastuzumab emtansine (TDM-1), a drug that demonstrates significant activity in the metastatic setting, compared with paclitaxel and trastuzumab in patients with stage 1 HER2-positive disease.[79] The RESPECT trial (clinicaltrials.gov identifier NCT01104935) is investigating survival end points in elderly patients with early HER2-positive breast cancer treated with trastuzumab versus trastuzumab with chemotherapy.

Pertuzumab

Pertuzumab is a monoclonal antibody against HER2 and human epidermal growth factor receptor 3 (HER3), which has demonstrated survival benefits for patients with metastatic HER2-positive breast cancer and has also been studied in the neoadjuvant setting.[80] The Neoadjuvant Study of Pertuzumab and Herceptin in an Early Regimen Evaluation (NeoSPHERE) study found that the addition of pertuzumab to trastuzumab and docetaxel improved pathologic complete response (pCR) rates from 29% to 45.8%.[81] A recent update reported at the 2015 ASCO Annual meeting suggested a trend for improved DFS with the combination of docetaxel, pertuzumab, and trastuzumab, but this was not statistically significant (HR 0.60, 95% CI 0.28–1.27).[82] The Trastuzumab Plus Pertuzumab in Neoadjuvant HER2 Positive Breast Cancer (TRYPHAENA) study compared the regimen of pertuzumab, trastuzumab, docetaxel, and carboplatin to two other pertuzumab-based regimens and showed an unprecedented pCR rate of 66.2% in the former arm.[83] Based on the results of NeoSPHERE and TRYPHAENA, the FDA granted provisional approval for the use of pertuzumab in the neoadjuvant setting. The results of the Adjuvant Pertuzumab and Herceptin in Initial Therapy of Breast Cancer (APHINITY) study will confirm whether the addition of pertuzumab improves survival outcomes in early HER2-positive breast cancer. Until then, the strict approval for pertuzumab in early breast cancer remains in the neoadjuvant setting, but the NCCN guidelines have made provisional statements to also consider its use in the adjuvant setting if a patient would have been eligible to receive pertuzumab preoperatively and did not (Fig. 55.1).[84]

Neoadjuvant Therapy

Adjuvant systemic therapy can improve recurrence and survival rates by killing cells that may have escaped the tumor bed via lymphatics and blood vessels. This initially led researchers to hypothesize that giving systemic therapy before surgery (neoadjuvant) might improve outcomes because it would destroy circulating cells; this was supported by preclinical data.[85,86] Therefore several studies were conducted to assess whether systemic therapy administered before or after surgery was superior in terms of DFS and OS for patients with early-stage breast cancer. The first large randomized trial that compared preoperative with adjuvant chemotherapy in patients with operable breast cancer was the NSABP B-18 trial.[87] This trial assigned 751 patients to receive preoperative AC and 742 patients to receive postoperative AC. In its most recent update and a follow-up of 16 years, there was no difference in DFS (HR 0.93, 95% CI 0.81–1.06, *p* = 0.27) or OS (HR 0.99, 95% CI 0.85–1.16, *p* = .90) between the two treatment arms.[88] A meta-analysis evaluating nine randomized studies including a total of 3946 patients found that neoadjuvant versus adjuvant therapy were equivalent in terms of death (summary RR = 1.00, 95% CI 0.90–1.12), disease progression (summary RR = 0.99, 95% CI 0.91–1.07), and distant disease recurrence (RR = 0.94, 95% I 0.83–1.06).[89] Although these analyses did not specify subtype of breast cancer nor did they include ant-HER2 therapy for those who were HER2-positive, these data are generally applicable to all subtypes of breast cancer. Nevertheless, a multidisciplinary approach and careful patient selection are required when considering patients for neoadjuvant systemic therapy.

Although initial evaluation may be performed by a surgical or medical oncologist, several additional factors should be considered during the initial assessment. In complex cases, the use of a multidisciplinary tumor board where pathologists, radiologists, surgical, medical, and radiation oncologists review the case can facilitate the development of a treatment strategy. Early referral to radiation oncology as part of the initial assessment should be considered to evaluate how response to treatment may affect radiation planning. Importantly, the neoadjuvant setting provides numerous opportunities for research and clinical trial participation, and these opportunities should be discussed with all eligible patients.

Advantages

The primary indication for neoadjuvant therapy has historically been to facilitate breast surgery.[84] Instances in which neoadjuvant therapy is indicated include patients with inoperable tumors that may become operable with reduction in tumor size, patients who desire breast conservation who are not candidates at diagnosis, and patients with inflammatory breast cancer. Patients desiring breast conservation who are not a candidate for this approach at the time of diagnosis, may expect overall breast conservation rates as high as 72.3% (OR 1.7, 95% CI 1.6–1.8).[90,91] Patients with a clinical diagnosis of inflammatory breast cancer may experience a survival benefit with neoadjuvant therapy, and neoadjuvant therapy is considered a standard of care for this population unless a contraindication exists.[92] If patients are not candidates for surgery at the time of diagnosis, neoadjuvant therapy can also be used to bridge patients to a point where they are more likely to be surgical candidates.

There are many other instances when neoadjuvant therapy may be considered, although a strict indication may not exist. Neoadjuvant therapy may be considered in patients with chemoresponsive breast cancer subtypes. Of all clinical breast cancer subtypes, HER2-positive and TNBCs are the most chemosensitive, therefore these subtypes are most amenable to neoadjuvant chemotherapy and indeed have the highest pCR rates.[93] Aggressive ER-positive subtypes and luminal B-like phenotype breast cancers tend to have higher pCR rates than the more indolent ER-positive subtypes (pCR 15% vs. 7.5%) and therefore may be suitable for neoadjuvant therapy as well.[94] Indeed, classic invasive lobular breast cancer tends to have inferior responses to neoadjuvant chemotherapy compared with invasive ductal carcinomas (pCR rate 11% vs. 25%, $p = .01$), thus less likely to benefit from neoadjuvant chemotherapy.[95] In patients with node-positive disease in whom chemotherapy remains the standard of care regardless of its sequencing, response to neoadjuvant treatment has the potential to affect locoregional management, including the extent of axillary surgery and radiation.

A key aspect of neoadjuvant therapy is that it may also be used in clinical research trials. As discussed subsequently, rates of pCR may be surrogates for survival end points, and thus drugs that increase pCR rates may improve survival rates. Furthermore, the neoadjuvant setting can be used to evaluate the biological effects of novel agents as tissue both before and after therapy because they are readily available and thus logistically more feasible.

Limitations

Routine use of neoadjuvant chemotherapy is not recommended for patients with stage I breast cancer, although there may be certain situations in which this could facilitate surgical or cosmetic options.[84] Use of neoadjuvant chemotherapy should particularly be scrutinized when the decision of whether to administer chemotherapy is not clear or where third- versus first- or second-generation chemotherapy regimens are being considered. In these cases, the final pathology from surgery is often essential to making decisions about the need for chemotherapy and the type of regimen. In the neoadjuvant setting, therapeutic decisions are largely based on clinical staging, including physical examination and imaging modalities, which may be less accurate than surgical staging. In particular, with regard to nodal staging, this may affect radiation therapy options.[96]

The extent of tumor defined by focality may affect breast conservation rates after neoadjuvant chemotherapy; indeed multifocal or multicentric tumors have lower chances of achieving breast conservation (unifocal 71.6%, multifocal 58.5%, multicentric 30%).[97] Patients with multicentric tumors, compared with unifocal, may have inferior DFS ($p < .001$) and OS ($p < .009$) after neoadjuvant chemotherapy, but this is abrogated if pCR is achieved.[97] There are insufficient data to support breast conservation after neoadjuvant chemotherapy in multicentric or multifocal disease, and therefore cases should be considered on an individual basis.[84]

Although most patients are still able to undergo surgery after neoadjuvant therapy, studies have reported that up to 12% of patients who start neoadjuvant chemotherapy were not able to undergo definitive surgery.[98] Even more uncommon, distant metastasis has been described in 4% of patients who experience progression of disease while receiving neoadjuvant chemotherapy.[98] Patients with subtypes of breast cancer that are relatively less chemosensitive, such as luminal A or classic invasive lobular breast cancer, may also be less likely to benefit from neoadjuvant therapy.[94,95]

Breast and Axillary Assessments

Locoregional assessment should be performed with careful physical examination and the use of mammography and ultrasound as recommended by the NCCN guidelines.[84,99] If clinical examination or breast imaging is notable for lymphadenopathy, a dedicated axillary ultrasound is recommended for further evaluation. Fine-needle aspirate (FNA) or core needle biopsy of any suspicious appearing lymph nodes should be performed.[84,100] The placement of a biopsy clip should be strongly considered at the time of performing an FNA or core needle biopsy because the presence of a biopsy clip can improve the success rate of surgical resection of biopsy-proven metastatic axillary lymph nodes. This allows for more accurate assessment of pathologic response in the axilla and decreases the false-negative rate when performing a sentinel lymph node (SLN) biopsy after neoadjuvant chemotherapy in patients with known axillary nodal involvement before systemic treatment.[101,102]

In certain cases, magnetic resonance imaging (MRI) of the breast may be helpful. MRI of the breast is more sensitive in determining the extent of the tumor but may also overestimate the tumor size.[103] MRI may be performed if there are other areas of concern on initial imaging, which may warrant additional evaluation.[104] A baseline MRI has been shown to decrease reexcision rates and also allows for assessment of the contralateral breast, where there is between 3% and 10% likelihood of synchronous disease.[105,106] The decision to pursue an MRI should be tailored to each patient's specific clinical situation and needs, particularly if breast conservation is desired.

For patients with clinically node-negative breast cancer at diagnosis, the role of performing a SLN biopsy before or after neoadjuvant chemotherapy is controversial. In the Sentinel Neoadjuvant (SENTINA) study, 35% of patients who were clinically node negative were found to have pathologically node-positive disease on SLN biopsy performed before neoadjuvant chemotherapy.[107] In these patients, repeat SLN biopsy after neoadjuvant chemotherapy detected additional SLNs in 61% of patients with a high false-negative rate of 51.6%. Thus the reliability of a SLN biopsy after excision of a positive node before neoadjuvant therapy is poor. In another study, SLN biopsy after neoadjuvant chemotherapy compared with the same procedure before treatment resulted in lower SLN identification rates (98 vs. 95%, before vs. after neoadjuvant therapy respectively, $p = .032$), but also to less frequent axillary dissections or radiation (45 vs. 33%, $p = .006$), therefore potentially reduced morbidity.[108] Furthermore, a key limitation of SLN biopsy before neoadjuvant therapy is that removal of affected nodes before treatment precludes the ability to assess pathologic response and decreases the significance of pCR.[109] With few compelling data to routinely perform SLN biopsy before neoadjuvant therapy, our preference is to perform SLN biopsy after neoadjuvant therapy in patients with a clinically node-negative axilla at presentation, but each case must be individualized.

Pathologic Complete Response

Individual patients who achieve a pCR defined as ypT0/is ypN0 are more likely to experience a survival benefit compared with those who are not able to achieve a pCR.[110] This has led to the hypothesis that a drug that increases the pCR rate in a population will translate into an improved survival outcome. It is important to distinguish these metrics and end points when considering neoadjuvant data.

The only instance in which improvements in pCR rates have resulted in improvements in survival outcomes in a large study is with trastuzumab. The addition of trastuzumab to chemotherapy has been demonstrated to increase pCR rates from 20% to 43% (RR for pCR 2.07, 95% CI 1.41–3.03, $p = .0002$) and decrease relapse rate from 20% to 12% (RR for relapse 0.67, 95% CI 0.48–0.94).[111] Survival data from the Neoadjuvant Herceptin (NOAH) study presented at the 2013 ASCO meeting also demonstrated that event-free survival (EFS) and OS were improved in those taking trastuzumab (HR 0.64 $p = .016$, and HR 0.66 $p = .055$, respectively).[112]

The success of lapatinib, a tyrosine kinase inhibitor targeting the intracellular domain of HER2, in the metastatic setting motivated several neoadjuvant studies investigating this drug in the neoadjuvant setting. The European Organization for Research and Treatment of Cancer (EORTC) 10054 study, NSABP B-41 study, and CALGB 40601 study, and Neoadjuvant Lapatinib and/or

Trastuzumab Treatment Optimization (NeoALTTO) investigators reported that the addition of lapatinib to trastuzumab-based neoadjuvant chemotherapy improved pCR rates by 4% to 21%.[113–116] For instance, the NeoALTTO study randomized patients to paclitaxel and either lapatinib, trastuzumab, or a combination of lapatinib and trastuzumab, after which they underwent definitive surgical treatment and then received adjuvant anthracycline-based chemotherapy. Although this study demonstrated a striking improvement in pCR rate with the addition of lapatinib to trastuzumab (30%–51% pCR rates comparing the trastuzumab arm with the trastuzumab and lapatinib arms, respectively), the combination arm was not associated with improved EFS (HR 0.78, 95% CI 0.47–1.28, $p = .33$) or OS (HR 0.62, 95% CI 0.30–1.25, $p = .19$). The study, however, was not powered to detect small differences in survival outcomes. The confirmatory Adjuvant Lapatinib and/or Trastuzumab Treatment Optimization (ALTTO) study, presented at the 2014 ASCO Annual Meeting, failed to demonstrate improved DFS by adding lapatinib to trastuzumab-based chemotherapy (HR 0.84, CI 0.70–1.02, $p = .048$, $p \le .025$ needed for statistical significance).[117] The discordant results between the NeoALTTO and ALTTO studies may be in part explained by the timing of the anthracycline-based therapy because in the NeoALTTO study, this regimen was given after surgery and therefore did not affect pCR rates. Although this informs future study designs, suggesting that all chemotherapy should be given upfront before surgery, these data demonstrate how an improvement in pCR rates by a drug do not necessarily correlate with improvements in survival end points.

With this consideration, the use of neoadjuvant pertuzumab should be scrutinized. The improvements in pCR in NeoSPHERE and TRYPHAENA have not correlated with improvements in survival as of yet. The 5-year analysis of NeoSPHERE demonstrated a trend to improvements in DFS (3-year DFS 85% vs. 92% favoring pertuzumab/trastuzumab/docetaxel vs. trastuzumab/docetaxel, HR = 0.60, 95% CI 0.28–1.27), but this difference between arms was not statistically significant.[82] We await results from the prospective APHINITY trial to see whether pertuzumab will demonstrate a correlation between pCR and survival end points.

Studies in TNBC have also not been able to demonstrate a consistent association with pCR rates and survival end points. Platinum agents studied in the neoadjuvant setting using various doses and schedules and in combination with various agents have consistently demonstrated improvements in pCR rates. The CALGB 40603 study found that rates of ypT0N0 pCR improved from 41% to 54% ($p = .0029$), the GeparSixto study found that in the TNBC cohort pCR rates improved from 36.9% to 53.2% ($p = .005$), and the iSPY2 study reported at the 2013 San Antonio Breast Cancer Symposium (SABCS) that pCR rates with carboplatin and velaparib were 52%.[110,118,119] Notably, these studies used various doses and schedules of carboplatin and in combination with nonstandard of care agents such as bevacizumab and velaparib. The addition of carboplatin is associated with significant toxicity in terms of myelosuppression and nausea. Grade III to IV hematological adverse events ranged from 59% to 82% in the GeparSixto study.[110] In the CALGB 40603 study, patients who received carboplatin were more likely to miss more than two doses of paclitaxel (36% vs. 16%), 20% of patients did not receive all planned doses of anthracycline and taxanes, and many patients required dose reductions.[118] This is an important factor to consider because anthracyclines and taxanes have robust long-term survival data.[18] Survival end points in the CALGB 40603 study were recently presented and did not demonstrate that the addition of carboplatin improved ERS (HR = 0.84, 95% CI 0.58–1.22, p = .36) or OS (HR = 1.15, 95% CI 0.74–1.79, p = .53).[120] The GeparSexto study also did not find in its general analysis including HER2-positive and TNBC that DFS was improved (HR = 0.81, 95% CI 0.54–1.21, p = .3115); however, in its TNBC subset, there was a benefit in DFS (HR = 0.56, 95% CI 0.33–0.96, p = .035).[121] In summary, the incorporation of carboplatin in the neoadjuvant setting requires additional studies using consistent doses and schedules, integration into standard regimens, and long-term survival data given its significant toxicity. Furthermore, adjuvant studies have been initiated to study the benefit of adding platinum for patients with early-stage TNBC powered to assess survival end points.

The addition of the antivascular endothelial growth factor receptor (VGEF) monoclonal antibody bevacizumab to chemotherapy has also been considered in numerous studies in the neoadjuvant setting. The German Breast Group (GBG) 44 study and the Avastin Randomized Trial with Neoadjuvant Chemotherapy for patients with Early Breast Cancer (ARTemis) found that in TNBC cohorts, the addition of bevacizumab improved the rates of ypT0N0 pCR by 11.4% (p = .003) and 14% (p = .03), respectively.[122,123] The Austrian Breast and Colorectal Cancer Study Group (ABCSG) 32 study and SWOG 0800 study have also reported improvements in pCR rates especially in TNBC.[124,125] The NSABP B-40 and CALGB 40603 studies found statistically significant improvements in ypT0Nx pCR in the breast with the addition of bevacizumab, but differences in ypT0N0 rates were not statistically significant (p = .08 and .057, respectively).[118,126] Although these neoadjuvant studies demonstrate improvements in pCR, three large randomized studies in multiple breast cancer subtypes in the adjuvant setting have failed to demonstrate a survival advantage.[127–129] These data demonstrate no role for

bevacizumab at this time in unselected populations in early-stage breast cancer.

In summary, the meaning of pCR for the individual patient who achieves it portends a favorable prognosis in terms of recurrence rates and survival; however, the ability of a drug to improve pCR rates in a population does not necessarily mean that survival will be improved. This is important as we interpret these studies with drugs that have significant potential for adverse events in the curative setting. Clearly, the anticancer potency of the drug under investigation matters, and perhaps the degree of change in pCR rate may also matter. When considering neoadjuvant therapy or extrapolation of neoadjuvant data into the adjuvant setting, a clinician must weigh the potential benefits of agents that do not have a proven survival benefit against the potential toxicity patients may experience.

Selected References

4. Perou CM, et al. Molecular portraits of human breast tumours. *Nature*. 2000;406:747-752.
9. Slamon DJ, et al. Use of chemotherapy plus a monoclonal antibody against HER2 for metastatic breast cancer that overexpresses HER2. *N Engl J Med*. 2001;344:783-792.
39. Rettig RA, et al. *False Hope: Bone Marrow Transplantation for Breast Cancer*. New York: Oxford University Press; 2007.
52. Gluz O, et al. West German Study Group Phase III Plan B Trial: first prospective outcome data for the 21-gene recurrence score assay and concordance of prognostic markers by central and local pathology assessment. *J Clin Oncol*. 2016.
81. Gianni L, et al. Efficacy and safety of neoadjuvant pertuzumab and trastuzumab in women with locally advanced, inflammatory, or early HER2-positive breast cancer (NeoSphere): a randomised multicentre, open-label, phase 2 trial. *Lancet Oncol*. 2012;13:25-32.

A full reference list is available online at ExpertConsult.com.

56

HER2-Positive Breast Cancer

GEORGE W. SLEDGE, JR.

HER2-positive breast cancer, in the course of a decade and a half, has gone from being the most feared to perhaps the most treatable of breast cancers. This sea change resulted from the recognition in the late 1980s that HER2 represented a potent driver of a small (15%–20%) fraction of breast cancers and the subsequent development of molecularly targeted therapies for HER2. The progressive application of these agents, first in the metastatic setting but subsequently in the adjuvant setting, has transformed the disease. Emerging therapies, currently under study in the adjuvant setting, have the potential to largely eliminate HER2 metastatic breast cancer as a public health threat.

This chapter reviews the biology of HER2, followed by a discussion of HER2 as a subject of pathologic analysis. It then discusses the role of HER2-targeted therapies in the adjuvant and metastatic settings and future prospects for HER2-targetd therapies.

HER2 Biology

HER2 (also known as c-erbB2 or *neu*) is an oncogenic driver of breast cancer growth, survival, invasion, and metastasis. A member of the Epidermal Growth Factor Receptor (EGFR) family of transmembrane receptor tyrosine kinases, it differs from other members of the family in that it lacks a functioning ligand-binding domain. The HER2 kinase is primarily activated by dimerization with other members of the HER family, with HER3 representing the preferential dimerization partner, although when HER2 is present in excess quantities, it may dimerize with other HER2 molecules. The tyrosine kinase portion of HER3 is defective, but HER3 is able to bind ligands of the neuregulin family and to transactivate other members of the family. HER2, in contrast, is incapable of ligand binding.[1]

After dimerization, kinase activation occurs and results in numerous downstream effects. These effects include activation of both proliferation and survival pathways, mediated via the PI3K/Akt/mTOR intracellular pathway and the mitogen-activated protein kinase (MAPK) pathway.[1]

In human breast cancer, HER2 pathogenesis occurs preferentially as a result of an amplification of a genomic region containing the HER2 gene on chromosome 17q12. HER2 is a constitutive protein present in organs throughout the body, but in HER2-positive tumors the amplification event results in significantly increased numbers of the HER2 molecule on the cancer cell surface. HER2-positive tumors can be either estrogen positive or estrogen negative, in roughly equal proportions. One consequence of HER2 activation is the downregulation of the estrogen

receptor (ER) via crosstalk with that receptor, and HER2-positivity and ER expression are therefore inversely correlated, rendering HER2-positive tumors relatively less sensitive to estrogen blockade.

Although the vast majority of HER2-driven tumors occur as a result of an amplification event, recent analysis of deep-sequenced primary breast cancers has suggested that a small fraction of these tumors harbor activating somatic mutations in HER2, perhaps in the 1% to 2% range.[2] These tumors are not positive through standard immunohistochemical or in situ hybridization testing, nor do they appear sensitive to standard monoclonal antibody therapies or to lapatinib, although preclinical trials suggest they may be sensitive to other investigational agents (e.g., neratinib), and there are at least anecdotal cases of response in this population.[3]

HER2 Pathology

HER2 amplification can be tested for in several ways. The HER2 cell surface protein may be evaluated by immunohistochemistry (IHC; using a 0, 1+, 2+, 3+ scoring system) or HER2 DNA copy number may be evaluated by fluorescence in situ hybridization (FISH). The American Society of Clinical Oncology (ASCO) and the College of American Pathologists (CAP) have published a joint guideline for the evaluation of HER2 that represent the current standard of care.[4] These guidelines (modified from Wolff and colleagues[4]) are shown in Box 56.1.

Immunohistochemical testing of HER2 has suggested the presence of heterogeneity in anywhere from less than 1% to 30% of tumors, although a carefully performed recent analysis suggests a rate of 5% for FISH. For HER2 testing by in situ hybridization, amplified cells can be present diffusely (the standard pattern) or as a minor population in either intermixed or clustered patterns.[4,5] Although there are limited data to suggest significant differences in outcomes between clustered and intermixed minority HER2 amplified cells, current CAP/ASCO HER2 testing guidelines recommend counting clustered cell populations separately.[4]

A common early problem with HER2 testing involved the lack of concordance seen between local and central laboratories, which occurs even in the hands of expert pathologists. An analysis of samples from three large adjuvant trastuzumab trials revealed 92% concordance among three expert pathologists for both IHC and FISH.[6] It is likely that results are worse in labs that do not routinely test for HER2 or have a pathologist that does not regularly evaluate HER2.

• Box 56.1 **American Society of Clinical Oncology/College of American Pathologists Guidelines for HER2 Testing**

Key Recommendations for Oncologists

- Must request HER2 testing on every primary invasive breast cancer (and on metastatic site, if stage IV and if specimen available) from a patient with breast cancer to guide decision to pursue HER2-targeted therapy. This should be especially considered for a patient who previously tested HER2 negative in a primary tumor and presents with disease recurrence with clinical behavior suggestive of HER2-positive or triple-negative disease.
- Should recommend HER2-targeted therapy if HER2 test result is positive, if there is no apparent histopathologic discordance with HER2 testing, and if clinically appropriate. If the pathologist or oncologist observes an apparent histopathologic discordance after HER2 testing, the need for additional HER2 testing should be discussed.
- Must delay decision to recommend HER2-targeted therapy if initial HER2 test result is equivocal. Reflex testing should be performed on the same specimen using the alternative test if initial HER2 test result is equivocal or on an alternative specimen.
- Must not recommend HER2-targeted therapy if HER2 test result is negative and if there is no apparent histopathologic discordance with HER2 testing. If the pathologist or oncologist observes an apparent histopathologic discordance after HER2 testing, the need for additional HER2 testing should be discussed.
- Should delay decision to recommend HER2-targeted therapy if HER2 status cannot be confirmed as positive or negative after separate HER2 tests (HER2 test result or results equivocal). The oncologist should confer with the pathologist regarding the need for additional HER2 testing on the same or another tumor specimen.
- If the HER2 test result is ultimately deemed to be equivocal, even after reflex testing with an alternative assay (i.e., if neither test is unequivocally positive), the oncologist may consider HER2-targeted therapy. The oncologist should also consider the feasibility of testing another tumor specimen to attempt to definitely establish the tumor HER2 status and guide therapeutic decisions. A clinical decision to ultimately consider HER2-targeted therapy in such cases should be individualized on the basis of patient status (comorbidities, prognosis, and so on) and patient preferences after discussing available clinical evidence.

Key Recommendations for Pathologists

- Must ensure that at least one tumor sample from all patients with breast cancer (early-stage or metastatic disease) is tested for either HER2 protein expression (IHC assay) or HER2 gene expression (ISH assay) using a validated HER2 test.
- In the United States, the American Society of Clinical Oncology/College of American Pathologists Guideline Update Committee preferentially recommends the use of an assay that has received Food and Drug Administration approval, although a CLIA-certified laboratory may choose instead to use a laboratory-developed test.

- Must report HER2 test result as positive if (a) IHC 3+ positive or (b) ISH positive using either a single-probe ISH or dual-probe ISH. This assumes that there is no apparent histopathologic discordance observed by the pathologist.
- Must report HER2 test result as equivocal and order reflex test on the same specimen (unless the pathologist has concerns about the specimen) using the alternative test if (a) IHC 2+ equivocal or (b) ISH equivocal using single-probe ISH or dual-probe ISH. This assumes that there is no apparent histopathologic discordance observed by the pathologist.
- Must report HER2 test result as indeterminate if technical issues prevent one or both tests (IHC and ISH) performed in a tumor specimen from being reported as positive, negative, or equivocal. This may occur if specimen handling was inadequate, if artifacts (crush or edge artifacts) make interpretation difficult, or if the analytic testing failed. Another specimen should be requested for testing, if possible, and a comment should be included in the pathology report documenting intended action.
- Must ensure that interpretation and reporting guidelines for HER2 testing are followed.
- Should interpret bright-field ISH on the basis of a comparison between patterns in normal breast and tumor cells, because artifactual patterns may be seen that are difficult to interpret. If tumor cell pattern is neither normal nor clearly amplified, test should be submitted for expert opinion.
- Should ensure that any specimen used for HER2 testing (cytologic specimens, needle biopsies, or resection specimens) begins the fixation process quickly (time to fixative within 1 hour) and is fixed in 10% neutral buffered formalin for 6 to 72 hours and that routine processing, as well as staining or probing, is performed according to standardized analytically validated protocols.
- Should ensure that the laboratory conforms to standards set for CAP accreditation or an equivalent accreditation authority, including initial test validation, ongoing internal quality assurance, ongoing external proficiency testing, and routine periodic performance monitoring.
- If an apparent histopathologic discordance is observed in any HER2 testing situation, the pathologist should consider ordering additional HER2 testing, conferring with the oncologist, and should document the decision-making process and results in the pathology report. As part of the HER2 testing process, the pathologist may pursue additional HER2 testing without conferring with the oncologist.
- Must report HER2 test result as negative if a single test (or all tests) performed in a tumor specimen show (a) IHC 1+ negative or IHC 0 negative or (b) ISH negative using single-probe ISH or dual-probe ISH.

CLIA, *Clinical Laboratory Improvement Amendments;* IHC, *immunohistochemistry;* ISH, *in situ hybridization.*
Modified from Wolff AC, Hammond ME, Hicks DG, et al. Recommendations for human epidermal growth factor receptor 2 testing in breast cancer: American Society of Clinical Oncology/College of American Pathologists clinical practice guideline update. J Clin Oncol. 2013;31:3997-4013.

HER2-Targeted Therapy

The realization that HER2 represents an important part of breast cancer biology led to the development of specific HER2-targeted therapies. Currently four US Food and Drug Administration–approved agents are in clinical practice in the neoadjuvant, adjuvant, and metastatic settings, and many other agents are currently in development. A listing of current FDA-approved HER2-targeting agents is provided in Table 56.1.

HER2 Metastatic Therapy

HER2-targeted therapy entered the therapeutic armamentarium in 1998 with the results of the pivotal Slamon trial.[7] This trial

randomized women with metastatic, previously untreated disease to either chemotherapy alone or chemotherapy plus trastuzumab. When the trial was initiated in the 1990s, doxorubicin represented the standard of care frontline metastatic chemotherapeutic agent. As the trial progressed, however, the increasing use of anthracyclines in the adjuvant setting, and the advent of taxanes in the metastatic setting, limited accrual of patients receiving frontline metastatic doxorubicin, leading to the amendment of the trial to allow the use of paclitaxel as the chemotherapeutic backbone.

This proved to be exceptionally fortunate, and not merely because of the increasing use of metastatic taxane therapy. Unbeknownst to the trial's investigators, the combination of doxorubicin and trastuzumab resulted in a large cardiotoxicity signal, with

TABLE 56.1	**Current FDA-Approved HER2-Targeting Agents**
Drug	**Indication(s)**
Trastuzumab	Adjuvant (with or after chemotherapy) Neoadjuvant (in combination with trastuzumab and docetaxel) Metastatic (first-line with a taxane; monotherapy after one or more chemotherapy regimens)
Pertuzumab	Neoadjuvant (in combination with trastuzumab and docetaxel) Metastatic (in combination with trastuzumab and docetaxel for frontline therapy)
Ado-trastuzumab emtansine	Metastatic (after prior trastuzumab and a taxane)
Lapatinib	Metastatic (in combination with (1) capecitabine, after prior therapy including an anthracycline, a taxane, and trastuzumab; or (2) letrozole in hormone receptor–positive, HER2-positive postmenopausal women

All indications assume the presence of HER2-positive disease; neoadjuvant pertuzumab represents an accelerated approval. Full label information can be accessed at http://www.fda.gov.

a significant increase in congestive heart failure. Subsequent work suggested that HER2 represents an important prosurvival/antiapoptosis signaling mechanism for cardiac myocytes, and interrupting that signaling in the setting of cardiac stress results in myocyte death and clinical congestive heart failure.[8] This is not, fortunately, an issue of similar concern when combined with taxanes.

Subsequent to the initial approval of trastuzumab for metastatic breast cancer, investigators spent much of the next decade studying secondary questions, including optimal therapeutic partners, treatment past first progression, and the role of HER2-targeted therapy in classically HER2-negative tumors.

To summarize what is now a relatively immense literature, trastuzumab may be combined safely with virtually every nonanthracycline chemotherapeutic agent used for the treatment of breast cancer. There is no convincing evidence that any particular chemotherapeutic "dance partner" is superior to any other, although phase III trials comparing chemotherapy/trastuzumab combinations are notable for their absence from the medical literature. An important exception involves paclitaxel itself, where weekly paclitaxel is superior to the initial every 3-week paclitaxel regimen when combined with trastuzumab.[9]

Roughly half of all HER2-positive patients are also ER positive, leading to the reasonable question of whether HER2-targeted therapy should be combined with ER-targeted therapy in the metastatic setting. This question has been asked in phase III trials with both trastuzumab and lapatinib. For both HER2-targeting agents, phase III trial data suggest that overall response rate and progression-free survival are improved by the addition of HER2-targeted therapy to ER-targeted therapy with an aromatase

inhibitor.[10,11] These trials, however, do not address an important question: is the combination of HER2-targeted therapy with ER-targeted therapy as good as the combination of chemotherapy and HER2-targeted therapy? Although we do not have an answer to this question, for the many patients who are intolerant of or unwilling to accept chemotherapy, the combination of HER2-targeted therapy plus an aromatase inhibitor represents a reasonable therapeutic option.

The question of treatment past first progression long vexed medical oncologists. Given the relative safety of trastuzumab in the metastatic setting, and the continuing presence of HER2 on the cell surface of tumors growing through trastuzumab-based therapy, many inclined to continue trastuzumab-based therapy. The question was not, however, successfully answered in the metastatic setting until von Minckwitz and colleagues compared capecitabine to the combination of capecitabine plus trastuzumab in patients progressing on frontline trastuzumab.[12,13] The combination was statistically superior to capecitabine monotherapy with regard to response rate and progression-free survival and numerically (although not statistically) superior for overall survival.

Trastuzumab was also evaluated in classically HER2-negative metastatic breast cancer. What to call "positive" for HER2 has represented a continuing source of disagreement among medical oncologists and pathologists. If one uses too strict criteria for HER2 positivity, one might well undertreat patients who would benefit from HER2 targeted therapy; in contrast, too loose criteria would result in overtreatment with an expensive (albeit relatively nontoxic) agent. However, in classically HER2-negative metastatic breast cancer, the addition of trastuzumab to paclitaxel failed to improve progression-free or overall survival in a phase III trial.[9] Whether this lesson also holds in the adjuvant setting is currently being studied in a phase III trial being conducted by the NRG cooperative oncology group.

Subsequent to the approval of trastuzumab for patients with metastatic breast cancer, three other HER2-targeting agents have entered routine clinical practice. These include a small molecule receptor tyrosine kinase inhibitor (lapatinib) and two novel HER2-targeting monoclonal antibodies (pertuzumab and T-DM1).

Lapatinib is a small molecule receptor tyrosine kinase inhibitor of HER1 and HER2. Preclinically the combination of lapatinib with trastuzumab was synergistic.[14] Early metastatic trials suggested significant single-agent activity similar to that seen with trastuzumab, as well as the suggestion of a combinatorial benefit.[15,16] A large phase III trial in patients progressing on trastuzumab compared the use of capecitabine alone with the combination of capecitabine and lapatinib in HER2-positive patients and demonstrated a significant improvement in progression-free survival, although ultimately no improvement in overall survival was seen.[17] This result led to the FDA's approval of lapatinib in combination with capecitabine in patients whose tumors had progressed while on trastuzumab-based therapy for metastatic disease. More recently, lapatinib was compared with trastuzumab in a large phase III randomized controlled trial as frontline therapy in the metastatic setting, where it demonstrated therapeutic inferiority.[18]

Pertuzumab is a monoclonal antibody that binds to the external membrane domain of HER2, where it interferes with HER2 dimerization and subsequent activation. Although not exceptionally effective as monotherapy in patients previously treated with trastuzumab, the combination of trastuzumab and pertuzumab showed significant combinatorial activity, and little added toxicity, in the metastatic setting.[19,20] Early phase I/II trial results led to a large phase III randomized controlled trial (the CLEOPATRA—Clinical Evaluation of Pertuzumab and Trastuzumab trial).

CLEOPATRA randomized patients with frontline metastatic breast cancer to receive docetaxel plus trastuzumab or docetaxel plus trastuzumab plus pertuzumab. Patients were eligible if they had not received previous chemotherapy or anti-HER2 therapy for their metastatic disease. The addition of pertuzumab to trastuzumab in this setting was associated with an impressive increase in both progression-free and overall survival. Updated data from this trial suggest that median overall survival was improved from 40.5 months in the control arm to 56.8 months[21] in the combination arm, an impressive increase with important implications for adjuvant trial design.

Although relatively devoid of clinical additive toxicity (in particular, there is no increased rate of congestive heart failure), the combination has significant financial toxicity. A recent cost-benefit analysis of the winning CLEOPATRA regimen suggested that the addition of pertuzumab cost $713,000 per quality-adjusted life year gained, an impressive and discouraging number that puts the combination in the unenviable position of being unaffordable over most of the planet.[22]

T-DM1 represents the other recently FDA-approved agent for metastatic HER2-positive breast cancer. T-DM1/ado-emtansine represents the linkage of trastuzumab to a maytansinoid plant poison, the latter working through its potent antimicrotubule effects. Trastuzumab carries the DM1 to the HER2-positive breast cancer cell, where the linkage is broken intracellularly through lysosomal action. The DM1 is then freed to damage the cancer cell's microtubules.

After initial phase I and II trials demonstrated relative safety and activity in previously treated patients,[23,24] the agent was tested in a phase III randomized controlled trial comparing the agent to the existing standard of capecitabine plus lapatinib.[25] The trial demonstrated that T-DM1 was more active than the combination of capecitabine plus lapatinib, with a median overall of 30.9 months versus 25.1 months. This benefit also combined with significantly less toxicity, leading to the FDA approval of T-DM1 and its rapid incorporation into standard practice in previously treated patients.

Subsequently, the combination of T-DM1 with pertuzumab has been compared with the combination of a taxanes plus trastuzumab for first-line metastatic breast cancer (the MARIANNE study; A Study of Trastuzumab Emtansine [T-DM1] Plus Pertuzumab/Pertuzumab Placebo Versus Trastuzumab [Herceptin] Plus a Taxane in Patients With Metastatic Breast Cancer). Regrettably, this combination did not prove superior to the standard taxanes + trastuzumab combination.[26]

Taken together, these trials suggest a strategy in the metastatic HER2-POSITIVE-positive stating in which patients initial receive the combination of a taxane with pertuzumab and trastuzumab (per the CLEOPATRA trial) followed by T-DM1. After T-DM1, things become murkier, with options including the lapatinib/capecitabine combination, the combination of a taxane with a nontaxane chemotherapeutic, or the combination of lapatinib and trastuzumab. No sufficiently well-sized studies exist to demonstrate the best path forward in such relatively refractory populations nor whether such combinations prolong survival in patients who have received prior pertuzumab or T-DM1.

Of note, it is worth mentioning that patients should be retested for HER2 expression at the time of development of metastatic disease. As reviewed by Penault-Llorca and coworkers, discordance for HER2 is approximately 8% to 10%, with HER2 gain (as measured by FISH) being more common than HER2 loss.[27]

Recent work in the clinic has focused on mechanisms of resistance to HER2 and their possible therapeutic implications. Preclinical data suggested that aberrant activation of the PI3K/Akt/mTOR intracellular signaling pathway (through loss of PTEN or mutations in PIK3CA, the catalytic subunit of PI3K) resulted in resistance to trastuzumab. This recognition led to the use of mTOR inhibitors as a therapeutic strategy. Everolimus, previously approved for use in ER-positive breast cancer, was examined in two separate phase III trials (BOLERO-1 and BOLERO-3, Breast Cancer Trials of OraL EveROlimus). In the former, patients were randomized to receive either 10 mg everolimus once a day orally or placebo plus weekly trastuzumab as frontline therapy.[28] For the overall group, progression-free survival was not significantly improved, although in the hormone receptor–negative, HER2-positive subpopulation, progression-free survival was improved by 7 months, a finding that should be considered exploratory and hypothesis generating. In the latter trial, patients with prior trastuzumab exposure were randomized to receive daily everolimus (5 mg/day) plus weekly trastuzumab (2 mg/kg) and vinorelbine (25 mg/m^2) or to placebo plus trastuzumab plus vinorelbine, in 3-week cycles.[29] Median PFS was 7 months with everolimus and 5.78 months with placebo (hazard ratio 0.78, $p = .0067$). In both studies, everolimus produced side effects similar to those seen in patients treated in the ER-positive setting.

HER2 Adjuvant Therapy

After the initial results of randomized controlled trials of HER2-targeted therapies, trials aimed at the treatment of micrometastatic disease were initiated. Several of these trials came to completion in 2005 and transformed the care of patients with early-stage HER2-positive disease.

Four large (and several smaller) adjuvant trials represented the first wave of therapy for micrometastatic disease. Collectively these trials approached the large question of whether HER2-targeted therapy improved overall therapeutic outcome in early-stage HER2-positive disease, although each trial asked this question in different ways, offering us a mosaic of findings.

With regard to the important question of whether HER2-targeted therapy improved outcome in HER2-targeted disease, the unequivocal answer was a resounding "yes." In each of the large trials, trastuzumab-based adjuvant chemotherapy significantly, even dramatically, improved disease-free survival, and subsequent follow-up from these trials has demonstrated an improvement in overall survival.[30–32] Long-term follow-up of the joint analysis of the National Surgical Adjuvant Breast and Bowel Project (NSABP) and North Central Cancer Treatment Group (NCCTG) trials has demonstrated that the initial benefit seen with adjuvant trastuzumab persists for at least a decade, with an improvement in 10-year overall survival from 75.2% to 84%.[33]

These benefits were seen whether trastuzumab was given in combination with chemotherapy (as was performed in the NSABP, NCCTG, and Breast Cancer International Research Group (BCIRG) trials or when given subsequent to adjuvant chemotherapy, as was performed in the HERA trial.[32] Whether trastuzumab is best given in combination with or after chemotherapy remains an open question. The NCCTG adjuvant trial performed a randomization of combination versus sequence as part of the larger trial, and although underpowered, the results suggest that combination may be superior to sequence.[34]

Similarly, the BCIRG-006 trial examined the role of anthracycline-based versus platinum-based chemotherapy. With regard to efficacy, both trials were compared with a nontrastuzumab-based control group, and the results are underpowered to demonstrate a difference, although the anthracycline-based arm is numerically but not statistically better. From a toxicity standpoint, the anthracycline-based arm has a slightly larger number of cardiac events (primarily congestive heart failure and ejection fraction decline), as would be suspected, although this did not translate to an increase in cardiac deaths. Both approaches have impassioned supporters.

Collectively the first generation of large adjuvant trials demonstrated that adjuvant trastuzumab could be given safely and could improve both disease-free and overall survival. Based on these results, adjuvant trastuzumab rapidly entered the oncologist's therapeutic portfolio and represents the appropriate standard of care on a global basis for patients with early-stage HER2-positive breast cancer.

Although this was accepted early on by physicians and regulatory authorities, several remaining questions were not answered by the initial suite of studies and, in some cases, remain unanswered today. These are discussed in the following sections.

Duration of Adjuvant Trastuzumab

The four large randomized trials all used a year's worth of trastuzumab, for totally arbitrary reasons. At the same time, the smaller Finland Herceptin (FinnHER) trial suggested that a relatively short course of adjuvant trastuzumab could be as beneficial as a year of therapy. Subsequent adjuvant trials, and longer follow-up of the initial HERceptin Adjuvant (HERA) trial, have compared the 1-year standard to either shorter (6 months) or longer (2 years) periods of therapy with adjuvant trastuzumab. Analysis of these trials suggests that 6 months is inferior to, and 2 years no different from, a year of adjuvant trastuzumab, which remains the standard of care.[35,36]

Predictors of Response to Adjuvant Trastuzumab

Because the initial large randomized trials all collected tissue specimens for subsequent analysis, several studies have been performed evaluating prediction of benefit or—the other side of the coin—resistance. In general, these analyses have proven frustrating or inconclusive, often due to lack of statistical power and other methodologic issues.

Recent data have suggested that the immune system may play an important role in trastuzumab's adjuvant efficacy. An analysis of tumor specimens collected in the NCCTG-9832 trial demonstrated that patients whose cancers expressed an immune signature were significantly more likely to receive adjuvant benefit.[37]

Although this marker of benefit is extremely interesting and may explain the lesser benefit of small molecule receptor tyrosine kinase inhibitors seen in the metastatic and adjuvant settings, it is not sufficiently advanced in development to recommend its routine use as a therapeutic biomarker.

Role of HER2 Variants

Although the initial suite of trials all required that patients be called HER2-positive (by either IHC or FISH), testing was performed both locally and centrally, allowing for exploration of several different issues. Again, in all of these analyses, the statistical powering was poor, leading to legitimate concerns over the results.

Some breast cancers demonstrate heterogeneity for HER2 expression, and analyses of these tumors suggested that tumors with foci of HER2-positive cells received adjuvant benefit similar to that seen with tumors that were relatively more homogenous.

Similarly, in cases where a tumor was called positive for HER2 based on local analysis but where subsequent central analysis suggested that the patient was not HER2-positive by standard criteria (e.g., a FISH ratio <2), patients still appeared to receive benefit from adjuvant trastuzumab. Although one possible explanation for these results is simple pathologic misclassification due to sampling error or misreading, the interest in and potential importance of this question led to the development of a large adjuvant trastuzumab trial (NSABP B-47) in patients with lesser HER2 expression (IHC 1–2+).

Role of Adjuvant Trastuzumab in Small, Lymph Node–Negative Tumors

The initial HER2 adjuvant trials were largely performed in patients with either larger or lymph node-positive tumors. As such, they left unanswered an important question: how low should one go with HER2-targetd adjuvant therapy? Numerous retrospective analyses have suggested that HER2 positivity increases risk of recurrence in smaller node-negative tumors. Given the relative safety of HER2-targeted therapy, should patients with smaller (<2 cm), lymph node–negative patients receive adjuvant trastuzumab?

Although no randomized controlled trials exist to answer this question definitively, Tolaney and colleagues performed a large registration trial in 406 patients with lymph node negative tumors up to 3 cm in size.[38] Patients received weekly treatment with paclitaxel (80 mg per square meter of body surface area) and trastuzumab for 12 weeks, followed by 9 additional months of every-3-week trastuzumab. The 3-year survival free from invasive disease was 98.7%, with only two distant metastases among the 12 recurring tumors. Relatively few (18.9%) patients entered in this trial had T1a (≤0.5 cm) tumors, rendering conclusions about this low-risk group uncertain. Nevertheless, the results reported support the use of adjuvant trastuzumab in combination with paclitaxel in small, node-negative HER2-positive cancers.

Future Directions in HER2-Targeted Therapy

Subsequent to the success of the initial wave of adjuvant trastuzumab trials, several adjuvant trials have explored the role of other HER2-targeted therapy, and results from these trials are now beginning to emerge.

First up for evaluation were small molecule receptor tyrosine kinase inhibitors such as lapatinib and neratinib. Lapatinib is an FDA-approved agent in the metastatic HER2-positive setting, and preclinical data suggested that it would be synergistic when combined with trastuzumab. This led to the development of the large, international Adjuvant Lapatinib And/Or Trastuzumab Treatment Optimisation (ALTTO) trial, which randomized patients to either a trastuzumab-based control arm (in which patients could receive HER2-targeted therapy in sequence after or in combination with chemotherapy) or to a lapatinib alone arm, an arm that combined trastuzumab with lapatinib, or in a final arm in which patients received trastuzumab and lapatinib in sequence. The results of this trial suggest that none of the experimental arms is obviously superior to the control trastuzumab-alone arm.[38a]

Neratinib is a small molecule inhibitor of HER2 developed subsequent to lapatinib. In the adjuvant setting, it was investigated in a randomized controlled phase III trial in which patients were randomized either to trastuzumab alone or to trastuzumab (administered for 1 year) followed by a year of neratinib. Initial results from this trial, presented in abstract form, have suggested a small but statistically significant improvement in disease-free survival favoring patients receiving late adjuvant neratinib, albeit with significant associated toxicity and with limited follow-up.[39]

More recent adjuvant trials have focused on novel antibody-based therapies. Pertuzumab and T-DM1 (discussed earlier in the metastatic therapy section) have entered large adjuvant randomized controlled therapeutic trials, with eagerly anticipated results. The Breast International Group's APHINITY (A Study of Pertuzumab in Addition to Chemotherapy and Herceptin [Trastuzumab] as Adjuvant Therapy in Patients With HER2-Positive Primary Breast Cancer) trial directly tests the role of pertuzumab in the adjuvant setting. Similarly, the KATHERINE (A Study of Trastuzumab Emtansine Versus Trastuzumab as Adjuvant Therapy in Patients With HER2-Positive Breast Cancer Who Have Residual Tumor in the Breast or Axillary Lymph Nodes Following Preoperative Therapy) and KAITLIN (A Study of Kadcyla [Trastuzumab Emtansine] Plus Perjeta [Pertuzumab] Following Anthracyclines in Comparison With Herceptin [Trastuzumab] Plus Perjeta and a Taxane Following Anthracyclines as Adjuvant Therapy in Patients With Operable HER2-Positive Primary Breast Cancer) trials are currently examining the role of T-DM1 in the adjuvant setting.

Of note, neoadjuvant trials with pertuzumab (administered in combination with trastuzumab and chemotherapy) have been performed in the preoperative/neoadjuvant setting. The Neo-Sphere (Neoadjuvant Study of Pertuzumab and Herceptin in an Early Regimen Evaluation) trial (a large, four-arm randomized phase II trial) showed a pathologic complete response rate of 45.8% in patients treated with docetaxel, pertuzumab, and trastuzumab, superior to the 29% pCR rate seen with trastuzumab and docetaxel.[40] These results, combined with the overall survival advantage seen in the metastatic setting with the addition of pertuzumab, led the FDA to approve the use of pertuzumab in the neoadjuvant setting. The National Cancer Comprehensive Network guidelines committee, in turn, extrapolated these results to the adjuvant setting.

Based on preclinical data suggesting that HER2-positive tumors overexpress Vascular Endothelial Growth Factor (VEGF), and that coinhibition of HER2 and VEGF had beneficial results in preclinical models, two phase III trials combining trastuzumab and bevacizumab in combination with chemotherapy were performed. These trials (AVEREL and BETH, Bevacizumab with Trastuzumab Adjuvant Therapy in HER2 + Breast Cancer) failed to demonstrate benefit for the addition of bevacizumab.[41,42]

As mentioned earlier, a small fraction of breast cancer patients lacking classic HER2 positivity (i.e., lacking an amplification event measurable by IHC or FISH) will have a somatic mutation for HER2 that is capable of serving as an oncogenic driver.[2] Clinical trials are currently underway evaluating the role of the small molecule receptor tyrosine kinase inhibitors, such as neratinib, as treatment for metastatic breast cancer in this population.[3]

Numerous other novel strategies are in the process of being evaluated in clinical trials. These include novel monoclonal antibodies with improved effector function (e.g., margetuximab; MGAH22),[43] novel tyrosine kinase inhibitors (e.g., afatinib),[44,45] and combinations with immune modulators of T-cell and natural killer–cell function (e.g., anti-PD-1 anti-CD137 monoclonal antibodies).[46] The coming years should see important changes in our ability to target this previously dreaded subset of breast cancer. It is reasonable to suggest that, in the not too distant future, HER2-positive breast cancer may cease to be an important public health issue.

Selected References

4. Wolff AC, Hammond ME, Hicks DG, et al. Recommendations for human epidermal growth factor receptor 2 testing in breast cancer: American Society of Clinical Oncology/College of American Pathologists clinical practice guideline update. *J Clin Oncol.* 2013;31:3997-4013.

7. Slamon DJ, Leyland-Jones B, Shak S, et al. Use of chemotherapy plus a monoclonal antibody against HER2 for metastatic breast cancer that overexpresses HER2. *N Engl J Med.* 2001;344:783-792.

21. Swain SM, Baselga J, Kim SB, et al. Pertuzumab, trastuzumab, and docetaxel in HER2-positive metastatic breast cancer. *N Engl J Med.* 2015;372:724-734.

33. Perez EA, Romond EH, Suman VJ, et al. Trastuzumab plus adjuvant chemotherapy for human epidermal growth factor receptor 2-positive breast cancer: planned joint analysis of overall survival from NSABP B-31 and NCCTG N9831. *J Clin Oncol.* 2014;32:3744-3752.

38. Tolaney SM, Barry WT, Dang CT, et al. Adjuvant paclitaxel and trastuzumab for node-negative, HER2-positive breast cancer. *N Engl J Med.* 2015;372:134-141.

A full reference list is available online at ExpertConsult.com.

57

Bisphosphonates in Early Breast Cancer

AJU MATHEW AND ADAM BRUFSKY

Bisphosphonates inhibit osteoclast-mediated bone resorption. As a result, bisphosphonates have several therapeutic roles. Primarily, they were used as an antiosteoporosis medications. Later these drugs were used to prevent or delay skeletal-related events such as fractures and bone pain in patients with metastatic cancers with disease in bones. Bisphosphonates are also used to prevent bone loss associated with aromatase inhibitors, which are used for adjuvant management of breast cancer in postmenopausal women and result in bone loss and hastened osteoporosis. Therefore in breast oncology, bisphosphonates are important supportive care medications in two indications: prevent or delay skeletal-related events in metastatic breast cancer involving bones, and prevent or treat aromatase inhibitor-induced bone loss.[1]

Bone is the commonest site of distant metastatic disease in breast cancer.[2] Tumor microenvironment plays an important role in cancer proliferation. Bisphosphonates alter the bone microenvironment and may have an anticancer effect.[3] Backed by preclinical studies that showed such an effect, secondary analyses of several adjuvant bisphosphonate clinical trials were conducted. In this chapter, we summarize these clinical trials (Table 57.1) and discuss the findings of an individual patient-level data meta-analysis aimed to evaluate the anticancer role of adjuvant bisphosphonates.

Bisphosphonates: Mechanism of Action

Bisphosphonates are pyrophosphate analogs that bind to bone hydroxyapatite.[4] Bone remodeling is mediated by osteoblasts and osteoclasts: the former ensure bone formation and the latter ensure bone resorption. In normal bone, the remodeling process works in equilibrium. Bone metastasis results in secretion of cytokines from cancer cells, which leads to a disproportionate activation of osteoclasts and a disruption in the osteoblast-osteoclast equilibrium. Bisphosphonates are internalized by osteoclasts and cause apoptosis of these bone-resorptive cells.

Types of Bisphosphonates

There are two types of bisphosphonates: aminobisphosphonates contain a nitrogen atom, and nonaminobisphosphonates do not contain the nitrogen atom.
- Aminobisphosphonates (*N*-containing) include alendronic acid (alendronate; oral), pamidronate (intravenous), risedronate (oral), ibandronate (oral and intravenous), and zoledronate (intravenous). The antiapoptotic effect is mediated by inhibition of farnesyl pyrophosphate synthase enzyme in the mevalonic acid pathway of cholesterol synthesis. Protein prenylation (posttranslational modification of GTP-binding proteins) is inhibited, resulting in apoptosis of osteoclasts.[5,6]
- Nonaminobisphosphonates (non-*N*-containing) include clodronate (oral and intravenous) and etidronate (oral). These are metabolized into hydrolysis-resistant analogs of adenosine triphosphate in the osteoclasts and cause apoptosis.

Rationale for an Anticancer Effect for Bisphosphonates

Breast cancer is a systemic disease, rather than a local problem. Patients with a distant site of metastatic breast cancer are thought to have had the disease from the time of initial diagnosis of primary breast cancer. The aim of adjuvant treatment using chemotherapy or hormonal agents is to kill cancer cells that may be hiding in a distant site, such as bone. Osteoclasts, immune cells, and stromal cells secrete cytokines and various growth factors, which in turn stimulate further production of osteoclasts. Bisphosphonates break this vicious cycle of osteoclast production in the bone.[7] By inhibiting osteoclasts, bisphosphonates produce a bone microenvironment that is less conducive for tumor cell adhesion, proliferation, and metastases. Apart from the effect on bone microenvironment, bisphosphonates may also have direct antitumor effects, such as impaired adhesion, inhibition of migration, induction of apoptosis, and inhibition of angiogenesis.[8] These direct and indirect effects of bisphosphonates on the tumor cell may help prevent or delay the incidence of bone metastases and improve breast cancer–related outcomes.

Clinical Trials on Adjuvant Bisphosphonates in Breast Cancer

Trials Using Clodronate

A study reported in 1998 randomized patients with primary breast cancer and tumor cells in bone marrow (n = 302) to clodronate for 2 years or observation (63% of participants were postmenopausal).[9] After 3 years of follow-up, incidence of distant metastases in the treatment arm was 13% compared with 29% in the observation group (*p* < .001). In contrast, Powles and coworkers reported in 2002 that in a trial of patients with early-stage breast cancer in which 60% of participants were hormone receptor–positive and 50% were postmenopausal, the use of clodronate did not result in decreased incidence of bone recurrence

TABLE 57.1 Adjuvant Bisphosphonate Trials in Early-Stage Breast Cancer

Study Details	Study Population	Study Arms	Primary End Point	Conclusions
Clodronate 1600 mg PO				
Diel et al.[9] 1998	Pre and postmenopausal (n = 302)[a]	Clodronate vs. standard care for 2 y	Incidence of distant metastasis	At 3 y of follow-up, distant metastases rate was 13% in clodronate group vs. 29% in control group (p < .001)
Powles et al.[10] 2002	Pre and postmenopausal (n = 1069)	Clodronate vs. placebo for 2 y	Incidence of bone metastasis	At 6-y follow-up, there was no difference in bone metastasis rates between the two groups
Saarto et al.[11] 2004	Pre and postmenopausal[b] (n = 299)	Clodronate vs. standard care for 3 y	Not specified	At 10-y follow-up, disease-free survival was lower in clodronate group vs. control (p = .01)
Paterson et al.[12] 2012 NSABP B-34 trial	Pre- and postmenopausal (n = 3323)	Clodronate vs. placebo for 3 y	DFS	At 7.5-y follow-up, there was no difference in DFS between two groups; subgroup analyses found benefit in older patients (≥50 y) with the secondary end points such as DFS and bone metastasis–free interval favoring clodronate arm of the study
Ibandronate 50 mg PO				
Von Minckwitz et al.[13] 2013 GAIN study	Pre- and postmenopausal (n = 2994)[c]	Ibandronate vs. standard care for 2 y	DFS	At 3-y follow-up, there was no difference in DFS between two groups
Zoledronate 4 mg IV				
Gnant et al.[14] 2015 ABCSG-12 study	Premenopausal (n = 1803)[d]	Zoledronate vs. standard care for 3 y	DFS	Final analysis after 8-y follow-up, showed improvement in DFS with the use of zoledronate (p = .042). These results were statistically significant at 5-y follow-up as well
Brufsky et al.[15] 2012 Z-FAST trial	Postmenopausal (n = 602)	Zoledronate: upfront vs. delayed for 5 y[e]	BMD[f]	At 5-y follow-up, disease recurrence or death rates were similar between the upfront vs. delayed groups (9.8% vs. 10.5%; p = .63)[g]
Coleman et al.[16] 2013 ZO-FAST trial	Postmenopausal (n = 1065)	Zoledronate: upfront vs. delayed for 5 y[e]	BMD[f]	At 5-y follow-up, upfront group had a decrease in incidence of DFS events vs. delayed zoledronate group (p = .0375)
Coleman et al.[17] 2014 AZURE trial	Pre- and postmenopausal (n = 3360)[h]	Zoledronate vs. standard care for 5 y[i]	DFS	At 5 y, there was no difference in DFS between the two groups (p = .30); zoledronate reduced the incidence of bone metastases and improved DFS in postmenopausal women

BMD, Bone mineral density; *DFS,* disease-free survival; *PO,* oral administration.

[a]All patients had tumor cells in bone marrow.
[b]Approximately 50% of patients received adjuvant chemotherapy.
[c]All patients received adjuvant chemotherapy.
[d]All patients received goserelin to suppress ovarian function, approximately 5% of patients received adjuvant chemotherapy.
[e]Delayed therapy was initiated when patient become osteopenic or develops pathologic fracture or has an asymptomatic vertebral fracture.
[f]Change in lumbar spine BMD, DFS was secondary end point.
[g]Approximately 25% of patients in the delayed group received zoledronate by 5 years.
[h]Approximately 95% patients received chemotherapy.
[i]Zoledronate 4 mg intravenous was given every 3 to 4 weeks for six cycles, then every 3 months for eight doses, followed by every 6 months for five cycles.

(hazard ratio [HR] 0.77; 95% confidence interval [CI] 0.56–1.08; $p = .1$)[10]; however, fewer deaths occurred in the group of patients who received clodronate ($p = .047$). A separate trial conducted in Finland also did not identify a decrease in incidence of bone metastases with the use of clodronate.[11] Finally, the National Surgical Adjuvant Breast and Bowel Project (NSABP) group conducted the NSABP B-34 trial to investigate the use of clodronate in improving disease-free survival in early breast cancer.[12] Their 2012 findings indicated that after 7.5 years (median) of follow-up, the study did not identify a survival benefit for the drug. However, a prespecified analysis in patients older than 50 years identified improvement in recurrence-free interval and bone metastasis-free interval with the use of clodronate.

Trials Using Ibandronate

The German Adjuvant Intergroup Node-positive (GAIN) study was a phase III 2 × 2 factorial design trial in node-positive women with early breast cancer (17% were older than 60 years of age) in which patients were randomized to either oral ibandronate for 2 years or observation.[13] The results were that the trial did not detect a significant difference in disease-free survival.

Trials Using Zoledronate

The Austrian Breast and Colorectal Cancer Study Group (ABCSG-12) study, published in 2012, was a 2 × 2 factorial trial in premenopausal women with hormone receptor–positive early-stage breast cancer. All patients received ovarian suppression using goserelin[14] and were randomized to tamoxifen or anastrozole in combination with either zoledronate 4 mg intravenously every 6 months for 3 years or observation. Only 5% of the study population received adjuvant chemotherapy. After a median follow-up of 5 years, zoledronate reduced the risk of recurrence (HR 0.68, 95% CI 0.51–0.91; $p = .009$) and noted a nonsignificant trend to an improvement in overall survival ($p = .09$).

The Z-FAST and ZO-FAST trials[15,16] investigated the use of adjuvant zoledronate in postmenopausal women with early-stage breast cancer receiving aromatase inhibitors. Patients were randomized to receive zoledronate 4 mg intravenously every 6 months either upfront for 5 years, from the beginning of adjuvant antiestrogen therapy or in a delayed manner, initiated after the incidence of osteopenia, pathologic fracture, or asymptomatic vertebral fracture. Approximately one-fourth of participants in the Z-FAST and ZO-FAST delayed groups eventually received zoledronate. After 5 years of follow-up, there was no difference in disease-free survival rates between the two groups in the Z-FAST trial.[15] In the ZO-FAST trial, there was significant improvement in disease-free survival rates for patients receiving zoledronate upfront versus in a delayed manner (HR 0.66; 95% CI 0.44–0.97; $p = .037$).[16] This beneficial effect for zoledronate was more pronounced on an exploratory analysis based on menopausal status at study entry, favoring older versus younger women.

The AZURE (BIG 01/04) phase III trial in women with stage II or III breast cancer investigated adjuvant zoledronate in combination with standard adjuvant systemic therapy versus standard therapy alone.[17] Zoledronate 4 mg dose was administered every 3 to 4 weeks for 6 doses, followed by every 3 months for 8 doses, followed by every 6 months for five cycles over 5 years. Forty-four of the study participants were premenopausal at study entry. Ninety-five percent of study participants received chemotherapy.

After 7 years of follow-up, there was no difference in disease-free survival rates between the two groups (HR 0.94, 95% CI 0.82–1.06; $p = .30$). In a prespecified subgroup analysis based on menopausal status, zoledronate improved invasive disease-free survival and bone metastases rates in women who were postmenopausal.

Based on the results of the ABCSG-12, ZO-FAST, and the AZURE trials, patients who were menopausal (induced by goserelin or naturally) benefitted from adjuvant zoledronate therapy. Taken together with the results of the NSABP B-34 and the GAIN trials, bisphosphonates appear to improve the standard of care therapy in women who were in a low estrogen state, that is, postmenopausal women and premenopausal women who undergo suppression of ovarian function.

Individual Patient-Level Data Meta-Analysis

In 2015 the Early Breast Cancer Trialists' Collaborative Group (EBCTCG) conducted an individual patient-level data meta-analysis of the various adjuvant bisphosphonate trials. The meta-analysis pooled data from 18,766 women with early-stage breast cancer who were treated with bisphosphonates.[18] There were borderline significant reductions with the use of bisphosphonates for distant recurrence, bone recurrence, breast cancer mortality, and all-cause mortality. On a subgroup analysis based on menopausal status, no benefit was seen in premenopausal women. In postmenopausal women, there were fewer bone recurrences at 10 years with the addition of bisphosphonates (6.6% vs. 8/8%, rate ratio [RR] = 0.72, 95% CI 0.60–0.86; $p = .0002$). The meta-analysis noted a significant improvement in breast cancer mortality with the addition of bisphosphonates (14.7% vs. 18.0%, RR = 0.82, 95% CI 0.73–0.93; $p = .002$). This benefit was independent of the type of bisphosphonate used, administration schedule, hormone receptor expression, nodal status, and use of adjuvant chemotherapy. There was no impact on the rate of visceral metastases, incidence of contralateral breast cancer or non–breast cancer mortality. In addition, bisphosphonates also reduced the risk of fracture (RR = 0.85, 0.75–0.97; $p = .02$).

Rationale for Bisphosphonate Benefit in Postmenopausal Women

Why would bisphosphonates protect the bones from developing metastasis in postmenopausal women but not in premenopausal women? In a well-conducted experiment designed to understand the interaction between reproductive hormones and bisphosphonates, it was observed that ovariectomized mice injected with disseminated MDA-231 breast cancer cells and treated with zoledronate had fewer detectable bone tumors than similarly treated sham-operated mice.[19] Zoledronate may be altering the bone microenvironment more effectively in ovariectomized mice (induced menopausal state). Another study investigated the prognostic effect of pyridinoline crosslinked carboxyterminal telopeptide of type I collagen (1CTP), a bone turnover marker, in women with primary breast cancer.[20] High levels of serum 1CTP were associated with poor prognosis only in postmenopausal women. The differential effect for bisphosphonates on development of bone metastasis may be related to the interactions among reproductive hormone levels (estradiol, inhibin, and activin), bone resorption rates, and alteration of bone microenvironment. Therefore there is a strong biological plausibility for the significant benefit of adjuvant bisphosphonates in early-stage breast cancer observed only in postmenopausal women (natural or induced) and not in premenopausal women.

Safety of Adjuvant Bisphosphonates

The major side effects for bisphosphonates are fever, infusion reactions, and bone pain. Rarely, patients may have gastrointestinal side effects with the use of oral clodronate or alendronate. There are rare reports of hypocalcemia, although it can be prevented with the use of supplemental calcium and vitamin D. There was no significant risk for renal dysfunction in the adjuvant trials. However, recommendations for bisphosphonate use in the setting of baseline renal dysfunction should be followed. Avoid bisphosphonate therapy if creatinine clearance is less than 30 mL/minute. In terms of the risk for osteonecrosis of the jaw, a pooled analysis of the zoledronate trials estimated the incidence at 1%.[21] Most cases of osteonecrosis of the jaw can be managed conservatively and could also be prevented with appropriate preventive dentistry. The adjuvant trials did not show an increase in atypical femur fractures, likely related to the shorter duration of use in this setting compared with its use in osteoporosis. Overall, bisphosphonates are well tolerated and safe for use in the adjuvant treatment of breast cancer.

When to Consider Adjuvant Bisphosphonates

Clearly, bisphosphonates have a significant benefit in early-stage breast cancer, but should all patients receive bisphosphonates? Which bisphosphonate should be used, and how? All postmenopausal women (natural or induced) on antiestrogen therapy should be considered for adjuvant bisphosphonate treatment. Patients who are on aromatase inhibitors and have baseline osteopenia or osteoporosis will potentially get double benefit from bisphosphonates—prevention of aromatase inhibitor induced-bone loss and the anticancer effect as described in this chapter. Patients who have normal bone mineral density at baseline should be counseled on the benefit of adjuvant bisphosphonates, which is small but significant and reflects a similar absolute risk reduction obtained with the use of polychemotherapy, and on the side

effects. It should certainly be strongly considered in women who have a higher risk for recurrence, such as those with node-positive disease. Based on the results of EBCTCG meta-analysis, a potent bisphosphonate such as zoledronate or clodronate (not available in the United States) could be considered. With regard to the dosing schedule, we recommend using the schedule described in the ABCSG-12 trial rather than the more intensive schedule used in the AZURE trial. As for duration of therapy, we recommend treating with zoledronate 4 mg intravenously every 6 monthly for at least 2 to 3 years.

Conclusions

Adjuvant bisphosphonate treatment has a beneficial role in reducing bone recurrence and breast cancer–related death in postmenopausal women, either naturally or induced through oophorectomy or ovarian suppression. The decision to treat early-stage breast cancer patients with adjuvant bisphosphonates should be individualized, as is the case in most areas of oncology.

Selected References

1. Mathew A, Brufsky A. Bisphosphonates in breast cancer. *Int J Cancer.* 2015;137:753-764.
14. Gnant M, Mlineritsch B, Stoeger H, et al. Zoledronic acid combined with adjuvant endocrine therapy of tamoxifen versus anastrozol plus ovarian function suppression in premenopausal early breast cancer: final analysis of the Austrian Breast and Colorectal Cancer Study Group Trial 12. *Ann Oncol.* 2015;26:313-320.
15. Brufsky AM, Harker WG, Beck JT, et al. Final 5-year results of Z-FAST trial: adjuvant zoledronic acid maintains bone mass in postmenopausal breast cancer patients receiving letrozole. *Cancer.* 2012;118:1192-1201.
17. Coleman R, Cameron D, Dodwell D, et al. Adjuvant zoledronic acid in patients with early breast cancer: final efficacy analysis of the AZURE (BIG 01/04) randomised open-label phase 3 trial. *Lancet Oncol.* 2014;15:997-1006.
21. Saad F, Brown JE, Van Poznak C, et al. Incidence, risk factors, and outcomes of osteonecrosis of the jaw: integrated analysis from three blinded active-controlled phase III trials in cancer patients with bone metastases. *Ann Oncol.* 2012;23:1341-1347.

A full reference list is available online at ExpertConsult.com.

58

Oncofertility Options for Young Women With Breast Cancer

LINDSAY F. PETERSEN,[a] MOLLY MORAVEK,[a] TERESA K. WOODRUFF, AND JACQUELINE S. JERUSS

Breast cancer is the most common cancer diagnosed in women in the United States.[1] Approximately 12% of breast cancers are diagnosed in women younger than 44 years of age.[2] The 5-year relative survival rate for early-stage breast cancer is approximately 98%,[3] yet younger women, diagnosed before age 40, have a 5-year relative survival rate closer to 85%.[4] Emerging treatments for breast cancer continue to result in improved outcomes, although some of these successful therapies have comorbidities, including long-term effects on the ovaries, resulting in premature ovarian failure and reduced fertility.[5] The concept of fertility preservation, or oncofertility, was first proposed with the goal of improving posttreatment reproductive outcomes for young patients diagnosed with cancer.[6] The interdisciplinary Oncofertility Consortium of physicians and scientists was consequently created and supported by the National Institute of Health. Currently, several societies including the American Society of Clinical Oncology (ASCO), the American Society of Reproductive Medicine (ASRM), and the National Comprehensive Cancer Network (NCCN) have guidelines advocating for counseling of young cancer patients regarding fertility preservation before the initiation of treatment.[7–9] Understanding ovarian biology in the context of a cancer diagnosis in young women and the existing and emerging options to protect hormonal and reproductive health is of importance to the patients and is reviewed in this chapter.

Oogenesis and Assessing Ovarian Reserve

Oogenesis

Although controversial, it is widely believed that women are born with a predetermined number of oocytes that do not have the ability to regenerate. The maximum number of oocytes, approximately 6 to 7 million, is observed in utero at 16 to 20 weeks' gestational age.[10] Throughout a woman's life span, oocyte numbers decline, secondary to atresia and degeneration, with approximately 1 million oocytes remaining at birth, 300,000 to 500,000 at puberty, and less than 1000 at menopause.[10–11] Throughout the reproductive years, oocytes mature, and ovulation occurs under the regulation of the hypothalamic-pituitary-ovarian axis. Supporting cells surrounding the oocytes respond to the pituitary

gonadotropins, follicle stimulating hormone (FSH) and luteinizing hormone (LH), leading to oocyte development and steroid hormone secretion that contributes to bone and other systemic organ health.

Each month, selected follicles develop, although most do not reach full maturity. Pituitary FSH stimulates a single follicle to outcompete the other developing follicles, and it becomes the dominant, rapidly growing structure. As the follicle grows, it produces increasing amounts of estradiol, which triggers a surge in LH. This hormone causes the breakdown of the follicle and the release of a now mature egg. This process is known as ovulation. If the oocyte is fertilized by sperm and successfully implants into the endometrium (the inner lining of the uterus), a pregnancy will result. Approximately 400 eggs will be ovulated during the reproductive life span of an individual, and the remaining follicles undergo apoptosis. It is both the rapidly dividing cells of the follicle and the oocytes that are damaged by chemotherapy and radiation. This fundamental description of follicle biology is important to convey to young women and their families.

Assessing Ovarian Reserve

Although the ovarian reserve is approximately 400,000 follicles, there are large differences in the rate of decline and starting number in the general population. Indeed some women will enter menopause 10 years earlier than the population-based average of 51.5 years, and others will have menses into their late 50s. We do not have a marker of the small "primordial" follicles that remain arrested in the outer cortex of the ovary and so have difficulty providing a personalized estimate even for healthy women. In the cancer setting, the number of follicles remaining is important for knowing whether women will be sterilized by the treatment (all remaining follicles will be damaged), will face infertility (difficulty achieving pregnancy), will have a cessation of menstrual cycles and then recover normal reproductive function. Despite this issue, we do have ways to assess follicles that have entered the growing population—the primary and secondary follicle stages—using imaging or hormone levels. The gold standard for follicle reserve is an *antral follicle count,* which is assessed by counting antral follicles (2–10 mm) via transvaginal ultrasonography. The presence of these follicles indicates ovarian activity and current ovarian reserve, but does not predict how long the ovary will continue to be active. Primary and secondary follicles also make hormones

---

[a]These authors contributed equally to this chapter.

like anti-müllerian hormone (AMH) and inhibin B and, as they develop further, produce increasing amounts of estradiol. The ovarian hormones feedback through endocrine loops to the pituitary and control FSH/LH production and release. If there are no ovarian follicles, AMH, inhibin B, and estradiol will be low or absent, pituitary hormone levels increase prodigiously, and high FSH represents a menopausal state. If follicles do become active after cancer treatment has completed, the ovarian hormones can restore pituitary FSH secretion to normal cyclical levels. AMH has been widely implemented to measure fertile potential after chemotherapy treatment and is a favorable assay because it does not vary significantly with the phase of the menstrual cycles or hormonal manipulation.[12]

These same gonadal hormones also regulate uterine function and the timing of the monthly menses. In the absence of cycling hormones, women develop amenorrhea (absence of menses). Because there is a complex relationship among gonadal hormones, follicle activation, follicle selection, the production of gonadal hormones and their effects on the pituitary and uterus, the absence of menses does not always mean a woman is infertile, nor does the presence of menses indicate that a woman is fertile.

These endocrine loops and the complexity of follicle selection is one of the reasons oncologists do not discuss the fertility outcomes with patients. Increasing the reproductive knowledge of providers, patients, and the public is a critical part of the oncofertility consortium mission, and more lay-friendly information can be found on myoncofertility.org. The information includes the basics of ovarian biology, effects of chemotherapy and radiation, and issues associated with sexuality and contraception, all of which should be part of a comprehensive oncofertility consult.

Gonadotoxicity of Cancer Therapies in Reproductive-Age Women

Breast cancer is treated is multimodal including surgery, chemotherapy, biological agents, endocrine therapy, and radiation. Many of these modes of treatment can have adverse effects on future fertility.

Surgery of the Breast

Surgery of the breast does not directly alter fertility, but future breastfeeding could be affected and should be carefully discussed with patients.[13] After breast conserving therapy, lactation may be conserved via the treated breast, although diminished.[14,15] The proximity of the lumpectomy incision to the areola and nipple, as well as dose and type of radiotherapy, may affect lactation.[16] After bilateral mastectomy, patients will not be able to breastfeed. However, patients with unilateral mastectomy generally can breastfeed well through the untreated breast without a decrease in capacity.[17] Evidence has suggested a decreased risk of breast cancer with ever having breastfed and with increased duration of breastfeeding.[18]

Impact of Radiation on Fertility

Radiation can be toxic to oocytes, based on age, dose, and treatment field. In historical studies, the median lethal dose required to destroy 50% of immature human oocytes was 2 Gy.[19,20] Nearly total loss of ovarian function occurs in 90% of patients who undergo abdominal radiation with 20 to 30 Gy and total body

irradiation with 15 Gy.[21] Reproductive-age oocytes are arrested in meiosis I (prophase) and are more resistant to radiation-induced damage compared with growing follicles, but DNA breaks in the oocyte result in rapid apoptosis of the damaged egg.[22,23]

Postmastectomy radiation therapy and whole breast radiation therapy are directed therapies, but some radiation may reach the ovaries. Pregnancy, as well as egg harvesting or in vitro fertilization procedures, should be avoided during radiation treatment.[24–26] Dose and type of radiotherapy may affect future breastfeeding, but lactation is possible in the irradiated breast approximately half of the time.[27] A radiation boost to the tumor bed may decrease the chances of successful lactation.[28]

Chemotherapy in the Breast Cancer Setting

Chemotherapy can be toxic to the ovaries as well, with its impact being age-, agent-, and dose-dependent.[29–32] The most common chemotherapy regimen used to treat breast cancer includes doxorubicin (an anthracycline) and cyclophosphamide, followed by a taxane (paclitaxel or docetaxel). An alternative and far less frequently used regimen includes cyclophosphamide, methotrexate, and 5-fluorouracil (CMF). Alkylating agents such as cyclophosphamide cause DNA breaks at any stage of the cell cycle and negatively affect both the oocytes and ovarian function. Treatment-associated mechanisms of oocyte depletion have been linked to damage to the granulosa cells or to the oocyte itself, resulting in follicular apoptosis, vascular damage, and fibrosis of the ovarian cortex.[33] In a study examining age and the impact of breast cancer chemotherapeutic regimens on menstrual function, for patients aged 40 and younger, the rate of amenorrhea for 6 months or longer after treatment with doxorubicin and cytoxan was 44%, and for those patients over 40 years, the amenorrhea rate was 81%. These age-related amenorrhea rates were higher for patients treated with doxorubicin, cytoxan, and a taxane. Permanent amenorrhea rates for patients receiving chemotherapy were 60% for patients aged 40 and younger, and 82% for patients over 40.[34]

For postpartum patients receiving chemotherapy, breastfeeding is discouraged. Chemotherapeutics can be excreted in breast milk. Neutropenia has been reported in an infant breastfed during maternal treatment with cyclophosphamide for lymphoma.[35]

Biological Agents Used in the Treatment of Breast Cancer

Trastuzumab is a monoclonal antibody and targeted treatment against Her2/neu overexpression, a transmembrane protein that is overexpressed in approximately 20% of patients with breast cancer. Cardiotoxicity is the most prominent aspect of the trastuzumab side effect profile. Trastuzumab is also a teratogen and is not recommended during pregnancy because birth defects including cases of oligohydramnios and anhydramnios have been reported.[36] Although trastuzumab may not cause problems with future fertility, the duration of trastuzumab treatment is 1 year, during which implementation of fertility preservation options should be delayed and contraceptive use encouraged.

Endocrine Therapy Used in the Treatment of Breast Cancer

For premenopausal women with hormone receptor–positive breast cancers, tamoxifen is the adjuvant regimen of choice. Tamoxifen therapy has been associated with amenorrhea of amenorrhea[37,38] and is also a teratogen.[39] Patients should avoid tamoxifen while attempting to conceive and during pregnancy. The current recommended duration of tamoxifen therapy is 5 to 10 years.[40,41] For breast cancer patients taking tamoxifen, sequencing tamoxifen treatment and fertility interventions, including delaying initiation to attempt pregnancy, or a tamoxifen hiatus to pursue pregnancy, may retain significant therapeutic benefit.[42-44] The prospective IBCSG POSITIVE trial to examine the impact of a tamoxifen treatment hiatus on pregnancy and disease-specific outcomes is ongoing.[45]

Fertility Preservation Options

Oocyte or Embryo Cryopreservation

For oocyte or embryo cryopreservation, daily injectable gonadotropins are administered to stimulate the growth of multiple ovarian follicles, and oocytes are ultimately retrieved transvaginally under ultrasound guidance. Mature oocytes are then either frozen without being fertilized or are fertilized with partner or donor sperm to create embryos. Embryos are generally frozen on either the day of fertilization or once they reach the blastocyst stage (5–6 days later), depending on laboratory preferences. For patients harboring genetic mutations, such as *BRCA*, day 5 or 6 embryos can undergo preimplantation genetic diagnosis, where embryos are biopsied and tested for a specific mutation before freezing. Oocytes and embryos are most commonly cryopreserved in an ultrarapid fashion called vitrification, which has decreased the damage rate seen in traditional freezing and has resulted in improved pregnancy rates.[46,47] Although the creation of embryos is the most mature technology with the highest likelihood of success, due to the rapid decisions necessary at the time of a cancer diagnosis and the profound emotional issues that accompany this news, creating embryos may not be the best course of action for all patients. Since approximately 2010, the methods for cryopreserving mature eggs have been developed and are now considered standard of care.[48] Currently, pregnancy rates from frozen oocytes approach those from fresh oocytes,[48] therefore, there is no longer a need for women without a male partner to select a sperm donor to preserve fertility. Overall pregnancy rates from oocyte cryopreservation are estimated to be 4.5% to 12% per thawed oocyte.[48] At the same time, success rates from both oocyte and embryo cryopreservation are dependent on the age of the patient at the time of cryopreservation, with better success found in younger patients. Reported live-birth rates for oocyte and embryo cryopreservation are listed in Table 58.1.[49,50] Importantly, live-birth rates for an embryo transfer cannot be directly compared with the rates reported for thawed oocytes. During an embryo transfer, multiple embryos may be included in what is considered a single event, and furthermore, the number of oocytes retrieved per developed embryo is also not commonly reported. As success rates for both oocyte and embryo cryopreservation increase with the number of oocytes retrieved, for older patients or patients with a lower oocyte yield, back-to-back stimulation cycles can be performed in an attempt to increase the cumulative number of oocytes available for potential fertilization and transfer.[51,52] Cancer patients need to be carefully counseled about the success rates of these assisted reproductive technologies so they can make well-informed decisions about pursuing fertility preservation.

For breast cancer patients, aromatase inhibitors, such as letrozole, have been used simultaneously with exogenous gonadotropins to minimize supraphysiologic estrogen levels during ovarian

TABLE 58.1 Live Birth Rates for Thawed Embryos and Oocytes

Age (y)	Live Birth Rates
Success Rates per Frozen Embryo Transfer in the United States[49]	
<35	44%
35–37	41%
38–40	36%
41–42	32%
>42	21%
Success Rates for Thawed Oocytes[50]	
30–36	8.2%
>36–39	3.3%

Data available for embryo transfers is national data and may vary among treatment centers. Additionally, multiple embryos may be transferred per embryo transfer, and the data in this table do not distinguish between transfers with only one embryo and transfers with multiple embryos. Furthermore, per embryo transfer data cannot be directly compared with per thawed oocyte data because the precise number of embryos and oocyte used per transfer is unknown.[49,50]

stimulation.[53,54] Letrozole with gonadotropins does not appear to reduce oocyte yield or fertilization rates, and women undergoing stimulation with letrozole and gonadotropins were shown to have equivalent oncologic outcomes compared with breast cancer patients who did not pursue fertility preservation.[55,56] Additionally, "random-start" protocols, in which gonadotropins are initiated as soon as possible irrespective of menstrual phase, instead of waiting for menses, have decreased the timeframe needed for fertility preservation-related procedures, without compromising oocyte yield or future pregnancy rates.[57,58] With implementation of this protocol, patients can begin cancer therapy an average of 2 weeks after initiation of hormone stimulation with gonadotropins.

Ovarian Tissue Cryopreservation and Transplantation

When hormonal stimulation is not possible, other biological options may provide fertility preservation after obtaining informed consent. As discussed earlier, because the ovary contains tens of thousands of dormant primordial follicles, the removal of ovarian tissue and cryopreservation of the outer cortical rim may provide a reserve population of follicles that are unaffected by radiation or chemotherapeutic damage.[59,60] Cortical ovarian tissue is surgically removed and cryopreserved for future use. The stored tissue can subsequently be thawed and autotransplanted either subcutaneously or into the peritoneal cavity. More than 60 live-births have been reported as a consequence of transplant with both hormone-induced follicle maturation and egg retrieval and natural pregnancies.[61,62] The risk of reexposure to latent cancer cells in the transplanted ovarian tissue is a significant concern.[63-66] As a result, research is evolving such that immature follicles may be retrievable from the ovarian cortical tissue, and then encapsulated in vitro follicle maturation (iIVFG) applied.[67] These techniques are considered experimental.

Mitigating the Risk: The Role of Ovarian Transposition and Medical Suppression

Surgical transfer of the ovaries can be performed to move them higher in the pelvis for increased protection during pelvic radiation, should this be necessary for other cancer types.[68–70] This procedure often results in the need for assisted reproductive technologies for future pregnancies secondary to the resulting distance of the ovaries from the uterus.[71] Additionally, the uterus cannot be moved outside the radiation field, and radiation-induced damage to the uterus can result in difficulties with implantation or carrying a pregnancy to term.

Ovarian suppression with gonadotropin0releasing hormone (GnRH) agonists is an experimental, medical option in which follicles may be protected from gonadotoxic agents by inhibitory effects of these agonists on the hypothalamic-pituitary-ovarian axis. Synthetic GnRH administration results in an initial surge of FSH and LH release, but chronic use results in down-regulation of FSH, LH, and GnRH receptors, which may suppress ovarian function. In a meta-analysis including premenopausal women with breast cancer, administration of a GnRH agonist concomitant with chemotherapy decreased the rate of premature ovarian failure in the first year but had no effect on resumed menses or spontaneous pregnancy rates.[72]

Contraception and Cancer Therapy

Pregnancy should be prevented while undergoing potentially teratogenic cancer therapy, and the different contraceptive options available in the United States are summarized in Table 58.2. In general, it is not clear whether modern formulations of hormonal contraceptives such as birth control pills, the transdermal patch, vaginal ring, and progestin-only implants stimulate the growth of hormone receptor–positive breast cancers or increase the risk of new breast cancers, yet most oncologists recommend the avoidance of these agents.[73] The Centers for Disease Control and Prevention (CDC) considers a diagnosis of breast cancer as a contraindication to hormone-containing contraception, and for patients with a history of breast cancer, the CDC states that the risks generally outweigh the benefits of this exogenous hormone exposure.[74] Furthermore, as patients with cancer are in a hypercoagulable state, hormonal forms of birth control, associated with an increased rate of venous thrombosis, are contraindicated.[75] The copper intrauterine device (IUD) is a nonhormonal implant that works by inducing an inflammatory reaction in the uterus that is hostile to sperm motility and also prevents fertilization of the oocyte and implantation of an embryo. IUD is favored as a contraceptive in breast cancer patients secondary to the ease of insertion and removal via an office procedure, high efficacy with a typical failure rate of 0.8%, and its rapidly reversible nature.[76]

Female Sexuality After Cancer Therapy

Breast cancer survivors have changes in their sexuality after treatment, which can include changes in body image, lack of libido, and dyspareunia. Surgery can alter the appearance of the breasts, resulting in physical and emotional insecurities. Chemotherapy can cause ovarian insufficiency and resultant hypoestrogenism, which can cause vasomotor changes, lack of libido, and dyspareunia. Medications such as tamoxifen and letrozole can result in hormone blockade, causing similar symptoms.[77,78] These symptoms are similar to those associated with menopause, but because

TABLE 58.2 Contraceptive Methods Available in the United States

Contraceptive Method	Hormonal Components	12-Month Failure Rate[76]
Rhythm method/natural family planning	None	24%
Withdrawal	None	22%
Female condom	None	21%
Male condom	None	18%
Diaphragm	None	12%
Combination oral contraceptives	Estrogen/progestin	9%
Progesterone-only pills	Progestin	9%
Contraceptive patch/ vaginal ring	Estrogen/progestin	9%
Depo-Provera injection	Progestin	6%
Copper intrauterine device	None	0.80%
Levonorgestrel intrauterine device	Progestin	0.20%
Etonogestrel implant	Progestin	0.05%
Female sterilization	None	0.50%
Male sterilization	None	0.15%

Methods with hormonal components are considered contraindicated in the setting of breast cancer.[76]

the effects are acute rather than through the gradual transition seen with traditional menopause, hot flashes, night sweats, vaginal dryness, weight and muscle changes, and impact on libido may be particularly severe.

Vaginal dryness and dyspareunia from hypoestrogenemia caused by breast cancer treatment can have adverse effects on sexuality and relationships, as well as decreased medication compliance. The American College of Obstetricians and Gynecologists recommends using nonhormonal treatments, such as lubricants or topical anesthetics, as first-line therapy for vaginal side effects, with vaginal estrogen reserved for those patients in whom nonhormonal remedies fail.[79] In general, local estrogen therapy to the vaginal lining in the form of creams, rings, or tablets, causes a minimal increase in circulating estrogen levels.[80] Thus although there have been concerns about an increased risk of breast cancer recurrence with oral hormone replacement therapy,[81] there is no evidence of increased risk with the use of vaginal products.[82–85]

Pregnancy in Cancer Patients and Survivors

Some concerns remain about the safety of pregnancy after treatment for breast cancer. Given the lack of randomized prospective data to address this issue and further concerns about selection bias and the healthy mother effect, much of the information on this question rests on findings from retrospective studies. To this end, recent retrospective studies suggest that pregnancy after breast cancer is safe.[86–90] The hormonal changes during pregnancy do not seem to have an effect on breast cancer prognosis.[91] To examine the effect of pregnancy after cancer with estrogen receptor–positive tumors, a recent multicenter retrospective cohort study was conducted.[92] No difference in disease-free survival was seen between pregnant and nonpregnant patients in the estrogen receptor–positive group or estrogen receptor–negative group.[92]

Talking With Patients and Families About Future Fertility

It is a priority to talk about future fertility with breast cancer patients and their families. Most young breast cancer patients report concerns about the development of infertility.[93] Unfortunately, fertility risks and preservation options are often not part of the routine medical oncology consultation.[94] During an initial patient encounter and history gathering, cancer providers can ask simple questions, such as, "Were you thinking about having a child?" or "Were you planning to have any more children?"[95] Breast oncologists should also be able to discuss the implementation of fertility preservation for breast cancer patients. Moreover, the oncologist or surgeon can provide the patient with information about the expected effects of the treatment on ovarian hormones independent of fertility concerns, for example "You may experience hot flashes or weight gain—these symptoms are likely associated with the loss of ovarian function" or "You may experience irregular or lost periods." Importantly, patients need to be informed that premature ovarian insufficiency can result in impaired bone and cardiovascular health and also be counseled about seeking care with a provider who is comfortable managing these issues for breast cancer survivors. After the discussion of the treatment plan, fertility preservation can be readdressed and the appropriate reproductive endocrinology referrals can also be facilitated.

Oncofertility in Clinical Practice

The necessary components of an oncofertility program include a multidisciplinary treatment team with good communication and awareness and access to timely fertility preservation procedures.[96] It is essential that oncologists are cognizant of fertility preservation options.[97] Oncologist should prioritize the management of cancer care while also addressing fertility preservation and referral to a reproductive endocrinologist. As surgery often precedes more fertility damaging treatments, fertility interventions

can be optimized during this window if effectively prioritized by physicians. Many oncofertility programs use a clinical coordinator to assist patients during the complex referral and treatment process, which often involves several different specialties. Additionally, mental health professionals that specialize in reproductive endocrinology can provide valuable guidance and support for cancer patients navigating the fertility preservation process. It is also important for medical centers to be equipped for temporary or long-term storage of harvested tissue and to have laboratory personnel with expertise in gamete and tissue preservation. A financial counselor can also be valuable for patients undergoing fertility preservation because most procedures are not covered by standard insurance.[98] Ultimately, fertility preservation has become a part of the multidisciplinary care plan for young patients with cancer, contributing to the overall goals of both cancer treatment and survivorship for young patients with breast cancer.

Acknowledgment

This work was supported by the Center for Reproductive Health After Disease (P50HD076188) from the National Institutes of Health/National Institute for Child Health and Human Development National Center for Translational Research in Reproduction and Infertility.

Selected References

2. Tomasi-Cont N, Lambertini M, Hulsbosch S, et al. Strategies for fertility preservation in young early breast cancer patients. *Breast*. 2014;23:503-510.
24. Jeruss JS, Woodruff TK. Preservation of fertility in patients with cancer. *N Engl J Med*. 2009;360:902-911.
37. Goodwin PJ, Ennis M, Pritchard KI, et al. Risk of menopause during the first year after breast cancer diagnosis. *J Clin Oncol*. 1999;17:2365-2370.
42. Llarena NC, Estevez SL, Tucker SL, et al. Impact of fertility concerns on tamoxifen initiation and persistence. *J Natl Cancer Inst*. 2015;107:djv202. doi:10.1093/jnci/djv202; https://jnci.oxfordjournals.org/content/107/10/djv202.full.pdf+html.
51. Turan V, Bedoschi G, Moy F, et al. Safety and feasibility of performing two consecutive ovarian stimulation cycles with the use of letrozole-gonadotropin protocol for fertility preservation in breast cancer patients. *Fertil Steril*. 2013;100:1681-1685.
A full reference list is available online at ExpertConsult.com.

59

Surgical Procedures for Advanced Local and Regional Malignancies of the Breast

OLUWADAMILOLA M. FAYANJU, PATRICK BRYAN GARVEY, MEGHAN S. KARUTURI, KELLY K. HUNT, AND ISABELLE BEDROSIAN

Surgery remains an integral part of the therapeutic plan for locally advanced breast cancer. Advances in systemic therapies have transformed the role of surgery for this population of patients from palliation to largely curative intent. Further, in the last decade, the integration of surgical care into the management algorithm of locally advanced breast cancer patients has also changed substantially with increasing use of neoadjuvant chemotherapy and more recently neoadjuvant endocrine therapy and targeted therapies for HER2-positive disease. Such neoadjuvant strategies have provided new opportunities to downsize the tumor burden and scope of surgical intervention. Advances in reconstructive techniques have also provided new opportunities to improve on quality of life of these heavily treated patients, although the need for radiation therapy in patients with locally advanced breast cancer remains an area of particular challenge for optimal timing of reconstruction.

Staging System Revisions and Implications

LABCs account for 10% to 15% of all newly diagnosed breast cancers, and they include tumors that are large or have extensive regional lymph node involvement and no evidence of distant metastatic spread on initial presentation. Patients with LABC have higher incidences of local and distant relapse and, concomitantly, worse survival than patients with early breast cancer. The term *locally advanced breast cancer* encompasses a heterogeneous group of breast neoplasms: locally recurrent (persistent) breast carcinoma, inflammatory breast carcinoma (T4d), and clinical stage IIIA, IIIB, and IIIC breast carcinomas, all of which have varying degrees and locations of lymph node involvement and some of which involve extension of cancer to the chest wall and/or skin (Fig. 59.1). Inflammatory and locally recurrent carcinomas are distinct biologic entities that are discussed elsewhere in this book.

Published in 2010, the 7th edition of the American Joint Committee on Cancer (AJCC) Staging Manual builds on the extensive revisions made to the breast cancer staging system in the 6th edition and reflects knowledge gained from improved and evolving application of sentinel lymph node biopsy, immunohistochemistry, molecular techniques, improved imaging modalities including

magnetic resonance imaging (MRI), and the results of clinical trials.[1] With regard to nodal staging, classification of isolated tumor cell clusters and single cells is now more stringent: small clusters of cells not greater than 0.2 mm and nonconfluent or nearly confluent clusters of no more than 200 cells in a single histologic lymph node cross section are classified as isolated tumor cells, that is, pN0 (i+). Likewise, in patients who have received neoadjuvant systemic therapy, posttreatment nodal metastases no greater than 0.2 mm are classified as ypN0 (i+), and these patients are not considered to have achieved a pathologic complete response (pCR). Furthermore, documentation of posttreatment response to neoadjuvant therapy must also describe the modality—physical examination, imaging (mammogram, ultrasound, MRI), or pathology (fine-needle aspiration [FNA], core needle biopsy, sentinel lymph node biopsy)—through which response to treatment is assessed. Finally, it has been clarified that the sentinel node modifier (sn) should be omitted if six or more sentinel nodes are identified on gross examination of surgical pathology specimens.[2] Given the prognostic significance of nodal disease burden in breast cancer, the increasingly refined assessment of both nodal involvement and clinical significance enabled by recent clinical trials and reflected in these staging guidelines has allowed clinicians to provide more multimodal and often less invasive treatment for patients presenting with LABC. The 8th edition of the AJCC staging system contains biological factors in addition to the anatomic designations of tumor (T), nodal (N), and metastasis (M).

Pretreatment Evaluation, Diagnosis, and Management

Establishing a tissue diagnosis is a priority for patients presenting with LABC. After thorough breast imaging, which includes bilateral diagnostic mammography and ultrasonography of the breast and nodal basins, core needle biopsy of the primary tumor should be performed to provide tissue for histopathologic examination and determination of hormone receptor status and HER2/neu expression. If breast conserving surgery (BCS) is being considered, a clip should be placed into the primary tumor site before initiation of any systemic therapy. Matted, fixed, or sonographically

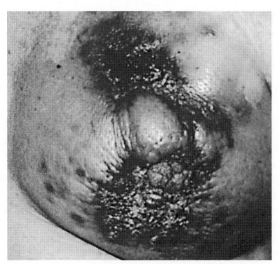

• **Fig. 59.1** Patient with locally advanced breast cancer involving the nipple-areola complex. Note the prominent skin retraction and nipple distortion caused by a large underlying primary tumor.

suspicious axillary, supraclavicular, infraclavicular, and even internal mammary lymph nodes should be subjected to FNA biopsy for more definitive staging by radiologists with the expertise to perform this procedure accurately and safely.[3] Core needle biopsy can also be performed and may be preferred when cytologic expertise is not available (Fig. 59.2).

A complete staging workup includes a thorough history and physical examination, a complete blood cell count with differential and platelet counts, a biochemical survey (i.e., comprehensive metabolic panel including electrolytes and liver enzymes), chest radiography, imaging for distant disease including a bone scan and abdominal cross-sectional imaging. Patients with bone pain, abnormal results on a bone scan, or elevated alkaline phosphatase levels should have pertinent bone radiographs obtained to rule out osseous metastases. Each patient should be evaluated in a multidisciplinary context with a team including surgical, medical, and radiation oncologists; radiologists; pathologists; and plastic surgeons. A consensus treatment plan should be presented to the patient initially and should be reviewed throughout the course of treatment in the context of response to neoadjuvant systemic therapy as well as postoperatively to review pathologic analysis of the surgical specimen.

Unimodal Treatment Approaches

As with early breast cancer, the most important outcomes used to assess treatment efficacy in patients with LABC are locoregional control and survival.

Surgery

Surgery is the oldest treatment for breast cancer, but enthusiasm for radical surgical resections has waxed and waned over the years. At the end of the 19th century, William Halsted described the radical mastectomy, which involved removal of the entire breast with en bloc removal of all axillary lymphatics, the chest wall musculature, and part of the sternum and ribs if they were involved with tumor. Despite this aggressive approach to locally advanced tumors, survival remained poor, ranging from 13% to 20% at 5 years.[4]

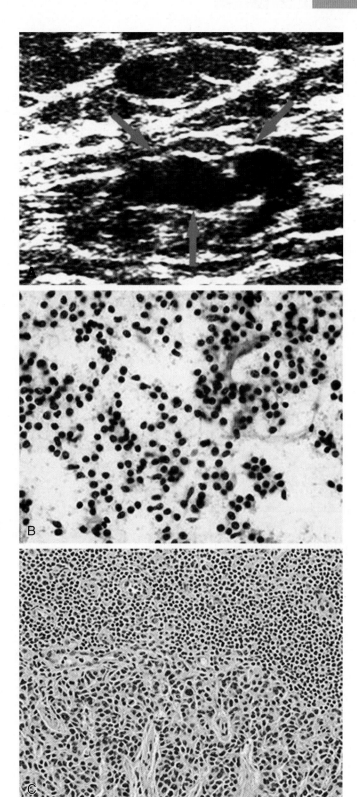

• **Fig. 59.2** (A) Ultrasound of the axilla showing an abnormal node with cortical thickening. (B) Fine-needle aspiration smear of the same lymph node shows benign lymphoid tissue. (C) The patient underwent a sentinel node biopsy, which demonstrated a metastatic focus.

Awareness of variations in biology (and therefore the effectiveness of therapy) of LABC stems from Haagensen and Stout's pioneering insights derived from nearly 30 years of cumulative experience in breast cancer management. On the basis of a review of 1135 breast cancer patients treated with radical mastectomy at Presbyterian Hospital in New York from 1915 to 1942, these authors observed that patients with certain features of LABC were beyond cure, even with radical surgery.[5] Haagensen's "grave signs" included edema of the skin of the breast, skin ulceration, chest wall fixation, an axillary lymph node greater than 2.5 cm in diameter, and fixed axillary nodes. Patients with two or more of these signs had a 42% local recurrence rate and a 5-year disease-free survival rate of only 2%.

McWhirter and colleagues demonstrated that less disfiguring surgery produced results similar to those seen with the more aggressive radical mastectomy, an idea that led to the recognition that treatment failure from breast cancer stemmed from systemic dissemination before surgery.[6,7] The Alabama Breast Project examined the efficacy of modified radical mastectomy versus radical mastectomy as unimodal therapy for stage III breast carcinoma in patients with a minimum of 10 years' follow-up.[8] In this study, patients with stage III disease who underwent modified radical mastectomy represented only 6% of the total study population but had 20% of the local recurrences. In contrast, patients with stage III disease who underwent radical mastectomy represented 5% of the total study population but had 6% of the local recurrences. Radical mastectomy significantly decreased the rate of local recurrence and improved survival compared with modified mastectomy, albeit with greater morbidity. The Alabama experience further supported the importance of exploring whether multimodal therapy might yield survival rates similar to those of radical mastectomy without the severely morbid sequelae of radical surgical interventions.

Radiotherapy

After Haagensen and Stout's publication of the criteria for inoperability, questions arose in the early 20th century surrounding the concept of radical en bloc ablation and whether radiation could be substituted for, or at least improve the results of, radical surgery. In 1949 Baclesse used radiotherapy alone to achieve local tumor control in select patients with advanced breast cancer.[9] In 1965, Fletcher and Montague from the University of Texas MD Anderson Cancer Center reported a 70% local control rate for advanced breast cancer treated with radiotherapy alone.[10] Distant metastasis occurred an average of 18 months later, and the 5-year overall survival rate was 25%. A 1976 retrospective review of the Joint Center for Radiation Therapy experience by Harris and associates reported a 54% rate of 5-year local tumor control and a 30% rate of 5-year overall survival using radical radiotherapy (dose >60 Gy) alone.[11] The National Cancer Institute in Milan, Italy, published its experience with "supervoltage" radiotherapy in the treatment of LABC in 1973.[12] This retrospective study reported an encouraging 50% control rate. However, 45% of the patients with "controlled" disease experienced relapse within 18 months of beginning radiotherapy, and 82% of those relapses occurred at a distant site. Overall, a 21% 5-year survival rate was achieved. However, the "supervoltage" radiotherapy, which included doses of 80 to 90 Gy, was not benign: fibrosis, skin ulceration, chest wall necrosis, pathologic fractures, cardiac and pulmonary complications, brachial plexus injury, and severe lymphedema of the ipsilateral arm were common and debilitating occurrences. In summary, early studies served to demonstrate that radiotherapy may be better suited as a component of the multimodal treatment algorithm for LABC rather than as monotherapy due to its dose-limiting side effects.

Multimodal Approaches

Experiences with unimodal therapy demonstrated that good local control rates achieved with surgery or radiotherapy alone did not correlate with good prognosis and long-term survival because hematogenous metastases were not being controlled. Consequently, by the late 1970s, systemic chemotherapy was an integral part of the primary management of LABC,[13] a development that occurred in large part as a result of several major prospective multimodal trials including the National Cancer Institute (Milan, Italy) trials in 1973 and 1975 and an MD Anderson Cancer Center trial in 1974.

Early Trials

In the first Milan trial, patients with stage IIIA or IIIB breast cancer were given four cycles of doxorubicin and vincristine, followed by 60 Gy to the breast and a 10-Gy boost to the area of residual tumor. Patients who demonstrated a complete response were randomized to either no further treatment or six more courses of chemotherapy. The objective response rate to this neoadjuvant chemotherapy regimen was 89%, the complete response rate was 15.5%, the major (≥50% tumor size reduction) response rate was 54.5%, and the minor (<50% tumor size reduction) response rate was 19%. Of the patients responding to neoadjuvant chemotherapy, 83% had a complete response with the addition of radiotherapy. This combined chemotherapy-radiotherapy approach resulted in an overall 3-year survival rate of 53%.[13]

In 1975, the Milan group began a second trial that ultimately enrolled 277 consecutive patients with stage IIIA and IIIB disease.[14] In this trial, patients received three courses of doxorubicin and vincristine preoperatively. They were randomized to radiotherapy or surgery (radical or modified radical mastectomy) followed by six additional cycles of chemotherapy. The best local control was achieved when surgery rather than radiotherapy was interposed between chemotherapy courses (82.3% vs. 63.9% complete local control rate). Freedom from disease progression was maintained for 5 years or longer in 25% of the patients who received chemotherapy and surgery but in only 4.9% of the patients who received chemotherapy and radiotherapy. Likewise, the overall 5-year survival rate was higher for the chemotherapy and surgery group (49.4% vs. 19.7%).

In 1974, a multimodality treatment protocol for LABC was initiated at MD Anderson Cancer Center to explore whether the combined use of chemotherapy, surgery, and radiotherapy would improve control of micrometastases and reduce local tumor burden in patients with stage III disease, thereby avoiding the need for either radical radiotherapy or radical mastectomy, both of which were standard of care for stage III patients at that time.[15] Between 1974 and 1985, 174 patients with stage III noninflammatory (operable and inoperable) breast cancer were initially treated for three cycles with combination systemic therapy consisting of 5-fluorouracil, doxorubicin (Adriamycin), and cyclophosphamide (Cytoxan) (FAC); up until 1978, bacillus Calmette-Guerin (BCG) was also included in this regimen.

After three cycles of neoadjuvant chemotherapy, patient response was assessed with a combination of clinical examination and mammography, and patients were assigned to one of three treatment arms based on clinical response: (1) those who had minimal or no residual disease (i.e., *complete responders*) were assigned to radiotherapy only (although it is important to note that in the early years of the trial, complete responders with large breasts sometimes underwent postchemotherapy, preradiation mastectomy to facilitate delivery of radiation); (2) those who had a moderate response (i.e., *moderate responders*) went on to modified radical mastectomy followed by radiotherapy (beginning in 1978, moderate responders also received adjuvant chemotherapy, the regimens for which varied over time, after undergoing surgery and before receiving radiation); and (3) those who had no response or progressive disease (i.e., *nonresponders*) went on to radiotherapy, with subsequent surgical resection if their disease was operable. In addition, although surgery alone was not a predetermined treatment arm, a subset of 40 patients underwent surgical resection alone for a variety of reasons including patient preference, patient comorbidities that precluded radiation, development of distant disease before receiving radiation, and provider preference or judgment.

With a median follow-up of 59 months, complete remission was achieved in 16.7% of patients and was more common in stage IIIA patients than in stage IIIB patients (17% vs. 8%); 70.7% of patients had a moderate response after the initial three cycles of neoadjuvant chemotherapy, again with higher rates of response among stage IIIA patients. All but 6 of the 174 treated patients were eventually rendered disease-free after neoadjuvant chemotherapy and local treatment; all 6 of the patients with residual/progressive disease had stage IIIB disease at presentation. Five-year overall and disease-free survival rates for stage IIIA patients were both 84%, whereas for stage IIIB patients, overall and disease-free survival rates were 44% and 33%, respectively. These findings demonstrated significant improvement over historical 5-year survival rates of 30% to 45% for stage IIIA and only 10% to 28% for stage IIIB patients and illustrated the efficacy of a multimodal approach in which systemic therapy mitigated the need for radical local therapy.

Chemotherapy

Neoadjuvant chemotherapy is an important component in the management of LABC. Although randomized trials have demonstrated that neoadjuvant chemotherapy and adjuvant chemotherapy are associated with similar recurrence-free and overall survival rates when the same regimen is applied,[16] neoadjuvant treatment nevertheless has many advantages over adjuvant therapy with regards to LABC.[17,18]

Neoadjuvant chemotherapy can (1) convert LABC from inoperable to operable, (2) increase the rate of BCS, (3) serve as an in vivo chemosensitivity test for a given tumor, and (4) allow treatment of micrometastatic disease at the earliest possible opportunity. Pathologic response to neoadjuvant systemic therapy in the breast and lymph nodes correlates with patient survival. A potential disadvantage rests in the loss of prognostic information provided by tumor size and nodal status in an untreated surgical specimen, but it has been shown that patients who have a complete clinical or pathologic response with neoadjuvant chemotherapy have improved overall and disease-free survival.[19] Multiple, large randomized trials have proven the safety of neoadjuvant chemotherapy in LABC and have shown objective response rates ranging from 60% to 80% as well as less morbidity than is observed with adjuvant chemotherapy.[20]

> • **BOX 59.1** MD Anderson Neoadjuvant and Adjuvant Chemotherapy Protocols

Regimens for HER2-Nonamplified Disease

- Paclitaxel × 12 weekly cycles followed by AC × 4 cycles (administered either as dose-dense every 2 weeks w/G-CSF support or every 3 weeks)[21]
  - TC × 4 cycles (administered every 3 weeks) with G-CSF support[22]

Regimens for HER2-Amplified Disease

- AC × 4 cycles (administered every 3 weeks) followed by THP × 4 cycles (continuation of trastuzumab to complete 1 year of therapy)[23–25,27,28]
- TCHP × 6 cycles (administered every 3 weeks with continuation of trastuzumab to complete 1 year of therapy)[23,25–28]

AC, Adriamycin (doxorubicin) 60 mg/m² IV + Cytoxan (cyclophosphamide) 600 mg/m² IV; G-CSF, Granulocyte colony stimulating factor; IV, intravenous; Paclitaxel, 80 mg/m² IV weekly; TC, Taxotere (docetaxel) 75 mg/m² IV + Cytoxan (cyclophosphamide) 600 mg/m² IV; TCHP, Taxotere (docetaxel) 75 mg/m² IV + carboplatin AUC (area under the curve) 6 mg/mL IV + Herceptin (trastuzumab) 8 mg/kg IV loading followed by 6 mg/kg IV maintenance + Perjeta (pertuzumab) 840 mg IV loading followed by 420 mg IV maintenance; THP, Taxotere (docetaxel) 75 mg/m² IV + Herceptin (trastuzumab) 8 mg/kg IV loading followed by 6 mg/kg IV maintenance + Perjeta (pertuzumab) 840 mg IV loading followed by 420 mg IV maintenance.

The response of patients to neoadjuvant chemotherapy in patients with LABC depends in large part on the agents or combination of agents used (Box 59.1).[21–28] Randomized trials have confirmed the superiority of anthracycline-based regimens over cyclophosphamide, methotrexate, and 5-fluorouracil in the treatment of early, locally advanced, and metastatic breast cancer.[29–31] The rates of pCR to neoadjuvant systemic therapy vary according to treatment regimen, ranging from 6% to 15% with anthracycline-based regimens to almost 30% with the addition of a taxane (Table 59.1).[32–34] The National Surgical Adjuvant Breast and Bowel Project (NSABP) B-27 trial randomized patients with resectable breast cancer into one of three neoadjuvant treatment arms: doxorubicin plus cyclophosphamide, doxorubicin plus cyclophosphamide and docetaxel, or preoperative doxorubicin and cyclophosphamide followed by postoperative docetaxel. The investigators observed a pCR rate of 26% associated with the addition of docetaxel to the preoperative anthracycline regimen.[35]

A retrospective study in Nottingham, England, compared outcomes in 106 consecutive patients with LABC who received one of two neoadjuvant chemotherapy regimens: an anthracycline-based regimen (5-fluorouracil, epirubicin/Adriamycin, cyclophosphamide; i.e., FEC/FAC) or a regimen consisting of mitoxantrone, methotrexate, and mitomycin (MMM). End points of locoregional recurrence, metastasis, and survival were analyzed after a median follow-up of 54 months.[18] All patients underwent neoadjuvant chemotherapy as part of a multimodal approach, which included subsequent mastectomy, radiotherapy, and adjuvant endocrine therapy if tumors were estrogen receptor (ER) positive. More patients in the anthracycline-based treatment group than in the MMM group had a complete clinical response (24% vs. 9%, $p = .035$). In addition, patients in the anthracycline group had a lower incidence of locoregional recurrence (6% vs. 19%) and distant metastasis (20% vs. 53%) and a higher survival rate (82% vs. 45%), findings that supported the use of anthracycline-based neoadjuvant regimens in LABC.

Although the effectiveness of anthracyclines and taxanes in treating breast cancer has now been demonstrated in multiple

TABLE 59.1	Clinical Trials Examining Neoadjuvant Protocols and Associated Rates of pCR		
Trial	**Population**	**Regimen: pCR Rate**	**Comments**
NSABP B-27[67]	802 patients 31% clinically node positive (N1), T1c–T3	AC → T: 63%	
TRYPHAENA[26]	225 patients Locally advanced/operable or inflammatory HER2+ breast cancer	TCHP × 6 cycles (n = 76): 47.5% in the HR+ subgroup (and 81.1% in the HR– subgroup FEC × 3 cycles → THP × 3 cycles (n = 75): 45.7% in the HR+ subgroup, 62.5% in the HR– subgroup	
NeoSphere[28]	417 patients Locally advanced/operative or inflammatory HER2+ breast cancer, primary tumor >2 cm	THP × 4 cycles (n = 107): 39.3% (treated with FEC × 3 cycles postoperatively)	
GEPARTRIO[68]	2090 patients with untreated breast cancer, of which 1390 responders randomized to receive four or six additional cycles	TAC × 8 cycles (n = 704) with clinical response of >50% reduction after initial two cycles): 23.5% TAC × 6 cycles (n = 686, with clinical response <50% after initial two cycles): 21%	pCR by subgroup: Age <50: 26.4% Age ≥50: 17.5% Ductal histology: 24% Lobular histology: 10.2% Grade 3: 31.5% Grade 1–2: 15.4% LN+: 23.4% LN–: 21.5% ER/PR–: 43.2% Other: 10% HER2+: 20.6%

AC → T, Adriamycin (doxorubicin) + Cytoxan (cyclophosphamide) followed by Taxotere (docetaxel); *ER*, estrogen receptor; *FEC*, 5-fluorouracil + epirubicin + Cytoxan (cyclophosphamide); *HER2+*, HER2/neu-amplified; *HR*, hormone receptor; *LN*, lymph node; *pCR*, pathologic complete response; *PR*, progesterone receptor; *TAC*, Taxotere (docetaxel) + Adriamycin (doxorubicin) + Cytoxan (cyclophosphamide); *TCHP*, Taxotere (docetaxel) + Carboplatin + Herceptin (trastuzumab) + Perjeta (pertuzumab); *THP*, Taxotere (docetaxel) + Herceptin (trastuzumab) + Perjeta (Pertuzumab).

trials, these agents are associated with significant morbidity including but not limited to neurologic and cardiac toxicities. Thus increasing attention has been devoted to maximizing cure at the population level while preventing overtreatment of the individual through a shift in focus from standardized chemotherapy treatment protocols to patient-specific treatments based on gene-expression signatures. This personalized approach to systemic therapy has been furthered greatly by the development and clinical use of commercially available genomic assays such as Onco*type* DX, MammaPrint, Mammostrat, and Prosigna, which were developed to assess the appropriateness of chemotherapy in the adjuvant setting in patients with early-stage breast cancer whose initial presentation did not suggest a need for chemotherapy. With increasing confidence in these genomic assays to tailor systemic therapy decisions among early-stage breast cancer patients, these assays are increasingly being tested for utility in tailoring treatment in patients with more advanced disease, in particular in those LABC patients with the ER-positive, HER2/neu nonamplified disease.

Developed in 2004, Onco*type* DX (Genomic Health, Redwood, CA) is a 21-gene recurrence score assay that has been validated in women receiving adjuvant tamoxifen with ER-positive, HER2/neu nonamplified (HER2-negative), node-negative breast cancer as being able to quantify both the likelihood of distant recurrence within 10 years (i.e., is *prognostic*) and also the likely magnitude of improved distant-recurrence-free survival that would occur with receipt of adjuvant hormonal and chemotherapy as opposed to only receiving hormonal therapy (i.e., is *predictive*).[36,37]

Onco*type* DX uses formalin-fixed, paraffin-embedded (FFPE) samples from surgical specimens to categorize patients into one of three groups based on recurrence scores—low (<18), intermediate (18–30), and high (≥31)—reflecting their likelihood of distant recurrence in 10 years. In the Trial Assigning IndividuaLized Options for Treatment (Rx), or TAILORx, women with a low recurrence score were found to have a less than 1% risk of recurrence in 10 years with receipt of endocrine therapy alone, thereby supporting a shift toward increasingly selective prescription of chemotherapy within the context of multimodal treatment for patients with ER-positive, HER2-negative disease.[38] The applicability of Onco*type* DX for prognosis for patients with more advanced disease is currently under investigation: the RxPONDER Trial (Rx for Positive Node, Endocrine Responsive Breast Cancer) was initiated in 2011 and is designed to determine whether ER-positive, HER2-negative patients with one to three involved axillary lymph nodes and low to intermediate Onco*type* DX scores would benefit from adjuvant chemotherapy and endocrine therapy versus adjuvant endocrine therapy alone. Another aim of this trial is to determine whether there is an optimal recurrence score cutoff point for these patients, above which chemotherapy should always be recommended.[39] Other genomic assays are the subject of ongoing investigation and validation in patients with invasive disease with varying combinations of biomarkers (e.g., Neoadjuvant Breast Registry Symphony Trial [NBRST]). The long-term results of these trials are eagerly awaited and hold great promise for the future of personalized management of breast cancer.

Endocrine Therapy

Endocrine therapy is a critical component of multimodal care for patients with ER-positive breast cancer. In a phase III trial launched by the European Organization for Research and Treatment of Cancer (EORTC), 410 patients with LABC were randomized to receive radiotherapy alone, radiotherapy plus chemotherapy, radiotherapy plus endocrine therapy, or radiotherapy plus endocrine therapy and chemotherapy. Endocrine therapy consisted of ovarian irradiation for premenopausal women and tamoxifen 10 mg twice daily for 5 years for postmenopausal women. After an 8-year follow-up, the combination of adjuvant chemotherapy with endocrine therapy produced a significant reduction in the risk of locoregional recurrence (from 60%–47%) and distant progression of disease. Although the combined treatments provided the greatest therapeutic effect, patients who received adjuvant endocrine therapy appreciated a significant improvement in survival with a 25% reduction in the death hazard ratio.[40] Thus, current recommendations dictate that premenopausal patients with hormone receptor–positive breast cancer receive at least 5 years of adjuvant tamoxifen, whereas postmenopausal women should receive an aromatase inhibitor, unless otherwise contraindicated based on each agent's described risk profile (discussed elsewhere in this book). It is important that the clinical team factor patient and tumor-specific features factor into the complex multimodal treatment equation.

In addition to tamoxifen and aromatase inhibitors, antiestrogen therapies including fulvestrant (which blocks ER and promotes its degradation) and aromatase inhibitors in combination with other agents (e.g., letrozole and palbociclib, a selective inhibitor of cyclin-dependent kinases [CDKs] 4 and 6) have been shown to improve progression-free survival in advanced breast cancer and are used in treatment of locally recurrent and/or treatment-resistant, hormone-sensitive cancers.[41,42] Furthermore, pharmacologic suppression of ovarian function has also proven to be an important component of endocrine therapy: results published in 2015 from the Suppression of Ovarian Function Trial (SOFT) trial demonstrated that in young women with ER-positive breast cancer who remained premenopausal (determined by estradiol levels) after receiving chemotherapy, ovarian suppression with triptorelin, a gonadotropin-releasing hormone (GnRH) agonist, given in combination with tamoxifen or with an aromatase inhibitor reduced the risk of recurrent breast cancer compared with tamoxifen alone.[43]

Primary endocrine therapy is increasingly used in the neoadjuvant setting and has been demonstrated to result in significant increases in breast conservation rates and improved postsurgical outcomes in patients with stage II and III ER-positive breast cancer.[44] Pathologic complete response rates are low compared with those observed with systemic chemotherapy; however, the Preoperative Endocrine Prognostic Index (PEPI score; ki67 proliferation biomarker, tumor size, nodal status and ER status) is a reliable predictor of prognosis after treatment with endocrine therapy.[44] Three to 4 months of therapy are typically administered and then treatment response is analyzed. In a phase III randomized trial in postmenopausal women, aromatase inhibitors, such as letrozole, had better efficacy compared with tamoxifen,[45,46] and the phase II American College of Surgeons Oncology Group (ACOSOG) Z1031 trial also demonstrated the efficacy of anastrozole, letrozole, and exemestane in the neoadjuvant setting for postmenopausal patients with ER-positive disease.[44]

The ALTERNATE (ALTernate approaches for clinical stage II or III Estrogen Receptor positive breast cancer NeoAdjuvant TrEatment in postmenopausal women) trial is an ongoing phase III study launched by the Alliance for Clinical Trials in Oncology in which postmenopausal women with clinical T2–4, node-positive, ER-positive, HER2-negative breast cancer are randomized to three endocrine therapies—(1) the ER downregulator fulvestrant, (2) the aromatase inhibitor anastrozole, and (3) the combination of fulvestrant and anastrozole—to help characterize the patients with hormone-responsive disease for whom adjuvant chemotherapy may be omitted and also to identify clinicopathologic characteristics of ER-positive, endocrine-resistant tumors that can be targeted in future therapeutic investigation.[47]

Targeted Therapy

The development of anti-HER2 targeted therapy has transformed HER2/neu amplified (HER2-positive) breast cancer from a disease with a poor prognosis to an opportunity for improved survival and cure. Multiple trials have now demonstrated improved rates of BCS, pCR, and survival when neoadjuvant trastuzumab is administered in conjunction with standard chemotherapy regimens.[23,48–50] Lapatinib has also been found to be effective in the treatment of HER2-positive breast cancer but has side effects that are generally found to be more severe than trastuzumab.[51,52] More recently, pertuzumab has emerged as a powerful adjunct to trastuzumab and docetaxel in the treatment of HER2-positive breast cancer, initially in the setting of demonstrably improved progression-free survival in patients with metastatic disease via the CLEOPATRA trial.[53,54] TRYPHAENA[26] and NEOSPHERE[28] are both randomized phase II trials that have demonstrated the efficacy of pertuzumab in improving rates of pCR in HER2-positive LABC without unacceptable cardiac toxicity when administered in conjunction with trastuzumab and docetaxel. The multinational phase III APHINITY trial will test whether the combination of pertuzumab and trastuzumab will result in improved disease-free survival in the adjuvant setting compared with single-agent adjuvant therapy with trastuzumab.

Adjuvant Radiotherapy

Postmastectomy radiotherapy (PMRT) as a component of multimodal therapy is considered standard of care for LABC patients. The 2016 National Comprehensive Cancer Network breast cancer guidelines recommend PMRT for patients with four or more positive lymph nodes. In addition, the guidelines urge practitioners to "strongly consider" PMRT in patients with one to three positive nodes and to "consider" PMRT in select patients with node-negative disease but with clinical features that put them at increased risk for local recurrence including tumor size 5 cm or greater and tumor size less than 5 cm but with less than 1 mm margins.[55] Most patients with LABC receive neoadjuvant chemotherapy, and it remains to be determined whether PMRT is beneficial in patients with LABC who experience pCR after neoadjuvant chemotherapy. A 2002 study at MD Anderson Cancer Center noted that the presenting stage of the disease is the most important predictor of locoregional recurrence and should factor into decision-making regarding adjuvant radiotherapy, even in patients who have a complete pathologic response to neoadjuvant chemotherapy.[56] NSABP B-51 is an ongoing phase III, randomized trial, the results of which will help provide more information about the most appropriate role for radiotherapy in the management of LABC after receipt of neoadjuvant chemotherapy, particularly in patients who experience pCR.[57]

In 2015, results from two randomized trials, the MA.20 study from Canada[58] and an EORTC trial on nonaxillary, regional nodal irradiation,[59] demonstrated that regional nodal irradiation could significantly improve outcomes for patients with LABC. In the MA.20 trial, 1832 women with node-positive (clinical N1 only) or node-negative, high-risk (i.e., T3 tumors; T2 tumors with <10 lymph nodes removed in axillary lymph node dissection and one or more factors of ER-negative status, grade 3 histology, or lymphovascular invasion) breast cancer were randomized from 2000 to 2007 to receive either whole breast irradiation only (i.e., the control group) or whole breast irradiation in conjunction with irradiation of the axillary, internal mammary, and supraclavicular lymph node basins. There was no difference between the two treatment arms in 10-year overall survival rates, but the group with nodal irradiation had higher disease-free survival (82% vs. 77%, $p = .01$) at 10 years as well as higher rates of grade 2 or higher acute pneumonitis (8.4% vs. 4.5%, $p = .001$). Notably, the improved disease-free survival seen in the group with nodal irradiation was in large part due to decreased recurrence in the lymph nodes, not decreased in-breast recurrence.

EORTC 22922/10925 was a phase III trial designed specifically to evaluate the potential benefit of adding internal mammary and medial supraclavicular radiation to the treatment of patients with central/medial breast cancers or with outer quadrant breast cancer and axillary involvement because both these sets of patients are at high risk for harboring microscopic extraaxillary regional disease. Between 1996 and 2004, 4004 patients, all of whom underwent axillary lymph node dissection, were randomized to receive either whole breast/chest wall irradiation only (i.e., the control group) or whole breast/chest wall irradiation with irradiation of the internal mammary and medial supraclavicular lymph node basins. At 10 years, the group with nodal irradiation had higher disease-free survival (72.1% vs. 69.1%, $p = .04$) and higher distant disease-free survival (78% vs. 75%, $p = .02$) as well as lower breast cancer–specific mortality (12.5% vs. 14.4%, $p = .02$), but there was no statistically significant difference between the two groups with regards to 10-year overall survival (82.3% vs. 80.7%, $p = .06$). The nodal irradiation group also had higher rates of pulmonary fibrosis. Thus these two trials demonstrated that nodal irradiation decreases the risk of locoregional—and perhaps even distant—recurrence but not without some additional morbidity.

Breast Conserving Surgery in Locally Advanced Breast Cancer

Although modified radical mastectomy has historically been the standard of care for LABC, BCS after neoadjuvant chemotherapy is increasingly performed for LABC in patients whose disease responds to systemic therapy. An early study from MD Anderson Cancer Center retrospectively analyzed surgical specimens from patients with stage IIIA and IIIB breast cancer after three cycles of neoadjuvant cyclophosphamide, doxorubicin, vincristine, and prednisone chemotherapy, citing complete and partial pathologic response rates of 16% and 84%, respectively. On the basis of criteria for breast conservation in early-stage breast cancer, they concluded that 23% of those patients could have undergone BCS after their neoadjuvant treatment.[60] Schwartz and colleagues retrospectively analyzed patients with stage IIB and III breast cancer

---

• BOX 59.2 Criteria for Breast Conservation Surgery After Induction Chemotherapy for Locally

Advanced Breast Cancer

- Resolution of skin edema (dermal lymphatic involvement)
- Residual tumor size for which resection would not render a cosmetically unacceptable postoperative appearance of the breast
- Absence of extensive intramammary lymphatic invasion
- Absence of extensive suspicious-appearing microcalcifications
- No known evidence of multicentric disease
- Patient's desire for breast preservation

---

who received induction chemotherapy and reported 5-year disease-free and overall survival rates of 56% and 67% for patients treated with mastectomy versus 77% and 80%, respectively, for patients treated with BCS; when patients were stratified according to age and degree of pathologic response; however, no difference in survival was seen between the two arms.[61] A 2004 report of the MD Anderson experience by Chen and associates analyzed locoregional recurrence rates in 130 women with stage IIIA–C breast cancer who underwent neoadjuvant chemotherapy and subsequent BCS. In-breast recurrence-free and locoregional recurrence-free survival rates of 95% and 91%, respectively, were reported at 5 years, demonstrating that BCS after neoadjuvant chemotherapy results in acceptably low recurrence rates in patients with LABC while citing the presence of N2 to N3 disease, residual tumor greater than 2 cm in size, multifocal disease, and lymphovascular invasion as predictors of increased recurrence.[62] Thus BCS is an acceptable option in terms of local control and survival for patients with LABC who experience a significant treatment response to neoadjuvant chemotherapy, and this option is offered to appropriate patients at our institution (Box 59.2).

Axillary Staging

Axillary Lymphadenectomy

Rationale

Level I and II axillary lymph node dissection (ALND) remains the standard of care in LABC, particularly in cases of biopsy proven axillary nodal metastases. ALND likely contributes little to overall survival but is crucial for staging and prognostic information as well as regional control.

Level I lymph nodes are located lateral to the pectoralis minor muscle, level II lymph nodes are located posterior to the pectoralis minor muscle. Level III lymph nodes are located medial to the pectoralis minor muscle and are not routinely dissected in breast cancer patients. Rotter nodes are located between the pectoralis major and minor muscles. As a rule, radiation therapy to the axilla is not used in conjunction with complete (level I/II with or without level III) ALND. In addition, the level I/II dissection avoids the functional and cosmetic difficulties that can result from axillary radiotherapy in an axilla that has already been completely dissected.[63] Because moderate doses of radiation therapy sterilize lymph nodes 1 cm or smaller, metastatic cancer in smaller, centrally located axillary lymph nodes (high level II and level III) are generally sterilized with radiation therapy. With use of such a combination of therapeutic modalities, the entire axilla is treated with minimal overlap of radiation portals with the surgically dissected portion of the axilla.

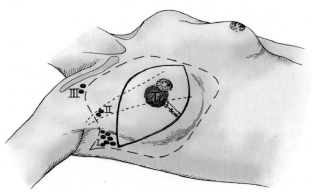

• **Fig. 59.3** Limits of dissection for the modified radical mastectomy *(dotted line)*. The dissection is inclusive of tumor and overlying skin, with an adequate skin margin to allow primary wound closure. Level I and level II nodes are dissected en bloc with the breast.

Technique

The technique of ALND is the same regardless of whether the patient is undergoing the procedure at the time of modified radical mastectomy or through a separate incision in cases of BCS. The technique of modified radical mastectomy is described elsewhere in this text. When ALND is performed as part of a modified radical mastectomy, the mastectomy incision is oriented so as to include the tumor mass, all involved skin, the nipple-areola complex, and previous biopsy sites as well as to allow easy access to the axilla. The arm is draped free so that the elbow may be flexed or extended and the arm adducted across the chest wall. Skin flaps for axillary dissection are developed superiorly to the level of the clavicle, medially to the medial half of the clavicle, and laterally to the deltopectoral triangle and cephalic vein. The lateral portion of the superior flap is developed until the anterior edge of the latissimus dorsi muscle is identified, at which point the superior flap is developed laterally and superiorly following the anterior edge of the latissimus dorsi muscle cephalad (Fig. 59.3). As the dissection continues toward the axilla, the major branch of the intercostobrachial nerve is identified. This nerve is composed of fibers from the lateral cutaneous branches of the second and third intercostal nerves and runs at right angles and anterior to the latissimus dorsi muscle. It can be sacrificed if multiple clinically positive lymph nodes are present, with the postoperative sequelae being paresthesias to the medial upper arm. The dissection is continued cephalad following the anterior border of the latissimus dorsi muscle until the white tendon of the latissimus dorsi muscle is identified. Immediately superior and anterior to this tendon, the axillary vein is identified and exposed.

Attention is then turned to dissection of the inferior flap. In elevating the skin flaps medially, the plane of penetration of the pectoralis major fascia by the perforating branches of the internal mammary vessel should be used as a guide for the medial extension of the dissection. The breast is dissected free from the pectoralis major muscle, beginning superiorly and medially and progressing inferiorly and laterally until the lateral border of the muscle is identified almost in its entirety.

The lateral border of the pectoralis major muscle is then retracted inferiorly and medially. Dissection is continued lateral and posterior to the pectoralis major muscle to identify the lateral border of the pectoralis minor muscle. The entire innervations of the pectoralis major and minor muscles can be preserved in this operation. The medial pectoral nerve is identified coursing lateral to (or penetrating) the pectoralis minor muscle at approximately the juncture between the superior one-third and inferior two-thirds of the pectoralis major muscle. The clavipectoral fascia lateral to the pectoralis minor muscle is opened, and the axillary vein is again identified. Working laterally along the axillary vein, the venous tributaries coursing inferiorly are divided and ligated. Laterally, the neurovascular bundle to the latissimus dorsi muscle is identified; this bundle contains the thoracodorsal nerve and major branches of the subscapular artery and vein. The lateral thoracic artery is usually identified just medial to it and is removed with the specimen. At the site of confluence of the thoracodorsal neurovascular trunk with the latissimus dorsi muscle, a venous tributary courses medially to join the chest wall. At this site, with meticulous dissection in a plane parallel to the long axis of the patient, the long thoracic nerve to the serratus anterior muscle (respiratory nerve of Bell) is best identified. The long thoracic nerve is traced superiorly until it exits the operative field posterior to the axillary vein.

The axillary contents are then removed from the serratus anterior muscle anterior and medial to the long thoracic nerve. The superior extent of the axillary dissection was previously defined by the axillary vein, and the medial extent of the dissection is represented by the lateral borders of the pectoralis major and minor muscles as well as the medial pectoral nerve and accompanying vascular structures. During surgery on a patient with stage IIIA, stage IIIB, or inflammatory (T4d) breast cancer who is to receive postoperative radiation therapy, any lymph nodes that are clinically positive should be removed from beneath the pectoralis minor muscle (within level II lymph nodes). The specimen is removed from the operative field and oriented for the pathologist, the wound is irrigated copiously with warm saline, and a closed-suction Silastic drain is placed in the dissected axillary space. The drain is sutured in place at the skin entrance site, and the wound is closed in two layers.

Role of Sentinel Lymph Node Biopsy

Patients with LABC routinely receive neoadjuvant chemotherapy as part of their multimodal treatment, and 30% to 40% of patients with LABC experience pCR in the nodal basin after neoadjuvant chemotherapy, with anti-HER2 therapy achieving even higher rates of pCR (as discussed earlier).[28,64-66] The accuracy of sentinel lymph node biopsy (SLNB) in this patient subset has been the subject of significant investigation, especially with regard to whether ALND can be omitted in patients who have clinical evidence of nodal response that is confirmed by a negative SLNB (Table 59.2).[26,28,67,68]

The ACOSOG Z1071 trial was launched in 2009 to investigate the false-negative rate of SLNB (with at least two nodes removed) after neoadjuvant chemotherapy in breast cancer patients with pretreatment nodal disease confirmed on needle biopsy; an acceptable false-negative rate was predetermined to be 10%.[66] Of 756 patients enrolled in the trial, 649 with clinical N1 (cN1) disease and 38 with clinical N2 (cN2) disease ultimately underwent SLNB and ALND after completing chemotherapy; 2 patients underwent SLNB only. Dual tracer technique was used in 545 of the 689 patients (79%) who received SLNBs. At least one sentinel node was found in 639 of these 689 patients (92.9%), with only one sentinel LN found in 78 patients (12%). Among the 525 cN1 patients in whom 2 or more SLNs were found, 215 (40.9%) had a complete nodal response. Of the remaining 310 patients found to have residual disease on ALND, 39 had a

TABLE 59.2	Clinical Trials Evaluating Sentinel Node Biopsy Following Neoadjuvant Chemotherapy in Clinically Node Positive Patients		
	ACOSOG Z1071[66,70] **(n = 637)**	**SENTINA (Arm C)**[33]	**SN FNAC**[34]
Nodal eligibility criteria	cN1–2	cN1–2	cN1–2
SLN identification rate	92.7%	87.8%	87.6%
Overall FNR (no IHC)	12.6%	14.2%	13.4%
FNR depending on Mapping agents			
One agent	20.3%	16%	16%
Dual agent	10.8%	8.6%	5.2%
FNR by number of SLNs			
1 SLN	31%	24.3%	18.2%
2 SLNs	21.1%	18.5%	≥2 SLNs =
≥3 SLNs	9.1%	4.9%	4.9%
FNR with IHC	8.7%	Not reported	8.4%

FNR, False-negative rate; *IHC*, immunohistochemistry; *SLN*, sentinel lymph node.

negative SLNB, yielding a false-negative rate of 12.6%, higher than the preset threshold for the trial of 10%.

SENTINA (SENTinel NeoAdjuvant) was a multicenter, prospective cohort study with more than 1000 patients from Austria and Germany conducted to determine the optimal timing of SLNB relative to neoadjuvant chemotherapy. Patients were accrued to one of several arms. Women with clinically node-negative (cN0) disease underwent SLNB before neoadjuvant chemotherapy were enrolled into Arm A. Arm B consisted of patients who were cN0 patients but found to have a positive SLNBs (pN1) and underwent a second SLNB after neoadjuvant chemotherapy. Women who presented with clinically node-positive disease (cN+) received neoadjuvant chemotherapy without preceding SLNB; those cN+ patients who went on to experience clinical pCR (i.e., became ycN0) received postchemotherapy SLNB and ALND (Arm C), whereas those who remained clinically node-positive (ycN+) undergoing ALND alone (Arm D). Compared with Z071, the false-negative rates of SLNB in SENTINA patients after neoadjuvant chemotherapy were higher. In Arm B patients, posttreatment SLNB had a false-negative rate of 51.6%, whereas Arm C patients with pretreatment cN+ disease that became ycN0, the false-negative rates of SLNB after chemotherapy were 24.3% for women who had one sentinel node removed and 18.5% for those who had two nodes removed.[69]

The findings from both ACOSOG Z1071 and SENTINA indicate that, given current practices and patient selection patterns, SLNB alone is not an appropriate alternative to ALND for axillary staging after neoadjuvant chemotherapy in patients with cN1 disease. However, there are adjunct clinical practices that could better identify patients in whom selective axillary surgery after neoadjuvant chemotherapy is more or less likely to be successful and sufficient. A secondary goal of ACOSOG Z1071 is a determination of axillary ultrasound (AUS) accuracy in LABC after completion of neoadjuvant chemotherapy. In a secondary analysis in which AUS images in 611 patients from this trial were reviewed, patients with axillary nodes that appeared suspicious on AUS had more positive nodes and larger nodal metastases compared with patients with sonographically normal appearing nodes. Thus a strategy in which SLNB was only performed on patients with nodes that appeared normal on AUS was modeled and projected to potentially reduce the false-negative rate among cN1 patients from 12.6% to 9.8%, that is, below the previously prescribed threshold of 10%.[70] However, these findings need further clinical validation before AUS is routinely adopted to screen patients at low risk for false-negative SLNB.

Another method of reducing the false-negative rate of selective axillary surgery after neoadjuvant chemotherapy is through targeted dissection of lymph nodes that had previously been found to harbor disease via pretreatment, ultrasound-guided FNA and that were marked with a clip at the time of biopsy. In a prospective study at MD Anderson, previously clipped nodes with pretreatment evidence of metastatic disease were localized with radioactive I-125 seeds and removed at the same time as sentinel nodes localized via traditional intraoperative mapping; ALND was subsequently performed. The combined excision of both sentinel and seed-localized clipped nodes, together known as targeted axillary dissection (TAD), yielded a false-negative rate of only 2%.[71]

Thus both AUS and TAD have the potential to shift the standard of care for LABC away from one in which ALND is mandatory for all patients and toward a more individualized approach in which ALND and its concomitant morbidity are safely avoided in selected patients. As of now, however, a complete level I and II ALND is still recommended for definitive staging and control of axillary disease for patients with LABC treated with neoadjuvant chemotherapy. Furthermore, although some centers continue to perform SLNB before commencing neoadjuvant systemic therapy, we recommend that AUS with selective FNA of suspicious nodes be performed for pretreatment axillary staging in LABC.

Timing of Therapies

There is a biological rationale for the sequence of modalities used to treat LABC. Neoadjuvant chemotherapy is used first in an attempt to achieve early control of distant micrometastases. Even though distant disease may be undetectable with current clinical diagnostic procedures, its presence is suggested by the high percentage of distant failures that occur even when complete local control is achieved with radiotherapy and surgery, as demonstrated by preliminary studies in the prechemotherapy era. In addition, the use of neoadjuvant chemotherapy may decrease primary tumor bulk sufficiently to convert some inoperable patients into candidates for mastectomy or BCS. Tumor responsiveness has also been shown to correlate with overall survival, and tumor responsiveness to neoadjuvant chemotherapy may serve as an in vivo chemosensitivity assay to indicate the potential effectiveness of individual agents.

If the tumor increases in size after an initial course of neoadjuvant chemotherapy, second-line chemotherapy is considered. If there is still no response to chemotherapy, surgical resection is considered if feasible. Otherwise, radiotherapy is used, followed by surgical resection. If the tumor has responded to neoadjuvant chemotherapy, surgery is then used as the second modality. At our institution, pathologic assessment of response to neoadjuvant chemotherapy is used as an indicator of prognosis. In addition, residual cancer burden (RCB), a prognostic index comprising primary tumor (size and cellularity) and nodal disease measures

Carcinoma

- The chest wall and peripheral lymphatics are treated to 50 Gy in 25 fractions.
- The chest wall is treated with either tangential photon-beam or electron-beam fields, depending on patient anatomy.
- When the chest wall is treated with tangents, a matched 15- to 20-degree obliqued electron field is used to treat the medial chest wall and internal mammary lymph nodes.
- A matched obliqued anterior photon field is used to treat the Rotter space, the level III axilla, and the supraclavicular lymph nodes. For patients with incomplete axillary dissection, a dose supplement is used to treat the level I and II axillary lymph node region. Three-dimensional treatment planning with contouring of structures/targets is used to ensure that targets are adequately covered by prescription dosages.
- The chest wall including the mastectomy scar and areas of gross undissected adenopathy receive a boost of 10–16 Gy.
- Patients with inflammatory carcinoma are treated on an accelerated, hyperfractionated (twice-daily) schedule unless they achieve a significant pathologic response to chemotherapy.

From Simona Shaitelman, MD, personal communication, 2016.

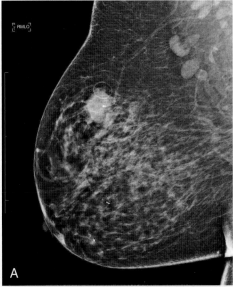

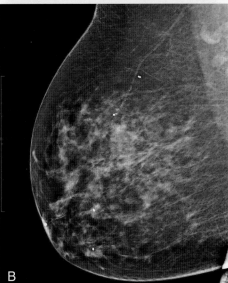

• **Fig. 59.4** Mammography before and after 12 weekly cycles of paclitaxel and 4 cycles of Adriamycin/Cytoxan. (A) Pretreatment mammogram showing a high-density mass in the upper aspect of the breast. (B) Mammogram after neoadjuvant chemotherapy, showing a complete radiographic response with only clip identified within tumor bed.

(number and size) derived from the surgical specimen, can lend granularity to the wide range of response that exists between pCR and chemoresistant disease by delineating categories of response— RCB-I (minimal RD), RCB-II (moderate RD), and RCB-III (extensive RD)—that correlate with likelihood of recurrence.[72] Thus pathologic review of the surgical specimen can help guide radiotherapy plans as well (Box 59.3). Radiotherapy is optimally performed at the completion of both surgical resection and chemotherapy, and the rationale for this sequence is further supported by the fact that radiotherapy and doxorubicin are poorly tolerated if given simultaneously.[15] In addition, local control is equally good with early or late radiotherapy, but more distant failures have been observed with postoperative radiotherapy given before adjuvant chemotherapy.

The issue of response versus progression of the primary tumor is assessed by physical examination and repeat imaging, which can include mammography, ultrasonography, and/or MRI (Fig. 59.4). Established criteria of the Union Internationale Contre le Cancer[73] are used to grade tumor regression. Surgical treatment consists of either total mastectomy or segmental mastectomy with level I/II axillary dissection as previously described. Surgical resection is generally performed 3 to 4 weeks after the last chemotherapy treatment to allow time for recovery from the myelosuppressive effects (e.g., granulocyte and platelet nadirs) observed in the 2 weeks after chemotherapy. In the event of prolonged myelosuppression, complete blood cell counts are followed until the granulocyte count is greater than 1500/mm³, at which time surgical resection is performed.

The surgical goal is to achieve the best possible local control on the chest wall and in the axilla to avoid the complex and difficult problem of chest wall recurrence. Surgery is performed before radiotherapy because having the tumor debulked surgically allows for better radiotherapeutic local control in the adjuvant setting.[67] No significant increases in postoperative infection or wound-healing problems have been noted in patients treated with this multimodal approach.[74]

Full-Thickness Chest Wall Resection Revisited

An accurate understanding of the natural biology of LABC, coupled with the ability to integrate extirpative and reconstructive surgery with the other available modalities, has radically improved our capacity to treat and even cure this formerly lethal disease. The efficacy of chemotherapy for control of distant disease has expanded the role of surgical intervention for palliation and local control of recurrent and progressive LABC. Patients with chest wall invasion often suffer from disabling symptoms of pain, bleeding, ulceration, thoracic deformity, soft tissue superinfection, and malodorous drainage. In many of these advanced cases, radical ablative procedures may be mandated because of extensive skin involvement or chest wall fixation. Data have emerged indicating that patients who develop chest wall recurrences after mastectomy are not, in fact, a homogeneous population with a uniformly dismal prognosis. A 2003 study from our institution analyzed factors associated with poor outcome, and after a 37-month follow-up, initial nodal status was found to be the strongest predictor of outcome by univariate and multivariate analyses. Patients presenting with initial node-negative disease who developed a chest wall recurrence after 24 months and received treatment with radiation had the best prognosis.[75]

Veronesi and associates reported low morbidity and mortality from full-thickness chest wall resection in patients with recurrent and locally advanced breast cancers. Partial or total sternectomy with resection of one or more ribs resulted in median overall and disease-free survival rates of 23.4 and 17.5 months, respectively, and only minor complications were observed.[76] Full-thickness chest wall resection is thus a valid option for symptom palliation and improvement in esthetic and functional outcomes, even in patients in whom standard multimodality treatment has failed.

Reconstructive Techniques

Reconstructive techniques are often used in patients with LABC to cover exposed vital structures, bring about timely wound closure, and avoid delay in commencing adjuvant therapy. In addition, in patients with advanced disease, reconstructive surgery may enhance the patient's quality of life by providing palliation of hygiene problems posed by bulky, necrotic tumors.

We examined a series of 90 patients with locally advanced or recurrent breast cancer (stage IIIB and IV) treated at the MD Anderson Cancer Center over a 12-year course who required immediate chest wall reconstruction as part of their surgical therapy. The majority of these patients received neoadjuvant and postoperative adjuvant chemotherapy and postoperative radiotherapy. The tumor size and chest wall defects were considerably large, with the average pathologic tumor size being 6.8 cm and the average defect size being 264 cm^2 (range, 70–900 cm^2). Reconstructive surgeons used various regional tissue transfers (most commonly rectus abdominis and latissimus dorsi) to reconstruct these defects, and 20% of these patients required multiple tissue transfers to achieve wound closure. Rigid or semirigid synthetic material such as methylmethacrylate cement and/or polypropylene mesh was used to restore chest wall integrity in 25% of the patients. In general, patients tolerated these procedures well, with a fourth of the patients developing primarily self-limited complications such as wound infections or delayed healing. The rate of total flap loss was just over 1%. Just over a quarter of the patients experienced cardiopulmonary medical complications such as pneumonia, congestive heart failure, or pleural effusion. No operative deaths occurred, the average hospital stay was 7 days (range 2–34 days), and patients had a mean survival of slightly more than 2.5 years. As previously reported in other series, survival was related to the stage of disease, not the complexity of the surgery, which supports a role for surgical palliation in advanced breast cancer.[77]

Timing of Breast Reconstruction

When postmastectomy breast reconstruction is being considered, careful attention must be paid to clinicopathologic factors such as breast cancer stage, sentinel lymph node status, preexisting scars, prior radiotherapy, planned or previous chemotherapy,

body habitus, and tobacco use because these factors influence not only the choice of reconstructive method but also the timing of reconstruction. The timing of breast reconstruction in relation to the primary surgery can be altered to allow appropriate delivery of radiation to the chest wall and optimize esthetic outcome. Although the chance of requiring PMRT can be forecasted preoperatively, the need for PMRT is not definitively determined until final pathologic review of the mastectomy specimen, both because nodal micrometastases are often not detected until final examination of the axillary contents several days after surgery and because the final pathologic tumor size can be larger than was measured by preoperative imaging. With the increasing application of PMRT as advocated by the results of the Danish and Canadian trials,[78,79] many centers in the United States now routinely recommend PMRT for patients with breast cancer and one to three positive lymph nodes, which adds to the complexity of selecting the appropriate reconstructive option.

Immediate Reconstruction

LABC was once thought to be a contraindication for immediate breast reconstruction because of the perceived potential for delays in commencing adjuvant therapy caused by wound complications, the perceived potential for increased incidence or delays in diagnosis of local recurrences, and the detrimental esthetic effects of PMRT.[80,81] Delayed reconstruction was thus favored in patients with LABC who underwent mastectomy, with immediate reconstruction reserved for patients at low risk for requiring PMRT (stage I breast cancer).

In our experiences at the MD Anderson Cancer Center, we have observed no increase in surgical complication rates in patients with stage IIB/IIIA breast cancer who undergo immediate breast reconstruction. Although a delay in commencement of adjuvant chemotherapy of up to 2 weeks has been observed in patients receiving immediate reconstruction, this does not appear to result in increased recurrence rates after a median follow-up of 58 months.[82,83]

Tran examined the long-term effects of radiation therapy on the outcome of breast reconstruction with the free transverse rectus abdominis musculocutaneous (TRAM) flap by comparing the outcome of immediate and delayed free TRAM flap breast reconstruction in patients who received PMRT. The incidence of early complications such as vessel thrombosis, partial or total flap loss, skin flap necrosis, and local wound-healing problems did not differ significantly between the two groups, although the incidence of late complications such as fat necrosis, volume loss, and flap contracture of the breast mound was significantly higher in the immediate reconstruction group than in the delayed reconstruction group (87.5 vs. 8.6%, $p < .0001$), with almost a third of the patients who underwent immediate reconstruction requiring an additional flap to correct postradiation flap distortions.[84] Garvey and colleagues found that modifications of the flap design from a deep inferior epigastric perforator (DIEP) to a TRAM had no effect on the rates of late flap complications, and that both DIEP and muscle-sparing free TRAM flaps experienced much higher rates of fat necrosis when radiated.[85]

Delayed Reconstruction

Delayed reconstruction may be preferable in patients known preoperatively to require PMRT because this avoids the difficulties associated with radiation delivery to an augmented (not flat) chest wall. Most patients with stage III breast cancer fall into this category. At the MD Anderson Cancer Center, we prefer to avoid implant-based breast reconstruction in patients who have received PMRT because of observed problems with wound healing and capsular contracture.[86] Esthetic outcomes of delayed reconstruction, although inferior to those achieved with immediate reconstruction, are acceptable, particularly when nonirradiated, autologous tissue is used. The retained, irradiated skin and mastectomy scar are excised at the time of reconstruction, and the inferior breast skin is replaced with the lower abdominal skin via a TRAM flap. The entire three-dimensional contour of the breast must be recreated because the skin envelope has been excised with the specimen, and thus more flap skin and soft tissue are needed to fulfill the anatomic requirements of the missing breast. The majority of the TRAM flap must often be used in this situation. We may use a bilateral perforator free flap for a unilateral breast reconstruction in such a clinical scenario to fully replicate the esthetic appearance of the native breast.[87,88] This may limit the ability to perform a bilateral autologous reconstruction from the lower abdominal wall, and patients must be counseled accordingly.[89] Up to a third of these patients require contralateral mastopexy to optimize symmetry between their native breast and their reconstructed breast (Fig. 59.5).

To address the loss of breast skin in delayed reconstruction, we performed a prospective trial of selected patients who were deemed preoperatively to be at a high risk for requiring PMRT.[90] Patients with T2 tumors, one biopsy-proven positive axillary lymph node, multicentric disease on ultrasound, or extensive microcalcifications by mammography were considered candidates for the clinical protocol examining a two-stage approach to reconstruction, which has been coined *delayed immediate reconstruction.*[91] Stage I consisted of a skin-sparing mastectomy with subpectoral placement of a tissue expander, which was completely filled to preserve the contour of the breast skin envelope, as allowed by the vascularity of the mastectomy skin flaps. If final pathology ruled against the need for PMRT, patients returned to the operating room as early as 2 weeks after their mastectomy to complete the second stage, which consisted of immediate reconstruction. If patients were deemed to require PMRT, the tissue expander was deflated to allow PMRT to be delivered to the internal mammary lymph nodes and a flat chest wall. Within 2 weeks after completion of PMRT (as tolerated by the resolving radiation skin changes), the tissue expander was rapidly refilled to as close as possible to the original dimension of the breast skin envelope and planned reconstructive result. A definitive flap reconstruction was then undertaken with preservation of a greater amount of the mastectomy skin, which should theoretically lead to a better esthetic result and permit harvest of a smaller flap.

The results of this approach did show promise. The overall complication rates for the delayed immediate patients were 21% for the first stage skin-preserving mastectomy and placement of the expander, 5% during postmastectomy radiotherapy, 25% for expander reinflation after radiotherapy, and 24% after the final skin-preserving delayed autologous reconstruction. Tissue expander loss rates were 32% overall in the delayed immediate group. The overall complication rate for standard delayed autologous reconstruction after PMRT was 38%. The 3-year recurrence free survival rates were 92% for the delayed immediate group versus 86% for the standard delayed group, which was not statistically significantly different. The authors concluded from this that the delayed-immediate reconstruction technique did not lead to increased locoregional recurrence risk and was associated with lower complication rates of definitive reconstruction.

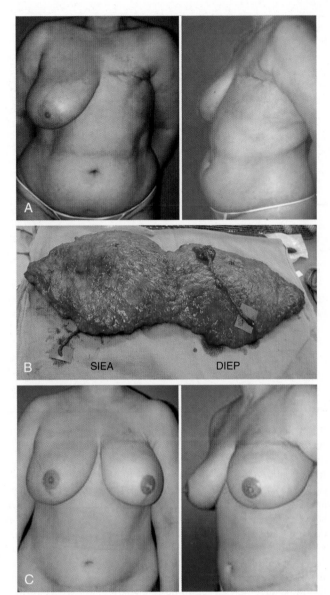

• **Fig. 59.5** Efficacy of bilateral flap to restore a large skin and large volume parenchymal deficit. (A) A 54-year-old woman after left modified radical mastectomy and postmastectomy radiation therapy for stage II (T2N1M0) breast cancer 4 years earlier, desiring delayed autologous reconstruction and symmetry with her contralateral breast. (B) Reconstruction with combined bilateral deep inferior epigastric perforator *(DIEP)* and superficial inferior epigastric artery *(SIEA)* free flaps was performed. (C) Four-year postoperative result after contralateral mastopexy and subsequent reconstruction of the nipple-areola complex. ([A and C] From Beahm EK, Walton RL. The efficacy of bilateral lower abdominal free flaps for unilateral breast reconstruction. *Plast Reconstr Surg.* 2007;120:41-54, with permission from Lippincott Williams & Wilkins.)

Options for Chest Wall Closure

The surgical options available for chest wall reconstruction are numerous. Factors that most strongly affect the reconstructive paradigm include the size and composition of the defect and the adequacy of donor and recipient tissues, which may have been compromised by prior surgery or radiotherapy. The patient's general medical condition and ability to withstand a lengthy

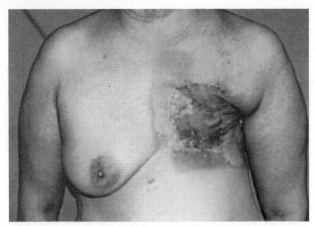

• **Fig. 59.6** Patient with a skin graft to the left chest wall. Note the thin cover and poor cosmetic appearance. (Courtesy Dr. Stephen Kroll.)

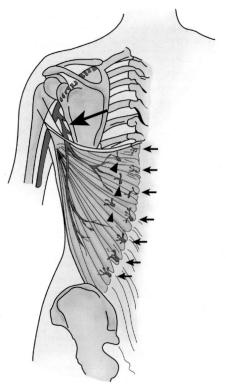

• **Fig. 59.7** Latissimus dorsi muscle: the vascular supply to the latissimus dorsi muscle. The thoracodorsal artery *(large arrow)*, a branch of the subscapular artery, is the dominant supply. Medially, the posterior intercostal vessels *(small arrows)* and laterally, the lumbar vessels *(arrowheads)* provide secondary segmental pedicles.

operative procedure, as well as the patient's overall prognosis and desires, must be considered. In addition, patient anatomy dictates the options available. Refinements in autologous tissue techniques and the increasing variety of prosthetic implants available have advanced the field of postmastectomy reconstruction and subsequent reconstructive outcomes.

Skin Grafts

If the defect is limited to the skin and subcutaneous tissue of the chest wall, and flap closure appears unwarranted due to donor site issues or the patient's medical status, a skin graft may be an appropriate choice for coverage. This straightforward maneuver closes the wound and usually tolerates postoperative radiotherapy once it has fully healed (Fig. 59.6). There are some disadvantages, however, in the application of skin grafts to the chest wall. A skin graft in this location is not as esthetically appealing and less durable than a vascularized flap. All grafts result in a certain degree of contracture, even if a full-thickness graft is used. Grafts also require time for both recipient and donor site healing. In addition, there may be compromise of skin graft take in an irradiated bed, and as such, skin grafts are not often used in chest wall reconstruction at our institution. A skin graft placed over an omental flap (see later discussion) may be a reasonable alternative for coverage of very large defects or if other options appear untenable.[71,85–94]

Myocutaneous Flaps

Latissimus Dorsi Musculocutaneous Flap

The latissimus dorsi musculocutaneous flap was first described in 1897 by the Italian surgeon Tansini.[95] The latissimus dorsi has a single dominant vascular pedicle from the thoracodorsal artery and multiple secondary segmental pedicles originating from the posterior intercostal arteries (Fig. 59.7).[96] In a standard flap incorporating the entire muscle, the dissection usually begins proximally, along the lateral aspect of the latissimus dorsi muscle, where the thoracodorsal vessels are identified and traced into the axilla, isolating the flap to its vascular pedicle. The thoracodorsal vessels in the axilla serve as the point of rotation in a latissimus pedicled flap. This arc of rotation may be increased by transection of the humeral insertion and/or transection of the vascular branches to the serratus muscle. This maneuver enables the flap to reach up

to the neck superiorly or medially to cross the midline. The muscular portion of the latissimus dorsi flap can be quite wide. The muscle supplies a broad skin territory that extends from the midaxillary line to the vestibular column in the posterior midline and from the axilla to the posterior iliac spine. As such, a variety of orientations of the skin paddle in this region is possible, including a complex fleur-de-lis or sickle shape used for breast reconstruction.[97] The size of the skin paddle harvested with a musculocutaneous latissimus flap is limited, however, by the need to achieve primary closure of the back after flap harvest. Primary closure of the latissimus flap donor site is considered imperative, because an open back wound is highly problematic and skin grafts on the back generally do not fare well. As such, although almost 20 cm of length may be harvested with a latissimus flap, it is rare that a skin paddle greater than 8 to 10 cm in width can be obtained and permit closure of the donor site, thus limiting overall musculocutaneous flap size.

Harvest of the latissimus muscle appears to be generally well tolerated.[98,99] Traditionally, it has been considered that patients notice little morbidity after a latissimus dorsi flap, perhaps because of similar actions by the teres major and minor.[100,101] More recent critical analyses using both dynamic and static testing, however, suggest that a significant reduction in strength develops in the affected extremity.[102] This decreased strength does not appear to preclude normal activities but must be considered in patients heavily reliant on shoulder girdle strength, such as patients who depend on crutches or walkers or athletes.

Perforator flaps based on the thoracodorsal vessels but sparing the latissimus muscle have been described.[103,104] Unfortunately,

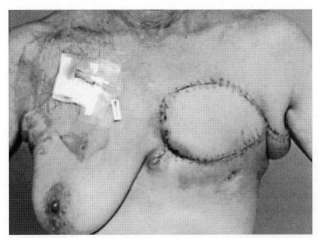

• **Fig. 59.8** Pedicled latissimus dorsi flap coverage of full-thickness chest wall defect. Note the improved esthetic appearance in comparison to a skin graft (see Fig. 59.7). (Courtesy Dr. Stephen Kroll.)

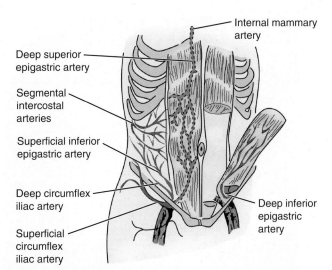

• **Fig. 59.9** Rectus abdominis. The vascular supply of the rectus abdominis flaps. The deep inferior and deep superior epigastric arteries communicate at the periumbilical watershed area. The deep inferior epigastric artery, the dominant blood supply to the muscle, is the most suitable pedicle for microvascular anastomosis. The deep superior epigastric artery, a branch of the internal mammary artery, provides the vascular basis for superiorly based rectus flaps. The muscle also receives direct vascular contributions from posterior perforating intercostal and internal mammary vessels.

perforator flaps generally exhibit a reduced flap vascularity compared with musculocutaneous flaps, and this limitation has hindered their application for chest wall reconstructions because delayed healing or flap compromise may have profound oncologic or medical repercussions. In cases in which the thoracodorsal vessels (which supply the latissimus) have been divided, it has been demonstrated experimentally that the flap can survive on the collateral flow between the thoracodorsal vessel and serratus branch.[105] Previous irradiation to the axilla is not a contraindication to the latissimus flap unless there has been prior division of the thoracodorsal pedicle, in which case it is postulated that flap loss may occur as a result of radiation, thereby limiting development of collateral circulation.[106]

The advantages of the latissimus dorsi flap for chest wall reconstruction include its general reliability and proximity to the defect, its large size, a long vascular pedicle, and a straightforward flap harvest. It represents a first-line choice for simple closure of chest wall defects after mastectomy for advanced breast cancer (Fig. 59.8). The disadvantages of this flap are relatively minor and include the additional operative time needed to move the patient into the lateral decubitus position and possible functional donor site morbidity.

Donor site complications are typically minor and include seroma formation (40%–50%)[107,108] Prolonged seroma formation after latissimus flap harvest is largely self-limited but can result in prolonged drainage, infection, or the need for serial aspirations. Attempts to surgically decrease the incidence of seroma have been investigated, and securing the flap to the underlying thoracodorsal fascia during donor site closure has been suggested to decrease seroma formation.[109,110]

Contraindications to latissimus dorsi flap reconstruction include prior lateral thoracotomy with division of the latissimus muscle, prior division of the thoracodorsal artery and vein, and prior irradiation to the ipsilateral posterior superior trunk.[111]

Rectus Abdominis Transposition and Free Flaps

Pedicled abdominal flaps based on musculocutaneous perforators from the muscle were used for a number of years before the introduction of the rectus abdominis island flap in 1977.[112] The rectus

abdominis musculocutaneous flaps have since become workhorse flaps in reconstructive surgery because of the ease of elevation, reliability, and the large size of the flap that may be harvested and still permit primary closure of the donor site.

The rectus abdominis muscle is supplied primarily by the deep inferior epigastric arteries, which communicate at the periumbilical watershed area with the superior epigastric arteries. The deep inferior epigastric artery, the dominant blood supply to the muscle, is the most suitable pedicle for microvascular anastomosis. The superior epigastric artery (a branch of the internal mammary artery) provides the vascular basis for superiorly based pedicled rectus flaps. The muscle also receives direct vascular contributions from posterior perforating intercostal and internal mammary vessels (Fig. 59.9). Because the rectus abdominis flap may be based on either of these vessels, numerous flap configurations are possible.

Vertical Rectus Abdominis Myocutaneous Flap

The vertical rectus abdominis musculocutaneous (VRAM) flap was the earliest of the rectus flaps to be described. Initially used for chest and abdominal wall reconstruction, this flap was subsequently applied to breast reconstruction by Robbins.[113] The VRAM is simple and quick to harvest and has the most robust vascularity of all the rectus abdominis flap configurations because the skin paddle is positioned directly over the muscle, where it is richly supplied by perforating vessels.[96,113] The drawbacks of the VRAM include a less esthetic donor site and a smaller available skin paddle in comparison to the TRAM flap. Nonetheless, often 15 cm or more of skin may be harvested with a VRAM flap because of the generalized skin laxity in an older population. Patients should be advised of a resultant off-center abdominal scar and umbilicus following reconstruction with a VRAM flap (Fig. 59.10).

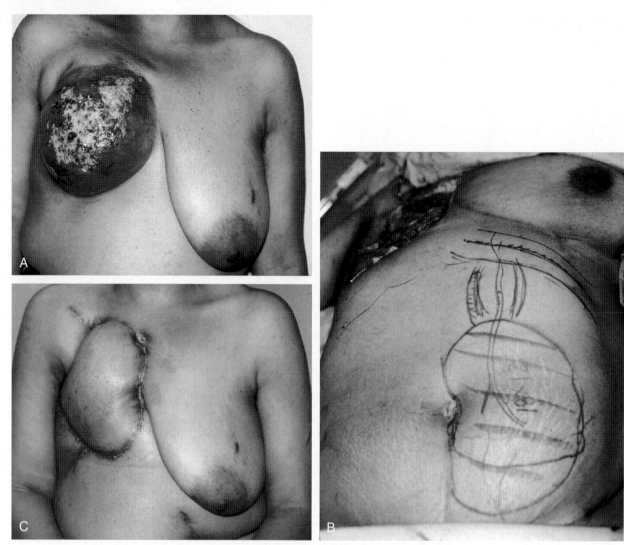

• **Fig. 59.10** Pedicled vertically oriented rectus abdominis myocutaneous flap. (A) A 32-year-old woman with locally advanced stage IIIB breast cancer. The tumor was excised leaving the underlying chest wall intact. (B) A vertical rectus abdominis myocutaneous flap based on the contralateral superior pedicle was planned due to an abdominal midline scar and sacrifice of the ipsilateral thoracodorsal and mammary vessels during the resection. (C) The vertical rectus flap and a local fasciocutaneous advancement flap provided stable coverage. The patient had an uncomplicated postoperative course but developed local and then distant metastasis 9 months postoperatively and succumbed to her disease.

Transverse Rectus Abdominis Myocutaneous Flap

Pedicled

The pedicled TRAM flap, with a transversely oriented skin island, is the most common flap used for autologous postmastectomy breast reconstruction.[114] It is suited for patients desiring autologous breast reconstruction from an abdominal donor site and patients with an inadequate skin envelope and/or ptotic contralateral breast to which they desire to achieve symmetry. The transverse orientation permits harvest of a generous skin paddle, and the donor scar, although long, is well positioned near the "bikini line" (similar to an abdominoplasty). If the flap is placed low on the rectus muscle, it has a long leash and a long axis of rotation, allowing the skin paddle to rotate quite far laterally or high into the axilla.

The single-pedicle, superiorly based TRAM flap is hindered by the less robust nature of its blood supply because a large part of the skin paddle does not lie directly over the muscle. As such, the flap is dependent on the integrity of a small number of perforating vessels and vascular anastomoses between the superior and inferior epigastric vessels and periumbilical (predominantly) vascular interconnections, which provide for blood flow from one vascular pedicle across both sides of the abdomen. The patterns of flap vascularity, coined angiosomes, have been extensively studied. The more distant the tissue is from the vascular pedicle, the less reliable the vascular supply.[115] In addition, pedicled TRAM flaps may be problematic in chest wall reconstruction because of damage of the internal mammary vessels, which form the dominant vascular pedicle to the flap. Although superior-based rectus flaps have been successfully based solely on the costal marginal (eighth intercostal) vessels, this is a less well-vascularized configuration, and in this

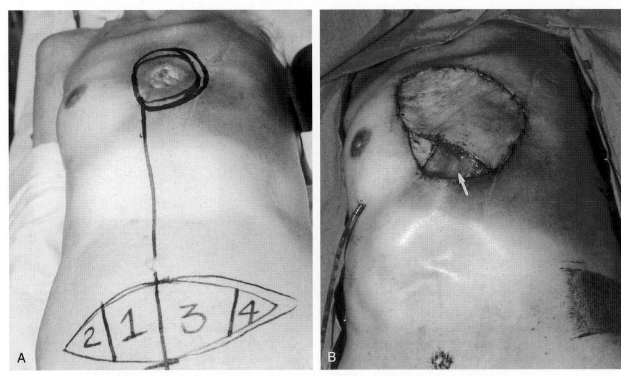

• **Fig. 59.11** Free transverse rectus abdominis myocutaneous (TRAM) flap. (A) A 48-year-old woman with osteoradionecrosis of the sternum and recurrent breast cancer. A superior-based pedicle TRAM flap based on the right superior epigastric vessels is planned, with the vascular zones of the TRAM illustrated. (B) The defect size necessitated skin grafting over a portion of the rectus muscle at the inferior wound edge *(arrow)*. The rotational course of the muscle into the wound may be seen. (Courtesy Dr. Robert Walton.)

situation a free-tissue transfer is preferable.[116] As such, if the defect is small or the chest wall is intact, the superior-based pedicled TRAM flap may be a reasonable choice (Fig. 59.11). In patients who smoke, are diabetic, or have multiple abdominal scars, however, circulation may be inadequate and may severely limit the size and viability of the flap. Accordingly, alternatives to the single-pedicle TRAM flap, such as the double-pedicle, "supercharged," "turbocharged," and free TRAM flaps, have been used as a means to enhance flap vascularity.

The double-pedicle TRAM flap is a variation of the single-pedicle TRAM flap in which the blood supply is doubled by basing the flap on both rectus abdominis muscles.[117] The enhanced blood supply of the double-pedicle TRAM flap permits safe harvest of a large flap. The inclusion of both muscles in the flap does, however, result in a much bulkier pedicle, limiting the arc of rotation. The decreased abdominal strength and reported increased risk of hernia (reported incidence, 1%–8%) that result from the loss of two rectus muscles are also significant disadvantages of this flap.[118–122] Patients generally tolerate the musculocutaneous flap donor sites well; however, in anticipation of potential abdominal wall compromise, we do not hesitate to use an inlay of synthetic or bioprosthetic mesh. At our institution, however, when the defect size or circumstances dictate the need for a larger flap, we most often favor use of the free TRAM flap or a free anterolateral thigh (ALT) flap over the bipedicled TRAM, not only because of donor site concerns but also because of enhanced vascularity and greater versatility in positioning the flap.

Free Rectus Musculocutaneous Flaps

The free rectus flap (either TRAM or VRAM) is based solely on the deep inferior epigastric vessels and necessitates microvascular anastomoses to reestablish blood supply to the flap.[123] During chest wall resections, a variety of recipient vessels are usually available for anastomoses. We have most commonly used the proximal portions of the internal mammary vessels and, less frequently, branches of the thoracodorsal vessels. Because a smaller amount of muscle is harvested in a free TRAM than with a pedicled TRAM, patients tend to have less postoperative pain, recover from surgery more quickly, and experience a lower incidence of hernia or abdominal bulge.[120] Criticisms of this technique include the need for microsurgical expertise, but most high-volume microsurgery centers realize a less than 1% free flap loss rate and feel comfortable with routine use of a free TRAM flap for chest wall reconstruction (Figs. 59.12 and 59.13).

The microsurgically enhanced ("supercharged" or "turbocharged") rectus flap may be seen as a compromise, providing the assurances of a pedicled flap and the enhanced vascularity of a free flap. With this approach, the inferior epigastric vessels are used to enhance the vascular supply of a pedicled flap by microvascular anastomoses of either the venous ("supercharged") or arterial and venous ("turbocharged") flap to suitable recipient vessels. This technique may also be helpful in salvaging a compromised or congested pedicled flap. We often dissect out and include a portion of the deep inferior or superficial inferior epigastric vessels during pedicle TRAM flap harvest to allow for this contingency. Table 59.3 summarizes the indications,

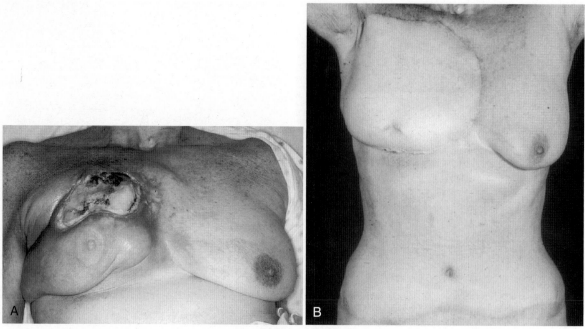

• **Fig. 59.12** Free transverse rectus abdominis myocutaneous (TRAM) flap. (A) A 62-year-old woman with recurrent breast cancer after prior segmentectomy and radiotherapy. (B) A full-thickness chest wall excision was performed, and the defect was reconstructed with a free TRAM revascularized with the internal mammary vessels. Note the large volume of tissue that can be transferred using the dominant inferior epigastric pedicle via microsurgical transfer.

contraindications, and characteristics for latissimus dorsi versus TRAM flap reconstructions.

Microvascular Composite Tissue Transplantation (Free Flaps)

Concerns stemming from abdominal donor site morbidity after standard TRAM reconstruction have prompted the increased use of perforator flaps for breast and other forms of reconstruction in many institutions, including our own.[124–128] Perforator flaps represent the most recent evolution of autologous flap reconstructions and theoretically permit transfer of tissue from numerous donor sites to almost any distant site with suitable recipient vessels for microsurgical anastomosis.

Deep and Superficial Inferior Epigastric Artery Perforator Flaps

The DIEP flap, like the free TRAM flap, uses the inferior epigastric vessels as its vascular supply. Microvascular anastomoses are typically performed to either the internal mammary or thoracodorsal vessels. Because the inferior epigastric artery is the dominant artery supplying the lower abdominal wall, this flap enables transfer of a sizeable amount of tissue. It is particularly suited for patients who smoke or have risk factors for postoperative complications such as morbid obesity or diabetes.[129] Perforator flaps are associated with less abdominal wall morbidity because perforator vessels from the inferior epigastric artery are dissected free without sacrificing the rectus abdominis muscle or rectus fascia. The superficial inferior epigastric artery (SIEA) flap derives its blood supply from the superficial inferior epigastric artery which originates from the common femoral artery. SIEA flaps are harvested without an abdominal wall incision, thus completely preserving abdominal wall integrity. However, a reliable superficial inferior epigastric artery is present in only half of the population, limiting the applicability of the SIEA flap.[126]

A recent retrospective study comparing reconstructive outcomes of the DIEP to the pedicled TRAM flap for postmastectomy breast reconstructions cites shorter hospital stays (4 vs. 5 days), longer operative times (5.5 vs. 4.5 hours), lower fat necrosis rates (17.7% vs. 58.5%), and lower incidences of abdominal wall hernias (1% vs. 16%) with the DIEP flap (all $ps < .001$).[130]

Contraindications specific to perforator flaps include history of previous suction-assisted lipectomy of the donor site or prior abdominoplasty in the case of a DIEP flap. Active smoking or the need for postoperative radiation represent relative contraindications to these flaps. Cases with prior chest wall radiotherapy should be approached with caution because radiation damages the recipient vessels and can increase the risk of fat necrosis or flap loss.[131]

Pectoralis Major Flap

The pectoralis major flap may be used as a rotational flap, based on its dominant thoracoacromial pedicle, or as a "turnover" flap, based on perforators of the internal mammary vessels that segmentally supply the muscle along its sternal border (Fig. 59.14A). A generous muscle flap may be harvested, and a skin paddle may also be incorporated with the flap. This flap has been used extensively for sternal and chest wall reconstruction.[77,132,133] The pectoralis major flap is particularly well suited to defects of the anterior and superior central chest. In the setting of reconstruction for advanced breast cancer, however, the ipsilateral pectoralis muscle is often involved in the disease process and resected with the tumor (see Fig. 59.14B). In our series, the pectoralis flap was used in only

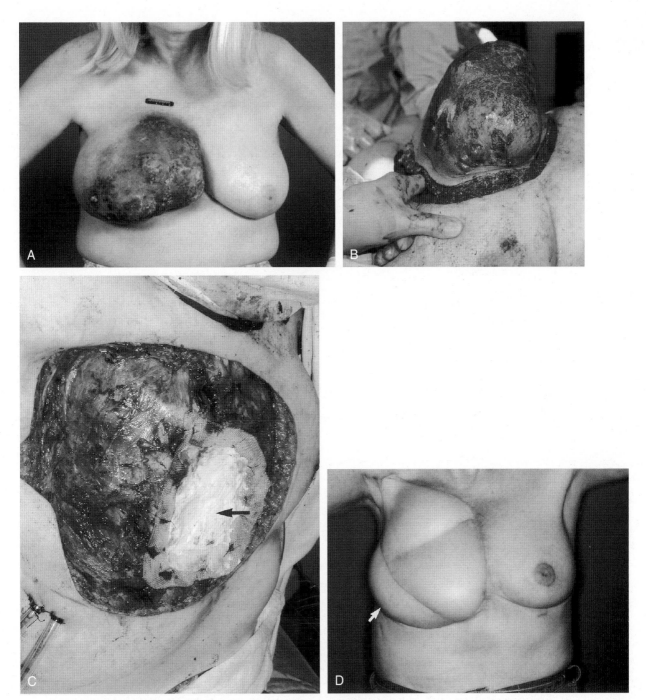

• **Fig. 59.13** Free transverse rectus abdominis myocutaneous (TRAM) and latissimus flap. (A) A 47-year-old with neglected locally advanced breast cancer responsive to neoadjuvant chemotherapy. (B) Tumor fixed to chest wall, excised with sternum and six ribs. Surgical margins were negative. (C) Resultant chest wall defect with sternum reconstructed with Marlex mesh and methylmethacrylate *(arrow)*. (D) Bilateral free TRAM and ipsilateral latissimus dorsi *(arrow)* myocutaneous flaps were used to close the wound. The patient had an uneventful recovery and is seen here 9 months after completion of radiation therapy.

10% of cases because of the location and size of the resultant defects.

External Oblique Flap

Although the latissimus dorsi and rectus abdominis musculocutaneous flaps can produce excellent cosmetic results, they are not feasible in some patient subgroups. Division of the thoracodorsal vessels during axillary node dissection can compromise the blood supply of the latissimus dorsi flap. In addition, raising this flap requires subsequent repositioning of the patient on the operative table. Previous abdominal surgery may render a rectus abdominis based flap unusable and prohibit its use in some patients. In such rare situations, the external oblique musculocutaneous flap is an

TABLE 59.3	Indications, Contraindications, and Characteristics for Latissimus Dorsi Versus Transverse Rectus Abdominis Myocutaneous Flap Reconstructions	
	Latissimus Dorsi	**TRAM**
Indications	Segmental mastectomy defects after BCS In conjunction with a TE for patients requiring salvage mastectomy Poor candidate for TRAM	Single-pedicled Compromised skin envelope with large breast size Desired abdominal donor site Double-pedicled Compromised skin envelope, damaged pectoralis muscle Less donor site fat/skin Large-mound reconstruction Free: same as pedicled but also smokers
Contraindications	Prior lateral thoracotomy with division of the latissimus muscle Prior division of the thoracodorsal artery and vein Prior irradiation to the ipsilateral posterior superior trunk Relative Plans for adjuvant PMRT Current smoker	Prior subcostal incision Prior abdominoplasty Relative Prior abdominal suction-assisted lipectomy Morbid obesity Current smoker
Advantages	Proximity to defect Minimal donor site morbidity	Hidden donor scar Double: very rich blood supply vs. single Free: versatility in positioning vs. pedicled Less postoperative pain Lower incidence hernia vs. pedicled Can harvest more tissue vs. pedicled
Disadvantages	Harvest requires patient repositioning	Single: Less robust blood supply Double: Bulky pedicle, limited arc Free: Microsurgery required
Mean OR time[a] (hours)	4	Single: 5.5 Double: 7 Free: 5–8
Coverage potential	10-cm skin paddle	Variable
Major complications[a]	Donor site seroma (incidence 40%–50%)	Single Abdominal hernia (6%–10%) Fat necrosis (10%) Free Fat necrosis (14%) Abdominal hernia (3%–12%)

BCS, Breast conservation surgery; *OR,* operating room; *PMRT,* postmastectomy radiation therapy; *TE,* tissue expander; *TRAM,* transverse rectus abdominis myocutaneous.
[a]All percentages represent patient incidences, and all means reflect those reported in the current literature.

alternative method of reconstruction after resection of a large, locally advanced breast carcinoma.

Lesnick and Davids first reported use of the external oblique musculocutaneous flap for lower abdominal reconstruction in 1952, and its use subsequently evolved for coverage of chest wall defects resulting from breast cancer.[134,135] The external oblique muscle is a large muscle that takes origin from the 6th to the 12th ribs and receives segmental blood supply from the lateral cutaneous branches of the inferior eight posterior intercostal vessels. Flap territory is large, extending from the midline of the abdomen to the anterior axillary line, enabling it to easily cover defects measuring 300 cm^2 (Fig. 59.15). The flap is elevated medially, with dissection between the internal and external oblique muscles, progressing laterally to the posterior midline with preservation of the perforating vessels, and rotated superiorly into the defect. Proponents of this flap cite straightforward flap harvest that obviates the need to intraoperatively reposition the patient, maintenance of abdominal wall integrity by sparing the rectus abdominis, and

reliable closure of large defects. Likewise, the flap harvest is straightforward, and complications are relatively uncommon, with superficial necrosis being the most frequently reported. Several successful series of the external oblique flap for chest wall reconstruction have been reported.[136–138] Segmental blood supply to the muscle, however, limits the useful arc of rotation. Although an extended modification to increase the flap reach has been reported, extensive dissection to facilitate flap rotation may compromise these segmental vascular pedicles. Lateral hernia formation is also a concern. These considerations have limited the use of the external oblique flaps for chest wall reconstruction at our institution.

Fasciocutaneous Flaps

A number of possible fasciocutaneous flap options exist for chest wall reconstruction, some of which may require free-tissue transfer. In general, these flaps are smaller than the TRAM or latissimus flaps, and are less commonly used for chest wall reconstruction.

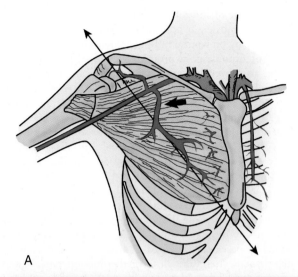

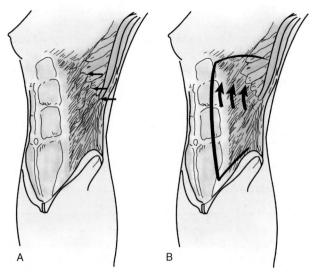

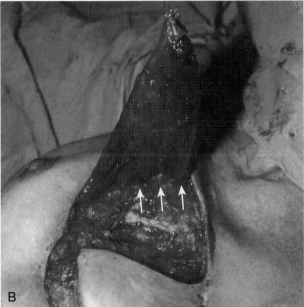

• **Fig. 59.14** Pectoralis major muscle. (A) Vascular supply of the pectoralis major flap. A muscle or myocutaneous flap may be based on the pectoral branch of the thoracoacromial artery *(arrow),* which is the dominant supply for the muscle. The pedicle may be found to lie at the junction of the midclavicular line and the xiphoacromial axis and is the dominant pedicle. A reverse or turnover flap can be based on the minor segmental pedicles (perforating branches of intercostal arteries 5, 6, and 7 and internal mammary perforating branches) and is useful for midline defects. (B) A contralateral turnover pectoralis muscle flap, based on the minor segmental perforating vessels *(arrows),* is used to cover a sternal defect.

The scapular and/or parascapular flaps based on the circumflex scapular vessels may be used alone or in combination with the latissimus dorsi.[139,140] We have used these flaps in relatively few cases, most commonly in combination with other flaps for very large defects or in situations in which the latissimus or TRAM territories were compromised.

The thoracoepigastric, or transverse abdominal, flap is based on the anterior midline overlying the upper portion of the rectus abdominis muscle and extending to the ipsilateral posterior axillary line. It is supplied by perforating vessels from the superior

• **Fig. 59.15** External oblique muscle. (A) The external oblique muscle, which arises from the lower eight ribs and inserts onto the anterior half of the iliac crest has a segmental blood supply, provided by the lateral cutaneous branches of the inferior eight posterior intercostal arteries *(arrows).* (B) The point of rotation of the external oblique flap is the costal margin at the anterior axillary line, which limits the flap utility in superior chest wall defects.

epigastric artery. The flap width is maximally 7 to 8 cm, with a length of 15 to 25 cm, and it is rotated superiorly 45 to 90 degrees for ipsilateral chest wall coverage. Although originally described for chest wall coverage and modified for use in breast reconstruction, this flap is limited to application in smaller defects by overall flap size, vascularity, and reach.[141,142]

Cutaneous and Local Flaps

Cutaneous flaps of the chest wall may be random or axial; the latter are based on perforating branches of the internal mammary and intercostal vessels. These flaps can play a role in smaller defects or in combination with regional or distant flaps, especially if the surrounding tissues are healthy. We do not favor their use if there is any potential compromise of these tissues by a prior history of radiation or tobacco use.

Omental Flaps

The highly vascularized greater omentum, which hangs from the greater curvature of the stomach, has been used for chest wall reconstruction for more than 30 years. Since then, the omentum has been used primarily as a pedicled flap covered by a skin graft to repair extensive thoracic defects.[94,143,144] Although either the right or left gastroepiploic artery may be used to supply the omental flap, the right gastroepiploic artery (a branch of the gastroduodenal artery) is the favored pedicle because it affords a 5- to 10-cm greater arc of rotation.

The omentum is relatively easy to harvest, is well vascularized, and typically provides a large flap. There are, however, some drawbacks to the use of this flap. Neither the thickness nor surface area of the available greater omental apron is possible to predict preoperatively, because it does not directly correlate with the patient's morphologic characteristics. The omentum, albeit well vascularized, is delicate and has an irregular surface. This may result in difficulties with fixation to the chest wall, retraction from defect edges, and instability of overlying skin graft. Harvest of the omental flap previously required a laparotomy, which held potential for a host of intraabdominal complications. Reports of laparoscopic flap harvesting procedures have demonstrated decreased postoperative complication rates and donor site morbidity.[145] In experienced hands, pedicled omentoplasty with meshed skin graft and VAC therapy has shown encouraging results for reconstruction of full-thickness chest wall defects.[146]

Full-Thickness Chest Wall Defects and Prosthetic Materials

Loss of chest wall integrity alters the reconstructive strategy. The spectrum of flaps used in these cases is comparable to those used when the chest wall is intact. The differences arise in that these defects are often larger and the reliability of the autologous tissue coverage is more critical than in the more superficial defects. Communication with the mediastinum or pleural cavity or exposure of any prosthetic materials used for chest wall stabilization can have profound and lethal consequences. The latissimus dorsi musculocutaneous flap is often the best choice for small defects that are within its arc of rotation. For defects lower on the chest wall that would be difficult to reach with the latissimus or for very large defects that the latissimus flap would not cover, the rectus abdominis flap in either the vertical or transverse configuration or the pedicled omental flap are good options. These flaps are quite reliable, and their bulkiness may help stabilize the chest wall and compensate for the loss of ribs. Rigid reconstruction of the rib cage is not typically necessary after resection of less than four ribs if good flap coverage and respiratory support are provided. For such defects, the chest wall defect is reconstructed with a prosthetic mesh like polypropylene or a bioprosthetic, xenograft acellular dermal matrix. If the mesh is completely covered by viable tissue, it is usually well tolerated and allows the patient to be weaned from the respirator and discharged from the hospital earlier than otherwise would be the case.[147] Because of the reliability of current prosthetic materials, materials or ribs are rarely used in this setting.[77] The use of rigid reconstruction of the chest wall or sternum with a polypropylene mesh and methylmethacrylate cement "sandwich" is typically used for defects encompassing four or more ribs.[148–150] (see Fig. 59.13C). Such larger chest wall defects require rigid stabilization to prevent paradoxical motion of the chest wall and avoid respiratory insufficiency. Although devastating infectious consequences can be associated with the use of prosthetic materials, these complications have not been generally manifest, provided that the overlying flap is well vascularized and that preexisting infection was not present. To ensure stable coverage and maximal vascularity, free-tissue transfer or microvascularly augmented flaps may be appropriate when prosthetic materials are used. In many of these large defects, multiple flaps are required for closure (see Fig. 59.13D).

Radiotherapy and Reconstruction

The increasing use of adjuvant radiotherapy has led to modifications in autologous tissue techniques, prosthetic developments, and the discovery of novel tissue substitutes and radioprotectors. Radiation therapy, whether administered preoperatively or postoperatively, complicates reconstruction of the chest wall due to tissue fibrosis and compromised wound healing. Radiation also compromises the quality of the recipient vessels for microvascular free tissue transfer. It appears that the deleterious effects of radiation therapy on wound healing are related to a chromosomal alteration of fibroblasts, a position supported by studies demonstrating an irreversible inhibition of replication and dysfunction in collagen formation and breakdown in fibroblasts after radiation.[151–153] At our institution, recent examination has demonstrated that more than 50% of patients who had mastectomy after radiation therapy for inoperable breast cancer manifested a wound complication (infection, dehiscence, necrosis), and some of these cases were so severe that the patients required flap coverage for salvage.[154] These findings suggest that a low threshold for flap coverage in radiated wounds may be prudent.

The use of preoperative radiotherapy is also problematic for chest wall reconstruction. Local tissues are compromised, and there is a greatly increased complication rate with reconstruction performed in previously radiated tissues.[77,131,155] The viability of radiated tissue is often difficult to predict intraoperatively, and as such, excision of all possible radiated tissue is helpful to minimize subsequent wound breakdown.[77] This increases the defect size and the invasiveness of the reconstruction. Total muscle necrosis has been reported when radiated muscles are transferred, so it is preferable to choose donor tissues out of the radiated field when possible.[92,93,131] Microsurgical transfer of flaps can bring nonradiated tissue to these compromised regions.

Reconstruction before radiotherapy, although technically easier, must take into consideration the subsequent impact of radiation on the transferred tissues. Radiation therapy after breast reconstruction has a complication rate of 30% to 87%.[84,131,156] Flaps may demonstrate contracture and fibrosis, fat necrosis, loss of skin grafts, or even partial flap loss after radiation. Some of these effects may be anticipated by the specific radiation dosage, ports, and boosts (e.g., supraclavicular tumor bed) used. In addition, each patient appears to have an individual response to radiation that is often unpredictable and leads to a spectrum of clinical manifestations.[131,155] Although fibrosis and scarring may be painful and unattractive, many of the pertinent issues in breast reconstruction are less important in cases of chest wall reconstruction. Concerns primarily focus on the stability of the tissues transferred for chest wall coverage, and fortunately, flaps are typically able to tolerate radiation and protect underlying structures.

Substances called radioprotectors, which may reduce some of the early and late effects of radiation, are under investigation. Amifostine (Ethyol) is a thiol synthetic compound and an oxygen free radical scavenger that has shown some promise in reducing morbidity and mortality in patients exposed to ionizing irradiation, yet it is associated with significant side effects. Recent research has focused on the development of radioprotective agents with lower toxicity and an extended window of protection. Natural compounds that exert their effect through antioxidant and immunostimulant activities are being evaluated as radioprotectants. Although recent agents have demonstrated lower efficacy, they have also exhibited lower toxicity, more favorable administration routes, and improved pharmacokinetics compared with the older thiol compounds.[157]

The management of patients seeking breast reconstruction in the setting of radiotherapy is highly controversial, poorly understood, and must be critically evaluated in terms of both oncologic and esthetic outcomes. Immediate reconstruction preserves more native breast skin, which is esthetically advantageous, provides a psychological benefit, and has a lower rate of short-term operative complications. Although the resulting fibrosis appears to be more severe if the flap itself is irradiated, there is an increased rate of flap-related complications in flaps placed in previously irradiated sites.[84,131,155,158–162] Furthermore, a large number of reconstructive flaps that have been subjected to postoperative radiation therapy appear to exhibit acceptable results.[163] There appears to be a wide variability in the clinical response to irradiation, leading to relatively minor changes in some flaps and severe deformation in others, which unfortunately cannot be accurately predicted from patient variables or radiation dosing. Objective evaluation of reconstructive results is limited by both the number and quality of the existing data in our study and similar studies.[84,160–162] Differences in outcomes may reflect patient variables, anatomy, surgical technique, experience, and surgeon preference and proficiency, all of which are problematic to control and assess. There are a number of technical nuances in the transfer of lower abdominal flaps for reconstruction with suggestions that one configuration, such as microsurgically transferred flaps, may tolerate insults such as radiation more favorably than other conventional (pedicled) flaps. Additionally, establishing esthetic outcome is by nature a highly subjective process and essentially impossible to quantify. There is significant discordance in outcome assessment between patients and their surgeons, with patients (fortunately) being more pleased than their respective reconstructive surgeons with the final esthetic result.

The flap-related conditions (fibrosis, firmness, and fat necrosis) that may result from radiation injury have no standardized measurement points in the literature and are limited to assessment by degrees of scale. Some authors, for example, describe fat necrosis as any firmness in the reconstructed breast, whereas others cite its presence only if surgical removal of the affected area is deemed necessary.[84,131,160] There are, however, consistent trends in the literature. Although each study has reported a variable amount of fat necrosis, fibrosis, and flap-related complications, they have all noted a statistically significant increase in complications and a higher percentage of unfavorable results in TRAM flaps treated with radiation therapy (10%–75%).[84,131,162,164,165] Many of these effects develop late and can insidiously progress even years after completion of treatment.[151,152,164–166] Accordingly, it is important to consider the follow-up period of any study that evaluates the effects of radiation therapy on breast reconstruction. In addition, such data should be presented with actuarial rather than crude statistics so that long-term estimations of effects can be generated.

A consensus treatment algorithm remains elusive for patients facing radiotherapy and desiring breast reconstruction. Currently, most plastic surgeons recommend delayed reconstruction if postoperative radiotherapy after mastectomy is planned due to the potential for an adverse operative outcome. A number of unanswered questions remain. From an esthetic standpoint, one must attempt to balance the degree of radiation-induced fibrosis with the loss of native skin and increase in flap-related complications that have been observed in delayed breast reconstruction. Although a large number of reconstructive flaps (≥70%) that have been subjected to postoperative radiotherapy appear to exhibit acceptable results, some do not fare as well. The differentiation between "acceptable" and "esthetic" in this instance is quite unclear, and herein lies the dilemma.

In terms of perspective, the overriding potential downside of immediate reconstruction concerns the question of whether the presence of a breast mound adversely affects the delivery of PMRT. For patients with advanced breast cancers, the radiation target volume should include a wide margin around the mastectomy site and the entire chest wall, the internal mammary lymph nodes, and the axillary apex and supraclavicular fossa. To treat these regional lymph nodes, multiple separate fields need to be geometrically matched, which can be more difficult over the sharply sloping contours created by a breast reconstruction. Motwani and colleagues found that immediate reconstruction led to a compromise in the radiation treatment planning in 52% of cases.[167] It is not known whether this actually affects patients' oncologic outcome because the article suggested a very low rate of local recurrence after radiation in patients with an immediate TRAM flap reconstruction. Although it is encouraging that these theoretical compromises in radiation planning do not seem to result in compromises in oncologic outcomes, this study and others like it are limited by small study population sample sizes.

If the presence of a flap or breast implant leads to significant compromise of the radiation therapy, then delayed breast reconstruction must be undertaken. It is important that surgical oncologists, radiation oncologists, and plastic/reconstructive surgeons work together to develop the best plan for an individual patient. Compromises in radiation treatments can often be avoided through minor modifications in reconstructive techniques, and at times, volume loss issues associated with radiation can be anticipated and planned for accordingly. Such multidisciplinary interactions also inspire confidence within patients and foster realistic expectations.

Multidisciplinary Approach

At our institution, we use a multidisciplinary approach to the management of LABC requiring chest wall reconstruction. The complex nature of these cases requires open communication between the ablative and reconstructive teams to optimally meet the oncologic imperative and preserve reconstructive options critical to successful closure of the defect. As with all joint surgical ventures, careful preoperative surgical planning is crucial. The treatment plan must include a realistic appraisal of the anticipated size, location, and composition of the defect, as well as the patient prognosis. In addition, the reconstructive surgeon must communicate the anticipated reconstructive strategy to the ablative surgeon, including any limitations of flap availability (e.g., related to prior surgery), preferred flaps, and recipient vessels to preserve these options, if possible. Because of the unpredictable nature of surgery, however, the reconstructive surgeon must plan for a number of alternative reconstructive strategies.

Algorithm for Chest Wall Reconstruction

Clinical experience supports a role for palliative procedures in patients with locally advanced or recurrent breast cancer.[77,132,148,149] There are, however, numerous challenges to the surgical management of extirpation and chest wall reconstruction for advanced breast cancer. These defects may be profound and complicated by prior surgery, radiotherapy, or patient-related variables. The reconstructive techniques used must neither encumber nor delay any necessary postoperative therapy, and they must not result in unacceptable morbidity or compromise quality of life. Our surgical approach to these cases requires a multidisciplinary team, and each operative plan is tailored to the individual patient. If the chest wall defect is superficial and small, local flaps or a skin graft may be a reasonable choice for wound closure. Chest wall defects resulting from extirpation of advanced breast cancer, however, generally require well-vascularized flaps. The pedicled latissimus dorsi flap is our choice for moderate ipsilateral defects, but it may also be used as a free flap. The rectus abdominis flaps provide an ample skin paddle and have been of great utility in larger defects.

Full-thickness chest wall defects pose an additional challenge. If four or fewer ribs are resected, a mesh or bioprosthetic matrix patch of the chest wall defect is appropriate, and rigid chest wall reconstruction is not required. Larger chest wall defects are best managed with a rigid prosthesis, such as a methylmethacrylate/ polypropylene "sandwich" technique. It is best to provide soft

tissue coverage of prosthetic materials with a well-vascularized flap rather than simply cover prosthetic materials with subcutaneous tissues, particularly if the patient will receive postoperative radiation therapy. We most frequently use a pedicled musculocutaneous flap such as the rectus abdominis or latissimus dorsi flap in chest wall reconstruction (Fig. 59.16), as these flaps provide reliable, durable, high-quality skin coverage that can reasonably tolerate postoperative radiation. Flap harvest does, however, necessitate

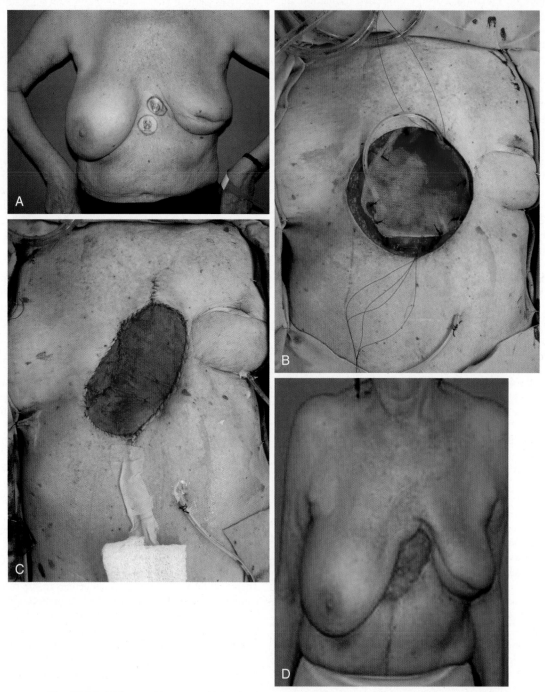

• **Fig. 59.16** A 66-year-old woman with local recurrence of breast cancer to the chest wall after previous failed latissimus dorsi flap with implant and subsequent pectoralis major flap for coverage. Patient had prior abdominal surgery that included aggressive ultrasonic liposuction, which limited the usable skin paddle for the abdominal territory. (A) Local recurrence to the chest wall manifesting as cutaneous nodules (noted by operative markings). (B) After wide resection of chest wall with reconstruction of full-thickness chest wall defect using prosthetic materials and a supercharged vertically oriented rectus abdominis myocutaneous flap. (C) With overlying split-thickness skin graft. (D) Four-month postoperative result.

a donor site with potential complications that should not be minimized. Our experience suggests that the donor site deformity from harvest of a musculocutaneous flap is generally well tolerated, and the benefits to these patients seem clearly to outweigh the risks.

Selected References

19. Kuerer HM, Newman LA, Smith TL, et al. Clinical course of breast cancer patients with complete pathologic primary tumor and axillary lymph node response to doxorubicin-based neoadjuvant chemotherapy. *J Clin Oncol.* 1999;17:460-469.

56. Buchholz TA, Katz A, Strom EA, et al. Pathologic tumor size and lymph node status predict for different rates of locoregional recurrence after mastectomy for breast cancer patients treated with neoadjuvant versus adjuvant chemotherapy. *Int J Radiat Oncol Biol Phys.* 2002;53:880-888.

75. Chagpar A, Meric-Bernstam F, Hunt KK, et al. Chest wall recurrence after mastectomy does not always portend a dismal outcome. *Ann Surg Oncol.* 2003;10:628-634.

81. Crisera CA, Chang EI, Da Lio AL, Festekjian JH, Mehrara BJ. Immediate free flap reconstruction for advanced-stage breast cancer: is it safe? *Plast Reconstr Surg.* 2011;128:32-41.

90. Kronowitz SJ, Lam C, Terefe W, et al. A multidisciplinary protocol for planned skin-preserving delayed breast reconstruction for patients with locally advanced breast cancer requiring postmastectomy radiation therapy: 3-year follow-up. *Plast Reconstr Surg.* 2011;127:2154-2166.

A full reference list is available online at ExpertConsult.com.

60

Solitary Metastases

JANE E. MENDEZ AND HENRY M. KUERER

Over the past 30 years, new and advanced breast cancer multimodality treatments have resulted in improved median survival times for patients with metastatic breast cancer.[1] Breast cancer most commonly metastasizes to bone, followed by lung, brain, and liver.[2] Until now, the treatment focus for metastatic breast cancer has been on palliative care rather than cure. However, a more aggressive treatment approach may be appropriate for patients with metastatic disease limited to a solitary lesion or to multiple lesions at a single organ site. Improved diagnostic, staging, and surgical techniques may allow curative surgery in these carefully selected patients with acceptable morbidity and very low mortality.[3] In addition, studies have shown that the molecular phenotype of breast cancer determines the timing, pattern, and outcome of metastatic disease and metastatic lesions may alter their receptor expression profile from their primary tumor.[4] The main goal of such curative surgery would be prolonged disease-free survival (DFS) and improved quality of life. Provided that the breast cancer primary is controlled, there is a long disease-free period, and the patient has a good performance status, surgery is an important component in the multimodality approach to breast cancer solitary metastases.

Liver

The liver is an uncommon site for solitary first metastasis in breast cancer, having been reported to occur only 3% to 9% of the time. Eventually, breast cancer liver metastases are found in 55% to 75% of autopsies performed on patients who died of breast cancer.[5] Hepatic metastases usually occur at later stages of disseminated disease and carry a poor prognosis, with a median survival of 6 months.[6] These patients are not candidates for resection and can be treated only with systemic therapy. Even with systemic chemotherapy, the median survival for patients with metastatic disease to the liver only or with limited disease elsewhere is approximately 19 months, using pretaxane chemotherapy regimens or 22 to 26 months with taxane-containing regimens.[7] Hormonal therapy is generally of limited use because most hepatic metastases are hormone receptor–negative; however, estrogen receptor–positive hepatic metastasis is not a rare phenomenon.[8] Hence, surgery has been proposed as a potential therapeutic tool for increasing survival in patients with isolated liver metastasis.[3]

Abbott and colleagues from the MD Anderson Cancer Center studied their institutional experience with 86 breast patients with metastases limited to the liver who underwent hepatic resection.[9] The primary aims were to document overall survival

(OS) and DFS and to identify predictors of survival that could be assessed preoperatively to optimize patient counseling, risk-benefit analyses, and outcome. Fifty-nine patients (69%) had estrogen receptor– or progesterone receptor–positive primary breast neoplasms. Fifty-three patients (62%) had a solitary breast cancer liver metastasis, and 73 (85%) had breast cancer liver metastases 5 cm or smaller. Sixty-five patients (76%) received prehepatectomy hormonal and/or chemotherapy. Four patients (6%) had progressive disease as the best response, and 19 patients (30%) had progressive disease before hepatectomy ($p < .001$). Seventy percent of patients who received preoperative chemotherapy or hormonal therapy had either response or stable disease immediately before hepatectomy. No postoperative deaths were observed. At a 62-month median follow-up, the DFS and OS were 14 and 57 months, respectively. On univariate analysis, estrogen receptor/progesterone receptor status of the primary breast neoplasm, best radiographic response, and preoperative radiographic response were associated with overall survival. On multivariate analysis, estrogen receptor–negative primary breast disease and preoperative progressive disease were associated with decreased overall survival. From their study, they concluded that resection of breast cancer liver metastases in patients with estrogen receptor–positive disease that is responding to chemotherapy is associated with improved survival. The timing of operative intervention may be critical; resection before progression is associated with a better outcome.

Van Walsum and colleagues on behalf of the Dutch Liver Surgeons Group evaluated the effectiveness and safety of resection of liver metastasis from breast cancer and to identify prognostic factors for overall survival.[10] A total of 32 female patients were identified. Intraoperative and postoperative complications occurred in 3 and 11 patients, respectively. There was no postoperative mortality. After a median follow-up period of 26 months, 5-year and median OS after partial liver resection was 37% and 55 months, respectively. The 5-year DFS was 19% with a median time to recurrence of 11 months. Solitary metastases were the only independent significant prognostic factor at multivariate analysis. Van Walsum and collaborators concluded that resection of liver metastases from breast cancer is safe and might provide a survival benefit in a selected group of patients. Especially in patients with solitary liver metastasis, the option of surgery in the multimodality management of patients with disseminated breast cancer should be considered.

Adam and associates offered hepatic resection to all patients with breast cancer liver metastases, provided that curative resection was feasible and extrahepatic disease was controlled with medical and/or surgical therapy.[11] The outcomes of 85 consecutive patients with breast cancer liver metastases treated from 1984 to 2004 were reviewed. Breast cancer liver metastases were solitary in 38% of patients and numbered more than three in 31%. After a median follow-up of 38 months, the median and 5-year survivals were 32 months and 37%. Median and 5-year DFS were 20 months and 21%. Study variables associated with a poor survival were failure to respond to preoperative chemotherapy, an R2 resection, and the absence of repeat hepatectomy. In addition, patients who were treated with repeat hepatectomy had a higher 5-year overall survival rate (81%), compared with patients with unresectable liver recurrences and patients without any hepatic recurrence after first hepatic resection but with extrahepatic metastatic disease. Their analysis determined that DFS was not an independent prognostic factor. Interestingly, the median survivals were longer in the group of patients treated from 1994 to 2004 versus 1983 to 1993. This improved survival might be a reflection of better diagnostic technology and surgical techniques. Adam and investigators concluded that favorable outcomes can be achieved even in patients with medically controlled or surgically resected extrahepatic disease, indicating that surgery should be considered more frequently in the multidisciplinary care of patients with breast cancer liver metastases.

Patient selection and operative criteria for hepatic resection are still controversial; however, important criteria are likely to be fewer than four metastases, no extrahepatic disease, and demonstrated disease regression or stability with systemic therapy before resection.[11] At a minimum, a patient should have a normal performance status and normal liver function tests.[3] Pocard and Selzner agreed that the size and number of hepatic metastasis was an important factor. Patients in whom liver metastasis was found more than 1 year after resection of the primary cancer had a significantly better outcome than those with early (<1 year) metastatic disease. The type of liver resection, the lymph node status at the time of the primary cancer resection, and the use of neoadjuvant high-dose chemotherapy had no significant impact on patient survival in their series.[12] Martinez and coworkers showed that survival was greater in patients with estrogen receptor–positive primary tumor and metastases, HER2/neu-positive metastases, two or fewer metastases, and age greater than 50 years at metastasectomy.[13]

The preference is for patients to receive chemotherapy before hepatic resection. Extensive preoperative staging evaluation before considering hepatic resection for breast cancer liver metastases is recommended. Diagnostic laparoscopy is recommended to avoid a nontherapeutic laparotomy if extrahepatic disease based on preoperative imaging is suggested. Hepatic resection is preferable if metastases can be safely removed with a negative surgical margin. Radiofrequency ablation should be reserved for those patients with tumors not amenable to safe resection or used as an adjunct to resection.[11] Radiofrequency ablation has been used for local control of breast cancer liver metastasis (BCLM); the reported series show a median survival of between 30 and 60 months, with no treatment-related deaths and only three serious treatment-related adverse events in 164 patients reported. Despite this, skepticism remains over the efficacy of BCLM ablation due to the heterogeneity of patient inclusion and selective nature of reporting. Randomized trials are needed to formulate robust evidence-based recommendations and direct the necessary allocation of health care resources.[14] Transarterial catheter embolization has emerged as a potential treatment option for direct liver delivery and possible better systemic toxicity profile.[15]

Lung

Isolated lung metastases have been reported to occur in 10% to 20% of all women with breast cancer. Approximately 3% of all women with breast cancer develop a solitary pulmonary lesion detectable by chest radiograph, of which 33% to 40% are breast metastases.[16,17] Considering the low morbidity and mortality rate, lung metastasectomy is the best treatment option in selected patients with lung metastases from breast cancer.

Meimarakis and colleagues investigated whether OS in patients with primary breast cancer is prolonged by pulmonary metastasectomy and which prognostic criteria may facilitate the decision in favor of thoracic surgical intervention.[18] The study assessed the median OS of 81 women after resection of pulmonary primary breast cancer metastases and matched patients who had not undergone resection from the Munich Tumor Registry served as controls.

In 81.5% of the patients R0 resection was achieved, which was associated with significantly longer median OS than occurred after R1 or R2 resection (103.4 months vs. 23.6 months vs. 20.2 months, respectively; $p < .001$). Multivariate analysis revealed R0 resection, number ($n \geq 2$), size (≥ 3 cm), and estrogen receptor and/or progesterone receptor positivity of metastases as independent prognostic factors for long-term survival. Presence of metastases in mediastinal and hilar lymph nodes correlated with decreased survival only in the univariate analysis. Matched pair analysis confirmed that pulmonary metastasectomy significantly improved survival. The investigators concluded that OS in patients with isolated pulmonary primary breast cancer metastasis is prolonged by metastasectomy. Patients with multiple pulmonary lesions or metastases with negative hormone receptor status are at greater risk of disease relapse and should be followed closely. Moreover, additive treatment tailored to the biological subtype defined by hormone receptor expression should be considered for this group.

Resection of pulmonary metastases is a common treatment in other primaries, but the role of breast cancer metastasectomy is still unclear. Welter and colleagues investigated the clinical outcome of operated patients with pulmonary breast cancer metastases and the different indications for metastasectomy.[19] Retrospective analysis of 47 patients with histologically proven pulmonary metastases from breast cancer showed the grading of the metastases was higher than the primary tumor in 26.7% and lower in 13.3% patients. R0, R1, and R2 resections were achieved in 27, 6, and 14 cases. The estrogen receptor status of the metastases differed from the primary tumor in 28.2% tested cases. HER2/neu receptor status differed in 4 of 16 tested patients. The histologic reports described a tumor spread around the metastasis in lymph or blood vessels in at least one resection specimen in 53.2% patients. The rate of major complications was 5.8%. The OS from the first pulmonary metastasectomy was 32 months with a 5-year survival of 36%. The main prognostic factor was the estrogen receptor status with a 5-year survival for receptor positive patients of 76% and 12.1% for receptor negative ones ($p = .002$). A similar survival difference was found for the status of HER2/neu receptor ($p = .037$). No prognostic influence could be demonstrated for age, number of metastases, initial tumor stage, complete versus incomplete resection, lymphatic spread, or lymph node or parietal pleural involvement. Welter and colleagues concluded that the gain in life expectancy in breast cancer patients with pulmonary metastases is based on chemotherapy and antihormone treatment. Tissue of the lung metastasis is needed to adjust medical therapy to estrogen receptor and HER2/neu expression and to reliably rule out primary lung cancer. In case of proven pulmonary metastases, the level of evidence for a curative approach is low, but some patients might benefit.

Friedel and colleagues evaluated the data from the International Registry of Lung Metastasis, including 467 patients who had lung metastases from breast cancer, with regard to long-term survival and prognostic factors.[20] In 84%, a complete resection was possible, with 5-, 10- and 15-year survival rates of 38%, 22%, and 20%, respectively. Positive prognostic factors were a disease-free interval of longer than 36 months, with 5-, 10-, and 15-year survival rates of 45%, 26%, and 21% respectively. Solitary lung metastasis was associated with a survival rate of 44% after 5 years and 23% after 10 and 15 years, but this was not statistically different compared with the outcome of patients undergoing resection of multiple metastases. In the Friedel study, there were no significant differences between the kind of resection used (wedge or segmental resection, lobectomy, pneumonectomy) in completely resected patients.

Kycler and associates reviewed retrospectively data for 33 patients who underwent 43 curative resections of breast cancer pulmonary metastases.[21] Potential prognostic factors affecting survival, namely survival after lung metastasectomy, assessed were disease-free interval (DFI), the number and location of lung metastases, the diameter (in millimeters) of metastases, and the extent of pulmonary resection. The median survival for 33 patients with pulmonary breast cancer metastatic lesions after metastasectomy was 73.2 months. Mean 5-year survival was 54.5%. There was a statistically significant difference in survival time with better prognosis for patients with DFI greater than 36 months ($p = .0007$), complete metastasectomy ($p = .0153$), unilateral pulmonary metastases ($p = .0267$), and for patients who underwent multiple operations ($p = .0211$). In multivariate analysis, there was significant influence for long-term prognosis for patients with DFI greater than 36 months ($p = .0446$) and for complete resection of the metastases ($p = .0275$). Analysis of the survival rates for patients with solitary pulmonary metastasis, with different size of tumors and after different types of pulmonary resection showed no significant differences. It was concluded that resection of lung metastases from breast cancer may offer a significant survival benefit for selected patients. The identified prognostic factor for survival after metastasectomy is DFI longer than 36 months and complete resection of the metastases. Also, the results showed that lung metastasectomy by conventional surgery is a safe procedure with low perioperative morbidity and mortality rate. Significant prognostic factors associated with survival include the number of metastases, DFI longer than 12 months, and complete resection.[22,23] Yoshimoto and coworkers demonstrated that the surgical approach to lung metastases from breast cancer may prolong survival in certain subgroups of patients to a greater extent than with systemic therapy alone. In addition, survival times were significantly longer for patients who initially presented with clinical stage I at breast surgery than those with stage II to IV.[24]

As part of the metastatic workup, it is important to obtain histologic diagnosis and differentiate between a metastatic lesion and a primary lung cancer. Early identification of the tumor is critical for appropriate treatment strategies. Proper aggressive evaluation can afford treatment of lung cancer and influence survival.[25] Rena and colleagues studied the role of surgery in the diagnosis and treatment of a solitary pulmonary nodule (SPN) in patients who had received previous surgery for breast cancer.[26] A total of 79 consecutive patients between 1990 and 2003 who had previously undergone curative resection for breast cancer and subsequently underwent surgery for an SPN were reviewed. Surgical diagnosis was obtained by open procedure before 1996 (37 cases), as well as by video-assisted thoracoscopic surgery (VATS) after 1996 (33 of 42 cases, nine open procedures) and intraoperative evaluation. Histology of SPN was primary lung cancer in 38 patients, pulmonary metastasis of breast cancer in 27, and benign condition in 14. The researchers concluded that VATS is a good procedure for diagnostic management and pathologic confirmation of peripheral SPN to determine appropriate surgical treatment.

Bone

Bone is the most common first site of metastases from breast cancer. Bone-only metastases have been reported to have a more favorable prognosis and an "indolent" course.[27] Patients with breast cancer with bone lesions and additional visceral metastasis have a poorer prognosis than patients with bone-only lesions. Patients with solitary bone lesions have a 39% chance of living after 5 years.[28,29] Bone metastases may result in considerable skeletal-related morbidity from bone pain, fracture, spinal cord compression, or hypercalcemia. In weight-bearing bones, this can lead to mobility problems. Spinal cord compression can be an acute life-threatening complication.[3] Multidisciplinary treatment is necessary for optimal care of these patients.

Greater understanding of the pathophysiology of bone metastases has led to the discovery and clinical utility of bone-targeted agents such as bisphosphonates and the receptor activator of nuclear factor kappa-B ligand (RANK-L) antibody denosumab.[30] With regard to prevention, there is no evidence that oral bisphosphonates can prevent bone metastases in advanced breast cancer without skeletal involvement. Several phase III clinical trials have evaluated bisphosphonates as adjuvant therapy in early breast cancer to prevent bone metastases. The current published data do not support the routine use of bisphosphonates in unselected patients with early breast cancer for metastasis prevention. However, significant benefit of adjuvant bisphosphonates has been consistently observed in the postmenopausal or ovarian suppression subgroup across multiple clinical trials, which raises the hypothesis that its greatest antitumor effect is in a low estrogen microenvironment. An individual patient data meta-analysis will be required to confirm survival benefit in this setting. The usual first treatment for bone metastases not at risk for fracture is systemic therapy, either endocrine- or chemotherapy-based treatment.

The incidence of metastatic bone disease is increasing as patients with cancer are living longer.[29] Local measures to treat bone metastases are limited in scope and benefit. The indications for surgical therapy include bone pain, prophylaxis for impending pathologic fracture, fixation of bony fractures, and spinal cord or nerve root compression.[31] A retrospective study of 59 breast cancer patients treated with radiation therapy for bony metastases reported pain relief and improved performance status in all patients.[32] Systemic administration of radioisotopes, such as strontium-89, has also been reported to relieve bone pain, but this treatment has limited use secondary to myelotoxicity.[33] Also, bisphosphonates present an important component of the treatment strategy for bone metastasis. Bisphosphonates are potent inhibitors of the osteoclastic bone resorption that is associated with skeletal metastases, with proven efficacy in reducing skeletal complications in metastatic breast cancer. Bisphosphonates may also prevent the development of bone metastases in newly diagnosed patients with no evidence of metastasis. A retrospective analysis of antitumor effects of zoledronic acid in breast cancer patients with bone-only metastasis showed that the zoledronic acid did not prolong progression-free survival or OS. In patients with bone-only metastasis, antitumor effects of zoledronic acid could not be demonstrated.[34]

Surgery is most frequently used for the treatment of long bone metastases and femoral fractures. The goals of relieving pain and restoring mobility may be accomplished by a variety of surgical techniques. Prophylactic surgical fixation for lytic lesions has been recommended for lesions of the cortex more than 2.5 cm in size, lesions involving more than 50% of the bone diameter, or lesions that are painful despite prior radiation treatment.[35] Weber and associates advocate using adjuvant radiation for all patients with surgically treated metastatic bone disease.[29] The standard radiation dose used is 30 Gy, with few side effects seen.[36] Postoperative radiation should start 10 to 14 days after surgery to allow wound healing. Epidural spinal cord compression is an oncologic emergency often heralded by increasing pain in a patient with known vertebral metastases. Early diagnosis is the key to maintaining neurologic function. Once neurologic deficit is present, surgery is rarely performed, and functional improvement is unlikely.[37]

Ahn and colleagues investigated the prognostic factors for patients with bone-only metastasis in breast cancer. The median time from the diagnosis of bone-only metastasis to the last follow-up or death was 55.2 months.[38] The Kaplan-Meier OS estimate at 10 years for all patients was 34.9%. In the multivariate Cox regression model, bisphosphonate treatment, estrogen receptor positivity, and solitary bone metastasis were significantly associated with longer OS in the bone-only recurrence group. Among the treatment modalities, only bisphosphonate treatment was identified as a significant prognostic factor. Noguchi and coworkers believe that sternal metastasis should be considered a different category from vertebral bone metastasis because the sternum lacks communication to the paravertebral venous plexus through which cancer cells spread easily to other bones.[29] Sternal metastasis seems to remain solitary for a longer time.

Shen and colleagues at MD Anderson Cancer Center investigated the role and outcome of radical surgery in contemporary multidisciplinary management of breast cancer patients presenting with isolated sternal or full-thickness chest wall (SCW) recurrence.[39] Seventy-six patients were identified, 44 treated surgically and 32 nonsurgically. OS at 5 years was not statistically different between patients who underwent surgery and those who did not (30.6% and 49.6%, respectively; $p = .52$), although patients selected for surgery presented with more advanced and biologically aggressive disease. Surgically treated patients were more likely to have triple-negative breast cancer at recurrence. Among surgical patients, 95% received preoperative systemic therapy. Clinical response with systemic therapy was significantly different, with surgically treated patients more likely to have responsive or stable disease (54% vs. 25%, $p = .04$). Complications related to radical surgical resection occurred in 25% of patients. For hormone receptor–positive recurrence, 5-year progression-free survival was significantly higher among surgical patients (46.3% vs. 14.5%; $p = .01$). The investigators concluded that among patients with isolated SCW recurrence, hormone receptor–positive recurrence is associated with improved survival. Systemic therapy should be the initial treatment, and clinical response can be used to help select patients who may benefit from radical resection.

Brain

Brain metastases are diagnosed in 15% of patients with metastatic breast carcinoma. Parenchymal brain lesions from breast carcinoma are frequently diagnosed in end-stage metastatic disease, but they may also be the first site of relapse. Metastases form in the brain tissue (parenchyma) or the leptomeninges. Breast cancer is the most common solid tumor to metastasize to the leptomeninges.[40] Unfortunately, a solitary brain metastasis is uncommon. In a retrospective study of breast cancer patients with brain metastases, 78% had multiple intracerebral metastases, 14% had solitary intracerebral metastases, and 8% had leptomeningeal disease.[41] Historically, the mean 1-year survival of patients with brain metastases has been only 20%.[42] The majority of patients with brain metastases die because of uncontrolled progression of the extracerebral systemic disease.[43]

There is a body of evidence suggesting that the incidence of central nervous system metastasis is increasing in patients with breast cancer, most likely because of the improved antitumor effects of newer chemotherapy regimens and targeted therapies (such as trastuzumab) in nonbrain metastases that do not cross the blood-brain barrier, allowing subsequent development of brain metastases.[44] The most widely accepted risk factors for the development of brain metastases are young patient age and estrogen receptor–negative primary tumors. Although young patients develop aggressive disease, the tropism for the brain suggests that inherent biological differences might be operative.[40,45] Metastasis to other sites also strongly predicted the development of brain metastases. HER-2 overexpression was also recognized to be a potential factor for increased risk in two other studies.

Chemotherapy has not generally been useful in the treatment of most brain metastases, in part as a result of the limitations on drug delivery imposed by the blood-brain barrier. Radiation, especially whole brain radiotherapy (WBRT), is a mainstay of therapy, especially for patients with multiple (>3) lesions. For patients with fewer lesions, surgical resection followed by WBRT has been shown to extend life and to minimize neurologic debility and death.[40] Surgery is especially useful in cases where few lesions are present; their location is favorable for resection and a rapid amelioration of the symptoms is needed.[46] In properly selected patients with brain metastases, stereotactic-guided radiosurgery (SRS, Gamma Knife) in association with WBRT confers a survival advantage over WBRT alone. This type of treatment is recommended for lesions equal to or smaller than 3 cm in diameter. For the lesions located in the deep cortical structures and cerebellar nuclei that cannot be safely resected, stereotactic surgery is the treatment of choice.[47] WBRT is commonly recommended after the complete resection of brain metastases. The rationale for this is that it helps eradicate micrometastases, which are too small to be visualized by computed tomography or magnetic resonance imaging.

The relative roles of SRS versus whole brain radiotherapy (WBRT) in the treatment of patients with brain metastases from breast cancer remain undefined. Kased and colleagues from the University of California San Francisco retrospectively reviewed 176 patients treated between 1991 and 2005 with Gamma Knife SRS for brain metastases from breast cancer.[48] The actuarial survival and freedom from progression end points were calculated using the Kaplan-Meier method. The median survival time was 16.0 months for 95 newly diagnosed patients and 11.7 months for 81 patients with recurrent brain metastases. In the newly diagnosed patients, omission of upfront WBRT did not significantly affect the median survival time, brain freedom from progression, or freedom from new brain metastases. Longer survival was associated with age less than 50 years, Karnofsky Performance Status (KPS) 70 or greater, primary tumor control, estrogen receptor positivity, and HER2/neu overexpression. No association was found between the number of treated brain metastases and the survival time. From these findings the authors concluded that upfront WBRT did not appear to improve brain freedom from progression, and a larger number of brain metastases was not associated with a shorter survival time.

Breast cancer might be distinct from other primary sites in terms of prognostic factors and the roles of WBRT and SRS for brain metastases. Lee and associates retrospectively analyzed the OS of 198 patients with brain metastases due to breast cancer.[49] The median age of the patients at the diagnosis of brain metastases was 45 years (range 26–78 years). Fifty-five patients (28%) had a single brain metastasis, whereas 143 (72%) had more than two metastases. A total of 157 (79.2%) patients received WBRT. A total of 7 (3.6%) patients underwent resection of solitary brain metastases, 22 (11%) patients underwent Gamma Knife surgery, 3 patients underwent intrathecal chemotherapy (1.5%), and 9 (4.6%) patients received no treatment. The overall median survival time was 5.6 months (95% confidence interval 4.7–6.5 months), and 23.1% of the patients survived for more than 1 year. The median overall survival time was 5.4 months for patients treated with WBRT, 14.9 months for patients treated with surgery or SRS Gamma Knife surgery only, and 2.1 months for patients who received no treatment ($p < .001$). The performance status, number of brain metastases, treatment modalities, and systemic chemotherapy after brain metastases were significantly associated with survival. The researchers concluded that patients with single-brain metastasis and good performance status deserve aggressive treatment. The characteristics of the primary breast tumor did not affect survival after brain metastasis.

Brain metastases–free survival (BMFS) differs between breast cancer subtypes. Berghoff and colleagues compared BMFS of breast cancer subtypes in patients treated between 1996 until 2010.[50] Data of 213 patients (46 luminal, 124 HER2, 43 triple-negative subtypes) with brain metastases from breast cancer were available for the analysis. BMFS differed significantly between breast cancer subtypes. Median BMFS in triple-negative tumors was 14 months compared with 18 months in HER2-positive tumors ($p = .001$) and 34 months in luminal tumors ($p = .001$), respectively. In HER2-positive patients, copositivity for ER and HER2 prolonged BMFS; in luminal tumors, coexpression of estrogen receptor and progesterone receptor was not significantly associated with BMFS. In patients with lung metastases, BMFS was significantly shorter. On the basis of the study, the authors concluded that the BMFS in triple-negative breast cancer and HER2-positive/ER-negative, is significantly shorter compared with HER2/ER copositive or luminal tumors, mirroring the aggressiveness of these breast cancer subtypes.

Dyer and colleagues studied the importance of extracranial disease status and tumor subtype for patients undergoing radiosurgery for breast cancer brain metastases.[51] Retrospective analysis of 51 patients who received SRS as part of the initial management of their brain metastases.

On multivariate analysis, triple-negative subtype, luminal B subtype, and omission of WBRT were associated with central nervous system progression. With respect to OS, KPS 80% or lower and progressive extracranial disease were significant on univariate analysis; progressive extracranial disease and triple-negative subtype were significant on multivariate analysis. Although median survival times were consistent with those predicted by the breast cancer–specific Graded Prognostic Assessment (Breast-GPA) score (a diagnostic tool to estimate survival for breast cancer patients with brain metastasis), the addition of extracranial disease status further separated patient outcomes. Tumor subtype is associated with risk of central nervous system progression after SRS for breast cancer brain metastases. In addition to tumor subtype and KPS, which are incorporated into the Breast-GPA, progressive extracranial disease may be an important prognostic factor for OS.

Breast cancer patients with solitary brain metastases at first site of metastasis constitute a subset of patients with a remarkable response to treatment and a relatively long survival, especially if they can be treated by surgery with postoperative radiation.[39] Several characteristics, including young age, optimal performance status, newly diagnosed metastasis, controlled or absent systemic disease, menopause status, postoperative radiation, and preoperative neurologic status, have been identified as significant prognostic factors.[40,41] Leptomeningeal carcinomatosis represents an uncommon but devastating manifestation of metastatic breast cancer. Intrathecal chemotherapy is being studied as a potential treatment option for patients with leptomeningeal involvement.[42]

It has been suggested that as the survival of cancer patients with disseminated disease is extended, and as adjuvant therapy becomes more effective, brain metastases will present a more frequent management issue.[43]

Summary

Improved breast cancer multimodality treatment has resulted in the increased median disease survival for patients with metastatic breast cancer. In selected patients with solitary metastases or multiple lesions at a single organ site, curative surgery should be considered provided the primary cancer is controlled, the patient has a good performance status, there has been a long disease-free interval, and negative margins can be achieved. Another important question that remains to be answered is the role of extirpation of the breast primary when the patient is diagnosed with stage IV solitary metastases at initial presentation. Curative surgery may also have a role in selected patients.

Selected References

3. Singletary SE, Walsh G, Vauthey JN, et al. A role for curative surgery in the treatment of selected patients with metastatic breast cancer. *Oncologist.* 2003;8:241-251.

9. Abbott DE, Brouquet A, Mittendorf EA, et al. Resection of liver metastases from breast cancer: estrogen receptor status and response to chemotherapy before metastasectomy define outcome. *Surgery.* 2012;151:710-716.

10. Van Walsum GA, de Ridder JA, Verhoef C, et al. Resection of liver metastases in patients with breast cancer:survival and prognostic factors. *Eur J Surg Oncol.* 2012;38:910-917.

18. Meimarakis G, Rüttinger D, Stemmler J, et al. Prolonged overall survival after pulmonary metastasectomy in patients with breast cancer. *Ann Thorac Surg.* 2013;95:1170-1180.

21. Kycler W, Laski P. Surgical approach to pulmonary metastases from breast cancer. *Breast J.* 2012;18:52-57.

30. Li BT, Wong MH, Pavlakis N. Treatment and prevention of bone metastases from breast cancer: a comprehensive review of evidence for clinical practice. *J Clin Med.* 2014;3:1-24.

39. Shen MC, Massarweh NN, Lari SA, et al. Clinical course of breast cancer patients with isolated sternal and full thickness chest wall recurrences treated with and without radical surgery. *Ann Surg Oncol.* 2013;20:4153-4160.

50. Berghoff A, Bago-Horvath Z, De Vries C, et al. Brain metastases free survival differs between breast cancer subtypes. *Br J Cancer.* 2012;106:440-446.

51. Dyer MA, Kelly PJ, Chen YH, et al. Importance of extracranial disease status and tumor subtype for patients undergoing radiosurgery for breast cancer brain metastases. *Int J Radiat Oncol Biol Phys.* 2012;83:e479-e486.

A full reference list is available online at ExpertConsult.com.

61

Locoregional Recurrence After Mastectomy

IRENE L. WAPNIR, JACQUELINE TSAI, AND STEFAN AEBI

Preventing locoregional failure of breast cancer is still a major objective of treatments today. Since the late 19th century, the effectiveness of mastectomy surgery has been judged by its success at controlling local disease. The use of adjuvant systemic treatments has improved overall outcomes and reduced the frequency of locoregional recurrence(s) (LRRs).[1-4] According to the US National Cancer Database, breast conserving surgery has now surpassed mastectomy, with or without nodal staging, as the most common operation performed for the treatment of early-stage breast cancer.[5] Advances in breast reconstruction have changed the mastectomy landscape with a shift toward skin- and nipple-areolar–sparing mastectomies and the increased use of contralateral prophylactic mastectomies.[6-10]

LRRs have been linked to a significantly elevated risk of distant metastases. Because most LRRs precede distant metastases by relatively short time intervals, it is argued that these events are significant indicators of occult disseminated disease. The CALOR (Chemotherapy as Adjuvant for LOcally Recurrent breast cancer) trial results have provided evidence-based rationale for the use of systemic treatments after LRR.[11] It is the first prospective randomized multicenter trial to show significant improvement in disease-free survival (DFS) and overall survival (OS) with physician selected chemotherapy after LRR. Thus essential management strategies for isolated LRR (ILRR) have evolved by addressing the likelihood of distant relapse in addition to refining definitive local interventions. The following sections of this chapter describe the prevalence, modes of presentations, prognosis, and management of LRR after mastectomy.

Definitions

Local failures can occur months to years after mastectomy surgery. In the words of William S. Halsted in 1894, "Local recurrence is the return of the disease in the field of operation."[12] Although the majority of LRRs occur in patients with a prior invasive cancer, approximately 1% arise in mastectomy-treated ductal carcinomas in situ.[13,14] Most LRRs present as isolated events and less frequently accompany or follow the diagnosis of distant metastasis.[15] The time interval between recurrences and the appearance of distant metastases can be brief, so it is plausible that these relapses are misclassified as either ILRR or distant metastases.[16,17]

An LRR can involve chest wall skin, subcutaneous tissues, chest wall muscles, or regional nodal areas of the ipsilateral breast (Figs. 61.1 through 61.3). Recurrent cancers are classified according to their anatomic location: skin, mastectomy scar, chest wall, regional lymph nodes (axillary, internal mammary, infraclavicular or Rotter, and supraclavicular), or extranodal recurrences. Contralateral nodal recurrences are excluded and have been defined by the Maastricht Breast Cancer Endpoints Consensus Panel as distant disease rather than a LRR.[18] From a management perspective, LRRs are classified as either operable or inoperable.

Incidence

The incidence of a LRR is influenced by the molecular characteristics of the primary cancer, stage of disease, extent of surgery, and adjuvant treatments.[19] Systemic regimens have significantly changed in the last few decades, resulting in a lower incidence of locoregional events in some cancer subtypes. Before routine HER2 testing, 3% to 32% of patients with stage I to III breast cancer developed a LRR within 10 years of mastectomy, either as a first event or accompanying distant disease.[2,16,17,20] Approximately 80% of these recurrences are detected within the first 5 years. Node-positive and hormone receptor–negative recurrences tend to present earlier than node-negative and hormone receptor–positive tumors.[21]

The radical mastectomy experience from the National Surgical Adjuvant Breast and Bowel Project (NSABP) provides a frame of reference for examining the incidence of first ILRR treated by surgery alone. In this setting, LRR events were less common than distant metastasis.[22] The 25-year follow-up of this trial found rates of local failure after radical mastectomy to be 5% and 8% and for regional recurrence 4% and 8% in node-negative and node-positive cancers, respectively.[23] In general, skin/chest wall recurrences were the most common, representing 49% to 83% of LRRs.[1,24] By comparison, nodal recurrences were less frequent constituting 15% to 52% of cases.

Higher disease stage, aggressive tumor biology or tumor subtype, and younger age are some of the prognostic factors associated with higher rates of local recurrence.[19,25-28] LRR rates in patients treated with neoadjuvant chemotherapy are similar to those who undergo surgery upfront. Although the literature on the subject is sparse at this time, the incidence of LRR is seemingly related to the degree of tumor response in breast or regional nodes.[29] This topic is discussed in greater detail later in the chapter.

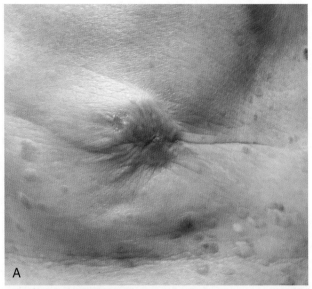

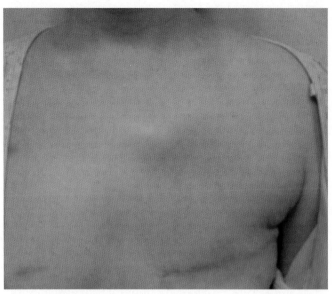

• **Fig. 61.2** Internal mammary visible node recurrence.

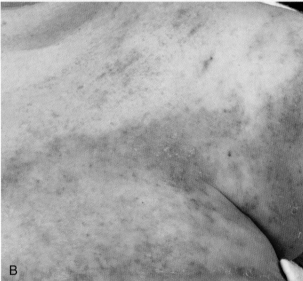

• **Fig. 61.1** Local recurrence. (A) Mastectomy scar raised mass-like recurrence. (B) Diffuse erythematous rash-like skin recurrence.

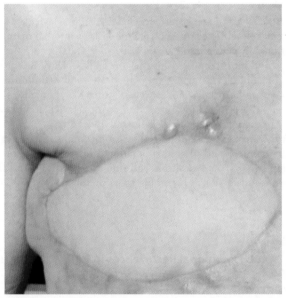

• **Fig. 61.3** Locoregional recurrence in native chest wall skin surrounding autologous tissue breast reconstruction.

Chest Wall Recurrences

In a pooled analysis of 5352 participants in International Breast Cancer Study Group (IBCSG) trials I through VII, 21.3% experienced a LRR event as a first relapse, and 53% of these were local or chest wall failures.[15] Another series spanning the years 1980 to 2004, reported a 10-year cumulative incidence of LRR for T1 and T2 node-negative cancers of 5.2% with 73% of these recurrences involving the chest wall.[28] However, in the absence of systemic treatments when risk factors such as larger tumor size, lymphovascular invasion, and positive margins are present, the incidence of LRR was 19.7%.

As mastectomy techniques have evolved to less disfiguring skin and nipple-sparing mastectomies, higher rates of LRR could have been expected but have not been found.[30–34] Specifically, in a study-level meta-analysis of nipple-sparing mastectomies, nipple recurrence were found to be acceptably low at 1.4% after 3 to 5 years.[10] These operative procedures are being extended to *BRCA1*

and *BRCA2* mutation carriers and to patients who have received neoadjuvant therapy.[35–37] Importantly, there is no indication that LRR rates are measurably higher with these more natural appearing mastectomy procedures.

Invasive locoregional skin or chest wall recurrences are uncommon in mastectomy-treated ductal carcinomas in situ.[13,14] In a series of 10 patients, recurrences were diagnosed 1 to 16 years after mastectomy. Not surprisingly, residual breast tissue was identified in half of these LRR.[38]

Nodal Recurrences

The extent of axillary nodal surgery has changed greatly since the era of radical mastectomy, when level I to III axillary node dissection was the norm. Regional recurrences ranged from 4% to 8%, with the bulk of these events occurring in the first 5 years.[23] In their pooled analysis of modified radical mastectomy-treated women in seven randomized trials, Wallgren and colleagues found that 26% of LRR involved supraclavicular/infraclavicular nodes compared with 13% in axillary nodes.[15]

Before sentinel node biopsy, recurrence rates were significantly higher when fewer axillary nodes are removed or in the presence of extranodal extension.[24,39] Weir and colleagues reported that when fewer than 6 nodes were removed during axillary dissection the rate of recurrence was 5% compared with 1%, when more than 10 lymph nodes were excised.[40] LRR are lower in node positive breast cancers as the number of uninvolved lymph nodes resected is higher.[41]

The management of the axilla has shifted toward a selective approach with the implementation of lymphatic mapping and sentinel node biopsy. Local recurrence rates of less than 2% have been reported in clinically node-negative breast cancers after sentinel node biopsy, which indicates that the incidence of recurrences in the axilla is comparable to that observed with axillary node dissections.[42–47] Lymphatic mapping and sentinel node biopsy after neoadjuvant therapy is gaining acceptance largely based on similar false-negative sentinel node identification rates.[48,49]

Extraaxillary nodal recurrences refer to supraclavicular, infraclavicular (level III or interpectoral nodes), or internal mammary locations. In newer studies, supraclavicular nodal recurrences are the second most common site after the axilla.[50] Until recent revision of clinical staging by the American Joint Committee on Cancer, supraclavicular nodes were considered synonymous with stage IV disease.[51] Clinical detection of infraclavicular and internal mammary nodal recurrences are rare (see Fig. 61.2). However, with the increasing use of new generation computed tomography (CT) scanners and the incorporation of magnetic resonance imaging (MRI) and positron emission tomography (PET)/CT subclinical detection is becoming more prevalent.

Prior Radiation Therapy

Local failure rates vary with the extent of adjuvant treatments administered for the primary cancer.[39,52–54] The Early Breast Cancer Trialists' Collaborative Group studied the effects of comprehensive adjuvant radiotherapy, defined as supraclavicular, axillary, and internal mammary nodal basins, using individual patient level data from 22 randomized trials.[55] There was no statistically significant effect on 10-year cumulative risk of ILRRs after mastectomy and axillary dissection for women with pathologically negative nodes. However, among the 3131 patients with positive nodes, postmastectomy radiation therapy decreased the overall rate of ILRRs from 26.0% (no RT) to 8.1% (RT), log-rank $2p <$ .00001. Radiotherapy significantly decreased first LRRs from 20.3% to 3.8% in the group with one to three positive nodes, and from 32.0% to 13.0% in those with four or more. Similarly, radiation improved local control in women who had axillary sampling instead of dissection, reducing the risk of LRR by 0.61.

In a retrospective analysis of 1000 patients from the Danish Breast Cancer Cooperative Group 82 b&c clinical trials, the greatest absolute reduction in LRRs was in the subgroup of patients with unfavorable prognostic characteristics.[56] Notably, in HER2-positive breast cancers, the rate of LRR with trastuzumab and postmastectomy radiation therapy was 0% at 5 years, indicating remarkable synergism between the two treatment modalities (Table 61.1).[54]

Prior Systemic Therapy

The risk of recurrence is determined by tumor biology and stage at presentation. The natural course of disease can be favorably altered by the use of adjuvant therapies tailored to tumor molecular markers. Chest wall recurrences occurred in 13% of patients who received adjuvant chemotherapy regimens but no radiation. However, the incidence was only 7.5% for those with one to three positive nodes, whereas it was 14% in those with four or more

---

TABLE 61.1   Locoregional Recurrences in HER2-Positive and Triple-Negative Breast Cancers

Author/Year/ Study Period	N	FU (y)	Receptor	T/N Stage	Systemic Tx	XRT (%)	LRR (%)
Peterson 2014[61] (1998–2009)	326	5	HER2+	T1–T2, N0	Without trastuzumab	0	2.6
					Trastuzumab		0.6
Lanning 2015[54] (1998–2007)	501	5	HER2+	T1–T4 49% N0	Without trastuzumab	25	6.5
							5.6
				T1–T4 35% N0	Trastuzumab	38	0
							2.8
Tseng 2015[60] (1997–2012)	1090	5	HER2+	T1–3 59.5% N0	Without trastuzumab	24.8	3.6
				T1–3 40.4% N0	trastuzumab	41.2	0.3
	695		TNBC	T1–3 55.2% N0	ChemoTx and/ or TAM	31.8	5.25
Zumsteg 2013[59] (1999–2008)	198	5	TNBC	T1–T2 N0	84% ChemoTx	0	5.4

ChemoTx, Chemotherapy; *FU,* follow-up; *LRR,* locoregional recurrence; *TAM,* tamoxifen; *TNBC,* triple-negative breast cancer; *Tx,* therapy; *XRT,* radiation therapy.

involved nodes.[24] In a combined analysis of 5758 patients with node-positive cancers treated with adjuvant therapies without postmastectomy radiation, 12.2% of patients presented with an ILRR compared with 43%, whose first failure event was distant metastasis.[17] The proportion of skin or chest wall recurrences was 56.9% compared with 22.6% supraclavicular, 11.7% axillary, and less than 1% parasternal and infraclavicular nodal recurrences. Predictive factors for local failure consisted of age less than 50, larger tumors, greater number of positive lymph nodes, and number of resected nodes. In this same study, the 10-year cumulative incidence of isolated regional failures was 3.5% or less, for women with one to three positive nodes, compared with 5.4% to 10.9% for those with four or more nodes, irrespective of tumor size.

Additional risk factors identified in a review of 12 studies involving 12,961 node-negative patients treated by mastectomy alone were less than 40 years of age, lymphovascular invasion, positive or close margins, and tumor size greater than 2 cm.[4] Additionally, tumor biology influences recurrence events. Specifically, higher rates of distant metastasis and LRR are reported for triple-negative breast cancers compared with non–triple negative tumors.[19,57–60]

Ma and colleagues reported different time intervals to LRR based on tumor receptors. The shortest median time interval to LRR was 18.2 months for HER2-positive cancers (largely without trastuzumab therapy), followed by 21.8 months for triple-negative and more than twofold longer for luminal A or B cancers.[21] In a pooled analysis of 162 nonirradiated mastectomy-treated T1–2 N0 HER2-positive cancers from the British Columbia Cancer Agency and Massachusetts General Hospital, 5-year LRR-free survival was 99.4% with anti-HER2 therapy compared with 97.4% for those who did not receive trastuzumab.[61] Similarly, patients with HER2 positive tumors experienced higher rates of LRR in the pre-trastuzumab era compared with those who received trastuzumab, wherein chest wall and nodal recurrence rates were cut by half (see Table 61.1).[54] Interestingly, the combination of adjuvant trastuzumab with postmastectomy radiation in this non-randomized retrospective series was associated with 0% LRR at 5 years.

Prior Neoadjuvant Chemotherapy

Patients with palpable breast cancers at presentation are increasingly directed toward neoadjuvant chemotherapy based on tumor molecular characteristics and disease stage. An LRR after neoadjuvant chemotherapy is highly associated with the pathologic response, with lower rate of relapse when a pathologic complete response (pCR) is attained. In a combined analysis of NSABP prospective randomized trials B-18 and B-27, tumor size greater than 5 cm (hazard ratio [HR] 1.58, $p = .0095$), clinical node-positive status (HR 1.53, $p = .017$), and pathologically residual nodal disease (HR 4.48, $p = .01$) were the most significant predictive factors for LRRs among 1071 mastectomy-treated patients without adjuvant radiation therapy.[29] The 10-year cumulative incidence of chest wall recurrences ranged from 0% to 2.2% for patients who had a breast pCR and negative nodes, regardless of their clinical presentation. In clinically node-negative cancers, regional recurrences were slightly higher, ranging from 0% to 6.2%. Among patients who were classified as clinically node-negative and were then found to have residual disease in axillary nodes, the overall rate of LRR ranged from 11.2% to 22.4%.

Genomic Characterization

Another proposed approach to predict locoregional failures among endocrine-responsive cancers is through genomic analysis. Mamounas and coworkers used the 21-gene Recurrence Score (RS) panel to examine LRRs among estrogen receptor–positive, node-negative mastectomy-treated patients on NSABP protocols B-14 and B-20.[62] Of these 505 nonirradiated mastectomy cases, 6.1% had LRRs: 18 chest wall or scar recurrences and 13 nodal or regional recurrences. A high RS was associated with a LRR in more than 10% of this subgroup compared with intermediate or low RS groups. Another study explored the utility of the 21-gene RS for predicting LRRs using the hormone receptor positive cohort of the NSABP B-28 protocol wherein anthracycline-based chemotherapy with or without paclitaxel was randomly assigned.[63] The risk of a LRR for mastectomy-treated subjects with one to three positive nodes was 6% or less in the low RS category versus 9.6% and 23.6% for the intermediate and high RS categories respectively. The predictive value of the RS has been described in other small series.[64] Similarly, EndoPredict, another genomic test, was investigated in the Austrian Breast Cancer Study Group trial 8. This test was prognostic for LRRs, with a 10-year local recurrence–free survival of 97.5% in the EndoPredict low-risk group versus 91% in the high-risk group.[65]

Detection and Diagnosis

The vast majority of LRRs are self-detected or found in asymptomatic patients on routine clinical examination.[66] A thorough clinical history and physical examination remain the best routine assessments. The median time interval from primary tumor surgery to LRR is usually 2.4 to 6.2 years.[2,11,39]

Most chest wall recurrences present as nodules or mass-like lesions in the vicinity of the mastectomy scar (see Fig. 61.1A and B).[2,67] Other presentations of local recurrences can be patchy or rash-like erythematous lesions, or as ulcerating masses involving the skin or subcutaneous tissues with or without invasion of chest wall structures. Fine-needle or core needle, skin punch, incisional, or excisional biopsies may be used to histologically evaluate clinically suspicious lesions. Pathologic confirmation and assessment of molecular markers are necessary to plan appropriate treatments.

Axillary node recurrences are usually detected on palpation but may be discovered during radiologic tests performed for other reasons. Less commonly, new-onset upper extremity lymphedema, pain, or discomfort on range of motion may herald the presence of a nodal recurrence. Imaging studies, such as CT, PET, or brachial plexus MRI, may be helpful in delineating the extent of disease, invasion into surrounding anatomic areas, and resectability. Nodal relapses are easily amenable to ultrasound guided fine-needle or core needle biopsy.

Once an LRR is suspected or diagnosed, imaging studies may be valuable for documenting the extent of local disease, determining operability, and ensuring the absence of distant metastases. CT and bone scan are the most accessible and affordable imaging studies. Fludeoxyglucose (FDG)-PET/CT is especially useful in assessing nodal disease and detecting distant recurrences. Lastly, MRI may be better suited for delineating operability and extent of metastases involving the brachial plexus.[68]

Routine radiologic screening of asymptomatic patients after breast cancer treatment is unproven and controversial. Detection of local failures in patients who received postmastectomy implant-based or autologous tissue reconstruction are perhaps more challenging because they can obscure physical examination but do not justify the routine annual use of either CT scans or MRI. The utility of mammography was prospectively studied in patients who underwent autologous reconstruction after mastectomy.[69] Compared with clinical examination, mammographic evaluations were not useful in detecting LRR. Clinically occult nodal recurrences were found in 1.1% of asymptomatic patients in a prospective study with PET-CT, but this represented a mere 0.67% of total imaging studies performed, calling into question the efficacy of such a screening policy.[70]

Nipple-sparing mastectomies have raised concerns of less complete mastectomies and higher LRR rates. It is assumed that the thoroughness of the mastectomy operation in skin-sparing procedures is the same as with standard non–skin sparing operations. Recurrences within the preserved nipple-areolar complex are clinically detectable. Therefore screening MRI or mammographic evaluations should not be considered unless there is heightened concern based on surgical technique.

Survival After Locoregional Recurrence

An LRR occurring within a short time interval of primary cancer is especially concerning and a poor prognostic indicator.[16] Historically, 5-year survival of patients with chest wall, axillary, or internal mammary recurrences ranged from 44% to 49%, whereas those with supraclavicular recurrences or nodal disease accompanying chest wall recurrences are lower, 21% to 24%.[71] In a series of 140 node-positive patients treated with adjuvant radiation therapy after mastectomy, the 10-year cumulative incidence of distant metastases for those with chest wall recurrences was 59% compared with 68% for those with relapse in regional nodes.[72] Patients with one to three positive nodes treated with mastectomy without radiation had a DFS of 49% and an OS of 75% on 4-year follow-up after LRR.[73] The 5-year mortality ranged from 39% to 50% after an isolated axillary recurrence.[74]

Differences in survival rates are also noted according to the location of the chest wall recurrence. Patients with subcutaneous LRRs compared with those involving the musculoskeletal structures, had better survival, 61% versus 45%, with a mean follow-up of 80.8 months.[75]

Local Treatment

Surgical resection is the standard treatment for operable LRRs, which is defined as tumor not fixed to the chest wall or limited skin involvement. The primary goal is to excise gross tumor to preferably microscopically clear margins. Unresectable recurrences are those that invade neurovascular structures, periosteum, intercostal muscles, or diffusely involving skin.

The local control achieved by surgery alone for operable recurrences is limited and associated with a risk of second local failures as high as 60% or greater.[74] Surgical excision and radiation improve local control after an LRR event and are associated with improved survival.[71,76] Specifically, the 5-year actuarial survival increased from 34% to 48% in patients who underwent surgical excision. The addition of radiation after excision of all gross disease improved local control.[77] In these patients, there was an overall 77% local regional control rate and a 55% OS rate at 5 years after management for the recurrence.

Multimodality therapies should be considered on patients with LRRs. No randomized clinical trial has been carried out to specifically demonstrate whether surgery and radiation therapy improve prognosis. The benefit of postmastectomy radiation has been extrapolated to patients with LRRs.[53,55] However, there is little doubt that the risk of local relapse is reduced.

Palliative surgery can be considered for ulceration, bleeding, or even pain in select circumstances. In the presence of metastatic disease, palliative local surgery may be indicated.[78] For example, tumor debulking may improve pain control or resection of an ulcerating tumor may improve local management of the disease. Extensive chest wall resections requiring complex reconstructive procedures have been reported but should be viewed as heroic undertakings with potentially only anecdotal benefit. These patients should be primarily managed with systemic treatments.

Repeat exploration of the axilla in patients who had prior axillary node dissections has been shown to be feasible.[79] Lymphatic remapping has been demonstrated after mastectomy both after previous sentinel node biopsy or axillary dissection. The Sentinel Node and Recurrent Breast (SNARB) cancer study was a multicenter registration effort in the Netherlands to evaluate repeat lymphatic mapping and sentinel node identification. Included were 35 women previously treated by mastectomy plus sentinel node biopsy and 26 who received mastectomy plus axillary dissection. Repeat lymphatic mapping was successful in 97.1% and 84.6% of these patients, respectively, with sentinel nodes identified in more than 76%.[80] However, the accuracy of this approach was not reported for the mastectomy subgroup alone. Of 31 lumpectomy and mastectomy-treated patients who underwent confirmatory axillary dissections and had negative sentinel lymph node biopsies, 2 were found to have macrometastases for a negative predictive value of 93.6% (95% confidence interval [CI] 78.4–99.0). It is controversial whether repeat lymphatic mapping and sentinel node biopsy should be considered in cases without clinical-radiologic evidence of concurrent axillary nodal disease. However, this approach may help identify occult axillary node disease and guide a completion axillary dissection if not previously performed.

Radiation Therapy

Radiation therapy has been one of the basic local treatment modalities used for breast cancer. In the primary setting, it has been shown to reduce local recurrence of disease and therefore logically, has a role in the treatment of LRR, especially if radiation has not been previously administered. Radiation dose for the treatment of a LRR depends on prior radiotherapy administration. Consideration for cumulative tissue toxicity is necessary when determining the dosage and extent of fields in those who have been previously radiated. As mentioned earlier, the use of multimodality treatment for LRR, including surgical excision and radiation, have been shown in several studies to improve local control and survival.[76,81] Curative intent with radiation achieved 100% local control using doses of 60 Gy or more. Better local control was attained with radiation to the entire chest wall. Even so, second chest wall recurrences occurred in 12% of the cases. In a study by Kuo and coworkers, patients who underwent tumor excision with entire-field radiotherapy had significantly better 5-year DFS and OS than patients who received radiation only (DFS 51% vs. 16%, $p = .006$; OS 62% vs. 37%, $p = .017$).[82] Increasing doses of radiation therapy from conventional 50-Gy dose with a 10-Gy boost to 54 Gy and a minimum of 12-Gy boost dose had no effect on 5-year DFS or OS, 39% versus 43%, $p = .3$ and 52% versus 57%, $p = .29$.[77] Brachytherapy can deliver higher doses and has been used as adjunct to salvage surgery in post mastectomy recurrences.[83] Heating tumor tissue or hyperthermia to 41°C to 43°C has been shown to enhance the effectiveness of repeat radiation for unresectable locoregional recurrences.[84] In this retrospective review of 414 patients in two Dutch institutions, local control of disease was achieved in 26% with a median time of 5 months (0–187 months).

Systemic Therapy

Whether LRR is a marker of occult metastatic disease or the origin and cause of later metastases has been debated. In either case, it was not clear whether systemic therapy added to local treatment of a LRR had any value. Few randomized clinical trials have been attempted to assess the importance of "secondary adjuvant" therapy after the complete resection of an isolated LRR (ILRR). A Cochrane review identified only three randomized clinical trials testing systemic therapy for LRR in women with breast cancer.[85] The largest of the three trials was the Swiss Group for Clinical Cancer Research (SAKK 23/82) study that randomized 167 patients with "good risk" ILRR (estrogen receptor positive in the ILRR, disease-free interval of >12 months, and ILRR consisting of ≤3 or tumor nodules, each ≤3 cm in diameter) to tamoxifen or no therapy. All patients underwent mastectomy for their primary cancer surgery and had no prior exposure to tamoxifen therapy. The ILRR was treated by complete surgical resection and radiation therapy (50 Gy) to the site of recurrence. At a median follow-up of 11.6 years, post-ILRR DFS was 6.5 years in the tamoxifen arm and 2.7 years with observation alone ($p = .053$). This difference was mainly due to reduction of second LRR events ($p = .011$). The median OS after ILRR was 11.2 and 11.5 years in the observation and the tamoxifen arms, respectively.[86]

Today the choices of endocrine therapy agents have expanded to include aromatase inhibitors and therefore are applicable in endocrine-responsive ILRR. The choice of the agents then depends on prior endocrine therapy use. Whether so-called targeted agents such as trastuzumab, everolimus, or palbociclib combined with endocrine therapy are effective remains to be investigated.

The CALOR prospective pragmatic trial studied the utility of systemic therapy in patients with ILRR.[11] A total of 162 subjects were randomized to receive investigator-selected chemotherapy or observation. The majority of patients received anthracycline or taxane-based treatments, and endocrine therapy was required for hormone-responsive ILRRs. Radiation therapy was also mandated for patients with microscopically involved surgical margins, and anti-HER2 therapy was optional. Five-year DFS was 69% with chemotherapy versus 57% without chemotherapy (HR 0.59, 95% CI 0.35–0.99; $p = .046$). Chemotherapy was significantly more effective for women with ER-negative ILRR (p interaction = .046); analyses of DFS according to ER expression of the primary tumor were not statistically significant. OS was significantly improved with chemotherapy (HR for death of any cause 0.41, 95% CI 0.0.19–0.89; $p = .024$) corresponding to a 5-year survival of 88% versus 76%. Estrogen receptor expression was not predictive of the effect of chemotherapy. Prior exposure to adjuvant chemotherapy did not negatively influence the efficacy

of chemotherapy for ILRR. This trial is not informative of the type of drug that is best used in the treatment of ILRR but does illustrate that it is possible to select effective chemotherapies based on the individual patient's primary therapy and current health status.

Trastuzumab and other HER2-directed therapies have not been assessed in a clinical trial for ILRR, but it is reasonable to extrapolate therapeutic regimens established in the metastatic setting to LRR. In general terms, it is likely that the biological properties of the relapse may be more relevant to the choice of therapy than the characteristics of the primary. Whether genomic profiling with contemporary tests such as the 70 gene (MammaPrint) or the 21 gene (Onco*type* Dx Recurrence Score) panels are useful is a matter of future research.

At present, systemic therapy for ILRR is recommended and should be guided by the drugs used for the primary breast cancer and individually tailored to the prior therapies received by the patient.

Conclusion

An LRR of breast cancer usually occurs as an isolated event that confers a poor prognosis because it is highly associated with an increased risk of developing distant disease. Definitive surgery and radiation followed by adjuvant systemic therapy tailored to the molecular characteristics of the disease have led to improved outcomes.

Selected References

11. Aebi S, Gelber S, Anderson SJ, et al. Chemotherapy for isolated locoregional recurrence of breast cancer (CALOR): a randomised trial. *Lancet Oncol*. 2014;15:156-163. doi:10.1016/S1470-2045(13)70589-8.
23. Fisher B, Jeong J-H, Anderson S, et al. Twenty-five-year follow-up of a randomized trial comparing radical mastectomy, total mastectomy, and total mastectomy followed by irradiation. *N Engl J Med*. 2002;347:567-575. doi:10.1056/NEJMoa020128.
29. Mamounas EP, Anderson SJ, Dignam JJ, et al. Predictors of locoregional recurrence after neoadjuvant chemotherapy: results from combined analysis of National Surgical Adjuvant Breast and Bowel Project B-18 and B-27. *J Clin Oncol*. 2012;30:3960-3966. doi:10.1200/JCO.2011.40.8369.
53. Whelan TJ, Julian J, Wright J, Jadad AR, Levine ML. Does locoregional radiation therapy improve survival in breast cancer? A meta-analysis. *J Clin Oncol*. 2000;18:1220-1229.
55. EBCTCG (Early Breast Cancer Trialists' Collaborative Group), McGale P, Taylor C, et al. Effect of radiotherapy after mastectomy and axillary surgery on 10-year recurrence and 20-year breast cancer mortality: meta-analysis of individual patient data for 8135 women in 22 randomised trials. *Lancet*. 2014;383:2127-2135. doi:10.1016/S0140-6736(14)60488-8.
79. Maaskant-Braat AJG, Voogd AC, Roumen RMH, Nieuwenhuijzen GAP. Repeat sentinel node biopsy in patients with locally recurrent breast cancer: a systematic review and meta-analysis of the literature. *Breast Cancer Res Treat*. 2013;138:13-20. doi:10.1007/s10549-013-2409-1.

A full reference list is available online at ExpertConsult.com.

62

Principles of Preoperative Therapy for Operable Breast Cancer

MELINDA L. TELLI

Coming of Age for Preoperative Systemic Therapy in Operable Breast Cancer

The concept of using preoperative or neoadjuvant systemic therapy was first put forth many decades ago for the treatment of locally advanced inoperable breast tumors. Early experiences showed that this approach enabled ultimate operability and resulted in highly effective local control.[1–6] In 1988, the National Surgical Adjuvant Breast and Bowel Project (NSABP) launched the B-18 clinical trial to evaluate preoperative systemic chemotherapy versus postoperative systemic therapy for the treatment of patients with stage I and II operable breast cancer.[7] The goals of the B-18 study were ambitious and aimed to determine whether preoperative chemotherapy results in improved disease-free survival (DFS) and overall survival (OS) compared with postoperative adjuvant therapy, if response to preoperative therapy was predictive of outcome, and also whether this approach could result in improved rates of breast preservation. More than 1500 patients were enrolled and randomly assigned to receive doxorubicin and cyclophosphamide for four cycles before or after surgery. The initial report from the B-18 study showed no difference between the two groups in regards to DFS or OS, and many more patients in the preoperative group underwent breast preservation surgery. After 16 years of median follow-up, no statistically significant differences between the two groups with regard to DFS and OS were observed (Fig. 62.1), although there was a trend toward better outcomes in women aged less than 50 years treated with preoperative therapy.[8] A subsequent meta-analysis of nine randomized trials including nearly 4000 patients with both operable and inoperable nonmetastatic breast cancer confirmed these findings, with the notable exception that locoregional relapses were increased among patients receiving preoperative therapy, particularly in studies where radiotherapy was given in the absence of surgery.[9]

These data helped to establish the safety and efficacy of preoperative systemic therapy in early-stage operable breast cancer. This approach is commonly used in clinical practice today for breast cancer patients with operable stage IIA (T2N0M0), stage IIB (T2N1M0 or T3N0M0), and stage IIIA (T3N1M0) breast cancer.[10] To deliver preoperative systemic therapy optimally in patients with operable early-stage breast cancer, appropriate patient selection and on treatment monitoring are paramount. This chapter reviews these principles of neoadjuvant systemic

therapy and highlights the current importance of this strategy as a platform for clinical trials and drug development (Box 62.1).

Rationale for Preoperative Systemic Therapy

In addition to demonstrating equivalent long-term outcomes with preoperative and postoperative systemic therapy and demonstrating improvement in rates of breast conservation, clinical experiences from clinical trials such as NSABP B-18 and others clearly demonstrated that the delivery of neoadjuvant therapy offers an important opportunity to assess therapy response in an individual patient. Importantly, it was observed that the attainment of a pathologic complete response (pCR) at the time of surgery is a strong surrogate for improved DFS in responders. In the recent Collaborative Trials in Neoadjuvant Breast Cancer (CTNeoBC) pooled analysis of 12 randomized neoadjuvant clinical trials including nearly 12,000 patients, event-free survival (hazard ratio [HR] 0.48; 95% confidence interval [CI] 0.43–0.54) and OS (HR 0.36; 95% CI 0.31–0.42) were higher in patients who achieved a pCR defined as an absence of invasive disease in the breast and axillary nodes at the time of surgery, irrespective of the presence of in situ disease.[11] Importantly, this analysis and others have demonstrated that the correlation between pCR and event-free survival varies by breast cancer subtype.[11,12] The strongest prognostic correlation exists for hormone receptor–negative, HER2-positive and triple-negative tumors. The correlation between pCR and long-term outcome is weakest for ER-positive disease. Tumor grade is another factor of significance influencing the likelihood of pCR, with high-grade tumors having significantly higher rates of pCR compared with low- and intermediate-grade tumors.[11]

On the basis of these observations, it was proposed that pCR could serve as a surrogate end point for prediction of long-term clinical benefit in early breast cancer. Until recently, our standard drug development strategy in breast cancer relied on testing novel agents first in the metastatic setting and later approving these agents in the adjuvant setting after completion of large and lengthy adjuvant studies. To accelerate drug development in high-risk early-breast cancer, an accelerated US Food and Drug Administration (FDA) approval pathway using the neoadjuvant platform in early-breast cancer was proposed by the FDA in 2012.[13] The idea was that an assessment of a novel agent's activity, when added to standard chemotherapy in early breast cancer, could be carried

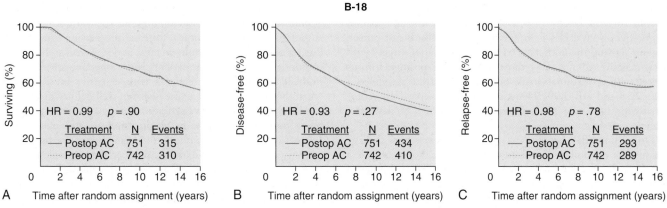

• **Fig. 62.1** Overall survival (A), disease-free survival (B) and relapse-free survival (C) with preoperative doxorubicin and cyclophosphamide (AC) versus postoperative AC in NSABP B-18. *HR,* Hazard ratio. (From Rastogi P, Anderson SJ, Bear HD, et al. Preoperative chemotherapy: updates of National Surgical Adjuvant Breast and Bowel Project Protocols B-18 and B-27. J Clin Oncol. 2008;26:778-785.)

• **Box 62.1** **Key Principles of Preoperative Systemic Therapy in Operable Breast Cancer**

- Preoperative therapy downstages primary breast tumors to enable breast conservation.
- Preoperative therapy provides an in vivo assessment of therapy response.
  - Association between pCR and prognosis is strongest in triple-negative and HER2-positive cancers.
- Accurate clinical staging at baseline is critical before embarking on preoperative therapy:
  - Possible overtreatment with systemic therapy if clinical stage is overestimated;
  - Possible undertreatment locoregionally with radiotherapy if clinical stage is underestimated; or
  - Patients with extensive in situ disease where the extent of invasive disease is unclear, those with nonpalpable tumors and those with a poorly delineated extent of tumor are noncandidates for a preoperative approach.
- Preoperative systemic therapy is an option for clinical stage IIA (T2N0M0), stage IIB (T2N1M0 or T3N0M0), and stage IIIA (T3N1M0) breast cancer, particularly in patients with
  - a large primary tumor relative to breast size in a patient who desires breast conservation or
  - Tumor subtypes associated with a high probability of response.
- On-therapy assessment of response to therapy is key.
  - Routine imaging is not advised.
  - Patients experiencing clinical progression should be taken immediately to surgery.
- A sentinel node biopsy or axillary lymph node dissection can be considered in patients with clinically positive nodes at baseline who convert to clinically negative posttreatment.
- Locoregional principles should be applied in the same manner as in patients treated with adjuvant therapy.
  - Decisions regarding the need for radiotherapy should be based on baseline clinical stage.

---

out in a smaller number of patients and over a much condensed time period compared with the standard adjuvant approach. A major goal of the CTNeoBC pooled analysis was to examine the potential of pCR as a surrogate end point for long-term outcomes. Although a correlation between pCR and long-term outcomes could be observed at the individual patient level, the pooled analysis could not establish a trial level correlation between pCR and long-term outcome. Despite this, the FDA took the position that if a novel agent produces a marked absolute increase in the frequency of pCR compared with standard therapy, that the agent could also be considered to be reasonably likely to result in long-term improvements in event-free and OS. On September 30, 2013, the FDA approved pertuzumab as part of a complete neoadjuvant regimen for patients with stage II–III early breast cancer. Pertuzumab was the first drug approved using this neoadjuvant approval pathway based on pCR end points from two phase II studies.[14]

In addition to providing a pathway to evaluate novel agents with the possibility of accelerated FDA approval of novel agents, the neoadjuvant setting offers additional clinical trial opportunities. Among patients with triple-negative or hormone receptor–negative, HER2+ breast cancer, for example, those patients who fail to achieve pCR have a significantly elevated risk of early relapse and death from breast cancer.[11,12,15] The CREATE-X clinical trial recently showed a DFS and OS advantage with capecitabine when delivered to high-risk HER2-negative early breast cancer patients with residual disease after standard neoadjuvant combination chemotherapy.[16] Current studies are underway to explore novel agents in the adjuvant setting when residual disease is detected after standard neoadjuvant chemotherapy. In addition, the neoadjuvant platform offers an opportunity for pre- and post-treatment tissue collection and enables the assessment of new tissue and imaging-based biomarkers. Finally, the results of neoadjuvant trials can help to inform the design and conduct of adjuvant studies, thus sparing time and costs associated with negative adjuvant studies.

In addition to the advantages already noted, for patients who will absolutely require systemic therapy, the use of preoperative systemic therapy may allow patients to begin their breast cancer therapy without excessive delays while waiting for results of genetic testing or in cases in which delays may be introduced due to planning required for breast reconstruction in patients electing to undergo mastectomy surgery. Recent data from a single institution suggest that a delay in time to chemotherapy can affect survival outcomes in stage I–III early breast cancer, particularly in those with high-risk breast cancer subtypes.[17] Specifically, initiation of chemotherapy 61 days or more after surgery was associated with adverse outcomes among patients with stage II (distant relapse-free survival HR 1.20; 95% CI 1.02–1.43) and stage III (overall survival HR = 1.76; 95% CI 1.26–2.46; and distant relapse-free survival HR 1.36; 95% CI 1.02–1.80) breast cancer. Patients starting chemotherapy 61 days or more after surgery with triple-negative tumors and those with HER2-positive tumors treated with trastuzumab had worse survival (HR 1.54; 95% CI 1.09–2.18 and HR 3.09; 95% CI 1.49–6.39, respectively) compared with those who initiated treatment in the first 30 days after surgery.

Other potential benefits of neoadjuvant systemic therapy include the possibility of sentinel lymph node biopsy only if a positive axilla is cleared with chemotherapy and the possibility of allowing for smaller radiotherapy ports or delivering less radiotherapy if axillary nodal disease is cleared with neoadjuvant therapy. This is currently being tested in the NRG 9353 (NSABP-51/RTOG 1304) trial where patients with clinical T1–3N1M0 breast cancer with biopsy-proven N1 nodal disease receive neoadjuvant chemotherapy and then, if axillary nodal involvement is negative at definitive surgery, are randomized to receive (1) postmastectomy radiotherapy versus not or (2) whole breast radiotherapy versus whole breast plus regional nodal irradiation.[18]

Patient Selection for Preoperative Therapy in Operable Breast Cancer

Although the neoadjuvant approach is commonly used in clinical practice today for breast cancer patients with operable stage IIA (T2N0M0), stage IIB (T2N1M0 or T3N0M0), and stage IIIA (T3N1M0) breast cancer, it is not appropriate for all patients.[10] Accurate clinical staging at baseline before initiation of preoperative systemic therapy is critical for selecting optimal candidates for this approach. Clinical stage should be calculated based on radiographic and physical examinations using the current *American Joint Committee on Cancer Staging Manual*.[10] National Comprehensive Cancer Network (NCCN) Breast Cancer Guidelines recommend that suspicious lymph nodes based on imaging or physical examination findings be biopsied by core biopsy or fine-needle aspiration to document clinical nodal stage before treatment.[19,20] In addition, marking of sampled lymph nodes with a tattoo or clip should be considered to allow verification that the biopsy-proven positive lymph node is removed at the time of definitive surgical resection. In patients with a clinically negative axilla, axillary ultrasound should be considered with biopsy by fine-needle aspiration or core of any lymph nodes suspicious on axillary ultrasound imaging before initiation of preoperative therapy. A core biopsy of the primary breast lesion is preferred to allow assessment of prognostic markers and an image-detectable marker or clip should be placed to demarcate the tumor bed for postsystemic therapy surgical planning. Areas suspicious for multicentric disease should be separately sampled before initiation of preoperative therapy if breast conservation surgery is being considered. For patients with clinical stage III disease or in those with clinical stage I–II disease with symptoms or signs of metastatic disease, systemic staging should be completed to rule out metastatic disease.

If clinical stage is overestimated, it is possible that the patient may be overtreated with systemic therapy. Conversely, if clinical stage is underestimated, it is possible that a patient can be undertreated locoregionally with radiotherapy. Ideal candidates for preoperative systemic therapy should have a palpable breast tumor that is easily clinically assessable. Patients with small, nonpalpable

tumors are not candidates for a preoperative approach because it is important that the tumor response be assessed during therapy. Although infrequent, clinical disease progression can happen during neoadjuvant systemic therapy, and it is critical that this be promptly identified and patients with operable disease taken immediately to surgery. Patients with extensive in situ disease when the extent of invasive disease is not well defined are also not candidates for preoperative systemic therapy and are better served by upfront surgery to gain better precision in pathologic staging. Likewise, patients with a poorly delineated extent of tumor preoperatively are not candidates for preoperative systemic therapy.

Candidates for preoperative systemic therapy include patients with inoperable breast cancer on the basis of having inflammatory breast cancer with skin involvement, bulky and matted N2 axillary nodes, N3 nodal disease, and those with noninflammatory T4 tumors. In patients with operable disease, patients with clinical stage IIA (T2N0M0), stage IIB (T2N1M0 or T3N0M0), and stage IIIA (T3N1M0) breast cancer are candidates for a preoperative systemic therapy approach, particularly if the breast primary tumor is large relative to breast size in a patient who desires breast preservation. In addition, this approach is generally favored in patients with breast cancer subtypes associated with a high likelihood of response such as those with triple-negative or HER2-positive disease. In these patients, response to therapy offers more powerful prognostic information compared with patients with hormone receptor-positive, HER2-negative disease.

Delivery of Optimal Preoperative Systemic Therapy

Preoperative Chemotherapy

Regarding the choice of preoperative systemic chemotherapy, many regimens have activity in the neoadjuvant setting. The NCCN Breast Cancer Guidelines recommend that chemotherapy regimens recommended in the adjuvant setting may be considered preoperatively.[19] For HER2-negative disease, preferred regimens include dose-dense doxorubicin and cyclophosphamide followed by dose dense or weekly paclitaxel and docetaxel and cyclophosphamide. For HER2-positive tumors, neoadjuvant chemotherapy incorporating trastuzumab for at least 9 weeks is recommended. Preferred regimens include doxorubicin and cyclophosphamide followed by paclitaxel plus trastuzumab ± pertuzumab (various schedules) and docetaxel, carboplatin, and trastuzumab ± pertuzumab.

As noted earlier, pertuzumab was the first drug granted accelerated FDA approval for the neoadjuvant treatment of HER2-positive breast cancer using a pCR end point. Per the FDA label, approved neoadjuvant pertuzumab-containing regimens include the following: (1) docetaxel, trastuzumab, and pertuzumab followed by adjuvant fluorouracil, epirubicin and cyclophosphamide (FEC; based on NeoSphere study); (2) neoadjuvant FEC followed by neoadjuvant docetaxel, trastuzumab, and pertuzumab (based on Tryphaena study); (3) neoadjuvant docetaxel, carboplatin, and trastuzumab (TCH) + pertuzumab for six cycles (based on Tryphaena study).[21–23] The FDA label currently states that there are no safety data with doxorubicin-containing regimens and that the safety/efficacy of pertuzumab for more than six cycles in early breast cancer has not been established.[24] These approved indications differ somewhat from regimens recommended by the NCCN. In addition, the NCCN guideline states that patients who have not received pertuzumab in the neoadjuvant setting can receive adjuvant pertuzumab (duration not defined).[19]

Although standard therapy today remains an anthracycline and taxane-based regimen for patients with estrogen receptor–negative, progesterone receptor–negative, and HER2-negative or triple-negative breast cancer (TNBC), to date there have been three randomized neoadjuvant studies examining the role of platinum as an "add-on" to standard anthracycline and taxane-based treatment. Initially, Alba and colleagues reported the randomized phase II neoadjuvant GEICAM/2006-03 study of epirubicin and cyclophosphamide for four cycles followed by docetaxel ± carboplatin area under the curve (AUC) 6 every 21 days for four cycles and found no improvement in pCR with the addition of carboplatin (pCR = 30% in both arms; n = 94).[25] Subsequently, two larger neoadjuvant TNBC platinum studies were reported which added important insights. The phase II GeparSixto trial from the German Breast Group provided important randomized data looking at a regimen of dose-intense anthracycline and taxane-based chemotherapy with bevacizumab ± carboplatin as neoadjuvant therapy for early-stage TNBC.[26] Unlike in GEICAM/2006-03, the GeparSixto study showed clear advantage in terms of pCR among 315 TNBC patients treated with 18 weeks of neoadjuvant weekly paclitaxel 80 mg/m^2, weekly nonpegylated liposomal doxorubicin 20 mg/m^2, and bevacizumab 15 mg/kg every 21 days who received carboplatin weekly AUC 1.5 compared with those that did not. Although a high proportion of patients discontinued in both arms due to adverse events, patients receiving carboplatin as a component of their neoadjuvant therapy achieved a pCR rate of 53.2% compared with 36.9% in patients who did not receive carboplatin. The randomized phase II neoadjuvant Cancer and Leukemia Group B (CALGB) 40603 study used a 2 × 2 study design to assess the role of standard anthracycline and taxane-based chemotherapy with or without carboplatin and with or without bevacizumab in patients with stage II–III TNBC.[27] All patients received 12 weekly doses of paclitaxel 80 mg/m^2 followed by dose-dense doxorubicin 60 mg/m^2 and cyclophosphamide 600 mg/m^2 (AC) every 2 weeks for four cycles. Patients were randomized to carboplatin AUC 6 every 3 weeks for four cycles concurrent with the paclitaxel versus paclitaxel alone and bevacizumab 10 mg/kg every 2 weeks for nine cycles concurrent during the paclitaxel and AC or not. In this study, the addition of carboplatin significantly increased the pCR rate (breast and axilla) by 13% (pCR with carboplatin = 54%; 95% CI 48%–61% and pCR without carboplatin = 41%, 95% CI 35%–48%; p = .0029). The addition of bevacizumab increased the rate of pCR but was not significant (pCR = 52% with bevacizumab, 95% CI 45%–58%; pCR = 44% without bevacizumab, 95% CI 38%–51%; p = .057). In this study, as in GeparSixto, the addition of carboplatin and/or bevacizumab led to increased rates of adverse events.

Recently both CALGB 40603 and GeparSixto reported on DFS outcomes. At a median follow-up of 35 months, the addition of carboplatin in GeparSixto was significantly associated with a DFS benefit (HR 0.56, 95% CI 0.33–0.96; p = .035) with 3-year DFS of 85.8% in patients receiving carboplatin and 76.1% in patients not receiving carboplatin.[28] At a median follow-up of 39 months, the CALGB 40603 study found that the addition of carboplatin did not significantly improve event-free survival (HR 0.84, 95% CI 0.58–1.22; p = .36) with a 3-year event-free survival of 76% among patients receiving carboplatin and 71% among patients not receiving carboplatin.[29] On the basis of these data, the routine addition of platinum to standard anthracycline and taxane-based neoadjuvant therapy is not recommended at this time because the results of GeparSixto and CALGB 40603 are inconsistent. Both studies were underpowered for survival outcomes, and both were potentially confounded by the inclusion of bevacizumab. NRG BR003 is currently enrolling patients to assess the role of carboplatin added to standard therapy in a definitive phase III adjuvant TNBC trial.[30]

Response-Adapted Preoperative Chemotherapy

Prior investigations into adapting preoperative chemotherapy based on response to therapy have been explored. The German Breast Group's GeparTrio study was a phase III study that enrolled more than 2000 patients with stage II–III breast cancer who were treated with an initial two cycles of docetaxel, doxorubicin, and cyclophosphamide (TAC). Clinical responders were then randomized to continuing the same therapy for four or six additional cycles, and nonresponders were randomized to continue the same therapy or sequence to an alternate chemotherapy combination of navelbine and capecitabine (NX) for four cycles. The primary end points of the study were to compare pCR rates in early responders and clinical response in early nonresponders. The primary results showed a nonstatistically significant difference in pCR among early responders treated with TAC × 6 compared with TAC × 8 (21% vs. 23.5%; p = .27)[31] and similar clinical responses were observed among early nonresponders with TAC × 6 compared with TAC-NX (50.5% vs. 51.2%; p = .008 for non-inferiority).[32] At a median follow-up of 62 months, DFS was significantly longer in early responders treated with TAC × 8 compared with TAC × 6 (HR 0.78; 95% CI 0.62–0.97; p = .026) and in early nonresponders treated with TAC-NX compared with TAC × 6 (HR 0.59; 95% CI 0.49–0.82; p = .001).[33] No significant difference in OS was observed in these two groups. Unexpectedly, looking at subsets within this study, response-guided therapy influenced DFS only in hormone receptor–positive and not hormone receptor–negative breast cancer. For patients with hormone receptor–negative disease achieving a pCR was associated with longer DFS, but response-guided therapy did not prolong DFS.

Endocrine Therapy

Rates of pCR after neoadjuvant chemotherapy in hormone-responsive breast cancer are uniformly low. In the CTNeoBC pooled analysis, rate of pCR among 1986 patients with hormone receptor–positive, HER2-negative, low- and intermediate-grade tumors was 7.5%.[11] This increased to a pCR rate of 16.2% among 630 patients with a tumor grade of 3. As these patients arguably receive their most important therapy, endocrine therapy, after chemotherapy, the focus of current neoadjuvant chemotherapy trials has shifted away from this group of patients in large part. Instead, neoadjuvant endocrine therapy strategies for these patients have gained greater traction. A number of studies have demonstrated that neoadjuvant endocrine therapy, similar to chemotherapy, can convert surgically inoperable breast cancers to operability and can effectively downstage larger primary breast tumors to avoid the need for mastectomy. Most of the data to date have focused on postmenopausal breast cancer,[34–38] with limited study of this approach in patients with premenopausal hormone-responsive disease.[39] In general, aromatase inhibitors are superior to tamoxifen in achieving tumor downstaging and longer duration of therapy is superior to shorter durations of treatment. The NCCN Breast Cancer Guideline supports the use of preoperative tamoxifen or an aromatase inhibitor with or without ovarian suppression. In postmenopausal women, an aromatase inhibitor is the preferred endocrine option.

On Treatment Monitoring and Posttreatment Management

When electing preoperative chemotherapy, it is recommended that all treatment be given before surgery. Pretherapy sentinel lymph node biopsy is discouraged. Tumor response should be routinely assessed by clinical examination and the primary tumor should be measured using calipers and documented at each visit. Imaging during preoperative systemic therapy should not be routinely performed but may be considered if tumor progression is suspected. Patients with operable breast cancer experiencing progression of disease during neoadjuvant therapy should be taken promptly to surgery. After neoadjuvant therapy has concluded, locoregional principles should be applied in the same manner as in patients treated with adjuvant therapy. If the axilla was positive at baseline, it should be restaged after neoadjuvant therapy. If the axilla is clinically positive posttherapy, an axillary lymph node dissection is appropriate. If the axilla is clinically negative posttherapy, the NCCN guideline supports the use of either sentinel lymph node biopsy of axillary lymph node dissection. Elevated false-negative sentinel lymph node biopsy rates have been observed in some studies in patients treated with neoadjuvant therapy.[40,41] This rate can be improved by marking involved nodes at baseline, using dual tracers, and removing more than two sentinel nodes.[42–44]

Some studies have reported an increased risk of locoregional recurrence in patients receiving preoperative therapy.[9] This increased risk of locoregional recurrence has been attributed to suboptimal delivery of definitive local therapy in patients treated in the preoperative setting. Importantly, decisions regarding the need for postoperative radiotherapy should be based on the baseline tumor stage.

Conclusions

Preoperative systemic therapy offers a number of advantages over adjuvant therapy, with in vivo assessment of tumor response and tumor downstaging to enable breast preservation ranking among the most important. It has been clearly established that long-term outcomes are similar whether treatment is given preoperatively or postoperatively and that a pCR at the time of surgery is associated with a very favorable outcome in all patients who achieve it. The neoadjuvant strategy has also shown great potential as a platform for drug development, and this has led the FDA to consider the rate of pathologic complete response (pCR) to neoadjuvant therapy as a surrogate end point for long-term outcomes to support accelerated drug approval in high-risk early-stage breast cancer.

Although the neoadjuvant approach is commonly used in clinical practice today for breast cancer patients with operable stage IIA (T2N0M0), stage IIB (T2N1M0 or T3N0M0), and stage IIIA (T3N1M0) breast cancer, it is not appropriate for all patients. Accurate clinical staging at baseline before initiation of preoperative systemic therapy is critical for selecting optimal candidates for this approach. Ideal candidates for preoperative systemic therapy should have a palpable breast tumor that is easily clinically assessable. Patients with extensive in situ disease when the extent of invasive disease is not well defined are not candidates for preoperative systemic therapy. Likewise, patients with a poorly delineated extent of tumor preoperatively are poor candidates for this approach. Although infrequent, clinical disease progression can occur during neoadjuvant systemic therapy, and patients with operable disease should be taken immediately to surgery. Regarding the choice of preoperative systemic chemotherapy, many regimens have activity in the neoadjuvant setting. The NCCN Breast Cancer Guidelines recommend that chemotherapy regimens recommended in the adjuvant setting may be considered preoperatively. Endocrine therapy as preoperative therapy is an option in hormone receptor-positive, HER2-negative breast cancer and is most appropriate for postmenopausal women because data in premenopausal women are limited. After neoadjuvant therapy has concluded, locoregional principles should be applied in the same manner as in patients treated with adjuvant therapy.

Selected References

1. Bonadonna G, Veronesi U, Brambilla C, et al. Primary chemotherapy to avoid mastectomy in tumors with diameters of three centimeters or more. *J Natl Cancer Inst.* 1990;82:1539-1545.
8. Rastogi P, Anderson SJ, Bear HD, et al. Preoperative chemotherapy: updates of National Surgical Adjuvant Breast and Bowel Project Protocols B-18 and B-27. *J Clin Oncol.* 2008;26:778-785.
11. Cortazar P, Zhang L, Untch M, et al. Pathological complete response and long-term clinical benefit in breast cancer: the CTNeoBC pooled analysis. *Lancet.* 2014;384:164-172.
22. Gianni L, Pienkowski T, Im YH, et al. 5-year analysis of neoadjuvant pertuzumab and trastuzumab in patients with locally advanced, inflammatory, or early-stage HER2-positive breast cancer (NeoSphere): a multicentre, open-label, phase 2 randomised trial. *Lancet Oncol.* 2016;17:791-800.
23. Schneeweiss A, Chia S, Hickish T, et al. Pertuzumab plus trastuzumab in combination with standard neoadjuvant anthracycline-containing and anthracycline-free chemotherapy regimens in patients with HER2-positive early breast cancer: a randomized phase II cardiac safety study (TRYPHAENA). *Ann Oncol.* 2013;24:2278-2284.

A full reference list is available online at ExpertConsult.com.

63

Locally Advanced Breast Cancer

RICARDO COSTA, NORA HANSEN, AND WILLIAM J. GRADISHAR

Locally advanced breast cancer (LABC) encompasses a wide array of breast tumors with poor prognoses (i.e., short disease-free [DFS] and overall survival [OS] rates) as a function of advanced stage upon diagnosis. Historically, a multidisciplinary approach and with the development of therapies such as chemotherapy, hormonal therapy, surgery, and radiation therapy (RT), outcomes have improved for patients with LABC. More recently, the introduction of HER2-targeted therapies has led to significant improvement in response rates and OS, not only for patients with metastatic breast cancer but also early stage (localized) and LABC. Breast tumors that are larger than 5 cm in diameter or that involve the chest wall or skin or with fixed axillary lymph nodes are generally classified as locally advanced. As a consequence, according to the 7th edition of the American Joint Committee on Cancer (AJCC) tumor, node, metastasis (TNM) staging system, breast tumors classified as T3 or T4 with any N stage or as N2 or N3 with any T stage are considered LABCs. Thus all patients with stage III disease and some patients with stage IIB disease (T3N0) meet the criteria for LABC.[1]

This chapter reviews the epidemiology, diagnosis and staging, prognostic factors, and treatment approaches for women with LABC. Of note, inflammatory breast cancer (IBC) is a rare and aggressive type of breast cancer, which is invariably either locally advanced or metastatic at diagnosis and has distinct clinical presentation, prognosis, and response to therapy.[2–5] Another chapter of this book will review current knowledge and clinical approaches to IBC.

Epidemiology

Among women who receive regular breast cancer screening with mammograms, less than 5% are diagnosed as having stage III disease.[6] Since the widespread adoption of screening mammography, the percentage of patients diagnosed with LABC has declined. Indeed, according to the Surveillance, Epidemiology, and End Results (SEER) data collected from 1976 through 2008, the incidence of breast cancer with nodal involvement declined among women 40 years of age or older by an absolute rate of approximately 8% (i.e., annual incidence of 78 cases per 100,000 in 2006–2008 compared with 85 cases per 100,000 in 1976–1978).[7] By contrast, according to incidence data collected by the SEER, the National Program of Cancer Registries; and the North American Association of Central Cancer Registries up to 31% of patients with breast cancer diagnosed between 2006 and 2012 had regional metastasis, likely as a function of low rates of regular screening mammograms in the general population.[8] The age distribution of

patients who have stage III disease at the time of diagnosis is similar to the age distributions for patients with breast cancer in other stages: approximately 1% of patients are 29 years of age or younger, 9% are 30 to 39 years of age, 22% are 40 to 49 years of age, 20% are 50 to 59 years of age, 19% are 60 to 69 years of age, 18% are 70 to 79 years of age, and 12% are 80 years of age or older. African American and Hispanic women are more likely to be diagnosed with advanced stage breast cancer (stage III and IV) than white women; however, interactions between race and socioeconomic characteristics on stage at diagnosis remain controversial.[9–13]

Survival

Patients with LABC are at high risk of relapse and death from recurrent, metastatic disease. The long-term outcome of these patients is rarely reported because this patient population usually represents a small subpopulation of trials enrolling patients with early-stage and LABC breast tumors. The National Cancer Database statistics show that patients with stage III disease who underwent modified radical mastectomy and both RT and systemic treatment have a 3-year relative survival rate of 68%, a 5-year relative survival rate of 50%, and a 10-year relative survival rate of 36%.[14] In a retrospective analysis the National Cancer Institute investigated the outcome of 61 patients with noninflammatory stage III breast cancer who received neoadjuvant chemotherapy (i.e., cyclophosphamide, doxorubicin, methotrexate, fluorouracil, leucovorin) and hormonal adjuvant treatment. Patients who had a complete response received definitive radiotherapy to the breast and axilla and patients with residual disease underwent mastectomy, lymph node dissection, and radiotherapy. The 15-year OS was 50% for stage IIIA and 23% for stage IIIB breast cancer.[15] In another series, 831 patients treated with neoadjuvant anthracycline-based chemotherapy regimens, the median follow-up duration was 69.9 months. Patients with LABC included 490 (59%) with inoperable disease at diagnosis. The 5-year recurrence-free and OS rates were 56% and 63%, respectively.[16] More recently 187 patients with HER2-negative LABC (i.e., clinical stage IIB or III) were treated with dose-dense doxorubicin combined with cyclophosphamide (AC), followed or preceded by nab-paclitaxel in the SWOG S0800.[17] After a median follow-up time of 3 years, the 3-year OS was 87%.

Importantly, LABC represents a heterogeneous group of tumors, with marked variations in biology, clinical patterns of presentation and recurrence, and response to therapy. For instance, the introduction of effective systemic targeted agents, such as trastuzumab, pertuzumab, and lapatinib, led to an improvement in outcomes in a subset of these patients (i.e., patients diagnosed with HER2-postive LABC).

Diagnosis and Staging

LABC can be detected during physical examination or with mammography followed by pathologic diagnosis established by a core needle biopsy. In all cases, estrogen receptor (ER) and progesterone receptor (PR) status, nuclear grade, and HER2 status, and ki67 should be determined on pathologic examination. As neoadjuvant chemotherapy with or without HER2-targeted therapy is considered at diagnosis it is important that radiopaque clips be placed at the time of biopsy to provide localization of disease for future surgical planning. The patient should undergo an imaging evaluation to establish the extent of locoregional disease before initiation of treatment. Diagnostic bilateral mammograms, ultrasonography, and breast magnetic resonance imaging (MRI) should be performed as clinically indicated. Of note, MRI in addition to mammography or mammography and ultrasound has been shown to more accurately delineate the extent of local disease and identify patients for whom breast conserving surgery would be contraindicated.[18–21] The routine use of MRI for the staging of patients with breast cancer has been limited by the lack of proven benefit for the end points of local recurrences and mortality reduction along with increased cost.[22]

All patients should undergo a thorough physical examination. Current guidelines recommend laboratory evaluation at diagnosis of LABC, including complete blood count, liver function tests, alkaline phosphatase, and chest imaging.[23] Patients in whom any abnormalities are detected on clinical evaluation should undergo imaging with computed tomography (CT) of chest abdomen and pelvis and bone scan. Other tests, such as CT of brain, MRI scans, and/or PET scans should be performed if indicated on the basis of clinical suspicion. Small studies have described the use of F-fluorodeoxyglucose positron emission tomography (FDG-PET) imaging in the staging of patients with LABC. The detection rates of confirmed distant metastatic disease ranged from 5% to 14%, and the rates of false-positive results in the studies ranged from 0% to 21%.[24–27] One should keep in mind that equivocal or suspicious sites identified by PET-CT scanning should prompt pathologic confirmation of diagnosis of distant metastatic disease whenever possible as the presence of distant metastatic disease may influence the treatment plan.

PET-CT is superior to CT in the detection of extraaxillary lymph node metastasis; however, the impact on patient outcome is not known.[28–30] Furthermore, a retrospective study comparing 132 paired bone scans with integrated FDG PET-CTs, in women with stages I–III breast cancer with suspected metastasis, showed a high concordance (81%) for reporting osseous metastases suggesting the a bone scan is not necessary in the setting of a positive PET-CT.[31] In sum, PET-CT could be considered more expensive alternative to CT scans for staging of LABC; however, there is insufficient evidence to support the use of PET-CT for the initial staging evaluation of unselected cases of LABC.[32,33]

Prognostic Factors

As is true for other types of breast cancer, increasing tumor size, site (i.e., axillary, infraclavicular, supraclavicular, or internal mammary) and number of lymph node metastasis all have independent correlation with disease recurrence and survival are important elements of the staging system.[34] Historical series support the strong correlation between breast cancer survival rates and number of involved nodes, with one study reporting 5-year survival of 73% for patients with metastases in one to three lymph nodes, compared with 46% for patients with metastases in four or more nodes.[35] This correlation is independent of tumor size. The vast majority of these patients did not receive chemotherapy. Increasing size of the primary tumor also has prognostic significance for patients with breast cancer, even in women with tumors larger than 5 cm in diameter.[36–38]

Tumor expression of ER and/or PR is generally considered a weak favorable prognostic factor and is highly predictive for response to hormonal treatment. Similar to early-stage disease, HER2-positive tumors have a worse outcome in both lymph node–negative and –positive disease.[39,40] Most importantly HER2 positivity is also a strong predictor of clinical benefit to trastuzumab in combination with chemotherapy.[41,42] Despite advances in the realm of biomarker-based studies for the adjuvant treatment of node-negative breast cancer, the American Society of Clinical Oncology (ASCO) guidelines do not recommend for the routine evaluation of novel tumor markers such as urokinase plasminogen activator (UPA) and plasminogen activator inhibitor (PAI)-1, p53, cathepsin, cyclin E, PAM50 recurrence score, 70-gene assay, and the Onco*type* DX assay for patients with lymph node–positive breast cancer due to lack of sufficient evidence in supporting changes in treatment for patients with LABC.[43]

Indeed, in light of poorer prognosis and the presumed benefit of chemotherapy treatment for all patients with LABC; this patient population remains minimally represented in prospective randomized trials and retrospective studies performed to evaluate the clinical utility of genomic predictions assays (e.g., 70-gene assay) in assessing the benefit from adjuvant chemotherapy treatment.[44]

Evolution of Local Therapy

The management of LABC has been challenging and has evolved over time. Initially most patients with LABC were treated with surgery alone and included resection of the breast, lymph nodes, and underlying muscle—the radical mastectomy. Although surgical intervention was possible in most patients, the majority of patients was not cured by surgery alone and ultimately developed metastatic disease, which eventually led to death.[45] For patients with inoperable disease, the role of RT to control the disease was investigated but this therapeutic modality led to many complications due to the high doses of RT needed to control the disease and did not lead to long-term survival.[46–48] It became clear that a multimodality approach was needed to treat patients with LABC. The emergence of adjuvant systemic therapies gave the physician another tool to treat these complex patients. Randomized trials suggested that adjuvant systemic therapy reduced the incidence of recurrence and death in patients with stage III breast cancer.[49] The effectiveness of systemic therapy varies greatly and is dependent on predictors of therapeutic benefit. A patient with a triple-negative or a HER2-positive tumor will likely respond better to systemic chemotherapy than an ER/PR-positive breast cancer. The ER-positive cancers often do respond to neoadjuvant therapy, but the rate of pathologic complete response (pCR) is not as high as the ER-negative/HER2-positive cancers.[50–53]

Neoadjuvant systemic therapy given before surgical intervention has increased over the past few decades and has become the standard approach to patients with LABC. It can potentially allow for breast conservation in a patient who was deemed not to be a

TABLE 63.1 **Randomized Clinical Trials of Neoadjuvant Versus Adjuvant Chemotherapy in Locally Advanced Operable Breast Cancer**

Study	Treatment	Study Population	N	BREAST CONSERVING SURGERY RATE		OVERALL SURVIVAL AT MEDIAN FOLLOW-UP	
				Neoadjuvant	Adjuvant	Neoadjuvant	Adjuvant
Institut Curie[59]	CAF × 4 → XRT ± S vs. XRT ± S → CAF × 4	T2–T3 N0–N1M0	414	82%	72%	86%	78%
Powles et al.[60]	Tam + 3M/2M × 4 → S ± XRT + 3M/2M × 4 vs. S ± XRT → 3M/2M × 8 + Tam	T1–T3 N0–N1M0	212	87%	72%	Not provided	Not provided
NSABP-18[58]	AC × 4 → S vs. S → AC × 4	T1–T3 N0–N1M0	1523	67%	60%	55%	55%
EORTC[55]	FEC × 4 → S ± XRT vs. S → FEC × 4 ± XRT	T1–T4b N–N1M0	698	Not provided	Not provided	82%	84%

3M, Mitomycin, mitoxantrone, methotrexate; *2M,* mitoxantrone, methotrexate; *AC,* doxorubicin, cyclophosphamide; *CAF,* cyclophosphamide, doxorubicin, 5-fluorouracil; *EORTC,* European Organization of Research and Treatment of Cancer; *FEC,* 5-fluorouracil, epirubicin, cyclophosphamide; *NSABP,* National Surgical Adjuvant Breast and Bowel Project; *S,* surgery; *Tam,* tamoxifen; *XRT,* radiation.

conservation candidate, and at times it can also make an inoperable candidate operable. The response rate in the primary tumor and regional nodes can vary with the best response seen in ER-negative and HER2-positive cancers.[52]

There have been no differences in DFS or OS in multiple neoadjuvant versus adjuvant therapy trials reassuring both patients and physicians that leaving the tumor intact during neoadjuvant therapy does not impart a worse outcome.[50,54,55]

Combined Modality Treatment

A combined modality approach that incorporates radiotherapy, surgery, or both; systemic therapy that includes chemotherapy and targeted agents such as trastuzumab, pertuzumab, and lapatinib; and hormonal therapy when indicated is currently widely used for the management of patients with LABC. This multimodality approach requires careful planning and coordination by a multidisciplinary team. The additional benefit of chemotherapy to surgery and RT was demonstrated in a randomized study of 120 patients with operable stage III breast cancer who were randomized after modified radical mastectomy to receive RT alone; vincristine, doxorubicin (Adriamycin), and cyclophosphamide (VAC) chemotherapy alone; or radiotherapy and VAC chemotherapy. The DFS was better with combined modality of RT and chemotherapy than with surgery alone (*p* < .001), and the 3-year OS rates were 57% for patients who received RT alone, 72% for those who received chemotherapy alone, and 90% for those who received both chemotherapy and RT therapy (*p* < .01).[56] These early findings supporting a role for adjuvant chemotherapy were confirmed by data from the Early Breast Cancer 2005 Trialists' Collaborative Group in their meta-analysis of worldwide experience with adjuvant chemotherapy versus no adjuvant chemotherapy in randomized clinical trials of approximately 150,000 women with early-stage cancer. These data demonstrated that adjuvant polychemotherapy produced highly significant reductions in mortality at 15 years of follow-up in women with node-positive breast cancer.[57]

Neoadjuvant chemotherapy is now preferred for patients with LABC because it can downstage tumors and thus increase the rate of breast conserving surgery. In cases of more advanced disease,

neoadjuvant chemotherapy can render inoperable tumors resectable. Equivalent OS has been shown for patients who receive neoadjuvant versus adjuvant therapy (Table 63.1).[55,58–60] The National Surgical Adjuvant Breast and Bowel Project (NSABP) B-18 study enrolled 1523 women with T1–T3, N0–N1, and M0 operable breast cancer who were randomized to receive either four cycles of AC given in the neoadjuvant setting or four cycles of the same regimen given as adjuvant therapy. At 16 years of follow-up, no significant differences between the two groups for DFS and OS end points continue to be observed (hazard ratio [HR] 0.93; 95% confidence interval [CI] 0.81–1.06; *p* = .27 and HR 0.99; 95% CI 0.85–1.16; *p* = .90, respectively).[58] Similar findings were confirmed by the European Organization for Research and Treatment of Cancer (EORTC) Breast Cancer Cooperative Group randomized trial of neoadjuvant versus adjuvant chemotherapy in patients with operable breast cancer using a fluorouracil, epirubicin, and cyclophosphamide (FEC) backbone.[55]

The optimal regimen, duration, and sequencing of neoadjuvant chemotherapy have not yet been determined. However, the National Comprehensive Cancer Network (NCCN) guidelines indicate a preference for neoadjuvant regimens that contain both an anthracycline and taxane for patients with LABC given the superior outcome of these regimens in the adjuvant setting for patients with lymph node–positive disease.[23,61,62] Among patients with HER2-positive tumors, neoadjuvant trastuzumab-, pertuzumab-, lapatinib, taxane-, and anthracycline-based regimens yield significantly higher clinical complete response (cCR) and pCR rates compared with chemotherapy alone.[63–65]

Adjuvant hormonal therapy with tamoxifen for premenopausal women[66] or aromatase inhibitors for postmenopausal women[67,68] improves DFS and is incorporated into the systemic management of patients with LABC as indicated based on the ER and PR status of the tumor. In addition, based on two recent randomized trials, consideration should be given to ovarian suppression combined with antiestrogen therapy for the treatment of premenopausal women with LABC. In the Suppression of Ovarian Function Trial (SOFT) 3066 women with hormone receptor–positive breast cancer were randomized to adjuvant treatment with 5 years of tamoxifen, tamoxifen plus ovarian suppression, or exemestane plus ovarian suppression.[69] After a median follow-up time of 67 months, the 5-year DFS rate of 86.6% in the tamoxifen–ovarian suppression arm and 84.7% in the tamoxifen group (HR 0.83; 95% CI 0.66–1.04; p = .10). For patients who received prior chemotherapy the 5-year rate of freedom from breast cancer was 85.7% in the exemestane–ovarian suppression group (HR for recurrence vs. tamoxifen, 0.65; 95% CI 0.49–0.87). Also in the combined analysis of 4609 premenopausal women treated in the SOFT and the Triptorelin With Either Exemestane or Tamoxifen (TEXT) trials (the latter also randomized premenopausal women to ovarian suppression combined with tamoxifen or exemestane for 5 years), the 5-year DFS was 91.1% in the exemestane-ovarian suppression group and 87.3% in the tamoxifen-ovarian suppression group (HR 0.72; 95% CI 0.60–0.85; p < .001).[70] Taken together, the results of these trials suggest that ovarian suppression combined with antiestrogen therapy for 5 years should be considered for women with high-risk breast cancer, such as hormonal receptor–positive LABC.

Furthermore, in the ATLAS trial, 12,894 women with early-stage breast cancer were randomized to continuation of tamoxifen for 5 years or to stop after completion of 5 years of tamoxifen.[71] Among women with ER-positive disease, allocation to continue tamoxifen reduced the risk of breast cancer recurrence (p = .002), and reduced breast cancer mortality (p = .01). Of note, only approximately 10% had tumors measuring more than 5 cm, and approximately 25% had N1–N3 disease. Similar results were observed in the UK Adjuvant Tamoxifen: To Offer More? trial (aTTom) trial.[72] Increased length of adjuvant treatment with tamoxifen from 5 to 10 years should be considered for premenopausal women with high risk of disease recurrence.[23]

The NCCN guidelines recommend postmastectomy RT for all patients with pathologic confirmation of four or more positive axillary lymph nodes, T_3 tumors, or clinical stage III disease.[23] For patients treated with neoadjuvant systemic therapy, indications for RT and treatment fields should be based on the maximum stage from the pretherapy clinical stage, pathologic stage, and tumor characteristics.

In a recent update the ASCO, American Society for Radiation Oncology, and Society of Surgical Oncology Focused Guideline recommend that patients with axillary nodal involvement after neoadjuvant systemic therapy should receive postmastectomy RT. Adjuvant RT should generally be administered to both the internal mammary nodes and the supraclavicular-axillary apical nodes in addition to the chest wall or reconstructed breast.[73] In a retrospective review of 150 patients (48% with stage IIIA or IIIB disease) treated with neoadjuvant chemotherapy followed by mastectomy at the MD Anderson Cancer Center, the 5- and 10-year rates of local-regional recurrence were both 27%. In patients with clinical stage III disease at diagnosis, the 5-year locoregional recurrence rate was 20%. In patients with clinical stage III disease who attained a pCR, the 5-year locoregional recurrence rate remained elevated at 33%. Increased pathologic tumor size and number of residual involved lymph nodes were associated with higher 5-year rates of locoregional recurrence.[74] Data from the NSABP B-18 and B-27 studies that randomized stage II and III patients to receive neoadjuvant or adjuvant chemotherapy prohibited the use of postmastectomy RT, and patients who underwent lumpectomy received breast RT only. In both studies, posttreatment pathologic lymph node involvement was a strong predictor of DFS and OS (p < .0001).[58]

There are no randomized studies evaluating the benefit of postmastectomy RT in patients treated with neoadjuvant chemotherapy. Huang and coworkers compared the outcome of 542

patients (73% with stage III disease) enrolled on several neoadjuvant chemotherapy trials who received mastectomy and RT with a cohort of 138 patients (46% with stage III disease) who received similar treatment but who did not receive RT. Patients who received postmastectomy RT had a lower 10-year rate of locoregional recurrence (8%) compared with those who did not receive RT (22%). RT also significantly improved the overall and cause-specific survival in patients with stage IIIB and IIIC disease and patients with four or more residual involved lymph nodes.[75] It is recommended that patients with baseline tumor characteristics that predict an increased risk of local-regional recurrence receive postmastectomy RT after neoadjuvant therapy regardless of clinical response.[23,76] This clinical practice requires the early involvement of the radiation oncologist in the multidisciplinary treatment planning of patients with locally advanced breast cancer.

Neoadjuvant Chemotherapy

Neoadjuvant chemotherapy for the treatment of breast cancer was introduced in the 1970s for patients with locally advanced disease. The terms *neoadjuvant, primary, preoperative,* and *induction* are all used to describe systemic chemotherapy given as initial therapy. Administering chemotherapy before other treatments has many theoretical advantages. Neoadjuvant chemotherapy can result in downstaging of tumors, thus increasing the rate of breast conserving surgery. In cases of more advanced disease, neoadjuvant chemotherapy can render inoperable tumors resectable. Other advantages of neoadjuvant therapy include the ability to obtain information on tumor response, which can be used to study the biologic effects of chemotherapy and determine long-term DFS and OS.[77]

The NCCN guidelines indicate a preference for neoadjuvant regimens that contain both anthracycline and taxane for patients with LABC.[23] Dieras and colleagues compared neoadjuvant AC and doxorubicin with paclitaxel (AP), and higher cCR and pCR rates were associated with AP (cCR 15%, pCR 16%) than AC chemotherapy (cCR 7%, pCR 10%). Breast conserving surgery was more frequent in the AP arm (58%) than the AC arm (45%; p value not provided).[78] Similar findings of a higher cCR and pCR were seen in the Anglo-Celtic Cooperative Oncology Group study that compared the combination of doxorubicin with docetaxel (AD) and AC. However, breast conserving surgery rates were equivalent (20%).[79] Steger and coworkers investigated whether six cycles of epirubicin and docetaxel (EC) resulted in a higher rate of pCR than three cycles of the same regimen in 262 breast cancer patients with stage II and III disease. Six cycles of EC compared with three cycles of EC resulted in a higher pCR (18.6% vs. 7.7%, respectively, p = .0045) and a trend toward a higher rate of breast conserving surgery.[80]

Several randomized studies have also investigated the sequential administration of taxanes after an anthracycline-based regimen and have shown higher rates of pCR. In the seminal NSABP B-27 study, which included 2344 patients with stages II and III breast cancer, all patients were assigned to receive four cycles of AC before surgery. Arm 1 received no further treatment, arm 2 received sequential neoadjuvant docetaxel for four cycles, and arm 3 received adjuvant docetaxel for four cycles. After surgery and RT for patients who underwent lumpectomy, all patients received tamoxifen regardless of age or ER or PR status. Eighty-six percent of patients who received neoadjuvant AC alone (arms 1 and 3) experienced a clinical response compared with 91% of patients who received neoadjuvant AC and sequential docetaxel chemotherapy ($p < .001$). The pCR rate increased from 13% to 26%. The improvement in pCR with the addition of docetaxel did not translate into an improvement in DFS or OS, although relapse-free survival favored the neoadjuvant docetaxel arm.[58] Similar findings were seen in the German Preoperative Adriamycin Docetaxel study, which randomized 904 patients with stage II and III breast cancer to receive four cycles of doxorubicin and docetaxel (AD) chemotherapy or four cycles of AC chemotherapy followed by four cycles of docetaxel. The arm that contained sequential administration of docetaxel resulted in a higher pCR (14.3%) compared with the combination arm (7%; $p < .001$).[81] The sequential administration of taxanes also provides benefit for patients who fail to respond to an anthracycline-based neoadjuvant regimen. In a study of 167 patients with LABC, responders to four cycles of neoadjuvant cyclophosphamide, vincristine, doxorubicin, and prednisolone (CVAP) chemotherapy were randomized to receive either four additional cycles of CVAP or four cycles of docetaxel; nonresponders were all treated with four cycles of docetaxel. Patients who received docetaxel showed significantly higher clinical and pathologic response rates and significantly better 3-year survival rates (97% vs. 84%, $p = .02$).[82]

The question of the potential benefit to the addition of antiangiogenic therapy to chemotherapy has also been addressed in clinical trials. In the GeparQuinto trial a total of 1948 women with HER2-negative, operable breast tumors were randomized to neoadjuvant treatment with epirubicin and cyclophosphamide followed by docetaxel, with or without concomitant bevacizumab (a vascular endothelial growth factor–directed antibody).[83] The pCR rate was 14.9% with epirubicin and cyclophosphamide followed by docetaxel and 18.4% with epirubicin and cyclophosphamide followed by docetaxel plus bevacizumab ($p = .04$). In parallel the NSABP B-40 trial assessed the efficacy of bevacizumab combined with docetaxel followed by treatment with AC in 1206 women with HER2-negative, operable tumors.[84] The addition of bevacizumab to the AC backbone significantly increased the pCR rate from 28.2% without bevacizumab to 34.5% with bevacizumab ($p = .02$). No survival advantaged was observed with the addition of bevacizumab to neoadjuvant chemotherapy in either trial.

The SWOG 0800 study was a phase II trial which accrued 215 patients with inflammatory or LABC.[17] In one arm of the study, patients were treated with nab-paclitaxel combined with bevacizumab followed by AC, which was compared with nab-paclitaxel followed or preceded by AC. The addition of bevacizumab significantly increased the pCR rate overall (36% vs. 21%; $p = .019$) and in triple-negative breast cancer (TNBC; 59% vs. 29%; $p = .014$) compared with chemotherapy alone, but not in hormone receptor–positive disease (24% vs. 18%; $p = .41$). A trend for improved event-free survival with bevacizumab was seen among patients with TNBC ($p = .06$). However, in light of the low magnitude of effect observed in these and other trials for increased pCR rates and the lack of improvement in DFS and OS with the addition of bevacizumab in the adjuvant setting, bevacizumab is not recommended for the neoadjuvant treatment of breast cancer.[85–87]

The clinical utility of the addition of non–cross-resistant chemotherapy agents to anthracycline-cyclophosphamide-taxane backbone has been studied by numerous trials.[84,88] For example, the previously described NSABP B-40 trial also assessed the efficacy of additional neoadjuvant therapy consisting of docetaxel, docetaxel plus capecitabine, or docetaxel plus gemcitabine for four cycles, with all regimens followed by treatment with AC for four cycles.[84] The addition of either capecitabine or gemcitabine to docetaxel therapy did not significantly increase the rate of pCR rates (30% and 32%, respectively, vs. 33%; $p = .69$).

Notwithstanding the lack of benefit of additional chemotherapy to unselected patients with nonmetastatic breast cancer the Cancer and Leukemia Group B (CALGB) 40603 trial showed increased pCR (i.e., absence of invasive disease in the breast or lymph nodes) in patients the operable TNBC treated with addition carboplatin.[89] The CALGB 40603 trial had a 2 × 2 factorial design trial in which 443 women with stage II to III TNBC received paclitaxel for 12 weeks, followed by AC for four cycles, and were randomly assigned to concurrent carboplatin once every 3 weeks for four cycles and/or bevacizumab once every 2 weeks for nine cycles. The addition of either carboplatin (60% vs. 44%; $p = .0018$) or bevacizumab (59% vs. 48%; $p = .0089$) significantly increased pCR in the breast alone, whereas only carboplatin (54% vs. 41%; $p = .0029$) significantly raised pCR in both breast and axilla. Likewise, in the GeparSixto, patients with stage II–III TNBC received neoadjuvant treatment with bevacizumab combined with weekly paclitaxel and pegylated liposomal doxorubicin ± carboplatin.[90] A total of 84 of 158 patients (53%, 95% CI 54.4–60.9) treated with carboplatin achieved a pCR compared with 58 of 157 (37%, 95% CI 29.4–44.5) without ($p = .005$). Grade 3 and 4 hematological and nonhematologic adverse events were more common among patients treated with carboplatin (i.e., neutropenia 65% vs. 27%, anemia 15% vs. one <1%, thrombocytopenia 14% vs. one <1%), and diarrhea 17% vs. 11%). These results along with the lack evidence of survival benefit with the addition of carboplatin to neoadjuvant treatment of breast cancer indicate that further studies are needed to establish the role of platinum agents for the treatment LABC.

Furthermore, caution should be taken when comparing the rates of cCR and pCR between neoadjuvant studies because of the different criteria used to define these outcomes.[51,91]

In recent meta-analysis of 12 randomized trials that pooled data from 11,955 patients undergoing neoadjuvant breast cancer treatment, absence of invasive disease from the breast and lymph nodes showed greater magnitude and strength of correlation with event-free survival (EFS) and OS than absence of invasive disease from the breast alone.[51] Patients with HER2-postive, hormone receptor–negative breast cancer treated with trastuzumab and TNBC who achieved a pCR (i.e., absence of invasive disease in the breast and lymph nodes) had significantly better outcomes; EFS: HR 0.15; OS: HR 0.08 and EFS: HR 0.24; OS: HR 0.16, respectively. In the overall HR-positive population the magnitude of correlation between pCR and EFS and OS was lower despite statistical significance (EFS: HR 0.49 and OS: HR 0.43). These results indicate that pCR indeed conveys prognostic information particularly in patients with aggressive tumors.

Neoadjuvant Anti-HER2-Based Therapy

Anti-HER2-targeted therapies have been integrated into the neoadjuvant setting in combination with chemotherapy for the treatment of patients with LABC. In the majority of studies, tumors were considered HER2-positive if the immunohistochemical (IHC) assay (DAKO) showed 3+ staining or there was gene amplification by fluorescent in situ hybridization (FISH). Because of concerns regarding the elevated rate of cardiac toxicity[92] associated with the combination of anthracyclines and trastuzumab, neoadjuvant studies have focused predominantly on combining trastuzumab with taxane-based regimens. Historically numerous small studies demonstrated promising increased efficacy of trastuzumab-based neoadjuvant chemotherapy regimens for patients with HER2-positive tumors.[63,64,93–96]

Indeed, in more recent larger randomized trials, efficacy of neoadjuvant treatment with trastuzumab-chemotherapy combinations was confirmed. The NeOAdjuvant Herceptin (NOAH) trial enrolled 235 women with HER2-positive LABC or IBC and randomized to neoadjuvant treatment with chemotherapy with or without trastuzumab. Trastuzumab was started with neoadjuvant chemotherapy and continued for a total of 1 year.[97] pCR rates were significantly higher in the trastuzumab-chemotherapy arm (38% vs. 19%; $p < .001$). After a median follow-up time of 5.4 years the 5-year EFS was 58% (95% CI 0.48–0.66) in patients in the chemotherapy/trastuzumab group and 43% (95% CI 0.34–0.52) in those in the chemotherapy alone group; the unadjusted HR was 0.64 (95% CI 0.44–0.93; $p = .016$). There was a trend toward an OS benefit with hazard ratio of 0.66 (95% CI 0.43–1.01; $p = .055$).[98] Of note, EFS survival was strongly correlated with pCR in patients given trastuzumab and only four cardiac events were considered to be drug related. These results indicate sustained benefit from neoadjuvant treatment with chemotherapy combined with trastuzumab in HER2-positive LABC.

More recently dual HER2-targeted therapy with trastuzumab combined with pertuzumab or lapatinib has shown increased pCR rates for the treatment of HER2-positive breast cancer compared with single-agent HER2 blockade with trastuzumab (Table 63.2). The NeoSphere trial was a randomized, phase II trial in which 417 women were randomly assigned to treatment with trastuzumab plus docetaxel every 3 weeks (arm A), or pertuzumab, trastuzumab plus docetaxel (arm B), or pertuzumab and trastuzumab (arm C) or pertuzumab plus docetaxel (group D).[52] Patients given pertuzumab and trastuzumab plus docetaxel (arm B) had a significantly improved pCR rate compared with those given trastuzumab plus docetaxel (group A) (45.8% vs. 29%; $p = .0141$). These data demonstrate the increased efficacy of dual HER2-targeted therapy combined with chemotherapy.

The TRYPHANEA trial was a phase II trial in which 235 women with operable, inflammatory, or LABC were randomized to neoadjuvant treatment with six neoadjuvant cycles of FEC combined with trastuzumab and pertuzumab followed by docetaxel combined with trastuzumab and pertuzumab (arm A), FEC followed by docetaxel combined with trastuzumab and pertuzumab (arm B); or docetaxel plus carboplatin combined with pertuzumab and trastuzumab (arm C).[65] The pCR rate was 61.6% (arm A), 57.3% (arm B), and 66.2% (arm C). During neoadjuvant treatment, two patients (2.7%; arm B) experienced symptomatic left ventricular systolic dysfunction and 11 patients (arm A: 4 [5.6%]; arm B: 4 [5.3%]; arm C: 3 [3.9%]) had declines in left ventricular ejection fraction of 10% points or more from baseline to less than 50%. The TRYPHAENA study was designed as a cardiac safety study and no indication of greater cardiac toxicity was evident with dual HER2 targeting with pertuzumab and trastuzumab.

Lapatinib, an oral tyrosine kinase inhibitor that targets the HER1 and HER2 oncoproteins, has also improved pCR rates when combined with trastuzumab. In the phase III NeoALTTO trial patients with HER2-positive tumors measuring more than 2 cm were randomized to neoadjuvant treatment with trastuzumab, lapatinib, or the combination given for 6 weeks, then added to paclitaxel for 12 weekly infusions.[99] A total of 154 patients received lapatinib, 149 trastuzumab, and 152 the combination. The pCR rate was significantly higher in the group given lapatinib and trastuzumab than in the group given trastuzumab alone (51% vs. 30%, $p = .0001$). There was no significant difference in pCR rate between the lapatinib and the trastuzumab groups. No major cardiac dysfunction was reported. The frequency of grade 3 diarrhea was higher with lapatinib (23%) and lapatinib plus trastuzumab (21%) than with trastuzumab (2%). After surgery, all patients received adjuvant treatment with FEC followed by 34 weeks of the same assigned anti-HER2 therapy. At median event follow-up time of 3.7 years, there was no significant EFS or OS difference between the groups.[100] Similarly, after 4.5 years of median follow-up, the adjuvant ALTTO study showed no difference in DFS with the combination of lapatinib and trastuzumab compared with trastuzumab alone. This phase III trial enrolled 8381 women who were randomized to adjuvant treatment with lapatinib combined with trastuzumab, lapatinib alone, trastuzumab followed by lapatinib or trastuzumab alone.[101]

Similarly, the NSABP B-41 was a phase III trial in which all 529 patients were treated with AC followed by weekly paclitaxel.[53] Concurrently with paclitaxel, patients were randomized to trastuzumab, lapatinib, or weekly trastuzumab plus lapatinib daily until surgery. Breast pCR rate was 53% in the trastuzumab group, 53% in the lapatinib group, and 62% in the combination group ($p = .095$). The most common grade 3 toxicity was diarrhea occurring in 2% of patients in the trastuzumab group, 20% in the lapatinib group, and 27% in the combination group ($p < .0001$). In the CALGB 40601 patients with HER2-positive stage II or III breast cancer had pCR rate of 56% when treated with 16 weeks of paclitaxel combined with lapatinib and trastuzumab compared with 46% when treated with trastuzumab and paclitaxel along ($p = .13$).[102]

Taken together these results suggest that neoadjuvant treatment of HER2-positive LABC should include dual HER2 blockade combined with chemotherapy to achieve the highest pCR. Lapatinib-based therapy is associated with higher rates of clinically important toxicities. However, current data do not demonstrate a survival benefit for the combination of trastuzumab with either pertuzumab or lapatinib.

Neoadjuvant Antiestrogen Therapy

The role of neoadjuvant antiestrogen therapy for patients with ER-positive and/or PR-positive cancers, large operable cancers, and LABC has been assessed in several studies, usually involving patients who were older and/or not felt to be candidates for neoadjuvant chemotherapy. Tamoxifen was first investigated as an alternative to surgery in elderly patients with large operable tumors with the goal of determining whether surgery could be avoided in a selected population of elderly patients. The results of the randomized studies of neoadjuvant tamoxifen alone versus surgery or neoadjuvant tamoxifen versus surgery plus tamoxifen conducted in elderly women not selected on ER-positive or PR-positive status are summarized in Table 63.3.[103–108] Local failure rates were higher in patients treated with tamoxifen alone, but none of the studies showed a benefit for surgery in decreasing the development of distant metastatic disease. These studies demonstrated that antiestrogen therapy is an effective alternative for elderly women with locally advanced disease who have a limited life expectancy and the results might have been more favorable for neoadjuvant endocrine therapy had the patient population been known to have tumors uniformly ER-positive.

Numerous trials have been reported evaluating different endocrine agents as preoperative therapy, but far fewer studies have

TABLE 63.2 Randomized Clinical Trials of Neoadjuvant Dual *HER2*-Targeted Therapies in Breast Cancer Including LABC

| Study | Treatment | Study Population | N | PCR RATE | | | | OVERALL SURVIVAL AT MEDIAN FOLLOW-UP | | | |
				Arm A	Arm B	Arm C	Arm D	Arm A	Arm B	Arm C	Arm D
TRYPHAENA[65]	A:[FEC]+ H + P × 3 → T + H + P x3 → S → H × 34 weeks vs. B: [FEC] ×3 → T + H + P ×3→ S → H × 34 weeks vs. C:T + C + H + P × 6 → S → 34 weeks	LABC (T2–3, N2 or N3, M0; T4a-c, any N, M0), or IBC (T4d, any N, M0) breast cancer, and a primary tumor size >2 cm	225	62%	57%	66%	NA	NR	NR	NR	NA
NeoSphere[52,189]	A:H + D × 4 → S → FEC × 3 + H × 40 weeks vs. B: H + P + D × 4→ S → FEC × 3 + H × 40 weeks vs. C: H + P × 4 → S → D × 4 + H × 12 weeks → FEC × 3 + H × 28 weeks vs. D:P + D × 4 → S→ FEC × 3 + H × 40 weeks	Breast tumors (T2–3, N0–1, M0), LABC (T2–3, N2–3, M0 or T4a–c, any N, M0), or inflammatory (T4d, any N, M0), Breast cancer, and primary tumors >2 cm	417	29%	46%	17%	24%	NR	NR	NR	NR
neoALLTO[99,100]	A: L + Tx ×12 →S → FEC × 3 → L × 34 weeks vs. B: T + Tx × 12 →S → FEC × 3 →T × 34 weeks vs. C: L + T + Tx × 12→S→ FEC × 3 → L + T × 34 weeks	Breast tumors >2 cm, M0	455	20%	28%	47%	NA	88%[a]	85%[a]	91%[a]	NA
NSABP B-41[53]	A:AC × 4 → Tx + T x 4→ S→ T × 52 weeks vs. B:AC × 4 → Tx + L ×4→ S→ T × 52 weeks vs. C: AC × 4 → Tx + T + L × 4→ S→ T × 52 weeks	Breast tumor > 2 cm; clinical stage T2 to T3, N0 to N2a, M0	529	49%	47%	60%	NA	NR	NR	NR	NA
CALGB 40601[102]	A: Tx + T × 16→S→ AC × 4 → T × 36 weeks vs. B: Tx + L × 16 → S → AC × 4 → T × 36 weeks vs. C: Tx + T + L × 16 → S → AC × 4 → T 36 weeks	Stage II or III, breast tumor ≥1 cm, M0	305	46%	32%	56%	NA	NR	NR	NR	NA

[a]At 3-year follow-up time (i.e., last women had been followed for at least 3 years).

AC, Doxorubicin, cyclophosphamide; *C,* carboplatin; *CALGB,* Cancer and Leukemia Group B; *FEC,* 5-fluorouracil, epirubicin, cyclophosphamide; *D,* docetaxel; *IBC,* inflammatory breast cancer; *LABC,* locally advanced breast cancer; *S,* surgery; *H,* trastuzumab; *L,* lapatinib; *NA,* not applicable; *NR,* not reported; *NSABP,* National Surgical Adjuvant Breast and Bowel Project; *P,* pertuzumab; *pCR,* pathologic complete response; *Tx,* paclitaxel.

TABLE 63.3	**Randomized Clinical Trials of Neoadjuvant Tamoxifen Versus Surgery or Surgery and Tamoxifen**					
Study	**Treatment**	**Study Population**	**Patient N**	**Local Failure (%)**	**Distant Failure (%)**
Gazet et al.[103]	Tamoxifen alone vs. surgery	Age >70 y, operable	200	25/38, p = ns	13/18, p = NS
Robertson et al.[104] and Kenny et al.[105]	Tamoxifen alone vs. wedge mastectomy	Age >70 y, operable	131	81/38, $p < 0.001$	24/19, p = NS
Fentiman et al.[106]	Tamoxifen alone vs. modified radical mastectomy	Age ≥70 y, operable	164	62/11, $p < 0.001$	23/20, p = NS
Mustacchi et al.[107]	Tamoxifen alone vs. surgery + tamoxifen	Age >70 y, operable	474	47/11, $p < 0.001$	22/25, p = NS
Bates et al.[108]	Tamoxifen alone vs. surgery + tamoxifen	Age >70 y, operable	381	35/21	Not provided

NS, Not significant.

been randomized. Several important questions that have been addressed include the following: (1) how does neoadjuvant chemotherapy compare with neoadjuvant antiestrogen therapy? (2) how does antiestrogen monotherapy compare with doublets of antiestrogen therapy in the neoadjuvant setting? and (3) how does antiestrogen therapy compare to antiestrogen therapy plus other targeted agents? Most of the trials that have been reported have been conducted in postmenopausal women with a much more limited experience in those with premenopausal disease.

A recent systematic review and meta-analysis of neoadjuvant endocrine therapy in patients with ER-positive disease puts these trial questions into perspective.[109] In this meta-analysis, 20 randomized clinical trials with a total of 3490 patients were analyzed. Three studies evaluated a comparison of neoadjuvant chemotherapy to neoadjuvant endocrine therapy. Endocrine therapy consisted of single-agent aromatase inhibitors if postmenopausal or a gonadotropin-releasing hormone (GNRH) agonist plus and aromatase inhibitor if premenopausal.[110–112] The chemotherapy regimens across the trials were somewhat different but all consisted of a taxane and anthracycline backbone. Although some patients were included had ER-negative tumors, the CR rate, radiologic response rate, pCR rate, and breast conservation rate were similar between those receiving endocrine therapy and chemotherapy. What was consistently different was significantly less toxicity, particularly grade 3–4 toxicity, in those receiving endocrine therapy.[110–112] These findings suggest that neoadjuvant endocrine therapy should be a consideration for women with ER-positive disease who are opposed to chemotherapy or are deemed not medically fit to receive it.

Another issue is whether one type of endocrine therapy is superior to another in the preoperative setting. Randomized trials have since been conducted comparing tamoxifen with the aromatase inhibitors in the neoadjuvant setting. Ellis and colleagues reported a randomized trial of tamoxifen versus letrozole in postmenopausal patients with hormone receptor–positive tumors who were not candidates for breast conserving surgery. Overall, 60% of patients treated with letrozole responded, and 48% underwent successful breast conserving surgery. In the tamoxifen arm, 41% of patients responded, and 36% underwent breast conserving surgery.[113] The superiority of letrozole over tamoxifen was also confirmed in the large BIG (Breast International Group) 1 to 98 adjuvant trial.[114] In the Immediate Preoperative Anastrozole, Tamoxifen or Combined with Tamoxifen (IMPACT) trial,

postmenopausal women with ER-positive operable and locally advanced potentially operable breast cancer were randomized to receive neoadjuvant tamoxifen, anastrozole, or a combination of the two agents for 3 months.[115] There was no significant difference in the approximately 36% clinical response rate among the three treatment arms. Patients who received anastrozole alone had a higher rate of breast conserving surgery (44%) compared with patients who received tamoxifen alone (31%).[115] The other important observation was that the combination of anastrozole and tamoxifen was no more effective than anastrozole alone mirroring the findings in the adjuvant ATAC trial (Arimidex, Tamoxifen, Alone or in Combination).[116] The Preoperative Arimidex Compared with Tamoxifen (PROACT) trial enrolled 451 postmenopausal women with ER-positive and/or PR-positive large operable and inoperable breast cancer. Patients could receive concomitant chemotherapy, and surgery was planned after 3 months.[117] The overall objective response rates were 39.5% with anastrozole versus 35.4% with tamoxifen. In patients who received neoadjuvant hormonal therapy alone, 43% and 31% treated with anastrozole and tamoxifen, respectively, were able to undergo breast conserving surgery.[117] In a premenopausal patient population, the STAGE study, compared tamoxifen and the GNRH agonist goserelin, to anastrozole plus goserelin.[118] Premenopausal women receiving anastrozole and 6 months of ovarian suppression with goserelin had a greater reduction in tumor size compared with those receiving tamoxifen and goserelin. These findings also are consistent with those reported in the recent SOFT and TEXT.[70] Although randomized studies have established the potential superiority of neoadjuvant aromatase inhibitor therapy for clinical response, the pCR rates for tamoxifen and the aromatase inhibitors are consistently low across all studies, ranging from 1% to 8%.

With expanded and more effective treatment options in the metastatic disease setting for patients with ER-positive breast cancer that include approved targeted agents like the CDK4/6 inhibitors palbociclib and ribociclib and the mechanistic target of rapamycin (mTOR) inhibitor, everolimus, the potential efficacy of neoadjuvant endocrine therapy may improve further.[119–121] These combinations are being evaluated in clinical trials in the neoadjuvant setting. Additionally, other CDK4/6 inhibitors, including abemaciclib, and PI3K inhibitors such as taselisib and buparsilib are in clinical trials in combination with endocrine agents in the neoadjuvant setting. Patient selection is ultimately important in deciding who is appropriate for an approach that includes neoadjuvant endocrine therapy. As better molecular tools become available that allow for selection of patients who are the optimal candidates for a neoadjuvant endocrine approach, clinical outcomes may be enhanced.

Assessment of Response to Neoadjuvant Chemotherapy

Accurate assessment of tumor response is a critical component of neoadjuvant therapy. Because clinical assessment of response to chemotherapy is sometimes inaccurate and subject to substantial interobserver variability, the role of imaging modalities such as mammography, ultrasonography, and breast MRI has been explored.[122–125] Herrada and colleagues found that the combination of physical examination and mammography increased the accuracy of the measurement of tumor dimensions.[124] Other authors have found that for the measurement of the primary tumor, ultrasonography is more accurate than either clinical examination or mammography alone.[123] Kuerer and colleagues studied the role of physical examination and ultrasonography in assessing axillary lymph node status in patients with locally advanced breast cancer treated with neoadjuvant chemotherapy.[126] The authors found that axillary sonography was more sensitive than physical examination in detecting axillary metastases (62% vs. 45%, $p = .012$). Small studies have reported an additional benefit of breast MRI for assessing response to neoadjuvant chemotherapy.[127–130] Yeh and coworkers evaluated 41 women with stage II and III breast cancer who received neoadjuvant chemotherapy. All underwent physical examination, ultrasound, mammography, and breast MRI before and after each cycle of treatment, and the agreement rates of clinical response were 32%, 48%, and 55%, respectively, for mammography, ultrasound, and breast MRI compared with clinical examination. The agreement rates of pathologic response were 19%, 26%, 35%, and 71% for clinical examination, mammogram, ultrasound, and MRI, respectively, compared with the gold standard, pathologic evaluation.[128] In addition, correlation between MRI accuracy measures and response to therapy are confounded by type of breast cancer and type of neoadjuvant therapy. For instance, high false-negative rates have been reported in HER2-negative patients, treated with bevacizumab.[131] ^{18}F-FDG PET-CT has also been studied as a tool of early prediction of response to neoadjuvant therapy in aggressive types of breast cancer (i.e., HER2-positive and TNBC) in small nonrandomized studies.[132,133] In the phase II AVATAXHER trial, 142 women with HER2-positive breast cancer received neoadjuvant docetaxel plus trastuzumab. Before the first and second cycles, ^{18}F-FDG PET-CT standardized uptake was measured and correlated with pCR. Patients who were predicted to be responders on PET–CT (i.e., variation in maximum standard uptake value of 70% or higher) continued to receive standard therapy.[134] Predicted nonresponders were randomly assigned to receive four cycles of docetaxel and trastuzumab plus bevacizumab (Arm A) or continue on docetaxel plus trastuzumab alone (arm B).[135] A total of 73 patients were predicted nonresponders and were assigned to arm A ($n = 48$) and arm B ($n = 25$). pCR were observed in 54% of PET responder and 44% of patients assigned to arm A. Among the 25 patients assigned to arm B, the pCR rate was 24%. Findings from this trial suggest that ^{18}F-FDG PET/CT may eventually help define appropriate neoadjuvant therapy in selected patients with breast cancer.

Predictors of Response to Neoadjuvant Therapy

Multiple studies have evaluated factors that may be predictive of a response to neoadjuvant chemotherapy or hormonal therapy. Smaller tumor size, poorly differentiated and hormone receptor–negative tumors are significantly more likely to respond to neoadjuvant chemotherapy than larger, well-differentiated, and hormone receptor–positive tumors.[136,137] TNBC (i.e., ER-, PR-, and HER2-negative status) is also a strong predictor for response to neoadjuvant therapy.[138] In an MD Anderson Cancer Center report of 1118 patients receiving neoadjuvant chemotherapy that included locally advanced and inflammatory breast cancers, patients with TNBC had significantly higher pCR rates (22%) than patients without TNBC (11%; $p = .034$).[139] In patients receiving neoadjuvant hormonal therapy, the degree of ER expression, HER2 status, and ki67 proliferation index scores have shown correlation with clinical response.[113,115] Whole genome analysis through next-generation sequencing (NGS) has allowed for identification of signatures with significant correlation with pCR in the setting of neoadjuvant breast cancer treatment. For example, in a study of 89 patients with LABC treated with neoadjuvant paclitaxel and doxorubicin, 24 genes that related to ER expression, proliferation, and immune regulation obtained using tumor DNA microarrays were associated with pCR.[140] Chang and colleagues evaluated 24 patients with LABC treated with neoadjuvant docetaxel chemotherapy and showed that differential expression of 92 genes correlated with response to treatment ($p = .001$).[141] Furthermore, NGS has also allowed for classification of breast cancer into intrinsic subtypes (i.e., luminal, basal-like, normal-like, and HER2-positive) based on expression profiles and were shown to have different prognoses.[142–144] In one series of 107 patients, 65 with stage III breast cancer, treatment consisted of neoadjuvant AC.[138] Tumors had the following IHC-based profile: 34 were basal-like, 11 were HER2 positive/ER negative, and 62 were luminal. pCR occurred in 36% of HER2-positive/ER-negative, 27% of basal-like, and 7% of luminal subtypes ($p = .01$). Despite initial chemosensitivity, patients with the basal-like and HER2-positive/ER-negative subtypes had worse distant DFS ($p = .04$) and OS ($p = .02$) than those with the luminal subtypes, indicating that correlations between pCR and improved outcomes are more likely to be tumor-type dependent. Greater chemosensitivity for basal-like and HER2-positive has also been reported by others.[145] Several small studies have shown significant correlation between expression of targeted and nontargeted gene signatures and increased pCR rates in realm of neoadjuvant treatment of breast cancer.[146–148] Nonetheless, more studies are needed to better define and clinical utility of genomic assays in tailoring treatment of LABC.

Breast Conserving Surgery

Patients with LABC can be poor candidates for operative intervention. Neoadjuvant chemotherapy was first used in LABC to make them operable candidates. Then the question became: "Can these patients eventually become candidates for breast conservation?" Many patients with LABC require the use of neoadjuvant chemotherapy to reduce the tumor burden with the hope of making them a breast conservation candidate. There have been several well-conducted randomized large trials that have demonstrated no difference in DFS or OS between neoadjuvant and adjuvant therapy. In addition, several trials have addressed the use of neoadjuvant and the subsequent breast conservation rate. The NSABP B-18 opened in 1988 and accrued 1523 patients at the time of its closure in 1993. Thirteen percent of patients in this study had tumors greater than 4.1 cm. Patients were randomized to receive four cycles of AC before surgery or four cycles of AC postsurgery. There was a statistically significant increase in breast conservation in patients who had neoadjuvant therapy implying that the neoadjuvant approach allowed more patients to undergo conservation and there was no statistically significant difference in DFS or OS.[54] A group at the MD Anderson Cancer Center looked at a set of 143 patients with LABC who were treated with neoadjuvant therapy and either a partial or complete clinical response. All patients had a mastectomy but they determined that 23% of these patients would have been conservation candidates.[149] The EORTC 10902 demonstrated a 23% breast conservation rate in their group of patients who were initially felt to be mastectomy candidates who underwent neoadjuvant therapy with FEC. However, it should be noted that those patients who did undergo breast conservation had a worse OS compared with those patients who were initially candidates for breast conservation implying a worse tumor biology.[55]

Neoadjuvant therapy also can reduce the axillary tumor burden, often making an axillary dissection unnecessary. It has also been shown that obtaining a pCR after neoadjuvant therapy imparts an improved outcome. Other studies have demonstrated similar results and have demonstrated an increased rate of breast conservation without significantly increasing the rate of ipsilateral tumor recurrence.[52,150-152]

The question of whether breast conservation in this group of LABC leads to a higher ipsilateral breast cancer recurrence rate has been addressed in many studies. Several studies in patients with large or LABC have shown acceptable local control in breast conserving surgery.[50,54,152] However, other large randomized trials have demonstrated a nonsignificant increase in breast recurrence in the conservation group.[54,55] In a recent meta-analysis of 14 trials with 5500 patients neoadjuvant therapy was found to increase local regional recurrence rates but there was no significant increase in studies where surgery was performed for all patients even after a complete clinical response reassuring one that breast conservation is safe in this patient population under certain clinical scenarios.[153] Patient selection is important and accurate preoperative imaging in needed to determine to which could conservation be offered.

Management of the Axilla: Historical Perspective and Current Recommendations

The management of patients with invasive breast cancer is constantly changing and can be challenging for physicians to stay up to date with all the new information. Tumor characteristics and molecular markers are becoming more important in treatment decisions but the status of the axilla remains one of the strongest prognostic indicators for patients with early-stage breast cancer. Over the past 25 years, there has been a dramatic change in the approach to the axilla. The routine use of a level I and II axillary lymph node dissection has now been replaced by sentinel node biopsy (SNB) for node-negative patients and even a subset of node-positive patients can now avoid the sequela of an axillary lymph node dissection. This change in management is likely related to advances in radiology, surgical technique, systemic

therapy, and radiotherapy. It is imperative for physicians to understand how to approach the axilla in early-stage breast cancer. To better understand how to best approach the axilla, it is important to understand how we have arrived at our current management strategies.

The incidence of axillary nodal positivity is dependent on tumor factors such as size, histologic type and grade, presence of lymphovascular invasion, and location. Studies have demonstrated that as the size and grade of the tumor increases, the risk of nodal positivity increases.[154,155]

Advances in imaging particularly the use of axillary ultrasound has led to improved clinical staging and identified node-positive patients before surgery.[156] This is an improvement over physical examination alone, which has notoriously been unreliable and the positive predictive value of physical examination alone has varied from 61% to 84% and the probability of no involvement after a normal examination has been 50% to 60%.[157]

Until the mid-1990s an axillary lymph node dissection was the standard of care for early-stage breast cancer and required removal of the level I and level II axillary lymph nodes. Removal of the axillary contents is not without morbidity and may result in lymphedema, axillary web syndrome, sensory morbidity, shoulder dysfunction, and infection.[158]

Management of the Axilla in Node-Negative Patients

The concept of a sentinel lymph node for patients with early-stage breast cancer was introduced in the early 1990s.[159-161] An SNB allows for accurate assessment of the nodal status, provides critical information for staging, and can help guide additional therapies. There have been several multicenter lymphatic trials that have confirmed the feasibility of a SNB as a staging procedure, and these trials have demonstrated high identification rates and low false-negative rates; this led to a change in the standard of care for node-negative patients. The largest of these studies were the American College of Surgeons Oncology Group (ACOSOG) Z010 and NSABP B-32.[162,163] The ACOSOG Z010 study enrolled 5210 patients who underwent an SNB, and if the SN was negative, no further axillary surgery was performed. The study reported a high SNB identification rate of 98.7% and an estimated false-negative rate of 0.3%. NSABP B-32 was a randomized study in which 5611 clinically node-negative patients were randomized to SNB followed by axillary node dissection (ALND) or SN alone if the SN was tumor free. The study reported a SNB identification rate of 97.1% and a false-negative rate of 9.8%, and there was no significant difference between the two groups with respect to OS, DFS, and regional control with a mean follow-up of 95.6 months. The majority of patients in this study received both systemic therapy and RT. The local recurrence rates were <1% in both arms despite a 10% false-negative rate in the ALND arm. There was no difference in local or regional recurrence or DFS and OS. Other studies have demonstrated similar findings and have shown that a SNB is a safe, less morbid procedure and has a low risk of nodal recurrences and therefore an ALND is no longer indicated.[164,165] A meta-analysis of 48 studies which looked at SNB-negative patients who did not have an ALND, the overall axillary recurrence rate was 0.3%—much lower than the published false-negative rate of SNB, implying that not all nodal positivity will be clinically relevant.[166] An SNB alone is also associated with decreased morbidity and an improvement in quality of life. The ALMANAC trial (Axillary Lymphatic Mapping Against Nodal

Axillary Clearance) addressed the issues of morbidity and quality of life in this trial. Women who had SN alone had significantly less lymphedema and sensory loss compared with those in the ALND group.[165] In light of all this information, ASCO guidelines, NCCN guidelines, and the St. Gallen Consensus group have acknowledged SNB alone as an acceptable treatment strategy for patients with a negative SN.[23,167,168]

Management of the Axilla in Node-Positive Patients

The role of axillary lymph node dissection in node-positive patients has come into question over the past decade. The concept of avoiding axillary surgery in node-positive patients is not new but one that has recently gained traction. The NSABP B-04 study was the first to look at the role of axillary surgery when women were randomized to total mastectomy versus total mastectomy with axillary lymph node dissection or axillary RT.[169] Although there was no difference is survival seen, critics found many faults with the study and its conclusions were overlooked and results of the study were not practice changing. The emergence of the SNB has reignited the debate and raised question as to the need for axillary lymph node dissection.

The use of SNB has led to the increase in detection of micrometastases, tumor deposit between 0.2 mm and less than 2 mm. In the early sentinel node (SN) trials, it was demonstrated that the use of serial sectioning of the SN and evaluation with both hematoxylin and eosin staining and cytokeratin IHC led to an increase in the detection of axillary metastasis in the SN. Giuliano and coworkers demonstrated a 42% axillary metastases rate in the SNB group versus 29% in the ALND group and this difference was largely related to the presence of micrometastases in the SN.[170] At the time of that publication, it was felt that these micrometastases were significant and the presence of these cells would impart a survival disadvantage to these patients. Since then we have learned much about the significance of micrometastases and how they affect survival and surgical management.

Several studies have now been published that evaluate the impact of micrometastases in the SN. The ACOSOG Z10 study was a prospective observational trial that enrolled 5210 clinical T1/T2 N0 patients.[162] All patients underwent a SNB; 24% were found to have a positive SN and underwent ALND. For the remainder of the patients who were found to be SN negative on hematoxylin and eosin staining, 10.5% of patients were found to have micrometastases based evaluation with immunohistochemistry at a central laboratory, and this information was blinded to both the physician and the patient. At a median follow-up of 6.3 years, there was no difference in DFS or OS between the node-negative patients and those with micrometastases. The NSABP B-32 study, which also examined the prognostic significance of IHC detected metastases, came up with slightly different findings. With 5 years of follow-up, the presence of micrometastases did impart a small but statistically significant decrease in both DFS and OS, but this decrease did not persist at 10 years of follow-up in OS.[163] The International Breast Cancer Study Group 23-01 study randomized 934 clinical T1/T2N0 patients with a micrometastases identified in the SNB to SNB alone versus ALND.[171] The majority of patients were postmenopausal and had favorable tumors with only 28% grade 3 tumors, and more than 80% were ER positive. There was no significant difference in DFS, OS, or axillary recurrence between ALND and SNB alone. Other groups have shown similar results with no differences in DFS or OS in

patients with low burden of disease in the SN defined as micrometastases who did not undergo completion ALND.[172] Avoiding ALND in patients with micrometastases in the SN is reasonable and the presence of micrometastases does not affect recurrence or OS. The use of IHC to find metastases is not warranted and should not be routinely used in the workup of a SN.

Because many of the decisions regarding adjuvant systemic or RT are no longer based on the number of positive axillary nodes, the need for an axillary dissection in SN-positive patients, or those with macrometastases, has come into question. There have been three recent trials that have tried to address this question. The ACOSOG Z11, the After Mapping of the Axilla: Radiotherapy or Surgery (AMAROS), and the National Cancer Institute of Canada Clinical Trials Group MA.20 trial all have addressed the issue of axillary management in the presence of nodal metastases.[173–175] The ACOSOG Z11 study was designed to address the question of the need for ALND in patients with no more than two positive SN. Women with clinical T1/T2 N0 with one or two positive SNs were randomized to either ALND or observation. The majority of patients in this study had macrometastases in the SN, but it should be pointed out that the majority of patients also had both systemic therapy and RT. All patients underwent breast conservation with whole breast radiation with some overlap of the axilla but were not supposed to have axillary specific RT. There was no difference in DFS or OS between the groups after a median follow-up of 6.3 years, and the axillary recurrence rates were very low in both treatment arms. There was a 27% incidence of additional nodal positivity in the ALND arm, and because this was a randomized study, it is reasonable to presume that the SNB only arm had a similar tumor burden in the axilla, which did not impart a survival disadvantage. Some have argued that the RT fields covered the axilla, so it was the added RT improved regional control.[173] Jagsi and colleagues performed a retrospective review of port films of 27% of the ALND group and 31% of the SN group. The majority of patients (81%) received tangent only RT, and 15% received supraclavicular irradiation. There was no difference between the two groups in the use of nodal RT or high tangents. Overall there was no significant difference between treatment arms in the use of protocol-prohibited nodal fields. It should also be noted that 11% of patients received no RT. Therefore with these data, it is unlikely that nodal irradiation affected the outcome in the ACOSOG Z11 study.[176] Although this study has been criticized by many for not meeting its target accrual, it has changed the practice pattern for women who meet the studies inclusion criteria. Several institutions have reported that 70% to 85% of their SN-positive patients met the Z11 criteria and were spared ALND.[177–179]

The AMAROS trial was designed to evaluate axillary RT as an alternative to surgery. Clinically node-negative patients with tumors less than 3 cm and a positive SN were randomized to either completion ALND or axillary RT. At a median follow-up of 6.1 years, the axillary recurrence rate in the ALND group was 0.54% compared with 1.03% in the RT arm. Although the noninferiority test was underpowered due to the low event rate, there were still no significant differences observed.[174] The majority of patients in this study had macrometastases and the morbidity in the RT arm was lower than the ALND arm. Not all patients in this study had breast conservation as in the ACOSOG Z11 study. To address concerns that the additional information gained in an ALND may affect treatment options, this group also looked at whether the additional information gained in the

ALND group influenced adjuvant therapy recommendations. In the first 2000 women enrolled in the study, the extent of nodal involvement was not significantly associated with the use of systemic therapy. The age of the patient, tumor grade, Multifocality, and the size of SN metastases were associated with the use of systemic therapy, implying that it is the information from the SN that is important, not the number of positive axillary lymph node.[180]

Finally, the MA.20 study evaluated the impact of nodal RT to patients undergoing ALND. Randomization was between RT with standard breast tangents and breast tangents plus regional nodal RT including the supraclavicular, infraclavicular, and internal mammary chains. Axillary fields were added in those patients with more than four positive nodes or those women who had less than 10 axillary nodes removed. Inclusion criteria included any node-positive patient or node-negative patients with tumors greater than 2 cm, fewer than 10 axillary LNs removed, and grade 3 histology, ER-negative, or lymphovascular invasion. At a median follow-up of 62 months, there was an absolute benefit of 2.3% in locoregional recurrence in the nodal RT group, and this led to a significant 5-year DFS benefit. There was a trend toward improved 5-year OS in the regional RT group, but it was noted that there was more morbidity in this group.[181]

Many studies have now shown us that despite leaving known axillary disease behind based on the axillary nodal positivity rate which ranges from 27% to 40%, the nodal recurrence rate in node-positive patients who do not undergo ALND is quite low and ranges from 0.9% to 15% and there was no significant difference in OS. This implies that not all nodal metastases are significant, and many will not progress or metastasize.[174,176,181]

The management of the axilla in node-positive patients has dramatically evolved since the mid-2000s. It is now accepted that completion ALND can be avoided in patients with micrometastatic disease in both breast conservation and mastectomy patients. Even before the published results of ACOSOG Z11, many surgeons in the United States were already abandoning ALND for low-risk node-positive patients.[182] For patients that fit the ACOSOG Z11 criteria ALND can be avoided in patients with one or two positive nodes who are undergoing breast conservation. It is difficult to know whether patients undergoing mastectomy can avoid ALND because the ACOSOG Z11 study did not include patients undergoing mastectomy. The AMAROS trial did include some patients undergoing mastectomy, but further study is needed to determine whether these patients can avoid ALND.

Management of the Axilla in Patients Undergoing Neoadjuvant Therapy

Traditionally neoadjuvant chemotherapy has been used in patients with locally advanced breast cancer, inflammatory cancer, and large cancers that required downsizing for breast conservation. More recently, however, early-stage breast cancer patients with smaller high-risk tumors with aggressive features are undergoing neoadjuvant therapy. Multiple neoadjuvant trials have demonstrated the ability to downstage the size of the primary tumor and can convert a node-positive patient to a node-negative patient. Despite the ability to downstage the tumor, there has been no benefit in DFS or OS in patients undergoing neoadjuvant therapy.[151,152,183] The role and timing of SNB in patients undergoing neoadjuvant chemotherapy has been a source of debate. If a SNB is done before neoadjuvant chemotherapy, then the results

can be adapted to the TNM staging system. This information can help direct the radiation oncologist in terms of need for postmastectomy RT and the plastic surgeon who may not offer the patient immediate reconstruction in the setting of postmastectomy RT. However, others would argue that an SNB done after neoadjuvant therapy may allow the patient to avoid undergoing an ALND. There have been multiple neoadjuvant trials looking at the identification rate of the SN and the false-negative rate of the SN after chemotherapy. Two meta-analyses found that the SN identification rate in clinically node-negative patients undergoing neoadjuvant therapy was 90% with a false-negative rate between 8.4% and 12%.[184,185] For those patients who were found to be node-positive before neoadjuvant therapy, the surgical recommendation was for an ALND after therapy was completed. Recently, this practice has been questioned because of improvements in nodal pCR, particularly for patients with triple-negative and HER2-positive tumors.

Several published trials have reported an acceptable false-negative rate of SNB for those node-positive patients who underwent neoadjuvant chemotherapy. The false-negative rate was 8% to 14%.[186-188] The ACOSOG Z1071 enrolled patients with T1–4, N1–2 who had biopsy-proven axillary metastasis and after neoadjuvant chemotherapy a SNB followed by ALND was performed. A total of 689 patients were evaluated. At least one SN was identified in 92.7% of patients, and the false-negative rate was 12.6% in those patients with clinical N1 disease. The false-negative rate dropped to 10.8% when dual tracer was used compared with 20.3% when a single agent was used. If three SN were identified, the false-negative rate dropped to 9.1%. If the known positive node that had been clipped before neoadjuvant chemotherapy was removed, the false-negative rate dropped to 6.8%. The prespecified end point in the study was a false-negative rate less than 10%, which was not met; however, this study did identify factors that would decrease the false-negative rate to an acceptable rate of less than 10%. These factors include the use of dual tracer as well as at least three SN identified.[186]

The SENTINA (SENTinel NeoAdjuvant) trial had similar goals to the ACOSOG Z1071 but included both clinical N0 and N1 disease. This was a prospective four-arm study that included 1737 patients from multiple institutions. The study concluded that a SNB is highly reliable before chemotherapy, but after neoadjuvant chemotherapy, there is a lower SN identification rate and higher false-negative rate. Overall the false-negative rate was 14.2%, but this decreased to 7.3% if more than three SNs were identified.[187] The Canadian Sentinel Node Biopsy Following Neo-Adjuvant Chemotherapy in Biopsy Proven Node Positive Breast Cancer (SN FNAC) had similar findings.[188] The ASCO Guidelines 2014 state that patients who have received neoadjuvant chemotherapy may be offered SNB. The NCCN guidelines also list this as an option for patients undergoing neoadjuvant chemotherapy.

The management of the axilla in early-stage cancer has gone through an evolution over the past 20 years from axillary dissection to SNB alone for node-negative patients, and the criteria to avoid ALND in SN-positive patients continues to evolve. We are continuing to strive to optimize and personalize treatment choices for patients with early-stage breast cancer, and as our treatment strategies continue to improve, along with our understanding of tumor biology, the microenvironment of the tumor, and genomics, there is no doubt that what is standard of care today will continue to evolve and improve outcomes for our patients with early-stage breast cancer.

Treatment Summary

LABC remains a difficult clinical problem, and even with optimal multidisciplinary treatment, breast cancer recurrence will occur in many patients. Current data support initiation of treatment with neoadjuvant systemic therapy because it increases the rate of breast conserving surgery and may render LABC resectable. Completion of all anthracycline-taxane-based chemotherapy with or without anti-HER2 therapy in the neoadjuvant setting increases the chance of a pCR and, when followed by surgical resection and consolidation RT, is a safe, effective, and well-tolerated approach. Furthermore, patients with HER2-positive tumors should be treated with dual HER2 blockade with trastuzumab (i.e., pertuzumab or lapatinib) combined with chemotherapy. Well-conducted randomized clinical trials consistently demonstrate increased pCR rates and favorable toxicity profile with this strategy. Tumors that respond to neoadjuvant treatment can be treated with lumpectomy or mastectomy and RT. Premenopausal patients with ER-positive and/or PR-positive LABC should be considered for adjuvant treatment with ovarian suppression combined with antiestrogen therapy (i.e., tamoxifen vs. aromatase inhibitor) for 5 years. Postmenopausal women are usually treated for 5 years with an aromatase inhibitor. The optimal duration of adjuvant endocrine therapy is covered elsewhere. Patients whose tumors do not respond to either an anthracycline-based regimen or a taxane can immediately undergo mastectomy if they have operable tumors. Patients with inoperable tumors should receive primary RT as a third-line approach to render the tumor resectable.

Patients in whom such treatment renders the tumor resectable would undergo surgery and should receive adjuvant hormonal therapy if indicated. Despite these advances, the need for better treatments remains, and all patients with LABC should be encouraged to participated in clinical trials.

Selected References

51. Cortazar P, Zhang L, Untch M, et al. Pathological complete response and long-term clinical benefit in breast cancer: the CTNeoBC pooled analysis. *Lancet.* 2014;384:164-172.
58. Rastogi P, Anderson SJ, Bear HD, et al. Preoperative chemotherapy: updates of National Surgical Adjuvant Breast and Bowel Project Protocols B-18 and B-27. *J Clin Oncol.* 2008;26:778-785.
65. Schneeweiss A, Chia S, Hickish T, et al. Pertuzumab plus trastuzumab in combination with standard neoadjuvant anthracycline-containing and anthracycline-free chemotherapy regimens in patients with HER2-positive early breast cancer: a randomized phase II cardiac safety study (TRYPHAENA). *Ann Oncol.* 2013;24:2278-2284.
109. Spring LM, Gupta A, Reynolds KL, et al. Neoadjuvant endocrine therapy for estrogen receptor-positive breast cancer: a systematic review and meta-analysis. *JAMA Oncol.* 2016;2:1477-1486.
173. Giuliano AE, McCall L, Beitsch P, et al. Locoregional recurrence after sentinel lymph node dissection with or without axillary dissection in patients with sentinel lymph node metastases: the American College of Surgeons Oncology Group Z0011 randomized trial. *Ann Surg.* 2010;252:426-432, discussion 432-3.

A full reference list is available online at ExpertConsult.com.

64

Inflammatory Breast Cancer

GEORGE SOMLO AND VERONICA JONES

Introduction and Historical Backdrop

Inflammatory breast cancer (IBC) was first described in 1814 by Sir Charles Bell as a "purple color on the skin over the tumor accompanied by shooting pains."[1] Thomas Bryant described the dermal lymphatic invasion as the cause for the inflammatory changes of the skin in 1887.[2] IBC was referred to as *mastitis carcinomatosa*,[3] *carcinoma mastoids,* and *acute carcinoma of the breast* before arriving at its current identifier *inflammatory breast cancer* coined by Lee and Tannenbaum in 1924.[4] Although the clinical presentation is what remains the cornerstone of diagnosis, what truly defines this disease as a distinct clinicopathologic entity is much more diverse and includes the explosive clinical course, a still not well-defined molecular profile, its response to current therapies, and ultimately its prognosis. In this chapter, we explore the characteristics unique to IBC and ways to capitalize on what we know about this disease to optimize treatment.

Epidemiology

IBC comprises 2.5% of all breast cancers and 7% of all breast cancer–related deaths in the United States. It is estimated that 6231 people will be diagnosed with IBC this year alone and 2862 will die of the disease.[5] The incidence of IBC has been reported to be higher in other countries, ranging from 5% in a series from Turkey to 17% of breast cancers diagnosed in a teaching hospital in Nigeria.[3] With a stricter definition of clinical criteria (at least two of the three features of erythema, edema, and peau d'orange) the true prevalence in regions such as North Africa (in Tunisia in particular), are likely to be lower than previously reported, at 5% to 7% versus more than 50%.[6] The mortality from IBC has decreased significantly over the past 2 decades with the 2-year disease free survival ranging from 62% for women diagnosed between 1990 and 1995, to 76% for women diagnosed between 2006 and 2010; but the median survival with IBC in that time period was only 2.9 years and remained inferior in comparison to 6.4 years for women presenting with locally advanced breast cancer.[6,7] The improvements for women with IBC are largely due to advances in chemotherapy; developments in targeted therapy, primarily human epidermal growth factor (HER2); targeted therapy; and the general acceptance of trimodality (systemic therapy, surgery, and radiation) therapy. Rueth and coworkers showed 5-year survival to be 55% in nonmetastatic IBC patients treated with trimodality therapy compared with 42.9% in those treated with chemotherapy and surgery and 40.7% in those treated with surgery and radiotherapy only (Fig. 64.1).[8] At the time of initial diagnosis, however, more than 30% of patients have

metastatic disease, most of whom will succumb to their disease.[9] Despite all improvements, the median overall survival for newly diagnosed IBC is less than 4 years, and 5-year survival rate is approximately 30%, although in previous decades IBC was considered an overwhelmingly fatal disease.[10,11]

Differences exist among races in the incidence and survival rates in IBC. It is more prevalent in African American, Hispanic American/Latina, and American Indian/Alaskan women than in Caucasian and Asian women. IBC has an earlier age of onset than noninflammatory breast cancer (non-IBC) with the majority of women being diagnosed between the ages of 40 and 59 years of age.[11] The age of onset is earliest in Hispanic American/Latina women with a mean age at diagnosis of 50.5 years compared with 55.2 in African American women and 58.1 in Caucasian women.[12] The median survival for Caucasian women is 47.6 months compared with 33.2 months in African American women and 43.1 months in Hispanic American women. Asian American women have the highest median survival of 49.7 months. The lowest median survival is found in American Indian/Alaskan women at 24.8 months.[13]

Besides race, other predictors of poor prognosis exist, including being single, having grade 3 tumors, having a higher stage at diagnosis, not receiving radiation treatment, undergoing a partial mastectomy, and obesity. Higher education seems to have been associated with lower incidence of estrogen receptor (ER) and progesterone receptor (PR) positive IBC. Older age at pregnancy has not been consistently linked to IBC in hormone receptor (HR)-negative breast cancer; however, many series show a higher proportion of IBC among pregnant and lactating women.[12] Additionally, premenopausal status has not been linked to IBC despite it being diagnosed more often in younger women than non-IBC.[3]

Diagnosis

Clinical Presentation

There are currently no known molecular or pathologic characteristics for a definitive diagnosis of IBC, and as such, IBC remains a clinical diagnosis. The current diagnostic definition as put forth by the American Joint Committee on Cancer is "a clinical-pathologic entity characterized by diffuse erythema and edema (peau d'orange) involving a third or more of the breast."[14] Physical examination may also reveal skin thickening and occasionally an underlying mass, although not consistently. IBC is categorized by the American Joint Committee on Cancer as a cT4d tumor and qualifies as at least a clinical stage III tumor. This definition is

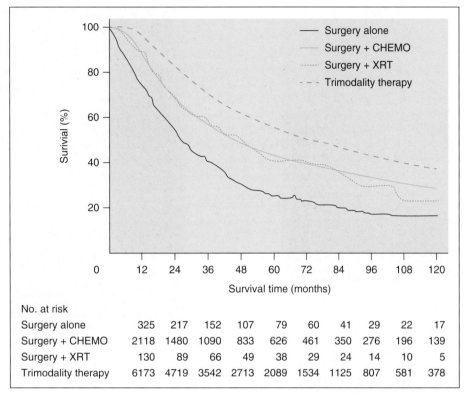

• Fig. 64.1 Survival curves associated with treatments for inflammatory breast cancer. Trimodality therapy has improved overall survival compared with other therapies alone or in combination.[8] *CHEMO,* Chemotherapy; *XRT,* radiation therapy. (Reprinted with permission from Rueth NM, Lin HY, Bedrosian I, et al. Underuse of trimodality treatment affects survival for patients with inflammatory breast cancer: an analysis of treatment and survival trends from the National Cancer Database. *J Clin Oncol.* 2014;32:2018-24.)

based primarily on the description put forth by Haagensen in 1971.[15] Patients with IBC complain of an abrupt onset of symptoms including pain, swelling, and redness of the breast that typically develops in less than 3 months (Fig. 64.2). The differential diagnosis includes mastitis with or without abscess, radiation change, locally advanced breast cancer, and primary breast lymphoma or other malignancies. Tissue diagnosis is necessary to document invasive carcinoma. History and physical examination are paramount in distinguishing this diagnosis from clinical mimickers. As a practical matter, because most IBC cases are first seen by health care providers not necessarily familiar with IBC, the absence of complete response to a trial of antibiotic therapy should heighten the clinician's suspicion of IBC and prompt further investigation.

Imaging

Diagnostic techniques used in IBC include mammography, ultrasonography, magnetic resonance imaging (MRI), and positron emission tomography with computed tomography (PET/CT). A retrospective review of 142 women diagnosed with IBC showed common findings seen on each modality.[16] The most common signs on mammography include thickening of the skin (84%), trabecular thickening (81%), asymmetric focal density (61%), and microcalcifications (56%) (Fig. 64.3). The increase in size of the skin thickness and trabecular thickening are often detected only compared with the contralateral side.[17] Other findings were nipple retraction and axillary lymphadenopathy. An associated breast mass was identified only 16%

of the time on mammography, and this is believed to be due to the increased breast density obscuring detection of a mass. Mammography is the least sensitive diagnostic tool available for IBC.[18]

Ultrasound is more reliable than mammography in detecting IBC. It can demonstrate skin thickening more than 90% of the time.[19] Detection of a mass was higher on ultrasonography (80%) than on mammogram, and it often appears as an irregular, hypoechoic mass with poorly defined margins. Even patients without a defined mass have extensive areas of parenchymal distortion seen on ultrasonography, which can be biopsied to make the diagnosis. Axillary, supraclavicular, and infraclavicular adenopathy is also detected on ultrasound in the majority of cases (93%, 50%, and 50% respectively).[17]

MRI can also show skin thickening and is more sensitive than mammography in detecting an underlying mass. Skin enhancement is also a common finding on MRI. In recent series, skin thickening and skin enhancement incidence ranged from 90% to 100%. A series published by Yang and coworkers showed a primary breast lesion was shown in every MRI obtained as either nonmass enhancement or masslike enhancement[18] (Fig. 64.4). Axillary involvement was seen in the majority of cases as well (80%). For these reasons, MRI can be helpful in guiding core biopsies to establish the diagnosis. However, MRI does have limitations, including its decreased specificity. It cannot reliably distinguish between IBC and other inflammatory conditions of the breast, such as mastitis. Furthermore, the small size of the enclosure and duration of examination make it intolerable for some patients.

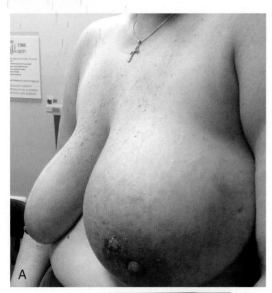

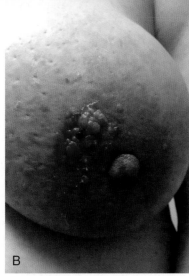

• **Fig. 64.2** (A and B) Inflammatory breast cancer with erythema and edema occupying the majority of the breast.

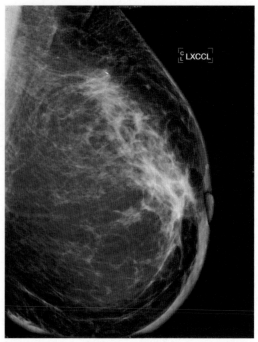

• **Fig. 64.3** Mammogram of inflammatory breast cancer. Notice the skin thickening and the lack of a well-defined mass.

PET/CT is emerging as an imaging modality for IBC. Yang and coworkers reported that PET/CT documented multicentric disease in 63% of patients, nodal disease in 88% of patients and distant metastasis with its treatment-driving implications in 38% of patients.[18] It can also detect dermal lymphatic invasion with prominent skin uptake.[20] The major limitation of PET/CT is its cost compared with other imaging modalities.

Pathology

Although the diagnosis of IBC is clinical, biopsy to confirm presence of invasive disease is mandatory, and image-assisted biopsy of the primary mass is needed. Although not necessary for the diagnosis of IBC, tumor infiltration (rather than the presence of tumor emboli) of the dermal lymphatics supports the diagnosis, and skin punch biopsy may be useful. Biological markers, such as ER and PR receptors (HRs), and HER2 status need to be determined. Because of the extensive and explosive nature of IBC, currently available multigene panel assays are not considered specifically useful.

The majority of IBC are ductal in nature.[21] They also often have a high histologic grade and are more likely HR negative. Only 44% of IBC were ER positive compared with locally advanced breast cancer (LABC), which had an ER-positive rate of 64%. PR positivity was 30% in IBC versus 51% in LABC.[22] More recent reviews reveal similar findings with IBC having ER-positive 56% and PR positive 45% compared with 67% ER positive and PR positive 54% in LABC, with higher prevalence of lymphovascular space invasion noted as well.[6,23] Among HR-positive IBCs, luminal A subtype occurs less frequently than in non-IBC.

Preclinical data do suggest alternative options for activating the estrogen signaling pathway in the absence of ER expression or alternative ER expressions such as the presence of ER α splice variants. One potential alternative pathway marker is GPR30, member of the G-protein-coupled receptor family implicated in bypassing the ER response and activating p-ERK 1/2.[24] There are ongoing attempts to better target variants/mutants of the ER receptor, and its downstream pathways. As expected, ER positivity has been linked to better survival rates with a median survival of 4 years in those with ER-positive tumors compared with 2 years in ER-negative tumors.[25]

HER2 positivity is found in 36% to 50% of IBC cases.[26] Although HER2-positive tumors in general are associated with more aggressive disease, HER overexpression has not been linked to a difference in outcome compared with HER2-negative or non-IBC HER2-positive tumors.[9] On the other hand, epidermal growth factor receptor (EGFR) is overexpressed in approximately 30% of patients with IBC and is associated with poor survival. Preclinical data suggest that the tumor microenvironment, specifically mesenchymal stromal cells may play a role increasing the expression of the EGFR receptors on the primary IBC cells and p-EGFR staining correlates between primary and stromal cells in patient samples. In xenograft experiments, and EGRF tyrosine kinase inhibitors do inhibit IBC metastasis.[27]

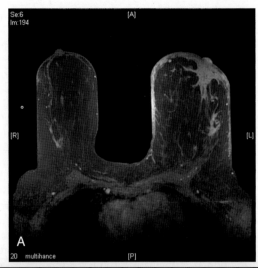

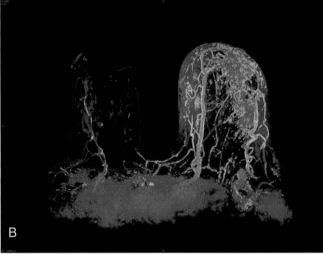

• **Fig. 64.4** (A) Magnetic resonance imaging showing thickened skin and increased enhancement within the left breast. (B) Dynamic contrast-enhanced magnetic resonance imaging showing the increased enhancement associated with inflammatory breast cancer within the left breast.

There seems to be a higher prevalence in epithelial cadherin (E-cadherin) expression and cancer stem cell markers characterized by CD44+/CD24 low expression in IBC, which may explain some of the differentiating clinical features in comparison to non-IBC.[28] Molecular drivers may also include the PI3K/AKT/mTOR and IL6/JAK2/STAT3 pathways, the latter of which is also involved in the proliferation of CD44+/CD24− breast cancer stem cells.[29]

Although their specific role in the pathophysiology is unclear (i.e., cause-effect or bystander), an increased fraction of proliferating endothelial cells and lymph endothelial cells with overexpression of angiogenesis-related (*KDR, bFGF, NAG1, TEI1,* and *TIE2*) and lymphangiogenesis-related (*VEGF-C, VEGF-D, FLT-4*) genes has been described.[30] More recently, interleukin 8 and its receptors CXCR1 and 2 have been found to regulate breast cancer stem cell activity, and their role, as well as that of other cytokines and their interactions with stem cell regulators, may bear further investigation in IBC.[31]

In one series, increased PDL1 expression was seen in 38% of 112 IBC samples out of the total of locally advanced 306 tumors tested. Comparatively, only 26% of non-IBC tested positive by messenger RNA assessment. PDL1 expression was a positive predictor for chemotherapy response in patients with IBC and was associated with a higher percentage of lymphocyte infiltration is such patients. There was greater degree of PDL1 expression seen in basal triple-negative and HER2-positive subtypes compared within ER-positive IBC.[32,33]

Genomic markers including mutations in the *p53* gene are also common in IBC and *p53* mutations have been linked to worse clinical outcomes even compared with matched subtypes.[23] Loss of WNT-inducible signaling protein 3 *(WISP3)* and the associated RHoC GTPase overexpression potentially acting as a transforming oncogene is also significantly more prevalent in IBC versus non-IBC.[34]

Current studies are directed toward identifying further molecular biomarkers specific to IBC that will aid in targeting therapy. A 79-gene signature developed for IBC and used by the World IBC Consortium was tested in IBC versus non-IBC and was able to distinguish IBC, but when assessed against The Cancer Genome Atlas (TCGA) database the panel identified IBC-like signatures in 25% of the TCGA breast cancer set, hence the degree of specificity is unclear. Genomic profiling of 53 IBC specimens was carried out to identify responses to targeted therapies and demonstrated that 96% of the specimens had a genomic alteration with TP53 being the most common (62%). Targetable mutations (*FGFR1, BRCA2,* and *PTEN* among others) have been noted in 51 of 53 IBC samples.[35] Further understanding of the genomic profile of IBC may lead to better targeted therapies.

Medical Management and Trials

The main indication of neoadjuvant therapy is to downsize the primary tumor for breast preservation, but in the setting of IBC, the role of such therapy is to allow for the feasibility of modified radical mastectomy without leaving positive margins behind, and in parallel, to avoid development of systemic metastases in patients presenting with such aggressive disease. Locoregional management alone is technically insufficient because positive margins are the likely outcome, followed by local recurrence. Hence, trimodality therapy is the standard of care for primary IBC. Pathologic complete response (pCR) has become a US Food and Drug Administration–accepted surrogate marker allowing for incorporation of new agents into the neoadjuvant sequence. Increasing the rate of pCR as a potential surrogate of better relapse-free and overall survival has been the accepted paradigm in sequential series of neoadjuvant regimens.

Over the past several decades, anthracycline-based, and more recently taxane-containing neoadjuvant regimens have become standard choices for IBC, aligned along the evolution of neoadjuvant treatments for non-IBC cases.[36] Prospective, randomized long-term data are not feasible in IBC alone, due to the rarity of the disease. However, in a large retrospective study, 15-year survival was the greatest (44%) in patients who accomplished pCR, versus 31% for those in partial response and 7% in those with less than partial response.[37] Pathologic complete response in the axilla is a predictor of better 10-year survival of 44% versus 25.4% for patients with residual disease in the axilla after neoadjuvant therapy.[38] The pCR rate after anthracycline-based chemotherapy is between 15% and 30%.[23] More recent trials of dose-dense versus conventional administration of anthracycline- and taxane-containing regimens included IBC. In 100 IBC patients enrolled in a prospective neoadjuvant randomized trial post hoc analysis revealed that dose-dense neoadjuvant therapy did not provide significant advantage for pCR (12% vs. 10%, p = nonsignificant), or for disease-free or overall survival at a median follow-up of 69 months, in contrast to 567 patients with non-IBC, who benefited from dose-dense therapy. Disease-free survival was 45% and overall survival was 59% with dose-dense versus conventional neoadjuvant therapy at the median follow-up. In a trial comparing weekly versus conventional dosing of doxorubicin and cyclophosphamide followed by taxane-, pCR was trending in IBC in favor of the continuous arm, but 5-year projected disease-free survival was inferior for IBC at around 45%.[39]

There is a higher reported percentage of HER2-overexpressing subtype among patients with IBC allowing for inclusion of HER2- targeting agents in the neoadjuvant regimen. In the HER2 setting, subset analysis of trastuzumab-containing neoadjuvant trials has shown a gradual increase in pCR rates in IBC as well as locally advanced breast cancer. Updated analysis of the randomized prospective NOAH trial testing the efficacy of trastuzumab in the neoadjuvant setting with a total of 10 cycles of chemotherapy with sequential anthracycline, taxane, and cyclophosphamide, methotrexate, and 5-fluorouracil, confirmed that pCR, particularly in HER2-positive locally advanced, and even more profoundly in IBC, is increased (36% pCR) versus chemotherapy alone. With trastuzumab then given in the adjuvant setting as well, the outcome at a median follow-up of 5.4 years was a 62% event-free survival in IBC (47 patients representing 20% of the patient population), even better than in 188 patients with locally advanced breast cancer.[40]

More recent data revealed 40% pCR with dual antibody therapy of pertuzumab and trastuzumab, given with docetaxel; pCR predicted for longer 5-year disease free survival versus patients without pCR (85% vs. 76% (hazard ratio of 0.54 (95% CI 0.29–1.00), but of note, patients also received an adjuvant anthracycline-containing treatment. However, only 7% (29/417) of patients in this trial were enrolled with IBC.[41,42] The rates of pCR vary depending on biological subtype. With longer duration of neoadjuvant therapy and with the inclusion of carboplatin with docetaxel, pertuzumab, and trastuzumab versus anthracycline-containing regimens, a high pCR of 62% was observed in the Tryphaena trial.[43] However, only 13 of 225 patients (6%) were enrolled with IBC. An interesting study describing pCR with anthracycline-containing and trastuzumab and bevacizumab-inclusive neoadjuvant therapy resulted in 63.5% pathologic complete response in 52 patients with IBC. Patients also received adjuvant trastuzumab and bevacizumab. On follow-up, the 3-year disease-free survival was 68%, and an association with pCR (80% vs. 53%) and with lack of circulating tumor cells (disease-free survival of 95% in patients with pCR and without circulating tumor cells at baseline) was noted.[44] Attempts to avoid anthracyclines and shorten the duration of treatment are ongoing with combinations of pertuzumab, trastuzumab, and a taxane in IBC and in trials allowing for enrollment of patients with IBC (clinicaltrials.gov identifiers NCT01796197 and 01730833).

Data on IBC with triple-negative (ER-, PR-, and HER2-negative) characteristics are limited, because most neoadjuvant trials excluded such patients. Therefore the efficacy of double stranded, DNA-targeting agents, and poly (ADP-ribose) polymerase (PARP) inhibitors is unknown in IBC, although data suggest that such agents may induce higher pCR rates in triple negative, locally advanced breast cancers. Data on the utility of antiangiogenic agents are also sparse, but at least one phase II prospective randomized trial suggested that the addition

of bevacizumab to anthracycline and taxane-based (in this case nab-paclitaxel) neoadjuvant therapy doubled the pCR rate to 30% (3 of 10 patients) versus 14.3% (2 of 14) among patients with IBC.[45]

The current array of promising therapeutic agents is broad. In the neoadjuvant and possibly in the postsurgical adjuvant settings, based on the phenotype and genotype, targeting the EGFR receptor by erlotinib, dual targeting by afatinib, or by other novel bispecific (EGFR and HER2) tyrosine kinase inhibitors are under evaluation.[41] Novel HER2-targeting agents such as neratinib, in addition to the currently available dual targeting with pertuzumab/trastuzumab or trastuzumab and HER2 tyrosine kinase inhibitor (TKI)-based strategy may contribute to better control of IBC with the potential to overcome HER2 mutations. Triple-negative, particularly DNA repair-deficient, IBC patients may benefit from platinum compounds and PARP inhibitors. An assessment of immunotherapeutic agents, including checkpoint inhibitors (PD1 or PDL1 inhibitors), particularly for PDL1 expressing patients, is needed. Targeted therapeutic agents based on molecular profiling of the tumor, and/or liquid biopsy samples (circulating tumor cells or cDNA)[46] might provide better selection guidance for individual IBC patients for phase II trials of the appropriate agents.

Finally, there needs to be further exploration of stem cell and stroma-targeting strategies. Agents under consideration include the JAK2 inhibitor ruxolitinib and others. Chemokine and chemokine receptor targeting agents (against CXCR4 and CXCR7 as examples), antibodies aimed at E-cadherin, and stem cell–targeting agents as well as pathway-specific TKI are under evaluation as part of the neoadjuvant IBC regimens. Although not used as primary neoadjuvant strategy in IBC, for ER-positive disease, in the postsurgical setting, the potential for developing mutations in the ER may call for testing selective ER downregulators and CDK 4/6 inhibitors earlier in the treatment course. The focus of this chapter is primary IBC, but the preceding strategies may provide much-needed help for patients presenting or relapsing with IBC, whose overall survival is under 3 years.[7]

Postneoadjuvant/Adjuvant Strategies

High-dose/dose-intense alkylator-containing therapies have yielded improved disease-free and overall survival, but the modality has not been tested sufficiently in a randomized prospective fashion, particularly in IBC, and is unlikely to be revisited.[25] Current therapeutic trials are particularly focused on adjuvant treatment strategies in patients with residual disease after neoadjuvant therapies. Such strategies are likely to be equally applicable for IBC and non-IBC locally advanced breast cancer, although the biological differences need further investigations in order to select appropriate strategies. Some of the trials already in progress are designed for specific subsets. As selected examples, in patients with HER2-positive locally advanced disease, TDM-1 is being compared with trastuzumab in the adjuvant setting after evidence of residual disease postneoadjuvant therapy (clinicaltrials.gov identifier NCT 01772472). Adjuvant cisplatin is being added with concurrent radiation for patients with residual triple-negative tumors (identifier NCT016748482). Also being tested is four cycles of adjuvant platinum therapy versus placebo (identifier NCT 02445391), the PARP inhibitor olaparib versus placebo (clinicaltrials.gov identifier 02032823), and cisplatin with or without the PARP inhibitor rucaparib (identifier NCT01074970) in *BRCA* carriers. Adjuvant immunotherapy with pembrolizumab versus placebo and the others listed are all ongoing or about to launch, albeit not specifically in IBC.

Surgical Management

The goal of surgical intervention in IBC is to achieve local control and thereby increase survival. In the 1970s and 1980s the standard treatment of IBC-included chemotherapy and radiation therapy only. Five-year overall and disease-free survival rates shown during this time period were 31% and 21%, respectively.[47] Addition of surgery to this treatment paradigm increased the overall survival and disease-free survival rates to 46% and 40%, respectively, showing that surgical intervention improves survival in IBC. Other studies have shown that the survival benefit is seen only in those patients that respond to neoadjuvant chemotherapy.[48] If response to chemotherapy is poor with residual skin changes seen, radiation therapy should be considered before surgical intervention.

Modified radical mastectomy (MRM) is the standard treatment for IBC,[49] although Bonev and colleagues showed breast conservation with axillary lymph node dissection to have comparable overall survival to modified radical mastectomy (57% vs. 59%, respectively) when preceded by neoadjuvant chemotherapy and followed with radiation in select patients. Median follow-up was 60 months, but locoregional recurrence rates were not reported.[50] In this series, dynamic contrast-enhanced magnetic resonance imaging (DCE-MRI) was used before initiation of neoadjuvant chemotherapy as well as at the conclusion of therapy to assess response. The breast conservation patients who achieved similar results to those treated with MRM had smaller-sized tumors. Additionally, the majority of patients were HER2-positive and received HER2-directed targeted therapy, which may account for the similar survival rates in each group.[50] Conversely De Boer and coworkers reported higher recurrence rates when breast conserving surgery was performed due to the inability to remove the full extent of disease and higher positive margin rates.[51]

Achieving negative margins is of paramount importance in improving survival regardless of the type of surgical intervention. Curcio and coworkers showed that positive margin status was associated with lower survival rates and higher recurrence rates and increased overall survival from 0% in those with positive margins to 47.4% among those with negative margins. In this study, margin status was shown to be a reliable prognostic indicator.[52] Because removal of all affected tissue is necessary to achieve local control, mastectomy is recommended by the National Comprehensive Cancer Network as the standard of care for treatment of IBC.[49]

A high proportion of patients with IBC will present with a clinically positive node and should also undergo complete axillary lymph node dissection. Sentinel lymph node biopsy is not recommended in cases of IBC.[53] This is because the dermal lymphatic invasion is thought to block the tracer from traveling through the lymphatic system and thereby decrease reliability of the sentinel lymph node identification. The sentinel lymph node identification and false-negative rates have been reported at 80% and 18.2%, respectively.[54] Stearns and colleagues report an even higher false-negative rate at 40%.[55] Because of this and a paucity of data on techniques to improve the identification rate of the sentinel lymph node in the setting of IBC, axillary lymph node dissection is the surgery of choice for all IBC patients for management of the axilla.

Reconstruction can be considered in this patient population. Hortobagyi and coworkers reported similar locoregional recurrence rates between patients who had reconstruction and those who had mastectomy alone.[56] Slavin and colleagues reported no difference in the detection of local recurrence when reconstruction had been performed.[57] As previously stated, achieving negative margins is of paramount importance to decrease recurrence and improve survival. For this reason, skin-sparing mastectomy is not typically possible, and this limits the type of reconstruction available to the patient. Another factor to consider is the need for postmastectomy radiation in these patients, which increases the complication rates associated with immediate reconstruction. Delayed reconstruction can be considered. Several studies have evaluated immediate reconstruction as a possibility in IBC patients. Chin and colleagues reported no difference in survival between the immediate reconstruction and the delayed reconstruction patients.[58] The majority of the patients had only autologous tissue reconstruction. Only 13% had implant-based reconstruction. Again, reconstruction must be considered only in the context of understanding that improvement in survival with IBC depends on multimodality therapy that includes excellent locoregional control with negative margins after surgery and radiation therapy.

The role of surgery in the metastatic setting is still being defined because no prospective randomized trials have been conducted particularly in the IBC population. Retrospective reviews have been encouraging, however, with respect to the role of surgery in these patients. Akay and coworkers showed significant improved overall survival and distant progression-free survival when surgery and radiotherapy were performed in both responders and nonresponders to chemotherapy with a median follow-up of 33 months. They recommend that trimodality therapy can be considered even in the metastatic setting.[59] Similarly, Warren and colleagues advocate for surgery in the metastatic setting to aide in locoregional control.[60] In their study, 5-year locoregional control was 83% when surgery and radiotherapy were given in the metastatic setting. Locoregional progression was more likely when metastatic disease was present in distant lymph nodes compared with other sites of metastasis. These studies indicate that in patients with more favorable histology and response to systemic therapy, surgery should be considered in the metastatic setting. Surgery can also be considered as palliation for those with symptom control such as bleeding or pain from their disease.

Radiation Management

Postmastectomy radiation is recommended in all patients treated with neoadjuvant chemotherapy and mastectomy for IBC. It is crucial to include preneoadjuvant images (photos and radiographs) and assess the patient in a multidisciplinary setting with the radiation oncologist, before initiating neoadjuvant therapy. Bristol and coworkers demonstrated that multimodality treatment including radiation therapy decreased the locoregional recurrence rate and improved disease-free and overall survival. Furthermore, they were able to stratify which patients benefitted from 66-Gy over 60-Gy doses in achieving locoregional control. These patients included those who had close or positive margins, those with less than partial response to neoadjuvant chemotherapy, and younger patients.[61] Brown and coworkers showed that once-daily radiation with high bolus achieved comparable control to the hyperfractionated regimens.[62] Dose escalation has also been shown to improve locoregional control.[63] Treatment to the skin, in particular, is paramount because this disease involves the dermal lymphatics.

Long-term data analysis suggests a survival benefit in breast cancer in general, with postmastectomy radiation.[64] The fields included in radiation treatment should include the chest wall, including the mastectomy scar, as well as the supraclavicular, infraclavicular, and internal mammary nodal basins. Locoregional failure can occur outside of the field of radiation when all areas are not treated. There is a role for radiation treatment to oligometastatic sites after response to neoadjuvant/induction chemotherapy as well, particularly when such are localized to lymph node areas.[65]

Despite the benefits of radiation in the treatment of IBC, it is underutilized. Loveland-Jones and coworkers showed that Medicare insurance, lower income, failure to receive other adjuvant therapies, treatment in the southern or western United States and treatment at lower-volume centers were all associated with less likelihood of receiving radiation treatment.[66]

Metastatic Disease

Distant metastasis is common at initial presentation with IBC and has been identified in 30% of patients. Development of distant metastasis during recurrence is also common and in one series occurred 43% of the time among stage III patients. The most common sites of distant metastasis were bone, central nervous system, lung and pleura, liver, chest wall, and regional lymph nodes.[67] Current treatment is in line of conventional therapies for stage IV disease, hence more specific and better options are needed because survival is under 3 years for such patients.

New Directions

Patients with IBC should be offered trimodality therapy as standard, and, if available, they should be offered participation in clinical trials. Besides the initial testing for ER, PR, and HER2 expression, the optimal selection of IBC patients for clinical trials should ideally be based on molecular assessment of the primary to identify targetable pathways. Ideally, serial tumor and liquid biopsies should be collected for assessment of the tumor and stroma, for quantitative and qualitative analysis of circulating tumor cells and circulating tumor DNA. IBC-specific phase II trials will hopefully provide guidance for improved therapies to increase the surrogate pCR rate leading to better survival. Better in vitro and patient-derived xenograft models are needed to further optimize therapies and in case of suboptimal response during neoadjuvant therapy, such models may help to direct us how to select the postsurgical therapy. Finally, emerging knowledge on the relationship between metabolomics, inflammatory processes, and IBC (including potential manipulation of cholesterol levels and interference with dyslipidemia through weight loss, exercise, and evoking statins) may provide adjunctive and even preventive tools to benefit our patients suffering from this most aggressive form of breast cancer.

Conclusion

Improved strategies inclusive of trimodality therapy for primary IBC, more effective targeting agents for non-IBC leading to incorporating such components into IBC-treatments, and better awareness and understanding of IBC has led to improvement in pCR and survival. International collaboration both in terms of sharing knowledge gained from preclinical studies and pooling resources to conduct and rapid complete clinical trials should lead to improved options for IBC patients.

Selected References

8. Rueth NM, Lin HY, Bedrosian I, et al. Underuse of trimodality treatment affects survival for patients with inflammatory breast cancer: an analysis of treatment and survival trends from the National Cancer Database. *J Clin Oncol.* 2014;32:2018-2024.
35. Ross JS, Ali SM, Wang K, et al. Comprehensive genomic profiling of inflammatory breast cancer cases reveals a high frequency of clinically relevant genomic alterations. *Breast Cancer Res Treat.* 2015;154:155-162.
40. Gianni L, Eiermann W, Semiglazov V, et al. Neoadjuvant and adjuvant trastuzumab in patients with HER2-positive locally advanced breast cancer (NOAH): follow-up of a randomised controlled superiority trial with a parallel HER2-negative cohort. *Lancet Oncol.* 2014;15:640-647.
46. Alix-Panabieres C, Pantel K. Clinical applications of circulating tumor cells and circulating tumor DNA as liquid biopsy. *Cancer Discov.* 2016;6:479-491.
55. Stearns V, Ewing CA, Slack R, et al. Sentinel lymphadenectomy after neoadjuvant chemotherapy for breast cancer may reliably represent the axilla except for inflammatory breast cancer. *Ann Surg Oncol.* 2002;9:235-242.
59. Akay CL, Ueno NT, Chisholm GB, et al. Primary tumor resection as a component of multimodality treatment may improve local control and survival in patients with stage IV inflammatory breast cancer. *Cancer.* 2014;120:1319-1328.

A full reference list is available online at ExpertConsult.com.

65

Neoadjuvant Chemotherapy and Radiotherapy

ISSAM MAKHOUL, ANGELA PENNISI, SANJAY MARABOYINA, AND
GWENDOLYN BRYANT-SMITH

Neoadjuvant chemotherapy (NACT) for breast cancer is the administration of systemic therapy to patients before surgery. It was initially used to downstage inoperable tumors but over time has become a useful tool to allow breast conservation surgery and a valid setting to assess the impact of new therapeutics on pathologic complete response (pCR), a surrogate end point for long-term survival. This chapter reviews the foundations of this treatment modality and the latest progress in the field. Two decades of progress in understanding the biology of breast cancer led to the classification of this disease into subtypes with distinct clinical behavior and response to treatment. The one-size-fits-all strategy was replaced by personalized treatments and a great opportunity to improve the eradication rate of this disease.

Historically, NACT was offered to patients with locally advanced breast cancer to downstage the tumor and improve surgical resectability[1] and sometimes as the only effective strategy to treat patients with inflammatory breast cancer (IBC). Later it was proposed as a treatment modality to increase breast conservation surgery in operable breast cancer and most recently as the preferred setting to test new drugs and combinations before embarking on long and costly adjuvant clinical trials.[2,3]

The need for systemic therapy emerged in the mid-20th century when increasingly aggressive surgical treatments failed to cure breast cancer patients who would succumb to systemic disease. This realization paved the way to adjuvant postoperative chemotherapy (ACT), leading to significant improvements of disease-free survival (DFS) and overall survival (OS) and proving the hypothesis suggesting that breast cancer cell dissemination occurs early in the course of the disease. The benefit of ACT was confirmed in multiple clinical trials using different chemotherapy agents and regimens that enrolled tens of thousands of patients; many of these trials were included in the Oxford overview.[4,5] As ACT became established, it was tempting to take the regimens that had proven efficacy in the adjuvant setting to the neoadjuvant setting. This led to a large number of clinical trials comparing ACT to NACT. Collectively, these trials proved that NACT was safe and results in equivalent long-term survivals compared with ACT (Table 65.1).[6–12] Another benefit of this treatment modality was the increase in the breast conserving surgery (BCS) rate without significant increase of local recurrences.

Two additional reasons for the use of NACT include the monitoring of response to chemotherapy for the individual patient that would allow its adjustment and also to test new drugs. Because in vitro chemosensitivity and resistance tests proved to be useless in routine clinical practice,[13] it was necessary to find a rapid and cheap way to test these drugs in vivo. The benefit of the NACT setting is the possibility to reach a quick conclusion (weeks or months) about the efficacy of new drugs compared with the ACT setting where the trials span over years and require much larger financial and human resources. The emergence of pCR as a predictor of DFS and OS has prompted the US Food and Drug Administration (FDA) to issue in 2014 an important memo titled "Guidance for Industry Pathologic Complete Response in Neoadjuvant Treatment of High-Risk Early Stage Breast Cancer: Use as an Endpoint to Support Accelerated Approval."[14] This document provides guidance to investigators and industry about the use of pCR as an end point for accelerated approval. This is discussed in detail in the following sections. Many investigators remain skeptical about the benefit of pCR, arguing that it selects for those who have chemosensitive disease that would have responded well to ACT anyway. However, when NACT is used as in vivo chemosensitivity test, it provides a unique opportunity for personalized treatment and represents a powerful research tool.[15]

Molecular Subtypes of Breast Cancer and Response to Neoadjuvant Chemotherapy

The first generation of neoadjuvant chemotherapy trials showed that different breast cancer subtypes responded differently to chemotherapy. Hormone receptor (HR) negativity and HER2 positivity were associated with more responsiveness, whereas HR positivity and HER2 negativity were associated with less responsiveness to chemotherapy. Other predictive markers of responsiveness included small tumor size, high ki67, high tumor grade, high tumor labeling index, and lymphovascular space invasion.[16–20]

The year 2000 was a turning point in our way of looking at breast cancer. The publication of a seminal paper "Molecular Portraits of Human Breast Tumors" by Perou and colleagues opened the field of molecular and genetic evaluation of this cancer and other solid tumors.[21] The main premise of the field is that

TABLE 65.1	Early Trials Comparing NACT to ACT						
Trial	Patient N	Tumor Size	Regimen	FU (Mo)	DFS IBTR	OS	BCS NAT vs AT
Fisher et al. 1998 NSABP B-18[10,a]	1523	All	AC × 4	96	=	=	68% vs. 60% p = .002
Van der Hage et al. 2001 EORTC 10902[160,a]	698	≥1 cm	FEC × 4	56	=	=	37% vs 21% p = NA
Taucher et al. 2008 ABCSG-7[11]	215	All	CMF × 3	NA	↑IBRT	=	NA
Scholl et al. 1994 S6[12]	414	3–7 cm	FAC × 4	66	=	=	82% vs. 77%

[a]These trials confirmed the safety and feasibility of this treatment modality with the increase of breast conserving surgery.

AC, Adriamycin (doxorubicin)/cyclophosphamide; *ACT,* adjuvant postoperative chemotherapy; *CMF,* cyclophosphamide/methotrexate/and fluorouracil; *DFS,* disease-free survival; *EORTC,* European Organisation for Research and Treatment of Cancer; *FAC,* fluorouracil/Adriamycin/cyclophosphamide; *FEC,* fluorouracil/epirubicin/cyclophosphamide; *FU,* follow-up; *IBTR,* ipsilateral breast tumor recurrence; *NACT,* neoadjuvant chemotherapy; *NA,* not available; *OS,* overall survival.

despite phenotypical similarities, breast cancers are different in terms of genes and pathways activated in each one and in their behavior and response to therapy. Using gene expression profiling, five intrinsic subtypes were identified: the basal-like, the HER2 positive, the luminal A and B, and the normal-like.[22,23] On the basis of this original work, the PAM50 and PAM50 risk of relapse (PAM50-ROR) assays were developed.[23] The first allows the classification of breast cancers into intrinsic subtypes, and the second provides important information about their prognosis. In the next decade, other gene expression profile (GEP)-based prognostic assays were developed, including the Onco*type* Dx and MammaPrint. All these assays generate a score that assigns a low, medium, or high risk of recurrence (PAM50-ROR, Onco*type* Dx) or good-bad prognosis (MammaPrint) to each individual cancer. Attempts at using a grouping of traditional classifiers such as HR, HER2, and ki67 yielded a good approximation of the intrinsic subtypes (luminal A: HR+/HER2−/ki67 low; luminal B: HR+/HER2−/ki67 high; luminal B: HR+/HER2+; HER2+: HR−/HER2+; triple negative: HR−/HER2−)[24] that fell short of fully recapitulating the subtypes defined by GEP.[25]

The intrinsic subtypes (basal-like, HER2 positive, luminal A and B, and normal-like) were able to describe the biological behavior and response to treatment. Indeed, pCRs after NACT were the highest for the first two and dropped sharply in the luminal subtypes and were nonexistent in the normal-like subtype (45%, 45%, 6%, and 0%, respectively).[22]

Eligibility for Neoadjuvant Chemotherapy or Neoadjuvant Radiation Therapy

The first reports of therapeutic effects of systemic chemotherapy appeared in the 1960s and of neoadjuvant therapy in the 1970s.[26] Historically, preoperative or NACT was offered to patients with locally advanced or inflammatory breast cancer.[27,28] Locally advanced breast cancer (LABC) is defined by tumor (T3, T4) or nodal (N2 or N3) stage (American Joint Committee on Cancer).[29] T3 tumors are those larger than 5 cm and T4 involve the chest wall (T4a), the skin (T4b) or both (T4c). N2 stage includes matted ipsilateral axillary lymph nodes (fixed to one another or

to other structures) (N2a) or clinically apparent ipsilateral internal mammary lymph nodes by imaging studies or clinical examination in the absence of ipsilateral axillary lymph node involvement (N2b). N3 stage includes metastases to ipsilateral infraclavicular (N3a), internal mammary and axillary (N3b) or to supraclavicular lymph nodes (N3c). IBC is defined clinically by the rapid onset (<6 months) of erythema and edema with palpable edges (peau d'orange) involving at least one-third of the breast (T4d) and confirmed by a breast biopsy.[30] Although the involvement of the dermal lymphatics with invasive breast cancer is considered the pathologic hallmark of this type, it is not specific nor is it required to make this diagnosis.[31] Lumping this form with LABC, which was frequently done in clinic trials in the past, is no longer justified according to new findings of biological and prognostic differences.[32] In LABC and IBC, upfront surgery may not be feasible and if done may leave large macroscopic disease in the tumor bed or axilla. NACT is likely to downstage the tumor and increase the likelihood of successful and complete surgical resection. Similar reasoning applies to situations in which the patient desires BCS but the tumor size is "large" relative to the breast, and upfront surgery is likely to lead to mastectomy.

Early animal studies have suggested a possible therapeutic advantage to NACT over ACT[8,33–37] based on the increase of labeling index in the residual tumor after removal of the primary tumor with the possibility to prevent this phenomenon if chemotherapy is given to the animals before tumor removal. This hypothesis was rejected when tested in humans. Trials comparing NACT to ACT showed that these two modalities had equal efficacy and safety (see Table 65.1).

Another advantage for the use of NACT in early-stage breast cancer is the assessment of in vivo sensitivity to chemotherapy because no in vitro sensitivity test could prove useful to predict chemotherapy efficacy in patients.[15,38] The many concerns that were raised against NACT (e.g., the fear of delaying curative local therapy, developing resistance by the metastases, or increasing the risk of subsequent surgery or radiation therapy [RT]) were not validated by the results of clinical trials. The advent of powerful imaging modalities such as magnetic resonance imaging (MRI) has mitigated the consequences of losing initial staging information.[37–39]

Evaluation of Candidates for Neoadjuvant Chemotherapy or Neoadjuvant Radiation Therapy

The initial evaluation of breast cancer patients helps the clinician assign a clinical stage and obtain precious information to direct the therapy (Box 65.1). The tumor size is measured by a caliper (in the sitting position using a horizontal and vertical axes or the longest diameter) and the presence of chest wall or skin involvement or inflammatory signs (edema, erythema, or peau d'orange sign) are documented; palpable lymph nodes should be evaluated for adhesion to the skin or axillary structures.[40] Mammography and ultrasound help determine the size of the cancer, the presence of multicentricity/mutifocality, diffuse microcalcifications, or synchronous contralateral breast cancer.[41] Ultrasound can also be used for monitoring of the size of the tumor during NAT.[42]

Many experts consider pretreatment MRI standard of care but its role compared with mammogram and ultrasound remains controversial. Its sensitivity in detecting occult contralateral breast cancers (approaching 94%–100%) is superior to mammography,[43,44] but the benefit from this high sensitivity is mitigated by low specificity (37%–97%).[45] The increased power of modern machines (from 1- or 1.5-T to 3-T MRI) adds to the sensitivity without improving the specificity.[46] Using diffusion-weighted MRI may increase specificity for small masses and non-masslike lesions.[43] MRI is not recommended for routine use before NACT in small operable breast cancers because of the high false positivity,[40] but its use is appropriate in locally advanced tumors and for response assessment and surgery planning. Two decades of experience with breast MRI allows the identification of MRI phenotypes that are predominantly associated with each biological subtype; this relationship between MRI phenotype and biological subtypes is not exclusive because all MRI phenotypes can be seen in any biological subtype.[47] Triple-negative breast cancer (TNBC) tends to be associated with unifocal masses, whereas HER2-positive breast cancers tend to be associated with multifocal masses. Nonmass or diffuse enhancements tend to be more common with HR-positive tumors (Figs. 65.1, 65.3, 65.5, 65.6, 65.8, 65.9, 65.11, 65.12, 65.14, and 65.15). The breast cancer team is interested in knowing the extent of the residual disease to help tailor surgical resection, especially if

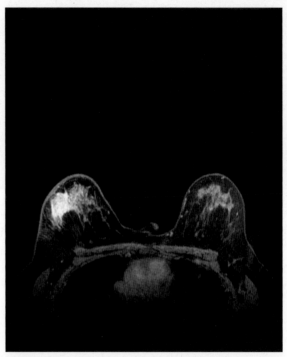

• Fig. 65.1 Pre–neoadjuvant chemotherapy estrogen receptor–negative, progesterone receptor–negative, HER2-positive invasive ductal carcinoma. Axial T1 fat-suppressed postcontrast image showing a unifocal enhancing mass in the right breast.

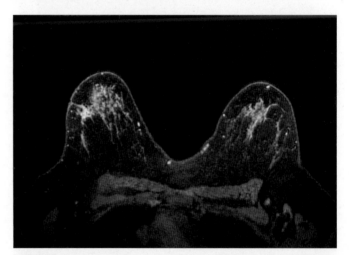

• Fig. 65.2 Post–neoadjuvant chemotherapy (NACT) estrogen receptor–negative, progesterone receptor–negative, HER2-positive invasive ductal carcinoma. Post-NACT axial T1 fat-suppressed magnetic resonance image postcontrast shows significant decrease in the original tumor in Fig. 65.1.

the patient is interested in breast conservation surgery. Responses to NACT and the accuracy of response assessment by MRI vary depending on the biological subtypes, with the best responses, and the most accurate assessments, being observed in TNBC and HER2-positive breast cancers compared with the HR-positive cancers, for which responses are poor and the MRI assessments are the least accurate (as was shown in the I-SPY study).[48] Indeed, underestimation of the size of residual tumor is observed more commonly (up to two-thirds of patients) in HR-positive cancers.[49] Positive predictive value, but not negative predictive value (NPV), of MRI is high and fairly accurate in these tumors (Figs. 65.2, 65.4, 65.7, 65.10, 65.13 and 65.16).

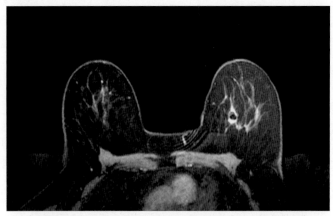

• **Fig. 65.3** Pre–neoadjuvant chemotherapy triple-negative invasive ductal carcinoma. Magnetic resonance axial fat suppressed T1-weighted image postcontrast shows a unifocal mass with a signal void from a clip postbiopsy in the left breast.

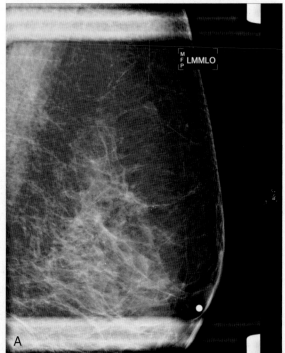

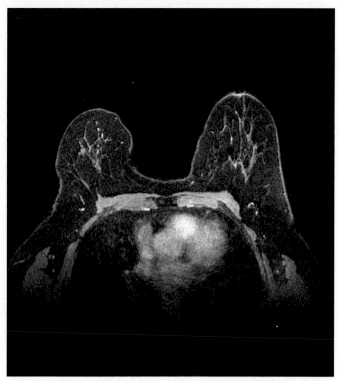

• **Fig. 65.4** Post–neoadjuvant chemotherapy triple-negative invasive ductal carcinoma. Magnetic resonance axial fat-suppressed T1-weighted image postcontrast shows a complete magnetic resonance imaging response after therapy with resolution of the mass previously noted in the left breast. No enhancement is now seen surrounding the clip.

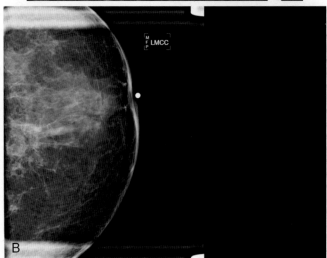

• **Fig. 65.5** Pre–neoadjuvant chemotherapy estrogen receptor–positive, progesterone receptor–positive, HER2-negative invasive ductal carcinoma. Malignant microcalcifications in the left superior breast on mammography. (A) Left magnified, mediolateral-oblique. (B) Left magnified, craniocaudal.

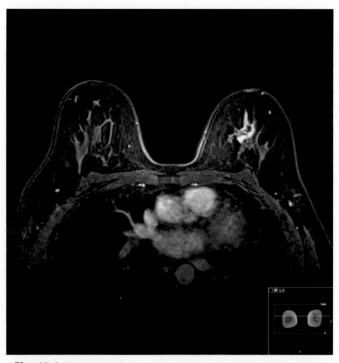

• **Fig. 65.6** Pre–neoadjuvant chemotherapy estrogen receptor–positive, progesterone receptor–positive, HER2-negative invasive ductal carcinoma. Axial postcontrast fat-suppressed T1-weighted image shows an irregular enhancing mass in the left breast.

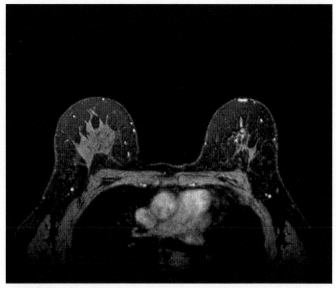

• **Fig. 65.7** Post–neoadjuvant chemotherapy estrogen receptor–positive, progesterone receptor–positive, HER2-negative invasive ductal carcinoma. Axial postcontrast fat-suppressed T1-weighted image shows resolution of the previously noted irregular enhancing mass in the left breast.

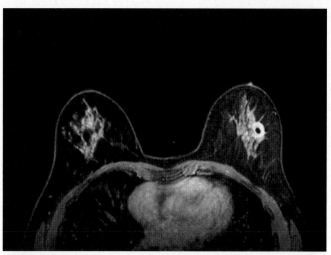

• **Fig. 65.9** Pre–neoadjuvant chemotherapy estrogen receptor–positive, progesterone receptor–positive, HER2-positive invasive ductal carcinoma. Axial fat-suppressed T1-weighted magnetic resonance image shows a unifocal mass in the left breast.

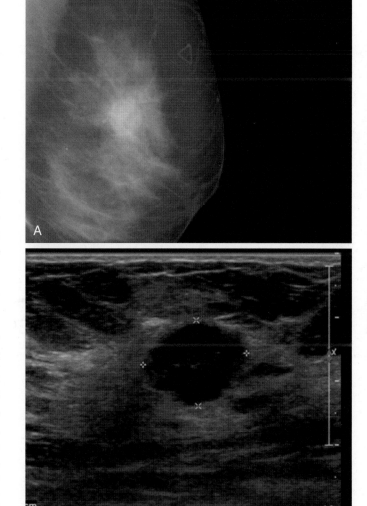

• **Fig. 65.8** Pre–neoadjuvant chemotherapy estrogen receptor–positive, progesterone receptor–positive, HER2-positive invasive ductal carcinoma. Unifocal mass noted on mammography (A) and ultrasound (B) in the left breast at 2:30.

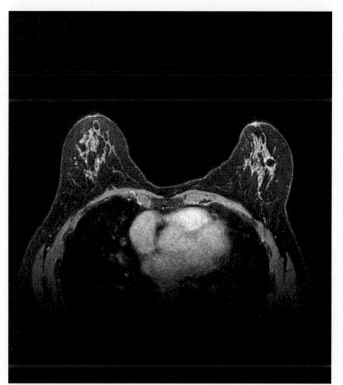

• **Fig. 65.10** Post–neoadjuvant chemotherapy estrogen receptor–positive, progesterone receptor–positive, HER2-positive invasive ductal carcinoma. Axial fat-suppressed T1-weighted magnetic resonance image shows almost complete resolution of the unifocal mass in the left breast.

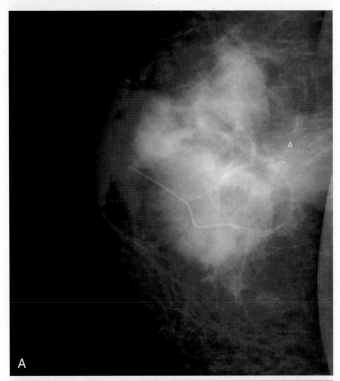

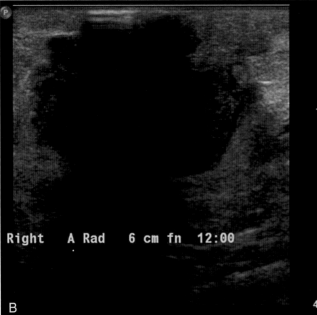

• **Fig. 65.11** Pre–neoadjuvant chemotherapy estrogen receptor–positive, progesterone receptor–negative, HER2-positive multifocal right breast invasive ductal carcinoma. Mammogram (A) and ultrasound (B) show multifocal disease in the right breast.

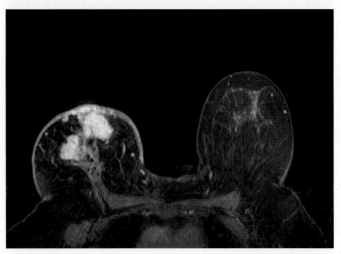

• **Fig. 65.12** Pre–neoadjuvant chemotherapy estrogen receptor–positive, progesterone receptor–negative, HER2-positive multifocal right breast invasive ductal carcinoma. Axial fat-suppressed T1-weighted image shows multifocal enhancing masses in the right breast with adenopathy and skin thickening.

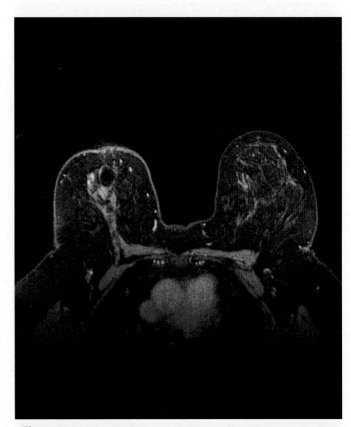

• **Fig. 65.13** Post–neoadjuvant chemotherapy estrogen receptor–positive, progesterone receptor–negative, HER2-positive multifocal right breast invasive ductal carcinoma. Axial fat-suppressed T1-weighted image shows significant improvement in multifocal enhancing masses in the right breast and improvement in adenopathy. Also, significant improvement in right breast skin thickening.

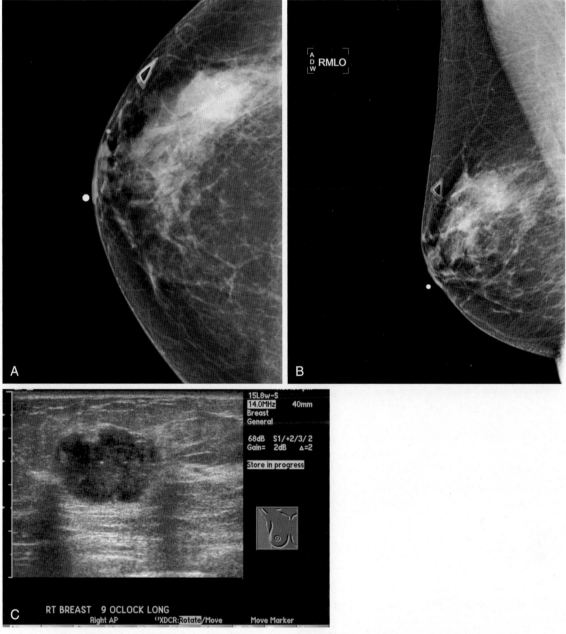

• **Fig. 65.14** Pre–neoadjuvant chemotherapy estrogen receptor–negative, progesterone receptor–negative, HER2-negative triple-negative right breast invasive ductal carcinoma. Mammogram ([A] craniocaudal view; [B] mediolateral view) and ultrasound (C) show a unifocal mass with associated pleomorphic microcalcifications.

One of the major challenges of the field is to identify those patients in whom radiologic complete response can predict pCR and may allow the patients to forgo surgery. Again, assessment with MRI is the most accurate in TNBC and HER2-positive breast cancers with NPV being the highest in these subtypes (60%–91% and 62%–95%, respectively).[50–54] These NPVs are still below the required cutoffs to forgo surgery because up to 40% of the patients would have false-negative MRI, and omitting surgery means that we would leave those patients with residual disease in the breast. Using diffusion-based imaging, Bufi and coworkers[54] reported NPVs of 100% in these two subtypes. These results need to be replicated. Thus the technology is not ready for wide clinical application because its performance needs to be improved and it must be validated by prospective clinical trials.

At least three core needle biopsies from the main lesion and one from any other lesion are considered standard procedure to obtain adequate tissue for full assessment of the tumor type and HR and HER2 status determination. Radiopaque clips may be placed during the same procedure to help with a future retrieval of the tumor.

Axillary lymph node status should be assessed clinically. Patients with clinically detectable lymphadenopathy should have a fine-needle aspiration biopsy or core biopsy from their lymph nodes. Clinically, nonpalpable lymph nodes can be assessed with

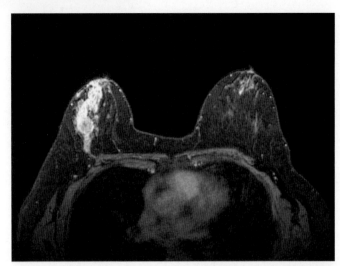

• **Fig. 65.15** Pre–neoadjuvant chemotherapy estrogen receptor–negative, progesterone receptor–negative, HER2-negative triple-negative right breast invasive ductal carcinoma. Axial fat-suppressed T1-weighted image shows a large area of nonmass enhancement involving the 9 o'clock axis of the right breast.

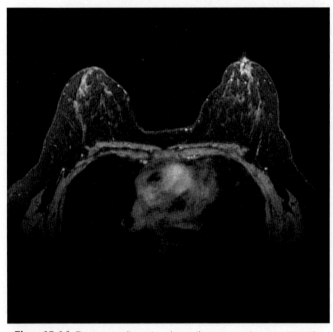

• **Fig. 65.16** Post–neoadjuvant chemotherapy estrogen receptor–negative, progesterone receptor–negative, HER2-negative triple-negative right breast invasive ductal carcinoma. Axial fat-suppressed T1-weighted image shows resolution of the large area of nonmass enhancement involving the 9 o'clock axis of the right breast.

sentinel lymph node procedure before or after NACT (as discussed later).

Outcomes and End Points of Neoadjuvant Therapy

Whereas phase III adjuvant trials address definitive end points of relapse and survival but are slow, require large samples, and are costly, neoadjuvant clinical trials use smaller populations and can rapidly test (usually in order of months) new drugs or schedules through surrogate end points likely to predict clinical benefit. Several clinical trials have shown favorable long-term DFS and OS rates for patients who achieved pCR after NACT.[55,56] The biological hypothesis behind these results is that clearance of the cancer from the breast translates into elimination of possible disseminated tumor cells or micrometastasis. Predictor of pCR after NACT are age less than 40 years, tumor less than 2 cm, ductal histology, high tumor grade, high proliferation index (assessed by ki67), negative estrogen receptor (ER) status and intrinsic subtype (basal-like or HER2-enriched).[16–20,57]

Interestingly, the National Surgical Adjuvant Breast and Bowel Project (NSABP) B-27 trial[58] failed to demonstrate that doubling of pCR with the addition of docetaxel to doxorubicin and cyclophosphamide (13.7 vs. 26.1 %; $p < .001$) translates into improvement of DFS or OS in the experimental arm but confirmed that patients who achieved pCR (defined in this trial as absence of invasive tumor in the breast only) had a better outcome irrespective of the regimen received.

On the basis of the accumulated evidence of the prognostic value of pCR, the FDA announced consideration for accelerated approval in early breast cancer for new drugs tested in neoadjuvant setting if the product "has an effect on a surrogate end point likely to predict clinical benefit"[59] and recommended pCR as such surrogate end point. Thus accelerated approval was granted in September 2013 to use pertuzumab as a part of neoadjuvant regimen for early-stage breast cancer expressing HER2 based on increased pCR achieved in the Neosphere[60] and TRYPHAENA[61] trials.

Despite the fact that pCR has been the primary end point for all recent NACT trials, the pathologic criteria to define pCR have been variable. The three most commonly used definitions of pCR are the following:

- **ypT0 ypN0:** absence of invasive cancer and in situ cancer in the breast and axillary nodes;
- **ypT0/is ypN0:** absence of invasive cancer in the breast and axillary nodes, irrespective of carcinoma in situ; and
- **ypT0/is:** absence of invasive cancer in the breast irrespective of ductal carcinoma in situ or nodal involvement.

It has been known that eradication of invasive carcinoma from lymph nodes after NACT carries a more favorable prognosis,[62] whereas residual carcinoma in situ in the breast does not significantly affect patient outcome.[63]

To investigate the relationship between pCR and long-term clinical benefit, the FDA established a working group known as the Collaborative Trials in Neoadjuvant Breast Cancer (CTNeoBC) that conducted a meta-analysis of twelve international large randomized neoadjuvant clinical trials with more than 12,000 patients enrolled.[64] Several lessons were learned from the CTNeoBC meta-analysis:

1. Individuals who achieved pCR by any of the three preceding definitions have a more favorable long-term outcome for both event-free survival (EFS) (hazard ratio 0.48, 95% confidence interval [CI] 0.43–0.54) and OS (hazard ratio 0.36, 95% CI 0.31–0.42).
2. Eradication of invasive cancer from both breast and lymph nodes (ypT0 ypN0 or ypT0/is ypN0) rather than in breast only (ypT0/is) was better associated with improved EFS (ypT0 ypN0: hazard ratio 0.44, 95% CI 0.39–0.51; ypT0/is ypN0: 0.48, 0.43–0.54; ypT0/is: 0.60, 0.55–0.66; and OS (ypT0 ypN0: hazard ratio 0.36, 0.30–0.44; ypT0/is ypN0: 0.36, 0.31–0.42; ypT0/is: 0.51, 0.45–0.58. On the basis of these

data, the FDA recognizes a definition of pCR for consideration for US marketing approval as the absence of residual invasive carcinoma in the complete resected breast specimen and all sampled regional lymph nodes irrespective of the presence or absence of residual ductal carcinoma in situ (DCIS) (ypT0/is ypN0 or ypT0 ypN0).

3. As expected, frequency of pCR was low in low-grade HR-positive tumors (hazard ratio 7.5%, 95% CI 6.3–8.7) but higher in the more aggressive subtypes: triple-negative (33.6%, 30.9–36.4), HER2-positive tumors treated with (50.3, 95% CI 45.0–55.5) or without (30.2%, 95% CI 26.0–34.5) trastuzumab, and grade 3 HR-positive/HER2-negative breast cancer (16.2%, 13.4–19.3). Improvement in long-term outcome was more significant in the aggressive cancer subtypes if pCR (defined as ypT0/is ypN0 based on findings described earlier) was achieved, with a reduction of the risk of death by 84% (95% CI 75–89), 92% (95% CI 78–97), 71% (95% CI 50–83), and 71% (95% CI 35–87), respectively. In contrast, the association between pCR and long-term outcome was weakest for HR-positive subtypes (particularly lower-grade cancers).

4. At a trial level, the CTNeoBC analysis demonstrated a weak association between pCR (ypT0/is, ypN0) and both EFS and OS. A potential explanation for the inability to demonstrate a clear correlation could be that the inclusion of heterogeneous populations in the pooled analysis may have obscured the association as the absolute improvements in the pCR rates between treatment arms was low (1%–11%). In contrast, when the improvement in pCR was high (20%) as in the case of the Neoadjuvant Herceptin (NOAH) trial comparing trastuzumab plus chemotherapy to chemotherapy alone in women with HER2-positive locally advanced breast cancer, a certain correlation was found between effect on pCR and long-term benefit. These results suggest that a correlation between pCR and long-term outcome might be identified in trials conducted in more homogeneous breast cancer populations and in more aggressive subtypes in which higher pCR rates are expected.

Switching nonresponders to a non–cross-resistant regimen did not result in increased rates of pCR. Indeed, there is no evidence that clinical response should be used to tailor subsequent treatment choices based on the results of the Aberdeen and the Gepar-Trio trials. The Aberdeen trial randomized patients who responded to four cycles of cyclophosphamide, vincristine, doxorubicin, and prednisone (CVAP) to receive either four cycles of the same regimen or four cycles of docetaxel. Nonresponders to four cycles of CVAP were switched to docetaxel. pCR doubled in responders who were switched to docetaxel (31% vs. 15%), whereas nonresponders had a modest pCR (2%) despite the addition of docetaxel.[65] The GeparTrio trial randomized nonresponders, defined as patients who did not achieve a decrease in size of their tumor by at least 50% after two cycles of docetaxel, doxorubicin, and cyclophosphamide (TAC), to four additional cycles of TAC or to four cycles of vinorelbine and capecitabine (NX).[66] Switching to NX did not improve pCR.

Because of the low rates of pCR after NACT and the weaker correlation between pCR and survival end points in HR-positive breast cancers, the neoadjuvant field has moved more generally toward strategies to omit chemotherapy in these subsets of patients. It is assumed that endocrine therapy acts through induction of cell-cycle arrest and changes in surrogates of cell proliferation could be considered a potential surrogate of response to neoadjuvant endocrine therapy (NET). One candidate is the nuclear nonhistone protein ki67, widely used as a marker for proliferation. Interestingly, changes in levels of ki67 in relatively small NET were able to anticipate outcomes from large adjuvant trials that showed the superiority of aromatase inhibitors (AIs) over tamoxifen[67–70] and equivalence between the three AIs[71,72] in postmenopausal women. The best time to assess ki67 response is not well defined, however. In the Immediate Preoperative Anastrozole, Tamoxifen, or Combined with Tamoxifen (IMPACT) trial, in which ki67 was measured as early as 2 weeks, the superiority of anastrozole over tamoxifen was confirmed based on a greater reduction in ki67 levels either after 2 or 12 weeks ($p = .013$ and $p = .0006$, respectively), despite the fact that the trial was negative for its primary end point (clinical response). Furthermore, in a multivariate analysis, ki67 expression at 2 weeks was significantly associated with recurrence-free survival (hazard ratio = 1.95; $p = .004$).[73]

One potential limitation of this early assessment of ki67 is the development of delayed or acquired resistance. Paradoxical increases in Ki67 in the surgical specimen compared with baseline (>5%) were seen in 12.3% of luminal A and 5.8%, luminal B patients included in American College of Surgeons Oncology Group (ACOSOG) Z1031 trial.[71] In addition, in IMPACT trial, the authors showed that 15% of patients who had early decreases in ki67 (on week two biopsy) on NET had increases in ki67 at the time of surgery (as assessed on surgical specimens), raising doubts about the optimal time points for assessment of this and other potential biomarkers. Currently, the advantage of measuring 2-week ki67 instead of pretreatment ki67 is being prospectively investigated in the large ($n = 4000$) Perioperative Endocrine Therapy for Individualising Care (POETIC) window-of-opportunity trial.[74]

Neoadjuvant Chemotherapy by Breast Cancer Subtypes

Chemotherapy is the first type of systemic therapy used neoadjuvantly. However, the introduction of endocrine and targeted therapies, based on better understanding of the disease, enriched our armamentarium in the recent years in this setting. The first chemotherapeutic agents used in this setting were the ones that had proven track records in the adjuvant setting such as cyclophosphamide, methotrexate, and fluorouracil (CMF). These were replaced by newer drugs such as anthracyclines and taxanes (Table 65.2).[75–80] Most neoadjuvant chemotherapy regimens in 2016 contain an anthracycline (doxorubicin or epirubicin), a taxane (docetaxel or paclitaxel), and cyclophosphamide. The addition of the vinorelbine, gemcitabine, and capecitabine in the adjuvant or neoadjuvant settings did not add more benefit.[66,81] Only the addition of platinum compounds in TNBC and HER2-positive cancers may have additional efficacy that is still being explored.[61,82]

It is now established that multiagent chemotherapy regimens are superior to single-agent regimens. Combinations of anthracyclines and taxanes are superior to each one alone and their efficacy is better when they are used sequentially rather than concurrently[15] (see Table 65.2). Dose-dense chemotherapy was also tested to increase pCR in a trial randomizing patients with LABC to fluorouracil, epirubicin, and cyclophosphamide (FEC) every 3 weeks or epirubicin/cyclophosphamide (EC) every 2 weeks. There was no difference in any of the end points evaluated (pCR, DFS, OS).[83] Five other trials were conducted with conflicting results.[84–88] A meta-analysis of all randomized trials showed significant 46.7%

TABLE 65.2 The Addition of Taxanes Resulted in Significant Increase in Pathologic Complete Response (pCR)

Trial	Patient N	Regimen	pCR (%)
Buzdar et al. 1999[75]	174	FAC × 4	16.4 (23)
		Paclitaxel × 4	8.1 (14)
Smith et al. 2002 (Aberdeen)[16]	104	CVAP	15
		CVAP-D	31
Dieras et al. 2004[76]	200	AC × 4	10
		AT × 4	16
Evans et al. 2005[77]	363	AC × 6	16 (24)
		AD × 6	12 (21)
Gianni et al. 2005[19]	451	AT × 4, CMF × 4	23
Green et al. 2005[78]	258	T Q3W × 4, FAC × 4	15.7
		T QW × 12 − FAC × 4	28.2
von Minckwitz et al. 2005 (GeparDuo)[79]	913	AD	11
		AC-D	22.3
Steger et al. 2007[80]	288	ED × 3	7.7
		ED × 6	18.6
Rastogi et al. 2008 (NSABP-B27)[55]	2411	AC	9.6 (13.7)
		AC-D	18.9 (26.1)
von Minckwitz et al. 2008 (GeparTrio)[65]	622	DAC × 6	5.3
		DAC × 2 -NX × 4	6
von Minckwitz et al. 2008[65] (GeparTrio)	1390	DAC × 6	21 v
		DAC × 8	23.5
von Minckwitz et al. 2010[81] (GeparQuatro)	1590	EC × 4, D × 4	22.3
		EC × 4, DX × 4	19.5
		EC × 4, D × 4, X × 4	22.3

Results of pCR in the breast only are in parenthesis. All the other results represent pCR in the breast and axillary lymph nodes.

A, Adriamycin; *C*, cyclophosphamide; *CVAP*, cyclophosphamide/vincristine/doxorubicin/prednisone; *D*, docetaxel; *DAC*, aka TAC (docetaxel/doxorubicin/cyclophosphamide); *E*, epirubicin; *F*, fluorouracil; *T*, paclitaxel; *X*, capecitabine.

improvement of pCR with dose dense but as expected, no impact on overall survival.[89]

Considering the heterogeneity of breast cancer, there is no single optimal chemotherapy regimen for all subtypes of this disease. Two schedules have been used to deliver chemotherapy; the first is the sandwich schedule in which patients receive some of the chemotherapy before and some after surgery, and the total preoperative schedule in which all the treatment cycles are given before surgery; the latter is considered the preferred modality to test the efficacy of the whole regimen and assess its impact on pCR.

Subset analyses of neoadjuvant chemotherapy trials showed unambiguously the low rates of pCRs in HR-positive breast cancer.[64,90] Patients with HR-positive breast cancer and those who cannot take chemotherapy may be offered neoadjuvant endocrine therapy. However, this modality (AIs and selective estrogen receptor modulators) results in much lower pCR rates compared with chemotherapy (pCR <2% and 15%–25%, respectively) and its effects are slower than the ones obtained with chemotherapy.[68,73,91,92]

Targeted Therapy

Anti-HER2 Therapy

The identification of HER2 as a major driver in breast cancer and the development of a monoclonal antibody (trastuzumab) that can specifically block it ushered in a new era in targeted therapy for breast cancer. Several small trials using trastuzumab in combination with chemotherapy in the neoadjuvant setting showed magnitudes of pCR, unseen before with chemotherapy alone[93–104] (Table 65.3). The high pCRs were achieved with the combination of trastuzumab and various chemotherapy regimens, but the optimal combination remains to be defined. Combinations of trastuzumab with anthracyclines were considered dangerous based on cardiac toxicity observed in the metastatic setting. Trastuzumab and different anthracycline (epirubicin) or novel formulations of doxorubicin (liposomal doxorubicin, pegylated or not) were also tested.[105–108] However, the lack of long-term safety data suggest that it is premature to use these combinations outside of the context of clinical trials (see Table 65.3). The GeparQuatro is a large neoadjuvant trial that enrolled 445 patients who received epirubicin/cyclophosphamide with trastuzumab followed by docetaxel with trastuzumab with or without capecitabine. The addition of trastuzumab led to 16% increment in pCR from 15.7% in historical control and HER2-negative cases to 31.7% in HER2-positive patients who received the drug. Buzdar and colleagues reinvestigated the role of concurrent administration of trastuzumab and anthracyclines in a phase III trial.[109] Concurrent administration of trastuzumab (T) and epirubicin (paclitaxel(P)/T followed by FEC-T vs. FEC followed by PT) resulted in no improvement of pCR, 56.5% (95% CI 47.8–64.9) vs. 54.2% (95% CI 45.7–62.6), respectively and additional cardiac toxicity in the concurrent arm as assessed at 12 weeks (2.9% vs. 0.8%, respectively). The authors concluded that concurrent use of trastuzumab and anthracyclines is not warranted. The HannaH trial explored the role of a subcutaneous (SQ) formulation of trastuzumab in a large phase III trial in patients with HER2-positive, operable, locally advanced or inflammatory breast cancer.[110] In this trial, patients were randomized to receive FEC × 4 − docetaxel × 4 with intravenous (IV; n = 299) or SQ trastuzumab (n = 297). Although the SQ arm pCR was not statistically inferior to the IV arm (40.7% vs. 45.4%, respectively), there was excess toxicity in the SQ arm.

A new generation of large trials explored the impact of adding trastuzumab to other anti-HER2 therapies such as the tyrosine kinase inhibitor lapatinib (Tykerb) or the anti-HER2 dimerization monoclonal antibody pertuzumab on pCR. The NeoALTTO trial is a large trial that explored the role of a combination of trastuzumab and lapatinib. The trial enrolled 455 patients who were equally divided between three arms: lapatinib (oral), trastuzumab (IV), or the combination, all given for 6 weeks followed by the addition of weekly paclitaxel for 12 weeks. After 4 weeks of rest the patients were taken to surgery, and all patients resumed their assigned anti-HER2 treatment for an additional period of 34 weeks.[111] There was no difference in pCR between the single agent arms (29.5% and 24.7% for the trastuzumab and lapatinib, respectively; *p* = .34), but pCR in the combination arm was

TABLE 65.3   Clinical Trials With HER2 Targeted Therapy

Trial	Patients N/Types	Regimen	Control	pCR Definition	pCR
Burstein et al. 2003[94]	40 HER2-positive (2+ or 3+ by IHC) stage II or III	T (4 mg/kg × 1, then 2 mg/kg/w × 11) with P (175 mg/m² Q 3 wk × 4)	None		18%
Buzdar et al. 2007[96]	42 (+22): Control 19 Chemo + T 23 (additional cohort 22) HER2-positive Stage II or IIIA	P Q 3 wk × 4: 225 mg/m² as a 24-h infusion plus T → FEC Q 3 wk × 4: F 500 mg/m² on day 1 and 4, C 500 mg/m² IV, day 1 and E 75 mg/m² day 1 plus T	P × 4 → FEC × 4	ypT0/is	Control 26.3% Chemo + T 23: 65.2% All 45: 60%
Sikov et al. 2009[102]	55 HER2-negative (37) and HER2+ (18) Stage IIA–IIIB	Carbo AUC 6 Q 4 wk P 80 mg/m² Q wk × 16 and T Q wk × 16 (only for HER2+)	Carbo AUC6 Q 4 wk P 80 mg/m2 Q wk × 16 for HER2–		HER– 31% HER2+ 76%
Untch et al. 2010 GeparQuattro[98]	1509 HER + or – HER2+ 445 Stages I–III	EC (90/600 mg/m²) Q 3 wk × 4 → D 100 mg/m² Q 3 wk × 4 (EC-T), *or* D 75 mg/m² plus X 1800 mg/m² Q 3 wk × 4 (EC-TX), or D 75 mg/m² Q 3 wk × 4 followed by X 1800 mg/m² days 1–14 Q 3 wk × 4 (EC-T-X). T 6 mg/kg (after loading dose of 8 mg/kg) Q 3 wk during all chemotherapy (8 or 12 cycles)	EC (90/600 mg/m²) Q 3 wk × 4 → D 100 mg/m² Q 3 wk × 4 (EC-T), OR D 75 mg/m² plus X 1800 mg/m² Q 3 wk × 4 (EC-TX), or D 75 mg/m² Q 3 wk × 4 followed by × 1,800 mg/m² days–14 Q 3 wk × 4 (EC-T-X)	ypT0/is, ypN0	HER2– 17.3% HER2+ 42%
Pierga et al. 2010[101]	340 HER2+ 120 Stage II and III	EC-D (E 75 mg/m², C 750 mg/m² Q 3 wk × 4 followed by D 100 mg/m² Q 3 wk × 4 T 8 mg/kg then 6 mg/kg IV Q 3 wk × 4 with D	EC-D (E 75 mg/m², C 750 mg/m² Q 3 wk × 4 followed by D 100 mg/m² Q 3 wk × 4	Chevallier classification grade 1 + 2 (= to ypT0/is, ypN0)	Control 19% Chemo + T 26%
Ismael et al. 2012; The HannaH study[110]		SQ D 75 mg/m² Q 3 wk × 4 → F 500 mg/m², E 75 mg/m², and C 500 mg/m² Q 3 wk × 4 Plus 600 mg fixed dose subcutaneous Q 3 wk × 8	IV D 75 mg/m² plus T 6 mg/kg (after loading dose of 8 mg/kg) Q 3 wk × 4 → F 500 mg/m², E 75 mg/m², and C 500 mg/m² plus T 6 mg/kg Q 3 wk × 4	ypT0/is, ypN0	SQ 40.7% IV 45.4%
Buzdar et al. 2013[109]	282 Concurrent 140 Sequential 142 HER2+ Stage II or IIIA	Concurrent P Q 1 wk × 12: 80 mg/m² plus T 2 mg/kg (after cycle 1 of 4 mg/kg) → FEC Q 3 wk × 4: F 500 mg/m² on days 1 and 4, C 500 mg/m² IV, day 1 and E 75 mg/m² day 1 plus T 2 mg/kg Q 1 wk × 12	Sequentil FEC Q 3 wk × 4: F 500 mg/m² on days 1 and 4, C 500 mg/m² IV, day 1 and E 75 mg/m² day 1 → P Q wk × 12: 80 mg/m² plus T 2 mg/kg (after cycle 1 of 4 mg/kg)	ypT0/is, ypN0	Concurrent 46.3% Sequential 48.3%

Continued

TABLE 65.3 Clinical Trials With HER2 Targeted Therap—cont'd

Trial	Patients N/Types	Regimen	Control	pCR Definition	pCR
Gianni et al. 2014; NOAH[100]	235	T 6 mg/kg Q 3 wk × 7, Q 4 wk × 3 (including a loading dose of 8 mg/kg) plus P150 mg/m² plus A 60 mg/m² IV Q 3 wk × 3, followed by P 175 mg/m² Q 3 wk × 4 followed by C 600 mg/m², M 40 mg/m², and F 600 mg/m² (on day 1, 8) Q 4 wk × 3 followed T 6 mg/kg Q 3 wk for up to 1 year	P 150 mg/m² plus A 60 mg/m² IV Q 3 wk × 3, followed by P 175 mg/m² Q 3 wk × 4 followed by C 600 mg/m², M 40 mg/m², and F 600 mg/m² (on days 1 and 8) Q 4 wk × 3	ypT0/is, ypN0	Control chemo 19.4% Chemo + T 38.4%
Chumsri et al. 2010[103]	33 Chemo: 14 Chemo + T: 19 Stage II and III HER2+	AC/P with T	AC/P without T	ypT0/is, ypN0 (?)	Chemo 28.6% Chemo + T 52.6%
Saracchini et al. 2013[104]	43 (39 evaluable) Stage II and III	NPLD (60 mg/mq IV) plus C 600 mg/m² IV Q 3 wk × 4 followed by D (35 mg/m² IV) plus T (4 mg/kg loading dose IV, then 2 mg/kg IV) Q 1 wk × 16	None	ypT0/is, ypN0	49%
Gavilá et al. 2015[106]	62 Stage II and III and inflammatory BC	TLC-D99 (50 mg/m²) day 1 Q 3 wk × 6, P (80 mg/m²) day 1 Q 1 wk × 18 and T (4 mg/kg as initial dose on day 1 and then 2 mg/kg Q 1 wk × 18	None	ypT0/is, ypN0	63%
Uriarte-Pinto et al. 2016[105]	30 HER2+ receptor and clinical stage IIa–IIIb	TLC-D99 (50 mg/m² on day 1 Q 3 wk), P (80 mg/m² Q 1 wk × 3) and T (8 mg/kg loading dose on day 1 followed by 6 mg/kg Q 3 wk)	None	Miller and Payne classification Grade 5 = ypT0/is, ypN0	40%

A, Doxorubicin; *AUC*, area under the curve; *C*, cyclophosphamide; *Carb*, carboplatin; *CX*, Capecitabine; *D*, docetaxel; *E*, Epirubicin; *F*, fluorouracil; *IV*, intravenous; *M*, Methotrexate; *P*, paclitaxel; *Q*, every; *T*, Trastuzumab; *TLC-D99*, nonpegylated liposomal-encapsulated doxorubicin.

significantly superior to the trastuzumab arm (51.3% vs. 29.5%; *p* = .0001). EFS was not different between arms (78%, 76%, and 84% for the lapatinib, trastuzumab, and the combination, respectively),[112] nor was overall survival at 3.84 years follow-up (93%, 90%, and 95% for the lapatinib, trastuzumab, and combination, respectively).[112] Further analysis of the results of this study showed that high HER2 protein expression correlated with increased benefit of adding lapatinib to trastuzumab, contrary to previous findings from the metastatic setting that correlated the benefit from lapatinib with p95HER2 (the truncated form of HER2).[113]

The NeoSphere trial is a phase II neoadjuvant trial that randomized HER2-positive breast cancer patients to one of four treatment arms: trastuzumab plus docetaxel (group A), pertuzumab plus trastuzumab plus docetaxel (group B), pertuzumab plus trastuzumab (group C), and finally pertuzumab plus docetaxel (group D); all treatments were given for four cycles at 3-week intervals. After surgery, all patients received three cycles of FEC and trastuzumab every 3 weeks for a total of 1 year.[60,114] pCR with the combination of trastuzumab/pertuzumab and docetaxel (group B) was 45.8%, significantly superior to the other groups (A; 29%; D: 24%; *p* = .0141). Ten to seventeen percent of patients on the A, B, and D arms had serious adverse events (neutropenia, febrile neutropenia, and leukopenia). Interestingly, group C, which received the biologically targeted agents without chemotherapy, had a pCR rate of 16.8% and only 4% of the patients in this group experienced serious adverse event. Five-year PFS was 81% for group A, 86% for group B, 73% for group C, and 73% for group D (hazard ratios 0.69 [95% CI 0.34–1.40] group B vs. group A; 1.25 [0.68–2.30] group C vs. group A; and 2.05 [1.07–3.93] group D vs. group B). DFS results were consistent with progression-free survival results and were 81% for group A, 84% for group B, 80% for group C, and 75% for group D.

Again, the value of achieving pCR was confirmed by this study with patients who achieved pCR having longer DFS compared with patients who did not (85% vs. 76%; hazard ratio 0.54 [95% CI 0.29–1.00]).[114]

In the TRYPHENA study, a multicenter, open-label phase II study, 225 HER2-positive breast cancer patients were randomized to two anthracycline-containing regimens: FEC/HP × 3 followed by docetaxel/HP for three cycles (arm A) or FEC for three cycles followed by docetaxel/HP for three cycles (arm B) or to a non–anthracycline-containing regimen: docetaxel/carboplatin and HP for six cycles (arm C). pCR (ypT0/is) was seen in 61.6% (arm A), 57.3% (arm B), and 66.2% (arm C) of patients.[115]

Antiangiogenic Therapy

The role of antiangiogenic therapy in the treatment of breast cancer remains controversial. After initial approval of bevacizumab, an anti–vascular endothelial growth factor (VEGF) monoclonal antibody, for the treatment of metastatic breast cancer in 2008 after the presentation of the results of E2100 the FDA decided to withdraw its approval in 2010 after the results of other trials did not confirm E2100 results.[116,117] The question of a possible role for the anti-VEGF bevacizumab at an earlier stage of breast cancer was tested in two large clinical studies using a combination of bevacizumab and different neoadjuvant chemotherapies, the NSABP B-40 and GeparQuinto.[118,119] Both clinical trials showed improved pCR, but interestingly, the group more likely to respond was different on each trial. The NSABP B-40 showed that effect of the addition of bevacizumab to chemotherapy (pCR 34.5% vs. 28.2%; $p = .02$) was more significant in the HR-positive disease. On the other hand, the GeparQuinto was also positive with smaller but statistically significant effect (pCR 24.6% with bevacizumab vs. 20.6% without bevacizumab; $p = .04$), but the group more likely to respond was the HR-negative breast cancer. Several phase II and phase III studies were published with a predominant effect of bevacizumab in TNBC.

Cao and colleagues (2015) and Ma and colleagues (2016) performed two meta-analyses of published trials.[120,121] Cao reviewed nine randomized controlled trials (RCTs) that enrolled a total of 4967 patients randomized on 1 : 1 ratio to bevacizumab plus chemotherapy or chemotherapy alone. The addition of bevacizumab to NACT increased the pCR rate (odds ratio [OR] = 1.34 [95% CI 1.18–1.54]; $p < .0001$) compared with chemotherapy alone. The effect of bevacizumab was more pronounced in patients with HER2-negative breast cancer (OR = 1.34 [95% CI 1.17–1.54]; $p < .0001$) and HR-negative cancer (OR = 1.38 [95% CI 1.09–1.74]; $p = .007$) compared with HER2-positive and HR-positive cancer. Additionally, the incidence of neutropenia, febrile neutropenia, and hand–foot syndrome was higher in patients who received bevacizumab.[120] Ma and colleagues reported in their meta-analysis on seven RCT and 5408 patients. Their results are consistent with Cao's results and conclude that the pooled OR for pCR was 1.48 [95% CI 1.23–1.78], $p < .0001$, in favor of bevacizumab administration.[121]

The mechanisms of action and predictive factors for response to bevacizumab remain under intense investigation. The mechanism of action of bevacizumab was postulated to be related either to collapsed blood vessels due to VEGF deprivation, which leads to tumor necrosis, or to normalization of blood vessels with the consequent delivery of higher concentration of chemotherapy to the tumor because the drug is not effective without combination with chemotherapy. Most neoadjuvant trials highlighted the exquisite sensitivity of TNBC. This subtype of breast cancer is characterized by high proliferation rate and active angiogenesis. Recent translational studies have shown the importance of increased microvessel density in predicting response to bevacizumab.[122] Other studies suggested that the more dependent the tumor on VEGF pathway, the more sensitive it would be to the effect of bevacizumab. Dependence on VEGF pathway is difficult to prove, but activation of rescue pathways may suggest the possibility of lack of dependence on VEGF pathway and hence lack of sensitivity to bevacizumab and vice versa.[123]

Neoadjuvant Radiation Therapy for Breast Cancer

The standard of care for radiation is to be delivered postoperatively (Box 65.2). In certain instances, patients with LABC that receive NACT may continue to have inoperable disease. In these cases, or neoadjuvant RT (NRT) may be added to improve local control to make the disease resectable or as a definitive treatment modality. Sometimes the combination of NRT and NACT is delivered preoperatively to achieve these goals.

Early RT/chemotherapy combination trials in the adjuvant setting with CMF showed improvement of local control and limited toxicity, but the effect of the combination on DFS and OS was not consistently shown.[124–126] As anthracyclines (doxorubicin,

---

• Box 65.2 Definitions for Response Evaluation

Clinical
- Partial: reduction of tumor area to ≤50% (cPR)
- Complete: no palpable mass detectable (cCR)

Imaging
- No tumor visible by mammography, ultrasound or magnetic resonance imaging (iCR)

Pathologic
- American Joint Committee on Cancer classification system
  - Only focal invasive tumor residuals in breast tissue (pPRinv)
  - Only in situ tumor residuals in breast tissue (pCRis, ypT0is)
  - No invasive or in situ tumor cells in breast tissue (pCR, ypT0)
  - No malignant tumor cells in breast tissue and lymph nodes (pCR breast and lymph nodes, ypT0, N0)

Miller and Payne Classification System
- Primary site response
  - Grade 1: Some alteration to individual malignant cells but no reduction in overall numbers compared with the pretreatment core biopsy
  - Grade 2: A minor loss of invasive tumor cells but overall cellularity still high
  - Grade 3: A moderate reduction in tumor cells up to an estimated 90% loss
  - Grade 4: A marked disappearance of invasive tumor cells such that only small clusters of widely dispersed cells could be detected
  - Grade 5: No invasive tumor, i.e., only in situ disease or tumor stroma remained
- Axillary lymph node response
  A: True axillary node negative
  B: Axillary node positive and no therapeutic effects
  C: Axillary node positive but evidence of partial pathologic response
  D: Initially axillary node positive but converted to node negative after primary systemic therapy

mitoxantrone, and epirubicin) were being introduced into the treatment of breast cancer, several trials using these agents in combination with RT were designed in the adjuvant setting.[127,128] Collectively, these studies showed improvement of local control with the combination but at the cost of increased skin toxicity, including recall reactions, and cardiac toxicity and, again, no improvement of DFS or OS compared with the sequential use of RT and chemotherapy. Finally, the combinations of taxanes and RT were also tested and found to improve local control but also to induce significant skin and pulmonary toxicity regardless of the schedule used (weekly or every 3 weeks).[129–133]

NRT alone or in combination with NACT have been investigated in patients with locally advanced breast cancer and in operable disease. Calitchi and colleagues investigated NRT alone as a preoperative single modality. Seventy-five patients were treated with NRT because breast conservation surgery was not feasible due to T2 and T3 disease. Eleven percent (11%) of patients achieved pCR and nine recurrences (12%) were observed on follow-up. In regard to cosmesis and late complications, 6% of patients had poor results.[134]

The concurrent use of chemotherapy as a radio-sensitizer in LABC has been tested but has not been accepted as a standard treatment modality due to toxicity and cosmesis concerns. Many agents were tested in this setting. 5-Fluorouracil and capecitabine were shown to potentiate the effect of NRT with acceptable toxicity, but their activity was modest.[135–137] Taxanes were used in different regimens, but the optimal schedule and dose are yet to be defined. The major issues with taxanes when used in combination with NRT are their toxicities that include skin reactions, pneumonitis, and postoperative complications.[138,139] Formenti and colleagues performed a phase I/II trial investigating the feasibility of NACT with twice-weekly paclitaxel and radiation given concurrently in LABC. Skin toxicity was seen in 7% of patients and 16% of patients had pCR after mastectomy and axillary lymph node dissection.[139] Skinner and colleagues conducted similar study using the weekly paclitaxel and radiation.[138] Forty-one percent (41%) of their patients experienced postoperative complications and 33% achieved pCR. In a larger study using the same taxane-based combination and schedule, Adams and colleagues reported a 23% pCR rate.[140]

The role of sequential chemotherapy followed by radiation then chemotherapy (sandwich neoadjuvant therapy) before surgery was also explored. Lerouge and coworkers studied prospectively NACT followed by NRT in noninflammatory LABC. Twenty percent of patients reached pCR. Low local failure rates were observed in patients without initial extensive nodal disease who responded to neoadjuvant therapy in the axilla and underwent mastectomy. High local failure rates were observed in patients with partial tumor response and those who underwent breast conservation therapy.[141] In another study by Jacquillat and colleagues using similar design (with different chemotherapy agents) in all stages of 250 breast cancer patients, the investigators identified tumor size and nodal status as major predicators of response and long-term DFS and OS.[142]

There are limited prospective data on the role of NRT in early-stage breast cancer. Accelerated partial breast irradiation (APBI) is a short course of radiation that can be completed within a week. APBI delivers radiation to the postoperative tumor bed. The advantage of APBI neoadjuvantly would be that a smaller volume would be treated compared with the postoperative tumor bed thus potentially minimizing acute and late complications. Van der Leij and coworkers performed a multicenter phase II trial studying preoperative APBI. Interim analysis of the first 70 patients showed limited fibrosis in a small volume and good to excellent outcome. Two patients had ipsilateral breast recurrences outside of the radiation field.[143]

The significance of achieving pCR with NRT or with the combination of NACT and NRT is not clear. Radiation therapy is considered a locoregional modality, and it is not clear that increasing local response would translate into systemic and long-term benefit. In the adjuvant setting, a large meta-analysis by the Early Breast Cancer Trialists' Collaborative Group (EBCTCG) showed that RT reduced local recurrence and improved long-term breast cancer survival in patients who had mastectomy and axillary dissection with one to three positive lymph nodes even when systemic therapy was given.[144] There may be a future role for NRT in the treatment of early and locally advanced breast cancer. As the use of neoadjuvant chemotherapy continues to expand, it is important to further study the addition of radiation to neoadjuvant therapy.

Response Assessment After Neoadjuvant Chemotherapy

Response assessment after NACT and the magnitude of residual disease will help decide on the best surgical option (Table 65.4).[145–149] The correlation between post-NACT pathologic response and clinical examination ($r = .42–.43$), ultrasonography ($r = .42–.612$), and mammography ($r = .41$) were mild to moderate. MRI resulted in much better correlations with post-NACT pathologic response ($r = .749–.896$).[150–153] MRI tend to provide much better assessment of the residual tumor compared with physical examination and ultrasonography that tend to overestimate the response to NACT.[152]

The predictive value of MRI depends on tumor biology and the type of chemotherapy. After NACT, the MRI predictive value of pCR is 95% and 50% in HER2-positive and HER2-negative breast cancer, respectively.[51] Epirubicin-based chemotherapy interacts positively, whereas docetaxel-based chemotherapy interacts negatively with the accuracy of MRI in predicting pCR.[154] To increase predictive value dynamic enhanced-contrast MRI (DCE-MRI) was tested.[155] Straver and coworkers showed that the positive and negative predictive values of post-NACT MRI were 90% and 44%, respectively. The risk of underestimating tumor size by more than 20 mm remained high leading to unjustified BCS in 13%. A predictive model using features from a multivariate analysis included tumors less than 30 mm on post-NACT MRI, the largest diameter of late enhancement on pre-NACT MRI, the reduction in tumor size after NACT and HR and HER2 status. The model had good predictive power, but it needed validation.

Surgical Management After Neoadjuvant Chemotherapy

Multiple factors help determine the most appropriate type of surgery, BCS versus mastectomy, after NACT. Anatomic factors include the extent of the disease before and the pathologic residual disease after NACT, multicentricity, the presence of DCIS, and the ability to achieve negative margins with good cosmesis.[40] Other factors include eligibility for RT, biological features of the tumor, and the patient's wishes.

TABLE 65.4 Neoadjuvant RT or RT and CT in Breast Cancer

	N	Stage	CT	RT Gy	AEs	cRR	pCR	MY/BCS
Kosma et al., 1997[136]	17	II–III, after failure of CT	F 500 mg/m^2 × 2/wk	75–90	P, G2 1 S, G2 1 PC, 1	70%	18%	3/0
Skinner et al., 2000[138]	29	IIB–III	Paclitaxel 30 mg/m^2 × 2/wk × 8 wk	45	PO, 41%	89%	33%	
Aryus et al., 2000[145]	73	LABC						29/45
	18		EC				6%	
	55		EC → CMF + RT	50			43%	
Calitchi et al., 2001[134]	74	II–III	—	45			11%	3/72
Formenti et al., 2003[146]	44	II–III	Paclitaxel 30 mg/m^2 × 2/wk		S, G3 7%	91%	16%	41/2
Lerouge et al., 2004[141]	120	IIIA–C						49/71
Kao et al., 2005[147]	16	IIIB–C	Bolus infusion vinorelbine (20 mg/m^2 day 1) plus CI (20–30 mg/m^2 QD × 4 days)	60–70	S, 8 H, 3	87.5%	44%	13/2
Bollet et al., 2006[148]	60	II–III	F 500 mg/m^2 QD days 1–5, and vinorelbine 25 mg/m^2 days 1 and 6		H, G4 22%		27%	18/41
Chakravarthy et al., 2006[149]	38	IIA–B, IIIA–B	Paclitaxel 30 mg/m^2 × 2/wk	45 + 14	S, G3 1 Fa, G3 3 LFT, G3 3 PO, 34		34%	21/16
Gaui et al., 2007[137]	28	IIB, IIIA, B, C, D After failure of anthracycline-based NACT	Capecitabine 850 mg/m^2 for 14 days	50	S, G2 3 PO, 1	25%	3.5%	23/0
Adams et al. 2010[140]	105	IIB–IIIC	Paclitaxel 30 mg/m^2 × 2/wk	45			23%	
van der Leij et al., 2015[143]	70	I and II	—	50 POPBI	S, G2, 1 PO, 11			1/68

AEs, Adverse events; *BCS*, breast conserving surgery; *C*, cardiac toxicity; *CT*, chemotherapy; *F*, fluorouracil; *Fa*, fatigue; *G*, grade; *H*, hematologic toxicity; *LABC*, locally advanced breast cancer; *LFT*, liver function tests abnormality; *MY*, mastectomy; *NACT*, neoadjuvant chemotherapy; *P*, pneumonitis; *PC*, pericarditis; *PO*, postoperative complications; *POPBI*, preoperative partial breast irradiation; *QD*, daily; *RT*, radiation therapy; *S*, skin toxicity.

In the absence of an accurate method to detect minimal residual disease, surgical removal of the tumor bed with all residual cancer to achieve negative margins and lymph node staging should be offered to every patient. A meta-analysis of nine randomized trials totaling 3946 patients and comparing NACT to ACT showed no statistically significant difference in survival, disease progression, or distant recurrence rates between patients who received NACT and those who received ACT.[9] However, the risk of locoregional recurrence (LRR) rate was higher with neoadjuvant therapy (LRR = 1.22; 95% CI = 1.04–1.43), especially if surgery was omitted in favor of RT (LRR = 1.53; 95% CI = 1.11–2.10). The uncertainty surrounding margin definition[156] and the volume to resect after NACT (the original volume vs. the post-NACT volume) are responsible for the limited effect of NACT on the rate of BCS. One-quarter of the patients deemed to need mastectomy before NACT ended up undergoing BCS after NACT on two large randomized trials (27% and 23% on the NSABP B-18 and European Organisation for Research and Treatment of Cancer 10902, respectively).[8,157] However, a meta-analysis that included 14 randomized NACT studies with a large total sample size of 5500 patients showed that BCS was performed only in 16.6% of patients who were initially eligible for mastectomy.[158]

Patterns of tumor shrinkage influence the decision to perform BCS or mastectomy. Concentric shrinkage lends itself more frequently to limited surgery with negative margins than the honeycomb shrinkage where limited resection is less likely to achieve clear margins as the tumor remains scattered over the same area as the original volume. Biological factors that determine the concentric pattern are high grade, ER negativity, HER2 positivity, and invasive ductal carcinoma.[22] High residual cellularity after NACT (defined as >5% of tumor area composed of invasive tumor cells) was seen in 74.7% and low residual cellularity (≤5% of tumor area composed of invasive tumor cells) in 25.3% of 396 patients who underwent NACT. Interestingly, intraoperative false-negative margin rate in patients with low residual cellularity was almost twice as high as in the group with high residual cellularity (23% vs. 13.8%), but the difference was not statistically significant (p = .210).[159] When patients are selected properly 5-year LRR and ipsilateral breast tumor recurrence (IBTR) in patients treated with BCS after NACT were 7% to 9%, and 4% to 5%, respectively.[160,161]

Several factors have been used to predict local recurrence, but there is no agreement on their nature. Beriwal and colleagues identified advanced nodal involvement at diagnosis, multifocal residual disease, residual tumor larger than 2 cm, and lymphovascular space invasion as predictors of LRR and IBTR,[160] whereas Chen and coworkers found that positive margins and advanced stage at diagnosis were the most important predictors for LRR.[161] Garimella and coworkers, on the other hand, found that vascular invasion was associated with overall recurrence but none of the factors identified by Beriwal and colleagues was associated with LRR.[162] The prognostic index score developed by the MD Anderson Cancer Center group (MDAPI) is based on these four features (pathologic, multifocal residual disease, residual pathologic primary size >2 cm, lymphovascular invasion, and the presence of clinical N2/N3 nodes). The MDAPI ranges from 0 to 4. In the retrospective study that done to develop the MDAPI, data from 815 patients who received neoadjuvant chemotherapy, surgery, and radiation were analyzed. Patients with low MDAPI of 0 or 1 had very low 10-year LRR rates that were not different between the mastectomy and BCS groups. Patients with a score of 3 to 4, LRR was significantly lower for those treated with mastectomy versus BCS (19% vs. 61%, p = .009).[163] The MDAPI was validated in an independent cohort of 551 patients by the same group.[164] Several attempts were made by other groups to validate this score. Some (smaller) studies showed similar findings for the size of residual tumor and N2 and N3 lymph node involvement,[165,166] whereas others have not been able to validate the MDAPI and identified ER status and multicentricity[167] or advanced stage at presentation, poor response to therapy, and LVI to be the most important predictors of LRR.[168]

Physical examination, mammography, ultrasound, and MRI are used for response assessment to guide surgical options. Physical examination tends to underestimate and mammography, US, and MRI tend to overestimate the size of residual tumors. However, MRI measurements appear to be the closest to pathologic measurements. Reasons for overestimating the size of residual tumor by MRI are reactive inflammation, fibrosis, or necrosis; DCIS; imaging artifacts; and partial volume effects.[169] Overestimation of residual tumor may lead to more radical surgery, whereas underestimation of residual tumor may lead to positive margins with increased risk of LRR. False-negative rate (FNR) used to be high with traditional MRI, which may also lead to increased risk of LRR if the patients undergo BCS.[152,153,170–172] Modern MRI scanners have resulted in significant improvement of MRI assessments of residual tumors. A recent meta-analysis of 19 studies totaling 958 patients evaluated the agreement between MRI, US, mammography, physical examination, and pathologic breast tumor size after NACT. MRI and US showed the lowest mean differences (MDs) in tumor size (MD: 0.1 cm) compared with pathologic tumor measurements. The overestimation of residual tumor size by mammography is much higher with MD of 0.4 cm. The underestimation by physical examination is also significant with MD at 0.3 cm.[169] A multifactorial MRI predictive model was developed and if validated will help triage patients who would benefit from BCS.[155]

Patients with IBC and those with large and multicentric disease on presentation should have mastectomy after NACT even if they had an excellent response to the treatment.[40]

Staging the Axilla and Sentinel Lymph Node Procedure

There is no unanimity regarding the best timing of sentinel lymph node biopsy (SLNB) relative to NACT. In clinical N0 disease, it can be performed either before or after NACT. The information obtained about the lymph node status if SLNB is performed before NACT helps design subsequent radiation and chemotherapy. If it is done after NACT, it provides information about the sensitivity to NACT. If the sentinel nodes are cancer free, full axillary lymph node dissection will not be necessary. Older studies of SLNB after NACT showed that SLN was identified in 85% to 90% of cases with FNRs that may range between 11% and 12%.[2,173–175] However, if lymph nodes are clinically positive, axillary lymph node dissection (ALND) remains the standard of care because only 40% may convert to node negative after anthracycline and taxane NACT, and the FNR is high, which precludes forgoing ALND.[175–177]

The timing of the SLNB relative to NACT has not been defined with certainty. The SENTINA (SENTInel NeoAdjuvant) trial is a large multicenter four-arm trial that enrolled 1737 patients who underwent NACT.[178] Patients who had clinical N0 breast cancer underwent SLNB before NACT. Patients with pN0 did not receive any further treatment to the axilla at the time of surgery after NACT (arm A), whereas those with N+ underwent a second SLNB at the time of the final surgery (arm B). Patients who had clinically positive lymph nodes were treated with NACT, and if they converted to clinical N0, they received SLNB and axillary lymph node dissection (arm C). Those who still had clinically positive axilla went directly to ALND. When the SLNB was performed before NACT, the sentinel lymph node was detected in 99.1% of the 1022 patients enrolled in arm A and B compared with 80.1% when the procedure was performed after NACT in patients who converted from cN+ to ycN− (arm C; 592 patients) with FNR of 14.2%. The FNR was higher when one lymph node was removed (24.3%) compared with two lymph nodes (18.5%). These results suggest that the best time to perform SLNB in patients with clinically negative axilla can be before or after NACT. However, if SLNB was performed before NACT and it was positive, SLNB after NACT has a low detection rate and high FNR, and the decision should be to proceed with ALND. Lee and colleagues had previously reached similar results.[179] However, the FNR in their study was low (at 5.6%) justifying their recommendation for SLNB before or after NACT.

ACOSOG Z1071 was designed to assess the FNR for SLNB after NACT in patients initially presenting with biopsy-proven clinically positive lymph nodes. Among the 663 evaluable and eligible patients, 649 underwent NACT followed by both SLNB and ALND with SLN identification rate (IR) of 92.9%. The SLN IR was 78.6% with blue dye alone; 91.4% with radiolabelled colloid. Patient factors (age, body mass index), tumor factors (clinical T or N stage), pathologic nodal response to chemotherapy, site of tracer injection, and length of chemotherapy treatment did not significantly affect the SLN identification rate.[180] Pathologic complete nodal response was of 41.0%. FNR was 12.6%, much higher than the threshold of 10% that the investigators considered safe to recommend SLNB after NACT.[181] Furthermore, FNR depended on the number of lymph nodes removed (31% if only one SLN was removed, 21.1% when two SLNs were examined and 9.1% when three or more SLNs were examined, p = .007) and the number of agents used for lymphatic mapping

(20% for isotope or dye alone and 10.8% for dual tracer). The American Society of Clinical Oncology (ASCO) clinical practice guideline update on SLNB for patients with early-stage breast cancer issued in 2014 stated that clinicians may offer the SLNB before or after NACT, although detection rate and accuracy of the procedure are decreased in post-NACT compared with pre-NACT.[182] In an attempt to decrease FNR, Boileau and colleagues improved the sensitivity of the SLNB by mandating the use of immunohistochemistry (IHC) and considering as positive any SN metastases of any size, including isolated tumor cells (ypN0[i+], ≤0.2 mm).[183] Using their method in 153 patients with biopsy-proven node-positive breast cancer, the authors showed SLN identification rate of 87.6% and the FNR of 8.4%. However, if SN ypN0(i+)s had been considered negative, the FNR would have increased to 13.3%. Using radioactive iodine seeds or clips to mark positive axillary lymph nodes before NACT was tried to increase detection rate and decrease FNR.[184,185] The identification rate in one study using radioactive iodine seeds was 97% and FNR was as low as 7%.[184] The National Comprehensive Cancer Network (NCCN) has recommended the use of a clip or radioactive seeds to mark positive LN before the initiation of NACT.[186]

The detection rate of the SLN on the SENTINA study was as low as 60.8% in patients who had a second SLNB after NACT with FNR at 51.6%. Patients with clinically N+ disease pre-NAT should be offered ALND even if they become cN− after NAT due to the high rate of false negativity with post-NAT SLNB. The ASCO Update Committee recommended against SLNB in patients with T4d/IBC who have received NACT due to the absence of safety data and in patients with T4abc due to insufficient safety data regardless of patients' clinical response.

Chemotherapy After Surgery

Until recently, there has been no evidence of benefit from additional chemotherapy in patients who do not achieve pCR. For example, MDAPI randomized patients who still had a residual tumor larger than 1 cm after NACT with three cycles of vincristine, doxorubicin, cyclophosphamide, and prednisone (VACP) to either a non–cross-resistant adjuvant therapy (five cycles of vinblastine, methotrexate with calcium leucovorin rescue, and fluorouracil [VbMF]) or to the same therapy. No significant difference in DFS and OS was achieved in patients who were randomized to the non–cross-resistant regimen.[187] There is no evidence that clinical response should be used to tailor subsequent treatment choices based on the results of the Aberdeen and the GeparTrio trials. The Aberdeen trial randomized patients who responded to four cycles of cyclophosphamide, vincristine, doxorubicin, and prednisone (CVAP) to receive either four cycles of the same regimen or four cycles of docetaxel. Nonresponders to four cycles of CVAP were switched to docetaxel. pCR doubled in responders who were switched to docetaxel (31% vs. 15%), whereas nonresponders had a modest pCR (2%) despite the addition of docetaxel.[65] The GeparTrio trial randomized nonresponders, defined as patients who did not achieve a decrease in size of their tumor by at least 50% after two cycles of docetaxel, doxorubicin, and cyclophosphamide (TAC), to four additional cycles of TAC or to four cycles of vinorelbine and capecitabine (NX).[66] Switching to NX did not improve pCR.

Toi and colleagues presented the results of their phase III study using capecitabine in breast cancer patients who had residual disease after NACT. The trial enrolled 910 HER2-negative breast cancer patients who received NACT that contained an anthracycline and/or a taxane followed by endocrine therapy as indicated. All patients had residual disease. Patients were randomly assigned to capecitabine or no additional therapy. Patients on the capecitabine arm (455) received eight 3-week cycles of capecitabine (1250 mg/m^2 twice a day for 2 weeks, followed by 1-week break). After a 2-year-follow up, patients who were assigned to capecitabine had a 31% decrease in their risk of recurrence compared with the no additional therapy arm. DFS was 87.3% for those assigned to capecitabine and 80.5% for those assigned to no additional therapy. Two-year median OS was 96.2% and 93.9% for the capecitabine and no additional therapy arms, respectively, but the difference was not statistically significant. Preliminary analysis suggested that the benefit is more pronounced in the HR-negative subtype.[188]

Radiation Therapy After Neoadjuvant Systemic Therapy

The role of RT in the adjuvant setting is established, but its role after NACT and surgery has not received as intense investigation as it did in the adjuvant setting. Patients who undergo BSC after NACT should receive adjuvant RT as per standard of care in the adjuvant setting. In this setting, RT decreases the risk of LRR and IBTR. The Early Breast Cancer Trialists Collaborative Group overview showed that for every four local recurrences, one breast cancer death is avoided at 15 years of follow-up.[188a] The radiation port should include the internal mammary lymph nodes only if they are involved. Women older than 70 years with hormone-sensitive stage I breast cancer may forgo RT and be offered tamoxifen after lumpectomy with excellent long-term results on local recurrence and survival.[189,190]

For those who undergo mastectomy, available guidelines suggest that decisions about RT should be based on maximal pre-NACT stage and tumor characteristics and/or postsurgical pathologic stage, regardless of response to NACT.[190a] It is clear that more clinical trials are needed to best address this question. The consensus statement released by the National Cancer Institute in 2008 suggested that RT after mastectomy after NACT should be offered to patients with clinical stage III disease (i.e., T4, N2–N3, or T3N1) or ypN+ disease.[40]

Despite methodologic limitations, important information may be derived from retrospective reviews on this question. Six consecutive neoadjuvant trials at the MD Anderson Cancer Center were reviewed by Huang and colleagues. The outcome of 542 patients who received RT after anthracycline-based chemotherapy and mastectomy with level I/II node dissection was compared with 134 patients' who received the same surgery and NACT but without RT. Actuarial LRR at 10 years was reduced from 22% to 11% (p = .0001) with the use of RT. The RT group enjoyed improved cancer-specific survival as well (hazard ratio for lack of radiation 2.0, 95% CI 1.4–2.9; p < .0001). Most of the benefit was seen in patients with pre-NACT, clinical T3 and T4 tumors, and post-NACT pathologic tumor size greater than 2 cm, or four or more positive lymph nodes. Achievement of pCR did not significantly affect survival but RT did.[191] On the basis of available evidence and expert opinion, Fowble and colleagues developed recommendations that classified patients into three risk groups based on the initial clinical stage, post-NACT pathologic stage, age, lymphovascular invasion, extracapsular extension, triple negativity, and number of involved lymph nodes. The low-risk group has a risk of locoregional failure of 10% or less, the intermediate risk group between 10 and less than 20%, and the high-risk group 20% or more. The authors suggest that the omission of RT for the low-risk group is reasonable and recommend it to those in the high-risk group. Recommendations for the intermediate-risk group are not clear.[192] Wright and coworkers reviewed the experience of the University of Miami on 464 patients who underwent NACT followed by mastectomy. Their conclusion was that pre-NACT stage, HR status, pathologic response to NACT, and omission of the supraclavicular field were significant risk factors for LRR in this setting.[193] However, Nagar and colleagues found that only post-NACT residual tumor and nodal status are predictive of LRR, not pretreatment staging. In their hands the risk of LRR was 16.1% without RT and dropped by 75% (hazard ratio 0.25) with RT. This improvement of LRR was also associated with improved 5-year DFS (91.3% vs. 64.8%).[194] This finding should be tempered by the finding reported by Huang and colleagues on their 33 patients with clinical stage III or higher who achieved pCR. Postmastectomy RT resulted in significant decrease in 10-year LRR (33% vs. 3%) and improved OS (33.3% vs. 77.3%).[191] Other investigators found that postmastectomy RT is not needed in patients who reached nodal pCR regardless of the pre-NACT clinical staging.[195,196]

It is clear that patients who present with N2 or N3 or stage T3 or T4 and those who are left with positive lymph nodes after NACT should be offered locoregional RT after mastectomy. Stage II patients (cT3, N0) who achieve pCR may forgo RT whereas those with stage II (T1–2, N1) who achieve nodal pCR, the answer is not clear, and enrollment in a clinical trial is an excellent decision if available.[197]

The NSABP B-51/RTOG (Radiation Therapy Oncology Group) 1304 phase III clinical trial (clinicaltrials.gov identifier NCT01872975; prospective randomized) and the RAPCHEM study (prospective, nonrandomized) are designed to answer whether regional radiotherapy improves local and systemic outcomes in patients with clinical N1 disease on presentation[198] (https://clinicaltrials.gov/ct2/show/NCT01279304). The NSABP51/RTOG 1308 trial randomizes patients with cT1–3 and pathologically proven N1 who achieve a nodal pCR after NACT and undergo mastectomy to either postmastectomy RT or no RT. In the RAPCHEM study patients with cT1–2 and/or pathologically proven N1 who receive NACT will undergo risk-adapted RT after surgery. No RT for patients who achieve nodal pCR after NACT.

The Neoadjuvant Setting for Research and Drug Development

In the past 3 to 4 decades, cancer drug development has been slow and extremely inefficient to bring new drugs to the clinic. Historically, the identification of potentially promising drugs from cell cultures and animal studies leads to the introduction of these drugs to patients in advanced metastatic stages. If successful, the drugs would be moved to early metastatic cancer, and if these trials show efficacy, it is only then that the drugs would be offered to patients in the adjuvant setting. Adjuvant trials require large number of patients (thousands) and run over many years for recruitment and follow-up to reach a conclusion about the final efficacy that is often modest. This process may take up to 2 decades and may cost between $1 and $2 billion per new drug.[199]

The discovery of breast cancer heterogeneity with specific markers linked to different subtypes allows the targeting of these subtypes more efficiently and by the same token may open the possibility to decrease the cost and time needed to validate new drugs. Progress in breast cancer screening resulted in the diagnosis of breast cancer at increasingly smaller sizes without necessarily decreasing the incidence of LABC that remains around 10% to 15% of all diagnoses and is responsible for a disproportionally large fraction of the mortality attributed to breast cancer.[200]

Taking advantage of the neoadjuvant setting and using pCR as a surrogate end point for long-term outcomes allows the rapid assessment of drug efficacy and quick transition from bench to bedside. Single arm and randomized multiple arm neoadjuvant studies were designed to accelerate this process. The design of these trials has changed over time from a blind pragmatic design to a new one informed by the biology of breast cancer and using a new statistical method called the Bayesian method.[201,202] The goal of this design is to obtain early information about treatment efficacy by modeling the relationship between pCR and baseline and longitudinal markers. Several profiles are established, and if their relationship to response is confirmed, they will be able to predict response to each drug. As the data accumulate over time, they instruct randomization to the arms in the trial by allocating the patients with a specific profile to the arm where maximal efficacy is noted. The I-SPY 2 trial is one of these modern adaptive designs.[203] The arms of the trials are designed based on biological characteristics: HR positive or negative, HER2 positive or negative, and two levels of MammaPrint scores. Drugs with high probability of being superior to standard treatment are graduated from the trial with their biological signature to be tested in small phase III trials. Drugs should have passed phase I safety studies and be of relevance to breast cancer. Two drugs have already been graduated and are being considered for phase III trials, neratinib in HER2-positive breast cancer, and veliparib in TNBC.[204,205]

Conclusion and Future Directions

Traditionally, neoadjuvant chemotherapy has been the standard of care for IBC and LABC. Recently its use for early-stage breast cancer has increased. When the same treatment is used in NACT and postoperatively, no difference in DFS and OS outcomes has been observed.

Absence of invasive tumor in the breast and axillary lymph nodes (not only in the breast) is the accepted definition of pCR by the FDA and the scientific community at large and is considered a valid end point to define efficacy of new drugs in future clinical trials for FDA approval; it is considered an appropriate surrogate end point for long-term survival especially in TNBC, HER2-positive, and high-grade HR-positive subtypes. pCR in low-grade HR-positive breast cancer does not correlate well with long-term DFS and OS. Future research should focus on the reasons for this finding and on new methods to increase pCR in the other subtypes where this end point is known to predict long-term survival.

Response should be assessed clinically and by imaging. Among the modern imaging methods currently in use, MRI is the most promising, but its lack of specificity precludes it from being the standard of care (when it shows complete response, up to 40% of patients may still have viable tumor in the breast or lymph nodes). Therefore, even if complete response is achieved by clinical or imaging methods, surgical resection is still indicated to complete local treatment. Future research should be directed toward finding a reliable method (new imaging technique, circulating DNA, or others) that is likely to detect minimal residual disease, or its absence thereof, with certainty. It is only then that patients may be able to forgo surgery.

In patients with clinically negative axilla, an SLN procedure can be performed before or after NACT. If it is performed before NACT and is found to be positive, ALND should be performed because of the low detection rate for a second SLNB. For patients with clinically positive axilla, ALND should be performed regardless of the response to NACT. Sampling three lymph nodes or more and using IHC on the lymph nodes may help decrease the risk of FNR to less than 10%, a threshold that is considered necessary to forgo ALND.

The rate of BCS is increased by approximately 25% after NACT. The achievement of negative margins is easier in TNBC and HER2-positive breast cancer due to their growth and shrinkage pattern, which is more often concentric. IBC and multicentric tumors will require mastectomy regardless of the response to NACT.

Considering the heterogeneity of the disease, there is no single optimal chemotherapy for all types of breast cancer. Combination regimens of dose-dense anthracyclines and taxanes used sequentially are superior to single-agent regimens. Non–anthracycline-containing regimens are frequently used today for HER2-positive breast cancer because of their lower cardiac toxicity and similar efficacy to the anthracycline-containing ones. Combination of biological HER2-targeted agents (trastuzumab and pertuzumab) with chemotherapy have improved both pCR and long-term DFS and OS in this subtype and have become standard of care. Targeting angiogenesis with bevacizumab continues being an area of investigation and results from large clinical trials are conflicting. The emerging consensus is that bevacizumab may be effective in the TNBC subtype of breast.

Progression on neoadjuvant chemotherapy is rare (<3%).[206] Nevertheless, frequent clinical assessment is required to detect the nonresponders and adjust surgical treatment plans. The use of NACT as "in vivo chemosensitivity test" has not been supported consistently by recent studies.

Indications for postsurgery RT are based on pretreatment stage and the pathologic results after surgery. This includes large tumors (T3, T4a–c), inflammatory breast cancer (T4d), persistent positive axillary lymph nodes, extranodal extension, and positive infraclavicular and supraclavicular and internal mammary lymph nodes.

Traditional clinical trial design has become obsolete because investigational agents are offered to all patients without consideration of the biological differences of their cancers; it requires a large number of patients and massive investment in resources and time without necessarily proving the efficacy of these novel treatments. Given the biological heterogeneity of breast cancer, it is expected that breast cancer patients would be divided into smaller, more homogenous groups with one or more common biological classifier that would also identify a common target for one of the new agents. Some of these groups may represent less than 5% of the total population. If not identified upfront for clinical trial designs, the effect of new agents may not be detected. The neoadjuvant setting is a perfect context to accelerate testing of new drugs to bring them quickly to the clinic. Trastuzumab is an illustration of the new paradigm. Its use in the neoadjuvant setting resulted in impressive responses that were later confirmed by large adjuvant trials. We owe this success to the foresight of the early investigators who understood the value of restricting the use of the drug to patients whose cancers depended on the amplification of HER2 gene for their survival. This is the model that needs to be generalized in future trials.

Selected References

14. US Food and Drug Administration. Guidance for industry pathological complete response in neoadjuvant treatment of high-risk early-stage breast cancer: use as an endpoint to support accelerated approval; 2014. http://www.fda.gov/downloads/drugs/guidancecomplianceregulatoryinformation/guidances/ucm305501.pdf.

58. Bear HD, Anderson S, Brown A, et al. The effect on tumor response of adding sequential preoperative docetaxel to preoperative doxorubicin and cyclophosphamide: preliminary results from national surgical adjuvant breast and bowel project protocol B-27. *J Clin Oncol.* 2003;21:4165-4174. doi:10.1200/JCO.2003.12.005.

90. Untch M, Harbeck N, Huober J, et al. Primary therapy of patients with early breast cancer: evidence, controversies, consensus: opinions of German specialists to the 14th St. Gallen International Breast Cancer Conference 2015 (Vienna 2015). *Geburtshilfe Frauenheilkd.* 2015;75:556-565. doi:10.1055/s-0035-1546120.

178. Kuehn T, Bauerfeind I, Fehm T, et al. Sentinel-lymph-node biopsy in patients with breast cancer before and after neoadjuvant chemotherapy (SENTINA): a prospective, multicentre cohort study. *Lancet Oncol.* 2013;14:609-618. doi:10.1016/S1470-2045(13)70166-9.

197. Kishan AU, McCloskey SA. Postmastectomy radiation therapy after neoadjuvant chemotherapy: review and interpretation of available data. *Ther Adv Med Oncol.* 2016;8:85-97. doi:10.1177/1758834015617459.

A full reference list is available online at ExpertConsult.com.

66

Detection and Clinical Implications of Occult Systemic Micrometastatic Breast Cancer

MARYANN KWA AND FRANCISCO J. ESTEVA

Breast cancer is the most common cancer type diagnosed among women in the United States with an estimated 232,000 new cases and 40,290 deaths in 2015; one in eight women will develop breast cancer during her lifetime.[1] The leading cause of death is complications from distant metastases. To date, surgical resection of the primary tumor followed by adjuvant systemic therapy remains the standard of care for early-stage breast cancer. Despite successful primary treatment leading to a significant decrease in breast cancer–related mortality, approximately 30% of women initially diagnosed with early-stage cancer will develop metastatic disease.[2] These relapses, many of which occur years after completion of adjuvant therapy, are often due to systemic micrometastatic tumor spread. Undetected micrometastasis can contribute to failure of primary treatment for breast cancer.

Single cancer cells may be shed by the primary tumor early in the course of disease, disperse throughout the body hematogenously and serve as a precursor for future metastatic growth at secondary sites. The importance of hematogenous dissemination of malignant cells from solid tumors was first recognized in the 19th century. In 1869, Thomas Ashworth described the presence of tumor cells in the peripheral circulation.[3] Stephen Paget developed the "seed and soil" hypothesis in 1889, describing the interaction between tumor cells and the microenvironment of secondary homing sites.[4] Unfortunately, the hematogenous spread of tumor cells from the primary tumor to distant sites cannot be detected by standard imaging methods. Therefore it is important to find new biomarkers that may effectively detect early development of systemic micrometastasis.

Detection of disseminated tumor cells (DTCs) in the bone marrow and of circulating tumor cells (CTCs) in the peripheral blood has become an important focus of translational research in breast cancer.[5] CTCs are rare cancer cells that are released from tumors into the bloodstream and are thought to play a key role in cancer metastasis. The bone marrow is a common homing organ for DTCs derived from epithelial tumors of different organs including the breast and may serve as a reservoir for DTCs with the ability to enter other distant organs. Analysis of bone marrow aspirates from breast cancer patients has provided important information on the prognostic relevance of DTCs. In 2005 a large meta-analysis of 4703 patients with early breast cancer (stages I–III) enrolled in nine clinical studies showed that bone marrow micrometastasis was detected in 30.6% of patients at the time of initial diagnosis.[6] Compared with women without bone marrow micrometastasis, patients with bone marrow micrometastasis had larger tumors, tumors with higher histologic grade, and were more often hormone receptor (HR)-negative and had frequent lymph node metastases ($p < .001$ for all variables). The presence of micrometastasis was found to be a significant independent prognostic factor for worse breast cancer–specific survival (BCSS) and overall survival (OS) ($p < .001$ for both outcomes).

A disadvantage of bone marrow sampling is the invasiveness of the procedure, and subsequent studies have focused on the evaluation of easily accessible CTCs in the peripheral blood. CTCs may be considered a surrogate marker for micrometastasis and can provide important prognostic and predictive information. In this chapter, we discuss the biological properties, detection methods, and prognostic relevance of CTCs, as well as their promising role in predicting and monitoring response to therapy in patients with early and metastatic breast cancer.

Gene Expression Profiling of Breast Cancer Cells

According to the traditional theory of carcinogenesis, metastasis arises from a small subpopulation of primary tumor cells that occur during later stages of tumor development.[7] This model predicts that multiple genetic and epigenetic changes underlie the initiation of tumor invasiveness and subsequent multistep progression to metastasis. As increasing information has become available on gene expression profiling studies of primary breast cancers, this theory has been challenged by another model in which the tendency to metastasize is determined by a poor prognosis gene expression signature present within the primary tumor.[8] In other words, cancer cells in a primary tumor may already possess a metastatic phenotype, and dissemination starts early in tumor development.

The theory of early metastasis is supported by gene expression studies, which reveal that patients with poorer prognosis can be identified before manifestation of overt metastases.[9] A study used gene expression profiling by DNA microarray analysis of primary breast tumors from 117 patients to predict clinical outcome by identifying a gene expression signature that was strongly predictive of short interval to distant metastases in patients without tumor involvement in local lymph nodes at time of diagnosis.[9] The poor prognosis signature consisted of genes regulating the cell cycle, invasion, metastasis, and angiogenesis. Another study demonstrated that dissemination of tumor cells in preclinical models of breast cancer, as well as from ductal carcinoma in situ in women, could occur in preinvasive stages of tumor progression.[10]

Additional genetic or epigenetic events and release from dormancy are critical for the metastatic growth of early-disseminated cancer cells. One study isolated single disseminated cancer cells from the bone marrow of breast cancer patients (n = 371) and performed single-cell comparative genomic hybridization.[11] The patients either underwent curative resection of the primary tumor (M0) or had overt metastases (M1); the disseminated cells were compared with the matched primary tumor. Disseminated cells from M0 patients had significantly fewer chromosomal aberrations compared with primary tumors or cells from M1 patients ($p < .008$ and $p < .0001$, respectively). A possible explanation may be that the disseminated cancer cells may have separated from the primary tumor at an early stage and evolved independently, suggesting an earlier dissemination.

The hypothesis that cells of primary tumors have metastatic capacity has also been supported by gene expression analyses that identified signaling pathways involved in dissemination of cancer cells to distant organs.[12] A study showed that primary hematogenous dissemination of breast tumor cells is a selective process associated with a specific molecular signature.[12] Expression analysis with DNA microarray showed distinct molecular profiles between primary tumors from patients with bone marrow micrometastasis compared with patients without. The differentially expressed genes in those with micrometastasis—in particular, dysregulation of *RAS* and the hypoxia-inducible factor 1α pathway *(HIF-1α)*—were involved in extracellular matrix remodeling, cell adhesion, and signal transduction. *RAS* activation is known to increase cellular proliferation, and *HIF-1α* is involved in hypoxia-related processes (e.g., angiogenesis, cellular metabolism, and proliferation) associated with metastasis. In addition, carboxypeptidase N (CPN) is a metallopeptidase that plays an important role in regulating vasoactive peptide hormones, cytokines, and growth factors by cleaving their C-terminal basic residues. Li and colleagues showed that the circulating peptides generated by CPN in the breast tumor microenvironment can serve as a biomarker of early disease onset and progression.[13]

Cancer Stem Cells

The biology of DTCs and CTCs remains not well understood. Characteristics include nucleated cells with expression of cytokeratin (CK) and absence of the leukocyte marker, CD45.[14] A subpopulation of CTCs—cancer stem cells—has been shown to harbor tumorigenic potential. The cancer stem cell theory describes the small population of tumor cells that are capable of quiescence, self-renewal, sustaining tumor formation, and differentiation into heterogeneous population of cancer cells.[15,16] Cancer stem cells are also often resistant to conventional treatments, such as chemotherapy and radiotherapy.[17,18] Breast cancer stem cells have mostly been associated with a CD44⁺CD24⁻/low phenotype[19] or by expression of aldehyde dehydrogenase 1 *(ALDH1)*.[20,21] Cells with this phenotype have been shown to be multipotent and retain

tumorigenic activity. CD44 is involved in cell-to-cell interactions, cell adhesion, and migration. CD24 is expressed in early stages of B-cell development and on neutrophils. ALDH is a detoxifying enzyme responsible for oxidation of intracellular aldehydes and is involved in early differentiation of stem cells through oxidizing retinol to retinoic acid.[22]

Esteva and colleagues investigated the relationship between serum concentration of CD44 and clinicopathologic features—in particular, human epidermal growth factor receptor 2 (HER2)—in 110 patients (of which 56 patients were HER2 positive) with breast cancer at a single institution.[23] Serum samples were collected before definitive surgery or before initiation of neoadjuvant chemotherapy (if indicated) for those with stage I to III breast cancer and before initiation of systemic therapy in patients with stage IV breast cancer. Serum CD44 concentration correlated with tumor stage ($p = .0308$), and serum CD44 levels were significantly higher in stage IV patients with liver metastases ($p = .0211$) than in those with distant metastases to other sites. The OS rate did not differ between patients with high CD44 concentration and patients with low concentration. However, serum CD44 concentration significantly predicted OS for patients with HER2-positive breast cancer, but not for patients with HER2-negative breast cancer, suggesting a role for serum CD44 as a prognostic marker in this subtype.

Many early-disseminated cancer cells detected in the bone marrow of breast cancer patients possess a cancer stem cell phenotype. Balic and colleagues evaluated bone marrow specimens from early breast cancer patients for cancer stem cells by immunohistochemistry and found that the majority of DTCs in the bone marrow (71%) had a putative stem cell phenotype (CD44⁺CD24⁻), compared with primary tumors where this phenotype represented a minor population (10%–20%).[24] Ginestier and colleagues showed that *ALDH1* is a common functional marker of both normal and malignant mammary stem cells.[20] In breast carcinomas, cells with high *ALDH1* activity contain the tumorigenic cell fraction, which is capable of self-renewal and the ability to generate tumors that recapitulate heterogeneity of the parental tumor. In a series of 577 breast carcinomas, high expression of *ALDH1* in the tumors was associated with poor clinical outcome.[20] The identification of normal and malignant stem/progenitor cells by the same *ALDH1* marker lend support to the cancer stem cell hypothesis and offer new possibilities for studying mammary stem cells and their role in tumorigenesis.

Methods for Analysis of CTCs

The capability to detect CTCs in the peripheral blood of breast cancer patients is promising, with many technologies developed in recent years. However, CTCs are rare and present in very low concentrations in the blood, typically 1 per 10^6 to 10^8 mononuclear cells, therefore their isolation presents a technical challenge.[25,26] CTCs can survive in a dormant state in the peripheral blood for many years, and overall, only a small fraction ever gives rise to distant metastases. A preclinical model showed that 2.5% of CTCs formed micrometastasis, most of which subsequently disappeared over time, and 0.01% of CTCs eventually formed macrometastases.[27] Because of their rarity, the identification and characterization of CTCs require highly sensitive and specific methods, which comprise an essential combination of enrichment (isolation) and detection (identification) procedures (Fig. 66.1).[26]

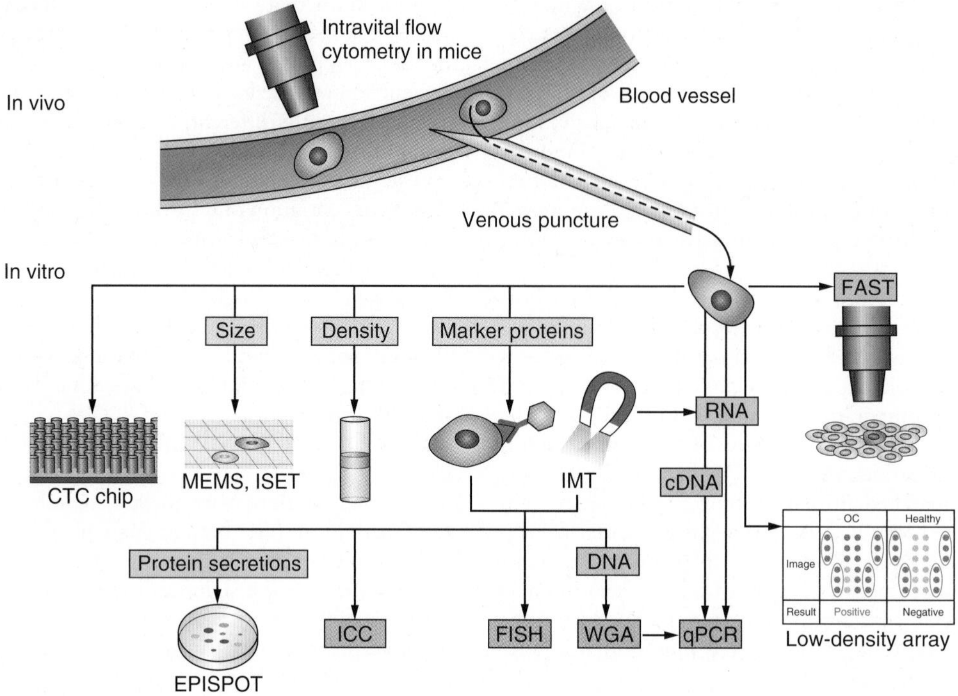

• **Fig. 66.1** Methods for circulating tumor cell (CTC) enrichment and detection. In vitro methods for processing CTCs have been established and approved in clinical trials. Enrichment methods are based on cell size (e.g., membrane microfilter devices such as MEMS; ISET), cell density, and marker protein expression or nucleic acid expression or mutation. Immunomagnetic bead techniques using antibodies to surface proteins, such as EpCAM, are most frequently applied. Enriched cells are further characterized by additional immunocytochemistry using antibodies for tumor-associated markers or on viable cells for protein expression by EPISPOT. Nucleic acid analyses are carried out on enriched cells as well as from total RNA or messenger RNA in the blood. Fluorescence in situ hybridization (FISH) is used for gene aberrations and quantitative real-time PCR (qPCR) for mRNA detection of tumor associated-target genes. Whole genome amplification (WGA) can be introduced into workflow to linearly increase amount of target DNA. High-throughput analysis has been promising with a colorimetric membrane complementary DNA (cDNA) array method using oligonucleotide probes and alkaline phosphatase for detection of mRNA of a small number of genes. The CTC chip uses a microfluidic platform that targets CTCs by antibodies to EpCAM that are coated on microposts. Aside from EpCAM-base separation, ultraspeed automated digital microscopy (FAST) and laser-printing techniques have been used to excite 300,000 cells per second to detect CTCs with fluorescence dye-conjugated antibodies. CTC detection was approached in vivo (in mice) by intravital flow cytometry. *FAST,* Fiber-optic array scanning technology; *ISET,* isolation by size of epithelial tumor cells; *MEMS,* microelectro-mechanical system. (From Pantel K, Brakenhoff RH, Brandt B. Detection, clinical relevance and specific biological properties of disseminating tumor cells. *Nat Rev Cancer.* 2008;8:329-340.)

CTC Enrichment

CTC enrichment strategies are based on technologies that can distinguish CTCs among the surrounding hematopoietic cells according to their physical (e.g., size, density, electrical charge, cell deformity) and biological (e.g., cell surface protein expression, viability) characteristics. Advantages and disadvantages of the main techniques are summarized in Table 66.1.

Physical Properties

A method for CTC separation based on physical properties (i.e., label-independent technologies) includes size separation through special filters (e.g., isolation by size of epithelial tumor cells, or ISET).[28] A limitation of filtration by size may be loss of smaller CTCs or clotting of filter pores by leukocytes. Another technique is based on density gradient separation (e.g., Ficoll, Onco-Quick).[17,29] Other methods based on physical properties of CTCs

include a biochip that uses differences in size and deformability of cancer cells compared with blood cells, a photoacoustic flow cytometer, a microfluidics device that combines dielectrophoresis (DEP) and multiorifice flow fractionation cell separation techniques, and a DEP field-flow fractionation method that isolates viable CTCs due to differences in response to DEP.[30–32]

Biological Properties

CTC separation methods based on biological properties (i.e., label-dependent technologies) primarily use immunologic techniques with antibodies directed against either tumor-associated antigens (positive selection) or CD45 (negative selection). Immunomagnetic assays target an antigen by an antibody coupled to a magnetic bead, and the antigen-antibody complex is subsequently isolated from the solution by exposure to a magnetic field. The majority of positive selection technologies are carried out with antibodies against the epithelial cell adhesion molecule (EpCAM),

TABLE 66.1   Advantages and Disadvantages of Main Enrichment and Detection Techniques for CTCs

Technique	Advantages	Disadvantages
CellSearch system	FDA approved High sensitivity Visual confirmation of CTCs Clinical relevance Semiautomated system	CTCs may be lost during enrichment that lack EpCAM expression (false negative) CTC determination is subjective Limited number of markers
Microfiltration (e.g., ISET)	Simple, fast, and inexpensive Can be used for EpCAM-negative CTCs	Smaller CTCs may be missed (low specificity)
Density gradient centrifugation (e.g., Ficoll, OncoQuick)	Simple, fast, and inexpensive Can be used for EpCAM-negative CTCs	Low specificity Low sample purity Cross-contamination of different layers (OncoQuick avoids this by incorporating a porous barrier)
CTC-chip	Visual confirmation of CTCs High sensitivity Additional molecular and genetic analysis possible	Dependent on EpCAM-positivity CTC determination is subjective
Immunocytochemistry	Morphologic analysis and quantification of CTCs Facilitates classical cytopathological review	CTC determination is subjective Time-consuming
Epithelial ImmunoSPOT (EPISPOT) assay	High sensitivity and high specificity Detects only viable cells	CTCs are not collected and subsequent cellular analysis cannot be performed Not an automated system
AdnaTest (RT-PCR)	High sensitivity Detects only viable cells	EpCAM and MUC1 dependent No morphologic analysis No quantification
CTCscope (RT-PCR)	High sensitivity Detects only viable cells	No morphologic analysis No visualization or quantification of CTCs

CTC, Circulating tumor cell; *EpCAM*, epithelial cell adhesion molecule; *FDA*, Food and Drug Administration; *ISET*, isolation by size of epithelial tumor cells; *MUC1*, mucin 1; *RT-PCR*, reverse transcription polymerase chain reaction.

which is frequently overexpressed by breast cancer and is absent from hematologic cells.[33]

Enrichment of CTCs by immunomagnetic capture has been the most successful and widely used approach to date, and among EpCAM-based technologies, the US Food and Drug Administration (FDA) has approved the CellSearch (Veridex) platform and the Ariol system.[34] The current gold standard remains the Cell-Search system, which combines semiautomated enrichment of EpCAM-positive cells using magnetic nanoparticles and characterization of CTCs by immunofluorescent staining of CK 8, 18, and 19, as well as the absence of CD45.[35] The system is based on enumeration of epithelial cells, which are separated from blood by antibody-coated magnetic beads and identified by fluorescently labeled antibodies against CK with a fluorescent nuclear stain.

The process for validation and qualification of CTC assays has been described by the Cancer Steering Committee of the National Institutes of Health Biomarkers Consortium.[36] CellSearch is the only CTC enumeration system to have been fully validated for reproducibility and performance characteristics.[37] It is used to aid in prognosis of patients with metastatic breast, colorectal, and prostate cancer.[38–40] The limitation of CellSearch, however, is that not all CTCs express EpCAM on their cell membrane or the expression may be weak.

Furthermore, cells undergoing epithelial to mesenchymal transition (EMT) may be missed during analysis. During this morphologic process, cells lose their epithelial characteristics and acquire a mesenchymal phenotype, endowing the cells with invasive properties and potential for metastasis.[41] This cellular phenotype can also cause increased resistance to common chemotherapies.[42] EMT is most evident in both the triple-negative breast cancer (TNBC) subtype and HER2-positive tumors and is less frequent in HR-positive tumors. Giordano and colleagues studied epithelial to mesenchymal transition-inducing transcription factors (EMT-TF) (*TWIST1, SNAIL1, ZEB1,* and *TG2*) and cancer stem cell features in 28 patients with HER2-positive metastatic breast cancer.[43] At least one EMT-TF mRNA was elevated in the CTCs of 88% of patients. *TWIST1* and *SNAIL1* transcripts were elevated in the CD326+ cell fractions, and *SNAIL1* and *ZEB1* transcripts were elevated in the CD45− cell fractions. Patients with EMT-TFs in their CTCs had more ALDH+CD133+ cancer stem cells.

Promising novel EpCAM-based enrichment technologies include microfluidic devices, notably the CTC chip,[44] Herringbone chip,[45] iChip,[46] and IsoFlux.[47] In 2007, Nagrath and colleagues initially described the CTC chip, a microchip technology on a microfluidic platform that separates CTCs from whole blood using microposts coated with an antibody against EpCAM under controlled laminar-flow conditions.[44] In a study of 116 patients, the CTC-chip technology successfully identified CTCs in the peripheral blood of 115 (99%) patients with metastatic breast, colon, lung, pancreatic, and prostate cancer.[44] The CTC-iChip is capable of sorting rare CTCs from whole blood at a rate of 10 million cells per second by using tumor antigen-independent microfluidic technology.[46] The MagSweeper (Illumina) is another automated device that positively enriches CTCs using a magnetic rod stirred through a blood sample that is prelabeled with anti-EpCAM antibody-coated magnetic beads.[48]

If a subset of CTCs undergoes EMT in which epithelial markers are downregulated, technologies reliant on EpCAM expression for CTC capture may fail to enrich an important subpopulation of cells. Increasing attention has therefore been dedicated to technology platforms that use marker-independent enrichment methods. Capturing CTCs without expression of EpCAM has involved antibodies against stem cell antigens and other epithelial cell surface antigens (e.g., HER2, epidermal growth factor receptor, and mucin-1) and mesenchymal antigens.[49,50]

CTC Detection

After enrichment, a substantial number of leukocytes still remain in the CTC fraction. CTCs need to be identified at the single-cell level by a method that can distinguish them from normal blood cells. Detection can be performed through cytometric strategies or nucleic acid–based techniques. Advances in the development of immunocytochemical and molecular assays enable the identification of individual disseminated tumor cells.

Protein-Based Strategies

Among cytometric techniques, classic immunocytochemistry is the most widely used immunologic approach. Immunocytochemical detection assays involve monoclonal antibodies that bind to tumor-associated or histogenic markers expressed on disseminated tumor cells but that are absent on the surrounding normal cells. The CellSearch system and many other CTC assays use the same identification step: cells are fluorescently stained for CK (positive marker), CD45 (negative marker), and a nuclear dye (4',6-diamidino-2-phenylindole, or DAPI). Through multicolor image analysis with a fluorescence microscope, CTCs are defined as CK$^+$/CD45$^-$/DAPI$^+$ cells. However, EpCAM-based methods do not recognize whether detected CTCs are viable or apoptotic cells, with only viable cells being able to contribute to metastasis. For detection of only viable CTCs, the newer functional Epithelial ImmunoSPOT (EPISPOT) assay can be added to any enrichment step.[51] The EPISPOT assay can determine cell protein secretion frequency and has been used to analyze peripheral blood and bone marrow samples in breast, colon, and prostate cancer. High-speed automated digital microscopy using fiber-optic array scanning technology has also been developed to detect CTCs that have been labeled by antibodies with fluorescent conjugates.[52]

Nucleic Acid–Based Strategies

Reverse transcription PCR (RT-PCR) assays that target specific mRNAs produced by viable CTCs have become the most widely used alternative to immunocytochemical assays. To detect most CTCs in breast cancer, a multimarker approach uses several cancer-related genes or epithelial markers (e.g., CK19, HER2, EpCAM, MUC1, CK18, mammaglobin, and c-MET). CK19 is one of the most frequently used mRNA markers in trials.[5,53] A study examined the detection of CK19 mRNA-positive cells by RT-PCR in the peripheral blood of a cohort of 148 patients with stage I and II breast cancer before the initiation of adjuvant systemic therapy.[54] Patients with CK19 mRNA-positive cells in the peripheral blood had a significantly reduced disease-free interval

($p = .0007$) and decreased OS ($p = .01$) compared with patients without detection.

The nucleic acid–based approach offers the highest sensitivity for CTC detection, although the specificity may decline if there is a high resemblance between mRNA markers of CTCs and those shed by normal blood cells, bone marrow cells, and other nontumor cells.[40] Despite high sensitivity, this approach can only determine whether a cell sample is positive for the specific marker and does not allow for cytomorphologic analysis or direct enumeration of CTCs. A commercially available RNA-based CTC assay is the AdnaTest (AdnaGen), in which CTCs are enriched by immunomagnetic beads labeled with antibodies to EpCAM and MUC1.[55] After enrichment, the mRNA of three markers (EpCAM, MUC1, and HER2) is amplified by multiplex PCR. It is a highly sensitive test with a detection limit of two tumor cells. The concordance rate of the CellSearch system and the AdnaTest has been reported to range between 70% and 90%.[56] Another promising technology is the measurement of single RNA molecules with the RNAscope technology used by CTCscope (Advanced Cell Diagnostics) for the detection of single CTCs from metastatic breast cancer patients.[57] This method requires minimal enrichment and is able to exclude apoptotic cells because they do not produce mRNA molecules.

Clinical Applications of CTCs

Metastatic Breast Cancer

CTCs can be detected in the peripheral blood of approximately 40% to 80% of patients with metastatic breast cancer.[58] The CellSearch system is the most commonly used method for analysis with a cutoff for positivity of five or more CTCs per 7.5 mL of blood. Several trials have demonstrated the independent prognostic significance of CTCs in metastatic disease. In 2004, the seminal prospective study by Cristofanilli and colleagues showed that among 177 patients with measurable metastatic breast cancer who had at least five CTCs per 7.5 mL of blood detected by CellSearch at baseline before treatment, there was significantly shorter progression-free survival (PFS) (2.7 months vs. 7.0 months; $p < .001$) and OS (10.1 months vs. >18 months; $p < .001$) compared with patients with fewer than five CTCs per 7.5 mL.[37] This difference between the groups persisted at the first follow-up (3–5 weeks) after initiation of treatment. Enumeration of CTCs both before and several weeks after initiating treatment was informative because maintaining or decreasing the number of CTCs to fewer than five indicated a treatment response and was predictive of improved PFS and OS. This pivotal study showed that the number of CTCs is an independent predictor of PFS and OS and subsequently lead to FDA approval of CellSearch in 2004 for prognosis and monitoring of treatment effectiveness for metastatic breast cancer.

Hayes and colleagues further expanded on the initial results of this cohort by demonstrating that CTC analysis at each consecutive follow-up time point (baseline, 3–5, 6–8, 9–15, and 15–20 weeks) during therapy predicted PFS and OS.[38] For patients with five or more CTCs per 7.5 mL, median PFS from each time point was significantly reduced compared with those with fewer than five CTCs, respectively. Median OS for patients with fewer than five CTCs from the five time points was greater than 18.5 months. For patients with five or more CTCs, median OS from these same time points was significantly shorter: 10.9, 6.3, 6.3, 6.6, and 6.7 months, respectively. In addition, patients who converted from elevated CTCs to nonelevated levels demonstrated PFS and OS similar to those with CTCs that were never elevated.

A pooled analysis of 1944 patients with metastatic breast cancer across 17 European centers confirmed the independent prognostic role of CTC count by CellSearch method on PFS and OS in metastatic breast cancer patients.[59] Patients who had a CTC count of five or more CTCs per 7.5 mL blood at baseline had decreased PFS (hazard ratio [HR] 1.92, 95% confidence interval [CI], 1.73–2.14; $p < .0001$) and OS (HR 2.78, 95% CI, 2.42–3.19; $p < .0001$) compared with patients with fewer than five CTCs per 7.5 mL. At both 3 to 5 weeks and 6 to 8 weeks after the start of treatment, increased CTC counts were significantly associated with shorter PFS and OS. The data provided strong evidence that CTC enumeration improved the prognostication of metastatic breast cancer when added to clinicopathologic prognostic models (e.g., tumor histologic subtype, histologic grade, number of prior lines of chemotherapy and hormonal therapy, presence of liver or visceral metastasis). In contrast, measurement of serum tumor markers—carcinoembryonic antigen (CEA) and cancer antigen (CA) 15-3—did not contribute significant information.

Other studies have shown that monitoring of CTC levels in the metastatic setting has been predictive of treatment efficacy. A strong association was demonstrated between CTC levels and radiographic disease progression in patients receiving chemotherapy or endocrine therapy for metastatic breast cancer.[60] Reduced CTC counts at weeks 3 to 5 on treatment correlated with radiographic response, and patients with fewer than five CTCs at weeks 3 to 5 and weeks 7 to 9 had an improvement in PFS. This supported the clinical utility of serial CTC enumeration in conjunction with standard radiographic imaging to improve the ability to accurately assess treatment benefit and to expedite identification of effective therapies for individual patients.

Early detection of disease progression with CTC count while on treatment could potentially allow for switching from less effective therapies to alternative regimens. In the prospective Southwest Oncology Group (SWOG) S0500 trial, patients receiving first-line chemotherapy for metastatic breast cancer were randomly assigned to continue current chemotherapy or start a new treatment regimen if they had five or more CTCs per 7.5 mL at baseline and after the first treatment cycle of 21 days.[61] The results, however, showed that for patients with persistently elevated CTCs at 21 days whose therapy was then changed to an alternative chemotherapy, both PFS and OS were not improved. The authors suggested that failure of treatment to reduce CTCs within the first cycle of starting first-line chemotherapy signifies a poor prognosis and may indicate resistance to chemotherapy.

After the SWOG S0500 trial, the ongoing CirCe01 trial (clinicaltrials.gov identifier NCT01349842) is studying whether patients whose CTC count does not decrease after the first treatment cycle benefit from a regimen switch. A total of 304 metastatic breast cancer patients with high CTC count before the start of third-line therapy will be randomized between a CTC-driven arm and a standard arm (i.e., chemotherapy management according to usual clinical and radiologic criteria). Recently the nonrandomized run-in phase of the CirCe01 trial was reported, which was designed to evaluate CTC changes and thresholds for other prognostic scores and establish CTC thresholds to be used in the randomized part of the study.[62] CTC count by CellSearch and other prognostic parameters were assessed in 56 metastatic breast cancer patients before the first cycle of third-line chemotherapy. Early changes in CTC count correlated with treatment outcome.

Independent prognostic markers in multivariate analysis were as follows: five or more CTCs per 7.5 mL, poor performance status, low serum albumin, and TNBC subtype. For patients with five or more CTC per 7.5 mL at baseline, a composite criteria of fewer than five CTC per 7.5 mL or a relative decrease of 70% or more of the baseline CTC count demonstrated improved prognostication for PFS ($p = .002$). Another study showed that analysis of CTCs before the second cycle of chemotherapy is an early and strong predictor of treatment outcome in metastatic breast cancer.[63] Several ongoing interventional studies evaluating the clinical utility of CTCs are described in Table 66.2.

Regarding the clinical value of CTCs in different subtypes of breast cancer, Giordano and colleagues retrospectively analyzed samples from 517 metastatic breast cancer patients and found that CTCs were strongly predictive of survival in all disease subtypes except for HER2-positive patients who had been treated with targeted therapy.[64] The authors postulated that the effectiveness of HER-2 directed therapy (trastuzumab and lapatinib) might eliminate a population of circulating epithelial cells with HER2 amplification or overexpression, thereby reducing the prognostic value of CTC enumeration. Other studies have shown similar results with CTCs losing prognostic value in metastatic HER2-positive tumors treated with targeted therapy.[65,66] In contrast, Liu and colleagues found that CTC analysis by CellSearch with a modified cutoff value of one or more but not five or more CTCs could serve as a useful prognostic factor for HER2-positive metastatic disease.[67] More studies are needed to determine an appropriate cutoff for this subgroup.

In TNBC, CTC enumeration has been shown to provide prognostic information.[68] The use of CTCs as a biomarker for monitoring response, disease progression, and survival may be particularly useful in this tumor subtype, which is associated with an aggressive biology and poor prognosis. Magbanua and colleagues compared two approaches for measuring CTCs—CellSearch and an alternative method called IE/FC, which uses EpCAM-based immunomagnetic enrichment (IE) and flow cytometry (FC)—in 102 metastatic TNBC patients participating in a prospective phase II clinical trial.[69] CTC enumeration was assessed at baseline and 7 to 14 days after initiation of treatment and was found from both assays to be highly concordant and significantly correlated with time to progression and OS.

Early Breast Cancer

Early diagnosis is a hallmark of successful management in breast cancer because it reduces morbidity and mortality. The follow-up of patients who are potentially cured is primarily based on clinicopathologic aspects of the tumor. Micrometastatic spread of tumor cells, however, may persist beyond initial surgery and adjuvant treatment and can serve as a surrogate marker for minimal residual disease. The monitoring of CTCs after therapy may permit assessment of individual treatment efficacy, as well as identify patients who may benefit from additional therapies and/or closer surveillance. CTCs have been reported to be detected in the peripheral blood of approximately 20% to 30% of patients with early breast cancer.[70,71]

A 2012 meta-analysis of the prognostic value of CTCs in approximately 3000 patients with early-stage breast cancer demonstrated that the presence of CTCs was significantly associated with shorter survival (DFS: HR 2.86; 95% CI 2.19–3.75; OS: HR 2.78; 95% CI 2.22–3.48).[72] A recent pooled analysis of 3173 patients with stage I to III breast cancer from five institutions also

TABLE 66.2 Ongoing Clinical Trials Investigating the Utility of CTCs in Breast Cancer

Trial Name (ClinicalTrials.gov Identifier)	Patients (n = Estimated Enrollment)	Description	Methodology	Estimated Primary Completion Date
CirCé01 (NCT01349842), France	MBC (n = 568)	Phase III evaluation of the use of CTCs to guide chemotherapy from the third-line chemotherapy for MBC	Patients with five or more CTCs/7.5 mL before the start of third-line chemotherapy are randomized between CTC-driven arm and standard arm.	January 2018
COMETI P2 (NCT01701050), United States	ER-positive, HER2-negative MBC (n = 121)	Phase II study of characterization of CTCs in MBC using the CTC-Endocrine Therapy Index (CTC-ETI) to identify patients who will progress	CTC-ETI is based on the expression of four markers (ER, BCL2, HER2, and ki67) and will be assessed on isolated CTCs to predict clinical response to endocrine therapy.	December 2016
CTC-CEC-AND (NCT02220556), France	Patients with solid tumors (including breast cancer) (n = 360)	Evaluation of different analysis methods for CTCs, circulating endothelial cells, and circulating tumor DNA	There will be 15 cohorts of patients, and each cohort will explore one analysis method and/or tumor type.	December 2015
CTC-EMT (NCT02025413), United States	MBC or metastatic prostate cancer (n = 80)	Isolation of CTCs using a novel EMT-based capture method	This is a nonrandomized study to evaluate mesenchymal-marker based ferrofluid (N- or O-cadherin–based) CTC capture method.	December 2016
DETECT III (NCT01619111), Germany	HER2-negative MBC patients with HER2-positive CTCs (n = 120)	Multicenter, open label phase III study to compare standard therapy alone ± lapatinib in HER2-negative MBC patients with HER2-positive CTCs	Patients will be randomized between standard therapy ± lapatinib. Those with bone metastases will be treated with denosumab in both arms. CTC clearance and survival end points will be analyzed.	March 2018
DETECT IV (NCT02035813), Germany	Patients with HER2-negative MBC and persisting HER2-negative CTCs (n = 520)	Multicenter, open-label phase II study that offers two treatment options for patients with HER2-negative MBC and HER2-negative CTCs	Patients with HR-positive MBC will receive endocrine therapy plus everolimus, and patients with triple-negative MBC or HR- positive MBC plus indication for chemotherapy will receive eribulin. CTC clearance and survival end points to be analyzed.	December 2019
STIC CTC METABREAST (NCT01710605), France	ER positive, HER2-negative MBC (n = 1000)	To evaluate the medicoeconomic value of CTCs in deciding on first-line therapy	Randomized, phase III study between clinician choice and CTC count-driven choice. In CTC arm, patients with five or more CTCs/7.5 mL will receive chemotherapy, and those with five or fewer CTCs/7.5 mL will receive endocrine therapy.	March 2016
Treat-CTC (NCT01548677), Europe	HER2-negative primary breast cancer with detectable CTCs (n = 2175)	Randomized phase II study of trastuzumab to treat patients who have one or more CTC/15 mL after completing (neo)adjuvant chemotherapy and surgery	Patients will be randomized 1 : 1 to either trastuzumab arm or observation arm.	December 2018

BCL2, B-cell lymphoma 2; *CTC*, circulating tumor cell; *EMT*, epithelial-mesenchymal transition; *ER*, estrogen receptor; *HER2*, human epidermal growth factor receptor 2; *HR*, hormone receptor; *MBC*, metastatic breast cancer.

provided strong evidence for the prognostic effect of CTCs.[73] CTCs were detected in 20% of patients who also had larger tumors, tumors with higher histologic grade, and increased involvement of lymph nodes, compared with patients without CTCs ($p < .002$ for all variables). The presence of CTCs was an independent prognostic factor for DFS (HR 1.82; 95% CI 1.47–2.26), distant DFS (HR 1.89; 95% CI 1.49–2.40), BCSS (HR 2.04; 95% CI 1.52–2.75), and OS (HR 1.97; 95% CI 1.51–2.59). In the German SUCCESS trial, CTCs were prospectively analyzed by CellSearch in 2026 patients with early breast cancer before adjuvant chemotherapy and in 1492 patients after chemotherapy; the patients were followed for a median of 35 months.[74] CTCs were detected in 21.5% of node negative and 22.5% of node positive patients before chemotherapy ($p < .001$). After completion of adjuvant chemotherapy, 22.1% patients (n = 330 of 1493) were CTC positive. These patients had a significantly shorter DFS (HR 2.11; 95% CI 1.49–2.99; $p < .0001$) and OS (HR 2.18; 95% CI 1.32–3.59; $p = .002$). CTCs that persisted after adjuvant chemotherapy negatively affected DFS (HR 1.12; 95% CI 1.02–1.25; $p = .02$) and OS (HR 1.16; 95% CI 0.99–1.37; $p = .06$). These results provide compelling evidence that CTCs can serve as a prognostic marker for survival before and after adjuvant chemotherapy. Other studies have also reported an association between CTC detection and survival in early-stage breast cancer patients.[53,75,76]

In the neoadjuvant setting, the achievement of a pathologic complete response (pCR) after neoadjuvant treatment is associated with favorable long-term clinical outcome. The presence of CTCs after neoadjuvant therapy may be a surrogate marker of therapy response and survival. Several neoadjuvant clinical trials have evaluated the correlation between CTC detection and pCR.[77–80] In the REMAGUS 02 study (n = 118), after a median follow-up of 70 months, detection of one or more CTC per 7.5 mL before chemotherapy was significantly associated with distant metastasis-free survival ($p = .04$) and OS ($p = .03$), whereas postchemotherapy CTC detection did not have a significant impact.[77,80] Of note, CTC positivity was the most predictive of survival during the first 36 to 48 months of follow-up. In the GeparQuattro trial that compared different chemotherapy with trastuzumab as neoadjuvant treatment for patients with HER2-positive tumors (n = 213), no association was found between tumor response to neoadjuvant chemotherapy and CTC detection.[78] HER2 expression on CTCs was also examined, and HER2-overexpressing CTCs were observed in 24% of CTC-positive patients, including eight patients with primary tumors who were HER2 negative. The HER2 status of CTCs may potentially be helpful for stratification of patients and monitoring of HER2-directed therapies. In addition, these results show that the phenotype of the primary tumor may not necessarily reflect the phenotype of CTCs, which has been described in other studies.[81]

Inflammatory breast cancer (IBC) is a rare and aggressive locally advanced breast cancer with poor survival. The BEVERLY-2 trial (n = 52) evaluated the efficacy of neoadjuvant chemotherapy with trastuzumab and bevacizumab in HER2-positive inflammatory breast cancer and found that the 3-year DFS rate was 68% and OS rate was 90%.[79] CTC detection at baseline independently predicted 3-year DFS (81% vs. 43% for patients with less than one versus one or more CTC per 7.5 mL, $p = .01$). Patients with a pCR had a 3-year DFS of 80%, whereas those with both a pCR and no CTCs detected at baseline had a 3-year DFS of 95%. Similarly, a prospective study analyzed CTCs from 63 stage III IBC patients who received primary systemic therapy, modified

radical mastectomy, and postmastectomy radiation.[82] One or more CTC was identified in 27% of patients after four cycles of primary systemic therapy. At a mean follow-up of 38 months, multivariable analysis showed that detection of one or more CTCs independently predicted shortened relapse-free survival (log-rank $p = .005$, HR 4.22, 95% CI 1.67–10.67, Cox $p = .002$) but not OS (log-rank $p = .54$, HR 1.53, 95% CI 0.41–5.79, Cox $p = .53$). The presence of CTCs after primary chemotherapy identified IBC patients at high risk for relapse; additional IBC studies are needed to better understand the mechanism underlying the metastatic potential of IBC.

Jung and colleagues studied whether altered plasma expression levels of microRNAs (miRNAs) were associated with sensitivity to trastuzumab in patients with HER2-positive breast cancer who were enrolled in a clinical trial of neoadjuvant trastuzumab-based chemotherapy.[83] At baseline before neoadjuvant therapy, circulating miR-210 levels were significantly higher in patients who had residual disease than in those who achieved a pCR ($p = .0359$). Expression of miR-210 was also significantly higher before surgery than after surgery ($p = .0297$) and in patients whose cancer metastasized to lymph nodes ($p = .0030$). To determine whether miR-210 variations were directly related to trastuzumab resistance, the mean relative expression levels were measured in trastuzumab-resistant BTR65 cells (clone 65 derived from HER2-overexpressing BT474 breast cancer cell line). The mean expression ratio for miR-210 was significantly higher in trastuzumab-resistant BT474 cells compared with wild-type BT474 cells that were sensitive to trastuzumab, suggesting that high relative expression levels for miRNA-210 in the plasma of HER-2 breast cancer patients are associated with trastuzumab resistance.

Role of CTCs as a "Liquid Biopsy" in Metastatic Disease

Tumor cell features may change over the course of the disease between primary and recurrent breast cancer. It has been shown that the genotype and phenotype may differ among the primary tumor, isolated tumor cells in secondary homing sites, and metastatic tumor sites.[84–86] Metastatic cells may gain genomic characteristics and develop independently over time from the primary tumor, or the metastatic subclone within the primary tumor may be small and easily missed. In particular, the status of the estrogen receptor (ER) and HER2 in the primary tumor may be discordant with the expression profile in CTCs and in metastatic sites.[87] Discordance rates in the ER, progesterone receptor (PR), and HER2 status have been reported to range from 10% to 40%.[88]

In the metastatic setting, such profiles should be determined in the metastatic tumor tissue; however, biopsies of metastasis are invasive and may present with technical difficulties (e.g., biopsy of bone metastasis). As a potentially less invasive alternative, the detection and characterization of CTCs in the peripheral blood may serve as a real-time "liquid biopsy." Fehm and colleagues compared HER2 status of CTCs in 254 patients with metastatic breast cancer at the time of first diagnosis or disease progression.[89] In this prospective, multicenter trial, HER2-positive CTCs were detected in 32% of HER2-negative tumors. Similarly, another study found an overall discrepancy of 31% between CTCs and primary breast tumors and 26% between CTCs and metastatic tumors with regard to HER2 status.[90]

The clinical value of CTCs in predicting the efficacy of HER2-directed therapy is currently being investigated in prospective randomized trials. The German DETECT III (clinicaltrials.gov identifier NCT01619111) is a phase III multicenter trial in which patients with a HER2-negative metastatic breast cancer but with HER2-positive CTCs are randomized to standard treatment alone or in combination with lapatinib. For patients with HER2-negative metastatic breast cancer with persisting HER2-negative CTCs, the role of everolimus in combination with endocrine therapies or eribulin on CTCs will be investigated in the DETECT IV trial (clinicaltrials.gov identifier NCT02035813).

Genomic alterations in solid tumors can be characterized by sequencing of circulating tumor DNA released from cancer cells into the plasma.[91,92] One study directly compared the measurement of circulating tumor DNA and other circulating biomarkers (CTCs and CA 15-3) and medical imaging for the noninvasive monitoring of 30 patients with metastatic breast cancer receiving systemic therapy.[93] Targeted or whole-genome sequencing was used to identify somatic genomic alterations, and personalized assays were designed to quantify circulating tumor DNA. Circulating tumor DNA was detected in 29 of the 30 women (97%) in whom somatic genomic alterations were identified, whereas CTCs and CA 15-3 were detected in 26 of 30 women (87%) and CA 15-3 in 21 of 27 women (78%), respectively. Compared with CTCs and CA 15-3, circulating tumor DNA provided the earliest measure of treatment response in 10 of 19 women (53%). Sampling of circulating tumor DNA as a liquid biopsy may therefore be a noninvasive option for sensitive and specific monitoring during the course of treatment and may identify mutations associated with drug resistance.

Moreover, DNA methylation studies have suggested the prognostic utility of methylated biomarkers for predicting outcome and monitoring treatment in breast cancer. Fackler and colleagues developed a quantitative multiplexed methylation-specific PCR assay, cMethDNA, for a panel of 10 genes.[94] This assay contains novel and known breast cancer hypermethylated markers, and after validation of the 10-gene panel in the TCGA (The Cancer Genome Atlas) breast cancer methylome database, the authors tested serum-specific prediction models in test and training sets from serum in patients with metastatic breast cancer. cMethDNA identified 91% of patients with recurrent metastatic breast cancers with a specificity of 96% ($p < .0001$) in the test set. Methylation levels reflected response to treatment, and circulating tumor DNA revealed a similar pattern of methylation as the solid tumor.

Conclusions and Future Directions

The evaluation of CTCs in the peripheral blood of breast cancer patients holds great promise with many new technologies being developed to better understand systemic micrometastatic disease. CTCs have emerged as a powerful independent prognostic indicator in both early and metastatic breast cancer and may aid in optimizing treatment strategies. In addition, the characterization of CTCs has helped contribute to improved understanding of the metastatic cascade. Further investigation should be performed on the molecular characterization of CTCs to better understand the genomic landscape of cancer cells to help guide treatment decisions and understand resistance to therapy. Additional study is also needed to evaluate CTC subpopulations including cancer stem cells and EMT populations and their alteration with treatment. The potential role of CTCs to individualize patient therapy should be investigated in prospective large-scale clinical trials to assess the effect of treatment decisions based on CTC analysis using standardized, sensitive, and reproducible methods. How CTC assessment may help guide therapy toward more efficient elimination of metastasis and decrease cancer mortality remains an important question. Overall, CTCs are an exciting area of translational research in breast cancer and can serve as novel biomarkers to help increase knowledge of metastasis, aid in prediction of treatment response, and potentially identify novel therapeutic targets.

Selected References

6. Braun S, Vogl FD, Naume B, et al. A pooled analysis of bone marrow micrometastasis in breast cancer. *N Engl J Med*. 2005;353:793-802.
9. van 't Veer LJ, Dai H, van de Vijver MJ, et al. Gene expression profiling predicts clinical outcome of breast cancer. *Nature*. 2002;415:530-536.
24. Balic M, Lin H, Young L, et al. Most early disseminated cancer cells detected in bone marrow of breast cancer patients have a putative breast cancer stem cell phenotype. *Clin Cancer Res*. 2006;12:5615-5621.
36. Parkinson DR, Dracopoli N, Petty BG, et al. Considerations in the development of circulating tumor cell technology for clinical use. *J Transl Med*. 2012;10:138.
37. Cristofanilli M, Budd GT, Ellis MJ, et al. Circulating tumor cells, disease progression, and survival in metastatic breast cancer. *N Engl J Med*. 2004;351:781-791.
38. Hayes DF, Cristofanilli M, Budd GT, et al. Circulating tumor cells at each follow-up time point during therapy of metastatic breast cancer patients predict progression-free and overall survival. *Clin Cancer Res*. 2006;12:4218-4224.
59. Bidard FC, Peeters DJ, Fehm T, et al. Clinical validity of circulating tumour cells in patients with metastatic breast cancer: a pooled analysis of individual patient data. *Lancet Oncol*. 2014;15:406-414.
72. Zhang L, Riethdorf S, Wu G, et al. Meta-analysis of the prognostic value of circulating tumor cells in breast cancer. *Clin Cancer Res*. 2012;18:5701-5710.
73. Janni W, Rack B, Terstappen LW, et al. Pooled analysis of the prognostic relevance of circulating tumor cells in primary breast cancer. *Clin Cancer Res*. 2016.
93. Dawson SJ, Tsui DW, Murtaza M, et al. Analysis of circulating tumor DNA to monitor metastatic breast cancer. *N Engl J Med*. 2013;368:1199-1209.

A full reference list is available online at ExpertConsult.com.

67

Management of the Intact Breast Primary in the Setting of Metastatic Disease

PATIENCE ODELE AND SEEMA A. KHAN

Approximately 6% of all breast cancer patients present with an intact primary and synchronous distant disease.[1] For these patients, overall survival is dictated by the systemic disease burden rather than the status of the primary tumor. Consequently, systemic therapy is first-line treatment, and resection of the intact breast tumor is generally not recommended because the expectation is that most patients succumb to their disease before they develop uncontrolled local disease (ULD). If surgical extirpation of an intact primary is undertaken, it is performed in an effort to avoid future complications of ULD or to palliate chest wall progression once it has occurred.

However, the clinical course of metastatic breast cancer is changing. Overall, patients with stage IV disease are living longer. In an analysis of temporal trends in survival for metastatic breast cancer patients, 724 patients who presented to three French centers with de novo stage IV breast cancer were divided by time periods. Those diagnosed in an earlier time period (1987–1993) had a 27% 3-year survival rate, whereas those diagnosed in a later period (1994–2000) had a 44% 3-year survival rate.[2,3] Similar trends are seen in data from the Surveillance, Epidemiology and End Results (SEER) registry.[4] Some of this difference may be attributable to lead-time bias from earlier diagnosis of metastases in the later time period, but much of it is related to improved therapy with targeted agents, and continued improvements in survival can be expected in the future as additional molecular targets are identified and manipulated for therapeutic gain. Several trials have shown that between 3% and 30% of patients with distant metastases treated with multimodality therapy can achieve long-term survival.[5,6] Thus improved systemic therapy and more sensitive imaging modalities both contribute to the fact that women live longer with known stage IV disease in the 21st century, many with a relatively small disease burden.[7]

As a result of these trends, recent analyses have examined the value of surgical approaches such as metastasectomy (lung, liver)[8–11] and resection of the intact primary in the management of patients with stage IV breast cancer. Metastasectomy has been studied in breast cancer patients with oligometastases and patients with multiple localized metastases that are amenable to surgical resection.[8–11] Nieto and colleagues reported on a highly selected series of 60 patients with oligometastases who were treated with surgical excision, with or without radiation, and adjuvant

chemotherapy.[12] At a median of 62 months, 51.6% of patients were alive and disease-free. These data and others are reviewed by Salama and Chmura.[13] The value of local therapy for limited metastatic disease, in addition to systemic therapy, is currently being evaluated in a randomized trial (clinicaltrials.gov identifier NCT02364557; NRG Oncology trial NRG-BR002).

The concept of elective (rather than palliative) resection of the intact primary in the setting of metastatic disease has not been widely discussed in the breast cancer arena until recently, but there is precedent in other malignancies, such as gastric, colon, and ovarian carcinoma. For example, in metastatic renal cell carcinoma, two prospective, randomized trials (Southwest Oncology Group [SWOG] and European Organization for Research and Treatment of Cancer) compared radical nephrectomy with nonoperative management of the primary tumor in patients treated with systemic therapy (interferon alfa-2β). Both trials demonstrated a statistically significant survival advantage for patients treated with surgery (11.1 vs. 8.1 months, $p = .05$; 17 vs. 7 months, $p = .03$, respectively).[14,15] A meta-analysis of patients with stage III and IV ovarian cancer found that maximal cytoreduction surgery was associated with improved survival.[16] There are several studies supporting a role for palliative gastrectomy in the setting of metastatic or advanced gastric cancer.[17–19] SEER analysis of over 8200 patients undergoing treatment for stage IV gastric cancer showed that those who had surgery had higher 3-year cancer-specific survival rates than nonsurgery patients (2.1% vs. 9.4% $p < .001$).[20] In a retrospective review of 105 patients with stage IV gastric cancer who were treated without surgery, with bypass surgery, or with surgical resection, there was a statistically significant difference in overall survival in the patients who had resection versus patients who did not (5.5 vs. 13.2 months, $p = .0006$).[21]

Along with clinical data, there have been new biological insights that suggest a unique role for the primary tumor in the continued dissemination of metastases. The identification of cancer stem cells and the recognition of their role in the metastatic process[22] lead to the suggestion that the intact primary is a particularly efficient source of these cells, and the continued presence of the primary tumor may facilitate the development of new metastases. Additionally, an increasing body of evidence suggests that there is molecular communication between the primary tumor and the premetastatic niche.[23] A specific role for

TABLE 67.1	Summary of Multicenter Studies Examining Primary Site Surgery or Radiotherapy in de Novo Stage IV Patients					
Author and Setting		Year	N (% Surgery/RT)	Outcome Measured	Difference (Surgery vs. No Surgery)	p Value for Main Effect
Khan, NCDB[29]		2002	16,023 (57%)	3-Year Survival	32% vs. 17%	.0001
Rapiti, Geneva Cancer Registry[31]		2006	300 (42%)	Disease-specific survival	HR 0.6 (CI 0.4–1)	.049
Gnerlich, SEER[32]		2007	9734 (47%)	Median survival	36 mo vs. 21 mo	.001
Ruiterkamp, Southern Netherlands Registry[33]		2009	728 (40%)	5-year survival	24.5% vs. 13.1%	<.0001
Cady, two-hospital database, Boston[34]		2008	622 (38%)	Median survival	36 mo vs. 24 mo	.0001[a]
Dominici, NCCN[35]		2011	551 (10%)	Median survival	42 mo vs. 36 mo	.29

CI, Confidence interval; *HR*, hazard ratio; *NCCN*, National Comprehensive Cancer Center Network; *NCDB*, National Cancer Database; *RR*, relative risk; *RT*, radiotherapy; *SEER*, Surveillance Epidemiology End Results.
[a]Attrition of significance was seen in some subsets with matched pair analyses.

mesenchymal stem cells that endow primary tumor cells with enhanced metastatic capacity provides a possible explanation for a beneficial role for resection of the primary tumor even in the setting of established distant disease.[24] Other hypotheses relating the presence of the primary tumor to the metastatic process implicate immune suppression caused by the primary tumor.[25,26] Conversely, laboratory data suggest that the presence of the primary tumor may restrain the growth of metastatic lesions,[27,28] although this has never been demonstrated in humans.

Prompted by the data from trials of metastatic renal cell carcinoma, the paradigm that surgical resection of an intact breast primary in the setting of metastatic disease has only palliative value has been questioned,[29] and multiple retrospective studies have evaluated the possibility of a survival benefit of primary site local therapy for stage IV breast cancer. These have shown a consistent association of the use of surgical resection of the intact primary with improved survival, leading to several randomized prospective trials. Two of these have been completed but thus far reported results have been null, showing no survival benefit for primary site local therapy (PSLT). These data are discussed at greater length next.

Retrospective Analyses of Primary Site Local Therapy

Surgical Resection of the Primary Tumor and Survival

Prompted by the results of SWOG 8949, which showed a survival advantage for stage IV renal cell carcinoma patients undergoing nephrectomy,[30] Khan and associates analyzed survival data on patients reported to the National Cancer Database (NCDB) of the American College of Surgeons.[29] Among 16,023 patients presenting with stage IV breast cancer in the NCDB from 1990 to 1993, surgical resection of the primary tumor was performed in 57%. The great majority of patients were treated with systemic therapy, but data on primary site radiation therapy was not available in the NCDB at that time. Surgical resection of the primary tumor was associated with a 39% reduction in the hazard of death from any cause. Other characteristics associated with overall

survival in multivariate analysis included the use of systemic therapy, the number of organ sites involved, and the presence of visceral disease.[29] In the NCDB report, the 3-year survival was 35 months in the surgically resected patients with free margins, compared with 26 months in women undergoing resection with involved margins and 17 months in the nonsurgical group.[29]

Subsequently, 18 retrospective analyses have evaluated the possible role of local therapy for the primary tumor, with the majority showing improved overall survival in women receiving treatment. The local therapy has consisted largely of surgery, although some studies have also addressed primary radiotherapy (RT). Six multiinstitutional studies (see Table 67.1) include a total of 27,000 patients, 14,443 of whom underwent surgical resection of the primary tumor. These analyses come from NCDB, the Geneva Cancer Registry, and the SEER database of the National Cancer Institute, the South Netherlands Eindhoven Cancer Registry, Massachusetts General Hospital and Boston Women's Hospital registries, and NCCN Breast outcomes database.[29–35] Thirteen additional studies come from single institutions, six from large academic institutions in the United States and seven from Europe and Asia, all of which are structured similarly and include data on 4000 patients, 1670 of whom had surgery (Table 67.2).[36–48] These single-institution studies provide detailed medical records so that questions regarding rates of positive margins, use of axillary surgery, RT, metastatic burden, and local control can be studied. More than half of these studies demonstrated a similar association between surgery and improved survival. Analyses of SEER data shows that surgically treated patients lived 11 to 15 months longer than those not receiving surgery ($p < .001$).[33,48] On the basis of this literature, Petrelli and Barni performed a meta-analysis that included 15 of these retrospective studies, with the goal of evaluating the relationship between survival and surgery or RT for the primary tumor and showed a hazard ratio (HR) of 0.69 (95% confidence interval [CI] 0.63–0.77, Fig. 67.1) associated with the use of surgery.[49] Survival benefit was independent of multiple factors such as age, tumor burden, type of surgery, margin status, site of metastases, hormone receptor status, and HER2 status.[49]

The role of axillary surgery on overall survival has been difficult to evaluate in the published retrospective analyses. A meta-analysis by Hartmann and colleagues[50] considered six retrospective studies[31,34,36,37,41,42] that gave information about whether

TABLE 67.2 Summary of Single-Center Studies Examining Primary Site Surgery or Radiotherapy in de Novo Stage IV Patients

First Author	Year	N (% Surgery/RT)	Outcome Measured	Difference (Surgery vs. No Surgery)	p Value for Main Effect
Babiera[36]	2006	244 (37)	Progression-free survival	RR .54 (CI .38–.77)	.0007
Blanchard[40]	2008	395 (61)	Median survival	27 mo vs. 17 mo	.0001
Hazard[41]	2008	111 (42)	Median survival	26 mo vs. 29 mo	NS
Fields[42]	2007	409 (46)	Median survival	32 mo vs. 15 mo	.0001
Bafford[39]	2009	147 (41)	Overall survival	HR 0.47[a]	.003[a]
Le Scodan[b,38]	2009	581 (55)	3-year survival	43.4% vs. 26.7%	.00002
Shien[44]	2009	344 (47)	Median survival	27 mo vs. 22 mo	.049
Leung[48]	2010	157 (33)	Median survival	25 mo vs. 13 mo	.06
Nguyen[43]	2012	733 (51.6)	5-year survival	21 vs. 14 mo	<.001
Perez Hidalgo[46]	2011	208 (59.1)	Overall survival	40.1 vs. 24.3 mo	<.001
Rashaan[47]	2012	171 (34.5)	Overall survival	HR 0.9 (0.59–1.37)	NS
Pathy[45]	2011	375 (37.1)	2-year survival	46.3% vs. 21.3	<.001
Neuman[37]	2010	186 (37)	Overall survival	RR .71 (CI 0.47–1.06)	NS

CI, Confidence interval; *HR,* hazard ratio; *NS,* nonsignificant; *RR,* relative risk.
[a]On subset analysis, those diagnosed with metastases postoperatively showed no survival advantage.
[b]Primary site therapy consisted of RT.

Study or Subgroup	log [Hazard ratio]	SE	Weight	Hazard ratio IV, random, 95% CI	Year
Khan 2002 R1	−0.286	0.028	10.1%	0.75 (0.71–0.79)	2002
Khan 2002 R0	−0.491	0.027	10.1%	0.61 (0.58–0.65)	2002
Rapiti 2006 R0	−0.511	0.261	2.8%	0.60 (0.36–1.00)	2006
Rapiti 2006 R1	−0.262	0.246	3.1%	1.30 (0.80–2.10)	2006
Babiera 2006	−0.693	0.443	1.2%	0.50 (0.21–1.19)	2006
Fields 2007	−0.635	0.119	6.7%	0.53 (0.42–0.67)	2007
Gnerlich 2007	−0.478	0.032	10.0%	0.62 (0.58–0.66)	2007
Blanchard 2008	−0.342	0.125	6.4%	0.71 (0.56–0.91)	2008
Hazard 2008	−0.226	0.354	1.8%	0.80 (0.40–1.60)	2008
Ruiterkamp 2009	−0.478	0.102	7.4%	0.62 (0.51–0.76)	2009
Bafford 2009	−0.75	0.25	3.0%	0.47 (0.29–0.77)	2009
Shien 2009	−0.117	0.06	9.1%	0.89 (0.79–1.00)	2009
Neuman 2010	−0.342	0.217	3.7%	0.71 (0.46–1.09)	2010
Perez-Fidalgo 2011	−0.654	0.202	4.0%	0.52 (0.35–0.77)	2011
Dominici 2011	−0.062	0.057	9.2%	0.94 (0.84–1.05)	2011
Booh Pathy 2011	−0.545	0.093	7.8%	0.58 (0.48–0.70)	2011
Rashaan 2012	−0.105	0.216	3.7%	0.90 (0.59–1.37)	2012
Total (95% CI)			**100.0%**	**0.69 (0.63–0.77)**	

Heterogeneity: $Tau^2 = 0.03$; $Chi^2 = 110.08$, df = 16 ($p < .00001$); $I^2 = 85\%$
Test for overall effect: Z = 7.15 ($p < .00001$)

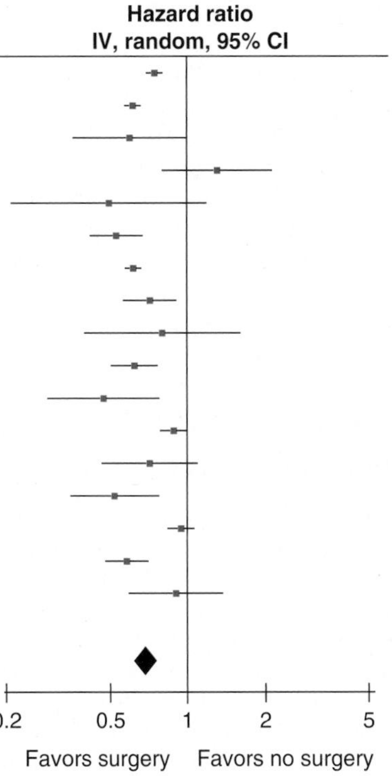

Favors surgery Favors no surgery

• **Fig. 67.1** Forest plot of meta-analysis by Petrelli and Barni, including 15 retrospective studies that examined the association between primary site local therapy and survival in de novo stage IV breast cancer patients. (From Petrelli F, Barni S. Surgery of primary tumors in stage IV breast cancer: an updated meta-analysis of published studies with meta-regression. *Med Oncol.* 2012;29:3282-3290.)

an axillary surgical procedure was performed in case of surgery. Of the patients reviewed, 42% had surgery. In the surgery group, 527 patients (69%) had axillary procedures. Only three studies investigated the impact of axillary surgery on survival, and did not find a benefit.[31,34] Given current concepts regarding the role and value of axillary dissection in nonmetastatic breast cancer, this procedure cannot be recommended in patients with metastatic disease.

Radiotherapy for the Primary Tumor and Survival

The use of primary RT for the primary tumor appears to show a survival benefit similar to that seen with surgical resection, although it is difficult to decipher individually because it is typically combined with surgery. Some patients in these series were treated with both surgery and RT, and the data suggest that the surgical group had higher rates of RT use. The larger RT studies have come mainly from single institutions in France and Canada. In 2009, Le Scodan and associates identified 581 patients with de novo stage IV breast cancer treated between 1984 and 2004; RT included both nodal fields and a boost to the tumor site for most patients. Of these patients, 320 received locoregional RT, 30 received only surgery, and 41 women received both surgery and RT. The 3-year overall survival rate was 43% versus 27% in the group receiving locoregional RT (LRT) versus those who did not, with an adjusted HR of 0.7 (95% CI 0.58–0.85).[38] Nguyen and colleagues have reported a series from British Columbia, evaluating the effect of LRT on survival in 733 patients presenting between 1996 and 2005. Of these, 378 patients had PSLT that consisted of surgery alone in 67% of patients, RT alone in 22%, and both in 11%. 355 patients had no local therapy. The 5-year overall survival rates were 21% in those who had PSLT compared with 14% in those who did not ($p < .001$).[43] The rates of locoregional progression-free survival were higher in those who had PSLT (72% vs. 46%; $p < .001$).[43] Patients who had both surgery and RT had a better 5-year overall survival of 32.5% compared with those who had surgery or RT alone (21 and 17%, respectively). A second French study of 239 patients comparing those who had surgery or RT alone showed a trend toward increased survival. However, no advantage was noted between either group after adjustment for prognostic factors, although RT alone did improve local control.[51]

Effect of Primary Site Local Therapy on Locoregional Control

The rationale for treatment of the primary tumor may relate to a need for palliation of a symptomatic tumor, or a fear of ULD. Clearly, a woman living with metastatic breast cancer will be further distressed if the primary site is uncontrolled. Chest wall outcomes are therefore important, but data regarding these is scant. The largest data set comes from a single-institution retrospective review, where chest wall control was related to use of surgery and to survival in patients with metastatic breast cancer and an intact primary tumor. Between 1995 and 2005, 111 patients were identified at Northwestern Memorial Hospital,[41] 42% of whom underwent surgical resection of the primary tumor within 6 months of diagnosis, in the absence of symptoms caused by the primary tumor. The nonoperative arm included patients who had delayed surgery secondary to symptomatic local progression or did not have surgery at all. Both groups were well matched, and all received systemic therapy. Local control was more often

maintained in patients treated surgically (82% vs. 34%; $p = .002$). Surgical resection was associated with longer time to first progression (adjusted HR 0.5, 95% CI 0.298–0.838), but there was no statistically significant difference in terms of overall survival. However, when survival was examined as a function of chest wall control, women who maintained a controlled chest wall survived significantly longer than those who developed symptomatic chest wall disease (i.e., skin nodules or ulceration) with better overall survival (HR 0.42, 95% CI 0.26–0.66; $p = .0002$).[41]

Similar questions regarding management of the primary site pertain to the scenario where metachronous distant recurrence is accompanied by an in-breast recurrence. Data regarding this come from a retrospective review of 5502 patients within the Danish Breast Cancer Group database, who had breast conserving surgery for stage I–II breast cancer from 1976 to 1998. Three hundred and seven patients were identified within breast tumor recurrence, and the role of surgical resection for recurrence was evaluated. Resection of the in-breast recurrence was shown to protect against both ULD and death.[52] After in-breast recurrence, patients treated nonoperatively had the highest rate of ULD (32%), followed by those treated with repeat breast conserving therapy (16%). Patients treated with salvage mastectomy had the lowest rate of ULD (10%; $p = .004$). The maintenance of local control was associated with longer survival duration compared with patients who developed ULD (5-year survival, 78% vs. 21%). Patients with the highest risk of ULD were patients with disseminated disease (odds ratio [OR] 12.7; $p < 0$) and patients treated nonsurgically (OR 5.6; $p = .003$).

Retrospective Studies Questioning the Benefit of Primary Site Local Therapy in De Novo Stage IV Breast Cancer

Contrary to the positive findings already discussed, a few studies have demonstrated only a trend toward improvement in survival or no improvement in survival.[33,35–37,41,48] The largest study showing a trend was a review by Cady and associates[33] in an analysis of 622 patients with de novo stage IV breast cancer, where surgically treated stage IV patients were matched to controls who did not receive PSLT. Matched-pair analysis lessened but did not eliminate the survival benefit associated with PSLT in all subsets. However, among women with visceral metastases only (100 patients), the matched analysis showed no significant survival benefit. A detailed review of medical records for 100 women within the study showed that tumor stage and surgical procedure were categorized inaccurately, which may have influenced results. The authors also noted benefits for patients who received surgery after systemic therapy, indicating that patients who had more favorable responses to systemic therapy were more likely to benefit from surgery.

Selection Biases in the Retrospective Analyses

Although these retrospective studies showed significant benefit and no worse outcome for patients undergoing surgical intervention, they suffer from substantial biases that lead to the question of whether the apparent survival benefit from PSLT is a cause-and-effect relationship or whether this is explained entirely by selection bias. These trends are demonstrated in the 15 trials included in the meta-analysis by Petrelli and Barni,[49] where a consistently better prognostic profile is seen in women receiving

TABLE 67.3	Randomized Trials Evaluating the Role of Surgery in Stage IV Breast Cancer						
Country	Clinical Trilas.gov Identifier	Accrual Period	N	Initial Therapy	Radiotherapy	Primary End Point
India	NCT00193778	2005–2012	450	CAF ± T	If indicated	Time to progression
Turkey	NCT00557986	2008–2012	281	Surgery	For BCT	Survival
Japan	JCOG1017	2011–2016	410	Systemic therapy	Not addressed	Survival
United States and Canada	NCT 01242800	2011–2015	383	Systemic therapy	Per standards for stage I–III	Survival
Austria	NCT01015625	2010–2015	93	Surgery	Per standards for stage I–III	Survival

Two additional trials were initiated, but closed with minimal accrual (Netherlands, NCT01392586 and Thailand, NCT 01906112).
BCT, Breast conserving therapy.

PSLT. The factors that significantly favor the PSLT groups range from younger age (in 10 of 15 trials), to smaller tumors (greater fraction of T1–T2 tumors in 10 of 11 trials where this is reported), greater frequency of single organ system metastases in 11 of 15 trials, significantly less frequent visceral disease in 11 of 15 trials, fewer comorbidities,[42] and better access to care.[32,40] Although these are recognizable biases that were adjusted for in statistical analyses, the possibility of unrecognized biases or incomplete adjustment remained. One bias that was recognized early on and particularly affects the data derived from tumor registries, is that of surgical timing. This relates to the fact that women who present with clinically nonmetastatic disease, do not undergo staging scans before resection of the primary tumor, then may be staged postoperatively and found to have metastases. Their metastatic burden is likely lower than that of women who present with symptomatic metastases; in both instances, however, they would be reported to the tumor registry as stage IV patients because this reporting typically occurs many weeks after surgery. This particular bias has been examined in several studies with mixed results. Rapiti and colleagues performed an analysis in which women diagnosed with metastases postoperatively were excluded and found a persistent association of the use of surgery with improved survival, although the effect was smaller.[31] In an analysis from MD Anderson, the optimal timing of surgery appeared to be 3 to 6 months after diagnosis, suggesting that these women were known to have metastases preoperatively, although this aspect is not specifically addressed.[53] In an analysis from Boston, the benefit of surgery appeared to be confined to the group who underwent resection before metastatic diagnosis.[39] In a second analysis, the same group used a case-control set from the NCCN with similar results, although the design of the study was difficult to interpret because women who underwent surgery before systemic therapy were compared with those who received no surgery, and women with known metastases who received systemic therapy before surgery were excluded.[35] The nonsurgery group comprised 236 patients versus 54 patients in the surgical group. Results showed that before matching, those in the surgery group were more likely to be younger, less likely to have more than one site of metastatic disease, and more likely to have received endocrine therapy. However, when matched for prognostic factors, there was no survival benefit to surgery when performed before systemic therapy. Survival was similar as well after adjusting for nonmatched factors such as presence of lung metastases, year of diagnosis, and use of trastuzumab.

Randomized Prospective Trials

As we have illustrated here, retrospective studies carry biases; whereas known biases can be adjusted for in analysis, unknown biases cannot. Therefore early in the course of this discussion, it was recognized that selection bias may be a strong driver of the apparent benefit of PSLT[54] and that randomized trials were needed to verify this effect. Several randomized trials were initiated, shown in Table 67.3; however, the trials in the Netherlands and in Thailand were terminated with minimal or no accrual, whereas the Austrian trial has closed after accrual of 93 patients (personal communication, Dr. Florian Fitzal, August 2016). The remaining four trials include one ongoing (Japan), one that has completed accrual with follow-up ongoing (USA/Canada), and two that have been completed with preliminary results reported (Turkey) and final results published (India).[55–59] These trials have a primary end point of overall survival but in addition will address questions about which subsets of patients may be particularly likely (or unlikely) to experience a benefit from primary site local therapy. The major secondary hypotheses relate to local control benefits, quality of life, and whether women with bone-only disease, whose disease biology likely favors longer survival, will benefit more or less than other subgroups.

Trials Requiring Induction Systemic Therapy

Three of these clinical trials included induction systemic therapy before randomization, with the idea that women whose distant disease is nonresponsive to first-line agents are unlikely to derive benefit from therapy directed to the primary tumor. These are shown in Table 67.3. The first to open was in India, at the Tata Memorial Cancer Institute in Mumbai in 2005 (clinicaltrials.gov identifier NCT00193778). The results were presented orally in 2013 and have since been published.[55] The participants were enrolled from a pool of 716 patients with de novo stage IV breast cancer of whom 25 had resectable primary tumors whereas the remainder did not. Those with unresectable tumors were treated with chemotherapy before registration to the trial; this consisted of anthracycline-based chemotherapy in 96%; taxanes were added in just under 5% of patients; 4% of participants received endocrine therapy. HER2-directed therapy was not available to HER2 positive patients (30% had HER2 positive tumors, and one patient received trastuzumab). Thus the induction systemic therapy was not directed to the presence of therapeutic targets (estrogen receptor or HER2), although the study arms were balanced with regard to systemic regimens used. After response assessment, 440 responders were registered, excluding those with involvement of more than two visceral sites, extensive hepatic metastases, and an expected survival of less than 1 year. From these, an additional 90 were excluded at randomization because they were unfit for surgery or declined further treatment, leaving 350 who were randomized to locoregional treatment consisting of surgery (with RT when indicated) versus continued systemic therapy. Primary outcomes were overall survival and disease-free survival. Secondary outcomes were locoregional progression-free survival, distant progression–free survival, and health-related quality of life. The trial was powered to detect a 6-month improvement in 2-year survival (from 18 to 24 months).

The two study arms were well balanced in terms of disease characteristics and demographics. There was relatively little crossover between arms, and locoregional therapy was, for the most part, delivered as randomized. Eight patients (5%) within the locoregional treatment group did not undergo locoregional treatment, and 18 (10%) within the no locoregional treatment group underwent subsequent surgical removal of the primary tumor for palliation of symptoms. Median duration of follow-up was 23 months with a total of 235 deaths at data cutoff date. Local progression-free survival was significantly better in the surgical group (80% at 5 years compared with 20% in the nonsurgical group ($p < .001$; Fig. 67.2A). The authors noted a shortening of time to first distant progression in the locoregional therapy arm (see Fig. 67.2B), but this did not lead to worse survival and may be a result of censoring of patients with earlier local progression in the systemic therapy arm. Median overall survival was 20.5% in the nonsurgical group and 19.2% in the surgical group at 5 years (HR 1.04, 95% CI 0.80–1.34; Fig. 67.2C). Additionally, no significant benefit was noted in survival outcomes after subset analyses evaluating factors such as hormone receptor or HER2 status of the tumor, number of metastatic lesions, and bone-only disease. Of note is that the median survival shown in this study is lower compared with the reported values in developed countries, as evidenced in the US Translational Breast Cancer Research Consortium patient registry.[60] This is likely due to differences in delivery of systemic therapy in India including lack of targeted therapy (92% of the 107 patients with HER2 positive tumors did not receive targeted therapy postoperatively) and financial constraints that made delivery inconsistent. Additionally, the majority of the patients had symptomatic disease, which suggests poor prognosis and likely a heavy metastatic burden. Overall the investigators concluded that there is no survival gain with surgical therapy for de novo stage IV breast cancer, and it should not be routinely used. It is important to note that in this population of women with unresectable disease, only 18 (10%) of 177 women in the no locoregional treatment group required palliative surgery during follow-up.[55] However, it is difficult to reconcile this low number with the large difference in locoregional progression in the two arms (HR 0.16, 95% CI 0.10–0.26).

The Japan Clinical Oncology Group (JCOG) 1017 trial also seeks to compare the efficacy of primary tumor resection plus systemic therapy versus systemic therapy alone. The trial began recruitment in June 2011 with an enrollment plan of 410 patients for randomization over a 5-year recruitment period. As of January 2017, it has registered 458 patients and randomized 307. After 3 months of systemic therapy, women who show no disease progression are randomized to undergo surgery or to continue systemic

therapy; RT is not required. The primary outcome is overall survival. Secondary outcomes are local recurrence rate and local control rate.[56]

In the United States and Canada, the Eastern Cooperative Oncology Group EA2108 (clinicaltrials.gov identifier NCT01242800) study closed July 2015 with 383 patients accrued. Patients received induction systemic therapy consisting of endocrine, cytotoxic, or biologic regimens appropriate to the patient's age and tumor type. Patients without progression of disease after 16 to 32 weeks of treatment were randomized to both surgery and RT or to continuation of systemic therapy. Randomization was stratified by type of induction systemic therapy (endocrine therapy, chemotherapy, or chemotherapy with anti-HER2 agents) because the choice of systemic therapy reflects the biologic subtype of the tumor. The study had a 15% built-in crossover rate. The primary outcome is survival; the trial is powered to detect an overall survival difference of 19% at 3 years (from 30% to 49%). The secondary outcomes are local progression-free survival and quality of life, and biological samples are being banked for correlative studies. This trial differs from JCOG 1017 with respect to the role of axillary clearance and radiation therapy, both of which are mandated to correspond to current standards for nonmetastatic breast cancer.[57] Follow-up is ongoing and results are expected in 2017.

Trials Requiring Randomization to Locoregional Therapy Before Systemic Therapy

In contrast, two additional trials considered the role of surgery upfront, before systemic therapy. The first trial with this design was opened by the Turkish Federation of Breast Diseases (MF07-01, clinicaltrials.gov identifier NCT00557986)[58,59] and has completed accrual, with a total of 274 patients evaluated. The design included randomization to surgery (mastectomy or lumpectomy followed by radiation therapy, with or without axillary dissection in patients with positive nodes) before systemic therapy, or systemic therapy alone. The trial was powered to detect a survival difference of 18% at 36 months. The primary outcome was 3-year survival, overall survival, with secondary outcomes related to progression-free survival, quality-of-life measures, and morbidity related to locoregional therapy. According to results reported at the 2016 American Society of Clinical Oncology (ASCO) meeting, there was no difference in survival at 36 months ($p = .5$). However, there was an improvement in survival with local therapy at 40 months median follow-up with a 9-month difference (46 vs. 37 months). Overall survival rate was 34% higher among women who received locoregional therapy, compared with women who did not (HR 0.66; 95% CI 0.49–0.88; $p = .005$).[59] Locoregional progression was also reduced in the locoregional therapy group (1%) versus the systemic therapy group (11%; $p = .001$).[59] In unplanned and exploratory subset analyses, the Turkish investigators found statistically significant higher rates of survival among women with hormone receptor positive–disease, HER2-negative tumors, patients younger than 55 years, and solitary bony lesions. Particularly for bone (unbiopsied) only metastasis, the median survival was 56 months in the locoregional group versus 42 months in the systemic therapy only group (HR 0.67; 95% CI 0.43–1.07; $p = .09$).[59] This result is difficult to interpret given the small number of such women, the imbalance between arms, the lack of biopsy confirmation, and the post hoc nature of the analysis, which was one among many other explorations of the data. This study suggests that patients with low burden or indolent disease derive a benefit from local therapy; however, longer follow-up is necessary to determine such benefit.

The POSYTIVE trial in Austria (clinicaltrials.gov identifier NCT01015625)[60,61] was designed similarly, with systemic therapy after randomization and completion of locoregional therapy versus systemic therapy alone, with a strong emphasis on biobanking. Patients with synchronous metastatic breast cancer were randomly assigned to receive local therapy to the primary tumor, consisting of primary tumor resection with axillary dissection, and optional radiotherapy, versus no local therapy to the primary site. Patients in the no surgery group could have surgery on demand.

Primary outcomes were median survival. Secondary outcomes included time to distant progression and time to local progression. The accrual goal was 254 patients. However, the study has closed after accrual of 93 patients (personal communication, Dr. Florian Fitzal, August 2016).

Prospective Registry Trial of de Novo Stage IV Breast Cancer Patients

Translational Breast Cancer Research Consortium (TBCRC) 0313 is a prospective multiinstitutional registry designed to gather

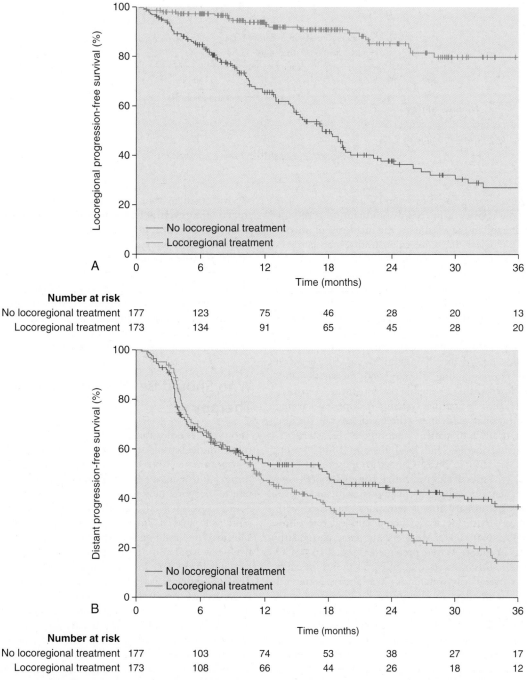

Number at risk

No locoregional treatment	177	123	75	46	28	20	13
Locoregional treatment	173	134	91	65	45	28	20

Number at risk

No locoregional treatment	177	103	74	53	38	27	17
Locoregional treatment	173	108	66	44	26	18	12

• **Fig. 67.2** Cancer outcomes of stage IV breast cancer patients treated with or without locoregional therapy of the primary breast tumor at Tata Memorial Center, Mumbai, India. (A) Locoregional progression-free survival. (B) Distant progression-free survival. *Continued*

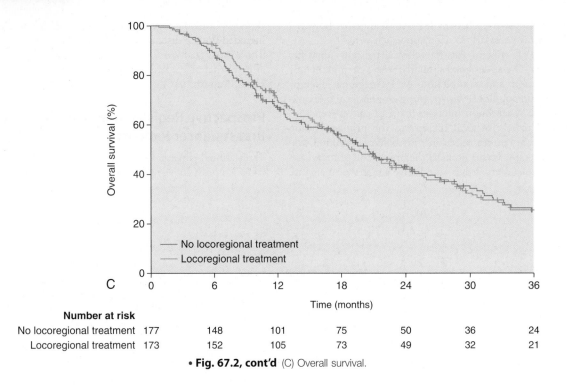

Number at risk

No locoregional treatment	177	148	101	75	50	36	24
Locoregional treatment	173	152	105	73	49	32	21

• **Fig. 67.2, cont'd** (C) Overall survival.

data on the modern management of stage IV breast cancer. The primary goal of the registry is to record information on the use of locoregional therapy in these patients, the incidence of uncontrolled disease, biological and molecular features of patient's tumors, and rate of surgical intervention for palliation for intact primary. Patients are categorized into cohorts of those with an intact primary (A, N = 112) or those with resected primary and metastases discovered within 3 months of surgery (B, N = 15). Local and distant disease is being carefully monitored, including the frequency of uncontrolled chest wall disease, and its effect on quality of life. Biopsy samples have been banked, and studies are planned to provide insight into biological interactions between responding and nonresponding primary and metastatic sites. Enrollment has closed with 127 eligible patients from 14 institutions. All patients received first-line systemic treatment according to standard institutional guidelines. Three-year overall survival was analyzed in relation to patient and tumor characteristics, response to systemic therapy and local therapy. Initial results presented at the San Antonio Breast Cancer Symposium in 2013 showed that at 2-year overall survival for all patients is 86% and was better for patients in cohort B (diagnosed with metastases within 3 months of primary tumor resection) compared with cohort A (diagnosed with metastases before surgical resection): 100% versus 84%, p = .03.[62] More recent data, particularly regarding patients in cohort A, were presented at the 2016 ASCO annual conference. This showed that after 54-month median follow-up, 3-year overall survival for is 70% and is better for patients who are responders to chemotherapy compared with nonresponders: 78% versus 24%, p = .001.[63] Forty-one percent of responders chose to have surgery, and these patients were more likely to have large tumors and single-organ metastasis and to have received first-line chemotherapy.[63] Among responders, no benefit was noted with surgery in 3-year overall survival (p = .85), and this was present regardless of tumor subtype, although HER2-positive status and response seems to provide longer survival (93%).[63] In addition, surgery did not affect progression-free

survival: median time to progression was 13 months in the no surgery group versus 12 months in those who had surgery.[63] This data also demonstrate that surgical palliation of the primary tumor is usually not required in the modern era because a majority (85%) of patients in this cohort are responders to first-line therapy. The results must be interpreted with caution due to the small sample size and the patients who had a benefit cannot be comparable to patients who were found to have metastases at diagnosis or responders to chemotherapy. It also highlights the need for extended follow-up in the studies investigating the role of surgery in patients with stage IV breast cancer.

Who Should Be Offered Locoregional Therapy

The present indication for locoregional therapy for the primary tumor in the setting of metastases continues to be the presence of a symptomatic tumor. For women with *asymptomatic* primary tumors, the mainstay of therapy remains systemic, and it is important to recognize (and to explain to patients) that medical therapy is in fact very effective at controlling the breast primary, in the same way that it controls distant disease. Thus both in the Mumbai/Tata randomized trial, and in the TBCRC registry, relatively few women in the systemic therapy group required surgery for palliation (10% in Mumbai and 5% in the TBCRC study). The notion that resection of the primary tumor is required to avert uncontrolled chest wall disease is not supported by these prospective data. Most important, the only mature clinical trial testing the survival value of primary site surgery[55] showed no hint of a survival advantage. Additionally, this study did not show a trend of benefit for the preplanned subset analyses, so that the subgroups that have been predicted to have higher likelihood of benefit from locoregional therapy (lower metastatic burden, osseous metastases, hormone receptor-positive disease) did not, in fact, demonstrate any advantage, although the caveat of differing medical therapy patterns in India remains. It is hoped that the possibility that there is a subset of patients who benefit from PSLT will be further elucidated in ongoing trials. Of note, none of the studies reported so far have found worse outcomes for women undergoing locoregional intervention.

A possible exception to the general rule that women with asymptomatic primaries should not be advised to undergo PSLT is the situation in which the distant disease is well controlled on medical therapy, but the primary tumor is progressing. This occurrence, although unusual, does present occasionally; in this setting, PSLT may be reasonable but with a full explanation that it is not known to improve survival. Another possible exception is the stage IV patient who has no evidence of evaluable distant disease after medical therapy, and the tumor in the breast is the only remaining site of disease. Such a patient would be rendered "stage IV NED (no evidence of disease)" by resection of the primary tumor, and retrospective data from highly selected patients who reach this state suggest that they may experience long-term survival.[64] If PSLT is decided upon following the preceding considerations, breast conservation (if feasible) is clearly the least harmful option. The role of RT in conjunction with surgery or as primary therapy should also be driven by palliative needs rather than therapeutic promise. There is no clear justification to offer PSLT to women with distant disease that is not well controlled (unless required for palliation). Even if both local and distant sites are well controlled, the rationale for PSLT is weak because the primary site is likely to remain well controlled for the patient's life span.

It is of utmost importance to consider the risks of locoregional therapy as well as the out of pocket cost it may render to the patient, particularly without Level I evidence suggesting a benefit. It is also important to be aware of the possible questions that may arise with providing surgery for the primary tumor, such as post-mastectomy reconstruction.

Conclusion

Improvements in breast cancer treatment have extended the life expectancy of stage IV patients beyond historic controls, so that considering optimal management of an intact primary tumor has become important. The possibility of a survival benefit from surgical extirpation of the intact primary is not supported by prospective data so far, but important questions remain that have enormous implications for the management of patients with in-breast disease and metastatic cancer. The results of the remaining ongoing trials will provide clarification on the role, extent, and timing of locoregional therapy for stage IV breast cancer. At present, locoregional therapy should only be offered to patients with stage IV de novo breast cancer with a clear understanding of the risks and costs of such therapy, and the lack of a demonstrated survival benefit.

Selected References

2. Andre F, Slimane K, Bachelot T, et al. Breast cancer with synchronous metastases: trends in survival during a 14-year period. *J Clin Oncol.* 2004;22:3302-3308.

15. Mickisch GH, Garin A, van Poppel H, et al. Radical nephrectomy plus interferon-alfa-based immunotherapy compared with interferon alfa alone in metastatic renal-cell carcinoma: a randomised trial. *Lancet.* 2001;358:966-970.

29. Khan SA, Stewart AK, Morrow M. Does aggressive local therapy improve survival in metastatic breast cancer? *Surgery.* 2002;132:620-626.

38. Le Scodan SR, Stevens D, Brain E, et al. Breast cancer with synchronous metastases: survival impact of exclusive loco-regional radiotherapy. *J Clin Oncol.* 2009;27:1375-1381.

49. Petrelli F, Barni S. Surgery of primary tumors in stage IV breast cancer: an updated meta-analysis of published studies with meta-regression. *Med Oncol.* 2012;29:3282-3290.

55. Badwe RA, Parmar V, Hawaldar R, et al. Locoregional treatment versus no treatment of the primary tumour in metastatic breast cancer: an open-label randomised controlled trial. *Lancet.* 2015;16:1380-1388.

56. Shien T, Nakamura K, Shibata T, et al. A randomized controlled trial comparing primary tumour resection plus systemic therapy with systemic therapy alone in metastatic breast cancer (PRIM-BC): Japan Clinical Oncology Group Study JCOG1017. *Jpn J Clin Oncol.* 2012;42(10):970-973.

57. Khan SA. A randomized phase III trial of the value of early local therapy for the intact primary tumor in patients with metastatic breast cancer http://www.cancer.gov/clinicaltrials/ECOG-E2108.

59. Soran A, Ozmen V, Ozbas S, et al. A randomized controlled trial evaluating resection of the primary breast tumor in women presenting with de novo stage IV breast cancer; Turkish study (protocol MF07-01) [presented at ASCO Annual Conference, 2016]. *J Clin Oncol.* 2016;34:suppl abstract 1005).

63. King TA, Lyman JP, Gonen M, et al. TBCRC 013: A prospective analysis of surgery and survival in stage IV breast cancer. *J Clin Oncol.* 2016;34:supplement abstract 1006, ASCO annual conference, 2016.

A full reference list is available online at ExpertConsult.com.

68

Management of Bone Metastases in Breast Cancer

URSA BROWN-GLABERMAN AND ALISON T. STOPECK

Bone is the most common site of first recurrence in patients with breast cancer; affecting up to 70% of patients with metastatic disease.[1] Patients with bone metastases are at high risk for developing clinically significant complications, often referred to as skeletal-related events (SREs), including radiation therapy or surgery to prevent or treat fracture and palliate pain, pathologic fracture (excluding major trauma), spinal cord compression, and hypercalcemia. If untreated, metastatic breast cancer patients experience an average of four complications per year related to bone metastases, with pathologic fractures and radiation therapy being the most commonly observed SREs.[2,3] Cancer registry data suggest that patients with metastatic breast cancer who develop SREs live significantly shorter than similar metastatic patients who do not develop skeletal complications.[4] Complications stemming from bone metastases can be life-threatening and are a major source of morbidity for patients, making their prevention and treatment a vital component of comprehensive oncologic care.

The development of bone metastases is common to all breast cancer subtypes but is especially prevalent in estrogen receptor–positive disease in which bone metastases are found in more than 80% of patients with distant relapse compared with 50% in patients with breast cancer negative for hormone receptor and HER2 expression (triple negative).[5] Up to 30% of patients with metastatic breast cancer relapse exclusively in the bone without visceral involvement (bone-only disease).[5,6] The most common skeletal sites affected, in decreasing order of frequency, are the spine, pelvis, skull, ribs, and femur.[7] The lumbar spine is the single most commonly involved site, accounting for up to 20% of osseous metastases. In the appendicular skeleton, the proximal femurs are the most common site of metastases, followed by the humeri.

This chapter addresses the pathophysiology, clinical presentation, diagnosis, and treatment of bone metastases with surgery, radiotherapy (RT), and systemic osteoclast inhibitors. Chapters 69 and 70 discuss chemotherapy and endocrine therapy options for patients with bone metastases, and are not discussed here. However, poor systemic disease control remains the greatest risk factor for progression of bone metastases and for the development of SREs, rendering traditional cytotoxic and targeted antitumor therapies essential in the management of all patients with bone metastases.

Pathophysiology

During physiologic conditions, bone is in a state of constant remodeling, maintaining a dynamic balance between osteoclastic (resorptive) and osteoblastic (bone-forming) activity. Bone resorption is mediated by osteoclasts, multinucleated giant cells derived from granulocyte-macrophage precursors. Bone formation is carried out by osteoblasts, which are derived from mesenchymal fibroblast-like cells. The receptor activator of NF-κB ligand (RANKL)-RANK pathway mediates osteoclast activity is a key regulator of bone metabolism. RANKL is produced by osteoblasts, bone marrow stromal cells, and other cells under the control of various proresorptive growth factors, hormones, and cytokines including parathyroid hormone (PTH), parathyroid hormone–related peptide (PTHrP), progesterone, prostaglandins, and interleukins. By binding to the RANK receptor expressed on osteoclasts and preosteoclasts, RANKL controls the development, formation, activation, and survival of osteoclasts and plays a primary role in stimulating osteoclast-mediated bone resorption. As the only known ligand for the RANK receptor, RANKL is indispensable for normal osteoclast activity. Osteoblasts and stromal cells also produce osteoprotegerin, a soluble decoy receptor that binds to and inactivates RANKL preventing osteoclast activation. The RANKL/OPG ratio is the primary determinant of osteoclast activity in physiologic as well as several pathologic conditions, including cancer.

In patients with metastatic bone disease, bone formation and resorption are uncoupled, leading to both osteoblastic and osteolytic lesions. Bone resorption can occur through tumor-mediated osteolysis in which cancer cells directly resorb local bone or, more commonly, through the direct activation and stimulation of osteoclasts via the secretion of RANKL as well as other osteoclast-stimulating factors. The process of bone resorption leads to the release of growth factors from the bone matrix including type I collagen, osteocalcin, insulin-like growth factors, transforming growth factor (TGF)-β, as well as calcium, which may stimulate cancer cells directly, leading to the hypothesized vicious cycle of bone destruction and progressive tumor growth.[8]

PTHrP is often the primary culprit responsible for RANKL release and bone destruction in breast cancer patients. This protein was originally identified as a hypercalcemic factor in several cancer types, including breast.[9] PTHrP has 70% homology to the first

13 amino acids of PTH, the major hormone responsible for calcium homeostasis and binds to the common PTH/PTHrP receptors. The binding of PTHrP to receptors on osteoblasts and marrow stromal cells results in the production of RANKL, causing increased osteoclast differentiation and activation and the initiation of the vicious cycle. Approximately 80% of hypercalcemic patients with solid tumors have detectable plasma PTHrP concentrations.[10]

The pathogenesis of osteoblastic metastases is less well understood than that of osteolytic lesions. As with osteolytic lesions, osteoblastic bone metastases are the result of dysregulated bone metabolism. Preclinical data suggest that in osteoblastic lesions, an initial phase of bone destruction may be followed by extensive bone formation, supported by the presence of elevated bone turnover markers in patients with prostate cancer metastatic to the bone.[11,12] Endothelin-1, a vasoconstrictor peptide produced by prostate and breast cancer cells, is thought to be a stimulator of the osteoblast proliferation contributing to the development and progression of blastic metastases.[8]

Clinical Presentation

Pain is the most common presenting symptom of bone metastases and is seen in up to 75% of patients.[13,14] Bone pain is also the most common cause of cancer-related pain in metastatic patients, rendering pain control an essential goal of therapy. The mechanisms of pain production are varied and depend on the location of the metastatic foci as well as the type of lesion causing the pain. Nociceptive pain is caused by the local release of cytokines and chemical mediators by tumor cells, periosteal irritation, and stimulation of intraosseous nerves. Neuropathic pain is produced by the direct destruction of nerve tissue by tumors, whereas mechanical pain is caused by pressure or mass effect of the tumor within the bone, leading to loss of bone strength. The use of pharmacologic therapies including nonsteroidal antiinflammatory drugs, opioid analgesics, gamma-aminobutyric acid (GABA) analogs, and corticosteroids are often an important and necessary adjuvant to nonpharmacologic therapies for pain control.

Other common presenting signs and symptoms in untreated patients include pathologic fractures, spinal cord compression, and hypercalcemia. Because bone metastases from breast cancer most frequently include a lytic component, pathologic fracture is the most commonly observed SREs, occurring in up to 60% of patients with metastatic breast cancer to bone in historical series.[3,15]

Spinal cord compression is also more common in breast cancer patients compared with other cancer types; however, it remains a relatively rare complication, occurring in only 3% to 5% of patients.[14,16] Cord compression most commonly occurs by direct extension of a hematogenously derived vertebral body metastasis into the epidural space with resultant compression of the spinal cord. Symptoms of spinal cord compression include pain, weakness, and sensory changes, with bowel or bladder dysfunction a late finding (see Chapter 73). Sixty percent of patients with back pain and an abnormal two-dimensional projection radiograph (plain radiograph) of the spine, have epidural disease on magnetic resonance imaging (MRI).[14]

Before effective treatment with bone-targeted and antitumor therapies, hypercalcemia was observed in up 20% of patients with metastatic breast cancer to bone.[10] More recent studies suggest that hypercalcemia of malignancy is a rarer condition, affecting less than 5% of patients with breast cancer.[17,18] Hypercalcemia of malignancy is thought to occur by several mechanisms, including direct skeletal destruction by tumor and via the release of humoral factors secreted by tumor cells, including PTHrP.[10] Hypercalcemia can also rarely occur as a complication of hormonal therapies, especially tamoxifen, as part of the flare response (see Chapter 70). Hypercalcemia may result in a variety of gastrointestinal, renal, neurologic, and cardiovascular complications including constipation, nausea, fatigue, lethargy, and death. The marked decrease in the incidence of malignant hypercalcemia is thought to be in part a result of the increased use of systemic osteoclast inhibitors including bisphosphonates and denosumab in patients with metastatic breast cancer.

Diagnosis

The diagnosis of bone metastases is suggested by the presence of symptoms, abnormal laboratory values (alkaline phosphatase and calcium), and imaging studies. Imaging studies may include plain radiographs, ^{99m}Tc bone scintigraphy (bone scan), MRI, computed tomography (CT), and positron emission tomography (PET) with or without CT or MRI. Plain radiographs are often the first test in the evaluation of bone pain because they are inexpensive and specific when abnormal albeit relatively insensitive (50%) for the detection of bone metastasis. Bone scans are more sensitive than plain radiographs, particularly for lesions with a blastic component as the radiolabeled diphosphonate preferentially accumulates in areas of osteoblastic activity. However, limitations in diagnostic specificity require confirmation of abnormal findings with plain radiographs, CT, MRI, or preferably biopsy. Bone scans are also less helpful for monitoring early responses because flare reactions can be observed for up to 8 months in responding lesions secondary to increased reparative osteoblastic activity. CT imaging provides additional information such as the presence of soft tissue masses and cortical integrity. MRI is superior for identifying spinal metastases, diagnosing radiologic spinal cord compression, and assessing bone marrow involvement.[19]

Fluorodeoxyglucose (^{18}F-FDG) PET/CT has shown higher sensitivity and specificity than bone scans for detecting osteolytic bone metastases because FDG uptake occurs predominantly in cancer cells providing for a more specific tumor tracer. However, PET scans may not be as sensitive as bone scans for detecting osteoblastic metastases, and in particular lesions originating from invasive lobular breast cancers. Recent studies suggest ^{18}F-FDG PET has improved sensitivity over bone scans in detecting early bone lesions as FDG uptake in metastatic tumor cells in the bone marrow may predate the osteoblastic activity required for detection by bone scan.[20,21] ^{18}F-FDG PET scans have limitations in certain parts of the body, such as the skull, where uptake from the brain may prevent visualization of skull metastases. PET offers an additional advantage for monitoring response to therapy as decreases in PET uptake (SUV_{max}) correlate with tumor responses and time to progression. ^{18}F-FDG PET/MRI has similar sensitivity as ^{18}F-FDG PET/CT but provides better anatomic delineation.

Fluorine-18–labeled sodium fluoride (F-fluoride) PET allows for the detection of bone metastases with high contrast and spatial resolution as ^{18}F-NaF is rapidly absorbed into areas of osteoblastic activity with subsequent incorporation into the bone mineral as a fluorapatite. F-fluoride PET has been shown to be more sensitive than bone scan as well as ^{18}F-FDG PET for detecting bone metastases; however, changes in SUV_{max} have not been consistently reported to correspond to tumor responses.[21] In addition, F-fluoride PET is useful only for the detection of bone metastases, whereas ^{18}F-FDG PET can be useful for detecting metastases in other organs and sites outside the bone.

Surgical Management

Surgery plays a vital role in the management of bone metastases, principally for lesions with a complete or impending pathologic fracture. It is also a consideration in patients presenting with spinal cord compression. The proximal femur is the most common metastatic location requiring surgical intervention in breast cancer.[22] The combination of frequent involvement, high stress and torque forces placed on the bone, and the significant morbidity associated with femur fractures justify the rate of surgical intervention. Disease metastatic to the humerus is better tolerated than disease in the lower extremity, unless the patient needs crutches for ambulation.

For both the upper and lower extremities, two operative strategies are commonly considered: (1) endoprosthetic reconstruction or (2) internal fixation with either intramedullary nailing or plate/screw fixation devices. Factors that favor endoprosthetic reconstruction over intramedullary stabilization include large periarticular lesions, involvement of the femoral neck, substantial bone loss, severe fracture comminution, and an oncologic benefit to resection.[23] Before surgically managing a completed or impending pathologic fracture, the entire bone in question should be imaged as other lesions in the vicinity may affect operative planning.

In a systematic review of 45 studies addressing the role of surgical management of bone metastases in multiple cancer types (including both prophylactic and after fracture), pain relief after surgical management was achieved in 91% to 93% of cases, and function was maintained or improved in 89% to 94%.[24] The pooled complication and mortality rates were 17% and 4%, respectively. The most commonly encountered complications in cancer patients include superficial surgical site infection and deep venous thrombosis.

Spinal cord compression from metastatic disease is considered a medical emergency because prompt treatment is essential to reverse neurologic symptoms. Metastatic breast cancer accounts for 15% to 20% of all cases of metastatic epidural spinal cord compression with the thoracic spine being the most common site affected followed by the lumbosacral and cervical spines. Corticosteroids, RT, and decompressive surgery are the established therapies with pain control and maintenance of function the goals of care. Indications for surgery include the need for tissue diagnosis; bone impinging into the spinal canal producing thecal compression; spinal instability with unremitting mechanical pain; radiculopathy with progressive or uncontrolled symptoms; and tumor growth unresponsive to RT or neurologic progression after RT. Randomized clinical trials support the use of early decompressive surgery for maintaining ambulation; however, age has emerged as an important variable in predicting preservation of function, and in patients over 65 years of age, marginal benefit was observed with surgery compared with radiation alone.[25]

Prophylactic Surgery

As a rule, if the patient undergoes surgery before fracture, the technical procedure is considerably simplified for the surgeon. In addition, patient morbidity and mortality are minimized because the patient does not suffer the intense pain associated with fracture or experience the complications inherent with the restrictions of immobilization associated with bed rest. The need for prophylactic surgery should be based on the estimated risk of fracture and the short-term prognosis of the patient.

Criteria historically used for selecting patients for prophylactic stabilization include lesions greater than 2.5 cm in greatest dimension involving the femur, lytic destruction of greater than 50% of the cortex of a long bone, avulsion of the lesser trochanter as seen on plain radiographs, and continued pain with weight bearing after radiation therapy.[22,26,27] If the patient has underlying osteoporosis, any defect in the cortex may weaken the bone sufficiently that fracture may occur with normal activity. Such pathologic or spontaneous fractures can occur with minimal stress, such as torque of the skeleton (twisting) when getting out of bed.

Scoring systems provide an objective method for estimating fracture risk. The Mirels Scoring System consists of a 12-point scale incorporating factors known to influence the risk of fractures such as the location of the lesion, severity of pain, degree of cortical destruction, and radiographic appearance (i.e., lytic, blastic, or mixed).[28] A score of 9 or higher defines an impending pathologic fracture for which prophylactic stabilization is recommended. This scale is widely used, has been validated in several studies, and in at least one series was found to be more sensitive than clinical judgment alone in assessing impending fracture risk.[29,30]

Pathologic Fractures

The main goals of surgery for pathologic fractures are to relieve pain and permit ambulation of the patient in the immediate postoperative period, to provide sufficient stability and bone apposition for a union to be achieved, and to debulk the tumor. Commonly used criteria for performing surgery are life expectancy of at least 1 month for a fracture of a weight-bearing bone, life expectancy of at least 3 months for a fracture of a non–weight-bearing bone, the ability to tolerate surgery, sufficient integrity of the surrounding bone to support the surgical device, and whether surgery will allow mobilization or facilitate general care in the context of the patient's overall performance status.[22] A single, definitive surgery is preferable because many patients with metastatic cancer will be unable or unwilling to undergo subsequent procedures.

Early operative stabilization of the pathologic fracture permits patients to ambulate quickly and decreases the risk of complications related to immobilization and pain medications. The most common factors associated with reconstructive failure after intramedullary fixation include tumor progression, nonunion, and hardware failure.[23] If osseous union is not achieved, internal fixation devices have a high risk of early failure. Resection of tumor, usually through intralesional curettement, is recommended to achieve local tumor control and allow surgical adjuvants, such as postoperative RT, to work more effectively. Removal of gross disease also permits the use of polymethylmethacrylate cement to fill the defect, leading to improved stability and faster time to weight bearing activity.

All patients should be evaluated for RT after operative stabilization to promote bone healing, reduce pain, and reduce the risk of subsequent fracture. A retrospective study from the University of Kansas by Townsend and colleagues found that postoperative RT was associated with improved function up to 12 months after surgery and decreased the need for further orthopedic procedures at the same site.[31,32]

Radiotherapy

Radiotherapy Alone

RT plays a primary role in the relief of painful bony metastases. The exact mechanism for the analgesic effect is unknown, although radiation-induced death of host macrophages that release chemical mediators of pain (e.g., prostaglandin E2) and interference with bone resorption by osteoclasts are the main hypotheses.

Older series have reported complete pain relief in approximately 50% of patients and partial pain relief in 80% to 90% of patients.[33–36] More recent studies using stricter criteria for pain response have reported complete response rates of 15% to 40% and partial pain relief in 60% to 80% of patients.[37,38] The incidence of pathologic fractures after RT has ranged from 2% to 18% in randomized trials.[39,40]

Multiple trials have examined various fractionation schedules for the treatment of painful bony metastases. In the Radiation Therapy Oncology Group (RTOG) 74-02 trial patients with bone metastasis were randomized to receive one of several radiation treatment plans with 15 to 40.5 Gy delivered in 5 to 15 fractions.[40] All schedules were equally effective in relieving pain. However, this trial has been widely criticized for the use of physician rather than patient assessment of pain, the inclusion of a wide range of primary sites and histologic types of cancer, and the failure to take narcotic use and incidence of retreatment into consideration.

To address some of these concerns, RTOG conducted trial 97-14, a study limited to patients with breast or prostate cancer, for a more homogeneous patient population, and more sensitive tools were used to assess pain and quality of life.[37] Patients were randomly allocated to receive either a single fraction of 8 or 30 Gy in 10 fractions over 2 weeks. At 3-month follow-up, a complete response as measured by pain control was achieved in 15% and 18% of patients in each arm, respectively ($p = .6$), and a partial response in 50% and 48% of patients, respectively. At 3 months, 33% of patients in both arms no longer required narcotic analgesics. There was no difference in the rate of pathologic fractures within or adjacent to the treatment field (5% and 4%, respectively). A significant difference between the two arms was observed in the rate of retreatment with twice as many patients in the 8-Gy arm receiving retreatment (18%) compared with the 30-Gy arm (9%). This discrepancy in retreatment rates has been found in numerous other studies comparing single-fraction to multiple-fraction regimens and is believed to be related to physician willingness to retreat patients who initially receive lower doses of RT, rather than differences in efficacy between the two arms, which are generally otherwise identical.[41]

Wu and associates at McMaster University performed a meta-analysis of dose-fractionation trials for the palliation of painful bone metastases.[38] They divided the studies into three groups: two trials comparing 4 Gy with 8 Gy, each given in a single fraction; eight trials of single-fraction versus multiple-fraction regimens; and six trials comparing different multifraction regimens. Overall response rates were significantly lower with 4 Gy compared with 8 Gy, although complete response rates were not significantly different. For the next comparison, 8 Gy was the most common single-fraction dose, and 20 Gy in five fractions or 24 Gy in six fractions were the most common schedules for the multifraction arms. The pooled intention-to-treat complete response rates were 33.4% for single-fraction treatment versus 32.3% in patients receiving a multifractionation treatment schedule ($p = .04$).

Overall response rates, 62.1% versus 58.7%, also favored single-fraction treatment ($p = .04$). No significant differences were found in response rates between the various multifraction regimens. The median duration of response and toxicity profile were also comparable between regimens.

Although there appears to be an equivalent pain response after single-fraction or multifraction RT, several studies suggest that other adverse events, including fracture rates and need for salvage surgery, may be more frequent with single-fraction RT schedules. The Dutch Bone Metastasis Study Group conducted a phase III randomized trial comparing single-fraction 8-Gy treatment to a multifraction regimen of 24 Gy in six fractions in 1171 patients with bone metastases.[39] There was no significant difference between the two arms with respect to pain relief, analgesic use, or toxicity. However, more fractures occurred in the single fraction arm compared with the multifraction arm (23% vs. 7%, respectively), and the median time to fracture was delayed in the multifraction arm. Similarly, in a retrospective series of patients receiving RT for uncomplicated spine metastasis without spinal cord compression or prior radiation or surgery, the rate of spinal adverse events (symptomatic vertebral body fracture, hospitalization resulting from uncontrolled pain at the previously irradiated spine site, interventional procedures for pain control at the spine site, salvage spinal surgery, new or deterioration in neurologic symptoms, or cord or cauda equina compression) were 6.8% versus 3.5% at 30 days, 16.9% versus 6.4% at 90 days, and 23.6% versus 9.2% at 180 days for single fraction versus multifraction, respectively.[42] Thus, although multifraction schedules are less convenient and more costly, they are appropriate for select patients, especially those with prolonged life expectancies.

Stereotactic body RT (SBRT) is an emerging method for the treatment of select patients with bone metastases. SBRT allows the delivery of a targeted ablative radiation dose in up to five fractions with subcentimeter precision. SBRT is useful for treating metastases to the spine, particularly in patients who have had prior radiation to the maximum allowable spinal cord dose, because it minimizes further irradiation of the spinal cord. In patients with metastatic breast cancer, SBRT often results in excellent pain control and local tumor control otherwise unavailable from simple (two-field) external beam radiation approaches.[43] However, the use of spinal SBRT may be associated with an increased risk of vertebral compression fracture, with the greatest risk observed in those treated with a single fraction of 20 Gy or greater and those with a baseline fracture, lytic tumor, or spinal deformity.[44] SBRT is being compared with traditional external beam radiation for the treatment of localized spinal metastases in the RTOG 0631 trial. SBRT is not suitable for patients with a limited life expectancy, extensive metastatic disease, or symptomatic spinal cord compression due to bone metastasis.

Postoperative Radiotherapy

When prophylactic surgery is necessary for stabilization, it should be performed before RT. Postoperative radiation should consider the nature and extent of the surgery when determining areas for treatment and at risk for recurrence. For example, the placement of an intramedullary fixation device or a long-stemmed cemented prosthesis exposes the entire intramedullary canal to tumor. In addition, tissue in the operative field can be contaminated with microscopic tumor. Thus radiation therapy for such a patient would be directed to all exposed regions and extend the full length of the involved bone. When RT is given without surgical stabilization, the risk of fracture in the short term may increase as a result of radiation-induced hyperemic response at the tumor periphery, which can weaken the adjacent bone.[22] Therefore the bone should be mechanically protected until adequate healing has occurred. Crutch walking is recommended if the lesion is in the lower extremity and should continue until pain resolution and a favorable response is observed on radiograph.

Side Effects

External-beam RT is well tolerated with side effects most frequently related to the treatment field. Nausea and vomiting can occur if the stomach is in the radiation field and can be minimized with prophylactic antiemetics. A "flare" reaction, or temporary increase in pain at the site of metastases, occurs in up to 40% of patients after external-beam radiation.[45] A phase III trial in patients with solid tumors undergoing single-fraction RT for painful bony metastasis randomized patients to 8 mg dexamethasone daily for 5 days starting 1 day before radiation therapy. Steroid treatment decreased the incidence of a painful flare reaction to 26% compared with 35% in the placebo group ($p = .05$).[45]

Other radiation-induced effects include skin reactions, which may require topical therapy, and edema when treating extremity lesions, which can be minimized by sparing a strip of soft tissue from the radiation portal. RT can also reduce osteoclast activity, causing brittle bones and potentially increasing the risk of fracture. However, differentiating a radiation-induced fracture from a pathologic fracture can be challenging in patients with metastatic bone disease.

Retreatment With Radiotherapy

For patients with recurrent pain stemming from bone metastases previously treated with RT, there are no standard guidelines regarding retreatment. Patients who responded to an initial course of RT are more likely to respond to reirradiation; however, a proportion of nonresponders may also respond. Several randomized trials comparing single-fraction RT to multifraction RT have shown higher retreatment rates in the single-fraction arms. However, many physicians are reluctant to retreat after multifraction RT due to concerns regarding excess toxicity—namely, fracture.[38]

The National Cancer Institute of Canada Clinical Trials Group completed a prospective randomized study (NCIC CTG SC20) of reirradiation in patients with solid tumors metastatic to bone including prostate, breast, and lung cancer.[46,47] Eight hundred and fifty patients were randomized to a single dose of 8 or 20 Gy in five daily fractions. The primary end point of the study was overall response rate at 2 months using the International Consensus schema, which combines the Brief Pain Inventory worst pain score (0–10 scale) with change in opioid analgesic use (using oral morphine equivalents). In the intent-to-treat analysis, the 2-month response rate was 28% with 8 Gy and 32% with 20 Gy ($p = .2$). There was a nonsignificant increased rate of pathologic fractures in the group treated with 8 Gy compared with 20 Gy, with 30 (7%) versus 20 (5%) pathologic fractures and 7 (1.6%) versus 2 (0.5%) spinal cord compression events, respectively. No difference in quality of life, as measured by the European Organisation for Research and Treatment of Cancer Quality of Life Questionnaire C30 scale, was observed between the arms suggesting reirradiation is a safe and effective option for select breast cancer patients with recurrent painful metastases. SBRT is an appealing option in patients requiring retreatment as it minimizes reirradiation of normal tissue. However, large clinical trials to guide its use are lacking.

Radiopharmaceuticals

Radiopharmaceuticals are intravenously administered radioactive agents that localize preferentially to reactive bone sites leading to the delivery of therapeutic radiation doses to multiple sites of bony metastatic disease simultaneously. Strontium-89 (Sr^{89}) and samarium-153 (Sm^{153}) emit beta particles and are the two most studied agents.[48] Most randomized trials evaluating Sr^{89} studied patients with prostate cancer; however, one small trial compared Sr^{89} to rhenium-186 in patients with metastatic breast cancer.[49] The primary end point of the study was pain palliation as assessed by the Wisconsin pain test at 2 months. Thirty-two percent of patients in both arms achieved a complete response in pain. In a study of Sr^{89} that included patients with various tumor types, the overall response rate for pain palliation in patients with breast cancer was 64%.[50] Several randomized trials of Sm^{153} in patients with bone metastases from a variety of tumor types, including breast cancer have similarly shown high response rates (50%–95%).[48] The primary toxicity associated with radiopharmaceutical administration is hematologic with grade III/IV thrombocytopenia reported in up to 32% of patients, and grade III/IV leukopenia reported in up to 14% of patients receiving radiopharmaceuticals as single agents and in up to 45% of patients when combined with chemotherapy.[48,49] Blood counts usually return to baseline levels 8 to 12 weeks after administration. In the United States, Sm^{153} is approved for the relief of pain in patients with confirmed osteoblastic bone lesions that enhance on radionuclide bone scan, whereas Sr^{89} is approved for the relief of bone pain in patients with painful skeletal metastases.

Radium-223 (R^{223}), the first in class alpha particle emitter, deposits high-energy radiation over an extremely short range (60–100 μm) to minimize toxicity to normal bone marrow while still providing therapeutic doses of radiation to the tumor cells. Radium-223 (R^{223}) has been approved by the US Food and Drug Administration for treatment of men with castration-resistant prostate cancer, symptomatic bone metastases, and no known visceral metastatic disease. There are limited case reports and small series regarding the use of R^{223} in patients with hormone-refractory bone-dominant metastatic breast cancer showing improvements in pain, evidence of biological activity in bone metastases, and a favorable safety profile in this patient population.[51]

Data on integrating radiopharmaceuticals with other treatments for bone metastases such as osteoclast inhibitors, chemotherapy, and external-beam RT are limited. Although radiopharmaceuticals appear to effectively palliate bone pain in breast cancer, the relative infrequency of bone-only metastatic disease in breast cancer compared with prostate cancer, the fear of potential marrow toxicity, and the plethora of other treatment options often limits this approach to breast cancer patients who refuse chemotherapy or with poor performance status and comorbidities that limit other treatment options.

Systemic Osteoclast Inhibitors

Bisphosphonates

Since the 1990s, bisphosphonates have been a mainstay of treatment for the prevention of skeletal-related events in patients with bone metastases. Bisphosphonates are pyrophosphate analogs with phosphorus-carbon-phosphorus central structures. They are rapidly incorporated into bone and are released during osteoclast-mediated bone resorption, where they impair the ability of osteoclasts to adhere to the bony surface and inhibit continued bone resorption. Bisphosphonates also decrease osteoclast progenitor development and recruitment and induce osteoclast apoptosis. The primary effect of bisphosphonates is on osteoclast inhibition; however, other potential direct antitumor effects have been suggested based on in vitro and preclinical models including induction of apoptosis and inhibition of tumor cell adhesion and invasion, as well as indirect mechanisms such as inhibition of angiogenesis.[52]

A number of bisphosphonates have been approved for use in patients with bone metastases with differing characteristics based on their long and short side chains (determining potency), route of administration, and pharmacokinetics (summarized in Table 68.1).[53–60] Clodronate, an oral non–nitrogenous-containing bisphosphonate currently unavailable in the United States, was shown in several placebo-controlled randomized trials to decrease skeletal-related events as well as pain.[53,54] The intravenous (IV) nitrogen-containing bisphosphonate pamidronate was the first therapy approved in the United States for the prevention of skeletal-related events in patients with metastatic breast cancer involving the bone. Two double-blind placebo-controlled trials

demonstrated a significant reduction in SREs and pain with monthly IV pamidronate compared with placebo.[55,56] Intravenous pamidronate was also found to be superior to oral clodronate for controlling pain in a small head to head trial.[61]

Ibandronate is a potent bisphosphonate, available outside the United States in oral and IV formulations, shown to have beneficial effects on bone pain and quality of life.[58,59] In 150 patients with breast cancer and bone metastases, treatment with intravenous ibandronate 6 mg over 15 minutes every 4 weeks for 24 months significantly reduced the proportion of patients who experienced an SRE compared with placebo (36% vs. 48%, $p = .027$).[59] Oral ibandronate at a dose of 50 mg daily has been shown to decrease the risk of SRE by approximately 40% compared with placebo in three randomized trials. However, compared with intravenous zoledronic acid in a phase III trial conducted in the United Kingdom, annual rates of SREs were 0.499 in the oral ibandronate arm compared with 0.435 in the zoledronic acid arm.[62] The authors thereby concluded that oral ibandronate is slightly inferior to zoledronic acid for preventing SREs, but its oral formulation provides a convenient option for patients without adequate venous access or who have a strong preference for oral treatment.

Zoledronic acid is a third-generation, intravenously administered, nitrogen-containing bisphosphonate that is 100 times more potent than pamidronate. It is the first drug in this class approved

TABLE 68.1 Commonly Used Bisphosphonates for Bone Metastasis[a]

Bisphosphonate (Administration Route)	Class	Potency	Approved in the United States for the Prevention of SRE	Dose	Efficacy Compared With Placebo[b]
Clodronate (PO)	• Non–nitrogen containing • First generation	+	No	1600 mg daily	• 30% relative risk reduction in SRE at 2 y (clodronate 29% vs. placebo 41%, $p < .001$) • Time to first SRE and incidence of fracture reduced[53,54]
Pamidronate (IV)	• Nitrogen containing • Second generation	++	Yes	90 mg every 3–4 wk	• 20% relative risk reduction in SRE at 2 y (pamidronate 51% vs. 64% placebo, $p < .001$) • Time to first SRE and incidence of fracture reduced • Time to progression of pain delayed[55–57]
Ibandronate (IV and PO)	• Nitrogen containing • Third generation	+++	No	6 mg every 3–4 wk (IV), 50 mg daily (PO)	• 25% relative risk reduction in SRE at 2 y (ibandronate 36% vs. placebo 48%, $p = .027$) • Time to first SRE and incidence of pain and fracture reduced[58,59]
Zoledronic acid (IV)	• Nitrogen containing • Third generation	++++	Yes	4 mg every 3–4 wk	• 40% relative risk reduction in SRE at 1 y (zoledronic acid 29.8% vs. placebo 49.6%, $p = .003$) • Time to first SRE and incidence of pain reduced[60]

[a]SRE rates exclude hypercalcemia of malignancy.
[b]In patients with metastatic breast cancer.
IV, Intravenous; *PO*, oral; *SRE*, skeletal-related event.

in the United States for use in all solid tumor patients with bone metastases as well as patients with multiple myeloma.[60,63-65] A large, multicenter, double-blind trial was conducted comparing IV monthly zoledronic acid (4 or 8 mg) with pamidronate (90 mg) in patients with metastatic breast cancer or multiple myeloma with bone lesions.[63] The primary end point was the proportion of patients with at least one skeletal-related event over 13 months, defined as pathologic fracture, spinal cord compression, RT, or surgery to bone. Both the primary end point and median time to first SRE was similar across all treatment arms. Toxicity was also similar in the 4-mg zoledronic acid and pamidronate arms. The 8-mg zoledronic acid dose was associated with an increased risk of renal dysfunction and discontinued. In patients with breast cancer, zoledronic acid appeared to be more effective than pamidronate at reducing the proportion of patients receiving RT to the bone, particularly for those receiving hormonal therapy. In addition, for those with osteolytic lesions, zoledronic acid was more effective than pamidronate, decreasing the risk of first SRE by an additional 17% ($p = .058$) and risk of multiple SREs (multiple event analysis) by an additional 30% ($p = .010$).[64]

Although randomized trials have demonstrated a reduction in pain in patients with bone metastasis treated with bisphosphonates, the effect on pain scores are often modest. Combining bisphosphonates with RT may be a more successful strategy for pain control. In a small trial examining opioid use in response to treatment with intravenous ibandronate and local RT, 24% of patients at 3 months and 8% of patients at 10 months required opioid analgesics compared with 84% at baseline.[66]

Despite optimal bisphosphonate administration, up to 40% of cancer patients with bone metastases still develop skeletal-related events while on bisphosphonate therapy.[60,65] Treatment-related side effects include gastrointestinal irritation with oral agents, nephrotoxicity with intravenous agents, and a flulike (or acute phase response) syndrome in up to 30% of patients receiving intravenous preparations, particularly zoledronic acid.[63-65] More significant complications are rare and include osteonecrosis of the jaw, atypical femur fracture, and hypocalcemia. Administration of both zoledronic acid and pamidronate result in an approximately 1% to 2% risk for the development of osteonecrosis of the jaw (ONJ).[67,68] ONJ is a serious and often difficult-to-treat complication characterized by exposed bone in the maxillofacial region that does not heal within 8 weeks after identification. Risk factors include poor oral hygiene, dental extractions, and oral infections, along with increased duration of IV bisphosphonate use. Attention to dental hygiene and regular dental examinations are recommended for all patients receiving systemic osteoclast inhibitor therapy.

IV bisphosphonates, and in particular zoledronic acid, carry a risk for renal toxicity that is dose and infusion time dependent. Monthly monitoring of renal function is recommended before zoledronic acid infusion. Because of the increased risk for renal toxicity, zoledronic acid is currently not recommended for use in patients with a creatinine clearance less than 30 mL/minute, requires dose reduction in patients with a creatinine clearance of less than 60 mL/minute, and should be used cautiously or not at all in patients receiving other nephrotoxic drugs.[69]

Several trials have examined lengthening the zoledronic acid dosing interval from 4 to 12 weeks in patients with metastatic breast cancer. The ZOOM and OPTIMIZE-2 trial in breast cancer patients and the Cancer and Leukemia Group B (CALGB) 70604 trial, which included 418 breast patients (47%) randomized patients to zoledronic acid on an every-4-week or 12-week dosing schedule.[70-72] In the ZOOM and OPTIMIZE-2 trial, patients completed an initial loading period of 9 to 15 monthly doses of zoledronic acid before randomization to the same or the extended every-12-week schedule while in the CALGB trial all patients were randomized with their first infusion. In these trials, the 12-week administration schedule was noninferior to the 4-week schedule, suggesting that less frequent dosing of these agents may be used in stable patients.

Denosumab

Denosumab is a fully human monoclonal antibody with high affinity and specificity for RANKL. It neutralizes the activity of both membrane-bound and soluble RANKL, thereby inhibiting osteoclast function, terminal differentiation, and survival. The initial phase I trials demonstrated that osteoclastic activity is almost completely eradicated while denosumab is in circulation.[73] As a monoclonal antibody, the effects of denosumab are long-lasting with a mean elimination half-life of 25 to 30 days. In addition, the effects on bone resorption are reversible after antibody clearance, and renal or hepatic impairment have little effect on clearance rates.

Denosumab is currently approved for the prevention of skeletal-related events in patients with bone metastases from solid tumors at a dose of 120 mg given subcutaneously every 4 weeks. It is additionally approved at a dose of 120 mg in patients with hypercalcemia of malignancy refractory to bisphosphonate therapy with a weekly dosing schedule (days 1, 8, and 15) in the first month of therapy. There have been three international, multicenter phase III randomized, double-blind, double-dummy, active controlled trials involving more than 5700 patients comparing denosumab with zoledronic acid for the prevention of skeletal-related events in patients with bone metastases.[68] The first published phase III trial randomized 2046 patients with metastatic breast cancer and radiologic evidence of at least one bone metastasis to either subcutaneous denosumab 120 mg or intravenous zoledronic acid 4 mg every 4 weeks.[74] The primary end point was time to first skeletal-related event (radiation to bone, pathologic fracture, surgery to bone, or spinal cord compression). Denosumab delayed the time to first on-study skeletal-related event by 18% compared with zoledronic acid (hazard ratio 0.82; $p = .001$ for noninferiority, $p = .01$ for superiority). Median time to first skeletal-related event was 26.4 months in the zoledronic acid group and 32.4 months in the denosumab arm.[75] Denosumab was also superior to zoledronic acid in several secondary end points, including pain prevention, opioid use, and quality of life.[76,77] The number of hypercalcemia events was also decreased in the denosumab arm compared with the zoledronic acid arm (rate ratio 0.48, $p = .036$).

Denosumab elimination is thought to occur through the immunoglobulin clearance pathway via the reticuloendothelial system, similar to that of other monoclonal antibodies. Dose reductions and renal monitoring are not required with denosumab therapy. However, there is a lack of safety data in patients with severe renal dysfunction. More frequent monitoring of serum calcium levels as well as ensuring adequate vitamin D levels before and upon initiation of denosumab therapy is recommended in patients with renal insufficiency as an increased incidence of hypocalcemia may be observed.

The major adverse events associated with denosumab therapy include hypocalcemia in up to 10% of patients and ONJ.[68] The patient-year-adjusted incidence of confirmed ONJ is approximately 1.1% during the first year of treatment, 3.7% in the second year, and 4.6% per year thereafter with a median time to ONJ of 20.6 months (range of 4–53 months) based on the phase III trials.[78] As with bisphosphonate use, good dental hygiene and regular dental examinations are recommended.

Tumor-induced osteolysis is associated with increased bone resorption markers such as urinary N-telopeptide of type I collagen (NTX) and serum bone-specific alkaline phosphatase. The use of antiresorptive agents including denosumab and zoledronic acid in patients with metastatic carcinoma of the breast significantly reduce markers of bone turnover.[74] The BISMARK trial attempted to dose zoledronic acid based on a patient's markers of bone resorption.[79] The trial was underpowered for its primary end point of noninferiority, but the marker-driven dosing arm had an increased number of SREs and higher proportion of patients with SREs compared with the standard monthly treatment, suggesting markers of bone turnover should not currently be used for determining dosing schedule. Elevated bone turnover markers have been consistently associated with worse prognosis and an increased risk of SRE in clinical trials. Recently it has also been demonstrated that patients with higher (above the median) levels of urinary NTX and serum bone-specific alkaline phosphatase after 3 months of antiresorptive therapy may also have worse clinical outcomes.[80]

The data strongly support the initiation of systemic osteoclast inhibitors in both asymptomatic and symptomatic patients with metastatic carcinoma of the breast involving bone for the prevention of SREs including hypercalcemia, improved pain palliation, and maintenance of quality of life. In breast cancer, systemic osteoclast inhibitor use has not been shown to affect overall survival or disease progression. Differences in efficacy, toxicities, administration, cost, and patient preferences should be considered when determining the most appropriate therapy (Table 68.2).[81] There are currently no data to support the combined use of a bisphosphonate with denosumab to further reduce the incidence of SREs. Because both agents are potent osteoclast inhibitors, the risk of increased toxicity with combination therapy, especially with regard to osteonecrosis of the jaw, hypocalcemia, and atypical femoral fractures are a concern.

There is no consensus with regard to duration of treatment with systemic osteoclast inhibitors. Current guidelines, including those from the American Society of Clinical Oncology and the European Society for Medical Oncology suggest treatment should be continued indefinitely until there is a substantial decline in the patient's performance status.[82,83] Reduced frequency of therapy may be reasonable for patients with well-controlled disease and/or normalized markers of bone resorption.

New Treatment Modalities

Novel treatments for bone metastases are under development. Percutaneous image-guided ablation, including radiofrequency ablation, cryoablation, and focused ultrasound have all been reported as effective in relieving pain and decreasing opioid use in patients with symptomatic bony metastases.[84] Vertebroplasty and kyphoplasty are other mechanical options for selected patients with painful compression fractures of the spine without epidural disease or retropulsion of bone fragments into the spinal cord.[85,86] Stereotactic body radiation is increasingly used in patients with limited skeletal involvement and may be particularly useful for treating the spine. Currently, there are few data on the long-term

TABLE 68.2 Systemic Osteoclast Inhibitors: Considerations for Clinical Decision-Making

Supporting Denosumab Use	Supporting Bisphosphonate Use
Improved efficacy in the prevention of SREs	Lower risk of hypocalcemia • Safer in patients unlikely to be compliant with oral vitamin D and calcium supplements
Better tolerability	Lower risk of osteonecrosis of the jaw, particularly for pamidronate and oral agents
Delays development of moderate or severe bone pain (better prevention of pain)	Lower cost
Safer in patients with progressive or baseline renal insufficiency • Patients receiving nephrotoxic chemotherapy • Patients with diseases more susceptible to renal dysfunction	Greater than 15 years experience with use in the medical community
Patients with intolerance to bisphosphonates	Patients with intolerance to denosumab
Patients currently receiving an intravenous bisphosphonate who experience an skeletal-related event	
Ease of subcutaneous administration • Patients without a central venous access device • Patients not receiving monthly chemotherapy infusion	

Modified from Brown-Glaberman U, Stopeck AT. Role of denosumab in the management of skeletal complications in patients with bone metastasis from solid tumors. *Biol Targets Ther.* 2012;6:89-99.

effectiveness of these interventions, and the completion of prospective clinical trials, such as RTOG 0631, comparing them with standard approaches are pending.

There is growing interest in understanding the bone microenvironment and in bone-specific tumor-host interactions. Increased research in the field will undoubtedly yield new targets for decreasing SREs, increasing bone strength, and improving therapies for patients with bone metastases.

Conclusions and Recommendations

Managing patients with bone metastases requires a multidisciplinary approach applying the expertise of orthopedic surgeons, radiation oncologists, medical oncologists, and radiologists. Small lesions can usually be successfully treated with RT alone, with subsequent surgical stabilization only for continued symptoms or fracture. Operative stabilization is recommended for lesions that are osteolytic, are painful, and comprise 50% or more of the bone diameter. Bones with diffuse, permeative destruction should be internally stabilized prophylactically if possible, followed by postoperative RT. Unless contraindicated, all patients with metastatic carcinoma of the breast with involvement of the bone should receive systemic osteoclast inhibitor therapy for the prevention of skeletal-related events, irrespective of pain symptoms or extent of disease. Future treatment modalities will further decrease the substantial morbidity associated with the development and progression of bone metastases.

Acknowledgment

We gratefully acknowledge the contributions of Judith L. Lightsey and Nancy P. Mendenhall, who authored this chapter in previous editions.

Selected References

8. Roodman GD. Mechanism of bone metastasis. *N Engl J Med.* 2004;350:1655-1664.

24. Wood TJ, Racano A, Yeung H, et al. Surgical management of bone metastases: quality of evidence and systematic review. *Ann Surg Oncol.* 2014;21:4081-4089.

39. Steenland E, Leer JW, van Houwelingen H, et al. The effect of a single fraction compared to multiple fractions on painful bone metastases: a global analysis of the Dutch Bone Metastasis Study. *Radiother Oncol.* 1999;52:101-109.

56. Lipton A, Theriault RL, Hortobagyi GN, et al. Pamidronate prevents skeletal complications and is effective palliative treatment in women with breast carcinoma and osteolytic bone metastases: long-term follow-up of two randomized, placebo-controlled trials. *Cancer.* 2000;88:1082-1090.

74. Stopeck AT, Lipton A, Body JJ, et al. Denosumab compared with zoledronic acid for the treatment of bone metastases in patients with advanced breast cancer: a randomized, double-blinded study. *J Clin Oncol.* 2010;28:5132-5139.

A full reference list is available online at ExpertConsult.com.

69

Chemotherapy and HER2-Directed Therapy for Metastatic Breast Cancer

ADRIENNE G. WAKS AND ERIC P. WINER

Although the past decades have seen great growth in the arsenal of breast cancer treatments, approximately 40,000 individuals still die each year from metastatic disease, which remains incurable in the vast majority of patients. In recent years, there has been significant progress made in the development of HER2-targeted therapies, dramatically improving the prognosis of this historically unfavorable disease subset. New agents such as mammalian target of rapamycin (mTOR) inhibitors and cyclin-dependent kinase (CDK) 4/6 inhibitors have been approved for the treatment of hormone receptor–positive disease, and many additional agents are in development. Despite major efforts in the development of smarter, less toxic targeted therapies, in 2016 cytotoxic chemotherapy remains a central component of treatment for most women with advanced breast cancer. Current research strives not only to develop new therapies but also to identify populations in whom existing agents will be most effective and to optimize the activity of newer therapeutic modalities such as targeted and immune-based therapy by combining them with a chemotherapy backbone. Overall, women living with metastatic breast cancer (MBC) have far more options than in the past, and there has been a modest prolongation in overall survival (OS) over the course of the 21st century.[1,2] Regardless the goal of cure remains unattained except in anecdotal cases, and ongoing progress is essential.

Epidemiology

Breast cancer remains the most common noncutaneous malignancy and the second leading cause of cancer death after lung cancer among women in the United States. In 2015 it was estimated that more than 230,000 new breast cancer diagnoses were made and that MBC was responsible for nearly 41,000 deaths.[2] For women aged 20 to 59, MBC remains the leading cause of cancer death and is therefore an important public health concern. Although only approximately 6% of women with breast cancer initially present with metastatic disease, many women with localized disease or locoregional spread at diagnosis go on to develop distant disease despite adjuvant therapy.[3] In patients diagnosed with MBC, 5-year survival is estimated to be 26%, and median OS is approximately 31 months, although this varies substantially based on disease characteristics.[4] As such, a significant number of women with advanced breast cancer survive for many years. This statistic stands in sharp contrast to many other solid malignancies

such as adenocarcinoma of the lung, pancreas, and stomach, in which 5-year survival remains less than 5%.[5] Nevertheless, there is an urgent need for better therapies.

Therapeutic Goals

Although there are rare anecdotes reporting cure or long-term remission in patients with MBC, in the overwhelming majority of cases, the goal of therapy is symptom control and prolongation in survival. Unfortunately, the vast majority of women with MBC will experience disease progression within 1 to 2 years of treatment initiation and only 1% to 2% will be alive 20 years from diagnosis of MBC.[6] Treatments should be selected to achieve three objectives simultaneously: prolong survival, control symptoms if present, and minimize therapy-associated toxicity. These goals are usually achieved through the administration of systemic therapy (hormonal therapy, chemotherapy, and targeted agents) with judicious use of both radiation therapy, and, less frequently, surgery.

Prognostication

Prognostic and predictive factors should be used to determine the most appropriate therapy for an individual. Although breast cancer was historically classified as a single disease, it is now known to be a heterogeneous group of diseases, all of which arise in the breast. Complex differences in tumor biology produce variable responses to therapy in individual patients. For this reason, the particular characteristics of a patient's tumor may help the clinician predict the pace of disease, likelihood of response to certain therapies, and OS.

In general, OS and disease-free intervals are longer for patients with estrogen receptor (ER)- and/or progesterone receptor (PR)-positive disease; this is likely the result of a more indolent natural history, and, even more important, the availability of a large armamentarium of active endocrine therapies that are generally used before the administration of chemotherapy. Similarly, given the development of multiple highly effective HER2-targeted therapies in recent years, more patients with HER2-positive disease are cured with adjuvant therapy, and median OS for HER2-positive metastatic breast cancer has improved dramatically. By contrast, patients with "triple-negative" tumors that do not express ER, PR, or HER2 typically have a shorter disease-free interval before the development of metastatic disease, as well as a shorter median OS from the time of diagnosis of metastatic disease.

Other disease-specific characteristics that may help predict prognosis include disease-free interval before the development of metastatic disease, number of disease sites, visceral versus bone-only metastases, and disease volume. On the basis of data assembled more than 2 decades ago from the MD Anderson Cancer Center, the 5-year survival for patients with isolated bone metastases is 23%, compared with only 13% for MBC patients with visceral metastases.[7] Patients with a prolonged relapse-free survival (>5 years) before diagnosis with MBC also have a more favorable prognosis. As a general rule, women with chest wall, nodal, bone, or soft tissue recurrences live longer than those with visceral or central nervous system (CNS) disease.[3]

The other component to prognosis rests in individual patient characteristics. Younger age, better performance status, fewer comorbidities, and lower burden of disease all predict a better prognosis. This may be partially a result of a patient's ability to tolerate toxic therapy and may also reflect differences in treatment approaches used for younger and older patients.[8] In addition, past response to therapy or lack thereof may predict future response to therapy with new agents. Although mechanisms of chemotherapy resistance have not been fully elucidated, historical information suggests that tumor resistance to one agent is associated with an increased likelihood of resistance to other chemotherapy agents.

Despite a broad survival range for patients with MBC, the median OS remains approximately 3 years.[3,4] Analysis of patients treated in the 1980s and 1990s suggests that independent of timing of detection of metastatic disease there has been an absolute improvement in prognosis for MBC patients, which has been largely attributed to the introduction of taxanes as first-line chemotherapy in the metastatic setting.[9] Multivariate analysis of patients treated throughout the 1990s demonstrates that for the period from 1991 to 2001, access to new therapeutic agents for MBC resulted in improved survival.[1] More recently, the slow uptrend in MBC survival has continued.[3,10] Although the therapeutic driver of this trend is not entirely clear, presumably some credit is due to the introduction of highly effective anti-HER2 therapies.

Medical Evaluation in the Metastatic Setting

Large randomized trials have shown that routine surveillance testing after adjuvant therapy does not improve survival or health-related quality of life.[11-13] As a result, the diagnosis of metastatic disease is typically made when a patient presents with new symptoms (e.g., bone pain, seizure, shortness of breath); has asymptomatic laboratory abnormalities; has a clinically detected local recurrence on the chest wall, in the regional lymph nodes, or within the breast itself; or has incidental findings on imaging performed for other purposes.

Once there is a suspicion for metastatic disease based on laboratory results, physical examination, or radiographs, it is generally important to biopsy a metastatic site to confirm that the lesion is consistent with breast cancer rather than another primary malignancy or some other benign process. It should be noted that there are multiple cases reported of women presenting with mediastinal lymphadenopathy on computed tomography (CT) scan that is assumed to be breast cancer but is found on biopsy to be sarcoidosis.[14] Rebiopsy at the time of diagnosis with metastatic disease also provides a unique opportunity to reassess receptor status before the initiation of therapy. Biopsy can determine whether the

patient's MBC has the same receptor expression as the original lesion because in some cases, these properties have been known to change. One prospective study demonstrated discordant receptor status between primary and metastatic lesion in 16%, 40%, and 10% of cases for ER, PR, and HER2, respectively.[15] In certain patients, the index of suspicion for MBC is high enough and/or the metastatic site is not amenable to biopsy, in which case one may choose to forgo biopsy. However, in almost all clinical scenarios, rebiopsy is feasible and recommended. Additionally, in the modern era, genomic profiling of metastatic biopsy tissue can have implications for clinical trial agent selection, and the use of molecular medicine will likely increase in the coming years.

Before initiation of therapy, one should assess the extent of disease with imaging of the chest and abdomen as well as with bone scan because bone involvement is quite common in MBC. The relative merits of fluorodeoxyglucose positron emission tomography (FDG-PET) scanning in this setting have been the subject of debate and at this time, PET scanning is an option but should not be considered essential. It is a sensitive imaging modality but not specific for malignancy, often resulting in findings that are difficult to interpret. Highly metabolic foci may be seen in inflammatory conditions such as rheumatologic disease or infection; FDG avidity may therefore result in unnecessary anxiety or inaccurate assumptions about the extent of disease. In patients with documented metastases, PET often does not offer enough clinical information over CT and bone scan to warrant the cost. With improvements in technology and changes in cost structure, recommendations may well evolve over time.

Imaging of the brain with contrast-enhanced CT or ideally gadolinium-enhanced magnetic resonance imaging (MRI) certainly should be performed in any MBC patient with focal neurologic findings or symptoms to suggest CNS involvement such as headaches, seizures, or cognitive changes. Given the high rate of CNS disease in women with HER2-positive breast cancer previously treated with trastuzumab and in triple-negative disease, there are some clinicians who advocate scanning asymptomatic patients with these disease subtypes, but there are no data to support that this approach improves survival or affects quality of life. In the absence of CNS signs and symptoms, brain imaging generally should not be performed when a patient is newly diagnosed with metastatic disease and is rarely required for clinical trial participation.

In addition to radiographic imaging, laboratory studies and a careful physical examination should also be performed. Physical examination should focus on identification of symptomatic foci such as bone tenderness, neurologic findings, chest wall disease, or lymphadenopathy. These findings may guide directed therapy with bisphosphonates or radiation and offer a baseline from which response to therapy may be assessed. Baseline laboratory studies can evaluate renal and hepatic function, electrolyte status, and bone marrow reserve in preparation for treatment with chemotherapy. Finally, serum tumor markers such as carcinoembryonic antigen (CEA) and cancer antigen (CA) 27-29 may be measured at the time of diagnosis and, if elevated, are often helpful in monitoring response to therapy. Tumor markers need to be used with caution because they do not always correlate with the course of the disease.

Local Therapy for Metastatic Breast Cancer

Although the general treatment paradigm for MBC is systemic therapy, there are unique clinical scenarios in which local therapy to a metastatic site may further the goals of therapy, namely symptom control and improvement in survival. Possible reasons to consider local therapy include oligometastatic disease, local symptoms that are unlikely to respond to systemic therapy, and impending local complications such as spinal cord compression, hydronephrosis, or bone fracture. Surgical interventions for metastatic disease may include resection of a CNS lesion, chest wall lesion, isolated pulmonary nodule, or isolated hepatic nodule, or drainage of a pleural effusion. Longitudinal data indicate that metastasectomy is becoming increasingly common in breast cancer and many other solid malignancies.[16] However, metastasectomy for reasons other than resection of a CNS lesion or other local palliation remains a nonstandard approach, and there are no prospective data demonstrating that it improves disease outcomes. Local radiation therapy is indicated in the event of cord compression or unstable bone lesions, although the need for radiation has been reduced by the widespread use of bone-modifying agents for lytic bone disease.

Breast Surgery in Patients With Metastatic Disease

The decision of whether to offer breast surgery to a woman presenting with metastatic disease has long been debated, and practice styles vary greatly. In general, local therapy to the primary tumor is not thought to have an impact on clinical outcome and offers only palliation in symptomatic patients. In a retrospective examination of the National Cancer Database from 1990 to 1993, more than 16,000 women presenting with stage IV disease were identified, and 42.8% of these patients did not undergo definitive resection of their tumors, whereas 57.2% of patients underwent partial or total mastectomy. Women treated with surgical resection in whom negative margins were achieved had a superior prognosis compared with women who did not receive surgery (hazard ratio [HR] 0.61).[17,18] Multiple smaller studies have reported similar results.[19,20] Another large study that addressed this question was a retrospective, population-based cohort study evaluating more than 9000 women with stage IV breast cancer from the Surveillance, Epidemiology, and End Results database. In this patient cohort, 47% underwent breast cancer surgery, and 53% did not. After controlling for confounding variables and propensity scores, patients who underwent surgery were less likely to die during the study period compared with women who did not undergo surgery (HR 0.63).[21] In retrospective studies, this benefit has only been seen in women whose tumors were resected with negative margins. Although these results suggest that local therapy may improve outcome, they likely also reflect a significant selection bias; women who underwent surgery were almost certainly different in ways that can and cannot be quantified from those in whom the primary tumor was not resected. Given the biases inherent in these retrospective analyses, this question can be answered only by prospective study.

Therefore numerous prospective evaluations have been undertaken, with inconclusive results thus far. The Turkish MF07-01 study was a phase III trial randomizing women with de novo MBC to systemic therapy with or without standard locoregional resection for their metastatic breast disease. The trial was powered to detect an 18% improvement in survival in the resection arm, and at a mean follow-up of 21.1 months, failed to demonstrate any difference in OS between the two groups. In a subgroup analysis, patients with solitary bone metastasis experienced significantly longer OS with surgery versus no surgery.[22] In a similar study

conducted in India, 350 women with de novo metastatic breast cancer and an objective response to initial chemotherapy were randomized to standard locoregional management, or no locoregional management. No significant OS difference was detected between the two groups at a median follow-up of 17 months.[23]

The Translational Breast Cancer Research Consortium study 013 prospectively followed metastatic breast cancer patients who had de novo metastatic disease and intact primary, or who developed metastatic disease within 3 months of primary breast surgery. In this nonrandomized design, patients who underwent breast surgery had significantly better 2-year OS than patients who did not undergo surgery. However, when the cohort was limited to patients with de novo metastatic disease and intact primary who responded to systemic therapy, there was no improvement in 2-year OS in patients who underwent elective breast surgery.[24] Overall, the therapeutic value of primary breast surgery in de novo MBC is still unclear, and many additional prospective studies of this question are underway. At present, the consideration of local resection in a woman with MBC should be managed on an individual basis.

Selecting Therapy for Metastatic Breast Cancer

Before initiating treatment in the metastatic setting, there are many factors to be weighed. The primary objective is to select the regimen that is most likely to yield a clinical response while minimizing toxicity and side effects. Tumor characteristics either from the original breast biopsy, or ideally from a metastatic site, determine which classes of agents are likely to be active against a given tumor. Chemotherapy is used invariably in the course of treatment for metastatic breast cancer of all subsets, but the appropriate time and context for its use varies by subtype (hormone receptor–positive vs. HER2-positive vs. triple-negative). ER-positive and/or PR-positive disease is often initially sensitive to endocrine therapy and cytotoxic agents are reserved for the scenarios outlined subsequently. HER2-directed therapies will form the backbone of all systemic therapy in HER2-positive disease but are generally used in combination with chemotherapy, as discussed later in the chapter. Lastly, in women with triple-negative cancers, cytotoxic therapy is the only treatment option with documented clinical activity and has a role in all lines of treatment, outside of a clinical trial.

In patients with hormone receptor–positive tumors, endocrine therapy should be the initial course of treatment unless they have extensive visceral metastases ("visceral crisis"), rapid disease progression, or symptoms that need rapid palliation (Fig. 69.1). Of course, the decision to use endocrine therapy also will be influenced by prior endocrine treatment in the adjuvant setting. Response rates to first-line treatment for ER-positive/PR-positive, ER-positive/PR-negative, and ER-negative/PR-negative tumors in patients who have never received endocrine therapy are approximately 70%, 40%, and 10%, respectively.[25–27] (Of note, the 10% response rate for ER-negative/PR-negative disease is based on old literature; this value has not been systematically evaluated with more accurate modern testing and is almost certainly far lower.) Although patients whose disease displays primary resistance to upfront endocrine therapy should usually proceed directly to treatment with chemotherapy, women with an initial response to endocrine therapy may receive multiple additional lines of endocrine therapy. Treatment options for women receiving endocrine therapy include tamoxifen, aromatase inhibitors, ovarian

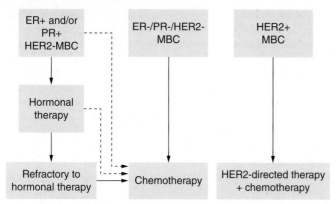

• **Fig. 69.1** General algorithm for the treatment of metastatic breast cancer. Endocrine-sensitive metastatic breast cancer (MBC) presenting with visceral crisis or impending organ dysfunction should be treated early with chemotherapy *(dashed lines)*. *ER*, Estrogen receptor; *PR*, progesterone receptor.

TABLE 69.1	MBC Response Rates to Single Chemotherapeutic Agents	
Agent	**RR (%): Prior Therapy**	**RR (%): No Prior MBC Therapy**
5-Fluorouracil	21	
Capecitabine	26–29	
Carboplatin		19–31ᵃ
Cisplatin		33ᵃ
Cyclophosphamide		35ᵇ
Docetaxel		34–35
Eribulin	12	
Doxorubicin		26
Gemcitabine	1–30	14–37
Ixabepilone	12	42
Liposomal doxorubicin		26
Paclitaxel	32	
Vinorelbine	32–36	34

ᵃTriple-negative breast cancer patients only. Some patients with one prior line of therapy in the metastatic setting.
ᵇSmall, historical study. Cyclophosphamide is seldom used as a single agent.
MBC, Metastatic breast cancer; *RR*, response rate.
Data are from references 32–45.

suppression with gonadotropin-releasing hormone (GnRH) agonists, fulvestrant, progestins, high-dose estrogens, and androgens. Aromatase inhibitors (letrozole, anastrozole, and exemestane)[28] are often used in the first-line setting for postmenopausal women given the low risk of "tumor flare" with agents such as tamoxifen and evidence that they offer superior time to progression (TTP) and response rates compared with first-line tamoxifen for MBC.[29] Recent evidence demonstrates that the combination of palbociclib (Ibrance, Pfizer, New York, NY), a cyclin-dependent kinase (CDK) 4/6 inhibitor, dramatically improves progression-free survival (PFS) when combined with both first- and second-line endocrine therapy in the treatment of metastatic disease.[30,31] Palbociclib gained US Food and Drug Administration (FDA) accelerated approval in 2016 and is currently standard of care in combination with endocrine therapy in women with hormone-responsive metastatic breast cancer.

In patients who have previously been treated either in the adjuvant or metastatic setting, shorter disease-free interval is a predictor of more aggressive disease. The degree of symptoms, tempo of disease, and extent of disease (visceral vs. bone-only involvement) are critical criteria for drug selection and timing of therapy in the palliative setting. Response to prior treatment has also been shown to be a predictor of response to the next line of therapy, so early relapse after adjuvant therapy is suggestive of resistant disease. If there is a short disease-free interval, generally defined as less than 1 to 2 years, strong consideration should be given to the use of new non–cross-resistant agents based on the presumption that the tumor is now resistant to drugs administered in the past. In general, women who have received anthracyclines in the adjuvant setting are not retreated with anthracyclines in the first-line setting for MBC, largely related to concerns about cumulative cardiac toxicity.

A final dimension to individualizing the treatment plan incorporates patient preference, performance status, and comorbidities. A patient's unique constellation of comorbidities, age, and general health status will likely predict her ability to tolerate a given treatment. The toxicity profile of a given agent may limit its use (e.g., avoiding anthracyclines in a patient with borderline cardiac function or risk factors for cardiac dysfunction or avoiding taxanes in a patient with preexisting neuropathy). In addition, patient preference regarding alopecia or concerns about toxicities (e.g., neurotoxicity), which may have an impact on occupation and quality of life, should also be considered in the decision-making process.

Selecting a First-Line Regimen in HER2-Negative Metastatic Breast Cancer

There is a panoply of chemotherapeutic agents known to be active in MBC, including anthracyclines, vinca alkaloids, antimetabolites, alkylating agents, and microtubule inhibitors (Table 69.1).[32–48] Selection of a first-line agent is often based primarily on a patient's previous treatment because likelihood of response is more a function of line of therapy than it is of the agent used. At this time, the National Comprehensive Cancer Network (NCCN) breast cancer panel does not recommend a specific first-line agent because there is no evidence to support the use of drugs in a particular sequence.[49] For this reason, treatment is tailored to the individual, as described previously. In patients who have received anthracyclines and/or taxanes in the adjuvant setting, agents with different mechanisms are chosen in the first-line setting for metastatic disease. Similarly, because no agent has been found to be superior, individualized therapy based on patient preference, comorbidities, and known drug toxicities is recommended. Multivariate analyses have demonstrated that the characteristics of the patient's tumor and pace of disease are better predictors of response and survival than the class of drug used.[50]

Single-Agent Versus Combination Chemotherapy in HER2-Negative Breast Cancer

It is a common and logical assumption that combination chemotherapy for MBC should result in superior response rates, as

TABLE 69.2   Controlled Trials of Combination Versus Sequential Single-Agent Chemotherapy

Study	Treatment Arms	RR (%)	TTP/TTF (mo)	OS (mo)	Superior QOL?	Crossover Permitted
Joensuu et al., 1998[52]	E→M	48→16	Equal	Equal	E→M	Y
	CEF→MV	55→7				
Norris et al., 2000 (MA8)[53]	AN	Equal	Equal	13.8	Equal	Y
	A			14.4		
O'Shaughnessy et al., 2002[54]	D	30	4.2	11.5	N/A	N
	XD	42	6.1	14.5		
Sledge et al., 2003 (ECOG 1193)[50]	A	36	5.8	18.9	Equal	Y
	T	34	6	22.2		
	AT	47	8	20.0		
Albain et al., 2004[55]	GT	41	6.1	18.5	GT	N
	T	26	4	15.8		
Martin et al., 2007 (GEICAM)[56]	GN	36	6	15.9	N/A	N
	N	26	4	16.4		

A, Doxorubicin; *C*, cyclophosphamide; *D*, docetaxel; *E*, epirubicin; *ECOG*, Eastern Cooperative Oncology Group; *F*, fluorouracil; *G*, gemcitabine; *GEICAM*, Spanish Breast Cancer Research Group; *M*, mitomycin; *N*, vinorelbine; *N/A*, not available; *OS*, overall survival; *QOL*, quality of life; *RR*, response rate; *T*, paclitaxel; *TTF*, time to treatment failure; *TTP*, time to progression; *V*, vinblastine; *X*, capecitabine.

well as improved palliation, disease-free survival, and OS. For many decades, it was theorized that combining drugs with non-overlapping toxicities and different mechanisms of action would overcome drug resistance in tumor cells via synergy. This approach has been successful in the treatment of lymphoma, leukemia, and germ cell tumors but has not been confirmed in MBC. Multiple clinical trials from the pretaxane era supported the superiority of polychemotherapy over monotherapy with respect to response rates, although improvements in OS were generally marginal at best.[51] It should be noted, however, that none of these trials that demonstrated even a modest improvement in survival compared combination chemotherapy with the same single agents used in sequence (Table 69.2).[52–56]

Dose reductions and missed doses are more common with polychemotherapy, and as a result, the total dose of each agent received over a given time period may be decreased. In addition, when more than one agent is used, it is difficult to determine which drug was effective when the time comes to dose-reduce or change lines of therapy.

An Intergroup trial (E1193) compared doxorubicin, paclitaxel, and the combination of doxorubicin and paclitaxel as first-line therapy in 739 patients with MBC. Patients receiving single-agent therapy crossed over to the other agent at the time of disease progression. Although a superior response rate and time to treatment failure were observed in the combination therapy arm, there was no significant improvement in median OS or quality of life compared with sequential single-agent therapy.[50]

In contrast to the findings of E1193, an international phase III trial comparing the efficacy and tolerability of docetaxel plus capecitabine (Xeloda, Hoffman-La Roche, Nutley, NJ) to single-agent docetaxel did demonstrate superior response rate, TTP, and OS in the combined treatment arm. It should be noted, however, that this study design did not facilitate crossover for the sequential use of the two agents as was done in the earlier Eastern Cooperative Oncology Group (ECOG) trial, so the two trials cannot be directly compared.[54] Indeed, only a small minority of the patients randomized to docetaxel went on to receive capecitabine, and in this subset, there was no suggestion of an improvement in OS with the combination therapy.[57]

The results of these and other similar studies[55] published over the past decade have helped address the controversy over combination versus sequential single-agent therapy. Combination therapy likely offers superior response rate and TTP but at the expense of increased toxicity and difficulty of customization. Because no known combination offers a substantial survival benefit, the general treatment paradigm in hormone-refractory MBC is to begin with sequential single-agent chemotherapy (Table 69.3).[35,37,58–72] In highly symptomatic patients or those with a large tumor burden, it is also valid and acceptable to select a strategy of combination therapy with the goal of more rapid and effective cytoreduction (Table 69.4).[54,55,73–75] It is unclear whether this aggressive approach offers a survival advantage, but on the basis of available data, it appears unlikely. As patients move beyond first-line therapy, they should generally be treated with single-agent chemotherapy; the likelihood of response decreases with each subsequent line of therapy, and toxicity with combination regimens is consistently higher than with single agents. Of note, the question of combination versus single-agent chemotherapy has not been adequately evaluated within biologically defined subgroups of women with MBC. It is conceivable, although unproven at this time, that combination therapy could be more effective than single-agent therapy in triple-negative disease.

Previous trials have explored the role of combination chemo-endocrine therapy in metastatic breast cancer, and have not shown significant improvement in response rates or in OS.[76] In 2009, a large randomized trial conducted in the adjuvant setting by the Breast Cancer Intergroup of North America demonstrated a trend toward worse breast cancer outcomes when tamoxifen was given concurrent with, as opposed to in sequence with, adjuvant chemotherapy.[77] After the publication of these data, standard practice has tended not to favor concurrent chemoendocrine therapy.

TABLE 69.3 Commonly Used Single-Agent Regimens in Metastatic Breast Cancer[a]

Drug	Dosing Schedule	Study
Albumin-bound paclitaxel	260 mg/m² IV q 3 wk *or* 100 mg/m² *or* 125 mg/m² IV, days 1, 8, 15 q 4 wk	Gradishar et al., 2005[58]
Capecitabine	1000–1250 mg/m² PO BID, days 1–14, q 3 wk	Bajetta et al., 2005[255]
Cisplatin	75 mg/m² q 3 wk	Silver et al., 2010[118]
Carboplatin	AUC 6 IV q 3–4 wk	Isakoff et al., 2016
Cyclophosphamide	50 mg PO daily, days 1–21, q 4 wk	Licchetta et al., 2010[60]
Doxorubicin	20 mg/m² IV q wk *or* 60–75 mg/m² IV q 3 wk	Gasparini et al., 1991[78] Chan et al., 1999
Epirubicin	60–90 mg IV q 3 wk	Bastholt et al., 1996[65]
Eribulin	1.4 mg/m² IV days 1, 8 q 3 wk	Cortes et al., 2011[66]
Gemcitabine	800–1200 mg/m² days 1, 8, 15, q 4 wk	Seidman et al., 1995[69]
Ixabepilone	40 mg/m² IV q 3 wk	Perez et al., 2007[68]
Paclitaxel	175 mg/m² q 3 wk *or* 80 mg/m² q wk	Seidman et al., 1995[69] Perez et al., 2001
Pegylated liposomal encapsulated doxorubicin	50 mg/m² IV q 4 wk[b]	Ranson et al., 1997[71] O'Brien et al., 2004[64]
Vinorelbine	25 mg/m² IV q wk	Zelek et al., 2001[72]

AUC, Area under the curve; *BID*, twice daily; *IV*, intravenous; *PO*, by mouth; *q*, every.
[a]Doses often need to be adjusted with all regimens based on individual toxicity and cumulative toxicity over time.
[b]Dose is often modified from 50 mg/m2 to 40 mg/m2 to minimize toxicity.

TABLE 69.4 Commonly Used Combination Chemotherapy for Metastatic Breast Cancer

Drug Combination	Dosing Schedule	Cycle Length (Days)	Study
AC	A:60 mg/m² IV day 1 C: 600 mg/m² IV day 1	21	Fisher et al., 1990[73]
FAC	F: 500 mg/m² IV days 1, 8 A: 50 mg/m² IV day 1 C: 500 mg/m² IV day 1	21	Hortobagyi et al., 1979
CAF	C: 500 mg/m² IV day 1 A: 50 mg/m² IV day 1 F: 500 mg/m² IV days 1 and 8	21	Smalley et al., 1977
FEC	F 500 mg/m² IV day 1 E: 60 mg/m² IV day 1 C: 500 mg/m² IV day 1	28	Blomquist et al., 1993
FEC	F: 400 mg/m² IV days 1, 8 E: 50 mg/m² IV days 1, 8 C: 500 mg/m² IV days 1, 8	28	Ackland et al., 2001[74]
Oral CMF	C: 100 mg/m² PO days 1–14 M: 40 mg/m² IV days 1, 8 F: 600 mg/m² IV days 1, 8	28	Bonadonna et al., 1976
IV CMF	C: 600 mg/m² IV day 1 M: 40 mg/m² IV day 1 F: 600 mg/m² IV day 1	21	Bonadonna et al., 1985
Docetaxel/ capecitabine	D: 75 mg/m² IV day 1 C: 1250 mg/m² PO BID day 14	21	O'Shaughnessy et al., 2002[54]
Paclitaxel/ gemcitabine	P: 175 mg/m² IV day 1 G: 850–1250 mg/m² IV days 1, 8	21	Albain et al., 2004[55]
Ixabepilone/ capecitabine	I: 40 mg/m² C: 1000 mg/m² PO BID days 1–14	21	Thomas et al., 2007[75]

A, Doxorubicin; *BID*, twice daily; *C*, cyclophosphamide; *E*, epirubicin; *F*, fluorouracil (5-FU); *IV*, intravenous; *M*, methotrexate; *PO*, by mouth.

Chemotherapy for Metastatic Breast Cancer

Anthracyclines

Before the advent of taxanes and the widespread use of anthracyclines in the adjuvant setting, doxorubicin was thought to be the drug with the greatest single-agent activity in MBC. It has long been known to be a very active drug for the treatment of MBC. Response rates for monotherapy in anthracycline-naive women are on the order of 35% to 50%. The likelihood of response in heavily pretreated patients is generally significantly lower. Phase II studies have shown that anthracycline rechallenge can be done with acceptable cardiac safety and reasonable activity, although given the multitude of available agents, retreatment with an anthracycline is often reserved for later in the course of disease treatment.

Epirubicin, a doxorubicin analog, is also a highly active drug for the treatment of MBC. In multiple randomized trials of every-week or every-3-week dosing, epirubicin and doxorubicin were found to have equivalent response rates and TTP. On a milligram-to-milligram basis, epirubicin is generally considered less toxic than doxorubicin, with a lower reported rate of gastrointestinal and cardiac toxicity.[78–80]

Anthracyclines can be safely combined with other agents as they are in the adjuvant setting. Well-studied combinations include doxorubicin/cyclophosphamide/5-fluorouracil (CAF/FAC) and epirubicin/cyclophosphamide/5-fluorouracil (FEC). In general, the inclusion of anthracyclines in these regimens increases toxicity but also raises objective response rates.

The major long-term toxicity seen with anthracyclines is myocardial damage, which can result in heart failure. The proposed mechanism for this is oxidative stress, which can cause arrhythmia, pericarditis, or myocarditis acutely, or death of cardiac myocytes chronically. Late-onset arrhythmias and ventricular dysfunction may be seen many years after treatment with anthracyclines. Risk of heart failure appears to be directly correlated with total lifetime dose, with a marked increase in risk of heart failure with cumulative doses greater than 400 to 450 mg/m^2 of doxorubicin as plotted on the Von Hoff dose-response curve.[81]

Multiple strategies have been devised to minimize anthracycline cardiac toxicity, including prolonged infusions, dose divisions, liposomal preparations, and the administration of cardioprotectant drugs such as dexrazoxane. Weekly dosing provides comparable efficacy with a lower rate of significant toxicity.[78] Liposomal preparations of doxorubicin such as pegylated liposomal doxorubicin (PLD/Doxil), nonpegylated liposome-encapsulated doxorubicin (NPLD; Myocet/D-99, Liposome Company, Elan Corporation, Princeton, NJ), and Evacet (TLC-99) have been shown to have at least equivalent response rates but less cardiac toxicity, allowing for the administration of greater cumulative doses. NPLD was studied in conjunction with cyclophosphamide for first-line treatment of MBC and found to have a safer therapeutic index than doxorubicin with a notable reduction in the rate of cardiotoxicity and grade 4 neutropenia.[82] PLD has been shown to be safe and effective in combination with cyclophosphamide, the taxanes, vinorelbine, gemcitabine, or trastuzumab. Patients treated with PLD have minimal alopecia, nausea, or vomiting but a high incidence of stomatitis and hand-foot syndrome (HFS), which can be ameliorated with alterations in dosing schedule. By contrast, the toxicity profile of NPLD is similar to that seen with conventional doxorubicin with the exception of cardiac toxicity.[83]

Although free radical scavengers such as dexrazoxane have been shown to lower the rate of adverse cardiac events in patients receiving both doxorubicin and epirubicin, most patients unfortunately have clinical progression before reaching cumulative doses concerning enough to warrant the drug's use. For this reason, it is rarely used in clinical practice.[84]

Of note, in the modern era anthracyclines are given less and less often for metastatic breast cancer. This is likely due to a combination of factors. As anthracycline-based regimens are used with increasing frequency for localized disease, less opportunity remains for additional dosing in the metastatic setting before the safety threshold for cumulative lifetime dose is reached, although in some patients there remains room for safe anthracycline rechallenge in later lines of therapy. Even in patients with metastatic disease and no prior anthracycline exposure, there is growing wariness about the issue of cardiac toxicity (with a reported incidence of approximately 3% in patients receiving 400 mg/m^2 of doxorubicin),[85] which has the potential both to impair patients' quality of life and to limit their eligibility for subsequent lines of standard and clinical trial-based therapy.

Taxanes

In the early 1990s, Holmes and colleagues first noted that paclitaxel resulted in objective response in 56% of patients with MBC.[86] This class of drugs generated great excitement not only because of its effectiveness but also because of its unique mechanism of action. Paclitaxel (Taxol, Bristol-Myers Squibb, Princeton, NJ), which is isolated from the bark of the Pacific yew tree (*Taxus brevifolia*), shifts the dynamic equilibrium in microtubule assembly from tubulin to microtubules, resulting in highly stable microtubules that are rendered dysfunctional.[87]

Docetaxel (Taxotere, Sanofi-Aventis, Bridgewater, NJ), which is synthesized from extracts of the needles of the European yew (*Taxus baccata*), was originally selected for development in the hope that it would improve on the efficacy of paclitaxel. It has a similar mechanism of action, which results in G2/M cell cycle arrest. Although similar, the effects of these drugs are not identical. In vitro, docetaxel has greater affinity for the tubulin binding site,[88] longer intracellular retention time, and higher intracellular concentrations in target cells.[89] In preclinical models, docetaxel has also been shown to both upregulate thymidine phosphorylase[90] and induce bcl-2 phosphorylation to a greater degree than paclitaxel, suggesting that it may have more potent antitumor apoptotic effects.[91] Nabholtz and associates conducted a phase III trial comparing docetaxel at 100 mg/m^2 every 3 weeks to mitomycin 12 mg/m^2 every 6 weeks plus vinblastine 6 mg/m^2 every 3 weeks. This demonstrated the efficacy of single-agent docetaxel for MBC with a response rate of 30% and a median survival of 11.4 months in patients with anthracycline-refractory disease.[32] Clinically, differences in pharmacokinetics and side effect/toxicity profiles have been observed between paclitaxel and docetaxel. When used in the commonly prescribed doses, neuropathy is more common with paclitaxel and fluid retention, myelosuppression, and fatigue are more commonly seen with docetaxel.[92] Paclitaxel is also more commonly associated with hypersensitivity reactions, although these remain quite rare.

Since taxanes were originally introduced, they have become a cornerstone of effective therapy for MBC and are now often administered before anthracyclines because they are perceived as a safer, equally effective alternative. A Cochrane meta-analysis indicated that for most patients, a taxane-containing regimen improved OS, TTP, and objective response rate compared with non–taxane-containing regimens. This was true for comparison with some, but not all, non–taxane-containing regimens.[93]

The schedule of administration of taxane chemotherapy has also been a topic of debate. Although paclitaxel was historically administered every 3 weeks, many heavily pretreated MBC patients develop neutropenia with this approach. Seidman and colleagues investigated and established the feasibility of weekly low-dose paclitaxel in this population.[70] Cancer and Leukemia Group B (CALGB) trial 9840 further addressed this question, comparing once-a-week to every-3-week paclitaxel in women with MBC. The study demonstrated that weekly paclitaxel is superior to standard (3-hour infusion) paclitaxel with respect to response rate (40% vs. 28%), TTP (9 vs. 5 months), and OS (24 vs. 16 months). Weekly paclitaxel was associated with more grade 3 sensory/motor neuropathy but less grade 3/4 neutropenia.[94] In the treatment of MBC, weekly paclitaxel is therefore the preferred schedule of administration.

The ideal dosing schedule for docetaxel has also been examined. A phase II randomized trial compared weekly to every-3-week docetaxel in 83 women with MBC. Grade 3 and 4 toxicities were more common in the every-3-week arm, but relatively more patients withdrew from the weekly treatment arm because of toxicity. The objective response rate, TTP, and median time to treatment failure were not significantly different between the two study arms.[95] Overall, it is generally believed that every-3-week docetaxel may be slightly more efficacious and less toxic than weekly treatment,[96] and thus every-3-week treatment is favored.

Attention has also focused on taxane dose intensity with the hope of achieving improved OS. In the metastatic setting, higher doses of docetaxel can improve response rates but not OS. Similarly, CALGB 9342 demonstrated that a higher dose of paclitaxel failed to improve outcome in women with MBC.[97] It should therefore be concluded that in the metastatic setting, lower doses are less toxic and probably more appropriate for achieving the goals of palliative chemotherapy.[98]

There is consensus on the efficacy of taxanes for MBC, but some debate remains as to whether paclitaxel and docetaxel have equal efficacy. A phase III randomized head-to-head trial comparing every-3-week docetaxel to every-3-week paclitaxel after an anthracycline for MBC found that docetaxel was superior in terms of OS, TTP, and objective response rate. However, both hematologic and nonhematologic toxicities, particularly pain, stomatitis, asthenia, and neurotoxicity, were greater in the docetaxel arm. Febrile neutropenia occurred in 14.9% of docetaxel-treated patients compared with 1.8% of patients in the paclitaxel arm. Quality of life was similar for patients treated with the two agents.[99] However, as discussed earlier, weekly administration is the optimal schedule for paclitaxel in the metastatic setting. The question of whether or not docetaxel is actually a superior drug to weekly paclitaxel in MBC can be answered only through a direct comparison with weekly paclitaxel, which has not been performed. Both paclitaxel and docetaxel remain reasonable options for the treatment of MBC. Of note, docetaxel is less influenced by multidrug resistance proteins and is incompletely cross-resistant with paclitaxel.[100] Therefore treatment with docetaxel is a consideration in patients who have previously been treated with paclitaxel, but there are generally equally effective and less toxic options available as well.

Common side effects/toxicities seen with taxanes include glove-and-stocking sensory/motor neuropathy, fluid retention, stomatitis, alopecia, myalgias, arthralgias, nausea/vomiting, nail disorders, and hypersensitivity/allergic reaction due to the vehicle, polyoxyethylated castor oil, and alcohol (Cremophor EL). The syndrome of arthralgias and myalgias usually begins 1 to 3 days after infusion and can last for 2 to 4 days. Neuropathy is a common toxicity and often results in dose reductions or treatment discontinuation, particularly during treatment with weekly paclitaxel. Preliminary studies have shown promise for some prophylactic neuroprotective agents, including glutamine, glutathione, vitamin E, and acetyl-L-carnitine, but final recommendations await prospective confirmatory studies.[101] Recent retrospective data suggest that venlafaxine may be an effective treatment for neuropathy secondary to taxane chemotherapy.[102]

Granulocytopenia is often seen with taxane therapy, particularly when every-3-week docetaxel is used. This toxicity can be mitigated by the use of prophylactic white blood cell–colony stimulating factors.[103] The NCCN recommends the prophylactic use of myeloid growth factors for any regimen with a greater than 20% risk of febrile neutropenia as has been documented with every-3-week docetaxel administration.[104] Toxicities more commonly ascribed to docetaxel are epiphora (excessive tearing) as the result of lacrimal gland stenosis and nail changes. The nail

changes are not merely cosmetic, with as many as one-third of patients reporting functional problems. In an effort to minimize this problem, a small trial in 45 patients used a gel-filled "frozen glove" with each infusion. This technique lowered the rate of both nail toxicity (51% vs. 11%) and skin toxicity (53% vs. 24%).[105] However, additional investigations have shown the "frozen glove" strategy to be minimally effective and uncomfortable for patients.[106] Hypersensitivity reactions are less common with docetaxel because it does not use the Cremophor vehicle but are still observed in a small percentage of patients.

In an effort to minimize the risk of taxane hypersensitivity reactions and eliminate the need for antiallergic corticosteroid premedication, nanoparticle albumin-bound (nab)-paclitaxel (Abraxane, Abraxis BioScience, Los Angeles, CA), an albumin-bound paclitaxel nanoparticle, was developed; it does not use Cremophor for drug delivery. In the absence of synthetic solvents, premedication with antihistamines and corticosteroids is not necessary. It offers additional convenience by shortening infusion duration from 3 hours to 30 minutes. Preclinical studies comparing nab-paclitaxel to paclitaxel in the standard, non–albumin-bound form demonstrated lower toxicity, with a maximum tolerated dose 50% higher for nab-paclitaxel.[107,108] Two subsequent multicenter phase II studies of nab-paclitaxel in MBC showed response rates at least equal to those seen with standard taxanes and an acceptable toxicity profile.[109,110] Numerous different doses and schedules of nab-paclitaxel have been examined, and phase II data indicate that nab-paclitaxel 150 mg/m^2 weekly for 3 of 4 weeks appears to be the most effective regimen in metastatic disease, although its side effect profile (particularly with regard to peripheral neuropathy) may prohibit long-term dosing.[111]

A phase III trial comparing every-3-week nab-paclitaxel to every-3-week standard paclitaxel in metastatic breast cancer patients demonstrated higher overall response rate and longer time to tumor progression with nab-paclitaxel.[58] On the basis of these data, albumin-bound paclitaxel was approved by the FDA for use in MBC after failure of combination anthracycline-containing chemotherapy. Nab-paclitaxel and docetaxel have also been compared head-to head in a phase II trial, which demonstrated significantly longer PFS and OS with nab-paclitaxel 150 mg/m^2 weekly.[33,111] However, more recent phase III data comparing weekly paclitaxel (the optimal paclitaxel dosing schedule in advanced disease) to nab-paclitaxel, in which both agents were given with bevacizumab in chemotherapy-naive advanced breast cancer patients, showed that nab-paclitaxel was nonsuperior to paclitaxel, with a trend toward inferiority. Moreover, toxicity (including both neuropathy and hematologic effects) was greater with nab-paclitaxel.[112] Therefore a standard role for nab-paclitaxel in the early lines of metastatic breast cancer treatment remains unclear. Data do indicate that nab-paclitaxel has some activity in patients previously treated with standard paclitaxel.[34] Therefore, like docetaxel, it is a therapeutic option in paclitaxel-refractory patients.

The combination of taxanes with other chemotherapeutic agents has been shown to improve response rates in advanced breast cancer. Data from ECOG 1193 discouraged the combination of taxanes with anthracyclines because of increased toxicity and no demonstrable effect on long-term survival.[50] The avoidance of this combination is further supported by the results of the Etude RegionAle dans le cancer du Sein MEtastatique (ERASME) 3 trial, which also combined anthracyclines and taxanes.[113] More convincing evidence is available to support the combination of taxanes with either gemcitabine or capecitabine. Randomized trials have shown modest gains with these combination regimens, again at the expense of added toxicity.[54,55,114] The decision to combine taxanes with other antineoplastics must carefully consider the risk/benefit ratio. Doublet therapy is generally reserved for patients who are very symptomatic or who have rapidly progressive disease in which the timing and degree of response are critical.

Alkylating Agents

The efficacy of alkylating agents in both the adjuvant and metastatic settings has been documented over many decades. Cyclophosphamide is the alkylating agent most commonly used in breast cancer because it is highly effective and can safely be combined with many other agents such as anthracyclines (e.g., doxorubicin) and antimetabolites (e.g., methotrexate). On the basis of data from the 1970s, single-agent cyclophosphamide was estimated to have a response rate between 10% and 50% in the first-line treatment of MBC. Estimated response rates in the modern era are difficult to calculate because cyclophosphamide is used commonly as a component of combination regimens in the adjuvant setting (AC, FEC, CMF) and rarely used in the first- or second-line setting for the management of metastatic disease.

Common toxicities seen with alkylating agents include nausea, vomiting, alopecia, and myelosuppression. The risk of hemorrhagic cystitis is quite low and nearly eliminated with the use of adequate hydration. Although the issue of secondary myelodysplasia or leukemia after treatment with alkylating agents is of concern in the adjuvant setting, this should not influence treatment decisions for patients with metastatic disease, given the risk/benefit ratio in the setting of shortened life expectancy.

In recent years, there has been increasing excitement about the platinum agents cisplatin and carboplatin for treatment of MBC, particularly in triple-negative disease. The use of platinums in MBC was originally investigated in the 1980s, when a small single-arm trial demonstrated a 47% response rate to cisplatin as first-line chemotherapy for MBC.[115] In the 1990s, carboplatin was found to have a response rate of 20% to 35% in relatively untreated breast cancer, and less than 10% in pretreated patients.[116,117] Because of concerns about the platinum agents' toxicity and the concurrent development of the taxanes, further development of single-agent platinum in breast cancer largely stalled after that point. However, in the last 10 years there has been a new recognition that platinums have significant activity specifically in triple-negative breast cancer. Platinums work through a mechanism of DNA cross-linking, which may be particularly effective in tumors with DNA repair defects conferred by BRCA mutations. Triple-negative breast cancers, in turn, share many features with BRCA mutant counterparts. A small study of neoadjuvant single-agent cisplatin in triple-negative disease demonstrated proof-of-principle for platinum efficacy in this cohort; 22% of patients achieved pathologic complete response, and 50% achieved good pathologic response by Miller-Payne criteria.[118]

In metastatic disease, a single-arm, phase II trial of cisplatin or carboplatin in first- or second-line treatment of triple-negative MBC demonstrated a response rate of 25.6%.[35] The randomized phase III TNT trial compared docetaxel to carboplatin in patients with metastatic or recurrent locally advanced triple-negative breast cancer; eligible patients had received no nonanthracycline chemotherapy for metastatic disease. Overall response rates were not statistically different (31.4% and 35.6% for carboplatin and docetaxel, respectively) in the overall population. Likewise, there were no significant differences in PFS or OS. There were significantly higher rates of grade 3/4 neuropathy and febrile neutropenia in the docetaxel arm. In the BRCA-mutant population specifically, there was a significantly higher response rate to carboplatin (68.0%, vs. 33.3% for docetaxel; p = .03).[59] The management of BRCA mutant patients is addressed later in this chapter. There is interest in developing genomic or genetic scores for BRCA-like phenotype in non-BRCA-mutant tumors, which could predict for platinum responsiveness; this pursuit is currently at an early stage.

Antimetabolites

Fluoropyrimidines

Fluoropyrimidines have been known for decades to be active in breast cancer and have been widely used in both the adjuvant and metastatic settings. Bolus 5-fluorouracil, both alone and in combination with leucovorin (LV), is known to be active in MBC and can be administered on various dosing schedules. In the past, 5-fluorouracil was preferred by some patients because of its low incidence of alopecia, nausea, and vomiting, and it was a reasonable choice in patients who had received multiple lines of therapy.[36,119] Infusional 5-fluorouracil is now rarely used because of the widespread availability of the oral agent, capecitabine.

Capecitabine (N4-pentyloxycarbonyl-5′-deoxy-5-fluorocytidine) is an oral fluoropyrimidine carbamate that was rationally designed to generate 5-fluorouracil preferentially in tumor tissue, mimicking the activity seen with infusional 5-fluorouracil. This agent is converted to 5-fluorouracil through a cascade of enzymes, the last of which is thymidine phosphorylase. It is believed that capecitabine selectively targets malignant tissue over healthy tissue because the former possesses higher thymidine phosphorylase activity.[120,121]

Multiple clinical trials have demonstrated the safety and efficacy of capecitabine in MBC that has progressed after treatment with anthracycline and taxane chemotherapies. In general, response rates of 20% to 29% are seen in the first-line setting,[122] and as one would expect in the first-line setting, median survival is consistently greater than 1 year.[37,123] Capecitabine's ease of administration and documented activity in heavily pretreated breast cancer make it a popular choice for the treatment of metastatic disease. Other available oral fluoropyrimidines include tegafur (Ftorafur) and uracil/LV (Orzel), but neither is commercially available in the United States.

The most common treatment-related toxicities seen with capecitabine are hand-foot syndrome (HFS), diarrhea, nausea, vomiting, and fatigue. Unlike many other chemotherapeutic agents, capecitabine has a low incidence of myelosuppression, facilitating its use in heavily pretreated patients, in the elderly, and in combination with other agents that do cause myelosuppression. HFS, characterized by erythema, numbness, tingling, and either dysesthesias or paresthesias of the palms or soles, is the dose-limiting toxicity in many patients and occurs in up to half of patients treated with capecitabine (Fig. 69.2). In severe cases of HFS, there can be painful swelling of the cutaneous tissues, and even desquamation, ulceration, or blistering. The syndrome may occur with initial courses of therapy or develop slowly over time. In a multicenter phase II study of capecitabine used to treat women with chemotherapy-refractory advanced breast cancer, 56% of patients developed HFS and 10% had severe HFS characterized by severe pain and/or skin breakdown.[123] Strategies that

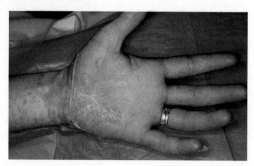

• **Fig. 69.2** Hand-foot syndrome related to 5-fluorouracil–based chemotherapy. Note the erythema, edema, rash, and early desquamation. Severe pain is associated with this toxic reaction. (From Skarin AT. *Atlas of Diagnostic Oncology: Expert Consult.* 3rd ed. Philadelphia: Mosby Elsevier; 2002.)

may be used to minimize toxicity include manipulation of the daily dose/dose schedule; prophylactic pyridoxine (50–150 mg orally each day) has been proposed as a prophylactic treatment to reduce HFS, but multiple small trials have failed to demonstrate its efficacy.[124] Topical emollients, particularly 10% urea cream, may prevent HFS[125] and may provide symptomatic relief when it occurs.[126]

Gemcitabine

Gemcitabine (Gemzar, Eli Lilly, Indianapolis, IN) is a nucleoside analog that replaces cytidine during DNA replication. This process arrests tumor growth, because new nucleosides cannot be attached to the "faulty" nucleoside, resulting in apoptosis. Response rates to gemcitabine in the metastatic setting vary from 14% to 37% in chemotherapy-naive patients to 1% to 30% in patients who have previously received a taxane and/or an anthracycline.[38] Although alopecia and gastrointestinal toxicity are generally mild, the drug's effects can be highly myelosuppressive, especially in patients who have received radiation or multiple lines of chemotherapy in the past. Flulike symptoms are reported in a small percentage of patients but are usually mild, transient, and treatable with acetaminophen. A rare but serious toxicity observed with gemcitabine is pulmonary toxicity (pneumonitis), which may occur more often when it is used in combination with a taxane.[127,128]

In a phase III trial of 529 patients treated with paclitaxel alone versus paclitaxel/gemcitabine for first-line therapy in the metastatic setting, the combination showed an OS improvement from 15.8 months to 18.6 months for paclitaxel versus gemcitabine/paclitaxel, respectively.[129] Of note, the paclitaxel was administered every 3 weeks. This trial led to the approval of gemcitabine for breast cancer in combination with paclitaxel. Subsequently, a trial of docetaxel alone versus docetaxel/gemcitabine in first- or second-line MBC showed no significant difference in response rate or OS.[39] A recent phase randomized phase III trial compared cisplatin/gemcitabine with paclitaxel (every-3-week)/gemcitabine first-line MBC treatment and showed that cisplatin/gemcitabine was both noninferior and superior to paclitaxel/gemcitabine in terms of PFS.[40] Gemcitabine also can be safely and effectively combined with a number of different agents in pretreated MBC, including taxanes,[130] vinorelbine,[131] and cisplatin.[132,133] In practice, gemcitabine is given infrequently in the first-line setting but is used as a single agent or as a component of doublet therapy in more refractory MBC.

Other Microtubule Inhibitors

Initially discovered in 1993, the epothilones are a class of nontaxane microtubule polymerizing agents obtained from the fermentation of myxobacterium *Sorangium cellulosum*. Similar to taxanes, epothilones cause cell cycle arrest at the G2/M transition leading to cytotoxicity; however, these novel agents retain a much greater toxicity against P-glycoprotein–expressing multiple drug-resistant cells.[134] Epothilones disrupt microtubule dynamics by stabilizing the microtubule from depolymerization, thereby enhancing microtubule polymerization. They compete for the same β-tubulin binding site as paclitaxel, but they are more powerful polymerizers of tubulin. Although they occupy the same binding site, they bind in a different fashion, compared with paclitaxel.[135,136] This may explain the lack of cross-resistance between these two drug classes.

Although the family of epothilone compounds comprises many compounds, the most clinically advanced is ixabepilone (BMS-247550). Preclinical data have shown that epothilones work through partially nonoverlapping mechanisms with taxanes. Phase I and II studies have shown epothilones to be active even in patients who have progressed through taxane therapy.[41,42,68] Ixabepilone (Ixempra, Bristol-Myers Squibb, Princeton, NJ) is a semisynthetic analog of epothilone B, which is a much more potent tubulin polymerizer in vitro than any of the commercially available taxanes. A phase III study of 752 patients with MBC who had previously received both an anthracycline and a taxane compared capecitabine monotherapy to capecitabine plus ixabepilone. The combined treatment arm had a longer median TTP (5.8 vs. 4.2 months) and an improved objective response rate (35% vs. 14%). Grade 3/4 treatment-related sensory neuropathy, fatigue, and neutropenia were more frequent with combination therapy.[75] A second randomized phase III study confirmed these findings, demonstrating improved response rate and PFS for ixabepilone/capecitabine compared with capecitabine alone in pretreated MBC, although with no OS difference.[43] Accordingly, ixabepilone was approved by the FDA in 2007 in combination with capecitabine to treat patients with metastatic or locally advanced breast cancer after failure of an anthracycline and a taxane. On the basis of a phase II trial demonstrating ixabepilone activity in patients with disease refractory to an anthracycline, taxane, and capecitabine, it was also approved as monotherapy.[68] Small trials have examined the use of every-3-week versus weekly ixabepilone dosing, and it appears that every-3-week dosing is associated with better activity, at the expense of increased toxicity.[137]

The toxicity profile of ixabepilone consists primarily of sensory neuropathy,[66] fatigue/asthenia, myalgias, nausea/vomiting, and cytopenias. Both the hematologic and nonhematologic side effects of ixabepilone are more common when the drug is administered in combination with capecitabine. Pretreatment with H1- and H2-antagonists is recommended because hypersensitivity reactions have been observed in patients receiving epothilones.

Eribulin mesylate is a second nontaxane microtubule inhibitor commonly used in MBC. Eribulin is a synthetic analog of halichondrin B, a natural product that is isolated from the marine sponge *Halichondria okadai*. The compound inhibits the growth phase of microtubules. In preclinical models, it retains activity in paclitaxel-treated cells.[138] After promising results in early-phase clinical studies, eribulin was investigated as a single agent for MBC in the phase III EMBRACE study.

In EMBRACE, patients who had received two to five prior chemotherapy regimens were randomized to either eribulin (administered on days 1 and 8 of a 21-day cycle) or treatment of the physician's choice. In the accrued cohort, 99% of patients had received prior anthracycline and taxane, and 73% of patients had received prior capecitabine. OS was significantly higher with eribulin, compared with treatment of physician's choice (13.1 months vs. 10.6 months, respectively). PFS was 3.6 months with eribulin versus 2.2 months with treatment of physician's choice. The most common side effects in both treatment arms were neutropenia (52% with eribulin, 30% with treatment of physician's choice) and asthenia/fatigue (54% with eribulin, 40% with treatment of physician's choice). Other notable potential side effects of eribulin include neuropathy and alopecia.[138] On the basis of these data, eribulin was FDA approved in 2010 for the treatment of MBC in the third line and beyond. Trials for its evaluation in earlier lines of therapy are ongoing.

Eribulin has also been formally compared with capecitabine in pretreated MBC. In a recent phase III trial, patients with locally advanced/MBC previously treated with up to three prior chemotherapy regimens, including an anthracycline and a taxane, were randomized to either eribulin or capecitabine treatment. There was no significant difference in OS or PFS between the two groups: 15.9 months versus 14.5 months for OS, and 4.1 months versus 4.2 months for PFS, for eribulin and capecitabine, respectively.[139] Therefore, although eribulin clearly has a role in the management of refractory MBC, its sequence with capecitabine remains at the treating physician's discretion.

Vinca Alkaloids

Vinorelbine (Navelbine, Pierre Fabre Pharmaceuticals, Parsippany, NJ), is a semisynthetic vinca alkaloid that prevents microtubule assembly (in contrast to taxanes, which stabilize microtubules). It has a well-established role in the treatment of MBC, demonstrating response rates of 16% to 50% depending on dosing and line of therapy; however, it has never been approved by the FDA for use in breast cancer.[44,45,140] Dose-limiting toxicity is generally bone marrow suppression, most notably neutropenia, although grade 1 or 2 peripheral neuropathy is also reported by many patients. Vinorelbine's side effect profile does not include cardiac toxicity, hypertension, or alopecia, thus making it an attractive agent for study in combination regimens as well as for use in the elderly. As has been the case with many other agents in MBC, the addition of a second chemotherapeutic agent to vinorelbine has not been shown to alter survival and generally increases toxicity.

An oral preparation of vinorelbine is also available for use in patients who prefer oral administration over intravenous infusion. Investigators in France have completed a phase II trial of first-line oral vinorelbine in women with locally advanced and MBC and have confirmed that it is both well tolerated and effective in this patient population. Data from clinical trials suggest that it is as active as the intravenous formulation. Of note, a higher incidence of gastrointestinal toxicity has been reported with the oral preparation. Despite its ease of administration, weekly blood counts must still be monitored given the risk of neutropenia; in the phase II trial, grade 4 neutropenia was seen in 17% of patients.[141]

Treatment of HER2-Positive Metastatic Breast Cancer

The epidermal growth factor family of receptors consists of four transmembrane proteins (HER1 [EGFR], HER2, HER3, and HER4); each has different properties, but all are involved in the regulation of cell proliferation. The *HER2* gene encodes the human epidermal growth factor receptor (HER2), which is known to be overexpressed in approximately 20% of all breast cancers.[142,143] These tumors are associated with many adverse prognostic markers, including high tumor grade, high rate of cell proliferation, increased rate of nodal metastases, and relative resistance to certain types of chemotherapy.[144] Retrospective studies suggest that HER2-positive disease is uniquely sensitive to anthracycline-based chemotherapy, and additional data support the efficacy of paclitaxel against this class of tumors.[145,146] HER2-overexpressing tumors are more aggressive, and amplification of this gene was an independent risk factor for shortened disease-free and OS before the advent of HER2-directed therapy with trastuzumab (Herceptin, Genentech, South San Francisco, CA).[143,147]

Trastuzumab is a humanized monoclonal antibody targeting the extracellular domain of the HER2 protein. Its exact mechanism is not certain but is thought to involve at least three main components: (1) attraction of immune cells to HER2-positive tumor cells through Fc domain interactions, resulting in antibody dependent cell-mediated cytotoxicity; (2) prevention of HER2 shedding, resulting in the inhibition of constitutive tyrosine kinase activity; and (3) internalization and degradation of HER2.[148] First studied in the metastatic setting, in HER2-overexpressing patients trastuzumab monotherapy exhibited response rates of 25%[149] in the first-line setting and 10% to 15% in previously treated MBC.[150,151] It is important to note that historically not all clinical trials have required fluorescent in situ hybridization (FISH) testing, and many early trials included patients with 2+ staining by immunohistochemistry (IHC). Therefore some of the patients entered into early trastuzumab trials may have had tumors that would today be regarded as HER2 nonamplified. The inadvertent enrollment of HER2-negative patients is likely to have attenuated some of the effects of targeted therapy observed in these large treatment trials.

Beyond its single-agent activity, trastuzumab is highly effective when administered in combination with chemotherapy for MBC. In vitro models have shown that trastuzumab has synergistic effects when used in combination with cisplatin,[152] carboplatin, docetaxel, and vinorelbine, and it has additive effects when administered with doxorubicin, cyclophosphamide, methotrexate, and paclitaxel.[153,154] Although trastuzumab monotherapy does yield clinical responses and is sometimes used in patients who cannot tolerate combined therapy, the likelihood of a meaningful response is greater with combination therapy.[155] For this reason, it is generally recommended that this HER2-directed therapy be administered in combination with chemotherapy to increase the likelihood of an objective response (Table 69.5).[156–167] Clinical data demonstrate that trastuzumab can be safely combined with many classes of drugs, including taxanes, vinorelbine, capecitabine,[162,168,169] platinum,[165] and ixabepilone.[166]

The landmark study of trastuzumab in HER2-positive MBC was published in 2001. This phase III trial randomized 469 patients with HER2-positive MBC to first-line therapy with either chemotherapy alone or chemotherapy plus trastuzumab. The addition of trastuzumab to chemotherapy was associated with a longer time to disease progression (7.4 vs. 4.6 months), a higher response rate (50% vs. 32%), longer duration of response (9.1 vs. 6.1 months), lower rate of death at 1 year (22% vs. 33%), and longer median survival (25.1 vs. 20.3 months). It is striking that a survival advantage was detected despite the crossover of 66% of patients in the chemotherapy-alone arm after disease progression.

TABLE 69.5	Commonly Used Therapeutic Regimens for HER2-Positive Metastatic Breast Cancer	
Agents	**Study**	**Regimen**
Docetaxel/trastuzumab/pertuzumab	Swain et al., 2015[156]	D: 75 mg/m^2 q 3 wk[a] + T: 8 mg/kg day 1 → 6 mg/kg q 3 wk + Pz: 840 mg/kg day 1 → 420 mg/kg q 3 wk
Paclitaxel/trastuzumab/pertuzumab	Dang et al., 2015[157]	P: 80 mg/m^2 q wk + T: 8 mg/kg day 1 → 6 mg/kg q 3 wk + Pz: 840 mg/kg day 1 → 420 mg/kg q 3 wk
T-DM1 (trastuzumab emtansine)	Verma et al., 2012[158]	T-DM1: 3.6 mg/kg q 3 wk
Paclitaxel/trastuzumab	Seidman et al., 2001[159]	P: 80 mg/m^2 q wk + T: 4 mg/kg day 1 → 2 mg/kg q wk
Docetaxel/trastuzumab	Marty et al., 2005[160]	D: 80–100 mg/m^2 day 1 + T: 4 mg/kg day 1 → 2 mg/kg q wk (q 3 wk)
Docetaxel/trastuzumab	Esteva et al., 2002[161]	D: 35 mg/m^2 days 1, 8, 15 + T: 4 mg/kg day 1 → 2 mg/kg q wk (q 4 wk)
Vinorelbine/trastuzumab	Burstein et al., 2001[162]	V: 25 mg/m^2 weekly + T: 4 mg/kg day 1 → 2 mg/kg q wk
Paclitaxel weekly/carboplatin/trastuzumab	Burris et al., 2004[163] Perez, 2004[164]	P: 70–80 mg/m^2 days 1, 8, 15 + C: AUC = 2 days 1, 8, 15 + T: 4 mg/kg day 1 → 2 mg/kg q wk (q 4 wk)
Paclitaxel q 3 wk/carboplatin/trastuzumab	Robert et al., 2006[165]	P: 175 mg/m^2 day 1 C: AUC = 6 day 1 T: 4 mg/kg day 1 → 2 mg/kg days 1, 8, 15 (q 3 wk)
Ixabepilone/trastuzumab	Tolaney et al., 2013[166]	I: 40 mg/m^2 q 3 wk + T: 8 mg/kg d1 → 6 mg/kg q 3 wk
Capecitabine/lapatinib	Geyer et al., 2006[167]	X: 1000 mg/m^2 PO BID days 1–14 L: 1250 mg PO QD days 1–21 (q 3 wk)

AUC, Area under the curve; *B,* bevacizumab; *BID,* twice daily; *C,* carboplatin; *D,* docetaxel; *L,* lapatinib; *P,* paclitaxel; *Pz,* pertuzumab; *q,* every; *QD,* daily; *T,* trastuzumab; *T-DM1,* trastuzumab emtansine; *V,* vinorelbine; *X,* capecitabine.
[a]At least six cycles of docetaxel are recommended.

The most common important toxicity seen was cardiotoxicity. New York Heart Association class III/IV cardiac dysfunction occurred in 16% of patients receiving trastuzumab/doxorubicin/cyclophosphamide compared with 3% of patients in the doxorubicin/cyclophosphamide arm. In patients who received taxanes, the rate of severe cardiac dysfunction was also higher with the addition of trastuzumab—2% in the paclitaxel/trastuzumab arm compared with 1% in those receiving paclitaxel monotherapy. Although the cardiomyopathy was severe and symptomatic in some cases, patients generally responded well to standard medical management. Clear benefit from the addition of trastuzumab was seen in both the anthracycline and the taxane subgroups.[170] Given the significant rate of cardiomyopathy when trastuzumab is administered in conjunction with anthracyclines, these agents should not be combined outside of a clinical trial setting. On the basis of the results of this seminal trial, trastuzumab was approved by the FDA to be used in combination with paclitaxel for first-line treatment of HER2-positive MBC. Multiple trials have confirmed the safety and efficacy of this combination, including trials in which both drugs were administered weekly.[159]

Similar clinical benefits were seen in a phase II trial combining trastuzumab with docetaxel for the first-line treatment of metastatic HER2-positive breast cancer. Patients receiving combination therapy had a superior response rate, OS, and TTP with minimal added toxicity, compared with docetaxel alone. Although grade 3 and 4 neutropenia, as well as febrile neutropenia, occurred more often in the combination arm, there was little difference in the number and severity of adverse events between the two arms.[160]

Multiple clinical trials have been designed to answer the question of which chemotherapy/trastuzumab combination is most effective and which, if any, will result in longest survival and TTP.[171] To determine the optimal trastuzumab-based chemotherapy regimen for HER2-positive MBC, the trastuzumab and vinorelbine or taxane (TRAVIOTA) study randomized patients to receive first-line trastuzumab with either weekly vinorelbine or a weekly taxane. Although underpowered due to poor accrual, the study evaluated responses in 81 women. Response rates for the vinorelbine/trastuzumab arm and the taxane/trastuzumab arm were 51% and 40%, respectively. The median time to disease progression was 8.5 months and 6 months for the vinorelbine and taxane-based arms, respectively. Although the trial confirmed that both combinations are safe and effective, neither combination was thought to be superior.[172] The Herceptin Plus Navelbine or Taxotere (HERNATA) study randomized patients with advanced HER2-positive breast cancer to first-line treatment with either vinorelbine/trastuzumab or docetaxel (administered every 3 weeks)/trastuzumab. In terms of efficacy, neither regimen was superior, with median time to progression of 12.4 versus 15.3 months, and a median OS of 35.7 months and 38.8 months for docetaxel and vinorelbine, respectively. There was significantly greater toxicity in the docetaxel arm, however.[173]

Coadministration of trastuzumab with standard anthracyclines is associated with an unacceptably high rate of cardiac toxicity; therefore, despite the fact that anthracyclines are known to be particularly active in HER2-positive MBC, this approach should be avoided in favor of other therapeutic combinations if possible.[174] Of note, there is evidence that concurrent use of trastuzumab and nonpegylated liposomal doxorubicin does not significantly increase cardiotoxicity rates, and therefore this combination could be considered in select circumstances.[175]

Approximately one-half of HER2-overexpressing breast cancers also express ER, and the optimal way to combine hormonal therapy with HER2-directed therapy in this population is a focus of ongoing investigation.[176] Molecular cross-talk between the HER2 and ER pathways has been demonstrated; experimental models suggest that HER2 upregulation leads to estrogen independence and resistance in ER-positive human breast cancer cells.[177] Therefore when endocrine therapy was well established and trastuzumab was early in its development, the randomized phase III TrAstuzumab in Dual ER-positive Metastatic breast cancer (TAnDEM) trial randomized 207 postmenopausal women with HER2-positive, ER-positive, and/or PR-positive MBC who wanted to avoid or postpone chemotherapy to anastrozole alone versus anastrozole plus trastuzumab. PFS was significantly longer (4.8 months vs. 2.4 months) in the patients who received anastrozole plus trastuzumab. No OS benefit was seen with trastuzumab, but this could have been due to a high percentage of Anastrazole-only patients crossing over to trastuzumab after trial completion.[178] A similar PFS benefit for the addition of lapatinib to letrozole in HER2-positive, hormone receptor-positive patients has also been demonstrated.[179] The absence of an OS benefit for the addition of trastuzumab to hormonal therapy raises some concern about combining the two therapies up front in patients with HER2-positive, hormone receptor–positive disease (given that combining trastuzumab with chemotherapy upfront results in a clear survival advantage).

Although evidence demonstrates that HER2-directed therapy (usually combined with chemotherapy) is effective in hormone receptor–positive tumors, the converse (that hormonal therapy is effective in HER2-positive tumors) is not necessarily true.[178] Accordingly, current clinical guidelines suggest that endocrine therapy alone may be considered only in a highly select subgroup of HER2-positive/hormone receptor–positive tumors (i.e., contraindication to HER2-directed therapy).[180]

There are unanswered questions about the optimal duration of trastuzumab in the metastatic setting, but prevailing evidence supports continuing therapy indefinitely for patients with a sustained clinical response in the absence of toxicity. Nonetheless, many clinicians question the need to continue trastuzumab indefinitely in some patients, particularly those who present de novo with low-volume disease and achieve a complete response to therapy. To date, no trial has compared continuation to discontinuation of trastuzumab in patients with stable or responsive disease. In patients with isolated CNS progression, it is generally assumed that the trastuzumab is active against systemic disease and that CNS progression results from failure of trastuzumab to cross the blood-brain barrier. Therefore in this clinical scenario, continuation of trastuzumab is considered a reasonable option.

There is evidence that continuing trastuzumab, with a different chemotherapy partner, beyond progression on prior trastuzumab-based therapy can result in maintained disease response. A retrospective review of 105 patients showed that patients derived benefit from continued trastuzumab therapy beyond disease progression.[181] The German Trastuzumab Beyond Progression (TBP) study was designed to address the question of whether patients continue to benefit from trastuzumab after initial disease progression. Women with HER2-positive locally advanced or MBC who had previously been treated with a trastuzumab-containing regimen were randomized to second-line therapy with either capecitabine alone or capecitabine plus trastuzumab. Although the trial closed early due to poor accrual, initial analysis revealed significantly better response rate and time to progression in patients who continued on trastuzumab.[182] There was no significant difference in OS, although this was an underpowered secondary end point. Subsequent post hoc analysis demonstrated a significant improvement in postprogression survival in patients who continued to receive anti-HER2 agents in the third line.[183] Thus the TBP study provides prospective, randomized data to support the continuation of trastuzumab beyond progression. Additionally, and discussed in-depth later in this chapter, there is strong evidence that alternative HER2-targeting agents such as trastuzumab emtansine (T-DM1) and lapatinib have significant activity, even in patients who have progressed on trastuzumab.

Trastuzumab is generally well tolerated and does not cause many of the toxicities or side effects seen with conventional chemotherapy; notably, it does not affect renal or hepatic function or cause nausea, vomiting, alopecia, or cytopenias. Mild infusion reactions are common during the loading dose; trastuzumab-associated lung injury is a rare complication that may manifest as bronchospasm, pleural effusions, pulmonary edema, and hypoxia.[184]

The greatest concern with trastuzumab is the development of a nonischemic cardiomyopathy, which usually responds well to medical management and is often reversible with drug discontinuation. HER2 is proposed to play a critical role in maintenance of cardiac contractility and myocyte survival. Multiple mechanisms are proposed to contribute to myocyte damage, including interference with survival signals, immune-mediated destruction of cardiac myocytes, augmentation of chemotherapy-induced cytotoxicity, and antagonism of the growth stimulation and repair properties of HER2.[185] Although this clinical syndrome may present with chest pain, shortness of breath, or palpitations, cardiac dysfunction is asymptomatic in many patients. In the four large adjuvant trials of trastuzumab after doxorubicin/cyclophosphamide, the rate of congestive heart failure was 1% to 4%, with 10% of patients experiencing a decrease in ejection fraction by echocardiography.[186]

Documented risk factors for trastuzumab cardiomyopathy include age older than 60 years and anthracycline use. Other suspected risk factors include past anthracycline therapy in excess of 400 mg/m^2, hypertension, preexisting cardiac dysfunction (baseline ejection fraction <60%), and a history of chest wall irradiation.[187] Data suggest that cardiac function can recover after drug discontinuation and may support the retreatment of these patients with trastuzumab, especially in the metastatic setting, where the risk/benefit ratio is heavily influenced by improvements in OS.[188] Baseline cardiac function should be evaluated with either echocardiogram or multiple gated acquisition scan before initiation of trastuzumab therapy. In addition, periodic cardiac evaluation should be performed during treatment, although there is no clear evidence-based consensus for when and how often. It has been suggested that because most cardiac dysfunction occurs in the first 16 weeks, additional follow-up imaging is not routinely required in the absence of new symptoms or physical examination findings.[189] Certainly, continued clinical assessment for congestive heart failure is required for patients receiving trastuzumab, and clinicians should maintain a low threshold for cardiac imaging at any point in the course of therapy.

As more patients are treated with trastuzumab-based therapy in the adjuvant and metastatic settings, the emergence of trastuzumab-resistant, HER2-positive MBC is a growing problem. Many mechanisms of trastuzumab resistance in HER2-positive tumors have been proposed, including the presence of different HER2 isoforms and aberrant signaling in alternative pathways such as the phosphoinositide 3-kinase (PI3K) pathway.[148] To circumvent this resistance, and improve the disease outcomes of HER2-positive breast cancer patients, multiple new HER2-targeted therapies have been developed. Since the early 2000s there has been explosive progress in this arena, leading to the FDA approval of novel anti-HER2 agents pertuzumab and T-DM1 in 2012 and 2013, respectively, for HER2-positive MBC. The multikinase inhibitor lapatinib has also been approved (in 2007) and has activity in trastuzumab-refractory patients. These developments have dramatically improved the prognosis of HER2-positive MBC and now offer clinicians a much broader set of tools for treating this patient cohort.

Pertuzumab (Perjeta, Genentech, South San Francisco, CA) is a humanized monoclonal antibody and the first in a class of agents known as HER dimerization inhibitors. It is known to block the interaction of HER2 with other receptors such as HER1 (EGFR), HER3, and HER4. Through this mechanism, it synergizes with trastuzumab to effect a more complete blockade of HER2 signaling.[156] The Clinical Evaluation of Pertuzumab and Trastuzumab (CLEOPATRA) trial was a phase III trial randomizing patients to either docetaxel/trastuzumab/pertuzumab or docetaxel/trastuzumab/placebo for first-line treatment of HER2-positive MBC. On this protocol, docetaxel was administered every 3 weeks for a recommended course of six cycles, and pertuzumab/trastuzumab were administered every 3 weeks until disease progression or unacceptable toxicity. In a prespecified analysis at 50 months' median follow-up, OS was significantly higher in the pertuzumab arm than in the comparator arm: 56.5 months versus 40.8 months, respectively, for a survival improvement of 15.7 months.

In terms of toxicities, no increased risk of cardiac adverse events with the addition of pertuzumab to trastuzumab was detected in this landmark phase III trial. The main toxicities that appeared numerically more common in the pertuzumab-treated patients were diarrhea, rash, pruritis, upper respiratory tract, and muscle spasm.[156] A small phase II trial has shown that the use of paclitaxel instead of docetaxel in this triplet regimen appears safe and effective.[157] In 2012, pertuzumab was FDA approved (in combination with trastuzumab and docetaxel, although in practice it is commonly given with paclitaxel as well) for the first-line treatment of HER2-positive MBC and is now standard of care.

T-DM1 is an antibody-drug conjugate of trastuzumab with a highly potent antimicrotubule agent (emtansine, or DM1), connected by a linker. As an antibody-drug conjugate, it is designed to target delivery of the cytotoxic agent specifically to HER2-overexpressing cells. In the randomized phase III EMILIA trial, patients with advanced HER2-positive breast cancer, previously

treated with trastuzumab and a taxane, were assigned to receive either T-DM1 or lapatinib plus capecitabine. T-DM1 was administered intravenously every 3 weeks. PFS was significantly longer for T-DM1 compared with lapatinib/capecitabine (9.6 months vs. 6.4 months, respectively), as was OS (30.9 months vs. 25.1 months, respectively). In addition, there were more grade 3 and higher adverse events with lapatinib/capecitabine than with T-DM1. The most common grade 3/4 adverse events seen with T-DM1 were thrombocytopenia (12.9% of patients) and transaminase elevations (approximately 3%–4% of patients). Cardiac events were rare and did not seem to differ between the two treatment arms; 97.1% of patients on T-DM1 maintained an ejection fraction of 45% or greater throughout study treatment.[158] On the basis of the EMILIA results, T-DM1 was FDA approved in 2013 for treatment of advanced HER2-positive breast cancer after trastuzumab and taxane therapy.

Combination regimens using T-DM1 and pertuzumab have also been explored. Preclinical and early-phase data suggested synergy between T-DM1 and pertuzumab in HER2-positive breast cancer patients, leading to the phase III MARIANNE study. In MARIANNE, metastatic HER2-positive breast cancer patients were treated in the first line with T-DM1 plus pertuzumab (experimental arm), T-DM1 alone (experimental arm), or taxane plus trastuzumab (control arm). Each experimental arm was compared with the control arm in two separate comparisons, and although both experimental arms were noninferior to taxane/trastuzumab in terms of PFS, neither was found to be superior. A comparison was also made between the two experimental arms (T-DM1 with or without pertuzumab), and no significant difference was shown; median PFS was 15.2 months for T-DM1 plus pertuzumab and 14.1 months for T-DM1 alone.[190] Therefore, although the combination of trastuzumab plus pertuzumab results in improved clinical outcomes, the data do not support use of combination T-DM1 plus pertuzumab.

Lapatinib is an oral small-molecule dual kinase inhibitor of both EGFR and HER2 that blocks the downstream signaling of HER2 homodimers as well as heterodimers of HER2 with EGFR (HER1). Its primary effect is believed to be mediated through inhibition of autophosphorylation sites on these receptors and by phosphorylation of the downstream modulator AKT (protein kinase B).[191] Its ease of administration as an oral tablet, low rate of cardiac toxicity, and incomplete cross-resistance with trastuzumab[192] make it an attractive option for patients who have advanced on first-line HER2-directed therapy. In phase I trials, lapatinib was generally well tolerated, with mild diarrhea and dermatitis/skin eruption as common toxic effects and a low incidence of cardiotoxicity. As a single agent, lapatinib has a response rate of 28% in trastuzumab-naive patients but yielded disappointing response rates in patients with trastuzumab-refractory disease.[193]

On the basis of the results of a pivotal phase III trial adding lapatinib to capecitabine, lapatinib was approved by the FDA in early 2007 for use in combination with capecitabine for the treatment of patients with MBC whose tumors overexpress HER2 and who have received prior therapy including an anthracycline, a taxane, and trastuzumab. In this phase III trial, patients with progressive HER2-positive disease after trastuzumab were randomized to capecitabine versus the combination of capecitabine and lapatinib. At interim analysis, the objective response rate was significantly improved (14% vs. 22%) and TTP nearly doubled (4.4 vs. 8.4 months) by the addition of lapatinib to chemotherapy (see Table 69.5).[167] As noted earlier, based on the results of the subsequent EMILIA study demonstrating superiority of T-DM1 over lapatinib/capecitabine in second line HER2-positive MBC, lapatinib is now more commonly used in highly refractory HER2-amplified disease.

Brain Metastases in HER2-Positive Breast Cancer

One of the greatest challenges faced in the management of HER2-positive MBC is management of CNS metastases. In a study of 319 women with breast cancer, HER2 overexpression was the strongest predictor of the site of first relapse with a 4.3% versus 0.4% incidence of brain metastases.[194] Innumerable trials and case series have reported a high incidence of CNS metastases in women treated with trastuzumab with rates on the order of 30% to 40%.[195,196] This is likely the result of an innate biological propensity for HER2-positive disease to travel to the CNS, as well as the failure, at least partially, of trastuzumab to cross the blood-brain barrier. HER2-directed therapy controls systemic disease in many women, thereby changing the natural history of HER2-positive MBC. The increasing frequency of both CNS metastases and progression after an initial course of radiation has left clinicians in search of new targeted therapies to control CNS disease.

Given their large molecular sizes, the antibody-based therapies trastuzumab, pertuzumab, and T-DM1 are thought to penetrate the intact blood-brain barrier poorly, decreasing their potential activity against CNS disease. Despite steric concerns that likely make direct access to CNS lesions difficult or impossible, clinical evidence suggests that trastuzumab and trastuzumab-based molecules maintain effectiveness even in patients with brain metastases.[197] In a retrospective exploratory analysis of patients with baseline or post-baseline CNS metastases in the EMILIA trial of T-DM1 versus lapatinib/capecitabine, T-DM1 maintained its OS benefit.[198] Additionally, in a follow-up analysis to the CLEOPATRA study, which randomized patients to docetaxel/trastuzumab/pertuzumab or docetaxel/trastuzumab/placebo, the median time to development of CNS metastases as first disease progression site was significantly longer in the pertuzumab-containing arm, although the incidence of CNS metastases did not differ between arms.[199] These data indicate that anti-HER2 antibody agents may improve disease outcomes even in the presence of CNS metastasis. Because the antibodies likely lack significant CNS penetration, improved outcomes could be due to improved extra-CNS control, and hence fewer tumor cells in the systemic circulation with potential to spread to the brain. There is interest in developing novel drug delivery strategies to facilitate access of large molecules, such as antibodies, to the CNS.[197] Direct intrathecal administration of trastuzumab for leptomeningeal carcinomatosis has been attempted in a small subset of cases, with potential indication of some clinical benefit.[200]

By contrast, as a small molecule, lapatinib's ability to cross the blood-brain barrier makes it a promising option for the management of HER2-positive brain metastases. Multiple phase II studies have shown it to have some limited activity in this setting. A National Cancer Institute (NCI)/Cancer Therapy Evaluation Program (CTEP) phase II pilot study of lapatinib monotherapy for brain metastases in HER2-positive MBC demonstrated modest activity, with 1 in 39 (2.6%) patients achieving a partial response and 7 in 39 (18%) patients being progression-free at both CNS and non-CNS sites at 16 weeks.[201] A much larger phase II trial in 242 patients confirmed the single-agent activity of lapatinib in women with recurrent brain metastases from HER2-positive breast cancer. Although no complete responses were

observed, 6% of women had a CNS objective response (50% or greater volumetric reduction), 21% of women had a 20% or greater volumetric reduction in CNS disease, and 53.5% of women were without disease progression at 2 months. The observed volumetric reductions and stabilization of CNS lesions reflect modest single-agent antitumor activity in the CNS with lapatinib alone. In an extension of the same phase II trial, 50 patients with HER2-positive CNS-metastatic disease were treated with lapatinib and capecitabine. In this doublet-treated group, 20% of patients achieved a CNS objective response, and 66.3% of patients were free of disease progression at 2 months.[202]

Finally, the single-arm phase II LANDSCAPE study investigated lapatinib plus capecitabine in patients with HER2-positive MBC and brain metastases not previously treated with whole brain radiation, capecitabine, or lapatinib. On this regimen, 29 of 45 patients (65.9%) achieved objective CNS partial responses; there were no complete responses.[203] Thus the combination of lapatinib plus capecitabine appears to have substantial activity in this difficult metastatic subset. In a phase I trial of lapatinib concurrent with whole brain radiation for patients with HER2-positive breast cancer metastatic to brain, a CNS objective response rate of 79% was seen; however, the combination was deemed infeasible from a toxicity standpoint on the basis of the authors' prespecified criteria. However, this dual-modality approach could be considered in a carefully selected patient population.[204] Overall, lapatinib-based therapy is currently the cornerstone of systemic management in HER2-positive CNS disease, but the identification and drug targeting of mechanisms leading to CNS metastasis is an area of active research[205] in which it is hoped that further progress is forthcoming.

Novel Agents in Metastatic Breast Cancer

Although the armamentarium of drugs active in MBC is large and continues to grow each year, there is an ongoing search for novel agents that may target pathways or mechanisms not affected by currently available cytotoxic chemotherapy, endocrine manipulation, and HER2-directed therapy. Some of the drug classes of greatest interest at this time include PI3K pathway inhibitors (including inhibitors of PIK3CA, AKT, and mTOR), CDK4/6 inhibitors, histone deacetylase (HDAC) inhibitors, poly(ADP ribose) polymerase (PARP) inhibitors, antiandrogen agents, novel HER2-directed tyrosine kinase inhibitors, novel antibody-drug conjugates, and immunotherapy (Table 69.6).[206–214]

Historical Treatments for Metastatic Breast Cancer

Antiangiogenic Therapy

Solid preclinical rationale supports the investigation of angiogenesis inhibitors in oncology. Laboratory evidence has shown a direct correlation between increased microvessel density and/or vascular endothelial growth factor (VEGF) expression, and poor clinical outcome in patients with cancer.[215] Antiangiogenic agents have demonstrated clinical activity in multiple metastatic cancers, most notably non–small cell lung cancer (NSCLC) and colorectal cancer. The best-studied antiangiogenic agent is bevacizumab (Avastin, Genentech, South San Francisco, CA), a humanized monoclonal antibody directed against the most potent proangiogenic factor, VEGF. Early-phase clinical studies in breast cancer

TABLE 69.6 Investigational Agents in Metastatic Breast Cancer

Drug Class	Patient Population of Interest	Example Drugs Under Investigation	Rationale for Use
PARP inhibitors	Triple-negative breast cancer; *BRCA* mutant breast cancer	Olaparib, niraparib, talazoparib	PARP enzymes are critical components of DNA damage repair
Cyclin-dependent kinase (CDK) inhibitors[a]	HER2-positive breast cancer	Palbociclib, abemaciclib, ribociclib	Cyclins regulate cell cycle progression; cyclin D1 is critical component of the HER2 pathway
Phosphoinositide 3-kinase (PI3K) inhibitors	Many	Taselisib, BKM120, BYL719, GDC0941	Activation of the PI3K pathway contributes to cell growth, cell cycle entry, cell survival, and cell motility.
Other PI3K pathway inhibition: mTOR inhibitors,[a] AKT inhibitors	Many	Everolimus, GDC0068	mTOR and AKT are key integrators of growth factor/cytokine signals in the PI3K pathway; they regulate cell growth, proliferation, and survival
Immunotherapy (i.e., checkpoint inhibitors)	Many	Pembrolizumab, MPDL3280A	Immune checkpoint proteins (such as PD-1 and PD-L1) diminish the antitumor immune response, and their inhibition can reconstitute antitumor immunity
ErbB tyrosine kinase inhibitors	HER2-positive breast cancer	Neratinib	Multiple receptor tyrosine kinases in the ERbB family (i.e. EGFR [HER1] and HER2) activate downstream effectors of cell growth
Antiandrogen therapies	Androgen receptor-positive breast cancer	Enzalutamide, bicalutamide	Androgen receptor signaling may regulate tumor growth in breast cancers that do not express ER or PR
Histone deacetylase (HDAC) inhibitors	Many	Entinostat	Modification of histones in the epigenetic environment may reverse resistance to standard therapies
Antibody-drug conjugates	Many	IMMU-132 (antibody: anti-Trop-2; cytotoxic: SN-38)	Antibody-drug conjugation allows targeting of cytotoxic compounds to tumor-specific antigens
p53 family signaling inhibition: WEE1 inhibitors, Chk1/2 inhibitors	Triple-negative breast cancer	AZD1775	p53 and its family members p63 and p73 are key regulators of tumor suppressive signaling pathways; p53 is the most commonly mutated gene in triple-negative breast cancer

ER, Estrogen receptor; *PARP*, poly(ADP ribose) polymerase; *PR*, progesterone receptor.
[a]At least one agent in this drug class is already approved by the US Food and Drug Administration in hormone receptor-positive breast cancer.
Table data from references 206–214.

demonstrated mild activity of bevacizumab in a combination regimen with chemotherapy.[216]

ECOG 2100 was the first large multicenter trial to explore the role of antiangiogenic agents in combination with chemotherapy in the first-line setting for MBC. This trial enrolled 722 patients with previously untreated, locally recurrent or MBC. Patients were treated with weekly paclitaxel either alone or in combination with bevacizumab. The addition of bevacizumab yielded a higher response rate (36.9% vs. 21.2%) as well as a 5.9-month improvement in PFS compared with chemotherapy alone (11.8 vs. 5.9 months, HR 0.60, *p* < .001). Overall survival, however, was not significantly affected by the addition of bevacizumab.[217] On this basis, the FDA granted accelerated approval in 2008 for bevacizumab in combination with paclitaxel in previously untreated, HER2-negative MBC.

However, in the subsequent Avastain and Docetaxel (AVADO) and Regimens in Bevacizumab for Breast Oncology (RIBBON-1) trials, PFS benefits of smaller magnitude (although still of statistical significance) were seen, and again no OS benefit was demonstrated. A meta-analysis of the three trials of first-line bevacizumab plus chemotherapy in MBC also failed to show an OS benefit for the addition of bevacizumab.[218] Given these follow-up data, in 2010 the FDA removed the breast cancer indication from bevacizumab's FDA label.[219] Investigation of receptor tyrosine kinases targeting the VEGF receptor, such as sunitinib and sorafenib, also have not yielded promising results in breast cancer patients.

Despite the revocation of FDA approval for bevacizumab in breast cancer, the potential activity of angiogenic blockade remains exciting, and antiangiogenic targeting has been fruitful in multiple other solid tumors. Therefore there is ongoing preclinical and clinical work evaluating antiangiogenic agents in combination with novel agents in breast cancer, such as immunotherapy. This work may yet yield a role for antiangiogenic therapy in breast cancer patients.

Treatment of Metastatic Bone Disease

More than 100 years ago, it was first noted that the bone and bone marrow microenvironment have unique properties that support the growth of tumor cells. When tumor cells metastasize to the bone, they corrupt normal bone physiology and result in skeletal destruction. This invasion of tumor cells drives the production and activation of osteoclasts, triggers angiogenesis through induction of VEGF expression, and forces osteoblasts to build disorganized woven bone. This bone resorption and production of "defective" bone results in instability, fracture, and pain. A cycle is established in which tumor growth stimulates bone resorption, and bone resorption triggers tumor growth.[220] The model is applicable to many cancers, including MBC, in which bone metastases are noted in up to 75% of patients at autopsy.[221] The mainstays of therapy at this time for the management of metastatic bone disease are second- and third-generation bisphosphonates (pamidronate and zoledronic acid), and denosumab, a receptor activator of NF-κB ligand (RANKL) inhibitor.

According to American Society of Clinical Oncology (ASCO) treatment guidelines, women with evidence of bone destruction should receive treatment with a bone-modifying agent, but women with a positive bone scan and the absence of bone destruction on other imaging (CT or MRI), should not be treated. As long as they meet the criteria defined previously, women who are asymptomatic from their bone disease should still receive treatment because they are likely to derive long-term benefit and palliation.[222]

A number of potential agents are now available for the management of bony metastatic disease. Bisphosphonates of the later generation have an amino group in the R2 side chain that targets the mevalonate pathway and blocks GTPase-mediated signaling. They have a very high affinity for bone's hydroxyapatite mineralized matrix and are incorporated into bone with high local concentrations at sites of active resorption. Once present in the bone, these agents interfere with osteoclast development and survival while promoting the survival of osteocytes.[168] There is also in vitro evidence that bisphosphonates have a direct cytotoxic effect on breast cancer cell lines and can block the growth of bone marrow metastases.[223,224]

Significant clinical evidence supports the use of bisphosphonates in breast cancer patients with bony metastases. A large, prospective placebo-controlled trial compared pamidronate to placebo in women with MBC and documented lytic bone lesions receiving systemic chemotherapy. The risk of osteolytic bone lesion complications was significantly decreased with monthly infusions of pamidronate, and this effect was maintained for at least 2 years. Median time to first skeletal complication was 14 months, compared with 7 months in the placebo arm. No effect on OS was observed.[225] Similar benefits from pamidronate have been observed in women with MBC receiving endocrine therapy.[226] In summary, the addition of pamidronate to standard chemotherapy or endocrine therapy produces a sustained reduction in skeletal complications in breast carcinoma patients with osteolytic bone metastases.[221] Zoledronic acid is a high-potency bisphosphonate that can be administered more quickly than pamidronate. It has also been shown in two large clinical trials to

decrease skeletal events in women with MBC and bone metastases.[227,228] Although effective in the prevention of skeletal-related events, bisphosphonates can cause troublesome side effects such as nephrotoxicity and flulike symptoms and cannot be used safely in patients with very low creatinine clearance.[229]

Denosumab is a fully humanized monoclonal antibody against RANKL, an important mediator of bone remodeling. RANKL regulates the generation, survival, and function of osteoclasts, the main effector cells of bone breakdown. By inhibiting RANKL, denosumab blocks the process of bone breakdown that allows bone metastases to survive and grow.[230] Denosumab has been compared head-to-head with zoledronic acid in a large randomized phase III trial of breast cancer patients. In this trial 2046 patients with breast cancer and at least one bone metastasis were randomized to either denosumab (administered subcutaneously every 4 weeks) or zoledronic acid (administered intravenously every 4 weeks). The primary end point of the study was time to first on-study skeletal-related event, and denosumab was significantly superior to zoledronic acid by this measure, with a hazard ratio of 0.82. Skeletal-related events were defined as pathologic fracture, bone radiation/surgery, or spinal cord compression.[229] Prevention of worsening pain was also improved with denosumab, compared with zoledronic acid.[231] OS and disease progression did not differ significantly between the two groups.[229]

The frequency of adverse events and serious adverse events was similar between the denosumab and zoledronic acid groups. Of 20 specific adverse events that differed significantly between the two groups, only 2 were more common with denosumab: toothache and hypocalcemia. Osteonecrosis of the jaw, the most feared complication of bone-modifying agents, occurred in 2.0% and 1.4% of patients in denosumab and zoledronic acid, respectively. These rates were not statistically different. Osteonecrosis of the jaw is not exclusively related to long-term use of a bone-modifying agent; the earliest occurrence of this complication on trial was within 6 months of randomization.[229] Another advantage of denosumab is that it does not require dose adjustment for renal function because it is not renally excreted, and unlike bisphosphonates, it is not associated with a risk of nephrotoxicity.[229,230] From a convenience standpoint, patients also tend to prefer denosumab because subcutaneous administration is faster than intravenous and does not require intravenous access.

The three main uses for bone-targeting agents in MBC are prevention or delay in bone complications (pathologic fracture, vertebral collapse, spinal cord compression, hypercalcemia, or need for bone-directed radiation or surgery) for women with bone metastases, palliation of bone pain, and direct cytotoxicity. Unfortunately, the prophylactic use of bisphosphonates in women without bone metastases has not been shown to decrease skeletal events or reduce the risk of developing skeletal metastases in multiple clinical trials.[232]

Treatment guidelines from ASCO in 2011 recommend every-3-to-4-week bone-modifying therapy (pamidronate, zoledronic acid, or denosumab) for women with bone metastases but note that there is insufficient evidence to support the use of one particular agent.[233] A recent large randomized noninferiority trial in patients with bone metastases from multiple malignancies (including breast cancer) compared the use of zoledronic acid monthly for 2 years (standard dosing) versus every 3 months for 2 years (experimental dosing). The experimental regimen was found to be noninferior, both in the overall population and in the breast cancer subset (n = 820), suggesting that less frequent dosing may be permissible.[234] A meta-analysis of the same question—monthly dosing versus increased interval dosing—in a breast cancer–specific population, including studies of pamidronate, zoledronic acid, and denosumab, also did not find a significant increase in skeletal-related events with every-3-month dosing.[235]

The optimal treatment duration for maximum benefit from bone-modifying therapy is not known at this time. Patients likely need to receive at least 1 year of therapy to see an improvement in skeletal events; however, some studies suggest that treatment well beyond 2 years is safe and offers meaningful palliation.[236,237] 2011 ASCO guidelines recommend use of bone-modifying agents until there is "substantial decline in a patient's general performance status."[233]

Despite the clear benefit seen with bone-modifying agents, many argue that additional therapies for metastatic bone disease are needed. The available drugs reduce but do not prevent skeletal destruction; as a result, many patients with MBC ultimately do experience skeletal-related events. Novel therapies with synergistic or alternative mechanisms to bisphosphonates and RANKL inhibition may prove helpful to better control bone destruction in MBC.[220]

Special Considerations

Treatment of Metastatic Breast Cancer in the Elderly

Age is a well-established risk factor for the development of breast cancer. Therefore, as the US population continues to age and average life expectancy increases, the number of cases of breast cancer is projected to rise accordingly. It is estimated that by 2040, persons older than 65 years of age will comprise more than 20% of the US population. Therefore this patient population deserves special consideration because patients older than 70 years of age often have comorbidities or a performance status that make treatment with chemotherapy more challenging.

Aging is a heterogeneous process, and thus chronologic age does not always predict physiologic status. There is a growing body of literature to show that elderly women with breast cancer are less likely to receive chemotherapy or to be enrolled in clinical trials, even when patients have an excellent functional status and harbor few comorbidities.[238,239] Kemeny and colleagues found that age itself was a major determinant of whether a clinical trial is offered to a patient with breast cancer, even after controlling for number of comorbidities, physical functioning, and disease stage.[240] This is postulated to be the result of clinician bias based in fear of harming patients with toxic therapies. There is also likely a contribution of "patient and family member bias" emerging from the belief that treatment is not worthwhile or too dangerous.[241] For these reasons, it is critical to highlight the available data on safe and effective treatment of MBC in the elderly so that care may be individualized accordingly. It is also important to note that physiologic age is likely more important than chronologic age as a determinant of how a geriatric patient will tolerate cancer therapy.

Although older women are more likely to present with more advanced disease, the disease biology tends to be less aggressive with a higher rate of endocrine sensitivity, lower proliferative rates, and less HER2 overexpression than is observed in younger patients. For these reasons, breast cancer survival in elderly women is similar to survival in the general population, irrespective of disease status.[242] When a patient is considered for treatment, the primary challenge is to identify patients who appear healthy but are at high risk for excessive chemotherapy-related toxicity, which can be life-threatening. The ideal tool to evaluate this is not established, although it has been suggested that the Comprehensive Geriatric Assessment may be useful to detect frail patients in whom supportive care may be the most appropriate choice.[243] A newer Geriatric Assessment Tool, which incorporates geriatric assessment variables, laboratory values, and patient, tumor, and treatment characteristics, has also demonstrated value for predicting chemotherapy toxicity in cancer patients aged 65 years and older.[244]

Most elderly patients who relapse or are diagnosed with metastatic disease have ER-positive disease, making them good candidates for endocrine therapy. An aromatase inhibitor should generally be considered first in this setting. Other active agents that can safely be used in older women include tamoxifen, fulvestrant (Faslodex, AstraZeneca Pharmaceuticals), and megestrol acetate.[245,246] In general, elderly patients on aromatase inhibitors should have careful monitoring of bone mineral density because these agents are known to accelerate bone loss, although, of note, no monitoring is needed in patients who are simultaneously receiving a bone-modifying agent for bony metastatic disease. Tamoxifen and megestrol acetate have been associated with thromboembolic events and fluid retention, respectively. They should therefore be used with caution in the elderly. Despite theoretical concerns about the use of tamoxifen in the elderly, it is quite safe in most elderly women. A subgroup analysis of elderly women (≥75 years) from the Breast International Group (BIG) 1-98 trial of letrozole versus tamoxifen for 5 years in the adjuvant setting failed to find an increased risk of thromboembolic or adverse cardiac events in the elderly women treated with tamoxifen.[247] As a general rule, similar to other age groups, endocrine therapy should be continued until there is convincing evidence of endocrine independence or until there is disease progression at a pace requiring the initiation of chemotherapy. The use of bisphosphonates for elderly women with lytic bone lesions is believed to be safe even for those in poor health as long as the dose is adjusted for renal function.

The decision to initiate chemotherapy in elderly women is often difficult. Because the goals are palliative, one should try to assess whether the treatment is likely to improve cancer-related symptoms and maintain or improve quality of life. The question of whether to use sequential single-agent or combination chemotherapy at the expense of increased toxicity and minimal or no effect on survival has also been asked in the elderly population. Given the lack of clear evidence that combination therapy prolongs survival and the increased risk of toxicity in this age group, single-agent regimens are generally the most appropriate choice for these patients.

The pharmacokinetics and pharmacodynamics of antineoplastic therapy are known to be altered in the elderly. Obstacles faced in patients receiving oral agents include altered gastrointestinal absorption and poor compliance. Because elderly patients have a greater percentage body fat, the volume of distribution of drugs may be altered, changing peak concentration and prolonging terminal half-life. In addition, altered metabolism by the P450 system may alter pharmacodynamics and increase the risk of drug interactions, particularly those metabolized by the CYP3A4 enzyme (Table 69.7). Finally, renal clearance is often overestimated in the elderly by serum creatinine due to loss of muscle mass. Because the Cockcroft-Gault equation is a less accurate estimates of glomerular filtration rate in the elderly, it has been

<table>
<tr><td colspan="3">

TABLE 69.7 Selected List of Common Inducers, Inhibitors, and Substrates for CYP3A4[a]

</td></tr>
</table>

Substrates	Strong Inhibitors	Inducers
Cyclophosphamide	Azole antifungals	Barbiturates
Docetaxel	Macrolide antibiotics	Carbamazepine
Doxorubicin	Grapefruit juice	St. John's Wort
Etoposide	Ritonavir (protease	Non–nucleoside reverse
Ifosfamide	inhibitor)	transcriptase
Paclitaxel		inhibitor
Tamoxifen		Phenytoin
Vinblastine		Rifampicin

[a]This is a selected list of agents commonly involved in the CYP3A4 pathways; many other agents have been cited in literature.
From http://en.wikipedia.org/wiki/CYP3A4.

suggested that the Wright equation be used instead.[248,249] The bone marrow reserve of older patients is also known to be compromised, further increasing the risk of toxicity in older patients receiving chemotherapy. To avoid adverse events, anemia should be treated promptly, and there should be a low threshold for the use of white blood cell colony–stimulating factors.

Although anthracyclines are generally very active in MBC, historically they were rarely used in the first-line setting for elderly women with MBC. Age is known to be the greatest risk factor for the development of doxorubicin-associated cardiomyopathy with the greatest incidence in patients older than 65 years of age who have received a lifetime dose of greater than 400 mg/m^2.[250] Li and Gwilt have explored the pathophysiology behind this toxicity and found that initial serum concentrations of doxorubicin are higher in the elderly as a result of decreased distribution clearance related to alterations in regional blood flow. These phenomena, in addition to higher rates of coronary artery disease and lower average cardiac reserve, likely explain older patients' predisposition to anthracycline toxicity.[251] However, in a randomized phase III trial of pegylated liposomal doxorubicin (known to have less cardiotoxicity than its nonliposomal counterpart) versus capecitabine as first-line chemotherapy in MBC patients aged 65 years and older, the efficacy and toxicity of the two regimens were not found to be significantly different. Only one grade 3 cardiac toxicity was seen among 40 patients in the pegylated liposomal doxorubicin treatment arm. On the basis of the results of this trial, both regimens were felt to be acceptable first-line options in elderly patients with MBC.[8]

Many other drugs commonly used to treat MBC, including taxanes, capecitabine, vinorelbine, and gemcitabine, have been studied in elderly patients and have been shown to have different response rates and toxicity profiles than are seen in younger patients.[252–254] For example, one study found that a lower dose (1000 mg/m^2 twice daily) of capecitabine yielded equivalent responses to typical dosing and was better tolerated compared with the standard dose (1250 mg/m^2 twice daily) group, in which two toxic deaths (7%) and frequent dose reductions (30%) occurred.[255] It was previously known that capecitabine requires dose reduction in renal dysfunction, but this study uncovered the benefits of lower doses even in elderly with apparently normal renal function. An Italian phase II trial of weekly paclitaxel in women 70 years of age or older with advanced breast cancer found a 15% rate of unacceptable toxicity but also an excellent response rate of 54%, likely because the trial included women with stage

IIIA/B disease. Toxicities reported include febrile neutropenia, severe allergic reaction, and cardiac toxicity, observed in 5 of the 46 patients. This trial supports the efficacy of weekly taxane administration in the elderly but also emphasizes the significant likelihood of life-threatening toxicity when chemotherapy is used at standard doses in this patient population.[256]

Data on the use of trastuzumab in the elderly are relatively limited as a result of poor enrollment of older patients into relevant clinical trials. Because age was an independent risk factor for trastuzumab-associated congestive heart failure in adjuvant treatment trials and older patients have a lower cardiac reserve on average, such patients must be screened carefully before initiation of HER2-directed therapy. In a prospective observational study that included 1014 patients aged 65 years and older with early-stage, nonmetastatic breast cancer treated with trastuzumab-based regimens, elderly patients appeared to have equivalent outcomes to younger age groups. The rates of cardiac adverse events, although numerically somewhat higher in older versus younger patients, were overall low.[257] Additional prospective clinical trials of trastuzumab as well as the newer agents pertuzumab and T-DM1 are underway in the elderly population.

It is postulated that the "fit elderly" can generally tolerate treatment when careful attention is paid to dose adjustment and drug-drug interactions. In contrast, the "frail elderly" may achieve a better quality of life and longer survival with palliative supportive care. "Frail elderly" have been defined as those with an excess decrease in lean body mass, poor mobility, poor tolerance of therapy, and excessive fatigue. Further development of cost-effective and easy-to-use assessment scales to aid clinicians in selecting patients most likely to benefit from antineoplastic therapy[249] will be helpful for optimizing the risk/benefit ratio of chemotherapy in elderly breast cancer patients. Fortunately, multiple dedicated clinical trials are now focused on developing safe and effective treatment strategies for this growing heterogeneous population.

Management of Metastatic Triple-Negative Breast Cancer

Triple-negative breast cancers do not express ER, PR, or overexpress the HER2 protein and are immunohistochemically characterized by staining for basal markers cytokeratin 5/6 and 17. Histologically they tend to be high grade with central necrosis.[258] Microarray expression profiling analyses have demonstrated that breast cancers can be systematically categorized into biologically and clinically distinct subgroups. Triple-negative tumors are mostly but not exclusively categorized as basal-like breast cancers in the "intrinsic" PAM50 classification scheme introduced in 2000 by Perou and colleagues.[259] They are so named because they arise from the outer (basal) layer of the breast duct, the myoepithelial cells.[258] On a molecular level, they demonstrate a high frequency of p53 mutations, deficiencies in homologous recombination DNA repair, and elevated levels of genomic instability.[206]

Clinically, triple-negative tumors represent 15% of all breast cancers and are associated with a poorer prognosis, even after correction for size, stage, grade, and age. After adjuvant therapy, these patients are more likely to experience local recurrence and distant relapse than women with non–basal-like cytokeratin expression. In women who exhibit relapse, the disease-free interval is often brief (<3 years), and the rate of relapse is higher than is seen in ER-positive and/or HER2-positive tumors treated with trastuzumab. Patients with triple-negative MBC are more likely to have visceral metastases and CNS involvement; OS is shorter in this subgroup of women. These cancers are particularly challenging to treat because they are insensitive to endocrine- and HER2-directed therapies, leaving cytotoxic chemotherapy as the only approved option at present.[258]

A cohort study of approximately 1600 Canadian women with breast cancer quantified the prognostic significance of triple-negativity. Of the 1601 patients, 180 (11.2%) had triple-negative breast cancer. At a median follow-up of 8.1 years, women with triple-negative breast cancer had an increased likelihood of distant recurrence (HR 2.6) and death (HR 3.2) within 5 years of diagnosis but not thereafter compared with other women with breast cancer. The pattern of recurrence was also qualitatively different; in the triple-negative group, the risk of distant recurrence peaked at 3 years and declined rapidly thereafter. In the remaining 89% of patients, the recurrence risk seemed to be constant over a longer time period.[260]

The pathogenesis of these highly aggressive lesions is not completely understood, although their epidemiology has been studied. Breast cancers in African American as well as African women and young premenopausal women are more likely to be triple-negative than cancers in the overall population.[206] Results from the Carolina Breast Cancer Study showed that 39% of premenopausal African American women diagnosed with breast cancer had basal-like disease, compared with 14% of postmenopausal African American women and 16% of non–African American women of any age.[261] Triple-negative breast cancers are also considerably increased in frequency among patients with germline BRCA

mutation, comprising 70% of tumors in BRCA1 mutant patients and 20% of tumors in BRCA2 mutant patients.[207]

At this time, there are no specific treatment guidelines for this patient population, and so most patients are treated on the basis of standard algorithms devised from clinical trials in which most women had luminal cancers. Triple-negative tumors tend to be initially more chemosensitive than their hormone-responsive counterparts.[259] Unfortunately, however, the genetic instability seen in triple-negative tumors probably results in an increased potential for the subsequent development of chemoresistance, making their management even more challenging.[262]

The triple-negative tumors, like breast cancer itself, represent a heterogeneous group of cancers with defects in a variety of molecular pathways. At some point in the future, molecular profiling of individual tumors may allow for matching drug mechanism to known targets in a given tumor; however, as of 2017, this strategy has not yet yielded significant clinical utility.[262] As discussed earlier in this chapter, given increasing recognition of the importance of DNA repair defects in many triple-negative tumors, DNA-damaging platinum chemotherapy is a particular focus of investigation in triple-negative breast cancer. In two important trials of metastatic triple-negative disease, platinum agents have shown significant activity in this patient subset.[35,54]

Additionally, early-phase clinical trials are currently examining a wide spectrum of potential targeted agents in advanced triple-negative disease, including inhibitors of PI3K or its downstream effectors AKT and mTOR, androgen receptor antagonists, and DNA damage-inducing PARP inhibitors (Fig. 69.3). Lastly, given

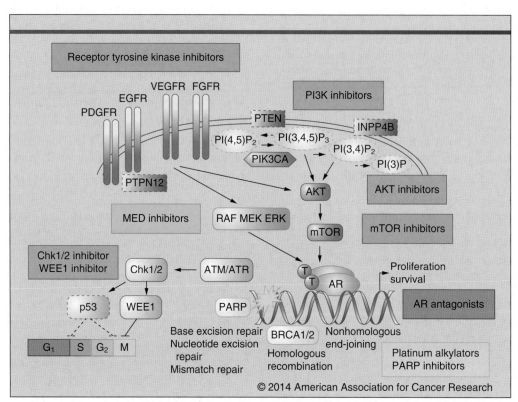

• **Fig. 69.3** Potential therapeutic targets in triple-negative breast cancer. *EGFR,* Epidermal growth factor receptor; *FGFR,* fibroblast growth factor receptor; *mTOR,* mechanistic target of rapamycin; *PARP,* poly(ADP ribose) polymerase; *PDGFR,* platelet-derived growth factor receptor. (From Mayer IA, Abramson VG, Lehmann BD, Pietenpol JA. New strategies for triple-negative breast cancer—deciphering the heterogeneity. *Clin Cancer Res.* 2014;20:782-790. Copyright American Association for Cancer Research.)

the hallmark genomic instability and inadequacy of current therapies for triple-negative MBC, it is the first breast cancer subtype in which immune checkpoint inhibition has been examined. Although no published data exist to date, reports of two phase I trials demonstrated a promising response rate of approximately 20% to immune checkpoint PD-1 or PD-L1 inhibition in refractory triple-negative breast cancer patients with tumor biopsies positive for PD-1 expression.[208,209] Phase III trials of checkpoint blockade in triple-negative disease are now underway. Overall, the median OS of metastatic triple-negative breast cancer remains on the order of 1 year,[35] whereas patients with advanced HER2-positive and hormone receptor–positive disease are seeing increasingly improved outcomes. Therefore there is a great need for rapid identification of effective therapies in the refractory triple-negative patient population.

Management of Metastatic Breast Cancer With Germline *BRCA* Mutations

The BRCA1 and BRCA2 proteins serve essential functions in the process of DNA damage repair by homologous recombination. Accordingly, patients with germline mutations in one allele of either *BRCA* gene are susceptible to tumorigenesis when the second allele is lost or altered in a somatic fashion, causing breakdown of normal DNA repair processes within the cell. As a result, a markedly increased risk of multiple malignancies, most notably breast and ovarian cancer, is clinically apparent in germline *BRCA* mutant patients. This oncogenic molecular mechanism motivated the development of PARP inhibitors for breast cancer patients with germline *BRCA* mutations. PARP family enzymes function in DNA damage repair, particularly base excision repair and single-stranded break repair. By inhibiting these repair pathways, PARP inhibitors render tumor cells that have also lost BRCA protein functionality nonviable, causing cell death due to the accumulation of abnormal, unrepaired DNA.[207]

Consistent with this biological rationale, in early-phase clinical trials multiple different PARP inhibitors have shown activity against refractory metastatic *BRCA* mutant breast cancers. Of note, the efficacy of PARP inhibitors was questioned briefly at one point, when, after a high-profile positive phase II result,[263] the reported PARP inhibitor iniparib failed to demonstrate significant activity in *BRCA* mutant breast cancers in a randomized phase III trial.[264] However, it was subsequently shown that iniparib lacked function as a PARP inhibitor, explaining its failure to produce clinical results in the definitive trial.

After this setback for the drug class, the development of true PARP inhibitors has resumed with success. The PARP inhibitor olaparib (Lynparza, AstraZeneca Pharmaceuticals, London, United Kingdom) produced tumor responses as a single agent in multiple refractory metastatic *BRCA* mutant cancers, including ovarian, breast, lung, pancreas, and prostate. Of breast cancer patients treated, 8 of 62 (12.9%) had a tumor response, and 47% had stable disease at 8 or more weeks.[265] Three randomized phase III trials of three different PARP inhibitor monotherapies (vs. physician's choice chemotherapy) are currently underway in germline *BRCA* mutant patients with MBC. If positive, an FDA label will be sought for this indication.[207]

Extending the observed efficacy of the DNA-damaging PARP inhibitors in *BRCA* mutant breast cancer, the activity of similarly DNA-damaging platinum chemotherapy has also been specifically examined in this patient subset. Platinum agents damage DNA via interstrand cross-linking, theoretically generating particular platinum sensitivity in DNA damage-deficient *BRCA* mutant cancer cells. Two recent studies have provided clinical support for this theory in *BRCA* mutant MBC patients. In a phase II single-arm trial of platinum for the first- or second-line treatment of triple-negative MBC, objective response rate was 54.5% in patients with germline BRCA mutations (n = 11).[35] In the phase III TNT trial, patients with *BRCA* mutations (n = 43) demonstrated a 68.0% objective response rate to carboplatin versus 33.3% to docetaxel, which was a highly significant difference. This difference was not observed among *BRCA* nonmutant patients.[59]

Given the sensitivity to DNA-targeting therapies in patients with germline BRCA mutation, there is growing effort to identify signatures of "BRCAness" that could predict this sensitivity in nonmutant patients.

Monitoring Response to Therapy

Patients undergoing treatment for MBC should be seen on a regular basis commensurate with the pace of disease, degree of symptoms, strength of support network, and degree of involvement from other physicians. Follow-up visits can be used to assess for progression of disease, response to therapy, and treatment-related toxicity. The tools used to evaluate response to therapy in MBC include serial physical examination, review of symptoms, laboratory studies, and radiographic imaging. The interval with which to repeat scans is patient dependent. Early in the course of disease, when the pace of progression is unclear, more frequent assessment is often warranted. In an asymptomatic patient with minimal visceral disease, it may be reasonable to reassess after three to four cycles of chemotherapy or every 3 to 6 months during endocrine therapy. It should be emphasized that repeating scans too early may fail to detect treatment response and inappropriately dismiss an active drug, especially in patients receiving endocrine therapy. By contrast, patients with new symptoms, clinical indicators of progressive disease, or those enrolled in clinical trials typically require more frequent imaging. Standardized guidelines for radiographic monitoring of patients with MBC are not established, and so the follow-up plan should be individualized for each patient. Given the limitations of these conventional measures, novel approaches to following disease progression and response have been proposed and include tumor markers, measurement of circulating tumor cells, and measurement of circulating cell-free tumor DNA.

Although tumor markers have not been shown to be helpful in surveillance after adjuvant therapy, they may be useful in the metastatic setting. Serum tumor markers, most notably CA 15.3 and CA 27.29, both products of the *MUC-1* gene, are elevated in many patients with MBC. If they are elevated initially, serial measurement may aid in evaluating response to therapy, particularly when other modalities such as CT are not helpful. These two markers correlate well with clinical disease course in 60% to 70% of patients. CEA, although elevated at a lower frequency and less specific for MBC, can be useful in a patient in whom *MUC-1* gene products are not elevated. At present, there are few data on the use of these serum markers, and so they should be interpreted in the context of other clinical and radiographic findings. Caution should be exercised in the interpretation of tumor marker values because spurious elevations can be seen in the first few months after treatment initiation ("marker flare") in up to 20% of patients and in patients with impaired hepatic function due to decreased clearance of these serum proteins.[266] Although it has been proposed that their use could lower medical expenditures by decreasing the need for radiographic imaging,[267] at present, their use does not supplant standard follow-up measures such as CT, physical examination, and laboratory studies.[268]

In more recent years, assessment of both circulating tumor cells and cell-free tumor DNA has gained attention as a potential tool for monitoring treatment response, with improved sensitivity and specificity over older methods. Circulating tumor cells (CTCs) are rare tumor cells found in the peripheral blood.[269] In a prospective study that measured serial circulating tumor cells in patients beginning a new line of therapy for MBC, the number of circulating tumor cells at the time of treatment initiation was found to be an independent predictor of prognosis. Patients with levels of five CTCs per 7.5 mL or more had a shorter median progression-free survival (2.7 vs. 7 months) and shorter OS (10.1 vs. longer than 18 months). In addition, continued elevation of CTCs at first interval follow-up after initiation of first-line therapy was closely associated with treatment failure.[270,271] A number of platforms, most notably the FDA-approved CellSearch system (Veridex, Warren, NJ), which identifies CTCs based on surface expression of the epithelial cell adhesion molecule (EpCAM), are available for the detection and quantification of circulating tumor cells in breast cancer patients. Clinical data suggest that levels of CTCs can be helpful for predicting patient outcome[269]; however, evidence has not yet been compelling enough to bring CTCs into standard clinical practice.

More recently, there has been increasing interest in using cell-free DNA as a treatment-monitoring tool for breast cancer of all stages, particularly metastatic disease. Cell-free DNA is nucleic acid derived from tumors and found circulating in small amounts in the blood, with many theoretical advantages over circulating tumor cells. It can be used as an indicator of somatic mutations in the tumor as they evolve over time, offering a potential window into mechanisms of treatment resistance.[269] For example, it has been used to detect the presence of mutations in genes such as *PIK3CA, TP53,* and *ESR1* in MBC patients.[272,273] Furthermore, it offers a noninvasive way to capture the genomic heterogeneity of multiple different sites of metastatic disease.[269] Compared with circulating tumor cells, cell-free DNA has shown improved sensitivity, greater dynamic range, and better correlation with tumor burden.[272] There is great interest in the further development of cell-free DNA as a widespread clinical tool for selecting treatments and after responses in MBC, without the need for serial biopsies. Although not yet adopted into clinical practice, so-called blood biopsies are now being incorporated into many clinical research efforts in breast cancer and may come to inform clinical decision-making.

Future of Systemic Therapy for Metastatic Breast Cancer

Although recent years have seen significant and rapid progress in the treatment of metastatic breast cancer, in 2017 this remains an incurable disease. Particularly important developments of the past 5 years include the introduction of two new, highly effective anti-HER2 therapies, pertuzumab and T-DM1, and the recognition that combination trastuzumab/pertuzumab as first-line therapy prolongs median OS by more than a year in patients with HER2-positive MBC. A new appreciation of the activity of platinum agents in triple-negative disease, and particularly in *BRCA* mutant patients, has been quite influential as well. Although important breakthroughs have been made in targeted therapy for MBC, with promising agents such as PI3K inhibitors, PARP inhibitors, and antiandrogen agents currently in later phase clinical trials, a curative role for single-agent targeted therapies remains elusive in advanced disease because the development of resistance is nearly ubiquitous.

Going forward, massive progress in the field of high-throughput sequencing technologies should be harnessed to improve our understanding of the mechanisms of response and resistance to therapy. The development of sensitive, specific biomarkers of both prognosis and treatment response will facilitate the design of novel therapies and allow smarter deployment of the many effective therapies already available. Thoughtful combinatorial treatment strategies will be essential to eliminate or prolong time until the development of treatment resistance. Lastly, the promise of immunotherapy, which has recently met with great success in a subset of melanoma, lung cancer, and renal cell cancer patients, is an exciting frontier in breast oncology. Ultimately, the success of new therapies in MBC will require a highly collaborative relationship between basic and clinical researchers to build a fast and efficient pipeline toward progress for the many patients living with MBC.

Although the main focus of this chapter has been on cancer-directed therapies for advanced breast cancer, it is also crucial for all clinicians to recognize the paramount importance of symptom management in this patient population. Many breast cancer patients will live for multiple years after a diagnosis of metastatic disease, and although cancer-related symptoms are common, toxicities of therapy are often uncomfortable as well. Therefore quality of life must be prioritized alongside quantity of life. An optimal patient-centered care approach will combine innovative thinking about therapeutic options with close attention to each patient's physical and emotional well-being.

Selected References

59. Tutt A, Ellis P, Kilburn L, et al. TNT: A randomized phase III trial of carboplatin (C) compared with docetaxel (D) for patients with metastatic or recurrent locally advanced triple negative or BRCA1/2 breast cancer. Presented at the San Antonio Breast Cancer Symposium 2014; abstract S3-01.

112. Rugo HS, Barry WT, Moreno-Aspitia A, et al. Randomized Phase III Trial of Paclitaxel Once Per Week Compared With Nanoparticle Albumin-Bound Nab-Paclitaxel Once Per Week or Ixabepilone With Bevacizumab As First-Line Chemotherapy for Locally Recurrent or Metastatic Breast Cancer: CALGB 40502/NCCTG N063H (Alliance). *J Clin Oncol.* 2015;33:2361-2369.

138. Cortes J, O'Shaughnessy J, Loesch D, et al. Eribulin monotherapy versus treatment of physician's choice in patients with metastatic breast cancer (EMBRACE): a phase 3 open-label randomised study. *Lancet.* 2011;377:914-923.

156. Swain SM, Baselga J, Kim SB, et al. Pertuzumab, trastuzumab, and docetaxel in HER2-positive metastatic breast cancer. *New Engl J Med.* 2015;372:724-734.

158. Verma S, Miles D, Gianni L, et al. Trastuzumab emtansine for HER2-positive advanced breast cancer. *New Engl J Med.* 2012;367:1783-1791.

A full reference list is available online at ExpertConsult.com.

70

Endocrine Therapy for Breast Cancer

KARI B. WISINSKI, AMYE J. TEVAARWERK, AND RUTH M. O'REGAN

History of Endocrine Therapy in Breast Cancer

Linking the Course of Advanced Breast Cancer to Female Reproductive Organs

In 1836, Sir Astley Cooper made one of the earliest known observations suggesting a role for endocrine therapy in treatment of breast cancer. He observed that advanced breast cancer appeared to wax and wane during the course of a woman's menstrual cycle.[1] In 1889, Schinzinger proposed making younger women "older" by removing their ovaries, noting that younger women with breast cancer had more aggressive disease than older women.[2] In 1895, Beatson extended this rationale into the arena of treatment by performing a bilateral oophorectomy for a woman who had developed recurrent breast cancer involving the chest wall 6 months after mastectomy. He reported that her chest wall disease resolved within 8 months of the bilateral oophorectomy and the patient remained disease free for 4 years.[3] Boyd subsequently reported a series of 54 patients who underwent bilateral oophorectomy as treatment for advanced breast cancer. Approximately one-third of patients had tumor regression and improved overall survival.[4] This ushered in an era of oophorectomy for the treatment of advanced breast cancer, although oophorectomy was eventually replaced by ovarian ablation techniques such as irradiation.[5]

Recognizing Hormone Dependency for Certain Human Tumors

Huggins and Bergenstal reported the beneficial effects of orchiectomy in men with prostate cancer, and subsequently, Huggins and Hodges showed that the effect of orchiectomy was mediated by reducing testosterone levels.[6,7] Block and associates contributed by demonstrating that the basal level of estrogen production was not reached for several months after ovarian radiation, correlating with the fact that breast cancers often did not regress until several months after ovarian radiation.[8] When synthetic corticosteroids became available in the early 1950s, bilateral surgical adrenalectomy also became feasible as a means of removing other sources of steroid hormones. In an early report by Huggins and Bergenstal, three of six patients with advanced breast cancer appeared to benefit from bilateral adrenalectomy.[9] Other investigators subsequently demonstrated objective response rates of 30% to 40% in advanced breast cancer patients after bilateral adrenalectomy.

Understanding Estrogen Action and Developing Antiestrogens

Modern drug development originated with the pioneering studies of Dodds, Lawson, and Noble in the 1930s and their discovery of the nonsteroidal estrogen diethylstilbestrol (DES).[10] In 1944, Haddow observed that women with advanced breast cancer responded to high-dose estrogen.[11] The women who responded tended to be older, but it was unclear why only some women responded to endocrine therapy. Similarly, responses to bilateral adrenalectomy had been noted to occur in premenopausal women, who had previously responded to oophorectomy.[12,13] Manipulation of female hormone levels was clearly unsuccessful in certain populations, but insight into the mechanism was lacking.

This clinical observation was correlated with mechanism when Jensen and Jacobson observed that radiolabeled estradiol localized to estrogen target tissues such as the uterus, vagina, and pituitary gland.[14] They proposed that a receptor must be present in these tissues to regulate response to estradiol. The estrogen receptor (ER) was subsequently identified. ER assays were then developed to predict which breast cancer patients would respond to endocrine therapy.[15,16] The response rate to endocrine therapy was 30% to 40% in unselected patients, compared with 60% or more in women with a positive ER assay.[15,17]

In 1958 Lerner, Holthaus, and Thompson reported the biological properties of the first nonsteroidal antiestrogen, MER-25.[18] The compound was found to be an antiestrogen in all species tested. MER-25 was initially studied as a contraceptive in laboratory animals. Unfortunately, the large doses needed for MER-25 to work were associated with unacceptable central nervous system side effects. A successor compound, MRL-41, or clomiphene, was a more potent antiestrogen and an effective antifertility drug in animals, although it paradoxically induced ovulation in subfertile women.[19] Clomiphene demonstrated modest activity in the treatment of advanced breast cancer, but further development stopped after the introduction of tamoxifen.[20]

The Modern Era of Endocrine Therapy

Similar to clomiphene, Harper and Walpole demonstrated that tamoxifen, a selective estrogen receptor modulator (SERM), had antiestrogenic and antifertility properties.[21] Tamoxifen was evaluated in a number of clinical scenarios, including as a contraceptive.[22] The first successful use of tamoxifen in treating advanced breast cancer was reported in 1971, with 10 of 46 patients (22%) demonstrating responses to therapy.[23] The response rates were similar to those with DES; however, side effects were significantly less with tamoxifen. Thus tamoxifen became the endocrine therapy of choice for advanced breast cancer in the 1970s. In 1986, tamoxifen was approved for adjuvant treatment of postmenopausal women with node-positive breast cancer. In 1990 tamoxifen was approved as an adjuvant treatment for pre- and postmenopausal women with node-negative disease.[24]

General Strategies for Targeting the Hormonal Axis

Hormone Assays

Approximately two-thirds of breast cancers express female hormone receptors (HR): either ER or progesterone receptor (PR), or both ER and PR. The decision to choose one endocrine therapy over another must take into consideration the comparative efficacy, ease of administration, and toxicity of therapy, as well as the menopausal status of the patient. There are multiple techniques available for determining the ER and PR status of tumors. The ER can be measured by a ligand-binding method after isolation from tumor sample.[25] This method has multiple shortcomings, including expense, requirement of fresh frozen tissue, and use of radioactive reagents. The development of monoclonal antibodies to specific to ER and PR and immunohistochemistry (IHC) techniques provided an alternative means of determining ER/PR status.[26] IHC is currently the most commonly used technique for assessing ER and PR status and overcomes many of the problems associated with ligand binding assays. One of the challenges of IHC is that the results are subjective and do not adequately quantitate the level of ER or PR expression. Newer techniques, such as reverse transcriptase polymerase chain reaction (PCR), tissue microarrays, and nanotechnology, are being investigated as alternatives to IHC, with improved quantitation of ER and PR levels.[27,28]

Predictive Power of ER/PR Status

The HR status of a tumor determines the likelihood that a patient will respond to endocrine therapy: 75% to 80% of patients with tumors positive for both ER and PR will respond to an initial endocrine therapy.[29] The response rates to endocrine therapy are lower for ER-positive/PR-negative tumors and ER-negative/PR-positive tumors at 25% to 30% and 40% to 45%, respectively.[29,30] However, patients with very low levels of ER and/or PR expression may still benefit from endocrine therapy.[31] Such findings led to the current American Society of Clinical Oncology (ASCO) guidelines that even patients with very low levels of ER or PR expression (≥1%) be recommended to receive endocrine therapy.[32] Patients whose tumors do not express either ER or PR at all typically do not benefit from endocrine therapy, although there is always a concern about false negativity of the assays especially when evaluating ER and PR status from a bone biopsy.[33]

The likelihood of expressing ER and/or PR increases with age and postmenopausal status. However, several other clinical factors other than menopausal status can be used to predict response to endocrine therapy. Patients with prolonged disease-free intervals after their initial diagnosis are more likely to remain HR positive. Additionally, patients with metastatic disease in soft tissue or bone, but not in visceral or central nervous system sites, are more likely to respond to endocrine therapy.[34]

Key Therapeutic Agents

As Table 70.1 demonstrates, there are now multiple drugs to prevent the development of breast cancer as well as to prevent and treat breast cancer recurrence. For a few decades, tamoxifen was considered the standard of care for first-line endocrine therapy for all women with metastatic breast cancer and was the only therapy in the adjuvant setting. This changed with the development of aromatase inhibitors (AIs). AIs prevent the peripheral conversion of androstenedione into estrogen, resulting in decreased levels of circulating estrogen.[35,36] AIs are not effective in the management of premenopausal breast cancer patients (in whom the ovaries are the main source of estrogen) although they are used in premenopausal women for fertility purposes.[37] Early nonselective AIs, such as aminoglutethimide, were poorly tolerated by patients and replaced by newer AIs developed in the 1990s. The selective AIs (anastrozole, letrozole, and exemestane) have proved to be active drugs for postmenopausal women with hormone-sensitive breast cancer.[38]

Selective Estrogen Receptor Modulators

Tamoxifen

Efficacy. Tamoxifen is currently US Food and Drug Administration (FDA)-approved for the treatment of all stages of hormone-responsive (aka HR-positive) breast cancer and for the prevention of breast cancer in high-risk women. As noted earlier, the efficacy of tamoxifen proved to be equivalent to that of androgens or high-dose estrogens such as DES in postmenopausal women, but the side effects of tamoxifen were mild in comparison. The efficacy of tamoxifen in both premenopausal and postmenopausal women has been demonstrated in multiple clinical trials.[23,39–43] Clinical benefit (defined as complete response plus partial response plus stable disease) is observed in 50% to 60% of HR-positive cancers. Duration of response ranges from 12 to 18 months, although select women may benefit for longer. For premenopausal women, tamoxifen is the first-line treatment of choice for hormone-sensitive advanced disease (see discussion later in the chapter on ovarian function suppression).

Side Effects. Tamoxifen has antiestrogenic effects on some tissues including the breast and has partial estrogenic effects elsewhere in the body. This complex mechanism of action results in side effects of treatment both beneficial and detrimental. In postmenopausal women treated with tamoxifen, clinical studies have shown an increase in trabecular bone density and a trend toward decreased loss of cortical bone density.[44,45] The National Surgical Adjuvant Breast and Bowel Project (NSABP) P-1 chemoprevention trial demonstrated fewer osteoporotic fracture events in women who received 5 years of tamoxifen compared with placebo; however, the results did not reach statistical significance. This reduction is mainly limited to postmenopausal women.[46]

Tamoxifen has been shown to have beneficial effects on the lipid profile. In adjuvant breast cancer trials, tamoxifen significantly lowers total cholesterol, mainly due to its effect on low-density lipoprotein (LDL) cholesterol.[47] Tamoxifen also lowers fibrinogen, lipoprotein(a), and homocysteine, all factors that contribute to cardiovascular risk.[48–50] However, until recently, no trial had demonstrated a reduction in cardiac events in patients taking tamoxifen. Extended follow-up of the Swedish tamoxifen adjuvant trial demonstrated reduced mortality from coronary heart disease in patients receiving 5 years of adjuvant tamoxifen, compared with those receiving 2 years of treatment.[51]

TABLE 70.1 **Endocrine Therapies Used to Prevent or Treat Breast Cancer**

Drug	Class	Menstrual Status Studied	Breast Cancer–Related FDA Indication(s)	Key Side Effects
Tamoxifen	SERM	Pre Post	Treatment of stage 0–4 HR+ breast cancer Prevention of breast cancer	Increased bone density Improved lipid profile Increased risk of endometrial dysplasia and cancer Increased risk of thromboembolism
Raloxifene		Post	Breast cancer prevention	Increased bone density Increased risk of thromboembolism
Toremifene		Post	First-line treatment of HR+ MBC	Not significantly different from tamoxifen
Anastrozole	AI	Post	First-line treatment of locally advanced or metastatic breast cancer (HR+ or unknown) Treatment of advanced breast cancer after disease progression on tamoxifen Adjuvant treatment of HR+ breast cancer	Decreased bone density Arthralgias Myalgias Vaginal atrophy Worsening of lipid profile Potential increased risk of cardiovascular disease[85]
Exemestane			Treatment of advanced breast cancer after progression on tamoxifen Treatment ER+ early breast cancer after 2–3 y of tamoxifen (for a total of 5 y)	
Letrozole			Adjuvant treatment of HR+ early breast cancer Extended adjuvant treatment of early breast cancer after 5 years of tamoxifen Treatment of advanced breast cancer after progression on antiestrogen therapy First- or second-line treatment of HR+ locally advanced or metastatic breast cancer	
Fulvestrant	SERD	Post	Treatment of advanced HR+ breast cancer after progression on antiestrogen therapy	Abnormal liver enzymes
Estradiol	Estrogen		Metastatic breast cancer, palliative treatment	Increased risk of endometrial dysplasia and cancer Hypercalcemia Increased risk of thromboembolism
Fluoxymesterone	Androgen		Metastatic breast cancer, palliative treatment:	Virilization Edema Abnormal liver enzymes
Megestrol acetate	Progesterone		Metastatic breast cancer, palliative treatment	Hypertension Adrenal insufficiency Increased risk of thromboembolism

AI, Aromatase inhibitor; *ER,* estrogen receptor; *HR+,* hormone-receptor positive; *MBC,* metastatic breast cancer; *SERD,* selective estrogen receptor downregulator; *SERM,* selective estrogen receptor modulator.

Tamoxifen has been associated with an increased incidence of endometrial carcinoma.[46,52] The relative risk of endometrial cancer in the tamoxifen-treated women from the NSABP P-1 prevention trial was 2.5. The increased risk was predominantly seen in women over age 50 in whom the relative risk was 4. All the endometrial cancers seen in the tamoxifen-treated women were International Federation of Gynecology and Obstetrics (FIGO) stage I. The tumors were of good prognosis, and none of the women treated with tamoxifen died from endometrial cancer. There was also an increased incidence of deep venous thrombosis in the tamoxifen-treated women in the NSABP P-1 trial. The relative risk of pulmonary embolism in the tamoxifen group was 3.0.[46]

Metabolism. The cytochrome P450 enzyme CYP2D6 catalyzes the formation of endoxifen and low to absent CYP2D6 activity due to common genetic variation significantly lowers the plasma concentration of endoxifen.[53] Goetz and coworkers first reported an association between endoxifen levels and benefit from tamoxifen by demonstrating that the presence of the CYP2D6*4 variant allele was an independent predictor of breast cancer relapse in postmenopausal women. They also showed that women with the variant allele had a lower incidence of hot flashes while taking tamoxifen.[54] Two additional studies of CYP2D6 and tamoxifen response had shown contradictory results, although differences in study populations made comparisons difficult.[55,56] The routine use of CYP2D6 testing to predict tamoxifen benefit is not currently recommended.[32]

Raloxifene

Efficacy. Raloxifene or keoxifene is another SERM that was initially developed as a treatment for breast cancer. Raloxifene has a shorter half-life than tamoxifen and has less estrogenic effects on the endometrium in preclinical models. Raloxifene was evaluated in patients with tamoxifen-refractory metastatic breast cancer.[57] There were no partial or complete responders, with only one patient achieving a minor response, indicating significant cross-resistance between raloxifene and tamoxifen. Another study evaluated a high-dose schedule of raloxifene at 150 mg twice daily as first-line therapy for HR-positive metastatic breast cancer.[58] The response rate was less than 20%, lower than what would be expected in this first-line setting. On the basis of these results, further development of raloxifene as a treatment for breast cancer was discontinued.

The Study of Tamoxifen and Raloxifene (STAR) trial was designed as a follow-up prevention trial to the NSABP P-1 trial. Postmenopausal women (n = 19747) who were considered high risk for developing breast cancer based on the Gail model were randomized to receive 5 years of tamoxifen or raloxifene. The rate of invasive breast cancers was not significantly different between the two treatment groups and was lower than what would have been expected in this population without treatment. Interestingly, there were fewer noninvasive cancers in the raloxifene-treated patients compared with the patients who received tamoxifen. The reason for this difference in noninvasive cancers is unclear but suggests the intriguing possibility that raloxifene is not preventing breast cancers but rather treating occult breast cancer. This theory was initially put forth to explain the results noted in the NSABP P-1 trial with tamoxifen. However, the sustained decrease in breast cancers noted with longer follow-up,[59] and the fact that tamoxifen was also noted to decrease benign breast lesions[60] places this theory into question. On the basis of the results of the STAR trial, raloxifene was approved as a chemopreventive in postmenopausal women at high risk of developing breast cancer. However, the fact that raloxifene has been developed in postmenopausal women only limits its use as a chemopreventive, given the rise of AIs as chemopreventives.[61,62]

Side Effects. In the STAR trial,[63] the rate of endometrial cancer was lower in patients treated with raloxifene compared with tamoxifen. The fact that this difference did not quite reach statistical significance may be partly explained by the fact that approximately 50% of women on the STAR study had hysterectomies before study entry. The Multiple Outcomes of Raloxifene Evaluation study randomized almost 8000 women with osteoporosis to placebo or one of two doses of raloxifene[64] and showed no increase in the rate of endometrial cancer in patients treated with raloxifene. Raloxifene was associated with a significantly reduced incidence of thromboembolic effects compared with tamoxifen, although there was no difference in the rate of cerebrovascular accidents. The rate of osteoporotic fractures was similar between the two groups.

In summary, raloxifene is currently approved for the prevention and treatment of osteoporosis and for the prevention of breast cancer in postmenopausal women. Raloxifene should not be used as an alternative to tamoxifen in patients with invasive breast cancer or ductal carcinoma in situ (DCIS) because there is currently no data at present to support its use in these settings. Additionally, raloxifene has not been evaluated in premenopausal women and should not be used as a chemopreventive in these women.

Toremifene

Efficacy. Toremifene is a chlorinated derivative of tamoxifen that is currently approved in the United States as an alternative to tamoxifen in the first-line treatment of hormone-responsive metastatic breast cancer. Toremifene was noted to have minimal activity in tamoxifen-refractory metastatic breast cancer,[65] indicating almost complete cross-resistance between the two SERMs. Five trials have compared toremifene at various doses with tamoxifen in the first-line treatment of hormone-receptor positive metastatic breast cancer. A meta-analysis of these trials[66] demonstrated equal efficacy and toxicity between the two SERMs. Toremifene is a reasonable alternative to tamoxifen in this setting. Of note, toremifene, unlike tamoxifen, has not been evaluated in premenopausal patients. Therefore, although toremifene can be considered a reasonable alternative to tamoxifen in postmenopausal patients with metastatic breast cancer, the widespread use of AIs in this group of patients limits its clinical importance.

Toremifene has been compared with tamoxifen as adjuvant therapy in patients with early-stage breast cancer.[67] Postmenopausal patients (n = 1480) with node-positive early-stage breast cancer were randomized between tamoxifen 20 mg and toremifene 40 mg daily for 3 years. At a follow-up of just over 3 years, the rate of recurrence was similar between patients treated with the two agents, 23% and 26% for patients treated with toremifene and tamoxifen, respectively (p = .31).

Side Effects. There was no significant difference in the side effects associated with either treatment, including the incidence of endometrial cancer.

Other Selective Estrogen Receptor Modulators

Other SERMs are in clinical use, such as ospemifene (Osphena), which is approved for women experiencing moderate to severe dyspareunia due to menopause. However, none of the SERMs in clinical practice or development appear to offer a significant advantage over tamoxifen in the treatment of breast cancer, with the possible exception of endoxifen, which is still being studied.

Aromatase Inhibitors

The primary source of serum estrogens in postmenopausal women is circulating androgens,[68] mainly in the adrenals but with a small contribution from the postmenopausal ovaries.[69,70] These androgens (mainly androstenedione) are converted into estrone, followed by reduction to estradiol (aromatization of circulating testosterone into estradiol contributes to a lesser degree). By preventing the conversion of androgens to estrogens via inhibition of the enzyme responsible, AIs lower serum estrogen levels. Over time, a series of AIs have been developed and studied. Fadrozole, formestane, aminoglutethimide, and vorozole were all studied and used to treat advanced breast cancer but are no longer clinically available. As a result, this section focuses on anastrozole, letrozole, and exemestane, which are currently available and in use. Initial studies conducted to evaluate the efficacy of third-generation AIs in patients with metastatic disease in the second-line setting compared these agents to megestrol acetate.

Steroidal Versus Nonsteroidal Aromatase Inhibitors

Anastrozole and letrozole are oral, substrate analogs of androstenedione, the normal substrate of the aromatase enzyme, and reversibly inhibits the enzyme.[71,72] Exemestane is an oral, irreversible steroidal inhibitor of the aromatase enzyme.[73] All three selective third-generation AIs potently inhibit aromatase activity and thus significantly reduce serum estrogen levels, although letrozole appears to be the most effective at reducing estrogen levels.[74] However, the clinically significant threshold for estrogen reduction is unknown. A consequence of aromatase inhibition can be an increase in serum androgen levels.[75]

Early Aromatase Inhibitor Trials

Buzdar and associates reported the results of two parallel, multicenter trials involving 764 women with metastatic, hormone-responsive breast cancer who had progressed after treatment with tamoxifen. Two doses of anastrozole, 1 mg and 10 mg daily, were evaluated compared with megestrol acetate (40 mg four times daily). At a median follow-up of 31.2 months, overall survival was significantly improved with anastrozole (1 mg: 26.7 months; 10 mg: 25.5 months vs. 22.5 months). This difference was statistically significant for the 1-mg dose of anastrozole. The improvement in survival was particularly interesting because there was no difference in response rates or time to progression between the AI and megestrol at either dose of anastrozole. Dyspnea, hypertension, weight gain, and vaginal bleeding were among the major side effects that were at least two times more common with megestrol acetate.[76] Subsequent trials with exemestane[77] and letrozole[78,79] versus megestrol demonstrated relatively similar results: improved efficacy and less toxicity.

A pooled analysis of the trials using second- and third-generation AIs in comparison with megestrol acetate after tamoxifen failure was conducted to determine whether there was a difference in efficacy between the two types of endocrine therapy. In this analysis, there was no significant difference in overall outcomes, and the efficacy was determined to be equivalent. However, there were notably more side effects experienced by patients treated with megestrol acetate, particularly increased weight gain, dyspnea, and peripheral edema.[80]

Aromatase Inhibitors Side Effects

Overall these agents are well tolerated. In general, there is little difference in the side effect profiles between AIs, although individual-level variations clearly exist in side effects experienced on one AI versus another. In clinical trials, the major side effects reported were hot flashes, musculoskeletal pain, vaginal dryness, and headache. AIs do not carry the association with thromboembolic disease seen with tamoxifen, as studies involving patients without a cancer diagnosis comparing AIs with placebo showed no increase in events.[81] Additional potential long-term side effects include bone loss and effects on lipid profiles.

The ATAC (Arimidex, Tamoxifen Alone or in Combination) trial[82] analysis also found the incidence of musculoskeletal disorders was significantly higher in the anastrozole-treated patients (35.6% vs. 29.4%, $p < .0001$). Conversely, the risk of endometrial cancer ($p = .007$), venous thromboembolic disease ($p = .0004$), vaginal bleeding or discharge, and hot flashes ($p < .001$ for all three) was lower in patients treated with anastrozole than tamoxifen. A bone substudy was conducted within the ATAC population.[83] This substudy found the mean decrease in bone mineral density (BMD) for women treated with anastrozole was 6.08% in the lumbar spine and 7.24% in the total hip. Women treated with tamoxifen, conversely, had a median gain in BMD of 2.77% in the lumbar spine and 0.74% in the total hip. Notably, among the patients with normal BMD at baseline, there were no cases of osteoporosis.

The rate of fractures seen in the BIG 1-98 trial was also significantly increased in women treated with letrozole compared with tamoxifen-treated patients (5.7% vs. 4%; $p < .001$). In the MA.17 companion study to evaluate the effect of letrozole on bone mineral density, 226 patients (122 letrozole and 104 placebo) were enrolled and prospectively evaluated for baseline BMD and changes in BMD over time. At 24 months, patients had significantly increased BMD loss in the total hip (3.6% vs. 0.71%; $p = .044$) and in the lumbar spine (5.35% vs. 0.70%; $p = .008$) compared with those receiving placebo.[84]

Adverse effects on lipid profiles have been suggested in some studies, but a clinically significant increase in risk of cardiovascular disease has not been seen in the major studies of AIs, although a meta-analysis suggests that there may be a small but statistically significant increase in cardiovascular events.[85] A study evaluated the effect of short-term therapy with 16 weeks of letrozole on plasma lipid profiles. This study did find a statistically significant increase in total cholesterol and LDL as well as unfavorable changes in the total cholesterol/HDL and LDL/HDL ratios.[86] Another study of patients treated with exemestane or placebo found a significant decrease of 6% to 9% ($p < .001$) in HDL levels and a 5% to 6% ($p = .004$) decrease apolipoprotein A1 levels. A slight increase in serum homocysteine levels was also noted. All of these changes were reversed within a year of withdrawing AI therapy.[87] A substudy of the MA.17 trial evaluated differences in plasma lipid profiles between 347 women enrolled in the study, from the letrozole (n = 183) and placebo (n = 164) arms, respectively. The study found no durable, significant change in plasma lipid profiles of patients treated with up to 36 months of letrozole compared with those receiving placebo.[88]

Selective Estrogen Receptor Downregulators

Fulvestrant is a steroidal analog of 17-beta-estradiol. It binds to the ER, preventing receptor dimerization and thus effectively downregulating the ER, as shown in both preclinical and clinical studies.[89] Fulvestrant is administered as an intramuscular injection because of poor oral bioavailability. Currently the only available agent in this class, fulvestrant was originally administered as a monthly intramuscular injection at a dose of 250 mg. However, later studies suggested that 500 mg monthly was more effective, with a 4.1-month improvement in overall survival.[90] Unfortunately, this result also causes some difficulties interpreting the results of earlier studies using 250 mg monthly. A double-blind randomized trial compared the efficacy of fulvestrant 250 mg to anastrozole in 400 women with advanced breast cancer whose disease has progressed on prior endocrine therapy. Fulvestrant was shown to be equivalent to anastrozole for time to progression (hazard ratio 0.92; $p = .92$), overall response rate (17.5% in both arms), and clinical benefit 42.2% vs. 36.1%, $p = .26$). Duration of response in patients who had a clinical response was significantly longer in the fulvestrant arm (19 months vs. 10.8 months).[91] A second study with a similar design enrolled 451 patients. In this study, fulvestrant 250 mg was as effective as anastrozole as second-line endocrine therapy for metastatic breast cancer, with regard to time to progression, overall response, clinical benefit rate, and duration of response.[92] It was on the basis of these trials that fulvestrant has been approved by the FDA for use in women with metastatic breast cancer that has progressed on previous endocrine therapy.

Fulvestrant has also been evaluated as a potential therapy for patients who have progressed on an AI. A phase II study conducted by the Swiss Group for Clinical Cancer Research (SAKK 21/00) evaluated two separate groups of patients, those who were AI-responsive (n = 70) and AI-resistant (n = 20).[93] In this study, all patients had previously received an AI, 84% had also been treated with tamoxifen or toremifene. Patients were treated with 250 mg of fulvestrant monthly until progression. Clinical benefit was obtained in 28% of patients with AI-responsive disease and 37% of patients with AI-resistant disease. Time to progression was similar in both groups at 3.6 and 3.4 months, respectively.

Both fulvestrant and exemestane have been evaluated as options in patients who have progressed on treatment with a nonsteroidal AI. A study compared fulvestrant to exemestane in this setting.[94] Patients with metastatic hormone-responsive breast cancer who had experienced recurrence or progression on treatment with a nonsteroidal AI were recruited and 693 eligible patients were enrolled. Patients were randomized to treatment with fulvestrant 250 mg injected monthly or exemestane 25 mg daily. Two-thirds of patients had been previously treated with two or more endocrine therapies. Median time to progression was 3.7 months for both groups. For fulvestrant and exemestane, the response rates (7.4% vs. 6.7%, $p = .736$) and clinical benefit rates (32.2% vs. 31.5%, $p = .853$) were similar. The median duration of benefit for fulvestrant was 9.3 months and for exemestane was 8.3 months. On the basis of this study, fulvestrant 250 mg is equivalent to exemestane as a treatment option for patients with metastatic disease who have progressed after therapy with a nonsteroidal AI. However, as noted here (see also "Advanced and Metastatic Breast Cancer: Treatment"), 500 mg monthly appears superior to 250 mg monthly.

Fulvestrant is a good treatment option for patients with metastatic hormone-sensitive breast cancer that has progressed on previous tamoxifen therapy. Additionally, fulvestrant is active in patients who progressed on treatment with an AI. More about fulvestrant for the treatment of metastatic disease can be found in "Advanced and Metastatic Breast Cancer: Treatment."

Fulvestrant Side Effects

In general, fulvestrant is well tolerated. Aside from injection site discomfort, hot flashes, elevations of liver enzymes, and arthralgias are possible.

Summary

Other agents such as high-dose estradiol, androgens, and progesterone agents are currently seldom used in the treatment of metastatic breast cancer, although they are included in Table 70.1 for the sake of completeness.

The most recent changes in endocrine therapy have been the inclusion of additional drugs to overcome primary and/or secondary resistance (reviewed in "Advanced and Metastatic Breast Cancer: Treatment"), and further insights into the optimal duration of therapy in the adjuvant setting (reviewed in "HR-Positive Invasive Breast Cancer: Adjuvant Treatment") and the benefits of ovarian function suppression for premenopausal women (reviewed in "HR-Positive Invasive Breast Cancer: Adjuvant Treatment").

Ductal Carcinoma in Situ

DCIS is noninvasive breast cancer, which remains confined by the basement membrane of the mammary duct. According to

the American Joint Committee on Cancer 7th edition staging criteria, it is classified as stage 0 breast cancer. Currently, DCIS accounts for 20% to 30% of mammographically identified breast cancers compared with less than 3% of all newly diagnosed breast cancers before mammograms.[95,96] Local treatment of DCIS involves either breast conservation typically followed by radiation or mastectomy.[97] After definitive local treatment of DCIS, there continues to be a risk for in-breast recurrences as well as contralateral new primary breast cancer. Because the majority of DCIS are HR-positive, endocrine therapy has been evaluated to reduce this risk. NSABP B-24 is a double-blind randomized controlled study of tamoxifen in women with DCIS who had completed lumpectomy and whole breast radiation therapy.[98] In this trial, 1804 pre- or postmenopausal women with resected tumors were randomized to tamoxifen 10 mg (n = 902) or placebo (n = 902) twice daily for 5 years. Stratification factors included age (≤49 or >49) presence of LCIS, and method of detection (mammogram, clinical examination, or both). Margins could be microscopically involved with tumor. The primary end point was the occurrence of invasive or noninvasive tumors in the ipsilateral or contralateral breast. At 5 years, the tamoxifen group had fewer breast cancer events than the placebo group (8.2 vs. 13.4%, hazard ratio 0.63; 95% confidence intervals [CI] 0.47–0.83; $p = .0009$). Subsequently, ER and PR were evaluated in 732 of the tumors: 76% had ER-positive DCIS.[99] Patients with ER-positive DCIS on tamoxifen had experienced a significant reduction in any breast cancer event (31% vs. 20%; hazard ratio 0.58; 95% CI 0.42–0.81; $p = .0015$) after a median follow-up of 14.5 years. After multivariate analysis, tamoxifen reduced the risk to time to any breast cancer as first event with a hazard ratio of 0.64 (95% CI 0.48–0.86; $p = .003$) in the ER-positive group. No difference was seen in the ER- group. Although this was an unplanned retrospective, subset analysis of B-24, the isolation of benefit to ER-positive DCIS is supported by data from large adjuvant endocrine trials for invasive breast cancer.[100]

The UK/ANZ randomized phase III trial used a 2 × 2 factorial design, in which women (n = 1701) with locally excised DCIS were randomized to radiation, tamoxifen, no adjuvant treatment or both.[101] Tamoxifen was administered 20 mg daily for 5 years. The primary end point of the study was any new breast cancer event, including invasive ipsilateral new events, DCIS and contralateral disease. After a median follow-up of 12.7 years, tamoxifen reduced the risk of incidence of all new breast events with a hazard ratio 0.71 (95% CI 0.58–0.88; $p = .002$), but had no effect on ipsilateral invasive disease ($p = .8$).

More recently, data have emerged regarding AIs in the setting of DCIS. The randomized, placebo-controlled phase III NRG Oncology/NSABP B-35 trial compared tamoxifen with anastrozole in postmenopausal women with HR-positive DCIS treated with lumpectomy and radiation.[102] Women (n = 3104) in this trial were randomized and stratified by age (<60 vs. ≥60) to tamoxifen 20 mg (n = 1552) once daily or anastrozole 1 mg (n = 1552) once daily for 5 years. The primary end point was breast cancer–free interval (BCFI), defined as time from randomization to any breast cancer event including local, regional, or distant recurrence or a diagnosis of contralateral invasive breast cancer or DCIS. With a median follow-up of 9 years, the 10-year point estimates for BCFI were 89.2% for tamoxifen and 93.5% for anastrozole (hazard ratio 0.73; $p = .03$). A significant interaction was seen between treatment and age group ($p = .04$) with benefit of anastrozole seen only in those women aged less than 60 years.

Ten-year overall survival was no different in the two groups at 92.1% and 92.5% (p = .48).

HR-Positive Invasive Breast Cancer: Adjuvant Treatment

Although the use of endocrine therapy has significantly improved survival for HR-positive breast cancer, many questions remain for this subset of breast cancer. Traditionally, the recommendation for adjuvant chemotherapy for ER and/or PR-positive tumors was based on patient age, tumor stage, and grade. However, this approach led to overtreatment of a large portion of women. Furthermore, it is now clear that HR-positive tumors can be divided into two groups, luminal A and luminal B,[103] which have differential prognoses and response to therapies. On the basis of this information, additional tests are now available to aid decisions about adjuvant chemotherapy. Furthermore, resistance to endocrine therapy continues to be a key challenge. Intrinsic or de novo resistance to endocrine therapy exists in nearly 50% of HR-positive tumors. Tumors can also acquire resistance during endocrine therapy. Here we describe the currently available tests that can be used to aid decisions about adjuvant chemotherapy and duration of endocrine therapy.

Predictive Tools for Use of Adjuvant Chemotherapy in HR-Positive Breast Cancer

21-Gene Recurrence Score (Oncotype DX Assay)

The 21-gene recurrence score (determined using the Onco*type* DX assay; Genomic Health, Redwood City, CA) measures the expression of 16 cancer-related genes and 5 reference genes in paraffin-embedded tissues using a quantitative PCR approach. The genes are primarily related to proliferation, invasion, and HER2 or estrogen signaling.[104] This assay reports scores as low risk (<18), intermediate risk (18–30), or high risk (≥31), although the TAILORx and RxPONDER trials used different cutoffs for recommending use of chemotherapy. Reviewed here are the studies supporting the 21-gene recurrence score as a prognostic test for endocrine-treated ER-positive breast cancers and as a predictive test for adjuvant chemotherapy.

The prognostic significance of the 21-gene recurrence score assay was analyzed in a retrospective prospective substudy of patients enrolled in NSABP B-14. In B-14, patients with node-negative, ER-positive tumors were randomized to receive tamoxifen versus placebo without chemotherapy.[105] Among the tamoxifen-treated patients, cancers with a high-risk recurrence score had a significantly worse rate of distant recurrence and overall survival.[104] Inferior breast cancer survival with a high recurrence score was also confirmed in a case-control series of node-negative, tamoxifen-treated patients.[106] The 21-gene recurrence score has also been demonstrated to be prognostic in tamoxifen-treated postmenopausal women with node-positive, ER-positive cancers.[107] In this retrospective subset analysis of the SWOG 8814 trial, patients with low recurrence score cancers had a significantly improved disease-free and overall survival even when stratified for number of nodes involved. Furthermore, the 21-gene recurrence score has similar prognostic results for the aromatase inhibitors. The ATAC trial compared adjuvant tamoxifen to anastrozole in postmenopausal women with HR-positive breast cancers. The retrospective subset analysis of the 21-gene recurrence score on

tumors from patients enrolled in this study demonstrated lower rates of distant recurrence with lower recurrence scores for both node-negative and node-positive patients. The prognostic value of the 21-gene recurrence score was similar in tamoxifen- and anastrozole-treated patients.[108]

Beyond the prognostic value of the 21-gene recurrence score in tamoxifen-treated patients, the predictive utility of this assay has also been evaluated. In NSABP B-14, a comparison of the placebo and tamoxifen-treated patients demonstrated that the 21-gene recurrence score was prognostic for 10-year distant recurrence-free survival in both groups.[109] It also predicted benefit from tamoxifen in cancers with a low- or intermediate-risk recurrence scores. In contrast, there was no benefit from the use of tamoxifen, compared with placebo, in cancers with high-risk recurrence scores. These data are intriguing and suggest that high-risk recurrence scores may predict for resistance to tamoxifen, and perhaps to other endocrine agents. Interestingly, the genes involved in the 21-gene recurrence score assay include ER, PR, HER2, and other genes associated with proliferation and invasion.

However, the greatest utility for the 21-gene recurrence score may be its ability to aid in decision-making regarding adjuvant chemotherapy in patients with node-negative and node-positive, ER-positive breast cancers. In the NSABP B-20 trial, adjuvant tamoxifen alone was compared with tamoxifen with chemotherapy in patients with node-negative tumors. A retrospective study of the 21-gene recurrence score in a subset of these tumors demonstrated that the benefit of chemotherapy was restricted to patients with breast cancers with higher recurrence scores.[110] Similarly, in node-positive tumors, chemotherapy benefit was only seen in those with high 21-gene recurrence scores in the SWOG 8814 trial that compared adjuvant tamoxifen to tamoxifen plus chemotherapy.[107]

Prospective studies are now underway to answer these questions more definitively. The TAILORx trial includes women with node-negative, HR-positive and HER2-negative tumors measuring 0.6 to 5 cm. The 21-gene recurrence score cutoffs were changed to low (0–10), intermediate (11–25), and high (≥26). Patients with high-score tumors were assigned to chemotherapy and endocrine therapy. Those with intermediate scores were randomized to chemotherapy or no chemotherapy followed by endocrine therapy. The results of these cohorts are still pending. However, results from the 1626 prospectively followed patients with low-risk tumors assigned to endocrine therapy alone demonstrated excellent outcomes with a 5-year risk of invasive disease-free survival of 93.8% and overall survival of 98%.[111] RxPONDER is evaluating women with one- to three-node positive, HR-positive, HER2-negative tumors. In the RxPONDER trial, women with 21-gene recurrence scores of 0 to 25 were randomized to adjuvant chemotherapy and endocrine therapy versus endocrine therapy alone. Those with scores of 26 or higher were assigned to chemotherapy and endocrine therapy. This study recently completed accrual. Of note, neither of these studies is investigating the lack of benefit of endocrine therapy in cancers with high recurrence scores. Finally, the role of the 21-gene recurrence score in understanding the risk for late recurrence and the optimal duration of endocrine therapy is being explored.

PAM-50

The PAM-50 (Prosigna) is a quantitative PCR assay initially used to identify the intrinsic breast cancer subtypes (luminal A, luminal B, HER2-enriched, and basal-like).[103] A newer Risk of Recurrence (ROR) score has been developed that includes this 50-gene expression profile using special weighting of a set of proliferation-associated genes as well as tumor size. In a series of node-negative or node-positive ER-positive breast cancers treated with adjuvant tamoxifen, the ROR score demonstrated prognostic utility.[112] In addition, the ROR was evaluated for its prognostic significance for distant recurrence in tumor samples from the previously described ATAC trial.[113] ROR correlated better with time to distant recurrence compared with the 21-gene recurrence score. However, it provided relatively similar information to IHC4 (ER/PR/HER2 and ki67). The prognostic utility of the ROR for distant recurrence was also demonstrated in an analysis of the ABCSG-8 study. In this study, postmenopausal women with ER-positive breast cancer received either adjuvant tamoxifen or anastrozole without chemotherapy. Those patients with a low ROR tumor score were found to have a very low risk for distant recurrence with 10-year DRFS of 96.7% (95% CI 94.6%–98%).[114] More recently, the ROR was evaluated in a combined analysis of the ATAC and ABCSG-8 studies to explore the ability of this test to identify individuals at risk for late recurrence of breast cancer. Of 2137 women who did not have recurrence 5 years after diagnosis, the ROR score was prognostic beyond a clinical treatment score (including nodal status, tumor size, grade, age, and treatment for the risk of distant recurrence in years 5 to 10.[115] A limitation of the PAM-50 data is the current lack of validation as a predictive biomarker. It has yet to be analyzed in randomized studies of chemotherapy with endocrine therapy versus endocrine therapy alone, or in trials comparing extended endocrine therapy to no extended therapy.

70-Gene Assay (MammaPrint)

The MammaPrint (Agendia, Amsterdam, The Netherlands) is a 70-gene DNA microarray assay that was developed for early-stage breast cancer. Initially, it was only available for fresh tissue analysis, but recent advances in RNA processing now allow for this analysis on formalin-fixed, paraffin-embedded (FFPE) tissue.[116] MammaPrint scores are classified as low or high risk and are associated with 5-year risk for distant recurrence prognosis for node-negative and node-positive breast cancers.[117] Comparisons of outcomes by MammaPrint for nonrandomized adjuvant chemotherapy with endocrine therapy or endocrine therapy alone cohorts of HR-positive breast cancers have reported that only high scores benefit from chemotherapy.[118] The utility of MammaPrint for adjuvant chemotherapy decision-making is being explored in the MINDACT phase III trial[119] in which patients with early-stage breast cancer (node-negative or up to three nodes positive) are treated based on clinicopathologic analysis and genomic risk using the MammaPrint 70 gene signature. Patients who had cancers that are high risk on the basis of both genomic and clinicopathologic analysis receive chemotherapy, in addition to endocrine and HER2-directed therapy where appropriate; patients who had cancers that are low risk by both criteria do not receive chemotherapy; patients with discordant results on either clinicopathologic or genomic criteria were randomized to receive chemotherapy or not. Almost 7000 patients were enrolled with 1800 having high-risk cancers and 2745 having low-risk cancers, using clinicopathologic and genomic criteria.[120] In the discordant groups, almost 600 were deemed low risk by clinicopathologic criteria but high risk by genomic analysis, and 1550 were deemed high risk by clinicopathologic criteria but low risk by genomic analysis. The use of genomic analysis rather than clinicopathologic criteria spared 14% of patients chemotherapy. As was noted in the TAILORx trial,[111] patients with cancers that were low risk by

both criteria had extremely favorable 5-year outcomes without the use of chemotherapy, with distant metastasis–free and overall survivals of 98% and 98%, respectively. Interestingly, there was no benefit for the use of chemotherapy in the two discordant groups, including for cancers that were deemed genomically high risk.

ki67

ki67 is a nuclear nonhistone protein, the expression of which varies in intensity throughout the cell cycle. ki67 has been used as a measurement of tumor cell proliferation.[121] A large meta-analysis demonstrated that a high ki67 is associated with a worse disease-free and overall survival in breast cancer.[122] ki67 has been reported as a clinical tool for classification of luminal A and B tumors.[123] In postmenopausal patients with ER-positive tumors who did not receive chemotherapy from the ATAC trial, the prognostic information from IHC4 (ER, PR, HER2, and ki67) was similar to that seen with the 21-gene recurrence score.[124] When IHC4 was compared with the ROR score in this cohort, ROR only improved upon IHC4 in the HER2-negative, node-negative cohort.[113] However, the ideal cutpoint for ki67 remains unclear, likely indicating it should be considered a continuous marker.[125] Furthermore, analytic validity and intraobserver variability in interpreting results remains challenging.[125] These issues continue to affect the clinical utility of ki67 for decision-making for adjuvant therapy.

ki67 has also been explored as an early predictive biomarker for neoadjuvant endocrine therapy. Changes in ki67 can occur early in response to the cytostatic effect of endocrine therapies and have been associated with improved recurrence-free and overall survival.[126] This is being investigated currently in the phase III ALTERNATE trial (clinicaltrials.gov identifier NCT01953588). This study is enrolling postmenopausal women with clinical stage II–III ER-positive breast cancer who are started on neoadjuvant endocrine therapy. An early biopsy evaluating ki67 is then used to determine whether patients will continue neoadjuvant endocrine therapy or change to neoadjuvant chemotherapy.

Breast Cancer Index (BCI)

BCI is an assay that consists of two gene expression biomarkers: molecular grade index (MGI) and *HOXB13/IL17BR*. BCI was validated as a prognostic test in blinded retrospective analysis of the Stockholm trial. In this prospective randomized study, node-negative, postmenopausal patients were treated with tamoxifen versus observation. When the BCI was evaluated in 588 ER-positive cases from this parent trial, there was a significant association with distant recurrence and breast cancer death. In tamoxifen-treated patients, cohorts at higher 10-year risk for distant recurrence were identified (risk up to 16.9%; 95% CI 7.2–25.6). However, more than 50% of the patients were able to be identified to have a very low risk of less than 3%, and chemotherapy avoidance may be considered for this low-risk population.[127] A subsequent analysis of tamoxifen-treated breast cancer cohorts demonstrated that BCI also was prognostic for late distant recurrences, occurring after 5 years of tamoxifen.[128] Further support for BCI as a potential predictive biomarker for extended endocrine therapy came from an analysis of MA.17, in which postmenopausal women were randomized to letrozole or placebo after completion of 5 years of adjuvant tamoxifen.[129] A prospective-retrospective case-control study (N = 249) showed that high *HOXB13/IL17BR* (H/I) ratio was associated with a decrease in recurrence-free survival from extended letrozole therapy (odds ratio = 0.35; 95% CI 0.16–0.75; *p* = .007). This remained significant when adjusted for clinicopathologic factors. Reduction in absolute risk of recurrence with letrozole was 16.5% in patients with a high H/I ($p = .007$). BCI was also compared with IHC4 and the 21-gene recurrence score in the TransATAC cohort from the large randomized phase III ATAC trial where it was found to have prognostic significance for both early (0–5 year) and late (5–10 year) recurrence.[130] Although further validation of BCI is needed, its potential use for both early decision-making regarding chemotherapy and late decisions regarding extended endocrine therapy is appealing.

Summary

The use of these biomarker assays can identify different subsets of HR-positive breast cancers. It is important to develop these tools to identify those patients who have tumors with an excellent prognosis and are sensitive to endocrine therapies and thus avoid the toxicities of chemotherapy in these patients. In addition, it is also critical to identify which patients remain at substantial risk for distant recurrence after 5 years of endocrine therapy for whom longer durations of endocrine therapy are rational. There continues to be development of multiple new assays to answer these clinical questions.

Adjuvant Endocrine Therapy for ER- and/or PR-Positive Breast Cancer

Premenopausal Women

In women under 45 years of age, tamoxifen for 5 years induces an absolute 15-year benefit of 10.6% in overall survival, reducing the 15-year breast cancer mortality from 35.9% to 25.3% (relative risk 0.71; 95% CI 0.61–0.83, $p = .00002$).[131] The landscape of endocrine therapy for premenopausal breast cancer is in a state of flux, with outstanding questions remaining about the optimal duration, use of ovarian function suppression (OFS), and best agent (tamoxifen versus AI + OFS). Current data and key questions are summarized in this section (see "Duration of Therapy" and "Ovarian Function Suppression").

Ovarian Function Suppression. OFS can be achieved medically (via chronic use of luteinizing hormone–releasing hormone [LHRH] agonists), surgically (via bilateral oophorectomy) or via radiation to the ovaries. When considering OFS in premenopausal HR-positive breast cancer, key questions include the following:

- What is the benefit (if any) of ovarian function suppression alone compared with tamoxifen alone?
- What is the benefit (if any) of ovarian function suppression plus tamoxifen compared with tamoxifen alone in premenopausal women?
- What is the best endocrine therapy agent (tamoxifen vs. an AI) to use in premenopausal women who receive ovarian function suppression? And are there other caveats?
- Does it matter how ovarian function suppression is achieved: Medically? Surgically? With radiation?
- What is the added toxicity of ovarian function suppression?

Table 70.2 summarizes key published trials.[132–138] Some answers have started to emerge but may need longer follow-up and further confirmation. SOFT (Suppression of Ovarian Function Trial) addressed the added value of ovarian function suppression combined with tamoxifen compared with tamoxifen alone, enrolling 2066 premenopausal women many of whom had also received chemotherapy but remained premenopausal despite this (a confounding factor in prior trials). SOFT results showed that there was no additional benefit in terms of disease-free or overall survival for adding OFS for premenopausal women as a whole.[132] At a median follow-up of 67 months, the 5-year disease-free survival

---

TABLE 70.2   Key Published Studies Addressing Ovarian Function Suppression in Premenopausal Women With Breast Cancer

Trial Name	Population (n, Key Inclusion Criteria)	Treatment Arms	Key Outcome
ABCSG-12[135,136]	n = 1803, premeno, stage I–II, HR+, <10 + nodes	Tam + Gos 3 y vs. AI + Gos 3 y (also randomized to ZA or not)	DFS: hazard ratio 1.08, $p = .591$ OS: hazard ratio 1.75, $p = .02$
E5188/INT 0101[137]	N+, HR+, premeno	After CAF, randomized to no treatment vs. Gos 5 y vs. Gos + Tam 5 y	Addition of Tam to improved TTR and DFS but not OS. There was no overall advantage for addition of Gos to CAF.
ZIPP[138]	n = 2076 age < 50 or premeno, Stage I–II	Randomized after primary therapy: no treatment vs. Gos 2y vs. Tam 2 y vs. Gos 2 y + Tam	In women who did not take Tam, there was a large benefit of Gos treatment on survival and recurrence. In women who did take Tam, there was a marginal potential benefit on these outcomes when Gos was added.
E3193[133]	n = 345 HR+, N–, premeno	Tam 5 y vs. Tam + OFS 5 y	DFS: 5-y rate: 87.9% vs. 89.7%; log-rank $p = .62$ OS: 5-year rate: 95.2% vs. 97.6%; log-rank $p = .67$
SOFT[132]	n = 2066, HR+, premeno	Tam 5 y vs. Tam + OFS 5 y (vs. AI + OFS 5 y)	DFS at 5 y: 84.7% vs. 86.6% (hazard ratio: 0.83; $p = .10$) OS
TEXT/SOFT[134]	n = 4690, premeno	Tam + OFS 5 yr vs. AI + OFS 5 yr	DFS at 5 y: 87.3% vs. 91.1% (hazard ratio 0.72; $p < .001$) OS at 5 y: 96.9% vs. 95.9% ($p = $ NS)

AI, Aromatase inhibitor; *CAF,* cyclophosphamide + adriamycin + fluoruracil; *CMF,* cyclophosphamide + methotrexate + fluoruracil; *DFS,* disease-free survival; *ER+,* estrogen receptor positive; *Gos,* goserilin; *HR+,* hormone receptor positive; *NS,* not significant; *OS,* overall survival; premeno, premenopausal; perimeno, perimenopausal; *N+,* node positive; *N–,* node negative; *Tam,* tamoxifen; *ZA,* zoledronic acid.

was 86.6% in the tamoxifen plus OFS and 84.7% in the tamoxifen group (hazard ratio 0.83; 95% CI 0.66–1.04; p = .10). However, among the subgroup under age 35 years who had received chemotherapy (only 233 women), the 5-year freedom from breast cancer was 67.7% (95% CI 57.3–76.0) in the tamoxifen alone versus 78.9% (95% CI 69.8–85.5) in the tamoxifen plus OFS group. Small numbers limit the ability to draw firm conclusions. Furthermore, SOFT and E3193 (an underpowered trial examining early-stage breast cancer treated with tamoxifen versus tamoxifen + OFS as the only adjuvant medical therapy) addressed the question of added toxicity over tamoxifen alone and demonstrate an increase in side effects (hot flashes, sexual dysfunction, bone health) resulting in decreased quality of life for the women receiving tamoxifen plus OFS.[132,133]

The combined results of SOFT and TEXT (Tamoxifen and Exemestane Trial) examine the questions of tamoxifen + OFS versus AI + OFS in 4690 premenopausal breast cancer patients.[134] After a median follow-up of 68 months, disease-free survival at 5 years was 91.1% versus 87.3% for AI + OFS versus tamoxifen + OFS (hazard ratio 0.72; p < .001), although overall survival at 5 years was 95.9% versus and 96.9% (p = not significant). An ASCO Panel issued updated guidelines in 2016, reflecting these new data.[139] At this time, the panel recommended that "high-risk" premenopausal women receive OFS in addition to endocrine therapy. Both tamoxifen and an AI are considered reasonable choices for endocrine therapy (even though the SOFT/TEXT studies did not demonstrate clinical benefit from adding OFS to tamoxifen). The panel currently considers the optimal duration of OFS to be 5 years in this setting. Routine estradiol measurement to assess for "adequate" OFS is not recommended. Premenopausal women were considered to have sufficient risk of recurrence to warrant the addition of OFS if they had stage I–III disease that would warrant the recommendation of chemotherapy. OFS was not recommended in women with stage I breast cancers that did not warrant chemotherapy or node-negative cancer with tumors less than 1 cm. Clarity is lacking in how best to treat patients with stage II disease who might not be recommended chemotherapy on the basis of a gene assay, even though chemotherapy would traditionally have been recommended on the basis of stage alone at the time of the SOFT and TEXT studies on which the guidelines are largely based. There are currently no data to guide the decision-making about OFS plus endocrine therapy for 5 years versus tamoxifen for 10 years. Finally, it is important to note the lack of data for OFS in HR-positive/HER2-positive cancers.

Postmenopausal Women

Tamoxifen has been the endocrine treatment of choice for breast cancer for more than 30 years; however, the partial estrogenic agonist effects of tamoxifen can cause an increased risk of endometrial cancer and venous thromboembolic disease.[52] Furthermore, tamoxifen resistance can develop, resulting in recurrences while on therapy.[140] Because of the success of AIs in the metastatic setting, studies were initiated to compare their efficacy to that of tamoxifen in the adjuvant setting. Initial trials of AIs in the adjuvant setting were restricted to postmenopausal women. A number of large randomized trials have addressed the question of whether AIs are effective as adjuvant therapy for HR-positive breast cancer. The studies directly compared AIs, both initially and sequentially after 2, 3, or 5 years of tamoxifen to tamoxifen alone. These studies are summarized in Table 70.3.[141–148]

The ATAC trial was a landmark study that compared the efficacy of anastrozole 1 mg daily to tamoxifen 20 mg daily or the

two combined. This study enrolled 9366 patients, with 3125 assigned to anastrozole, 3116 to tamoxifen, and 3125 to the combination. The patients included in the study were postmenopausal women with operable breast cancer who had completed their primary therapy. At the time of study design, HR status was not routinely checked. As a result, the study did not limit enrollment to patients with HR-positive breast cancer. However, a preplanned analysis of efficacy in patients with known HR status was included in the protocol. Early results showed no benefit from the combination with outcomes similar to the tamoxifen alone arm.[149] The most recent analysis was after a median follow-up of 100 months. The primary endpoint of DFS was significantly better with anastrozole than tamoxifen in the intention-to-treat and HR-positive populations. In the HR-positive population, DFS was 71.1% for the tamoxifen arm compared with 74.2% with anastrozole (hazard ratio 0.85, 95% CI 0.76–0.94; p = .003), and the rate of distant metastases was also superior with the anastrozole (hazard ratio 0.84; p = .022).[141] However, no survival benefit was seen. The side effect profiles of the two agents were quite different with statistically significant increases in vaginal bleeding, venous thromboembolic events, and hot flashes with tamoxifen versus arthralgias and fractures with anastrozole.[82]

Letrozole was also been shown to be superior to tamoxifen as initial adjuvant therapy for early-stage breast cancer in the Breast International Group 1-98 (BIG 1-98) study.[62] Also designed as a randomized, double-blind study, the BIG 1-98 study enrolled 8028 postmenopausal women, with HR-positive early breast cancer. Patients were randomized to treatment with letrozole 2.5 mg daily or tamoxifen 20 mg daily. At a median follow-up of 76 months, a significant benefit in DFS of 85.6 with letrozole versus 82.6% with tamoxifen (hazard ratio 0.88; p = .03) was seen. Overall survival differences were not significant.[142] The differences in adverse events were similar to those seen in the ATAC trial.

Subsequent AI studies evaluated switching strategies. The landmark Intergroup Exemestane Study (IES) evaluated the steroidal AI exemestane. IES evaluated postmenopausal women with ER-positive or unknown tumors who had completed 2 to 3 years of tamoxifen.[150] Patients were randomized to continued tamoxifen or switching to exemestane 25 mg daily. This trial was one of the first studies to demonstrate an improved DFS with switching to an AI. In the intention-to-treat population, after a median follow-up of 30.6 months, the 3-year DFS with exemestane was 91.5% versus 86.8% (hazard ratio 0.68; 95% CI 0.56–0.82; p < .001). Longer follow-up of a median 55.7 months continued to show improved DFS (hazard ratio 0.76; p = .0001). In the ER-positive patients, overall survival was also modestly improved (hazard ratio 0.83; p = .05).[143] Additional switching studies have evaluated anastrozole and letrozole and shown similar improvements in DFS (see Table 70.3). In addition to the comparison of 5 years of tamoxifen versus letrozole, the BIG 1-98 trial also investigated the importance of AI and tamoxifen sequencing. The four arms in this trial included tamoxifen once daily for 5 years, letrozole once daily for 5 years, tamoxifen for 2 years followed by 3 years of letrozole, or letrozole for 2 years followed by 3 years of tamoxifen. After a median follow-up of 71 months, DFS was not significantly improved with either sequential regimen compared with letrozole alone.[142] At this time point, DFS from letrozole for 5 years did remain superior to tamoxifen only.

Initial reports suggested that there could be potential differences in breast cancer outcomes among the AIs. The MA.27 trial addressed this concern. In this study, postmenopausal women with ER-positive early breast cancer were randomized to exemestane

TABLE 70.3 Major Adjuvant Aromatase Inhibitor Studies in Postmenopausal Women[a]

Trials	Median Follow-Up	Treatment Regimen	No. of Patients	Disease Free Survival	Hazard Ratio
Trials of Aromatase Inhibitor vs. Tamoxifen × 5 Years					
ATAC[141]	100 mo	Anastrozole	2618	74.2%	0.85 (0.76–0.94; p = .003)
		Tamoxifen	2598	70.1%	
BIG 1-98[142]	76 mo	Letrozole	2463	85.6%	0.88 (0.78–0.99; p = .03)
		Tamoxifen	2459[b]	82.6%	
Switching Trials Up to 5 Years Total Duration					
BIG 1-98[142]	71 mo	Tamoxifen 2 y → Letrozole 3 y	1548	86.2%	1.05 (0.84–1.32; p = NS)
		Letrozole 2 y → Tamoxifen 3 y	1540	87.6%	0.96 (0.76–1.21; p = NS)
		Compared with Letrozole × 5 y	1546	87.9%	
IES[143]	55.7 mo	Tamoxifen (2–3 y) → Exemestane	2352	85%	0.76 (0.66–0.88; p = .0001)[c]
		or			
		Tamoxifen	2372	80.9%	
ARNO95/ABCSG[146]	28 mo	Tamoxifen (2 y) → Anastrozole	1618	95.9%[d]	0.60 (0.44–0.81; p = .0009)
		or			
		Tamoxifen	1606	93.2%	
ITA[147]	64 mo	Tam (2–3 y) → Anastrozole	223	82.5%[d]	0.57 (0.38–0.85; p = .005)
		or			
		Tamoxifen	225	72%	
TEAM[148]		Tamoxifen (2–3 y) → Exemestane	4875	85%	0.97 (0.88–1.08; p = .60)
		or			
		Exemestane	4904	86%	
Extended Aromatase Inhibitor Therapy After 5 Years of Tamoxifen					
MA.17[144]	30 mo	Letrozole	2593	94.4%	0.58 (0.45–0.76; p < .001)
		Placebo	2594	89.8%	
NSABP B-33[145]	30 mo	Exemestane	799	91%	0.68; p = .07
		Placebo	799	89%	

[a]Hormone receptor–positive data shown for all studies.
[b]Includes 619 patients with selective crossover to letrozole.
[c]Intention-to-treat population results reported including estrogen receptor unknown.
[d]Event-free survival reported.
NS, Not significant.

25 mg daily versus anastrozole 1 mg once daily.[151] At a median follow-up of 4.1 years, 4-year event-free survival was 91% for exemestane and 91.2% for anastrozole (hazard ratio 1.02; 95% CI 0.87–1.18; p = .85). Distant disease-free survival was also similar. Rates of discontinuation were high overall in the study (31.6%), but with similar rates of hot flashes, arthralgias and myalgias, and fragility fractures between the groups. Thus current data suggest similar outcomes and adverse event profiles among the AIs.

On the basis of these studies, anastrozole, exemestane, and letrozole have been approved in the United States for initial adjuvant treatment of HR-positive early-stage breast cancer. It is reasonable to interpret that the exact sequencing of AI, and tamoxifen therapy is less important than that postmenopausal women receiving an AI for at least 2 to 3 years of their adjuvant endocrine treatment. This is supported by a meta-analysis of individual data from 31,920 postmenopausal women with ER-positive early-stage breast cancer who participated in randomized studies.[152] The primary outcome was any recurrence of breast cancer. The AIs reduced recurrence rates by approximately 30% compared with tamoxifen, but only during the duration of time when treatments differed and not thereafter. Treatment with 5 years of an AI compared with 5 years of tamoxifen reduced 10-year breast cancer mortality by 15%.

Extended Duration of Endocrine Therapy

Another key challenge in HR-positive breast cancer is related to the protracted risk of recurrence for HR-positive tumors even after 5 years of adjuvant endocrine therapy.[153] Thus, personalizing the optimal duration of endocrine therapy remains a pertinent issue.[100] The use of assays to help clarify duration has already been reviewed earlier. This section focuses on clinical trial results.

There have been multiple trials investigating the optimal treatment duration of adjuvant tamoxifen in both pre- and postmenopausal women. Given the lower risk of recurrence and improved overall survival demonstrated in trials comparing 2 versus 5 years of tamoxifen, 5 years existed as the standard of care for many years.[154–157]

Trials comparing 5 years of adjuvant tamoxifen to extended tamoxifen treatment duration now support longer durations of tamoxifen. Initially, in both the NSABP B-14 trial and the Scottish Adjuvant Tamoxifen trial, there was no additional benefit in continuing tamoxifen beyond 5 years. In the NSABP study, there was actually a slight advantage in progression-free survival to patients who discontinued the tamoxifen. Furthermore, in both studies, the incidence of endometrial cancer increased with extended tamoxifen therapy.[158,159] In contrast to the NSABP and Scottish trials, the Easter Cooperative Oncology Group (ECOG) 4181/5181 trial studying indefinite tamoxifen therapy in node-positive patients showed a trend toward improvement in DFS.[160] The first data clearly supporting longer tamoxifen came from the adjuvant Tamoxifen Treatment—offer more? (aTTom) and Adjuvant Tamoxifen—Longer Against Shorter (ATLAS) trials. Both compared 5 years with 10 years of tamoxifen in pre- and postmenopausal women. Among the 12,894 women on the ATLAS trial, 6846 had known ER-positive disease. The cumulative risk of recurrence during years 5 to 14 was 21.4% in the group continuing tamoxifen compared with 25.1% in the control group with a relative risk for breast cancer recurrence in the study of 0.84 (95% CI 0.76–0.94; p = .002). Breast cancer mortality was also improved by the longer duration of tamoxifen.[161] Similar outcomes were observed in the 6953 patients with ER-positive or unknown cancers who received 10 years of tamoxifen on the aTTom trial.[162] Interestingly, in both trials, most of the benefit was seen after subjects completed 10 years of tamoxifen, most likely due to a carryover effect of the 5 years of tamoxifen. The risk of endometrial cancer and venous thromboembolic events was increased in the women who received 10 years of tamoxifen.[161,162] The different results from the NSABP B-14 trial, compared with the ATLAS and aTTom trials, may be perhaps explained by the larger number of patients and also the proportion with higher-risk disease on the latter two trials.

In addition, a number of trials have shown the benefit of extending adjuvant endocrine therapy with sequential tamoxifen and AI therapy to 10 years (see also Table 70.3). The National Cancer Institute of Canada Clinical Trials Group MA.17 trial was designed to study the efficacy of 5 years of letrozole therapy after completion of 4.5 to 6 years of tamoxifen adjuvant therapy.[163] The study enrolled 5187 postmenopausal women with HR-positive breast cancer who had completed tamoxifen within 3 months of enrolling in the study. Patients were randomized to receive 5 years of letrozole therapy or placebo. A significant benefit was seen in the primary end point of disease-free survival in patients treated with letrozole after a median follow-up of 30 months. Four-year disease-free survival was 94.4% with letrozole compared with 89.8% with tamoxifen (hazard ratio 0.58; 95% CI 0.45–0.76; p < .001). There was no overall survival benefit in the intent-to-treat population, but for the subset with node-positive disease, there was a statistically significant benefit in overall survival (hazard ratio = 0.61, 95% CI 0.38–0.98; p = .04).[144] The results of this first interim analysis resulted in an unblinding of the study and

crossover from placebo to letrozole was allowed. Subsequent analyses were conducted to determine whether duration of therapy or delayed initiation of letrozole had an influence on outcome. At 48 months of follow-up, a longer duration of letrozole therapy was associated with greater benefit in the extended adjuvant setting.[164] Furthermore, at a median follow-up of 5.3 years, disease-free survival was better in patients who changed from placebo to letrozole (n = 1579) than those who stayed on placebo (n = 804) with a hazard ratio of 0.37 (95% CI 0.23–0.61; p < .0001) Two other studies have also investigated extended therapy with an AI after 5 years of tamoxifen. ABCSG 6a was a small study of 856 patients but demonstrated that 3 years of anastrozole resulted in an improvement in risk of recurrence (hazard ratio 0.62, 95% CI 0.40–0.96; p = .031).[165] NSABP B-33 did not show a statistically significant benefit but was limited by lack of full accrual due to early termination after results of MA.17 were available.[145]

Recently the first extended study of an aromatase inhibitor beyond 5 years was reported. MA.17R was a phase III randomized study that enrolled 1918 postmenopausal women who had received 4.5 to 6 years of prior adjuvant aromatase inhibitor with completion of the initial AI within the previous 2 years.[166] Patients were randomized 1 : 1 to letrozole or placebo for 5 years. Of note, 70% of participants had 5 years of adjuvant tamoxifen before the AI. Patients were stratified by lymph node status, prior adjuvant chemotherapy, interval since last dose of the AI, and duration of prior tamoxifen. The primary end point was DFS, which was defined as time from randomization to recurrence of breast cancer (in breast, chest wall, nodal, or metastatic) or development of a new breast cancer. Occurrence of another type of cancer or death without breast cancer recurrence were not included as events. With a median follow-up of 6.3 years, the 5-year disease-free survival rate was 95% with letrozole and 91% with placebo (hazard ratio 0.66; CI 0.48–0.91; p = .01). However, it is notable that distant recurrence was 4.4% versus 5.5% of events compared with contralateral breast cancer in 1.4% versus 3.2% of events, respectively, for letrozole and placebo. Overall survival was not different between the two cohorts. Of note, fractures were higher in the letrozole group (14 vs. 9%; p = .001), but no difference in cardiovascular events were noted.

Taken altogether, it is reasonable to consider extended adjuvant therapy on an individual patient basis. If a patient remains premenopausal after completing 5 years of tamoxifen, one should consider extending tamoxifen treatment for an additional 5 years based on results from the ATLAS and aTTom trials. If a patient becomes definitively postmenopausal during the first 5 years of tamoxifen, switching to an AI for 5 additional years is a reasonable option, although this strategy has not been directly compared with continuing tamoxifen for a total of 10 years.[167] In postmenopausal women treated with upfront 5 years of AI or with tamoxifen followed by 5 years of an AI, extending the AI up to 10 years can be now considered, but the effect on distant recurrence is small. Thus the risks and benefits should be individualized for the patient. Of note, there are no current data regarding using extended endocrine therapy with tamoxifen after 5 years of an AI.

On the basis of the current literature for adjuvant endocrine therapy in postmenopausal women, the 2014 ASCO Clinical Practice Guidelines recommend the following options: (1) tamoxifen for 10 years, (2) AI for 5 years, (3) tamoxifen for 5 years and then switching to an AI for up to 5 years (total duration up to 10 years) or tamoxifen for 2 to 3 years and then switching to an AI for up to 5 years (total duration up to 7–8 years).[32] See the preceding section "Ovarian Function Suppression" for a discussion of the 2016 ASCO Clinical Practice Guidelines regarding premenopausal women and ovarian suppression. It is anticipated that these guidelines will be updated to include AI for up to 10 years, to integrate the recent MA.17R data.

Neoadjuvant Endocrine Therapy for HR-Positive Breast Cancer

Although well established as adjuvant therapy for HR-positive breast cancer, the role of neoadjuvant endocrine therapy continues to be evaluated. Clinical responses and pathologic complete responses (pCR) to neoadjuvant chemotherapy in HR-positive breast cancers is low.[168] Furthermore, a meta-analysis of chemotherapy treated-patients demonstrated that pCR was not prognostic in the luminal A subgroup (defined as grade 1–2, HR-positive, HER2 negative). Clinical responses to neoadjuvant endocrine therapy are seen in 35% to 55% of HR-positive tumors with higher breast conservation rates when AIs are used.[169–171] Longer durations of endocrine therapy may also influence response.[172] However, the key challenge is identifying which HR-positive tumors are most likely to respond to preoperative endocrine therapy versus chemotherapy.

The American College of Surgeons Oncology Group Z1031 and the IMPACT trials have evaluated suppression in ki67 as a predictive biomarker for neoadjuvant endocrine therapy.[171,173] The Z1031B was a preoperative study in which postmenopausal women with stage II–III HR-positive breast cancer received anastrozole or letrozole. If the ki67 remained greater than 10% after 4 weeks, patients were switched to chemotherapy. Of the 245 women enrolled on this study, 35 had a ki67 greater than 10% and were switched to chemotherapy. Two of 35 (5.7%) had a pCR to the chemotherapy.[174] This feasibility study has led to the large preoperative ALTERNATE trial, which uses ki67 at 4 weeks to determine switch to chemotherapy versus continued endocrine therapy. Other ongoing studies are also examining the 21-gene recurrence score as a predictive biomarker for endocrine therapy.[175] Lastly, neoadjuvant endocrine therapy in combination with targeted therapies directed at HER2, cyclin-dependent kinase (CDK)4/6, and the PI3-kinase/mechanistic target of rapamycin (mTOR) pathways are all being evaluated.

Advanced and Metastatic Breast Cancer: Treatment

First-Line Therapy

Before the development of third-generation AIs, tamoxifen was the standard of care for first-line treatment of HR-positive metastatic breast cancer. Because of the favorable toxicity profile of AIs and at least equivalent efficacy results compared with megestrol acetate in patients who had progressed on first-line tamoxifen, studies were initiated to evaluate AIs as first line therapy for MBC. The largest trial randomized more than 900 patients with between tamoxifen or letrozole.[176] At a median follow-up of 32 months, letrozole was superior to tamoxifen with a significant improvement in time to progression of 9.4 months as opposed to 6 months for tamoxifen. There was no significant difference in overall survival likely because 50% of patients crossed over to the opposite agent at the time of progression (Table 70.4). Similar trials comparing anastrozole to tamoxifen have also shown improved outcomes with an AI in the first-line setting.[177]

Fulvestrant was initially compared with anastrozole in patients with metastatic HR-positive breast cancer who had progressed on first-line tamoxifen. These studies showed that fulvestrant was equivalent to anastrozole in time to progression, response rate, and

TABLE 70.4	Outcomes From Randomized First-Line Trials in Patients With Hormone Receptor–Positive Metastatic Breast Cancer					
Trial	Patient N	Control Arm	PFS/TTP (Months)	Comparison Arm	PFS (Months)	*p* Value
P025[176]	916	Letrozole	9.4	Tamoxifen	6.0	<.0001
TARGET[177]	353	Anastrozole	11.1	Tamoxifen	5.6	.005
Howell et al.[178]	587	Fulvestrant	6.8	Tamoxifen	8.3	.088
SWOG0226[179]	694	Anastrozole	13.5	Anastrozole + Fulvestrant	15.0	.007
FACT[180]	514	Anastrozole	10.2	Anastrozole + Fulvestrant	10.8	.91
FIRST[181]	205	Anastrozole	13.1	Fulvestrant	23.4	.01
PALOMA-1[182]	165	Letrozole	10.2	Letrozole + Palbociclib	20.2	.0004
Paul et al.[183]	120	Letrozole	11	Letrozole + dasatinib	22	.05
HORIZON[186]	1112	Letrozole	9.0	Letrozole + Temsirolimus	8.9	.9
LEA[184]	380	Endocrine therapy[a]	13.3	ET[a] + bevacizumab	17.6	.434
CALGB[185]	350	Letrozole	16	Letrozole + bevacizumab	20	.016

[a]Letrozole or fulvestrant.
PFS, Progression-free survival; *TTP*, time to progression.

| TABLE 70.5 | Outcomes From Randomized Trials in Patients With Hormone Receptor–Positive Metastatic Breast Cancer Who Received Prior Therapy With Nonsteroidal AIs |

Trial	Patient N	Control	PFS/TTP (Months)	Comparison Arm	PFS/TTP (Months)	P Value
EFECT[94]	693	Exemestane	3.7	Fulvestrant	3.7	.65
BOLERO-2[190]	724	Exemestane	2.8	Exemestane + everolimus	6.9	<.001
TAMRAD[192]	111	Tamoxifen	4.5	Tamoxifen + everolimus	8.6	.002
CONFIRM[90]	736	Fulvestrant SD[a]	5.5	Fulvestrant HD[a]	6.5	.006
FERGI[193]	168	Fulvestrant	3.7	Fulvestrant + pictilisib	7.4	.096
BELLE-2[194]	1147	Fulvestrant	5.0	Fulvestrant + buparlisib	6.9	<.001
PALOMA-3[195]	521	Fulvestrant	3.8	Fulvestrant + palbociclib	9.2	<.001
ENCORE[198]	130	Exemestane	2.3	Exemestane + entinostat	4.3	.055

[a]SD = standard dose, 250 mg every 4 weeks; HD = high dose 500 mg every 4 weeks after loading schedule of 500 mg on days 1 and 15 in cycle 1.

PFS, Progression-free survival; *TTP*, time to progression.

clinical benefit rate.[91,92] On the basis of these trials, fulvestrant was approved, at a dose of 250 mg every 4 weeks, by the FDA for use in postmenopausal women with metastatic breast cancer who had experienced disease progression on previous hormonal therapy. Fulvestrant at this dose was subsequently compared with tamoxifen in the first-line setting but showed equivalent outcomes (see Table 70.4).[178] Given the relative modest activity of fulvestrant at this dosing schedule, subsequent trials were designed to evaluate alternative dosing schedules. A pivotal trial that accrued patients with HR-positive metastatic breast cancer who had received prior endocrine therapy demonstrated superiority of a higher dose fulvestrant schedule (500 mg every 4 weeks with a loading schedule of 500 mg on day 1 and day 15 of cycle 1) compared with the original FDA-approved dosing schedule (Table 70.5).[90] On the basis of these results, the FDA approved this higher dosing schedule of fulvestrant, which has now become standard of care. Fulvestrant at the higher dose schedule was demonstrated to be superior to anastrozole in the first-line treatment of HR-positive metastatic breast cancer with median time to progression of 23 months, compared with 13 months, in the FIRST trial (see Table 70.4). Overall survival was improved from 48 months with anastrozole to 54 months with fulvestrant.[179] The FALCON trial is a randomized phase 3 trial designed to confirm the results noted in the FIRST trial.

The combination of fulvestrant and anastrozole in the first-line setting has been compared with anastrozole in two trials with somewhat conflicting results. A SWOG trial showed improved median progression-free survival with the combination arm compared with the anastrozole arm (13.5 months vs. 15.0 months; hazard ratio 0.80; p = .007).[180] In contrast, the Fulvestrant and Anastrozole in Combination Trial (FACT) trial[181] did not show a significant improvement in median time to progression with the combination, compared with anastrozole alone (10.8 months versus 10.2 months, p = .99; see Table 70.4). The conflicting results in these two trials may be attributed to differences in the size of the trials and differences in patient populations, with more patients with de novo metastatic disease in the SWOG trial. The median progression free survival was longer in the anastrozole only arm in the SWOG trial, compared with the FACT trial,

suggesting that a higher proportion of patients in the SWOG trial had endocrine-sensitive disease.

Palbociclib is an oral inhibitor of CDK4/6 proteins involved in regulating cell cycle progression (Fig. 70.1). Preclinical data showed activity for palbociclib in HR-positive breast cancer cell lines. PALOMA-1 was a phase II trial in which 165 patients were randomized to letrozole alone versus the combination of palbociclib and letrozole as first-line therapy for HR-positive advanced breast cancer.[182] Median progression-free survival was 20.2 months in the combination arm compared with 10.2 months for the letrozole alone arm hazard ratio = 0.49; p = .0004). With these promising results, palbociclib was approved with letrozole in the first-line setting for patients with HR-positive metastatic disease. Results from the confirmatory PALOMA-2 phase III randomized (2 : 1) trial were shown at ASCO 2016 with a median PFS of 24.8 versus 14.5 months (hazard ratio 0.58; 95% CI 0.46–0.72; p < .000001). The most common side effects of palbociclib include neutropenia and infection. Thus it is recommended that patients have white blood count checks at the start of each cycle as well as midway through the first cycle. There are currently no biomarkers available to determine which patients require palbociclib in the first-line setting, and it is certainly possible that some patients would do well with endocrine therapy alone.

A number of other agents have been evaluated with variable success in the first-line HR-positive metastatic setting. The addition of the SRC inhibitor, dasatinib, to letrozole has been demonstrated to significantly prolong progression-free survival compared with letrozole alone, from 11 to 22 months.[183] Two trials recently demonstrated an improved progression- free survival with the addition of bevacizumab to endocrine therapy in the first-line setting. In the LEA trial,[184] the addition of bevacizumab to either letrozole or fulvestrant in the first-line setting improved progression-free survival from 13.3 to 17.6 months, although the difference was not statistically significant. The Cancer and Leukemia Group B (CALGB) 40503 trial[185] evaluated the addition of bevacizumab to letrozole in the first-line setting and noted a marginally significant improvement in progression-free survival from 16 to 20 months. Given the significant toxicity associated with bevacizumab, it is unclear, however, whether this

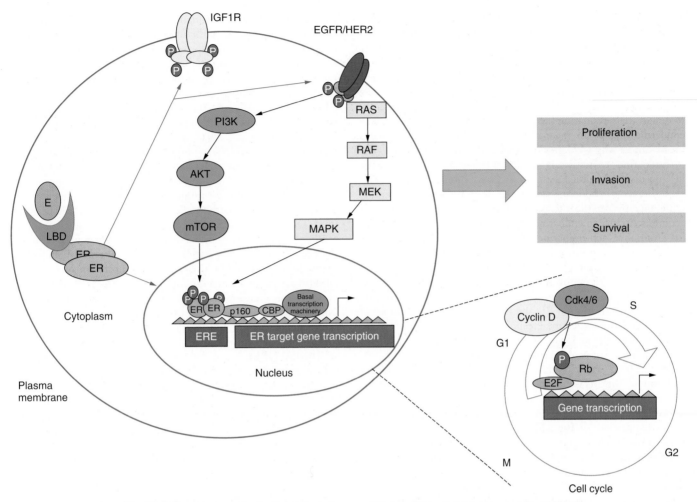

• **Fig. 70.1** Estrogen receptor function in breast cancer. Estrogen (E)-bound estrogen receptor (ER) acts as a ligand-activated transcription factor in the nucleus. Upon translocation to the nucleus, ER binds as a homodimer to promotor regions of target genes either directly through estrogen response elements (ERE) and recruiting a large coactivator complex (p160 and CREB-binding protein [CBP]). ER can also act indirectly via interactions with other transcription factor in the nucleus. Outside the nucleus, ER can interact with growth factor receptor tyrosine kinases (RTKs) such as epidermal growth fact receptor [EGFR], HER2, and insulin-like growth factor 1 receptor [IGF1R]) in a nongenomic mechanism. These interactions activate downstream signaling pathways (e.g., PI3-kinase [PI3K]/AKT and Ras/RAF/MEK/MAPK), which then phosphorylate nuclear transcription factors and coregulators, including components of the ER pathway. Overall, these activities of ER result in proliferation, invasion and survival of the breast cancer cells. Cyclin D and the cyclin dependent kinase 4/6 (CDK4/6) are integral for the G1 (cell growth period) to S (DNA replication) transition in the cell cycle. CDK4/6 forms a complex with cyclin D, phosphorylating the tumor suppressor retinoblastoma (Rb) protein. pRb releases the transcription factor E2F, activating gene transcription and allowing for cell cycle progression. Elements associated with resistance to endocrine therapy include activating mutations in the ligand binding domain (LBD) of ER, cyclin D1 overexpression, and upregulation of growth factor signaling pathways.

will become a widely used approach, especially considering the less toxic therapeutic options available. Addition of the mTOR inhibitor, temsirolimus, to letrozole did not improve outcome for patients with HR-positive metastatic breast cancer treated in the first-line setting.[186]

In the absence of a clinical trial, decisions on the optimal first-line endocrine therapy for patients with HR-positive disease should be made on the basis of prior therapy in the adjuvant setting. The combination of fulvestrant and anastrozole is reasonable but should probably be reserved for patients with de novo metastatic disease or those patients who have a long disease-free interval from initial diagnosis. Biomarkers are needed to

determine the optimal approach for patients with newly diagnosed metastatic breast cancer. For example, the 21-gene recurrence score appears to be prognostic, and perhaps predictive, for outcome in patients with metastatic HR-positive breast cancer.[187]

Prior Treatment With Nonsteroidal Aromatase Inhibitor

The Evaluation of Faslodex versus Exemestane Clinical Trial (EFECT) randomized patients with HR-positive metastatic breast cancer who had received prior therapy with nonsteroidal AI to exemestane versus fulvestrant. Time to progression was identical at just under 4 months in each arm, and there was no significant difference in any of the other trial end points (see Table 70.5).[94] This trial suggests that no single endocrine agent appears superior to another in this setting. Additionally, the short time to progression (<6 months) suggests that the majority of patients accrued had endocrine-resistant disease (all had previously received at least a nonsteroidal AI). The EFECT trial has been used subsequently to design trials evaluating the addition of other targeted agents to endocrine therapy in the patients with HR-positive metastatic breast cancer who were previously treated with nonsteroidal AIs.

Endocrine resistance is a critical issue for patients with HR-positive metastatic breast cancer. Some tumors harbor intrinsic resistance to endocrine agents and do not benefit from endocrine therapy. In the metastatic setting, all tumors ultimately acquire resistance to endocrine therapy. The mechanisms underlying resistance to endocrine therapy are complex. However, enhanced signaling through growth factor receptor pathways has been demonstrated in preclinical and clinical studies.[188] The PI3-kinase/Akt/mTOR pathway is a signaling cascade that can be regulated by ER. Activation of this pathway can lead to estrogen-independent activation of ER and has been associated with resistance to endocrine therapy. Preclinical data showed that mTOR inhibition can restore sensitivity to endocrine therapy and induce apoptosis in breast cancer cells.[189]

BOLERO-2 was a randomized phase III trial evaluating the addition of the mTOR inhibitor everolimus to exemestane in patients with HR-positive metastatic breast cancer who had experienced disease progression on or recurrence after treatment with a nonsteroidal AI.[190] The addition of everolimus to exemestane led to a significant improvement in progression-free survival (6.9 vs. 2.8 months by local assessment, $p < .001$; 10.6 vs. 4.1 months by central assessment, $p < .001$; see Table 70.5). Interestingly, there is no significant difference in overall survival between the two arms on BOLERO-2.[191] Additionally, the addition of everolimus was associated with increased toxicities. The most common grade 3 or 4 adverse events were stomatitis, fatigue, hyperglycemia, anemia, and pneumonitis. On the basis of the results of BOLERO-2, the FDA approved everolimus in combination with exemestane for HR-positive, HER2-negative, postmenopausal, advanced breast cancer patients. Everolimus has been studied in combination with other endocrine agents. The TAMRAD trial was a phase II trial that compared the combination of tamoxifen and everolimus to tamoxifen alone.[192] The primary end point of clinical benefit rate was significantly improved in the combination arm (61% vs. 42%, $p = .045$). Time to progression was additionally improved in the combination arm (8.6 vs. 4.5 months). The toxicities observed in TAMRAD were similar to BOLERO-2.

Other agents targeting the PI3-kinase pathway are in development for HR-positive metastatic breast cancer in patients who have experienced disease progression after prior endocrine therapy. The FERGI trial[193] evaluated the addition of the PI3-kinase inhibitor, pictilisib, to fulvestrant in patients with HR-positive metastatic breast cancer who had received prior treatment with nonsteroidal AI. Progression-free survival was improved from 3.7 to 7.4 months with the addition of the PI3-kinase inhibitor (see Table 70.5). The larger BELLE-2 trial[194] randomized more than 1100 postmenopausal patients with HR-positive metastatic breast cancer, with prior disease progression on nonsteroidal AIs to fulvestrant alone or fulvestrant in combination with buparlisib, an oral pan class 1 PI3-kinase inhibitor, that targets all four isoforms of PI3-kinase. In the overall population, progression-free survival was improved from 5 to 6.9 months (hazard ratio 0.78, $p < .001$).

In a planned analysis evaluating the addition of buparlisib to fulvestrant in patients with tumors with activated PI3-kinase, there was no significant improvement in progression-free survival in the buparlisib arm (6.8 vs. 4 months for the control arm, hazard ratio 0.76, $p = .014$; see Table 70.5). However, a significant improvement in progression-free survival was noted with the addition of buparlisib to fulvestrant when PI3-kinase mutations were detected using circulating tumor (ct) DNA (7 vs. 3.2 months, hazard ratio 0.56, $p < .001$), whereas no such increase was noted in patients with ctDNA without mutant PI3-kinase. The most common toxicities were elevated liver function tests, hyperglycemia, rash, depression, and anxiety.

At the time of disease progression on endocrine therapy and everolimus, it is currently unclear whether the cancer has developed resistance to the endocrine agent, everolimus, or both. Studies are underway to evaluate the potential benefit of continuing everolimus beyond progression with an alternative endocrine agent. Inhibition of PI3-kinase signaling upstream of mTOR is currently being evaluated among patients who have disease progression on everolimus. BELLE-3 (clinicaltrials.gov identifier NCT01633060) is an ongoing phase III trial randomizing patients between fulvestrant and the combination of fulvestrant and buparlisib.

The PALOMA-3 trial evaluated the addition of palbociclib to fulvestrant in patients with HR-positive metastatic breast cancer with prior disease progression on nonsteroidal AIs.[195] Patients treated with fulvestrant plus palbociclib had a significant improvement in disease progression, compared with fulvestrant alone, from 3.8 to 9.2 months ($p < .000001$; see Table 70.5). Response rates were low and not significantly different between the arms, but clinical benefit rate was improved from 19% to 34% with the addition of palbociclib to fulvestrant. Overall survival results are not yet mature. There are several ongoing studies evaluating other CDK inhibitors in HR-positive metastatic breast cancer.

Preclinical data support the concept that histone deacetylase (HDAC) inhibitors may play a role in reversing resistance to endocrine therapy.[196,197] The ENCORE trial evaluated the addition of entinostat, a HDAC inhibitor, to exemestane in patients with HR-positive metastatic breast cancer, with prior disease progression on nonsteroidal AIs.[198] Although there was no significant improvement in progression-free survival (see Table 70.5), a significant improvement in overall survival was noted. The FDA has given entinostat breakthrough designation and the results of the ENCORE trial will be confirmed in the ongoing ECOG 2112 trial (clinicaltrials.gov identifier NCT02115282).

In summary, resistance to endocrine agents remains a critical issue for patients with HR-positive metastatic breast cancer. Recent trials demonstrate improved disease control with the addition of targeted agents, including mTOR inhibitors and CDK inhibitors, in patients with HR-positive metastatic breast cancer who have previously received endocrine therapy. It remains unclear whether all patients treated outside of the first-line setting need the addition of these targeted agents, given the added toxicity and expense. Further correlative studies will need to address this issue. Given that HR-positive cancers change at a molecular level as endocrine resistance develops, it is essential to correlate the activity of targeted agents with the cancers in real time, which is not generally possible without serial biopsies. The advent of "liquid biopsies" evaluating circulating tumor cells and circulating DNA should allow a more accurate assessment of why a given targeted agent may or not work in real-time, and further correlative studies should focus in this area.

Selected References

82. Howell A, Cuzick J, Baum M, et al. Results of the ATAC (Arimidex, Tamoxifen, Alone or in Combination) trial after completion of 5 years' adjuvant treatment for breast cancer. *Lancet.* 2005;365:60-62.

90. Di Leo A, Jerusalem G, Petruzelka L, et al. Final overall survival: fulvestrant 500 mg vs 250 mg in the randomized CONFIRM trial. *J Natl Cancer Inst.* 2014;106:djt337.

134. Pagani O, Regan MM, Walley BA, et al. Adjuvant exemestane with ovarian suppression in premenopausal breast cancer. *N Engl J Med.* 2014;371:107-118.

182. Finn RS, Crown JP, Lang I, et al. The cyclin-dependent kinase 4/6 inhibitor palbociclib in combination with letrozole versus letrozole alone as first-line treatment of oestrogen receptor-positive, HER2-negative, advanced breast cancer (PALOMA-1/TRIO-18): a randomised phase 2 study. *Lancet Oncol.* 2015;16:25-35.

191. Piccart M, Hortobagyi GN, Campone M, et al. Everolimus plus exemestane for hormone-receptor-positive, human epidermal growth factor receptor-2-negative advanced breast cancer: overall survival results from BOLERO-2. *Ann Oncol.* 2014;25:2357-2362.

A full reference list is available online at ExpertConsult.com.

71

Immunologic Approaches to Breast Cancer Therapy

SASHA E. STANTON, ERIK RAMOS, AND MARY L. DISIS

The emergence of the prognostic importance of tumor immune infiltrates in breast cancer, the essential role of the immune system in contributing to the response to chemotherapy, and the generation of clinical responses with emerging therapies including vaccines and immune checkpoint inhibitor monoclonal antibodies have clearly demonstrated that breast cancer is immunologically active.[1-3] In the future, therapies that harness the immune system will be used in all stages of breast cancer treatment, including the possibility of stimulating immunity for breast cancer prevention.[4] This chapter provides an overview of the current immunologic approaches to develop predictive and prognostic assays in breast cancer, novel and clinically effective immune therapy, and will overview considerations of new directions in breast immuno-oncology for the future.

Immunity and Breast Cancer

The human immune system is generally categorized as providing either an innate immune response or an adaptive immune response. Innate immune cells are the body's first responders to a foreign insult, and the innate immune response does not require recognition of proteins or antigens. The innate response is short-lived; no immunologic memory is generated. Adaptive immunity does require antigen recognition and is a slower response because antigens have to be processed and presented to T cells by innate immune cells. Immunologic memory can be elicited in an adaptive response so that protective immunity can be generated in anticipation of a future threat by the same organism.

Some cells of the innate immune system demonstrate antitumor activity. Natural killer T cells (NK T cells) respond to stress signals, including loss of major histocompatibility complex (MHC) class I expression and can both trigger direct cytotoxicity of tumor cells and release cytokines that promote adaptive immunity.[5] Increased tumor-infiltrating NK T cells and the presence of NK T-cell–associated gene expression patterns in tumors have been shown to predict improved outcome for breast cancer patients.[6] Other cells of the innate immune system suppress potentially functional immunity. Macrophages are antigen-presenting cells and are needed for displaying immunogenic proteins to the cells of the adaptive immune system (lymphocytes). In response to environmental signals, macrophages also release cytokines that influence the phenotype of the evolving adaptive immune response. M1 macrophages secrete type I lymphocyte-activating cytokines (including interferon gamma [IFN-γ],

interleukin [IL]-2, and IL-12) that promote the generation of a CD8$^+$ T-cell (cytotoxic T lymphocytes, CTL) response. M2 macrophages secrete type II cytokines including transforming growth factor-beta (TGF-β), IL-4, and IL-13 that inhibit proliferation of CD8$^+$ T cells and facilitate antibody formation. Intratumoral macrophages in breast cancer are predominantly M2 and have been associated with poor prognosis. In a study of 216 breast cancer samples, increased proliferating macrophages (CD68$^+$, a macrophage marker, and PCNA$^+$, an anti–proliferating cell nuclear antigen, a proliferation marker) in breast tumors were associated with an increased risk of death (hazard ratio [HR] 1.75, 95% confidence interval [CI] 1.0–3.0; $p = .048$).[7] An investigation in almost 200 patients with locally advanced breast cancer demonstrated patients whose tumors did not express a macrophage-associated gene signature enjoyed a greater clinical benefit after chemotherapy and improved survival compared with patients whose tumors displayed such a signature ($p = .0009$).[8]

Another innate immune cell type that is associated with tumor progression and advanced stages of breast cancer is the myeloid-derived suppressor cell (MDSC). MDSCs are a population of immature myeloid cells that trigger immune suppression by producing reactive oxygen species and secrete immune-suppressive cytokines.[9] The presence of MDSCs has been shown to predict an unfavorable prognosis in breast cancer, with an increase in circulating peripheral blood MDSCs associated with progression of disease. The highest levels of circulating MDSCs are found in metastatic breast cancer.[10] MDSCs may be particularly important in enhancing the development of bone metastasis. MDSCs have been proposed to be osteoclast progenitors contributing both to bone resorption and modification of the bone immune environment in a manner that promotes increased breast cancer metastases.[11] The cells of the innate immune system play a critical role in helping to define the immune microenvironment for a particular tumor and can significantly influence the adaptive immune response that develops in breast cancer.

Adaptive immunity requires interaction with a specific antigen (Fig. 71.1). Many antigens are available for immune recognition. These include tumor-associated antigens that are not very different from self (see Fig. 71.1B) and antigens that may be mutated or phosphorylated to appear more dangerous to the immune system (see Fig. 71.1C). Interaction with antigen displayed in the MHC is the first signal to the immune system of the strength of the immune response needed upon antigen recognition. Adaptive immunity is defined by the presence of lymphocytes, either T or

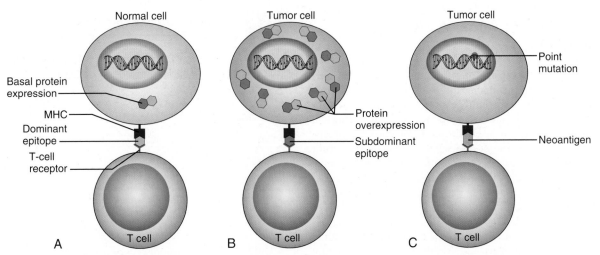

• **Fig. 71.1** Recognition of tumor antigens by T cells. (A) Epitopes of self-proteins presented in the major histocompatibility complex *(MHC)* do not trigger T-cell recognition. "Dominant" epitopes are tolerizing. (B) Epitopes derived from aberrantly overexpressed self-proteins are termed subdominant and when presented in the MHC do stimulate T cells. These peptides have not been available to the immune system for recognition and are not tolerizing. (C) Epitopes that are presented that contain a mutation can be seen as "neo-antigens." Mutational sequences are unique to the immune system and can elicit a T-cell response.

B cells, and includes both CD8⁺ cytotoxic T cells that are the effector cells that directly destroy tumor cells, CD4⁺ helper T cells that regulate CD8⁺ T-cell and B-cell function, and B cells that present antigen and produce antibodies. Type 1 (Th1) CD4⁺ T helper cells secrete cytokines that support the function of CTL. Type 2 (Th2) CD4⁺ helper T cells secrete cytokines that support B-cell proliferation and antibody production. Regulatory CD4⁺ helper T cells (Tregs) are a third type of T cell that modifies the tumor immune environment. Tregs secrete cytokines that dampen an inflammatory response and play a role in preventing autoimmunity. Tregs are defined by Forkhead box P3 (FOXP3) expression and are operative in cancer as many immunogenic proteins are nonmutated self-antigens that are aberrantly expressed. Antigen-specific Tregs have been defined that function to prevent immunity to self as a mechanism of limiting potential autoimmunity. Recent studies have suggested that Th1 immunity is needed for cancer eradication. In examining 20 tumor types, including breast cancer, increased Th1/CD8⁺ tumor immune infiltrates predicted improved clinical outcomes whereas increased Th2/Treg tumor immune infiltrates predicted inferior outcomes.[12] In breast cancer, Th1 tumor-infiltrating T cells, as defined by the expression of Tbet, have been shown to impart a favorable prognosis. In a study of more than 600 tumors derived from breast cancer patients, a lack of Tbet positive cells in the tumor was associated with a reduced disease-free survival compared with Tbet high tumors in multivariate analysis (relative risk [RR] 5.62, 95% CI 1.48–50.19, $p = .0027$).[13] However, the majority of breast tumors display a Th2 immune environment including Th2 and Treg cells that inhibit CD8⁺ T-cell function and dampen the antitumor immune response.[14,15]

B cells present in the tumor environment indicate an evolving adaptive humoral immune response. B cells develop into plasma cells that release antibodies against an antigen. Autoantibodies against oncogenic proteins can be detected in patients before cancer diagnosis and are indicative of immune recognition of the tumor.[16] Tumor antigen–specific antibodies have been isolated from the peripheral blood of patients and been shown to have potential antitumor activity. Endogenous HER2-specific antibodies can bind the extracellular domain of HER2, inhibit cell signaling, and limit the growth of breast cancer in culture.[17] In a transgenic mouse model of mammary cancer, stimulating antibody immunity against multiple intracellular oncoproteins resulted in complete disease regression.[18] Furthermore, several studies have also shown increased tumor-infiltrating B cells to predict improved outcome in breast cancer. In one gene expression study, the B-cell metagene was associated with improved metastasis-free survival in three independent patient populations totaling 558 patients (first validation cohort n = 286, HR 0.78, 95% CI 0.6–0.8, $p = .034$; second validation cohort n = 302, HR 0.83, 95% CI 0.7–0.9, $p = .021$).[19] A second study of 37 breast cancers found a B-cell metagene to be associated with improved distant relapse–free survival in high proliferating hormone receptor positive breast cancer (HR 4.29, 95% CI 2.0–9.0, $p = .001$) and triple-negative breast cancer (HR 3.34, 95% CI 1.6–7.0, $p = .001$).[20] In ovarian cancer, improved outcome with tumor-infiltrating B cells have not been associated with increased autoantibodies, but rather their role in presenting tumor antigens to the tumor-infiltrating T cells. Furthermore, tumor-infiltrating B cells may help facilitate Th1 CD4⁺ T-cell memory.[21,22] However, the presence of tumor-infiltrating B cells has also been linked with chronic inflammation and immunosuppression promoting a Th2 immune environment and tumor progression. B cells have been found to be elevated in 70% of solid tumors, with some studies associating increased tumor-infiltrating B cells with poor prognosis in several cancer types including breast cancer. Furthermore, the presence of certain autoantibodies has been associated with poor prognosis in breast cancer; for example, in 61 patients with breast cancer, high titers of p53 autoantibodies was associated with a lower 5-year survival than patients with lower titers.[23–25] Defining the elements of a successful immune response in breast cancer has led to a greater understanding of how to harness immune system cells for diagnostic and prognostic purposes.

Diagnostic Role of Tumor-Associated Autoantibodies

The immune system is capable of responding to abnormal cells that develop early in the malignant transformation of breast cancer. Overexpressed or aberrantly expressed proteins present in breast cancer elicit an immune response and are antigenic. Immune recognition can be assayed by the detection of autoantibodies directed against tumor-associated proteins in the serum of women who have breast cancer compared with non–tumor-bearing controls. Investigations of antibody immunity against single antigens have demonstrated that the presence of such antibodies can be a reflection of oncogenic protein expression in breast cancer. The HER-2/neu (HER2) protein is overexpressed in about 25% of breast cancers and is one of the most commonly studied breast cancer antigens. In an evaluation of 107 recently diagnosed breast cancer patients and 200 women who did not have breast cancer, HER2 autoantibodies could be detected in the serum of 11% of the breast cancer patients but none of control samples. Furthermore, the presence of HER2 autoantibodies correlated with HER2 overexpression as 20% of HER2-positive patients had detectable autoantibodies compared with 5% of HER2-negative breast cancer patients.[26] The likelihood of developing humoral immunity to HER2 has been shown to increase with increasing HER2 protein overexpression in the tumor. An assessment of HER2 antibodies in 104 women with breast cancer demonstrated that 82% of patients with 3+ HER2 expression in their tumors had detectable HER2 autoantibodies compared with 18% of patients with 2+ tumor HER2 expression, and 0% of patients with 1+ tumor HER2 expression as measured by immunohistochemistry (IHC) ($p < .001$). Furthermore, there was an increase in the magnitude of the HER2 antibody response with increasing levels of overexpression of the HER2 protein ($p = .02$).[27] The p53 protein is found in abundance in the tumors of approximately 50% of breast cancer patients. Studies have shown that autoantibodies to the p53 protein can be detected in up to half of all women with breast cancer. In one analysis of 82 patients with stage I–II breast cancer, 48% of patients had detectable autoantibodies to p53.[28] Similarly, an investigation of 24 non-metastatic breast cancer patients demonstrated 47% had evidence of p53 autoantibodies at initial diagnosis.[29] The decline in p53 antibody titer paralleled treatment in some patients, whereas an increase in titers preceded relapse in others. A recent evaluation of more than 100 breast cancer patient sera identified autoantibodies to Breast Cancer Susceptibility Gene *(BRCA)1* in 19% of serum samples and 37% of samples contained detectable antibody titers to *BRCA2* reflecting disease pathogenesis.[30]

There are many tumor-associated proteins that elicit autoantibodies in breast cancer patients, and these few examples demonstrate that breast cancer patients mount antibody responses to the oncogenic proteins that are present their disease. Investigations of antibody immunity to single antigens, however, demonstrate that only a minority of breast cancer patients develops autoantibodies to a particular antigen expressed in their tumor. Common examples are shown in Table 71.1.[31–38] Furthermore, each breast cancer subtype is likely to have significant variability in the types of tumor-associated antigens expressed, thus the use of single antigens as diagnostic biomarkers may not be the optimal method of exploiting the humoral immune response for breast cancer detection. Investigators have therefore begun to assess autoantibody panels for breast cancer diagnostics.

TABLE 71.1	Common Autoantibodies Expressed in Breast Cancer	
Autoantibody	% Patients With Antibody Response	%Tumors Overexpressing Antigen
MUC1	24[31]	38[32]
SURVIVIN	24[33]	65[34]
P53	48[28]	43[35]
SOX2	18[36]	33[37]
HER2	11[26]	30[38]

Unlike circulating tumor cells or tumor DNA that are typically detected in the presence of bulky tumor, serum autoantibodies can be detected in the presence of small or even preinvasive lesions. Breast cancer–associated autoantibodies have been identified in women with preinvasive breast cancer and have also been detected retrospectively in the serum of women before a breast cancer diagnosis.[39,40] These observations and the understanding that humoral immunity is a reflection of the malignant antigenic repertoire has led to the exploration of the use of panels of autoantibodies to diagnose breast cancer. The evaluation of panels of tumor-associated autoantibodies has been shown to improve diagnostic sensitivity and specificity over the assessment of individual antigens alone. In a study of 184 advanced-stage breast cancer patients and 134 control individuals, p53 specific antibody immunity could not discriminate between the two populations (area under the curve [AUC] 0.48, $p = .538$). A combination of the detection of p53 and HER2 specific antibodies increased both sensitivity and specificity to distinguish breast cancer patient sera from controls (AUC 0.61, $p = .006$). If four antigens (p53, HER2, topoisomerase 2 [TOPO2A], and insulin-like growth factor-binding protein 2 [IGFBP2]) were assessed, breast cancer patient sera could be more readily identified with an AUC 0.63 ($p = .001$).[41]

Several studies have now shown the potential for autoantibody panels to detect breast cancer. In one investigation evaluating 137 patients and testing for six antibodies (p53, mucin 1 [MUC1], c-myc, New York Esophageal Cancer-1 [NY-ESO-1], BRCA2, and HER2), 64% of patients with early invasive breast cancer and 45% of patients with ductal carcinoma in situ (DCIS) were positive for at least one of the antigens providing a sensitivity of 85%, despite positivity to single antigens ranging from 3% to 34%.[42] A study of 60 patients with primary breast cancer, 82 patients with DCIS and 93 controls demonstrated the detection of five autoantibodies (peptidylprolyl isomerase A [PPIA], peroxiredoxin 2 [PRDX2], FK506 binding protein 4 [FKBP52], heat shock protein family D [HSP60], and MUC1) could discriminate invasive breast cancer (AUC 0.73, 95% CI 0.60–0.79) and DCIS (AUC 0.80, 95% CI 0.71–0.85) from control sera.[43] A second autoantibody panel could discriminate DCIS sera from samples derived from patients with invasive breast cancer. This study used protein microarray analysis to identify overexpressed immunogenic proteins in DCIS versus invasive breast cancer serum samples. Five autoantibody targets (recombination signal binding protein for immunoglobulin kappa J region [RPBJκ], high mobility group nucleosome binding domain 1 [HMGN1], proline/serine rich coiled coil 1 [PSRC1], cold inducible RNA binding protein [CIRBP], and ethylmalonyl-CoA decarboxylase 1 [ECHDC1]) could distinguish DCIS from invasive breast cancer with AUC 0.794 (95% CI 0.674–0.877). Among patients with DCIS, higher antibody levels against these antigens could differentiate higher grade (grade 3) from low and intermediate grade (grade 1 and 2) DCIS (AUC 0.749, 95% CI 0.581–0.866) as well as identify patients who had inferior relapse-free survival ($p = .011$).[44]

Retrospective studies provide evidence that autoantibodies against tumor-associated proteins can be detected well before the diagnosis of breast cancer. Using serum collected from a longitudinal analysis of the Women's Health Initiative, panels of autoantibodies have been able to differentiate serum samples derived from women who eventually developed breast cancer from samples collected from women who did not develop breast cancer. In an evaluation of a panel of three autoantibodies (HER2, p53, and cyclin B1), samples from women who would develop breast cancer could be distinguished from control serum samples drawn more than 150 days before a cancer diagnosis with AUC 0.60 (95% CI 0.46–0.73).[40] Serum proteomic evaluation of similar serum samples identified numerous autoantibodies associated with the glycolysis and spliceosome pathways that provided AUCs of 0.68 (95% CI 0.59–0.78) and 0.73 (95% CI 0.63–0.82), respectively, to predict those women who would eventually develop breast cancer.[45] These data suggest humoral immunity is operative early in the course of breast cancer and that autoantibody panels may be useful to diagnose breast cancer either as a single modality or in conjunction with other forms of screening such as mammography. Large-scale validation trials are needed to fully assess the utility of the approach.

Prognostic Role of Tumor-Infiltrating Lymphocytes

The cellular immune infiltrate found in the stroma surrounding a breast cancer as well as infiltrating the tumor parenchyma indicates the immune system has recognized the cancer and has mounted an immune response against that tumor. The presence and levels of tumor-infiltrating lymphocytes (TILs) have been shown to predict both prognosis and response to therapy across many tumor types, including breast cancer. Initial studies of the importance of TILs to influence response to chemotherapy in breast cancers have focused on the evaluation of patients undergoing neoadjuvant chemotherapy. In the neoadjuvant setting, the development of a pathologic complete response (pCR) after treatment is used as a surrogate end point for improved survival.[46,47] An evaluation of TILs in 1058 patients undergoing neoadjuvant chemotherapy for locally advanced breast cancer demonstrated that some patients' tumors contained greater than 60% lymphocytic infiltrate and were termed "lymphocyte predominant." Those patients with lymphocyte-predominant breast cancer (LPBC) were more likely to obtain a pCR by multivariate analysis both in a test (42% pCR with LPBC and 3% pCR without LPBC, HR 1.38, 95% CI 1.08–1.78, $p = .012$) and validation set (40% pCR with LPBC and 7% pCR without LPBC HR 1.21, 95% CI 1.08–1.35, $p = .001$). Tumors of patients with the triple-negative subtype of breast cancer had the highest percentage of LPBC.[48] This observation has been confirmed in a second trial of 580 patients with triple-negative and HER2-positive disease in which increased pCR was associated with LPBC (HR 1.2, 95% CI 1.16–1.36, $p < .001$).[49]

The prognostic role of TILs predicting improved overall and disease-free survival in breast cancer has also been evaluated in several large adjuvant chemotherapy trials. In these studies, the beneficial role TILs in predicting improved overall survival was seen only in the triple-negative breast cancer subtype. In one study of node positive patients, enrolled in the Breast International Group (BIG) 02-98 adjuvant study, for every 10% increase in TILs in the tumors of patients with triple-negative breast cancer, there was a 17% decrease in risk of recurrence and 27% decrease risk of death. Triple-negative breast cancer patients whose tumors demonstrated LPBC enjoyed a 5-year disease-free survival of 92% (compared with 62% if there was <10% TILs, $p = .018$) and a 5-year overall survival of 92% (compared with 71% if there was <10% TILs, $p = .036$). The improvement in overall and disease-free survival associated with LPBC was not observed for hormone receptor–positive, HER2-negative, or HER2-positive breast cancers.[50] Very similar survival benefits in triple-negative breast cancer have been validated in subsequent large clinical cohorts receiving adjuvant chemotherapy. In one study of 481 triple-negative breast cancer patients who received adjuvant chemotherapy, each 10% increase in stromal TILs was associated with a 14% reduction in risk of recurrence (HR 0.84, 95% CI 0.74–0.95, $p = .005$) and 19% increase in overall survival (HR 0.79, 95% CI 0.62–0.92, $p = .003$).[51] These retrospective analyses demonstrate that, for triple-negative breast cancer, the benefit of TILs is not only in tumors with the highest immune infiltrate but that there is an additive effect on prognosis with each increase of 10% of TILs in the tumor. The location of TILs in breast cancer is not as critical as has been reported in other tumor types. Both intraepithelial and stromal TILs have been shown to be prognostic. Because stromal TILs appear to be found in more abundance than intratumoral TILs, many studies only report the number of lymphocytes that are present at the stromal barrier.

The phenotype of the immune response generated is also important in prognosis. Although increased Th1 TILs have consistently predicted improved prognosis in breast cancer, the benefit has been primarily observed in the triple-negative breast cancer subtype. One large study of 1334 breast cancers demonstrated that an increased level of CD8+ tumor T-cell infiltrate predicted improved overall survival across all breast cancers (HR 0.55, 95% CI 0.39–0.78, $p < .001$). When the subtypes were evaluated separately, however, breast cancer–specific and disease-free survival benefit was only observed for triple-negative tumors.[52] In one small study of 102 HER2-positive breast tumors, presence of the Th1 transcription factor Tbox transcription factor 21 (Tbet) in TILs predicted a survival benefit when increased after trastuzumab therapy, but this marker has not been consistently evaluated in larger data sets.[53] The presence of FOXP3+ Treg TILs is associated with an unfavorable prognosis.

An evaluation of 237 breast cancers revealed increased Treg tumor infiltrates, defined by FOXP3 expression on the lymphocytes, was associated with inferior progression-free survival (HR 2.15, 95% CI 1.10–4.17, $p = .03$) and overall survival (HR 2.4, 95% CI 1.07–5.38, $p = .03$) in hormone receptor–positive tumors.[54] This result has been confirmed in a second study of 1270 breast cancers, which showed that FOXP3+ TIL infiltrate greater than the median predicted worse progression-free (HR 1.90, 95% CI 1.12–3.22, $p = .018$) and overall (HR 1.53, 95% CI 1.04–2.25, $p = .029$) survival.[55] Data suggest that subtype-specific differences can affect tumor immune recognition and may affect the composition of TILs. The triple-negative subtype is most likely to contain the greatest amount of lymphocytic immune infiltrate of any of the subtypes.[56] Hormone receptor–positive tumors tend to have the fewest tumors with LPBC and the greatest number of patients with no lymphocytic infiltrate. However, patients with HER2-positive tumors have similar levels of TILs to triple-negative breast cancer and yet have not experienced the same survival benefit seen with increasing levels of TILs in triple-negative breast cancers.[57] Future studies of TILs should evaluate breast cancer subtypes separately when examining the effect of specific tumor-infiltrating immune cell populations on prognosis.

More work is needed to determine whether an evaluation of TILs should be added to the standard staging system for breast cancer. An international consortium has developed recommendations for the enumeration of breast cancer TILs, which include the locations of TILs to be examined, how to quantitate TILs, the number of tissue sections to be evaluated, and the instruction that TILs be assessed as a continuous parameter.[58] In the future, the evaluation of the existing tumor immune infiltrate at diagnosis may provide important prognostic information or even act as a guide as to whether a patient will benefit from the addition of immune therapy to standard treatment regimens.

Immunologic Effects of Standard Breast Cancer Therapies

Breast cancer treatments with immunologically mediated mechanisms of action are currently the standard of care for HER2-positive breast cancer. Monoclonal antibodies induce antibody-dependent cell-mediated cytotoxicity (ADCC) that results in the activation of NK T cells, macrophages, and dendritic cells.[59–61] Activation of cells of the innate immune system leads to the secretion of Th1 cytokines, enhanced antigen processing, and presentation of endogenous tumor antigens to T cells eliciting an adaptive immune response. These immune effects are evident in studies of patients receiving trastuzumab. In an analysis of 38 HER2-positive patients, the use of trastuzumab resulted in increased NK T cells both infiltrating the tumor ($p = .0532$) and in the surrounding tissue ($p = .0097$) compared with the patients not receiving the monoclonal antibody.[59] Furthermore, in a similar evaluation of 26 metastatic breast cancer patients, increased NK T-cell activity was associated with increased progression-free survival ($p = .024$).[62] Patients treated with trastuzumab also demonstrate increased TILs compared with those not receiving monoclonal antibody therapy. Patients treated with trastuzumab (n = 38) increased both intratumoral CD4$^+$ T-cell infiltrate ($p = .02$) and stromal CD8$^+$ T-cell infiltrate ($p = .05$) compared with patients not treated with trastuzumab (n = 23). Furthermore, CD8$^+$ T-cell infiltration predicted pCR in the trastuzumab-treated arm ($p = .05$).[59] There is increasing evidence that trastuzumab therapy results in the development of HER2-specific adaptive immunity. In 40 patients with stage I–III HER2-positive disease receiving adjuvant chemotherapy plus trastuzumab, patients with pCR (n = 16) had increased levels of circulating IFN-γ secreting HER2 specific CD4$^+$ T cells compared with those without pCR (98% vs. 33%, $p = .0002$). In addition, the HER2-specific Th1 response was independently associated with pCR by multivariate analysis (odds ratio [OR] 8.82, 95% CI 1.50–51.83, $p = .016$).[63] These data indicate the immune response elicited by trastuzumab potentially improves clinical outcome. Early studies suggest that a quantitative assessment of HER2 specific Th1 immunity may be a marker of the therapeutic efficacy of the drug.

TABLE 71.2	Immunologic Effects of Common Chemotherapeutic Agents Used in Breast Cancer Treatment
Chemotherapy	**Immunologic Effects**
Doxorubicin[64,71]	Increases antitumor immune recognition through TLR4-like stress signals
Taxanes[53,66,67,74]	Increases antitumor CD4$^+$ tumor infiltrate by increasing expression of Th1 cytokines and decreases intratumoral Th2 regulatory T cells
Cyclophosphamide[76]	Decreases peripheral circulating Th2 regulatory T cells without affecting circulating Th1 immune cells at low doses
Gemcitabine[68]	Increases MHC class 1 expression on tumors
Cisplatin/carboplatin[69,70]	Increases MHC class 1 expression and decreases MDSC and Th2 regulatory T cells in the tumor
Trastuzumab/pertuzumab[59,63]	Increases ADCC NK T-cell recruitment to tumors by recognition of FC portions of the targeted antibody therapy

ADCC, Antibody-dependent cell-mediated cytotoxicity; *FC,* fragment crystallizable region; *MDSC,* myeloid-derived suppressor cell; *MHC,* major histocompatibility complex; *NK,* natural killer; *Th1,* type 1 CD4$^+$ T helper cells; *Th2,* type 2 CD4$^+$ T helper cells; *TLR4,* toll-like receptor 4.

Therapeutic chemotherapy regimens have been selected for the cytotoxic effect of specific drug combinations against rapidly dividing cancer cells. Other cell types with high turnover rates are also adversely affected by chemotherapy, such as cells in the gastrointestinal tract and hematopoietic cells. The ability of chemotherapy to significantly reduce numbers of immune cells resulting in immune suppression in some cases has led to the wide-held belief that cytotoxic chemotherapy generally depresses immunity. There is emerging evidence that certain forms of chemotherapy may actually increase immune recognition and aid in the development of effective antitumor immunity through specific immunologic mechanisms (Table 71.2).[64–70] For example, the immune system is variably triggered by different forms of cell death. Normal apoptotic cell turnover induces immune tolerance whereas infection and inflammation triggers cellular stress receptors that induce immune activation. These stress signals are recognized through toll-like receptors (TLR) and other pattern recognition receptors in dendritic cells causing dendritic cell activation, maturation, antigen processing, and T-cell activation. Some chemotherapeutic agents have been shown to trigger immune recognition of the tumor by induction of specific proteins released during cell death. Doxorubicin, for example, induces the secretion of a protein called high-mobility-group box 1 (HMGB1) by dying cancer cells. HMGB1 binds to TLR-4 on dendritic cells resulting in the secretion of IFN-γ, antigen presentation, and activation of T cells.[71] The resulting adaptive immune response may be a major mechanism of effective clinical responses after doxorubicin treatment. A TLR-4 genetic polymorphism, Asp299Gly, has been shown to decrease the binding of HMGB1 thereby decreasing IFN-γ secretion by 50% ($p < .05$) in in vitro assays. In an evaluation of 280 breast cancer patients treated with adjuvant anthracycline, 40% of the patients carrying the TLR-4 Asp299Gly polymorphism developed metastatic disease in 5 years compared with 27% of patients that did not bear the polymorphism (RR 1.53, 95% CI 1.1–3.59, p = .03). Similarly, preapoptotic release of calreticulin induces immunogenic cell death not only for anthracyclines but for oxaliplatin and cisplatin as well.[72]

Specific chemotherapy use is associated with an increased influx of immune system cells into the tumor. Anthracyclines are cornerstones of breast cancer neoadjuvant and adjuvant chemotherapy and, in preclinical mouse models, have been shown to increase CD8[+] tumor T-cell infiltrates. When evaluating gene expression panels from breast cancer patients, 1062 patients who did not receive chemotherapy and 114 patients who received anthracycline monotherapy, the CD8 (HR 0.72, 95% CI 0.59–0.82, p = .005) and IFN-γ (HR 0.56, 95% CI 0.56–0.89, p = .016) tumor expression predicted improved pCR only in the patients who had been treated with an anthracycline.[73] This study suggests that some of the clinical efficiency of anthracycline-based chemotherapy may be due to the enhanced immune infiltration. Similar results have been observed when examining CD8[+] tumor T-cell infiltrate by immunohistochemistry in 368 triple-negative breast cancer patients were improved from 31% to 74% (95% CI 2.49–16.08, p < .0001) when patients were treated with anthracyclines and demonstrated CD8[+] TILs. However, pCR was not dependent on tumor-immune infiltrate in non–anthracycline-containing regimens.[74]

Some standard chemotherapies have the potential to induce more effective immunity by limiting the outgrowth of cells that suppress the adaptive immune response. This inhibitory effect may occur at much lower doses than what is used for cytoreduction. Very low doses of paclitaxel have recently been shown to decrease the accumulation of MDSC that limit T-cell activation in a preclinical melanoma model.[75] The use of low-dose paclitaxel reduced the chronic inflammation seen with growing malignancy and enhanced CD8[+] T-cell effector functions. Similarly, low-dose cyclophosphamide can deplete regulatory T cells without affecting levels of effector T cells.[76] In a study of 12 metastatic breast cancer patients, low-dose oral cyclophosphamide (50 mg daily) resulted in a short-term 40% reduction in peripheral Tregs (p = .002). Depletion of Tregs was associated with an increase in circulating tumor-specific T cells (p = .03) that remained elevated throughout treatment and were associated with both disease stabilization (p = .03) and overall survival (p = .027).[77] The current evidence suggests that common chemotherapies may affect the tumor immune environment in different ways and that many of the cornerstone drugs used in breast cancer treatment are associated with enhancing immunity which may be linked to improved clinical outcomes.

Breast Cancer Vaccines

The goal of a breast cancer vaccine is to educate the patient's immune system to recognize the cancer and elicit an antitumor immune response capable of destroying any current tumor and providing durable immune surveillance to prevent disease recurrence. Most of the early studies of breast cancer vaccines focused on glycosylated antigens that were ubiquitously expressed on most breast cancers. Antigens such as MUC1 or sialyl-TN were constructed as vaccines using a variety of adjuvants and studied for immunogenicity and clinical efficacy in a number of settings in breast cancer but the results of phase III studies were not

encouraging. A double-blind randomized phase III trial of sialyl-TN with keyhole limpet hemocyanin (KLH) as an adjuvant versus KLH alone enrolled 1028 women with metastatic breast cancer. There was no difference in time to progression or overall survival between vaccinated and nonvaccinated patients.[78] A pilot phase III study of a mannan-MUC1 vaccine construct demonstrated that although the vaccine could generate antibody immunity in majority of patients vaccinated, few individuals developed T-cell immunity potentially needed for tumor eradication.[79] These two studies underscore the pitfalls of early vaccines: the vaccines were poorly immunogenic and the glycosylated antigens were more likely to induce antibodies of the immunoglobulin (Ig)M subtype that are short-lived and incapable of further activating immunity. Newer approaches to vaccinating with carbohydrate-based vaccines are focusing on methods to increase the conversion of IgM to IgG antibodies, which are more potent in triggering innate immune cells, leading to cross-priming for tumor-specific T cells.[80]

Most current phase II and III vaccine trials are targeting non-mutated self-proteins that are immunogenic and tumor associated. Many of these proteins are markedly overexpressed in cancer compared with tissues that express basal levels of these proteins. Studies in autoimmune disease have demonstrated that overexpression of self-proteins results in a unique MHC-peptide repertoire display associated with unmasking of subdominant epitopes that have not been previously available for immune recognition.[81] Thus, overexpression of cancer-associated proteins can allow the T-cell response to be selective to the cancer tissues because of the higher expression of subdominant epitopes.[82] One of the most commonly studied vaccine targets in breast cancer is the HER2 protein. The degree of HER2 overexpression can trigger both increasing antibody and T-cell responses.[26,27,83] Several HER2 vaccines have been shown to be safe, immunogenic, and have evidence of clinical response in early trials. In a study of 22 HER2-positive metastatic breast cancer patients receiving a peptide-based HER2 vaccine targeting class II MHC binding epitopes with granulocyte macrophage colony stimulation factor as an adjuvant, 74% of the patients developed new or augmented HER2-specific Th1 immunity. Both intramolecular and intermolecular epitope spreading developed, with 71% of evaluated patients developing augmented Th1 immunity to oncogenic proteins other than HER2. In this trial, the median progression-free survival was 33% at 3 years with overall survival of 86% at 4 years. Increased HER2 specific T-cell responses trended to improved overall survival (p = .08) suggesting that development of immunity may be a factor for the improved outcomes.[84] HER2-specific vaccines have been explored in the adjuvant setting as well in patients with early-stage breast cancer. In a pooled analysis of phase I/II studies that evaluated immunization with a short peptide vaccine targeting a HER2 epitope that has been shown to induce cytotoxic T cells in human leukocyte antigen (HLA) A2/A2 positive patients (E75), a 24-month landmark analysis demonstrated that disease-free survival was 94.3% in the vaccinated group and 86.8% in the control group (p = .08).[85] In a subset analysis, the beneficial outcome was associated with receiving the optimal dose of the vaccine, having a grade 1 or 2 tumor, and the presence of positive lymph nodes. Furthermore, those patients with the lowest levels of HER2 expression on their tumors as measured by IHC (1–2+) appeared to have a more favorable outcome than those who demonstrated 3+ overexpression. Whether this observation was due to the more aggressive nature of tumors that highly express HER2 was not explored.

The E75 vaccine, now called NeuVax, is in the final stages of a phase III study to prevent disease recurrence. HER2 vaccination has also been evaluated for the treatment of DCIS.[86] Patients with DCIS were vaccinated with a HER2 peptide-based vaccine. The majority of patients vaccinated developed significant levels of HER2-specific CD4[+] and CD8[+] T cells. Seven of 11 evaluable patients also showed decreased HER2 expression in the surgical tumor specimen, often with measurable decreases in HER2 expression in residual DCIS. These early data, using similar vaccines against a single antigen, suggest a potential role for vaccination in all stage of HER2-positive breast cancer to improve clinical outcomes.

Other self-antigens have also been used in breast cancer vaccination. Mammaglobin-A is overexpressed in 80% of hormone receptor–positive breast cancer, and a trial was performed using a DNA vaccine that stimulated antigen-specific CD8[+] T cells in 57% of patients (8 of 14) with metastatic breast cancer. Vaccinated patients had an improved progression-free survival at 6 months of 53% compared with 33% ($p = .011$) in patients who were unable to be vaccinated based on HLA phenotype but otherwise met trial enrollment criteria.[2] Studies have also been performed using vaccines to enhance chemotherapy. The PANVAC vaccine is a poxvirus vaccine that expresses carcinoembryonic antigen (CEA) and MUC1 as epitopes, along with costimulatory molecules B7.1, intracellular adhesion molecule 1 (ICAM1), and lymphocyte associated antigen-3 (LFA-3).[87] A phase II study of 48 patients with metastatic breast cancer evaluated docetaxel with and without PANVAC. There was a trend toward improved progression-free survival of 7.9 months compared with 3.9 months (HR 0.65, 95% CI 0.03–1.14, $p = .09$) in patients who received both vaccine and docetaxel. These studies demonstrate newer methods of vaccination are effective in eliciting cellular immunity and that vaccines may be potentiated when combined with chemotherapy. Finally, there is much work being done to define patient-specific mutations that may encode neo-antigens that may have never been exposed to the immune system. Mutated proteins that occur in cancer may truly be cancer specific because mutations would not be present in normal tissues. Although mutations may be identified in a patient's tumor, whether those mutations can be processed and presented in the MHC for T-cell recognition is unknown. The development of mutation specific vaccines for the treatment of breast cancer is an area of intense investigation.

Data from all breast cancer vaccine clinical trials to date suggest vaccines are safe and well tolerated with primarily grade 1 and 2 toxicities and no evidence clinically significant autoimmune toxicities. HER2 targeting vaccine studies show the majority of toxicities were grade 1–2 injection site reactions. Furthermore, none of the HER2 vaccines tested have had evidence of the cardiac toxicity seen with other HER2 directed therapies such as trastuzumab.[84,88] The Mammaglobin-A vaccine similarly demonstrated a favorable toxicity profile with no grade 3 toxicities and mainly infusion site grade 1 toxicities.[2] Low-risk toxicity profiles have been consistent across published breast cancer vaccine studies and will be particularly beneficial when combining vaccine therapies with other typically less well-tolerated therapies. Vaccination as monotherapy tends to be less effective in patients with a large tumor burden as advanced breast cancer display an immune suppressive tumor environment that can serve as an antigen sink, drawing the vaccine-activated immune cells to the tumor but then inactivating them and preventing effective function.[89] Therefore, vaccine therapy may show the most benefit in the adjuvant setting where there is no evidence of cancer and therefore the immune response mounted to the vaccine can acutely target minimal residual disease. For patients with more advanced disease, vaccine therapy may be more effective if used in combination with other therapies such as chemotherapy, adoptive T-cell therapy, or checkpoint inhibitor monoclonal antibody therapy.

Adoptive T-Cell Therapy

Patients with treatment-refractory metastatic breast cancer may not have the ability to mount an appropriate immune response, and any antitumor T cells present may have undergone anergy or exhaustion. T-cell exhaustion is a natural response to continued immune activation in the face of chronic antigen exposure and is meant to prevent damage from continuous inflammation. In cancer, the continued activation of T cells by tumor antigens leads to increased immune suppressive signals including increased levels of programmed death-1 (PD-1), T-cell immunoglobulin domain and mucin domain 3 (TIM3), and leukocyte activation gene 3 (LAG3), extension of the effector phase of T-cell activation preventing the development of memory T-cells, and increased immunosuppressive cytokine release in the tumor causing the antitumor T-cells present to be unable to function properly.[90] Adoptive T-cell therapy is a therapeutic strategy that expands large numbers of T cells that have been activated outside the body to avoid anergy and then infuses those cells back into the patient providing a high concentration of activated, tumor-specific T cells that may traffic to all sites of disease. Adoptive T-cell therapy does not require the patient's immune system to mount a response but rather is a passive therapy that gives back patients' expanded and activated antitumor T cells with the goal that these cells will destroy established tumors.[91] Cancer-specific T cells can be isolated from TILs, developed through immunization with antigen-specific vaccines, or produced through genetic modification of existing T cells to be highly functional against a particular tumor antigen (chimeric antigen receptor [CAR] T-cell therapy).[92] Most trials have evaluated adoptive T-cell therapy using either CD8[+] or CD4[+] T cells or a combination of both, although there are some studies showing clinical benefit by infusion other immune cell populations including NK T cells and gamma delta T cells.[93]

In tumors such as melanoma that have robust T-cell infiltrates, antitumor T cells can be identified in TILs, expanded and activated, and reinfused into the patients. Melanoma-specific T cells have demonstrated significant tumor regressions in more than 50% of treated patients.[94] However, in breast cancer, there are fewer intratumoral T cells, and therefore peripheral T cells either activated with tumor ex vivo or stimulated by vaccination are more commonly used. In a trial of 16 metastatic breast cancer patients, autologous T cells were collected from the patient's bone marrow and then activated against the breast cancer cell line MCF7 ex vivo. In this study, 44% (7 of 16) of treated patients had tumor-reactive T cells in their peripheral blood after adoptive therapy, and the patients who demonstrated immune responses displayed improved survival compared with the patients where infused T cells did not persist (58.6 compared with 13.6 months, $p = .009$).[95] Furthermore, vaccination before T-cell collection and expansion was used in a study of seven HER2-positive breast cancer patients immunized with a peptide vaccine specifically designed to stimulate HER2-specific Th1 CD4[+] T cells. In this study, 66% (4 of 7) patients had increased levels of HER2-specific T cells up to 70 days after T-cell infusion, and partial clinical responses were observed in 43% of the patients (three of seven).

This study used low-dose cyclophosphamide to decrease circulating Tregs before infusion of the expanded T cells.[96] None of the published adoptive T-cell therapy trials in breast cancer have demonstrated the dramatic durable responses observed after T-cell infusions in melanoma, suggesting that further modifications are needed for the transferred T cells to show maximal function and benefit.

CAR T-cell therapy is a subset of adoptive T-cell therapy that attempts to overcome the limitations of relying on isolating tumor-infiltrating T cells or the patient producing antitumor T cells through vaccination. CAR T cells are engineered to be tumor specific, highly avid, and self-activating. A CAR T cell includes both a segment that recognizes the tumor-associated antigen and typically two activation domains that can include induced by lymphocyte activation (41BB, 137), tumor necrosis receptor super family member 4 (OX40, CD134), inducible T-cell costimulator (ICOS, CD278), or CD28 that allows optimal activation.[97] A CAR T cell designed to target HER2 included activation signal moieties to 41BB, CD28, and CD3ζ. This construct was used to treat a patient with refractory HER2-positive metastatic colon cancer. On the first infusion of the CAR T cells, the patient developed cytokine storm due to the highly activated T cells with respiratory and hemodynamic failure and eventual death.[98] The high avidity of these cells for antigen can also result in nonspecific binding of the activated T cells to normal tissues expressing basal levels of HER2. Indeed, off-target effects are a major limitation of CAR T-cell therapy in solid tumors because there are few antigens that are unique to cancer cells with no expression in normal tissues. Studies of intratumoral injections of CAR T cells, a strategy meant to limit toxicity, are currently being evaluated for therapeutic efficacy in breast cancer.[99] Moreover, CAR T cells directed against specific mutations present in a patient's tumor may allow selectivity of the T cells to the tumor and not to normal tissues. The development of mutation specific CAR T cells may mediate some of the significant toxicity associated with infusions.

Some of the causes of only limited clinical responses after adoptive T-cell therapy in breast cancer include the inability of antigen-specific T cells to completely infiltrate solid tumors because of tumor stromal barriers, lack of appropriate chemokine receptor expression on metastatic tumors, and inadequate activation of the T cells to allow tumor trafficking.[100] CAR T cells have been associated with significant toxicity due to off-target binding, and the generation of the cells may take months to develop for a particular patient. Furthermore, in many cases, CAR T cells are short-lived and do not persist for long periods of time in vivo after infusion.[101] Future studies will continue to modify adoptive T-cell transfer techniques to identify the most appropriate immune cells and to identify methods to ensure that the T cells will home to and penetrate all tumors. CAR T cells are also being designed with control elements that can modify their function and life span.[102] Adoptive T-cell therapy has the potential to become an effective immunotherapeutic in the advanced disease setting.

Immune Checkpoint Inhibitor Therapy

The activity and function of a T-cell requires a series of costimulatory signals to either maintain self-tolerance or augment the amplitude and duration of an immune response. A family of these costimulatory proteins, referred to as *immune checkpoints,* requires interactions from receptors both on the T cell and an antigen-presenting cell or tumor cell. Signals generated from the interaction of receptors include both activating and repressing costimulatory signals that affect the function of the T cell.[103] Targeted monoclonal antibodies that block inhibitory T cell signals including cytotoxic t-lymphocyte-associated protein 4 (CTLA-4, CD152) and PD-1 on the T cell or programmed death ligand-1 (PDL-1) on the tumor cell have shown marked clinical responses in subsets of patients with metastatic cancers including melanoma, bladder cancer, and lung cancer.[104–106] Breast cancers have been shown to express increased levels of checkpoint inhibitor proteins, particularly high-grade tumors and the triple-negative subtype.[107,108]

Expression of PDL-1 has been associated with increased TILs in the tumor (HR 0.268, 95% CI 0.099–0.721, $p = .009$).[107] A study that evaluated 105 breast cancers for both PDL-1 and TILs demonstrated that PDL-1 expression was found in 30% of the tumors and was associated with the presence of TILs. This study also evaluated pCR after neoadjuvant chemotherapy and found that both increased PDL-1 and increased TILs correlated with improved pCR.[109] The upregulation of PDL-1 protein, in the presence of TILs, reveals the dynamic nature of this immune receptor and the role of inflammation in influencing both PDL-1 and PD-1 expression. This observation underscores the difficulty of the use of PDL-1 protein expression to identify patients likely to respond to immune checkpoint inhibitor therapy.[110]

In early trials, treatment with immune checkpoint inhibitor–specific monoclonal antibodies has been modestly effective in the treatment of breast cancer. Initially, anti-PD-1 therapy was thought to be ineffective in breast cancer because none of the breast cancer patients included in the initial anti-PD-1 trials showed any response to treatment.[104] Furthermore, in a study of tremelimumab, an anti-CTLA-4 monoclonal antibody, and exemestane in metastatic breast cancer, the only clinical response was stable disease with a duration of a minimum of 12 weeks in 42% (11 of 26) of patients.[111] Recently data have emerged that demonstrate clinical activity with the use of immune checkpoint inhibitor therapy in breast cancer. In a trial of 168 patients receiving the anti-PDL-1 monoclonal antibody, avelumab, which included 43% hormone receptor–positive, 35% triple-negative, and 16% HER2-positive breast cancers (7% unknown subtype), there was a 28% disease control rate including a 4.8% overall response rate (95% CI 2.1–9.2). Disease control included one complete response and seven partial responses as well as 23% of patients with stable disease after a median follow-up of 10 months. Although the majority of clinical responses were in triple-negative breast cancer, 3% were found in HR-positive disease, and 4% were found in HER2-positive disease.[112] When evaluating the triple-negative breast cancer subtype alone, overall responses to anti-PD-1 therapy are better than that seen in any of the other subtypes. In one study of 27 patients with tumors that overexpressed PDL-1, there was an 18.5% overall response rate to pembrolizumab (an anti-PD-1 monoclonal antibody). These responses included one complete response (4%), four partial responses (15%), and seven patients with stable disease (26%).[3] Addition of nab-paclitaxel chemotherapy to the checkpoint inhibitor atezolizumab (an anti-PDL-1 monoclonal antibody) in 24 patients with triple-negative breast cancer demonstrated a confirmed overall response rate of 42% (95% CI 22.1–63.4) as well as five patients with stable disease after 12 months on the study.[113] However, despite most clinical data showing triple-negative breast cancer with the best response to immune checkpoint inhibitor therapy, one study of 25 patients with hormone receptor–positive breast cancer that overexpressed PDL-1 reported an overall response rate of 12% (95% CI 2.5–31.2) to pembrolizumab (3 partial responses and no complete responses) and 4 patients with stable disease (16%).[114] These data suggest that there may be a role for immune checkpoint inhibitor therapy in all subtypes of breast cancer. Currently, there are other immune checkpoint therapies now in clinical trials beyond anti-CTL-4 and anti-PD-1/PDL-1 therapies including coactivation therapies OX40, OX40 ligand, and 41BB.[115,116] These coactivation antibodies have been shown to inhibit mammary tumor growth in preclinical models and several clinical trials are currently ongoing.[117–119] In breast cancer, immune checkpoint inhibitor therapy will most likely have the greatest efficacy when used in combination with other immunomodulatory approaches focused on increasing TILs so that blocking immune checkpoint inhibitor proteins will augment both the number and function of tumor-infiltrating T cells to the clinical benefit of the patient.

Immuno-Prevention of Breast Cancer

Increased immune infiltrate is seen in breast lesions from the earliest evidence of atypia suggesting that the immune system recognizes and mounts an immune response against preinvasive breast disease.[120] Unfortunately, similar to invasive breast cancer, the immune infiltrate that most commonly develops in preinvasive breast cancer is a Th2 infiltrate that may inhibit a cancer lytic immune response.[4] Immune infiltrates have been shown to predict outcome in lesions as limited as DCIS. In a study of 62 DCIS tumors, lesions that demonstrated increased FOXP3+ TILs (mean 4 per high-power field, $p = .01$) compared with normal breast (mean 0.5 per high-power field) and patients with FOXP3+ TIL infiltration higher than the mean had worse disease-free survival (HR 2.81, 95% CI 0.99–7.99, $p = .05$) and increased risk of recurrence ($p = .04$).[54] Similarly, in gene expression studies evaluating DCIS, genes associated with Th1 immunity predicted improved relapse-free survival.[121] These data indicate that adaptive immunity is operative at the earliest stages of the malignant transformation in breast cancer setting the stage for immune intervention to prevent the development of the disease. Two methods of breast cancer immuno-prevention include drug therapy and prophylactic vaccines. Both modalities can increase the immune system's ability to recognize and destroy developing breast cancer cells before developing invasive disease.

The most effective chemoprevention agents in breast cancer have been tamoxifen and aromatase inhibitors. The use of these agents in the prophylactic setting can provide up to a 65% relative reduction in the incidence of breast cancer.[122,123] The clinical efficacy of aromatase inhibitors may have an immune component as estrogen has been shown to decrease the expression of the IFN-γ inducible MHC receptors on tumor cells preventing antitumor immune recognition of the tumor. In human breast cancer cell lines, treatment of the cells with estradiol decreased HLA DRα expression by increasing estrogen receptor-α (ERα) even with IFN-γ stimulation. Furthermore, degradation of ERα allowed increased HLA DRα even when treated with estradiol.[124] In a phase II trial conducted in locally advanced, hormone receptor–positive postmenopausal breast cancer patients, letrozole as a single agent could reduce the levels of FOXP3+ Tregs in 82% of patients ($p = .0001$). Decreased Tregs were associated with the development of a clinical response ($p < .03$).[125] Other well-studied chemoprevention agents, potentially effective in breast cancer prophylaxis, have also been shown to have immunologic mechanisms of action. The use of aspirin is established for the prevention of

colon cancer; however, a meta-analysis of case-control studies in breast cancer suggests a role for aspirin in breast cancer prevention. Routine low-dose aspirin was found to decrease the risk of breast cancer (OR 0.81, 95% CI 0.71–0.93 evaluating 196,087 patients).[126] Cyclooxygenase 2 (COX2) has been found to be overexpressed in both breast cancer (43% of 42 tumors) and DCIS (63% of 16 tumors) and is associated with aggressive disease.[127] In vitro data have demonstrated that prostaglandin E2, which is increased by COX2 expression, can induce monocyte differentiation to MDSC and increase the immune inhibitory effect of regulatory T cells.[128–130] Therefore aspirin and/or COX2 inhibitors may decrease the function of immune suppressive cells, improving immune recognition of developing tumor. Metformin has also been associated with a reduced risk of developing breast cancer in a meta-analysis (RR 0.88, 95% CI 0.75–1.03, $I^2 = 60\%$, 13 studies).[131] Metformin can both increase Th1 memory T cells through 5′ adenosine monophosphate-activated protein kinase (AMPK) activation and MHC class I expression in evolving tumor cells and enhance the interaction of CD8+ T cells with antigen.[132,133] A pharmacologic approach to breast cancer prevention depends on the patient's adherence to taking daily medication often for prolonged periods of time. Compliance with daily drug dosing can be a major barrier to effective prevention.[134,135] Vaccines that could elicit immunologic memory may provide protection from breast cancer for an extended period of time after limited short-term dosing.

Therapeutic breast cancer vaccines have been shown to be well tolerated and may also provide durable immune surveillance without requiring daily compliance to medications.[84,86,88] Furthermore, use of vaccines as a monotherapy should be effective in breast cancer prevention because preinvasive disease is slow growing, the patients have a low tumor burden, and the patient's immune system has not been suppressed either by tumor or chemotherapy.[136] The goal of a prophylactic breast cancer vaccine would be stimulate T-cell memory against appropriate antigens, which would be presented to the immune system at the earliest stages of breast cancer transformation. Proof of concept has been demonstrated in transgenic mouse models of mammary carcinogenesis. Transgenic FVB mice that overexpress human HER2 spontaneously develop tumors by a median of 45 weeks; every-2-week vaccination with a chimeric human-rat anti-HER2 DNA vaccine for the lifetime of the mouse was able to prevent tumor development in 65% of the animals up to 90 weeks and to reduce the number of tumors in the mice that did develop mammary tumors.[137] Furthermore, vaccinating with an anti-α lactalbumin DNA vaccine in transgenic mice that overexpress rat neu (TgMMTV_neu) and develop spontaneous tumors were able to completely protect the mice from tumor development at 10 months ($p = .0004$).

The protein α lactalbumin has been found overexpressed the majority of breast cancers but otherwise is only expressed in lactating breasts.[138] An additional investigation vaccinated transgenic mice that overexpress both polyomavirus middle T and the oncogene MUC1 and where all animals spontaneously develop mammary tumors within a median of 15 weeks. Dendritic cells fused with tumor cells overexpressing MUC1 were used for immunization. This whole tumor vaccine prevented tumor development in 60% of mice at 180 weeks.[139] Another example vaccinates transgenic mice with multiple antigens using a tri-antigen vaccine targeting HER2, IGFBP2, and IGF1R in the TgMMTV_neu model. All three of these proteins are overexpressed in both DCIS and invasive breast cancer, and that overexpression is associated with progression to invasive cancer.[140–142] The mice were vaccinated at 18 weeks when the majority of the mice already had hyperplastic premalignant breast lesions. The vaccine prevented tumor development in 65% of the mice compared with adjuvant alone. Even the mice that developed tumors after immunization had a longer overall survival and slower tumor growth with increased intratumoral CD8+ T-cell infiltration. In combination with bexarotene, vaccination resulted in protection from mammary cancer in more than 95% of mice with pathologic examination showing no evidence of DCIS. The use of three antigens together resulted in a longer disease-free survival than vaccination with any of the individual antigens alone.[143] This vaccine is now in clinical trials in early-stage breast cancer.

Most currently contemplated prophylactic breast cancer vaccine approaches focus on immunization with antigens that have been defined in patients with existing disease. Studies are ongoing to identify the earliest tumor antigens that can be used to develop vaccines for primary prevention. The lack of a uniform precursor lesion in breast cancer is a challenge for antigen discovery. Further concerns that must be addressed for breast cancer prevention vaccines, including long-term toxicity; specifically the risk of autoimmunity and any potential effects on fertility. These concerns are particularly relevant because a vaccine may be aimed at younger women in their childbearing years (e.g., women at a genetically high risk of developing breast cancer).

Conclusion

Breast cancer is an immunogenic tumor and, as has been shown from the benefit of high levels of TILs, improved immune recognition may improve clinical outcomes. Moving forward, it will be essential to assess a patient's tumor immune microenvironment at the time of diagnosis for both prognosis as well as therapeutic planning.[144] Combination immune checkpoint inhibitor therapy and chemotherapy is demonstrating significant clinical efficacy in advanced stage patients even in the second- and third-line setting and will most likely show similar efficacy in combination in the adjuvant setting.[113] Vaccines and other forms of immune modulation may provide a means by which all breast cancer patients can develop high levels of TILs. Finally, our increasing

understanding of lesions that put women at a high risk for breast cancer will facilitate the discovery of cancer-driving proteins that can be targeted by immunomodulation for breast cancer prevention.

Acknowledgments

MLD was supported by a Komen Leadership Grant, an American Cancer Society Clinical Research Professorship and the Athena Distinguished Professorship for Breast Cancer Research. SES was supported by the Institute of Translational Health Sciences, National Institutes of Health grant KL2TR000421.

Conflict of Interest

MLD is a stockholder in EpiThany and VentiRx and receives grant support from Celgene, EMD Serono, VentiRx, Jansen, and Seattle Genetics. SES and ER have no conflicts to disclose.

Selected References

4. Marquez JP, Stanton SE, Disis ML. The antigenic repertoire of premalignant and high-risk lesions. *Cancer Prev Res (Phila)*. 2015;8:266-270.
12. Fridman WH, Pages F, Sautes-Fridman C, et al. The immune contexture in human tumours: impact on clinical outcome. *Nat Rev Cancer*. 2012;12:298-306.
21. Nelson BH. CD20+ B cells: the other tumor-infiltrating lymphocytes. *J Immunol*. 2010;185:4977-4982.
58. Salgado R, Denkert C, Demaria S, et al. The evaluation of tumor-infiltrating lymphocytes (TILs) in breast cancer: recommendations by an International TILs Working Group 2014. *Ann Oncol*. 2015;26:259-271.
64. Galluzzi L, Senovilla L, Zitvogel L, et al. The secret ally: immunostimulation by anticancer drugs. *Nat Rev Drug Discov*. 2012;11:215-233.
71. Apetoh L, Ghiringhelli F, Tesniere A, et al. Toll-like receptor 4-dependent contribution of the immune system to anticancer chemotherapy and radiotherapy. *Nat Med*. 2007;13:1050-1059.
91. Rosenberg SA, Restifo NP. Adoptive cell transfer as personalized immunotherapy for human cancer. *Science*. 2015;348:62-68.

A full reference list is available online at ExpertConsult.com.

72

Diagnosis and Management of Pleural Metastases and Malignant Effusion in Breast Cancer

NICHOLAS D. TINGQUIST AND MATTHEW A. STELIGA

Pleural metastases and malignant pleural effusion may occur with metastatic breast cancer. Presentation can vary widely from an incidental finding on imaging to a large effusion with severe dyspnea. Any pleural effusion in a breast cancer patient can be suspected to be a malignant effusion until proven otherwise. The focus of the clinician should be to provide the most efficient, accurate diagnosis with the least risk of complication and pain for the patient. Overall, malignant pleural effusions account for approximately 20% to 25% of all effusions. Infectious or postinfectious etiologies are the most common cause of exudative effusion and pleural malignancies, both primary and metastatic, are the second leading cause of exudative pleural effusions,[1] estimated to number approximately 150,000 annually in the United States.[1,2] Breast cancer is second only to lung cancer as the leading cause of all pleural metastases and thus accounts for approximately one-fourth of all malignant effusions.[3,4] In women, it is the most common cause of a malignant effusion, accounting for up to 40%.[5] In this chapter, we review the magnitude and presentations of pleural metastases and malignant pleural effusion (MPE) in breast cancer, their biochemical profiles, and methods of diagnosis and management. A similar related clinical entity, malignant pericardial effusion (MPCE), is also covered.

The estimated incidence of malignant pleural involvement in breast cancer ranges from 2% to 12%.[4,6–8] Although cancer cell–positive effusions have been noted as the initial presentation of a malignancy, this is not commonly reported as the initial diagnosis of breast cancer.[9,10] Conversely, malignant breast cancer pleural metastases are a common initial presentation of disease progression or recurrence, occurring in 42% to 43% of patients.[8,11] Overall, in advanced breast cancer, pleural metastases are a common occurrence and are found in 36% to 65% of advanced disseminated diseases.[12–15] The time of initial breast cancer diagnosis to the development of malignant pleural involvement varies but averages 35 to 42 months.[10,11] The contribution of malignant pleural involvement by breast cancer toward the overall mortality and morbidity of the disease depends on the number of metastatic disease sites, total tumor burden within the pleural space, and underlying pulmonary reserve of the patient.

Pathogenesis

Although MPE can be a significant problem for those affected, the details of its pathogenesis are not clear. It appears to be a combination of factors leading to an overall increase in pleural fluid production that overwhelms its removal, thereby causing an accumulation manifest as MPE. Interestingly, pleural effusion does not occur in every patient with pleural metastases. Current research has shed light on the fact there may be certain genetic characteristics or "secretomes" carried by these tumors that do cause effusions. Tumor cells may produce vascular endothelial growth factor (VEGF) along with a host of concomitant factors. These factors interact with inflammatory cells in the mesothelium and endothelium leading to capillary leak into the pleural space that overwhelms the lymphatic system's ability to reabsorb. There is also some thought that direct tumor invasion of the lymphatics may disrupt this drainage system as well.[16]

Clinical Presentation

Symptoms associated with breast cancer pleural metastases may be related to local and systemic effects. Unlike primary pleural tumors, metastatic cancers to the pleural space, including breast cancer, rarely present as bulky metastases without pleural effusion.[17] Dyspnea is, in general, the most common presenting symptom and is often related to the size of the pleural effusion. However, up to one-fourth of patients may be asymptomatic at presentation.[4]

Pleural metastases from breast cancer result in dyspnea by causing a restrictive pulmonary physiology and gas-exchange abnormalities. The incompressible pleural fluid collection and the limited outward chest wall excursion result in compression and atelectasis of the underlying lung parenchyma. The reduction in vital capacity reduces the effective gas exchange. Although the pulmonary circulation has an adaptive hypoxic vasoconstrictive response, this is incompletely effective when there is a large effusion and when an atelectatic lobe or lung leads to significant shunting and ventilation/perfusion mismatching. Other causes of subjective dyspnea without significant hypoxemia include

Atelectasis of lung parenchyma resulting from malignant pleural effusion
Inflammatory pleurisy and chest wall pain leading to splinting
Lung parenchymal metastases
Pneumonia obscured by effusion
Pulmonary thromboembolism
Pneumonitis secondary to radiation
Left ventricular dysfunction leading to pulmonary edema
Cardiotoxicity due to antineoplastic agents
Malignant pericardial effusion and tamponade
Anemia secondary to advanced cancer or antineoplastic therapies

TABLE 72.1 Causes of Paramalignant Pleural Effusion

Cause	Transudates	Exudates
Congestive heart failure from all causes, especially bilateral effusions	++++	Rarely
Parapneumonic effusions	—	++++
Pulmonary thromboembolism	+++	+
Postobstructive atelectasis	++++	—
Hypoalbuminemia resulting from cachexia	++++	—
Associated with ascites, malignant or cirrhosis	+++	+
Chylothorax resulting from thoracic duct obstruction	—	++++
Mediastinal adenopathy, including compression of pulmonary arteries	+	+++
Superior vena cava syndrome	++++	—
Status post chest wall or mediastinal radiation	—	++++
Drug-induced pleural reactions (bleomycin, cyclophosphamide, methotrexate, mitomycin, procarbazine)	—	++++

mediastinal shifting and reflex stimulation of the chest wall and lungs as a result of altered compliance (Box 72.1).[18]

Aside from the aforementioned causes of dyspnea, other concomitant factors may contribute to breathlessness. Anemia reduces the oxygen-carrying capacity and systemic oxygen delivery and may induce a hyperdynamic cardiac response and strain. Patients are generally older and may have underlying degrees of congestive heart failure, which is often manifested as dyspnea. Risks of pulmonary thromboembolism are increased secondary to hypercoagulable states of cancers, effects of hormonal therapy, and the decreased mobility of many cancer patients. Pulmonary embolism (PE) is listed as the fourth most common cause of pleural effusions by some authors[1] and must be considered in the differential diagnosis of a "paramalignant effusion" (Table 72.1). One-fourth of PE-associated effusions may be transudative, but three fourths of them are exudative and may confound the diagnosis of a breast cancer–associated malignant effusion.

Malignant pericardial involvement should be suspected in a patient with persistent dyspnea after drainage of MPE. The patient with an MPCE may or may not have hemodynamic instability. The true incidence of MPCE associated with all breast cancer patients is unclear, but it has been reported as high as 19% in an autopsy series.[19] Of the subgroup of patients with known metastatic pleural breast cancer with pericardial spread of disease, 63% to 100% also have lung and pleural metastases at the time of MPCE diagnosis.[20,21] These patients with both breast MPE and MPCE appear to have a higher frequency of bilateral malignant effusions.[21] Dyspnea may also be a result of antineoplastic therapies. Pulmonary parenchyma can be quite radiosensitive, and radiotherapy directed against breast cancer may scatter and lead to subacute radiation pneumonitis and delayed fibrosis with restriction. Some cytotoxic chemotherapy agents have associated pulmonary toxicities, or cardiotoxicity. In addition to intrinsic lung dysfunction, cytotoxic and radiation-induced immunosuppression with concomitant structural lung damage may predispose patients to pulmonary infections. In a clinicopathologic review of the pattern of metastatic diseases and cause of death in breast cancer patients, the pulmonary system is the number one or two site of metastases, and infections account for about one-fourth of the deaths.[13,19]

Other nonspecific chest symptoms attributable to pleural metastases often include cough and, much less commonly, pleurisy and chest wall pain. Tachypnea, tachycardia, and cyanosis may be related to impaired gas exchange and hypoxemia. A large pleural effusion may transmit increased pressure to the pericardium and rarely cause a tamponade-like effect; in general, however, hypotension is not expected. Likewise, fever and hemoptysis

should prompt a search for concomitant processes such as empyema, pneumonia, sepsis, pulmonary thromboembolism, or endobronchial metastases.

Diagnosis

Radiographic Findings

Plain chest radiography is the most common radiographic means of identifying malignant pleural involvement. There is opacification of various extent of the hemithorax, ranging from blunting of the costophrenic angle on the frontal view and posterior gutter on the lateral view to complete opacification of the hemithorax, with or without a midline shift of the mediastinal structures.[22] Decubitus films to confirm a free-flowing liquid layer may be used to follow up suspicious blunting without the classic meniscus fluid sign. With the ready availability of computed tomography (CT) scans that provide superior discrimination of tissue versus fluid, advanced three-dimensional imaging can help direct diagnosis and treatment. Contrast enhancement of the parietal pleural is useful in separating exudative from transudative effusions.[23] More specific features of malignant pleural involvement include pleural nodularity and irregularity and pleural thickness greater than 1 cm.[24] Pleural surfaces thus assessed with CT scanning have a sensitivity of 87% and specificity of 100% for malignant involvement, although the sensitivity is lower for metastatic cancers versus primary pleural cancers.[24] A large pleural effusion normally shifts the mediastinum away toward the contralateral

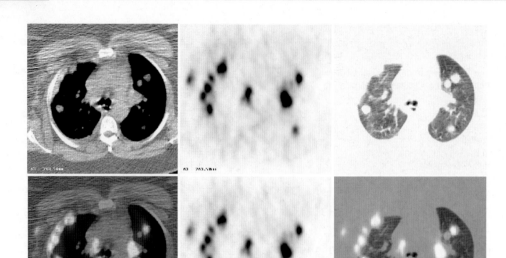

• **Fig. 72.1** Computed tomography (CT), 18-fluorodeoxy glucose positron emission tomography (FDG-PET) and fused PET-CT images of pleuropulmonary metastases from breast cancer. Disseminated stage IV breast cancer with bilateral pulmonary, mediastinal (right paratracheal and left para-aortic) nodal, right anterior pleural, right chest wall disease. Note the absence of FDG uptake in the bilateral small dependent pleural effusions but clear activity in the right anterior nodular pleural lesions. (A) Soft tissue window (*top*); fused soft tissue window (*bottom*). (B) FDG-PET. (C) Soft tissue window of the lung (*top*); fused lung and soft tissue windows (*bottom*). (Courtesy R. Wahl and C. Cohade.)

chest, sometimes causing critical compression of vascular and conducting airway structures. Therefore a midline undeviated mediastinum or even ipsilaterally deviated mediastinum in the presence of a large effusion suggests central airway obstruction leading to complete atelectasis of the lung. This should prompt an airway examination to look for endobronchial obstruction resulting from tumor or volume loss resulting from inspissated mucus. Ultrasound can complement chest films and/or CT scans to guide bedside sampling and drainage of fluid pockets, especially when these are small or may have become loculated, or when the patient physiology and physiognomy such as chronic obstructive pulmonary disease and obesity will increase the risk of complications from thoracentesis.

Most metastatic pleural effusions from breast cancer are unilateral and arise in the hemithorax ipsilateral to the initial site of disease 50% to 83% of the time.[11,25,26] Although bilateral pleural effusions have usually been attributed to left ventricular dysfunction and congestive heart failure, up to 10% of patients may have bilateral malignant effusions.[11] It should be qualified that these studies are from the era before CT scans were routinely used to assess disease progression or to identify pleural pulmonary involvement. The routine use of CT scanning may detect many smaller pleural effusions. Distribution of metastatic implants on the pleural surfaces have been studied in vivo during diagnostic and therapeutic thoracoscopy,[27,28] and this has demonstrated that a majority of the visible lesions stud the visceral pleura and the parietal pleura.[28] Given the differential blood supply and lymphatic drainage of the visceral and parietal pleural surfaces, this suggests that most pleural metastases occur in combination with and perhaps subsequent to hematogenous and lymphangitic spread of disease to the lungs. Canto-Armengod[27] observed a preponderance of ipsilateral pleural metastases studding the costal

pleura, whereas metastases to the contralateral pleura more commonly affect the mediastinal pleura.

18-Fluorodeoxy glucose positron emission tomography (FDG-PET) is accepted as an effective metabolic imaging adjunct to help characterize abnormal-appearing tissue as likely being neoplastic, inflammatory, or benign. FDG-PET has high sensitivity and specificity rates in the imaging of primary pleural cancers, as in mesothelioma.[29] FDG-PET is superior to CT alone scanning in the detection of pleural metastases in primary bronchogenic carcinoma, with a sensitivity approaching 90% and a specificity and accuracy of 94.1% and 91.4%, respectively.[30] In terms of breast cancer, FDG-PET has been used for imaging and staging of primary breast cancer, although the results for axillary and mammary nodal staging vary and depend on nodal size and the tumor proliferation index.[31] In its evaluation of disseminated metastatic disease in breast cancer, FDG-PET is at least as effective as Tc[99m]-MDP bone scanning,[32] but with regard to the pleural space, although there are case reports,[33] its efficacy in detecting metastatic disease has not been formally evaluated.

An example of FDG-PET positive pleural, lung parenchymal, and extrathoracic soft tissue metastases in a breast cancer patient is presented in Fig. 72.1. The use of PET-CT scanners with fused PET-CT imaging facilitates the localization of pleural metastases and help distinguish these from metastases to the lung periphery, chest wall osseus, and soft tissue structures.

Tissue Confirmation

Thoracentesis and Studies on the Pleural Fluid

The radiologic advances outlined earlier have greatly improved our ability to detect earlier and characterize the extent of possible pleural metastases from breast cancer. However, the broad

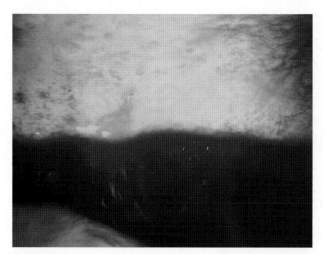

• **Fig. 72.2** Thoracoscopic view of a pleural cavity with malignant pleural effusion and nonspecific pleuritis of the parietal pleura.

differential of possible paramalignant effusions generally makes it necessary to obtain a tissue diagnosis to confirm regional spread of disease before proceeding with appropriate regional and/or systemic therapy.

Because the presentation of malignant pleural metastases from breast cancer is most often a pleural effusion (Fig. 72.2), symptomatic or otherwise, the initial diagnostic step is removal and analysis of fluid for diagnosis and as needed for the relief of symptoms. Thoracentesis can be performed "blind," without real-time radiologic guidance, after review of a chest film or CT scan; however, beside ultrasonography by physicians can be a valuable tool, especially in patients with smaller or loculated effusions. The diagnostic yield of pleural fluid cytology varies and ranges from 40% to 90%,[2] depending on the tumor type, tumor burden, and number of thoracentesis performed. Breast cancer appears to have a higher pleural cytologic yield than metastatic lung cancer.[34] There is debate as to whether a large volume of fluid improves diagnostic yield; practice currently varies from sending only 10 to 20 mL to more than 1 L.[35] Furthermore, local laboratory practice differs as to whether only a small aliquot is processed as a smear or a cytospin slide or whether a larger volume is processed into a cell block. There is evidence that the preparation of a cell block increases the diagnostic yield from 11%[35] to 38%.[36] An additional advantage of a cell block is having additional material available for immunostaining. Routine tests performed on the pleural fluid include chemistries to distinguish an exudate from a transudate. Glucose, pH, lactate dehydrogenase (LDH), and cultures may be ordered to rule out an infected or complicated postobstructive parapneumonic effusion, one of the several causes of a paramalignant effusion (see Table 72.1).[1,2,17] A malignant effusion with low glucose, low pH, and a high LDH generally portends a worse prognosis,[38] but it should not discourage the clinician from attempting to drain and sclerose the affected space for palliation.

Immunohistochemistry

Given the rich source of tumor markers associated with adenocarcinomas, and markers with greater specificity for breast cancer in particular, there have been ongoing attempts to improve on the diagnostic sensitivity and prognostic value of identifying a malignant breast effusion with such molecular markers. The 2007 American Society of Clinical Oncology (ASCO) recommendations for the use of tumor markers include the measurement of steroid hormone receptors (estrogen and progesterone receptor status) and HER2/neu status of the primary tumor.[38] Although metastatic effusions from breast cancer also have a high frequency of positive estrogen receptor (ER) and progesterone receptor (PR) staining (72% and 52%, respectively), so do ovarian metastatic effusions, thus limiting the specificity of ER and PR staining.[39]

Biomarkers of tissue proliferation have also been looked for in suspicious pleural fluid, both as an aid to diagnosis and, perhaps in the future, as a target for specific therapy. Ki67 is a human nuclear antigen present in cycling but not resting cells, and positive immunohistochemical labeling of suspicious but cytologically negative effusions may obviate more invasive surgical procedures.[40] VEGF has been found and measured in various malignant serous effusions, including pleural effusions, and reaches levels 10 times higher than that in matched sera. The use of anti-VEGF neutralizing antibodies in in vitro systems point the way toward possible future targeted therapy.[41]

Tissue Biopsies

Pleural needle biopsy with a variety of needles had been performed "blind" after confirming entry into a pocket of pleural fluid with a finder 21-gauge or smaller needle or directly with ultrasound. The yield of pleural needle biopsy is generally lower than that provided by fluid cytology.[2,34] Unlike diffuse granulomatous inflammation, sampling the patchy pleural metastases, and especially the finding of predominantly visceral pleural implantation (Fig. 72.3), including the inaccessible mediastinal pleural surfaces,[27,28] may explain the low additional yield. Given the potential risk of parenchymal lung puncture, occasional life-threatening bleeding, and the availability of more accurate minimally invasive image-guided procedures, blind pleural needle biopsies are generally of historical interest and unwarranted.

Surgical approaches for tissue diagnosis may be required when repeated thoracentesis with or without image-guided pleural biopsy fails to provide a tissue confirmation or when the initial presentation suggests a multiloculated complex malignant effusion. Thoracoscopic approaches, either with simple single-entry thoracoscopy with the patient under local anesthesia and conscious sedation or video-assisted thoracic surgery (VATS) with the patient under general anesthesia, have 86% to 100% diagnostic accuracy in diagnosing a malignant pleural effusion.[27,28,42,43] Confirmation of malignant pleural involvement based on histologic examination of fresh-frozen tissue or the appearance under visual examination may expedite long-term management of the involved pleural space by pleurodesis at the end of the case, either by mechanical or chemical means.

Treatment: Indications, Approaches, and Complications

Intervention and management of patients with malignant pleural effusion from metastatic breast cancer should be guided by a few general principles. Because the presence of malignant cells in the pleural space implies metastatic and hence incurable disease, the goal of therapy is primarily to palliate symptoms and to anticipate and thus avoid complications caused by pleural involvement (Box 72.2). As a rule, the development of malignant pleural involvement, especially if it is one of multiple sites of metastases, portends more aggressive disease, a higher tumor burden, and hence

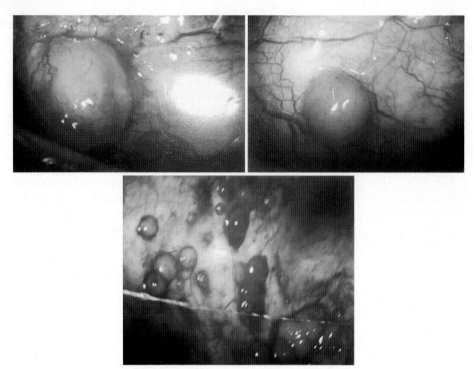

• **Fig. 72.3** Macroscopic view of tumor implants on the visceral pleura.

• BOX 72.2 **Management of Malignant Pleural Effusions From Breast Cancer**

Therapeutic Thoracentesis
Rapid relief, easily done with local anesthetic
Incomplete drainage, frequent recurrence

Percutaneous Drain Placement
Rapid relief, often complete drainage, easily done with local anesthetic, image guidance can improve efficacy
Frequent recurrence once drain is removed

Tube Thoracostomy (Chest Tube)
Rapid relief, often complete drainage, able to administer sclerosant (talc slurry) through tube
Significant pain

Indwelling Pleural Catheter
Can be placed at bedside or in operating room; allows patient to drain fluid as needed outside of hospital
External catheter requires care

Pleuroperitoneal Shunting
Generally abandoned in favor of indwelling pleural catheter
Can be associated with abdominal complications and tube malfunction

Thoracoscopy (Video-Assisted Thoracic Surgery)
Ability to biopsy when diagnosis is questioned, ability to break up loculations and allow more thorough drainage
Insufflation of talc is possible; at the same time, pericardial effusions can be addressed simultaneously
Requires conscious sedation or general anesthesia

Open Surgical Approaches
Generally abandoned in favor of thoracoscopy; greater pain and longer hospital stay

---

worse outcome.[44] However, given the varied responses patients may have to cytotoxic, hormonal, and biologic agents, treatment must be tailored for the individual patient, taking into account the patient's overall functional status, comorbidities, prior exposure to treatment, and finally the nature and extent of the pleural involvement.

Systemic cytotoxic chemotherapy, hormonal therapy, and biologic and immune therapy are covered elsewhere in detail. Suffice it to say, there are select cases of MPEs that have responded to systemic therapy alone, although the specific rates of response are unknown. Therefore, for asymptomatic or minimally symptomatic metastatic breast cancer effusions in patients who are scheduled for follow-up systemic therapy, it may be reasonable to defer immediate local pleural interventions.

The exception here is terminally ill patients with large MPEs who are not active enough to elicit symptoms. If large effusions that compress the lung are not controlled, the lung can develop fibrinous peel and/or tumor deposits that encase it and prevent reexpansion, even when the fluid is drained. The patient suffers from the so-called trapped lung and a decline in pulmonary function secondary to mechanical compression of the lung.[45] In addition, the residual space is prone to infection from contamination during frequent procedures, and clearance of infection in that space can be incredibly challenging. Similarly, malignant pleural effusions that develop multiple loculations are often difficult to treat. Therefore symptomatic MPEs that do not respond to systemic chemotherapy require drainage of the pleural fluid and obliteration of the pleural space.

Pleural Space Drainage

Thoracentesis

Thoracentesis is often the first step in both the diagnosis and treatment of MPEs from breast disease. It is not definitive, however, because the mean recurrence interval is within 4.2 days, and the overall recurrence rate is 98% within 30 days.[3] In the case of MPE, thoracentesis is more useful as a diagnostic technique because there is no mechanism to prevent recurrence of fluid accumulation or continued drainage. Despite its short therapeutic duration, a thoracentesis not only confirms the cause of the effusion but also can usually ascertain whether the fluid can be removed and whether the lung is able to reexpand. Drainage of up to as much as 1 to 2 L at the initial thoracentesis is warranted. Although the sudden evacuation of more than 1.5 L of pleural fluid of a chronically collapsed lung has been associated with unilateral reexpansion pulmonary edema,[46] this complication is rare.[47,48] Large volume thoracentesis may be better tolerated if allowed to drain slowly or drain to gravity rather than rapid evacuation with suction. In practice, we terminate the procedure at the onset of excessive coughing and pleuritic chest pain. Any residual fluid is aspirated at a later date. Repeated thoracentesis is reserved for those with acute life-threatening problems, patients who are waiting on the effects of systemic chemotherapy, and those who are poor operative risks (Karnofsky score <30%).[49] Repeated thoracentesis has the potential risks of inducing hypoproteinemia, empyema, pneumothorax, and can produce intrathoracic loculations of pleural fluid. Although chemical pleurodesis can theoretically be administered after thoracentesis with a needle or a small-caliber drainage catheter, it is generally more effective when done with VATS drainage with sclerosant insufflation or tube thoracostomy.

Indwelling Pleural Catheter

With the advent of readily accessible bedside imaging modalities such as ultrasound, placement of indwelling pleural catheters (IPC) to an effusion is now a safe and efficient method for continued symptomatic relief of MPE. This method has been shown to be superior to repeated thoracentesis in a variety of ways. It is generally safer than repeated thoracentesis and has a higher success rate, specifically with smaller or loculated pleural fluid collections.[50,51] In a recent case series of 80 patients with MPE, ultrasound-guided catheter placement was met with success in 87% of the patients.[51] This method is often found to be better tolerated from a patient care standpoint. It does not require a large skin incision or blunt dissection to accommodate a large-bore chest drain as used in the tube thoracostomy method discussed next and has been shown to have fewer insertion-related complications.[51,52] Also in this case series of 124 patients with various etiologies of pleural effusions, larger bore size chest tube was not found to have an improved benefit on treatment of the symptomatic effusion.[51] One common pleural drainage system is the PleurX drain (Denver Biomaterials, Golden, CO), a tunneled pleural catheter with a fabric cuff that promotes ingrowth and is suitable for permanent placement. It is easily inserted either in the operating room or with local anesthetic at the bedside. These systems offer continued drainage of the refractory pleural effusion as well as being smaller, more comfortable, and more portable than the traditional chest tube. The catheter can be easily used at home by home health nurses, family members, or by the patient themself. It is easily connected to disposable plastic evacuated bottles to drain the effusion whenever it becomes symptomatic. Repeated drainage can improve dyspnea and promote symphysis of the visceral pleura to the parietal pleura thus obliterating the space for recurrent effusions to develop. If no longer desired, the catheters can be removed at the bedside with local anesthetic if removal is desired, but permanent placement is also common.

Tube Thoracostomy

Classically, tube thoracostomy was employed as the first-line treatment of MPE that did not resolve after thoracentesis drainage and systemic therapy. This painful method is not well tolerated by the conscious patient at the bedside and has not been shown to be superior to image-guided drain placement of small-bore catheters.[51,52] With increasing availability of ultrasound or CT guided drainage, indications for large bore chest tube placement are decreasing. One possible indication may be a patient presenting to an emergency department in distress, without availability of percutaneous drainage. In this case a 20- to 24-French chest tube is inserted at the bedside, usually with the patient under intravenous sedation and local analgesic infiltration. The chest tube is placed to water seal drainage reservoir, serial chest radiographs obtained, and chest drainage recorded. Pleurodesis can then be performed through the tube if the lung has reexpanded and the pleural drainage has been sufficiently low (<200 mL per 24 hours, as is typical of our practice). Pleurodesis can be successful only if the lung is completely reexpanded so that the parietal and visceral pleura can oppose, otherwise pleurodesis will further "trap" the lung in a partly collapsed state, and sclerosing agent such as talc could become infected, which would present a clinical challenge.

Pleurodesis

Pleurodesis can be accomplished by a variety of methods with the introduction of the IPC and VATS but has classically been accomplished via tube thoracostomy. A 2016 Cochrane review of the different management options for MPE with regard to pleurodesis compared 16 agents with a variety of methods for instillation and administration showed that the most effective single agent was talc. The best improvement in subjective dyspnea scores at 30 days posttreatment was with talc slurry administered through an IPC.[53] This was associated with better patient tolerance of the procedure and equivalent postprocedural fever.

Once the drainage is sufficiently reduced to allow chemical pleurodesis, the patient is premedicated with a narcotic analgesic and up to 4 mg/kg of lidocaine 1% is instilled in the tube first. Then 50 mL saline is mixed with 5 g sterile talc sclerosant into a slurry. The talc slurry is then instilled into the chest tube, and the tube held in an elevated position (typically taped over the bed rail) on water seal for 4 hours to allow the slurry to stay in the chest. Rotation in the patient's body position is generally unnecessary to achieve distribution of the sclerosant within the pleural cavity. After 4 hours, the tube is brought to a dependent position and suction reapplied. The chest drainage is monitored on suction for at least 48 hours. When drainage falls to less than 100 mL per 24 hours, the chest tube is removed. The process can be repeated if needed. Median hospitalization for patients with tube thoracostomy and successful pleurodesis is approximately 6 days.[54–56] If the chest drainage does not fall below 150 mL per 24 hours after 4 days, the sclerosant agent is readministered and the procedure repeated. Further failure to respond to therapy qualifies as a failure of conservative therapy.

It is well accepted to use small-bore (10- to 16-French) percutaneous catheters instead of standard large-bore (24- to 32-French) chest tubes in the drainage and sclerotherapy of malignant pleural effusions. Standard chest tubes limit patient mobility and are often a source of significant discomfort. Chest tubes not only have higher pain with placement but can also be a source of ongoing pain while the tube is in place. Furthermore, some patients can have chronic intercostal neuralgia. In prospective and retrospective studies, smaller catheters are better tolerated, have minimal complications, and exhibit few major differences in outcomes such as probabilities of recurrence.[57–60]

"Spontaneous pleurodesis" without sclerosant has been observed with the use of a chronic, small-bore indwelling pleural catheter (Pleurx, Denver Biomaterials).[61,62]

Surgical Intervention: Video-Assisted Thoracoscopic Surgery, Pleural Decortication, Pericardial Drainage

If diagnosis is in question, or pleurodesis has failed and a malignant pleural effusion recurs, thoracoscopy (VATS) is a useful diagnostic and therapeutic tool. VATS offers a magnified view of the hemithorax, thus the extent of pleural metastases, including the degree of tumor encasement of the lung, can be determined. Options for therapeutic maneuvers include lysis of adhesions, limited decortication, pleurectomy, mechanical and chemical pleurodesis, and visual positioning of drainage tubes.[55] Complete decortication is difficult and not likely of significant benefit, but limited decortication with VATS can allow lung expansion in some with loculated effusions. Insufflation with talc (i.e., *talc poudrage*) then follows. Mechanical pleurodesis with an abrasive pad can be done to achieve pleurodesis, but as tumor deposits may be vascularized, this could result in unnecessary oozing or bleeding and should be considered with caution. Bilateral effusions can be treated with sequential VATS plus pleurodesis. The operative mortality of VATS for pleurodesis in patients with advanced malignant pleural effusions is approximately 5%.[63,64]

A less common, but often more urgent, clinical scenario referred for surgical evaluation is pericardial effusion in either a patient with known or suspected metastatic breast cancer. This may vary from incidental finding of pericardial effusion on imaging to a patient with hemodynamic instability and impending cardiac tamponade. It is of paramount importance to understand the patient's overall clinical condition and goals of care to provide the best treatment for MPCE. Options for treatment include the following: ultrasound-guided pericardiocentesis, ultrasound-guided pericardial drain placement, surgical pericardial drainage, and pericardial window. Pericardiocentesis can be rapidly achieved at the bedside, as can ultrasound-guided drain placement. Unfortunately, recurrence is common and results in the same clinical scenario. A more durable palliation may be achieved with open drainage of the pericardial sac if the patient is able to undergo surgery. Subxiphoid drainage may be the fastest surgical route in a hemodynamically unstable patient. In the more stable patient, other options exist. One common approach is to perform thoracoscopy to drain pleural effusion, and during the thoracoscopy, the pericardium is widely opened so the pericardial effusion may drain into the pleural space, and an IPC can then be placed in the pleural space, which may help relieve both MPE and MPCE with one drain.

Surgical Pleurectomy

With modern-day therapies available for MPEs, pleurectomy is largely anachronistic. This procedure, with its high operative morbidity and mortality, cannot be justified as a palliative measure and has been replaced by interventions with lower morbidity rates.

Patients With Trapped Lung

If the effusion has not been controlled or is loculated, the lung could be trapped (>25% pleural dead space). Similarly, the lung can become trapped as a result of encasement by extensive tumor involvement, and the tumor implants cannot be removed during surgery. A trapped lung that cannot expand leaves pleural dead space that will rapidly reaccumulate fluid and nullify any attempts at pleurodesis. A pleuroperitoneal shunt, usually the Denver shunt (Codman and Shurtleff, Randolph, MA), has been placed as an alternative.[65,66] These shunts are placed in the pleural space and the peritoneum and have a pumping chamber that sits in a subcutaneous pocket at the anterolateral costal margin. Patients must actively pump this chamber, often up to 25 times every 4 hours; thus, patient compliance is an important issue. Another obvious issue with this is the distribution of malignant cells and/or infection from the pleural space into the peritoneal space. The inconvenience and complications of this type of drain, including abdominal complications, have led most to abandon it in favor of a tunneled IPC, which is drained externally. In general, patients with a trapped lung present difficult management problems, and proper selection of the most appropriate palliative option must be done on an individual basis.

Sclerosing Agents

Many agents have been used to affect pleural symphysis.[2,17,37,67,68] Most have a direct irritant effect, usually eliciting an intense pleural inflammation and subsequent fibrosis. A number of antineoplastic agents have also been administered locally into the pleural space, with the purported dual cytotoxic and fibrotic action on the involved pleural surfaces.[14,69,70] Most of these reports consist of small case series without a comparator arm. The results appear encouraging from some studies, such as with mitoxantrone in two small case series of 18 and 6 patients, with a 72% to 100% response (complete response and partial response), with a prolonged median survival of 17 months as measured against historical survival of less than 12 months from the time of pleural metastases.[67,70] Other compounds, such as radioactive phosphorus, thiotepa, and 5-fluorouracil, either offered no additional benefit over drainage alone or required concomitant sclerosants to be effective.[71]

Because of its efficacy, ready availability, and relative lesser expense, talc remains the agent of choice for chemical pleurodesis.[55,56,64,72–79] The route of administration, either talc slurry or thoracoscopic talc insufflation, was evaluated in a randomized trial of 482 patients with MPE due to a variety of primary tumors. Methods were similar in efficacy overall; however, the subgroup with MPE due to lung or breast primary had higher success with thoracoscopy compared with talc slurry through a tube (82% vs. 67%).[80] There remain safety concerns regarding the episodic development of posttalc instillation respiratory complications, ranging from transient hypoxemia to acute respiratory distress syndrome (ARDS), with some patient deaths.[81–83] The pathophysiology of this posttalc syndrome remains unclear, and the frequency and severity of response may be related to the dosage and talc particle size used in pleurodesis.[37,84] Current recommendation is to limit the amount of talc used to 5 g per instillation. Research has demonstrated a reduction in talc-related ARDS with administration of "graded" or "large particle" talc showing reduced systemic uptake which has been the suggested method of its pathogenesis.[53,85] Sclerosis of the pericardial space with talc is not advised for concerns of pericarditis, but thiotepa has been reported as an effective sclerosing agent for MPCE.[86]

Prognosis

The development of malignant effusion in a breast cancer patient generally portends a poor prognosis, with a median survival time of 5 to 15.7 months.[11,25,26,44,74] Patients with metastatic pleural disease as the solo manifestation of relapse have a significant survival advantage over those with more widespread disease: 48 months versus 12 months in one series.[44] The concomitant presence of invasion into other mesothelium-lined cavities, including the pericardium and peritoneum, are especially ominous signs.

Summary

Malignant involvement of the pleural space by breast cancer is a common occurrence late in the course of progressive disease and may be a major cause of morbidity. Because of the broad differential causes of pleural effusions, including contralateral or bilateral effusions, a tissue diagnosis should be obtained rather than assuming a malignant cause. If a malignant cause has been ascertained, it is certainly a sign of incurable disease and further management should be focused on symptom control and patient comfort.

Diagnosis should first be attempted through the use of thoracentesis. Samples should be sent for fluid cytology as well as chemistry studies to determine whether they are exudative. A cell block should be requested and will improve the diagnostic yield of fluid cytology. A second attempt at pleural fluid cytology may be attempted, or the patient may be referred for diagnostic thoracoscopy. Closed pleural needle biopsy is seldom warranted, although it may be performed by experienced practitioners during the second thoracentesis, especially if diagnostic thoracoscopy is not readily available. Thoracoscopy has a very high diagnostic yield and can allow simultaneous therapeutic drainage of effusion and effective pleurodesis by mechanical means or by talc insufflation. Open surgical biopsy or drainage thoracotomy is seldom necessary. More recently, indwelling pleural catheters have shown great promise for MPE management and have been shown to be highly effective with talc administration as a sclerosant agent for pleurodesis.

Selected References

1. Light RW. *Pleural Diseases.* 3rd ed. Baltimore: Williams & Wilkins; 1995.
2. Anthony VB, et al. Management of malignant pleural effusions: official statement of the American Thoracic Society. *Am J Respir Crit Care Med.* 2000;162:1987.
16. Stathopoulos GT, Kalomenidis I. Malignant pleural effusion: tumor-host interactions unleashed. *Am J Respir Crit Care Med.* 2012;186:487-492.
50. Daniels CE, Ryu JH. Improving the safety of thoracentesis. *Curr Opin Pulm Med.* 2011;17:232-236.
51. Abusedera M, Alkady O. Ultrasound-guided pleural effusion drainage with a small catheter using the single-step trocar or modified Seldinger technique. *J Bronchol Intervent Pulmonol.* 2016;23:138-145.
53. Clive AO, Jones HE, Bhatnagar R, Preston NJ, Maskell N. Interventions for the management of malignant pleural effusions: a network meta-analysis. *Cochrane Database Syst Rev.* 2016;(5):CD010529.
62. Putnam JB Jr, et al. Outpatient management of malignant pleural effusion by a chronic indwelling pleural catheter. *Ann Thorac Surg.* 2000;69:369.
80. Dresler CM, Olak J, Herndon JE II, et al. Phase III intergroup study of talc poudrage vs talc slurry sclerosis for malignant pleural effusion. *Chest.* 2005;127:909-915.
86. Cozzi S, Montanara S, Luraschi A, et al. Management of neoplastic pericardial effusions. *Tumori.* 2010;96:926.

A full reference list is available online at ExpertConsult.com.

73

Management of Central Nervous System Metastases in Breast Cancer

RICARDO COSTA AND PRIYA KUMTHEKAR

Incidence

In 2016, there was an estimated 246,660 new cases of breast cancer in the United States alone, and 40,450 women died of this disease.[1] A subset of these patients succumbed to brain metastasis as their primary cause of death. Population-based studies support that the cumulative incidence of brain metastasis in 5 years is approximately 5.0% in patients with breast cancer in general.[2,3] The true incidence of metastatic breast cancer (MBC) to the brain remains to be determined because postmortem autopsy series report higher prevalence.[4] Each year in the United States an estimated 170,000 cancer patients are diagnosed with brain metastasis.[5] Overall breast cancer is the second most common cause of brain metastasis, second only to lung cancer and accounting for approximately 20% of the cases of brain metastases.[6] Breast cancer brain metastases are commonly a late occurrence, with a median time from diagnosis of breast cancer to brain metastasis identification of 2 to 3 years.[7] The median age of diagnosis of metastatic disease to brain is approximately 45 years.[8]

Leptomeningeal metastatic disease (LMD) is rarer than brain parenchyma disease. In one series of 4079 patients with breast cancer and 1809 patients with recurrent disease, LMD was present in 0.86% of patients with breast cancer and 1.9% of patients with recurrent disease.[9] The median age of incidence ranges from 45 to 57.[9,10]

The 5-year cumulative incidence of metastatic epidural spinal cord compression (ESCC) preceding death of breast cancer was reported at 5.52% among 35,197 cases of breast cancer analyzed in Ontario, which is in harmony with results from other series.[11,12] At diagnosis its prevalence was estimated at 0.11%.[11] The median age at diagnosis is of ESCC is 51 years.[12]

Risk Factors

Results from a population-based studied conducted in the United States among 51,898 women supports that age less than 40 and African American women correlated with higher risk of central nervous system (CNS) involvement among patients with early-stage breast cancer.[3] Evans and coworkers reported a case series in which 219 patients in which 43% of women diagnosed with MBC would eventually develop brain metastsis.[13]

Stage at the time of diagnosis is a determinant risk factor for CNS brain metastasis. This is a rare event in women undergoing breast conserving surgery for early-stage breast cancer with 5-year cumulative incidence as low as 1.7% reported in patients with clinical stage I–II tumors.[14] Axillary node metastasis also seems to increase the risk of CNS relapse compared with axillary node–negative disease.[15] Patients presenting with increased number of metastatic sites are at increased risk for occult CNS disease.[16] In addition, in one series multivariate modeling supported a hazard ratio (HR) of 4.3 for CNS metastasis when patients had pulmonary involvement.[17] These findings indicate that tumor burden is most likely a continuous variable, which correlates positively with the risk CNS involvement in either early- or late-stage disease.

Tumor biological variables are also predictive of increased risk of CNS disease in patients with breast cancer. HER2 overexpression, which is observed in up to 25% to 30% of patients diagnosed with breast cancer, confers poor prognosis in the localized and metastatic settings.[18–20] The advent of targeted therapies against HER2 overexpressing breast cancer amounted to significant improvement in overall survival (OS) and disease-free survival.[21–26] The median OS for patients presenting HER2-positive MBC and treated with the combination of trastuzumab, pertuzumab, and docetaxel is now estimated at 56.5 months 95% CI (49.3 to not reached) in the first-line setting.[22] In light of improved management and prolonged survival, brain metastasis were found to be a common event in patients with presenting with metastatic HER2-positive breast cancer with a risk ranging from 35% to 50% over the course of their disease.[27–29] For patients presenting with early-stage disease, HER2-positive breast cancer, CNS-only recurrence is a rare event regardless of trastuzumab adjuvant therapy with cumulative risk less than 3% reported in different studies.[30,31] Nonetheless, it is important to highlight that late recurrences diagnosed several years from the diagnosis of breast cancer are also more prevalent in HER2-positive/HR-negative tumor compared with other subtypes.[32]

Lack of estrogen receptor (ER) overexpression has also been correlated with increased risk of CNS recurrence in early breast cancer, whereas ER-positive tumors seem to have a lower risk of CNS involvement.[13–15,33]

Furthermore, most recently next-generation sequencing has clustered breast tumors according to variation in genomic transcriptional patterns resulting in different prognostic subtypes.[34,35] In one series of 1434 consecutive patients with stage I–II invasive breast cancer with a median follow-up of 85 months, Arvold and coworkers stratified patients according to immunohistochemistry approximate genomic subtypes; the 5-year cumulative risk of brain metastasis was 0.1% for luminal A, 3.3% luminal B, 3.2%

for luminal HER2, and 7.4% for triple-negative breast cancer (TNBC) tumors.[14]

Other pathologic features of the primary breast tumor associated with increased risk of CNS relapses include expression of cytokeratin 5/6 and 14, epidermal growth factor receptor (EGFR), p53, elevated S-phase fraction, DNA ploidy, tumor size, tumor grade, and invasive ductal histology.[36–40]

LMD is more common among lobular carcinoma of the breast compared with ductal histology.[9,41] Small series conducted in the pre-HER2 era suggest that LMD may be more prevalent the hormone receptor–negative tumor population.[10] Finally, small case series suggest that ESCC is more common in patients with tumors overexpressing hormonal receptors.[12]

Methods of Spread and Distribution

Among 400 women with breast metastatic to the CNS reported by Kim and colleagues, approximately 80% of patients presented with brain metastases confined to the brain parenchyma, 7.5% had LMD only, and 13% had both. Furthermore, more than 95% of women presented with CNS involvement as a late manifestation of disease.[42] Intracerebral metastases at presentation are five times more common compared with solitary lesions.[13] Brain recurrence as the first site of recurrence is a rare event accounting for up to 12% of cases with CNS metastasis.[43] Patients presenting with locally advanced or inflammatory breast cancer seem to have higher risk of recurrence in the CNS as their first site of disease recurrence.[39] Likewise, LMD is a late complication of breast cancer and usually associated with concomitant systemic disease.[10] The median latency period from breast cancer diagnosis and LMD is 25 to 38 months.[10,44] In one small series, LMD was the first manifestation of recurrent disease in 4 of 25 patients and another 1 of 44 patients.[10,44]

Clinical Presentation

Brain Metastasis

Signs and symptoms from brain metastases are varied and are caused by the displacement or destruction of structures within the brain. Possible symptoms include headache, focal neurologic dysfunction, cognitive decline, encephalopathy, seizures, and strokes.[45] A cross-sectional study published by Posner and colleagues evaluated 111 patients with either primary or metastatic tumors to the brain and their presenting symptoms.[46] Headaches were present in up to 48% of patients and equal for primary and metastatic brain tumors. The typical headache was bifrontal but worse ipsilaterally to the metastatic lesion(s) and was the worst symptom in only 45% of patients. Unlike true tension-type headaches, brain tumor headaches were worse with bending over in 32%, and nausea or vomiting was present in 40% of patients. The "classic" early-morning brain tumor headache was uncommon. Nausea, vomiting, an abnormal neurologic examination, or a significant change in prior headache pattern suggests that the headache may be caused by a tumor. The high prevalence of headache in patients with metastatic or primary brain tumor has been observed in other studies.[47] Encephalopathy alone is a rare presentation of metastatic brain tumors and is often secondary to systemic toxic metabolic encephalopathy.[48] Up to 18% of patients present with seizures as the first manifestation of brain metastatic disease.[49] Intracranial bleeding is a recognized complication of metastatic tumors to the brain and clinical presentation depends on location of the event.[50] Although hemorrhage can be seen, anticoagulation is otherwise safe for medical indications in patients with brain metastases as long as patients have not had active bleeding of their metastases.

Leptomeningeal Metastasis

Most commonly LMD presents with headache and involvement of cranial nerves, often particularly to the cranial nerves that control extraocular muscles.[9,44] In addition symptoms of LMD can be caused by the following pathophysiologic mechanisms: (1) mass effect resulting in cerebrospinal fluid (CSF) obstruction and hydrocephalus and/or increased intracranial pressure, (2) tumor involvement of the cranial nerves or spinal roots, (3) invasion of brain parenchyma via Virchow-Robin spaces, and/or (4) disruption of the blood-brain barrier (BBB). The clinical hallmark of LMD is a constellation of signs and symptoms caused by multifocal involvement of the neuraxis (i.e., cerebrum, cranial nerves, and spinal roots). Because LM is a disease of cancer cells in the subarachnoid space and CSF, there is frequent cranial nerve and spinal nerve involvement along with other classic meningitis signs. In a study of 102 patients with LMD, 33%, 39%, and 13% of patients had signs and symptoms involving one, two, or all three levels of the neuraxis, respectively.[51]

Rarely do patients present with a single neurologic symptom, and often careful neurologic examination reveals other neurologic dysfunction such as ocular muscle paresis, facial weakness, diminished hearing, optic neuropathy, trigeminal neuropathy, hypoglossal neuropathy, blindness, and diminished gag reflex.[52] Other findings include seizures, hemiparesis, cerebellar dysfunction (manifested as difficulty walking), nausea, and vomiting. Another common symptom from cranial nerve involvement is facial numbness, particularly involvement of the third division of the trigeminal nerve. This cranial nerve neuropathy results in numbness of the chin and is referred to as the *numb chin syndrome*.[53] Spinal root invasion often causes symptoms of weakness, paresthesias, back and neck pain, radicular pain, and/or bowel and bladder dysfunction. Meningeal signs of nuchal rigidity and pain on straight leg raises are common. Symptoms of hydrocephalus and/or increased intracranial pressure, which include headache, nausea, vomiting, and dizziness, occur in 50% of patients.

Epidural Spinal Cord Compression

Epidural Spinal Cord Compression (ESSC) is a medical emergency and should be promptly recognized and treated. In one case series of 70 patients, the most common presenting symptoms with spinal cord compression were pain (94%), muscle weakness (96%), sensory loss (79%), and sphincter dysfunction (61%); at least one of these symptoms was present in 100% of the patients.[12] In one series of 100 patients with known breast cancer presenting with signs/symptoms of radiculopathy or myelopathy, epidural metastasis were diagnosed in 54% of the cases, indicating the diagnostic workup should be initiated with no delay in this patient population.[54]

The most common presentation for ESCC is complaint of severe lower back pain that progressively worsens. The pain is worse when lying supine; this occurs because of distension of the epidural venous plexus. The pain may also result from disruption of the periosteum, the cauda equina, the spinal cord, or paravertebral soft tissue. Over time, the pain may develop into a radicular quality.[55] Abrupt worsening of back pain may be a sign of a compression fracture.

Up to 85% of patients have partial weakness or paresis at presentation.[54–59] ESCC generally produces symmetric bilateral extremity weakness. A superimposed radiculopathy can occur with lateralized epidural lesions. Associated hyporeflexia is seen with ESCC at the level of the cauda equina, whereas hyperreflexia is seen with a lesion at or above the conus medullaris. If treatment is not initiated promptly, which is common, the weakness will progress to cause difficulty with ambulation and, eventually, paralysis. Most patients (60%–70%) have difficulty with ambulation at the time of diagnosis.[54,56–59] Sensory deficits also occur in the majority of spinal cord compression patients on presentation.[54–59] The most frequent symptom is ascending paresthesias. On physical examination, the sensory deficit corresponds closely to the dermatome level. "Saddle anesthesia" is a common sensory deficit in patients with cauda equina syndrome. Lhermitte sign (an electrical sensation down the spine elicited by neck flexion) is rarely seen with ESCC and more frequently seen in LMD.[60]

Autonomic dysfunctions such as urinary hesitancy, retention, and incontinence are relatively uncommon.[54,55] These symptoms usually occur as a late manifestation of myelopathy. Isolated painless ataxia secondary to spinocerebellar tract dysfunction caused by ESCC has also been reported.[61]

Unfortunately, the diagnosis of ESCC is often delayed. A prospective study of 301 patients examining the delay in presentation, diagnosis, and treatment of spinal cord compression observed a median delay of 14 days (range, 0–840 days) between onset of symptoms and treatment.[56]

Diagnostic Evaluation

Diagnosis of CNS metastases can often be made based on clinical history, presentation, and/or imaging findings. However, a biopsy and/or CSF sampling may be helpful.

Brain Metastases

The differential diagnosis for a brain lesion includes primary brain tumor, infectious abscess, progressive multifocal leukoencephalopathy, demyelination, cerebral infarction or bleeding, and radiation necrosis (if the patient has had prior radiation therapy [RT] to the brain).

Gadolinium-enhanced magnetic resonance imaging (MRI) is the best method for detecting and localizing brain metastases with increased sensitivity compared with contrast-enhanced computerized tomography (CT) scan.[62–64] MRI also has increased sensitivity in detecting posterior fossa and cortical lesions.[64] Sensitivity and specificity of 18 fluorodeoxyglucose positron emission tomography (FDG-PET) was tested against MRI as the gold standard in one series of 40 patients with suspected brain metastatis.[65] Twelve patients with brain metastasis were identified on FDG-PET with a sensitivity of 75% and specificity of 83%. Small lesions were particularly difficult to diagnose on FDG-PET. In another cross-sectional study of 50 patients with suspected brain metastasis assessed the accuracy of combining FDG-PET fused with CT imaging.[66] Seventy cerebral metastasis were diagnosed on MRI in 20 patients and FDG-PET/CT's sensitivity of detection of all 70 lesions was only 20%. These results indicate that MRI should remain the preferred radiologic test for the evaluation of suspected brain metastasis.

Brain metastases are usually located at gray-white junctions and have well-circumscribed boundaries. The majority of patients with diagnosis of cancer present with multiple lesions, and a significant amount of edema may surround a metastasis that is disproportionate to the size of the tumor mass.[67] On a CT scan, breast cancer metastases are usually isodense to the surrounding brain with enhancement after contrast infusion.[68] Calcification within a metastasis is rarely seen. On MRI studies, the metastasis is usually hypointense to the brain on T1-weighted images and hyperintense to the brain on T2-weighted images.[63,67] After contrast administration, most brain metastases strongly enhance on both CT and MRI. A solid homogeneous enhancement pattern is typical, but a ring-enhancing pattern may be seen. Cystic and heterogeneously enhancing breast cancer brain metastases are seen less frequently with few cases reported in the literature.[69] Newer imaging modalities such as MRI spectroscopy and FDG-PET may prove to be helpful in the diagnoses of brain metastases. Currently, they are used to help differentiate between tumor recurrence and radiation necrosis.

A biopsy is warranted if the diagnosis of brain metastases is ever in doubt, especially if a patient presents with a single brain metastasis. In one prospective study of 54 patients with a history of primary cancer and a single mass lesion seen on both CT and MRI, 6 (11%) of those patients had nonmetastatic lesions, including two glioblastomas, one low-grade astrocytoma, two abscesses, and one nonspecific inflammatory reaction.[70] Therefore, biopsy should be strongly considered before RT if complete surgical resection of a single lesion is not planned or if there is doubt about the diagnosis. Cerebral abscesses are especially problematic because they can mimic metastases clinically and radiographically, and treatment of an abscess with RT would be detrimental. Modern stereotactic cerebral biopsy is a highly effective technique to obtain a tissue diagnosis and can be performed with low morbidity. In one series of 500 cases with predominant target locations within the cerebral centrum-basal ganglia (284 cases) and diencephalic-mesencephalic regions (129 cases) in which stereotactic biopsy was formed for diagnostic and therapeutic objective the observed mortality was 0.2% and morbidity was 1%.[71] Possible complications from the procedure include intracerebral hemorrhage and infection.

Leptomeningeal Metastases

The differential diagnosis for LMD includes infectious etiologies (i.e., bacterial meningitis, Lyme disease), autoimmune disorders (i.e., vasculitis, sarcoidosis), and artifact (i.e., post-RT changes). The diagnosis of LM is based on obtaining a detailed history and identifying neurologic signs on physical examination that suggest multifocal involvement of the neuraxis. Combining contrast-enhanced MRI scans with CSF cytology enhances the diagnostic accuracy of LM. CSF cytology has 100% specificity and a sensitivity of 75% for single analysis.[72] The probability of disease detection with CSF cytology can be affected by not only by tumor dependent variables but also by the amount of CSF collected, site of CSF sampling, and processing time. Sensitivity of CSF analysis correlates with number of collections and has been reported to be 98% with four collections.[73] MRI of symptomatic area (axial imaging of the brain or sagittal imaging of the spine) has been reported to be as sensitive and CSF cytology with sensitivity of 76% and specificity of 77%.[72]

Radiologic evaluation of possible LMD should be performed through MRI brain imaging. CT scan has limited clinical utility

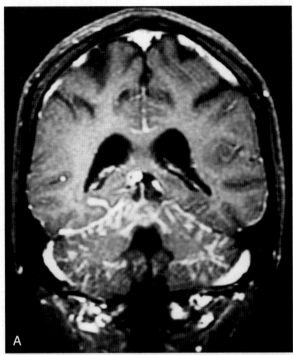

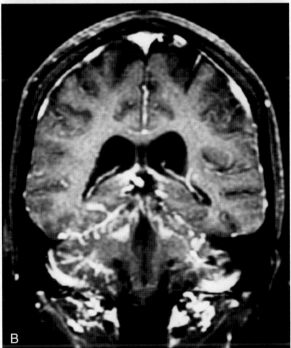

• **Fig. 73.1** (A and B) Magnetic resonance images showing cerebellar leptomeningeal enhancement secondary to metastatic breast cancer.

in diagnosing LMD insofar as it has been reported to have a sensitivity as low as 40% compared with up to 100% for MRI in a small series of 41 patients with LMD.[74]

Nearly all LMD enhances dramatically after contrast administration for an MRI scan (Fig. 73.1). Typical MRI findings in the brain include thin, diffuse leptomeningeal enhancement, multiple nodular or plaque-like deposits adherent to the dura, and tumor masses with or without hydrocephalus. On MRI, the entirety of the spinal cord, as well as the cauda equina, exhibits linear

enhancement. Nodular deposits may be seen on spinal nerve roots and on the cauda equina.

Before a lumbar puncture is performed, increased intracranial pressure should be ruled out via an ophthalmic examination for papilledema. The typical CSF findings for LM are elevated opening pressure, elevated protein content, decreased glucose concentration, elevated white blood cell count, and xanthochromia. Elevation of tumor markers (i.e., CEA, CA-15.3, CA-125, CA19.9) in the CSF may corroborate the diagnosis of LM in breast cancer patients.[75,76]

Spinal Cord Compression

The differential diagnosis when considering ESCC includes benign musculoskeletal disease, spinal abscess, and radiation myelopathy. To diagnose ESCC, the metastatic tumor must extrinsically compress the thecal sac. Neurologic examination may lead to the clinical suspicion, but ultimately, this should be radiographically confirmed. Plain radiographs are insufficient to observe this compression, so MRI of the spine with and without contrast or myelography are the diagnostic tools of choice. These tests should be ordered promptly in patients with known breast cancer presenting with myelopathy/radiculopathy syndrome given the high prevalence of ESCC in this patient population.[54]

The sensitivity and specificity of radiography for ESCC have been estimated at 91% and 86%, respectively, in patients with presenting with symptoms.[77] False positives can occur, and MRI should be performed once ESCC is suspected for therapeutic planning as well. CT scanning is more sensitive than plain films but is not as sensitive or as specific as MRI.[78,79]

A CT does not accurately distinguish the epidural space or spinal cord but is commonly used to direct percutaneous biopsies and help plan surgery. Isotope bone scans with Tc^{99m} are more sensitive than plain films for detecting bony metastases[79] but not for judging the integrity of the epidural space and thecal sac. Thus a bone scan should not be used for diagnosing ESCC.

The best radiographic techniques for visualizing the epidural space and thecal sac, and therefore diagnosing ESCC, are myelography or MRI. Myelography has the following disadvantages: (1) it requires a lumbar puncture, (2) it is contraindicated if there is increased intracranial pressure or coagulopathy, (3) it is contraindicated if the subarachnoid space at the level of the spinal cord is obstructed, and (4) it does not provide soft tissue resolution. However, myelography is quick and thus more tolerable for a patient in pain, and CSF sampling can be performed at the time of lumbar puncture. Myelography followed by CT scanning (i.e., CT myelogram) provides additional information regarding spinal cord and root compression, but such information is not as useful as that provided by MRI, which has become the definitive imaging study for the evaluation of ESCC because of its widespread availability. MRI scans the spinal cord and column in multiple planes, thus providing unsurpassed visualization of intramedullary, intradural, extradural, and paraspinal lesions (Fig. 73.2).[78,80,81] Because of its clear superiority in sensitivity and specificity, any patient with known breast carcinoma who develops persistent back, neck, or radicular pain should have an MRI scan.

Treatment

Although brain metastases are almost uniformly fatal, several possible treatment modalities can ameliorate symptoms and possibly

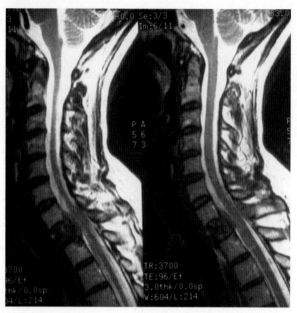

• **Fig. 73.2** Magnetic resonance imaging: sagittal views of a T1 spinal metastasis from breast cancer with impingement of the spinal cord.

TABLE 73.1	RTOG Recursive Partitioning Analysis Prognostic Classes				
RPA Class	Age	KPS	Primary Tumor	Extracranial Disease	Median Survival (Months)
1	<65	≥70	Controlled	Absent	7.1
2	≥65	≥70	Uncontrolled	Present	4.2
3	Any	<70	Either	Either	2.3

KPS, Karnofsky Performance Score; *RPA,* recursive partitioning analysis; *RTOG,* Radiation Therapy Oncology Group.
From Gaspar L, Scott C, Rotman M, et al: Recursive partitioning analysis (RPA) of prognostic factors in three Radiation Therapy Oncology Group (RTOG) brain metastases trials. *Int J Radiat Oncol Biol Phys.* 1997;37:745-751.

improve survival. These include corticosteroids, chemotherapy, RT alone or combined with surgical resection, and radiosurgery.

Prognosis

Historically patients with CNS metastases have a poor prognosis with medial OS ranging from 4 to 5.5 months with treatment.[36,82] Without therapeutic intervention, life median OS is estimated at 1 to 2 months.[82,83] For patients presenting with CNS recurrence neurologic disease is the cause of death and a major contributing factor to it in 68% of the cases as demonstrated in one series.[84] Patients presenting with solitary lesions have better prognosis compared with patients with multiple brain metastases.[84,85]

A prognostic prediction rule has been fostered in patients with brain metastases from solid tumors indicating that poor performance status and age over 65 years at diagnosis, along with uncontrolled extracranial disease, are variables that correlate with shorter median OS. Gaspar and coworkers reported data analysis of 1200 patients from three Radiation Therapy Oncology Group (RTOG) trials.[86] Patients who had Karnofsky performance scores (KPS) less than 70 were classified in RPA class 3. To be classified into recursive partitioning analysis (RPA) class 1, a patient has to satisfy the following criteria: age less than 65 years, KPS greater than or equal to 70, primary site under control, and no extracranial metastases. According to this analysis, only 20% of brain metastases patients were classified as RPA class 1, whereas 65% and 15% were RPA classes 2 and 3, respectively (Table 73.1). Other favorable prognostic factors identified by the study included a primary diagnosis of MBC ($p = .001$) and having a single lesion ($p = .021$). Aggressive treatment with surgery, RT, and chemotherapy should be used in patients with favorable prognoses (RPA class 1). Whole-brain RT (WBRT) alone should be used in patients with poor prognosis. These findings were in independently validated in a different data set.[87,88] Another and more recent prognostic prediction rule, graded prognostic assessment (GPA), has been analyzed in an even larger data set of database of 1960 patients with brain metastasis from five RTOG clinical

trials.[89] The new index, the GPA, was derived from the database after analysis of many possible prognostic factors. These included age, sex, KPS, histologic characteristics, interval from initial diagnosis to time of presentation with brain metastases, and patients with brain and bone-only metastases. GPA classification was able to provide patient prognostic classification comparable to RPA but easier to use. Different data sets used to validate this new index yielded similar results.[90–92]

The TNBC subtype also correlated with worse prognosis. In one series of 136 patients with breast cancer brain metastasis treated with stereotactic radiosurgery (SRS), multivariate analysis showed an HR for death of 2.0 ($p = .006$) in patients with TNBC even after controlling for number of lesions and activity of extracranial disease.[85] Breast cancer with HER2 positivity and brain metastasis seem to have a better prognosis compared with historical controls. In one series of 377 with HER2-positive MBC and CNS metastasis, the estimated median OS was 26.3 months.[28] Of note 53.9% of patients presented with more than one site of metastasis and 9.6% with LMD. Given that trastuzumab has negligible CNS penetrance, the improved prognosis could be secondary to improved systemic control with HER2-targeted therapy.[93] In addition, retrospective clinical data support that patients with HER2-positive MBC and CNS metastasis, when treated with trastuzumab before or at the time of CNS metastasis diagnosis, live longer compared with patients not treated with trastuzumab.[94] More recently a retrospective analysis of 1552 cases of breast and metastatic disease to brain showed that HER2 status, number of CNS metastasis, age at diagnosis, and performance status all have independent prognostic significance in RPA analysis.[95]

Corticosteroids

Corticosteroids should be the first treatment administered for any patient with symptomatic CNS metastases in brain parenchyma and LMD. For ESCC, higher doses of corticosteroids are a mandatory part of initial management. Corticosteroids reduce vasogenic edema by decreasing capillary permeability and reduce inflammation by suppressing the migration of polymorphonuclear leukocytes, thereby decreasing pain and maintaining or improving neurologic function. A loading dose of 10- to 100-mg intravenous dexamethasone followed by maintenance dosing of 4 to 24 mg orally or intravenously every 6 hours has been commonly used. Steroid therapy is tapered during or after the course of treatment. High-dose corticosteroids have been studied with varied results, and there is no clear advantage to high-dose corticosteroids over standard dosing.[59,96,97] Gastric prophylaxis with either an H2-receptor antagonist or a proton pump inhibitor should be given to all patients. *Pneumocystis carinii* pneumonia prophylaxis should be considered in patients who receive long-term corticosteroids. Corticosteroids may not be needed in asymptomatic patients with CNS metastases discovered by screening or in patients whose only symptoms are seizures, which may be best palliated with anticonvulsants.

Anticonvulsants

Seizures are a common manifestation of brain metastases. In a series of 195 patients with brain metastasis, approximately 18% of brain metastases patients present with seizures and an additional 10% develop seizures after diagnoses of a brain metastasis.[49] The diagnosis of a seizure disorder is usually made clinically, and an electroencephalogram may be helpful if the diagnosis is in doubt. Seizure disorder secondary to brain metastases should be treated with first-line anticonvulsants such as levetiracetam, valproic acid, and/or carbamazepine among others. If the patient is receiving chemotherapy, anticonvulsants that do not induce hepatic cytochrome P450 enzymes should be considered (i.e., levetiracetam, lamotrigine, or topiramate). Treatment should be initiated with a single agent to increase compliance and avoid side effects associated with multidrug treatment. Prophylactic anticonvulsant therapy should not be used in brain metastases patients without seizure disorders. A meta-analysis of randomized trials that assessed the use of prophylactic anticonvulsant therapy in brain tumors found that there was no evidence to support prophylactic anticonvulsant therapy.[98] The American Academy of Neurology recommends that prophylactic anticonvulsant therapy should not be used for brain metastases patients.[99] Perioperative anticonvulsant therapy is often used after neurosurgery for patients with brain metastases without a diagnosis of a seizure disorder because of concerns that surgery increases the risk of seizure. A meta-analysis failed to show a statistically significant benefit to the use of prophylactic anticonvulsant therapy after craniotomy.[100] The American Academy of Neurology recommends that anticonvulsant therapy should be tapered within 1 week after neurosurgery in patients who do not develop a postoperative seizure disorder.[99]

Anticonvulsant therapy may impair neurocognitive function and quality of life[101] and as such should be used only in patients with known seizures. Prophylactic anticonvulsant therapy should not be used in newly diagnosed brain metastases patients who do not have a seizure disorder, and anticonvulsant medications should be promptly discontinued in the perioperative setting.

Whole-Brain Radiation Therapy

WBRT is considered the standard of care in patients with more than three brain metastases. The role of RT in the management of brain metastases has been well established. By the mid-1950s, it was recognized that WBRT improved survival and symptoms in patients with brain metastases.[102] According to one series, WBRT improved neurologic symptoms in 74% of patients treated, and two-thirds of these patients had lasting improvement until death.[103] The complete response rate for brain metastases from breast cancer, assessed by CT, treated with 3000 cGy in 10

fractions has been reported to be 35% among 46 patients, which indicates brain metastases are responsive to palliative radiation therapy.[104] Several retrospective studies have shown that patients with brain metastases from breast cancer typically have a median survival of 4 to 6 months and a 70% to 90% improvement in symptoms with WBRT alone.[105,106] However, 31% to 68% of the patients die of neurologic complications.[84,107,108] Prognostic factors identified in these studies were KPS, radiation dose, and extracranial disease. It is difficult to assess improvement of symptoms after WBRT because the evaluation is subjective and may be influenced by the patient's general well-being and use of corticosteroids. The RTOG reported a 70% to 80% improvement in the patients' palliative index (a four-point functional activity index) after radiation. Several retrospective studies and a randomized trial have established the role of adjuvant WBRT after resection of a single brain metastasis in solid tumors including breast cancer.[109-115] The use of adjuvant WBRT is discussed in the surgical treatment of brain metastases section.

Treatment Technique and Dose Fractionation

Radiation is delivered through opposed lateral fields designed to treat the cerebrum, cerebellum, brainstem, and upper spinal cord (usually down to C1–C2). The most common fractionation regimen used in the United States is 3000 cGy in 10 fractions.[116] However, because brain metastases are almost always associated with incurable disease, many investigators have sought radiation treatment regimens that would ease the burden of therapy in these patients.[116] Using larger fraction sizes and a shorter overall treatment time may decrease the patient's time away from family and friends, achieve a greater biological effect, and minimize the use of medical resources.

The RTOG published three studies evaluating different fractionation regimens in patients with brain metastases.[107,117] Patients in these studies were assigned to 4000 cGy in 20 fractions, 4000 cGy in 15 fractions, 3000 cGy in 15 fractions, 3000 cGy in 10 fractions, or 2000 cGy in 5 fractions. Patients with breast cancer accounted for 16% to 18% of the participants in these studies. The overall response rate for symptom palliation (75%–80%) and median survival (15–18 weeks) were similar for all the dose fractionation schedules. Breast cancer patients had a mean survival of 21 weeks. A subsequent study compared 3000 cGy in 10 fractions with 5000 cGy in 20 fractions and saw no survival difference with a median survival of only 17 weeks.[118] Only 7% of these patients had breast cancer. The RTOG has also investigated dose escalation and accelerated fractionation schedules, but to date neither has shown an improvement in survival.[118-120]

A French study compared WBRT of 1800 cGy in three fractions with or without an additional 2500 cGy in 10 fractions.[121] In this study, 29% of the patients had breast cancer. No significant difference was noted in survival. Another study from the United Kingdom compared 3000 cGy in 10 fractions over 2 weeks with 1200 cGy in 2 fractions separated by 1 week. Although there was a significant survival difference in favor of the longer fractionation regimen (84 vs. 77 days), many prefer the shorter regimen, given the questionable clinical significance of 7 days survival.[122]

On the basis of available data, no dose fractionation schedule is superior. The standard and most often prescribed dose fractionation schedule for WBRT is 3000 cGy in 10 fractions. One may consider shorter (2000 cGy in 5 fractions) or longer dose (4500 cGy in 20–25 fractions) schedules based on the patient's projected prognosis and/or severity of symptoms.

Toxicity of Whole-Brain Radiation Therapy

During WBRT, side effects are mild and generally tolerable. Possible acute toxicities include alopecia, serous otitis media, radiation dermatitis, nausea and vomiting, and myelosuppression. Radiation dermatitis and partial or complete alopecia are common. A dose-response relationship for the hair follicle has been reported to correlate with permanent alopecia and previous chemotherapy may increase the risk of radiation-induced alopecia.[123] Nausea and vomiting are infrequent, as is myelosuppression. Occasionally, a patient's neurologic symptoms can worsen during WBRT secondary to worsening cerebral edema. If a patient's neurologic symptoms should acutely worsen, corticosteroids should be started; if the patient is already on corticosteroids, the dose should be increased in the short term. Acute encephalopathy may occur with fraction sizes larger than 300 cGy. The patient has symptoms of severe headache, nausea, drowsiness, and focal neurologic deficits and fever. The physiologic mechanism is thought to be radiation damage to the BBB resulting in cerebral edema. Death may occur secondary to cerebral herniation. The incidence of acute encephalopathy is low; in one series from 1970s, 6% of patients were dead 48 hours after receiving a single fraction of 1000 cGy with cobalt-60.[124] Diffuse enhancement is often seen on brain MRI scans; it is not correlated with acute toxicity and resolves after WBRT.

Possible late toxicities include somnolence syndrome, radiation necrosis, and neurocognitive impairment. Somnolence syndrome is a subacute effect of cranial irradiation that occurs more commonly in pediatric patients 1 to 6 months after WBRT and is characterized by extreme sleepiness and signs of increased intracranial pressure (i.e., headache, nausea, vomiting, anorexia, and irritability). Somnolence syndrome is rare in adults; it resolves spontaneously and does not result in late effects. Radiation necrosis and neurocognitive impairment are possible late effects (>90 days after completing WBRT). Radiation necrosis is highly unlikely with standard dose fractionation schedules used for palliative WBRT (i.e., 3000 cGy in 10 fractions) and is uncommon with doses less than 5000 cGy in 25 fractions.[125] The risk of radiation necrosis increases with increasing dose and fraction size as well as the use of subsequent chemotherapy.[125] The incidence of radiation necrosis is 5% with doses of 5500 to 6000 cGy, although these doses are not typically used for WBRT. Radiation necrosis is more common after SRS. The rate of necrosis in patients treated with SRS with or without WBRT is 4% to 6%.[126]

Some have argued, based on retrospective data, that neurocognitive function and quality of life decline after WBRT and that therefore SRS is preferable to WBRT. Neurocognitive dysfunction is often multifactorial and distinguishing the cause of a patient's mental deterioration may be difficult. The brain metastasis(es) itself, progressive disease, neurosurgical procedures, anticonvulsants, steroids, narcotic medications, chemotherapy, and/or RT can all contribute to neurocognitive dysfunction. Several other variables may influence the development of neurocognitive dysfunction, including total radiation dose, fraction size, volume of brain irradiated, concurrent chemotherapy, age, and presence of diabetes mellitus. The pathophysiologic mechanism is thought to be vascular damage and demyelination from RT. A phase III randomized trial that assessed the efficacy of motexafin gadolinium in brain metastases patients receiving WBRT documented that 90% of brain metastases patients have baseline neurocognitive impairment before any therapy.[127] Higher baseline neurocognitive function correlated with improved survival. A subsequent analysis of 208 patients from this trial showed that patients who

had a good response (>45% tumor shrinkage) had better neurocognitive function preservation.[128] Those with progressive disease in the brain had worsening neurocognitive function. A question also remains regarding the feasibility and risks of sparing the subgranular zone of the hippocampus during WBRT for brain metastases as a strategy to reduce the risk of neurocognitive decline.[129] Despite the provocative results of small studies using hippocampal sparing WBRT with cancer CNS metastases indicating stable scores of neurocognitive function, further validation of this new approach is warranted.[130,131]

Furthermore, in the RTOG 0214 patients with stage III non–small cell lung cancer treated with prophylactic WBRT to total dose of 30 Gy/15 fractions once daily compared with observation had no significant differences in global cognitive function (Mini–Mental State Examination [MMSE]) or quality of life after prophylactic WBRT, but there was a significant decline in memory at 1 year.[132]

Hyperfractionated RT has been used to spare normal tissues, and its ability to spare neurocognitive function has been tested. RTOG 94-01 tested whether accelerated hyperfractionation (160 cGy twice daily to 5440 cGy) improved neurocognitive outcome in brain metastases patients receiving WBRT. The patients treated with accelerated hyperfractionation did not have significantly different neurocognitive outcomes compared with the patients treated with 3000 cGy in 10 fractions.[133] Furthermore, the rate of decline in neurocognitive function at 3 months was smaller for those whose brain metastases were radiologically controlled compared with those with uncontrolled brain metastases ($p = .02$). Aoyama and colleagues published an analysis of neurocognitive function in patients with one to four brain metastases in a randomized trial comparing WBRT plus SRS with SRS.[134] The 1-, 2-, and 3-year actuarial free rate of a three-point drop in MMSE scores was 76.1%, 68.5%, and 14.7%, respectively, in the WBRT plus SRS arm versus 59.3%, 51.9%, and 51.9%, respectively, in the SRS-alone arm. The average duration until MMSE deterioration was longer in the WBRT plus SRS patients (16.5 vs. 7.6 months, $p = .05$). Tumor progression was found to be the cause of neurocognitive decline more often in patients treated with SRS alone, meaning that neurocognitive decline is most likely caused by brain metastases progression and not radiation damage to the brain. However, survival is limited in patients with brain metastases, and they may not survive long enough to develop RT-induced neurocognitive impairment.

A smaller randomized trial evaluating SRS alone versus SRS + WBRT was stopped after the first 58 patients.[135] WBRT was prescribed to a total dose of 30 Gy given in 12 daily fractions of 2.5 Gy per day. There was a high probability (96%) that patients randomly assigned to receive SRS plus WBRT were significantly more likely to show a decline in learning and memory function (mean posterior probability of decline 52%) at 4 months than patients assigned to receive SRS alone (mean posterior probability of decline 24%). At 4 months there were four deaths (13%) in the group that received SRS alone, and eight deaths (29%) in the group that received SRS plus WBRT. Seventy-three percent of patients in the SRS plus WBRT group were free from CNS recurrence at 1 year, compared with 27% of patients who received SRS alone ($p = .0003$).

Finally, recent meta-analysis of randomized controlled trials comparing surgery or SRS plus WBRT with surgery or SRS alone for treatment of brain metastases failed to capture the potential negative impact for WBRT on neurocognitive function and health-related quality of life.[136]

TABLE
73.2 **Randomized Trials for Surgery and WBRT**

	Patient n	Arms	Local Recurrence	Distant Recurrence in Brain	Median OS	Neurologic Death	Median Time to Neurologic Death
Patchell, 1990[70]	48	WBRT vs. WBRT + surgery	52% vs. 20% (*p* < .02)	13% vs. 20% (*p* = .52)	14 vs. 40 wk (*p* < .01)	NS	26 vs. 62 wk (*p* < .0009)
Vecht, 1993; Noordijk, 1994[137,138]	63	WBRT vs. WBRT + surgery	NS	NS	24 vs. 40 wk (*p* = .04)	NS	NS
Mintz, 1996[139]	84	WBRT vs. WBRT + surgery	NS	NS	22 vs. 25 wk (*p* = .24)	NS	NS
Patchell, 1998[115]	95	Surgery vs. WBRT + surgery	46% vs. 10% (*p* < .001)	37% vs. 14% (*p* < .01)	43 vs. 48 wk (*p* = .39)	44% vs. 14% (*p* = .003)	81 vs. 115 wk (*p* = .03)

NS, Not stated; *WBRT,* whole-brain radiation therapy.

Surgery

Surgery can rapidly relieve neurologic symptoms from the mass effect of a brain metastasis and provide local control and a histologic diagnosis. Before recommending surgery, oncologists must consider the patient's age, KPS, status of extracranial disease, location of the brain metastasis, and the number of brain metastases. If surgery is necessary, perioperative anticonvulsant therapy should be considered.

Surgical Intervention for Single Metastasis

There is considerable randomized evidence suggesting that surgical resection of brain metastasis before WBRT improves quality of life and lengthens survival.[70,115,137,138] These data have been confirmed by multiple clinical trials, three which compared WBRT to WBRT plus surgical resection,[70,137–139] and one which compared WBRT plus surgery to surgery alone[115] (Table 73.2).

Patchell and colleagues published the first randomized trial comparing WBRT versus WBRT plus surgery in patients with a single brain metastasis.[70] Adding surgical resection of a single brain metastasis decreased local recurrence and lengthened both OS and time to neurologic death. The percentage of patients who developed a recurrence at the site of the original metastasis was only 20% in the WBRT plus surgery arm versus 52% in the WBRT arm (*p* < .02). Of the patients with recurrences at the site of the original metastasis, the length of time from treatment to recurrence was a median of 59 weeks in the WBRT plus surgery arm versus a median of 21 weeks in the group treated with WBRT alone (*p* < .001). There was no difference in recurrences elsewhere in the brain (13%–20%, *p* = .52). When deaths from only neurologic causes were used as end points, the surgical group had a median neurologic survival of 62 weeks, whereas the group treated with WBRT alone had a neurologic survival of only 26 weeks (*p* < .0009). The median OS was longer in the WBRT plus surgery arm (40 vs. 14 weeks, *p* < .01). The surgical group maintained KPS ratings of more than 70% for a median of 38 weeks, whereas the group treated with RT alone maintained a functionally independent level for a median of only 8 weeks (*p* < .005). The treatment morbidity and mortality were similar. One caveat to applying the findings of this study to patients with MBC is that only 3 of the 48 patients (6%) studied had breast

carcinoma as their primary tumor; 37 (77%) of the patients had non–small-cell lung carcinoma.

A randomized Dutch trial also showed an OS benefit from adding surgery to WBRT.[137,138] Investigators from this study randomized 63 patients (19% with breast primaries) with a single brain metastasis to either WBRT alone or WBRT plus surgery. The median OS was 24 weeks in the WBRT-alone arm and 40 weeks in the WBRT plus surgery arm (*p* = .04). Furthermore, the median OS was 5 months for both arms if the patients had active extracranial disease. A Canadian multicenter randomized trial failed to show a survival benefit from adding surgery to WBRT.[139] Eighty-four patients were randomized, and the median OS was 22 weeks in the WBRT-alone arm and 25 weeks in the WBRT plus surgery arm (*p* = .24). The authors suggest that patient selection may have negated the survival benefit seen in the two aforementioned trials.[140] The Canadian trial included patients with a lower baseline median KPS; a higher proportion of them (50%) had extracranial metastases. In addition, 10 of 43 patients randomized to the WBRT-alone arm received surgical resection.

These trials have established that adding surgical resection before WBRT improves survival and quality of life in cancer patients with a single brain metastasis. Patchell and colleagues completed another randomized trial to assess the benefit of WBRT after resecting a single brain metastasis.[115] Ninety-five patients were randomized to surgery alone or WBRT plus surgery. Adding postoperative WBRT reduced local recurrence, distant brain recurrences, and neurologic death. The absolute reduction of any brain failures, either local or distant, was 50% when giving WBRT after surgical resection of a single brain metastasis (*p* < .001). Neurologic deaths were also fewer in the WBRT plus surgery arm (14% vs. 44%, *p* = .003). However, OS was not significantly different between the two arms (43–48 weeks, *p* = .39). On multivariate analysis, the use of WBRT predicted for better neurologic survival (*p* < .009). There was no difference in median time to KPS decline below 70 (35–37 weeks). There were more deaths from systemic disease in the WBRT plus surgery arm, probably because of the higher rates of neurologic death in the surgery-alone arm. Taken together, the results of these trials support that WBRT in conjunction with surgery leads to better clinical outcomes than WBRT alone for good performance patients with solitary metastatic intracranial lesions. With recent advances and concern for quality-of-life detriment with WBRT, SRS has been increasingly used in brain metastases patients including in patients with more than three metastases

Surgery for Multiple Metastases

The role of surgery for multiple brain metastases is controversial, and the data are limited to single-institution retrospective series. Bindal and coworkers conducted a retrospective review of 56 patients who underwent surgery in the setting of multiple cerebral metastases.[141] These patients were divided into two groups: one in which one or more brain metastases were left unresected (n = 30) and another in which all the brain metastases were resected (n = 26). An additional group of patients treated with complete surgical resection of a single metastasis was also evaluated (n = 26). All three groups were matched on the basis of important clinical factors. The group with multiple metastases and at least one metastasis left untreated had a median survival of 6 months, and the two groups with complete resection of their multiple or single metastases each had a median survival of 14 months (p > .5). Thus the median OS was significantly worse in the patients who had one or more unresected brain metastases (p < .05). Recurrence of brain metastases was similar for patients who had complete resection(s) of their multiple or single brain metastases (31%–35%, p > .05). The complication rate for patients undergoing multiple craniotomies was 8% to 9%, and it was 8% for patients undergoing a single craniotomy. The 30-day mortality rate was 3% to 4% for patients with multiple brain metastases and 0% for patients with a single brain metastasis. The authors concluded that resection of all lesions in selected patients with multiple brain metastases resulted in a prognosis similar to that of patients undergoing surgery for a single brain metastasis. Of note, only 11 patients in this series had breast cancer.

In another retrospective series, 70 breast cancer patients with brain metastases had surgery as part of their treatment.[142] Fifty-four patients had single brain metastases and 16 had multiple brain metastases; there was no statistical difference in survival between these groups of patients (median survival, 13.9–14.8 months, p = .28). The median survival of 22 patients with positive hormonal receptor ER or progesterone receptor (PR) was significantly longer than the median survival of 20 patients with negative ER/PR (21.9 vs. 12.5 months, p < .05).

These retrospective studies should be interpreted with caution because they may have included highly selected patients. No prospective trial evaluating surgery for multiple metastases has been performed; therefore the role of surgery for these patients is not clearly defined. Furthermore, these studies were not designed to address the fundamental question of breast cancer subtype and the value of surgical approach to CNS brain metastases. Surgical decision should be individualized based on pattern of disease progression, control of systemic disease, number, size and location of brain metastasis (es) and patient performance statues, comorbidities, and expectations.

Stereotactic Radiosurgery

SRS was developed by the Swedish neurosurgeon Lars Leksell in the 1950s and has become increasingly popular for the treatment of single or a limited number of brain metastases.[143] SRS is a noninvasive option to neurosurgery, especially for brain metastases in difficult to access areas or for patients who cannot have traditional surgery, and it can be combined with WBRT. Through the use of multiple convergent beams, SRS delivers a large dose of radiation in one or a few fractionated treatments to a limited target volume. The hallmark of SRS is the rapid dose falloff with increasing distance from the target, which allows for the sparing of nontarget normal tissues in the brain. SRS can be delivered with high-energy x-rays from linear accelerators (i.e., LINAC, CyberKnife), gamma rays from multiple cobalt-60 sources (i.e., Gamma Knife), or via charged particles such as protons. Compared with fractionated RT, SRS has a radiobiological advantage. The delivery of a single high dose of radiation results in a higher proportion of cellular death and cell cycle arrest. Brain metastases must be less than or equal to 3 cm and adequately distant from the optic apparatus for SRS. Doses may range from 1500 to 3500 cGy. Studies have shown that SRS for a single brain metastasis results in a 1-year local control rate of 80% to 95% and median survival of 7 to 13 months.[126,144–146]

Stereotactic Radiosurgery Versus Surgery

There are several advantages to using SRS instead of surgery. First, SRS is a noninvasive, outpatient procedure that can be used to treat single or multiple metastases. It can also be used to safely treat surgically inaccessible brain metastases or brain metastases that result in significant neurologic morbidity when surgically resected. Also, SRS has been reported to be more cost-effective than surgery.[147,148] Mehta and colleagues analyzed the total cost of treatment for WBRT, WBRT plus surgery, and WBRT plus SRS. The average cost per week of survival was $310 for WBRT, $524 for WBRT plus surgery, and $270 for WBRT plus SRS. However, symptomatic patients with surgically accessible lesions are best treated by surgery, because surgery allows for immediate decompression and symptom relief. Also, neurologic complications and local failures increase for brain metastases greater than 3 cm treated with SRS.

There are no randomized trials comparing SRS with surgery, but some retrospective series have suggested that SRS is as effective as surgical resection. Most of these studies analyzed patients treated with WBRT plus SRS. Auchter and colleagues reviewed 122 patients (10% with primary breast tumors) who had only one brain metastasis and were candidates for surgical resection followed by WBRT but were treated with WBRT and SRS.[144] The median follow-up and survival were 123 weeks and 13 months, respectively. The median SRS and WBRT doses were 1700 and 3750 cGy, respectively. The overall local control rate for the areas treated with SRS was 86%. Twenty-seven patients (22%) had distant intracranial recurrences. The median duration of functional independence was 10 months. These results are comparable to WBRT plus surgery arms in the trials published by Patchell and colleagues[70] and Noordijk and colleagues[138] Another retrospective study compared patients with a single brain metastasis who were eligible for surgical resection or SRS.[149] In this investigation, 74 patients who had surgery were compared with 24 patients who had SRS. Also, 82% of the surgery patients and 96% of the SRS patients were treated with WBRT (p = .172). There was no difference in survival (median survival of 12 months; 1-year survival of 56% for the SRS patients and 62% for the surgery patients, p = .15). There were no local failures for the patients treated with SRS, whereas 19 (56%) patients treated with surgery had local failures. Bindal and colleagues performed a similarly matched comparison between patients treated with surgery versus SRS.[150] The median SRS dose was 2000 cGy. They observed a significantly worse median survival for patients treated with SRS on multivariate analysis (7.5 months for SRS vs. 16.4 months for surgery, p = .0009). The authors stated that the worse survival in

TABLE 73.3   Randomized Trials for Stereotactic Radiation Therapy

	No. of Patients	Arms	One-Year Local Control	Median Overall Survival	Distant Recurrence in Brain	Neurologic Death
Kondziolka 1999	27	WBRT vs. WBRT + SRS	0%[a] vs. 91%	7.5 vs. 11 mo (p = .22)	NS	NS
RTOG 9508	333	WBRT vs. WBRT + SRS	71% vs. 82% (p = .0132)	5.7 vs. 6.5 mo (p = .1356)[b]	NS	31% vs. 28% (p = NS)
Chougule 2000	109	SRS vs. WBRT + SRS vs. WBRT	87% vs. 91% vs. 62% (p = NS)	7 vs. 5 vs. 9 mo (p = NS)	43% vs. 19% vs. 23% (p = NS)	NS
JRSOG-9901	132	SRS vs. WBRT + SRS	72.5% vs. 88.7% (p = .002)	8 vs. 7.5 mo (p = .42)	63.7% vs. 41.5% (p = .003)	19.3% vs. 22.8% (p = .64)

NS, Not stated; *SRS*, stereotactic radiation therapy; *WBRT*, whole-brain radiation therapy.
[a]This includes patients who died before 1 year and those still living, all with tumor progression.
[b]Survival advantage was seen in patients with a single brain metastasis treated with WBRT + SRS (6.2 vs. 4.9 mo, p = .0393).
Data from references 146, 155, 158, 159.

patients treated to SRS was the result of a greater progression rate of the radiosurgically treated lesions (p = .0001). One additional study retrospectively analyzed 206 patients (19% had breast cancer) in RPA classes 1 and 2 who had one or two brain metastases.[105,151] The authors compared patients treated with SRS alone to those treated with surgical resection and WBRT. Comparison of the two groups showed no significant difference for OS (p = .19), brain control (p = .52), or local control (p = .25).

Most recently, Yamamoto and colleagues conducted a prospective observational study of 1194 patients with untreated multiple brain metastases.[152] Patients with 1 to 10 newly diagnosed brain metastasis (<3 cm in longest diameter) and a KPS score of 70 or higher were enrolled. Ten percent of the patients had MBC. Tumor volumes smaller than 4 mL were irradiated with 22 Gy at the lesion periphery and those that were 4 to 10 mL with 20 Gy. The primary end point was OS. Median OS after stereotactic radiosurgery was 13.9 months (95% confidence interval [CI] 12.0–15.6) in the 455 patients with one tumor, 10.8 months (95% CI 9.4–12.4) in the 531 patients with two to four tumors, and 10.8 months (95% CI 9.1–12.7) in the 208 patients with 5 to 10 tumors. The results suggested that stereotactic radiosurgery without WBRT in patients with 5 to 10 brain metastases is noninferior to that in patients with two to four brain metastases.

These results have supported the use of SRS as an upfront treatment approach for patients with increasing number CNS metastatic disease with less than 3 cm greatest dimension. Per National Comprehensive Cancer Network guidelines, WBRT remains indicated for patients with more than three metastases; however, in clinical practice, SRS is becoming more widely used for more than three lesions.[153] These new parameters are largely determined institutionally until national guidelines change to match this evolving perspective.

Whole-Brain Radiation Therapy Versus Whole-Brain Radiation Therapy Plus Stereotactic Radiosurgery Boost

Given that SRS has a similar efficacy to that of surgical resection, investigators have studied the possible benefit of adding SRS to WBRT. A multiinstitutional retrospective review was conducted comparing patients treated with WBRT alone to those treated with WBRT and SRS,[154] and 502 patients were eligible and

stratified according to RPA class. The addition of SRS increased survival. The median survival rates for patients treated with WBRT plus SRS versus WBRT alone stratified by RPA class were 16.1 versus 7.1, 10.3 versus 4.2, and 8.7 versus 2.3 months for classes 1, 2, and 3, respectively (p < .05).

Two randomized trials have compared WBRT to WBRT plus SRS boost. Kondziolka and coworkers published a randomized trial of 27 patients (14 to WBRT alone and 13 to WBRT plus SRS; Table 73.3).[146] Patients had two to four brain metastases. Fifteen percent of the patients in this study had primary breast cancer. The WBRT dose was 3000 cGy in 12 fractions, and the SRS dose was 1600 cGy. The trial was stopped early after the interim analysis,[146] which revealed a significant benefit in the rate of local tumor control after WBRT plus SRS (p = .0016). The local failure rate at 1 year was 100% in the WBRT-alone arm versus 8% in the WBRT plus SRS arm, with a corresponding median time to local failure of 6 and 36 months (p = .0005). Survival was not statistically different between the two arms: patients who received WBRT alone lived a median of 7.5 months, whereas those who received WBRT plus SRS lived 11 months (p = .22).

The RTOG conducted a multiinstitutional phase III trial comparing WBRT alone to WBRT plus SRS boost for patients with one to three unresectable brain metastases.[155] In this study, 333 patients were randomized, 10% of whom had primary breast cancer, and patients were stratified according to the number of brain metastases (one vs. two and three). The WBRT dose was 3750 cGy in 15 fractions, and the SRS doses were 2400 cGy (≤2 cm), 1800 cGy (>2 cm but ≤3 cm), and 1500 cGy (>3 cm but ≤4 cm). The overall median survival for the WBRT group was 5.7 months, and for the WBRT plus SRS group, it was 6.5 months (p = .1356). The median survival for patients with a single brain metastasis treated with WBRT plus SRS boost was significantly better at 6.5 versus 4.9 months (p = .0393). On multivariate analysis, RPA class I predicted better survival than RPA class II (p < .0001). The 1-year local control was better for patients treated with WBRT plus SRS (82% vs. 71%, p = .0132). Local recurrence was 43% more likely in the WBRT-alone arm (p = .0021). Patients in the WBRT plus SRS arm were more likely to have a stable or improved KPS at 6-month follow-up than were patients allocated to the WBRT-alone arm (43% vs. 27%, respectively, $p = .03$) and were able to taper steroid use sooner. Acute toxicities of grade 3 or greater were reported in 3% of the WBRT plus SRS patients versus none of the WBRT patients. Late toxicities of grade 3 or greater were reported in 6% versus 3% of WBRT plus SRS and WBRT patients, respectively. The authors concluded that WBRT plus SRS should be the standard treatment for patients with an unresectable single brain metastasis and considered for patients with multiple brain metastases.

Stereotactic Radiosurgery Versus Whole-Brain Radiation Therapy

Some have argued that because of the possible neurocognitive impairment caused by WBRT, SRS alone could be used for selected patients with WBRT reserved for salvage treatment.[145,156] Numerous retrospective studies have compared SRS alone to WBRT alone.[157] These studies have shown that survival is similar between patients treated with SRS alone versus WBRT alone but that local and distant failures in the brain are higher in patients treated with SRS alone. Two randomized trials have compared SRS alone to WBRT plus SRS.[158,159] Chougule and colleagues randomized 109 patients with three brain metastases or fewer to Gamma Knife (GK) radiosurgery, GK plus WBRT, or WBRT alone.[159] Currently data are published only in abstract form. The majority of patients in this study had primary breast cancer (62 patients, 57%). The radiation doses for the three arms of the study were as follows: GK-alone arm, 3000 cGy; WBRT plus GK arm, 3000 cGy WBRT and 2000 cGy GK boost; and WBRT-alone arm, 3000 cGy. Of note, 51 patients (47%) had surgical resections of large, symptomatic brain metastases before randomization. The median OS was similar for each treatment arm: 7, 5, and 9 months for the GK, GK and WBRT, and WBRT-alone arms, respectively. Local control appeared to be better in the GK arms: 87%, 91%, and 62% for GK, GK plus WBRT, and WBRT-alone arms, respectively. The incidence of new brain metastases was lower in the two arms that received WBRT: 43%, 19%, and 23% for GK, GK plus WBRT, and WBRT-alone, respectively.

A multiinstitutional phase III randomized trial from Japan (JRSOG-9901) reported results of treating 132 patients with one to four brain metastases (each ≤3 cm) with either SRS alone or WBRT plus SRS.[158] The radiation dose for the SRS-alone arm was 2200 to 2500 cGy for lesions 2 cm or smaller and 1800 to 2000 cGy for lesions greater than 2 cm. In the WBRT plus SRS arm, the SRS dose was 30% lower. The WBRT dose was 3000 cGy in 10 fractions. Only nine (7%) patients in this study had breast cancer. The median follow-up was 7.8 months. The primary objective was survival; however, the trial was terminated early because of the significant difference in brain metastasis recurrence rates. Thus criticisms of this trial are that it was insufficiently powered to observe a potential survival difference and that 805 patients would have to be enrolled to detect a significant difference in survival. There were no differences in median survival (8 vs. 7.5 months) or neurologic death (19.3% vs. 22.8%, $p = .64$). The multivariate survival analysis revealed that age less than 65 years, stable primary tumor status, stable extracranial metastases status, and KPS score 90 to 100 significantly predicted better survival. The 1-year local control rate was significantly higher for the WBRT plus SRS arm than for the SRS-alone arm (88.7% vs. 72.5%, $p < .001$). The 1-year distant brain recurrence rate was lower for patients treated with WBRT plus SRS: 41.5% versus 63.7% ($p = .003$). On multivariate analysis, receiving WBRT plus SRS, having stable extracranial metastases, and having a KPS score

of 70 to 80 predicted fewer distant brain recurrences. The number of brain metastases did not predict for survival or distant brain recurrence. Salvage treatment for progression of brain tumor was required significantly more frequently in the SRS-alone group (29 patients) than in the WBRT plus SRS group (10 patients, $p < .001$). Neurologic preservation (maintenance of KPS ≥70) was the same for each arm. There was one grade 3 or greater acute neurotoxicity reported in the WBRT plus SRS arm and two in the SRS-alone arm. There were four grade 3 or greater late neurotoxicities in the WBRT plus SRS versus two in the SRS-alone arm.

In another prospective study, 58 patients with one to three newly diagnosed brain metastases were randomly assigned to SRS plus WBRT or SRS alone.[135] The trial was stopped in light of significantly more decline in learning and memory function in the WBRT plus SRS group compared with the SRS only cohort.

These results favor the use of SRS for patients with asymptomatic oligometastatic disease to brain with less than 3 parenchymal lesions compared with WBRT.

Chemotherapy

Historically, the main treatment of brain metastases has been radiation. Chemotherapy was not thought to be effective given the belief that hydrophilic drugs and/or large molecules could not pass the BBB. The multidrug-resistance gene (P-glycoprotein) is known to be highly expressed by the endothelium of brain capillaries. It was typically thought that only small lipid-soluble molecules could pass the BBB, but this theory has been questioned.[160] Metastatic tumors are known to have abnormal vascular supply in both function and anatomy, and thus the BBB may not be functioning normally. Some investigators have used BBB-disruption agents in conjunction with cytotoxic chemotherapy.[161,162] A list of chemotherapy agents that can or cannot cross the BBB can be found in Table 73.4. A problem with all of the phase I and II trials assessing chemotherapy in brain metastases patients is that the patient populations in these trials have been heavily pretreated and often the shortcoming of treatment is not necessarily BBB penetrance but rather aggressive disease biology from more resistant cancers.

Box 73.1 lists the reported active chemotherapy regimens for CNS metastases from breast cancer. Commonly used drugs include anthracyclines, taxanes, alkylating agents, antimetabolites, and vinca alkaloids. The largest series by Rosner and coworkers included 100 patients treated with a variety of regimens, most commonly cyclophosphamide, fluorouracil, and prednisone, or cyclophosphamide, fluorouracil, prednisone, methotrexate, and vincristine.[163] Ten patients had a complete response (CR), 40 had a partial response (PR), 9 had stable disease, and 41 had no response (NR); thus 50% of the patients responded to systemic chemotherapy. The median survival for patients having CR, PR, and NR was 39.5 months, 10.5 months, and 1.5 months, respectively. Franciosi and colleagues prospectively analyzed 56 breast cancer patients with brain metastases treated with platinum and etoposide for a median of three cycles.[164] None of the patients received RT or other chemotherapy between the time of the diagnosis of brain metastases and treatment. The authors reported an objective response rate (ORR) of 38%. The median duration of response and time to progression was 8 months. There was a median survival of 8 months and a 1-year survival rate of 32%. Investigators from the Netherlands reported a 59% response rate at 6 months in 22 breast cancer patients with brain metastases treated with cyclophosphamide, doxorubicin, and fluorouracil

TABLE 73.4 Chemotherapeutic Agents That Cross the Blood-Brain Barrier

Agent	Crosses Blood-Brain Barrier?
Temozolomide	Yes
Tamoxifen	Yes
Idarubicin	Yes
Liposomal doxorubicin	Yes
Methotrexate	Yes
Temozolomide	Yes
Fluorouracil	Yes, but limited
Carboplatin	Yes, but limited
Cisplatin	Yes, but limited
Cyclophosphamide	No
Doxorubicin	No
Daunorubicin	No
Paclitaxel	No
Docetaxel	No
Vinorelbine	No
Etoposide	No
Fulvestrant	No
Trastuzumab	No
Capecitabine	Unknown

Modified from Lin NU, Bellon JR, Winer EP. CNS metastases in breast cancer. *J Clin Oncol.* 2004;22:3608-3617.

• BOX 73.1 Chemotherapeutic Regimens With Reported Activity Against Breast Central Nervous System Metastases

Cyclophosphamide, fluorouracil, and prednisone
Cyclophosphamide, fluorouracil, prednisone, methotrexate, and vincristine
Methotrexate, vincristine, and prednisone
Cyclophosphamide, methotrexate, and fluorouracil
Cyclophosphamide, doxorubicin, and fluorouracil
Bendamustine
Temozolomide
Temozolomide + whole-brain radiation therapy
Capecitabine
Cisplatin and etoposide
Tamoxifen
Megestrol acetate
Anastrazole
Letrozole
Temozolomide

Modified from Lin NU, Bellon JR, Winer EP. CNS metastases in breast cancer. J Clin Oncol. 2004;22:3608-3617.

(CAF) or cyclophosphamide, methotrexate, and fluorouracil (CMF).[165] The median duration of response, median survival time, and 1-year survival rate were 7 months, 6 months for the whole group (16 months for responders), and 25%, respectively. The authors showed that these results compared favorably with results from matched historical controls treated with RT alone. However, the response rate of 34% and median survival of 2.5 months in their radiation-only historical controls are much lower than commonly reported in the WBRT literature.

Antifolate inhibitors have been studied in metastatic CNS disease. A retrospective study of 31 women (29 with breast cancer) treated with high-dose intravenous methotrexate (3.5 g/m^2) for CNS parenchymal or leptomeningeal metastases showed an objective radiographic response and stable disease were each observed in nine patients (28%), and 13 (44%) patients progressed. Prior treatment with low-dose MTX for systemic disease did not affect response ($p = .8$). The median OS (n = 32) was 19.9 weeks. Myelosuppression and elevated serum hepatic transaminases were the most common acute toxicities.[166] Also, prospective trials assessed pharmacokinetics and efficacy of pemetrexed in patients with brain parenchymal metastasis and LM metastatic disease.[167] Twenty-one patients (13 with breast cancer) were treated with pemetrexed. The median number of cycles was 3 (range 1–14). Responses included 1 partial response, 10 stable disease cases, and 10 progressive disease cases. Median time to progression and survival was 2.7 and 7.3 months. No major toxicities were seen.

Because malignant gliomas can be successfully treated with concurrent RT and temozolomide, interest has developed for using temozolomide as a treatment for brain metastases.[168–173] Temozolomide has been shown to be able to cross the BBB. In a phase II trial published by Antonadou and colleagues,[168] 53 patients with brain metastases (5% or 10% of whom had breast cancer) were randomized to oral temozolomide (75 mg/m^2/day) concurrent with 4000 cGy in 20 fractions of WBRT versus 4000 cGy WBRT alone. The group receiving temozolomide and RT continued temozolomide therapy (200 mg/m^2/day) for 5 days every 28 days for an additional six cycles. The ORR was significantly ($p = .017$) improved in patients receiving temozolomide and WBRT versus WBRT alone. Twenty-three patients (96%) in the temozolomide plus WBRT arm had an objective response, including 9 (38%) with CRs and 14 (58%) with PRs. With RT alone, 14 (67%) of 21 assessable patients responded, including 7 (33%) with CRs and 7 (33%) with PRs. The proportion of patients requiring corticosteroids 2 months after treatment was lower in the temozolomide group compared with RT alone (67% vs. 91%, respectively). Daily temozolomide concurrent with RT was generally well tolerated; however, greater than grade 2 nausea (48% vs. 13%, $p = .13$) and vomiting (32% vs. 0%, $p = .004$) were significantly increased in the temozolomide group. Another similarly designed phase II trial enrolled 82 patients and showed that progression-free survival (PFS) at 90 days was better in patients who received temozolomide plus WBRT (54% for WBRT vs. 72% for WBRT and temozolomide, $p = .03$).[173] Thirteen (16%) patients in the study had breast cancer. The median OS has been reported to be 8 to 13 months for patients with brain metastases treated with WBRT plus temozolomide.[171,172,174] Temozolomide has been evaluated as monotherapy in phase II trial among 157 patients with solid tumor with metastasis to the brain.[175] Patients received temozolomide 150 mg/m^2/day (days 1–7 and 15–21 every 28- or 35-day cycle) and the partial response rate in the 51 patients with diagnosis of breast cancer was 4% only with a median PFS of 58 days.

Others have combined temozolomide with other cytotoxic chemotherapy agents.[176-178] A phase I trial treated breast cancer patients with brain metastases with temozolomide and capecitabine.[178] All but one patient had been treated with up to three different chemotherapy regimens before entry on this trial. A total of four (18% ORR) patients responded; three were PRs and one was a CR. The median response duration was 8 weeks (range, 6–64 weeks), and the median time to progression in the brain was 12 weeks (range, 3–70 weeks). A phase II trial combining temozolomide and cisplatin treated 32 patients with brain metastases (47% had primary breast cancer).[177] Six of the breast cancer patients had a PR and none had a CR. Only one patient died from neutropenia/septicemia. The authors concluded that temozolomide combined with cisplatin can act against brain metastases and is well tolerated. Iwamoto and colleagues concluded from a phase II trial that adding vinorelbine to temozolomide did not improve response rates compared with trials that used single-agent temozolamide.[176] Freedman and colleagues conducted a phase II study of sagopilone, an epothilone B analog that crosses the BBB, in patients with breast cancer brain metastases. Women were treated with 16 mg/m^2 or 22 mg/m^2 intravenously every 21 days.[179] Of 15 women in the study only 2 achieved PR and the estimated median PFS was 1.4 months indicating the modest activity of the agent.

Overall, investigators report response rates of 38% to 59%, median survivals of 8 to 15 months, and 1-year survivals of 30% to 55% in patients with brain metastases treated with chemotherapy with or without RT.[82,163-165,180,181]

Patients with TNBC have high risk of CNS metastasis. Lin and coworkers reported the estimated risk to be as high as 46% in one series of 116 with metastatic TNBC.[182] These patients also tend to have brain metastasis earlier in the course of metastatic disease. In one series patients with metastatic TNBC had a median brain metastases–free survival of 14 months compared with 34 months in hormonal receptor positive patients.[183] In recent years, efforts have been initiated to improve the unmet need for improved therapeutic options in patients presenting with TNBC and CNS metastasis. Anders and colleagues conducted a phase II trial in which 37 patients with TNBC and concomitant brain metastasis were treated with irinotecan 125 mg/m^2 intravenously days 1 and 8 of each 21-day cycle.[184] When the study opened, iniparib was dosed at 5.6 mg/kg intravenously (IV) on days 1, 4, 8, and 11 of each 21-day cycle. In 2011, based on emerging data in primary brain tumors, the dose of iniparib was raised to 8 mg/kg on the same schedule. Of note, more than 50% of the cohort had received prior WBRT and chemotherapy. Median TTP was 2.14 months and median OS was 7.8 months. Intracranial response rate was 12% indicating modest activity of the regimen.

Because up to 30% to 50% of HER2-positive, MBC patients will develop a CNS metastasis, the use of a targeted therapy directed against the HER2 receptor is desirable.[27-29] Dijkers and colleagues reported a feasibility study to determine the optimal dosage and time of administration of the monoclonal antibody zirconium-89 ((89)Zr)-trastuzumab to enable PET imaging of HER2-positive lesions.[185] PET scanning after administration of (89)Zr-trastuzumab allowed for visualization of brain metastasis in three patients indicating BBB penetration of trastuzumab. In a retrospective study of 251 patients with HER2-positive breast cancer and brain metastases, patients who had received trastuzumab had longer time to death from brain metastases compared with patients who did not (median 14.9 vs 4.0 months, p = .0005).[186] Multivariate modeling, however, suggested that

improved time to death from brain metastasis was secondary to extracranial disease control (HR 8.4, 95% CI 4.9–142; p < .0001). In addition, a retrospective, exploratory analysis of the EMILIA trial identified 95 patients with HER2-positive, metastatic disease to the brain.[187] Among patients with CNS metastases at baseline, a significant improvement in OS was observed in the T-DM1 arm compared with the capecitabine arm (HR 0.38; p = .008; median, 26.8 vs. 12.9 months).

In an ongoing phase II trial (PATRICIA), patients with CNS metastases secondary to HER2-positive MBC will receive pertuzumab in combination with high-dose trastuzumab. Pertuzumab will be given as 840 mg during the first IV infusion, followed every 3 weeks thereafter by a standard dose of 420 mg. Trastuzumab will be given as 6 mg/kg once weekly via IV infusion without a loading dose.[188]

Lapatinib is an orally active small-molecule inhibitor of the EGFR (also called erbB-1) and HER2 (erbB-2) that can cross the BBB. A phase III randomized trial has shown that adding lapatinib to capecitabine as a second-line treatment for locally advanced breast cancer that has progressed through anthracycline-, taxane-, and trastuzumab-based therapy is more effective than capecitabine alone. Also, there are fewer cases with CNS involvement at first progression (four patients, or 2%, in the lapatinib and capecitabine arm versus 13 patients, or 6%, in the capecitabine arm, p = .045).[189,190]

Bachelot and colleagues published the seminal multicenter phase II trial in which patients had HER2-positive MBC with brain metastases not previously treated with WBRT, capecitabine, or lapatinib.[191] Treatment was given in 21-day cycles: patients received lapatinib (1250 mg, orally) every day and capecitabine (2000 mg/m^2, orally) from days 1 to 14. The primary end point was the proportion of patients with an objective CNS response, defined as a 50% or greater volumetric reduction of CNS lesions in the absence of increased steroid use, progressive neurologic symptoms, and progressive extra-CNS disease. A total of 45 patients were accrued, and 29 had an objective CNS response (65.9%, 95% CI 50.1–79.5); all were partial responses. Of all 45 treated patients, 22 (49%) had grade 3 or 4 treatment-related adverse events, of which the most common were diarrhea in nine patients (20%) and hand-foot syndrome in nine patients (20%). Fourteen patients (31%) had at least one severe adverse event; treatment was discontinued because of toxicity in four patients. No toxic deaths occurred. With a median follow-up of 21.2 months (range 2.2–27.6), OS at 6 months was 90.9% (95% CI 77.6–96.5), and the median OS for the 44 patients who were assessable for efficacy outcomes was 17.0 months. Although results were encouraging, this treatment was associated with a 49% grade 3 to 4 toxicity rate, which is greater than that seen in the short-term with radiation therapy using either WBRT or SRS.

The American Society of Clinical Oncology (ASCO) practice guidelines for the treatment of HER2-positive MBC to the brain state that if patients have asymptomatic, low-volume brain metastases and have not received radiation therapy, upfront therapy with lapatinib and capecitabine is an option, although radiation therapy in this setting is still the standard option.[192]

Lapatinib has been tested in combination with temozolomide in a phase I trial.[193] Sixteen patients with HER2-positive progressive brain metastasis were enrolled, fourteen of whom had had prior WBRT. For the 15 remaining assessable patients, stable disease was achieved in 10 patients (67%) and progression of disease in 5 patients (33%). The most common adverse events (AEs) were fatigue, diarrhea, and constipation.

TABLE 73.5 Ongoing Clinical Trials for HER2-Positive Breast Cancer With Brain Metastasis

Agent	Phase of Study	Clinicaltrial.gov Identification No.
Everolimus/vinorelbine/ trastuzumab	II	NCT01305941
BKM120/trastuzumab/ capecitabine	Ib/II	NCT01132664
Lapatinib/whole-brain radiation therapy	II	NCT01622868
Neratinib/capecitabine	II	NCT01494662
Afatinib/vinorelbine	II	NCT01441596
ARRY-380/trastuzumab	I	NCT01921335
GRN1005/trastuzumab	II	NCT01480583
ITC trastuzumab/ITC pertuzumab	I	NCT02598427
Cabozantinib/trastuzumab	II	NCT02260531
Irinotecan/trastuzumab	II	NCT00303992
Capecitabine/everolimus/ capecitabine	II	NCT01783756
Pertuzumab/trastuzumab	II	NCT02536339

From http://www.clinicaltrials.gov; accessed November 2015.

A phase II trial reported by Lin and coworkers in patients with HER2-positive metastatic disease to the brain evaluated lapatinib as monotherapy after WBRT.[194] Patients received lapatinib 750 mg orally twice a day. Tumor response was assessed by MRI every 8 weeks. Thirty-nine patients were enrolled. All patients had developed brain metastases while receiving trastuzumab; 37 had progressed after prior radiation. One patient achieved a PR (objective response rate 2.6%). These results taken together indicated the response rates are low after WBRT progression.

In light of the risk of CNS metastasis in patients presenting with metastatic HER2-positive breast cancer, several clinical trials with novel agents are being developed (Table 73.5).

Radiation Sensitizers

Radiation sensitizers, such as motexafin gadolinium and efaproxiral, have been tested with WBRT for brain metastases.[195] A phase III trial randomized 401 patients (19% of whom were breast cancer patients) to WBRT or WBRT with concurrent motexafin gadolinium.[195] There was no significant difference in median survival (5.2 months for WBRT plus motexafin gadolinium vs. 4.9 months for WBRT alone, $p = .48$) or time to neurologic progression (median, 9.5 vs. 8.3 months, respectively, $p = .95$). Efaproxiral (RSR13) is an allosteric modifier of hemoglobin that reduces the binding affinity of hemoglobin for oxygen, thereby increasing the partial pressure of oxygen in the blood and tissue. Radiobiologically, hypoxic tumor cells are more resistant to radiation, and the use of efaproxiral may reoxygenate tumor cells and make them more sensitive to RT. A phase III trial evaluated whether efaproxiral improved survival in patients with brain metastases

treated with WBRT.[196] There were 515 patients (21% had breast cancer) randomized in this trial to WBRT alone or WBRT plus efaproxiral. With a median follow-up of 15.2 months, there was no difference in median survival: 5.4 months for the efaproxiral arm versus 4.4 months for the control arm (HR 0.87, $p = .16$). However, an exploratory analysis by primary tumor type showed that the largest efaproxiral treatment effect was observed in the 107 patients with brain metastases from breast cancer (HR 0.51, $p = .003$). On multivariate analysis, the HR for breast cancer brain metastases was 0.59 (0.42–0.84, $p = .01$). In a follow-up subgroup analysis of the 107 breast cancer brain metastases patients in this trial, the authors reported that the median survival time was 4.47 months in the WBRT arm and 9 months in the WBRT plus efaproxiral arm (unadjusted $p = .004$). On multivariate analysis, the addition of efaproxiral to WBRT reduced the death rate by 46% ($p = .0086$) after adjusting for other prognostic factors. Because of the positive results in the breast cancer patients, a confirmatory trial for breast cancer patients has been initiated.

Lin and coworkers also tested lapatinib as radiosensitizer in a phase I trial.[197] In this study, 27 patients with HER2-positive breast cancer and one or more brain metastasis received lapatinib 750 mg twice on day one followed by 1000, 1250, or 1500 mg once daily. WBRT (37.5 Gy, 15 fractions) began 1 to 8 days after starting lapatinib. Lapatinib was continued through WBRT. Overall, 7 of 27 patients at 1250 mg (maximum tolerated dose) had DLTs: grade 3 rash (n = 2), diarrhea (n = 2), hypoxia (n = 1), and grade 4 pulmonary embolus (n = 2). Among 28 evaluable patients, the CNS ORR was 79% (95% CI 59%–92%) by prespecified volumetric criteria; 46% remained progression free (CNS and non-CNS) at 6 months. However, the study did not meet predefined criteria for feasibility because of toxicity.

Chargari and coworkers recently reported results of prospective clinical trial of 31 patients presenting HER2-positive MBC to brain treated with WBRT and trastuzumab.[198] The patients received trastuzumab 2 mg/kg weekly (n = 17) or 6 mg/kg repeated every 21 days (n = 14). In 26 patients, concurrent WBRT delivered 30 Gy in 10 daily fractions. In 6 patients, other fractionations were chosen because of either poor performance status or patient convenience. After WBRT, radiologic responses were observed in 23 patients (74.2%), including 6 (19.4%) with a complete radiologic response and 17 (54.8%) with a partial radiologic response. No grade 2 or greater toxicity was observed. The authors concluded that these results warrant additional validation.

Recurrent Brain Metastasis

Treatment options for recurrent brain metastases after initial therapy are surgery, SRS, or WBRT. Careful patient selection must be made when considering salvage treatment. Patients younger than 65 years of age and those with stable extracranial disease, good performance status, and one to a few recurrent lesions have the best prognosis after salvage treatment. The salvage treatment chosen depends on the initial treatment. If the patient has had only surgery as their initial treatment, RT is the salvage treatment of choice. Most patients, however, have had WBRT for their initial treatment, and reirradiation with WBRT would result in unacceptable toxicity. In this scenario, if the patient has a limited number of recurrent lesions, SRS would be a good option. Breneman and associates reported on 84 patients with brain metastases treated with SRS, 93% of whom were treated with SRS for recurrent brain metastases after initially receiving WBRT.[199] The median survival from time of SRS was 43 weeks. Patients with one or two brain metastases or stable extracranial disease survived longer. Two patients developed radiation necrosis. If SRS was the initial treatment of a patient's brain metastases, then WBRT would be an option for retreatment. Several researchers have reported on the use of a second course of WBRT after failure from the initial WBRT treatment.[200,201] The median survival after reirradiation with WBRT in these retrospective series ranges from 8 to 16 weeks. Wong and coworkers reported on 86 patients who were retreated with WBRT for recurrent or progressive brain metastases.[202] The median dose for the first course of WBRT was 3000 cGy and for their second course of WBRT it was 2000 cGy. Retreatment was delivered as WBRT in 65 patients, partial brain irradiation in 18 patients, and WBRT followed by a boost in 3 patients. Twenty-three patients (27%) had resolution of their neurologic symptoms, 37 (43%) had partial improvement of their neurologic symptoms, and 25 (29%) had either no change or worsened after reirradiation. The median survival after reirradiation was 4 months (range, 0.25–72 months). The majority of patients had no major toxicities; only one patient had leukoencephalopathy.

Reoperation may be considered for selected patients. One study found that reoperation could be performed with acceptable morbidity and mortality and appeared to confer a significant survival and quality-of-life benefit compared with historical controls.[203] This study reported the outcomes of 48 patients who underwent reoperation for cerebral metastasis recurrence after complete surgical resection at the initial diagnosis. The recurrence was local in 30 (63%) patients, distant in 16 (33%) patients, and local and distant in 2 (4%) patients. The median interval from initial craniotomy to diagnosis of recurrence in the brain was 6.7 months. At the time of recurrence, 42 (88%) patients had a solitary lesion and the remainder had two lesions. The median survival after reoperation was 11.5 months. Additional treatment options to consider after reoperation are brachytherapy and local chemotherapy delivery by biodegradable polymer wafers in addition to systemic therapy.[204,205]

Brain Metastases: Conclusions

Brain metastasis is a life-threatening disease that develops in roughly 20% of breast cancer patients. Fortunately, brain metastases respond to a range of palliative therapies. For single lesions amenable to surgery, resection followed by WBRT is standard treatment. SRS with or without WBRT is an alternative treatment for smaller lesions when there are no substantial symptoms of mass effect. WBRT alone may be appropriate when life expectancy is less than 3 months or if there are multiple or large metastases. WBRT might be withheld in carefully selected patients with a single brain metastasis when the development of additional brain lesions is less likely. The patient can be retreated if there is a new metastasis or a recurrence. This approach may avoid the long-term toxicity of WBRT in patients with a prolonged survival.

Treatment of Leptomeningeal Metastases

The median survival time after multimodality treatment of LM is much shorter than for the treatment of brain metastases. Without treatment, the median survival for breast cancer patients with LM is 3 to 6 weeks.[44,205,206] With treatment, the median survival is 2 to 6 months, with a 1-year survival of 11% to 25%.[10,44,206–211] Approximately 29% to 69% of breast cancer patients with LM die of its complications.[10,208] For breast cancer patients with LM that responds to treatment, the median survival is 7.5 months.[208] Systemic and intrathecal chemotherapy (ITC) are the mainstays of treatment. RT is used to treat bulky sites of disease for neurologic symptom relief. Surgery is typically not used except for minor procedures, such as ventricular drain placement, which alleviates obstructive hydrocephalus. Breast cancer LM appears to be more responsive to treatment than other solid tumors.[212,213] Between 60% and 80% of patients achieve symptomatic improvement with therapy.[52,207]

Medical Management

Steroids should be started early if there are signs of increased intracranial pressure and symptoms related to edema. A ventriculoperitoneal shunt may be needed to manage obstructive hydrocephalus, but one must weigh the morbidity, mortality, and complications associated with this procedure, particularly because the peritoneal cavity may be seeded with cancer cells if ventriculoperitoneal shunt is placed in a patient with active LMD. Before administering ITC, a CSF flow study with a radionuclide cisternogram may be done to assess for any CSF flow blockage if there is suspicion of flow obstruction. ITC will not be homogenously distributed if there is LM obstructing normal CSF flow. RT to areas of obstruction may help improve CSF flow, even if there is no corresponding abnormality on MRI. Glantz and colleagues studied CSF flow obstructions using Tc^{99m}-diethylenetriamine pentaacetate ventriculography in 31 patients with LMD.[214] Nineteen of these (61%) patients had CSF flow obstructions, and RT relieved the obstruction in 11 of these 19 (58%) patients. The areas most often obstructed were the skull base, spinal canal, and above the convexities. Follow-up CSF sampling is required to assess for response. Samples of CSF should be obtained from the ventricular and lumbar areas. Most trials require two consecutive negative CSF cytologies from each location to document a response. Obtaining ventricular CSF fluid can be problematic if an Ommaya reservoir is not present. The CSF should be monitored during and after therapy.[215]

Chemotherapy

Intrathecal Chemotherapy. ITC is the treatment of choice in the management of LMD. The most commonly used drugs for ITC are methotrexate (MTX), liposomal cytarabine, and thiotepa. ITC is usually administered in three phases: induction, consolidation, and maintenance. Chemotherapy is administered either directly into the lateral ventricle through a subcutaneous reservoir and ventricular catheter (Ommaya reservoir) or into the lumbar thecal sac via a lumbar puncture. ITC is more effective for small leptomeningeal deposits and cells floating in the CSF than for bulky tumor deposits. ITC cannot adequately diffuse into bulky tumor deposits.

Studies have shown that chemotherapy distributes better in the CSF when administered intraventricularly than via a lumbar puncture, which does not allow the drug to reach the subarachnoid space 10% to 15% of the time.[215,216] Furthermore, administration of ITC via the lumbar thecal sac requires multiple lumbar punctures, which cause the patient repeated discomfort. This discomfort can be avoided by using the Ommaya reservoir. This ventricular access device consists of a Silastic catheter inserted into a lateral ventricle of the cerebrum and attached to a Silastic dome-shaped reservoir positioned deep in the scalp and secured to the pericranium of the skull. The reservoir dome can be accessed percutaneously for CSF withdrawal and for installing chemotherapeutic agents. This device obviates the need for repeated lumbar punctures to access the intrathecal space. The Ommaya reservoir can be placed with minimal morbidity. The procedure carries a small risk of intracerebral hemorrhage along the track of the ventricular catheter, but these hemorrhages are usually not significant. There is also a small risk of infection. After the insertion procedure, it is recommended that appropriate placement of the ventricular catheter be confirmed with a CT scan before administering any chemotherapeutic agents. However, because ITC agents do not get distributed systemically, they are associated with minimal systemic side effects.

The most commonly used ITC agent is MTX. It has a response rate of 40% to 80% based on small series.[52,207,208] Boogerd and coworkers reported in the only randomized clinical trial in breast cancer patients with LM.[217] In this trial, 35 patients with LM and breast cancer were randomized to ITC treatment arm and non-ITC arm. In both arms, patients received similar administration of involved-field RT, and systemic therapy was encouraged in both groups. In the ITC arm, patients were treated with MTX at 10 mg of MTX twice weekly until the disappearance of tumor cells from four consecutive ventricular CSF samples, subsequently 10 mg of MTX once every 4 weeks for 3 months, 10 mg of MTX once every 6 weeks for 3 months, and 10 mg of MTX once every 4 months. Median survival of ITC patients was 18.3 weeks and 30.3 weeks for non-ITC patients (difference 12.9 weeks; 95% CI −5.5 to 34.3 weeks; $p = .32$). Neurologic complications of treatment occurred in 47% ITC versus 6% non-ITC ($p = .0072$) and delayed leukoencephalopathy are reported in up to 10% of cases. The small sample size of this randomized trial does not support firm conclusion on the efficacy of ITC in patients with breast cancer and LMD. Finally, a recent systematic review published in 2015 further illustrated the unmet need for clinical trials in patients with LMD from breast cancer, which supported that only five prospective studies have been published in this patient population,[218] four of which encompassed multiple primary tumors presenting with LMD. The standard dosage of MTX is usually considered to be 10 to 20 mg delivered two to three times per week. The duration and frequency of ITC depends on the patient's clinical response and CSF cytology. It is not necessary to calculate the dose of ITC by body mass because the volume of CSF is relatively constant across populations. Thiotepa is another systemic agent for managing LM that has comparable response rates to MTX.[219] The Eastern Cooperative Oncology Group (ECOG) performed a study randomizing patients with LM to receive intrathecal MTX or thiotepa.[219] Although 40% of the entire population had primary breast cancer, these patients were unequally distributed between the two arms of the study. The authors found no significant difference in overall toxicity or efficacy between these two agents. A third agent, cytarabine (Ara-C), is commonly used to manage LMD from lymphoma or leukemia but is believed to have little efficacy in solid tumors.[215] Researchers have challenged this belief in recent studies.[220,221] In a randomized study reported by Glantz and coworkers,[221] patients with LM of solid tumor origin, 36% of whom had primary breast tumors, received intrathecal MTX twice weekly or intrathecal sustained-release liposomal Ara-C once every 2 weeks.[221] There was no significant difference in median survival, but there was a significant increase in median time to neurologic progression in patients treated with sustained-release liposomal Ara-C. The advantage

to using liposomal Ara-C over MTX is the reduced frequency of administration.

The use of multiagent ITC has not been extensively tested, and thus its superiority over single-agent ITC has not been established. No survival or disease control advantage has been seen with the use of combined chemotherapy in the management of LM.[6,215,222] In a Japanese series of 55 patients with LM (13 breast patients, 24%), half of the patients received single-agent intrathecal MTX and the other half received intrathecal MTX, hydrocortisone, and Ara-C until a cytologic response was obtained. The cytologic response rate to ITC was significantly higher in the multiagent group than in the MTX group (38.5% vs. 13.8%, $p = .036$). The median survival was 18.6 weeks in the multiagent arm and 10.4 weeks in the MTX arm ($p = .029$). Other ITC agents tested are etoposide, dacarbazine, nitrosoureas, busulfan, trimetrexate, melphalan, and topotecan. The use of intrathecal trastuzumab (20–25 mg per week) in patients with HER2-positive breast cancer with LM has been reported in a few cases.[223–225] In these patients, intrathecal trastuzumab resulted in partial clinical and radiographic responses. In a recent systematic review and pooled analysis of patients presenting with LMD and HER2-positive breast primary, only 17 cases were reported.[226] There was clinical improvement observed in 66.7% of the patients. This approach remains investigational with an ongoing national multicenter trial evaluating its efficacy.

Systemic Chemotherapy. Controversy exists over the necessity of ITC. Data support the belief that intravenous chemotherapy is as efficacious as ITC depending on the chemotherapeutic agent in question. There are advantages to administering chemotherapy intravenously as well as intrathecally and treatment decisions are made on a case-by-case basis. It is important to keep in mind the potential toxicities with intrathecal therapies. For example, the increased frequency of chemical meningitis of with intrathecal cytarabine or the delayed leukoencephalopathy seen with ITC methotrexate administration.[217,221] By using the IV route, the potential risks and complications from surgical placement of an Ommaya reservoir can be avoided. Systemic chemotherapy may provide better drug distribution to bulky lesions because chemotherapy would be delivered via the arterial circulation and CSF. Systemic high-dose MTX with leucovorin rescue is the most common alternative to ITC. Glantz and colleagues showed a significant survival advantage for high-dose IV MTX compared with standard IT MTX.[227] The dosage for high-dose MTX was one to four courses (mean 2.3 courses) of 8 g/m^2 over 4 hours and leucovorin rescue. Cytotoxic CSF and serum MTX concentrations were maintained much longer in patients treated with high-dose IV MTX. Negative CSF cytology was seen in 81% of the patients treated with high-dose IV MTX compared with 60% of the patients treated intrathecally ($p = .3$). Median survival in the high-dose MTX group was 13.8 months versus 2.3 months in the IT MTX group ($p = .003$). Bokstein and colleagues compared two prospective series in which patients were treated with IV chemotherapy with or without ITC.[209] In this retrospective review, in which 60% of the patients had primary breast cancers, both cohorts had a median survival of 4 months. Neurotoxicity was delayed in the intravenous chemotherapy-only group. A prospective randomized study comparing IV with ITC would be of great interest. Although ITC is considered the standard, these studies suggest that IV chemotherapy may suffice and therefore is worthy of further investigation. Other agents that have been investigated include high-dose cytarabine, capecitabine, trastuzumab, and lapatinib.

Radiation

RT is the single most effective treatment for LM. However, it can be associated with significant toxicity. RT is more effective than ITC at improving neurologic symptoms. RT is given to treat symptomatic sites and bulky disease or to relieve CSF obstruction before administering ITC. Patients with cranial nerve signs and symptoms are often treated with WBRT, whereas those with evidence of CSF obstruction or bulky disease can be treated with smaller, more localized fields. Patients with lower extremity weakness and/or bowel and bladder dysfunction can receive significant symptomatic relief with lumbosacral irradiation. To avoid myelosuppression, cranial-spinal irradiation should be avoided. The standard palliative RT dose is 3000 to 3600 cGy at 300 cGy per fraction. Most studies in LMD are retrospective and contain few RT details. Fractionation regimens range from 3000 cGy in 10 fractions to 2400 cGy in eight fractions.[52,210,228] Care must be taken when delivering RT in conjunction with ITC. Leukoencephalopathy may be especially prominent when RT is administered before or concurrent with IT or systemic chemotherapy, particularly MTX. Local RT produces few major side effects, is well tolerated by patients, and appears to be efficacious for relieving symptoms and flow obstructions.[52]

Toxicity of Therapy

Early side effects of therapy include aseptic meningitis (acute meningoencephalopathy), infection, and trauma associated with placement of the Ommaya reservoir. Aseptic meningitis can occur within hours of administering IT MTX and is characterized by headache, fever, nuchal rigidity, change in mental status, and nausea and vomiting. This condition is typically self-limiting and resolves in 72 to 96 hours. Absorption of MTX from the CSF into the plasma may lead to mucositis and myelosuppression. These side effects can be alleviated by administering folic acid. Acute headaches and epidural hemorrhage are also possible toxic effects of ITC injections. Ommaya reservoir infections are uncommon.[206,208]

Late side effects observed in long-term survivors result most commonly from necrotizing leukoencephalopathy. Leukoencephalopathy is characterized by progressive dementia, seizures, and quadriparesis, and it is associated with white matter changes on brain imaging scans, often after prolonged therapy.[215] Leukoencephalopathy occurs in 2% to 25% of patients treated for LM and may be fatal.[10,52,209] It is reported to occur more commonly when ITC is given after or concurrent with radiation, although this has not been demonstrated unambiguously.[10,206,207,229] In an ECOG study, radiation in 300-cGy fractions was delivered concurrently with IT MTX to 53% of 28 patients, 60% of whom had primary breast cancers. Only one patient developed leukoencephalopathy after 16 weeks of therapy, and it was unclear whether this patient also received radiation. Ongerboer de Visser and colleagues reported that 2 of 33 breast cancer cases developed leukoencephalopathy[207]; again, it was unclear whether these two patients also received radiation. In a study by Wasserstrom and colleagues,[52] 4 of 90 patients developed leukoencephalopathy; all had received chemotherapy and radiation, survived longer than 6 months, and had prolonged drug exposure with a median dose of 140 mg of MTX. These authors suggest that the development of leukoencephalopathy is a result of prolonged treatment time and total dose of intrathecal MTX and thus is more commonly seen in long-term survivors who continue therapy. Boogerd and colleagues,[10] who reported that 11 of 17 breast cancer patients with LMD who survived longer than 4

months developed leukoencephalopathy, have also supported this theory.

Conclusions

LMD can be devastating and has a poor prognosis. The standard treatment is ITC with single-agent MTX. Localized palliative RT should be used to relieve symptoms caused by bulky disease and to relieve CSF obstruction before administering ITC. There are anecdotal reports of clinical improvement in patients with HER2-positive MBC treated with ITC trastuzumab.

Treatment of Epidural Spinal Cord Compression

Prompt diagnosis of ESCC is of the utmost importance because, if left untreated, ESCC will inevitably lead to paresis or paralysis. Treatment delay must be avoided to preserve neurologic function. The single most important prognostic factor is pretreatment neurologic status. Steroids and RT are the standard treatment.

Prognosis

The median survival after diagnosis of ESCC is 2 to 6 months.[230–232] However, the median survival for breast cancer patients diagnosed with ESCC has been reported to be longer, up to 20 months in one retrospective series.[233] Rades and associates identified the prognostic factors for functional outcome, recurrence, and survival for 335 breast cancer patients with ESCC treated with RT.[233] Factors that predicted for better functional outcome after RT were the ability to ambulate before treatment and slower development of motor deficits before RT ($p < .001$). Age, number of involved vertebral bodies, performance status, or radiation schedule had no effect on functional survival. On multivariate analysis, patients treated with a longer course of RT predicted fewer in-field recurrences ($p < .008$). Survival was negatively affected by the presence of visceral metastases ($p < .001$), the rapid development of motor deficits before RT ($p = .044$), reduced performance status ($p < .001$), and deterioration of motor function after RT ($p < .001$). The 2-year OS for patients with and without visceral metastases was 0% and 66%, respectively. The ability to ambulate before RT approached significance for favorably predicting survival (2-year OS of 57% vs. 20%, $p < .06$). All of the patients with deteriorating motor function after RT were dead at 2 years, whereas those with improved motor function had a 2-year OS of 63%. In summary, patients who are ambulatory before treatment, have a slow onset of motor deficits, have good performance status, and do not have visceral metastasis have the best outcomes after treatment.

Corticosteroids

Corticosteroids should be initiated immediately in patients with ESCC. Corticosteroids reduce inflammation and edema caused by tumor compression of the thecal sac, reduce pain, and restore and preserve neurologic function. A randomized trial assessed the use of high-dose dexamethasone versus no dexamethasone as an adjunct to RT for the treatment of ESCC.[212] Fifty-seven patients (two-thirds had breast cancer) participated. Dexamethasone was administered as an IV bolus of 96 mg intravenously, followed by 96 mg orally for 3 days and then tapered over 10 days. At the end of the study and at 6 months after treatment, 81% and 59% of the patients in the dexamethasone group were still ambulatory, compared with 61% and 33% in the no dexamethasone group. A subgroup analysis of breast cancer patients showed similar results. The authors observed significant side effects in 11% of the patients treated with dexamethasone. Heimdal and coworkers reported their results from using high-dose dexamethasone, including a serious side effect rate of 14.3% (one fatal stomach ulcer, one rectal bleeding, and two bowel perforations).[234] They subsequently abandoned the high-dose regimen and started using the standard-dose regimen of 4 mg, four times a day, titrated to zero over 14 days. There were no serious side effects for the patients treated with the standard-dose regimen, and the number of patients able to ambulate after treatment was similar to the patients treated with high-dose dexamethasone. Another study randomized 37 patients to either an initial bolus of 10 mg IV (conventional treatment) or 100 mg IV (high dose) followed by 16 mg daily orally and observed no difference in pain, ambulation, or bladder function.[235]

The standard-dose regimen is a loading dose of 10 mg of IV dexamethasone followed by a maintenance dose of 4 mg orally every 6 hours, which should be tapered during the course of RT or shortly thereafter. High-dose dexamethasone can be used, but the clinician should monitor the patient for side effects.

Radiation

Radiation is the main treatment modality in the management of ESCC. It can be used as primary treatment or after surgical decompression.

Treatment Technique and Dose Schedule. The radiation portal is centered on the spine approximately 8-cm wide, encompasses the transverse process at the involved vertebral level, and extends to one vertebral body above and below. Cervical spine lesions can be treated with opposed lateral fields to minimize radiation-induced odynophagia. Thoracic spine lesions are often treated with a single posterior field, and lumbar spine lesions may best be treated with anteroposterior and posteroanterior fields to ensure an adequate dose distribution.

Several fractionation schedules have been studied.[236–238] A prospective observational study of 214 patients compared 3000 cGy in 10 fractions to 4000 cGy in 20 fractions.[238] The efficacy was similar for both regimens, and the authors recommend that 3000 cGy in 10 fractions should be used because of its shorter treatment course. A retrospective study conducted by the same authors showed no benefit to escalating the dose above 3000 cGy in 10 fractions.[239] Maranzano and colleagues published a randomized trial of 300 patients with ESCC and compared a short course of 1600 cGy (two fractions of 800 cGy) to a split course of 3000 cGy (three fractions of 500 cGy, a break, then five fractions of 300 cGy).[236] There were no differences in efficacy or toxicity. A large retrospective study (1304 patients) compared five RT schedules for ESCC: (1) 800 cGy in 1 fraction, (2) 2000 cGy in 5 fractions, (3) 3000 cGy in 10 fractions, (4) 3750 cGy in 15 fractions, and (5) 4000 cGy in 20 fractions.[237] Among the five regimens there was no difference in improvement of motor function or posttreatment ambulatory rates. The in-field failure at 2 years was lower in the prolonged treatment schedules: 24% for 800 cGy, 26% for 2000 cGy, 14% for 3000 cGy, 9% for 3750 cGy, and 7% for 4000 cGy ($p < .001$). There was no statistical difference for in-field failure when comparing 3000 cGy, 3750 cGy, and 4000 cGy ($p = .71$). The authors recommended 800 cGy in one fraction for patients with poorly predicted survival and 3000 cGy in 10 fractions for other patients.

The standard RT schedule is 3000 cGy in 10 fractions to 4000 cGy in 20 fractions. One fraction of 800 cGy is also acceptable.

Efficacy of Radiation Therapy. Numerous studies clearly show a symptomatic benefit with radiation for most patients. RT results in relief of pain in 50% to 60% of patients, and 60% to 70% of patients are able to ambulate after treatment.[236–238] In addition, 20% to 40% of patients have improved motor function.[237,238] Patients who are ambulatory before treatment have an 80% to 100% chance of being able to ambulate after RT. Of those who are nonambulators before RT, approximately one-third of patients with paraparesis regain function, as do 2% to 6% of paraplegic patients. Zaidit and colleagues reported on 139 patients with ESCC treated with steroids and RT.[240] At presentation, 55 patients (40%) could not ambulate and, after RT, 20 of these patients regained the ability to ambulate; thus 37% of the nonambulatory patients regained function. Among the nonambulatory patients, starting treatment less than 12 hours after loss of walking ability increased the likelihood of patients regaining ambulation with treatment compared with treatment begun more than 12 hours after loss of walking ability ($p < .001$).

Radiation and Surgery

Surgical decompression may be performed in carefully selected patients. Surgery is indicated in patients with predicted prolonged survival with a limited area of ESCC. Surgical decompression should be followed by adjuvant RT. Surgery is also recommended for recurrent or progressive ESCC after RT. Laminectomy is not as effective as vertebral body resection with stabilization because most ESCCs are located anterolaterally. The aim of surgery in this setting is to decompress the neural elements to minimize the instability of the bony spine. A posterior approach through a laminectomy is the least morbid approach but has the disadvantage of limited visualization of the vertebral body, the most frequent origin of the epidural compression. In addition, a laminectomy weakens the posterior supporting elements of the bony spine; this can be detrimental because the anterior supporting elements are already weakened by tumor involvement. An anterior approach through a laparotomy or thoracotomy provides the most direct route to the vertebral body and allows the anterior elements to be stabilized with instrumentation. The disadvantage of the anterior approach is the added morbidity of a thoracotomy or laparotomy. Posterolateral and retroperitoneal approaches have been developed to combine the advantages and minimize the disadvantages of the anterior and posterior approaches.

Several retrospective series and a small randomized trial have compared laminectomy with RT to RT alone and found no difference in efficacy.[58,59,241–243] As discussed previously, laminectomy may not be the appropriate surgery for epidural decompression. Patchell and coworkers conducted a multiinstitutional randomized trial evaluating direct decompressive surgery with postoperative RT and RT alone.[244] Patients eligible for this study had biopsy-proven cancer, MRI evidence of ESCC, at least one neurologic sign or symptom (including pain) and had not been paraplegic for longer than 48 hours before study entry. Patients with multiple discrete compressive lesions or ESCC of the cauda equina or nerve roots were excluded. Of the 101 patients randomized, 13 had biopsy-proven ESCC caused by breast cancer. All patients were given 100 mg dexamethasone immediately, then 24 mg every 6 hours, and then another reduced dose until completion of RT. Patients were stratified according to ambulatory status. The RT dose for each arm was 3000 cGy in 10 fractions. Those randomized to receive surgery had an immediate direct circumferential decompression of the spinal cord. RT was given within 14 days after surgery. The primary end point was the ability to walk after treatment; secondary end points were urinary continence, muscle strength and functional status, the need for corticosteroids and opioid analgesics, and survival time. The trial was stopped early, after the interim analysis showed that surgery plus RT was superior. Significantly more patients were able to walk after surgery and RT than after RT alone: 84% versus 57%, respectively ($p = .001$). Maintaining the ability to walk was better in the surgery arm of the study (median, 122 days vs. 13 days, $p = .003$). Thirty-two patients in this study were unable to ambulate before treatment. Surgery plus RT improved the chances of ambulation in these patients; 10 of 16 (62%) patients in the surgery group regained the ability to walk compared with 3 of 16 (19%) in the RT-alone group ($p = .01$). The maintenance of urinary continence, muscle strength and functional status, and survival were significantly better in the surgery group. Also, these patients substantially reduced their use of corticosteroids and opioid analgesics.

Toxicity

Surgical morbidity is reported to be 5% to 30% and mortality 3% to 14%; both are mostly associated with spinal instability.[58,245] The acute side effects of radiation for ESCC are transient and easily managed with medication. The most devastating late effect of therapy is the development of radiation-induced myelopathy, which typically occurs 6 to 20 months after treatment and depends on total dose, fraction size, and the length of the spinal cord treated. The true tolerance of the spinal cord is uncertain. The most commonly used dose limit for the spinal cord is 4500 cGy in 25 fractions. A recent study has suggested that the probability of myelopathy at 4500 cGy is 0.03% and at 5000 cGy it is 0.2%; the dose for a 5% myelopathy rate is 5930 cGy.[246] These data were predominately based on regimens with a single fraction per day. Maranzano and colleagues reported that in a group of patients with ESCC treated with hypofractionated regimens (with similar biologic effective doses), only 1 of 13 long-term survivors (median survival time, 69 months) developed radiation-induced myelopathy.[247] Because the median survival in patients diagnosed with ESCC is 6 to 9 months,[54,230,248] many patients may die before the development of radiation-induced myelopathy. Breast cancer patients tend to have a longer median survival time, and they may be at greater risk of developing radiation-induced myelopathy after palliative RT for an ESCC than individuals with other tumor types. Late side effects such as radiation-induced myelopathy are more likely to occur with larger fraction sizes, so a more standard fractionation regimen may decrease the chance of this devastating late toxicity.

Recurrence

Local recurrence develops in about 10% to 20% of patients.[249–251] The median time to recurrence is 3 to 6 months. A prospective study documented the occurrence and details of recurrent spinal epidural metastasis (SEM) in a group of 103 patients (54% of whom had breast cancer).[251] Recurrent SEM occurred in 21 of the 103 patients (20%) after a median interval of 7 months, and

a second recurrence occurred in 11 patients (11%) after treatment. The recurrent SEM occurred at the same level in 55% of the recurrent patients. As patients lived longer, the chance of recurrence increased: 50% of the patients surviving 2 years and nearly all patients surviving 3 years or longer developed recurrent SEM. The ability to ambulate was preserved despite retreatment.

Reirradiation is not usually recommended for fear of radiation-induced myelopathy; however, given its time to development, the short median survival, and lack of other therapeutic options, reirradiation should not be categorically dismissed. Schiff and colleagues published a series in which favorable results were achieved with reirradiation[249]; 69% of the patients who developed an SEM recurrence after radiation regained the ability to ambulate after a second course of radiation. Rades and associates reirradiated 62 patients with recurrent SEMs.[250] None of the patients developed myelopathy, 25 patients (40%) showed improvement of motor function, and of the 16 previously nonambulatory patients, 6 (38%) regained the ability to walk. Intensity-modulated RT and/ or stereotactic body RT may offer a therapeutic option in place of conventional RT techniques, because they can better minimize the dose to the spinal cord.

Conclusions

ESCC can cause paralysis and even death. Prompt diagnosis and treatment before the development of paralysis or paresis is associated with a better prognosis. Patients who present with cord compression without paresis can be adequately treated with RT alone (with or without corticosteroids). Patients who present with paresis or paralysis are less likely to regain neurologic function and have a worse prognosis. These patients require urgent evaluation and may be best treated with immediate decompression through surgery followed by postoperative RT.

Selected References

23. Cameron D, Casey M, Oliva C, et al. Lapatinib plus capecitabine in women with HER-2-positive advanced breast cancer: final survival analysis of a phase III randomized trial. *Oncologist.* 2010;15:924-934.
28. Brufsky AM, Mayer M, Rugo HS, et al. Central nervous system metastases in patients with HER2-positive metastatic breast cancer: incidence, treatment, and survival in patients from registHER. *Clin Cancer Res.* 2011;17:4834-4843.
70. Patchell RA, Tibbs PA, Walsh JW, et al. A randomized trial of surgery in the treatment of single metastases to the brain. *N Engl J Med.* 1990;322:494-500.
152. Yamamoto M, Serizawa T, Shuto T, et al. Stereotactic radiosurgery for patients with multiple brain metastases (JLGK0901): a multi-institutional prospective observational study. *Lancet Oncol.* 2014;15:387-395.
158. Aoyama H, Shirato H, Tago M, et al. Stereotactic radiosurgery plus whole-brain radiation therapy vs stereotactic radiosurgery alone for treatment of brain metastases: a randomized controlled trial. *JAMA.* 2006;295:2483-2491.

A full reference list is available online at ExpertConsult.com.

74

Management of Pericardial Metastases in Breast Cancer

THOMAS AVERSANO

The pericardium consists of parietal and visceral surfaces and is composed of relatively inelastic collagen fibers.[1] The pericardium protects the heart from pathologic conditions involving adjacent structures such as the lung, fixes the heart within the thorax, and imposes a physical limitation on the acute expansion of heart volume that may occur with abrupt aortic or mitral regurgitation. The space between the parietal and visceral pericardium contains up to 50 mL of fluid[1] that serves as a lubricant between the two surfaces, which are in constant motion in relation to one another. This space is drained primarily by lymphatics.

This chapter reviews the pathophysiology, clinical presentation, useful diagnostic studies, and available treatments for breast cancer–associated pericardial disease. Treatment of pericardial involvement in breast cancer is aimed primarily at providing comfort and improved quality of life rather than at prolonging survival.

Pericardial Effusion in Breast Cancer

The hemodynamic effect of excess fluid in the pericardial space depends primarily on its volume and rate of accumulation. Because the parietal pericardium is relatively noncompliant, small increments of pericardial fluid that accumulate abruptly (e.g., myocardial rupture) above approximately 200 mL rapidly affect systemic hemodynamics and lead to tamponade. Slow accumulation of fluid (e.g., with metastatic disease) allows the parietal pericardium to stretch[1] to accommodate a substantial increase in volume. Volumes in excess of 1000 or 2000 mL can be accommodated with minimal symptoms if the process is sufficiently slow. It is unusual for the patient with breast cancer to present with acute tamponade and small-volume effusions and much more common for these patients to present with subacute or chronic pericardial effusion associated with moderate to large effusion volume.

Pathology

Metastases from breast cancer most commonly spread to the pericardium via the lymphatic channels, although hematogenous spread and local extension can also occur.[2] In autopsy studies, approximately 20% of patients dying with breast cancer have pericardial metastases,[3–5] yet clinically apparent pericardial disease develops in only a small subset of these patients. Most commonly, pericardial metastases result in production of a serosanguineous fluid, which, if a sufficient volume collects more rapidly than can be reabsorbed in the confined pericardial space, results in the accumulation of pericardial effusion.

Importantly, nonmalignant involvement of the pericardium is seen in up to 50% of patients with metastatic breast cancer and pericardial effusion.[6] Exposure to chemotherapeutic agents such as doxorubicin[7] or to radiation can cause pericardial effusion. In the patient with breast cancer, pericardial effusion can result from inflammatory or infectious causes as well.

Pathophysiology

The pathophysiology of pericardial tamponade is reviewed in detail in many general cardiology texts.[8] Regardless of etiology, at some point during accumulation of fluid, the parietal pericardium can no longer stretch to accommodate additional volume and pressure within the pericardial space rises. As a result, ventricular filling pressure rises while ventricular volume is constrained secondary to elevated pericardial pressure (Fig. 74.1). Clinically, increased filling pressure leads to dyspnea, and reduced stroke volume leads to tachycardia—and ultimately to reduced cardiac output and systemic hypotension. In dehydrated patients, effusions of relatively smaller volume causing less elevation of intra-pericardial pressure can be hemodynamically significant (termed *low-pressure tamponade*).

Clinical Presentation

Pericardial effusion is not infrequently first detected as an incidental finding in an asymptomatic patient. Effusion can be identified in a chest computed tomography or magnetic resonance imaging scan or in an echocardiogram (ECG) performed for another reason.

Clinical symptoms and signs associated with pericardial effusion depend on the pressure of the effusion on surrounding structures (e.g., lung, trachea, esophagus, nerves) and the degree to which ventricular filling pressure is increased and cardiac output is impaired.

A common symptom is dyspnea, which may result from multiple causes including elevated ventricular filling pressure and potentially compression of the lung, trachea, or bronchi. Fatigue is also a common symptom, resulting from reduced cardiac output. A decreased stroke volume typically leads to tachycardia (to maintain cardiac output), which in turn can lead to a sense of

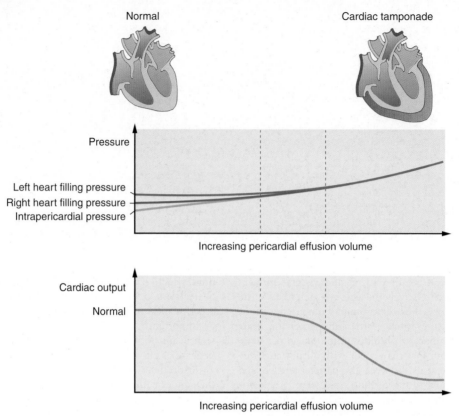

Normal   Cardiac tamponade

• **Fig. 74.1** Relationship between intracardiac filling pressures and intrapericardial pressure and cardiac output in cardiac tamponade. (From Roy CL, Minor MA, Brookhart MA, Choudhry NK. Does this patient with a pericardial effusion have cardiac tamponade? *JAMA.* 2007;297:1810-1818.)

a "rapid heartbeat" or palpitations. Other less common symptoms include dysphagia resulting from esophageal compression, hiccups resulting from vagal or phrenic nerve involvement, and hoarseness resulting from recurrent laryngeal nerve involvement.[8] Hemodynamic collapse secondary to cardiac tamponade is a still less common but potentially fatal presentation.

Tachycardia is the most common sign in tamponade. In addition, pulsus paradoxus, an exaggeration of the normal inspiratory decline in systolic blood pressure, is greater than 10 mm Hg in tamponade. Marked elevation of the jugular venous pulse is often present on examination of the neck veins but may be absent in the dehydrated patient. The lung fields are typically clear and heart sounds may be normal or diminished in intensity.

Diagnostic Evaluation

The chest x-ray may reveal a classic "water-bottle" enlargement of the heart with clear lung fields. The ECG is not specific but with very large effusions, and, particularly with tamponade, QRS complex amplitude is reduced and electrical alternans is an occasional finding (Fig. 74.2). The echocardiogram (Fig. 74.3) is useful in qualitatively defining the volume and hemodynamic significance of pericardial effusion even before tamponade is apparent clinically. Diastolic collapse of the right atrium and ventricle (Fig. 74.4), marked and 180-degree out-of-phase respiratory variation in mitral and tricuspid diastolic inflow velocity (E velocity; Fig. 74.5), and dilatation of the inferior vena cava and absence of respiratory variation in its diameter are all echocardiographic features of actual or impending tamponade.

Because pericardial effusion is often nonmalignant, obtaining routine laboratory studies such as a complete blood count, liver function studies, thyroid studies, and erythrocyte sedimentation rate are often useful. Other studies (e.g., antinuclear antibody titer) are guided by clinical presentation.

Treatment

A guiding principle in the management of pericardial effusion in the patient with breast cancer is the assessment of the risks and benefits of any potential therapy considered in the context of the patient's prognosis, wishes, and comfort.

In patients with known breast cancer, an asymptomatic pericardial effusion with no echocardiographic features suggesting hemodynamic significance does not require pericardiocentesis or other treatment.[9] Close monitoring of the patient's symptoms and signs with periodic echocardiographic evaluation is warranted. Exceptions to a wait-and-see approach to asymptomatic effusions include those that may be the only indication of otherwise undiagnosed metastatic disease or those associated with persistent fever and no obvious source that might indicate an infectious cause.

At the other extreme of presentations, tamponade is a medical emergency. Symptoms are so severe and so uncomfortable for the patient, and the risks and discomfort of pericardiocentesis so small,[10] that there are few, if any, reasons not to proceed with prompt pericardiocentesis. Before the procedure, an immediate measure that augments systemic blood pressure is expansion of intravascular volume. This is of particular importance in this group of patients because relative dehydration may result from reduced

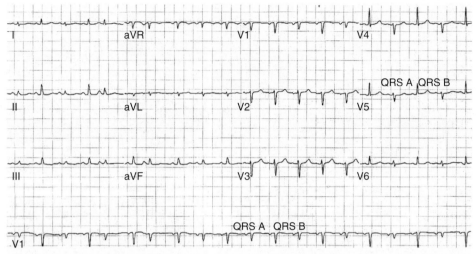

• **Fig. 74.2** Twelve-lead electrocardiograph showing electrical alternans (QRS A and QRS B). (From Billakanty S, Bashir R. Echocardiographic demonstration of electrical alternans. *Circulation*. 2006;113:e866-e868. Copyright American Heart Association.)

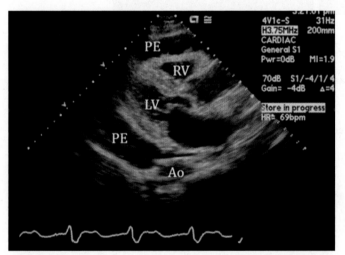

• **Fig. 74.3** Two-dimensional echocardiogram demonstrating a large, circumferential pericardial effusion. *Ao,* Descending aorta; *LV,* left ventricle; *PE,* pericardial effusion; *RV,* right ventricle. (From Anaya-Cisnerosa M, Tongb MS, Calvoc AR. Effusive-constrictive pericarditis secondary to primary pericardial lymphoma: a case report. *World J Oncol.* 2012;3:87-90.)

oral intake of fluids related to their underlying disease or its treatment. Vasoactive agents can also be used as a temporizing measure to augment blood pressure while definitive treatment is arranged.

Definitive therapy requires removal of pericardial fluid. This is probably best accomplished in the cardiac catheterization laboratory using fluoroscopic, electrocardiographic, and echocardiographic guidance. Removal of even a small amount of fluid can result in a dramatic increase in blood pressure. As much pericardial fluid is removed as possible, but as reaccumulation is common, a multiholed drainage catheter is left in the pericardial space to allow for drainage over several days.[11] Once drainage has decreased to less than 25 mL per 24-hour period, the drain can be removed.[12] Most patients with breast cancer, particularly those who can be treated systemically for their disease, will not have a recurrence with this simple procedure. Pericardial biopsy is rarely necessary.

The complications of echocardiographically guided pericardiocentesis and drainage are extremely low, and the procedure itself is well tolerated. Major complications such as pneumothorax, right ventricular perforation requiring surgery, or infection occur in less than 2% of patients.[11] Even minor complications, including supraventricular tachyarrhythmias, clinically insignificant cardiac chamber perforation, clinically insignificant pneumothorax, and vasovagal reactions, occur in less than 4% of patients.[11] The resolution of the patient's symptoms is so dramatic, rapid, and complete (see Fig. 74.3) and complications so rare that treatment rarely should be withheld.

Postpericardiocentesis Diagnostics and Therapeutics

Fluid removed from the pericardial space is sent for cytologic, microbiologic, hematologic, and chemical examination. Detection of malignant cells in the effusion not only may determine prognosis but can affect treatment.[12] Among patients with malignant pericardial effusion, cytology is diagnostic in 60% to 80%. Newer methods, such as molecular imaging,[13] may improve sensitivity and specificity for identification of malignant cells in the future. Microbial causes are identified using aerobic, anaerobic, tuberculous bacterial, and fungal cultures of pericardial fluid. Simple blood tests, including complete blood count, thyroid studies, and erythrocyte sedimentation rate, may also provide clues to etiology. In a significant number of patients, the exact etiology remains obscure and the cause labeled idiopathic.

If cytologic analysis demonstrates a malignant cause of effusion, and if systemic therapy options are available, a therapeutic approach that includes removal of the pericardial fluid by one of the aforementioned techniques combined with appropriate systemic therapy can be considered.

Clinically significant (i.e., symptomatic) effusions that cannot be associated with malignancy, such as those caused by inflammation or infection, are best treated with removal of pericardial fluid and treatment aimed at the underlying offending agent. If inflammation is caused by a drug or radiation, the offending agent is removed (if possible), and treatment with antiinflammatory

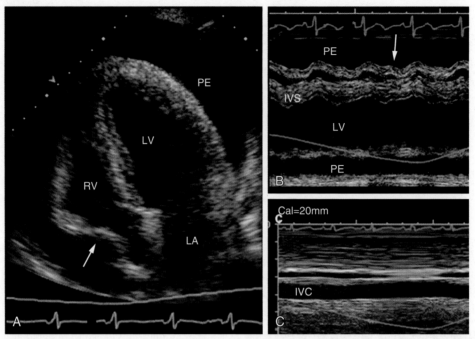

• **Fig. 74.4** (A–C) Two-dimensional echocardiogram showing diastolic collapse of the right atrium *(arrow in left panel)*. Right ventricular diastolic collapse is shown in the M-mode echocardiogram in the upper right panel *(arrow)*. Right ventricular and atrial collapse are features of tamponade, as is dilatation and lack of respiratory variation in diameter of the inferior vena cava *(lower right panel)*. *IVC,* Inferior vena cava; *IVS,* interventricular septum; *LA,* left atrium; *LV,* left ventricle; *PE,* pericardial effusion; *RV,* right ventricle. (From Troughton RW, Asher CR, Klein AL. Pericarditis. *Lancet.* 2004;363:717-727.)

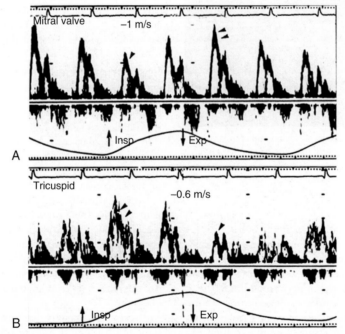

• **Fig. 74.5** (A and B) Exaggerated (>25%) respiratory variation of mitral and tricuspid Doppler flow velocity in pericardial tamponade. At the start of inspiration mitral inflow velocity (E velocity) falls >25% compared with peak mitral inflow velocity. Note that at the lowest tricuspid inflow velocity (E velocity) occurs at the onset of expiration, 180 degrees out of phase with mitral E variation, and is also more than 25% lower than peak tricuspid inflow velocity. These are echocardiographic features of tamponade and can be identified before tamponade is clinically apparent. (From Cosyns B, Pleiin S, Nihoyanopoulos P, et al. European Association of Cardiovascular Imaging (EACVI) and European Society of Cardiology Working Group (ESC WG) on Myocardial and Pericardial diseases. European Association of Cardiovascular Imaging (EACVI) position paper: multimodality imaging in pericardial disease. *Eur Heart J Cardiovasc Imaging.* 2015;16:12-31.)

agents may be appropriate. If an infectious cause is identified, removal of the purulent pericardial fluid can be accompanied by administration of appropriate systemic antibiotic agents.

The prognosis of patients with pericardial effusion depends on the underlying disease process rather than the effusion or its treatment.[12,14,15] Most series report a median survival of about 12 months,[12,14,15] although longer-term survival is possible if systemic treatment options are available.

Recurrent Pericardial Effusion

For most breast cancer patients, pericardiocentesis followed by several days of drainage is the only therapy required for malignant effusions.[11] In some patients, however, the effusion can recur. Several strategies are available for treatment of recurrent malignant effusions, including sclerotherapy or the creation of a pericardial window, either with balloon pericardiotomy or with one of a number of available surgical procedures.

In sclerotherapy, the space between the visceral and parietal pericardium is obliterated by introducing agents that inflame these structures, leading ultimately to their fusion. After sclerotherapy, success (measured as the lack of recurrence at 30 days in surviving patients) ranges from 75% to 90%. The most common agents used for sclerotherapy are the antibiotic doxycycline[16] or the chemotherapeutic agents bleomycin and thiotepa.[17] The complications of sclerotherapy are few and include pain, fever, supraventricular arrhythmias, and infection.

Creation of a pericardial window that prevents accumulation of pericardial fluid by creating a fenestration in the parietal pericardium is an alternative to sclerotherapy. A number of methods are available, including pericardiotomy via a transthoracic approach, which is a major procedure that requires use of general anesthesia or a subxiphoid approach, which is less invasive and can often be accomplished with the patient under local anesthesia.[18] Balloon pericardiotomy has been used in the past[19] but has fallen into some disfavor in our institution because of its relatively high failure and complication rates. Another common approach to recurrent pericardial effusions in breast cancer patients in our institution is video-assisted thoracoscope pericardiectomy.[20] Success rates are extremely high, and the most gravely ill patient can undergo the procedure with little or no morbidity.

The choice among these approaches to recurrent malignant pericardial effusion depends on the patient's prognosis and wishes, available therapeutic options, and local expertise.

Pericardial Constriction in Breast Cancer

In addition to fluid accumulation, the pericardial space can become obliterated, the visceral and pericardial surfaces fused, and the pericardium becomes fibrotic or calcified. In the context of breast cancer, this most often occurs as a consequence of radiation. Compensation for the slow development of pericardial constriction begins as elevation of right- and left-sided heart filling pressures, leading ultimately to signs and symptoms of right- and left-sided heart failure.

Pericardial constriction in breast cancer patients is much less common than pericardial effusion and is usually associated with prior radiation therapy. The effects of radiation on the pericardium (and other cardiac structures) can be delayed for years after treatment. A combination of both effusion and constriction can also occur, albeit rarely, referred to as effusive-constrictive pericarditis.

Pathology

Radiation injury can affect all elements of the heart, including the coronary arteries, conduction system, myocardium, and pericardium.[21] Pericardial injury can result in acute pericarditis, typically within a few months from the onset of radiation therapy, and in chronic, constrictive pericarditis, that can occur years after treatment.[22]

In constrictive pericarditis, the parietal and visceral pericardium fuse because of radiation-induced injury, ultimately becoming a single, thickened structure that encases the heart in a stiff shell.

Pathophysiology

Pressures required to fill both the left- and right-sided cardiac chambers increase, accounting for most of the signs and symptoms of constrictive pericardial disease. There is a marked rise in right-heart pressure, distending neck veins and causing hepatic congestion, ascites, and lower extremity edema. Because left ventricular volume is fixed and cannot use Starling's law to increase stroke volume, increasing heart rate maintains and augments cardiac output. Pressure required to fill the left ventricle rises and cardiac output cannot increase as required.

Clinical Presentation

Signs and symptoms of pericardial constriction are not related to primary myocardial disease but rather to the heart's encasement in a stiff pericardium.

Frequently, the presentation includes lower extremity edema and abdominal swelling and discomfort due to elevated right heart pressure, as well as fatigue and breathlessness due to limited cardiac output and the rise in left ventricular filling pressure.

Tachycardia is a common sign, and systemic blood pressure may be low. Other characteristic clinical features include lower extremity edema, ascites, enlarged and tender liver, and distended neck veins.[17] Kussmaul sign is occasionally present, with a paradoxical increase (rather than the usual decrease) in jugular venous pressure during inspiration—a result of severe restriction of right-sided chamber filling. Despite dyspnea on exertion and fatigue, the lung fields are usually clear.

Diagnostic Studies

The chest x-ray and ECG are usually normal or show nonspecific abnormalities. Although echocardiography can demonstrate a thickened or calcified pericardium, the physiology of pericardial constriction is demonstrated using Doppler interrogation of the left ventricular diastolic flow velocity and mitral annulus tissue velocity (Fig. 74.6). In constrictive pericardial disease, early diastolic filling of the left ventricle is rapid and normal (E velocity) but ends abruptly once the limit of ventricular volume, restricted by the pericardium, is reached. Late diastolic filling (A velocity, associated with atrial contraction) is markedly diminished or absent because of pericardium-restricted ventricular filling. The resulting markedly increased E/A ratio (>2) is characteristic of constrictive pericardial physiology, although not specific because it can also be seen in restrictive cardiomyopathy. However, mitral annular velocity is usually normal in patients with constrictive pericardial disease, but markedly diminished in restrictive cardiomyopathy, distinguishing these two pathophysiologic states. Although rarely performed, right heart catheterization shows equalization of

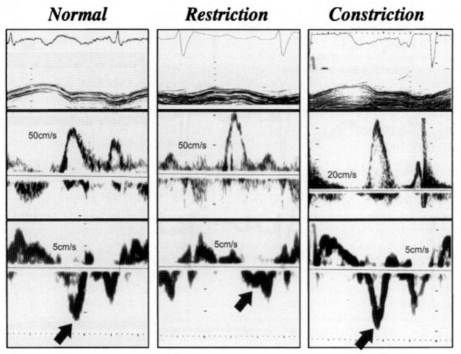

• **Fig. 74.6** Mitral flow velocity *(middle panels)* and mitral annular velocity *(lower panels)* in constrictive pericarditis. Not that early mitral inflow (E) velocity is high in both restriction and constriction *(middle panels)*, leading to a very high E/A ratio (>2), but in constriction mitral annular velocity *(lower right panel, arrow)* is normal. This distinguishes restrictive physiology from constrictive physiology because, in restriction, mitral annular velocity is markedly reduced *(lower middle panel, arrow)*. (From Garcia MJ, Thomas JD, Klein AL. New Doppler echocardiographic applications for the study of diastolic function. *J Am Coll Cardiol.* 1998;32:865-875.)

end-diastolic pressures and, in the right ventricular pressure tracing, the characteristic "square root sign" corresponding to the rapid increase in diastolic pressure associated with restriction of ventricular volume by the pericardial "shell."[18] Magnetic resonance imaging and computed tomography scanning are superior to cardiac ultrasound in detecting and quantifying pericardial thickening, which, if sufficient (e.g., >3.5 mm) can assist in both making the diagnosis and planning for possible surgery[8] (Fig. 74.7).

Treatment

The treatment of pericardial constriction is surgical. Although avoiding dehydration and medications that may impair ventricular filling (e.g., preload reducing agents such as nitrates or morphine) are helpful, the only way to correct constrictive physiology is to remove the pericardium from the myocardium. This, of course, requires thoracotomy and technical expertise, particularly if the visceral pericardium must be removed. For this reason, the patient's underlying prognosis and physiologic state are important determinants of whether to proceed with definitive treatment.

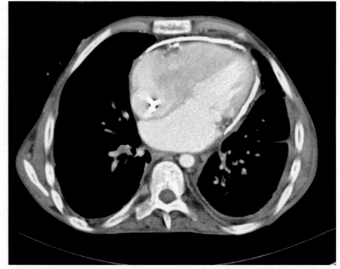

• **Fig. 74.7** Computed tomography scan showing calcific constrictive pericarditis. (From http://radiopaedia.org/cases/calcific-constrictive-pericarditis-1; accessed March 10, 2016.)

Selected References

1. Karam N, Patel P, deFilippi C. Diagnosis and management of chronic pericardial disease. *Am J Med Sci.* 2001;322:79.
2. Chiles C, et al. Metastatic involvement of the heart and pericardium: CT and MR imaging. http://www.rsna.org/education/rg_cme.html. Accessed 2001.
7. Shanholtz C. Acute life-threatening toxicity of cancer treatment. *Crit Care Clin.* 2001;17:483.

8. Spodick DH. Pericardial diseases. In: Braunwald E, ed. *Heart Disease: A Textbook of Cardiovascular Medicine.* 6th ed. Philadelphia: WB Saunders; 2001.
10. Tsang TS, et al. Consecutive 1127 therapeutic echocardiographically guided pericardiocenteses: clinical profile, practice patterns, and outcomes spanning 21 years. *Mayo Clin Proc.* 2002;77:429.
A full reference list is available online at ExpertConsult.com.

75

Bilateral Breast Cancer

ANDREA V. BARRIO AND HIRAM S. CODY III

In 1945 Foote and Stewart[1] memorably stated that "the most frequent antecedent of cancer of one breast is the history of having had cancer in the opposite breast." In fact, among breast cancer survivors, a contralateral breast cancer (CBC) is the most frequent second-cancer event.[2] The incidence of CBC among breast cancer survivors has traditionally been reported as a constant incidence rate of 0.5% to 1.0% per year.[3,4] CBC risk is even higher among carriers of *BRCA1* or *BRCA2* mutations and noncarriers with a significant family history of breast cancer.[5–7] However, recent studies have shown a favorable decline in CBC in the United States since 1985,[3] which is largely due to the widespread adoption of tamoxifen in the mid-1980s for the adjuvant treatment of breast cancer.[8] The Early Breast Cancer Trialists' Collaborative Group's (EBCTCG) overview of 12 randomized trials demonstrated a 39% reduction in CBC development among women with estrogen receptor (ER)-positive or ER-unknown breast cancers who took tamoxifen for 5 years.[9] Despite the documented declining incidence of CBC, a dichotomous shift toward more aggressive surgical therapy with contralateral prophylactic mastectomy (CPM) has occurred. A review of the Surveillance, Epidemiology and End Results (SEER) database demonstrated that CPM rates more than doubled from 1998 to 2003.[10] Reasons for this aggressive approach are multifactorial and include an overestimation of CBC risk among patients, increasing use of breast magnetic resonance imaging (MRI), availability of postmastectomy reconstruction, and overestimation of benefit of CPM. In the era of modern systemic therapy, the subject of bilateral breast cancer, and, in particular, CBC, is of particular importance when considering the appropriate management and counseling of patients with unilateral breast cancer.

In this chapter, we review risk factors for CBC, including age at diagnosis, genetic risk assessment, family history, prior radiation exposure, invasive lobular histology, and a personal history of lobular carcinoma in situ (LCIS). We also discuss the impact of advanced imaging on detection of synchronous CBC and discuss the effects of adjuvant systemic therapy on declining CBC risk. We review prognosis among breast cancer patients who have developed a CBC. Finally, we discuss the CPM epidemic that has developed in the United States since the early 2000s, and we review the benefits and risks associated with more aggressive surgery.

Risk Factors for Bilateral Breast Cancer

Age

Studies from the 1970s, before the availability of genetic testing, initially demonstrated an association between young age at first breast cancer diagnosis and CBC risk. The results of large population-based studies from England[11] and Connecticut[12] (and the large personal experience of Haagensen)[13] demonstrated the greatest risk of CBC in the youngest patients. However, lack of knowledge of genetic mutations in these patients limits the findings in these early studies. A recent report from the Women's Environmental Cancer and Radiation Epidemiology (WECARE) Study demonstrated that among noncarriers of *BRCA1* and *BRCA2* mutations with no family history, the 10-year cumulative risk of CBC was approximately 4.6% (95% confidence interval [CI] 4.0%–5.1%) in women 25 to 54 years of age at first diagnosis. This was substantially lower than the 18.4% 10-year cumulative risk of CBC among *BRCA1/BRCA2* mutation carriers or the 15.6% 10-year cumulative risk of CBC in noncarriers with a family history of bilateral breast cancer in the same age group[7] (Table 75.1). Furthermore, among young breast cancer patients, molecular phenotype also contributes to risk of CBC. In a population-based study using SEER data, Nichols and coworkers demonstrated that current age-specific CBC rates (per 100/year) for an ER-positive cancer were 0.45 for first cancers diagnosed before age 30 compared with 1.26 for ER-negative cancers.[3] Although young age at first diagnosis may be an indication for genetic testing, young women who are noncarriers with no family history can be counseled that their risk of CBC is low, particularly among women with ER-positive first breast cancers.

Hereditary Breast Cancer

Approximately 5% to 10% of breast cancers are hereditary and associated with an inherited germline mutation. Mutations in the tumor-suppressor genes *BRCA1* and *BRCA2* account for most hereditary breast cancers and confer a 36% to 84% lifetime risk of first primary breast cancer.[6] The risk of CBC after a first primary breast cancer among *BRCA1* or *BRCA2* mutation carriers is substantially higher than the risk in sporadic breast cancer survivors. A recent population-based, nested case-control study

| TABLE 75.1 | Cumulative 10-Year Risk of Contralateral Breast Cancer According to Family History and Age at First Breast Cancer Diagnosis |

Age at First Diagnosis (Years)	NONCARRIERS WITH NO FAMILY HISTORY		NONCARRIERS WITH BILATERALLY AFFECTED FIRST-DEGREE RELATIVE		*BRCA1* OR *BRCA2* MUTATION CARRIERS	
	10-Year CBC Risk (%)	95% CI (%)	10-Year CBC Risk (%)	95% CI (%)	10-Year CBC Risk (%)	95% CI (%)
25–29	6.3	4.4–8.7	21.7	11.1–42.3	28.2	16.0–50.0
30–34	7.0	5.4–8.7	23.7	12.8–44.2	30.7	18.4–51.5
35–39	5.2	4.1–6.3	18.1	9.8–33.4	23.7	14.3–39.3
40–44	4.2	3.3–5.1	14.8	8.0–27.2	19.4	11.8–32.1
45–49	4.5	4.1–5.6	15.1	8.2–27.7	12.2	6.5–22.9
50–54	4.0	3.6–4.9	13.4	7.3–24.7	10.2	5.8–20.3
All ages (25–54)	4.6	4.0–5.1	15.6	8.5–28.5	18.4	16.0–21.3

CBC, Contralateral breast cancer; *CI,* confidence interval.

Modified from Reiner AS, John EM, Brooks JD, et al. Risk of asynchronous contralateral breast cancer in noncarriers of BRCA1 and BRCA2 mutations with a family history of breast cancer: a report from the Women's Environmental Cancer and Radiation Epidemiology Study. *J Clin Oncol.* 2013;31:433-439.

of CBC risk among 705 patients with CBC and 1398 controls with unilateral breast cancer (from the WECARE study) demonstrated that *BRCA1* and *BRCA2* mutation carriers had a 4.5-fold (95% CI 2.8-fold–7.1-fold) and 3.4-fold (95% CI 2.0-fold–5.8-fold) increased risk of CBC, respectively, compared with noncarriers. Furthermore, the relative risk of CBC among *BRCA1* carriers increased as age at first diagnosis decreased, with an 11-fold increased CBC risk among women first diagnosed before 35 years of age, compared with 2.6-fold increased risk in women 45 to 54 years of age at first diagnosis.[6] Similar risk estimates were reported in a retrospective, multicenter, cohort study evaluating CBC risk in 978 *BRCA1* and *BRCA2* positive families. The cumulative risk of CBC at 25 years after first diagnosis was 48.1% (95% CI 38.3%–57.9%) in *BRCA1* patients and 47.1% (95% CI 28.9%–65.3%) in *BRCA2* patients. *BRCA1* patients younger than 40 years of age at first diagnosis had a 25-year CBC incidence of 62.9% (95% CI 50.4%–75.4%) compared with 43.7% (95% CI 24.9%–62.5%) in women 41 to 50 years of age and 19.6% (95% CI 5.3%–33.9%) in women older than 50 years.[5] This substantial risk of CBC among *BRCA1* and *BRCA2* patients, particularly in women younger than 40 years at first diagnosis, should be considered at the time of first diagnosis when counseling women regarding surgical treatment options.

Multigene, or panel testing, has led to the identification of additional breast cancer genes, although the magnitude of breast cancer risk for many of these mutations remains poorly understood.[14] Among patients with non-*BRCA* deleterious mutations, the most common pathogenic mutations include *PALB2, CHEK2,* and *ATM,* with a prevalence of 1.3%, 0.9%, and 0.8%, respectively.[15] There is strong evidence that protein-truncating mutations in these three genes are associated with a moderate breast cancer risk among unaffected carriers,[14] with mutations in PALB2 conferring the highest risk.[16] However, data regarding reliable risk estimates for CBC in these patients are lacking, and it is not clear that surveillance strategies or surgical treatment should be altered in these patients on the basis of the presence or absence of the mutation alone. Patients with moderate penetrance genes should be counseled on CBC risk according to their individual personal

risk factors and family history of breast cancer; more importantly, decisions for risk-reduction strategies in these patients should be individualized because the magnitude of risk for future breast cancer is far less clear than in patients with high-penetrance genes.

Multigene panel testing has also identified variants of uncertain significance (VUS) in which the predicted amino acid sequence of a protein has been altered, without information as to whether this genetic variant impairs the function of the protein. As a result, these variants are not clinically actionable, and VUS results should not be used in isolation to counsel patients about breast cancer risk or CBC risk and should not alter patient management.[17]

Family History

A family history of breast cancer is a well-established and significant risk for breast cancer, even in the absence of a known genetic mutation. Seventy-four studies before 1997 link family history to the risk of breast cancer and are the subject of a comprehensive meta-analysis.[18] Taken together, these studies confirm increased breast cancer risk based on a family history in any relative (relative risk [RR] 1.9), a mother (RR 2.0), a sister (RR 2.3), a daughter (RR 1.8), a mother and sister (RR 3.6), and a second-degree relative (RR 1.5).[18]

CBC risk among non-*BRCA* women with a family history of breast cancer was assessed in the WECARE study. Those with a first-degree relative with breast cancer had an almost two-fold greater risk of developing CBC (RR 1.9, 95% CI 1.4–2.6) compared with women without a family history. Risk of CBC was also influenced by the age at diagnosis of the affected individual, age at diagnosis of the family member, and the nature of the family history (see Table 75.1; Fig. 75.1).[7] Notably, a history of bilateral breast cancer in an affected relative was one of the most important predictors of CBC risk, with a 10-year cumulative risk of CBC of 15.6%. This CBC risk in women with a first-degree family history of bilateral breast cancer was similar to the 10-year risk seen in *BRCA* mutation carriers (15.6% vs. 18.4%, respectively),[7] suggesting that these women should be considered for preventive counseling at first diagnosis of breast cancer.

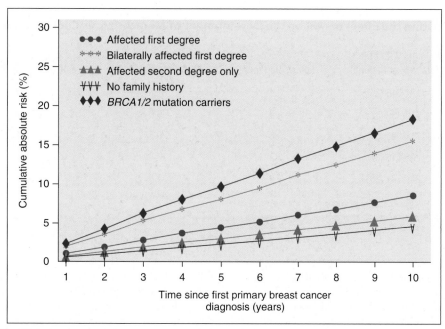

• **Fig. 75.1** Cumulative absolute risk of contralateral breast cancer according to family history and *BRCA* mutation status. (From Reiner AS, John EM, Brooks JD, et al. Risk of asynchronous contralateral breast cancer in noncarriers of BRCA1 and BRCA2 mutations with a family history of breast cancer: a report from the Women's Environmental Cancer and Radiation Epidemiology Study. *J Clin Oncol.* 2013;31:433-439.)

Radiation Exposure

Increasing use of conservative surgery plus radiotherapy (RT) for early-stage breast cancer has raised concern about the possibility of CBC induced by low-dose radiation scatter. This has not been observed. A 20-year follow-up of the National Surgical Adjuvant Bowel and Breast Project (NSABP) B-06 trial comparing total mastectomy, lumpectomy, and lumpectomy and irradiation demonstrated no difference in CBC rates among the treatment groups (8.5% [total mastectomy] vs. 8.8% [lumpectomy] vs. 9.4% [lumpectomy plus irradiation]).[19] Another large breast conservation trial from Milan, Italy, showed no statistically significant difference in the 20-year cumulative incidence of CBC among women treated with radical mastectomy compared with breast conservation therapy (*p* = .5).[20]

These data do not absolutely rule out an effect of RT on the risk of CBC. In the 2005 EBCTCG overview[9] (a meta-analysis of 46 randomized trials of RT vs. no RT and 17 trials of RT vs. more surgery, in 32,800 patients), the incidence of CBC at 15 years was marginally but significantly higher in the RT arm than in the control arm (9.3% vs. 7.5%, *p* = .002). Notably, the absolute difference in CBC between the two groups was small. Furthermore, these data do not take into account the increased precision of contemporary RT techniques or the effects of current systemic treatments (chemotherapy and/or hormonal) in reducing the incidence of CBC, which is addressed elsewhere in the chapter.

A striking exception to the preceding findings is the increased risk of breast cancer noted in young women after mantle RT for Hodgkin's lymphoma. Early reports from Aisenberg and colleagues suggested the following: (1) that a relationship existed between age at RT exposure and risk of breast cancer, with an RR of 56 (95% CI 23.3–107) for those 19 years of age or younger at the time of treatment compared with an RR of 0.9 (95% CI 0–5.3) for those 30 years of age and older, and (2) that breast cancer onset occurred approximately 11 to 25 years after initial chest irradiation.[21] Recently, a longitudinal cohort study of childhood cancer survivors demonstrated that the cumulative incidence of breast cancer was 30% by 50 years of age among 1230 female childhood cancer survivors who received chest irradiation,[22] which is similar to the incidence of breast cancer in *BRCA1* carriers (estimated cumulative risk: 31% by age 50). Furthermore, women treated with mantle RT have a higher risk of bilateral breast cancer, with Yahalom and colleagues and Basu and colleagues reporting an incidence of bilaterality of 22% and 34%, in their respective studies.[23,24] Basu and colleagues additionally reported that the time to bilateral breast cancer after first primary breast cancer was short (12–34 months) in their patient cohort. The incidence of bilaterality among female patients treated with mantle RT is substantially more common than in sporadic breast cancer cases, and treatment of first primary breast cancer in these patients should include discussion regarding risk for CBC.

Invasive Lobular Carcinoma

On the basis of data before the routine use of adjuvant systemic therapy for the treatment of breast cancer, lobular histology was believed to be an independent risk factor for metachronous CBC (compared with ductal histology).[25] More recent data from the SEER registry comparing CBC incidence in 134,501 women with unilateral breast cancer showed no difference in CBC rates based on histology of the index cancer; specifically, actuarial rates of CBC at 5, 10, 15, and 20 years were 2.6%, 6.0%, 9.1%, and 12.1% for invasive ductal cancers (IDCs) compared with 3.2%, 6.4%, 9.0%, and 11.7% for invasive lobular cancers (ILCs), respectively.[26] Similarly, a single-institution review of a consecutive cohort of 1182 patients with breast cancer demonstrated no difference in the incidence of metachronous CBC between patients with ductal (12 of 1011; 1%) and lobular (2 of 171; 1%)

TABLE 75.2	Studies Evaluating the Effect of MRI on the Development of Metachronous Contralateral Breast Cancer				
Reference	Patients With MRI/ Total No. of Patients	Follow-Up (Years)	CBC Rates: MRI (%)	CBC Rates: No MRI (%)	P Value
Fischer 2004[34]	121/346 (35%)	3.4	1.7	4.0	<.001
Solin 2008[38]	215/756 (82%)	8.0	6.0	6.0	.39
Kim 2013[35]	1771/3094 (57%)	3.8	0.5	1.4	.02
Ko 2013[36]	229/615 (37%)	5.7	2.2	1.3	.51
Pilewskie 2014[37]	596/2321 (26%)	4.9	3.5	3.5	.86

CBC, Contralateral breast cancer; *MRI*, magnetic resonance imaging.
Modified from Pilewskie M, King TA. Magnetic resonance imaging in patients with newly diagnosed breast cancer: a review of the literature. *Cancer.* 2014;120:2080-2089.

histology (*p* = not significant) at a median follow-up of 4 years.[27] In contrast to metachronous CBC, the incidence of synchronous bilateral breast cancer is reported to be slightly higher in patients with ILC[27,28]; however, a modern study using the Netherlands Cancer Registry demonstrated the absolute difference in CBC within 6 months of diagnosis of the index lesion in patients with lobular versus ductal histology was only 0.6%, and did not justify the routine use of preoperative breast MRI in patients with ILC to evaluate the contralateral breast.[29] On the basis of the aforementioned studies, imaging evaluation and surgical recommendations for the contralateral breast in women with ILC should be no different from that for women with IDC.

Lobular Carcinoma in Situ

Women with LCIS have a 7- to 10-fold increase in breast cancer risk compared with the general population.[30] The classic studies of Haagensen[13] and Rosen and colleagues[31] both document an invasive breast cancer risk in patients with LCIS of approximately 30% at 20 to 25 years' follow-up, with half of the cancers in the ipsilateral breast and half in the contralateral breast. In a study of 4853 patients with LCIS from the SEER database, Chuba and colleagues report a slightly lower but similar risk of invasive breast cancer of 11.1% at 15 years.[32] In one of the largest single-institution experiences with almost 30 years' follow-up, King and colleagues reported on 1060 patients with LCIS; the annual cancer development rate was 2% per year for the first 6 years after LCIS diagnosis, with an overall 15-year cumulative cancer incidence of 26%. Twelve percent of the cancers were bilateral; importantly, breast cancer incidence was significantly reduced with chemoprevention (10-year cumulative risk: 21% no chemoprevention; 7% with chemoprevention) highlighting the effect of systemic therapy on breast cancer risk reduction in high-risk patients.[30]

Impact of Advanced Imaging and Adjuvant Therapy on Bilaterality

Magnetic Resonance Imaging and Contralateral Breast Cancer Detection

In women with newly diagnosed breast cancer, synchronous CBC is reported in 1% to 3% of patients.[33] MRI, with its reported high sensitivity, can improve detection of mammographically occult

CBC, which would allow both (ipsilateral and contralateral) tumors to be treated simultaneously. A meta-analysis by Brennan and colleagues evaluating CBC detection rates by MRI among 3253 women with unilateral breast cancer demonstrated that MRI detected occult synchronous CBC in 4.1% (95% CI 2.7%–6.0%) of women.[33] Logically, we could surmise that by identifying more synchronous disease, MRI also has the potential to decrease metachronous CBC rates. However, most retrospective series have shown little to no difference in metachronous CBC rates in newly diagnosed breast cancer patients with and without MRI (Table 75.2).[34–38] It is important to note that the two studies reporting a significant difference between CBC rates found an absolute difference of 1% to 2% in the MRI and no-MRI groups.[34,35] Furthermore, results from the study by Fischer and colleagues are limited by the fact that statistical adjustments were not performed to account for differences between the groups.[34] Overall, CBC development rates in all these studies were low (0.5%–6.0%) in both groups.

Although there is little doubt that the use of MRI increases CBC detection rates in newly diagnosed breast cancer patients, its routine use in the era of systemic therapy with documented declining CBC rates is difficult to justify, particularly when data demonstrating improved outcomes with MRI are lacking.

Chemotherapy

Several studies address the impact of adjuvant chemotherapy on the risk of a CBC. In a prospective cohort study of 4660 breast cancer patients by Bernstein and colleagues,[39] treatment with chemotherapy significantly reduced the risk of a CBC (RR 0.56, 95% CI 0.33–0.96). Similarly, Bertelsen and coworkers demonstrated a lower risk of CBC with chemotherapy (RR 0.57, 95% CI 0.42–0.75) versus no chemotherapy among 1792 women from the WECARE (matched, case-control) study.[40] The benefit of chemotherapy in reducing CBC risk is not limited to sporadic breast cancer patients. In a subset analysis of the WECARE study, chemotherapy was associated with a substantial reduction in CBC risk among *BRCA1* and *BRCA2* mutation carriers after their first diagnosis of breast cancer (RR 0.5; 95% CI 0.2–1.0).[41] Finally, the 2005 EBCTCG overview,[9] evaluating the effect of systemic therapy for early breast cancer on recurrence, demonstrated a marginal reduction in the incidence of CBC before any other recurrence with the use of polychemotherapy (0.5% vs. 0.6%/ year, 2*p* = .05).[9]

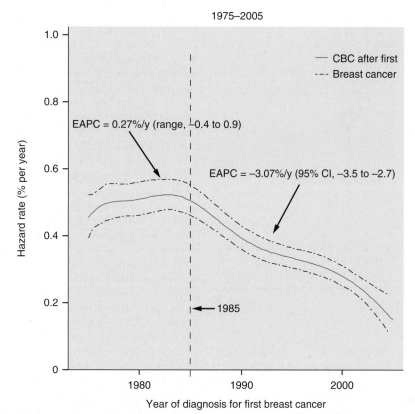

1975–2005

• Fig. 75.2 Temporal trends in contralateral breast cancer over time (1975–2005). *CBC,* Contralateral breast cancer; *CI,* confidence interval; *EAPC,* estimated annual percentage change. (From Nichols HB, Berrington de Gonzalez A, Lacey JV Jr, et al. Declining incidence of contralateral breast cancer in the United States from 1975–2006. *J Clin Oncol.* 2011;29:1564-1569.)

Tamoxifen

The widespread adoption of tamoxifen as adjuvant therapy for breast cancer in the 1980s resulted in a decline in the incidence of CBC, particularly among patients with ER-positive first breast cancers. The 2005 EBCTCG overview[9] demonstrated a reduction in CBC of about one-third in women who received adjuvant tamoxifen for 5 years compared with those who did not (4 vs. 6 per 1000 per year; $p < .00001$). This benefit was limited to women who had ER-positive (or ER-unknown) disease and had little effect on CBC rates among women who had originally ER-poor disease (RR 0.99, 95% CI 0.70–1.36).[9] Recent data from the Adjuvant Tamoxifen: Longer Against Shorter (ATLAS) trial demonstrated a further reduction in CBC development among ER-positive breast cancer patients taking 10 years of tamoxifen compared with 5 (RR 0.88; 95% CI 0.77–1.0; $p = .05$), although the incidence of pulmonary embolus, ischemic heart disease, and endometrial cancer also increased with longer therapy.[42]

Aromatase inhibitors are more effective than tamoxifen in preventing CBC. In the most recent report of the Arimidex, Tamoxifen, Alone or in Combination (ATAC) trial, the hazard ratio (HR) at 100 months for CBC was significantly lower for Arimidex than tamoxifen (HR 0.60, 95% CI 0.42–0.85; $p = .004$), and persisted beyond the 5-year treatment period. At 9 years' follow-up, the absolute CBC rates were 2.5% in Arimidex-treated patients versus 4.2% in tamoxifen-treated patients (compared with an expected 6.3% CBC rate with no systemic therapy).[43] A patient-level meta-analysis of 9885 women treated with 5 years of an aromatase inhibitor compared with 5 years of tamoxifen demonstrated a

significant reduction in risk of CBC with aromatase inhibitors (RR 0.62; 95% CI 0.48–0.80; $2p = .0003$).[44] Cumulatively, these data demonstrate a significant reduction in CBC in ER-positive patients treated with hormonal therapy for their index cancer.

Declining Incidence of CBC

Taken together, the widespread use of systemic therapy in the treatment of early-stage breast cancer has resulted in a dramatic decline in CBC development. Nichols and colleagues examined temporal trends in CBC incidence after first breast cancer using the United States SEER database from 1975 to 2006. Before 1985, CBC rates were stable with an estimated annual percentage change (EAPC) of 0.27% per year, after which they declined with an EAPC of −3.07% per year (Fig. 75.2).[3] This trend was primarily seen in women whose original cancer was ER positive, with a marginally significant rise in CBC among women whose first breast cancer was ER negative (EAPC 1.68%/year).[3] The widespread adoption of hormonal therapy in the treatment of early-stage breast cancer has likely contributed to the favorable decline in CBC among ER-positive patients and may explain why ER-negative patients continue to have a substantial incidence of CBC.

Prognosis of Bilateral Breast Cancer

As prognosis for first primary breast cancer has improved, attention has been drawn to prognosis in women who develop a metachronous CBC. Hartman and colleagues reviewed prognostic

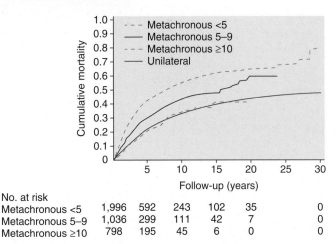

• **Fig. 75.3** Breast cancer-specific mortality after contralateral breast cancer stratified by time since diagnosis of first breast cancer. (From Hartman M, Czene K, Reilly M, et al. Incidence and prognosis of synchronous and metachronous bilateral breast cancer. *J Clin Oncol.* 2007; 25:4210-4216.)

No. at risk						
Metachronous <5	1,996	592	243	102	35	0
Metachronous 5–9	1,036	299	111	42	7	0
Metachronous ≥10	798	195	45	6	0	0

features of bilateral breast cancer among 123,757 women from the Swedish Cancer Registry. Overall, 6550 women developed bilateral breast cancer. Women with bilateral breast cancer had a worse prognosis than women with unilateral breast cancer; however, the lowest mortality from breast cancer was observed in women with the longest disease-free interval between the first and second cancer (Fig. 75.3),[45] suggesting that prognosis is largely linked to a more favorable response to systemic therapy. The development of an early CBC may suggest a relative resistance to systemic therapy, which would result in a worse overall prognosis for the patient.

Similar findings were noted in a study by Liederbach and colleagues; utilizing SEER data, 83,001 patients with newly diagnosed breast cancer were identified from 1998 to 2005. Overall, 2.6% developed a CBC, with half developing within 5 years and half more than 5 years after the first diagnosis. Patients who developed a CBC 4 years or less after the initial cancer had a worse disease-specific survival (DSS) compared with patients with unilateral cancer (HR 1.36, 95% CI 1.03–1.79). Patients who developed CBC 8 years after the initial breast cancer had improved DSS (HR 0.37, 95% CI 0.20–0.67).[46] A major limitation of the study by Liederbach and colleagues is the lack of information in the SEER database regarding adjuvant systemic therapy (chemotherapy or hormonal therapy). It is possible that patients with early CBC had no systemic therapy for their primary cancer or had a poor response to systemic therapy, which predisposed the patient to early CBC development. Without knowledge of systemic therapy data in this study, causality between CBC and worse survival cannot be established.

Contralateral Prophylactic Mastectomy

Despite a declining incidence of CBC related to the widespread use of systemic therapy for treatment of the first primary breast cancer, rates of CPM are increasing in the United States among patients with invasive cancer and ductal carcinoma in situ. Using SEER registry data, Tuttle and colleagues demonstrated that the rates of CPM increased by 150% for all stages of invasive breast cancer between 1998 and 2003.[10] Similarly, among women with

ductal carcinoma in situ (DCIS) undergoing mastectomy, the CPM rate increased by 188%, from 6.4% in 1998 to 18.4% in 2005.[47] Although CPM has been demonstrated to reduce the risk of CBC among women with unilateral invasive breast cancer (risk reduction of approximately 90%–97%),[48–50] the effect of CPM on overall survival (OS) is questionable.

In a large cohort study of 50,000 patients, Herrinton and coworkers demonstrated a reduction in risk of death from breast cancer (HR 0.57, 95% CI 0.45–0.72) in patients with CPM compared with no CPM. However, the CPM cohort also had a lower all-cause mortality (HR 0.60, 95% CI 0.50–0.72),[48] suggesting that selection bias, with healthier patients choosing CPM, was responsible for the improvement in survival seen in this study. More compelling data from Portschy and colleagues modeling OS outcomes from CPM showed a less than 1% survival benefit to CPM.[51] Reasons that CPM would not confer a survival benefit are related to the low and declining incidence of CBC among sporadic breast cancer patients as well as the inherent risk of distant metastases and death from the index breast cancer. In a population-based study of 107,106 women with breast cancer treated with mastectomy between 1998 and 2003, the rate of CBC in women less than 50 years of age with ER-positive stage I and II cancers was 0.5% compared with a breast cancer–specific mortality of 6.8% (related to the index lesion). In women with ER-negative tumors, these figures were 0.9% and 13.5%, respectively.[52] Removal of the "normal" contralateral breast would have no impact on the risk of death from the index lesion, which outweighs any small benefit related to CPM in average-risk women. Even compared with women undergoing breast-conserving surgery, CPM appears to add no benefit. In a recently published large population-based cohort study of 496,488 women with unilateral invasive breast cancer, Wong and colleagues found no significant improvement in breast cancer–specific survival (BCSS) or OS for women undergoing CPM compared with breast-conserving therapy (BCSS: HR 1.08, 95% CI 1.01–1.16; OS: HR 1.08, 95% CI 1.03–1.14), regardless of age or hormone receptor status,[53] reinforcing that aggressive risk-reducing surgery does not eradicate the risk of distant metastases from the primary breast cancer.

The decision to undergo CPM is complex and confounded by the fact that the majority of women undergoing CPM are at low risk for CBC. In a single-institution study of almost 3000 early-stage breast cancer patients treated with mastectomy, King and coworkers observed that the increased use of CPM did not appear to be associated with identification of patients at higher risk of CBC, but rather a combination of patient- and treatment-related factors which contributed to its increased frequency.[54] Well-documented clinical factors associated with the receipt of CPM include family history of breast cancer, invasive lobular histology, young patient age, and MRI, to name a few.[54,55] One of the most commonly cited social reasons patients choose CPM is to achieve "peace of mind"[56] and to reduce risk of future breast cancer, a concern which seems disproportionate to the actual risk of CBC. Reduced surveillance, an overestimation of benefit related to CPM, and the wide availability of postmastectomy reconstruction[57] are additional reasons why patients elect for CPM. Furthermore, patients are often biased by friends or family members who encourage the "do-everything" approach, which is further endorsed by stories of media celebrities undergoing "lifesaving" CPM.

These psychological and social drivers of CPM need to be balanced with the added morbidity and complications associated with more aggressive surgery. Miller et al reviewed their single-institution experience with CPM and reported that among 600 patients treated with either unilateral mastectomy or unilateral mastectomy + CPM, CPM patients were 1.5 times more likely to have any complication (OR 1.53; 95% CI 1.04–2.25, p = .029) and 2.7 times more likely to have a major complication compared with unilateral mastectomy patients (OR 2.66; 95% CI 1.37–5.19, p = .004). In a retrospective, single-institution analysis, Eck and colleagues similarly demonstrated that CPM conferred additional morbidity in one in eight women, resulting in an increased need for reoperation.[58]

The CPM epidemic highlights the needs for physicians to appropriately counsel patients regarding the low absolute risk of CBC and how this risk is influenced by increased utilization of systemic therapy. Patients should also be counseled about options that are less extreme than CPM. Enhanced surveillance may detect a breast cancer in its early stages, allowing for conservative treatment. Adjuvant hormonal therapy for ER-positive cancers also significantly reduces the risk of CBC,[3] and the magnitude of that benefit should be fully explained to patients. Patients should also be aware of the potential morbidity associated with additional surgery, without significant added benefit, and that the "do-everything" approach does not necessarily result in improved survival from breast cancer.

CPM remains an appropriate treatment for a small subset of breast cancer patients, primarily those with an extremely high-risk family history, *BRCA1* or *BRCA2* mutation carriers, and those with a personal history of mantle radiation before age 30. For those patients, the risk of CBC after diagnosis of a first primary breast cancer is substantial and warrants consideration of risk-reduction measures.

Recommendations and Future Directions

Any decisions regarding the normal contralateral breast must be made considering the following: (1) the prognosis of the first cancer (which usually carries the greater risk), (2) the factors predisposing to bilaterality, and (3) contralateral risk reduction from required adjuvant therapy (chemotherapy and/or tamoxifen and/or aromatase inhibitors).

Some challenges remain. The first challenge relates to risk assessment. No single variable, including *BRCA* status, is sufficient to accurately predict the occurrence of a breast cancer or a CBC. Risk assessment is complex, taking into account individual patient factors, family history, and genetic testing. The increased use of multigene, or panel, testing has also created some challenges. Half of the genetic mutations identified today occur in moderate penetrance genes; currently, there are no guidelines as to how patients with these mutations should be managed, and concern for overtreatment exists. The second challenge relates to breast imaging and its effect on local therapy. The added sensitivity of MRI results in detection of additional foci of ipsilateral and contralateral disease, which may not be clinically relevant and may be adequately treated with systemic therapy. The evolution of breast-conservation surgery has taught us that subclinical multicentricity is well controlled by adjuvant therapies, does not invariably result in local failure, and is not an indication for mastectomy. Logically, the same principle can be applied to subclinical disease in the contralateral breast. Despite a higher incidence of synchronous cancers detected with MRI, outcome studies have failed to demonstrate a clinically significant reduction in metachronous CBC with MRI use. The final challenge is with respect to the CPM epidemic. As we evolve from more to less radical surgical approaches with equivalent cure rates, it is incumbent on the surgical community to educate breast cancer patients about the equivalent effectiveness of risk reduction with chemoprevention. Ironically, patients are more willing to consider aggressive surgery with CPM than risk-reduction measures with tamoxifen or aromatase inhibitors because patients consistently overestimate side effects associated with medical therapy and underestimate side effects associated with surgery. Ultimately, the patients' autonomy to make a decision about CPM must be respected, but the patient's decision should be made with full knowledge regarding the risk-benefit ratio of the additional procedure.

Selected References

7. Reiner AS, John EM, Brooks JD, et al. Risk of asynchronous contralateral breast cancer in noncarriers of BRCA1 and BRCA2 mutations with a family history of breast cancer: a report from the Women's Environmental Cancer and Radiation Epidemiology Study. *J Clin Oncol*. 2013;31:433-439.

9. Early Breast Cancer Trialists' Collaborative G. Effects of chemotherapy and hormonal therapy for early breast cancer on recurrence and 15-year survival: an overview of the randomised trials. *Lancet*. 2005;365:1687-1717.

10. Tuttle TM, Habermann EB, Grund EH, et al. Increasing use of contralateral prophylactic mastectomy for breast cancer patients: a trend toward more aggressive surgical treatment. *J Clin Oncol*. 2007;25:5203-5209.

15. Lerner-Ellis J, Khalouei S, Sopik V, et al. Genetic risk assessment and prevention: the role of genetic testing panels in breast cancer. *Expert Rev Anticancer Ther*. 2015;15:1315-1326.

19. Fisher B, Anderson S, Bryant J, et al. Twenty-year follow-up of a randomized trial comparing total mastectomy, lumpectomy, and lumpectomy plus irradiation for the treatment of invasive breast cancer. *N Engl J Med*. 2002;347:1233-1241.

22. Moskowitz CS, Chou JF, Wolden SL, et al. Breast cancer after chest radiation therapy for childhood cancer. *J Clin Oncol*. 2014;32:2217-2223.

A full reference list is available online at ExpertConsult.com.

76

Male Breast Cancer

SARIKA JAIN AND WILLIAM J. GRADISHAR

Epidemiology

Male breast cancer (MBC) is a rare disease worldwide. As a result of its rarity, it is treated similarly to female breast cancer, but important differences exist. In the United States, it was estimated that 2600 men were diagnosed with breast cancer and 440 died from this disease in 2016. MBC accounts for less than 1% of all breast cancers and less than 0.5% of all male cancer deaths in the United States.[1] Globally, the highest male incidence rate was observed in Israel at 1.24 per 100,000 man-years followed closely by the Philippines, Italy, and France. The lowest male incidence rate was recorded in Thailand at 0.16 per 100,000 man-years followed by Japan, Singapore, and Colombia.[2]

The worldwide female-to-male incidence rate ratio of breast cancer is 122:1.[2] MBC compared with female breast cancers occur later in life with higher stage, higher grade, and more estrogen receptor (ER)-positive tumors. The median age of onset of MBC is 72 years of age, compared with 61 years in women.[3] According to the US Surveillance, Epidemiology, and End Results (SEER) registry database, the incidence rates of MBC were slightly increasing from 1975 to 2004 (0.9–1.2 cases per 100,000 men at risk). A rapid increase in female breast cancer incidence was observed in the mid-1970s to mid-1990s in the United States and Europe largely due to the greater use of mammographic screening. Mortality rates in the late 1980s and 1990s tended to be lower than 3 decades earlier, likely owing to advances in diagnostics and therapeutics.[4] The most recent SEER database analysis shows a decrease in breast cancer incidence and mortality in both men and women, but the trends were greater for women. Comparing patients diagnosed from 1996 to 2005 versus 1976 to 1985 and adjusting for age, stage, and grade, MBC death declined by 28% among men and 42% among women[5] (Figs. 76.1 and 76.2).

Racial/ethnic differences also exist. In the United States the ratio of female-to-male breast cancer is approximately 100:1 in whites and 70:1 in blacks. Age-adjusted incidence rates per 100,000 men are highest in blacks (1.65), intermediate in whites (1.31), and lowest in Hispanics (0.68) and Asian/Pacific Islanders (0.66). Blacks are also diagnosed at an earlier age and at a more advanced stage compared with other ethnicities.[6] Similar to black women, black men have an increased breast cancer–specific mortality even after adjustment for clinical, demographic, and treatment factors.[7]

The distribution of tumor subtypes is also different across racial/ethnic groups. In the largest population-based study evaluating breast tumor subtypes in 606 patients with MBC, 82.8% of white men (95% confidence interval [CI] 79.3%–86.4%) had hormone receptor–positive tumors, 14.6% had HER2-positive tumors (95% CI 11.3%–18%), and 2.6% had triple-negative breast cancer (95% CI 1.1%–4%). In contrast, among blacks, 73.3% had hormone receptor–positive tumors (95% CI 60.4%–86.3%), 17.8% had HER2-positive tumors (95% CI 6.6%–29%), and 8.9% had triple-negative tumors (95% CI 0.6%–17.2%); among Hispanics, 77.6% had hormone receptor–positive tumors (95% CI 67.6%–87.6%), 16.4% had HER2-positive tumors (95% CI 7.6%–27.5%), and 6% had triple-negative tumors (95% CI 0.3%–11.6%). Among the patients with hormone receptor–positive tumors, black and Hispanic men were more likely to have progesterone receptor (PR)-negative tumors than white men. No statistically significant differences in survival were observed according to tumor subtype ($p = .08$). Among hormone receptor–positive patients, blacks experienced the worse survival.[8]

Risk Factors

Several risk factors are associated with the development of MBC, including endocrine, nutritional, and genetic factors (Box 76.1). In a large retrospective review of a US Veterans Affairs database assessing 642 cases of MBC, conditions associated with increased risk of MBC included diabetes, orchitis/epididymitis, Klinefelter syndrome, and gynecomastia. Among blacks, cholelithiasis emerged as a significant risk predictor.[9] A large prospective study found family history, history of bone fracture, obesity, and low physical activity to be positively associated with MBC. Some of these identified risk factors are common to female breast cancer and suggest an importance of hormonal mechanisms.[10]

The strongest risk factor for MBC is Klinefelter syndrome.[9] This rare condition results from the inheritance of an additional X chromosome (XXY). Men with this condition have atrophic testes, gynecomastia, high serum levels of gonadotropins (follicle-stimulating hormone, luteinizing hormone), and low plasma levels of testosterone. It is hypothesized that the increased estrogen-to-testosterone ratio could, in turn, lead to abnormal hormonal stimulation of cell proliferation in mammary ductal epithelium. Of the few epidemiologic studies conducted in this area, the largest cohort study of 3518 men with cytogenetically diagnosed Klinefelter syndrome found 19- and 58-fold increases in incidence of and mortality from MBC, respectively, compared with the general population. Alteration of hormone levels, particularly the elevated ratio of estrogen-to-testosterone, administration of exogenous androgens, gynecomastia, and genetic factors are possible explanations for the high risk. Additional studies are needed to delineate which patients with Klinefelter syndrome are at increased risk for MBC, and the importance of patient education, self-examination, and regular examinations should be enforced.[11]

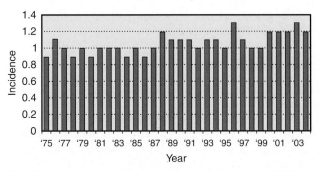

• **Fig. 76.1** Surveillance, Epidemiology, and End Results (SEER) incidence rates for male breast cancer from 1975 to 2004.

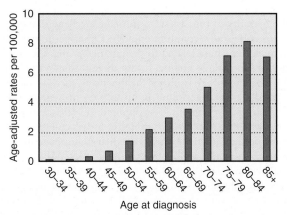

• **Fig. 76.2** Surveillance, Epidemiology, and End Results (SEER) age-specific rates for male breast cancer from 1975 to 2004.

• BOX 76.1 Risk Factors Associated With Male Breast Cancer

Endocrine
Gynecomastia
Testicular conditions
Liver disease
Diabetes mellitus
Nutritional/lifestyle
Obesity
Low physical activity
Alcohol use
Genetic
Family history
Klinefelter syndrome
BRCA carrier (BRCA2 > BRCA1)
Cowden syndrome
Li-Fraumeni syndrome
Hereditary nonpolyposis colorectal cancer (Lynch) syndrome

Chronic liver diseases such as cirrhosis, chronic alcohol injury, and schistosomiasis have been associated with an increased risk of MBC. Cirrhosis limits the ability of the liver to metabolize endogenously produced estrogen, leading to a relative hyperestrogenic state with an imbalance in the estrogen-to-testosterone ratio.[12] Similarly, ethanol, which has been associated with an increased risk of breast cancer in females, is a metabolic modifier for mammary epithelium and may promote the most carcinogenic pathway of estradiol metabolism to catechol estrogen. Very few

cases of MBC have been documented in patients with chronic liver diseases, possibly due to the shortened life span associated with these disorders. Results from some studies have not found an association between liver cirrhosis and MBC.[9]

Gynecomastia, when related to states of estrogen excess, has been associated with MBC. Gynecomastia is most often drug related, and several medications that cause gynecomastia have been associated with an increased risk of MBC. Breast cancer has been described in three men who were prescribed finasteride, a drug approved for the treatment of benign prostatic hyperplasia. Cases of MBC have also been reported with digoxin, thioridazine, and spironolactone, and in male-to-female transsexuals who were castrated and given high doses of estrogen.[13] Testicular conditions have also been associated with an increased risk of MBC. These include orchitis, undescended testis (cryptorchidism), and testicular injury. Other conditions associated with an increased estrogen-to-testosterone ratio such as thyroid disease and marijuana use have not firmly established a link to MBC.

Experimental evidence suggests that prolactin may promote tumorigenesis in animal models; however, physiologic states of prolactin excess in humans (e.g., multiple pregnancies) do not confer an increased risk of breast cancer and may be protective. Several case reports have described the development of MBC in association with a prolactinoma, a setting in which low plasma testosterone levels are often observed.[14] The association between prolactin excess and MBC remains unclear.

Androgens may convey a protective effect by inhibiting cell proliferation in breast tissue. In some reports, mutations in the DNA-binding domain of the androgen receptor (AR) gene have been implicated in the development of MBC. Conversely, a pathologic case study that analyzed tumor material from two series of patients with MBC without clinical evidence of androgen insensitivity reported no AR gene mutations. In a study of 43 MBC patients, AR expression by immunohistochemistry inversely correlated with survival.[15]

Approximately 5% to 10% of female breast cancer cases are thought to be hereditary, with the majority of these cases associated with mutations in two genes: breast cancer type 1 and 2 susceptibility genes (BRCA1 and BRCA2). These genes are inherited in an autosomal dominant pattern and confer a lifetime risk of female breast cancer ranging from 50% to 85%. Approximately 15% to 20% of MBC is associated with a positive family history for the disease compared with only 7% of the general male population.[16]

BRCA2 mutations are more frequent than BRCA1 mutations. In an Italian series of 50 BRCA carriers, 92% harbored the BRCA2 mutation compared with 8% with the BRCA1 mutation.[17] Inherited mutations in BRCA do not increase the risk of breast cancer to the same degree in males as in females. The breast cancer risk also appears to be higher with BRCA2 mutations as opposed to BRCA1. Men who carry a BRCA2 mutation have an approximate 6.5% cumulative risk for breast cancer by age 70, which is 100-fold higher than the general male population. A paucity of data exists correlating the risk for MBC in BRCA1 carriers. One Dutch and one American family have been described that carried the BRCA1 mutation; each had one case of MBC as well as multiple associated female breast cancer cases. A report from the National Cancer Institute Cancer Genetics Network suggests that the cumulative risk of breast cancer by age 70 in men harboring a BRCA1 mutation is 1.2% (95% CI 0.22%–2.8%) (Fig. 76.3).[16]

The classification of molecular subtypes based on immunohistochemical profiles as proposed in female breast cancer is still

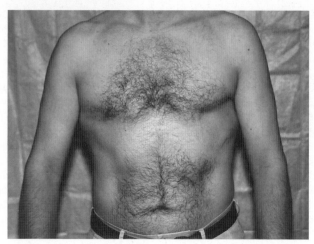

• **Fig. 76.3** A 51-year-old man diagnosed with stage I left breast cancer at age 46. A strong family history of breast cancer led to genetic testing, identifying a *BRCA1* genetic mutation. He subsequently underwent a prophylactic right mastectomy.

controversial in MBC. In one report of 382 MBC cases including 50 *BRCA* carriers, the immunophenotypic profiles differed between 4 *BRCA1*- and 19 *BRCA2*-asssociated patients, in whom complete ER, PR, and HER2 status were available. Of the 4 *BRCA1*-related MBC cases, 3 showed a luminal A subtype, and 1 a triple-negative tumor. Of the 19 *BRCA2*-related MBCs, 7 were luminal A, 9 luminal B, and 3 HER2-positive. Notably, all 7 triple-negative tumor cases were *BRCA2*-mutation negative. In a multivariate logistic model, *BRCA2*-associated MBCs showed positive association with high tumor grade (odds ratio [OR] 4.9, 95% CI 1.0–23.9) and inverse association with PR expression (OR 0.19, 95% CI 0.04–0.92), suggesting that the *BRCA2* subgroup is characterized by a more aggressive phenotype.[17]

Genetic mutations other than *BRCA* may predispose males to developing breast cancer. Cowden syndrome, an autosomal dominant cancer susceptibility syndrome, is associated with germline mutations in the tumor suppressor gene *PTEN* located on chromosome 10. This syndrome is characterized by multiple hamartomas and an increased risk for both male and female breast cancer and thyroid malignancies. Two cases of MBC have been reported with germline *PTEN* mutations and the Cowden syndrome phenotype. Other hereditary syndromes associated with MBC include Li-Fraumeni syndrome, caused by the *TP53* mutation, and hereditary nonpolyposis colorectal cancer (Lynch) syndrome, caused by mutations in the mismatch repair genes.[18]

Recent genome-wide association studies (GWAS) identified common single nucleotide polymorphisms (SNPs) that influence female breast cancer risk. A GWAS study of MBC compromising 823 MBC cases and 2795 controls were genotyped and validated in an independent sample set, and the SNP RAD51B was found to be significantly associated with MBC risk.[19] Other studies have found genetic variants that influence susceptibility to breast cancer, which differ between male and female breast cancer.

Guidelines from the National Comprehensive Cancer Network (NCCN) recommend that genetic testing be offered to men who develop breast cancer as well as to families with a known *BRCA* mutation, a case of MBC, or the presence of female relatives with a history of breast or ovarian cancer that suggests the presence of an inherited breast or ovarian cancer syndrome. Furthermore, adherence to recommended screening guidelines for prostate

cancer is advised because males with *BRCA2* mutations have an elevated risk of prostate cancer.

Clinical Features

Similar to women, MBC typically presents as a painless lump. The mass is usually subareolar and less often in the upper outer quadrant. A slight predilection exists for the left breast. Nipple involvement is a fairly early event, occurring in 40% to 50%, with retraction in 9%, discharge in 6%, and ulceration in 6%. Bilateral MBC is rare with a reported incidence of 1.5% to 2% of all MBCs.[20] Infrequently, MBC presents as an axillary nodal metastasis without a palpable breast lump. Other findings on examination for malignancy include fixation to skin or muscle and breast tenderness.[21]

The majority of breast lesions in males are benign, with gynecomastia as the most common etiology. Other pathologic lesions in the male breast are related to the cutaneous and subcutaneous tissue and can include lipoma, breast abscess, metastatic lesion to the breast, and other primary malignancies such as sarcoma.[22] Gynecomastia has been found in up to 55% of male breasts in a series of autopsy specimens.[21] As opposed to MBC, gynecomastia usually presents as bilateral, symmetric breast enlargement with irregular borders in the absence of axillary lymphadenopathy or fixation to the chest wall. On mammography, MBC is usually subareolar and eccentric to the nipple. In contrast, gynecomastia appears as a round or triangular area of increased density positioned symmetrically in the retroareolar region. Calcifications are rarer and coarser than those occurring in female breast cancer. Because of the low incidence of MBC in the general population, there is no role for screening mammograms in men. One report described a male *BRCA2* carrier who was diagnosed with breast cancer by screening mammography; clear guidelines have not been established for this population.[23]

Diagnosis

The first step in the evaluation of a suspicious breast mass in a male is mammography. A mammogram can usually distinguish between malignancy and gynecomastia and is abnormal in 80% to 90% of MBCs. Mammographic features of malignancy include a dense mass generally without calcifications and often with spiculated, indistinct, or microlobulated margins. Sonography usually reveals an irregularly shaped hypoechoic mass, as seen in female breast cancers. Any cysts that are discovered on imaging should be sampled because simple cysts are rare in men and are associated with neoplastic papillary lesions. Likewise, radiologic features such as a well-defined lesion that would suggest a benign finding in a female are unreliable in men and require biopsy. In one series, MBC was manifested as a well-defined mass in 15% of cases using mammography and in 23% using sonography.[24]

Several studies have suggested that mammography added no diagnostic information to the combination of physical examination and pathologic evaluation. In one retrospective analysis of 134 male patients with a history of a breast lump between 2001 and 2003 and undergoing mammographic imaging, only four cases of breast cancer were diagnosed. All four patients presented with a painless lump, for a mean duration of 7 months, in whom breast cancer was suspected by clinical examination and confirmed by biopsy.[25] The use of breast MRI has not been widely studied in MBC, and no prospective data exist for its use in screening or diagnosis of MBC.

Once a suspicious breast mass is identified, biopsy is required to confirm the diagnosis and to assay for ER, PR, and HER2 status. Fine-needle aspiration (FNA) is a reliable procedure, which has been shown to avoid surgical biopsy in 59% of cases. However, in one report of 153 FNAs of the male breast, 13% did not provide sufficient tissue for diagnosis.[26] Compared with FNA, core needle biopsy offers a more definitive histologic diagnosis, avoids inadequate samples, and usually distinguishes between invasive and in situ cancer.

Pathology

The most common histopathologic type of MBC is invasive ductal carcinoma, similar to female breast cancer, and accounts for 85% of all MBC cases. Conversely, invasive lobular carcinoma is much less frequent in males compared with females, constituting only 1.7% of MBCs.[27] The rarity of lobular carcinoma in males may be due to the lack of acini and lobules in normal male breast tissue. The very rare cases of lobular carcinoma have occurred in men with Klinefelter syndrome, transsexuals taking estrogens, and men with prostate cancer. Ductal carcinoma in situ (DCIS) accounts for 20% to 25% of all cases of female breast cancer. In contrast, the frequency of DCIS in men ranges from 0% to 17%, with an average of 7%. Few case reports of lobular carcinoma in situ (LCIS) exist in the published literature. Paget disease of the breast has a higher incidence in males (5%) compared with females (1%–4%) and appears to have a worse 5-year survival in men.[28] Likewise, invasive papillary carcinoma is more common in males (2%–4%) than in females (1%). All other subtypes of breast cancer, including inflammatory breast cancer, have been reported in men.[29]

Immunohistochemical and molecular characteristics of MBC have shown a greater incidence of hormone receptor positivity and significantly less frequent overexpression of HER2/neu. In females with breast cancer, tumors are ER-positive in 77% of patients compared with 92% of ER-positive tumors in males. The incidence of HER2 overexpression is only 2% to 15% in MBC; approximately 18% to 20% of all female breast cancers overexpress HER2.[30]

More information has become available regarding molecular markers in MBC. In a series of 134 cases of MBC, tumor samples were analyzed for ER, PR, HER2, AR, the proto-oncogene p53, the cell cycle regulatory protein cyclin D1, a marker of apoptosis bcl-2, among others. According to immunohistochemically defined molecular subtypes, the vast majority of cases were classified as luminal A (75%), whereas 21% of tumors were luminal B. No HER2-driven cases were identified; all HER2-positive cases (3%) showed ER positivity and were classified as luminal B. The remaining 4% of cases were basal-like.[31] Expression of AR (81%), bcl-2 (75%), and cyclin D1 (77%) were very common, in line with previous studies. Approximately half of the tumors were positive for p21 (48%) and BRST2 (56%). p21, the most important downstream effector of p53, is a universal cyclin/cyclin-dependent kinase inhibitor which inhibits proliferation and has been associated with worse disease-free survival. Overexpression of p21 has been seen more frequently in MBC than in female breast cancer. In contrast, p53 accumulation (15%) was rare, somewhat lower than other reports in which up to 54% of samples were p53-positive. Expression of the basal markers CK5/6 (9%), CK14 (1%), and EGFR (12%) were encountered infrequently. This study also elucidated the clinical relevance of several biomarkers in MBC. PR-positive and bcl-2-positive tumors showed favorable histologic features, whereas HER2-positive, ki67-positive, and p21-positive tumors correlated with higher grade and mitotic count. p53 and BRST2 significantly predicted the presence of lymph node metastases, and PR negativity and p53 accumulation emerged as independent predictors of decreased survival.[32]

Treatment of Localized and Locally Advanced Disease

Surgical Management

The treatment of localized invasive early-stage breast cancer in men follows the same general principles as in women. The current operative procedure of choice in MBC is a total mastectomy with sentinel lymph node (SLN) biopsy. Traditionally, the preferred approach was a modified radical mastectomy (MRM). Although randomized studies have not been conducted in men, retrospective data suggest the equivalence of radical mastectomy and MRM in terms of local recurrence and survival, and studies in women also support the equivalence of these two procedures. The only exception is extensive chest wall muscle involvement in which radical mastectomy may be of benefit if neoadjuvant chemotherapy does not sufficiently reduce the tumor burden. Breast conserving therapy (lumpectomy followed by breast irradiation) is a possible option for men with breast cancer. However, the lack of adequate surrounding breast tissue and the central location of tumors precludes this approach in some. Per the SEER database for the 1777 men with stage I–II, T1–2, N0 breast cancer, 83% received mastectomy, and 17% underwent breast conserving therapy. MRM alone had an actuarial 5-year cause-specific survival (CSS) of 97.3% for stage I and 91.2% for stage II, compared with 100% CSS in the BCT regardless of stage.[33]

The literature suggests that MRM is used in approximately 70% of male patients, followed by radical mastectomy (8%–30%), total mastectomy (5%–14%), and lumpectomy with or without radiation (1%–13%). Radical mastectomy was more commonly used in older series, likely reflecting practice patterns as well as later stage at diagnosis.[30] In a review of more recent data from the SEER database, of 1541 cases of MBC, almost 20% were treated with breast conservation. Although these SEER data do not include information on local recurrence rates, in one retrospective study of seven patients treated with breast conserving therapy with a median follow-up of 67 months, there were no local recurrences.[34]

Management of Regional Nodes

Axillary nodal involvement is a strong predictor of both local recurrence and metastatic risk and is present in approximately 50% of men with breast cancer. As such, surgical assessment of the axillary nodes is an essential component of primary treatment. In early-stage breast cancer in women, SLN biopsy has emerged as a less morbid alternative to a full axillary lymph node dissection.[35] In an experienced center, the SLN accurately predicts the status of the remaining regional nodes, and a negative SLN eliminates the need for a complete axillary node dissection. In an effort to understand the predictive value of SLN biopsy in men, several retrospectives studies have been carried out. The European Institute of Oncology (IEO) investigated 32 MBC patients with clinically negative axillary lymph nodes who underwent a SLN biopsy.

Preoperative lymphoscintigraphy and subsequent imaging successfully identified the SLN in all patients, with a mean number of 1.5 SLN removed per patient. A total of 26 patients (81%) had negative SLN; lymph node metastases were found in 4 patients and micrometastases in the remaining 2 patients. After a median follow-up of 30 months, no axillary recurrence events occurred.[36] Memorial Sloan-Kettering Cancer Center reported their experience in 78 patients with MBC. SLN biopsy was successful in 76 (97%), yielding a similar failure rate as in female breast cancer. Negative SLNs were found in 39 of 76 (51%) patients. Of these, three (8%) were found to have a positive non-SLN during intraoperative palpation. Positive SLNs were found in 37 of 76 (49%) patients. The two patients who failed SLN biopsy underwent a complete axillary node dissection. At a median follow-up of 28 months, there were no axillary recurrences.[37] Data from the American College of Surgeons Oncology Group Z0011 study suggest that patients with clinically staged T1N0 or T2N0 breast cancer with fewer than 3 positive sentinel lymph nodes can forgo completion axillary node dissection, as long as adjuvant therapy and whole-breast irradiation are part of the treatment plan. Although this study did not include men, there are case reports in men utilizing this technique.[38] These retrospective and single institution experiences with SLN biopsy in men are comparable to those in women. A joint expert panel of the Breast International Group and the North American Breast Cancer Group concluded that total mastectomy with SLN biopsy is the established standard of care.[30] An expert panel convened by the American Society of Clinical Oncology (ASCO) concluded that the use of SLN biopsy in MBC was "acceptable."

Locally Advanced Disease

Men with locally advanced disease (T3N0 or stage III disease) or inflammatory breast cancer are treated similarly to women. Neoadjuvant chemotherapy followed by mastectomy should be considered for these individuals because randomized trials of neoadjuvant therapy followed by surgery versus primary surgery followed by adjuvant chemotherapy, as studied predominantly in female breast cancer, show high rates of clinical response and improved cosmesis without compromising survival outcomes.

Adjuvant Radiation Therapy

There are limited data assessing the role for and clinical impact of adjuvant radiation therapy in men. In several series, postoperative radiation therapy was administered to some patients, but the technical aspects of radiotherapy varied between series and over time, making any assessment of clinical impact difficult. Men are more likely to be offered postmastectomy chest-wall radiation therapy (PMRT) due to concern of adequate surgical margins even in small tumors and the higher incidence of nipple or skin involvement. Prospective studies of PMRT have demonstrated a survival advantage in women with node-positive breast cancer, although their generalizability to MBC is unclear. In one series with 75 MBC cases, 29 (39%) did not undergo PMRT and 46 (61%) completed PMRT. Patients who received PMRT demonstrated no benefit in overall survival but significantly better local recurrence-free survival compared with those who did not receive radiation therapy.[39] A retrospective study from Johns Hopkins suggests that similar indications for PMRT should be applied to both men and women with breast cancer.[40] As with female breast cancer, PMRT is recommended for men with four or more positive lymph nodes (N2/N3) or locally advanced (T3/T4) primary tumors.

There is less agreement on radiation treatment for fewer positive nodes. Data from a combined analysis of two Danish trials and the National Cancer Institute of Canada Clinical Trials Group MA.20 trial demonstrated a survival benefit from PMRT in patients with fewer than four positive nodes. Therefore radiation therapy should also be considered in men with one to three positive lymph nodes.

Adjuvant Systemic Therapy

Recommendations for adjuvant endocrine therapy, chemotherapy, or biological therapy after surgical resection of the primary tumor in MBC are based largely on the benefits derived from these interventions in women with early-stage breast cancer. The low incidence of MBC precludes robust clinical trial development and timely completion to assess the efficacy of adjuvant therapy.

Because most MBCs are hormone receptor–positive, adjuvant tamoxifen for 5 years is often recommended. Prospective trials to confirm this approach are not available; however, retrospective studies support a survival benefit from tamoxifen in MBC. In one report, 39 patients who received tamoxifen demonstrated improved 5-year actuarial survival and disease-free survival compared with a historical control group who underwent mastectomy alone (61% vs. 44% and 56% vs. 28%, respectively).[41]

Tamoxifen is generally well tolerated, but several studies indicate that a large proportion of men discontinue treatment before 5 years. A recent retrospective review from MD Anderson Cancer Center evaluating 64 MBC patients treated with adjuvant tamoxifen demonstrated a high rate of adverse events. At a median follow-up of 3.9 years, 34 (53%) patients experienced one or more toxicities, most commonly weight gain (22%) and sexual dysfunction (22%). Thirteen (20.3%) patients discontinued tamoxifen due to toxicity, including ocular complaints (1 patient), leg cramps (1), neurodegenerative deficits (2), bone pain (2), sexual dysfunction (3), and thromboembolic events (4).[42] In a study of 116 men, adherence to tamoxifen decreased from 65% at year 1% to 18% at year 5. Factors associated with low adherence were lack of social support, age 60 years or younger, and side effects. Compared with men who were adherent to tamoxifen, those with low adherence had significantly diminished overall survival (98% vs 80%, respectively, $p = .008$) and disease-free survival (95% vs 73%, respectively, $p = .007$). Sixty-four patients experienced side effects, including fatigue, anxiety, sleep disorders, decreased libido, and weight gain.[43] Conversely, in a recent large population-based study of 158 cases of MBC, adjuvant tamoxifen was prescribed to 109 patients, and only 14 (11.7%) patients discontinued therapy due to toxicity, similar to a matched female control group.[44]

Aromatase inhibitors are an established adjuvant treatment for postmenopausal female breast cancer and have been shown to be more effective than tamoxifen in preventing recurrence. In a retrospective study of 257 men with hormone receptor–positive breast cancer, overall survival was significantly better with tamoxifen compared with an aromatase inhibitor at a median follow-up of 42.4 months. After adjusting for patient and tumor characteristics, aromatase inhibitor treatment was linked to a 1.5-fold increase in risk of mortality compared with tamoxifen (HR 1.55; 95% CI 1.13–2.13, $p = .007$). These findings may be related to insufficient suppression of estrogen levels in men by aromatase inhibitors because 20% of estrogen is produced by the testes. Moreover, aromatase inhibitors lead to an increase in follicle-stimulating hormone and testosterone level, which may in turn increase the rate of aromatization.[45] As such, tamoxifen remains the preferred agent in MBC when hormone therapy is indicated.

Studies concerning adjuvant chemotherapy are similarly limited in MBC. One report of 11 patients with stage II–III MBC treated with adjuvant cyclophosphamide, methotrexate, and 5-fluorouracil (CMF) showed favorable outcomes compared with historical controls. At the National Cancer Institute (NCI), 31 patients with axillary node-positive, stage II MBC were treated with adjuvant CMF chemotherapy for up to 12 cycles. At a follow-up of 20 years, the overall survival was shown to be 65% at 10 years, 52% at 15 years, and 42% at 20 years.[46] There are no data on the benefit of anthracyclines or taxanes in men with breast cancer.

The Onco*type* DX breast cancer 21-gene assay using standardized quantitative reverse transcriptase polymerase chain reaction was validated in women with early-stage, node-negative hormone receptor–positive breast cancer to estimate the likelihood of chemotherapy benefit. In a genomic study of 347 male and 82,434 female breast cancer patients with ER-positive tumors, the patterns of expression of the Onco*type* DX genes were more similar than different between males and females. The proportion of tumors with low risk of recurrence based on the Recurrence Score was 53.6% in males versus 53.4% in females, intermediate risk of recurrence was 35.2% in males versus 36.3% in females, and high risk of recurrence was 11.2% in males versus 10.3% in females. Of note, mean expression of ER, PR, and proliferation genes (*ki67, MYBL2, Survivin, Cyclin B1,* and *STK15*) were higher in males. In conclusion, current recommendations for adjuvant chemotherapy options in women with early-stage breast cancer should be considered in men.

Trastuzumab, a humanized monoclonal antibody directed against the HER2 protein, was associated with a significant survival benefit in women with HER2-positive breast cancer, when combined with chemotherapy. The incidence of HER2 overexpression/amplification in MBC appears to be low, and there are no prospective data evaluating survival outcomes with adjuvant trastuzumab in MBC. In a study with 147 stage I–III MBC cases, 9 patients were known to overexpress HER, and only 5 of these patients received trastuzumab with chemotherapy.[43] Nonetheless, its use should be considered in men with HER2-positive breast cancer.

Treatment of Metastatic Disease

Hormonal manipulation has played a central role in the initial management of metastatic MBC because of the high incidence of hormone receptor positivity. Multiple reports of orchiectomy as treatment of metastatic MBC indicate response rates between 32% and 67%, with a median survival of 56 months in responding patients versus 38 months in nonresponding patients. Other ablative surgical procedures have been evaluated in metastatic MBC, either as primary treatment or at the time of disease progression after orchiectomy. Adrenalectomy and hypophysectomy are associated with response rates of 76% and 58%, respectively. These surgical procedures are rarely used today because of the associated morbidity and the introduction of medical management of metastatic disease.[47]

Tamoxifen is the endocrine treatment of choice in metastatic disease. Objective response rates as high as 81% have been reported in ER-positive MBC with tamoxifen treatment.[48] Other agents including aminoglutethimide, megestrol acetate, androgens, antiandrogens, steroids, and luteinizing hormone–releasing hormone (LHRH) analogs are associated with 50% to 70% response rates in ER-positive MBC.

Aromatase inhibitors are very active in women with hormone receptor–positive metastatic breast cancer, but its role in men is less clear. One study of 15 patients treated with an aromatase inhibitor reported a complete response in 2 patients, partial response in 4 patients, and stable disease in 2 patients (response rate of 40%); activity correlated with significant reductions in estradiol levels.[49] Current data suggest that aromatase inhibitors may be considered after progression on tamoxifen. The German Breast Group will conduct a prospective, randomized multicenter phase II study (GBG-54 MALE) evaluating tamoxifen with and without an LHRH analog versus an aromatase inhibitor with an LHRH analog in MBC. The role of fulvestrant, a selective estrogen receptor downregulator, is less clear. One case series described 14 men treated with fulvestrant in the second to fourth-line setting. In all cases, fulvestrant was well tolerated. Partial response was noted in 3 (21%) patients, stable disease in 7 (50%) patients, with a median overall survival of 62 months.[50]

Treatment with chemotherapy should be considered for patients with ER-negative tumors, for those with rapidly progressing disease, and in patients refractory to hormone therapy, similar to principles for initiating chemotherapy in women. HER2-directed therapies including trastuzumab, pertuzumab, and lapatinib have not been formally studied in metastatic MBC. Using these agents in HER2-positive metastatic MBC is reasonable considering the significant survival benefit seen in women with metastatic breast cancer.

Prognosis

Male and female breast cancers are staged according to the American Joint Committee on Cancer Staging System. Similar to women with breast cancer, stage, tumor size, and axillary lymph node status are important factors influencing outcome. This was illustrated in a report derived from the SEER database of 1541 men with breast cancer. The breast cancer–specific mortality increased by stage: 1% in situ, 5% stage I, 15% stage II, 38% stage III, and 57% stage IV.[51]

Molecular subtyping of breast cancer has emerged as a significant predictor of outcome in women. Because MBC is rare, large series elucidating the significance of molecular subtyping is lacking. Some studies have found the distribution of tumor subtypes in MBC to be different compared with female breast cancer, which may point to important differences in biology and outcomes.[31] Furthermore, in one study of 197 patients, HER2 positivity was not associated with poorer outcome, even though the majority of patients had not received adjuvant chemotherapy or trastuzumab. Larger studies are required to validate these findings.

The risk of a contralateral breast cancer and second primary nonbreast cancers appears to be increased in men with breast cancer. In a review of 4873 MBCs from the SEER database, 93 (2%) were identified with a second MBC and 1001 (21%) with a second primary cancer. This underlines the importance of continued long-term surveillance for a second breast cancer and appropriate screening for nonbreast cancers in men.

Some reports have suggested that MBC has a worse prognosis than female breast cancer. From the SEER database, 6157 cases of MBC were compared with 877,885 cases of female breast cancer from 1973 to 2008. Survival was significantly higher in female breast cancer compared with MBC but improved over time in MBC (1 year, 96% vs. 91%; 3 year, 85% vs. 80%; 5 year, 77% vs. 68%, respectively).[3] Conversely, in a case-control study of 144 patients (72 female, 72 male) with early-stage breast cancer, male patients received comparable systemic therapy as their female counterparts. Disease-free and overall survival were similar, suggesting that male sex is not a poor prognostic factor for treatment outcomes.[52]

Race/ethnicity may also influence breast cancer prognosis and treatment. It is known that black women have poorer survival compared with white women. From the SEER data, one report illustrated that black and Asian men had lower 1- to 5-year survival compared with white men, despite similar treatment modalities. Notably, black and Asian men had a higher incidence of poorly differentiated histology compared with white men (19%, 20%, and 13%, respectively).[3] In an analysis of 510 MBC cases (456 white, 34 black), black men were approximately 50% less likely to undergo consultation with an oncologist and subsequently receive chemotherapy; however, results did not reach statistical significance. After multivariate analysis, breast cancer–specific mortality hazard ratio was shown to be more than triple for black versus white men.[7]

Survivorship Issues and Surveillance

Scant research exists on the psychological and social impact in men treated for breast cancer. Several common themes include emasculation, psychological distress associated with living with a feminized illness, negative body image, changes in sexuality, and cancer-specific stress such as fear of recurrence and anxiety. In one study with 161 men with breast cancer, clinical levels of depression and anxiety as measured with the Hospitalized Anxiety and Depression Scale were present in 1% and 6%, respectively, whereas 23% reported high levels of cancer-specific distress. Risk factors appeared to be younger age, altered body image, more frequent use of avoidance coping, and uncertainty about the future. These data support that men treated for breast cancer experience significant long-term issues, which require further study.[47] All male patients should be followed longitudinally after completing treatment for breast cancer. Although guidelines do not exist specifically for MBC, extrapolation from the follow-up of women is reasonable. The role of mammography as part of surveillance in men remains unclear.

Management Summary

- A suspicious breast mass in a man must be evaluated by tissue sampling. Needle biopsy is the preferred method of diagnosis.
- A diagnosis of male breast cancer should prompt a referral to genetic counseling and *BRCA* testing.
- Total mastectomy with SLN biopsy is the established surgical approach for most male cancers.
- Chest wall and regional lymph node irradiation should be given using the same criteria developed for use in women.
- Adjuvant systemic therapy recommendations are similar to those for women with the same stage of disease. For hormone receptor–positive tumors, adjuvant tamoxifen with or without chemotherapy should be recommended. Current recommendations for adjuvant chemotherapy options in women with early-stage breast cancer should be considered in men. Trastuzumab is indicated for HER2-positive MBC.
- For locally advanced disease, neoadjuvant chemotherapy followed by mastectomy should be considered.
- In patients with metastatic disease, tamoxifen should be used as first-line treatment in hormone receptor–positive metastatic disease. The role for aromatase inhibitors and fulvestrant remains unclear. Chemotherapy should be recommended for rapidly progressing disease, hormone receptor–negative, or hormone-refractory disease. HER2-directed therapy should be used in HER2-positive advanced breast cancer.

Selected References

8. Chavez-MacGregor M, Clarke CA, Lichtensztain DY, Hortobagyi GN, Giordano SH. Male breast cancer according to tumor subtype and race: a population based study. *Cancer*. 2013;119:1611-1617.

30. Korde LA, Zujewski JA, Kamin L, et al. Multidisciplinary meeting on male breast cancer: summary and research recommendations. *J Clin Oncol*. 2010;28:2114-2122.

38. Bratman SV, Kapp DS, Horst KC. Evolving trends in the initial locoregional management of male breast cancer. *Breast*. 2012;21:296-302.

45. Eggemann H, Ignatov A, Smith BJ, et al. Adjuvant therapy with tamoxifen compared to aromatase inhibitors for 257 male breast cancer patients. *Breast Cancer Res Treat*. 2013;137:465-470.

52. Rushton M, Kwong A, Visram H, et al. Treatment outcomes for early stage male breast cancer: a single centre retrospective case-control study. *Curr Oncol*. 2014;21:e400-e407.

A full reference list is available online at ExpertConsult.com.

77

Local Recurrence, the Augmented Breast, and the Contralateral Breast

BHARTI JASRA, ASTRID BOTTY VAN DEN BRUELE, D. SCOTT LIND, AND EDWARD M. COPELAND III

As the number of women undergoing treatment for breast cancer increases, more patients will experience local recurrence or develop a second primary breast cancer. The exponential increase in breast augmentation has led to more women potentially developing cancer in a previously augmented breast requiring a unique management approach. After mastectomy or breast conserving surgery, recurrence of disease can be local, regional or distant.

Local recurrence refers to reappearance of the original cancer in the ipsilateral treated breast or chest wall, whereas regional recurrence implies tumor recurring in the regional lymph nodes such as the ipsilateral axillary, supra/infraclavicular, or internal mammary lymph nodes.

This chapter addresses complex conditions requiring comprehensive multidisciplinary planning and treatment, such as locoregional recurrence (LRR) after mastectomy with or without reconstruction, LRR after breast conserving therapy (BCT), breast cancer in the augmented breast and breast cancer risk in the contralateral breast.

Locoregional Recurrence After Mastectomy

Although most women with breast cancer can be treated with BCT, some women still require or desire mastectomy. *Locoregional recurrence after mastectomy* refers to the reappearance of breast cancer in the skin flaps, in the mastectomy scar on the chest wall, or in the ipsilateral regional lymphatics (axillary, internal mammary, and supraclavicular lymph nodes). Locoregional postmastectomy recurrences are usually detected by physical examination and they represent a heterogenous group of lesions ranging from a small, solitary tumor nodule in the surgical scar to diffuse *carcinoma en cuirass* involving the entire chest wall and regional lymphatics (Fig. 77.1).

In the last several decades, the number of breast cancer survivors has increased due to earlier diagnosis and more effective treatments. It is estimated that there are over 3.5 million women living in the United States with a history of breast cancer and approximately one-quarter million women will be newly diagnosed this year.[1] There remains, however, considerable controversy regarding the appropriate follow-up after the initial breast cancer treatment. Logically, one would expect that intensive posttreatment surveillance would lead to earlier detection of recurrences and improved survival. However, expensive diagnostic tests to detect occult metastatic disease, such as serum markers, computed tomography (CT), magnetic resonance imaging (MRI), and positive emission tomography scans have not been shown to improve survival.[2] Recent versions of the American Cancer Society,[1] American Society of Clinical Oncology,[3] and National Comprehensive Cancer Network (NCCN)[4] guidelines for follow-up of breast cancer recommend that asymptomatic patients be followed with a detailed history, physical examination, and mammography. Furthermore, a recent Cochrane review examined all randomized controlled trials evaluating the effectiveness of follow-up strategies after the primary treatment of breast cancer.[1] The findings of this review confirmed the conclusions of an earlier review[5] that demonstrated that follow-up programs based on regular physical examinations and yearly mammography are as effective as more intensive approaches with respect to detection of recurrence, overall survival, and quality of life. The frequency of breast cancer follow-up is also not evidence-based. The American Society for Clinical Oncology recommends breast cancer patients be seen by a healthcare provider every 3 to 6 months for the first 3 years after initial treatment, every 6 to 12 months for years 4 and 5, and then annually thereafter.[3] In addition to breast cancer–specific follow-up recommendations, clinicians should be aware of the NCCN guidelines for cancer survivorship that provide screening, evaluation, and management recommendations for all cancer patients after their initial treatment.[6]

The coordination of care among providers managing breast cancer survivors is also important. One study from the United Kingdom demonstrated improved patient satisfaction when breast cancer follow-up was performed by a family practitioner compared with a specialist, but this satisfaction difference may have been due to patient familiarity with their family physician.[7] In addition, the recent Cochrane review also concluded that follow-up care performed by general practitioners working in an ambulatory practice setting had comparable effectiveness to that delivered by hospital-based specialists.[2] In summary, breast cancer follow-up necessitates an organized, team-based approach emphasizing health promotion, surveillance, screening, physical and psychosocial concerns, and care coordination.

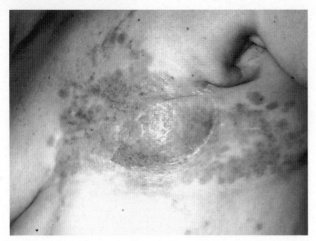

• **Fig. 77.1** Diffuse local recurrence involving the entire chest wall. The patient had a latissimus dorsi flap reconstruction, and the underlying implant was removed to facilitate the delivery of chest wall radiation.

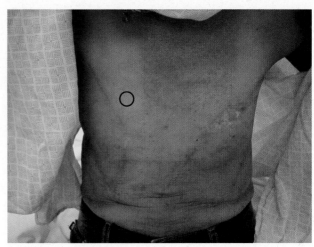

• **Fig. 77.2** Patient with breast cancer developing in breast tissue *(circle)* remaining in the mastectomy flaps 25 years after bilateral mastectomy.

The incidence of local recurrence after mastectomy varies from 7% to 32%[8–11] depending on several factors, including tumor biology, the initial extent of disease (e.g., tumor size, lymph node, and margin status), the type of primary therapy (e.g., hormonal, chemotherapy, and/or radiotherapy), the length of follow-up, and the method of detection.[8] The majority of chest wall recurrences appear within the first 2 years after mastectomy, and 90% occur within 5 years.[10] Some solitary local recurrences result from incompletely excised tumor or tumor cells deposited at the time of surgery. Rarely, a new primary cancer develops in residual breast tissue remaining in the skin flaps at the time of mastectomy (Fig. 77.2). In this circumstance, long-term disease-free survival may be possible with appropriate local therapy.

Recently gene expression studies have identified four major biological breast cancer subtypes: (1) luminal A (estrogen receptor [ER]/progesterone receptor [PR]–positive, HER2-negative, low/intermediate-grade), (2) luminal B (ER/PR-positive, HER2-negative, high-grade), (3) HER2-positive, and (4) triple-negative (ER-, PR-, HER2-negative) breast cancer.[12] These breast cancer subtypes are associated with prognosis, response to therapy, and recurrence. Some evidence suggests that molecular profiling can stratify patients with respect to LRR more precisely than traditional determinants that focus on initial tumor burden. In a recent meta-analysis of 5418 patients undergoing mastectomy, patients with triple-negative cancers had a much higher relative risk of LRR compared with patients with non–triple-negative cancers.[13] Patients with HER2-positive tumors treated with the anti-HER2 monoclonal antibody trastuzumab (Herceptin) have a lower risk of LRR. Interestingly, this fundamental difference in the risk of LRR based on hormone receptor and HER2 status remains present even in tumors less than 1 cm.[13] Time to recurrence is also correlated with breast cancer molecular subtype with LRR in triple-negative and HER2-overexpressing cancers occurring within the first 5 years of diagnosis, and cancers with ER expression having a more prolonged time to LRR.[9]

Gene expression profiling has also led to several commercially available predictive assays that may identify subgroups of patients who benefit from adjuvant endocrine treatment alone, avoiding the toxicity and risks associated with chemotherapy. For example, the 21-gene expression assay (Onco*type* DX-Genomic Health)[14] or a 70-gene expression assay (MammaPrint-Agendia)[15] can be used to predict the risk of recurrence in node-negative, ER/PR-positive tumors. However, the most recent updates of the NCCN breast cancer guidelines (Version 1. 2017) state that multigene assays may be used to help predict the risk of recurrence but have not been validated to predict the response to chemotherapy.[4] Therefore, future clinical trials should incorporate molecular profiling when examining local and systemic treatment strategies.

Patients with advanced stage at initial diagnosis develop LRR more rapidly than do patients who present with earlier stage disease. Since most chest wall recurrences after mastectomy are detected by physical examination, patients must understand the importance of careful evaluation of the chest wall and axilla and bring any self-detected changes to a provider's attention. Any suspicious lesion mandates a thorough evaluation and biopsy. If recurrence is confirmed histologically, the tissue must also be examined for hormone receptor status and HER2 overexpression because these factors may influence the type of systemic therapy. The majority of locoregional recurrences are isolated to the chest wall, whereas some chest wall recurrences also include a regional component in the lymphatic basin (i.e., axillary, internal mammary, and supraclavicular). Some patients present with concomitant distant disease at the time of locoregional recurrence, and therefore complete restaging is necessary at the time of locoregional recurrence.

The treatment of an isolated chest wall recurrence should include the combined modalities of surgery, radiation, and systemic therapy. Ideally, these patients should be presented at a multidisciplinary breast cancer conference for comprehensive multimodal treatment planning. Complete excision with negative margins and chest wall radiation, if possible, is the preferred local therapy. In some cases, skin grafting or flap coverage may be required to close the defect resulting from resection. Rarely, a formal chest wall resection and reconstruction may be required to achieve tumor-free margins. The functional consequences to the patient must be carefully considered before entertaining such radical resection. When surgical therapy is not possible or is too major, systemic therapy may be given first to downstage the recurrent disease before resection.

Regional recurrence refers to the return of breast cancer in the ipsilateral regional lymphatics that drain the breast (axillary, internal mammary, or supraclavicular nodes). The axilla is the primary site of drainage for most breast cancers and therefore the most common site for regional recurrence. Most axillary lymph node recurrences are discovered as a palpable mass on routine follow-up examination. Rarely, axillary recurrence presents with brachial plexopathy symptoms or lymphedema without palpable lymphadenopathy. Patients with these symptoms should undergo CT scan or MRI to determine whether the cause of these symptoms is radiation fibrosis or axillary recurrence.

The risk of axillary recurrence is also dependent on many factors including tumor size, the number and extent of nodal involvement, the type of axillary surgery and whether radiation was given. Historical data suggest the axillary recurrence rate is approximately 17% for patients with a clinically negative axilla who receive no axillary treatment, whereas the axillary recurrence rate after an axillary lymph node dissection (ALND) is 1% to 3%.[16] Axillary recurrences are divided into three main categories: isolated axillary recurrence, axillary recurrence concurrent with a breast recurrence, and axillary recurrence simultaneous with distant disease. Isolated axillary recurrences are rare, and they are more commonly a component of chest wall recurrence. The potential morbidity of an untreated axillary recurrence is significant, and symptoms resulting from brachial plexus involvement include intractable pain, motor and sensory impairment, decreased arm mobility, and lymphedema.[17] Unfortunately, the treatment of axillary recurrence after axillary dissection is often palliative. In one study involving 145 patients with LRR treated with combined modality therapy, the 5-year survival rate for those patients with an isolated axillary recurrence was 50%. In another study, de Boer and associates[18] identified 59 patients with an axillary recurrence treated with a combination of chemotherapy, hormonal therapy, radiotherapy, and surgery. Complete surgical eradication was achieved in only 34 patients (58%), and the overall 5-year actuarial survival rate was 39%.

Sentinel lymph node (SLN) biopsy has essentially replaced axillary dissection in the management of most patients with breast cancer. Several studies suggest axillary recurrence rates are low in women who undergo SLN biopsy with no axillary dissection.[19,20] The American College of Surgeons Oncology Group (ACOSOG) Z0011 trial prospectively examined the LRR and overall survival of patients with SLN metastases undergoing BCT randomized to undergo ALND after SLN biopsy or no further axillary specific treatment.[21,22] At a median follow-up of 9.25 years, there was no statistically significant difference between the two groups in local recurrence-free survival. The 10-year cumulative locoregional recurrence was 6.2% with ALND and 5.3% with SLND alone. Therefore SLND without ALND provides excellent local-regional control for selected patients with early-stage breast cancer treated with BCT and adjuvant systemic therapy.

The incidence of internal mammary (IM) node metastasis is primarily dependent on tumor size and location in the breast (i.e., inner vs. outer quadrants) and the histology of the axillary lymph nodes.[23,24] Routine removal of the IM nodes does not have an impact on LLR or overall survival for patients with breast cancer.[25–28] However, the emergence of SLN biopsy led to a renewed interest in the clinical significance of the IM lymph nodes. Lymphoscintigraphy studies demonstrate that between 18% and 35% of patients have breast lymph drainage to the IM nodes, but isolated IM nodal drainage occurs in only 5% to 8% of patients.[29–32] The incidence of IM nodal drainage is also dependent on the site of radionuclide injection with peritumoral injections have a much higher likelihood of IM nodal drainage than subareolar or subdermal injections.[33] The recent revision of the eighth edition of the American Joint Commission on Cancer (AJCC) tumor, lymph node, and metastasis (TNM) staging manual for breast cancer does not have any major changes to N classification.[34] A positive IM node found by SLN biopsy and not by imaging is given an N1 designation, whereas a positive IM node found by preoperative imaging (excluding lymphoscintigraphy) is given an N2 designation. If a positive IM node is found in conjunction with a positive axillary node, an N3 designation is given. The clinical outcome for patients with isolated positive IM nodes is similar to those patients with isolated positive axillary lymph nodes. In a multiinstitutional study by Krag and associates,[35] the IM node was the only positive sentinel node in 3% of patients. Most patients with tumor-containing IM nodes also have concurrent involved axillary nodes.[36] Patients with metastasis to the axillary and IM nodes have a worse overall survival than patients with metastasis to a single lymphatic basin.[37] In a study by Sugg and coworkers,[28] 65 of 72 (90.2%) patients with involved IM nodes also had accompanying metastasis to axillary nodes.

The status of the IM nodes does not alter the treatment recommendations for the vast majority of breast cancer patients.[38] However, a subset of patients with small breast tumors with tumor-free axillary nodes may have treatment recommendations altered by a positive IM node biopsy. In the study by Sugg and coworkers, less than 2% of patients fell into this specific subgroup.[28] The concealed location of the IM lymph nodes in the intercostal space behind the sternal border makes detection of recurrence by physical examination difficult. Internal mammary nodal recurrence presents as a parasternal mass, swelling, or pain. Isolated IM node recurrences are uncommon, and CT scan or MRI may detect them. In a study by van Rijk and colleagues,[39] only 1 of 803 patients with a sentinel node biopsy recurred solely in the IM lymph nodes. In a similar study by Cranenbroek and associates,[40] nearly 6000 breast cancer patients were followed for recurrence, and only 6 patients developed isolated IM nodal metastases.

Supraclavicular lymph node metastasis as a first site of recurrence of breast cancer is also relatively uncommon, occurring in less than 2% of patients after mastectomy.[41] The supraclavicular space is defined by the internal jugular vein, the omohyoid muscle and tendon, the clavicle, and the subclavian vein. In the eighth edition of the AJCC TNM staging system for breast cancer, supraclavicular nodal involvement was classified as N_3 disease.[34] This classification was changed based on data suggesting that patients with supraclavicular metastases who undergo aggressive multimodal treatment have similar outcomes to patients with stage III locally advanced disease. The majority of patients with metastasis to the supraclavicular lymph nodes also have positive axillary lymph nodes. Patients with more than four positive axillary lymph nodes have radiation fields expanded to include the supraclavicular region.[42] Isolated supraclavicular recurrence is unusual, and it is usually simultaneous with local or distant recurrence. A study by van der Ploeg and coworkers[43] followed 748 patients with breast cancer who had a tumor-free sentinel node and found that only 2 patients (0.25%) developed isolated supraclavicular nodal metastases. In a study by Chen and colleagues, the 5-year overall survival in patients treated for supraclavicular lymph node metastases was 33.6%.[44] Similar to other LRR, the treatment of supraclavicular nodal metastases requires a combination of surgery, chemotherapy, and radiation.

The heterogeneity of patients with LRR after mastectomy complicates the design of prospective randomized trials examining this group. Therefore, most studies examining locoregional recurrence after mastectomy have been small, single-institution, retrospective series.[8–10,45] In these retrospective studies, patients have received diverse adjuvant therapies, making any comparison between studies difficult. Historically, local recurrences after mastectomy have carried a poor prognosis, with an overall 5-year survival rate of approximately 35% from the time of recurrence after mastectomy. Because locoregional recurrence is an independent predictor of simultaneous or subsequent distant metastases, patients with locoregional recurrence after mastectomy require a metastatic workup. Multiple local recurrences that arise after a short disease-free interval may represent hematogenous spread of tumor cells to the mastectomy site. Therapy in this group of patients tends to be palliative, but efforts toward locoregional control even in patients with metastatic disease should be maximized.

In selected patients with isolated chest wall recurrences (i.e., ribs, intercostal musculature), radical chest wall resection may be indicated to provide palliation and long-term disease-free survival. Recently, Shen and colleagues from the University of Texas MD Anderson Cancer Center reported the largest contemporary experience for patients with isolated chest wall recurrences. They identified 76 patients, of whom 44 were treated surgically and 32 nonsurgically. The 5-year overall survival was approximately 40%, and complications related to radical surgical resection occurred in 25% of patients. Surgically treated patients were more likely to have triple-negative breast cancer at recurrence, and 95% received preoperative systemic therapy. For hormone receptor–positive recurrence, 5-year progression-free survival was significantly higher among surgical patients.[46] These data are similar to other historical[47-49] and contemporary series[50] of radical resection for isolated chest wall recurrences. Both Shah and Urban[47] and Toi and associates[48] reported a 5-year survival rate of 43% and 47%, respectively, using full-thickness chest wall resection for isolated chest wall recurrences. Some investigators have demonstrated a significant difference in survival rates after chest wall resection between patients with greater than a 2-year disease-free interval versus patients with less than a 2-year disease-free interval.[49] Large anterior chest wall resections involving multiple ribs and/or the sternum require stabilization with prosthetic material to prevent paradoxical chest wall motion. Soft tissue coverage may be achieved after chest wall resection through the use of pectoralis, latissimus, or rectus muscle flaps. In summary, patients with isolated chest wall recurrences requiring radical resection are best treated at centers with multidisciplinary teams experienced in performing complicated resections and sophisticated reconstructions.

Recent data support the hypothesis that reducing the rate of locoregional failure for breast cancer improves overall survival.[51] In addition, because locoregional recurrence after mastectomy is associated with such a poor outcome, prevention of locoregional recurrence at the time of initial treatment is an important goal. Postmastectomy radiation therapy has been shown to significantly decrease the rate of locoregional recurrence in high-risk patients.[52–54] Historically, indications for postmastectomy radiation have included four or more tumor-containing lymph nodes, tumor size 5 cm or greater, inadequate margins, or skin invasion. However, data from randomized prospective trials conducted in Canada and Europe demonstrate that postmastectomy radiation in women with one to three positive lymph nodes improves not only local control but also survival.[55–57] The magnitude of the survival benefit from postmastectomy radiation in these studies was similar to the survival benefit seen from adjuvant chemotherapy in previous studies. Questions remain, however, regarding the generalizability of these data because of differing surgical and radiotherapy techniques. In addition, the survival benefit specific to postmastectomy nodal irradiation needs to be further defined by ongoing studies. CT-assisted treatment planning may limit the cardiopulmonary toxicity associated with postmastectomy radiation. Finally, the optimal integration of postmastectomy radiation with systemic therapy and reconstructive surgery requires additional investigation.

If locoregional recurrence is often a manifestation of systemic disease and chemotherapy affects systemic relapse, then chemotherapy should also affect locoregional relapse. Despite this line of reasoning, the effect of chemotherapy on locoregional recurrence has been difficult to prove because of selection and other confounding factors. Patients with locally advanced disease who have a good response to preoperative chemotherapy have a significantly reduced risk of local recurrence. Because patients with locally advanced disease are also treated with mastectomy and chest wall radiation therapy, it is difficult to sort out the impact of chemotherapy alone on local recurrence. The optimal sequence and timing of adjuvant radiation and chemotherapy in the overall management of breast cancer remain to be defined. Although radiation oncologists emphasize the importance of adjuvant radiotherapy in achieving optimal local disease control, medical oncologists argue that potential gains in terms of local control may be at the expense of increased distant relapse. The integration of these modalities requires individual patient assessment to maximize locoregional control and minimize distant relapse. Delaying radiation therapy until after the completion of chemotherapy in patients at greatest risk for systemic relapse appears to have little negative effect on local control.

The recent publication of the results of the CALOR trial (Chemotherapy as Adjuvant for LOcally Recurrent Breast Cancer) validated the use of adjuvant chemotherapy for patients with completely resected isolated local or regional recurrence of breast cancer.[58] In this multicenter, randomized trial, 85 patients with histologically proven and completely excised LRR were randomized to investigator-determined, multidrug chemotherapy or no chemotherapy. Patients with ER-positive LRR received adjuvant endocrine therapy, radiation therapy was required for patients with microscopically involved surgical margins, and anti-HER2 therapy was optional. At a median follow-up of 4.9 years, adjuvant chemotherapy increased the risk of disease-free and overall survival by 41% and 59%, respectively. In this study, adjuvant chemotherapy was most effective in patients with ER-negative recurrences, whereas longer-term follow-up was required for patients with ER-positive recurrences.

In summary, local relapse after mastectomy should be treated aggressively for palliation and improved survival (Fig. 77.3). Prior staging procedures, local and systemic treatments significantly influence the multimodal management of these patients. For example, the use of SLN biopsy during initial therapy requires axillary restaging at the time of recurrence. In addition, with the increasing use of postmastectomy chest wall irradiation, many postmastectomy recurrences occur in previously irradiated patients. Patients with recurrence after mastectomy who have not previously received radiation should receive radiation therapy in addition to surgery to decrease the risk of another local relapse. The high risk of simultaneous or subsequent distant metastases in the setting of isolated locoregional recurrence after mastectomy

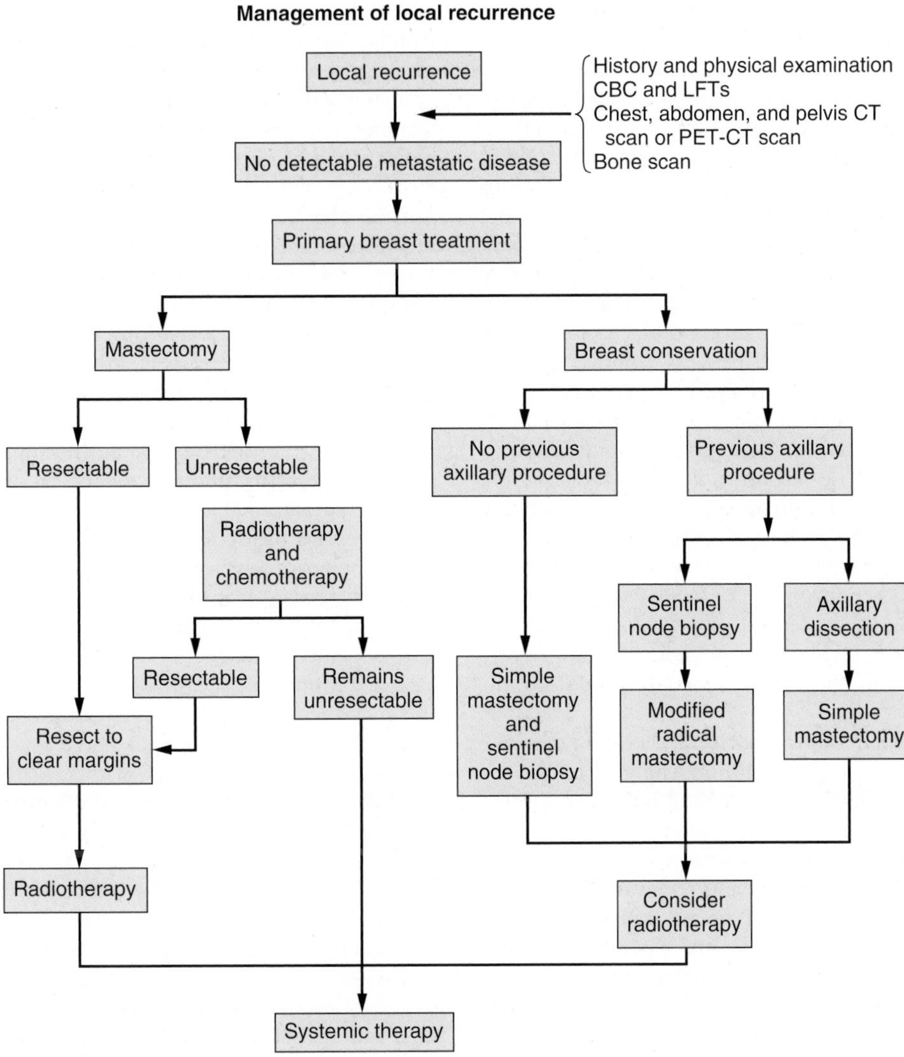

Management of local recurrence

• **Fig. 77.3** Algorithm for the management of local recurrence of breast cancer. *CBC,* Complete blood count; *CT,* computed tomography; *LFTs,* liver function tests.

justifies the administration of systemic chemotherapy. The type, dose, duration, and response to any initial systemic therapy must be carefully reviewed in the treatment planning of patients with LRR. Finally, the sequencing of treatment modalities should be determined through careful multidisciplinary evaluation of each patient.

Recurrence in the Reconstructed Breast

Over the past several decades, advancements in plastic surgery have revolutionized breast reconstruction for patients undergoing mastectomy. Overall, approximately 40% of patients having a mastectomy in the United States undergo breast reconstruction and the rate of immediate reconstruction appears to be increasing. Breast reconstruction can be performed with prosthetic implants, autologous tissue or a combination of both techniques. Approximately 60% of breast reconstructions involve the combination of tissue expanders and implants, whereas 16% are implants only, and 25% employ autologous tissue transfer.[59] In the past decade, there has been a trend toward higher proportions of breast conserving surgery–eligible patients undergoing mastectomy, breast reconstruction, and bilateral mastectomy. Kummerow and

colleagues recently studied more than 1.2 million adult women treated at centers accredited by the American Cancer Society and the American College of Surgeons Commission on Cancer to determine trends in mastectomy for early-stage breast cancer. They found that from 2003 to 2011, the use of mastectomy increased 34%, and from 1998 to 2011, rates of breast reconstruction increased from 11.6% to 36.4% and rates of bilateral mastectomy for unilateral disease increased from 1.9% to 11.2%.[60]

Despite these recent data, controversy continues regarding the optimal timing of reconstruction. Historically, an empirical 2-year interval between mastectomy and reconstruction was recommended based on the assumption that most local recurrences occurred during this critical time interval. That assumption has been challenged by studies demonstrating that chest wall recurrence rarely occurs in the first 2 years postoperatively in patients with stage I disease.[61–63] Other skeptics of immediate breast reconstruction were fearful that delaying postmastectomy radiation therapy after reconstruction might increase local recurrence rates and that the reconstructed breast might mask the signs and symptoms of a recurrence. Many studies have since shown no increase in the rate of locoregional recurrence or distant metastasis in patients who undergo immediate breast reconstruction and that the postradiation effects on the reconstructed breast are well tolerated and easily managed.[64]

Advocates of immediate breast reconstruction cite potential benefits such as improved self-image, superior cosmetic results, elimination of subsequent surgeries and anesthetic risks, and an overall decrease in cost as reasons not to delay reconstruction.[64] Along with these benefits, potential problems and conflicting reports must be considered regarding the timing of breast reconstruction. For instance, the complication rate after immediate breast reconstruction has been reported in one study to be as low as 15%, with only 9% of patients undergoing autologous tissue transfer requiring additional operative procedures.[65] On the other hand, one retrospective review of 50 patients reported a much higher complication rate of 50%, prolonged hospitalization, and a more frequent need for blood transfusions associated with immediate breast reconstruction.[66] Potentially, wound-healing complications after immediate reconstruction may also significantly delay the initiation of adjuvant therapies, but several studies have found this delay to be of no statistical significance with regard to recurrence or mortality rates. In a recent comprehensive meta-analysis of 31 studies involving 139,894 patients, Zhang and associates found no difference in disease-free/overall survival or LRR between women undergoing immediate breast reconstruction after mastectomy and those undergoing mastectomy alone.[67]

The surgical management of breast cancer has evolved over the past century from radical resections to more conservative procedures with equivalent oncologic outcomes and improved cosmesis. In 1991 Toth and Lappert[68] first reported the technique of a skin-sparing mastectomy (SSM) that included resection of the nipple-areola complex, the biopsy scar, and removal of the breast parenchyma with preservation of the breast skin envelope to improve cosmetic outcome. Since that initial report, SSMs with or without nipple preservation have gained acceptance as an option for immediate breast reconstruction because this technique preserves the skin envelope and thereby provides the best cosmetic outcome. In patients without locally advanced or large tumor burdens, an SSM with immediate reconstruction has proven to be an oncologically safe operation with no increased rate of locoregional recurrence.[68,69]

Investigators at the University of Alabama examined the factors associated with local recurrence in 173 patients with invasive breast cancer who underwent SSM and immediate breast reconstruction over an 11-year period.[45] The locoregional relapse rate after SSM and immediate breast reconstruction was 4.5%, and the median follow-up was 73 months. Factors associated with locoregional recurrence were tumor stage and differentiation. The authors concluded that locoregional relapse was an independent predictor of survival after SSM, but it is a function of tumor biology rather than surgical modality, supporting the practice of less aggressive oncologic resections. A more recent study from the University of Texas MD Anderson Cancer Center examined the rates of local, regional, and systemic recurrence, and survival in 1810 breast cancer patients who underwent SSM or conventional mastectomy (CM) The local, regional, and systemic recurrence rates did not differ significantly between the SSM and CM groups. After adjusting for clinical TNM stage and age, disease-free survival rates between the SSM and CM groups did not differ significantly.[70]

There are conflicting data regarding the effect of radiation therapy on reconstructed breasts. Some studies have demonstrated high rates of flap necrosis requiring additional surgery and impaired cosmetic outcomes related to capsular contractures in women that undergo prosthetic reconstruction,[71–73] whereas other investigations have shown no difference in outcome.

Liang and colleagues reviewed 191 patients receiving postmastectomy radiation therapy from 1997 to 2001 and found that 82 patients had a transverse rectus abdominis muscle (TRAM) flap reconstruction and 109 patients received no reconstruction. In general, the indications for postmastectomy radiation therapy included tumor size of more than 5-cm, involved lymph nodes, and positive or close surgical margins. The patients were followed for a median time of 40 months, and complications, recurrence, and distant metastasis were observed. The researchers found no statistical differences between patients who had received postmastectomy radiation, whether they underwent a TRAM reconstruction or had no reconstruction. They concluded that immediate TRAM flap reconstruction could be considered a feasible treatment for breast cancer patients requiring postmastectomy radiotherapy.[74]

Immediate breast reconstruction may also interfere with the design of postmastectomy radiation fields. The contour of the reconstructed breast may lead to an inability to cover all treatment targets within the radiation fields and increase the volume of normal tissue irradiated. Therefore radiation given to patients who have had immediate breast reconstruction may not be as effective and may increase the risk of radiation-related complications. As an intermediate compromise, some reconstructive surgeons have suggested a staged approach, with initial placement of a tissue expander followed by conversion to autogenous flap reconstruction after completion of all oncologic therapy.[75]

While the use of autologous fat transfer or lipofilling to correct volume/contour defects and asymmetry after breast cancer surgery has increased dramatically, oncological concerns remain. While most clinical studies fail to point out a significant increase in LRR in patients who receive fat transfer after breast cancer surgery, more prospective studies are needed with a sufficient follow-up time and analysis of critical factors involved.[76]

In summary, immediate breast reconstruction is best offered to patients who are anticipated to be at lower risk for postoperative adjuvant therapies. However, evidence is growing that such reconstruction is an acceptable component of the multimodality treatment for breast cancer with similar outcomes and complication risks. The coordination of the multidisciplinary breast team, including the medical, radiation, and surgical oncologist as well as the reconstructive surgeon, is essential to provide optimal care to the patient with breast cancer.

Recurrence After Breast Conserving Therapy

BCT consists of resection of the primary cancer with a margin of normal-appearing tissue followed by adjuvant radiation therapy. For many women with early invasive breast cancer (stage I, IIA, and IIb) BCT is preferable to total mastectomy. BCT produces equivalent survival rates while preserving the breast, thereby enhancing cosmesis and patient satisfaction. Several randomized prospective studies have identified that BCT results in disease-free and overall survival rates equal to mastectomy.[77,78] Although breast conservation rates vary geographically, approximately 60% of women with newly diagnosed breast cancer in the United States will be treated with BCT.[79] This translates to approximately 110,000 partial mastectomies yearly that have the corresponding potential to develop locoregional recurrence. Improvements in systemic therapy together with the increasing use of neoadjuvant chemotherapy, partial breast irradiation, and SLN biopsy may impact the incidence of ipsilateral breast tumor recurrence (IBTR) after BCT and also influence the subsequent management of these patients.

Early detection of local recurrence after BCT is important. IBTR after BCT is detected as a palpable mass on physical examination or as an abnormality on follow-up mammography. Because the lumpectomy scar and radiation fibrosis may produce radiographic distortion, a baseline mammogram is required approximately 6 months posttreatment. Patient migration may complicate the continuity of follow-up care; therefore an experienced examiner is required to follow the irradiated breast. Any change detected on breast examination should be thoroughly evaluated, and, similar to the situation with a mass in a previously untreated breast, the presence of a mass within a normal mammogram should still be investigated for the possibility of a local recurrence or second primary cancer. Rarely, local recurrences after breast conserving surgery can present with inflammatory breast changes such as warmth, erythema, and peau d'orange and are often misdiagnosed as postoperative infection (Figs. 77.4 and 77.5).

There are differences in the time to recurrence and clinical characteristics of locoregional failures after BCT versus mastectomy. Local recurrences tend to occur later after breast conserving surgery, particularly if patients initially received chemotherapy or hormonal therapy. Although most local recurrences after mastectomy are detected by physical examination, local recurrences after lumpectomy are detected solely by mammography approximately 40% to 75% of the time, by physical examination alone in 10% to 30%, a combination of mammography and physical examination in 10% to 25%, and by other imaging modalities such as MRI in 5% of cases.[80] In general, locoregional recurrence after mastectomy has a worse prognosis than recurrence after breast conserving surgery.

In the 20-year follow-up data from the National Surgical Adjuvant Breast and Bowel Project Protocol B-06, the local recurrence rate was 39% for lumpectomy alone but decreased to 14% when lumpectomy was followed by radiation therapy.[81] Women who received radiation had their recurrences later in their postoperative course, with 31% developing after 10 years. These data are in contrast to the lumpectomy-only group, with 73% of local recurrences occurring within the first 5 years after surgery. The Early Breast Cancer Trialists' Collaborative Group meta-analysis of 36 breast cancer trials, which involved more than 17,000 women, showed an isolated breast tumor recurrence rate of 6.7% after BCT.[82] It has been difficult in the past to determine a subgroup of women who might not require radiation after lumpectomy. Prospective data suggest that women 70 years of age or older with small ER-positive tumors treated with lumpectomy with tumor-free margins plus an aromatase inhibitor without breast irradiation experience a locoregional recurrence rate of less than 5%.[83]

The majority of local recurrences in the ipsilateral breast after breast conserving surgery occur in the proximity of the primary excision. It can be difficult, however, to distinguish a late local recurrence from a metachronous second primary breast cancer after breast conserving surgery. Local recurrences can develop in or near the lumpectomy site, whereas second primary cancers develop in other breast quadrants. If the initial tumor was an invasive cancer then the majority of subsequent recurrences will be invasive, however, if the initial tumor was noninvasive or in situ cancer, then 50% of the recurrences will be invasive and the remainder will be noninvasive recurrences. Genomic profiling may provide a useful tool to distinguish a recurrence of the original lesion from a metachronous tumor. Local recurrence after BCT may be a marker for aggressive disease at the time of lumpectomy. Predetermined tumor biology should not, however, lessen the importance of careful patient selection and meticulous surgical technique to minimize the risk of local recurrence.

The rate of local recurrence has been shown to be dependent on a multitude of factors, including patient age, tumor size, stage, grade, method of detection, and family history.[84] In patients receiving preoperative chemotherapy, poor clinical response and residual axillary disease after chemotherapy have been shown to be independent predictors of local recurrence.[85] Other factors that may favor recurrence after lumpectomy include positive surgical margins at the time of lumpectomy, lymphatic invasion, anaplasia, associated in situ disease in both the primary cancer and surrounding parenchyma, tumor necrosis, invasive lobular carcinoma, inadequate radiation dose, and a delay of radiation therapy after lumpectomy.[86] Because many of these variables are interrelated, it is difficult to establish independent prognostic factors for local recurrence. In addition, studies that attempt to identify risk factors for local recurrence after breast conservation suffer from patient heterogeneity and treatment selection biases.

Until recently, the lack of an accepted definition of a positive margin and a failure to standardize pathologic assessment of the surgical margin made it difficult to precisely define the impact of

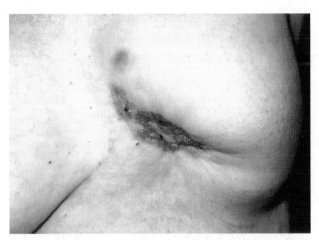

• **Fig. 77.4** Patient with local recurrence after lumpectomy.

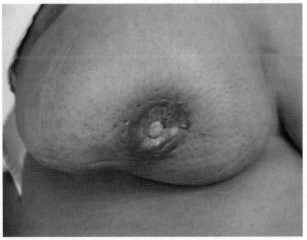

• **Fig. 77.5** Patient with inflammatory local recurrence after lumpectomy.

a positive margin on local recurrence after breast conserving surgery. However, a recently published report from a consensus panel convened by the Society of Surgical Oncology and the American Society for Radiation Oncology states that "no ink on tumor" should be the standard pathologic margin assessment for patients treated BCT. This recommendation was based on a meta-analysis of 33 studies, with a median follow-up of more than 6.5 years where a positive margin defined "as ink on tumor" was associated with a greater than twofold increase local recurrence. Interestingly, wider margins were not associated with a lower recurrence rate.[87] Regardless of the definition of a positive margin, it is important to ensure that all suspicious microcalcifications have been removed on postexcision mammography before administering radiation therapy. If margins are positive or close, factors to consider when contemplating reexcision include patient age, the extent of the close margin (focal vs. diffuse disease), differences between radiographic and pathologic tumor size, and the morbidity involved with a reexcision lumpectomy. Again, these patients should be presented at a multidisciplinary tumor board to determine the need for additional surgery. At the University of Florida, the use of frozen section of shaved margins performed during lumpectomy resulted in lower reexcision rates and a local recurrence rate of 2% for invasive cancer with a median follow-up of 5.6 years.[88]

The relationship between extensive intraductal component and local recurrence is also controversial. If one assumes that tumor cells spread locally via the breast ducts, then a greater intraductal component might increase the risk of local recurrence. Reports indicate that the presence of extensive intraductal component alone is not, however, a contraindication to breast conserving surgery, but its presence may require a more extensive resection to achieve uninvolved margins. In addition, the relationship between infiltrating lobular histologic subtype and risk of local recurrence after mastectomy is unsettled. Lobular cancers are diffusely infiltrative, with individual tumor cells being difficult to identify pathologically at the tumor margin. Mammography also tends to underestimate the pathologic extent of invasive lobular cancer. Therefore it may be more difficult to obtain histologic tumor-free surgical margins for patients with invasive lobular cancer. Several reports have documented, however, that select patients with invasive lobular cancer can be treated with lumpectomy, axillary dissection, and radiotherapy with an acceptable local recurrence rate.[89-91] Therefore lobular histology by itself is not a contraindication to breast conserving surgery. Breast MRI may be particularly helpful in selecting patients with invasive lobular cancer for breast conserving surgery.

Preoperative or neoadjuvant chemotherapy may be used to downsize tumors that are too large to meet the criteria for BCT. Before chemotherapy, the placement of a radiopaque clip using mammographic or ultrasound guidance should be employed to identify the tumor site should the patient experience a complete clinical response. Studies demonstrate that breast conservation rates are higher after preoperative chemotherapy but that there is no survival advantage over postoperative adjuvant chemotherapy. At the University of Texas MD Anderson Cancer Center, a prognostic index was developed to predict local recurrence for patients undergoing breast conservation surgery after neoadjuvant chemotherapy. This index included four factors previously found on retrospective analysis to be significant: clinical N2 or N3 disease, residual pathologic tumor size less than 2 cm, multifocal residual tumor, and lymphovascular invasion. Unfortunately, three of these factors are discovered postoperatively in

the pathology report and therefore are not useful in preoperative decision-making.[92]

The treatment of local recurrence after BCT is dependent on the type of recurrence as well as the initial treatment of the primary tumor. Salvage mastectomy is considered the standard treatment for local recurrence after breast conserving surgery. Doyle and associates found a 10-year survival of 64% for 93 patients with local recurrences after breast conserving surgery treated with salvage mastectomy for recurrent invasive cancer. Of these patients with recurrence, 44% were free of systemic metastasis.[93] These data compare favorably to series reported by other investigators in which local recurrence after breast conservation was treated with mastectomy.[94,95] Several series have recently demonstrated that repeat lumpectomy with salvage radiotherapy to the bed of the recurrent tumor is well tolerated and provides reasonable local control.[96,97] A study by Alpert and colleagues[98] compared outcomes of salvage mastectomy to salvage breast conserving surgery in 166 women who experienced an IBTR. With a median length of follow-up of 13.8 years, patients who underwent repeat lumpectomy had outcomes comparable to those who underwent salvage mastectomy but remain at continued risk for IBTR. Other studies have provided further support for repeat lumpectomy for patients with IBTR after breast conserving surgery. A recent analysis by Jobsen and colleagues[99] demonstrated a pattern in risk of IBTR over time, with 2 peaks, first at approximately 5 years and a second, much higher peak at approximately 12 years, especially for women ≤40 years old. They also noted that the absence of adjuvant systemic therapy and the presence of lymphovascular invasion were independent prognostic factors of IBTR for women ≤40 years old with tumor-free resection margins. For women >40 years old, the presence of lymphovascular invasion and the presence of lobular carcinoma in situ were independent risk factors. The introduction of newer local radiation techniques such as partial breast irradiation and combined hyperthermia and radiation may provide new opportunities in the local management of IBTR.

There are limited data addressing the role of chest wall or regional lymphatic radiation after mastectomy for postlumpectomy recurrence. Postmastectomy radiation may be considered for patient with recurrences greater than or equal to 5 cm in size, close or positive margins after mastectomy, or four or more positive nodes.

The management of the axilla in patients who experience local recurrence after breast conserving surgery depends on several factors, including whether the recurrence is noninvasive or invasive, previous axillary surgery, radiation therapy, and whether the status of the axillary nodes will change treatment decisions. If clinically suspicious axillary nodes are present, then ultrasound-guided fine-needle aspiration of the lymph nodes is appropriate. If the axilla is clinically negative, then repeat axillary staging with lymphatic mapping and sentinel lymph node biopsy is appropriate. Surgeons from the Memorial Sloan Kettering Cancer Center recently reported[100] reoperative SLN biopsies performed in patients suffering a local recurrence after BCT. They concluded that reoperative SLN biopsy is feasible in the setting of local recurrence after previous lumpectomy and radiation. In addition, lymphoscintigraphy identified more sites of nonaxillary drainage; the number may be greater in the setting of reoperative SLN biopsy than in the initial sentinel lymph node procedure.

Immediate reconstruction should be used with caution and is best offered to patients who are anticipated to be at lower risk for postoperative adjuvant therapies. If immediate breast reconstruction is considered after salvage mastectomy, autogenous tissue transfer (i.e., TRAM flap, deep inferior epigastric perforator [DIEP] flap) is preferable compared with placement of an implant in an irradiated field.

The value of systemic adjuvant therapy in patients suffering an IBTR after BCT remains unproven. If IBTR is in fact a marker for increased risk of distant failure and death, then one would assume that chemotherapy would be indicated. Unfortunately, few well-designed studies have addressed this important topic.

Breast Cancer in the Augmented Breast

Breast augmentation is the most commonly performed cosmetic procedure performed in the United States. More than 300,000 augmentation mammoplasties are performed annually, which represents an 800% increase since the 1990s.[101] Because approximately 1 in 8 women will develop breast cancer, it is obvious that many women with breast implants will also develop breast cancer. It has been estimated that approximately 45,000 women undergoing augmentation every year will develop breast cancer sometime during their lives. Therefore the safety of implants and concern over the ability to detect breast cancers and recurrences in augmented breasts has been at the forefront of discussion.

Although studies in the 1940s found that foreign bodies could produce sarcomas in rodents, subsequent studies have shown that the subcutaneous implantation of silicone does not give rise to malignancy, does not increase the risk of breast cancer, and may actually have a protective effect against breast cancer.[102] The earliest cohort study was conducted by Deapen and coworkers,[103,104] who reviewed the records from 35 plastic surgeons in the Los Angeles area in an effort to follow more than 3000 women with implants. Those women who developed breast cancer were identified through a population-based cancer registry (the Los Angeles County Cancer Surveillance Program). With a median follow-up of 14.6 years, the number of women with implants in whom breast cancer developed was significantly less than expected. In a Canadian study,[105] researchers who followed more than 11,000 women with implants found that at an average of 10.2 years after the procedure, breast cancer had developed in a lower than expected 41 women. A more recent meta-analysis provided additional confirmation of a lack of association between breast implants and cancer.[106] Therefore, based on a significant body of literature, women with implants can be assured that they are not at increased risk for developing breast cancer.

Although breast implants do not increase breast cancer risk, concerns have been raised that they might delay breast cancer detection. It is well established that silicone implants are radiopaque and obscure some portions of breast tissue from mammographic visualization. This can potentially increase the risk of late detection; however, studies have been conflicting because of methodological flaws and the small numbers of patients implants developing breast cancer thereby limiting statistical power.

Cahan and colleagues[107] retrospectively reviewed 22 patients in whom cancer developed after prosthetic augmentation mammaplasty and found no difference in mean tumor size, preinvasive cancer, or axillary lymph node involvement in these patients compared with more than 600 nonaugmented control breast cancer patients or Surveillance, Epidemiology, and End Results (SEER) data. Silverstein and associates[108] updated their results from a previous study to examine the data from 4082 women with breast cancer treated between 1981 and 2004; of these patients, 129 breast cancers occurred in augmented patients. The authors had previously found that the augmented group had an overall worse prognosis, no occult or in situ lesions, and a higher percentage of positive axillary lymph nodes compared with the nonaugmented group. In the updated study, they found that there was no significant difference in stage at diagnosis and prognosis between the two groups. Significantly more augmented patients present with palpable cancers, suggesting that implants may actually facilitate the detection of breast tumors on physical examination.

Silicone breast implants can affect mammography by making breast compression more difficult and by distorting adjacent breast architecture. During mammography, the average nonaugmented breast can be compressed to a thickness of 4.5 cm, whereas the average augmented breast can be compressed only to a thickness of 7 cm.[109] Capsular contracture and implant position also play a role in the reduction of mammographically visualized breast parenchyma.[110] These radiographic limitations have led to special mammographic techniques such as the Eklund push-back technique, along with the use of other breast imaging modalities such as ultrasound and MRI. Retromammary implants may compress the breast parenchyma against the skin, which may obscure the normal parenchymal pattern. Capsule contracture and scarring may present as an indistinct mass on physical examination and produce a false-positive mammogram. Silicone granulomas may also be palpably indistinguishable from carcinoma, and they may appear as a calcified mass on mammogram (Fig. 77.6). Although some clinicians initially feared that primary breast cancer in augmented women might present as an en cuirass mass surrounding the retromammary implant, reports to date demonstrate that these cancers tend to be mobile and not attached to the implant capsule. These issues are concerning, but the use of radiolucent implants and further advances in breast imaging techniques will undoubtedly improve our ability to detect breast cancer in women with augmented breasts.

Additional studies suggest that the stage of breast cancer at the time of detection is no different in women with augmented breasts.[111] Furthermore, some evidence suggests that women with breast implants practice breast self-examination more regularly, allowing for earlier detection of primary cancers or recurrences.[112] Some investigators argue that the implant provides a firmer surface against which to feel breast masses, making detection easier. In the Canadian study noted earlier, the stage at diagnosis and the 5- and 10-year survival rates of the 41 women with implants in whom breast cancer developed were not statistically different from those of the more than 13,000 control women with breast cancer from the Alberta Cancer Registry.[113] In addition, Deapen and coworkers[103,104] have provided similar results and showed the 5-year survival rate in their study was comparable to those established by the National Cancer Institute's SEER program. In 2001 Hoshaw and colleagues performed a comprehensive meta-analysis and estimated a relative risk for breast cancer in women who have had augmentation mammoplasty to be 0.72 (95% confidence interval 0.61–0.85). There has been a wide range of speculation to offer as an explanation, including enhanced immunologic response, tissue compression resulting in decreased blood supply, and even reduced temperature.

Lymph node status is the single most important prognostic indicator for women with breast cancer, and the advent of SLN biopsy has been a major breakthrough in breast cancer treatment and diagnosis. Successful sentinel node identification depends on intact lymphatic channels from the breast to the axilla. Implants placed via a transaxillary or periareolar incision are more likely to interfere with lymphatic flow to the axilla than are implants placed

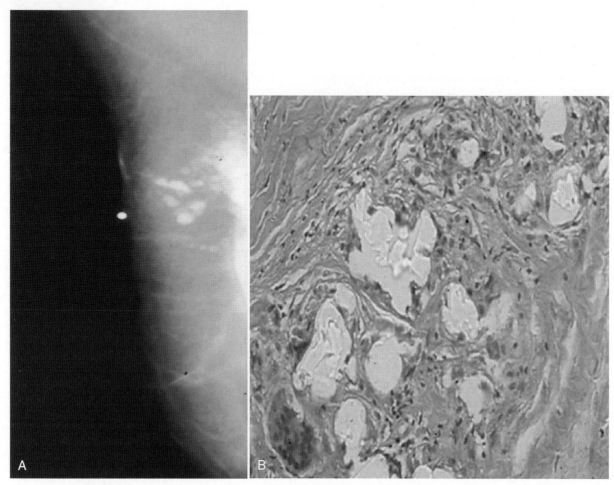

• **Fig. 77.6** (A) Mammogram demonstrating silicone granuloma. Radiopaque skin marker delineates palpable mass. (B) Histologic section through the silicone granuloma in A.

through an inframammary or transumbilical approach. Similarly, retroglandular implants would be more likely to disrupt the lymphatic drainage pathways of the breast and cause a false-negative SLN biopsy result than are submuscular implants. Although this theoretical concern is logical, further data regarding the use of SLN biopsy in women with implants are essential.

Another concern regarding breast augmentation is that it may interfere with the delivery of radiation therapy. Despite this concern, published studies demonstrate that radiation therapy can be effectively delivered to women with implants because neither saline nor silicone gel–filled implants attenuate x-rays.[114,115] Radiation therapy can cause capsular contracture and impair cosmetic outcome, but in 1994, Guenther and colleagues[116] showed that good to excellent cosmetic results were achieved in 85% of patients with implants who received radiation therapy. The location of the implant affected cosmetic outcome in that all patients who had retromuscular implants showed excellent results. Handel and others[71] studied 33 women who had undergone prosthetic augmentation and who had breast cancer treated with BCT. More than 50% developed capsular contracture on the irradiated side, and almost half of these patients required corrective surgery. These authors also expressed concern that capsular contracture may impair the ability of mammography to detect recurrences. Therefore long-term follow-up is required before BCT can be accepted as standard treatment for breast cancer that develops in women with breast implants.

In summary, the bulk of available evidence suggests that breast implants do not (1) cause breast or other cancers, (2) delay the detection of breast cancer, (3) result in advanced stage of breast cancers once detected, or (4) impair overall breast cancer survival rates.

Breast Cancer After Skin-Sparing Mastectomy

Genetic testing and the use of mathematical models have significantly improved our ability to more accurately define breast cancer risk. Preventive options for women at increased risk for breast cancer currently include increased screening efforts, chemoprevention, and risk-reduction surgery. Recent data confirming the efficacy of risk-reduction mastectomy for patients at high risk for breast cancer has led to a renewed interest in this risk-reduction strategy.[117] There remains, however, no clear consensus on the indications for risk-reduction mastectomy.

The breast procedures that reduce breast cancer risk include total mastectomy, skin-sparing mastectomy, and subcutaneous mastectomy. Total mastectomy refers to removal of the skin overlying the breast: the breast tissue and the nipple-areola complex. SSM includes resection of the nipple-areola complex, the biopsy scar, and removal of the breast parenchyma. Subcutaneous mastectomy involves removal of most of the breast tissue with preservation of the nipple-areola complex. Subcutaneous mastectomy can be performed as an open procedure through an incision in the inframammary crease or via a minimally invasive or endoscopic approach. Although subcutaneous mastectomy preserves nipple sensitivity and is cosmetically superior to total or SSM, preservation of the nipple-areola complex necessitates leaving retroareolar breast tissue at theoretical risk for subsequent cancer. In addition, there may be significant variability in the technique of subcutaneous mastectomy related to the aggressiveness in removing as much breast tissue as possible. This may be particularly important in patients with inherited breast cancer mutations, such as *BRCA1* or *BRCA2*, because these germline mutations are present in every cell.[118] It also remains to be proved whether the reduction in breast cancer risk is proportional to the amount of breast tissue removed. There are numerous reports of breast cancer developing in women after subcutaneous mastectomy.[119] Furthermore, cancers occurring after subcutaneous mastectomy are often detected at an advanced stage, perhaps a result of a false sense of security in women who believed that their risk of developing breast cancer had been eliminated. Subcutaneous mastectomy was historically performed by plastic surgeons for risk reduction. In the past decade, breast surgeons have begun performing nipple sparing mastectomy (NSM) for patients with early-stage breast cancer. Single institutional series have demonstrated acceptable outcomes with short follow-up. To provide multi-institutional data with longer follow-up, the American Society of Breast Surgeons has begun an NSM registry to follow these patients.[119a]

In a frequently quoted, retrospective cohort analysis from the Mayo Clinic,[117] 639 women with a family history of breast cancer underwent bilateral prophylactic mastectomies from 1960 to 1993. In the 639 women in this study, 575 had subcutaneous procedures and 64 had total mastectomies. This study demonstrated a reduction of approximately 90% in the risk of breast cancer. All seven women in whom breast cancer subsequently developed had previously undergone bilateral subcutaneous mastectomies, whereas no breast cancers were detected in the women who underwent total mastectomy. The difference in risk reduction between subcutaneous and total mastectomy in this study was not statistically significant, however, because of the small number of events (only seven cancers). A direct comparison of subcutaneous versus total mastectomy has not been performed, and case reports have documented the occurrence of breast cancer after either total mastectomy. Given the available evidence, however, subcutaneous mastectomy should be considered suboptimal as a risk-reduction strategy for breast cancer. Although no operation ensures the removal of all breast tissue, the best method of complete extirpation of all breast tissue is via total mastectomy. Some authors have even recommended frozen section analysis to ensure removal of all breast tissue during simple mastectomy.[120]

Recent studies demonstrate a considerable interest for prophylactic mastectomy among high-risk women and their physicians,[121] but current practice patterns show that prophylactic mastectomy is not being performed on a large scale in certain geographic areas.[122] The benefits of prophylactic mastectomy over alternative strategies (surveillance and chemoprevention) remain to be proved and must be weighed against the irreversibility and psychosocial sequelae of the procedure. In young, high-risk women with mammographically dense breasts, prophylactic mastectomy may be preferable to lifelong surveillance with physical examination and mammography or chemoprevention.[123] The decision to perform prophylactic mastectomy must be collaborative and multidisciplinary, with active patient participation.

Further research is required to answer the many remaining questions regarding risk-reduction surgery.

Cancer Risk in the Contralateral Breast

Although the risk of developing breast cancer in the contralateral breast has been discussed in many chapters in this text, a brief summary is provided here. Environmental, genetic, morphologic, and biochemical factors implicated in breast carcinogenesis affect each breast equally. Because the number of women who have been treated for breast cancer is increasing, more and more women are at risk for developing breast cancer in the opposite breast. The risk of contralateral breast cancer depends on the duration of follow-up and the method of detection. When a combination of physical examination and mammography is used for follow-up, a contralateral primary breast cancer develops in 4% to 15% of surviving breast cancer patients, a risk two to six times higher than that for the general population. This risk remains relatively constant throughout the lifetime of the patient.[124] In a study of 292 women who developed contralateral breast cancer, Horn and colleagues[125] found that factors associated with an increased risk in the opposite breast were lobular histology, a positive progesterone assay in the initial primary cancer, and AB blood type. Interestingly, adjuvant chemotherapy significantly lowered the risk. However, the influence of adjuvant chemotherapy on the development of contralateral breast cancer must be interpreted with caution, because patients receiving chemotherapy are more likely to have more advanced disease in the initially affected breast, and their death from recurrent disease removes the risk of developing contralateral breast cancer. In addition, patients with metastatic disease may not be intensively evaluated for contralateral breast cancer. There is also strong evidence to indicate that adjuvant hormonal therapy significantly reduces the risk of contralateral breast cancer. The Early Breast Cancer Trialists' Group meta-analysis reported that 5 years of adjuvant tamoxifen was associated with a 47% reduction in the risk of contralateral breast cancer. In this overview, there was no benefit from adjuvant tamoxifen on contralateral breast cancer risk in women whose first breast cancer was ER negative.

The risk of metachronous contralateral breast cancer is even higher for patients with a family history of breast cancer. Fowble and associates at the Fox Chase Cancer Center found the 10-year cumulative incidence of contralateral breast cancer was 7% in 1253 women treated with conservative surgery and radiation. In this study, young age and positive family history were significantly associated with an increased cumulative risk of contralateral breast cancer.[126]

Women found to be *BRCA1* and *BRCA2* carriers are at high risk for early-onset breast cancer and bilateral disease. One study[127] found the risk of contralateral breast cancer to be as high as 5.2% per year or 20% to 31% at 5 years in women identified to be carriers of *BRCA1* or *BRCA2* mutations. Because normal *BRCA1* and *BRCA2* function may be associated with DNA repair, radiation-induced breast cancer is a possibility in carriers of *BRCA1* and *BRCA2* treated with breast conservation and radiation. Haffty and others[127] from Yale University recently reported a 42% rate of contralateral breast cancer at 12 years for women with deleterious mutations in *BRCA1* and *BRCA2* treated with breast conserving surgery followed by radiotherapy. None of these women had received tamoxifen or had undergone prophylactic oophorectomy. The risk of contralateral breast cancers in this group was not higher than the risk of contralateral cancers in carriers of *BRCA1* and *BRCA2* who underwent mastectomy without radiotherapy. Although longer follow-up is necessary, these data suggest that there is no increased risk of radiation-induced breast cancers in *BRCA1* and *BRCA2* carriers. The effect of tamoxifen or oophorectomy on the rate of ipsilateral or contralateral events in *BRCA1* and *BRCA2* carriers choosing conservative surgery and radiotherapy needs further study.

A plan for follow-up management of the contralateral breast in patients with in situ breast cancer is difficult to obtain from reports in the literature. Data on bilaterality often include patients with a previous or synchronous breast cancer and greatly overestimate the actual risk of cancer developing in a normal contralateral breast. For example, in one of the earliest reports of a large series of patients with minimal breast cancer followed for up to 20 years,[128] 59% of patients with lobular carcinoma in situ (LCIS) had bilateral breast cancer, yet none of the patients with a normal contralateral breast at risk developed subsequent breast cancer; 5% of patients with intraductal carcinoma in situ and the opposite breast at risk developed a subsequent invasive breast cancer. Likewise, in a report by Baker and Kuhajda,[129] 6% of patients who initially had invasive lobular carcinoma developed a subsequent cancer in the contralateral breast. LCIS was not a reliable marker for predicting the presence of either synchronous or metachronous invasive cancer in the opposite breast. The combination of both invasive lobular carcinoma and LCIS, however, may portend a significant increase in the expected incidence of contralateral breast cancer.[130] The actual incidence of invasive carcinoma occurring in either breast at the time of diagnosis of LCIS is about 5%.

Estimates of bilateral multicentricity of LCIS range from 25% to 69%, and subsequent development of breast cancer in either breast ranges from 4% to 67%.[131] More than half of these invasive lesions develop more than 15 years after the LCIS is diagnosed.[132] Therefore in those clinical series in which a large percentage of patients have LCIS, only a few breast cancers ever develop.

The treatment for the contralateral breast in a patient with LCIS would seem to be careful surveillance throughout the remainder of the patient's life. In fact, most investigators now recommend only close follow-up for the ipsilateral breast. Because both breasts are at equal risk for the development of invasive cancer, the treatment for both breasts should be the same. Thus if total mastectomy is the selected surgical therapy, it should be applied bilaterally.

Studies on the bilaterality of intraductal carcinoma are inconclusive. Reports indicate an incidence as high as 26%, yet long-term follow-up data on the opposite breast yield an actual breast cancer incidence of only 4% to 7%.[133] Consequently, most investigators recommend close follow-up with physical examination and mammography, just as is done for invasive breast cancer.

For some women with breast cancer, contralateral prophylactic mastectomy may be the preferred strategy. McDonnell and coworkers[134] followed a cohort of 745 women with both a personal and a family history of breast cancer who had a contralateral mastectomy at the Mayo Clinic between 1960 and 1993. Eight women developed a contralateral new primary breast cancer despite prophylactic mastectomy. Their results support a 90% reduction in contralateral breast cancer risk with prophylactic mastectomy. Using SEER data, Tuttle and colleagues have recently reported that the rate of contralateral prophylactic mastectomy for breast cancer had more than doubled from 1998 to 2003.[135] In this study the rate of prophylactic mastectomy was particularly high in young women and those patients with lobular histology.

Frequently, however, the perceived risk of cancer in the contralateral breast is exaggerated, and in many patients the risk of systemic metastases from the original breast cancer exceeds the risk of contralateral breast cancer. In addition, complications resulting from contralateral mastectomy may delay chemotherapy or radiation therapy after surgery. Prophylactic simple mastectomy for the contralateral breast should probably be reserved for patients who have multiple associated risk factors, such as florid LCIS and invasive lobular carcinoma in the ipsilateral breast, multiple first-degree relatives with breast cancer, *BRCA1* or *BRCA2* mutation carriers, or a contralateral breast that is difficult to follow clinically because of the density and nodularity of the breast tissue.

Selected References

1. Runowicz CD, Leach CR, Henry NL, et al. American Cancer Society/American Society of Clinical Oncology Breast Cancer Survivorship Care Guideline. *CA Cancer J Clin*. 2016;66:43-73.
22. Giuliano AE, Ballman K, McCall L, et al. Locoregional recurrence after sentinel lymph node dissection with or without axillary dissection in patients with sentinel lymph node metastases: long-term follow-up from the American College of Surgeons Oncology Group (Alliance) ACOSOG Z0011 randomized trial. *Ann Surg*. 2016;264:413-420.
52. Early Breast Cancer Trialists' Collaborative Group (EBCTCG), Darby S, McGale P, et al. Effect of radiotherapy after breast-conserving surgery on 10-year recurrence and 15-year breast cancer death: meta-analysis of individual patient data for 10,801 women in 17 randomised trials. *Lancet*. 2011;378:1707-1716. doi:10.1016/S0140-6736(11)61629-2.
58. Aebi S, Gelber S, Anderson SJ, et al. Chemotherapy for isolated locoregional recurrence of breast cancer (CALOR): a randomised trial. *Lancet Oncol*. 2014;15:156-163.

A full reference list is available online at ExpertConsult.com.

78

Carcinoma of the Breast in Pregnancy and Lactation

MARY L. GEMIGNANI AND DAMIAN MCCARTAN

Pregnancy-associated breast cancer is defined as the diagnosis of breast cancer during the gestational period, within 1 year of pregnancy or anytime during lactation.[1] It is the second most common malignancy occurring in pregnancy, after carcinoma of the cervix. The incidence of pregnancy-associated breast cancer is 1.3 to 3.7 per 10,000 deliveries.[2,3] The estimated probability of developing breast cancer within the next 10 years is 1 in 225 for a woman 30 years of age, increasing sharply to 1 in 69 for a woman 40 years of age.[4] The median age at diagnosis of breast cancer in pregnancy is 33 years.[5]

Epidemiologic studies have shown that pregnancy is associated with a reduced lifetime risk of developing breast cancer. However, this protective effect is neither immediate nor constant. These studies have shown that the greatest degree of protection is conferred by pregnancy at a younger age.[6] As women delay childbearing for a variety of personal and professional reasons, the possibility of encountering the diagnosis of breast cancer occurring during pregnancy increases. A transient increase in breast cancer risk seen after pregnancy is more conspicuous in women with late age at first birth.[7]

The diagnosis and treatment of breast cancer during pregnancy encompasses many diagnostic and therapeutic dilemmas, and the input from a multidisciplinary team is of paramount importance for therapeutic planning during this difficult time.

Prognosis and Historical Perspective

Reports of outcomes after treatment for pregnancy-associated breast cancer from the early decades of the 20th century were dismal. Five-year survival rates of 17% were reported by Kilgore and Bloodgood in 1929,[8] and of 15% by Harrington and coworkers in 1937.[9]

Over the next several decades, published studies began reporting variations in outcomes stratified by differences in nodal status at presentation. More than 70% of patients with pregnancy-associated breast cancer in these studies presented with axillary nodal metastases. The prognosis associated with pregnancy-associated breast cancer was worse overall, both in node-positive and node-negative patients.[10–12]

Studies in the 1980s and 1990s were mostly single institution and retrospective that collected patients over several decades.[13–15] These case-control studies compared pregnancy-associated breast cancer cases with nonpregnant controls. When these patients were grouped by stage, there was no statistical difference identified between pregnant and nonpregnant patients.[1] Petrek and colleagues compared 56 stage I–III pregnancy-associated breast cancers with nonpregnant controls treated between 1960 and 1980. Sixty-one percent of the patients with pregnancy-associated breast cancer had positive nodes, compared with 38% of the nonpregnant controls. Overall, 5-year survival for node-negative patients was identical for both groups at 82%. All patients had a radical or modified radical mastectomy. For node-positive patients, the 5-year overall survival of 47% for pregnancy-associated breast cancer was not statistically inferior to the 59% seen in nonpregnant patients. A delay in diagnosis because of pregnancy is thought to play an important factor in the late stage at presentation of many of these patients, thus accounting for the worse prognosis.

However, both meta-analyses and data from national cancer registries point toward a poorer prognosis for patients with pregnancy-associated breast cancer. A 2012 meta-analysis incorporated studies from 1969 to 2009 and—as expected given the disparate definitions, matching criteria, and outcome reports—significant heterogeneity was noted in the pooled analyses. After a series of adjustments, an estimated hazard ratio of 1.4 was calculated for the negative effect of pregnancy on overall survival. On subgroup analysis, patients diagnosed in the postpartum period had a clearer trend toward worse overall survival.[16] Reports from US and Swedish cancer studies bolster this finding, as both identified that patients with a diagnosis of breast cancer within 1 year of giving birth had a lower overall survival.[17,18] Neither of these studies adjusted for differences in tumor subtypes.

More recent studies, including a large international registry of German and Belgian patients, provide some grounds for optimism. With contemporary multimodality therapy, when adjusted for stage, patients with pregnancy-associated breast cancer did not have a worse prognosis than age- and stage-matched nonpregnant patients. This cohort of 311 patients reported a 5-year overall survival of 78%.[19]

Diagnostic Evaluation and Staging During Pregnancy

During pregnancy, the breasts undergo physiologic hypertrophy and proliferative changes in response to high levels of estrogen and progesterone that stimulate and prepare the breast for lactation. These changes mean that physical examination of the breasts becomes gradually more difficult as the pregnancy progresses due to increases in both breast mass and density.[20] These changes continue into the postpartum period in women who are breastfeeding. The ideal time for a thorough examination of the breasts is during the first trimester when the breasts have undergone the least change. Any abnormality encountered should be promptly evaluated at this time.

Delays in diagnosis are thought to play a significant role in pregnancy-associated breast cancers, and the often late stage at diagnosis that is encountered. A multiinstitutional study of 192 patients in Japan found that the average time from symptom development to diagnosis was just over 6 months, 1 month longer than in a series of age-matched controls.[13] In keeping with other reports, patients with pregnancy-associated breast cancer had larger primary tumors and a higher burden of axillary nodal disease compared with the nonpregnant patients. These characteristics all contributed to an overall worse prognosis in patients diagnosed during pregnancy or lactation. Contemporary reports continue to point to delays in presentation as a common occurrence in pregnancy-associated breast cancer.[21] These delays can be on the part of the patient not bringing a palpable mass to medical attention or on the part of the physician due to a reluctance to proceed with imaging and biopsy during pregnancy for fear of complications.

Imaging Studies During Pregnancy

The index of suspicion for cancer must be high for women who present with a breast mass during the gestational or lactational period. The majority of these breast lumps will prove benign. The differential diagnoses encompass a spectrum of benign and lactating entities, including, but not limited to, fibroadenoma, lactating adenoma, galactocele, cystic disease, lobular hyperplasia, breast abscess, and lipoma.

Mammograms are typically not obtained during pregnancy despite the fact that the average glandular dose to the breast for a two-view mammogram of 0.4 HmSv equates to a negligible radiation exposure to the developing fetus.[22] The radiation exposure to the fetus can be further reduced by up to 50% by abdominal lead shielding.[23] However, the increased parenchymal density of the breasts that accompanies the pregnant state reduces the sensitivity of mammography.[24] Mammography may be useful in determining the extent of disease including multifocality and multicentricity and should be considered in any patient with a highly suspicious mass seen on ultrasound or when a diagnosis of pregnancy-associated breast cancer has been made. Lactating patients should be encouraged to nurse or express immediately before mammography to decrease parenchymal density related to retained milk products.[25] Ultrasound is more sensitive than mammography in evaluation of a solid mass in pregnancy or lactation and should be the first modality used in evaluating a pregnant or lactating patient who presents with a breast mass.[26,27] Ultrasound in this setting has a high reported negative predictive value for exclusion of malignancy[26] and also allows for prompt biopsy of any suspicious lesions identified.

Although magnetic resonance imaging (MRI) has been used in the obstetric patient both for fetal imaging and for evaluation of maternal conditions such as appendicitis,[28] its reported use for breast evaluation in pregnancy is limited. Breast MRI requires contrast-enhanced imaging with gadolinium. The use of gadolinium contrast agents is avoided during pregnancy because of the potentially long half-life in the fetus, its association with teratogenicity in animal studies, and the paucity of data on its safety in pregnancy. Its use may be considered in women who are postpartum, even if lactating, at the time of diagnosis if it is felt that additional information beyond that provided by mammography and ultrasound is required. The American College of Radiology guidelines do not require that patients discontinue breastfeeding. Images obtained on MRI may be difficult to interpret during the pregnant or lactating state. Increased enhancement from hypervascularity may pose a challenge when trying to differentiate lactational changes from suspicious findings.[29]

Once the diagnosis of breast cancer has been made, many routine systemic staging studies use ionizing radiation. The most sensitive period for radiation-associated malformations is in the first 8 weeks of the pregnancy (organogenesis). As noted earlier, pregnancy-associated breast cancer tends to present at a later stage, but the indications for systemic staging should follow National Comprehensive Cancer Network guidelines as for nonpregnant patients. Patients with clinical stage III (cT3N1 or any ≥ N2) or stage IV disease or symptoms suggestive of distant metastases should prompt a systemic evaluation. The risks and benefits of obtaining these imaging examinations during pregnancy need to be carefully evaluated.

Chest x-rays are considered to be safe during pregnancy because the dose with abdominal lead shielding is relatively low. Chest or abdominal computed tomography (CT) scans are generally avoided because of the large cumulative radiation dose. Although less sensitive than MRI or CT, ultrasound is a safe first-choice modality for liver imaging in the pregnant patient. If brain metastases are suspected, MRI is the most sensitive imaging technique. Bone remains the most common site of breast cancer metastases. Alkaline phosphatase levels increase during normal pregnancy and cannot be used as an indicator of bone metastases. Bone scintigraphy is reported as safe during pregnancy and is associated with a 0.02-cGy dose of radiation exposure to the fetus. Modifications of the technique, including adequate maternal hydration, that result in a lower fetal radiation exposure have been described.[30] The use of positron emission tomography (PET) in pregnancy is very limited. Estimates of fetal radiation dose from ^{18}F fluorodeoxyglucose (^{18}F-FDG) have been provided, but there is no evidence to support its use. The amounts of ^{18}F-FDG excreted in breast milk after a PET scan are low, and guidelines would suggest the only adjustments that a nursing mother should make after a PET scan are to avoid close contact with the infant for up to 12 hours.

Breast Biopsy During Pregnancy

Any breast mass during pregnancy that is suspicious on either clinical or ultrasound evaluation requires biopsy. Core biopsy is the most accurate means of establishing a diagnosis. These biopsies can be performed under local anesthesia with subcutaneous lidocaine, and patients should be reassured that this has no known harmful fetal effects. The formation of a milk fistula after core needle biopsy has been reported, but the literature contains only sporadic case reports, and it would therefore appear that the overall rate of milk fistula formation is low. The risk is higher with an open surgical biopsy and for more centrally placed lesions.[31,32]

Fine-needle aspiration (FNA) can be used for the diagnostic evaluation of a breast mass in pregnancy. However, reports have highlighted the difficulties of interpreting the cytologic findings.[33,34] There are potential pitfalls in the cytologic interpretation of even physiologic changes in the breast. Because of the increased cellularity and frequent mitosis that can be seen accompanying pregnancy, it is important to have an experienced cytopathologist who is familiar with the cytologic appearances of physiologic changes of breast in pregnancy. One study of 214 aspirates from pregnant or lactating women noted that none of the patients with a benign biopsy developed cancer in the follow-up period of 1.5 to 2 years. All cases of cancer on cytology were confirmed on surgical excision.[33,35]

In the postpartum period, risks of milk fistula formation, bleeding, and infection can be minimized by the cessation of breastfeeding before the biopsy, prophylactic antibiotics, and ensuring adequate hemostasis.[36]

Pathologic Findings

As in nonpregnant women, the majority of pregnancy-associated breast cancers are invasive ductal carcinomas. Clinically, women with pregnancy-associated breast cancer are more likely to have larger tumors and present with axillary nodal metastasis.[13,37] Pregnancy-associated breast cancers exhibit a range of pathologic features that underline their propensity for a more aggressive course. These tumors are frequently of high nuclear grade (approximately 50%) and exhibit lymphovascular invasion (LVI); more than 60%).[38]

The receptor profile also differs with a shift toward tumors that are estrogen and progesterone receptor negative. It should be acknowledged that breast cancers in younger women who are not pregnant also exhibit many of these unfavorable pathologic characteristics such as high grade and hormone receptor negativity. Two retrospective, national case-control studies from France and Japan have included age-matched controls. The cumulative rate of estrogen receptor negative tumors in the pregnancy-associated breast cancer patients was 55% compared with 40% in the nonpregnant patients.[13,22,37] Both studies also found consistently lower rates of progesterone receptor positivity in pregnancy-associated breast cancer. Only a handful of studies have examined human epidermal growth factor receptor 2 (HER2) positivity in women with pregnancy-associated breast cancer. The average rate of HER2 positivity in eight recent reports with a total of 275 patients with pregnancy-associated breast cancer is 31%.[39–46] This is almost identical to the 32% HER2 positivity reported in a 2013 International Registry study that included 311 pregnant patients.[19] These studies have not included age-matched controls, so no adequate conclusions can be reached regarding whether HER2 positivity is more prevalent in pregnancy-associated breast cancer. Most recent case series have not found an increase in the rate of inflammatory breast cancer in pregnant or lactating patients.

A full family history is an important part of assessment for these patients. Given the aforementioned tendency toward estrogen receptor–negative disease in a young age group, genetic counseling should certainly be offered to patients with a pregnancy-associated breast cancer. The probability of detecting a germline mutation in a young patient with a triple-negative breast cancer is approximately 20%.[47]

Treatment

Surgery

Historically, mastectomy was considered the standard surgical procedure for the local management of pregnant patients with breast cancer. However, mastectomy is not mandatory, and when appropriate patient and tumor factors are taken into consideration, breast-conserving therapy may be appropriate if lumpectomy is performed in the third trimester and radiotherapy is given postpartum. A delay in postoperative radiotherapy has been associated with increases in local recurrence in nonpregnant patients, and thus lumpectomy in the first or early second trimester with long delays to radiotherapy are often not advised.[48] Recent commentary has suggested that because the majority of these patients will receive chemotherapy—some in the neoadjuvant setting—incorporation of this time period may allow consideration of breast conservation for patients in the second trimester without a delay to radiotherapy if the patient is being treated with neoadjuvant chemotherapy. In patients in the third trimester or those who are postpartum, this potential delay to radiotherapy is not an issue. Therefore a breast-conserving operation is an option if the same factors that determine suitability for breast-conserving therapy in nonpregnant patients apply, such as tumor size, tumor location, and tumor-to-breast–size ratio as well as adjuvant therapy. A number of small studies support the safety and feasibility of breast conservation in terms of local control.[49–51]

General anesthesia during pregnancy is of concern because of the physiologic changes that accompany pregnancy in the later stages of pregnancy. General anesthesia has not been reported to increase the risk of congenital anomalies in published reports. Spontaneous abortion has been reported in women undergoing surgery in the first and early second trimesters of pregnancy.[52,53] All general anesthetic drugs cross the placenta. The anesthetic management of pregnant patients requires a balanced consideration of both maternal and fetal physiology, as well as pharmacology. Avoidance of maternal hypoxia or hypotension are key tenets in ensuring a favorable outcome for both mother and fetus.[54]

In nonpregnant patients, sentinel lymph node biopsy (SLNB) is the gold standard axillary staging procedure. Recent studies suggest SLNB can be performed safely for both the mother and the fetus. The use of isosulfan blue dye in pregnancy (a US Food and Drug Administration category C drug) as a mapping agent is not recommended because of the low but potentially very harmful underlying risk of a maternal anaphylactic reaction as well as very limited data on potential teratogenic effects of isosulfan blue.

Although the radiocolloids used for sentinel node mapping do emit a radiation dose, the administration of the agent is locoregional as opposed to systemic. Studies have demonstrated that the doses absorbed by the fetus are less than the National Council on Radiation Protection and Measurements limit for a pregnant woman.[55,56] It is advisable to inject the technetium radiocolloid on the morning of surgery to minimize the exposure to radiation. A number of studies have demonstrated accurate and safe lymphatic mapping in pregnant patients with the use of 99m-Tc, including the description of a low-dose technique for lymphoscintigraphy.[57–60]

In patients who are deemed node positive preoperatively, on the basis of either clinical assessment or ultrasound, an axillary lymph node dissection should be performed.

To date, only one report has documented short-term outcome with immediate breast reconstruction after mastectomy in pregnancy-associated breast cancer. No major surgical complications were noted in 13 patients who underwent a two-stage procedure with tissue expander insertion. In all cases, the final implant exchange took place after delivery and completion of adjuvant chemotherapy and radiotherapy.[61] The authors concluded that it was best to allow a longer time (median 15 months) from insertion to final implant exchange. In that manner, it enabled the size and shape of the contralateral breast to stabilize, and 7 of the 13 patients underwent a contralateral symmetrizing procedure at the time of implant exchange.

Systemic Chemotherapy

Many of the agents used for the systemic treatment of breast cancer in nonpregnant women are safe to administer after the first trimester of pregnancy. Systemic chemotherapy for primary breast cancer is typically recommended in premenopausal women with node-positive breast cancer or when the primary tumor size is larger than 1 cm. Therefore a large number of women with pregnancy-associated breast cancer would qualify for adjuvant systemic therapy. The decision for chemotherapy should be taken based on the tumor biology and prognostic factors taken into consideration in nonpregnant patients.

Although administering chemotherapy during pregnancy may trigger concerns, the clinician should caution the patient against delaying therapy, especially in cases of locally advanced or poor-prognosis breast cancer, as delays in starting chemotherapy are associated with significantly worse outcomes.[62,63]

Pregnant women receive weight-based doses of chemotherapy that are similar to the doses received by women who are not pregnant.[64] There is little published information on specific pharmacokinetics of cytotoxic agents in the pregnant patient.[65] A number of physiologic changes of pregnancy, such as increased blood volume coupled with brisker renal and hepatic clearance, may be anticipated to reduce effective drug concentrations. Reduced albumin levels may increase the levels of the unbound drug, an effect that may be offset by the actions of estrogen increasing other plasma proteins. The absorption of orally administered drugs may be affected by the decreased gastric motility that accompanies pregnancy.[64,66]

The use of chemotherapy is contraindicated in the first trimester of pregnancy due to a well-established higher risk of fetal malformations.[67] This critical period of organogenesis carries the greatest risk for development of congenital abnormalities, chromosomal abnormalities, stillbirth, and miscarriage. The reported rate of major malformations in the general population is 3%.[68] The studies that have recorded outcomes after first trimester exposure to chemotherapy have estimated the rate fetal malformation between 14% and 18%.[69–71] Initiation of chemotherapy should not be before 14 weeks gestation.

Chemotherapy in the second or third trimester is associated with a risk of fetal malformation of less than 2%, the same as population norms,[69] but is still linked to other adverse outcomes such as intrauterine growth restriction, prematurity, and low birth weight.[64,72,73]

Anthracyclines, cyclophosphamide, and taxanes are the standard adjuvant or neoadjuvant combinations used in nonpregnant patients. The most commonly used regimens in pregnant women with breast cancer are doxorubicin plus cyclophosphamide (AC) or 5-fluorouracil, doxorubicin, and cyclophosphamide (FAC). The limited studies of administration of chemotherapy in the second and third trimesters suggest that the major cause of undesirable fetal outcome appears to be from premature delivery rather than from a direct chemotherapy effect. Hahn and colleagues reported a study of 57 pregnant breast cancer patients treated with FAC in the adjuvant (n = 32) or neoadjuvant (n = 25) setting.[74] All patients who delivered had live births with

follow-up identifying one child with Down syndrome and 2 with congenital anomalies (club foot; congenital bilateral ureteral reflux). Of 162 exposures to doxorubicin across a number of cancers, including some in the first trimester, complications included preeclampsia, midtrimester miscarriage, and transient neonatal neutropenia with sepsis and intrauterine growth restriction.[64] Doxorubicin is favored over other anthracyclines such as epirubicin that have been associated with neonatal cardiotoxicity (Table 78.1).[75–79]

Anthracyclines have been linked to dose-related cardiotoxicity in children and adults. Whether in utero exposure to anthracyclines is cardiotoxic to the developing fetus is unknown. One small study of 10 cases assessed maternal echocardiogram as well as amniotic fluid index; fetal Doppler and cardiac function determined that anthracycline exposure did not result in acute maternal and fetal cardiac dysfunction.[80]

Studies have shown that dose-dense treatment leads to better outcomes than conventional regimens, and this approach does seem to be an acceptable option during pregnancy.[45]

Taxanes are non-DNA damaging agents, and the transplacental transfer rate is low.[81] A recent update from an International Registry of mainly German and Belgian patients includes 311 patients treated between 2003 and 2011. Only 4 patients did not receive chemotherapy. In those treated with chemotherapy, one-third were treated with neoadjuvant chemotherapy and 47% received taxanes.[19] A collation of 16 studies with a cumulative 50 patients treated with taxanes reported in 2013. A completely healthy infant was born in 77% of cases. The treatments were generally well tolerated with granulocyte colony-stimulating factor administration used in only in 8% of cases. Intrauterine growth restriction was reported in 13% of cases. Thirty children were followed up for more than 1 year. The three cases with reported persistent health problems included one child with recurrent otitis media, one child with immunoglobulin A deficiency, and one child with mild constipation. A 2010 international consensus meeting provided a comprehensive overview of published data on the clinical diagnosis, treatment, and outcomes in patients with breast cancer during pregnancy, including supplemental individual study data.[82] They concluded that "the use of taxanes during the second and third trimesters appears possible with limited risk for both the mother and the fetus."

Platinum derivatives may have a role in the treatment of triple-negative breast cancer.[83] Carboplatin may occasionally be considered during the second and third trimesters in such cases, although there are no specific data in pregnancy to support its use. One small clinical study has shown low platinum values in the fetoplacental unit at the time of delivery in 21 patients receiving neoadjuvant chemotherapy for cervical carcinoma during pregnancy.[84] The use of platinum derivatives, mainly cisplatin, has been reported in the setting of cervical cancer, with all 48 newborns (1 miscarriage) having a reported favorable outcome at 1 year.[85]

The success of targeted therapy directed against HER2 has represented one of the major advances in breast cancer in recent times, especially when administered concurrently with cytotoxic chemotherapy.[86] However, there are very few data pertaining to its safety during pregnancy. A 2013 study analyzed 18 reports using trastuzumab during pregnancy. The rate of oligohydramnios and anhydramnios was 61% and mostly self-limiting when therapy was discontinued. The average duration of trastuzumab use was 14 weeks with a mean gestational age at delivery of 34

TABLE 78.1	Case Series Reporting Use of Chemotherapy During Pregnancy								
Author	Year	Country	No. of Patients	Regimens Used	Patients Treated With NACT, %	Median Gestation at Start of Chemotherapy	Median No. of Cycles	Median GA at Delivery (Weeks)
Ring[75]	2005	UK	24	AC (46%), EC, CMF	30%	20	6	37
Hahn[74]	2006	US	57	FAC	44%	23	4	37
Azim[76]	2008	Italy	26	Anthracycline Most E	35%	Second trimester	4	35
Peccatori[77]	2009	Italy	20	Epirubicin	0%	19	12	35
Cardonick[78]	2010	US, Europe, Australia	120	AC (59%) Others: FAC, FEC, single-agent T	23%	20	4	36
Meisel[45]	2013	US	74	AC (8% with T)	22%	81% second trimester	4	56% <37
Amant[19]	2013	Europe	311	47% T	32%	—	—	—
Murphy[79]	2012	US	99	83% anthracycline 66% T	—	—	—	—

A, Doxorubicin; *C*, cyclophosphamide; *E*, epirubicin; *F*, 5-fluorouracil; *GA*, gestational age; *M*, methotrexate; *NACT*, neoadjuvant chemotherapy; *T*, taxane.

weeks. However, 4 of the 18 births did not survive beyond 5 months. Given this association with serious adverse events on both the pregnancy and fetus, the international consensus guidelines recommend that prolonged exposure to trastuzumab should be avoided.[82]

An area of concern associated with in utero exposure to antineoplastic agents is their potential effect on normal childhood development, fertility, and carcinogenic potential. To date, the follow-up of children is reassuring, although it is short. The largest individual series reported on the survey assessed outcomes of 63 children who had been exposed in utero to chemotherapy (5-fluorouracil, doxorubicin, and cyclophosphamide) for breast cancer at a median age of 7 years. Most responders considered their children to be healthy overall. A variety of minor health issues were reported, such as developmental milestone delay in 12%, but no significant cognitive abnormalities were reported.[87]

For patients with estrogen receptor–positive and/or progesterone receptor–positive tumors, the use of tamoxifen or other selective estrogen receptor modulators should be avoided during pregnancy and delayed until after delivery due to the risk of associated vaginal bleeding, spontaneous abortion, birth defects, and fetal death.[88–90] Delaying adjuvant hormonal treatment until after delivery will not reduce the efficacy, and given that the majority of these patients will receive systemic chemotherapy, tamoxifen can be commenced after completion of chemotherapy as in nonpregnant patients.

Consensus guidelines on the use of supportive medications, such as those for nausea and vomiting, have been published.[91] Obstetric review every third week should occur during pregnancy to allow an ultrasound assessment of the fetus, umbilical artery flow, and amniotic fluid. If abnormal findings are identified, a more intense fetal monitoring or even (preterm) delivery may be required. A 2- to 3-week period between the last dose of chemotherapy is recommended to support bone marrow recovery. Chemotherapy should not be administered after 35 weeks due to the higher likelihood of spontaneous labor after this time. Term delivery should be aimed for because prematurity and low birth weight can both negatively affect the emotional and cognitive development of the newborn. If preterm delivery is inevitable, steps should be taken to ensure fetal lung maturation. The mode of delivery is managed as per normal obstetric practice for the specific case, and, although reported rarely, the placenta should be analyzed to exclude the possibility of placental metastases.[92]

Many cytotoxic drugs, including cyclophosphamide and doxorubicin, are excreted in breast milk, and patients should be advised that breastfeeding is contraindicated while receiving chemotherapy.[93,94]

Radiation Therapy

Radiation therapy for breast cancer is part of the treatment for women who undergo breast-conserving surgery. It is also indicated postmastectomy in certain cases, such as a primary cancer of 4 cm or greater in size, in all cases of axillary nodal metastases with involvement of more than three lymph nodes, and in certain cases with one or two lymph nodes involved.[95] Although there are reports of successful employment of radiotherapy for breast cancer during pregnancy,[96–98] radiation therapy has traditionally been contraindicated during the gestational period because of the risks associated with fetal radiation exposure.[99,100]

Radiation therapy poses the risks of teratogenicity to the developing fetus as well as the risk of induction of childhood malignancies. The amount of radiation to which the fetus is exposed is dependent on the source of irradiation, as well as the size of the treatment fields and their proximity to the fetus, which varies with stage of pregnancy.[101] With a standard 50-Gy therapeutic course, the estimated level of fetal exposure varies from around 0.1 Gy in the first trimester to 2 Gy toward the end of pregnancy.[36,96,102]

The biological effects of radiation on the fetus depend both on the gestational age and on the dose of radiation. Before implantation, irradiation will lead to spontaneous abortion.[103–105] During organogenesis (gestational weeks 2–8), exposure to radiation above a threshold dose of 0.1 to 0.2 Gy can cause fetal malformations. Intrauterine growth retardation, microcephaly, and mental retardation are potential results of exposure.[106] Prenatal radiation exposure also seems to increase the risk of childhood cancer and leukemia by approximately 40%. However, the absolute risk remains low (3–4 per 1000[103,107]). At this time, there are no reports on the use of intraoperative radiation therapy for pregnancy-associated breast cancer, and its use cannot be recommended.

Considering that the majority of patients with pregnancy-associated breast cancer will have a clear indication for systemic chemotherapy on the basis of tumor stage and/or biological subtype, in practical terms, the timing of adjuvant radiotherapy should be planned for after delivery. Pregnant women with early-stage breast cancer who are diagnosed in the late second or early third trimester can undergo breast-conserving surgery followed by adjuvant chemotherapy, or, alternatively, if no adjuvant systemic therapy is planned, surgery can be performed in the third trimester, with radiation therapy deferred until after delivery, because delays in locoregional radiation for up to 6 months to accommodate adjuvant chemotherapy, or up to 4 months when no adjuvant systemic therapy is planned, do not seem to compromise local control.[108,109] For pregnant patients with locally advanced-stage disease, neoadjuvant chemotherapy can be offered at presentation before definitive breast surgery later in the pregnancy, or surgery postpartum followed by radiation therapy.[74]

Some authors state that in certain pregnancy-associated cancers, given the lower level of fetal exposure in early pregnancy when the uterus remains in the pelvis, radiation therapy with appropriate techniques and shielding may be a treatment option during the first and second trimesters of pregnancy.[82]

Irradiation of the breast can affect lactation by causing lobular atrophy, periductal and perilobular fibrosis with ductal shrinking, and cytoplasmic loss.[110] A small percentage of patients have successfully breastfed after whole breast irradiation. However, because of the risk of mastitis, which may prove difficult to manage, coupled with the risk of lymphedema, women with breast cancer are advised against breastfeeding from the irradiated breast.[110,111]

Special Issues

Therapeutic Abortion

The decision to continue or terminate the pregnancy is a difficult one for the individual and should be made by a properly informed and counseled patient. There are a number of factors that are involved, including, but not limited to, the potential effect of any systemic treatment on future fertility, the level of family support, and prognosis of the breast cancer, as well as a discussion on the possibility of fetal complications from exposure to treatments in utero. There is no evidence that early termination of pregnancy improves the outcome of pregnancy-associated breast cancer.[102]

Studies that have reported an overall worse prognosis for patients who had a therapeutic abortion involve important selection biases that abrogate such conclusions.[112]

BRCA Mutations and Pregnancy-Associated Breast Cancer

Studies have suggested that because of their relatively younger age at diagnosis, *BRCA* mutation carriers may be particularly susceptible to the transient increase in the risk of breast cancer associated with the hormonal changes that accompany pregnancy.

A 1998 study from Sweden identified that of 265 women who developed breast cancer before age 40 years, the rate of pregnancy-associated breast cancer was 6.6% in *BRCA* mutation carriers and 5.7% of nonmutation carriers. The study separately examined the occurrence of pregnancy-associated breast cancer in the pedigrees of 39 known *BRCA* families and identified that pregnancy-associated breast cancer was more likely in families with a *BRCA1* germline mutation than *BRCA2* families.[113]

Cullinane and colleagues matched 1260 *BRCA* mutation carriers (74% *BRCA1*) with a history of breast cancer to mutation carriers with no personal history of breast cancer. In *BRCA1* mutation carriers, there was a small reduction in the breast cancer risk in the 2 years after a pregnancy. However, in *BRCA2* mutation carriers, the risk of breast cancer in the 2 years after a birth was moderately increased compared with nulliparous controls.[114]

It is commonly thought that early age at first pregnancy is protective for risk of developing breast cancer. Two matched case-control studies have examined whether early pregnancy is protective against the development of breast cancer *BRCA* mutation carriers,[115,116] and in both studies, *BRCA1* or *BRCA2* mutation carriers with a history of breast cancer were matched to mutation carriers who had not developed breast cancer. Both studies found that a later age at first full-term birth in mutation carriers did not confer an increased risk of breast cancer. One of these studies did find that compared with nulliparous mutation carriers, carriers of *BRCA1* and *BRCA2* mutations who have children were more likely to develop breast cancer by age 40.[115]

Follow-up of 128 *BRCA* mutation carriers who were diagnosed with breast cancer while pregnant or who became pregnant after a diagnosis of breast cancer has shown that 15-year survival estimates were not inferior to those in mutation carriers with breast cancer who did not become pregnant.[117]

Conclusion

There are no randomized trials addressing the range of issues presented by pregnancy-associated breast cancer. The doctrine of characteristics and management strategies of pregnancy-associated breast cancer have, up until recently, been established on small case series collected over many decades. It appears that outcomes for women with pregnancy-associated breast cancer are similar, stage for stage, to outcomes for nonpregnant women.

It is crucial that recent advances in breast cancer care are adapted for pregnant patients. The establishment of national and international case registries with rigorous follow-up represents one potential means of navigating the deficit of randomized trials to evaluate outcomes with pregnancy-associated breast cancer. Examples of particular areas that warrant further study include the implications of the seemingly high rate of HER2 positivity in these cases and how to safely translate the success of targeted anti-HER2 therapies to pregnant patients, the safety and efficacy of neoadjuvant chemotherapy, the role of SLNB in axillary staging, and the prevalence of inherited germline mutations in these women diagnosed with breast cancer at a young age.

Prompt evaluation of any mass encountered in pregnancy is important to avoid potential delays in diagnosis. The treatment of pregnancy-associated breast cancer is complex and requires a multidisciplinary team approach. Counseling is a crucial component of this treatment. Treatment is dependent on the gestational age of the pregnancy because some treatments will be of potential harm to the developing fetus. Weighing the benefits of treatment to the mother, in the context of a developing fetus, is crucial.

Selected References

19. Amant F, von Minckwitz G, Han SN, et al. Prognosis of women with primary breast cancer diagnosed during pregnancy: results from an international collaborative study. *J Clin Oncol.* 2013;31:2532-2539.

45. Meisel JL, Economy KE, Calvillo KZ, et al. Contemporary multidisciplinary treatment of pregnancy-associated breast cancer. *Springerplus.* 2013;2:297.
64. Cardonick E, Iacobucci A. Use of chemotherapy during human pregnancy. *Lancet Oncol.* 2004;5:283-291.
78. Cardonick E, Dougherty R, Grana G, et al. Breast cancer during pregnancy: maternal and fetal outcomes. *Cancer J.* 2010;16:76-82.
79. Murphy CG, Mallam D, Stein S, et al. Current or recent pregnancy is associated with adverse pathologic features but not impaired survival in early breast cancer. *Cancer.* 2012;118:3254-3259.

A full reference list is available online at ExpertConsult.com.

79

Unknown Primary Presenting With Axillary Lymphadenopathy

KATE I. LATHROP AND VIRGINIA KAKLAMANI

Breast cancer can rarely present as isolated axillary adenopathy without any evidence of a primary breast mass creating many diagnostic and therapeutic challenges. Occult breast cancer is defined as isolated axillary adenocarcinoma without detectable tumor in the breast by either physical examination or with imaging such as mammogram, ultrasound, or magnetic resonance imaging (MRI). Occult breast cancer, although rare, has been acknowledged for more than 100 years. It was first described by Halsted in the *Annuals of Surgery* in 1906.[1]

Incidence

Occult breast cancer with axillary metastasis is rare and likely accounts for less than 1% of all newly diagnosed breast cancers (Fig. 79.1).[2] It is difficult to determine the exact incidence because the case series are small and imaging techniques have improved. With improving sensitivity of breast imaging, including the addition of MRI imaging, it is a reasonable assumption that more primary breast lesions will be identified before surgery.[3]

Diagnosis

The majority of patients presenting with isolated axillary adenopathy will subsequently be diagnosed with benign reactive adenopathy (Fig. 79.2). Within the setting of malignancy, lymphoma is a more common cause of isolated axillary adenopathy than an occult breast cancer. Other cancers that can present as occult metastatic disease include lung, colon, gastric, and melanoma.[4] In one recent study, the pathology was reviewed for 65 patients who presented with isolated axillary lymph node swelling between 2005 and 2011 and subsequently had an axillary lymph node excisional biopsy. Only 24% (16) of the biopsies were malignant, and of the malignant biopsies, 10 were consistent with a breast primary.[5]

Selected Imaging

Diagnostic workup generally starts with a core needle biopsy of the axillary node consistent with adenocarcinoma or carcinoma not otherwise specified (Fig. 79.3). On the basis of current National Comprehensive Cancer Network (NCCN) guidelines, mammography should be the first imaging study[6] (Fig. 79.4). A nonpalpable breast mass may be successfully identified with mammography in approximately 10% to 20% of cases. However, small tumor size and high breast density can lead to false-negative findings on mammography.[7] In one small case series, mammogram was able to detect a primary breast mass in 10 of 17 patients presenting with axillary adenopathy and a clinically normal breast examination.[8] If mammography is nondiagnostic, then ultrasound and MRI of the breast are indicated (Fig. 79.5). Systemic imaging should include computed tomography (CT) scans of the neck, chest, and abdomen. A bone scan should be considered in patients with elevated alkaline phosphatase or if they have symptoms concerning for bone lesions.[6]

Systemic imaging with CT scans and specific immunohistochemical stains can often help diagnose the primary malignancy in the case of metastatic disease from a site other than the breast. Primary tumors of the breast that are located in the axillary tail of the breast can be incorrectly classified as axillary adenopathy. Routine breast imaging such as mammogram and ultrasound can assist the clinician in determining whether the mass is located in the axillary tail.[7]

MRI of the breast can help find occult breast cancers and can potentially help select patients who are most likely to benefit from a mastectomy. One study by Olson and coworkers found that in 40 patients with biopsy-proven breast cancer in the axilla and an either negative or indeterminate mammogram, MRI was successful in identifying a primary breast lesion in 70% of the patients.[9] In this review, all patients had mammograms, ultrasounds, and MRI imaging without gadolinium. Positive MRIs were then compared with histologic findings at the time of surgery. MRI was successful in identifying the primary lesion in 28 of the 40 women. In this small series, 34 women proceeded with some form of breast surgery as part of their treatment. A total of 18 were treated with MRM, and 16 (47%) were treated with breast conserving therapy. Although a single and small study, this shows that breast MRI can successfully identify a primary breast lesion that was not apparent with other imaging modalities and may allow the opportunity for breast conversation surgery.

There is not sufficient evidence to support positron emission tomography (PET) CT imaging in the diagnostic workup of occult axillary breast cancer (Fig. 79.6). There are case reports of PET imaging successfully identifying a primary breast lesion that was not apparent with mammography.[10] PET-CT imaging has been successful in the diagnosis of carcinomas of unknown primaries as a whole and finding asymptomatic metastatic disease but has not been extensively studied specifically in occult breast cancers.[11] It is uncertain what additional diagnostic utility PET

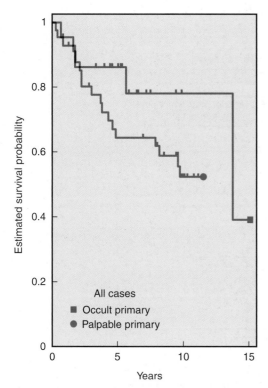

• **Fig. 79.1** Survival of women (n = 22) with occult primary breast cancers whose mastectomy specimens contained measurable invasive tumor compared with patients presenting with palpable primary tumors matched on tumor size, number of involved lymph nodes, tumor type, and age at diagnosis. (From Rosen PP, Kimmel M. Occult breast carcinoma presenting with axillary lymph node metastases: a follow-up of 48 patients. *Hum Pathol.* 1990;21:518-523.)

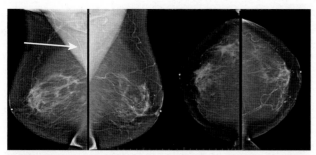

• **Fig. 79.2** Imaging study from a 55-year old woman with biopsy-proven poorly differentiated carcinoma extensively replacing a lymph node in the upper outer right breast. Mediolateral oblique *(left)* and craniocaudal *(right)* mammograms showing a postsurgical scar in the right low axillary region *(arrow),* related to an excision biopsy of a metastatic lymph node. No primary breast lesion was detected.

CT scanning can contribute in the setting of mammography, ultrasound, and MRI imaging of the breast.

Pathologic Evaluation

Accurate pathologic assessment is essential for proper management, and a core needle biopsy is usually required. The diagnosis should not be made based on fine-needle aspiration sampling alone.[12] With occult breast cancer, the histology is usually either adenocarcinoma or poorly differentiated carcinoma. The standard immunohistochemical markers include estrogen receptor (ER),

progesterone receptor (PR), and human epidermal growth factor receptor 2 (HER2). Elevated ER and/or PR levels provide strong evidence for a primary breast cancer. However, the absence of estrogen and progesterone markers does not rule out a breast primary. In a small series from 1987 of 10 patients with axillary nodal metastasis of unknown origin, 7 biopsies were either estrogen or progesterone positive. All patients were subsequently found to have a primary breast mass. This small series is therefore consistent with the known prevalence rate of about 30% for ER and PR negative breast cancers.[13] Other important immunohistochemical markers include carcinoembryonic antigen (CEA), cytokeratins (CK) 7 and 20, mammaglobin, thyroid transcription factor-1 (TTF-1), and CA125. None of these markers individually can make a definite diagnosis of breast cancer, but patterns can emerge that help rule in or rule out breast cancer as the etiology of axillary metastatic disease.

CEA is a sensitive marker for adenocarcinomas in general and can be positive in malignancies arising from the breast, gastrointestinal tract, or lung. Different expression patterns of cytokeratins such as CK7 and CK20 can help separate these histologies. CK7 is usually expressed in tumors of the breast, lung, ovaries, and endometrium. Whereas CK20 is most commonly expressed in tumors arising from the lower gastrointestinal tract and urothelium. Therefore an immunohistochemical pattern of CEA and CK7 positive and CK20 negative would be consistent with a breast primary. TTF-1 is a useful marker in ruling out the breast as a primary, as it is rarely positive in the breast and positive in 70% to 80% of nonsquamous cancers arising from the lungs.

Mammaglobin and CA125 can both be positive in breast primary tumors. Although CA125 is most common in ovarian cancers, it can be positive in approximately 10% of breast tumors. Mammaglobin is sensitive for breast cancers but is not specific. It can be positive in many other tumor types including ovarian, lung, urothelial, colon, and hepatobiliary tumors.[14]

Management

For patients with no sign of metastatic disease and breast-specific imaging and pathology most consistent with a breast primary, treatment should be in accordance to currently established guidelines for stage II/III breast cancer. Specifically, occult breast cancers are staged as T0N1, stage IIA, if adenopathy is movable and positioned in level I or II, or T0N2, stage IIIA, if nodes are clinically fixed or matted based on the 2016 NCCN staging guidelines.

Recommendations for management of patients with axillary primaries are generally based on a limited number of retrospective studies involving small numbers of patients. Traditionally, women were treated with a mastectomy and axillary dissection. However, surgical management has shifted since the early 2000s to treating with axillary nodal dissection only, followed by locoregional radiation therapy. One retrospective review of patients treated at Rosewell Park Cancer Institute between 1997 to 2004 found 10 cases of patients with occult breast cancer. All patients were treated with an axillary nodal dissection. Management of the ipsilateral breast varied in that series with eight patients managed with radiotherapy alone, one with a wide local resection followed by radiotherapy and one patient treated with a mastectomy. After a median of 57 months of follow-up, none of the patients had evidence of recurrent disease.[15]

A group in Milan reported on their experience with 50 cases of occult breast cancer. After extensive workup, 27 patients had

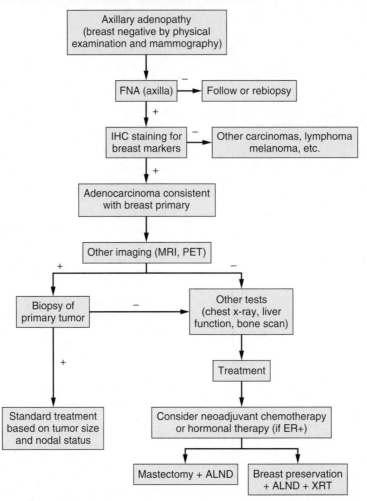

```
Axillary adenopathy
(breast negative by physical
examination and mammography)
        │
        ▼
   FNA (axilla) ──── − ──▶ Follow or rebiopsy
        │
        + │
        ▼
  IHC staining for ──── − ──▶ Other carcinomas, lymphoma
  breast markers              melanoma, etc.
        │
        + │
        ▼
Adenocarcinoma consistent
   with breast primary
        │
        ▼
  Other imaging (MRI, PET)
   +  │         │  −
      ▼         ▼
  Biopsy of ─ − ─▶ Other tests
  primary tumor    (chest x-ray, liver
                   function, bone scan)
      │                │
      +                ▼
      │            Treatment
      │                │
      ▼                ▼
Standard treatment   Consider neoadjuvant chemotherapy
based on tumor size  or hormonal therapy (if ER+)
and nodal status          │
                    ┌─────┴─────┐
                    ▼           ▼
              Mastectomy + ALND  Breast preservation
                                 + ALND + XRT
```

• **Fig. 79.3** Treatment algorithm for patients presenting with axillary adenopathy without an obvious primary tumor. *ALND,* Axillary lymph node dissection; *ER,* estrogen receptor; *FNA,* fine-needle aspiration; *IHC,* immunohistochemistry; *MRI,* magnetic resonance imaging; *PET,* positron emission tomography; *XRT,* radiation therapy.

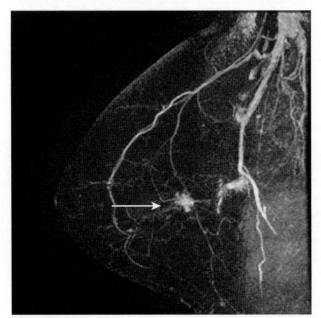

• **Fig. 79.4** Sagittal maximum intensity projection image of the breast magnetic resonance imaging examination showing an irregular enhancing 1.5-cm mass *(arrow)* that is suspicious for a carcinoma, in the same patient as picture in Fig. 79.2.

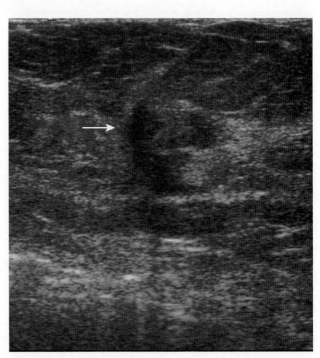

• **Fig. 79.5** "Second-look" ultrasound of the right breast performed after the magnetic resonance imaging examination, in the same patient as picture in Fig. 79.2, showing an irregular hypoechoic 1.2-cm mass with posterior shadowing *(arrow).* Poorly differentiated invasive carcinoma was identified by ultrasound-guided core biopsy.

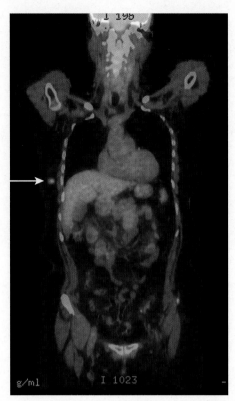

• **Fig. 79.6** Frontal fused positron emission tomography/computed tomography image showing a fluorodeoxyglucose-avid lesion in the right breast *(arrow)*, in the same patient as picture in Fig. 79.2.

no evidence of a breast primary and were therefore treated with a complete axillary dissection and radiotherapy to the ipsilateral breast. Of the original group of 50 patients, 27 received adjuvant chemotherapy alone, 5 received hormonal therapy alone, and 18 received both hormonal therapy and chemotherapy. At a median follow-up of 41 months, disease-free survival was 84%, with two patients alive with local recurrence and five patients having died of metastatic disease but with no evidence of in-breast recurrence.[16]

Another case series included 45 patients with occult breast cancer diagnosed between 1951 and 1998 at MD Anderson Cancer Center of which the majority of the patients were treated with breast conservation therapy. Of the 13 patients (29%) who had mastectomies, only one primary breast mass was identified. The remaining 32 patients (71%) were treated with axillary lymph node dissection (ALND) alone and locoregional radiotherapy. There was no significant difference on locoregional recurrence, development of metastatic disease, or 5-year survival in the patients treated with breast conservation compared with

mastectomies with ALND. The number of positive axillary lymph nodes was predictive of risk of recurrence and development of metastatic disease with a 5-year overall survival of 87% with one to three positive axillary lymph nodes compared with 42% 5-year overall survival with four or more positive axillary lymph nodes.[17]

A recent meta-analysis of seven studies with a combined 241 patients explored the locoregional recurrence, distant metastasis, and mortality rates for patients with occult breast cancer.[18] The aim of the analysis was to compare mastectomy with less invasive surgical modalities. Patients included in the meta-analysis were classified into three groups: group 1 had ALND with radiation, group 2 had ALND with mastectomy, and group 3 had ALND alone. On the basis of the findings of this analysis, the addition of mastectomy to ALND did not improve locoregional control, distant metastases, or overall survival compared with ALND combined with breast radiation. Also, this study demonstrated that patients undergoing ALND with irradiation had statistically significant better locoregional recurrence rates compared with ALND alone (34.3 vs. 12.7%). The authors of this analysis note a trend toward improved mortality rates in the patients treated with ALND and irradiation compared with ALND alone, although it was not a statistically significant difference.

On the basis of these small case series and this recent meta-analysis, it appears that breast conservation with radiation therapy after ALND can be considered as appropriate local management for women presenting with occult breast cancer in the axilla. In regard to systemic therapies, patients should be treated according to current guidelines for T1N1 and T2N1 tumors and modified based on ER, PR, and HER2 status. Prognosis remains good, and the 5- and 10-year survival rates are essentially the same as patients who present with a primary breast mass.[19]

Selected References

2. Rosen PP, Kimmel M. Occult breast carcinoma presenting with axillary lymph node metastases: a follow-up study of 48 patients. *Hum Pathol.* 1990;21:518-523.
3. Pentheroudakis G, Lazaridis G, Pavlidis N. Axillary nodal metastases from carcinoma of unknown primary (CUPAx): a systematic review of published evidence. *Breast Cancer Res Treat.* 2012;119:1.
9. Olson JA, Morris EA, Van Zee KJ, et al. Magnetic resonance imaging facilitates breast conservation for occult breast cancer. *Ann Surg Oncol.* 2000;7:411-415.
15. Varadarajan R, Edge SB, Yu J, et al. Prognosis of occult breast carcinoma presenting as isolated axillary nodal metastasis. *Oncology.* 2006;71:456-459.
18. Macedo F, Eid J, Flynn J, et al. Optimal surgical management for occult breast carcinoma: a meta-analysis. *Ann Surg Oncol.* 2016;23:1838-1844.

A full reference list is available online at ExpertConsult.com.

80

Clinical Management of the Patient at Increased or High Risk

THERESE B. BEVERS AND PARIJATHAM S. THOMAS

For a number of years, there has been a steady decline in the number of women dying of breast cancer.[1] This has been attributed to a combination of early detection from mammographic screening and improved treatment strategies.[2,3] The decline in the use of hormone replacement therapy (HRT), due in large part to published data from the Women's Health Initiative showing an association between HRT and breast cancer,[4] is a probable contributing factor.[5–8] A possible contributing factor is the use of raloxifene since 1999 for osteoporosis prevention and treatment because it has also been shown to reduce the incidence of breast cancer.[9]

There are now interventions to reduce a woman's chance of being diagnosed with breast cancer as well as strategies for the screening of increased or high-risk women. It is essential that clinicians in primary care settings recognize women at increased or high risk of breast cancer due to personal risk factors, medical conditions, or family history, so that appropriate screening activities can be encouraged, appropriate risk reduction interventions offered, and/or referral made to specialists for cancer risk assessment and counseling.

The intent of this chapter is to bring the components of breast cancer risk assessment, risk reduction, and screening, the specifics of which are discussed in depth in other chapters, into a clinical perspective. A practical approach to identifying breast cancer risk, the components of the risk assessment process, and recommendations for the clinical management of women at increased and high risk for breast cancer are reviewed.

Breast Cancer Risk Assessment

Breast cancer risk assessment involves identifying a woman's breast cancer risk factors and determining her probability of developing breast cancer. It serves as a basis for recommendations on appropriate preventive interventions and screening strategies based on her level of risk.

Qualitative Breast Cancer Risk Assessment

Numerous risk factors for the development of breast cancer have been identified[1] (Box 80.1). Being female and becoming older are the most common risk factors. However, these risks apply to all women and are not clinically useful because they provide no ability to discriminate the breast cancer risk of one woman compared with another. The lifetime risk of breast cancer in the

United States is 1 in 8 (about 12%).[1] This commonly quoted lifetime risk estimates populational risk, not individual cancer risk.

Somewhat more helpful are age-specific risks because this focuses a woman's attention on risks of women in her age range[1] (Table 80.1). However, these categories include women at minimal risk and those at very high risk. The actual risk to any individual woman may be very different. Age-specific incidence rates increase dramatically beginning at 40 years of age.

Quantitative Breast Cancer Risk Assessment

Mathematical models have been developed to quantitate a woman's risk of developing breast cancer. The National Cancer Institute (NCI) Breast Cancer Risk Assessment Tool (BCRAT) assesses breast cancer risk using nongenetic factors. The hereditary/familial models (e.g., Claus, Tyrer-Cuzick, and BRCAPRO models) assess genetic and familial risk of breast cancer. The clinical implications of these models are discussed in this chapter, but the specifics pertaining to the models are reviewed in Chapter 17.

Risk Assessment Models Based on Nongenetic Factors

The BCRAT, or Gail model, (www.cancer.gov/bcrisktool) provides a risk estimate of developing breast cancer for the next 5 years and an estimate of lifetime risk.[10] Women with a 5-year risk of 1.7% or greater are considered to be at increased risk of developing invasive breast cancer and can be considered for preventive therapy. This is the risk estimate used for the major breast cancer prevention trials and is supported by NCCN Breast Cancer Risk Reduction guideline.[11]

The BCRAT was initially developed based on a cohort of white women in the Breast Cancer Detection and Demonstration Project (BCDDP).[12] The model has been updated to provide adjusted estimates for African American and Asian and Pacific Islander women.[13,14] Risk estimates for other populations of women (e.g., Hispanic women) are subject to greater uncertainty; this should be considered when counseling women about their breast cancer risk. Although the BCRAT has been shown to have good predictive capability in large cohorts of women, it has only modest discriminatory ability in an individual woman.[15] It should be noted that for any two women with identical risk factors except

• BOX 80.1 Breast Cancer Risk Factors

Female gender
Age
Race/ethnicity
Family history
    Sporadic
    Familial
    Hereditary (e.g., *BRCA1*, *BRCA2*, Li-Fraumeni and Cowden syndromes)
    Ashkenazi Jewish heritage
Reproductive/hormonal
    Early menarche (<12 years)
    Late menopause (>55 years)
    Late age of first live birth (>30 years)
    Nulliparity
    Parity
    Never breastfed a child
    Recent use of hormonal contraception
    Recent and long-term use of hormone replacement therapy
Medical history
    Personal history of breast cancer
    Personal history of endometrial, ovarian, or colon cancer
    Atypical hyperplasia
    Lobular carcinoma in situ
    Therapeutic thoracic radiation between 10 and 30 years of age
    Increased breast density
    Increased bone density (postmenopausal)
Lifestyle
    Adult weight gain
    Obesity (postmenopausal)
    Physical inactivity
    Alcohol consumption
    High socioeconomic status

Modified from American Cancer Society. Breast Cancer Facts & Figures 2015–2016. Atlanta, GA: American Cancer Society, Inc.; 2015.

• BOX 80.2 Variables Used for Risk Calculation in the Modified Gail Model

Age
Age at menarche
Age at first live birth or nulliparity
Number of first-degree relatives with a history of breast cancer
Number of breast biopsies and if any biopsy identified atypical hyperplasia
Race

Data from National Cancer Institute: Breast Cancer Risk Assessment Tool. Available at: www.cancer.gov/bcrisktool.

TABLE 80.1 Age-Specific Probabilities of Developing Invasive Breast Cancer[a]

Current Age	Probability of Developing Breast Cancer in the Next 10 Years
20	0.1% (1 in 1674)
30	0.4% (1 in 225)
40	1.4% (1 in 69)
50	2.3% (1 in 44)
60	3.5% (1 in 29)
70	3.9% (1 in 26)
Lifetime risk	12.3% (1 in 8)

[a]Among women free of cancer at beginning of age interval. On the basis of cases diagnosed between 2010 and 2012. Percentages and "1 in" numbers may not be numerically equivalent due to rounding.
From American Cancer Society. Breast Cancer Facts & Figures 2015–2016. Atlanta, GA: American Cancer Society, Inc.; 2015.

age, the 5-year risk is greater for older women than for younger women. Conversely, the lifetime risk is greater for younger women than for older women.

The BCRAT is not applicable to women with breast cancer, ductal carcinoma in situ (DCIS), or lobular carcinoma in situ (LCIS). It uses a limited number of risk factors (Box 80.2) and does not take into account risk factors such as current or former use of HRT, breast density or previous radiation therapy to the chest in females 10 to 30 years of age. The model does not consider any paternal family history; maternal family history other than first-degree relatives; personal or family history of ovarian cancer; or other familial factors of concern for an inherited mutation such as male breast cancer, bilateral breast cancer in a relative, and an early age of diagnosis of breast cancers in the family. As a result, the model may significantly underestimate breast cancer risk, especially for women with a known or suspected genetic predisposition, and should not be used to estimate their risk.

In an analysis by the Mayo Clinic, the BCRAT model has been shown to underestimate the risk of breast cancer in women with atypical hyperplasia (AH).[16] They suggest that women with AH have a 1% per year risk of developing breast cancer.[17] Additionally, Hartmann and colleagues[18] and Collins and coworkers[19] have shown that the risk of women with atypical hyperplasia was not further increased by a family history of breast cancer. They hypothesized that atypical hyperplasia is a biological manifestation of the woman's overall breast cancer risk, which includes family history. In the BCRAT, family history has an additive effect when factored with atypical hyperplasia thus the estimate is likely an overestimation of breast cancer risk when both variables are incorporated.

Even with these limitations, the BCRAT provides valuable information and serves as a starting point in the evaluation of breast cancer risk in women without a known or suspected genetic predisposition to breast cancer; a personal history of breast cancer, DCIS, or LCIS; or a history of thoracic radiation under 30 years of age. One of the values of the BCRAT is its simplicity and ease of implementation in a primary care setting.

Risk Assessment Models Based on Family History and Genetic Factors

The Claus model is useful in understanding a woman's risk of breast cancer based on familial factors. This model was developed based on population-based data from the Cancer and Steroid Hormone study.[20] It is applicable only to women with a family history of breast cancer who do not have a personal history of the disease. This model includes information on up to two first- and/ or second-degree relatives with invasive breast cancer along with specification as to maternal or paternal lineage, age of the patient, and age of relatives at the time of breast cancer diagnosis. A family history of DCIS and LCIS as well as personal and family history of ovarian cancer are excluded from risk calculations in the Claus model and likely result in an underestimation of actual risk for some women. The Claus model does not include data on race/ethnicity; history of breast biopsy, including the presence of atypical hyperplasia or LCIS; other medical history; or reproductive/hormonal factors for breast cancer.

The Tyrer-Cuzick model is another model that can be used to evaluate breast cancer risk in women with a significant family history of the disease. This model was developed using cancer incidence rates of the general population from the United Kingdom national statistics and cancer incidence in daughters of mothers who had breast cancer.[21,22] Similar to the Claus model, the Tyrer-Cuzick model takes into account first- and second-degree relatives with invasive breast cancer including maternal or paternal lineage as well as age of relatives at time of diagnosis. The model also includes personal risk factors such as the woman's reproductive risk factors, history of atypical hyperplasia or LCIS, menopausal status, and use of hormone replacement therapy.[23] The Tyrer-Cuzick model provides information on both the 10-year and lifetime risk of developing breast cancer as well as the risk of having a *BRCA1* or *BRCA2* mutation. This model can identify women for preventive therapy (10-year breast cancer risk ≥5%) and women eligible for supplemental screening with breast MRI (lifetime risk ≥20%). The Tyrer-Cuzick model also provides an estimate of a *BRCA1* or *BRCA2* mutation, which can identify women in whom genetic testing should be considered. Although it is the most comprehensive of the breast cancer risk assessment tools, its application in a busy clinical practice, especially in a primary care setting, is limited by the time needed to complete the breast cancer risk survey.

In addition to estimating risk of developing invasive breast cancer, there are models that are available to estimate an individual's risk of carrying deleterious mutations in BRCA1 and BRCA2 (e.g., BRCAPRO). The BRCAPRO model is a theoretical model that uses Bayesian analysis to estimate an individual's chance of having a *BRCA1* or *BRCA2* mutation.[24] This model fully considers family history and relevant factors for determining *BRCA1* or *BRCA2* carriers, but its use is limited to these two mutations and is best utilized in the genetic counseling session.

Breast Cancer Risk Assessment in the Clinical Setting

Perception of risk has been evaluated in several studies, and women consistently overestimate their risk of breast cancer.[25–27] The intent of risk counseling is to provide information, education, and clarification of risk with the hope that it will decrease anxiety and increase the use of screening practices and other measures to decrease breast cancer risk.

All women should be provided risk counseling, especially those who perceive themselves to be at increased risk for breast cancer and want assistance in understanding and dealing with this risk. Appropriate concerns to be addressed include not only the level of risk but also other health care decisions such as medical or surgical measures for risk reduction, screening practices, or the use of HRT.

Nongenetic Breast Cancer Risk Counseling

Before breast cancer risk assessment is initiated, any significant comorbid conditions that limit life expectancy or therapeutic

---

> ● **BOX 80.3** Features Indicating an Increased Likelihood of a Genetic Predisposition Toward Breast Cancer

Personal history of breast cancer diagnosed ≤45 years of age
Personal history of triple-negative breast cancer diagnosed ≤60 years of age
Family history of multiple cases of early-onset breast cancer
Personal history of ovarian cancer with a family history of breast or ovarian cancer
Breast and ovarian cancer in the same woman
Bilateral breast cancer
Ashkenazi Jewish heritage
Male breast cancer

From the University of Texas MD Anderson Cancer Center, Genetic Counseling Referral Criteria, 2015.

---

intervention should be considered. Risk reduction strategies and screening may not be appropriate in women with a life expectancy of less than 10 years or in whom comorbidities prohibit risk management interventions.

Absent this concern or a personal history of breast cancer, risk should be assessed for all woman 35 years of age or older. Risk assessment may need to be performed earlier if the patient has a strong family history of breast cancer, especially if the onset of the disease is early (i.e., age <50 years), a history of therapeutic thoracic radiation between the ages of 10 to 30 years, or if there is a personal history of proliferative breast lesions (AH or LCIS).

An ordered approach to breast cancer risk assessment helps to ensure that risk is not underestimated. A logical order for determining how best to identify a woman's risk includes the following:
1. Review family history for features that indicate an increased likelihood of having a *BRCA* mutation (Box 80.3) and refer for genetic counseling.
2. Identify women known to be at increased risk for breast cancer. Women with a personal history of AH,[1] LCIS,[1] or a personal history of thoracic radiation between 10 and 30 years of age[28–31] have an increased risk of developing the disease, but their risk is not calculated by the NCI Breast Cancer Risk Assessment Tool.
3. Calculate the risk for the women not excluded in the first two steps using the BCRAT.

Breast cancer risk assessment in a busy clinical practice can be daunting. The key to initiating the risk assessment process is to involve the nursing staff. The nurse can identify the appropriate approach to determine the woman's breast cancer risk, whether it is referral for genetic counseling (based on preidentified criteria; see Box 80.3) or risk calculation using the BCRAT. The nurse can place the genetic consultation request or the BCRAT calculation on the chart for review and discussion by the physician. Women at increased risk can be provided educational materials to read while waiting for the physician so as to streamline the initial risk discussion as well as strategies for risk reduction and screening recommendations.

Training for the nursing staff is critical for this process to be successful. In addition to outlining the three-step process for the nursing team, two variables in the BCRAT are often not well understood and should be explained to avoid inclusion of incorrect variables in the model. When determining a woman's age at first live birth, it is critical to realize that this may not be the woman's first pregnancy, if the first pregnancy ended in a spontaneous or induced abortion. Additionally, it is important to realize that a therapeutic cyst aspiration (done to relieve pain, not diagnose) does not count as a breast biopsy, and a needle biopsy that results in surgical excision, whether elective or to further define the breast lesion, counts as a single biopsy because it is the same process.

Breast cancer risk should periodically be reassessed because it is not static. Risk should be recalculated by the BCRAT at least every 5 years if the initial risk calculation was less than 1.7% because age is a variable in the risk estimate, with increasing age associated with an increased risk of breast cancer. Women at increased risk who declined risk reduction therapy should have their risk recalculated if any significant change in risk factors should occur, such as a new diagnosis of atypical hyperplasia or the report of a new first-degree relative with breast cancer, because the event and the higher risk estimate may change their initial decision regarding preventive therapy. Depending on the family history, a new diagnosis of breast cancer in the family may warrant reevaluation for a genetic predisposition.

Genetic Breast Cancer Risk Counseling

Individualized genetic counseling is a time-consuming process. Women concerning for a genetic predisposition are best served by referral to a comprehensive breast program with dedicated genetic counselors.

The length of the counseling process depends on the issues of concern. The initial session is spent collecting information for review and taking a history (if not done before the visit) as well as providing general information about breast cancer risk and cancer genetics and providing the risk assessment. If genetic testing is recommended, the benefits, risks, and limitations of testing are reviewed. Follow-up sessions are indicated to disclose results of genetic testing and clinical implications.

In certain situations, women may have previously had genetic testing with negative results. Because this field is constantly changing with discoveries of new mutations of significance, it is important to periodically review what genetic testing has been completed for the patient in the past and if further evaluation for extended testing may be warranted for the patient. Multigene panels are more frequently used and may be considered in patients that previously had negative genetic testing. Further genetic counseling and testing may be warranted in individuals that have a change in their family history with a new diagnosis of breast or ovarian cancer, especially in a relative at a young age.

Risk Management in the Clinical Setting

Breast cancer risk management options should be tailored to a woman's level of breast cancer risk with an understanding of her anxiety as well as her therapeutic goals. A number of increased or high-risk categories can be identified for which individualized risk reduction and screening interventions are recommended:

1. High-risk women with a known or suspected genetic predisposition.
2. High-risk women with a history of radiation to the chest between 10 and 30 years of age or a personal history of AH or LCIS
3. Women identified as being at increased risk of breast cancer by BCRAT 5-year risk of 1.7% or greater.

Management options available to women identified as being at increased or high risk for breast cancer include earlier or more frequent screening with clinical breast examination (CBE), mammography and breast magnetic resonance imaging (MRI) as well as medical interventions such as selective estrogen receptor modulators (SERMSs, e.g., tamoxifen or raloxifene), aromatase inhibitors (AIs, e.g., anastrozole or exemestane) or risk-reducing surgery (e.g., bilateral prophylactic mastectomy [BPM] and risk-reducing salpingo-oophorectomy [RRSO]) to decrease breast cancer risk.

Women who are considered at increased risk may be particularly concerned about risk potentially posed by use of hormonal contraceptives and menopausal hormones. The link between hormones and breast cancer has been long established (see Chapter 15). Women considering HRT (estrogen alone or estrogen plus progesterone) need to carefully weigh the benefits against the risks. Because the benefits are commonly quality-of-life issues, the role of the clinician is to be sure that the woman fully understands alternative nonhormonal therapies to manage her symptoms. In counseling women about how hormones affect their cancer risk, some interesting facts emerge regarding the use of hormones in women with an intact uterus. The combination of estrogen and progesterone has been shown to increase breast cancer risk, whereas women taking estrogen alone do not have an increased risk of breast cancer.[32,33] However, those with an intact uterus who use unopposed estrogen have an increased risk of uterine cancer. This risk is negated by the addition of progesterone. The Million Women Study provides some information on the balance of the risk between these two cancers. Women with a uterus who took estrogen alone had fewer cancers (breast and uterine combined) than women who took progesterone in addition to estrogen.[34] Bottom line, either approach (estrogen alone or estrogen plus progesterone) increases the risk of developing a cancer. The decision is which cancer, breast or uterine, the woman (and the clinician) is willing to risk incurring. Clearly, the facts and the decisions are complex.

Risk Reduction Options Based on Level of Risk

Studies exploring whether modification of lifestyle factors can reduce breast cancer risk have yielded inconsistent findings. Because they can lead to better overall health and have been suggested to reduce breast cancer risk, healthy lifestyle changes are recommended for women at all risk levels.

American Institute of Cancer Research recommendations on nutrition to reduce cancer risk include the following[35]:

1. Be as lean as possible without becoming underweight.
2. Avoid sugary drinks. Limit consumption of energy-dense foods.
3. Eat more of a variety of vegetables, fruits, whole grains, and legumes such as beans.
4. Limit consumption of red meats (such as beef, pork, and lamb) and avoid processed meats.
5. If consumed at all, limit alcoholic drinks to 2 for men and 1 for women a day.
6. Limit consumption of salty foods and foods processed with salt (sodium).

American College of Sports Medicine recommendations on physical activity are[36]:

1. Aim for at least 150 minutes of moderate physical activity each week or 75 minutes of vigorous physical activity each week
2. Include muscle strengthening at least 2 days per week.

High-Risk Women Secondary to Premalignant Lesions and Elevated Gail Risk

Both SERMs and AIs have been shown to significantly reduce the risk of developing breast cancer. The evidence supporting their use is described in Chapter 16.

Tamoxifen is the only agent approved to reduce breast cancer risk in premenopausal women at increased risk of the disease.[37] Although both premenopausal and postmenopausal women obtained a similar reduction in their breast cancer risk with tamoxifen, the adverse events were increased only in women older than 50 years of age. Thus premenopausal women obtain the benefits of tamoxifen without incurring risks making this group of increased-risk women ideal candidates for preventive therapy.

Postmenopausal women now have a number of options. Tamoxifen and raloxifene provide similar breast cancer risk reduction while on therapy, but the benefits of tamoxifen are more durable once therapy has been discontinued.[9,38] Both agents reduce the risk of osteoporotic bone fractures equally, but only raloxifene is US Food and Drug Administration (FDA) approved for this indication. Raloxifene is associated with fewer risks than tamoxifen, especially for women with an intact uterus. For some women, the greater long-term risk reduction associated with tamoxifen makes it a more attractive option than raloxifene. Conversely, women desiring to reduce their breast cancer risk but incur minimal risks may elect raloxifene. Although not FDA approved for breast cancer risk reduction, 2 AIs (exemestane and anastrozole) have been shown in small trials to provide greater risk reduction with fewer serious risks than either tamoxifen or raloxifene for postmenopausal women.[39,40] Off-label prescription of these medications is an option for breast cancer risk reduction, especially for women with contraindications to the use of a SERM (e.g., prior thromboembolic event).

Women with AH or LCIS are at extremely high risk of developing breast cancer and their reduction in breast cancer risk with preventive therapy is substantial (e.g., a 75% long-term reduction in risk with tamoxifen in women with AH).[41] These women, absent an absolute contraindication to therapy, warrant prescription of preventive therapy. In other women at increased risk of breast cancer, the decision to initiate preventive therapy should be approached in a shared decision-making manner. The discussion should include a consideration of the individual's overall health status, an understanding of the absolute and relative breast cancer risk reduction achieved with the preventive intervention, and a thorough discussion of the risks of each suitable option with an emphasis on age-dependent risks and identification of any contraindications to therapy.

Before initiating risk reduction therapy, a review of the medical history should ascertain that there are no contraindications for use of the selected agent. This should include a history of deep vein thrombosis, pulmonary embolism, thrombotic stroke, or transient ischemic attack. Women on anticoagulant therapy are not appropriate candidates for risk reduction therapy. These agents should not be used in pregnant women or women planning to become pregnant. The current use of HRT is a contraindication to the use of any of these agents. An effective nonhormonal method of contraception should be used to prevent pregnancy in premenopausal women taking tamoxifen. Women with severe or worsening osteoporosis may not be optimal candidates for AI therapy.

Women on risk reduction therapy are typically seen every 6 months to monitor therapy and for recommended screening. At each visit, a symptom assessment should be performed. This includes inquiries about thromboembolic or gynecologic symptoms. Women taking tamoxifen should be educated about gynecologic symptoms and the need to promptly report any abnormal vaginal bleeding. Any abnormal vaginal bleeding should be evaluated with transvaginal sonography, endometrial biopsy, or other procedures as the clinical situation dictates. There is currently no indication for routine endometrial screening, either by transvaginal sonography or endometrial biopsy, of asymptomatic women taking tamoxifen. Women on AIs should be routinely monitored for the development of osteoporosis/osteopenia with bone mineral density testing.

The common side effects of preventive therapy have been well defined. Hot flashes can be associated with preventive therapy. They are more common in women near the age of menopause and in women who have just discontinued estrogen replacement therapy; however, hot flashes can occur in women of any age. They can usually be managed with education about avoidance of triggers (caffeine, spicy foods, alcohol, hot showers, etc.) and lifestyle changes (sleepwear should be cotton, not nylon; availability of fans and cold/ice water; etc.) because the symptoms diminish with time in most patients. Some patients report symptomatic relief with vitamin E or evening primrose oil.[42] Prescription medications that may be of benefit include paroxetine (Paxil) and venlafaxine (Effexor), which have been shown in randomized controlled trials to reduce the frequency and intensity of hot flashes.[42] The use of paroxetine in some women on tamoxifen may interfere in the metabolism of tamoxifen to the active metabolite endoxifen.[43] The clinical significance of this is uncertain. Other agents that may be of benefit in managing hot flashes include clonidine and gabapentin, a nighttime dosing of which may be helpful in women also experiencing problems with sleep.[42]

Women experiencing vaginal dryness are first managed with education and nonhormonal over-the-counter remedies (e.g., Astroglide, Replens). Estrogen creams should be avoided because of the sustained systemic absorption seen with such preparations. However, Estring, a slow-release estrogen vaginal ring, and Vagifem were allowed in the STAR trial. Arthralgias seen with the use of AIs can be managed with over-the-counter nonsteroidal antiinflammatory drugs.

High-Risk Women Secondary to Genetic Predisposition

Surgical options for women at substantially increased risk of breast cancer include BPM and RRSO (see Chapter 31). Although BPM is an aggressive surgical procedure with many physical and psychological ramifications, it confers a significant 90% risk reduction in women at high risk of breast cancer.[44,45] Prophylactic mastectomy should be undertaken only after extensive counseling so that the patient has a thorough understanding of her breast cancer risk and other available risk-reduction strategies. The irreversibility of the surgical procedure, options for breast reconstruction, and the effect of the procedure on body image and sexuality should be addressed. An important counseling point is the limitation of the procedure in regard to breast cancer risk reduction. Many women contemplating the procedure do so under the mistaken impression that by undergoing the prophylactic mastectomy, they have eliminated their risk of developing breast cancer. It is important to point out that the 90% risk reduction associated with this procedure means that a residual 10% risk of developing a breast cancer remains. For women contemplating risk reduction surgery, presurgical evaluations at comprehensive cancer centers are recommended. A multidisciplinary approach encompassing a breast surgeon, plastic surgeon, genetics professional, and psychologist helps ensure that patients fully understand their personal breast cancer risk and the potential benefits and harms of the risk-reducing surgery.

RRSO reduces the risk of breast cancer by about 53% to 68% and decreases the risk of ovarian cancer, which may be elevated in mutation carriers, by 80% to 95%.[46–51] The benefit is greater in women with *BRCA1* mutations.[48] If performed after age 40 years, the reduction in breast cancer risk is not as dramatic.[48] RRSO has implications on a woman's childbearing decision-making; for this reason, experts in reproductive health and gynecologic oncology should be involved in the decision-making process.

The benefits of risk reduction therapy in women with a known or suspected genetic predisposition are uncertain. Subset analyses of the Breast Cancer Prevention Trial (BCPT) participants were conducted to better understand potential benefits for women with a *BRCA1* or *BRCA2* gene mutation.[52] The findings demonstrated a nonsignificant reduction in the risk of developing breast cancer in women with *BRCA2* mutation (relative risk [RR] 0.38, 95% confidence interval [CI] 0.06–1.56), whereas no benefit was seen in women with *BRCA1* mutations (RR 1.67, 95% CI 0.32–10.70). Understanding that tamoxifen affects only hormone receptor–positive breast cancer and that women with *BRCA2* mutations are more likely to develop a hormone receptor–positive breast cancer than *BRCA1* mutation carriers is helpful in understanding the potential differences seen with tamoxifen in these two groups. In women that do not opt for BPM or RRSO, tamoxifen can be considered for risk reduction therapy, preferably in *BRCA2* carriers.

Risk-Based Screening Recommendations

Recommendations for breast cancer screening have been outlined in the NCCN Breast Cancer Screening and Diagnostic Guideline based on breast cancer risk category.[53] Women at increased risk may undergo more frequent screening with clinical examinations every 6 months, earlier initiation of mammographic screening, or supplemental screening with breast MRI.

Although most breast cancers are slow growing, women at increased or high risk of breast cancer are at risk for the development of an interval cancer because their tumors tend to be more aggressive than that seen in the general population. In addition, mammographic screening is known to be less sensitive in younger women when the breasts are more dense. The use of breast MRI as an added screening modality at alternating 6-month intervals with the annual mammogram may have added value for this population of women. The current American Cancer Society (ACS) recommendations for use of breast MRI as a screening test are outlined in Box 80.4.[54] Potential risks and benefits of breast MRI imaging should be reviewed with patients. As more is understood about the role of breast MRI, other populations that may benefit from this screening modality will likely be identified.

> ## • BOX 80.4 American Cancer Society Recommendations for Breast MRI Screening as an Adjunct to Mammography
>
> Recommend annual MRI screening (based on evidence[a])
> BRCA mutation
> First-degree relative of BRCA carrier, but untested
> Lifetime risk of approximately 20%–25% or greater, as defined by BRCAPRO or other models that are largely dependent on family history
> Recommend annual MRI screening (based on expert consensus opinion[b])
> Radiation to chest between age 10 and 30 years
> Li-Fraumeni syndrome and first-degree relatives
> Cowden and Bannayan-Riley-Ruvalcaba syndromes and first-degree relatives
> Insufficient evidence to recommend for or against MRI screening[c]
> Lifetime risk of 15%–20%, as defined by BRCAPRO or other models that are largely dependent on family history
> Lobular carcinoma in situ or atypical lobular hyperplasia
> Atypical ductal hyperplasia
> Heterogeneously or extremely dense breast on mammography
> Women with a personal history of breast cancer, including ductal carcinoma in situ
> Recommend against MRI screening (based on expert consensus opinion)
> Women at less than 15% lifetime risk
>
> [a]*Evidence from nonrandomized screening trials and observational studies.*
> [b]*Based on evidence of lifetime risk for breast cancer.*
> [c]*Payment should not be a barrier. Screening decisions should be made on a case-by-case basis, because there may be particular factors to support MRI. More data on these groups are expected to be published soon.*
> MRI, *Magnetic resonance imaging.*
> From Saslow D, Boetes C, Burke W, et al. American Cancer Society guidelines for breast screening with MRI as an adjunct to mammography. CA Cancer J Clin. 2007;57:75-89.

High-Risk Women Secondary to Elevated Gail Risk, Prior Thoracic Radiation at an Early Age, or Premalignant Lesions

In women with a BCRAT predicted 5-year breast cancer risk of 1.7% or greater, annual screening mammogram and CBE every 6 to 12 months should be started at the age of identified increased risk, unless other higher priority risks factors exist.[53]

Women who received thoracic radiation therapy between the ages of 10 to 30 years are at increased risk for developing breast cancer beginning 8 to 10 years after treatment. For this reason, the NCCN recommends that 8 to 10 years after radiation therapy, women obtain CBE every 6 to 12 months and annual screening mammograms alternating with screening breast MRIs. Although the CBE could be performed at younger ages, the imaging should not be initiated before 25 years of age.[53]

Women with AH or LCIS should have CBE every 6 to 12 months and annual screening mammograms from the time of diagnosis but not before age 30. On the basis of emerging evidence of substantial risk in this population of women, the NCCN states that breast MRI, beginning at diagnosis but not before age 30, may be a consideration for supplemental screening.[53] Because the ACS currently categorizes these women in the "insufficient evidence" category, there may be limitations on insurance coverage for MRI[54] (Box 80.4).

High-Risk Women Secondary to Known or Suspected Genetic Predisposition

NCCN guidelines for women with a known genetic predisposition recommend annual breast MRI beginning at age 25; beginning at age 30, annual screening mammograms are recommended.[55]

For women with a strong family history concerning for a genetic predisposition, CBE every 6 to 12 months and annual screening mammography alternating with breast MRI should begin 10 years before the age at diagnosis of the youngest breast cancer case, but not before age 30.[53]

Conclusions

Breast cancer risk assessment and management is now an integral part of the paradigm of breast cancer management. Because a significant portion of this activity takes place in the primary care setting, tools and educational materials should be used to facilitate the conduct of this activity in the clinical setting. Women with a gene mutation or a family history of concern for an inherited predisposition, prior thoracic radiation therapy, or high-risk lesions (AH or LCIS) have complex management issues and are best referred to a multidisciplinary breast program for care.

Selected References

10. National Cancer Institute: Breast cancer risk assessment tool. <http://www.cancer.gov/bcrisktool>. Accessed 21 November 2015.

11. The NCCN Clinical Practice Guidelines in Oncology (NCCN Guidelines®) Breast Cancer Risk Reduction (Version 2.2015). © 2015 National Comprehensive Cancer Network, Inc. < https://www.nccn.org/professionals/physician_gls/f_guidelines.asp>. Accessed 29 November 2015.

17. Hartmann LC, Radisky DC, Frost MH, et al. Understanding the premalignant potential of atypical hyperplasia through its natural history: a longitudinal cohort study. *Cancer Prev Res (Phila)*. 2014;7:211-217.

23. Tyrer J, Duffy S, Cuzick J. A breast cancer prediction model incorporating familial and personal risk factors. *Statist Med*. 2004;23:1111-1130.

38. Vogel VG, Costantino JP, Wickerham DL, et al. Update of the NSABP Study of Tamoxifen and Raloxifene (STAR) P-2 Trial: Preventing Breast Cancer. *Cancer Prev Research*. 2010;3:696-706.

41. Fisher B, Costantino JP, Wickerham DL, et al. Tamoxifen for the prevention of breast cancer: current status of the National Surgical Adjuvant Breast and Bowel Project P-1 study. *J Natl Cancer Inst*. 2005;97:1652-1662.

53. The NCCN Clinical Practice Guidelines in Oncology (NCCN Guidelines®) Breast Cancer Screening and Diagnosis (Version 2.2015). © 2015 National Comprehensive Cancer Network, Inc. <https://www.nccn.org/professionals/physician_gls/f_guidelines.asp>. Accessed 29 November 2015.

54. Saslow D, Boetes C, Burke W, et al. American Cancer Society guidelines for breast screening with MRI as an adjunct to mammography. *CA Cancer J Clin*. 2007;57:75-89.

55. The NCCN Clinical Practice Guidelines in Oncology (NCCN Guidelines®) Genetic/Familial High-Risk Assessment: Breast and Ovarian (Version 2.2015). © 2015 National Comprehensive Cancer Network, Inc. <https://www.nccn.org/professionals/physician_gls/f_guidelines.asp>. Accessed 29 November 2015.

A full reference list is available online at ExpertConsult.com.

81

General Considerations for Follow-Up

ISSAM MAKHOUL, RAJESH BANDERUDRAPPAGARI, AND ANGELA PENNISI

Most women treated for early-stage breast cancer will be long-term survivors. In 2016 more than 3.5 million breast cancer survivors were expected in the United States alone and millions more worldwide.[1] Breast cancer and its treatment can have a heavy impact on a woman's physical, psychological, social, vocational, and spiritual well-being beyond the immediate time frame of active therapy. After treatment of breast cancer, regular follow-up with a health care provider is prudent to ensure prompt recognition of recurrences or second primary cancers as well as to adequately assess for complications of treatment, foster adherence to recommended therapy and screening, and provide psychosocial and decision-making support. Relatively few studies have evaluated the risks and benefits, let alone cost-effectiveness, of surveillance and intervention modalities in breast cancer survivors. Nevertheless, several recommendations can be made based on available evidence and expert consensus. Box 81.1 details current recommendations for standard follow-up care based on an evidence-based review conducted by an expert panel convened by the American Society of Clinical Oncology (ASCO) and the American Cancer Society (ACS).[2] These recommendations can also be adopted for men with a history of breast cancer, recognizing that data are limited in this population.

Surveillance for Locoregional Recurrences or New Primary Disease

Monitoring for local recurrence or for development of a new primary breast cancer is an important component of follow-up care for breast cancer survivors. Unlike the rate of distant metastases, which peaks in the second year after diagnosis at 5% then it declined progressively until the eighth year, the rate of local recurrences remains steady for up to 10 years at 1% per year, especially with hormone receptor–positive disease.[3–5] Risk factors include young age, lymphovascular invasion, multicentricity, and more advanced stage.[6–8] In a meta-analysis of 12 studies with a total of 5045 women who underwent a mix of local and systemic therapies, more extensive lymph node involvement and more advanced stage of disease were associated with the 378 locoregional recurrences reported.[7] Several studies have revealed the association between young age and increased risk of local recurrence. In one trial testing the utility of boost radiation, younger women were found to have higher risk of recurrence, with the absolute benefit from the addition of a boost found to be the greatest in the youngest patients. At 10 years' median follow-up, boost radiation reduced risk of recurrence from 23.9% to 13.5% in those younger than 40 years of age, from 12.5% to 8.7% in those 41 to 50 years of age, and from 7.8% to 4.9% in those 51 to 61 years of age, and from 7.3% to 3.8% in those older than 60 years of age.[8] The impact of patient age (≤45 years vs. >45 years) and the type of surgery were evaluated in a cohort of 813 Danish lymph node–negative breast cancer patients diagnosed between 1989 and 1998 and treated with mastectomy ($n = 515$) or breast conservation therapy (BCT; lumpectomy with whole-breast radiation therapy; $n = 298$) and no adjuvant systemic treatment. Twenty-year local recurrence (LR) risk was 20% and developed throughout the entire 20-year period after BCT, whereas LR after mastectomy was 8.7% and developed within the first 10 years after mastectomy. Younger patients' 20-year LR risk was higher than older patients' (19% vs. 5%, $p < .001$) and was significantly associated with distant metastasis (DM; hazard ratio [HR] = 2.7, 95% confidence interval [CI] 1.8–4.2) and 20-year breast cancer mortality (HR = 2.7, 95% CI 1.7–4.4). BCT was associated with higher 20-year breast cancer mortality (HR = 1.5, 95% CI 1.0–2.4) and higher 20-year all-cause mortality (HR = 1.7, 95% CI 1.2–2.5) than mastectomy. In older patients, LR was not associated with DM, and breast cancer mortality was similar for BCT and mastectomy.[9]

LRs, which account for only 10% to 30% of recurrences, are associated with reduced survival, especially in younger patients.[9–11] The risk of death from breast cancer after ipsilateral breast tumor recurrence (IBTR) depends on the initial stage at diagnosis, with 15-year breast cancer mortality rate being at 16% for women with ductal carcinoma in situ, 32% for women with stage I, and 59% for women with stage II breast cancer.[12] Several types of IBTR were described on the basis of the distance from the primary lumpectomy scar, the presence of in situ tumor, and the margin status.[13] IBTRs close to the scar with in situ lesions and a negative surgical margin of the primary cancer behave as new primaries (NP) by this classification and have a distant disease–free survival similar to that of new primaries away from the scar or in the opposite breast. In contrast, IBTRs that occur close to the scar without in situ lesions (true recurrence) had significantly poorer prognosis than NP (Table 81.1).

However, it is not known whether earlier detection of recurrences lengthens life for these patients. Locoregional recurrences

• BOX 81.1 2016 ASCO and ACS Recommendations for Follow-Up for Breast Cancer Survivors

Target population: Female adult breast cancer survivors

Target audience: Primary care providers, medical oncologists, radiation oncologists, and other clinicians caring for breast cancer survivors

Methods: An expert panel was convened to develop clinical practice guideline recommendations based on a systematic review of the medical literature

Surveillance for Breast Cancer Recurrence

History and Physical Examination

Recommendation 1.1: It is recommended that primary care clinicians (a) should individualize clinical follow-up care provided to breast cancer survivors based on age, specific diagnosis, and treatment protocol and as recommended by the treating oncology team (LOE = 2A); and (b) should make sure the patient receives a detailed cancer-related history and physical examination every 3–6 months for the first 3 years after primary therapy, every 6–12 months for the next 2 years, and annually thereafter (LOE = 2A).

Screening the Breast for Local Recurrence or a New Primary Breast Cancer

Recommendation 1.2: It is recommended that primary care clinicians (a) should refer women who have received a unilateral mastectomy for annual mammography on the intact breast and, for those with lumpectomies, an annual mammography of both breasts (LOE = 2A); and (b) should not refer for routine screening with MRI of the breast unless the patient meets high-risk criteria for increased breast cancer surveillance as per ACS guidelines (LOE = 2A).

Laboratory Tests and Imaging

Recommendation 1.3: It is recommended that primary care clinicians should not offer routine laboratory tests or imaging, except mammography if indicated, for the detection of disease recurrence in the absence of symptoms (LOE = 2A).

Signs of Recurrence

Recommendation 1.4: It is recommended that primary care clinicians should educate and counsel all women about the signs and symptoms of local or regional recurrence (LOE = 2A).

Risk Evaluation and Genetic Counseling

Recommendation 1.5: It is recommended that primary care clinicians (a) should assess the patient's cancer family history; and (b) should offer genetic counseling if potential hereditary risk factors are suspected (e.g., women with a strong family history of cancer [breast, colon, endometrial] or age 60 years or younger with triple-negative breast cancer; LOE = 2A).

Endocrine Treatment Impacts, Symptom Management

Recommendation 1.6: It is recommended that primary care clinicians should counsel patients to adhere to adjuvant endocrine (antiestrogen) therapy (LOE = 2A).

Screening for Second Primary Cancers

Cancer Screenings in the Average-Risk Patient

Recommendation 2.1: It is recommended that primary care clinicians (a) should screen for other cancers as they would for patients in the general population; and (b) should provide an annual gynecologic assessment for postmenopausal women on selective estrogen receptor modulator therapies.

Assessment and Management of Physical and Psychosocial Long-Term and Late Effects of Breast Cancer and Treatment

Body Image Concerns

Recommendation 3.1: It is recommended that primary care clinicians (a) should assess for patient body image/appearance concerns (LOE = 0); (b) should offer the option of adaptive devices (e.g., breast prostheses, wigs) and/or surgery when appropriate (LOE = 0); and (c) should refer for psychosocial care as indicated (LOE = IA).

Lymphedema

Recommendation 3.2: It is recommended that primary care clinicians (a) should counsel survivors on how to prevent/reduce the risk of lymphedema, including weight loss for those who are overweight or obese (LOE = 0); and (b) should refer patients with clinical symptoms or swelling suggestive of lymphedema to a therapist knowledgeable about the diagnosis and treatment of lymphedema, such as a physical therapist, occupational therapist, or lymphedema specialist (LOE = 0).

Cardiotoxicity

Recommendation 3.3: It is recommended that primary care clinicians (a) should monitor lipid levels and provide cardiovascular monitoring, as indicated (LOE = 0); and (b) should educate breast cancer survivors on healthy lifestyle modifications, potential cardiac risk factors, and when to report relevant symptoms (shortness of breath or fatigue) to their health care provider (LOE = I).

Cognitive Impairment

Recommendation 3.4: It is recommended that primary care clinicians (a) should ask patients if they are experiencing cognitive difficulties (LOE = 0); (b) should assess for reversible contributing factors of cognitive impairment and optimally treat when possible (LOE = IA); and (c) should refer patients with signs of cognitive impairment for neurocognitive assessment and rehabilitation, including group cognitive training if available (LOE = IA).

Distress, Depression, Anxiety

Recommendation 3.5: It is recommended that primary care clinicians (a) should assess patients for distress, depression, and/or anxiety (LOE = I); (b) should conduct a more probing assessment for patients at a higher risk of depression (e.g., young patients, those with a history of prior psychiatric disease, and patients with low socioeconomic status; LOE = III); and (c) should offer in-office counseling and/or pharmacotherapy and/or refer to appropriate psycho-oncology and mental health resources as clinically indicated if signs of distress, depression, or anxiety are present (LOE = I).

Fatigue

Recommendation 3.6: It is recommended that primary care clinicians (a) should assess for fatigue and treat any causative factors for fatigue, including anemia, thyroid dysfunction, and cardiac dysfunction (LOE = 0); (b) should offer treatment or referral for factors that may impact fatigue (e.g., mood disorders, sleep disturbance, pain, etc) for those who do not have an otherwise identifiable cause of fatigue (LOE = I); and (c) should counsel patients to engage in regular physical activity and refer for cognitive behavioral therapy as appropriate (LOE = I).

Bone Health

Recommendation 3.7: It is recommended that primary care clinicians (a) should refer postmenopausal breast cancer survivors for a baseline DEXA scan (LOE = 0); and (b) should refer for repeat DEXA scans every 2 years for women taking an aromatase inhibitor, premenopausal women taking tamoxifen and/or a GnRH agonist, and women who have chemotherapy-induced, premature menopause (LOE = 0).

Musculoskeletal Health

Recommendation 3.8: It is recommended that primary care clinicians (a) should assess for musculoskeletal symptoms, including pain, by asking patients about their symptoms at each clinical encounter (LOE = 0); and (b) should offer one or more of the following interventions based on clinical indication: acupuncture, physical activity, and referral for physical therapy or rehabilitation (LOE = III).

Pain and Neuropathy

Recommendation 3.9: It is recommended that primary care clinicians (a) should assess for pain and contributing factors for pain with the use of a simple pain scale and comprehensive history of the patient's complaint (LOE = 0); (b) should offer interventions, such as acetaminophen, nonsteroidal

• BOX 81.1 2016 ASCO and ACS Recommendations for Follow-Up for Breast Cancer Survivors—cont'd

anti-inflammatory drugs, physical activity, and/or acupuncture, for pain (LOE = I); (c) should refer to an appropriate specialist, depending on the etiology of the pain once the underlying etiology has been determined (e.g., lymphedema specialist, occupational therapist, etc; LOE = 0); (d) should assess for peripheral neuropathy and contributing factors for peripheral neuropathy by asking the patient about their symptoms, specifically numbness and tingling in their hands and/or feet, and the characteristics of the symptoms (LOE = 0); (e) should offer physical activity for neuropathy; and (f) should offer duloxetine for patients with neuropathic pain, numbness, and tingling (LOE = IB).

Infertility
Recommendation 3.10: It is recommended that primary care clinicians should refer survivors of childbearing age who experience infertility to a specialist in reproductive endocrinology and infertility as soon as possible (LOE = 0).

Sexual Health
Recommendation 3.11: It is recommended that primary care clinicians (a) should assess for signs and symptoms of sexual dysfunction or problems with sexual intimacy (LOE = 0); (b) should assess for reversible contributing factors to sexual dysfunction and treat, when appropriate (LOE = 0); (c) should offer nonhormonal, water-based lubricants and moisturizers for vaginal dryness (LOE = IA); and (d) should refer for psychoeducational support, group therapy, sexual counseling, marital counseling, or intensive psychotherapy when appropriate (LOE = IA).

Premature Menopause/Hot Flashes
Recommendation 3.12: It is recommended that primary care clinicians should offer selective serotonin-norepinephrine reuptake inhibitors, selective serotonin reuptake inhibitors, gabapentin, lifestyle modifications, and/or environmental modifications to help mitigate vasomotor symptoms of premature menopausal symptoms (LOE = IA).

Health Promotion
Information
Recommendation 4.1: It is recommended that primary care clinicians (a) should assess the information needs of the patient related to breast cancer and its treatment, side effects, other health concerns, and available support services (LOE = 0); and (b) should provide or refer survivors to appropriate resources to meet these needs (LOE = 0).

Obesity
Recommendation 4.2: It is recommended that primary care clinicians (a) should counsel survivors to achieve and maintain a healthy weight (LOE = III); and (b) should counsel survivors if overweight or obese to limit consumption of high-calorie foods and beverages and increase physical activity to promote and maintain weight loss (LOE = IA, III).

Physical Activity
Recommendation 4.3: It is recommended that primary care clinicians should counsel survivors to engage in regular physical activity consistent with the

ACS guideline[a] and specifically: (a) should avoid inactivity and return to normal daily activities as soon as possible after diagnosis (LOE = III); (b) should aim for at least 150 minutes of moderate or 75 minutes of vigorous aerobic exercise per week (LOE = I, IA); and (c) should include strength training exercises at least 2 days per week and emphasize strength training for women treated with adjuvant chemotherapy or hormone therapy (LOE = IA).

Nutrition
Recommendation 4.4: It is recommended that primary care clinicians should counsel survivors to achieve a dietary pattern that is high in vegetables, fruits, whole grains, and legumes; low in saturated fats; and limited in alcohol consumption (LOE = IA, III).

Smoking Cessation
Recommendation 4.5: It is recommended that primary care clinicians should counsel survivors to avoid smoking and refer survivors who smoke to cessation counseling and resources (LOE = I).

Care Coordination/Practice Implications
Survivorship Care Plan
Recommendation 5.1: It is recommended that primary care clinicians should consult with the cancer treatment team and obtain a treatment summary and survivorship care plan (LOE = 0, III).

Communication With Oncology Team
Recommendation 5.2: It is recommended that primary care clinicians should maintain communication with the oncology team throughout the patient's diagnosis, treatment, and posttreatment care to ensure care is evidence-based and well-coordinated (LOE = 0).

Inclusion of Family
Recommendation 5.3: It is recommended that primary care clinicians should encourage the inclusion of caregivers, spouses, or partners in usual breast cancer survivorship care and support (LOE = 0).

Additional Resources
More information, including a data supplement with additional evidence tables, is available with the online version of this article at asco.org/guidelines/breastsurvivorship and asco.org/guidelineswiki; patient information is available at onlinelibrary.wiley.com/doi/10.3322/caac.21319/pdf; journal-based continuing education is available at acsjournals.com/ce

[a]Rock CL, Doyle C, Demark-Wahnefried W, et al. Nutrition and physical activity guidelines for cancer survivors. CA Cancer J Clin. 2012;62:243-274.
ACS, American Cancer Society; ASCO, American Society of Clinical Oncology; DEXA, dual-energy x-ray absorptiometry; GnRH, gonadotropin-releasing hormone; LOE, level of evidence.
From Runowicz CD, Leach CR, Henry NL, et al. American Cancer Society/American Society of Clinical Oncology breast cancer survivorship care guideline. CA Cancer J Clin. 2016;66:43-73.

---

reflect either that the primary therapy failed to eradicate the cancer (in the majority of cases) or that, because of a predisposition, whether due to genetics or environmental exposure, an entirely new cancer has developed in the residual breast tissue. Patients with chest wall recurrences after mastectomy have very poor prognoses. After lumpectomy, new primaries are more likely in those who have *BRCA1* or *BRCA2* mutations, younger age at diagnosis, and possibly in those with lobular histology.[14-16] Patients who have developed breast cancer after exposure to ionizing radiation (e.g., therapeutic mantle irradiation for Hodgkin disease) also carry a higher risk of new primary cancers in the radiation field. For the average breast cancer survivor, the risk of new contralateral breast cancer is doubled, making absolute risk 0.5% to 1% per

year, which is reduced in women who receive adjuvant endocrine therapy. This risk is higher in premenopausal than postmenopausal women.[17]

Given the evidence of benefit of screening mammography in lower risk women, annual mammogram of remaining breast tissue combined with regular history and physical examination is recommended for surveillance for locoregional recurrence and new primary disease in breast cancer survivors.[18] Despite this recommendation, in a study of 391 women with early-stage breast cancer in Los Angeles; Washington, DC; and Kansas, it was found that 40% did not get a mammogram in the year after diagnosis.[19]

There has been interest in breast magnetic resonance imaging (MRI) in survivors. In a study of 969 women with a recent

TABLE 81.1	Classification of Ipsilateral Breast Tumor Recurrences (IBTRs)		
	Surgical Margin of Primary Cancer	In Situ Lesion of IBTR	Cause of IBTR
IBTR occurred far from primary lumpectomy scar (FS group)	+/–	+	NP
	+/–	–	TR
	–	+	NP
IBTR occurred close to primary lumpectomy scar (CS group)	+	–	TR
		–	TR

CS, Close to the Scar group; FS, Far from the Scar group; NP, new primary; TR, tumor recurrence.

Modified from Sakai T, Nishimura S, Ogiya A, et al. Four types of ipsilateral breast tumor recurrence (IBTR) after breast-conserving surgery: classification of IBTR based on precise pathological examination. *Pathol Int.* 2015;65:113-118.

TABLE 81.2	American Cancer Society Recommendations for Breast Magnetic Resonance Imaging (MRI) in General Population	
Level of Recommendation for Annual MRI Screening	Population	
Insufficient evidence to recommend[a]	Personal history of breast cancer. Heterogeneously or extremely dense breast on mammography	
Yes, based on evidence[b]	BRCA mutation, first-degree relative of BRCA carrier (herself untested). Lifetime risk 20%–25% of breast cancer	
Yes, based on expert opinion[c]	Radiation to chest between 10 and 30 y of age. Li-Fraumeni, Cowden, and Bannayan-Riley-Ruvalcaba syndromes, as well as first-degree relatives with other rare genetic syndromes	
No, based on expert opinion	Women at <15% lifetime risk of breast cancer	

[a]Payment should not be a barrier. Screening decisions should be made on a case-by-case basis.
[b]Evidence from nonrandomized screening trials and observational studies.
[c]Based on evidence of lifetime risk for breast cancer.
From Saslow D, Boetes C, Burke W, et al. American Cancer Society guidelines for breast screening with MRI as an adjunct to mammography. *CA Cancer J Clin.* 2007;57:75-89.

diagnosis of unilateral breast cancer without mammographic or clinical evidence of contralateral disease, breast MRI detected contralateral cancer in 30 women (3.1%). However, biopsies were conducted in 121 women, 75% of which were negative for cancer (9% of total number of women screened).[20] There is no evidence that early detection with MRI improves outcomes, and false-positive findings using this expensive technology may be associated with significant physical and psychological morbidity. For women who are at greater than 20% risk of new primary disease, such as women with predisposing genetic mutation (e.g., *BRCA1* or *BRCA2*) or history of radiation to the chest, MRI screening is recommended (Table 81.2).[21] MRI may also be considered for women with dense breasts and for those whose initial breast cancer was not seen on mammography, although there are no data to suggest that a woman whose first cancer was missed by mammography will have a second that is missed by mammography or that survival will be improved by MRI surveillance.[22] The lack of evidence for benefit of MRI for early detection of future locoregional breast cancer events precludes recommending it as a standard surveillance modality in follow-up for average risk patients.

The utility of high-resolution ultrasound (US) suffers from operator dependence, but one small study (27 patients) suggested a benefit when suspicious lesions are detected by examination or mammogram.[23] When used in routine screening, US led to comparable cancer detection rate to mammography, with a greater proportion of invasive and node-negative cancers among US detections. However, false positives were more common with US screening.[24] The addition of US to mammography in the evaluation of 2809 women, with at least heterogeneously dense breast tissue, yielded an additional 1.1 to 7.2 cancers per 1000 high-risk women, but it also increased the number of false positives.[25] Hence, US should not be used in routine evaluation of woman with average risk. Recently tomosynthesis in combination with digital mammogram was associated with a decrease in recall rate and an increase in cancer detection rate and should be offered to patients whenever available.[26]

Although breast self-examination did not improve survival in a large randomized study of unscreened healthy Chinese women, the efficacy of breast self-examination in survivors has not been rigorously evaluated.[27] In light of the fact that the majority of locoregional recurrences are detected first by the patient herself, it is generally recommended that survivors consider regular breast self-examination, and at a minimum, be familiar with their own breasts and chest wall in order to be able to bring any concerns or changes to the attention of a health care provider.[7]

The ASCO and the ACS updated their guidelines for follow-up of breast cancer survivors[2] (see Box 81.1). Similar recommendations were suggested by the second international consensus guidelines for breast cancer in young women.[28]

Detecting Distant Relapse

Distant relapse is more common than locoregional recurrence or second primary cancers.[10] The occurrence of a distant relapse implies that the cancer had already spread by hematogenous, lymphatic, or serosal routes beyond the breast before definitive locoregional therapy, and that it was resistant to adjuvant therapy. Conventional predictors of risk of distant recurrence are similar to those for locoregional recurrence and include more advanced stage, higher grade and other markers of increased proliferation rate, hormone receptor negativity, HER2 positivity (although this is less clear now with the advent of trastuzumab adjuvant therapy), and younger age at diagnosis.[29] More recently, evaluation of genetic signatures has provided additional prognostic and predictive information in some settings.[30,31] Rates of distant recurrence are highest in the first few years after diagnosis but continue for at least 15 years, particularly for women with hormone receptor–positive disease.[5,32] One study of 647 patients with stage II or III breast cancer found that the hazard curve for recurrence peaked at 3 years then fell abruptly for estrogen receptor (ER)-negative disease, but for ER-positive disease, peak recurrence rate was at 4 years and decline thereafter was slow.[4] Specifically, 1-, 3-, 5-, and 10-year hazard rates for recurrence for ER-negative disease were 0.10, 0.10, 0.05, and 0.02, whereas rates for ER-positive disease were 0.05, 0.08, 0.06, and 0.03. Subtypes of breast cancer are also associated with location of recurrence. For example, HER2-positive metastatic disease is more likely to recur in the viscera and the central nervous system, whereas ER-positive recurrences are more likely to involve the bones, and lobular carcinomas may preferentially recur at serosal surfaces.[33–35] ER-negative relapses tend to be visceral.[4]

The majority of distant recurrences are detected by regular clinical evaluation (history and physical examination) or by patient reporting of symptoms prompting evaluation.[36,37] When a patient reports new bone pain, dyspnea, jaundice, neurologic complaints, or any other symptom that may be attributable to metastatic disease, prompt evaluation for recurrence should be undertaken. The particular imaging used should be targeted to the symptom of concern. For example, in the setting of bone pain, a bone scan is a reasonable first step. If findings are suspicious of recurrent disease, additional imaging such as a chest, abdomen, and pelvic computed tomography (CT) scan or a positron emission tomography (PET)/CT can be done to assess the full burden of disease and evaluate for an optimal site to biopsy for confirmation of the diagnosis if possible. Blood work to evaluate for organ dysfunction should include complete blood count, chemistries including calcium, and liver function tests. When locoregional recurrence is detected, regardless of additional symptoms, thorough clinical staging is appropriate to assess for metastatic disease as the risk of synchronous metastatic disease is significant in this setting. In a medical record review of 2233 women treated in Milan in the 1970s and 1980s, local recurrence was found to be a risk factor for distant recurrence, especially when the local recurrence occurred in the first 2 years after diagnosis.[3] In one older study, CT scanning of the chest revealed occult intrathoracic metastases in two-thirds of those with locoregional recurrence.[38]

Two large randomized trials conducted in Italy have evaluated whether early diagnosis of metastatic disease affects survival.[36,37] In the Interdisciplinary Group for Cancer Care Evaluation (GIVIO) study, 1300 women were randomized to receive either standard follow-up consisting of yearly mammograms as well as physical examinations every 3 months for 2 years and then every 6 months for the next 3 years or to receive standard follow-up plus blood tests at the time of each physical examination, annual bone scan and liver US, and chest x-ray every 6 months for 2 years and then annually. No difference was found between the groups in overall survival, disease-free survival, or health-related quality of life.[36] In the second multicenter trial, 1243 women were randomized to either a control group that received the same standard follow-up procedures as in the GIVIO trial or to an intervention group that underwent screening chest x-ray and bone scan every 6 months in addition to standard follow-up. No difference was found in disease-free or overall survival between the two groups.[37] A recent meta-analysis of five randomized trials involving a total of 4023 women supports these findings. None of these trials used newer imaging techniques such as CT or MRI, however, and none followed tumor markers. As more effective therapies for metastatic breast cancer (e.g., trastuzumab, aromatase inhibitors [AIs], and taxanes) are introduced into practice, it will be important to reinvestigate the role of more intensive imaging in the follow-up period. Modern imaging modality may allow early detection of

relapse at a time when tumor burden is still small, which may help improve overall survival (OS) of these patients. Gioia and coworkers studied 813 patients with MRI and/or PET/CT and tumor markers (CEA and CA15-3) and were able to detect 29 MBC, 7 of which (24.1%) with limited disease (≤3 metastases to a single organ). Comparing overall survival in accordance to extent of MBC, the 3- and 5-year overall survival of patients with limited disease were 71.4% and 53.6%, and those with disseminated disease (56.7%) and (34.8%), respectively, but this difference was not significant.[39]

At present, patients can be educated regarding the fact that any diagnostic test or procedure carries not only cost but also the 10% to 50% possibility of false-positive results, with ensuing anxiety, expense, and risk of complications from subsequent investigation.[18] Therefore, routine screening for distant recurrence with imaging or blood work is not recommended, but patients are encouraged to report new symptoms.

Managing Long-Term and Late Effects of Cancer Treatment

The diagnosis of breast cancer and subsequent treatment may result in substantial long-term and late medical and psychosocial repercussions for survivors. Table 81.3 lists common late effects after surgery, radiation, and/or systemic therapy for early breast cancer. With careful follow-up, awareness, and attention to potential complications, patient health and comfort may be optimized, and psychological distress may be minimized. There are limited data regarding many of these potential sequelae of breast cancer therapy, particularly in the very long term and in younger patients, making survivorship research a priority for this population.

Lymphedema and Other Local Sequelae

Lymphedema of the upper extremity is a sequela of ipsilateral breast irradiation and of axillary surgery. Some women also suffer persistent chest wall pain after mastectomy, as well as continuing local difficulties subsequent to breast reconstruction. The risk of implant infection or skin breakdown declines over time, but discomfort may persist. Risk of lymphedema rises with increasing intensity of axillary surgery or radiation, obesity, and trauma to the arm.[40–42] With the advent of sentinel node biopsies allowing many women to forgo full axillary dissections, the incidence of significant lymphedema has decreased. In the American College of Surgeons Oncology Group Z0011 prospective trial randomizing clinically node-negative women with positive sentinel lymph node biopsies to axillary dissection or no axillary dissection, there were higher rates of wound infections ($p = .0016$), axillary seromas ($p = .0001$), paresthesias ($p = .0001$), and lymphedema ($p = .0001$) in the group that received full axillary dissection. Reported 12-month rates of subjective lymphedema were 2% in those who underwent only sentinel node biopsy and 13% in those who also underwent full axillary dissection.[43] By arm measurement, 12-month lymphedema rates were 6% versus 11%, respectively, again favoring sentinel node biopsy alone. The advent of a novel procedure that spares the lymph nodes draining the arm, Axillary reverse mapping (ARM), is promising for further decrease in the risk of lymphedema without compromising the quality of the evaluation of axillary lymph nodes.[44] Other investigators were not able to confirm these results, however.[45]

| TABLE 81.3 | Common Long-Term and Late Effects of Breast Cancer Treatment |

Effect	Management Options
Surgical	
Cosmetic effects	Plastic surgery
Functional disability of arm or chest wall, pain	Physical therapy
Scarring/adhesions	Plastic surgery
Lymphedema	Physical therapy, avoid trauma to involved arm
Radiation	
Second malignancies	Image masses arising near radiation field
Xerophthalmia, cataracts	Regular visits to ophthalmologist
Hypothyroidism	Check thyroid-stimulating hormone if symptoms of hypothyroidism
Pneumonitis, pulmonary fibrosis	Symptomatic management
Cardiac damage	Lifestyle risk reduction (diet, exercise)
Lymphedema	As above
Systemic Therapy	
Second malignancies (myelodysplasia and leukemia)	Check complete blood count if symptoms of leukemia arise
Ototoxicity (e.g., cisplatin)	Symptomatic management
Cardiomyopathy (e.g., anthracyclines)	Symptomatic management
Renal toxicity (e.g., cisplatin)	Symptomatic management
Premature menopause and infertility (e.g., alkylating agents)	Referral to infertility specialist
Menopausal symptoms and sexual dysfunction	SSRI, SSNRI, gabapentin, counseling
Osteoporosis (e.g., hormonal therapy, chemotherapy)	Calcium, vitamin D, exercise, bisphosphonate
Neuropathy (e.g., taxanes and platinums)	Symptomatic management
Cognitive dysfunction, weight gain, fatigue	Exercise, rule out depression and anemia

SSNRI, Selective serotonin norepinephrine reuptake inhibitor; *SSRI,* selective serotonin reuptake inhibitor.

From Hayes DF. Clinical practice. Follow-up of patients with early breast cancer. *N Engl J Med.* 2007;356:2505-2513.

Management of lymphedema may include elevation of an affected body part, compression garments, massage and physical therapies, and, more rarely, surgery and diuretics.[46] Before beginning any treatment for lymphedema, it is important to consider and evaluate for the possibility of tumor recurrence, infection, or venous thrombosis in the axilla. To minimize the chances of lymphedema, protection of the affected limb from infection, compression, venipuncture, exposure to intense heat, and abrasion may be prudent, although the utility of such measures has not been formally evaluated.[47] Furthermore, because obesity is a risk factor for lymphedema, maintenance of a healthy weight and weight loss as needed may prevent or treat lymphedema. Ongoing studies are evaluating the role of local compression (i.e., compression sleeves) and exercise for lymphedema prevention.

Osteoporosis

Postmenopausal women on AIs and premenopausal women who become amenorrheic due to chemotherapy or who are receiving hormonal therapy are at risk for osteoporosis. In a randomized trial of exemestane versus placebo in 147 postmenopausal women with early breast cancer, the femoral neck bone density loss was 2.72% per year in the exemestane group and only 1.48% per year in the placebo group.[48] In the National Cancer Institute of Canada Clinical Trials Group MA.17 trial of letrozole versus placebo after 5 years of tamoxifen, prevalence of lumbar spine osteoporosis after 2 years was 4.1% in those receiving letrozole versus 0% in those on placebo ($p = .064$), but these results are confounded by the fact that more women in the placebo group were treated with bisphosphonates.[49] In the Anastrozole and Tamoxifen Alone or in Combination (ATAC) trial, median 5-year changes in lumbar spine bone mineral density were −6.08% in the anastrozole group and +2.77% in the tamoxifen group.[50]

Although tamoxifen appears to improve bone density in postmenopausal women via its proestrogenic effects, in premenopausal women, it has been associated with decreased bone mineral density.[51] Ovarian suppression reduces bone mineral density in premenopausal women as well.[52] However, the clinical significance of reduced bone mineral density in premenopausal women remains unclear because most studies have been done in the postmenopausal population. It has been recommended that bone density be monitored in survivors at risk for osteoporosis at baseline and every 1 to 2 years, although definitive evidence regarding the optimal frequency of monitoring is not available.[53] Lifestyle modifications, including weight-bearing exercise, smoking cessation, and supplementation of dietary calcium and vitamin D, are also recommended for those at risk for osteopenia.

Bisphosphonate (BP) therapy has been demonstrated not only to reduce fractures in those with osteoporosis but also to limit bone loss in patients with normal bone mineral density who are starting on AIs.[54] It is standard of care that anyone with osteoporosis receives bisphosphonate therapy, but prophylactic bisphosphonate treatment for those on AIs is more controversial because of the potential side effects, including jaw osteonecrosis.[55] Despite encouraging results in postmenopausal or ovarian-suppressed women from many clinical trials suggesting a protective effect of BPs against recurrent or new primary breast cancer, they have not become widely used.[56,57] The use of oral BP in women treated with tamoxifen showed no protective effect in a large database from Kaiser Permanente.[58] Another large database study showed improvement in breast cancer–specific survival in postmenopausal women who used oral BP for at least 18 months after the diagnosis of breast cancer.[59] The role of BP was reviewed by the Early Breast Cancer Trialists' Collaborative Group (EBCTCG) in a meta-analysis that included 26 trials and

18,766 participants. Using BP therapy had no apparent effect on any outcome in premenopausal women, but among 11,767 postmenopausal women, it produced significant reductions in recurrence (relative risk [RR] 0.86, 95% CI 0.78–0.94; $2p = .002$), distant recurrence (0.82, 0.74–0.92; $2p = .0003$), bone recurrence (0.72, 0.60–0.86; $2p = .0002$), and breast cancer mortality (.82, 0.73–0.93; $2p = .002$).[60] On the basis of these data, a panel of European experts recommended the use of BP (intravenous zoledronic acid or oral clodronate) in postmenopausal women as a part of the adjuvant therapy for early-stage breast cancer, but no similar recommendations have been made in the United States to date.[61]

Although raloxifene, a selective estrogen receptor modulator like tamoxifen, is used to prevent and treat osteoporosis in women without breast cancer and also to prevent breast cancer in those who have never previously been afflicted, it is not used in breast cancer survivors because it has not proven as effective as tamoxifen in treating breast cancer.[62] Furthermore, raloxifene is not used in conjunction with tamoxifen because its action is so similar and may interfere with benefits or exacerbate risks of tamoxifen.

Musculoskeletal Complaints

Chemotherapy-induced neuropathy (CINP) is common during and after treatment with taxanes or platinum agents. Permanent hearing loss can occur with cisplatin, and peripheral neuropathy is particularly frequent with taxane therapy. Prevention clinical trials of the antiepileptic agents gabapentin, lamotrigine, and the antidepressants nortriptyline and amitriptyline have shown modest to no effect.[63] Treatment options are limited, although physical therapy can help improve function, and there have been reports of some success with lessening neuropathy with glutamine and amitriptyline.[64] Available data support the use of duloxetine, but they are inconclusive regarding tricyclic antidepressants (such as nortriptyline), gabapentin, and a compounded topical gel containing baclofen, amitriptyline HCL, and ketamine. However, considering the paucity of options for CINP, these agents may be offered on the basis of data supporting their utility in other neuropathic pain conditions.[63,65]

Joint pains and generalized aches can continue after treatment with cytotoxic agents and are a tremendous problem for some women on hormonal therapies, especially AIs.[66] Arthralgias due to AIs are usually symmetrical; often involve the hands, arms, knees, feet, pelvic bones, and back; and may be more severe in the morning. It is not known whether rates are higher with certain members of this drug class than others. Exercise and analgesics may improve arthralgia, and pain usually resolves within weeks of stopping an AI.[67] A recent cross-sectional survey of 200 women receiving adjuvant AI therapy found that 47% reported joint pain and 44% reported joint stiffness. Body mass index of 25 to 30 kg/m² and prior tamoxifen therapy were found to be associated with a reduced likelihood of joint symptoms. Patients who had previously received a taxane were four times as likely as those who had not to report joint symptoms.[68]

Chemotherapy-Related Amenorrhea, Ovarian Dysfunction, and Infertility

Infertility is a dreaded consequence of breast cancer treatment for some young women with the disease. It is recommended that providers address the possibility of infertility with patients treated during their reproductive years soon after their diagnosis and be prepared to discuss possible fertility preservation options or refer appropriately.[69] For young women with breast cancer, adjuvant cytotoxic chemotherapy carries a risk of chemotherapy-related amenorrhea (CRA), associated ovarian dysfunction, and permanent cessation of menses (menopause) that increases with increasing patient age. Rates of CRA also vary based on regimen, with higher doses of alkylating agents increasing the likelihood of ovarian damage. A prospective study of 25- to 40-year-old women with breast cancer found that menstrual cycles persisted more often after regimens containing lower cumulative doses of cyclophosphamide.[70] For women concerned about their risk of infertility, fertility-sparing efforts are available, including embryo cryopreservation, gonadotropin-releasing hormone agonists, and other techniques including cryopreservation of oocytes or ovarian tissue.[69–71] Embryo freezing and oocyte cryopreservation require ovarian stimulation and may delay cancer treatment.[72] Unfortunately, all these methods suffer from limited efficacy and safety issues.

Many young breast cancer survivors are interested in determining their menopausal status and their fertility potential in follow-up. Available measures for ovarian function in breast cancer survivors are limited and imprecise. Although the presence or absence of regular menses may reflect whether ovulation is occurring, some women menstruate without ovulating, and others ovulate without menstruating. There is also evidence that some women who initially regain menses after adjuvant chemotherapy go on to experience premature menopause in a few years.[73] Less often, some women who assume they are postmenopausal after adjuvant chemotherapy because they do not menstruate for several years later resume menstruating. In a study of 45 women who were treated with an AI after at least 6 months of CRA at the Royal Marsden Breast Unit, 10 resumed menses while taking the AI, 1 became pregnant, and 1 had a biochemical recovery of plasma estradiol to greater than 1500 pmol/L.[74] It is therefore important not to transition women from tamoxifen to AI on the basis of CRA alone.[75] Ovarian ultrasounds to measure antral follicle count and ovarian volume may play a role in determining whether follicular development is occurring, as may measurement of serum hormones such as estradiol, follicle-stimulating hormone, and luteinizing hormone, although these parameters also fluctuate substantially in survivors. Newer markers of ovarian reserve, including anti-müllerian hormone and inhibin B, may be more reliable measures of potential fertility.[76–78]

Pregnancy

Many women diagnosed during childbearing years may be interested in having a subsequent pregnancy after breast cancer.[79] There have been concerns that pregnancy increases the risk of recurrence of hormone receptor–positive tumors because of the high hormonal levels surrounding a pregnancy. However, the available evidence does not reveal any negative effect of subsequent pregnancy on the prognosis of young women with breast cancer. A Finnish study compared the survival of 91 women who had given birth more than 10 months after breast cancer diagnosis with 471 controls (matched by year of diagnosis, stage, and age). The controls were found to be 4.8 times (95% CI 2.2–10.3) more likely to have died in the years after the breast cancer diagnosis than were those who had given birth to a live child.[80] Likewise, a comparison of more than 400 American women who gave birth more than 10 months after their breast cancer diagnosis to nearly

3000 matched controls who did not give birth after their diagnosis found that the pregnancies were associated with a decreased risk of death (RR 0.54, 95% CI 0.41–0.71).[81] A similar trend was found in the Danish Breast Cancer Cooperative Group evaluation of outcomes of all women who became pregnant out of 5725 women younger than 45 years of age with breast cancer with 35,067 total patient-years of follow-up. The 173 women with subsequent pregnancy had a statistically nonsignificant trend toward reduction in risk of death compared with those who did not become pregnant (RR 0.55, 95% CI 0.28–1.06).[82] Moreover, a study of the International Breast Cancer Study Group database reported that 94 patients who had a total of 137 pregnancies after breast cancer at 35 years of age or younger had better 5- and 10-year survival rates than 188 age-matched controls (92 ± 3% vs. 85 ± 3% for the 5-year data and 86 ± 4% vs. 74 ± 4% for the 10-year data). There were recurrences in 23% of those who became pregnant and in 54% of those who did not.[83] A meta-analysis of 14 retrospective or population studies confirmed that women who become pregnant after breast cancer diagnosis had a 41% reduced risk of death compared with women who did not become pregnant (RR: 0.59, 90% confidence interval 0.50–0.70). This difference was seen particularly in women with history of node-negative disease.[84] All of these studies may suffer from the "healthy mother bias," which reflects the fact that the women who become pregnant may be at lower risk of recurrence at baseline than women who do not become pregnant.[80] At present, women who do desire future pregnancies can be reassured by the lack of harm found in the existing limited data. Prospective research is ongoing.

It is commonly recommended that women wait at least 2 years after breast cancer treatment is completed before attempting conception to get through the period of highest risk of disease recurrence. Women who are taking tamoxifen or other hormonal therapy are urged to complete 5 years of therapy, during which pregnancy is contraindicated. Because rates of recurrence are significant long beyond the 2-year point and fertility wanes with aging, some women, particularly those at low risk of recurrence, may elect to pursue pregnancy soon after cancer treatment is completed. Young *BRCA* mutation carriers who are planning prophylactic oophorectomy in the future may be particularly eager to complete childbearing. Although it is important that providers and patients approach decisions about fertility preservation with caution, for some young women with breast cancer, a threat to the possibility of having a future biologic child has major psychosocial and developmental consequences.[85] Many young women with breast cancer struggle with the competing interests of optimizing personal survival and the desire to become pregnant. Oncology providers should strive to provide accurate unbiased information and psychosocial assistance to young survivors facing such challenging situations.

There is no evidence for an increased rate of congenital abnormalities in children conceived from the eggs of patients exposed to chemotherapy in the past. In three large studies including nearly 4000 offspring of both male and female survivors of childhood cancer, when clearly hereditary cancers such as retinoblastoma were excluded, no statistically significant increase in cancers or malformations was detected in the offspring.[86] Recently, a report from the Childhood Cancer Survivor Study that analyzed cases of congenital anomalies among 4699 children of female and male childhood cancer survivors, showed that the children of cancer survivors are not at significantly increased risk for congenital anomalies from their parent's exposure to mutagenic cancer treatments.[87] It is generally recommended that there be a minimum of several months between last dose of chemotherapy and conception.

Hormonal Symptoms and Sexual Dysfunction

Menopausal symptoms, including hot flashes, genitourinary problems, and sexual difficulties are common among breast cancer survivors due to the use of hormonal agents, development of CRA, and concerns about hormone replacement therapy in women who have been treated for breast cancer.[88] In postmenopausal women after breast cancer therapy, a survey regarding menopausal symptoms revealed rates for the following conditions: hot flashes 65%, vaginal dryness 48%, night sweats 44%, difficulty sleeping 44%, depression 44%, and dyspareunia 26%.[89] In a survey of 371 women who had been treated for breast cancer at or under 40 years of age, 77% of whom were premenopausal and 49% of whom were taking tamoxifen, responders reported the following menopausal symptoms: hot flashes 46%, vaginal dryness 51%, night sweats 46%, early awakening 52%, and dyspareunia 39%.[90] It is important for physicians to ask women about dyspareunia and libido as well as about hot flashes and vaginal dryness.[48] A randomized controlled trial of usual care versus treatment with assessment, education, counseling, and interventions directed at severe menopausal symptoms in 76 breast cancer survivors found that the treatment group reported improved menopausal symptoms ($p = .004$) and sexual functioning ($p = .04$) compared with the usual care group.[91] Hormone replacement is not a recommended option for treatment of bothersome symptoms in these women. A Swedish randomized, noninferiority trial (HABITS) compared hormone replacement therapy with nonhormonal management. After a median follow-up of 4 years, 39 of the 221 women in the hormonal therapy arm and 17 of the 221 women in the control arm experienced a new breast cancer event (HR = 2.4, 95% CI = 1.3–4.2).[92] Even in those with hormone receptor–negative disease, there is concern that the likelihood of a second primary cancer may be increased by hormonal exposure.[93] Furthermore, even in prospectively randomized healthy women, the overall health risks of exogenous hormones have been shown to exceed benefits.[94]

Nonestrogenic treatments for hot flashes and night sweats are believed to be safer than hormonal replacement.[95] Among nonhormonal treatments, antidepressants (serotonin and norepinephrine reuptake inhibitor [SNRIs], selective serotonin reuptake inhibitor [SSRIs]), clonidine, gabapentin, and pregabalin have been proven to be efficacious in randomized controlled trials. Antidepressants, such as the SNRI venlafaxine, significantly reduce hot-flash frequency and intensity in women with breast cancer compared with a placebo.[96,97] Venlafaxine (37.5–150 mg/day), paroxetine (10–20 mg/day), or citalopram (10–30 mg/day) are the most effective in reducing hot-flash frequency (from 14% to 58%) and severity compared with placebo.[98] Some SSRIs, such as paroxetine, may deleteriously reduce serum levels of the active metabolite of tamoxifen, but venlafaxine and citalopram do not appear to affect these levels significantly.[99,100] Gabapentin (300–900 mg), pregabalin (50–150 mg) and clonidine (0.1 mg) have also been shown to reduce hot flashes substantially.[100–102] In addition, vitamin E has been shown to have modest effectiveness on vasomotor symptoms in women with breast cancer, but the placebo effect is also significant in most of these studies.[103] Black cohosh and different formulas containing various phytoestrogens were tested in randomized trials with no proven benefit in controlling hot flashes in breast cancer patients.[104]

For vaginal dryness caused by treatment-induced menopause or AI therapy, water-based lubricants are the first-line therapy. Women with vaginal atrophy or stenosis may benefit from vaginal dilatation as well as lubricants. Intravaginal estrogen therapy with estrogen creams or estrogen-impregnated rings may relieve genitourinary symptoms and may be associated with minimal systemic absorption of estrogen, but the potential risk that this estrogen therapy may increase likelihood of recurrence of a hormone receptor–positive tumor has not been well explored. Vaginal lubrication may improve libido indirectly, and behavioral counseling and psychotherapy may also be helpful. Transdermal testosterone was not found to improve libido in one randomized trial of postmenopausal female cancer survivors.[105]

Fatigue

Fatigue is a common complaint in breast cancer survivors. Cancer-related fatigue (CRF) is often underreported, underdiagnosed, and undertreated. A multicenter study by Eastern Cooperative Oncology Group, designed to describe the prevalence and severity of CRF and its interference with daily living showed 52% incidence of moderate to severe fatigue in breast cancer survivors less than 5 years from treatment and 18% incidence in those who are more than 5 years from their treatment.[106] ASCO and National Comprehensive Cancer Network, recommend screening for CRF after completion of primary therapy, as clinically indicated and at least annually.[107] Evaluation and treatment of potential causes of fatigue, including pain, malnutrition, hypothyroidism, anemia, insomnia, and depression, is recommended. In those for whom no treatable cause is found, nonpharmacologic interventions such as energy conservation, exercise, psychotherapy, mindful meditation, and yoga are preferred over pharmacologic interventions. mindfulness-based stress reduction has been shown to improve mood, quality of life, and well-being more effectively than standard care in a randomized trial.[108] Yoga has shown to improve sleep quality and reduce sleep medicine use in a randomized controlled trial.[109] Psychostimulants such as modafinil and dextroamphetamine have shown mixed results in individual randomized studies, though Cochrane based review showed a small but significant improvement in fatigue with methylphenidate over placebo.[110] Finally, a large meta-analysis was recently published by Mustian and colleagues that included 113 unique studies and enrolled 11,525 participants. Exercise, psychological, and exercise plus psychological interventions improved CRF during and after primary treatment, whereas pharmaceutical interventions did not.[111]

Cognitive Impairment

Cognitive impairment during and after chemotherapy is of significant concern to many women. In a comparison of 31 women receiving chemotherapy, 40 women who had received chemotherapy in the past, and 36 healthy control participants, impaired cognition was found more frequently in women on active treatment than in control participants.[112] Another study of cognitive dysfunction 2 years after chemotherapy was completed showed that rates were higher in the 34 who had received high-dose chemotherapy (32%) than the 36 who received standard-dose chemotherapy (17%), with the lowest rates (9%) seen in the 34 who never received chemotherapy.[113] Interestingly, although more patients in the chemotherapy groups complained of difficulty with concentration, memory, thinking, or language, there was no significant correlation between self-report and objective measures of cognitive dysfunction in this study.[113] A study of patients who received chemotherapy or local therapy for breast cancer (n = 70) or lymphoma (n = 58) 5 years earlier suggests that cognitive deficits may not completely resolve over time. Neuropsychiatric test scores were lower in those treated with chemotherapy in the past ($p < .04$), especially with regard to verbal memory and psychomotor functioning.[114] However, most deficits were subtle, with scores still in the normal range. A meta-analysis of cognitive functioning in breast cancer survivors who were treated with chemotherapy showed that observed cognitive deficits are small in magnitude and limited to the domains of verbal ability and visuospatial ability.[115] The rate and severity of cognitive impairment experienced by breast cancer survivors may vary based partly on the type of treatment received.[116,117]

Nonpharmacologic and pharmacologic treatments have been tried to improve cognitive functioning and quality of life in cancer survivors. A recent systematic review concluded that current evidence does not favor the pharmacologic management of cognitive alterations associated with breast cancer treatment.[118] A single-arm pilot study of a cognitive-behavioral treatment called Memory and Attention Adaptation Training (MAAT) found that 29 women complaining of difficulties with memory and attention at a mean of 8 years after chemotherapy for stage I or II breast cancer experienced improvements in their symptoms immediately after the intervention and at 2-month and 6-month follow-ups.[119] MAAT consisted of four monthly visits, a telephone call in between each visit, and a workbook. Cognitive function, quality of life, and standard neuropsychological test scores rose as women were educated regarding memory attention, taught self-awareness and self-regulation (relaxation, scheduling, and pacing), and instructed in compensatory strategies.[119] A randomized controlled trial evaluated the efficacy of training in memory or speed of processing for improving cognitive function in breast cancer survivors. Both interventions improved self-reported measures of cognitive function, symptom distress, and quality of life.[120] There are limited data on efficacy of central nervous system stimulants in improving cognitive impairment. Agents that are under study include l-carnitine, modafinil, bupropion, and SSRIs.[121] Preliminary data suggest that modafinil may lessen symptoms of "chemo brain," such as memory problems and difficulties concentrating.[122] In a randomized study examining the effects of modafinil on fatigue, a secondary analysis to assess the effect of modafinil on cognitive function was performed. The results showed that modafinil improved cognitive performance in breast cancer survivors by enhancing some memory and attention skills.[123] However, a multicenter randomized controlled trial in brain cancer patients showed that modafinil did not exceed the effect of placebo[124] and double-blind randomized trial of D-methylphenidate during chemotherapy was found to have no beneficial effect on cognitive functioning.[125]

Psychosocial Concerns

It is common for breast cancer survivors to experience psychosocial distress in follow-up. Distress can result from the fear of recurrence or secondary to physical, psychological, or social, problems.[126] In a study of rates of depressive and anxiety disorders in 202 early-stage breast cancer patients younger than 60 years of age, prevalence of one or both conditions averaged 48% over the first year after diagnosis, twice that in the general population.[127] After the first year, rates were found to return to the same as in the general population. Risk factors for psychosocial distress in women with breast cancer include young age at diagnosis and menopausal transition with therapy.[128] Other risk factors include history of psychiatric disorders, cognitive impairment, and social problems like family or caregiver conflict or financial problems.[129,130] Protective factors against persistent psychological strain in survivors of a variety of cancers have been found to include emotionally supportive relationships, active coping strategies, and emotional expression.[128] Whether surveillance visits themselves provide psychological benefit is controversial and probably patient specific.[131] Fear of recurrence is often a dominant psychological sequela to cancer. However, the inconvenience and often discomfort of surveillance testing, as well as the stress of waiting for test results and visits with clinicians can themselves generate anxiety.[132] Randomized trials of surveillance after breast cancer have not found any overall positive psychological effects with more intensive surveillance strategies.[36]

Antidepressant and antianxiety medications, individual and group psychotherapy, and relaxation and meditation therapy have all been found to improve psychosocial distress in survivors of cancer.[128] Management of patients with clinical psychiatric diagnoses such as anxiety, depression, or posttraumatic stress disorder is generally similar to that in patients without a history of cancer. An important component of follow-up care for breast cancer survivors is evaluation for distress as well as referral to counseling, support groups, stress management, or mental health providers when appropriate.

Thrombosis

Tamoxifen predisposes to clots, particularly in postmenopausal women. The risk of venous thromboembolism (VTE) is increased approximately threefold by tamoxifen,[133] and some, but not all, studies have reported an increased risk of stroke as well.[134–136] In a large breast cancer cohort comprising 13,202 patients, Walker and coworkers showed that VTE risk is the highest in the first 3 months after initiation of tamoxifen (a significant fivefold increased risk compared with non–tamoxifen users) then it drops to a nonsignificant twofold thereafter.[137] Aromatase inhibitors are not associated with increased risk of VTE. Therefore a history of VTE or stroke is a relative contraindication to the use of tamoxifen and an indication for an AI. In the same study, the adjusted HR for VTE during chemotherapy was 10.8 (95% CI 8.2–14.4) compared with no chemotherapy and dropped to 8.4 (95% CI 4.9–14.2) in the month afterward.[137] The risk of surgery-related VTE is 2.2 compared with patients who do not undergo surgery, regardless of the type of surgery. Because of the additionally elevated risk of clot after an operation, some providers ask patients to stop taking tamoxifen for 2 weeks before an elective surgery, particularly if there will be a substantial period of inactivity after the surgery.[22]

Cardiac Disease

Mortality from breast cancer and cardiovascular disease (CVD) in women treated for breast cancer was compared in a cohort of 1413 breast cancer patients matched with same age controls. Compared with women without breast cancer, survivors of breast cancer are at higher risk for CVD-related mortality, but this risk seems to be time-dependent.[138] Indeed, the authors of this study found that the risk of CVD death was lower among breast cancer survivors in the first 7 years (HR: 0.59, 95% CI 0.40–0.87; *p* <

.001), whereas breast cancer survivors had nearly twice the risk of CVD mortality compared with those without breast cancer (HR: 1.9, 95% CI 1.4–2.7) after 7 years of their treatment. Because this study excluded anthracycline-induced cardiomyopathy the question of the other causes that may have been responsible was raised. Early menopause,[139] with its associated lipid and clotting abnormalities,[140–142] is one of the most important factors, which explains well the higher incidence of CVD in premenopausal women. However, other studies do not support this view.[143] Coronary artery disease, conduction system disease, and valvular disease may result from chest wall radiation, although cardiac exposure is much reduced by newer techniques of irradiation. Studies using old radiation techniques in the 1970s and 1980s showed a significant association between radiation and cardiovascular mortality.[144] These techniques exposed more of the heart and carried a 20% to 30% increased risk of cardiovascular disease.[11] With current breast irradiation techniques including optimizing cardiac shielding, rates of cardiac compromise due to radiation are thought to be much lower. A recent large Surveillance, Epidemiology, and End Results/Medicare study found no increased risk of myocardial infarction in women diagnosed with left-sided versus right-sided breast cancers between 1992 and 2000, suggesting that modern radiation does not significantly add to cardiac toxicity.[145] Some large European studies of patients treated in the 1990s concurred with these conclusions,[146] but others from the United States and Europe found no difference between the rate of radiation-induced cardiac disease in those treated before or after 1990 and slight increase of risk in those who received radiation to the left breast especially if fields were accidentally set too deep (which occurred more often with those who had a body mass index >25).[147–150]

The risk of congestive heart failure (CHF) with anthracyclines is well known to be cumulative dose–dependent, with risk approximately 5% at 400 mg/m^2, 16% at 500 mg/m^2, and 26% at 550 mg/m^2 (from a retrospective review of three clinical trials done during 1980–1990).[151] These rates are significantly higher than what was previously reported on studies done in the 1970s by Von Hoff and colleagues.[152] Lower cumulative doses of 200 to 300 mg/m^2 are associated with a risk of CHF in 0.5% to 2% of patients. CHF occur relatively early in the first 5 years after treatment. Late CHF is uncommon. In a published analysis of 10- to 13-year follow-up data from Southwest Oncology Group S8897, breast cancer patients who had received doxorubicin-containing chemotherapy no longer demonstrated reduced ejection fractions compared with the 5- to 8-year follow-up evaluation.[153] Similar results on incidence of late left ventricular dysfunction (LVD) after more than 10-year follow-up on breast cancer patients were published by Murtagh and coworkers.[154] Although a drop of left ventricular ejection fraction (LVEF) was observed in 1.9% of the patients, no LVD was seen. These data may underestimate rates of cardiac damage, however, because those studied were a selected observational subgroup consisting only of those who were alive and without recurrence.

Risk factors for anthracycline-induced cardiomyopathy are lifetime cumulative dose (exceeding 400–550 mg/m^2 of doxorubicin and 900–1000 mg/m^2 of epirubicin), age, radiation therapy to the chest, preexisting coronary and hypertensive heart disease, diabetes mellitus, peripheral vascular disease, and chronic obstructive pulmonary disease.[155–157] Careful patient selection before anthracycline administration, liposomal formulation of doxorubicin, the use of less cardiotoxic anthracyclines (epirubicin), and continuous monitoring of heart function are likely to decrease the incidence of these toxicities.[158] Slow infusion of doxorubicin instead of bolus infusion remains controversial.[159,160] Recently, several investigators suggested the use of genetic testing to identify the patients at increased risk for doxorubicin-induced cardiac toxicity.[161,162]

Trastuzumab heightens the risk of cardiac toxicity. In a meta-analysis including eight studies and involving 11,991 patients, Moja and colleagues found that trastuzumab significantly increased the risk of CHF defined as New York Heart Association class III or IV (2.5 vs. 0.4%; RR 5.11; 90% CI 3.00–8.72; $p < .00001$) and LVEF dysfunction (range 7.1%–18.6%; RR 1.83; 90% CI 1.36–2.47, $p = .0008$).[163] Older age, lower ejection fraction at beginning of therapy, and antihypertensive medications predicted higher risk of cardiac dysfunction in the trastuzumab-treated patients.[164] When trastuzumab was combined with paclitaxel or docetaxel, the incidence of CHF did not exceed 0.5% and 0.4%, respectively.[165,166] All these studies suggested that trastuzumab-induced heart failure might be reversible.[164,167] The standard protocol used to monitor heart function during trastuzumab treatment consists of a baseline evaluation of LVEF that is repeated every 3 months. Trastuzumab treatment is held if there are symptoms of heart failure, if LVEF drops below normal limits, or there is a drop of 16 or more percentile points. If LVEF returns to baseline on follow-up, it is considered safe to resume the treatment with close surveillance. The current surveillance guidelines during treatment were recently called into question because they do not have a strong evidence to support their use, nor is there any proof to support their utility.[168] No screening or prophylaxis for cardiac damage is currently recommended in the follow-up period, and management of heart failure or coronary disease is the same as that in people who do not have a history of cancer. All patients should be advised to exercise regularly, avoid tobacco, and control lipid and blood pressure.

Treatment-Related Cancers

Breast cancer survivors are at risk for several types of treatment-related cancers such as myelodysplasia (MDS) or acute myeloid leukemia (AML) due to chemotherapeutics; uterine cancer, including endometrial cancer, or, more rarely, sarcoma due to tamoxifen; and lung cancer or angiosarcoma secondary to chest radiation.

Chemotherapy-induced MDS and AML are well known long-term side effects of chemotherapy, especially alkylating agents and topoisomerase II inhibitors. AML associated with topoisomerase-II inhibitors occurs within 5 years after treatment and is frequently associated with 11q23 cytogenetic abnormality, whereas AML after alkylating agents is often associated with abnormalities in chromosomes 5 and 7 and typically develops after 5 years of completing the treatment and has a poor prognosis.[169] Anthracyclines (doxorubicin, epirubicin, and mitoxantrone) have both alkylating and topoisomerase-II inhibition functions to different degrees, which explains their variable leukemogenic potential. A large case-control study showed that the risk of mitoxantrone-containing regimens is dose dependent and significantly much higher than the other anthracycline-containing regimens. The risk was the highest in women younger than 65 years of age, with 4-year leukemia rate of 0.63% for cumulative doses of mitoxantrone less than 12 mg/m^2 and 3.89% for cumulative doses greater than 56 mg/m^2. These regimens are no longer in use these days.[170,171] The risk of the other anthracyclines is lower but nonetheless real. Five of 2305 breast cancer patients (0.2%) treated with doxorubicin and cyclophosphamide at different doses developed leukemia within 5 years of therapy in the National Surgical Adjuvant Breast and Bowel Project B-22 study.[172] A higher rate was seen in another trial, in which 5 of 351 patients receiving high doses of cyclophosphamide-epirubicin-fluorouracil developed acute leukemia within 5 years of chemotherapy.[173] Patients who were administered cumulative doses of epirubicin and cyclophosphamide higher than those used in standard regimens (≤720 and ≤6300 mg/m^2, respectively) had an 8-year cumulative probability of developing AML/MDS of 4.97% (95% CI 2.06–7.87) compared with 0.37% (95% CI 0.13–0.61) for patients who received standard doses of these drugs.[174] Furthermore, the addition of radiation therapy increases the risk of leukemia. In 3093 women who underwent curative breast surgery for cancer between 1982 and 1996, 12 women developed leukemia, all of whom had received radiotherapy and 10 of whom had also received chemotherapy.[171] Thus the true rate of anthracycline-induced AML or MDS has been estimated to be 0.1% to 1.5% at 5 to 10 years, with radiation adding to the risk.[175] Taxanes have the safest profile. No or rare cases of leukemia were reported with docetaxel-[176] or with paclitaxel-containing regimens.[177] The leukemogenic effect of granulocyte colony-stimulating factor (G-CSF) remains controversial.[178–180] A systematic review of the effect of G-CSF in 25 randomized controlled trials showed an estimated RR of AML/MDS at 1.92 (95% CI 1.19–3.07; $p = .007$) in breast cancer patients treated with high-intensity therapy with growth factor compared with the less intense regimens and no growth factor.[181] The relative contribution of dose intensity and growth factors is difficult to sort out in this context.

The risk of type 1 uterine cancer is also heightened by 2.5-fold due to the estrogen-agonistic property of tamoxifen in postmenopausal women.[182–184] Type 1 endometrial cancer is the most common type and is estrogen dependent contrary to the uncommon type 2.[185] The condition of the endometrium before initiation of tamoxifen was thought to determine the response of the endometrium to the drug. Thin endometrium (consistent with inactive atrophic histology) suggests a low chance of stimulation, whereas the presence of a benign endometrial polyp increases the incidence of atypical endometrial hyperplasia.[186] However, the association of benign endometrial polyps with endometrial cancer was not found to be higher than with other benign conditions of the uterus. Hence, the presence of benign hyperplastic endometrial polyp should be considered a surrogate marker for endometrial activity rather than a precursor of cancer. The risk of tamoxifen-associated endometrial cancer is increased by the length of the treatment and does not abate after its cessation.

The notion that tamoxifen-associated endometrial cancer has a good prognosis has been called into question in recent years with long-term follow-up studies. Large retrospective studies (39,451 patients) have suggested a greater risk of aggressive uterine sarcomas (malignant mixed müllerian tumors [MMMT]) on tamoxifen relative to other histologic types of endometrial cancer.[187] More recent and larger studies (85,930 patients) have refuted this notion and showed that there is increased risk of MMMTs in breast cancer patients in general regardless of the treatment with tamoxifen.[188] However, in the absence of prospective assessment of this rare cancer, the issue remains unsettled, with studies showing results to support both assertions.[189–191] Considering the role of estrogen and estrogen-like compounds in promoting endometrial cancer, it is recommended to use an AI instead of tamoxifen whenever possible and switch patients who received tamoxifen to an AI after 3 to 5 years of treatment to minimize the risks of this complication.

Menstrual cycle irregularities are common on tamoxifen, and cessation of periods may occur with or without continued ovarian function. The patient should be advised to use a reliable nonhormonal contraceptive method even if periods have ceased. Vaginal bleeding in postmenopausal women should be investigated by a gynecologist and with vaginal US. Routine regular screening has been proposed in asymptomatic patients on tamoxifen. However, the false-positive rate of vaginal US in this population is unacceptably high, and thus it is not recommended.[192,193] Breast cancer therapy is not known to increase rates of ovarian cancer, but tamoxifen can cause benign ovarian cystic growths in postmenopausal women.[194] Women who have strong family histories of breast or ovarian cancer or who are known to carry a BRCA mutation are at increased risk of ovarian cancer, and prophylactic oophorectomy is considered.

A larger cohort of 16,705 women treated for nonmetastatic breast cancer between 1981 and 1997 found significantly more sarcomas and lung cancers in the 13,472 who had received radiation compared with the 3233 who had not ($p = .02$).[195] In a recent overview of the published literature on radiation-induced sarcoma (RIS), the incidence rate was low at 0.2% of women with breast cancer treated with radiation.[196] The treatment consists of wide surgical excision to negative margins with or without radiation. No adjuvant therapy is available nowadays for this cancer.

Age-appropriate routine cancer screening (e.g., for cervical and colon cancer) is recommended for breast cancer survivors, but no additional screening for non–breast cancers is recommended in a breast cancer survivor unless she is known to carry a genetic cancer mutation (such as BRCA).

Non–Cancer-Related Care

Although some oncologists are willing and able to act as a primary care physician, surveys have shown that most would prefer not to.[197] Maintenance of a relationship with a primary care physician has been a strong predictor of a patient receiving high-quality general medical care.[198] Surviving cancer provides several opportunities to actually improve health. First, if a hereditary predisposition to cancer is suspected, genetic counseling and testing may lead to interventions that could prevent future cancers in the cancer survivor and the survivor's relatives. Second, breast cancer survivors usually have more medical contacts than people without a history of cancer and consequently have more opportunity to receive recommended health maintenance interventions such as screenings (e.g., cholesterol, bone density, checks for other cancers) and immunizations.[199] Patients faced with a life-threatening illness may be more receptive to messages about improving health behaviors, making the development of cancer a potential "teachable moment."[66] In particular, physicians can counsel patients at surveillance visits on lifestyle modifications such as smoking cessation, ending alcohol abuse, and decreasing sun exposure. A study in which 450 women were randomized to usual care or recommendation by an oncologist to exercise showed modest improvement in self-reported exercise in the group who received the recommendation.[200] Preexisting conditions such as arthritis, chronic obstructive pulmonary disease, and cardiovascular disease should be taken into account before exercise is recommended to patients.[201] There is actually emerging evidence that lifestyle factors such as diet and exercise may play a role in preventing recurrence, perhaps particularly for those

with hormone-negative tumors. The Women's Intervention Nutrition Study, which randomized 2437 postmenopausal women to a usual diet versus a low-fat diet (15% of calories from fat) found a nonsignificant trend toward reduced breast cancer recurrence rates.[202] The Women's Healthy Eating and Living Study tested the efficacy of more intensive dietary change.[203] The adoption of a diet that was very high in vegetables, fruit, and fiber and low in fat did not reduce additional breast cancer events or mortality during the 7.3-year follow-up period of the study. Nevertheless, patients should be encouraged to follow ACS dietary recommendations, including the following: maintain a normal weight (lose weight if overweight); seek out vegetables, fruits, and unrefined grains; and avoid excessive saturated fat, sugar, and refined grains.[204]

Given that breast cancer survivors account for nearly one-fourth of the 10 million cancer survivors in the United States—and that number will grow as the population ages—optimizing the provision of health care after breast cancer is important.[205] A multicenter, randomized, controlled trial investigated whether long-term outcomes of breast cancer were different when patients received follow-up care in the cancer center instead of the primary care clinic. Nine hundred sixty-eight patients who had been diagnosed with early-stage breast cancer 9 to 15 months earlier were randomized to follow-up with their family practitioner or with their oncologist. Rates of recurrence (11.2% in the family practice group vs. 13.2% in the cancer center group) and death (6% vs. 6.2%, respectively) were not significantly different between the groups. Likewise, no differences were detected between the groups in recurrence-related serious clinical events (3.5% in the family practice group vs. 3.7% in the oncologist group) or health-related quality of life.[206]

Survivorship Care Planning

The Institute of Medicine established a committee to examine adult cancer survivorship issues and make recommendations to improve the health care and quality of life of cancer survivors. Four survivorship priorities were identified, including prevention (of recurrent and new cancers and other late effects), surveillance (for cancer and medical or psychosocial effects of treatment), intervention (to improve medical and psychosocial outcomes), and coordination (among care providers). One of the committee's recommendations was that those completing primary therapy should be provided with a clearly written survivorship care plan including an individualized comprehensive care summary and follow-up outline. Such a plan would aim to help patients and to improve communications between oncologists and patients' other health care providers.[207] Recently, the ASCO Survivorship Task Force and experts from around the country have coordinated efforts to design and implement templates that can be tailored to individual patients, which can be found at www.asco.org. The efficacy of these survivorship care plans in breast cancer has yet to be tested rigorously. It is hoped that comprehensive multidisciplinary or breast cancer–specific survivorship programs, in which cancer centers create a team of providers who focus primarily on issues that arise after treatment, will facilitate improved care.[208]

Conclusions and Future Directions

The number of breast cancer survivors continues to grow in the United States and worldwide. Follow-up care presents several challenges, not the least of which is routine attention to unique issues facing breast cancer survivors and coordination of care among multiple providers. Chemotherapeutic and hormonal treatment regimens change as clinical trials provide evidence for adoption of more effective treatments, some of which will undoubtedly alter the care women require in the follow-up period. Research to investigate both the utility and cost-effectiveness of various strategies of surveillance, intervention, and overall delivery of survivorship care is necessary from both individual and societal perspectives. Attention to long-term survivorship care planning will also be important to optimize communication with patients and health care practitioners to provide the highest quality of care to breast cancer survivors.

Selected References

28. Paluch-Shimon S, Pagani O, Partridge AH, et al. Second international consensus guidelines for breast cancer in young women (BCY2). *The Breast*. 2016;26:87-99.

43. Lucci A, McCall LM, Beitsch PD, et al. Surgical complications associated with sentinel lymph node dissection (SLND) plus axillary lymph node dissection compared with SLND alone in the American College of Surgeons Oncology Group trial Z0011. *J Clin Oncol*. 2007;25:3657-3663.

60. Early Breast Cancer Trialists' Collaborative Group. Adjuvant bisphosphonate treatment in early breast cancer: meta-analyses of individual patient data from randomised trials. *The Lancet*. 2015;386:1353-1361.

80. Sankila R, Heinävaara S, Hakulinen T. Survival of breast cancer patients after subsequent term pregnancy: "healthy mother effect." *Obstet Gynecol*. 1994;170:818-823.

138. Bradshaw PT, Stevens J, Khankari N, et al. Cardiovascular disease mortality among breast cancer survivors. *Epidemiology*. 2016;27:6-13. doi:10.1097/EDE.0000000000000394.

A full reference list is available online at ExpertConsult.com.

82

Management of Menopause in the Breast Cancer Patient

NEIL MAJITHIA, CHARLES L. LOPRINZI, AND KATHRYN J. RUDDY

American women enter menopause at the average age of 51 years and spend one-third of their lives after menopause. More than 40 million women are now in or past menopause, and another 20 million will enter menopause over the next decade.[1] With advances in oncologic diagnosis and treatment, breast cancer survivors constitute a growing proportion of these women. Also, treatment for breast cancer can speed the onset of menopause and increase the severity of menopausal symptoms.

This chapter explores menopause and discusses management of menopausal symptoms in breast cancer patients. The safety of hormone therapy (HT) for treatment of vasomotor and vulvovaginal symptoms in breast cancer survivors is explored, as are alternative treatments. Finally, menopause-related depression, osteoporosis, and cardiovascular disease are discussed with special consideration of the needs of breast cancer survivors.

What Is the Experience of Menopause in Women With Breast Cancer?

In the United States, more than 240,000 women are diagnosed with breast cancer annually.[2] Approximately 25% are premenopausal at the time of diagnosis,[3] and most of these women will lose ovarian function earlier than they would have otherwise, in many cases during chemotherapy.[4] In premenopausal women with localized breast cancer, older age and more gonadotoxic chemotherapy are associated with a higher risk for amenorrhea 1 year after treatment.[5] Only 30% of women diagnosed with breast cancer between 40 to 49 years old resume menstruation after receipt of standard adjuvant chemotherapy,[6] although regimens that do not contain alkylating agents may be less likely to induce menopause.[7] The risks of amenorrhea and associated menopausal symptoms with newer chemotherapy regimens requires further study because these can influence patient perceptions of the cost-to-benefit ratio of specific cancer treatments (thereby better informing decision-making).

The most widely acknowledged symptom of menopause is the hot flash, occurring in about 75% of all menopausal women.[8] There is increasing evidence that hot flashes are a physiologic response to a change in the hypothalamic set point.[8] During menopause, decreases in gonadal hormones appear to cause fluctuations in levels of norepinephrine and serotonin that, in turn, alter thermoregulation. In women without breast cancer, hot flash frequency and severity may be worsened by obesity, smoking, and stress. Hot weather, confining spaces, and ingestion of caffeine, alcohol, or spicy foods are acute triggers for some women.

Hot flashes can be objectively measured as diminished skin resistance. Duration ranges from 30 seconds to several minutes, and frequency and severity can vary substantially. Some women also experience palpitations and feelings of anxiety.

Most women remain symptomatic for more than a year.[9] There is wide variability in the distress associated with hot flashes, with some women reporting hot flashes that disrupt sleep and adversely affect quality of life. For breast cancer survivors, hot flashes tend to be more frequent, more severe, and more persistent than in age-matched controls.[10] The menopausal transition may last only weeks to months as chemotherapy and/or oophorectomy can cause estrogen levels to plummet, triggering the abrupt onset of vasomotor symptoms. Both tamoxifen and aromatase inhibitors can incite or exacerbate hot flashes,[11] and in one report, 20% of women discontinued or considered discontinuing adjuvant antiestrogen therapy because of intolerable side effects.[12] As in all menopausal women, hot flashes and night sweats in breast cancer survivors are associated with poor quality sleep and increased fatigue.[13]

Vulvovaginal symptoms usually begin 3 to 5 years after natural menopause but may occur within months of primary treatment for breast cancer. As estrogen levels decline, the vulva loses most of its collagen, adipose tissue, and water-retaining ability, becoming flattened and thin. The vagina shortens and narrows, and the vaginal walls become thinner, less elastic, more friable, and less able to produce lubricating secretions during intercourse. Vaginal pH becomes more alkaline, predisposing to colonization with urogenital pathogens. Symptoms include vaginal dryness, dyspareunia, vaginal bleeding, increased vaginal infections, urinary incontinence, and urinary tract infections. As potent suppressors of estrogen synthesis, aromatase inhibitors are associated with a high rate of urogenital symptoms. By contrast, tamoxifen may have estrogenic effects on the vagina, similar to the estrogenic effect it exerts on the uterus and bones.

Is Hormone Therapy an Option for Women With Breast Cancer?

Estrogen effectively controls hot flashes in perimenopausal women. Double-blind, placebo-controlled trials of HT demonstrate a significant reduction in symptoms compared with placebo

(75% vs. 57%).[14–18] Duration of therapy usually ranges from 1 to 3 years. In women with an intact uterus, a progestin is routinely added to curtail increasing endometrial cancer risk.

Listed among the absolute contraindications to estrogen use is a personal history of breast cancer. Although a 2001 systematic review suggested that HT does not increase the risk of recurrence in breast cancer survivors,[19] the Hormonal Replacement Therapy after Breast Cancer Diagnosis—Is it Safe? (HABITS) trial did support the concept that HT was detrimental in survivors. This study recruited women with a history of up to stage II breast cancer and menopausal symptoms of sufficient severity to require treatment. Subjects received either 2 years of HT or nonhormonal, symptomatic treatment, with a primary end point of development of new breast cancers. The HT regimen was directed by local practice.[20] After a safety analysis in 2003, the HABITS trial was terminated early, at which time follow-up data were available for 345 women, with a median follow-up of 2.1 years. New breast cancer events were reported in 26 women in the HT group compared with only seven in the non-HT group (relative hazard 3.3, confidence interval [CI] 1.5–7.4). Subgroup analyses for hormone receptor status, tamoxifen use, and prior HT use did not change the results.

In contrast, the Stockholm Randomized Trial reported that HT did not increase risk of breast cancer recurrence. This study enrolled women with a history of primary operable breast cancer and randomized them to either 5 years of standardized HT or no HT.[21] After early termination related to safety concerns and poor accrual, new breast cancers were reported in 11 of 188 women in the HT group compared with 13 of 190 in the control group over a median follow-up of 4.1 years (hazard ratio [HR] 0.82, CI 0.35–1.9).

Differences in study design and between the study populations offer a partial explanation for these discrepancies. HABITS enrolled a higher proportion of lymph node–positive patients and fewer patients taking tamoxifen. It is important to note that HT may be both less dangerous and less effective at controlling vasomotor symptoms in women concomitantly taking selective estrogen receptor modulators, which may saturate the estrogen receptor.[22] The Stockholm trial limited the use of continuous combined HT, which was hypothesized to stimulate breast cell proliferation, and it favored cyclic therapy, which was hypothesized to downregulate growth factors. This is consistent with findings from both the Women's Health Initiative (WHI)[2] and the Million Women Study (a prospective cohort study of HT and incident invasive breast cancer),[23] in which progestin-containing regimens were associated with a higher risk of breast cancer (Table 82.1).

An updated review of HT in breast cancer survivors included the HABITS trial, but data from the Stockholm trial were not available. There was no increased risk of breast cancer recurrence for all studies combined, but there was significant heterogeneity. The pooled relative risk for observational studies was 0.64 (CI 0.50–0.82) compared with 3.41 (CI 1.59–7.33) for randomized trials. The authors concluded that given limitations in the observational studies, only randomized trials would provide a reliable estimate of risk.[24]

On the basis of current knowledge of the risks and benefits of HT, its use in breast cancer survivors remains questionable, and HT should be considered only for refractory and severe symptoms. If it is prescribed to a breast cancer survivor, HT should be used only at the lowest effective dose for the shortest duration possible. Informed consent is essential, and women need to be counseled on the lack of safety data.

TABLE 82.1 Hormonal Agents and Risk of Breast Cancer

Hormone	Risk
Estrogen alone	Lower risk of breast cancer compared with placebo in a large prospective, randomized trial of hysterectomized postmenopausal women but failed to achieve statistical significance[143]
Estrogen plus progestin	Higher risk of breast cancer compared with placebo in a large prospective, randomized trial of postmenopausal women[144]
Megestrol acetate	Safety in breast cancer unknown[61]
Tibolone	Increased risk of breast cancer compared with never use of hormone therapy in one large observational trial of postmenopausal women[23] No recurrence at 1 year in a small prospective, randomized, placebo-controlled trial of women with early breast cancer[145]
Soy phytoestrogens	Safety in breast cancer unknown[146]

Alternatives to Estrogen-Based Therapy for Management of Vasomotor Symptoms

Antidepressants

In the 1990s, both SSRI (selective serotonin reuptake inhibitor) and SNRI (serotonin and norepinephrine reuptake inhibitor) antidepressants were anecdotally noted to decrease hot flashes. These observations were independently seen with venlafaxine, paroxetine, fluoxetine, and sertraline, leading to the conduct of four trials (Table 82.2).[25–28]

The first of these studies to be published was a randomized, placebo-controlled trial evaluating three doses of venlafaxine and reported significant reduction in hot flashes among patients receiving this SNRI.[29] The study supported a starting dose of 37.5 mg daily for a week, with subsequent increase to a target dose of 75 mg daily. An editorial accompanying this article acknowledged that this approach appeared to be helpful for hot flashes in breast cancer survivors but questioned whether it would be beneficial in patients without a history of breast cancer.[30]

After the publication of this initial study, three additional randomized, placebo-controlled trials evaluating paroxetine, citalopram, and escitalopram were conducted; results indicated that these antidepressants were similarly helpful for decreasing hot flashes in women with breast cancer.[28,31,32] Studies of fluoxetine and sertraline suggested comparatively limited efficacy of these particular SSRIs for hot flashes in this setting.[33,34]

Subsequent studies have been performed to assess the efficacy of both SNRIs and SSRIs as treatment for hot flashes in women without a history of breast cancer, with results providing further support for use of these agents.[35–47] A pooled analysis considered the impact of breast cancer history and tamoxifen exposure on the effectiveness of antidepressants; it reported that these

TABLE 82.2	Select Non-Hormonal Therapies for Treatment of Menopausal Hot Flashes	
Agent	**Recommended Target Dose**	**Notes**
Venlafaxine[29,147,148]	75 mg/day	Acute toxicity (nausea/vomiting) and withdrawal require careful dose escalation and tapering
Desvenlafaxine[35,36,44,149,150]	150 mg/day	Similar results as seen with other listed antidepressants
Paroxetine[45,73,151]	7.5 mg/day	Only FDA-approved agent for treatment of hot flashes; should be avoided in patients taking tamoxifen due to CYP2D6 blockade
Citalopram[37,42]	20 mg/day	Appropriate first-line agent for most patients
Escitalopram[39,152]	20 mg/day	Appropriate first-line agent for most patients
Gabapentin[52,54–56]	900 mg/day	Can be particularly helpful for women with predominantly nighttime symptoms
Pregabalin[53]	300 mg/day	More expensive and less well studied than gabapentin

FDA, US Food and Drug Administration.

nonestrogenic therapies were helpful in reducing hot flashes, irrespective of etiology.[48]

None of the preceding medications were initially developed for treating hot flashes. Nonetheless, in 2013, the US Food and Drug Administration approved paroxetine for the treatment of moderate to severe vasomotor symptoms associated with menopause.[49] A recent review addressed the practical approach to use of these antidepressants, concluding that paroxetine, citalopram, and escitalopram are reasonable first-line options.[50] Currently, paroxetine and citalopram are most cost-effective. Importantly, paroxetine should be avoided in combination with tamoxifen because paroxetine may inhibit cytochrome P450 CYP2D6, which metabolizes tamoxifen into endoxifen, and endoxifen is thought to confer much of the therapeutic benefit of the drug.[51]

Gabapentinoids

Gabapentin and pregabalin reduce hot flashes to a similar degree as the newer antidepressant agents, irrespective of breast cancer history.[48,52–55] A randomized, crossover, clinical trial that evaluated patient preferences between these agents found that patients preferred venlafaxine over gabapentin by a 2:1 margin, despite similar relief of vasomotor symptoms with the two agents.[56] When switching from an antidepressant to gabapentin, it is recommended to continue the antidepressant for an overlap period of a couple weeks because abrupt discontinuation of the antidepressant is associated with increased side effects.[57] These side effects likely reflect withdrawal symptoms, as opposed to gabapentin toxicity. Combination therapy with these agents does not confer a benefit in terms of hot flash reduction. When used for this purpose, the recommended target dose is 900 mg for gabapentin and 300 mg for pregabalin.

Clonidine

This centrally acting alpha-adrenergic agonist, used for management of hypertension, is associated with dry mouth, insomnia, constipation, and drowsiness. In a crossover trial, 116 women receiving tamoxifen for breast cancer and experiencing at least seven hot flashes per week received transdermal clonidine (equivalent to 0.1 mg orally) or placebo for 4 weeks. Those taking clonidine reported a 20% reduction in hot flash frequency compared

with placebo.[58] In a second trial, 194 women taking tamoxifen for breast cancer received oral clonidine 0.1 mg/day or placebo for 8 weeks. Women taking clonidine reported a 37% decrease in hot flash frequency at 4 weeks compared with 20% for placebo. At 8 weeks, there was a 38% reduction in frequency with clonidine compared with 24% for placebo.[59] This drug is not often used for treating hot flashes because of the availability of alternative agents that are more efficacious and better tolerated.

Progesterone Analogs

In a crossover trial, 97 women with history of breast cancer and 66 men with prostate cancer treated with androgen deprivation therapy received either megestrol acetate 20 mg twice daily or placebo for 4 weeks. The megestrol group experienced an 85% reduction in hot flash frequency compared with 21% for placebo. In this study, 71% of the megestrol group experienced a 50% decrease in hot flash frequency compared with only 24% for placebo. There was a significant carryover effect from megestrol to placebo, and data could not be interpreted for the second treatment period. Vaginal bleeding was reported in 31% of women after withdrawal of megestrol.[60] At 3 years of follow-up, 18 women were still using megestrol, and five experienced abnormal vaginal bleeding.[61] Medroxyprogesterone acetate can be administered as a single intramuscular shot with about a 50-day half-life and decreases hot flashes to a similar degree as megestrol acetate.[62] This provides a convenient dosing option, which can relieve hot flashes for months.

The long-term safety of progesterone analogs has not been evaluated in breast cancer survivors. Although the results from the WHI and Million Women Study suggest that progestins carry a higher risk for breast cancer when combined with estrogens, the implications of their use in isolation are unknown. Both megestrol acetate and medroxyprogesterone have been used in the past for treatment of metastatic breast cancer at higher doses; however, it is important to acknowledge and discuss with patients that the impact of this therapy on breast cancer prognosis is uncertain.

Complementary and Alternative Methods

Even before publication of WHI data, there was significant interest in complementary and alternative therapies for treatment of vasomotor symptoms, with 22% of menopausal women in one study reporting their use.[63] Women with breast cancer are no exception. In a survey of women with recently diagnosed early-stage breast cancer, 28% reported new use of alternative therapies.[64]

Vitamin E at a dose of 800 IU daily appears to have a marginal effect on hot flash frequency, with a reduction of less than one hot flash daily compared with placebo.[65] A systematic review of randomized controlled trials found no data to support the effectiveness of red clover.[66] Studies of black cohosh produced conflicting results.[67] A systematic review of black cohosh in cancer patients included four studies in women with breast cancer. The authors concluded that in light of conflicting results and significant methodologic flaws, black cohosh does not appear to be effective.[68] Soy phytoestrogens have also garnered considerable interest, but a review of 30 controlled trials concluded that there was no evidence to support their use for vasomotor symptoms of menopause.[69]

A review of exercise for management of vasomotor symptoms could draw no conclusions because of a lack of trials.[70] Other behavioral interventions, such as paced respirations[71] and comprehensive support programs,[72] have been shown to reduce symptoms but may be difficult to replicate outside of research settings. Newer studies have supported that hypnosis can reduce hot flashes,[73,74] but this approach is not readily available to most patients.

Acupuncture has not been established as a means to decrease hot flashes, despite multiple attempts to address this subject.[75–82] Pilot trial reports and a small double-blinded randomized trial support that stellate ganglion blocks can be helpful for treating hot flashes, although this approach is not commonly used in practice.[83–103] There are also pilot data to support that oxybutynin, an agent commonly used for the treatment of urinary incontinence, can alleviate hot flashes, although no double-blinded placebo-controlled trials have been published to demonstrate success with this approach.[104]

Are Topical Estrogens an Option for Women With Breast Cancer?

Oral and transdermal HT are no longer indicated for treatment of vulvovaginal atrophy in the absence of vasomotor symptoms. Vaginal estrogens are appealing because they are perceived to cause little systemic absorption. A review of intravaginal estrogens across 19 randomized trials concluded that creams, tablets, and rings were all effective. In this review, creams were most commonly associated with systemic absorption, whereas rings had the lowest absorption. A progestin was recommended for women with an intact uterus using creams at a dose greater than 0.5 mg estradiol daily. The ring had the highest acceptability, followed by tablets. Limitations of this review include short duration of treatment, small numbers of participants, exclusion of women with breast cancer, and heterogeneity in pooled results. Only seven trials were placebo controlled.[105] Newer data support that all vaginal estrogen products are systemically absorbed to varying degrees.[106] Safety data for vaginal estrogens in women with a history of breast cancer are sparse. A cohort study of 69 women previously treated for breast cancer (including those with estrogen receptor–positive tumors) who used low-dose topical estrogens for 1 year had no increased risk of recurrence, but the study was underpowered to detect such differences.[107]

A prospective study of six women taking aromatase inhibitors for early-stage breast cancer showed a significant rise in serum estradiol after 2 weeks of daily therapy with vaginal estradiol 25-μg tablets for severe atrophic vaginitis. After 2 weeks, when dosing decreased to twice-weekly (as recommended by the manufacturer), estradiol levels dropped to pretreatment levels in only two of the six women.[108] Given that effectiveness of aromatase inhibitor therapy relies on suppression of estrogen stimulation, it is reasonable to conclude that vaginal estrogens should not be used with aromatase inhibitors.

Alternatives to Topical Estrogens for Vulvovaginal Atrophy

Continued sexual activity, with its increase in blood flow, is thought to help maintain vaginal tissues. Water-based lubricants can decrease discomfort during intercourse. Women should avoid products such as detergents that may cause contact dermatitis. Polycarbophil-based moisturizers are hydrophilic polymers that bind vaginal epithelial cells and release fluid until sloughed. Such products induce epithelial cell maturation and restore normal pH[109] and were shown to be as effective as vaginal estrogen in a randomized trial.[110] In a randomized, double-blind, crossover study of 45 breast cancer patients, those using a polycarbophil product reported that symptoms of vaginal dryness decreased by 64% and dyspareunia by 60% after 4 weeks. Relief was comparable to a moisturizing placebo, which was not inert.[111]

Data support that dehydroepiandrosterone (DHEA) decreases vaginal dryness and reduces sexual activity–associated discomfort without causing increased systemic estrogen levels in women with vaginal dryness who do not have breast cancer.[112,113] In women with a history of cancer, a randomized, double-blind, placebo-controlled clinical trial, supported that DHEA is safe and helpful in women with vaginal dryness and/or dyspareunia.[114,115] Additional work in this area is needed.

Depression

Evaluation for and treatment of depression are important components for the comprehensive care of the woman with breast cancer (Box 82.1). The prevalence of depression is as high as 50% in the first year after a breast cancer diagnosis.[116,117] Risk factors include

---

• BOX 82.1 Evaluation and Treatment of Depression in the Menopausal Breast Cancer Patient

Prevalence as high as 50%
Risk factors
    Difficulty coping with cancer diagnosis
    Difficulty tolerating cancer treatments
    Work and family issues
    Sexual dysfunction
Menopause also associated with increased risk of depression
    Hot flashes and night sweats
    Other factors may also play a role
Screening for depression; positive response should prompt formal evaluation
Treatment: antidepressants, although women may be reluctant to take
    additional drugs, and some agents may interfere with tamoxifen therapy
Counseling

difficulty coping with a cancer diagnosis, difficulty tolerating cancer treatments, work and family issues, sexual dysfunction, and a history of depression.[118] The menopausal transition may contribute to these mood symptoms as well.[119,120] Hot flashes and night sweats can cause sleep disturbances in both healthy women and breast cancer patients. Research suggests that the role of sleep disturbance in psychological distress is significant, but in both groups of women, it does not fully explain the effect of menopause on mood.[10]

Although there are many screening questionnaires for depression, the following two Patient Health Questionnaire—2 (PHQ-2) questions may be sufficient for survivors:

1. Over the past 2 weeks, have you felt down, depressed or hopeless?
2. Over the past 2 weeks, have you felt little interest or pleasure in doing things?

The response options for these two questions are "Not at all" (scored 0), "Several days" (scored 1), "More than half the days" (scored 2), and "Nearly every day" (scored 3). A total score of 3 or greater for these two items warrants a formal evaluation for depression (http://www.cqaimh.org/pdf/tool_phq2.pdf).

Treatment of depression in a menopausal breast cancer survivor should be based on the history of any previous psychological disorders and medications used, as well as knowledge of the patient's current breast cancer therapy, menopausal symptoms, work and family stressors, and sexual dysfunction. SSRIs and SNRIs can be extremely beneficial and cost-effective partly because of potential to reduce vasomotor symptoms (with the caveat that some of these drugs could interfere with the efficacy of tamoxifen, as described earlier in the section Antidepressants). Short-term counseling, such as cognitive or behavioral therapy, can also be helpful.

Osteoporosis

Growing evidence indicates that bone health is of particular concern for women with breast cancer. Data from the WHI Observational Study, a prospective, longitudinal cohort of postmenopausal women, demonstrated a 31% higher risk of fracture in women with breast cancer.[121] The cessation of HT use, the onset of chemotherapy-induced premature menopause, and the use of aromatase inhibitors and/or ovarian function suppressing medications all accelerate loss of bone and speed the development of osteoporosis. Chemotherapy itself may also adversely affect bone density, independent of any endocrine-mediated effect.

In a prospectively designed substudy of the Arimidex, Tamoxifen, Alone or in Combination (ATAC) trial, bone mineral density (BMD) was assessed in 308 postmenopausal early-stage breast cancer patients at baseline and over 2 years of therapy. Anastrozole was associated with significant loss of BMD at the lumbar spine and total hip (median loss 4.1% and 3.9%, respectively), whereas tamoxifen was associated with BMD improvements (median increase 2.2% and 1.2%, respectively). The effect of anastrozole was most marked in women within 4 years of menopause.[122] Fracture data were available for the full study population of 6186 women who completed 5 years of therapy. Three hundred and forty fractures (11%) were reported in the anastrozole group versus 237 (7.7%) in the tamoxifen group (odds ratio 1.49, CI 1.25–1.77).[123] All three available aromatase inhibitors seem to affect bone turnover to a similar degree.[124]

The American Society of Clinical Oncologists therefore recommends regular counseling about and screening for osteoporosis in

---

• BOX 82.2 Guidelines for Osteoporosis Screening in Women With Nonmetastatic Breast Cancer

Counsel all women about adequate calcium and vitamin D intake, weight-bearing exercise, and smoking cessation

Assess bone mineral density annually by dual-energy x-ray absorptiometry scan if woman is:

- 65 years or older
- 60–64 years with other risk factors (family history of osteoporosis, low body weight, history of nontraumatic fracture, other risk factors)
- receiving aromatase inhibitor therapy
- has treatment-related premature menopause

From Hillner BE, Ingle JN, Chlebowski, RT, et al. American Society of Clinical Oncology 2003 update on the role of bisphosphonates and bone health issues in women with breast cancer. J Clin Oncol. 2003;21:4042-4057.

---

women with nonmetastatic breast cancer (Box 82.2).[125] As for women without breast cancer, treatment (Table 82.3) is recommended for those with osteoporosis (T score −2.5 or lower). For women with osteopenia (T score between −1.00 and −2.49), treatment decisions should be based on an individual's fracture risk.

The use of bisphosphonates for survivors of breast cancer has increased dramatically in recent years, thanks to data from several trials showing that bisphosphonates protect against aromatase inhibitor–induced bone loss.[126–128] Data suggesting that adjuvant zoledronic acid infusions may also reduce risk of breast cancer recurrence in postmenopausal women have further increased enthusiasm for this approach. In addition, zoledronic acid also appears to prevent bone loss and possibly improve disease recurrence risk in premenopausal women who are receiving a gonadotropin-releasing hormone agonist as part of their adjuvant therapy. In the randomized, open-label, four-arm ABCSG-12 trial comparing adjuvant tamoxifen/goserelin and anastrozole/goserelin with or without zoledronic acid, twice-yearly zoledronic acid was found to preserve BMD at 3 years in the lumbar spine in 401 premenopausal patients with hormone-responsive early-stage breast cancer. BMD loss was greatest in the anastrozole/goserelin group (−17.3%) followed by the tamoxifen/goserelin group (−11.6%). No fractures were reported, but the median age of subjects was less than 50 years.[129] After 94.4 months of median follow-up, relative risks of disease progression (HR = 0.77; 95% CI 0.60–0.99; p = .042) and of death (HR = 0.66; 95% CI 0.43–1.02; p = .064) were lower in the patients who received zoledronic acid (although the trend toward an improved overall survival was not statistically significant).[130]

An increased risk of osteonecrosis of the jaw has raised concern over use of bisphosphonates. On the basis of reports of spontaneous osteonecrosis of the jaw submitted to manufacturers, the reporting rate is estimated at one event per 100,000 person-years of exposure, although these data have significant limitations.[131] Dental trauma is an important risk factor, with 60% occurring after a tooth extraction or other dentoalveolar procedure.[132] Good oral hygiene with regular dental care is the best way to reduce risk of osteoporosis of the jaw in breast cancer survivors taking bisphosphonates.[133]

Cardiovascular Disease

Cardiovascular disease (CVD) is a major cause of mortality and morbidity for women in the United States (Box 82.3).[134] Many

TABLE 82.3	**Drug Treatment for Postmenopausal Osteoporosis**	
Drug	**Dosage**	**Comments**
Bisphosphonates		
Alendronate Oral tablets and solution	Prevention: 5 mg/day or 35 mg/week Treatment: 10 mg/day or 70 mg/week	Alendronate and risedronate decrease risk of fracture at all sites by 50% in osteoporotic women[a]
Ibandronate Oral tablets	Prevention/treatment: 150 mg/month	Ibandronate not shown to reduce risk of hip fracture
Risedronate Oral tablets	Prevention/treatment: 5 mg daily or 35 mg weekly or 75 mg on 2 consecutive days (two tablets per month)	Zoledronic acid decreases risk of fracture by 70% at the vertebrae, 41% at the hip in osteoporotic women[b] Case reports of jaw osteonecrosis
Zoledronic acid IV infusion	Prevention: 5 mg yearly	Contraindicated in renal insufficiency Tablets contraindicated if esophageal abnormality or dysmotility
Selective Estrogen Response Modifier		
Raloxifene Oral tablet	Prevention/treatment: 60 mg/day	Theoretical concern for estrogen receptor modulation if concurrent or sequential use with tamoxifen[c]
Hormones		
Calcitonin nasal spray Solution for injection	Treatment: 200 IU/day intranasally or 100 IU every other day by SC or IM injection; also effective for acute fracture pain	Decreases risk of vertebral fracture Less potent antiresorptive effect than alendronate Consider for women unable to tolerate bisphosphonates
Teriparatide (parathyroid hormone) Solution for injection	Treatment: 20 µg/day by SC injection	Theoretical concern for stimulation of micrometastases in bone Not recommended after radiation therapy due to reports of osteosarcoma in animal studies[d]

IM, Intramuscular; *IV,* intravenous; *SC,* subcutaneous.

[a]Guyatt G, Cranney A, Griffith L, et al. Summary of meta-analyses of therapies for postmenopausal osteoporosis and relationship between bone density and fracture. *Endocrinol Metab Clin N Am.* 2002;31:659-679.

[b]Black DM, Delmas PD, Eastell R, et al. Once-yearly zoledronic acid for treatment of postmenopausal osteoporosis. *N Engl J Med.* 2007;356:1809-1822.

[c]O'Regan RM, Gajdos C, Dardes RC, et al. Effects of raloxifene after tamoxifen on breast and endometrial tumor growth in athymic mice. *J Natl Cancer Inst.* 2002;94:274-283.

[d]Vahle JL, Sato M, Long GG, et al. Skeletal changes in rats given daily SC injections of recombinant human parathyroid hormone (1-34) for 2 years and relevance to human safety. *Tox Pathol.* 2002;30:312-321.

patients and physicians are not aware that more women die every year from CVD than from breast cancer.[135] The majority of women with acute CVD are older than their male counterparts.[136] The delay in the development of coronary disease in women has long been attributed to the effects of circulating estrogen before menopause. Endogenous estrogen is known to have beneficial effects on cholesterol, vascular tone, and clotting factors. However, the risk of coronary disease increases after menopause and equals that of men by 80 years of age. Traditional cardiac risk factors (diabetes, hypertension, elevated cholesterol, smoking, family history) influence cardiac risk in women, but the magnitude of these effects may differ. Assessment of CVD risk in an asymptomatic postmenopausal breast cancer survivor should mimic that in any postmenopausal woman and should include a detailed history and physical examination with measurement of body mass index and blood pressure, as well as fasting lipid profile and glucose level, as dictated by American Heart Association Guidelines.[137] Women with a history of breast cancer may be especially motivated to engage in lifestyle change. Lifestyle modifications including achievement of optimal weight and regular exercise should be recommended to reduce risk of cardiovascular disease, as well as recurrent breast cancer, in survivors.[138]

There are special cardiovascular concerns for breast cancer survivors, including early menopause and the toxicities of some oncologic treatments. The effect of early menopause on CVD risk has not been well studied in any group of women, and it is unclear whether breast cancer survivors who receive ovarian function suppressing medication or who enter early menopause after chemotherapy or oophorectomy are at increased risk for coronary disease.

The effect of endocrine therapy on cardiovascular risk remains poorly studied as well. Tamoxifen is known to increase the risk of clotting but does not increase the risk of cardiac events, and it does not appear to significantly affect serum cholesterol in breast cancer survivors.[139] Aromatase inhibitor therapy does not affect clotting, but it may adversely affect lipid profiles. One study compared 3 months of letrozole to 3 months of exemestane in 246 postmenopausal breast cancer survivors and found that exemestane reduced high-density lipoprotein levels whereas letrozole increased low-density lipoprotein levels (but only in those who had previously been taking tamoxifen).[140] Another smaller study of patients with metastatic breast cancer showed that letrozole only increased low-density lipoprotein for the first 6 months of therapy, and levels returned to baseline thereafter.[141,142] Likewise, the SABRE trial suggested that lipid profiles did not change between baseline and 12 months in patients treated with adjuvant anastrozole.[142]

Conclusions

In women with breast cancer, menopause can significantly affect quality of life and long-term health. Alternative nonhormonal

---

• BOX 82.3 Women and Cardiovascular Disease

One in three women develop CVD
One in two women die of CVD
Endogenous estrogen levels appear protective until menopause
Traditional risk factors for men play a similar role in women
Unclear if breast cancer survivors are at increased risk for CVD
CVD risk assessment includes:
- Detailed history and physical examination
- Screening for hyperlipidernia, diabetes, and renal disease with fasting lipid profile, fasting glucose, and urinalysis
- Prompt referral to primary care provider or cardiologist for any abnormalities

Prevention of CVD includes:
- Regular exercise (30 minutes on most days of the week)
- Smoking cessation
- Limiting alcohol consumption to no more than four to seven drinks per week
- Low-dose aspirin is effective for stroke prevention but not myocardial infarction in women

CVD, Cardiovascular disease.

---

treatments, including certain antidepressants and gabapentinoids for hot flashes, and DHEA or nonhormonal topical preparations for vaginal dryness, should be used as first-line therapies. Although effective for symptom control, HT raises substantial safety concerns for women with a history of breast cancer, and its use is therefore limited to the management of severe, refractory vasomotor symptoms. Addressing the symptoms most bothersome to the patient is central to individualized care.

With advances in diagnosis and treatment, most women can expect to survive a diagnosis of breast cancer. Comprehensive care of breast cancer survivors must include screening for depression, osteoporosis, and CVD. Early detection and appropriate treatment will increase the likelihood that survivors will enjoy a longer, healthier life.

Selected References

7. Ruddy KJ, Guo H, Barry W, et al. Chemotherapy-related amenorrhea after adjuvant paclitaxel-trastuzumab (APT trial). *Breast Cancer Res Treat.* 2015;151:589-596.
20. Holmberg L, Anderson H. HABITS (hormonal replacement therapy after breast cancer—is it safe?), a randomised comparison: trial stopped. *Lancet.* 2004;363:453-455.
22. Sestak I, Kealy R, Edwards R, et al. Influence of hormone replacement therapy on tamoxifen-induced vasomotor symptoms. *J Clin Oncol.* 2006;24:3991-3996.
23. Beral V. Breast cancer and hormone-replacement therapy in the Million Women Study. *Lancet.* 2003;362:419-427.
24. Col NF, Kim JA, Chlebowski RT. Menopausal hormone therapy after breast cancer: a meta-analysis and critical appraisal of the evidence. *Breast Cancer Res.* 2005;7:R535-R540.
27. Loprinzi CL, Sloan JA, Perez EA, et al. Phase III evaluation of fluoxetine for treatment of hot flashes. *J Clin Oncol.* 2002;20:1578-1583.
48. Bardia A, Novotny P, Sloan J, et al. Efficacy of nonestrogenic hot flash therapies among women stratified by breast cancer history and tamoxifen use: a pooled analysis. *Menopause.* 2009;16:477-483.
51. Jin Y, Desta Z, Stearns V, et al. CYP2D6 genotype, antidepressant use, and tamoxifen metabolism during adjuvant breast cancer treatment. *J Natl Cancer Inst.* 2005;97:30-39.
56. Bordeleau L, Pritchard KI, Loprinzi CL, et al. Multicenter, randomized, cross-over clinical trial of venlafaxine versus gabapentin for the management of hot flashes in breast cancer survivors. *J Clin Oncol.* 2010;28:5147-5152.
63. Newton KM, Buist DS, Keenan NL, et al. Use of alternative therapies for menopause symptoms: results of a population-based survey. *Obstet Gynecol.* 2002;100:18-25.
69. Lethaby AE, Brown J, Marjoribanks J, et al. Phytoestrogens for vasomotor menopausal symptoms. *Cochrane Database Syst Rev.* 2007;(4):CD001395.
104. Sexton T, Younus J, Perera F, et al. Oxybutynin for refractory hot flashes in cancer patients. *Menopause.* 2007;14:505-509.
105. Suckling J, Lethaby A, Kennedy R. Local oestrogen for vaginal atrophy in postmenopausal women. *Cochrane Database Syst Rev.* 2006;(4):CD001500.
106. Wills S, Ravipati A, Venuturumilli P, et al. Effects of vaginal estrogens on serum estradiol levels in postmenopausal breast cancer survivors and women at risk of breast cancer taking an aromatase inhibitor or a selective estrogen receptor modulator. *J Oncol Pract.* 2012;8:144-148.
110. Nachtigall LE. Comparative study: Replens versus local estrogen in menopausal women. *Fertil Steril.* 1994;61:178-180.
114. Barton DL, Sloan J, Shuster LT, et al. Impact of vaginal dehydroepiandosterone (DHEA) on vaginal symptoms in female cancer survivors: Trial N10C1 (Alliance). *J Clin Oncol.* 2014;32(suppl 5).
118. Ganz PA. Breast cancer, menopause, and long-term survivorship: critical issues for the 21st century. *Am J Med.* 2005;118(suppl 12B):136-141.
121. Chen Z, Maricic M, Bassford TL, et al. Fracture risk among breast cancer survivors: results from the Women's Health Initiative Observational Study. *Arch Intern Med.* 2005;165:552-558.
122. Eastell R, Hannon RA, Cuzick J, et al. Effect of an aromatase inhibitor on bmd and bone turnover markers: 2-year results of the Anastrozole, Tamoxifen, Alone or in Combination (ATAC) trial (18233230). *J Bone Miner Res.* 2006;21:1215-1223.
125. Hillner BE, Ingle JN, Chlebowski RT, et al. American Society of Clinical Oncology 2003 update on the role of bisphosphonates and bone health issues in women with breast cancer. *J Clin Oncol.* 2003;21:4042-4057.
129. Gnant MF, Mlineritsch B, Luschin-Ebengreuth G, et al. Zoledronic acid prevents cancer treatment-induced bone loss in premenopausal women receiving adjuvant endocrine therapy for hormone-responsive breast cancer: a report from the Austrian Breast and Colorectal Cancer Study Group. *J Clin Oncol.* 2007;25:820-828.

A full reference list is available online at ExpertConsult.com.

83

Rehabilitation

SAMMAN SHAHPAR, PRIYA V. MHATRE, AND SONAL OZA

According to the National Cancer Institute and National Coalition for Cancer Survivorship, an individual is considered a cancer survivor from the time of cancer diagnosis through the balance of his or her life. With improved diagnostics and treatment plans, the "balance of life" has been steadily increasing with an estimated 2.975 million female breast cancer survivors in the United States in 2012.[1] As a result of breast cancer and its treatment, survivors often develop impairments. Impairments may be classified as short-term when occurring during treatment, long-term when occurring at the time of diagnosis or treatment and then persisting, or as late effects that may manifest after treatment has completed or as currently unrecognized toxicities. A survivor's experiences are unique and involve factors that are disease-specific (cancer type, location, presence of metastases), treatment-specific (surgery, chemotherapy, radiation, endocrine therapy), and individual-specific (precancer medical and functional status, precancer psychosocial status). Consequently, breast cancer survivors often do not feel quite the same as they have before diagnosis and may experience a decline or loss of function, impeding their ability to perform job-related, recreational, and other daily activities.

Cancer rehabilitation can be defined as any evaluation or intervention assisting in restoration of maximum function and ability in any survivor with cancer at any point in the disease continuum. The rehabilitation team is best led by a physiatrist, who is a specialist in physical medicine and rehabilitation (PM&R) and responsible for patient's overall functional health. Although there is no formal subspecialty of cancer rehabilitation, there are physiatrists that focus their clinical and research interests specifically on this population, whereas many others often have experience working with cancer survivors. Other members of the rehabilitation team include physical therapists, occupational therapists, speech language pathologists, exercise physiologists, and rehabilitation nurses. Each member of the rehabilitation team brings a unique skill set and training background that survivors may benefit from. Not unlike an oncology team, individualized care should be developed based on an individual survivor's current and future potential impairments.

Multiple studies have demonstrated a high prevalence of physical impairments amenable to rehabilitation in the breast cancer populations.[2,3] Thus it is clear that cancer rehabilitation should be an important component of a survivor's care plan. However, this is not always the reality.[4] This chapter highlights the need for rehabilitation care to be involved in the care breast cancer survivors' care from the time of diagnosis throughout the balance of his or her life.

Deconditioning

Deconditioning can be defined as multiple, potentially reversible changes in body systems brought about by physical inactivity and disuse. It is a cumulative multifactorial phenomenon, resulting in functional decline in multiple body systems. It is not an "all or nothing" decline but occurs across a spectrum depending on length and frequency of inactivity. It is important to understand that the changes that occur due to deconditioning are separate from any change due to other underlying medical or surgical issues. Breast cancer survivors often have a decrease in their activity level before, during, and after treatment secondary to the physical, psychological, and social stressors on their lives. It is important for all clinicians to be aware of potential effects that may occur due to those activity changes. This section reviews the major changes seen in the musculoskeletal and cardiovascular systems, and Box 83.1 highlights some of the other effects that can be seen throughout the body.

Musculoskeletal System

With strict bedrest, skeletal muscle strength declines by 1% to 1.5% per day[5,6] and with cast immobilization, up to 1.3% to 5.5% decline in strength per day can be seen.[7,8] The loss of strength is noted to be greatest within the first week of immobilization, decreasing up to 40%.[9,10]

Muscle atrophy is another complication with the reduction of muscle protein synthesis and whole body protein production as likely main contributors.[11,12] Type 1 muscle fibers are affected more than type 2 muscle fibers, and the lower limbs are affected more that upper limbs.[13,7] There is evidence that these processes can be minimized with activity, including as little as resisted leg exercise greater than 50% of maximum effort every second day.[14,15] A potential treatment target is the inhibition of myostatin, which is a growth factor-beta protein that inhibits muscle synthesis and known to increase during bed rest.[16] Although there are no current available treatments for humans, there are ongoing animal studies.

It is also important to be aware of sarcopenia, which is an age-related loss of muscle mass and strength. Despite society's acceptance of loss of muscle mass and strength with age, sarcopenia has been shown to be reversible with high-intensity resistive exercise.[17]

Cardiovascular System

With bedrest, immobilization tachycardia can occur, and with 3 weeks of bed rest, it has been shown that resting heart rate can

• BOX 83.1 Effects of Deconditioning

Increase risk of deep vein thrombosis
Impaired balance and coordination
Perceptual impairment
Restlessness
Decreased pain tolerance
Sleep disturbance
Insulin resistance
Decreased bone density
Urinary retention/incomplete bladder emptying
Decreased diaphragmatic movement with decreased strength and endurance
    of intercostal, axillary respiratory muscles leading to atelectasis, hypostatic
    pneumonia
Reflux esophagitis
Decreased peristalsis/constipation

• BOX 83.2 ICD-10 Criteria for Cancer-Related Fatigue

The following symptoms have been present every day or nearly every day during the same 2-week period in the past month:
A. Significant fatigue, diminished energy, or increased need to rest, disproportionate to any recent change in activity level, plus five or more of the following:
    1. Complaints of generalized weakness, limb heaviness
    2. Diminished concentration or attention
    3. Decreased motivation or interest to engage in usual activities
    4. Insomnia or hypersomnia
    5. Experience of sleep as unrefreshing or nonrestorative
    6. Perceived need to struggle to overcome inactivity
    7. Marked emotional reactivity to feeling fatigued
    8. Difficulty completing daily tasks attributed to feeling fatigued
    9. Perceived problems with short-term memory
    10. Postexertional fatigue lasting several hours
B. The symptoms cause clinically significant distress or impairment in social, occupational, or other important areas of functioning
C. There is evidence from the history, physical examination, or laboratory findings that the symptoms are a consequence of cancer or cancer therapy
D. The symptoms are not primarily a consequence of comorbid psychiatric disorders such as major depression, somatization disorder, or delirium

ICD-10, International Classification of Diseases, 10th Revision.
From Cella D, Davis K, Breitbart W, et al. Cancer-related fatigue: prevalence of proposed diagnostic criteria in a United States sample of cancer survivors. J Clin Oncol. 2001;19:3385-391.

increase 10 to 12 beats per minute.[18] After just 24 hours of bed rest, plasma volume can decrease with a correlated drop in cardiac output and stroke volume.[19,20] With these changes, and additionally a blunted sympathetic response with limited vasoconstriction, orthostasis can occur.[21] The body's normal response from rising up from supine may be completely lost after 3 weeks and make take weeks to months for recovery.

Cardiopulmonary Fitness

Cardiopulmonary fitness, which is a key predictor for mortality in all populations, can be measured in metabolic equivalents (METs) or maximal oxygen consumption ($VO_{2max} = mL \cdot kg^{-1} \cdot min^{-1}$, 1 MET = 3.5 mL $O_2 \cdot kg^{-1} \cdot min^{-1}$). In part, due to the effects already discussed, deconditioning causes a significant reduction of cardiopulmonary fitness. With 20 days of bed rest, VO_{2max} can decline by 27%.[22,23] However, this may be counteracted with even low levels of physical activity (see Box 83.1).[24]

Fatigue

Cancer-related fatigue (CRF) is one of the most common and concerning symptoms for breast cancer survivors during treatment, but often persists in disease-free survivors.[25,26] CRF is defined by the National Comprehensive Cancer Network (NCCN) as a persistent, subjective sense of physical, emotional, and/or cognitive tiredness or exhaustion related to cancer or cancer treatment that is not proportional to recent activity and interferes with usual functioning.[27] CRF may clinically present as sensory, physical, affective, and/or behavioral complaints with fatigue often further classified as peripheral or central in nature depending on a survivor's symptoms. This multidimensional nature is evident in the *International Classification of Diseases,* 10th Revision (ICD-10) definition of CRF (Box 83.2).[28]

The pathophysiology of CRF is not well understood. Recent research has begun to connect fatigue symptoms with inflammation and inflammatory pathways. It is still not clear what triggers the initial inflammatory process, although it is suspected to be related to the underlying malignancy and the various oncologic treatment interventions stimulating a neuroendocrine, immune, and/or biopsychological response.[29] Studies have demonstrated increased inflammatory biomarkers in breast cancer survivors with fatigue initially posttreatment and persisting years after treatment has been completed.[30–32]

Screening and Diagnosis

According to NCCN guidelines, the recommendation for standard of care includes all patients being screened for fatigue at the initial visit as well as regularly during and after cancer treatment with the use of interdisciplinary teams for management.[30] Although there is an ICD-10 criterion for the diagnosis, there is no clear objective assessment tool. However, CRF can be evaluated and monitored by using one of the available patient reported outcome measures, such as Patient-Reported Outcomes Measurement Information System (PROMIS) Fatigue Short Forms or Brief Fatigue Inventory (BFI).

Treatment

Breast cancer survivors may also have other numerous potential contributing etiologies for CRF (Box 83.3). Many of the underlying factors are treatable, including anemia, endocrine dysfunction, sleep disturbances, poor nutrition/hydration, pain, mood disturbances, and deconditioning. Beyond addressing these factors, pharmacologic interventions include the use of stimulants, such as methylphenidate and modafinil, although currently evidence is limited to survivors undergoing active treatment or with advanced disease.[33] Cytokine antagonists, which disrupt initiation and continuation of the suspected underlying proinflammatory pathways, have also shown promise in improving CRF in cancer survivors, although data are quite limited thus far.[34,35] There is better evidence that exercise interventions can improve CRF.[36,37] In addition, exercise has well-accepted benefits on muscle strength, cardiopulmonary fitness, aerobic capacity, quality of sleep, pain, and mood disturbances. Studies also support psychological interventions, such as a cognitive behavioral therapy and relaxation therapy, as well as education. However, these positive research findings are limited in widespread applicability due to study population and intervention variability.

In summary, breast cancer survivors with CRF should be evaluated for physical activity, rehabilitation, and psychological interventions as well as have treatable contributing factors and concurrent symptoms addressed.[38]

Upper Quadrant Dysfunction

Breast cancer survivors are at heightened risk to develop upper quadrant (neck, upper thorax, axilla, and arm) dysfunction. This dysfunction can manifest during the treatment period and may persist for months to years. Studies have reported upper extremity pain and limited upper quadrant flexibility and strength at up to 10 years posttreatment completion.[39,40] Upper extremity impairment and pain suggests an underlying musculoskeletal or neuromuscular disorder. Cited postsurgical effects include axillary web syndrome, lymphedema, postmastectomy pain syndrome, paresthesias, and decreased glenohumeral range of motion (ROM) due to rotator cuff disease or shoulder impingement syndrome. There is a significant association among pain, disability, and scapulothoracic dysfunction.[41] Left unaddressed, these conditions reduce function; impede one's ability to participate in daily activities and to reintegrate fully into the community. The following is a summary of upper extremity biomechanics, observed treatment-related effects, the impact on daily life, and methods to identify individuals with upper extremity limitations.

Pretreatment Upper Quadrant Function

Musculoskeletal disorders of the neck and shoulder are known to occur with age. Preoperative upper extremity ROM, level of activity, and pain may be predictors of long-term functional outcome.

The incidence of preoperative impairments such as mobility and pain varies. One study revealed that 40% of more than 2000 breast cancer survivors with shoulder symptoms at 5-year follow-up postsurgery and postradiation had also reported symptoms at baseline.[42] Additionally, it has been demonstrated that survivors with pectoralis tightness either at preoperative baseline or 3 months after had a higher prevalence of rotator cuff disease at 1 year posttreatment.[43] Because these survivors may be more susceptible to further injury after surgery and radiation therapy, appropriate screening before surgical intervention could prevent further decline.

Biomechanics: Range of Motion, Scapular Control, Muscle Strength

Breast cancer survivors often exhibit reduced shoulder flexion, shoulder abduction, and lateral rotation.[40,41,44–46] Some have reported up to 68 degrees of decreased ROM reported in individuals posttreatment.[40] A review of more than 5000 breast cancer survivors demonstrated decreased abduction, forward flexion at 1 month postsurgery and decreased abduction, internal rotation, and strength at 2 years.[47] Furthermore, the limited mobility may persist for more than 5 years in 20% to 80% of survivors.[42,48] Even in survivors with intact range of motion, a thorough strength assessment often reveals weakness with dynamic movement.

The preceding findings suggest that cancer and its treatment alter shoulder mechanics. Three-dimensional motion analysis has revealed significant asymmetry in humeral movement and differences in the anterior and posterior tilt between the treated and the normal side.[41] Changes in muscle size and recruitment likely contribute to this reduced scapular stability. Dynamic studies have shown an ipsilateral weakened and smaller pectoralis minor muscle as well as decreased recruitment of the upper trapezius, rhomboid and serratus anterior. The pectoral shortening can cause anterior posturing. Interestingly, the decreased activity of upper trapezius and rhomboids suggests altered muscle activity in areas indirect to the treatment field. Weakened, stiffened shoulder girdle muscles are associated with increased susceptibility to rotator cuff injury, winged scapula, brachial plexopathy and axillary web syndrome and dropped shoulder syndrome.[41] As already described, the weakened shoulder stabilizing muscles affect upper extremity function.

Correlation of Surgical Intervention and Upper Quadrant Dysfunction

Proposed causative factors for altered upper quadrant biomechanics include the type of surgical procedure, use of radiation therapy and decreased use of the treated side. Depending on the degree of tissue removal, the resulting asymmetry in mass alters scapulohumeral movement as previously described.[49] Furthermore, tumor resection or lymph node removal involves interventions proximal to critical neural structures. Axillary nerve injury during the axillary lymph node dissection (ALND) even without nerve dissection can result in symptoms in addition to potentially affecting the nearby thoracodorsal, long thoracic, and intercostal brachial nerves.

The type of surgery affects impairment. In a systematic review, women had a 5.67 times greater odds for shoulder restriction postmastectomy.[40] Additionally, ALND appears to be associated with greater shoulder morbidity than sentinel lymph node biopsy (SLNB).[39,50–52] Studies have found that 10% to 80% of participants post ALND demonstrated decreased ROM versus 0% to 41% post SLNB.[48,53,54] These individuals also exhibit a higher prevalence of pectoral tightness. Although many improve or return to premorbid function after 6 months to 1 year, a growing number of studies show reduced mobility in the ALND group after 5 to 10 years. Individuals with SLNB typically present with less arm pain swelling, and decreased incidence of paresthesias compared with those post-ALND.[48,53–55]

It should be considered that individuals who undergo ALND likely had more extensive disease and may have undergone additional treatments affecting physical health. Regardless, the finding serves as a way to identify individuals at risk and presents an objective way to measure function.

Impact of Impairments on Daily Activities

Many daily activities require shoulder mobility and coordination. Overall, impaired mobility, altered mechanics, and weakness affects activities requiring some force or impact or free arm movement.[56] Decreased upper trapezius and serratus muscle activity is significantly associated with pain while performing activities such as placing an object on a shelf or pushing an object.[41] Individuals acknowledged difficulty also with opening a jar, ironing, and carrying groceries.[44,56]

Relationship to Physical Activity Level

Pain when using the arm and ROM restriction has been found to be significant predictor of activity level up to years posttreatment. Multiple long-term analyses cite grip strength, elbow strength, and shoulder abduction mobility as predictors of subsequent impairment and function.[44,51] These predictors persist over a time, with one study citing significance at up to 7 years.[57] Conversely, less physically active individuals before surgery have a propensity to develop shoulder morbidity or limitations. Older, obese, and less educated are also more likely to report limitations (Fig. 83.1).[58]

Screening

Upon evaluation of a breast cancer survivor, given the prevalence and associated comorbidities, screening should be performed for upper quadrant dysfunction. The history should attempt to elicit any history for upper quadrant or shoulder injuries and dysfunction. The physical examination should at least include range of motion assessment with shoulder flexion, extension, abduction as well as internal and external rotation, observation for signs of scapular asymmetry or winging at rest and with range of motion activities, grip strength, and assessing for signs of lymphedema or axillary cording. In addition, several validated self-reported questionnaires area available to assess upper quadrant dysfunction in breast cancer survivors. The questions address the ability to carry out daily activities, level of pain, and quality of life (Box 83.4).

Treatment

Treatment for upper quadrant dysfunction depends on the diagnosis. Generally, a multimodality approach is used that includes medications, physical and/or occupational therapy. Evaluation by a physiatrist will guide the individualized treatment plan to restore function. Specific therapy interventions involve soft tissue scar massage, stretching, scapular stabilization and postural exercises, strength training, and myofascial release.[59] Strategies to retrain upper quadrant proprioception improve coordination. For individuals whose pain limits mobility and strength, nonsteroidal antiinflammatory drugs are the recommended first-line agent. For more severe or nonremitting pain, individuals should undergo evaluation for a steroid injection; however, this should be in conjunction with physical therapy.[60] For those with lymphedema, massage, compression wrapping, and special garments help to redirect fluid. Individuals would benefit from a referral to a certified lymphedema specialist.

In summary, upper quadrant dysfunction is a combination of reduced mobility, decreased strength and endurance and altered mechanics. Although some of the impairments may not be caused solely by cancer treatment, it is important to assess for underlying musculoskeletal conditions to determine who may be susceptible to further progression. Because of the effects of upper quadrant limitations on daily activities and physical activity, the interplay of musculoskeletal pathology, function, and quality of life have emerged as key issues in survivorship care.

Neuropathy

The treatment of breast cancer can cause both short- and long-term effects on the peripheral nervous system, leading to pain and loss of function.

Mononeuropathies

Upper extremity mononeuropathies are common in the general population and also affect breast cancer patients, both during and after treatment.

Carpal tunnel syndrome (CTS) is classified by compression of the median nerve at the wrist level. Affected individuals initially

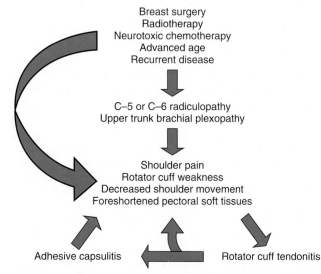

• **Fig. 83.1** Algorithm for predictors of shoulder mobility limitations. (From Stubblefield MD, Keole N. Upper body pain and functional disorders in patients with breast cancer. *PM R.* 2014;6:170-183.)

> • **BOX 83.4** **Self-Reported Questionnaires to Assess Upper Quadrant Dysfunction**
>
> American Shoulder and Elbow Surgeons Shoulder Score
> DASH (Disabilities of the Arm, Shoulder, and Hand questionnaire)
> Kwan's Arm Problem Scale
> Pennsylvania Shoulder Score
> Shoulder Disability Questionnaire

present with paresthesias within the median nerve distribution of the palmar surface of the hand; symptoms can progress to include sensory changes and motor weakness. It has been previously proposed that lymphedema related to breast cancer is a risk factor for development of CTS, but a recent retrospective study by Stubblefield and coworkers found that there was no association between presence or severity of lymphedema and CTS.[61]

Other mononeuropathies, such as cubital tunnel syndrome (ulnar nerve entrapment at the elbow) or radial neuropathy can also be seen breast cancer patients but are overall less common.

Radiculopathy

Cervical radiculopathy is a commonly encountered diagnosis in both the general and breast cancer populations, leading to neck and arm pain, as well as arm weakness. Compression occurs most often secondary to herniation of the intervertebral disc, but in breast cancer patients, other etiologies such as instability or tumors should also be considered. Symptomatic radiculopathies can also develop or worsen during chemotherapy treatment.[62]

Patients typically present with neck pain radiating into the upper extremity, with symptoms typically following a dermatomal or myotomal distribution. Weakness is expected but may not be present if only the dorsal nerve root is affected.[60] On physical examination, cervical spine range of motion should be assessed; lateral rotation or bending toward the affected side may reproduce symptoms. Evaluation of strength, sensation, and reflexes will also assist in the identification and localization of affected nerve roots.

Brachial Plexopathy

Brachial plexopathy may be seen in survivors of breast cancer, but is typically not seen at time of initial diagnosis unless disease is already advanced.[62] Brachial plexopathy is frequently seen from either local tumor invasion or as a complication of radiation therapy.

In all cancer survivors, the frequency of neoplastic brachial plexopathy is 0.43%, but in breast cancer survivors, this number can be as high as 1.8% to 4.9%.[63] Tumors have a tendency to invade the lower plexus initially and present with pain (localized to shoulder and axilla with radicular symptoms into the arm/hand).[63] Horner syndrome (ptosis, miosis, and anhidrosis) may also be present.

In breast cancer specifically, radiation therapy (RT) can lead to radiation-induced brachial plexopathy (RIBP), with injury localized to the axillary-supraclavicular region. Delayed progressive RIBP can occur months to decades after treatment.[64,65] The overall incidence of RIBP has drastically declined with advances in radiation therapy; from 15% of those receiving total dose of 57.75 Gy and 73% of those receiving total dose of 63 Gy,[66] to current incidence of less than 2% of women irradiated for breast cancer.[65,67]

Survivors typically present with sensory changes such as paresthesias, with eventual progression to hypoesthesia; neuropathic pain is rare. Survivors develop motor weakness, which progressively worsens, and can eventually lead to upper limb paralysis. Skin and muscle atrophy may also occur. The overall prognosis for delayed progressive RIBP is poor.

Less commonly, survivors can develop early transient RIBP within the first year after irradiation. Those with early transient RIBP have better prognosis; 80% will have complete resolution

of symptoms. Symptoms are initially similar to delayed progressive RIBP, with distal paresthesias but also with proximal pain. Motor impairments can occur immediately or within a few months and progressively worsen. Symptoms typically regress within 3 to 6 months.[64]

Chemotherapy-Induced Peripheral Neuropathy

Chemotherapy is a frequently used treatment modality in breast cancer, and chemotherapy-induced peripheral neuropathy (CIPN) is a common adverse effect experienced by cancer survivors.[68] CIPN is classified by damage or dysfunction to the peripheral nerves and can include motor, sensory, and autonomic nerves of the upper and lower extremities.[60,69] Survivors often present with sensory symptoms such as paresthesias, numbness, cold sensitivity, or pain; less commonly, motor symptoms such as weakness may be seen. Several chemotherapy agents have been implicated in the development of CIPN.

Taxanes

Taxanes are an established treatment regimen for both early and metastatic breast cancer but are well known to cause neuropathy; incidence of taxane-associated CIPN ranges from 11% to 64% overall for docetaxel to 57% to 83% for paclitaxel.[69] The mechanism of action of taxanes is to affect microtubules, an essential component of both mitotic spindles and also axonal structures of nerves; axonal damage, therefore, is a common side effect.[70] The solvents used in various taxanes can be an additional source of neurotoxicity; the solvent of paclitaxel, for example, has been shown in preclinical studies to lead to axonal degeneration and demyelination.[71] The neurotoxic effects of taxanes appear to be dose dependent, with higher or more frequent doses associated with higher incidence of neuropathy. Persistent neuropathy can be a dose-limiting factor for treatment of breast cancers with taxanes, in turn affecting survival rates.[69–71] Taxane-related CIPN is managed with dose delays or reductions; discontinuation is recommended for patients who develop severe neuropathy.[71] Symptoms can present as early as within the first 24 hours of infusion, and may improve or resolve within 3 to 6 months of discontinuation in mild to moderate cases, but more severe cases of neuropathy are less likely to resolve.[69,72]

Platinum Derivatives

Platinum derivative chemotherapy agents have also been implicated in causing CIPN, primarily because platinum compounds deposit within dorsal root ganglion cells, leading to neurotoxicity. The incidence of CIPN from cisplatin, one platinum derivative, ranges from 10% to 28%.[69] Symptoms include numbness, tingling and paresthesias in the upper and lower extremities as well as ataxia.[72,73] Platinum-induced CIPN can be associated with worsening neuropathy symptoms after discontinuation of treatment, known as "coasting."[69,72,73]

Vinca Alkaloids

Vinca alkaloids can also lead to CIPN. Similar to taxanes, these chemotherapy agents target the microtubules, and lead to adverse effects in axons.[73] The incidence of CIPN secondary to vinca alkaloids ranges from 30% to 47%.[69] Vinca alkaloids generally lead to a sensory neuropathy but can also cause ataxia (although less frequently than platinum derivatives). These agents can also lead to severe autonomic impairment, including bladder dysfunction and constipation.[72]

Risk factors for developing CIPN regardless of agent used include diabetes mellitus, prior exposure to neurotoxic chemotherapy, and radiculopathy.[69]

Diagnosis

Many neuropathies can be diagnosed through history and physical alone. Electrodiagnostic studies (electromyography and nerve conduction studies) can also be helpful for diagnosing mononeuropathies (such as CTS), brachial plexopathy, and peripheral neuropathy. Advanced imaging such as magnetic resonance imaging can be used for evaluation for cervical radiculopathy (to evaluate for disc herniation or tumor invasion) as well as brachial plexopathy (to rule out tumor recurrence).

Treatment

Unfortunately, no agents exist to prevent the development of neuropathies associated with breast cancer. Treatment is targeted toward symptomatic management. Recent guidelines from the American Society of Clinical Oncology recommend use of duloxetine for management of pain associated with chemotherapy-induced peripheral neuropathy.[74] Other agents, such as tricyclic antidepressants (such as amitriptyline or nortriptyline), gabapentin, antiepileptics (such as lamotrigine), may be considered but do not have robust evidence at this time (Table 83.1).[72]

TABLE 83.1	Selected Pharmacologic Agents Evaluated for Treatment of CIPN	
Pharmacologic Agent	Neurotoxic Chemotherapy	Recommendation
Acetyl-l-carnitine		Not recommended—prevention trial associated with increased CIPN
Duloxetine	Taxane or platinum	Recommended—positive trial for oxaliplatin or paclitaxel neuropathy
Gabapentin	Vinca alkaloids, platinum, or taxanes	Not recommended—negative trial, but effective in other forms of neuropathy
Lamotrigine	Vinca alkaloids, platinum, or taxanes	Not recommended—negative trial
Nortriptyline/amitriptyline	Vinca alkaloids, platinum (cisplatin), or taxanes	Not recommended—small trials, not powered but favor treatment arms
Topical (amitriptyline, ketamine, ± baclofen)	Vinca alkaloids, platinum, taxanes, or thalidomide	Not recommended—suggestion of improvement in active treatment arm, but not statistically significant

CIPN, Chemotherapy-induced peripheral neuropathy.
From Hershman DL, Lacchetti C, Dworkin RH, et al; American Society of Clinical Oncology. Prevention and management of chemotherapy-induced peripheral neuropathy in survivors of adult cancers: American Society of Clinical Oncology clinical practice guideline. *J Clin Oncol.* 2014;32:1941-1967.

Acupuncture

Acupuncture is becoming an increasingly common modality to treat acute and chronic pain, including CIPN. It may be administered with or without electrical stimulation (called electroacupuncture). Although the exact mechanism of action has not been identified, proposed pathways include stimulating the release of endogenous opioids and neurotransmitters, inhibiting proinflammatory pathways, and improving nerve conduction velocity[75,76,77] The treatment is fairly well tolerated, with one study evaluating more than 31,000 acupuncture consultations demonstrating the most common side effects of bleeding at the needling site, pain, and aggravation of symptoms, none of which persisted.[78] Case series and small prospective trials have demonstrated the benefit of acupuncture in improving symptoms of CIPN[79,80,81]; however, systematic reviews have concluded there is insufficient evidence to evaluate the effectiveness of acupuncture due to small sample sizes in studies.[76,82] Given the limited evidence of any efficacious treatment for CIPN, acupuncture should still be considered as a primary or adjuvant treatment modality as the potential benefits appear to outweigh risks.

Pain

As described earlier, breast cancer survivors experience pain due to the tumor, posttreatment effects, and the effect of other medical comorbidities. Pain can be classified as nociceptive, neuropathic, or mixed. Nociceptive pain is related to damage to body tissues and being further broken down into somatic pain, which is from the body surface or musculoskeletal tissues, and visceral pain, which is from pain receptors of internal organs and may cause referred pain. Neuropathic pain is caused by dysfunction in the nervous system.

The frequency and intensity of pain varies among survivors. Overall the discomfort and dysfunction decreases with time, and studies have shown that most survivors returned to baseline by 3 months.[83] However, a number of survivors report moderate levels of pain months to years postsurgery with one study indicating 30% of individuals reporting pain at rest at 5-year follow-up (Box 83.5).[84]

Screening

In 2015, the American Cancer Society and American Society of Clinical Oncology published guidelines for the assessment of breast cancer survivors. The guidelines highlight the recommendation for clinicians to assess for musculoskeletal symptoms, including pain, by asking patients about their symptoms at each clinical encounter and, when appropriate, offer interventions, including acupuncture, physical activity, and referral for physical therapy or rehabilitation.[85] Although pain measurement is subjective, a focus on correlation to function effectively guides management. Asking about pain at rest, during activity, and interference with daily function helps to elicit this information. Rehabilitation and pain experts suggest a multidisciplinary approach: medication, physical therapy, exercise, and psychosocial interventions.[86]

Treatment

Similar to pain in noncancer survivors, providers should carefully assess the etiology of pain and attempt to treat modifiable factors. When determining the use of medications, the World Health

---

• BOX 83.5 Chronic Pain Syndromes

Surgery
Intercostal neuralgia
Lymphedema
Neuroma pain
Pain related to implants, reconstruction
Phantom pain
Postmastectomy pain

Radiation
Chest pain/tightness
Fibrosis of skin or myofascia
Myelopathy
Osteoradionecrosis
Peripheral nerve entrapment
Plexopathies

Hormonal Therapy
Arthralgia/myalgia
Muscle cramp/spasm
Carpal tunnel syndrome
Trigger finger

Chemotherapy
Arthralgia/myalgia
Osteoporosis
Osteonecrosis
Chemotherapy-induced peripheral neuropathy
Muscle cramps

Steroids
Osteoporosis
Osteonecrosis (avascular necrosis, typically femoral head, knee, humeral head)

Bisphosphonate
Osteonecrosis of the jaw

Modified from Stubblefield MD, Keole N. Upper body pain and functional disorders in patients with breast cancer. PM R. 2014;6:170-183.

• BOX 83.6 Key Points of 2008 Physical Activity Guidelines for Americans

Avoid inactivity; some physical activity is better than none.
Adults should do at least 150 minutes of moderate-intensity aerobic activity or 75 minutes of vigorous-intensity aerobic activity per week.
Further health benefits are gained by engaging in physical activity beyond the recommendations.
Muscle-strengthening activities involving all major muscle groups should also be include in the exercise program on 2 or more days a week for additional health benefits.

From 2008 Physical Activity Guidelines for Americans. U.S. Department of Health and Human Services. <http://health.gov/paguidelines/pdf/paguide.pdf>; October 2008.

Organization recommends a three-step approach, often referred to as the analgesic ladder. The first step is the initiation of nonopioid pain medications for mild pain with or without adjuvant medications to treat symptoms such as anxiety, depression, or insomnia as well neuropathic symptoms. If the pain is not relieved or is moderate in severity, then addition of weak opioids should be considered. If the pain is still not relieved or increases in severity, a strong opioid may be trialed. Individuals should be closely followed to adjust the regimen as appropriate. If oral medications continue to lack efficacy, then interventional measures should be considered, although these may be used earlier if a clear amenable etiology is identified.

The use of therapy services and modalities is often indicated and should be used in conjunction with medication management. As discussed earlier, upper quadrant dysfunction and musculoskeletal related conditions are amenable to treatment with a therapy program. For neuropathic pain, desensitization and transcutaneous electrical stimulation units may provide relief. Specific therapy modalities vary depending on the patient and specific etiologies of pain, but manual stretching and massage, progressive resistance training, myofascial release, and neuromuscular reeducation have been shown to alleviate symptoms.

Exercise

Physical activity has been described as any body movement requiring energy expenditure; it can be an activity of daily life or recreational. Exercise also is defined as movement but is more structured and has measurable parameters, including body fat, range of motion, muscle strength, endurance, and cardiovascular capacity.[87,88] Often, clinicians and patients may use the terms interchangeably, but the structure and measurability of exercise are key differentiating components and important when attempting to address medical and functional impairments.

Exercise had been postulated to modulate certain cellular pathways, inhibiting the process of carcinogenesis and promoting the body's own immune response.[89] In addition, there are indirect effects for cancer prevention in ways such as helping achieve a health ideal body weight, decreasing insulin resistance.[90,91]

Exercise may also be able to assist in controlling tumor recurrence and progression in conjunction with standard oncologic therapies. This has been demonstrated in mice models using estrogen receptor–negative and estrogen receptor–positive tumor cells implanted orthotopically and randomly assigned to exercise or sedentary control groups. The exercise group demonstrated statistically significantly reduced tumor growth, increased apoptosis compared with the sedentary group.[92]

Although deconditioning plays a role in reducing cardiopulmonary fitness as discussed earlier, breast cancer survivors have been shown to have a VO_{2max} 21% to 27% lower than agematched healthy sedentary women prior the adjuvant treatment.[93,94] This decline in VO_{2max} has been to shown to become more significant during adjuvant chemotherapy and even persist up 7 years after treatment as completed.[94,95] When considering that prior studies have shown a reduction of death by 17% in women for every 1 MET increase in aerobic capacity, this impairment of cardiopulmonary fitness is even more concerning.[96] There is evidence that exercise can not only prevent this decrement in cardiopulmonary fitness but also creates improvements, even during cancer treatment.[97,98]

Given the proven positive effects of physical activity and exercise, American College of Sports Medicine published its Exercise Guidelines for Cancer Survivors in 2010. The guidelines concluded that exercise training is not only safe during and after cancer treatments but also recommended cancer survivors follow the 2008 Physical Activity Guidelines for Americans with adaptations, if needed, given the benefits on physical functioning and quality of life (Box 83.6).[99]

Cognitive Dysfunction

Cognitive dysfunction after treatment of breast cancer is common, with prior studies showing that at least 19% of patients may be affected before or after chemotherapy treatment, or both. A definitive cause has not been identified as the etiology of pretreatment cognitive decline, although inflammatory cascades and altered cognitive/brain reserves have been proposed.[100] There has been an association noted between postchemotherapy cognitive dysfunction and the dose of chemotherapy administered: those exposed to high dose chemotherapy are more likely to demonstrate impairments on neuropsychological testing.[101] Endocrine therapy has also been implicated as a cause of cognitive decline. Cognitive changes can be seen in the realms of attention, concentration, memory, and executive function and may persist up to 20 years after treatment.[102]

Screening

The gold standard to evaluate for cognitive impairment is neuropsychological testing; testing, however, can be time-consuming and must be administered by a trained psychologist.[103] Several questionnaires have been developed to screen for cognitive dysfunction and can be administered during physician clinic visits. The Cognitive Failures Questionnaire is a 25-item survey that assess cognitive changes in the past 6 months and has been shown to have good validity.[104] Other computer-based tests, such as CogHealth and Headminder, are able to assess realms including reaction time, memory, and executive function; these tests have also been validated for use in non-English-speaking individuals.[103]

Treatment

The treatment of cognitive dysfunction can include medications or therapy. Medications that have been used include gingko biloba and methylphenidate, although studies have not been conclusive on positive effects with long-term use. Cognitive rehabilitation therapy can include specialized treatments by speech language pathologists in the outpatient setting, or computerized training programs to focus on memory and executive function.[101]

Vocational Rehabilitation

A number of breast cancer survivors are diagnosed with cancer during their working years and often cannot anticipate how their work life may change. Many health care providers may not have discussed how the cancer and treatment could prevent them from functioning at the same capacity at work.

The rate of return to the same or different employer varies from 30% to 93% in cancer survivors.[105] Cancer survivors may be 1.4 times more likely to be unemployed.[106] A number of factors limit return to work in this population. In breast cancer survivors, those post-ALND with limited ROM had a greater percent decrease in return to work.[53] Additionally, CRF, impaired mobility, and cognitive changes may affect work performance and productivity. Work environment factors such as the nature of the occupation, time commitment, and employer knowledge, and support greatly affect one's ability to return to work.[107]

Employment provides a number of personal and societal benefits. Psychologically, it provides a sense of purpose and fulfillment. It may be associated with improved health recovery in cancer survivors and enables the pursuit of financial stability while contributing to society's economic health. Additionally, survivors often need to continue with their employment to maintain adequate insurance coverage to offset the costs of their cancer care.

Vocational rehabilitation is a multipronged approach to facilitate employment. It involves interactions with the patient and employer. Conversations with the employer entail understanding the physical work environment as well as work hours and potential modifications while facilitating communication between the employer and health care providers as appropriate.[105] With the patient, interventions such as stress management, coping mechanisms and problem-solving suggestions serve to empower individuals. For those with health-limiting factors, it directs patients toward appropriate medical providers. Through these, the rehabilitation program assesses one's capacity to work and implements targeted vocational counseling. Vocational counselors can also assist with navigating legal and benefits issues.

Conclusion

Breast cancer survivors may experience a multitude of impairments that affect quality of life, participation in daily activities, physical activity and exercise, and employment status. In conjunction with the oncology team, the rehabilitation team led by a physiatrist can empower individuals with cancer to navigate and to take control of their new lives as survivors. Given that these impairments may occur at any point in the disease continuum, early involvement of the rehabilitation team has the potential to prevent severe impairments and decline in performance while improving quality of life by implementing targeted interventions.

Acknowledgment

We gratefully acknowledge the contribution of Dr. Thomas A. Gaskin III, who authored this chapter in previous editions.

Selected References

2. Cheville AL, Beck LA, Petersen TL, Marks RS, Gamble GL. The detection and treatment of cancer-related functional problems in an outpatient setting. *Support Care Cancer.* 2009;17:61-67.

3. Schmitz KH, Speck RM, Rye SA, DiSipio T, Hayes SC. Prevalence of breast cancer treatment sequelae over 6 years of follow-up: the Pulling Through Study. *Cancer.* 2012;118:2217-2225.

37. Mitchell SA. Cancer-related fatigue: state of the science. *PM R.* 2010;2:364-383.

94. Jones LW, Courneya KS, Mackey JR, et al. Cardiopulmonary function and age-related decline across the breast cancer survivorship continuum. *J Clin Oncol.* 2012;30:2530-2537.

99. Schmitz KH, Courneya KS, Matthews C, et al. American College of Sports Medicine Roundtable on exercise guidelines for cancer survivors. *Med Sci Sports Exerc.* 2010;42:1409-1426.

A full reference list is available online at ExpertConsult.com.

84

Psychosocial Consequences and Lifestyle Interventions

KARISHMA MEHRA, ALYSSA BERKOWITZ, AND TARA SANFT

Psychosocial Aspects of Breast Cancer

As early detection and treatment of breast cancer have improved, survival rates have increased to the extent that 89% of individuals with breast cancer now survive 5 years beyond diagnosis and 83% of individuals survive at least 10 years.[1] The majority of women are diagnosed with early-stage cancer localized to the breast, and the 5-year survival rate for this group is 99%.[1] As of January 2014, more than 3.1 million women were living with the diagnosis of breast cancer in the United States.[2] Additionally, approximately 2600 men are diagnosed with breast cancer annually.[1] The diagnosis of breast cancer generates significant distress in the lives of patients and their families because cancer is often considered synonymous with death, pain, and suffering.[3] The first section of this chapter provides an overview of methods to assess distress in individuals with breast disease throughout the continuum of the disease and provides an overview of options for psychosocial intervention with special attention to certain groups of patients. The second section of the chapter examines lifestyle interventions, a growing area of investigation for breast cancer patients, survivors, and women at risk for the disease. This section provides an overview of the rationale behind studying the impact of lifestyle factors on breast cancer risk and prognosis, summarizes the interventional studies in this area, and highlights future research directions.

Distress in Breast Cancer

Distress is defined as a multifactorial unpleasant emotional experience of a psychological (cognitive, behavioral, emotional), social, and/or spiritual nature that may interfere with the ability to cope effectively with cancer, its physical symptoms, and its treatment.[4] Distress extends along a continuum, ranging from common normal feelings of vulnerability, sadness, and fears to problems that can become disabling, such as depression, anxiety, panic, social isolation, and existential and spiritual crisis. All patients experience some level of distress associated with the diagnosis and treatment of cancer at various stages of the disease.[5] In 2004, the Canadian Strategy for Cancer Control designated emotional distress as the sixth vital sign to highlight the importance of distress as a marker of well-being and its reduction as a target outcome measure.[5]

Research has demonstrated that across the trajectory of the illness (from the time of diagnosis through treatment, termination of treatment, survivorship, or recurrence and palliation), the incidence of emotional distress in people diagnosed with cancer ranges from 35% to 45%.[6-11] Evidence suggests that among women undergoing breast cancer treatment, psychological distress is associated with adverse physical symptoms such as pain, fatigue, and nausea.[12-14] In some studies, elevated distress has also been linked to poorer health outcomes such as higher mortality, greater morbidity, nonadherence to treatment, and poorer immune functioning.[15,16] Furthermore, other outcomes such as medical expenditures and occupational functioning may be adversely affected in patients experiencing serious psychological distress.[17,18] Addressing distress may affect outcomes; a recent Cochrane review determined that psychological interventions were effective in improving survival at 12 months in metastatic breast cancer.[19] Additionally, there is evidence that early intervention in treating depression and anxiety can improve treatment adherence and reduce medical costs by 25%.[20] Many other studies have been conducted to examine the efficacy of distress screening in improving patient outcomes. A recent systematic review showed that 17 of the 24 studies reviewed reported statistically significant benefits of distress screening on outcomes such as quality of life (QOL), distress, and patient-clinician communication.[21]

In 2007, the Institute of Medicine (IOM) report *Cancer Care for the Whole Patient* stated that the failure to address the very real psychosocial health needs of cancer patients and their caregivers is a failure to effectively treat that patient's cancer.[22] The IOM report supported the National Comprehensive Cancer Network (NCCN) Distress Management guidelines first released in 1999 and most recently updated in 2015.[4] The American College of Surgeons Commission on Cancer (CoC) echoed the importance of psychological distress screening and required cancer centers to implement screening programs for psychosocial distress by 2015 in order to acquire or maintain accreditation.[23]

Unfortunately, despite the documentation that distress occurs, and the benefit of timely psychological intervention, the initial assessment of a patient's distress is often delayed or goes unnoticed by oncology professionals.[24] In 2013, a study showed that less than half of the 70 CoC-accredited institutions surveyed had begun distress screening.[25] Another study found that compliance with the Distress Screening guidelines varied across clinics with 47% to 73% of eligible patients being screened at least once during their treatment.[26] Barriers to screening included lack of buy-in among key cancer center staff including oncologists, lack of training on how to implement screening, discomfort with the amount of time required to address concerns, and lack of competence on how to refer patients when significant distress was identified. Other issues include budget and availability of appropriate support staff.[20,25]

Although traditional psychosocial services are available on a referral basis from the health care team, these referrals are commonly made only when a patient reaches a crisis. This type of reactive approach may jeopardize the patient's relationship with the health care team as well as effective participation in treatment. At a minimum, psychosocial screening can provide the opportunity to identify and predict which patients are more at risk for distress and are more unlikely to adapt to the many stressors associated with a cancer diagnosis and its treatments.

Screening for Distress

The NCCN standards for managing distress suggest that all patients should be screened to ascertain their level of distress at the initial visit, at appropriate intervals, and as clinically indicated, especially when changes occur in disease status (remission, recurrence, progression, or treatment-related complications).[4] A number of identified risk factors may place an individual at increased risk for distress, and these factors should be assessed during the initial evaluation. Risk factors for distress include younger age, female gender, living alone, having young children, education level, severe comorbid disease, experiencing uncontrolled symptoms, having other sources of stress, history of

psychiatric disorder or depression, cognitive and/or communication barriers, and a history of alcohol or substance abuse.[4]

Oncology clinicians often fail to recognize patient distress in clinical encounters underscoring the need for standardized screening methods.[27] Various tools exist to screen for distress in cancer patients. These include the distress thermometer (DT),[28,29] Hospital Anxiety and Depression Scale (HADS),[30,31] and the Brief Symptom Inventory (BSI).[32] Only a few instruments have been developed specifically for breast cancer patients. These include the Breast Cancer Chemotherapy Questionnaire (BCQ),[33] the Functional Assessment of Cancer Therapy—Breast (FACT-B),[34] and the European Organization for Research and Treatment of Cancer core questionnaire and breast module (EORTC QLQ-C30/+BR23).[35] The FACT-B and the EORTC QLQ-C30/+BR23 are designed for use in breast cancer patients in a wide range of disease stages, undergoing different treatments to detect clinically meaningful changes in QOL over time. Both the FACT-B and the EORTC QLQ-C30/+BR23 combine a generic core questionnaire with site-specific modules that have been internationally validated.[34,35] These instruments do take time to complete and interpret, and therefore they are not useful for screening for distress in a busy clinical setting.

The DT (Fig. 84.1) is a one-item, self-reporting, nonstigmatizing tool that is both easy to administer and to score and interpret; it is endorsed by the NCCN Distress Management guidelines for use in all oncology settings.[4] The DT is a thermometer-like Likert scale that asks the patient to circle the number (0 = no distress

Screening tools for measuring distress

Instructions: First please circle the number (0–10) that best describes how much distress you have been experiencing in the past week including today.

Extreme distress — 10
9
8
7
6
5
4
3
2
1
No distress — 0

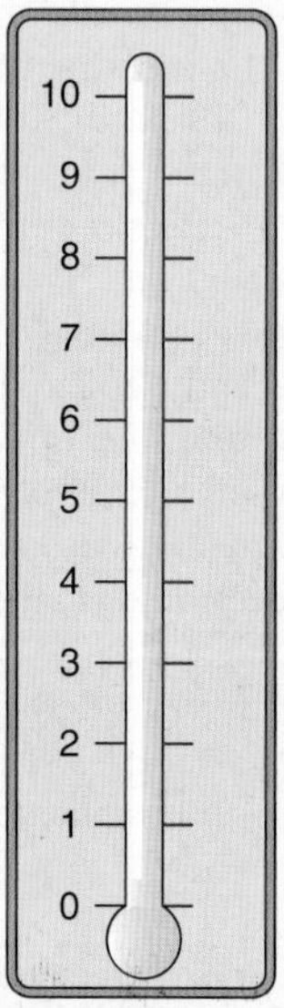

Second, please indicate if any of the following has been a problem for you in the past week including today. Be sure to check YES or NO for each.

YES NO **Practical Problems**
☐ ☐ Child care
☐ ☐ Housing
☐ ☐ Insurance/financial
☐ ☐ Transportation
☐ ☐ Work/school

Family Problems
☐ ☐ Dealing with children
☐ ☐ Dealing with partner

Emotional Problems
☐ ☐ Depression
☐ ☐ Fears
☐ ☐ Nervousness
☐ ☐ Sadness
☐ ☐ Worry
☐ ☐ Loss of interest in usual activities

☐ ☐ Spiritual/religious concerns

YES NO **Physical Problems**
☐ ☐ Appearance
☐ ☐ Bathing/dressing
☐ ☐ Breathing
☐ ☐ Changes in urination
☐ ☐ Constipation
☐ ☐ Diarrhea
☐ ☐ Eating
☐ ☐ Fatigue
☐ ☐ Feeling swollen
☐ ☐ Fevers
☐ ☐ Getting around
☐ ☐ Indigestion
☐ ☐ Memory/concentration
☐ ☐ Mouth sores
☐ ☐ Nausea
☐ ☐ Nose dry/congested
☐ ☐ Pain
☐ ☐ Sexual
☐ ☐ Skin dry/itchy
☐ ☐ Sleep
☐ ☐ Tingling in hands/feet

Other Problems: _____

_____

• **Fig. 84.1** Screening Tools for Measuring Distress.

| TABLE 84.1 | Screening Tools for Distress and Related Conditions |

Instrument Name	Dimensions Assessed	Score Range	Score Warranting Intervention	Comments
Distress Thermometer (DT)	Distress	0–10	≥4	Developed by the NCCN Distress Management Panel. Administered with a problem list covering various aspects of a patient's life.
Patient Health Questionnaire-4 (PHQ-4)	Depression, anxiety	0–12 (0–6 for each subscale)	≥3 in either scale	Combination of two-item depression (PHQ-2) and two-item anxiety (GAD-2) scale. Grades symptom burden as mild (3–5), moderate (6–8), and severe (9–12).
General Health Questionnaire (GHQ-12)	Current mental health	0–36	≥5	Abbreviated from the original 60 questions version. Focuses on two major areas: the inability to carry out normal functions and the appearance of new and distressing experiences.
Hospital Anxiety and Depression Scale (HADS)	Depression, anxiety	0–42 (0–21 on each subscale—anxiety and depression)	≥14 on total scale. ≥11 on HADS-Depression and ≥ 11 on HADS-Anxiety.	Widely used and validated by many studies. Total score indicates general distress.
Brief Symptom Inventory-18 (BSI-18)	Global Severity Index (GSI); subscales: Depression, Anxiety, Somatization	0–72	Total score ≥63, score ≥50 for cancer survivors	Based on Symptom Checklist-90—Revised (SCL-90-R) and BSI-53, which have additional domains.

NCCN, National Comprehensive Cancer Network.

and 10 = extreme distress) that best describes how much distress the patient has been experiencing in the past week including that day. A level 4 or higher signifies clinically significant distress and warrants a member of the oncology team performing a review of the problem list and conducting an evaluation to identify and execute appropriate referrals. Distress levels less than 4 may be mild and the oncology team may choose to address those through usual supportive care in the clinic.[4]

DT has been tested against the Patient Health Questionnaire depression module (PHQ-9) and was found to be an effective tool for detecting depression in newly diagnosed breast cancer patients in a clinical setting.[36,37] Table 84.1 includes some examples of screening instruments that have been validated and are applicable to individuals with cancer.

Sources of Psychological Distress in Breast Cancer

Hereditary Breast Cancer

Although hereditary breast cancers make up only a small proportion of all breast cancer cases, those individuals who do carry the *BRCA* mutation often experience significant amounts of distress

related to their risk of developing breast cancer.[2] Genetic risk assessment can be a complex process for patients and their families, involving different stages, including extended counseling, specialist screening, and genetic testing for mutations. Although most people undertaking cancer genetic risk assessment do so with minimal emotional sequelae,[38] approximately 25% report high levels of distress during the process of risk assessment and gene testing.[39,40] Factors that may predict distress during this process include the anticipation of future problems after a positive test outcome such as the consideration of prophylactic surgery (mastectomy and/or salpingo-oophorectomy) and being a carrier of a mutation. Additionally, being pessimistic, age less than 50 years, having a large number of relatives with breast or ovarian cancer, having a parent pass away from cancer, and high levels of baseline anxiety are predictors of distress.

For women who test positive or negative for the *BRCA1/2* mutation and who do not have a strong family history, the interpretation of the results and subsequent recommendations are well defined. Women who have a family history of breast cancer and test negative for a *BRCA1/2* mutation receive an uninformative negative result because although they know that *BRCA1/2* has not caused breast cancer in their family, this does not mean that they have the same risks as the general population.[41,42] Accumulated data on associations between distress and actual *BRCA1/2* testing have been mixed. A recent study showed that *BRCA1/2* mutation carriers with known maternal transmission and whose mother was deceased report higher perceived stress and anxiety, lower quality of life, and bereavement scores correlated with psychological measures.[43] Conversely, a review of the literature concluded that in individuals with no personal cancer history, *BRCA1/2* carriers are not adversely affected, and noncarriers may even derive some psychological benefits from the test results.[44]

In addition to distress concerning genetic testing, women who are found to carry *BRCA1/2* mutations are also faced with decisions regarding prophylactic surgery. Because prophylactic surgery is an irreversible procedure that is performed in healthy high-risk women on parts of the body that are conceivably related to self-image and sexual attractiveness, emotional distress can be expected.[45] Compounding this distress is the belief among some patients that prophylactic surgery must be done quickly after the presence of a *BRCA1/2* mutation is discovered.

Another aspect of genetic testing is direct-to-consumer genetic testing in which patients and relatives are able to test for underlying mutations directly through the company. There is concern that without involvement of a health care professional, positive results from these tests may cause further distress. However, a recent survey showed that even when patients received unexpected positive results, they did not report extreme anxiety; some patients experienced moderate anxiety, but this was transient. Positive tests, however, led to these subjects seeking medical attention, undergoing prophylactic surgeries, and encouraging other family members to undergo screening.[46]

Diagnostic Process

The process of detecting and diagnosing breast cancer often creates a great deal of uncertainty and anxiety among woman. This distress often begins as early as an abnormal screening mammogram. Several studies have shown that an abnormal screening result causes significant increases in anxiety associated with waiting for the next test and its results.[47,48] The manner in which a patient is informed of an abnormal screening is an important factor in the patient's emotional response. Pineault found that women who were more satisfied with the information provided to them by clinicians experienced less anxiety while waiting for their next tests and results.[48] Providing patients with adequate information about their results is important not only to help alleviate anxiety but also to increase adherence to follow-up appointments.[49,50] In a study of follow-up after abnormal screening mammograms among low-income minority women, Allen and coworkers found that many women did not even realize their results were abnormal. Some women stated that they thought a "positive finding" was good news and that they did not understand the need for a second mammogram after just having their routine one.[49]

Breast biopsy, the next step of the diagnosis process, provides the only definitive diagnosis for breast cancer. In the United States, more than 1.6 million breast biopsies are performed annually, and approximately 80% of these findings are benign.[1] Uncertainty regarding the potential diagnosis results in distress that can interfere with the ability to obtain necessary health care. Patients have reported that they postponed follow-up appointments in fear of receiving a cancer diagnosis. If diagnosed with cancer, distress related to the biopsy can increase postoperative discomfort,

impair decision-making ability and lower immune function.[49,51,52] Research has shown that the anxiety continues through the peridiagnostic period; women with a benign diagnosis reported lingering anxiety regarding continued detection practices.[53] Unfortunately, many of these biopsies are ordered by primary care providers who do not have sufficient resources to screen women or educate them before such procedures, and distress often goes unrecognized and untreated by the health care team. Similar to the mammography process, women who are adequately informed about their cancer risk and the tests they are undergoing have been found to experience less distress, cope better with the possibility of having cancer, participate in decision-making, and have a greater trust in the health care team.[54]

Cancer patients commonly report feeling overwhelmed at the time of diagnosis. For individuals with breast cancer, the first year after a breast cancer diagnosis is accompanied by intense challenges that cut across the physical, psychological, social, and spiritual domains of life. There are a number of stressors throughout the illness trajectory: awaiting diagnosis, anticipating the outcome of metastatic evaluations, surgery, adjuvant therapy, coping with side effects, and facing the risk of recurrence. The period immediately after diagnosis is usually filled with complex decision-making for primary therapy and, for many women, adjuvant therapy that will take place over the ensuing 4 to 6 months.[55] During this time, there may be an increased sense of vulnerability, confusion, uncertainty, loss of control, and existential concerns. This is often exacerbated by inadequate information, scheduling conflicts with various providers (surgeon, medical oncologist, radiation oncologist, plastic surgeon), and the need to make decisions based on the recommendations of a new team of physicians and caregivers.

Surgery

Women with early-stage breast carcinoma generally have the choice of three equally effective surgical options: breast conserving surgery (BCS), mastectomy, or mastectomy with reconstruction. Although BCS as an alternative to mastectomy has gained popularity with time and has become the standard of care for many patients with T1 and T2 tumors, mastectomy is still a commonly used procedure[56,57] Several factors influence which procedure a woman decides to undergo, including perceived chance of survival; concerns about breast loss, local tumor recurrence, and radiotherapy; and the patient's perception of the surgeon's preference.[56,58] Although numerous studies have evaluated QOL among women who undergo BCS, mastectomy, or mastectomy with reconstruction, a meta-analysis of the literature revealed that one procedure has not been clearly demonstrated to provide a better QOL.[56] Recent studies have found that patients who make informed decisions based on their personal beliefs, values, and expectation are more likely to be satisfied postsurgery. Women who were dissatisfied with the information provided in the decision-making process were more likely to experience surgery decision regret.[57] Additionally, women who felt that their role in the decision-making process met their desired role were more likely to be satisfied with the decision, regardless of the procedure.[59]

Adjuvant Therapy

Adjuvant treatments including radiation therapy, chemotherapy, and antiestrogen therapies generate additional physiologic and psychological difficulties that further affect body image, sexuality, and family. Acute adverse reactions and symptoms associated with each treatment can significantly challenge patients.

Chemotherapy causes an array of symptoms including fatigue, nausea and vomiting, skin changes, and alopecia. A meta-analysis found that alopecia is often listed as one of the top three important side effects of chemotherapy among breast cancer patients and describe their hair loss as a traumatizing event.[60] Although dramatic improvements have occurred in the supportive care and management of many symptoms, alopecia and fatigue can exacerbate the negative effects treatment has on body image and overall QOL. Women taking aromatase inhibitors (AI) often report musculoskeletal symptoms, vaginal dryness and pain with intercourse, and increased cognitive problems[61]; because the duration of endocrine therapy varies and can be up to 10 years in some cases, these side effects can be long term.

Cancer Survivorship

Breast cancer survivors constitute 22% of the estimated 14.5 million cancer survivors in the United States.[62] Because an increasing number of breast cancer patients are now either cured of their disease or live for many years with it, they face the complex process of adjusting to life long after cancer treatment ends. The first year after primary treatment, the "reentry" phase,[63] is characterized by physical, emotional, and social recovery. Women report high unmet care needs and have to cope with lingering physical and emotional symptoms of treatment, fear of recurrence, decreasing social support, losing the safety net of care providers, and resuming professional and recreational activities.[64–66] Cancer is a disease that can substantially affect several physical and psychological aspects of the survivor's life years later. Many patients report heightened anxiety leading up to regular checkups or follow-up tests (e.g., mammograms, tumor markers, bone scans) that may uncover a recurrence of the cancer. Patients may also report hypervigilance to physical changes or minor aches and pains; this may be especially pronounced when medical monitoring becomes increasingly less frequent.

Zampini and Ostroff[67] identified four critical life domains in which cancer survivors may experience challenges: physical health, psychological and social well-being, maintenance of adequate health insurance coverage, and employment. Many survivors actively strive to meet these challenges by maintaining their physical health through preventive regimens of diet, exercise, stress reduction, and smoking cessation. These activities restore some sense of control to the cancer survivor in the realm of physical health. Psychological and social well-being of survivors may be challenged on a number of fronts including frustration with the constant intrusion that residual symptoms and follow-up visits have on their lives and their desire to move forward and return to a normal life.

The maintenance of adequate health coverage is very important, and survivors often worry about the threat of policy cancellations or reductions in coverage. Furthermore, the link between employment and insurance in the United States creates difficulties for survivors who feel compelled to retain their current employment rather than risk the possibility of losing their health care coverage. There may also be issues related to job opportunities, for promotions, negative attitudes toward cancer from coworkers or supervisors, and the possibility of dismissal because of poor performance or absenteeism related to residual symptoms or ongoing surveillance appointments.

Cancer Recurrence or Progression

Cancer recurrence or progression presents a somewhat different set of challenges for patients and health professionals. Fear of cancer recurrence is one of the most commonly reported factors of distress among cancer survivors.[68] Younger age, higher level of education, and female gender have been associated with increased fear of recurrence.[69] The fear of recurrence is common and associated not with actual risk of recurrence but with perception of risk.[70]

When disease recurs, the emotional trajectory for women with recurrent disease is somewhat unclear, and there are discrepancies in the current literature regarding psychosocial outcomes. Some studies report that recurrence among survivors increases distress and other studies report that it does not.[71–73] These discrepancies may be attributed to several factors, including variance in measures used, the control group used, time since recurrence, and the nature of the recurrence.[74] Patients with metastatic disease may experience more distress than those with local cancer recurrence (i.e., recurrent disease on the chest wall after mastectomy).[75] Psychosocial responses to cancer recurrence include depressive symptoms, such as the loss of hope for recovery, anxieties and fears of death, and difficulties with disability. Specifically, Brothers and Anderson[6] found that high levels of hopelessness after a breast cancer recurrence was predictive of increased depressive symptoms. Other issues may include uncontrolled pain, appetitive difficulties, and poor body image.

Special Consideration

Males With Breast Cancer

Male breast cancer (MBC) makes up about 1% of all breast cancer cases in the United States.[1] Although it is similar to breast cancer in women in many ways such as pathology, risk factors, and treatment options, MBC is usually diagnosed at a later stage and is twice as likely to have lymph node involvement. The low incidence of MBC has so far hindered the efforts made by investigators to develop randomized prospective trials, and therefore treatment decisions are made based on the data for women.[76]

The vast majority of men are unaware that breast cancer can affect males, and this likely contributes to delays in diagnosing MBC. Studies show that even when men had a genetic family history of breast cancer, they were only first made aware of MBC when diagnosed.[76,77] The lack of MBC awareness can also cause tension in the physician-patient relationship. Many men reported that their clinical team did not adequately answer questions they had regarding treatment and side effects by stating they had "no case reference" to answer the question or by simply acknowledging their lack of experience with MBC. This created a sense of illegitimacy as breast cancer patients among the men.[78]

The labeling of breast cancer as a "woman's disease" creates a stigma around MBC due to its effects on traditional gender roles and masculinity. Men have stated that diagnosis of breast cancer would make them question their masculinity, and about 30% are embarrassed to see their doctor.[79]

Disclosing a breast cancer diagnosis is difficult for many men, with some likening the experience to the coming-out process.[78] Although women will actively seek support for their struggle with breast cancer, men are more likely to use concealment or avoidance as a coping strategy and are less likely to join support groups, regardless of whether the groups were all male or mixed gender.[79] It should be noted that men, in general, are less likely to seek out social support.[80] So although these behaviors may not be uncommon for many males coping with cancer, it is important that breast cancer clinicians who are accustomed to treating a primarily female population be aware of the differences in health-seeking behaviors between genders.

Finding relevant information about breast cancer is another challenge because most often resources include female-specific topics such as bra fittings and female reproductive health. Given the lack of male-specific or gender-neutral literature, men reported receiving most of their information verbally instead of through patient information literature, resulting in many men to be unprepared for the esthetic and physical changes brought about by mastectomy.[76]

About 20% of men discontinued adjuvant hormonal therapy due to various side effects including sexual dysfunction, loss of libido, hot flashes, weight gain, and neurocognitive dysfunction.[81] Moving forward, it is important that health care providers be educated on MBC to help them be more attuned to the physical and psychological needs of men so that the provider may respond appropriately.

Very Young Breast Cancer Patients

Another group of patients requiring special attention is women under age 40 with breast cancer. Although this group makes up less than 10% of all breast cancer cases in the Unites States, breast cancer is the leading cause of cancer-related death in women 20 to 39 years old. Compared with older cohorts, younger women more frequently present with higher-grade and hormone receptor–negative tumors, as well as more advanced disease, usually resulting in more aggressive treatment.[82] These factors, combined with the stage of life at diagnosis, puts younger woman at increased risk of psychosocial distress.[83] Specific issues of concern for younger women include fertility and family planning, sexual functioning, body image, financial burden of care, launching or sustaining careers, and child care.[83] Although the aim of treatment for younger women should be to decrease the risk of recurrence, it is important that clinicians thoughtfully consider important QOL determinants such as fertility, premature menopause, sexual dysfunction, body image, weight gain, and other long-term medical complications including cardiovascular and cognitive health and risk for secondary malignancies. Appropriate early referrals to fertility clinics, mental health providers, genetic counseling, and supportive services are essential in this population of patients.

Psychosocial Intervention

Breast cancer is often described as a traumatic life event that can lead to high levels of distress and disruption, some of which can be long lasting. On the other hand, the experience of a major life event, such as breast cancer, can lead to adaptive changes that may improve well-being and life satisfaction. Failure to recognize and treat distress may lead to several problems including nonadherence to treatment, trouble in making medical decisions, increased visits to physician's office or emergency room that can lead to increased stress within the oncology team, and strain in the doctor-patient relationship.[9] Psychosocial interventions can provide a relatively quick and safe method of decreasing distress and improving QOL in cancer patients and their families.

Timing of Intervention

The Distress Management guidelines issued by the NCCN focus on ensuring that no patient with distress goes unrecognized and untreated.[4] All patients should be screened to ascertain a level of distress at the initial visit and at appropriate intervals as clinically indicated especially when there is a change in disease status. The screening should identify the nature and level of distress and be treated accordingly.

There are certain situations during the course of disease in which psychosocial interventions play a crucial role. At the time of initial diagnosis, education about the disease and assistance with treatment-related decisions (e.g., type of surgery, adjuvant treatment, and preparation for side effects) are frequent needs. When communication is done well at diagnosis, the stage is set for future positive trusting encounters. Younger women may also need assistance in explaining the diagnosis and subsequent changes to their young children. Presurgical interventions also help women prepare for the changes in their body after surgery as well as decisions about type of surgery and breast reconstruction. Another important time for psychosocial intervention is when a patient is diagnosed with metastatic or recurrent disease. Managing pain, decreasing or controlling adverse side effects, and dealing with issues of loss typically become the new focus and need to be addressed appropriately.

Types of Intervention

The application of nonpharmacologic, psychosocial interventions with cancer patients and their families has gained increased support and recognition over the past two decades. The increased awareness of the psychosocial issues associated with cancer, along with increased patient demand for supportive services, has led to an increase in the development and utilization of psycho-oncologic interventions. The NCCN Distress Management Guidelines[4] provide a resource for the oncology health care team in terms of management and referral options. It is important that patients with a positive distress screen are provided with appropriate referrals or interventions because lack of appropriate aftercare is the most significant barrier to screening success.[21]

A variety of psychosocial interventions aim to decrease distress and improve QOL in women dealing with the stress and disruption associated with a diagnosis of cancer. In general, research has shown that breast cancer patients randomized to receive psychosocial or psychoeducational interventions show less distress,[84] improved body image,[85] greater control,[86] increased optimism, and improved ability to derive meaning from their cancer experience (positive benefit finding)[87,88] than those who did not receive an intervention.

Pharmacologic Interventions. Pharmacotherapy is used to assist in several conditions. Unfortunately, the number of randomized controlled trials using antidepressants to treat depression in cancer are limited. Several studies have shown benefit in use of antidepressants and antianxiety drugs in the treatment of depression and anxiety in adult patients with cancer. Fluoxetine has been shown to lower the level of depressive symptoms in patients with advanced cancer compared with placebo.[89] Paroxetine and amitriptyline have also been shown to effectively decrease depressive symptoms.[90] Alprazolam has been compared with progressive muscle relaxation, and patients who receive the drug showed slightly more rapid decrease in anxiety and a greater reduction in depressive symptoms.[91] Therefore benzodiazepines and selective serotonin reuptake inhibitors (SSRIs) are most commonly used to treat anxiety and depression in patients with cancer.

Psychostimulant drugs such as methylphenidate and modafinil have shown promise to treat fatigue in cancer patients, but additional trials are required to show efficacy.[92] Nonopioid and opioid analgesics are used to treat cancer-related pain and associated psychological symptoms.

Psychosocial Interventions

Cognitive Behavioral Therapy. Cognitive behavioral therapy (CBT) explores the connections among thoughts, behaviors, and emotions to help individuals identify and challenge maladaptive thoughts and behaviors. This form of therapy allows patients to focus on their current issues while developing pragmatic strategies to address them. In randomized trials, CBT has been shown to effectively reduce anxiety, depression, pain, and fatigue.[93] A randomized study using a brief CBT intervention called Memory and Attention Adaptation Training (MAAT) showed that the intervention was able to improve verbal memory performance and spiritual well-being in patients with early-stage breast cancer after adjuvant chemotherapy.[94]

Supportive Psychotherapy. Different types of group psychotherapy have been evaluated in clinical trials among patients with cancer. Supportive–expressive group therapy encourages participants to express their feelings about their illness and its impact on their life and has been found to improve quality of life and reduce psychological symptoms and self-reported levels of pain in patients with metastatic breast cancer.[95] Meaning-centered group therapy, designed to help patients with advanced cancer sustain or enhance a sense of meaning, peace, and purpose in life, has also been shown to reduce psychological distress among patients with advanced cancer.[96]

Psychoeducation. Education regarding specific psychological and physical conditions associated with cancer has also shown to reduce distress. A randomized control trial examining the effects of a psychoeducational intervention in women with early-stage breast cancer showed that attending an eight-session education program improved mental and physical health for up to 6 months after the intervention.[97] A meta-analysis examining psychoeducational interventions in 3857 cancer patients showed significant long-term improvement in quality of life.[98]

Social Work Services. These are essential to assist patients with practical problems such as employment, financial assistance, and transportation and help with activities of daily living. Social workers and counselors can also assist patients adjusting to their illness and help with family conflicts, social isolation, and concerns about advance directives and end-of-life care.

Spiritual Services. Religious and spiritual support has been associated with improved satisfaction of medical care. Studies have found that more than three-fourths of patients with cancer have had spiritual needs and that patients whose spiritual needs were not met reported lower satisfaction with their care. There is evidence that providing spiritual care has a positive effect on patient-provider relationships and improves emotional well-being of patients.[99,100]

Family and Couples Therapy. When a family member is diagnosed with cancer, all members of the family are affected in some way. Psychosocial interventions aimed at patients and their families together might lessen distress more effectively than individual interventions.

Lifestyle and Breast Cancer

A large number of interventional studies in breast cancer patients have focused on lifestyle behaviors, such as dietary intake and physical activity patterns. Although initial studies focused on QOL and other psychosocial outcomes, data suggest that lifestyle behaviors may influence breast cancer risk and prognosis as well. The US Department of Agriculture (USDA), The American Cancer Society (ACS), and the World Cancer Research Fund/American Institute for Cancer Research (WCFR/AICR) have recommended lifestyle modifications to lower the risk of breast cancer recurrence and mortality.[101–103] Dietary recommendations include a diet high in vegetables, fruits, and whole grains; avoidance of sugar-sweetened beverages; and limited consumption of processed food, red meat, and alcohol. Physical activity recommendations include 150 minutes per week of moderate-intensity aerobic exercise (or 75 minutes/week of vigorous-intensity exercise), two strength training sessions per week, and decreasing sedentary time.[101–103] These recommendations are based on the growing data that diet, physical activity, and weight loss improve breast cancer risk and outcomes.

Epidemiologic Evidence Linking Breast Cancer and Lifestyle Factors

Physical Activity

A recent meta-analysis demonstrated that among women diagnosed with breast cancer, increased physical activity is associated with 34% lower risk of breast cancer death, 41% lower risk of all-cause mortality, and 24% lower risk of breast cancer recurrence.[101] In the Nurses' Health Study cohort, patients who engaged in more than 9 metabolic equivalent (MET)-hours per week of physical activity, equivalent to walking at a 2.0 to 2.9 mph average pace for 3 hours per week, had a 50% lower risk of breast cancer recurrence, breast cancer death, and all-cause mortality than women who were inactive.[104] In the Collaborative Women's Longevity Study,[105] the risk of breast cancer–specific death was 15% less for each 5 MET-hour-per-week increase in moderate activity. In the Women's Healthy Eating and Living study,[106] women who both consumed five or more servings of fruits and vegetables per day and completed at least 9 MET-hours of physical activity each week had a mortality of 4.8% versus 11.5% in participants who had low physical activity and low intake of fruits and vegetables. Thus modest amounts of physical activity are associated with both a significant decrease in breast cancer risk and a significant improvement in breast cancer outcomes.

Diet

Differences in dietary patterns around the world have long been thought to contribute to geographic variations in breast cancer incidence. Although individual studies have often shown an association between a specific dietary element and breast cancer risk, the only consistent relationship that has been seen to date is a modest increase in breast cancer risk associated with regular consumption of alcohol.[107,108] The relationship between fat consumption and breast cancer risk has been studied significantly; however, no significant association has been found. Similar results were seen in analyses of carbohydrates, fruit and vegetables, soy products, antioxidants, dairy products, and green tea.[107] Studies have also shown that fruit and vegetable intake and moderate alcohol consumption do not appear to be related to breast cancer prognosis.[109] It is possible that difficulties in accurately assessing dietary patterns, or focusing studies on diet later in life, has obscured the influence of diet on breast cancer, most of the available data do not support a strong association between dietary intake and either breast cancer risk or prognosis.

Body Weight

The relationship between body weight and breast cancer risk is highly dependent on menopausal status. Premenopausal women who are overweight or obese have been shown to have a lower risk of breast cancer compared with leaner women, whereas the opposite is true in postmenopausal women. A pooled analysis of seven prospective cohort studies,[110] including 337,819 women and 4385 incident cases of breast cancer, demonstrated that premenopausal women with a body mass index (BMI) greater than 31 kg/m^2 had a relative risk (RR) for breast cancer of 0.54 (95% CI 0.34–0.85) compared with those with a BMI less than 21 kg/m^2. In postmenopausal women, those with a BMI greater than 28 kg/m^2 had a RR of 1.26 (95% CI 1.09–1.46) compared with women with a BMI less than 21 kg/m^2. Some studies have suggested that the excess risk of breast cancer in obese postmenopausal women may be especially pronounced in those who gain a significant amount of weight during adulthood.[111] Excess weight at diagnosis has been associated with poor prognosis in both premenopausal and postmenopausal women.[112,113] The impact of lifestyle on cancer risk and mortality has been studied extensively. The Vitamin and Lifestyle (VITAL) study showed that breast cancer risk was reduced by 60% in women who met the WCRF/AICR recommendations compared with those who did not meet the recommendations.[114] McCullough and colleagues found a 24% lower cancer mortality risk among 6613 women enrolled in the Cancer Prevention Study II who adhered to the lifestyle guidelines (RR = 0.76, 95% CI 0.65–0.89).[115] Despite numerous groups communicating these guidelines, in this study, only 4% of women met the lifestyle recommendations. Similarly, in the DIANA trial, at baseline, only 7% of breast cancer patients with metabolic syndrome (and 13% of breast cancer patients without the metabolic syndrome) met the recommendations,[116] and the Iowa Women's Health Study found that only 34% of the 2193 female cancer survivors met the recommendations,[117] indicating that there is still a large percentage of breast cancer survivors who could benefit from these recommendations.

Research has suggested that providing patients with tailored information or programs can increase the number of lifestyle behaviors practiced at recommended levels. In FRESH START, 519 patients with newly diagnosed early-stage breast or prostate cancer were randomized to a 10-month, tailored, mail-based intervention designed to increase fruit and vegetable intake, decrease fat intake, and/or increase physical activity, or to a control group that received nontailored information about diet and exercise. Both groups significantly changed diet and exercise behaviors, but the tailored intervention group increased physical activity to a greater extent (an increase of 59.3 min/week vs. 39.2 min/week in the control group, $p = .02$). The intervention group also significantly increased intake of fruits and vegetables (1.1 serving increase vs. 0.6 in controls, $p = .01$) and decreased fat intake (4.4% decrease vs. 2.1% in controls, $p < .0001$).[118]

Mechanisms

The biological mechanisms underlying the relationship between lifestyle factors and breast cancer are being extensively studied. In postmenopausal women, obesity is associated with higher estrone and estradiol levels due to increased peripheral aromatization of adrenal androgens in adipose tissue.[119] Obesity also leads to lower levels of sex hormone–binding globulin (SHBG), leading to higher levels of free estradiol in circulation. However, in premenopausal women, preoperative estradiol levels are not related to risk of breast cancer recurrence or death, suggesting that obesity must affect prognosis through some mechanism other than estradiol levels in this population.[120]

One hypothesis regarding the biological mechanism that underlies the link between obesity and breast cancer mortality focuses on insulin. Insulin promotes proliferation of malignant breast cells in vitro,[121] raises free estradiol levels by decreasing SHBG, and is a structural homolog of insulin-like growth factor-1, which has been demonstrated to have mitogenic properties in vitro and is associated with an increased risk of premenopausal breast cancer.[122] Higher levels of fasting insulin have been associated with a two- to threefold increase risk of mortality in women diagnosed with breast cancer.[123,124]

In addition to insulin, many other biomarkers have been evaluated to study the relationship between obesity and breast cancer. Increased C-reactive protein has also been associated with higher risk of breast cancer mortality.[125] Adipose cells produce many hormones and biologically active substances, such as leptin, adiponectin, and hepatocyte growth factor. These proteins, known as adipocytokines, are involved in modulating insulin sensitivity, and preclinical studies have implicated several of them in breast cancer pathogenesis, especially leptin and hepatocyte growth factor, which have been shown to stimulate growth of breast cancer cell lines in vitro.[126] Epidemiologic studies have also demonstrated that high levels of leptin and low levels of adiponectin are associated with breast cancer risk.[107]

The recently published Lifestyle, Exercise and Nutrition (LEAN)[127] study examined whether or not lifestyle changes could affect specific biomarkers. Breast cancer survivors were randomized to one of three cohorts: in-person counseling, telephone counseling, and usual care. The counseling sessions focused on reducing caloric intake, increasing physical activity, and participating in behavioral therapy; both the in-person and telephone groups received the same lifestyle intervention. Women in the intervention arms experienced a 30% decrease in their C-reactive protein levels. Additionally, they found that a weight loss of 5% or more was associated with decreased levels of insulin, leptin, and interleukin-6.[127]

Preliminary data studying the effect of exercise on DNA methylation levels of certain genes show that exercise lowers DNA methylation of the lethal 3 malignant brain tumor L1 (*L3MBTL1*) tumor suppressor gene, which is associated with breast cancer. High levels of *L3MBTL1* may lead to decrease expression of this tumor suppressor gene leading to cell proliferation and tumor progression.[128] Telomere shortening due to repeated cell divisions may also be associated with increased breast cancer risk and mortality; lifestyle interventions may alter telomere length, suggesting a possible mechanism mediating a relationship among diet, exercise, and breast cancer mortality.[129,130]

Lifestyle Interventions With Quality of Life Outcomes

A meta-analysis of 78 exercise interventional trials in cancer survivors showed that exercise interventions resulted in clinically significant improvements in quality of life that continued after the completion of intervention.[131] Another study showed that cancer survivors had significantly reduced cancer-related fatigue levels with evidence of a linear relationship to the intensity of resistance exercise.[131,132] Trials have also shown that physical activity is not only safe but actually reduces the incidence and severity of lymphedema.[132,133] Arthralgia is a common adverse effect of women taking AIs, with 50% of women reporting the symptom within 6 months of starting AI treatment and can result in discontinuation of the therapy[134,135] The Hormones and Physical Exercise (HOPE) study examined the effect of exercise on AI-induced arthralgia by randomly assigning 121 symptomatic women taking an AI to the exercise arm, consisting of resistance training and aerobic exercise or usual care group. At 12 months, women in the exercise group reported a 29% decrease in joint pain, whereas those in usual care had a 3% increase.[136]

Multiple studies have enrolled breast cancer patients to study the effect of exercise interventions with and without dietary components on QOL outcomes. In Project Leading the Way in Exercise and Diet (LEAD),[137] 182 older (age >65 years) breast and colorectal cancer survivors were randomized to a 6-month mail- and telephone-based diet and exercise intervention or to an attention control group that received general health information. Dietary quality significantly improved in the intervention group compared with controls (p = .003), but there were no significant differences in physical functioning or physical activity between groups.

In the Reach out to ENhancE Wellness (RENEW) trial[138] 641 overweight long-term survivors of colorectal, breast, and prostate cancer over the age 65 were randomized to the intervention which provided participants with tailored material to promote increased physical activity, a healthy diet, and modest weight loss or a delayed intervention control group. Of the 641 participants, 289 were breast cancer survivors. At 12-month follow-up, mean physical function scores declined less rapidly in the intervention arm versus the control (−2.15 vs. −4.84, p = .03). Moreover, changes in the intervention arm were significantly more favorable in terms of lessened pain and enhanced vitality, overall health, social functioning, mental health and physical and emotional roles. The recently published Exercise and Nutrition Enhance Recovery and Good Health for You (ENERGY) trial[139] randomized 692 breast cancer survivors to a yearlong intensive intervention consisting of a combined 52 group and telephone counseling sessions versus a nonintensive (control) arm consisting of two in-person counseling sessions. Patients were followed for a 2-year period. Although significant decreases in physical function were seen in the control group at 6 and 12 months, the intervention arm sustained their baseline levels of physical function. Additionally, the intervention arm reported improvements in vitality and body image that were statistically significant compared with the control arm. These differences diminished over time, however, and depressive symptoms worsened in the intervention group at 24 months (p = .0308). Therefore although improvement in QOL has been reported in trials with lifestyle interventions with short-term follow-up, this trial suggests that these benefits may diminish over time.

Lifestyle Interventions With Disease End Points

Several large-scale randomized trials have been done to examine the impact of diet on breast cancer risk and prognosis, including the Women's Health Initiative (WHI) Dietary Modification Trial,[140] the Women's Interventional Nutrition Study (WINS),[141] and the Women's Healthy Eating and Living (WHEL) study.[142] Although these three studies all aimed to lower fat consumption, the dietary goals, intervention structure, and eligibility criteria between the studies vary. WINS focused exclusively on reducing dietary fat, through an intervention based on individual and group meetings with dieticians. The study enrolled women with newly diagnosed early-stage breast cancer who consumed at least 20% of their daily calories from fat. The WHI study also focused primarily on lowering fat intake through in-person group sessions with dieticians but restricted enrollment to postmenopausal women who consumed at least 32% of their daily calories from fat. The WHEL Study focused equally on reducing fat consumption and increasing intake of fruits and vegetables through a telephone-based intervention program and in-person cooking classes. Participation was not restricted based on baseline diet, and women could enroll in the study up to 4 years after breast cancer diagnosis.

All three studies significantly affected dietary intake: in WINS, fat consumption was 20 g per day lower in intervention patients versus controls at 60 months (33 vs. 51g/day, p < .001)[104]; in WHI, fat consumption was 8.1% lower in the intervention group compared with controls at 6 years[105]; and in WHEL, intervention participants consumed 65% more vegetables, 25% more fruit, and 13% less fat at 6 years Of the three trials, only WINS showed a statistically significant impact of the dietary intervention on disease outcomes, with a 20% reduction in subsequent breast events in the intervention group. Although WINS was the only trial to show statistical significance, the nonsignificant trends from WHI suggest that an extended follow-up period on the participants would yield a more definitive comparison between the two groups. Therefore the question remains whether decrease fat intake and weight loss are associated with improved outcomes in breast cancer.

The Lifestyle Intervention Study in Adjuvant (LISA)[143] trial was designed to study the association between breast cancer outcome and weight loss through changes in diet and physical activity. The study was prematurely terminated due to loss of funding, and only 338 of the 2150 planned patients were enrolled. This study, however, did show that patients receiving standardized telephone-based lifestyle interventions that included diet and physical activity had significantly greater weight loss compared with the other control arm that received mail-based delivery of general health information (4.3 vs. 0.6 kg at 6 months, 3.1 vs. 0.3 kg at 24 months, p < .001).

There are currently two trials in progress studying effects of lifestyle interventions versus medications on breast cancer outcomes (a four-arm trial of weight loss with or without metformin and a four-arm trial of exercise with or without metformin) that are being conducted as a part of the National Cancer Institute funded Transdisciplinary Research of Energetics and Cancer Initiative.[144] Table 84.2 has a summary of trials which looked at lifestyle interventions with disease end points.

Conclusion

The diagnosis of cancer affects every aspect of an individual's life. Each step in the cancer continuum presents itself with new challenges, both physical and psychological, often generating a great deal of distress. If not detected and addressed, this distress can have a negative impact on the patient's medical decision-making, QOL, adherence to treatment, and even the effectiveness of treatment. Identifying and addressing distress in patients is an essential part in developing a therapeutic relationship between the patient and the oncology team and is now considered a quality measurement for cancer centers. Although the NCCN has guidelines for distress management, the onus lies on all members of the team to identify the patients who are at risk and intervene as appropriate.

TABLE 84.2 Randomized Trials of Lifestyle Interventions With Disease End Points			
	Women's Health Initiative (WHI)	Women's Intervention Nutrition Study (WINS)	Women's Healthy Eating and Living Study (WHEL)	Lifestyle Intervention Study for Adjuvant (LISA) Treatment of Early Breast Cancer
Study population	Postmenopausal women	Stage I–IIIa breast cancer ≤1 y from diagnosis	Stage I–IIIa breast cancer ≤4 y from diagnosis	Stage I–IIIa, hormone receptor–positive breast cancer Receiving letrozole ≤15 mo from diagnosis
No. of patients	48,835	2437	3088	388 of the planned 2150
Lifestyle eligibility criteria	≥32% calories from fat	≥20% calories from fat	None	Body mass index: 24–40 kg/m²
Primary end point	Breast cancer incidence	Relapse-free survival	Invasive breast cancer event Overall survival	Disease-free survival (not met)
Type of intervention	Dietary	Dietary	Dietary	Weight loss
Intervention goal	<20% calories from fat	<15% calories from fat	8 servings of fruits/vegetables, 15%–20% fat calories	10% Body weight loss
Median follow-up	8.1 y	60 mo	7.3 y	24 mo
Summary	No significant reduction in breast cancer risk, however, a nonsignificant trend was seen.	Low-fat dietary interventions can influence body weight and decrease breast cancer recurrence.	Dietary changes did not decrease the risk of breast cancer recurrence or change overall survival.	Significant weight loss in the intervention arm at 6 and 24 months.

Various epidemiologic studies have shown that lifestyle factors affect not only the risk of developing breast cancer but also the prognosis and risk of recurrence. However, the lack of randomized controlled trials assessing the impact of lifestyle changes especially weight, physical activity, and diet on breast cancer has made it difficult to make standardized recommendations to patients at risk or suffering from breast cancer. Given existing data, patients should be counseled on healthy behaviors, which include the recommendations for diet and exercise as outlined by the USDA, WICR/AICR, and ACA.

Acknowledgments

We gratefully acknowledge the contribution of Giselle J. Moore-Higgs and Jennifer A. Ligibel, who authored this chapter in previous editions.

Selected References

4. National Comprehensive Cancer Network. *NCCN Clinical Practice Guidelines in Oncology: Distress Management V.3.2015.* Fort Washington, MD: National Comprehensive Cancer Network; 2015.

22. Adler NE. *Cancer Care for the Whole Patient: Meeting Psychosocial Health Needs.* Washington, DC: National Academies Press; 2008.

37. Hegel MT, Collins ED, Kearing S, et al. Sensitivity and specificity of the Distress Thermometer for depression in newly diagnosed breast cancer patients. *Psychooncology.* 2008;17:556-560.

101. Rock CL, Doyle C, Demark-Wahnefried W, et al. Nutrition and physical activity guidelines for cancer survivors. *Cancer.* 2012;62:243-274.

102. US Department of Agriculture; US Department of Health and Human Services. Dietary Guidelines for Americans 2010; 2010. http://health.gov/dietaryguidelines/dga2010/DietaryGuidelines2010.pdf.

A full reference list is available online at ExpertConsult.com.

85

Breast Cancer Survivorship

HOLLY J. PEDERSON AND JENNIFER R. KLEMP

Background

The diagnosis and treatment of breast cancer includes imaging, biomarker-driven targeted therapies, and genetic and genomic testing used to stratify risk and response to treatment. The treatment plan requires personalization, and the same degree of personalization is now suggested for patients who have completed therapy to optimize quality of life and oncologic outcomes.[1,2] An individual is considered a cancer survivor from the time of diagnosis through the balance of his or her life. Family, friends, and caregivers are also affected by an individual's treatment for breast cancer.[3] Standards for survivorship care should include prevention of new and recurrent cancers and other late effects, surveillance for cancer spread, recurrence or second cancers, assessment of late psychosocial and physical effects, intervention for consequences of cancer treatment, and coordination of care between primary care providers and specialists to ensure that all of the survivor's health needs are met.[4] National mandates are pushing the delivery of a treatment summary and long-term care plan after treatment, which requires the ability to develop and deliver this tool and the necessary health care delivery model to manage the unique needs of each cancer survivor. Navigation and care coordination across the continuum to assess needs, meet those needs, and outline and manage expectations are essential. Plans for survivorship care require transparency and clear communication among the cancer team, the patient, and the primary care provider. Necessary components of care include identification and management of late and long-term effects of breast cancer and its treatment and understanding cancer risk and management strategies. A process must be in place that meets those needs and monitors outcomes. Survivorship care is a specific approach that addresses patients' long-term needs according to evidence-based American Society of Clinical Oncology (ASCO) guidelines.[5] The National Comprehensive Cancer Network has also released recommendations for survivorship care.[6] Ideally this care is delivered in a collaborative, patient-centered model among multiple subspecialties.[7] Because a majority of cancer care occurs in a community setting, challenges to delivery of care include successful navigation, communication, and clear delegation of responsibilities by providers, survivors and community support organizations, and sufficient time and resources to deliver survivorship care. Having access to guidelines and recommendations promotes the delivery of patient-centered, coordinated care, and requires ongoing evaluation of outcomes.

Identification and Management of Late and Long-Term Effects of Breast Cancer and Treatment

Late and long-term effects of breast cancer and treatment include both physical and psychosocial issues. Later effects can appear months or even years after treatment (Box 85.1).

Physical effects include pain, fatigue, sleep disorders, weight gain, pulmonary toxicity, bone loss, cardiac toxicity, sexual dysfunction, menopausal symptoms, and fertility issues. Factors that increase the risk of late effects include age at diagnosis (older and younger patients are at highest risk), family history, type and cumulative dose of treatment, and lifestyle factors (e.g., tobacco use, alcohol use, weight, and physical activity). Patient-reported outcomes addressing late and long-term effects of cancer and its treatment should be part of continuity of care for breast cancer survivors. This chapter targets some of the major issues that breast cancer survivors face.

Fatigue

Breast cancer and its treatment are associated with cancer-related fatigue (CRF), which is the most common, and possibly most disabling, symptom of breast cancer survivors. CRF is different from fatigue in otherwise healthy individuals, whose fatigue can be resolved with rest.[8,9]

CRF is defined by the National Comprehensive Cancer Network (NCCN) as "a distressing, persistent, subjective sense of physical, emotional and/or cognitive tiredness, related to cancer or cancer treatment that is not proportional to recent activity and interferes with usual functioning."[1] Approximately 25% to 30% of breast cancer survivors experience persistent fatigue for 1 or more years after the completion of cancer treatment, and it is rarely addressed to the satisfaction of the survivor. Risk for severe fatigue increased with higher stage of disease, and risk decreased in breast cancer survivors who reported having a partner and in those who did not receive chemotherapy, but only surgery with or without radiation[10–12] CRF can affect daily activities, work performance, and overall quality of life.

Breast cancer survivors may worry that fatigue might be a sign of disease progression, but they need to be reassured that fatigue is common both during and after treatment. Understanding the onset and presentation of fatigue is vital to establish the pattern, duration, and intensity. In addition, a comprehensive assessment

---

• BOX 85.1 **Late and Long-Term Effects of Cancer Treatment**

Chemotherapy

- Cardiotoxicity/heart problems
- Cataracts/vision changes
- Cognitive impairment
- Endocrine dysfunction
- Early menopause/menopausal symptoms
- Increased risk of recurrence and second cancers
- Infertility
- Liver problems
- Lung problems
- Mouth/jaw problems
- Nerve damage
- Osteoporosis
- Pain
- Reduced lung capacity

Radiation Therapy

- Cataracts
- Cavities and tooth decay
- Fatigue
- Heart and vascular problems
- Hypothyroidism
- Increased risk of other cancers
- Infertility
- Intestinal problems
- Lung disease
- Lymphedema
- Memory problems
- Osteoporosis
- Pain
- Skin changes

Surgery

- Disfigurement and body image concerns
- Fatigue
- Lymphedema
- Mobility problems
- Pain

From Klemp J. Optimizing survivorship care with a team approach. Health Monitor Medical Update. 2015:5-6.

• BOX 85.2 **Cancer-Related Fatigue Management**

I. Patient and family education: providing information and reassurance regarding cancer-related fatigue (CRF) both during and after treatment
  a. Standard screening
  b. Survivor and family education, counseling, and intervention as needed
  c. Self-monitoring
II. Nonpharmacologic strategies for managing CRF
  a. Energy conservation and activity management (ECAM)—modest benefit
  b. Prioritize activities: structure and routine, delegate activities, focus on time of day, postpone nonessential activities, pace and intensity, limit naps to not interfere with sleep quality
  c. Physical exercise and movement: address limitations due to stage of disease, surgical management, and comorbid conditions
    i. Meta-analyses found relief with exercise
    ii. Encourage initiation or maintaining exercise program as appropriate for level of activity and with a focus on safety:
      1. Use cancer-specific exercise programs or meet with a cancer-certified trainer
      2. American College of Sports Medicine and the American Cancer Society recommend 150 minutes of moderate aerobic activity
      3. Walking, jogging, swimming, yoga, light resistance training
    iii. Consider cancer rehabilitation
    iv. Massage therapy by a cancer-specific trained therapist
  d. Psychosocial interventions
    i. Cognitive behavioral therapy
      1. Cognitive restructuring and distraction techniques
    ii. Manage anxiety and depression
  e. Nutrition
  f. Sleep: address sleep hygiene and consider cognitive behavioral therapy for insomnia (CBT-I) or bright white light therapy
III. Pharmacologic strategies for managing CRF
  a. Treat pain, anemia, thyroid dysfunction, sleep
  b. Manage anxiety and depression
    i. Antidepressants
  c. Psychostimulants

Modified with permission from the NCCN Clinical Practice Guidelines in Oncology (NCCN Guidelines®) for Cancer-Related Fatigue V.1.2017. © 2016 National Comprehensive Cancer Network, Inc. All rights reserved. The NCCN Guidelines® and illustrations herein may not be reproduced in any form for any purpose without the express written permission of NCCN. To view the most recent and complete version of the NCCN Guidelines, go online to NCCN.org. The NCCN Guidelines are a work in progress that may be refined as often as new significant data becomes available. National Comprehensive Cancer Network® (NCCN®) makes no warranties of any kind whatsoever regarding their content, use, or application and disclaims any responsibility for their application or use in any way.

---

should include pain, emotional distress (depression and anxiety), anemia, sleep disturbance, lifestyle (diet and exercise, alcohol consumption), review of medications, and comorbidities.[1] One common comorbid condition found in breast cancer survivors that can result in fatigue is hypothyroidism, especially in older breast cancer survivors. Thyroid function should be monitored on a regular basis regardless of treatment modalities.[13]

Numerous strategies have been evaluated to address cancer-related fatigue. Box 85.2 outlines management strategies for CRF.

Cognition

Breast cancer– and cancer treatment–related effects on cognitive function are common concerns for breast cancer survivors.[14] A number of factors may contribute to the development and experience of cognitive impairment for breast cancer survivors, including age, education level, menopausal status, psychological distress, type and dose of chemotherapy, endocrine therapy, time

since radiation therapy, and time since general anesthesia.[15–21] The majority of breast cancer survivors report some degree of cognitive dysfunction after completion of chemotherapy.[20] A subset of cancer survivors (17%–34%) who receive chemotherapy appear to experience long-term cognitive impairment.[22] Long-term cognitive sequelae have been documented as late as 20 years after the completion of therapy for women with breast cancer.[23]

Breast cancer survivors describe cognitive changes such as forgetfulness, absentmindedness, and an inability to focus when performing daily tasks.[24] Complaints also include difficulty with short-term memory, word-finding, reading comprehension, driving/directional sense, and concentration.[15] A variety of mechanisms have been proposed for the development of cognitive impairment, including cytokine-induced inflammatory response, deficits in DNA repair mechanisms, genetic predisposition,[22] chemotherapy-induced anemia, chemotherapy-induced menopause,[25] and injury to neural progenitor cells involved in white matter integrity and adult hippocampal neurogenesis.[26] Cognitive impairment experienced before receiving treatment for cancer has been hypothesized to be due to the release of cytokines associated with tissue damage from the tumor.[27,28] Cognitive impairment perceived before treatment for breast cancer may also be influenced by the impact of the cancer diagnosis on mood states (such as anxiety and depression) and the resultant effects on the capacity to direct attention.[16] Results of previous research also suggest relationships between perceived cognitive impairment (PCI) and fatigue, sleep disturbance, and neuropathy for survivors who have received chemotherapy.[15]

The potential role of inflammatory cytokines as a causal mechanism for cancer and cancer treatment-related cognitive complaints is intriguing. Chronic inflammation is associated with a negative effect on the neural systems involved in cognition and memory and has been linked to obesity.[29,30] Obesity is a risk factor for breast cancer, disease recurrence, and poor prognosis.[31] Weight gain is common for women receiving chemotherapy for breast cancer.[32,33] The chronic inflammatory state associated with obesity may contribute to the risk of cognitive changes in this population as has been seen preclinically[30] and in populations with other disorders such as the metabolic syndrome, which is linked to cardiovascular risk factors.[34]

Exercise is a strategy employed by some breast cancer survivors to attempt to decrease PCI,[15] and evidence is building in support of exercise as an intervention for cancer-associated cognitive complaints.[35] Numerous organizations have published guidelines and recommend regular exercise and strength training for cancer survivors and recently added routine exercise as one of the general strategies for management of cancer-associated cognitive dysfunction.[36]

Challenges in supporting the right types of interventions have to do with study design and assessment tools used in previous research. There is modest correlation between objective and subjective testing. The capacity for comprehensive testing is limited in most cancer care facilities, and no sensitive brief screening tool for cancer-related dysfunction has been accepted as the gold standard. Education and validation of the survivor-reported cognitive dysfunction is a first step. Survivors should be reassured that cancer-associated cognitive dysfunction is common but usually transient.

On the basis of clinical assessment, management strategies to address cognitive dysfunction include[6] the following:

- Support engaging in enhanced organizational skills including the use of lists, calendaring, smart devices, GPS, and consistent behaviors such as putting keys in the same place.
- Reinforce the need to be realistic about what can be accomplished during and after treatment. Trying to maintain pretreatment levels of activity might not be realistic and can be frustrating to the survivor.
- Encourage behavioral techniques to reduce stress and for relaxation.
- Manage anxiety, depression, sleep disturbance, fatigue, pain, and other comorbidities.
- Encourage lifestyle modification including increasing exercise, healthy diet, and limiting alcohol consumption.

Formal neuropsychological evaluation and referral for cognitive rehabilitation are recommended to address unresolved cognitive dysfunction. Cognitive rehabilitation is a behavioral intervention that strives to train or retrain cognitive functions or to compensate for specific cognitive deficits. This emerging area of clinical research explores how to optimally guide survivors on how to cope with cognitive complaints and dysfunction.[35] Outcomes of cognitive rehabilitation research support objective improvements in overall cognitive function, visuospatial constructional performance, and delayed memory and subjective improvements of cognitive impairment and psychosocial distress.[37,38] If these strategies are not effective, then psychostimulants can be considered under the direction of a licensed practitioner.[6]

Since the establishment of the International Cognition and Cancer Task Force in 2003, there has been a multidisciplinary consensus of neuropsychologists, clinical and experimental psychologists, neuroscientists, imaging experts, physicians, and patient advocates who participate in regular workshops on cognition and cancer. This group strives to advance our understanding of the impact of cancer and cancer-related treatment on cognitive and behavioral functioning in adults with noncentral nervous system cancers.[39] Ongoing investigation to further explore the mechanisms of action, validate clinically meaningful screening, and understand the effects of hormone therapy will enhance the current understanding and management of a common issue experienced by breast cancer survivors.

Cardiac Dysfunction

As a significant number of breast cancer survivors live with and through their disease, attention to cardiovascular morbidity and mortality is an essential part of breast survivorship care. In long-term breast cancer survivors over age 66 with early-stage disease, cardiovascular disease (CVD), is the most common cause of death.[40] In all breast cancer survivors receiving adjuvant treatment, cardiovascular disease is the third most common cause of mortality after breast cancer recurrence and second primary tumor.[41] A recent comparison between women with and without a diagnosis of breast cancer revealed that breast cancer survivors were at greater CVD-related mortality, and this risk manifested approximately 7 years after diagnosis.[42]

There are a number of established preexisting risk factors for CVD: age, obesity/body mass index, sedentary lifestyle or difficulties with exercise tolerance, comorbid medical conditions (diabetes, dyslipidemia, hypertension, stroke), family history, tobacco use, chronic kidney disease, and poor cardiorespiratory fitness.[43] Thus, many women diagnosed with breast cancer are already at elevated risk for CVD before any treatment, and issues should be addressed before the initiation of treatment. Collecting CVD risk factors during an initial consult and throughout ongoing care is supported by the National Cancer Institute Community Cardiotoxicity Task Force[44] and the International CardiOncology Society.[45] These experts support cardio-oncology as a growing field and promote collaboration between highly specialized professionals and primary care.

Breast Cancer Treatment–Specific Cardiovascular Disease Risk Factors

Anthracyclines are agents that directly cause cardiac damage. The likely target are cardiomyocytes, which have a poor antioxidant defense system.[46] It is thought that anthracycline exposure leads to myocyte apoptosis and damage is irreversible, resulting in an increase in CVD-related morbidity and mortality.[47,48] The incidence of anthracycline-induced cardiotoxicity is dose dependent and can result in heart failure.[49] Breast cancer survivors who have received treatment that includes anthracycline (e.g., doxorubicin >250 mg/m^2, >epirubicin 600 mg/m^2) should be considered at high risk for developing cardiac dysfunction.[50] Predictors of anthracycline-induced cardiotoxicity include high doses and symptoms that occur within the first year after the initiation of treatment. The clinical course is often dependent on the left ventricular ejection fraction (LVEF) at the end of treatment.[51]

A 10% or greater decrease in LVEF or LVEF less than 50%[52] is considered significant. By this point, permanent damage has likely occurred.[53] Before the introduction of HER2-directed therapies, the incidence of anthracycline-induced cardiac dysfunction (median dose of doxorubicin at 390 mg/m²)[54] had been previously reported to be 2.2%, with rates highest in those receiving anthracycline-based regimens combined with a taxane.[55] In a retrospective cohort study of 12,500 women diagnosed with breast cancer, 20% to 25% exhibited amplification of HER2 and received trastuzumab, and approximately 30% received an anthracycline-based regimen.[56] After adjusting for age, comorbidities, stage, year of diagnosis, radiation therapy, the cumulative incidence of heart failure or cardiomyopathy at 5 years after treatment was 4.5% for anthracyclines, 12.1% for trastuzumab and 20.1% receiving the combination.[56,57] Survivors who received a combination therapy including an anthracycline and trastuzumab were generally younger, healthier, and presumably at lower risk for CVD.[57]

Another striking finding is the high rate of subclinical dysfunction among breast cancer survivors. Kalyanaraman and coworkers found that doxorubicin-induced subclinical cardiomyopathy affects approximately one in four breast cancer survivors.[58] With the increase in disease-free survival in breast cancer survivors, many may already have or will acquire traditional CVD risk factors. These findings highlight the long-term need to monitor breast cancer survivors.[57]

Trastuzumab, a HER2-directed targeted therapy, indirectly causes cardiac damage that will typically have a significant delay of months to years from the time of treatment until cardiac dysfunction is detectable. Exposure to trastuzumab can have a cumulative dose-dependent effect that is often reversible.[59] This result can be an independent exposure or a result of the combined toxicity with an anthracycline.[60]

Radiation therapy has long been a concern for cardiac dysfunction, especially if treating a left-sided breast cancer. Radiation exposure is associated with risk of ischemic heart disease in breast cancer survivors based on the dose and lag time of up to 20 years.[61] More recent findings using modern techniques of computed tomographic guidance and respiratory gating for left-sided breast cancer result in lower cardiac doses. Unfortunately, the long-term effects of low-dose radiation are unclear.[62]

Exercise has been shown to provide benefit to those with and without CVD.[56] Exercise has been studied extensively in breast cancer survivors but has not yet been shown to mitigate cardiotoxicity. Organizations including the American Cancer Society and the American College of Sports Medicine recommend 150 minutes per week of moderate-intensity exercise with the inclusion of resistance training.[63,64]

Current practice guidelines are limited in the long-term management of cardiac dysfunction in breast cancer survivors. The assessment of risk will be aided by the development of risk prediction models that will stratify breast cancer survivors.[65,66] By categorizing breast cancer survivors into high or moderate risk, appropriate follow-up can be recommended. The types of ongoing surveillance are under review. The inclusion of serum biomarkers, cardiac imaging with echo/multigated acquisition scan or cardiac

magnetic resonance imaging (MRI), the use of strain (which represents the magnitude and rate of myocardial deformation), and referral to a cardio-oncologist will all be part of follow-up guidelines.[67,68]

Efforts should be made to identify risk factors and interventions that can be employed during this brief window to reduce the excess burden of CVD in this vulnerable population. Clinicians need information to screen high-risk patients and prevent cancer treatment–related cardiotoxicity, to balance effective cancer treatment and cardiac risk assessment in treatment decision-making, and to manage long-term cardiac risks.

Sexual Health, Body Image, and Relationship Issues

Sexual quality of life is an important issue, and sexuality ranks high on surveys of unmet survivorship needs.[69] Issues are most commonly due to the toxicities of cancer treatment.[70] Sexual problems after cancer are linked with menopause, depressed mood, poor quality of life, and decreased intimacy. The impact of breast surgery on body image and self-esteem, both important in sexual health, are well characterized.[71–73] Chemotherapy may result in side effects (fatigue, nausea, etc.) that may limit a woman's sexual interest or ability to become aroused. Chemotherapy-induced menopause may lead to vasomotor symptoms, urogenital symptoms (vaginal dryness), atrophy-related urinary symptoms, and decreased libido. Hormonal therapy to treat breast cancer also affects sexuality. Although both tamoxifen and the aromatase inhibitors may affect sexual function, the risk may be higher with the aromatase inhibitors with regard to lubrication issues, dyspareunia, and global dissatisfaction with one's sex life.[74] One recent cross-sectional survey assessing 129 women during the first 2 years of aromatase inhibitor therapy showed that 93% scored as dysfunctional on the Female Sexual Function Index and 75% of dysfunctional women were distressed about their sexual problems. Twenty-four percent stopped having sex, and 15.5% stopped aromatase inhibitor therapy.[75] Women who receive radiation therapy may experience cosmetically detrimental skin changes affecting body image.[76]

Women should be asked about sexual function at regular intervals. Patients are not likely to bring up sexual concerns spontaneously. Providers should ensure that engaging patients directly in conversations regarding sexual health address concerns. Direct conversations are a sign for patients that the provider is open to discussing sexual issues, and this might enable patients to raise these issues in the future should they arise. The NCCN Survivorship Guidelines Version 2.2015[6] recommends a brief sexual symptom checklist for women as a primary screening tool.[77] Past and present sexual activity should be reviewed including a discussion about how cancer treatment has affected sexual functioning and intimacy. In addition, treatment-associated infertility should be discussed, if indicated, with appropriate referrals.[78] For a more in-depth evaluation of sexual dysfunction, consider the Female Sexual Function Index (FSFI),[79] which has been validated in cancer patients and/or the PROMIS sexual function instrument.[80] It is important to remember that complete sexual recovery may not be possible during or after cancer treatment. In creating a care plan, one must build from where the patient is and focus on creating a "new normal," using the specific concerns of the patient to guide treatment. By highlighting positive changes and new attitudes, many patients will find equally if not more meaningful sexual experiences posttreatment.

When dealing with the multiple stressors that can be associated with a diagnosis of breast cancer, body image can also be a negatively affected. Hair loss, body disfigurement due to surgery or lymphedema, radiation therapy, and weight gain can have profound effects on breast cancer survivors. There also may be partner issues that can affect whether a breast cancer survivor undergoes breast reconstruction. Intimacy is commonly affected.

Recognizing that female sexuality and relationship satisfaction is often driven by psychological and psychosocial influences, Basson elaborated on our understanding by incorporating intimacy as a driver for desire and sexual activity.[81] For couples, Manne and Badr, proposed the Relationship Intimacy Model, which characterizes the recovery from cancer treatment as multifactorial.[82] Beyond instruments aimed to query sexual function, other questionnaires are available to help evaluate other aspects of sexual health including body image,[83] quality of relationships[84] and intimacy within relationships.[85] Of course, the status of the relationship and satisfaction with intimacy for a couple before the breast cancer diagnosis is important in evaluating subsequent concerns.

First-line therapy for addressing sexual health may include gynecologic care (vaginal moisturizers, lubricants, vaginal dilators, vibrators, relaxation techniques, or exercises. Second-line therapy including topical estrogen therapy (if not contraindicated) may be considered if first-line therapies do not adequately provide relief. Encourage ongoing partner communication and identify resources for psychosocial dysfunction with appropriate referrals for psychotherapy or sexual/couples counseling. Vaginal dryness due to antiestrogen therapy commonly leads to dyspareunia. Women may feel disinterested due to fear of pain with intercourse. Vaginal estrogen is an effective treatment for dryness, but concerns exist about detectable increases in serum estrogen levels.[86] A recent study, however, that included 13,000 women with breast cancer found no increase in the recurrence risk in women treated with endocrine therapy whether or not local estrogen therapy was administered.[87] A systematic comprehensive review of minimally absorbed vaginal estrogen products is provided by Pruthi and coworkers.[88] Low-dose vaginal 17-beta estradiol tablets (10 mcg) are associated with a typical estradiol level of 4.6 pcg/mL and a maximum annual delivered dose of 614 mcg. Estring vaginal ring inserted vaginally every 3 months has a typical serum level of 8.0 pcg/mL and an annual delivered dose of 2.74 mg. Prospective long-term safety data are lacking, and the use of estrogen for vaginal atrophy in the breast cancer survivor remains controversial. A prospective trial is underway at Memorial Sloan Kettering Cancer Center examining follicle-stimulating hormone and estradiol levels, sexual function and quality of life in breast cancer patients receiving an aromatase inhibitor and 10 mcg of 17-beta estradiol vaginal tablets.[89] A phase III randomized clinical trial of 216 postmenopausal women without breast cancer given dehydroepiandrosterone showed improvement in all domains of sexual function without significantly increasing serum estrogen, testosterone, or androgen levels.[90] A nonhormonal vaginal moisturizer, hyaluronic acid vaginal gel (Hydeal D), was recently studied and showed improvement in vaginal and sexual health issues.[91] Regular sexual activity has also been found to be useful in preventing vaginal atrophy.[92] Survivors should engage in informed decision-making regarding hormone therapy, including coordination with the treating oncologist, discussing the pros and cons, and a summary of data to date.

Vasomotor symptoms include hot flashes and night sweats (which do not always occur at night).[93] Numerous strategies have been evaluated to manage this common complaint in breast cancer survivors. Nonhormonal management strategies that have been reported to provide relief include: selective serotonin reuptake inhibitors, serotonin norepinephrine reuptake inhibitors, gabapentin, acupuncture, and exercise (including yoga).[94–96]

Psychosocial Issues and Healthy Lifestyle

Psychosocial issues occur at all stages across the breast cancer continuum. Addressing issues related to survivorship including fear of recurrence, anxiety and depression, body image concerns, relationship issues, and financial sequela is vital for all patients. Psychosocial consequences and lifestyle interventions are covered specifically in Chapter 84 of this text. Fear of recurrence may be persistent. More than one-third of cancer survivors report a high fear of recurrence, which may lead to decreased quality of life, greater pain and fatigue, and higher utilization of medical services.[97] These feelings last beyond 5 years, particularly in breast cancer survivors.[98]

Promotion of healthy lifestyle is important for all survivors. Large meta-analyses have shown increased breast cancer–specific and overall mortality in obese survivors.[99] Additionally, overweight and obese survivors report higher levels of cancer-related symptoms and poorer physical functioning.[100]

Fertility and Menopause

Young women at the time of diagnosis are faced with many decisions that are clouded by uncertainty. Trying to determine the best option for fertility preservation while concurrently getting expert opinion on clinical management is overwhelming. The fear of breast cancer often trumps the desire to have a family at diagnosis; however, the risk of premature menopause, infertility, and the suitability of fertility preservation approaches need to be discussed in a multidisciplinary setting with all eligible women before the start of cytotoxic therapies.[101] Fertility preservation is an important concern both at the time of diagnosis and posttreatment. The American Society of Clinical Oncology has incorporated a discussion on fertility preservation into the Quality Oncology Practice Initiative (QOPI) standards. In 2016, 5% to 7% (up to 17,266 cases) of cases of invasive breast cancer in the United States were in women under age 40 at diagnosis. Approximately 25% of live births in the United States occur between the ages of 30 and 40; therefore, many women diagnosed with breast cancer in this decade may not have the ability to bear children. Current estimates suggest that less than 10% of women under age 40 will have children after a diagnosis of breast cancer,[102–104] despite the fact that 50% desire to, and there appears to be no unfavorable effect on breast cancer outcome of a subsequent pregnancy after adjuvant breast cancer therapy.[101] One reason is that women under age 40 often receive alkylating agents, which is associated with a low birth rate after a diagnosis of breast cancer. In addition, an estimated two-thirds of women under age 40 are hormone receptor positive and will receive 5 to 10 years of antihormonal therapy with or without a gonadotropin-releasing hormone agonist. The goal is ovarian suppression. Therefore childbearing will be delayed at least 5 years before attempting childbearing.[105] Depending on the treatment and age of the patient, there is a 10% to 40% rate of chemotherapy-related amenorrhea. This is directly linked to the dose of the alkylating agent. This relationship is not seen in HER2-positive patients receiving trastuzumab.[105]

Women making decisions regarding family planning have several options before initiating treatment, including embryo cryopreservation and mature oocyte cryopreservation, and there are several additional methods still under investigation.[106] There are organizations to assist patients in accessing providers and in obtaining discounts for unreimbursed services. In addition, it is important for breast cancer survivors to understand that there are other mechanisms to complete their family including surrogacy and adoption.[107,108]

Fertility preservation should be part of early conversations for those women newly diagnosed with breast cancer or posttreatment. Patients report that their concerns are often not managed, and this can result in feelings of grief and regret.[109–111] One way to start this conversation is to ask, "Have you started or completed your family?" Including this question as part of a navigation intake or initial consultation will give permission to discuss an important topic to many young women with breast cancer.

Understanding Cancer Risk and Management Strategies

An important component of survivorship includes understanding cancer risk and management strategies. Germline genetic testing may be indicated for many survivors, and genomic testing may be useful in prognosis. Adherence to hormonal therapy and ongoing surveillance for recurrence is important, and screening for other cancers must be addressed.

Identification of patients with heritable cancer syndromes is a vital tool for risk stratification that has an impact on surgical decision-making, treatment, risk management, and care of families. A careful personal and family history is key to identifying those patients whose cancer may be associated with heritable predisposition. Heritable syndromes account for only about 5% to 10% of breast cancers, but women who harbor pathogenic variants in highly penetrant genes have a very high risk for the development of cancer. Every year, more eligible patients are missed than tested. Of newly diagnosed cancer patients who meet NCCN criteria for genetic testing, about 44.5% are captured.[112–114] Different models will be important to improve detection of high-risk individuals going forward. At Cleveland Clinic, with a genetic counselor embedded in the Breast Center, more patients were referred (odds ratio [OR] 1.49; confidence interval [CI] 1.16–1.94, $p = .003$), and more patients followed through with genetic counseling if they were referred (OR 1.66; CI 1.02–2.71; $p = .042$).[115]

Germline mutations in highly penetrant genes increase the risk of malignancies of the breast and of other tissues. These mutations are inherited in an autosomal dominant fashion. The most common of these syndromes is hereditary breast and ovarian cancer syndrome (HBOC), caused by germline mutations of the BRCA1 or BRCA2 genes. NCCN criteria for identifying patients who may have heritable cancers and referring them for cancer genetics consultation include early age at onset (≤50), "triple-negative breast cancer" (estrogen receptor negative, progesterone receptor negative, and HER2 negative), ovarian cancer at any age, male breast cancer, a known familial mutation in a breast cancer susceptibility gene, multiple affected relatives or being from a population at increased risk (e.g., women of Ashkenazi Jewish descent).[114] Clearly, identification of BRCA carriers allows for the

opportunity for risk-reducing salpingo-oophorectomy, but discussions about contralateral breast cancer risk are also influenced by testing. BRCA mutation carriers are at a higher risk of a second primary breast cancer and of subsequent contralateral breast cancer, and risk increases with length of time since diagnosis.[116]

The recent introduction of multigene testing for hereditary forms of cancer has rapidly altered the clinical approach to testing at-risk patients and their families. Using next-generation sequencing technology, a set of genes that are associated with a specific family cancer phenotype or multiple phenotypes is simultaneously analyzed. Multigene panels identify rare germline mutations in genes such as in CDH1 and PTEN and more frequently identified mutations in "intermediate" penetrant (moderate risk) genes such as CHEK2, ATM, and PALB2. For many of these moderate-risk genes, there are limited data on the degree of cancer and management guidelines are evolving. For example, for carriers of ATM, CHEK2, and PALB2 mutations, MRI screening is now recommended, and for carriers of PALB2 mutations, a discussion about risk-reducing mastectomy is now recommended.[117] Cancer genetic risk assessment by genetic experts ensures that the correct genetic testing is offered to the most appropriate patients, with personalized interpretation of results and provision of future management recommendations including the individual's personal and family history.[118] With increasing focus on value-based health care, genetic counseling with appropriate testing will become even more important.[119] The appropriate choice for a genetic test can be discussed with the patient, and counseling provides an opportunity for shared decision-making around focused versus extensive genetic testing depending on personal and family history and patient preference (Box 85.3).

Multigene panel testing will identify more patients at risk for hereditary syndromes than single syndrome testing and may have an impact on screening for other cancers as well, but challenges exist including payment for follow-up and a trained workforce

---

> ## BOX 85.3 Types of Genetic Testing
>
> **Single-Site Testing**
> To confirm presence of a known familial germline mutation
>
> **Multisite Three Testing**
> Focused testing in individuals of Ashkenazi Jewish descent for the three most common mutations seen in the Jewish population: BRCA1 185delAG, BRCA1 5382insC, and BRCA2 6174delT
>
> **Integrated BRCA1 and BRCA2 Testing (Comprehensive BRCA1 and BRCA2 Testing With Large Rearrangement)**
> Aimed to identify the most common highly penetrant gene mutations in BRCA1 and BRCA2 while avoiding the complexities and implications of multigene testing and variants of uncertain significance
>
> **Multiplex Panel Testing of Highly Penetrant Gene Mutations**
> Testing for known pathogenic variants in highly penetrant genes for which there are information and guidelines about penetrance, associated risks, and management
>
> **Multiplex Panel Testing of Highly Penetrant Gene Mutations and Moderate-Risk Gene Mutations**
> Testing for known pathogenic variants in highly penetrant genes for which there are information and guidelines about penetrance, associated risks, and management as well as testing for variants in moderate-risk genes

with the time and expertise to manage high-risk patients. Studies report a 4% to 16% prevalence of mutations other than *BRCA1* and *BRCA2* among patients who met evidence-based practice guidelines for *BRCA* testing, with a high rate (15%–88%) of variants of uncertain significance, particularly in moderate-risk genes which lack actionability.[120] A patient experience study from Kurian and colleagues failed to demonstrate an increase in distress or uncertainty after multigene panel testing.[121] Bradbury and coworkers reported increased knowledge and decreased general anxiety and uncertainty after pretest counseling and disclosure of results of multiplex panel testing, but an increase in cancer worry after result disclosure.[122] In general, genetic results predict the risk of future cancers and potential prevention strategies more than they guide treatment options for the diagnosed disease.

As genomic testing continues to evolve, these tests may also be useful in survivorship planning. Prognostic assessment provided by molecular signature testing may provide peace of mind for low-risk patients and serve as the basis for ongoing surveillance in higher-risk patients. Molecular signature testing may also influence decisions about the duration of hormonal therapy. Tests predicting risk of recurrence in long-term follow-up may be helpful in separating patients into risk groups who could be spared or potentially benefit from extended hormonal therapy beyond 5 years of treatment but still require larger randomized studies to demonstrate their efficacy.[123] The use of risk stratification for recurrence and major toxicities was nicely described by McCabe and colleagues.[124] Survivorship services should be based on the risk of long-term and late effects, cancer recurrence, and second primaries. Establishing risk categories of low, moderate, or high risk provides the basis for surveillance, intervention, and overall need. Genetic testing may guide surveillance and screening protocols, and routine health care maintenance cannot be forgotten.

Imaging and Breast Cancer Survivors

With regard to breast imaging, women treated with breast conserving therapy should have their first posttreatment mammogram no earlier than 6 months after definitive radiation therapy. Subsequent mammograms should be obtained every 6 to 12 months for surveillance of abnormalities. Mammography should be performed yearly if stability of mammographic findings is achieved after completion of locoregional therapy.[125] Breast MRI is not recommended for routine breast cancer surveillance except in germline mutation carriers, but it may be more sensitive in detecting recurrences than mammography alone in this population. A study by Weinstock and coworkers identified women under the age of 65 with a history of breast cancer and at least one follow-up MRI performed along with a mammogram done within 6 months of the MRI. Overall, MRI had a sensitivity of 84.6% (95% CI 54.6–98.1) and a specificity of 95.3% (95% CI 93.3–96.9); mammography a sensitivity of 23.1% (the 95% CI 5.0–53.8) and a specificity of 96.4% (the 95% CI 94.5–97.8).[126]

Development of Breast Cancer Survivorship Care: Program Development and Outcomes

Comprehensive breast cancer survivorship care requires engagement by providers, the survivor, caregiver/family, and community support organizations to address and manage late and long-term effects. Without evidence supporting outcomes, there is not a standard model that will work even within a single organization. Organizations should begin or grow the development of a survivorship program by evaluating what aspects of survivorship care already exist within or outside the organization. This inventory will identify many aspects of care that should be integrated and accessible to cancer survivors and providers. The next step is to identify what elements of survivorship care require process improvement or need to be developed to meet the goals of comprehensive survivorship care including managing posttreatment effects and addressing risk, screenings, and preventive care.[127] The Survivorship Care Plan (SCP) has been suggested as a solution to improve communication between providers and to guide survivor care. The SCP should include the following[128]:

- A summary of an individual's cancer diagnosis and treatment information
- An overview of both physical and psychosocial effects of diagnosis and treatment
- A detailed follow-up plan that outlines surveillance for recurrence and potential late effects as well as recommendations for health-promotion strategies
- Referrals and resources for physical, psychosocial, and practical needs

Requirements to meet national accreditation standards include treatment summaries and care plans, which has posed a daunting task for most cancer care teams.

Example Organizations Requiring the SCP:
- The American College of Surgeons Commission on Cancer[129]
- The National Accreditation Program for Breast Centers (NAPBC)[130]
- ASCO Quality Oncology Practice Initiative[131]

Time and reimbursement are two of the major challenges in the delivery of survivorship care. Barriers include integration into the electronic medical record and time commitment; it has been shown to take 45 to 90 minutes or longer of unreimbursed time to prepare for and to complete a survivorship treatment summary.[132] A recent study of an auto-populated SCP in a population of endometrial cancer survivors showed no evidence of a benefit of SCPs on satisfaction with information and care. Furthermore, SCPs increased patients' concerns, emotions, symptoms, and the amount of cancer-related contact with the primary care physician.[133] This highlights the need for future clinical research focused on meaningful clinical, psychosocial, and economic outcomes and may fit nicely into an oncology patient-centered medical home model. Challenges for most practices in delivering survivorship care are that it costs money to the organization and to the providers, without evidence-based outcomes or financial return on the investment. To encourage the growth of survivorship care, we must see that patient care is improved and patient outcomes are better, with consistently high patient satisfaction, all at an equal or lower cost than a local comparator group.[134]

Conclusions

The development and implementation of survivorship care into a shared care practice model faces barriers and opportunities. National mandates are pushing the delivery of a Survivorship Care Plan for all survivors, which require the ability to develop and deliver this tool and the necessary health care delivery model to manage the unique needs of each cancer survivor. Health systems research will provide outcomes-based guidelines for development of best models for delivery and ongoing evolution of risk-stratification tools to identify cancer survivors at the highest risk. This will provide further personalization of care. Incorporating survivorship care into an oncology patient-centered medical home may provide the coordination and reimbursement requirements necessary for the ongoing management of cancer survivors. Working across disciplines will require a change in training programs and professional development. To prepare the current and future workforce in the management of cancer survivors, we must prioritize multidisciplinary education caring for the cancer patient from diagnosis through their life span.[2]

Selected References

4. From Cancer Patient to Cancer Survivor: Lost in Transition. Committee on Cancer Survivorship: Improving Care and Quality of Life, Institute of Medicine and National Research Council; 2006.

http://www.nap.edu/catalog/11468.html. Accessed 12 November 2015.

6. NCCN Survivorship Guidelines Version 2.2015. http://www.nccn.org/professionals/physician_gls/pdf/survivorship.pdf. Accessed 12 November 2015.

99. Chan DS, Vieira AR, Aune D, et al. Body mass index and survival in women with breast cancer-systematic literature review and meta-analysis of 82 follow-up studies. *Ann Oncol.* 2014;25:1901-1914.

117. NCCN Genetic/Familial High-Risk Assessment: Breast and Ovarian Guidelines Version 1.2016. http://www.nccn.org/professionals/physician_gls/pdf/genetics_screening.pdf. Accessed 1 November 2016.

118. Smith M, Mester J, Eng C. How to spot heritable breast cancer: a primary care physician's guide. *Cleve Clin J Med.* 2014;81:31-40.

A full reference list is available online at ExpertConsult.com.

86

Delayed Diagnosis of Symptomatic Breast Cancer

KENNETH KERN

The delayed diagnosis of symptomatic breast cancer remains a leading source of error in clinical practice. Diagnostic errors in breast disease are but one component of the overall problem of diagnostic errors in medicine leading to liability. Based on a recent 25-year analysis of the US National Practitioner Data Bank, diagnostic errors, in general, occur at a rate of approximately 4000 per year (n = 100,249 liability claims for diagnostic error over 25 years).[1] More specifically, diagnostic errors related to both asymptomatic and symptomatic breast cancer remain among the top 10 conditions leading to medical negligence lawsuits, according to the most recent analysis of 2157 closed claims carried out in 2013 by the Physicians Insurers Association of America (PIAA).[2] Diagnosis of asymptomatic breast cancer occurs during population screening using mammography, or occasionally other radiologic methods. In contrast, diagnosis of symptomatic breast cancer applies to the patient presenting to a physician with detectible breast signs and symptoms. This chapter focuses solely on the delayed diagnosis of symptomatic breast cancer, which has a direct impact on physicians who are asked to evaluate the wide variety of signs and symptoms of benign and malignant breast disease. The problem of delayed diagnosis of symptomatic breast cancer is a worldwide problem, affecting all physicians in developed countries who evaluate breast disease.[1,3]

It is important to distinguish delays in the diagnosis of asymptomatic breast cancer from those of symptomatic breast cancer because the two scenarios provide vastly different diagnostic strategies to the physician faced with evaluating breast lesions. Diagnostic delay in the asymptomatic patient relates to misinterpretation of screening mammograms (or other screening imaging modalities) in which the hallmarks of breast cancer are truly present but the images are misread as "normal." This scenario might be better termed "the delayed diagnosis of radiographic-*detectable* breast cancer" and is largely confined to radiologists. In contrast, in the delayed diagnosis of symptomatic breast cancer, radiologic (e.g., mammographic) hallmarks of breast cancer are almost never present, and therefore radiographic images are read correctly as "normal." This is truly a setting of radiographic-*undetectable* breast cancer. Unfortunately, in this setting, no further diagnostic studies beyond an unremarkable mammogram are usually undertaken, and so the patient's symptomatic condition (e.g., unilateral breast

mass, unilateral thickening, or isolated and focal breast pain) is labeled as "normal." This distinction is critical because it is the absence of radiographic detectability in certain settings of symptomatic breast disease that is the driving force behind misdiagnosis. Knowing this distinction enables physicians to understand why relying on mammography as the sole diagnostic tool in the symptomatic setting leads to the delayed diagnosis of breast cancer.

Delays in diagnosis of symptomatic breast cancer involve prematurely labeling breast lesions as benign when in fact these lesions are later shown to be malignant. It is surprising that delays in diagnosis occur so frequently because there are a limited number of diagnostic elements used in the "diagnostic cycle of symptomatic breast disease." The diagnostic cycle in symptomatic breast disease begins with a history and physical examination, continues with the use a variety of imaging modalities, and ends in biopsy of one type or another (fine-needle aspiration [FNA], core-cutting biopsy, or open biopsy). Although extremely short-term observation of breast lesions for 6 weeks or less may, in some cases after more thorough imaging studies, be interspersed in this diagnostic algorithm, this approach is fraught with hazard if the definitive diagnosis reveals breast cancer. It is the goal of this chapter to highlight for physicians that delays in the diagnosis of symptomatic breast cancer occur when the diagnostic cycle of symptomatic breast disease is interrupted prematurely, at the radiographic imaging stage. Fundamentally, the biology of symptomatic breast cancer differs from that of screen-detectable disease in the asymptomatic setting. Ultimately, the prevention of diagnostic delay in symptomatic patients requires completion of the diagnostic cycle by biopsy, regardless of normal findings on radiologic imaging. It is axiomatic that only tissue sampling by biopsy can definitively rule out breast cancer in the symptomatic setting.

Given the limited number of diagnostic components—in essence, only the physician's physical findings, the reports of imaging (mammogram, sonogram, or magnetic resonance imaging [MRI]), and a decision regarding biopsy—one might presume that errors in diagnosis should occur infrequently. Yet historically, before introduction of radiologic screening technology, breast diagnosis experts such as Haagensen recognized the difficulties inherent in preventing the delayed diagnosis of breast cancer.[4] Reflecting on his own 1% rate of diagnostic errors in breast cancer examinations over a 30-year interval, Haagensen's writings emphasized that diagnostic errors occurred chiefly because many of the symptoms of breast cancer closely mimicked benign conditions, including masses, infections, and skin rashes. "The price of skill in the diagnosis of breast carcinoma is a kind of eternal vigilance," Haagensen wrote, "based upon an awareness that any indication of disease in the breast may be due to carcinoma."[4]

Paradoxically, the advent of widespread radiographic screening for breast cancer has raised the diagnostic error rate in the symptomatic cancer setting far beyond the 1% reported by Haagensen. The PIAA 2013 report documents that the delayed diagnosis of breast cancer accounted for 22% of all indemnity claims in their database.[2] Of these claims, nearly two-thirds (59%) were breast conditions labeled as benign that later proved to be malignant disease.[2] Unfortunately, the modern area of breast imaging has been accompanied by an increased rate of delays in diagnosis of symptomatic breast cancer, despite the promises to the public of improved detection rates for breast cancer. This fact is not well known to physicians involved in the diagnosis of breast disease. When 400 expert physicians (pathologists, medical oncologists, and surgical oncologists) were recently surveyed as to what top five cancers they believed were most frequently misdiagnosed, they ranked breast cancer as number two on the list.[5] Surprisingly, these expert physicians felt that significant delays in the diagnosis of cancer occurred only rarely, at rates of less than 10% of presenting cases. The missed diagnosis of symptomatic breast cancer is often thought of as simply the result of substandard medical care by "bad physicians." However, the events that lead to misdiagnosis are far more complex, and the numbers of diagnostic errors far too numerous, to be ascribed solely to individual physician competency. In fact, underlying misdiagnosed symptomatic breast cancer are unique features of the disease, and misunderstood uses of radiologic imaging, that make delays in diagnosis not only possible but, under certain conditions, highly probable. For example, delayed diagnosis of breast cancer almost always involves a specific category of patients, an identifiable specialty of physicians, and a reproducible set of clinical circumstances. These three factors interact to produce delays in diagnosis that are frequent, and often lengthy. This chapter attempts to outline in more detail the individual components leading to high-probability scenarios for diagnostic error in symptomatic breast cancer.

Because delays in diagnosis of symptomatic breast cancer occur repeatedly under certain clinical conditions, it follows that the circumstances producing diagnostic failures should be predictable and that diagnostic delays should be avoidable. A thorough understanding of the causes and consequences of the delayed diagnosis of symptomatic breast cancer is central to risk management for clinicians managing breast disease. Ultimately, an analysis of the determinants of delayed diagnosis of breast cancer in the symptomatic setting is an important and useful tool in defining the limits of the perceptual, cognitive, and radiologic detection of breast cancer, by patients and clinicians alike.

Magnitude of the Problem

In terms of all diagnostic errors among providers of primary health care to women, the delayed diagnosis of breast cancer ranks among the top three misdiagnoses, as shown in Box 86.1. This list was created from data compiled in 1995 and 2001 by the PIAA.[6,7] The PIAA is an insurance trade association of 25 domestic insurance companies that provide malpractice insurance to more than 90,000 physicians in the United States. The data

> ### • BOX 86.1 Top Three Errors in Diagnosis Resulting in Claims for Medical Malpractice by Physician Specialty
>
> **General Surgery**
> 1. *Breast cancer*
> 2. Appendicitis
> 3. Spinal fracture
>
> **Family Practice**
> 1. Myocardial infarct
> 2. *Breast cancer*
> 3. Appendicitis
>
> **Internal Medicine**
> 1. Lung cancer
> 2. Myocardial infarct
> 3. *Breast cancer*
>
> **Obstetrics/Gynecology**
> 1. *Breast cancer*
> 2. Ectopic pregnancy
> 3. Pregnancy
>
> **Radiology**
> 1. *Breast cancer*
> 2. Lung cancer
> 3. Spinal fracture

represent indemnity claims over the 16-year interval from January 1985 to December 2000.

More recently, The Doctors Company, the nation's largest physician-owned insurance company with 77,000 insured member-physicians, published data on 1877 specialty-specific, diagnosis-related claims closed between 2007 and 2013.[8] The delayed diagnosis of breast cancer ranked between first and third on the list of top five diagnostic errors in the specialties providing health care to women: obstetrics and gynecology (first most common, 21.4% of 98 claims); general surgery (second most common, 9.8% of 143 claims); family medicine (third most common, 4.1% of 417 claims). The 2013 PIAA study (1a) of more than 2000 breast cancer malpractice claims closed between 2002 and 2011 noted the following rank order of physician specialty involved in diagnostic delays: radiology, 43%; obstetrics and gynecology, 16%; general surgery, 12%; family practice, 8%; internal medicine, 8%; and other, 13%.

A recent study of 4793 claims filed against 2680 radiologists documented that failure to diagnose breast cancer was the most common source for liability claims, occurring at a rate of 4.13 claims per 1000 person years.[9] In 2015, The Doctors Company partnered in a liability study with CRICO Strategies, which is the medical malpractice insurer for the Harvard medical community and other non–Harvard-affiliated hospitals located across the United States.[10] These liability companies jointly analyzed 562 breast cancer malpractice claims from 2009 to 2014. These claims were drawn from an overall database of 300,000 medical malpractice claims from more than 500 hospitals and 165,000 physicians across the United States.

In the CRICO study, of 342 malpractice claims involving failure to diagnose breast cancer, the following key factors were noted. First, 48% of cases (163) involved radiologists, and 39%

of cases (135) involved physicians in family practice and obstetrics and gynecology. Second, the misreading of mammograms as "normal" when hallmarks of cancer were truly present accounted for 49% (162) of cases. Third, in 27% of cases (94 claims), the medical records showed that diagnostic delay resulted from a failure to order any diagnostic testing beyond physical examination alone. Fourth, the failure or delay in obtaining additional opinions from experts in breast disease accounted for 17% (57) cases. And last, the severity of outcomes for 69% of patients sustaining diagnostic delays (239 cases) was "severe" (death, permanent grave or major harm), with 13% of delays associated with death (43 cases). These studies confirm earlier claims data analyses reporting that 24% (44 of 181 claims) of diagnostic delays in the ambulatory medical setting were related to breast cancer.[11]

Physicians and their medical malpractice insurers bear a heavy financial burden resulting from the delayed diagnosis of symptomatic breast cancer. In general, malpractice claims related to diagnostic errors account for 30% to 40% of liability payments, and average approximately $300,000 per claim.[12] More specifically, the delayed diagnosis of breast cancer is the second most expensive area of claims to indemnify by liability carriers. Tables 86.1 and 86.2 demonstrate these findings and compare the delayed diagnosis of breast cancer with four other common and expensive conditions resulting in malpractice actions. The 2013 PIAA liability study reported that the average indemnity payment for breast cancer claims of "severe" harm and death was $350,000 and $500,000, respectively.[2]

TABLE 86.1	Most Prevalent Conditions Resulting in Claims of Medical Malpractice		
Condition		**No. of Patients**	**Average Cost Per Case**
Breast cancer		3370	212,894
Brain-damaged infant		3308	487,839
Pregnancy		2656	159,922
Acute myocardial infarction		2336	180,506

This table represents claims closed by payment between January 1985 and December 2000 (16 years).
Data from Physician Insurers Association of America (PIAA). *Data Sharing Reports, Executive Summary (2001)*. Washington, DC: PIAA; 2001.

TABLE 86.2	Most Expensive Conditions to Indemnify for Medical Malpractice		
Condition		**No. of Patients**	**Total Paid (Millions)**
Brain-damaged infant		3308	$754.20
Breast cancer		3370	$295.80
Acute myocardial infarction		2336	$155.90
Pregnancy		2657	$122.40

This table represents claims closed by payment between January 1985 and December 2000 (16 years).
Data from Physician Insurers Association of America (PIAA). *Data Sharing Reports, Executive Summary (2001)*. Washington, DC: PIAA; 2001.

For example, in 1990, the PIAA noted that the delayed diagnosis of cancer, in general, accounted for 2956 claims out of a total of 15,356 claims for diagnostic errors.[13,14] Indemnity payments for misdiagnosed cancer approached $200 million annually, or approximately 30% ($194 million out of $698 million) of paid-out liability claims for medical misadventures. Even by 2001, indemnification of misdiagnosed cancer continued to represent almost 8% of the 16-year liability payout by insurers ($8.5 billion).[6,7] A third study by the PIAA, published in 2003, continued to document that the delayed diagnosis of breast cancer remained the leading cause of malpractice claims against physicians.[15]

Kern corroborated the frequency and expense of misdiagnosed breast cancer using data derived from our own nationwide medicolegal study of 338 cases of misdiagnosed cancer occurring in 13 major organ sites, as shown in Fig. 86.1.[16] This histogram illustrates that breast cancer ranked first in misdiagnosed cancer, accounting for 127 of 338 cases. The delayed diagnosis of breast cancer exceeded the next most common organ site involved in diagnostic delays, colon cancer, by more than twofold (38% vs. 15%). Kern's study demonstrated that the expense of liability claims for misdiagnosed breast cancer totaled more than $50 million, or 38% of the combined total, for all 13 organ sites, of $133 million. In Kern's 1995 article reviewing 711 negligence claims in the field of general surgery, breast cancer claims again ranked first on this list, with 172 cases (24%) of the total caseload of 711 liability claims.[17] Despite the frequency with which general surgeons evaluate and treat breast cancer, misdiagnosis of this condition ranks first in diagnoses resulting in negligence litigation against general surgeons.

Other studies have supported these findings. In 1988 the St. Paul Fire and Marine Insurance Company, a large medical liability carrier, reported that failure to diagnose cancer was the third most frequent allegation against physicians. Of these diagnostic delays, one-third focused on breast cancer.[18] In 1963 Harper reviewed 1000 cases of litigation while serving as a medicolegal defense consultant to California insurers. The delayed diagnosis of cancer was reported in 1.4% of negligence cases (42 of 1005 cases), equally divided among cancers of the rectum, breast, and cervix.[19] In a study of 1371 malpractice claims from an insurance survey in New Jersey, Kravitz and collaborators[20] noted that breast operations accounted for 9% (26 of 304) of general surgery operations resulting in negligence claims. In 2006 Gandhi and colleagues reviewed 181 malpractice claims in the ambulatory setting. The most common misdiagnosis was cancer (59%, 106 of 181 cases), and the most common cancer misdiagnosed was breast cancer (24%, 44 of 106).[21] In 2007 Singh and associates performed a comprehensive analysis of published literature in the field of diagnostic errors, which also supported the finding that breast cancer is the most frequently misdiagnosed cancer.[22]

The frequency of delayed diagnosis of breast cancer is not a direct result of the high incidence of breast cancer in the population. Data tabulated in our 1994 study of delayed diagnosis of cancer nationwide[16] illustrate that the frequency of delayed diagnosis of breast cancer is twice as great, on a proportionate basis, as the frequency of breast cancer in the US population. The mortality rate of breast cancer patients from this medicolegal study was no different from that of breast cancer patients in the 1973 to 1987 Surveillance, Epidemiology, and End Results (SEER) Program of the National Cancer Institute, when calculated on a proportionate basis (the absolute difference in mortality rates was 1.2 between delayed diagnosis cases and SEER cases).

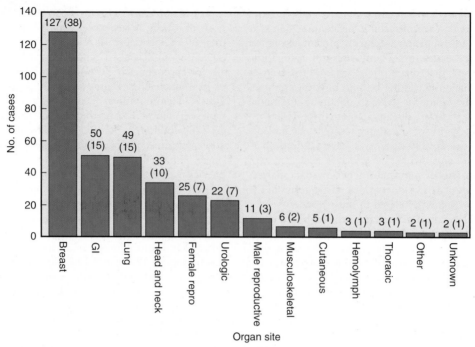

• **Fig. 86.1** Histogram illustrating the frequency distribution of the delayed diagnosis of breast cancer, by organ site, plotted for 338 cases of malpractice litigation nationwide. The data represent 338 jury verdicts surrounding misdiagnosed cancer from 42 states, covering the years 1985 to 1990. The 338 cases are divided into 13 principal organ sites. Four cancer sites accounted for nearly 80% (259 of 338, 77%) of the claims frequency against physicians: breast (38%, n = 127), gastrointestinal *(GI)* (15%, n = 51), lung (15%, n = 50), and head and neck cancers (10%, n = 33). (Data from Kern KA. Medicolegal analysis of the delayed diagnosis of cancer in 338 cases in the United States. *Arch Surg.* 1994;129:397.)

The proportionate mortality rate of breast cancer patients with delayed diagnosis was 13% (17 deaths in 127 cases of delayed diagnoses), compared with a mortality rate of 11% for the SEER breast cases (24 deaths from breast cancer per 105 population/212 breast cancer events per 105 population).

The 2013 PIAA study[2] also showed a discrepancy between the US incidence rates for breast cancer and the rank order of 2157 closed liability claims involving breast cancer. Whereas breast cancer is the second most common cancer reported in the National Program of Cancer Registries (122 cases per 100,000 women), it ranks first in the number of closed liability claims compared with nine other common malignancies (including prostate, lung, colorectum, uterine, bladder, lymphoma, melanoma, and renal cancer). There is something truly unique about the diagnostic approach to symptomatic breast cancer that results in this disease occupying the number one position for frequency of liability claims against physicians.

Unfortunately, there is strong evidence that many clinicians do not fully understand the correct approach to promptly diagnosing symptomatic breast cancer. This evidence is derived from medical malpractice claims for failure to diagnose breast cancer, as described in the preceding discussion. When stratified by which actions on the part of physicians are most costly to malpractice carriers, manual examination of the female breast ranks 9 out of 20, accounting for $38 million (162 claims out of 8234 total malpractice cases, or 2%).[6–14] An approximate calculation of the number of misdiagnosed breast cancers resulting in litigation may be derived from findings accrued by the PIAA. This group defends approximately 300 cases of misdiagnosed breast cancer each year among its 100,000 insured physicians (encompassing a wide range of specialties). Because there are about 1 million physicians in the United States, with roughly one-third caring for adult women, it can be estimated that there may be as many as 1000 cases per year of misdiagnosed breast cancer undergoing evaluation for medical negligence (average, 20 cases per state). This represents 0.5% of the new cases of invasive breast cancer (180,000) diagnosed each year.

Several factors contribute to persistence of errors in the delayed diagnosis of breast cancer. First, breast cancer and benign breast disease are common, and both may adopt similar signs and symptoms. The American Cancer Society reported that nearly 232,000 new cases of invasive female breast cancer occurred in 2015, or approximately 123 cases per 100,000 females, were diagnosed in 2015.[23] Estimates of the number of breast biopsies performed in the United States are reflective of the volume of benign breast disease, which includes 250,000 open surgical procedures and 37,000 needle biopsies of palpable breast lesions.[24] Second, clinically occult, undetectable breast cancer is present in up to 10% of women. Holford and coworkers[16] showed that the percentage of women with breast cancer at autopsy in whom the diagnosis was overlooked antemortem ranged between 3% and 11%. Both contralateral biopsy and prophylactic contralateral mastectomy have revealed an incidence of occult breast cancer of 5% to 10%.[25–27] Thus, some fraction of women presenting with breast symptoms who do not have a biopsy performed initially (for defensibly correct reasons) will later be diagnosed with breast cancer that was detected incidentally. Finally, many physicians evaluate breast complaints. In the absence of specialists in the field or well-defined clinical practice guidelines, errors in diagnosis are bound to occur. In particular, failure to biopsy a breast mass is a leading source of error.[6,7,15,28,29] Indeed, the failure to biopsy is one category of "errors of omission" leading to malpractice in oncology, in which physicians are being sued for "not doing something right" (as opposed to "doing something wrong").[30]

Definition of Delayed Diagnosis of Breast Cancer

Delayed diagnosis of breast cancer may be classified in several ways because the terminology applied to diagnostic delays is not standardized. Specific classifications of delayed diagnosis of breast cancer are based on who is primarily responsible for the delay: the physician, the patient, or the medical system itself. This chapter focuses on the general categories of patient- and physician-associated delays in the diagnosis of breast cancer.

Patient-Associated Delays in Diagnosis

Studies of Patient-Associated Delays in Diagnosis

Regardless of the type of cancer under review, studies of the delayed diagnosis of cancer have shown that most delays occur before medical consultation.[31] This finding has been noted for more than 60 years. For example, in 1943 Harms and colleagues[32] studied 158 cancer patients and reported that the median interval between the onset of symptoms and treatment was 8.5 months. Breast cancer had the second longest delay time in presentation to a physician, surpassed only by cancer of the skin.

While studying a wide range of cancers, Mor and colleagues[33] showed that 25% of cancer patients delayed seeking medical consultation for more than 3 months. Other studies have shown similar results, with 35% to 50% of cancer patients delaying more than 3 months before seeking medical attention.[34] Hackett and coworkers[35] in a study of 563 cancer cases from the Massachusetts General Hospital with a wide range of diagnoses, showed that 15.6% of cancer patients delayed their presentation to a physician for more than 1 year. Hackett reported that between the years 1917 and 1970, only modest decreases in the length of delayed diagnosis of cancer of all types were appreciated. In the years 1917 to 1918, delays averaged 5.4 months; between 1921 and 1922, the average delay was 4.6 months; and by 1930, the delay interval remained at 4.8 months. The median time to presentation was 3 months.

Hackett and coworkers created a kinetic curve describing the rate of presentation for medical evaluation versus time. These investigators demonstrated that the half-time rate of delay for patients presenting to physicians with a variety of cancer types was slightly greater than 2 months.[35] Based on this kinetic analysis, it can be predicted that 10% to 20% of cancer patients will never consult their physician about their symptoms. These results serve as a mathematical predictor that a group of patients will demonstrate extraordinarily long symptomatic intervals before presenting to a physician for diagnosis.

Clinical studies have confirmed this mathematical prediction. For example, Aitken-Swann and Paterson[36] reported a series of patient interviews with British cancer patients. In this study, approximately 50% of cancer patients with a variety of tumors delayed seeking advice for 3 months or more, and 25% of cancer patients delayed seeking treatment for a year or more after first noticing symptoms. In a subset of women with breast cancer,

Wool[37] confirmed that symptomatic delays could reach extraordinarily lengthy intervals, with some patient-associated delays approaching 2 to 3 years.

Historically, studies specific to the delayed diagnosis of breast cancer have shown that diagnostic delays were usually long. Nonetheless, a chronologic analysis demonstrates that delays have been steadily decreasing over time. In 1892 Dietrich (as reported by Bloom and Richardson[38]) reported that only 23% of breast cancer patients presented within 6 months of discovering their breast tumor. Over the next 50 years, the proportion of patients sustaining lengthy delays continued to decrease.[39] By 1910 to 1914, Harrington,[39] at the Mayo Clinic, reported that 33% of breast cancer patients were treated within 6 months of discovery of a breast tumor and 54% were treated in less than 1 year. By the late 1930s, these proportions had increased to 50% and 70%, indicating earlier diagnosis of these cases. Lewis and Reinhoff[40] in the late 1930s, and later, Eggers and deCholnoky[41] in the 1940s, reported less optimistic findings, with only 34% of patients seeking medical advice within 6 months, and 55% seeking advice within 1 year. By the 1950s, Bloom and Richardson[38]; Bloom[42]; and Bloom, Richardson, and Harries[43] reported on a series of 406 patients and showed that 65% of the patients sought treatment within 6 months of the first symptom, and 85% of patients presented for evaluation within 1 year. Hultborn and Tornberg[44] reported 517 cases from the years 1930 to 1955. Thirty percent of the patients presented for treatment in less than 1 month, 37% in less than 6 months, and 22% in less than 1 year. Between 1930 and 1955, there was no change, on a proportionate basis, in the rate at which patients presented for diagnosis.

In 1959 Waxman and Fitts[45] reported on 740 patients with breast cancer and showed that, between the years 1940 and 1951, the number of patients reporting their symptoms to a physician within 1 month of self-discovery increased 10%. The authors attributed this effect to increased publicity about breast cancer. Robbins and Bross[46] compared the range of pretreatment symptom delays in 3802 patients treated with radical mastectomy between 1940 and 1955. Patients were divided into two groups: those treated between 1940 and 1943 and those treated between 1950 and 1955. In the patients from the 1940s, delays of less than 2 months were present in 42.9% of patients, compared with 47.5% of the patients in the 1950s. Delays exceeding 6 months were present in 30.8% of the 1940s group, and 27.7% of the 1950s group. Between the two time periods, the median delay for delayed presentation of symptoms dropped by only 0.8 month. Tumor sizes at presentation in these same time periods showed a shift downward at diagnosis in 2% to 10% of patients. For patients in the 1940s (1281 patients), T1 tumors (<2 cm) were present in 20%; T2 tumors (<4 cm), 46.7%; and T2 tumors (>4 cm), 33.3%. In the 1950s group (2168 patients), these same figures were T1, 28.4%; small T2, 48.7%; and larger T2, 22.9%.

More recent studies have shown a continued decline in the time to presentation for medical evaluation after the appearance of the first symptom of breast cancer. In 1971 Sheridan and associates[47] reported that in 1860 women in Western Australia, 24% had delayed seeking treatment for 1 to 4 weeks, 32% delayed 1 to 3 months, 18% delayed 3 to 6 months, and 6% delayed more than 6 months. A small fraction of patients (2%) sustained lengthy delays in presentation of 4 years or more. Only 5% of patients visited a physician within 1 week of symptoms. Nichols and coworkers[48] confirmed that 23% of women delayed consultation for more than 3 months. Gould-Martin and associates[49] reported that in a study of 275 women 40 to 65 years of age who had breast cancer, 7% of patients delayed for more than 6 months before seeking medical attention. Waters and colleagues[50] and Cameron and Hinton[31] noted that 20% to 30% of patients delayed presentation to a physician for more than 3 months. Pilipshen and associates[51] reported in 1984 that 63% of breast cancer patients treated at Memorial Hospital in New York delayed for less than 2 months. Robinson and coworkers[52] studied 523 women with breast cancer and noted a mean delay from symptoms to diagnosis of 5.5 months (median, 4 months). Mor and coworkers[53] studied nearly 500 breast cancer patients and showed that one-third of patients delayed presentation to a physician after the onset of symptoms for more than 3 months. Rossi and colleagues[54] demonstrated that the median symptom-delay time was 2 months, with 35% of women waiting more than 3 months before presenting to a physician.

Keinan and coworkers[55] noted that typical delays for American and Canadian women from symptoms to diagnosis were 3 to 6 months. Katz and associates,[56] in a study of women in Washington State and British Columbia, noted that 16% to 17% of patients had a symptom-delay time of 3 months and 13% had a symptom-delay time of 6 months. Diagnosis-delay times of 3 months were present in 4.6% of Canadian patients and 13.1% of American patients; patient-associated diagnostic delays exceeding 6 months were present in 3.5% and 11.4% of Canadian and American patients, respectively. In 1995 Andersen and Cacioppo[57] confirmed that the mean delay time from a patient first noticing a symptom to clinical evaluation by a physician was 3 months. In a subset of women, delays can be extreme, approaching 2 to 3 years.[37] Given the large number of new cases of breast cancer diagnosed in American women in 2003 (211,000), it has been estimated that in that time frame, more than 70,000 American women will sustain patient-associated diagnostic delays exceeding 3 months.[58]

Patient-associated delays approximating 3 months from the onset of symptoms to presentation to a physician appear to be universal throughout the developed world. In a study of Australian women, Margarey and colleagues[59] confirmed that 25% of patients delayed presentation to a physician for more than 4 months. In a study of 48,000 women from Sweden, Mansson and Bengtsson[60] noted that the average delay from symptom detection to visiting a physician was 5 months and that only 40% of women visited a physician within 1 month of symptoms. In the developing world, delays may extend over a far greater period. Goel and associates[61] noted that in India, the average patient-delay time was 6.7 months. Ajekigbe[62] noted similar results in Nigeria, and Chie and Chang[63] confirmed lengthy patient-associated diagnostic delays in Taiwanese patients.

Physician-Associated Delays in Diagnosis

Compared with patient-associated delays, the many factors accounting for physician-associated delays in diagnosis are less well studied. Facione[58] noted that the true extent of provider delay is underresearched and underestimated. However, since the 1930s, it has been recognized that physicians are responsible for the majority of delay in the time from symptom detection to the diagnosis of breast cancer. In 1926 Lane-Claypon[64] reported that in a series of 670 breast cancer cases, the average interval from first medical consultation to treatment averaged 6 months. Pack and Gallo,[65] in a series of 1000 patients, stated that physicians were solely responsible for 17% of delays in diagnosis. These authors proposed that an equal number of delays resulted from the combination of patient and physician delays. Rimsten and Stenkvist,[66] confirming earlier reports of Leach and Robbins,[67] noted that physicians were responsible for diagnostic delays in 28% of patients; physicians contributed to the combination of patient-physician responsibility in another 11%. In a series of 400 patients, Kaae[68] noted that physicians were responsible for delays in diagnosis in 12% of cases. As will be discussed later, these diagnostic delays were often related to the patient's age: women 40 years of age or younger were twice as likely to sustain delays in diagnosis compared with women older than age 50.

The relationship between the age of patients and delays in diagnosis of breast cancer has been noted since the 1940s. Harnett[69] found that in a series of 2000 patients with breast cancer, biopsy was delayed in 7% of patients because of a physician's missed diagnosis. More than 25% of these biopsy delays occurred in patients younger than age 50. Rimsten and Stenkvist[66] noted that 25% of women younger than age 50 sustained a delay in diagnosis ranging from 4 months to 2 years and that physicians were solely responsible for these delays in nearly 25% of patients. Nichols and colleagues[48] noted that 10% of malignant breast diseases were delayed in their diagnosis by physicians for more than 1 month. Robinson and coworkers[52] noted that physician-associated delays in diagnosis occur in 8% to 30% of patients.

Physician Factors in Delayed Diagnosis of Breast Cancer

Interval of Diagnostic Delay

Physician-associated errors in diagnosis tend to follow reproducible and predictable patterns. Kern found that the average length of a delay in diagnosis of breast cancer was 15 months, with a median length of diagnostic delay of 11 months (90th percentile, 24 months).[16,70] Others have confirmed this average length of diagnostic delay in breast cancer.[6,13,71–73] In a 1992 study,[70] Kern found that the range of diagnostic delay in 37 cases was 1 to 60 months from the time of the patient's presentation to the biopsy-proven diagnosis of breast cancer. Broken down on a yearly basis, 67% (25 of 37) of patients were diagnosed as having breast cancer within 1 year, 78% (29 of 37) of patients within 2 years, and 95% (35 of 37) of patients within 3 years.

A comparison of intervals of diagnostic delay in breast cancer to 10 other cancers was also performed by Kern in a 1994 study.[16] The mean length of diagnostic delay for 212 cases was 17 months, with a median of 12 months (90th percentile, 33.5 months). This comparison shows surprisingly similar lengths of median diagnostic delay among the 13 types of cancers, including cancer of the colon (11 months),[74,75] thyroid cancer (12 months),[76] and cancer of the lung (15 months).[16]

In a study of 338 misdiagnosed cancers nationwide,[16] Kern found that 156 cases were recorded with a death or terminal condition (46%, or 156 of 338). These cases were not all breast cancers. In 88 of the fatal cases, the length of diagnostic delay was known and averaged 16 months, with a median length of delay of 12 months (90th percentile, 25 months). This length of delay was not different statistically from the 17-month average delay of the entire group of 212 cases. Kern also analyzed the lengths of diagnostic delays for 296 cancers overall in relation to the outcome of subsequent malpractice litigation. No statistical difference was found in the average lengths of diagnostic delays between defense verdicts (14 months, n = 64), plaintiff verdicts (19 months, n = 61), settlements out of court (17 months, n = 83), and all deaths (16 months, n = 88). In addition, the data demonstrated similar lengths of diagnostic delay between patients who died, patients who succeeded in their lawsuit, patients who lost their lawsuit, and patients who settled their negligence lawsuits out of court.

A frequency distribution by 3-month intervals of the delayed diagnosis of breast cancer, derived from my previous civil court study,[70] demonstrated a bimodal distribution of diagnostic delays, with the first peak at 7 to 9 months and a second later peak at 31 to 33 months of delay. Kern analyzed the diagnostic delays in 273 cases from the PIAA 1990 study of misdiagnosed breast cancer, grouping delays in 5-month intervals.[13] Here, a single peak at 6 to 11 months of delay was found, with a long tail to the frequency distribution curve, extending out to 72 to 77 months. On the basis of these data, it appears that most cancers make their presence known after misdiagnosis within 1 year; however, a smaller fraction continues to go undiagnosed for lengthy periods.

On the basis of the data from my nationwide study of 338 cases, the outcomes of litigation were correlated versus the lengths of diagnostic delay, categorized by 3-month intervals, as shown in Fig. 86.2. The 205 verdicts were divided into 65 defense verdicts (32%), 59 plaintiff verdicts (29%), and 81 settlements out of court (40%). At less than 3 months, the 11 jury verdicts largely favored the defense in the following proportion: 64% defense verdicts (7 of 11), 9% plaintiff verdicts (1 of 11), and 27% settlements out of court (3 of 13). At 4 to 6 months, the proportion of defense verdicts decreased to 42% (13 of 31), plaintiff verdicts rose to 29% (9 of 31), and settlements also rose to 29% (9 of 31). By 7 to 9 months, defense verdicts decreased further still but stabilized at the level of 26% (7 of 27), plaintiff verdicts remained roughly the same at 22% (6 of 27), and settlements stabilized at

52% (14 of 27). Grouped by 3-month intervals thereafter (10–12 months, 13–15 months, 16–18 months, 22–24 months, and more than 25 months), the proportion of verdicts remained roughly the same. With diagnostic delays of more than 25 months, the verdicts were 26% (7 of 27) for the defense, 33% (9 of 27) for the plaintiff, and 41% (11 of 27) for settlements out of court.

How juries view delays in diagnosis as negligent is a complex and incompletely understood process. Experimental research on jury decision-making has focused on criminal cases, and little is known about how juries in civil trials of medical negligence allocate liability among parties or assess compensatory and punitive damages.[77] One theory, derived from basic research on human judgment, suggests that juries reach decisions through an information-integration model, in which evidence is mentally averaged until a decision threshold is reached.[78,79] Thereafter, exact statistics are disregarded in favor of the mentally weighted average. This model best explains the decline in number of defense verdicts at 3 months and the stabilization of these verdicts after 6 months. Apparently, juries view 6 months of diagnostic delay as the threshold for negligent delay in diagnosis. Beyond this point, the length of diagnostic delay, or survival of the patient, appears to be irrelevant to the jury's final deliberation. Others have suggested that defensibility of breast cancer malpractice falls dramatically at 12 months of diagnostic delay.[29]

Specialty Training of Physicians

The specialty distribution of physicians involved in diagnostic delay from Kern's 1992 study was obstetricians and gynecologists in 21 of 42 cases (50%), family practitioners in 15 of 42 cases

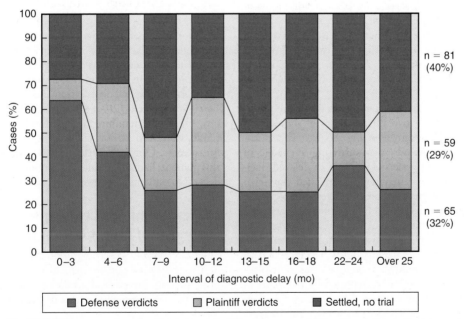

• **Fig. 86.2** Histogram comparing the outcomes of litigation versus the lengths of diagnostic delay, categorized by 3-month intervals, for 205 cancer cases of different types. Breast cancer accounted for more than 100 cases. The *blue bars* represent jury verdicts in favor of the physician being sued for negligent delay in diagnosis. The *yellow bars* indicate jury verdicts in favor of the patient. The *red bars* indicate a settlement before trial, where no blame is assigned to the physician. When the length of diagnostic delay exceeds 3 months, verdicts in favor of the physician decline rapidly and plaintiff verdicts and settlements increase in number. After 6 months of diagnostic delay in cancer, the combination of settlements out of court and jury verdicts against the physician account for two-thirds of the case decisions. (Data from Kern KA. Medicolegal analysis of the delayed diagnosis of cancer in 338 cases in the United States. *Arch Surg.* 1994;129:397-403.)

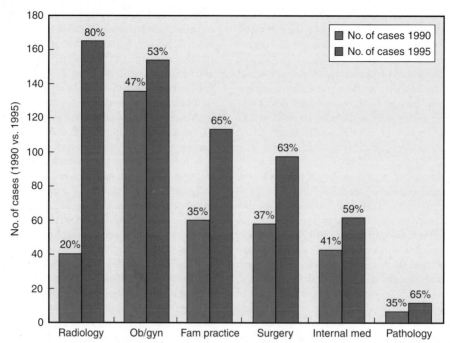

• **Fig. 86.3** Comparative distribution of specialty training of physicians involved in the delayed diagnosis of breast cancer, derived from Physician Insurers Association of America (PIAA) reports in 1990 compared with those of 1995. The *blue bars* represent the distribution of specialties in the PIAA 1990 study; the *red bars* represent the distribution in 1995. There is a marked increase in the number of radiologists named in lawsuits in the 5-year interval between studies. (Data derived from Physician Insurers Association of America (PIAA). *Breast Cancer Study 1995.* Washington, DC: PIAA; 1995.)

(36%), general surgeons in 12 of 42 cases (29%), radiologists in 4 of 42 cases (10%), and internists in 2 of 42 cases (5%). The numbers of physicians involved in these 42 cases ranged from one to four in each case. The distribution of physicians involved in these cases was one physician in 27 cases, two physicians in 10 cases, three physicians in 3 cases, and four physicians in 2 cases.

A frequency distribution of the specialty training of physicians, created from data from two PIAA studies of the delayed diagnosis of breast cancer, is shown in Fig. 86.3.[2,4] This histogram compares two time periods, demonstrating a change in the specialty distribution of physicians involved in delayed diagnosis. In 1990 the three most frequently implicated physician specialties in the delayed diagnosis of breast cancer, in rank order, were obstetricians and gynecologists, family practitioners, and general surgeons. This distribution in 1990 was consistent with my findings, published in 1992. A reassessment of data reported by the PIAA in 1995 showed that radiologists had increased in frequency of misdiagnosis from 20% of the total cases to involvement in 80% of the cases. In 487 cases reported by the PIAA in 1995, 917 physicians were involved in delayed diagnosis. On average, two physicians were involved in each case. The increase in radiologists involved in diagnostic delays between 1990 and 1995 suggests that more emphasis is being placed on mammographic interpretation of breast findings suggestive of cancer. When the diagnosis of detectable breast cancer is delayed, both the radiologist and other primary care providers to the patient might be named in any negligence lawsuit. More recent data from the 2013 PIAA claims study confirms an increase to 43% in involvement by radiologists in the delayed diagnosis of breast cancer.[2]

Diagnostic Workups Requested by Physicians

Studies by Kern in 1992 and 1994[16,70] determined that the diagnostic workup of patients who were misdiagnosed was largely inadequate, reflecting the mistaken idea that these women with breast masses could not have breast cancer. For example, 51% (23 of 45) of patients in Kern's 1992 study had no workup of breast masses beyond visual observation and physical examination alone. Forty-four percent (20 of 45) of patients underwent mammography. Of the 20 mammograms performed, 80% (16 of 20) of the results were read as normal, despite the presence of a malignant breast mass. Only one patient (2%) underwent FNA biopsy, but this patient had a false-negative result, leading to a diagnostic delay. No patients underwent ultrasonographic evaluation.

Clinical Scenarios Leading to the Delayed Diagnosis of Breast Cancer by Physicians

There are several well-recognized clinical scenarios that lead to delays in diagnosis on the part of physicians. The following sections present the clinical scenarios leading to these inadequate workups of symptomatic breast disease.

Triad of Error for Delay in Diagnosis of Breast Cancer

In several previous publications, Kern has proposed that women are at the highest risk for receiving a delayed diagnosis of breast cancer when they fulfill these three criteria: (1) they are 45 years of age or younger; (2) they present to their physician with a self-discovered, unilateral breast mass; and (3) they undergo "screening" mammography as an attempted diagnostic tool, which results in a false-negative study (the mammogram fails to image their breast mass).[16,70,80-89] To help clinicians remember these elements,

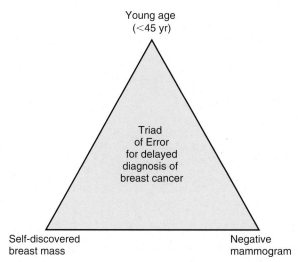

• **Fig. 86.4** The "Triad of Error" for misdiagnosed breast cancer describes women at the highest risk for a delayed diagnosis of breast cancer. The three legs of the triad are (1) women younger than age 45, with (2) a self-discovered breast mass, and (3) a negative mammogram. Women who fulfill these criteria account for more than two-thirds of patients sustaining the delayed diagnosis of breast cancer.

Kern has named them the *Triad of Error* for misdiagnosed breast cancer, succinctly stated as follows: Young age, Self-discovered breast mass, and Negative mammogram (Fig. 86.4).[83] Patients who harbor this triad sustain misdiagnosis of breast cancer in more than three-fourths of cases. These patients are believed to be too young to develop breast cancer, and their mammograms, if obtained, are often read as negative, despite the presence of a breast malignancy. An analysis of actual medical malpractice litigation reveals that physicians are lulled into the misdiagnosis of breast cancer by the young age of patients, not by vague findings or difficult diagnostic situations. Data from medicolegal studies show that in more than 80% of misdiagnosed breast cancers, a physical finding clearly compatible with breast cancer is present. Because of the relative youth of these patients, physicians are not aggressive enough in pursuing a diagnosis beyond mammography. Unfortunately, in this setting, physicians often believe a negative mammogram is sufficient proof of benign disease, even in the presence of a breast lump. This is the classic clinical scenario leading to the delayed diagnosis of breast cancer and subsequent cases of medical malpractice. Much of the evidence for the Triad of Error comes from Kern's studies of the delayed diagnosis of breast cancer and its attendant malpractice litigation. Medicolegal data were analyzed from several perspectives, including a clinical,[16,70] historical,[82] and risk prevention viewpoint.[83,86] The following paragraphs evaluate each of the legs of the Triad individually.

Young Age. Most patients in whom the diagnosis of breast cancer is delayed are young, with a median age of 42 years.[16,70,71] In Kern's previous 20-year review of the delayed diagnosis of breast cancer,[70] 45 cases of breast cancer malpractice litigation tried in the US federal and state civil court system between 1971 and 1990 were critically analyzed. In 21 cases in which a patient's age could be identified, the patients were young, with a mean age of 40 years (range, 22 through 59 years). When cases were grouped by 10-year intervals, the ages of patients were as follows: 4 (19%), 20 to 29 years; 8 (39%), 30 to 39 years; 5 (30%), 40 to 49 years; and 4 (19%), 50 to 59 years. Of the patients with known ages,

4 (19%) were younger than 29 years of age; 11 (52%), younger than 39 years of age; 16 (76%), younger than 49 years of age; and all patients younger than 59 years of age. The menopausal status of the patients was identified in 25 (55.5%) of cases. Of these 25 women, 68% were hormonally active, 15 (60%) were known to be premenopausal, and 2 (8%) were pregnant. Postmenopausal women made up only 5 (11.1%) members of the group. The PIAA 1995 Breast Cancer Study[6] noted the average age of misdiagnosed patients was 46 years, an increase of 2 years over the average age of 44 years reported in their previous 5-year study.[13]

More current claims studies have continued to demonstrate the extraordinarily young age of misdiagnosed breast cancer patients. In the 2013 PIAA claims review of 2157 cases,[2] the median age range was 40 to 49 years, which constituted 32.7% of all cases. Patients aged 30 to 39 comprised 15.9% of cases, and those under age 30 comprised 4.1% of cases. Those patients 50 to 59 years accounted for 26.3% of cases, followed by those 60 to 69 years (11.6% of cases), with those greater than 70 years of age comprising 4.9% of cases.

Perhaps the most important finding from my Kern's medicolegal study was that misdiagnosed breast cancer patients are on average 20 years younger than the median age of breast cancer patients in the US SEER/NCI database, which is 63 years.[16] This same finding of misdiagnosed patients being younger than those reported in cancer databases holds true for other types of misdiagnosed cancer as well. Fig. 86.5 illustrates the age differential in misdiagnosed cancer patients from our study of delayed diagnosis in 13 different organ sites. For all organ sites, a delayed diagnosis occurred in patients at a younger age than the typical age of presentation in the SEER population. The difference in median ages between diagnostic delays and the SEER database ranged from 8 to 27 years. On average, patients with diagnostic delays were younger than SEER patients by 16.2 years (standard error, 2 years).

Kern refers to the age differential in misdiagnosed cancer as a *litigation gap* rather than an age gap, because the young age of cancer patients, in general, leads to delays in biopsy and specialized radiographic imaging, which often results to malpractice litigation. As it relates to breast cancer, other studies have confirmed these findings that misdiagnosed patients are younger than the typical population at risk. Diercks and Cady[71] also confirmed a median age of 42 years for 57 patients in Massachusetts in whom the diagnosis of breast cancer was delayed. Max and Klamer[90] studied 120 women younger than 35 years of age who had breast cancer. In this group of women, who had a mean age of 31 years, 9.1% were pregnant or lactating. Delays in diagnosis were common: in 7% of patients, physicians delayed more than 2 months before recommending a biopsy. In this study, 61% presented with a painless lump; mammography was done in 61% of patients, and in 52% of this group, mammography was negative. In 11% of patients, mammography was equivocal and did not lead to biopsy. Pregnancy-associated delays in diagnosis are discussed more completely later in this chapter but are mentioned here to emphasize the importance of young age as a cause of misdiagnosis. The average age of pregnant patients with breast cancer is 32 to 38 years. However, pregnant patients harboring breast cancer can be extremely young, and some have been described to be as young as 16 to 18 years of age.[91] This is in contrast to nonpregnant patients, in whom breast cancer before age 20 to 25 is extraordinarily rare. In a series of 95 adolescent girls with breast masses, Hein and coworkers[92] showed there were no breast cancers in these young women, who had an average age

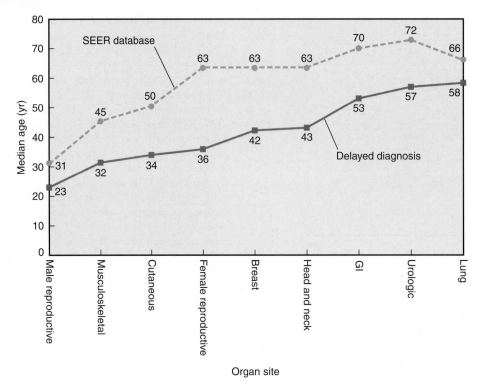

• Fig. 86.5 Line chart comparing the ages of patients with misdiagnosed cancer in nine organ sites with the median age of patients presenting with cancer derived from the Surveillance, Epidemiology, and End Results (SEER) Reporting Program of the National Cancer Institute database. Patients receiving a delayed diagnosis of cancer are younger than the median age for cancer in the SEER population, by intervals ranging from a minimum of 8 years (male reproductive cancer) to a maximum of 27 years (female reproductive cancer). For the delayed diagnosis of breast cancer, the difference in age between those misdiagnosed and the SEER population is 21 years. This age differential is called a litigation gap because it is the most common cause of misdiagnosis leading to malpractice litigation. GI, Gastrointestinal. (From Kern KA. The anatomy of surgical malpractice claims. Bull Am Coll Surg. 1995;80:34-49.)

of 15.9 years (range 12–20 years). However, the authors noted two cases of cystosarcoma phyllodes.

The young age of patients with the delayed diagnosis of cancer is a unique aspect of negligence litigation in malignant disease. Generally, elderly women are more likely to sustain negligence-related, adverse medical events not related to breast cancer. For example, in one study, patients older than 64 years were twice as likely to experience legally compensable complications during hospitalization as patients younger than 45 years of age.[93] Many physicians are unaware that nearly one-fourth of all breast cancer deaths occur in women whose age is not usually associated with the presence of breast cancer. Two percent of breast cancers occur in women between 15 and 34 years of age, 10% occur in those younger than 40 years of age, and 21% occur in women between 35 and 54 years of age.[94–96] A recent study of the rates of breast cancer in women 30 years of age or younger with breast masses found the incidence of cancer was 2.5%.[97] McWhirter[98] calculated that each general practitioner in England is likely to see a case of breast cancer in women younger than 40 years of age only once in every 15 years of his or her working life.

Self-Discovered Breast Mass. Palpable masses are often present in misdiagnosed women with breast cancer. In Kern's civil court analysis of 45 cases of misdiagnosed breast cancer,[70] definite physical findings were present in 82% (37 of 45) and included the following: painless mass, 64% (29 of 39); painful mass, 9% (4 of 45); and nipple discharge (bloody or green) or rash, 6% (3

of 45). Thus 73% of misdiagnosed breast cancer patients presented with a self-discovered breast mass.[70] This finding was confirmed in a larger series of 127 breast cancer cases, in which 61% of patients presented with a breast mass.[16] In the 1990 PIAA study of misdiagnosed breast cancer,[13] the findings at physical diagnosis were reported. In 273 cases, 62.1% (159 of 273) presented with a mass without palpable axillary nodes, and 9.8% (25 of 273) presented with a mass and palpable nodes. Thus 72% of patients with delayed diagnosis of breast cancer originally presented to a physician with a self-discovered breast mass. Abnormal physical findings exclusive of breast masses were present in a smaller percentage of patients: 5.9% (15 of 273) presented with bleeding or nipple discharge, 3.5% (9 of 273) presented with palpable axillary nodes only, and only 16% (41 of 273) presented with no physical findings. Summing up these figures, 81.3% (208 of 273) of patients presented with a physical finding compatible with breast cancer. In these litigated cases, only 72.9% (199 of 273) of patients received a mammogram, only 19.8% (54 of 273) underwent a fine-needle biopsy or aspiration, and only 2.9% (8 of 273) received an ultrasound examination. These studies show that a physical abnormality was detected and was documented by physicians on initial presentation in more than three-fourths of patients in whom the diagnosis of breast cancer was delayed.

Unfortunately, the physical abnormalities detected initially in patients with misdiagnosed breast cancer are misinterpreted as benign disease, largely because further workups of these breast abnormalities are either inadequate (relying solely on mammography) or are not performed at all. From medicolegal studies as noted, Kern suggests that isolated, unilateral masses of the breast in women older than age 25, which, on ultrasound evaluation are either solid or are not simple cysts, receive a cytologic or histologic diagnosis (with FNA biopsy, core biopsy, or open excisional biopsy). Such lesions cannot be accurately diagnosed based on visual observation, physical examination, or mammography alone. Even ultrasonography without needle aspiration or biopsy has been accompanied by breast cancer malpractice litigation. In the 2013 PIAA claims study,[2] 4% of cases (87 of 2157) involved diagnostic ultrasound that incorrectly diagnosed a malignant breast lesion as benign.

Unfortunately, before the definitive diagnosis of breast cancer is made in misdiagnosed patients, a benign label is applied to their breast condition, without attempts to obtain a histologic diagnosis. In 1992 Kern reported the prediagnostic labels for 29 cases of misdiagnosed breast cancer.[70] The benign labels were as follows: fibrocystic disease was diagnosed in nine cases, a simple or premenstrual cyst was diagnosed in four cases, abnormal milk gland or galactocele was diagnosed in four cases, mastitis was diagnosed in four cases, a "hormonal" mass was diagnosed in four cases, and an intraductal papilloma was diagnosed in four cases. None of these diagnoses were confirmed by the results of biopsy.

Other studies have confirmed that palpable breast lesions presenting as isolated breast masses are commonly misdiagnosed. Nichols and coworkers,[48] in a study of the National Health Service and breast cancer evaluation, reported that 25 of 57 women with discrete lumps were not referred immediately for evaluation. Many errors are related to the initial inability of a physician to palpate a mass detected by the patient. Deschenes and colleagues[99] reported the high frequency of mislabeling of breast cancers in middle-aged women as benign fibroadenomas. Reintgen and associates[100] studied the threshold of physical detection of breast cancers. From a study of 509 breast cancers at a university breast clinic, they determined the following: (1) the threshold of clinically detected breast cancer is 5 mm, (2) the median detection limit (50% of cancers detected) occurs at 11 mm, and (3) experienced clinicians do not detect more than 80% of breast cancers until the cancer is larger than 16 mm. Because the absolute threshold of detection of breast cancer by patients has never been specifically evaluated, one explanation for physician error in physical examination is simply that patients can detect breast masses at smaller sizes than physicians are able to detect.[101]

False-Negative Mammogram. The role of diagnostic mammography in women with symptomatic breast disease is a subject of controversy because it has been linked to the creation of diagnostic delays by physicians. This chapter does not address the issue of screening mammography in asymptomatic women, which has been shown through a variety of clinical studies to improve survival in women older than 50 years and perhaps those younger as well.[102-104] Instead, this section addresses the question of failure to image symptomatic or palpable breast cancers.

Errors in reading mammograms include technical errors in 5%, observer errors in 30%, and nonimaging of breast tumors because of dense or dysplastic breast parenchyma.[105] Nonimaging because of dense or dysplastic breast parenchyma is an age-related phenomenon and the greatest cause of mammographically associated delays in diagnosis.[6,7,16,70,71] In most cases, diagnostic delays in women with symptomatic breast cancer are a result of false reassurance to physicians that the mammogram does not show breast cancer (i.e., false-negative mammography). Although the

threshold size for detection of breast cancer (the minimum size required to consistently see the lesion) is thought to be approximately 2.3 to 2.6 mm,[105,106] this applies to women with optimal breast tissue for imaging, which generally occurs in women older than 50 years of age. For women younger than 50 years of age, the threshold size of tumor visualization may be considerably greater; it may not be reached until 2 cm or greater, particularly in the youngest of women. Thus despite the presence of an obvious breast mass, the mammogram may show nothing suspicious. In such women, the cancer may have grown to a size allowing metastasis long before it can be imaged with modern mammography. By the time a tumor has reached only 2 mm in size, it contains 4 million cells and has undergone 22 net cell doublings. Tumor angiogenesis, a mandatory process before metastases can reach the systemic circulation, is thought to occur much earlier, at 13 net cell doublings or 0.3 mm in size.[107,108] Tumor size alone, however, is not the sole determinant of metastases. The role of histologic determinants of prognosis and the future role of molecular genetic determinants of metastases remain central to any discussion regarding the timing of metastatic spread of disease.[109] As yet, our understanding of the interaction between tumor growth, local nodal spread, and systemic spread of metastases is incomplete.

The high frequency of false-negative mammograms in middle-aged women with breast masses is unappreciated by many physicians. Although the false-negative rate for mammography is generally reported as being 7% to 20%,[16,70] this figure applies to women older than 50 years of age; the actual false-negative rate increases greatly in younger women. For example, the false-negative rate of mammography approaches 80% in Kern's studies.[16,70] Other medicolegal studies have shown similar high false-negative rates of mammography.[71] In both the 1995 and more recent 2002 PIAA studies of breast cancer lawsuits, 70% to 79% of diagnostic mammograms were falsely read as negative (or less commonly, equivocal results).[6,15] Thus a breast mass was documented by physicians on initial presentation in almost three-fourths of patients. However, evaluation by physicians rarely proceeded beyond a negative mammogram, resulting in the delayed diagnosis of breast cancer.[6]

In another study of women younger than 30 years of age with an isolated breast mass, 74% of these masses did not produce an image on mammography.[80] In the Breast Cancer Detection and Demonstration Project involving 280,000 women, mammographic results were falsely negative in 36% of patients 40 years of age compared with 9% of women 75 years of age.[82,83] Woods and coworkers[110] reported that the average age of those with palpable breast lesions and false-negative mammograms was 44 years. This was significantly less than the average age of those with positive mammograms of 57 years.[110] Mann and associates[111] reviewed 36 women with palpable breast cancer and false-negative mammographic results. The average age of patients was 45 years. The subsequent delays in diagnosis ranged from 3 to 24 months. They noted that 52% of women younger than 45 years had normal mammograms despite a malignant breast mass. Bennett and colleagues[112] reported a false-negative mammography rate in 227 women with symptomatic breast cancer of 24% (8 of 33 cancers). The reported delay caused by false-negative mammography was 8 months. Max and Klamer[90] noted that 52% of mammograms were falsely negative in women younger than 35 years of age who had palpable breast cancers. Walker and Langlands[113] and Walker, Gebski, and Langlands[114] noted a false-negative rate of 30.7% in a group of 230 women with a median age of 50 years. The false-negative report led to a mean treatment delay of 12.7 months, ranging between 3 and 60 months. Joensuu and coworkers[115] reported that the false-negative rate in women younger than 50 was 35% in a study of 306 women with invasive cancer. This was significantly different than the rate of 13% in women older than 50 years of age ($p < .0001$). In those with a false-negative mammogram, 30% had delays of 6 months or more. For those with true-positive mammograms, no patients were delayed 6 months.

Others have reported that false-negative mammography is common in middle-aged women.[72,73] Thus the woman with a breast mass who is 45 years of age or younger faces two perils in the diagnostic process. First, physicians assume that she is too young to have breast cancer. Second, given the difficulties inherent in imaging premenopausal breast tissue, mammograms may not provide useful diagnostic information about the mass. Kern reported that of the 44% of patients (20 of 45) who underwent mammography, studies were negative in 80% (16 of 20). Only one patient (2%) underwent FNA of a breast mass, which proved to be falsely negative.[70] As in palpable masses, the reason for false-negative mammography is related to the increased breast density of younger women, which makes x-ray penetration more difficult.[116]

The impact of false-negative mammograms on the delay in diagnosis was studied by Burns and colleagues.[117] In a group of 80 women with negative mammograms, 50 (63%) presented with palpable breast masses. The negative mammogram resulted in a delay in diagnosis in this group of 1 month to 5.4 years; it averaged 11 months. Burns and associates[117] pointed out the irony that although women were being urged to learn breast self-examination and more than 80% of breast cancers are found on palpation by the patient herself, false-negative mammography was creating delays in diagnosis after patients presented to a physician with a self-discovered breast mass.

Others have also noted the curious anomaly that the introduction of mammography into clinical practice as a technique for the early detection of asymptomatic breast cancer has resulted in delayed diagnosis because of its widespread use as a diagnostic tool in symptomatic women. Max and Klamer[90] noted, in a study of 120 women with breast cancer with an average age of 31 years (range, 22–35 years), that in 7% of women who contacted a physician immediately after the onset of symptoms, the physician delayed for more than 2 months before recommending biopsy. Locklear and Langlands[118] noted that in a study of 735 women with breast cancer, 13% had false-negative mammograms, resulting in a diagnostic delay of 11.2 months, ranging from 2.5 to 48 months. Age played a significant role in the rate of false-negative mammographic results. Of the women with false-negative mammographic results, 73% were premenopausal, compared with 38% in the no-delay group.

Others have reported that delays in diagnosis occur in almost 50% of premenopausal women because of false-negative mammography.[111] Although some authors have argued that it would take 80 biopsies of benign palpable lesions in this age group to detect four misdiagnosed breast cancers,[118] Kern believes it is unlikely that patients will accept these probabilistic arguments as a reason not to seek a timely diagnosis of mammographic abnormalities. Minimally invasive breast biopsy techniques, such as FNA biopsy or ultrasound-guided core biopsy, are accompanied by extremely low morbidity rates. The safety of these approaches negates any arguments suggesting that these types of biopsies are "unnecessary surgery." Katz and coworkers[56] reported that in a series of women in British Columbia and Washington State, the preponderance of diagnostic delays was the result of

nonsuspicious, false-negative mammograms. Tennvall and colleagues[119] demonstrated that women with both negative or inconclusive mammograms and negative FNA cytology of palpable breast masses were found to be 11 years younger than the group with combined positive findings. In these young patients, negative cytology and negative mammography led to extended diagnostic delays. Delays in diagnosis, even when the end result is benign, can have significant adverse psychological impact on patients.[120]

The high rate of false-negative mammograms in young women has led some to recommend that diagnostic mammography simply not be used in symptomatic women.[88,121] Mahoney and Csima[121] studied 302 women with breast cancer and found 87%, or 263 women, had false-negative mammograms. Mahoney noted that mammography is most productive when used as a routine screening study in women older than 50 years of age with clinically normal breasts. These workers noted that 53% of palpable breast cancers did not image in women younger than 45 years of age. The mean age for a false-negative mammogram with a palpable breast cancer was 49.3 years; for a positive mammogram with a palpable cancer, it was 58 years. The mean size for a negative mammogram was 2.1 cm, and for a positive mammogram, it was 3.3 cm. Mahoney recommended three rules related to mammography and breast cancer: (1) use mammography as a screening study in older women with normal breasts; (2) never delay biopsy of a breast lump that is solid on aspiration because of a negative mammogram; and (3) mammography in symptomatic women younger than 35 years of age is unrewarding and should not be used.

Barratt and coworkers used a telephone survey to evaluate women's expectations of mammography in a subpopulation of women (n = 115) completing a larger, comprehensive breast health survey (n = 2935).[122] Unrealistically high expectations of the ability of mammography to detect disease were present in these women, many of whom favored litigation despite the known, reported false-negative rate for mammography. Inadequate education on the true ability of mammography to detect disease in a variety of settings and patient age groups is one important contributor to the malpractice problem in breast cancer. Chamot and Perneger came to similar conclusions, suggesting that the patient's lack of understanding of the ability of mammography to detect breast cancer is one key factor in litigation.[123] The widespread use of mammography in symptomatic breast cancer comes at a high cost, as noted previously. The indemnity cost of misdiagnosed breast cancer, based on errors in mammographic readings, averaged about $230,000 per case in 2005 and had grown to more than $300,000 in 2015.[2,124]

Langlands and Tiver[125] reviewed 1433 consecutive patients undergoing mammography and found a false-negative rate in those with palpable abnormalities of 30%. In 16% of these patients, the false reassurance of mammography directly contributed to diagnostic delays ranging from 2 to 24 months. Langlands and Tiver[125] used a statistical argument to show that the use of diagnostic mammography in women with a palpable breast lesion of any age is inappropriate for two reasons: (1) the low probability of imaging the lesion in the young and (2) the inability to make definitive statements about a cancer diagnosis without a confirmatory biopsy, even in older women. In this series, diagnostic delays as a result of false-negative mammography ranged from 2 months to 3 years.

Some authors have disputed the rate of false-negative mammography. Cregan and coworkers[126] studied the extent of delay in 219 women and found that only 11% of women had false-negative mammography. This led to a delay in diagnosis of 1 to 3 months in 10% of women (3 of 32 cases). These authors pointed to the value of mammography in women as young as 25 years of age (in whom early signs of familial cancer may be detected, such as irregular, clustered microcalcifications), especially in those with a family history of breast cancer in which early onset is the rule. Bassett and associates[127] argued for a tailored mammographic examination in women younger than 35 years of age with localized breast symptoms, particularly those without a palpable lump. In a study of 1016 women younger than 35 years of age with breast cancer, Bassett evaluated a group of 454 women with palpable breast masses. He noted that two women sustained delays of 4 months and 10 months because mammograms did not image palpable lesions of 2 cm and 1.5 cm; these lesions were labeled as fibroadenomas without biopsy confirmation. In terms of nonlump symptoms in a group of 53 patients, one 34-year-old patient with localized breast tenderness was diagnosed with architectural distortion on tailored mammogram, leading to an immediate breast biopsy and cancer diagnosis. One 26-year-old patient with unilateral discharge had a negative mammogram and sustained a delay of 6 weeks before a biopsy was performed. On the basis of these results, Bassett reminded readers that a negative mammogram should not preclude biopsy of a palpable, solid mass. Blichert-Toft and colleagues[128] in a series of 167 patients in a Danish breast clinic, showed that immediate workup of vague symptoms or unilateral palpable findings by needle aspiration biopsy or open biopsy prevented delayed diagnosis, despite false-negative mammograms in eight patients (5%).

Screening mammograms that show highly suspicious lesions in younger women with no palpable breast abnormalities may diagnose breast cancer with great accuracy and with a detection rate as high as 40%.[129] However, when mammograms are read as nondiagnostic, indeterminate, or not suspicious, the rate of missed cancers approaches 5% (6 of 127).[129] Erickson and colleagues[130] showed that 2% of patients observed because of an indeterminate mammogram, without the presence of symptoms, were later diagnosed as having cancer. Of the 114 women in the study group, 3 sustained delays of 3, 12, and 15 months, respectively. Nonetheless, with an average delay of 10 months, patients had no progression in stage, as measured by the rate of positive axillary nodes.

The introduction of three-dimensional mammography and other computerized techniques to enhance mammographic imaging has resulted in concerns that mammograms read without these advanced technologies might expose radiologists to a greater degree of malpractice risk. However, until such time as advanced methods to computerized or enhance breast imaging is the generally accepted standard of care, the impact of these techniques in reducing the delayed diagnosis of breast cancer, and subsequent litigation, remains unknown.[131]

Delays Related to Pregnancy-Associated (Gestational) Breast Cancer

Diagnostic delays in gestational breast cancer are frequent for two reasons. First, the incidence in clinical practice is low, leading to inexperience on the part of physicians. Second, the physiologic changes in the gestational breast are similar to those of malignancy.

Although only 1% to 2% of cases of breast cancer overall are diagnosed during pregnancy,[132–134] the number of pregnancies that are complicated by breast cancer ranges from 0.03%[125] to 3.1% for women in the childbearing age group of 15 to 45 years.[132,133]

Others have estimated the rate of gestational breast cancer to be between 1 case per 1360 deliveries[135] and 1 case per 6200 deliveries.[136] Donegan[132,133] has provided a table of age-specific frequency that demonstrates a rate for women in the United States during 1970 as having gestational breast cancer ranging between 0.25 to 2 cases per 100,000. As cited by Scott-Connor and coworkers,[137] other reviewers have placed this rate at 10 to 39 gestational breast cancers per 100,000 women. Because there are approximately 3.4 million live births in the United States annually,[138] the author estimates the number of gestational breast cancers to range from 350 to 1400 cases yearly. The average obstetrician manages between 150 and 250 pregnant women yearly, and thus the chance that an individual obstetrician will see gestational breast cancer in any one practice is extremely low. A large multiphysician group that delivers more than 3000 infants yearly might expect to see one to three cases of gestational breast cancer each year. Because of its rarity, it is important for clinicians managing pregnant women to understand the potential for pregnancy and breast cancer. Special attention should be given to high-risk groups, such as women in breast cancer–prone families, who may develop gestational breast cancer.

In the 1950s, McWhirter[98] pointed out that pregnant patients were often given wrong advice when presenting with a breast mass. Instead of being advised to undergo diagnostic biopsy, they were often asked to do what McWhirter believed were potentially harmful maneuvers such as massaging the lump or applying a poultice. As noted by Bottles and Taylor,[136] delayed diagnosis in gestational pregnancy presents a paradox because pregnant patients are seen many more times than usual by physicians compared with nonpregnant patients. In 1958 Treaves and Holleb[139] reported from a study of 108 patients with gestational breast cancer that the median delay in diagnosis in pregnant women was 4 months, which was twice as long as that for nonpregnant women. In one report, 50% of gestational breast cancers were not diagnosed until 3 weeks after delivery.[138] Petrek[140,141] has shown that fewer than 20% of patients with gestational breast cancer were diagnosed during pregnancy. Others have shown that the duration of symptomatic breast cancer before diagnosis in pregnant women ranges between 2 and 15 months.[134–136,140–144] Byrd and coworkers[145] noted that two-thirds of women with a breast cancer first detected during pregnancy were advised to defer biopsy until after delivery, on the incorrect assumption that their breast masses were benign. Supporting this finding, Donegan[132] has shown that only one-third of pregnant women are admitted to the hospital for definite treatment of breast cancer within 6 months of discovery of a breast mass. Donegan also determined that the delay in diagnosis of breast cancer in pregnant women averages 13 months. Deemarsky and Semiglazov[135] confirmed that the delay in diagnosis of breast cancer in pregnant women ranges between 11 and 15 months. Gallenberg and Loprinzi[91] noted that delays in diagnosis of breast cancer generally exceed 5 months. Treves and Holleb[139] reported that physicians watched an abnormal breast mass for an average of 2 months longer than they normally would in nonpregnant patients.

Given the frequent diagnostic delays until final diagnosis, gestational breast cancer is often in advanced and late stages. This finding of late disease has been attributed to delay in diagnosis, largely by physicians.[37,140,141,144,146] Zinns[147] concluded that delay in diagnosis is "the most significant, controllable factor in the patient's prognosis." Westberg[144] stated that "it would seem thus that pregnancy has no very great effect on prognosis of breast cancer, apart from the fact that patients delay in consulting a physician, and the physician is inclined to postpone surgery." Many other authors believe that delay in diagnosis is the sole factor accounting for the diminished survival of pregnant patients with breast cancer[37] because stage-for-stage survival is equivalent in the two groups.[137,140,148–151] In contrast, other authors cite the unfavorable biological factors favoring rapid tumor growth and early dissemination in gestational breast cancer, such as the high nutrient hormone levels and relatively low host immunity during pregnancy.[140,141,146]

Barnavon and Wallack[143] used a comprehensive review of the world literature to demonstrate that regardless of diagnostic delay, pregnant patients with breast cancer fare worse overall than their nonpregnant, premenopausal counterparts. Typically, gestational breast cancers are large, with the median size in one study of 3.5 cm.[138,140,141] Gestational breast cancers are often associated with positive axillary nodes; up to 70% to 89% of patients are node positive.[134,152,153] Byrd and colleagues[145] reported that pregnant patients with involved axillary lymph nodes had a longer delay from first symptom to definite diagnosis, nearly twice that of nonpregnant patients (7.4 vs. 3.1 months). Guinee and coworkers[152] have shown that the odds ratio of a pregnant patient dying of breast cancer is threefold that of a woman with breast cancer who has never been pregnant.

Given the high risk of misdiagnosis of gestational breast cancer, the use of fine-needle biopsy has been advocated to diagnose any dominant or suspicious breast abnormality in the pregnant or lactating woman,[136,137] particularly when the patient believes the abnormality appears or feels different than usual. Great caution should be used in interpreting FNA biopsy results. Any cytologic atypia should be followed by open breast biopsy because atypical changes in breast tissue are not caused by pregnancy and suggest the presence of malignant disease.[154] Kern advocates a core-cutting needle biopsy to decrease the rate of equivocal or misleading cytology seen with a fine-needle approach. Open breast biopsy is safe when performed with the patient under local anesthesia, and it should not be delayed in the pregnant woman with an isolated, dominant mass that has either clinically suspicious characteristics or has undergone needle aspiration and been found to contain cytologic atypia, an indeterminate diagnosis, or frank cancer.

Delays in Diagnosis Related to Male Breast Cancer

Delays in the diagnosis of male breast cancer are common.[98,155,156] In males, more advanced stages of disease are present at final diagnosis,[116,155–158] and this is hypothesized to be the result of a combination of delay in diagnosis and anatomic factors. In males, there is less intervening tissue between the breast, skin, and chest wall. Bounds and colleagues[147] noted that only 1% of cases of breast cancer occur in males. Of all male cancers, only 0.2% take the form of breast cancer.[155] The incidence of male breast carcinoma in the United States is 1 per 100,000, nearly 150 to 200 times less frequent than breast cancer in females. The median age of patients has been reported to vary between 63 years[156] and 70 years. Because of its infrequent nature and presentation in elderly patients who often exhibit typical senile gynecomastia, delays in diagnosis by physicians (and delayed recognition of symptoms by patients) are common.[156,158] This is believed to be one factor accounting for the percentage of patients with positive axillary nodes on diagnosis (50%) and metastatic disease (80%). Stierer and colleagues[156] documented that the delay

in diagnosis from the first onset of symptoms and the onset of therapy ranged from 1 week to 84 months, with a median delay of 3 months. Tumor size correlated with the median delay; small T1 tumors had a median delay of 2 months, whereas large T3 and T4 tumors had a median delay of 10 months. The investigators[156] believe that diagnostic delays are so common that they establish proof that early diagnosis is virtually never reached in male breast cancer.

Delays in Diagnosis Related to False-Negative Fine-Needle Aspiration Biopsy

FNA biopsy plays an important role in the rapid diagnosis of palpable breast masses and other palpable abnormalities of the breast.[159] Svensson and associates[159] demonstrated the ability of FNA biopsy to diagnose malignant tumors in women as young as 20 years of age, an age generally not recognized as being prone to breast cancer development. In a series of more than 3000 FNA biopsies, Gupta evaluated 691 women younger than 30 years of age. The false-negative FNA rate was 0.4% (3 of 691).[152,160,161]

The introduction of FNA has been shown to decrease the rate of excisional biopsies in dedicated breast clinics.[162] However, FNA biopsy may be accompanied by false-negative studies. Giard and Hermans[163] reviewed 29 articles containing information on more than 31,000 aspiration biopsies and could not determine a reproducible accuracy rate for FNA biopsy. Bates and colleagues[162] showed that a delay in diagnosis of more than 50 days occurred in 6.9% in a series of more than 1000 women evaluated in a dedicated breast clinic in Great Britain. Although the rate of excisional biopsies fell by more than 50% (from 238 to 110 annually), the rate of delayed diagnosis did not change over a 2-year interval. However, the group of patients affected by delay did change. In the interval before the initiation of FNA, the median age of patients sustaining a diagnostic delay was 47 years; after the introduction of FNA, the age of patients misdiagnosed dropped to a median of 40. The type of symptom associated with diagnostic error during this time frame changed from isolated breast mass to an area of asymmetric thickening, which often resulted in nondiagnostic FNA biopsies. Thus FNA biopsy has its best role in the diagnosis of isolated, dominant breast masses. The young patient with indefinite thickening of nodularity may need open biopsy, despite negative FNA findings. Sonographic evaluation of breast masses is a key intervening step before open excisional biopsy. If sonography confirms a simple cyst with smooth internal walls, and no internal septations, then aspiration and follow-up is a satisfactory diagnostic course. However, any sonographic evidence of septations, wall thickening, or irregular internal structures should be followed by excisional biopsy. Breast sonography allows for more accurate FNA biopsy and may even allow vacuum-assisted biopsy with removal of tissue sections large enough for formalin-fixation and standard histologic reading.[164]

Kern advocates that FNA biopsy should always be followed by total excisional biopsy to confirm the diagnosis before initiating cancer therapy. In Kern's 1992 study of 45 malpractice cases related to the delayed diagnosis of breast cancer, one patient who underwent FNA biopsy had a false-negative result. In addition, a jury trial in New York resulted in a $1.5 million verdict against a surgeon, pathologist, and internist for failure to diagnose breast cancer, based on an erroneous FNA biopsy. In this instance, a 37-year-old homemaker with a breast mass underwent FNA biopsy, which was read incorrectly by a pathologist as being benign. Because of this falsely negative report, the mass was not excised. Sixteen months later, the mass grew larger and excisional biopsy revealed invasive breast cancer. Despite mastectomy and chemotherapy, the patient died 33 months after initial misdiagnosis (*Smith v. Dutkewych*, No. 88-1980 [Madison Cty. Sup. Ct. N.Y. June 8, 1992]). Brenner has discussed in detail the medical and legal issues associated with FNA biopsy.[165]

Miscellaneous Factors Leading to the Delayed Diagnosis of Breast Cancer

Several other conditions are typically associated with the delayed diagnosis of breast cancer. Paget disease of the nipple is commonly misdiagnosed as eczema, breast infection, or psoriasis.[1,166,167] Surgical biopsy errors, particularly needle localization biopsy in which the actual tumor mass cannot be identified on follow-up mammograms, are potential risks for the surgeons. The failure to perform yearly follow-up mammography of the surgically treated breast to detect metachronous breast cancer, which may occur many years after initial therapy, is also an error. In one study, delays in diagnosis of second metachronous breast cancers contributed to larger tumor sizes and more lymph node involvement.[168] Scar-associated breast cancer may present many years after a breast biopsy, and in this setting, the surgeon mistakes the thickening of the tumor for the presumed thickening of the scar. FNA biopsy would prevent this dilemma. The potential problem for masking of breast cancers after silicone implant breast augmentation is a phenomenon being evaluated and prevented by displacement of the prosthesis on a screening mammogram[169–172] or by use of MRI.[173]

Influence of Delayed Diagnosis of Breast Cancer on Survival

Medical liability in breast cancer diagnosis has its origin in the workers' compensation system begun in the early 1900s.[82] At that time, because of a limited understanding of cancer epidemiology based largely on anecdotes, trauma was thought to initiate cancer de novo. On the basis of this incorrect biological concept, the random association of workplace trauma with subsequent breast cancer was thought to be causally linked, a situation calling for compensable legal remedies. Later, with the maturation of scientific knowledge and the acceptance that breast cancer was a spontaneous cellular aberration and not associated with single episodes of acute, limited trauma, workers' compensation cases disappeared from the civil justice system. However, in their place arose cases alleging that a delayed diagnosis of breast cancer breached the standard of medical care because it led directly to injury through diagnostic delay itself; therefore, delayed diagnosis cases were equivalent to legally compensable injuries. Here, the biological basis of litigation rests on a theoretical but critically dependent relationship between the timing of diagnosis, cancer progression, and cancer metastases. Although much debate surrounds the workings and details of this theory, it lies at the core of the medicolegal controversy surrounding all liability in the delayed diagnosis of cancer.

The influence of a delayed diagnosis of breast cancer on prognosis, including staging and patient survival, has been the subject of study for more than 60 years. The following section traces chronologically the influence of a delay in diagnosis on the prognosis and survival from breast cancer.

Studies Showing an Adverse Effect of Diagnostic Delay on Survival

In the 1930s Luff[174] noted a progressive increase in mortality in a group of 1500 patients with delayed diagnosis of breast cancer derived from case files of the British Medical Association. Those patients with a delay of 1 to 3 months had a 4-year survival rate of 31% compared with patients with delays of greater than 12 months, who had a survival rate of only 16%. Referring to this analysis, in 1950 Cade[175] stated that "the mortality of cancer of the breast in England and Wales could be reduced from 7000 yearly to 1000, if all cases were adequately treated in the first month of the appearance of the disease." Other investigators in the 1930s to 1940s confirmed the detrimental effect of a delayed diagnosis of breast cancer. Haagensen and Stout[176] reported a series of patients from 1915 to 1934 and showed a 12% difference between those presenting within less than 1 month from discovery of symptoms compared with patients with symptomatic intervals exceeding 6 months. Those presenting within 1 month had positive axillary metastases in 56.5% of cases, compared with those with lengthier delays, in which 68.8% of cases had positive axillary nodes. Hoopes and McGraw,[177] in the 1940s, found that the percentage of 5-year survivors after radical mastectomy decreased slightly with increased duration of symptoms before treatment. In a series of 240 patients undergoing the Halsted radical mastectomy, patients with negative axillary nodes and symptoms of 1 month or less had 5-year survival rates of 71.4% compared with a survival rate of 65.6% in those with delays exceeding 6 months. When axillary metastases were present, 5-year survival with delays of 1 month or less were 34.6% and dropped to 25.8% when delays exceeded 6 months. The number of patients with positive axillary nodes increased when delays in symptoms increased from less than 1 month (55%) to more than 6 months (63%).

During this same era, MacDonald,[178] in 1942, demonstrated that the highest rate of survival in a large series of breast cancer patients was found in those treated within 2 months of discovery of the tumor. Paradoxically, as delays exceeded 1 year, survivals began to increase. Eggers and coworkers[41] confirmed these findings. They noted a 5-year survival rate of 76% for patients operated on within 1 month of symptoms, compared with a 20% 5-year survival rate for delays of 1 to 2 years. Yet as delays increased beyond 2 to 3 years, survivals rose to 41%. In the 1950s, Smithers and associates[179] analyzed 846 English breast cancer patients and demonstrated a shift in anatomic staging dependent on the length of diagnostic delay. When patients had symptomatic intervals of less than 6 months, 64% were stage I or II, whereas when delays exceeded 12 months, only 32% were stage I or II; at more than 18 months, the percentage of early tumors dropped to 18%. The percentage of advanced stage III and IV tumors doubled as delays exceeded 12 months, from 31% (for delays <6 months) to 65%.

Robbins and Bross[46] evaluated the significance of diagnostic delay in 1281 patients undergoing radical mastectomy between 1940 and 1943. Later, Robbins and coworkers[180] compared the results of the initial study with those of 2168 patients treated between 1950 and 1955. In the initial series, as delays in diagnosis increased from less than 1 month to more than 12 months in node-positive women, 5-year survival rates decreased from 55% to 30%. In node-negative patients, as delays increased to more than 12 months, survival decreased from 88% to 70%. An analysis of variance was undertaken in patients who delayed more than 6 months in an effort to determine the relative importance of several factors influencing survival. Three factors were found to account for 89% of the variance in the results between patients without diagnostic delay and those delaying for more than 1 year: (1) spread to lymph nodes (62% of variance), (2) tumor size (23% of variance), and (3) delay in presentation (4% of variance).

On the basis of these data, Robbins reasoned that a delay in diagnosis contributed to decreased survival but at a very low level of importance on a hierarchy of prognostic factors, as demonstrated by its minimal contribution to the variance in results. Using this same analysis of variance, Robbins demonstrated a correlation between a delay in treatment and node involvement but at a nonstatistical level of significance. In patients who stated they delayed 1 month or less before receiving surgery, 45.2% had negative nodes, compared with patients who delayed 1 year or more, in which only 25% had negative nodes. This effect was only noted for level I and II nodes; there was no correlation between level III nodes and duration of symptoms. Robbins concluded the following:

We have not found any report offering any data on a preoperative clinical or laboratory procedure that will predict the growth rate of any specific breast cancer. Until such testing is available, it is important and imperative to institute definitive therapy with a minimum delay in all cases of proved operable cancer.

In 1959 Robbins and coworkers[180] also compared results of a similar study in women treated between 1950 and 1955. Patients in both groups reporting long delays had a 50% increase in the number of large cancers compared with those patients with shorter delays. However, 95% of the changes in stage appeared to be independent of the duration of pretreatment symptoms. At most, Robbins hypothesized that delay in presentation for treatment of cancer accounted for 5% of changes in clinical stage and survival. Robbins concluded that more could be gained from a search for asymptomatic lesions than by a drive for less delay in treatment. He believed that it would be easier to persuade patients and physicians alike to search for asymptomatic lesions through radiographic screening studies because of reticence to change practice patterns and because of emotional factors induced by cancer-related fears in patients.

In 1959, Waxman and Fitts[45] demonstrated a direct correlation between survival and the length of diagnostic delays in a group of 740 patients. The 5-year survival rates of patients according to length of diagnostic delay were as follows: (1) delays of less than 1 month, 67%; (2) 1 to 2 months, 60%; (3) 3 to 5 months, 55.8%; (4) 6 to 9 months, 44.8%; and (5) more than 10 months, 37.1%. Waxman and Fitts concluded that patients who reported cancer symptoms early had a better chance of survival. In a study of 549 patients younger than 35 years of age, Treaves and Holleb[139] demonstrated that there was a loss of 7% in 5-year survival rate and an increase of 12% in axillary node positivity rate when delays in diagnosis increased from less than 1 month to more than 12 months. In a subset analysis of 116 patients seen within 6 months, the clinical 5-year cure rate was 42% and the positive axillary node rate was 58.3%. In 65 patients seen after 6 months of symptoms, the 5-year cure rate was 33.8% and the incidence of metastatic disease to the axilla was 64%. Treaves and Holleb concluded that delays in diagnosis had an adverse effect on survival but only at a modest level of significance (5%–10%).

In several important studies of the influence of delay in diagnosis on the natural history and prognosis of breast cancer, Bloom[181] demonstrated that delays decreased survival in grade I breast cancers and, to a lesser extent, in grade II tumors.

High-grade breast cancers were not affected by delays in diagnosis of up to 3 years. In his study of 1411 cases from the Middlesex Hospital in London, England, 1200 cases were treated with radical mastectomy and followed for 20 years. Overall, for all grades combined, Bloom demonstrated no difference in survival over 20 years for any length of diagnostic delay. Here, the distribution of tumor grades counterbalanced the influence of delay on survival. However, when Bloom categorized tumors by their degree of cellular differentiation, he demonstrated that patients with tumors of intermediate- and low-grade histology may lose years of life because of diagnostic delay. Bloom was the first to demonstrate that the effect of delay on survival can be understood only when the degree of tumor differentiation is taken into account.[38] He therefore concluded that "early treatment must be the undoubted principle for all cases."

In 1970 Brightmore and colleagues[94] demonstrated, in a series of 101 women younger than 35 years, that 5-year overall survival rates were correlated with length of diagnostic delays. For delays of less than 1 month, the survival was 43%; for delays of 3 to 7 months, the survival was 26%, and for delays of more than 1 year, the survival was 22%. Delays in diagnosis may not completely explain the poorer survival of young women with breast cancer. Chung and colleagues[182] reported that women younger than 40 years have more advanced anatomic stages than their older counterparts. In an analysis of 3000 women with carcinoma of the breast in Rhode Island, the majority of women younger than 40 years had stage II lesions; this is in contrast to the usual finding that approximately one-third of women overall present with stage II disease (personal communication, Connecticut Tumor Registry, 2002).

In 1971 Anglem and Leber[183] studied a group of 47 patients treated with radical mastectomy who had an extremely short duration of preoperative symptoms (1 week). The 10-year survival rate for this group was 79% compared with a poorer survival rate for patients with a duration of symptoms of more than 1 week. Of patients dying within 5 years of diagnosis, only 6% had a short duration of symptoms of 1 week or less; 96% of those patients dying within 5 years had longer delays in diagnosis. Anglem and Leber concluded that these findings were a "natural argument" in support of the great importance of an early diagnosis of breast cancer.

Sheridan and associates[47] demonstrated that the effect of delayed diagnosis was stage dependent. Patients with stage I breast cancer had no effect on 5-year survival despite delays ranging from 1 week to more than 6 months. Paradoxically, in patients with stage I disease, survival was 74% for those with less than 4 weeks of delay but rose to 85% for patients with 6 to 9 months of delay. This improvement with increasing delay suggests that stage I tumors form a unique classification of tumor types, characterized by indolent and nonaggressive biologic behavior. In contrast, the stage II tumors demonstrated a decreased 5-year survival rate with increasing intervals of diagnostic delay. When the treatment was less than 4 weeks from the first symptoms, the survival rate was 65.8%; at 5 to 12 weeks, it was 55.9%; at 3 to 6 months, it was 59.5%; and at more than 9 months, it was 46.8%.

In 1973 Balachandra and coworkers[184] analyzed 5549 cases of radical mastectomy treated at Memorial Hospital between 1940 and 1965. These investigators determined delay in diagnosis from symptoms to treatment and correlated these findings with the tumor size and degree of node positivity in several groups of patients (the groups of patients were divided into 15- to 20-year time intervals). In the 25-year intervals between 1940 and 1943 and 1960 and 1965, the distribution of tumor sizes shifted to a greater proportion of smaller tumors: of 1281 patients treated in 1940 to 1943, 20% had tumors smaller than 2 cm, whereas in 1960 to 1965, 38% of the 2100 patients treated had tumors smaller than 2 cm. These investigators found a similar effect regarding the distribution of positive axillary nodes, although the magnitude of the effect did not approach the nearly twofold difference regarding tumor size. In the 20-year study interval, the percentage of patients with positive axillary nodes decreased from 55.5% to 46.4%. Balachandra and coworkers[184] believed decreases in time to presentation were responsible for this improved anatomic staging in patients from the 1960s. In 1940 to 1943, 42.9% of patients had delays of less than 2 months and 30.8% of patients had delays of more than 6 months. Twenty years later, 60.5% of patients were treated in less than 2 months and 25.6% of patients were treated in less than 6 months. During this same time interval, the 10-year overall survival from breast cancer treated with radical mastectomy increased from 51.6% to 74.2%. Although these differences in tumor size, node involvement, and survival ranged only between 5% and 23%, these investigators concluded that earlier detection of breast cancer results in improved anatomic staging; they linked this improved anatomic staging to improved overall survival. The difference in delay in diagnosis between those operable and inoperable was threefold. Differences in operative technique, postoperative radiotherapy, and chemotherapy were not discussed.

In 1974 Say and Donegan[185] reported on 1344 patients from the Ellis Fishel State Cancer Hospital treated with radical mastectomy between 1940 and 1965. The data showed that smaller tumors had less frequent node metastases. Because these investigators believed that tumor size on presentation was decreasing over the years of the study as a result of public health campaigns regarding breast cancer, they concluded that decreased delay in diagnosis led to smaller tumor size at presentation. From this reasoning, they extrapolated that node metastases would be less frequent and therefore survival would increase. This indirect argument begs the question of how delay in diagnosis and outcome are related because the entire argument is based on an untested, indirect chain of reasoning.

Wilkinson and colleagues[186] evaluated 1784 cases from Roswell Park Memorial Institute and confirmed a significant relationship between the length of delay and the extent of disease, the length of survival, and age. Delay by patients was found to affect survival through the influence on extent of disease at diagnosis. Wilkinson and colleagues proposed that a 2-month symptom delay time should be a standard time in which patients should recognize their symptoms, and physicians should act on these findings through referral for definitive treatment. Patients with less than a 2-month symptom delay time demonstrated a better survival rate ($p < .001$) compared with those sustaining delays of more than 3 months. The extent of disease was directly related to the length of delay: for delays of less than 2 months, local disease was seen 53% of the time, but it was seen only 27% of the time when the delay was more than 6 months. Regional disease increased from 41% to 50% when delays increased to more than 6 months. Distant metastatic disease also increased from 6% to 24% as delays increased to more than 6 months. Even when controlling for the stage of disease, delays of more than 3 months resulted in greater numbers of patients with regional and metastatic disease. This effect was not seen in patients with stage I disease. Wilkinson emphasized that the problem of delayed

diagnosis is not an "either/or" phenomenon. Both delay and the biological nature of breast cancer are important in determining survival.

Others have also shown that delays in diagnosis of breast cancer have an adverse effect on prognosis. In an attempt to answer the question of whether prompt diagnosis of breast cancer improves survival as assessed from the date of the first symptom, Elwood and Moorehead[187] studied 1059 women in British Columbia with histologically confirmed primary breast cancer. Patients with long delays in diagnosis had a poor average survival from the date of diagnosis, with an overall average relative survival rate at 5 years of 57% compared with 70% in those with short delays. For patients with delays in diagnosis of 1 month or less, survival at 5, 10, 15, and 20 years was 65%, 55%, 50%, and 45%, respectively. However, for patients with delays of more than 12 months, overall survival decreased by 15% to 20% for each length of follow-up. Barr and Bailey[188] showed that tumors with short delays had an average diameter of 1.6 cm, whereas those with longer delays had an average size of 3.1 cm.

Gould-Martin and associates[49] confirmed that increased intervals of symptom delay from self-discovery of a breast cancer were associated with more frequent instances of positive axillary lymph nodes. In a group of 2299 cancer patients, Robinson and coworkers[189] demonstrated delays of more than 6 weeks from the onset of symptoms to diagnosis were associated with decreased survival in carcinoma of the breast but not in other tumor types. Porta and colleagues[190] analyzed 1247 cases of cancer from five sites: lung, breast, stomach, colon, and rectum. They found that only breast cancer showed a distinct pattern of increasing anatomic stage of disease with increasing delays between symptoms and diagnosis. Overall, the average symptom-to-diagnosis interval in this study was 7.4 months. Correlating stage and delay in diagnosis demonstrated significant differences in the extent of disease versus the length of delay: for localized breast cancer, the symptom-to-diagnosis interval was 2.5 months; for regional disease, it was 3.4 months; and for disseminated disease, it was 4.2 months. The difference in the symptom-to-diagnosis interval between localized disease and more advanced stages was significant at the $p < .01$ level. The probability of survival decreased linearly with increasing stage of breast cancer.

Dohrmann and associates[191] studied 435 breast cancer patients and compared staging when symptom duration increased from 1 week to more than 6 months. They found that there was a significant difference in the distribution of advanced tumors in patients with lengthy symptom duration. In this study, 12% of patients had delays of less than 1 week, 26% of 1 week to 1 month, 33% of 1 month to 6 months, and 21% of 6 months or more. Compared with patients with symptom durations of less than 1 week, those with symptoms of more than 6 months had increased numbers of stage III lesions (8% vs. 19%). During the same period, the number of stage I lesions decreased from 39% to 26%. The differences in the number of stage IV tumors also increased with delays of more than 6 months, with a significance level of $p < .003$. Survival rates were greater by 18% for patients with symptoms of less than 1 week, compared with those with symptoms of 6 months or more (82% vs. 64%, $p < .007$).

Feldman and associates[192] studied 664 patients in 15 hospitals in New York and were able to demonstrate the biologic heterogeneity of breast cancer and associated diagnostic delays. These investigators categorized tumors as relatively small, nonmetastatic tumors (5 cm with negative lymph nodes, termed class I) and large, aggressive tumors associated with cancers larger than 5 cm with positive axillary lymph nodes (termed class III). Whereas class I tumors had 4-year survival rates that increased from 83% to 91% after 12-month delay in diagnosis, the class III tumors had a 50% decrease in survival rate after a 12-month diagnostic delay. In class III tumors, ominous changes in breast symptoms occurred more frequently after lengthy delays. For example, skin changes doubled from 4.2% to 7.8%; nipple discharge rose from 3.3% to 7.8%; nipple changes, from 3.3% to 6.9%; and two or more grave signs, from 9.4% to 18.6%. These findings were interpreted to demonstrate that breast cancer can be divided into two biological subgroups. One group (Feldman class I) includes slow-growing, nonmetastasizing tumors that remain in class I even after a delay of 12 months. According to this study, in another subgroup of relatively fast-growing, metastatic tumors, delay in treatment appears to be harmful, leading to reduced survival rates. By the time grave symptoms begin to show during the delay, the prognosis is reduced further still.

Pilipshen and coworkers[51] reviewed a large series of patients from Memorial Hospital and determined that patients delaying more than 6 months before presentation with breast symptoms had twice the chance of having tumors of at least 4 cm compared with those with symptom delays of less than 6 months. Patients with delays of less than 2 months had T1 tumors (<2 cm) in 35% of cases, whereas patients with delays of more than 6 months were diagnosed with T1 tumors in only 17% of cases. Patients with long diagnostic delays were 40% more likely to have positive axillary nodes than those with short delays. Yet if tumor size were held constant, delay in diagnosis had no impact on the presence of positive axillary nodes. For example, T1 lesions were accompanied by positive axillary nodes in 21% of cases in which the delay was less than 2 months and in 24% of cases in which the delay was more than 6 months. T2 tumors (>4 cm) had 65% positive axillary nodes for delays of less than 2 months and 69% positive axillary nodes for delays greater than 6 months.

Charlson and Feinstein studied 685 women treated between 1962 and 1969.[193–196] They noted that patients with less than 3 months' duration from symptoms to treatment had better survival rates than those with longer delays. At 10 years of survival, patients with less than 3 months delay had a 60% survival rate, compared with a 50% survival rate in those with greater than a 6-month delay. The patients with the shorter delays fared better than those with longer delays because they had a more favorable distribution of clinical stages. With increasing delay, there was a stepwise increase in the proportion of patients in more advanced stages III or IV. In patients with less than a 3-month delay, 76% were stage I or II, compared with only 46% with more than 6 months of delay.

Charlson[193–196] identified a subset of patients who demonstrated adverse changes during the diagnostic delay (termed a change in clinical state) and demonstrated a poorer prognosis than the group that remained clinically stable during the delay. Despite breaking delays into 3-month intervals, those without changes in clinical state had a 10-year survival of 61%. Despite longer delays in diagnosis in patients with prolonged and stable breast symptoms, the survival rates were as good as, or better than, those patients with similar symptoms but short delays in diagnosis. However, patients developing adverse clinical signs during the delay—for example, skin and nipple retraction, ulceration, axillary adenopathy, pain, or edema—demonstrated a significantly worse outcome in overall and stage-specific survival. Nonetheless,

only a limited number of patients were ultimately affected by delays in diagnosis because most patients remained clinically stable during the interval of delay. Charlson estimated that 5.5% of patients (37 of 685) were adversely affected by diagnostic delays. This number was estimated to be the maximum amount of potentially preventable deaths that would result from prevention of the delayed diagnosis of breast cancer. Charlson concluded that decreased survival resulting from the delayed diagnosis of breast cancer is related to an increase in the stage of the disease; however, the impact of delay is limited to a subset of patients who had biologically active and aggressive disease during the interval of diagnostic delay.

In a study of 179 patients, Robinson and coworkers[52] demonstrated that patients with delays exceeding 6 weeks from the onset of symptoms had 43% stage I tumors, compared with 66% stage I tumors in a group without diagnostic delay. Stage III tumors increased from 44% to 80% as delays increased past 6 weeks. In another study, Robinson and colleagues[189] evaluated 523 patients with delays in diagnosis of breast cancer. She determined that patients who delayed presentation past 6 weeks incurred upstaging to a more advanced stage of cancer in 10% to 15% of cases. Stage III disease was more frequently found in those with delays, whereas stage I disease was found most commonly in those patients without diagnostic delays.

Neale and associates[197] studied 1261 women at the MD Anderson Hospital between 1949 and 1968, and they correlated the duration of symptoms with the relative risk of surviving 10 years from diagnosis. Women with less than 3 months of symptom delay had a relative risk of dying within 10 years of 0.8 (indicating a slightly improved survival rate compared with a group with intermediate delays); when the delay was 3 to 6 months, the relative risk of dying within 10 years was 1.1 (virtually the same as a standard population); and when the delay was greater than 6 months, the relative risk of dying within 10 years was increased by 50%, to an odds ratio of 1.5. In this pairwise analysis of the relative risk of dying in relation to diagnostic delays, the inverse relationship was statistically significant at $p = .001$. In addition, the three categories of delays were statistically different from each other. Nearly 50% of those with little or no delay in seeking treatment were living after 10 years. Only about half as many patients who waited more than 6 months to seek medical attention survived 10 years. The researchers proposed that diagnostic delay decreased survival by leading to more advanced clinical stages of disease.

The Italian Group for Cancer Care (GIVIO)[198] conducted a study at 63 Italian general hospitals to determine the effect of diagnostic delays in 1110 women. They noted a doubling of the stage III and IV cancers in women with more than a 3-month delay in diagnosis (34% vs. 17%). At 6 months of diagnostic delay, the size of the tumors increased, as demonstrated by the odds ratio for a T3 or T4 tumor of three to four times those with no delay. The relative risk of node positivity in patients with a delay of greater than 6 months was twice that of patients without diagnostic delay.

In a study of 596 breast cancer patients, Machiavelli and associates[199] demonstrated that a larger proportion of patients with delays in diagnosis of more than 3 months had advanced stage III and IV disease. At 10 years of survival, there was a 10% difference in survival, for the group as a whole, between patients with less than 3 months versus those with more than 6 months of delay (33% vs. 22%). In patients with stage I or II lesions, survival was 68% at 10 years for those with less than 3 months' delay versus

50% for those with longer delays. Machiavelli and associates[199] calculated that 51 patients, or roughly 10% of the group, were affected by diagnostic delays through upstaging to stage III or IV disease. These stage shifts resulted in 30 excess deaths. Interestingly, the negative influence of delay was almost exclusively demonstrated in the patients older than 50 years of age. This is the same age group of patients demonstrated by mammographic studies, such as the Health Insurance Plan of New York (HIP) study, to benefit from early diagnosis from mammographic screening.[200–202]

Rossi and coworkers[54] studied 189 women and correlated symptoms, age, tumor grade, and diagnostic delay with prognosis. Delays were divided into groups of less than 1 month, 1 to 3 months, 3 to 6 months, and 6 months to 1 year. A consistent and direct relationship was found between delay and tumor size, nodal involvement, and presence of metastases. As delays increased from 1 month to 1 year, there was a 46% increase in the number of T4 tumors and a 50% decrease in the number of T1 tumors. Lymph node metastases were present in 37% of patients with delays of less than 1 month, in 62% of patients with delays of at least 3 months, and in 100% (12 of 12) of patients with delays of greater than 1 year. Systemic organ metastases increased from 5% of cases to 25% of cases as delays increased from 1 month to 1 year. Survival rates decreased with longer delays: those with less than 1 month of delay had a 90% survival at 3 years, whereas those with more than a 3-month delay had a 66% survival at 3 years; for patients with more than 1 year of delay, the survival was only 56%.

Tennvall and associates[119] also recently showed that patient delay and age adversely affected survival through a shift in anatomic staging. For 273 patients studied, the mean age was 56 years. Stage I tumors had an average delay of 1 month or less, and patients averaged 49 years of age. Stage II tumors also had a delay averaging 1 month, with an average patient age of 56 years. Stage III tumors had an average delay time of 2 months, with an average patient age of 63 years. Stage IV tumors had an average delay time of 6 months, with an average patient age of 70 years.

Afzelius and colleagues[203] studied the prognostic implications of patient and physician delay in primary operable breast cancer in 7068 patients in Copenhagen, Denmark. A long patient delay was associated with an unfavorable stage and poor survival compared with a short delay. If the patient delay was more than 60 days, the mortality rate was 24% higher than that for a shorter delay. A long patient delay of more than 60 days was associated with larger tumors, more positive lymph nodes, and decreased rate of survival. For example, only 8% of patients with short delays had tumors larger than 5 cm, compared with 19% in patients with long delays (>60 days). The number of node-negative patients dropped from 62% to 51% as the delay increased. Those with more than four positive lymph nodes increased from 12% to 20% with long delays. Afzelius and colleagues hypothesized that delay times reflect biological characteristics of breast cancer and its presentation. One unusual aspect of this study was that long physician delay times were associated with better survival because tumors were smaller and less anaplastic. This factor suggests that physicians recognized aggressive and rapidly growing tumors and diagnosed them promptly. In comparison, smaller, more indolent tumors may have presented in a more subtle fashion and were more difficult to diagnose. Although the delays in recognizing these tumors were longer, a negative impact on stage brought about by a delayed diagnosis could not be demonstrated.

Studies Showing No Effect of Diagnostic Delay on Survival

Several series of patients treated with radical mastectomies in the 1940s to 1950s have shown that delay in diagnosis does not increase mortality from breast cancer; indeed, in some series, those with longer delays exhibit improved survival.

In 1944 Hawkins[204] evaluated the duration of disease before treatment in white and black women. For white women, the mean duration of disease before treatment was 15.2 months, and for black women, it was 22.6 months. The duration of disease was not correlated with survival rates when corrections were made for stage of disease. Hawkins explained this finding by noting that the biology of breast cancer is highly variable; some tumors may grow slowly and metastasize rarely, whereas others may grow rapidly and metastasize early. To understand the true impact of a delayed diagnosis of breast cancer on survival, it would be necessary to understand more precisely these three factors: (1) the actual time of onset of the disease, (2) the rate of growth of the disease, and (3) the inherent tendency of breast tumors to metastasize.

In 1941, Eggers and colleagues[41] reported 5-year survival rates in 235 patients with surgically treated breast cancer. Although delays in treatment of up to 2 years were associated with decreases in survival rates from 76% to 20%, the survival rate increased to 41% for a subgroup of 22 patients with diagnostic delays exceeding 3 years. Beginning in the 1940s, MacDonald[178,205,206] developed his theory of biological predeterminism to explain the variability and unpredictability of breast cancer prognosis. To explain the difficulty of diagnosing and curing breast cancer, MacDonald postulated that the events that determine survival occur in the very early preclinical phase of the tumor, long before the tumor itself is detectable. This theory of biological predeterminism, constructed in the 1940s, is the forerunner of the modern-day alternative theory of breast cancer pathophysiology, which emphasizes that breast cancer is often a systemic disease from its inception. During the preclinical phase, the predetermined biological aggressiveness of the cancer directs the timing and extent of occult metastases, which will later overwhelm the host. In this regard, MacDonald believed that it was the influence of natural selection of aggressive clones of malignant cells rather than the timing of treatment that determined the end results of breast cancer therapy.

The evidence for the theory of biological predeterminism rested largely on the finding from MacDonald's 1951 study.[205] In this study, 56% of tumors that were 1 cm or smaller had metastasized to the nodes of the axilla, whereas 23% of tumors greater than 5 cm had not metastasized. MacDonald then argued that although there was a correlation between the spatial size of the tumor increasing with longer duration of symptoms (tumors of 1 cm decreased in number from 19% to 5% when duration of symptoms increased from 1 month to >12 months), there was no direct relationship between metastatic spread of disease to the axilla and tumor size. MacDonald demonstrated that as tumors increased in size from 1 to 5 cm, there was no increase in the rate of regional node disease.

MacDonald was one of the first investigators to posit that the average breast cancer is invisible to detection by radiologic studies from the time of its inception to its eighth year of growth, at which time it would appear to be 1 cm in size. The remainder of a breast cancer's clinical phase would last approximately 4 years. The calculations for these tumor dimensions were based on tumor doubling times averaging 100 days. The variability in the life cycle of breast tumors would depend on the wide range in tumor doubling time, which others have shown ranges between 42 and 944 days.[105,207–213] Heuser and coworkers[211] analyzed serial mammograms from 23 women selected from the Breast Cancer Detection Demonstration Project of 10,120 women undergoing screening mammography. They reported that the average tumor volume doubling time in 23 breast cancers was 325 days, with several tumors either growing too fast between mammogram intervals to be measured or, in 9 of 23 cases, not growing at all. Fast-growing tumors had an incidence of positive nodes at surgery of 34%, and slow-growing tumors were accompanied by positive nodes at surgery in 15% of cases.[211] Thus tumors that metastasize in the preclinical, nondetectable phase would lead to an ultimately fatal outcome, despite the apparent efficacy of an early diagnosis. Spratt has emphasized the importance of recognizing the silent interval of potential tumor spread and of recognizing the limitations of anatomic staging without taking into account the malignant potential of tumors.[107,108]

As early as 1942 Haagensen and Stout[176] also identified from retrospective clinical reviews two groups of women who responded differently to diagnostic delays. In a group of 623 women who underwent radical mastectomies for breast cancer, Haagensen noted that one group had an adverse effect on survival with up to 35 months of delay. Thereafter women with diagnostic delays exceeding 36 months had increased survival compared with the group as a whole. For example, women with delays of 2 weeks or less had 5-year survival rates of 54%; at 1 year of delay, the 5-year survival rate was 28%; and at 24 to 35 months of delay, the 5-year survival rate was 22%. However, after 36 months of delay, no further decline in survival rate was noted; instead, the overall survival increased to 42%. Axillary node metastases increased 18% (from 50% to 68%) in patients with diagnostic delays that increased from 1 month to more than 6 months. Explaining the paradox in these survival figures for patients with very long delays, Haagensen concluded that this represented a subgroup of women who manifested indolent, nonmetastatic breast cancer. This provided an explanation for the paradox of why early diagnosis and treatment seemed to be important factors increasing the survival of some women, whereas other women had poor survival rates despite entering treatment soon after diagnosis.

In 1951 Park and Lees[214] summarized current knowledge about diagnosis and survival from breast cancer. They concluded that the difference in survival between those operated on without diagnostic delay and those with lengthy diagnostic delays exceeding 3 years was only 7.5%. Commenting on the fact that the difference between treated and untreated patients at the time (when adjuvant chemotherapy was rarely used) was only 20%, these investigators believed early treatment was simply selecting out slow-growing, smaller (and therefore favorable) tumors for treatment. In 1953 Harnett[69] evaluated 2880 cancer patients overall for relationship between length of delay, stage, and survival. In a group of 660 breast cancer patients divided into those with delays in diagnosis ranging between 0 and 12 months, there was no difference in survival among the groups when all stages I through III were combined. In 53 patients with untreated breast cancer, the actual duration of survival averaged 35.9 months, with a decrease in the percentage of normal life expectancy of only 27% (a somewhat surprising finding in the absence of any therapy).

In the 1950s Bloom[42] reported a series of 406 breast cancer patients and noted that regardless of the duration of symptoms (from <6 weeks to >12 months), diagnostic delays had no influence on survival. Five-year survival rates at 6 weeks of delay were 50%, whereas survival rates at 12 months or more of delay were 52%. In a more detailed analysis, Bloom demonstrated that as the duration of symptoms increased, the clinical stage of the patients progressed: for patients with delays of 3 months or less, 37% were stage I, whereas with delays of 1 year or more, only 25% were stage I. Those patients with advanced stage III breast cancer increased from 19% with short delays to 44% with delays longer than 1 year. Paradoxically, longer duration of symptoms was also correlated with increasing numbers of grade I tumors: 24% of patients with grade I tumors were present in the group with a 6-week delay versus 38% of patients having grade I tumors in the group sustaining a 1-year delay. In addition, longer delays correlated with decreasing numbers of grade II tumors (45% for 6-week delay vs. 34% for a 1-year delay) and grade III tumors (31% for a 6-week delay versus 28% for a 1-year delay). From an analysis of grade and survival, Bloom concluded that grade III tumors presented earliest, had the shortest mean duration of symptoms (7.1 months), and were not influenced in terms of 5-year survival rates by delays in diagnosis of any time interval (29% with a 6-week delay vs. 21% with a 1-year delay). In contrast, grade I tumors had the latest presentation, had the longest duration of symptoms (mean, 10.1 months), and were affected by delays in diagnosis (92% with a 6-week delay vs. 78% with a 1-year delay). Ultimately, Bloom concluded that outcome in mammary carcinoma was largely a function of histology and growth rate rather than of the promptness of treatment.

In 1952 Smithers and associates[179] determined that prognosis in a group of 846 British breast cancer patients was related to a clinically determined rate of tumor growth. The rate of growth was said to be slow when the tumor changed less than 1 cm in 6 months, and these patients had 5-year survival rates of 84%. When the tumor changed no more than 1 cm in 6 months, growth was said to be moderate, and survival rates decreased to 64%. Tumor growth was said to be fast when the tumor changed more than 1 cm in 6 months, in which the survival rate was 18%. Smithers and associates[179] also documented a paradoxical increase in survival in patients with a symptom duration exceeding 18 months. In a study of 846 British patients with breast cancer, those with a duration of symptoms of less than 6 months (364 cases) demonstrated a 5-year absolute survival of 43%. When the duration of symptoms was less than 12 months, the survival rate dropped to 26% but rose again to 41% when the duration of symptoms exceeded 18 months.

In 1955, McKinnon[215,216] raised the important issue that stage I breast cancer is not synonymous with short-duration or earlier diagnosed breast cancer. Rather, stage I breast cancer is more reflective of a unique type of breast cancer biology, one that holds low metastatic potential and low lethality for the patient. McKinnon made the prescient point that the wide variations in survival of patients with cancers of other stages also reflect the wide variations in malignancy in these stages that are not accurately revealed by histopathology. Only advances in the newer fields of molecular oncology, which will reveal the genetic determinants of malignancy, will be truly predictive of tumor behavior and patient prognosis.

In 1957 McWhirter,[98] in a study of 1000 patients in England, noted that there was no correlation between the size of primary breast cancer and the duration of symptoms as stated by the patient. Indeed, comparing patients with delays of more than 1 year with those with delays of 1 month, the number of tumors smaller than 1 cm was roughly the same as the number of tumors larger than 6 cm. The 5-year survival rate of patients who delayed for more than 1 year was slightly higher than that of patients who delayed for less than 3 months (a 1-year delay resulted in a 61% survival rate vs. a 58% survival rate in <3 months' delay). Yet when all groups of patients were combined, including the inoperable group and the group of patients with locally advanced carcinoma, the survival rate declined from 49% to 40% with delays of more than 1 year compared with those of less than 3 months. McWhirter explained this effect as resulting from the additive effect of poor prognosis in patients with metastatic disease because these patients increase in number if delays are greater than 1 year. In 1960 Hultborn and Tornberg[44] reported that the duration of symptoms in 517 patients with breast cancer gave no significant information of prognostic value. Postoperative survival curves showed no difference for patients with pretreatment delays of less than 1 month versus delays of increasing intervals up to 2 years.

In one of the first kinetic analyses of breast cancer growth related to survival, Humphrey constructed a "coefficient of growth rate" from a large group of breast cancer patients and correlated this number with their overall 5-year survival rate. Initially, Humphrey and Swerdlow[217] reported that the overall survival rate at 5 years for a group of breast cancer patients was decreased by 10% when delays exceeded 30 days from diagnostic biopsy to radical mastectomy (47% vs. 36.8%). Despite this finding, the duration of tumor symptoms had no effect on the 5-year survival rate, except for those with symptomatic delays between 7 and 9 months, in whom the survival rate was 36.4%. This is in comparison to the other groups of patients with delays ranging up to 1 year, in whom the 5-year survival rate was 50%. To clarify this issue, Humphrey used the coefficient of growth rate, defined as the ratio of tumor size in centimeters to duration of symptoms in months. When the coefficient was 0.1 to 0.5 (indicating either a very small tumor or a tumor whose delay far exceeds its size), the 5-year survival rate was 62%. When the coefficient of growth was 0.6 to 1 (indicating a larger tumor, or a tumor whose growth rate is beginning to exceed its duration of symptoms), the 5-year survival rate fell to 38.5%. This finding suggests that the duration of symptoms can be interpreted prognostically only when the biology of tumor growth is integrated into the analysis.

In 1967 Devitt[218,219] challenged the idea that advanced stages of breast cancer result from the disease having been present and untreated for increased periods. Devitt studied 1440 patients from the Ottawa Clinic in Ontario, Canada, from 1946 to 1961. Correlating the stage of breast cancer with the length of pretreatment symptoms, he found that the distribution of patients with stages I and II lesions, in terms of the symptomatic interval, was identical. Although the distribution of patients with stage III and IV lesions was increased with longer pretreatment symptomatic intervals, he believed this finding was not enough to account for the vastly different 5- and 10-year survival rates. For example, those with 1 month or less of delay comprised 31% of patients with stage I disease; 26% of patients with stage II disease; 18% of patients with stage III disease, and 13% of stage patients with stage IV disease. With delays of 4 to 6 months, 17% were stage I, 16% were stage II, 17% were stage III, and 8% were stage IV. At symptomatic intervals before treatment of greater than 1 year, 12% were stage I, 16% were stage II, 35% were stage III, and 49% were stage IV. However, survival rates did not change with increasing intervals of treatment delay. For delays of 1 month or less, the 5-year survival rate for those with stage I lesions was 75%;

with stage II, 56%; and with stage III, 20%. For delays of 1 year or more, survival for patients with stage I lesions at 5 years was 80%; with stage II, 54%; and with stage III, 21%.

Devitt's study showed that survival rates were independent of the time before treatment, regardless of the clinical stage. The shapes of the survival curves for each clinical stage described the rate of dying from systemic disease; each of the curves was different for the three stages described. The yearly death rate for stage I breast cancer was 6%; for stage II breast cancer, 12%; and for stage III, 21%. On the basis of these different behaviors, Devitt proposed that tumor biology, not diagnostic delay, was the central determinant of the tumor stage and its prognosis. Using a simplified mathematical formula, Devitt proposed that the tumor stage at the time of definitive diagnosis was not simply defined by growth rate × time. Instead, tumor size and spread were more closely approximated by an equation that adjusts for tumor biology and the tumor-host interaction, which Devitt proposed could be schematically stated as follows:

$$\text{Tumor stage at diagnosis} = \text{Tumor growth potential} \div \text{Host resistance} \times \text{Time}$$

Further support for the importance of the tumor-host interaction and tumor biology comes from a study by Devitt of the survival times for patients diagnosed with metastatic disease after primary treatment for breast cancer. Those patients who originally presented with stage I primary breast cancers lived longer, even after developing metastases, than those patients who presented initially with primary tumors of stage II or more. For example, if the patient had an osseous recurrence and her primary cancer stage was stage I, her median time to death was 10 months. This is twofold greater than the median time to death (5 months) of a patient whose primary tumor was stage III at the time of diagnosis. These data support the idea that presenting clinical stage was a measure of the tumor-host interaction as much as a measure of the chronologic age or physical extent of the tumor.

In 1968 Brinkley and Haybittle[220] reported a 15-year follow-up study of patients treated for breast cancer in England. They reported that for a given clinical stage and age group, the length of pretreatment history did not significantly affect survival rates. This finding suggested that the growth rate of the tumor was not of primary importance in determining prognosis. However, they noted that longer clinical histories of breast cancers were associated with later clinical stages and poorer survival rates.

In 1971 Alderson and coworkers[221] performed a multivariate analysis of 21 prognostic factors in 272 cases of breast cancer treated with radical mastectomy. The duration of symptoms in the months preceding initial hospital treatment was evaluated for its predictive power in estimating 5-year survival both as an independent and dependent predictor of local and systemic recurrence. The correlation coefficient between duration of symptoms and survival was 0.09, not a statistically significant relationship. Indeed the total contribution of the factor "duration of symptoms" to the variance in survival determined by 22 prognostic factors was only 0.4%. Thus delay in diagnosis, or length of pretreatment symptoms, had no predictive power or statistical significance as an independent prognostic factor of survival. In contrast, the three factors—axillary node metastases, clinical stage, and pathologic size of the primary tumor—were highly predictive of future survival. All of these factors are critical elements defining the inherent biology of a breast cancer.

Dennis and colleagues[222] studied 237 patients with breast cancer treated with mastectomy. The average symptom delay was 4.8 months and was not correlated with race, age, or socioeconomic group. When the length of survival versus the length of delay was plotted, no correlation was noted between the two. The average time to recurrence throughout the group ranged between 20 and 24 months, and there was no difference between less than 1 month of delay, 3 months of delay, or more than 12 months of delay. Patients free of disease at 5 years and those with recurrent disease had similar symptom delay times (5.8 ± 1.4 months) and physician delay times (0.56 ± 0.15 months). There was no correlation between delay in diagnosis and the number or presence of positive axillary lymph nodes.

Fisher and coworkers[223-225] noted that delays in diagnosis were correlated with a significant increase in grave signs of breast cancer, including skin changes, nipple irregularities and discharge, and nodal disease. As the duration of symptoms increased from 1 month to more than 9 months, tumor sizes and grave signs increased: the number of tumors larger than 1 cm increased from 63% to 78%; the frequency of clinically positive nodes increased from 31% to 41%; nipple involvement was present more commonly, increasing from 9.8% to 17.5%; and skin involvement was found more often, increasing from 2.3% to 11.4%. The number of positive axillary nodes did not correlate strongly with length of delay: at 9 months of delay, the incidence in patients with more than four positive nodes increased slightly from 30.1% to 32.9%, and in those with no positive nodes, it decreased from 48% to 43%. Consistent with the findings from several studies reviewed earlier, Fisher and colleagues showed that the number of treatment failures decreased as symptoms increased beyond 9 months of diagnostic delay.

In 1979 Fox[226] reported a similar analysis of survival in women with breast cancer. Fox identified two populations of cancer patients with different kinetic rates of death from breast cancer. One population died at a yearly rate exceeding 2.5%. A second population died at a much slower rate, more closely akin to the rate of death in the normal population. Fox raised the possibility that what has been labeled as a single disease under the heading of breast cancer should be considered as representing two or more distinct populations with different biological behaviors.

Further studies on the prognostic usefulness of clinical changes seen over time in a breast cancer, and as an estimate of its growth rate, are derived from Boyd and coworkers,[227] who studied 756 patients from 1965 to 1972 at the Princess Margaret Hospital. These investigators characterized, by clinical means, transition events during the diagnostic delay interval of patients. Transition events were defined as changes in the symptoms in the breast reflecting structural or anatomic progression of disease. These events included a change in size of the breast mass, a change in consistency of the mass, the development of other masses, skin changes, contracture or a change in the size or shape of the breast itself, retraction of the skin, pain, or edema. Patients with transition events and a delay in diagnosis measured in months were categorized as having fast-growing tumors. Such patients had a relative death rate twice that of those with slow-growing tumors, defined as those with no transition events and a lengthy symptomatic interval. Boyd and coworkers concluded that differences in the clinical history of a breast cancer's growth rate correspond to true biologic differences, which can be classified according to clinical characteristics. For example, in this study, the relative risk of having more than four positive lymph nodes

was nearly 10 times greater in women with fast-growing tumors (1.87 relative risk) than in those with slow-growing tumors (0.2 relative risk). In separate investigations, Cummings and associates[228] also noted the importance of the relationship of tumor growth rate to survival. In 160 breast cancer patients with a variety of pretreatment delays, fast-growing tumors appeared to be unaffected by diagnostic delays. For the group as a whole, the overall survival was better in patients with shorter diagnostic delays.

Heuser and coworkers[211] noted two groups of breast cancer growth rates during an evaluation of 10,120 women in the Breast Cancer Detection Demonstration Project over a 5-year interval. These investigators noted fast-growing cancers that surfaced between yearly mammographic screenings. These tumors were characterized by aggressive biological characteristics, including higher mitotic index, poor cellular differentiation, and larger tumor size. These tumors tended to occur in young women, demonstrating lymphatic invasion around the tumor and accompanied by a higher proportion of axillary metastases. Patients with fast-growing tumors had a cumulative 5-year survival rate of 74% compared with a 94% survival rate in patients with cancers found on screening that developed over more than 1 year.

Mueller[229,230] brought attention to the different mortality kinetics in breast cancer, described by the half-time death rate and annual death rate. These two mortality figures were not the same in stage I and stage II disease. Studying the kinetics of breast cancer mortality in the National Surgical Adjuvant Breast and Bowel Project and from the Tumor Registry of Connecticut, Mueller identified a small but statistically different result between stages I and II for both half-time death rates and annual death rates. This differential mortality for stages I and II ranged between 3% and 5%. For example, stage I breast cancer had a half-time death rate of 11.8 to 12 years, with an annual death rate of 4.7% to 5%. In contrast, stage II disease has a half-time death rate of 7.4 to 8.5 years and an annual death rate of 8% to 9%. These data suggest that stages I and II breast cancers are not the same disease as reflected by a direct progression from early to intermediate stages. Instead, these data appear to reflect three populations of breast malignancies: stage I, an overlap between stages I and II, and a separate stage II population. Mueller proposed the following:

> Women with stage II breast cancer are not those who seek medical care later but are instead those who have a tumor that is more aggressive, whose axillary lymph node metastases are more obvious, whose distant metastases show themselves sooner, whose local recurrences are more frequent, and whose death is therefore likely to occur earlier.

In essence, patients who are going to die of breast cancer after surgical treatment and local radiation already have micrometastases at the time of treatment. One hypothesis to link the factors of tumor size and poor prognosis is related to an increase in metastatic cell clones as tumors increase in size. Larger tumors may become multiclonal and thereby have an increased potential to metastasize. Small tumors are likely to be monoclonal and are likely to behave in an indolent and controllable fashion. With an increase in tumor size, a breast cancer may lose its monoclonal features, and its behavior becomes more erratic, leading to greater chances for metastases.

Neave and colleagues[231] studied 1675 women in New Zealand who sustained delays in diagnosis of 6 weeks or more. There was no difference in survival based on diagnostic delay, although variables in tumor size, skin attachment, and nipple retraction were worse in the group with longer delays. A 5% to 10% difference in tumor size and grave signs of malignancy accompanied delays of more than 6 weeks. For example, tumors larger than 5 cm were present in 17% of those who sustained delays, compared with 12% of those without a delay; nipple retraction was present in 87% of those with delayed diagnosis, compared with 81% of those without a delay. However, the number of positive axillary nodes was no different between the two groups. Interestingly, Neave and colleagues found an adverse prognostic significance to a group with short delay. This included a group of women whose tumors had grade III histology and negative estrogen receptors. If patients with these tumors presented quickly for diagnosis, prognosis was decreased compared with other groups. The researchers ascribed this finding to a particularly aggressive biology in these tumors. Clayton[232] supported the prognostic implications of biological aggressiveness as determined by high mitotic count in breast cancer.

In a different approach to the problem using an analysis of lawsuits for failure to diagnose breast cancer in Massachusetts, Diercks and Cady[71] demonstrated biological differences indicating a more benign clinical course in a subpopulation of patients sustaining long diagnostic delays. These investigators compared patients with delays in diagnosis of 18 months with patients with less than 6 months of delay. The tumor sizes in the long-delay group were smaller (average 3 cm in 8 cases) compared with patients with shorter delay (average 5 cm in 18 cases). Furthermore, compared with patients with an 18-month delay, patients with less than a 6-month delay had a 10% increase in positive axillary nodes (72% vs. 62%). Patients were found to have more than five positive axillary nodes 50% of the time in less than 6 months of delay but only 40% of the time with more than 18 months of delay. Thus the data from lawsuits in Massachusetts suggest that there are two groups of patients with breast cancers of different degrees of biological aggressiveness.

Rudan and collaborators[233] studied node-positive patients and correlated survival with delays of less than 1 month, 1 to 3 months, 3 to 6 months, and more than 6 months. The average delay was 4.6 months. The influence of delay on 5-year survival was not significant, even in patients with less than 6 months of delay, compared with those with more than 24 months of delay. A similar study[234] in patients with metastatic disease showed no influence of delay on survival.

Kern[16,70] addressed the issue of the impact of a delayed diagnosis of breast cancer on prognosis by using data derived from US civil trials. Actual tumor sizes and data on lymph node status were extracted from legal databases of completed malpractice trials. The data on tumor stage and size versus diagnostic delay were plotted, making it possible to determine the relationship between delay and tumor behavior in this select group of patients. No correlation was found between tumor, node, metastasis (TNM) stage, or tumor size and the length of diagnostic delay. Linear regression analysis was nonsignificant ($p = .91$) for the relationship between months of delay and tumor stage and for the relationship between months of delay and tumor size (plotted as natural log of tumor diameter). Importantly, virtually all cases were stage II or greater. It is possible that once a tumor is stage II, delay has a limited impact on survival. At what point these tumors became stage II during the interval of delay is unknown.

The lack of correlation between diagnostic delays and survival time reported by the studies reviewed earlier probably reflects the fact that other factors, such as cell kinetics, rate of growth, immune response, hormone factors, and patient age, may also play a role in survival.[109,235-237] Spratt and Spratt[107] have argued that the duration of symptoms represents only a small fraction of the life span of the tumor; therefore events influencing survival are occurring in a time at which the tumor is occult and nondiagnosable by present technology.

Conclusion: How to Prevent the Delayed Diagnosis of Breast Cancer—Synopsis of Clinical Risk Prevention

Limited attempts to prevent errors in breast cancer diagnosis by codifying clinical pitfalls have been undertaken previously. More than 20 years ago, Haagensen[4] gave an excellent account of problems related to breast diagnosis. In his 1971 edition of *Diseases of the Breast*, he noted that since 1926, the percentage of carcinomas of the breast discovered by physicians on routine breast examination had increased nearly 20-fold to 17%. However, errors in the diagnosis of breast cancer remained common. In his personal series of 1433 patients with breast cancer, 19% (270 patients) sustained misdiagnoses before referral to him, resulting in an average diagnostic delay of 14 months. In 19% of these cases, two or more physicians had examined the breast and missed the diagnosis of breast cancer. On the basis of the experience with these patients, Haagensen classified diagnostic errors in breast disease into nine types, all related to a failure to biopsy a breast lesion in a timely fashion:

1. Failing to examine a breast containing an obvious tumor while treating the patient for an unrelated disease
2. Failing, during palpation of the breast, to feel the tumor that the patient had discovered and for which she came for consultation
3. Mistaking a carcinomatous tumor of the breast for a breast infection
4. Wrongly diagnosing a carcinomatous tumor of the breast as a benign lesion and failing to recommend a biopsy or excision
5. Disregarding a history of acute and sharp pain in the breast
6. Disregarding a definite retraction sign
7. Failing to determine the cause of a nipple discharge
8. Relying on negative aspiration biopsy
9. Relying on mammography rather than palpation

Haagensen further analyzed his own diagnostic errors, which occurred at a rate of 1% (17 misdiagnosed breast cancers in 1669 women studied between 1935 and 1967). He highlighted pitfalls in diagnosis based on his personal errors as a breast diagnostician and presented solutions to these problems, as follows:

- Ignoring the patient's statements that a mass is present, even if the physician cannot initially palpate it. Ask for the location of the mass and search again for it.
- Ignoring the statements of referring physicians that a mass is present. If not detected initially, ask for a revisit soon thereafter.
- Failing to ask patients with a nipple discharge, but no obvious cause, for revisits and frequent examinations until the cause is found. Monthly revisits may be necessary.
- Rushing and examining patients under inadequate conditions, with less than optimal time spent in the examination.
- Failing to perform a biopsy on benign-appearing masses in women older than 25 years of age, even if they appear to be fibroadenomas on clinical evaluation.

- Assuming new masses in the breast of patients with previously biopsied benign lesions are also benign. For women 25 years of age or older, aspiration and biopsy of solid breast masses is mandatory.
- Allowing patients with nodularity to go without reexamination for 6 months or more. Every 2 months is mandatory.
- Failing to impress on patients the need to keep follow-up appointments, even at frequent intervals, until a definite diagnosis is determined.

Haagensen's analysis of diagnostic errors in breast disease continues to provide a valuable contribution and excellent clinical guide to preventing errors in the diagnosis of breast cancer. Perhaps Haagensen's greatest contribution, however, was something not stated explicitly in his solutions to diagnostic dilemmas, but one he demonstrated by example. To avoid the delayed diagnosis of symptomatic breast cancer requires the physician to make a personal commitment to expending the time and thought required to reach an accurate diagnosis. Haagensen stated the following:

It is a heavy responsibility that we, as physicians, bear in the diagnosis of lesions of the breast. Each one of us must set for [ourself] the highest standard of exactitude in the diagnosis of lesions of the breast, always seeking to improve our personal clinical skill and to discipline it by the pathologic diagnoses in our patients. We must also improve our medical education in regard to the diagnosis of breast lesions.[1]

Selected References

1. Tehrani ASS, Lee HW, Mathews SC, et al. 25-year summary of US malpractice claims for diagnostic errors 1986–2010: an analysis from the National Practitioner Data Bank. *BMJ Qual Saf.* 2013;22:672. http://qualitysafety.bmj.com/on October 16, 2015—Published by group.bmj.com.
2. Physician Insurers Association of America (PIAA). *Breast Cancer Study 2013. MPL (Medical Professional Liability) Cancer Claims Miniseries.* Vol. 1. Rockville, MD: PIAA; 2013.
8. Troxel DB. *Diagnostic Error in Medical Practice by Specialty. The Doctors Advocate (Third Quarter, 2014).* Napa, CA: The Doctors Company; 2014.
11. Gandhi TK, Kachalia A, Thomas EJ, et al. Missed and delayed diagnoses in the ambulatory setting: a study of closed malpractice claims. *Ann Intern Med.* 2006;145:488-496.
12. Singh H, Sethi S, Raber M, Petersen LA. Errors in cancer diagnosis: current understanding and future directions. *J Clin Oncol.* 2007;25:5009-5018.

A full reference list is available online at ExpertConsult.com.

Index

Page numbers followed by f indicate figures; b, boxes; t, tables; e, online content.